REPLACEMENT OF RENAL FUNCTION BY DIALYSIS

REPLACEMENT OF RENAL FUNCTION BY DIALYSIS

A textbook of dialysis

Third edition

Updated and enlarged

Edited by

JOHN F. MAHER

KLUWER ACADEMIC PUBLISHERS

DORDRECHT / BOSTON / LANCASTER

Library of Congress Cataloging-in-Publication Data

Replacement of renal function by dialysis: a textbook of dialysis /
    edited by John F. Maher. – 3rd ed., updated and enl.
        p.   cm.
    Includes bibliographies and index.
    ISBN 978-94-010-6979-3
    1. Hemodialysis. 2. Chronic renal failure – Treatment. 3. Maher, John F. (John Francis), 1929–
    [DNLM: 1. Hemodialysis.   WJ 378 R425]
    RC901.7.H45R46 1988
    617′.461059 – dc19
    DNLM/DLC
    for Library of Congress
    ISBN 978-94-010-6979-3   88-13539
                                                                              CIP

First edition 1978
Second, revised and enlarged edition 1983
Third edition, updated and enlarged 1989

Cover illustration: the characteristic chromatogram showing peak 7C from the studies
of Dr. J. Bergström and Dr. J. Fürst.

Published by Kluwer Academic Publishers
P.O. Box 17, 3300 AA Dordrecht, Holland.

Kluwer Academic Publishers incorporates the publishing programmes of
D. Reidel, Martinus Nijhoff, Dr W. Junk and MTP Press.

Sold and distributed in the U.S.A. and Canada
by Kluwer Academic Publishers,
101 Philip Drive, Norwell, MA 02061, U.S.A.

In all other countries, sold and distributed
by Kluwer Academic Publishers Group,
P.O. Box 322, 3300 AH Dordrecht, Holland.

To Marge

It is difficult to say what is impossible,
for the dream of yesterday is the hope of
to-day and the reality of to-morrow.

ROBERT H. GODDARD

FOREWORD TO THE THIRD EDITION

BELDING H. SCRIBNER

The foreword to this edition is more difficult for me to write than that for the first edition because we are just entering a new era in the use of hemodialysis to treat end-stage kidney disease. This new era results from a substantial increase in our knowledge of the pathophysiology of renal failure and its therapy (see below). Consequently, I feel I must become bolder in my speculations.

Last spring (1987), the second patient to enter the Seattle hemodialysis program which began in 1960, died suddenly of a myocardial infarction on a golf course in Palm Springs, California. He was in his 28th year of renal replacement therapy, having received a transplant from his mother in 1968. Patient #5 of the original Seattle group remains on dialysis and is beginning his 27th year. Dr. Robin Eady, an academic dermatologist in London, began dialysis in Seattle in February of 1963. After 25 years on dialysis, he recently had his first renal transplant at Oxford. He had waited four and one-half years for a negative cross match. Since he reacted to 100% of the test panel, this successful transplant exemplifies the great advances being made in transplant immunology.

These three patients are among the several hundred worldwide who have survived more than 20 years on renal replacement therapy. Based on the unexpectedly long survival of these original patients and considering the fact that by today's standards their dialysis therapy during the first 5 years was terrible, one can entertain the following important prediction: A patient with end-stage renal failure who is in the 20 to 50 year age range and is otherwise well who starts renal replacement therapy in the 1980's *should have a nearly normal life expectancy*. There are, however, two caveats that must be fulfilled: 1) circulatory access must be maintained and 2) hypertension must be controlled beginning with the onset of chronic renal failure.

The subject of control of hypertension raises immediately my concern over the long-term effects of so called 'high flux' dialysis. That term, from the patients' perspective, translates into less time on dialysis which accounts for the current enormous popularity worldwide and its enthusiastic promotion by the manufacturers of the numerous devices needed to provide the required technology. On the plus side, I must admit that I am amazed that urea can be removed at these high transfer rates without causing CNS complications. After all, the neurosurgeons used to use urea to shrink the brain. Nevertheless, very high urea clearances and dialysis times as short as 120 min seem to be well tolerated with less post-dialysis morbidity. The latter benefit could be due to the fact that the membranes used for high flux dialysis cause less immunologic insult as discussed below.

The down side of high flux dialysis lies in two areas. The first is a concern over the increase in morbidity and mortality that seems inevitable as a result of placing the required 'high tech' equipment in inexperienced hands. Any time you push a system toward its technological and physiological limits, the chance of malfunction increases dramatically. I fear that such malfunction may increase as the use of high clearance dialysis becomes widespread. Of even greater concern is the adverse effect that shortening dialysis time has on extracellular fluid removal and hence adequate control of blood pressure. In the February 1983 issue of *Nephron*, Bernard Charra and his colleagues presented a classic paper that is yet to be fully appreciated. They showed that by using long, slow 'low flux' dialysis, blood pressure control was excellent, toxic anti-hypertensive drugs could be eliminated, and the risk of accelerated atherosclerosis was reduced to near zero. High flux dialysis represents the opposite end of the spectrum. One simply cannot remove enough fluid to achieve good control of blood pressure in so short a time, especially in patients who have poor compliance with a low salt diet. The net result is either poor control of blood pressure or high doses of anti-hypertensive medication or both, which in my view, in the long-term represents a dangerous trend.

The above prediction of a nearly normal life expectancy for patients on renal replacement therapy, even if it is overly optimistic, has important implications for the future.

Unfortunately, the economic implications head the list. Longer survival means that the total number of patients on renal replacement therapy (dialysis plus renal homografts) will continue to increase for several more decades. At the same time, the percent of the gross national product devoted to health care continues to increase, at least in the United States, despite serious efforts to reverse the trend. A conflict between these two trends appears inevitable and will not be easy to resolve. One possibility is a return to 'do it yourself' home hemodialysis but with easy to use, fully automated equipment. Home peritoneal dialysis with on-line preparation of the dialysis fluid at the bedside, may become another good alternative.

The implications of long survival for a patient's chances of obtaining a kidney transplant are more difficult to predict. On the one hand, longer survival translates into more demand for grafts. On the other hand, as Dr. Eady's case demonstrates, improvement in transplant matching and immunotherapy undoubtedly will increase the number of successful grafts as well as their longevity, decreasing the need for second transplants. Therefore, the situation probably will remain indefinitely as it is today, namely, a chronic shortage of renal homografts. Hence, various forms of dialysis will continue to carry the major burden.

A NEW ERA FOR DIALYSIS THERAPY

About 20 years after the discovery of insulin, the various degenerative complications of diabetes became manifest. It, therefore, is an interesting historical parallel that beginning in 1980 as we passed the 20-year mark for the use of dialysis to treat end-stage renal disease, several problems began to emerge that were new and unexpected. Two have been particularly worrisome. The first, chronic aluminum intoxication, is covered in depth in this edition, and shows promise of being prevented in the future. The second, dialysis amyloid syndrome, first was described by Laurent and colleagues in 1981. This complication also is dealt with in detail herein. However, we are just beginning to understand the possible relationship between this disease and the hemodialysis process itself. Indeed, a whole new area of investigation, the immunologic impact of the hemodialysis process, is just now being investigated and much of the early work is covered in this edition.

I am not an immunologist, so I will try to summarize the current situation as I understand it in clinical terms because I believe the implications for the future are very great indeed.

Each time a patient undergoes hemodialysis, the immunologic systems are stimulated by at least three factors: 1) blood-membrane interaction, 2) acetate infusion and 3) pyrogens in dialysis fluid. There may be additional factors as yet unidentified. The consequences of this stimulation include the familiar sequestration of leukocytes in the lung, increased production of β_2 microglobulin and a newly discovered severe catabolic reaction in skeletal muscle. This catabolic reaction was described by Jonas Bergström in a landmark presentation at the International Congress of Nephrology in London last summer (1987). Bergström and his colleagues demonstrated that sham dialysis in normal individuals caused destruction of skeletal muscle. The effect occurred at the end of the 2 h sham dialysis and persisted for at least 2 additional hours; it could account for the postdialysis fatigue syndrome. This catabolic effect was prevent-

ed when dialysis membranes that do not stimulate the immune system were substituted for cellulose membranes.

Closely related to Bergström's observation are the unpublished data from Seattle of Robertson and Ahmad. They have demonstrated a remarkable muscle weakness in even the healthiest dialysis patients. Using the maximum exercise test, they showed that muscle weakness was the limiting factor to exercise, unlike normal individuals for whom cardiac output is limiting. Furthermore, they found that curing the anemia with erythropoietin did not fully correct exercise ability, providing further confirmation of the marked degree muscle weakness of the hemodialysis patient.

Since the factors in a dialysis that are known to stimulate the immune response are all amenable to correction, they will be altered in the future provided costs per dialysis can be kept down. Thus, using compatible membranes that do not stimulate the immune system will help reduce β_2 microglobulin production and also, unlike cellulose membranes, will remove some β_2 microglobulin with each dialysis. These new membranes also will reduce the catabolic effect of each dialysis on skeletal muscle. Switching to bicarbonate dialysate and making it pyrogen-free also may further reduce the immune response to a dialysis.

The question of whether or not reducing the immune response to dialysis will help in the long run to prevent the amyloid problem, improve muscle strength and perhaps benefit the patient in other as yet unidentified ways will undoubtedly be answered in the pages of the 4th edition of this book. However, other developments of this new dialysis era already are underway and are sure to improve the quality of life of the dialysis patient by correcting hormonal deficiencies of chronic renal failure. The first of these, the introduction of $1,25-(OH)_2$ vitamin D_3, which has so greatly improved management of renal osteodystrophy is covered in detail in this edition. The second more recent development, the introduction of the renal hormone, erythropoietin, will have a major impact on patients' well being, as described in the chapter by Eschbach. As this volume goes to press, the magnitude of that impact is not yet fully appreciated because so little time has elapsed since human recombinant erythropoietin became available. Suffice it to say that the combined impact of all these developments of this new dialysis era could be so beneficial to the quality of life of dialysis patients that the decision to go for a transplant, especially a second transplant, could become very difficult indeed.

FOREWORD TO THE FIRST EDITION

BELDING H. SCRIBNER

The year was 1942 and William Kolff was hard at work perfecting the device that would not only revolutionize the treatment of renal failure, but more importantly point the way to the development of the entire field of extracorporeal devices in general and cardiac bypass devices in particular.

The enormity of the impact that Kolff's contribution was to have on medicine was revealed retrospectively to me when I recalled that in that same year, 1942, I was a second year medical student at Stanford University, taking among other things, P.J. Hanzlik's required course in pharmacology. I have two memories of that course. One was the requirement that we students learn to recognize 64 old time drugs by appearance, smell and taste. For better or worse, almost all of the 64 have disappeared from the scene. The other memory is the more pertinent one. I can still visualize the scene in the small classroom in the attic of the old red brick Stanford Lane building at Webster and Sacramento Streets. Professor Hanzlik had a pigeon for a 'patient' and had planned a dramatic demonstration. I can still hear him command one of my fellow students to 'Seize the patient!', which the student did in fear and uncertainty as the poor bird struggled against its fate. Hanzlik then proceeded with great flair and ceremony to inject some drug intended for intravenous use into the poor pigeon, where upon the bird promptly expired and Hanzlik drove home the point that intravenous therapy of any kind was dangerous and should be avoided at all costs. This 'conservative' attitude was quite consistent with that prevailing throughout the practice of medicine in that era. If intravenous therapy was dangerous, then a device for extracorporeal circulation must be an invention of the devil! Indeed, for the decade after the first clinical dialysis in Europe and Canada, acceptance was painfully slow and often resisted by all the usual techniques of those in power. During the early 60's, we encountered exactly the same kind of resistance to the concept of chronic dialysis. But as has happened over and over again in all of science, the heresy of one decade becomes the practice of the next – a phenomenon that the young heretics among the third generation readers of this volume should not forget.

And so, today Drukker, Parsons and Maher have successfully undertaken the very difficult task of bringing together in one volume all the diverse elements of dialysis therapy. The size of the volume reflects not only the magnitude of the interdisciplinary effort that brought about the technical and clinical advances, but also the many clinical and other ramifications of dialysis therapy.

In 1977, this therapy will cost the United States taxpayer nearly one billion dollars as the number of dialysis patients in the United States soars above 30,000, while the projection of the ultimate number increases from 40,000 to 60,000 and the cost projection to two billion per year by 1985. Concurrently, in the United States, the percentage of patients on home dialysis has dropped from a high of 41% in 1973 to just under 15%. This trend away from home dialysis cost the United States taxpayer an additional 150 million dollars in 1976. In an effort to control costs, the United Kingdom has increased the percentage of patients on home care to nearly 70%. In addition, the United Kingdom and perhaps other Western countries are beginning to exert subtle but effective cost control on dialyses by limiting the numbers of dialysis patients (1). In contrast, in the United States in 1977, there is no cost control on dialysis. What this contrast means to me is that dialysis is having an impact on Western medicine far beyond its significant impact on the patients, family, physicians and staff who are directly involved.

The nature and enormity of this impact began to become apparent to me in 1962 when magazine writer Shana Alexander came to Seattle to do a story on the artificial kidney. I shall always remember how incredulous I was that she did not want to see or hear about the patients whose lives had been saved – no interest there. She wanted to find out all about the 'life and death committee'. As a result, her article on the Seattle Life and Death Committee appeared in *Life Magazine* that fall (2) and set off discussion and controversy that have persisted to the present (3); indeed, the current British versus American approach to chronic dialysis is but a dramatic extension to international medicine of the basic 'who shall live' issue that was raised by the Seattle Life and Death Committee. I believe that what has happened is that dialysis has greatly accelerated the process of bringing to the forefront a basic issue in Western medicine that up to now has been kept hidden. That issue is *priorities*. Can the United States really afford to spend two billion dollars per year on dialysis? If not, who will decide to curtail expenses, and how will the decision be implemented? Significant curtailment already is being implemented in the United Kingdom by limiting the dialysis population (1). The question is how are they able to 'get away with it', and if the real truth were known, could they get away with it?

To put this issue in a different context, I believe the rapid development of dialysis marks the beginning of the end for unrestrained expansion of expensive medical technology – just as surely as the energy crisis tells us that unlimited expansion of a petroleum based Western civilization is about to come to an end. I believe that the energy crisis poses the greatest threat to democracy that has ever been posed in peacetime because the basic inability of the democratic process to cope with decisions about priorities in times of crises. Does dialysis and other very expensive technology pose a similar threat to medical free enterprise as still practiced mainly in the United States? Unless we put our house in order, I believe it does.

Let us take a brief look at another example of costly medical technology that already has overtaken dialysis in terms of total cost. Coronary by-pass surgery is currently costing Americans nearly two billion dollars per year. Preston, in a just published critique of the operation (4), points out that not only is its efficacy unproven, but he makes a strong case for the point that the economic incentives of the free enterprise system rather than medical efficacy explain why in 1975 the operation was performed on 28 patients/100,000 population in the United States in contrast to 2.1 patients/100,000 population in Western Europe.

Dialysis doctors can take comfort in the fact that at least the question of efficacy is not an issue with our expensive technology. But important and unresolved issues nag at our conscience with respect to the cost-benefit ratio of dialysis. These issues are far too complex to be resolved during the life-time of the first generation of readers of this volume and pose the ultimate challenge to the younger generations. The clinical and technological aspects of dialysis must not remain static at the state of the art level described in this volume while the demand for costly services increases. Rather, we must build on the knowledge reviewed in this book to improve the cost-benefit ratio of our services. Meanwhile, we function as our technological advances create new social problems. And so my advice to all three generations is to try and understand and cope with a new responsibility that dialysis, because of its high cost, has introduced into the basic doctor-patient relationship. How can each of us fulfill our basic responsibility to our patients while at the same time doing everything possible to reduce the overall cost to society of this very expensive treatment?

REFERENCES

1. Distribution of nephrological services for adults in Great Britain. Report of the Executive Committee of the Renal Association. *Br Med J* 2: 903, October 16, 1976
2. Alexander S: They decide who lives, who dies. *Life Magazine*, p. 102, November 9, 1962
3. Fox RC, Swazey JP: *The courage to fail – A social view of organ transplants and dialysis.* Chapters 8, 9 and 10. University of Chicago Press, 1974
4. Preston TA: *Coronary by-pass surgery: A critical review.* Raven Press, New York, 1977

PREFACE

In this rapidly evolving field it is appropriate to update frequently our state of the art knowledge of uremia therapy. Hence, this third edition of *Replacement of Renal Function by Dialysis* appears before many of its predecessors have been destroyed by normal wear and tear over 11 and 6 years of use, respectively.

The first two editions of this book were designed to be integrated comprehensive reviews of the pertinent aspects of dialysis and related fields with sufficient clarity for the novice to learn, yet adequate depth for the expert to rely on them as encyclopedic desk references on renal replacement therapy. Based on the favorable readers' comments and reviewers' opinions these editions achieved their goal. The success of those editions is a tribute to the expertise of the authors and to the skill and dedication of my coeditors Dr. William Drukker and Dr. Frank M. Parsons, with whom it was an honor, an education and a pleasure to associate (Figure 1). When Dr. Drukker and Dr. Parsons announced their retirements, I was somewhat reluctant to undertake the task of editing this text again, especially without their capable association. Nevertheless, I felt that it was important to proceed with another edition as new information

developed. When I did not identify European colleagues who had the expertise who could expend the time and with whom I could work so smoothly, I began alone.

Although I was tempted to ask all the same authors as had written so well previously to contribute again, I realized that the new edition must be revitalized. Accordingly a fraction of the authors changed, some new topics have been added and others have been deleted. The multinational character of authorship has been maintained. Existing chapters have been rewritten thoroughly, and new authors have provided as requested a full discussion and bibliography in keeping with the previous editions.

As previously, the first half of the book emphasizes the techniques and procedures for blood purification, while clinical considerations of various types follow in the latter pages. This edition begins with a description of uremia toxicity and includes the classical chapters on the history of dialysis, now updated. New chapters dealing with technical aspects of renal replacement therapy are those on continuous arteriovenous hemofiltration, short treatment, single-needle hemodialysis and continuous ambulatory peritoneal dialysis. Other new chapters relate to the complement sys-

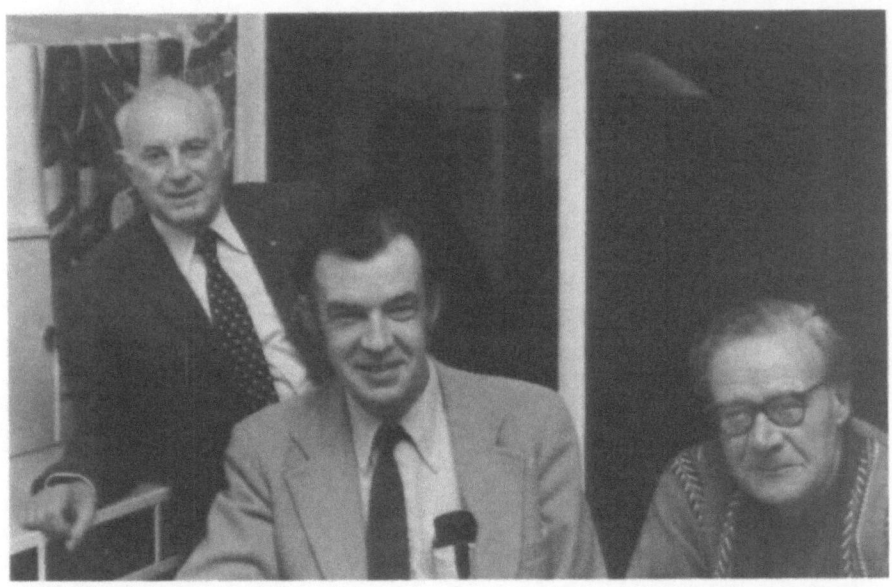

Figure 1. Dr. Drukker (standing), Dr. Parsons (sitting right), and Dr. Maher (center) during an editorial meeting in Amsterdam in 1981.

tem, acid-base homeostasis and pulmonary, gastrointestinal and oral aspects of renal failure and dialysis. The changing dialysis patient population can be appreciated by the chapters devoted to long-term survivors of dialysis treatment, diabetes mellitus, and acquired immunodeficiency syndrome. Importantly, a chapter has been added about the prevention of end-stage renal failure. Nephrologists should all strive to prevent uremia, the treatment of which provides their income.

The editor acknowledges with gratitude the excellent contributions of over 100 distinguished colleagues without whom the book would not be a reality. Included among the authors are a group of peers who have enlightened me considerably about these topics over the past few decades, as well as some younger colleagues who provide fresh insights.

The characteristic chromatogram showing peak 7C from the studies of Dr. Jonas Bergström and Dr. Peter Fürst has been kept as the symbolic cover illustration. It represents the success of our therapy and advances in our knowledge of uremia as well as the limitations of our insights and the need for further research.

The production and publication by Kluwer Academic Publishers (Martinus Nijhoff) has also been integral to the success of the book and is appreciated. Mr. B.F. Commandeur has been primarily responsible for this effort which has assisted the editor appreciably.

My colleagues, particularly Dr. P. Hirszel and Dr. E. Marks, graciously abided the distractions that editing created.

I am especially grateful to Mrs. Barbara Fitzgerald who provided outstanding secretarial assistance throughout the preparation of this edition.

Finally, adding an editing task to an already full agenda takes personal time from those who are most giving and understanding, from family. Thus, the patience, tolerance, encouragement and devotion of my wife, Marge, is most appreciated, for without it this publication would not have occurred.

JOHN F. MAHER

TABLE OF CONTENTS

CONTRIBUTING AUTHORS

Michael Adler, M.D.
Associate Professor
Department of Gastroenterology
Université Libre de Bruxelles
Chef de Clinique
Department of Gastroenterology
C.U.B. Hôpital Erasme
Brussels, Belgium
Chapter 39

Allen C. Alfrey, M.D.
Professor of Medicine
University of Colorado
Chief of Renal Section
Veterans Administration Medical Center
Denver, CO USA
Chapter 49

Anthony J.F. d'Apice, M.D., FRACP, FRCPA
Assistant Director
Department of Nephrology
Royal Melbourne Hospital
Victoria, Australia
Chapter 27

Conrad A. Baldamus, M.D.
Professor, Internal Medicine and Nephrology
Medizinische Universitätsklinik I
University Hospital
Cologne, FRG
Chapter 14

Claudio Bazzi, M.D.
Assistant, Division of Nephrology
San Carlo Hospital
Milan, Italy
Chapter 30

Christopher R. Blagg, M.D., FRCP
Professor of Medicine
University of Washington, Seattle
Director Northwest Kidney Center
Seattle, WA USA
Chapter 33

Juan Bosch, M.D.
Professor of Medicine
Director of Renal Diseases
George Washington University Medical Center
Washington, DC USA
Chapter 15

Michel J.C. Broyer, M.D.
Professor of Pediatrics
Necker's School of Medicine
Université Paris V
Director, Pediatric Nephrology
Hôpital des Enfants Malades-Necker
Paris, France
Chapter 32

Felix P. Brunner, M.D.
Professor of Medicine
University of Basel
Department of Internal Medicine
Kantonsspital
Basel, Switzerland
Chapter 31

Hans O.A. Brynger, M.D., Ph. D.
Associate Professor of Surgery
University of Göteborg
Director Transplant Unit
Sahlgren's Hospital
Göteborg, Sweden
Chapter 31

Vardaman M. Buckalew, Jr., M.D.
Professor of Medicine and Physiology
Chief of Nephrology
Department of Medicine
Bowman Gray School of Medicine
of Wake Forest University
Winston-Salem, NC USA
Chapter 55

John M. Burkart, M.D.
Assistant Professor of Medicine
Bowman Gray School of Medicine
of Wake Forest University
Medical Director, Piedmont Dialysis Center
Winston-Salem, NC USA
Chapter 55

Cyril Chantler, M.A., M.D., FRCP
Professor Paediatric Nephrology
Evelina Children's Department
United Medical and Dental Schools of
Guy's and St. Thomas's Hospitals
Guy's Hospital
London, England
Chapter 32

Stefano Chiaramonte, M.D.
Associate of Clinical Nephrology
Department of Nephrology
St. Bortolo Hospital
Vicenza, Italy
Chapter 37

Jack W. Coburn, M.D.
Professor of Medicine
University of California, Los Angeles
Nephrology Section
Veterans Administration Wadsworth Medical Center
Los Angeles, CA USA
Chapter 44

Jean Crosnier, M.D.
Professeur
Université René Descartes
Faculte de Médecine Necker Enfants-Malades
Clinique Néphrologique
Hôpital Necker
Paris, Cedex, France
Chapter 42

Nancy Boucot Cummings, M.D.
Associate Director for Research
and Assessment, NIDDK
National Institutes of Health
Bethesda, MD USA
Chapter 57

Giuseppe D'Amico, M.D.
Professor of Medicine
University of Milan
Head, Division of Nephrology
San Carlo Hospital
Milan, Italy
Chapter 30

Norman Deane, M.D.
Chairman, Section on Nephrology
Doctors Hospital
Director Manhattan Kidney Center
New York, NY USA
Chapter 18

Wilfried A. De Backer, M.D.
Pulmonary Medicine Division
University Hospital Antwerp
Antwerp, Belgium
Chapter 38

Marc E. De Broe, M.D., Ph. D.
Professor of Medicine
University of Antwerp
Director Nephrology Division
University Hospital Antwerp
Antwerp, Belgium
Chapter 38

Françoise Degos M.D.
Service d'Hépatologie
Hôpital Beaujon
Clichy, France
Chapter 42

Barbara G. Delano, M.D.
Associate Professor of Clinical Medicine
Director-Home Dialysis Program
State University of New York
Health Science Center at Brooklyn
Brooklyn, NY USA
Chapter 29

Raymond A. Donckerwolcke, M.D.
Pediatric Nephrologist
Department of Pediatrics
University of Utrecht
Director, Dialysis and Transplant Program
Wilhelmina Children's Hospital
Utrecht, The Netherlands
Chapter 32

William Drukker, M.D.
Formerly Reader in Dialysis
Department of Medicine Queen Wilhelmina
University Hospital, Amsterdam
Emeritus Director Department of Nephrology and Dialysis
St. Lucas Hospital, Amsterdam
Present Address: De Lairessestraat 75
1071 NV Amsterdam, The Netherlands
Chapters 3, 19, 22

Sheila R. Dykes
Administrator
EDTA Registry
St. Thomas Hospital
London, England
Chapter 31

Joseph W. Eschbach, M.D.
Clinical Professor of Medicine
Division of Nephrology
Department of Medicine
University of Washington
Seattle, WA USA
Chapter 40

Aldo Fabris, M.D.
Associate of Clinical Nephrology
Department of Nephrology
St. Bortolo Hospital
Vicenza, Italy
Chapter 37

Winfried Fassbinder, M.D.
Professor of Nephrology
University Hospital
Frankfurt am Main
Head, Department of Nephrology
Städtische Klinikum
Fulda, FRG
Chapter 31

Mariano Feriani, M.D.
Associate of Clinical Nephrology
Department of Nephrology
St. Bortolo Hospital
Vicenza, Italy
Chapter 37

Eli A. Friedman, M.D.
Professor of Medicine
Chief, Renal Diseases Division
State University of New York
Health Science Center at Brooklyn
Brooklyn, NY USA
Chapter 54

Peter W. Gardner, B.S.
Chief Research Technician
Dialysis Unit, Nephrology Section
Medical Service, Wadsworth Division
West Los Angeles Veterans Administration Medical Center
Los Angeles, CA USA
Chapter 16

Ram Gokal, M.D., FRCP
Consultant Nephrologist
Honorary Lecturer
University of Manchester
Manchester Royal Infirmary
Manchester, England
Chapter 25

Frank A. Gotch, M.D.
Associate Clinical Professor of Medicine
University of California, San Francisco
Medical Director
Dialysis Treatment and Research Center
Davies Medical Center
San Francisco, CA USA
Chapter 4

Hans J. Gurland, M.D.
Professor, Director Nephrology Division
Medical Department I. Klinikum Grosshadern
University of Munich
München, FRG
Chapter 21

Robert W. Hamilton, M.D.
Associate Professor of Medicine
Bowman Gray School of Medicine
of Wake Forest University
Medical Director, Dialysis Unit
North Carolina Baptist Hospital
Winston-Salem, NC USA
Chapter 55

Lee W. Henderson, M.D.
Professor of Medicine
University of California, San Diego
Veterans Administration Medical Center
San Diego, CA USA
Chapter 13

Robert J. Heyka, M.D.
Medical Director – CCF West Side Dialysis Center
Department of Hypertension/Nephrology
The Cleveland Clinic Foundation
Cleveland, OH USA
Chapter 34

Nicholas A. Hoenich, Ph.D.
Lecturer in Clinical Science
Department of Medicine
Medical School
Newcastle upon Tyne, England
Chapters 5, 17

Peter Ivanovich, M.D.
Professor of Medicine
Section of Nephrology
Northwestern University Medical School
Director of Hemodialysis
Department of Medicine, Section of Nephrology
Veterans Administration Lakeside Medical Center
Chicago, IL USA
Chapter 6

Stefan Jacobson, M.D., Ph.D.
Assistant Professor, Institute of Medicine
Karolinska Institute
Associate Physician
Division of Nephrology, Department of Medicine
Karolinska Hospital
Stockholm, Sweden
Chapter 26

Frans G.I. Jennekens, M.D.
Senior Neurologist
Head of the Laboratory for Neuromuscular Diseases
Department of Neurology
University Hospital Utrecht
Utrecht, The Netherlands
Chapter 46

Aagje Jennekens-Schinkel, M.D.
Neuropsychologist, Department of Neuropsychology
University Hospital Leiden
Leiden, The Netherlands
Chapter 46

Paul Jungers, M.D.
Départment de Néphrologie
Hôpital Necker
Paris, France
Chapter 42

William F. Keane, M.D.
Professor of Medicine
University of Minnesota School of Medicine
Division of Nephrology
Hennepin County Medical Center
Minneapolis, MN USA
Chapter 41

Prakash R. Keshaviah, Ph.D.
Senior Research Associate
University of Minnesota, Department of Medicine
Director of Dialysis Regional Kidney Disease Program
Hennepin County Medical Center
Minneapolis, MN USA
Chapters 7, 12

Carl M. Kjellstrand, M.D., FACP
Professor of Medicine and Surgery
University of Minnesota
Chief, Division of Nephrology
Department of Medicine
Karolinska Hospital
Stockholm, Sweden
Chapter 26

Franciszek Kokot, M.D.
Professor of Medicine
Department of Nephrology
Silesian School of Medicine
Katowice, Poland
Chapter 45

Giuseppe La Greca, M.D.
Professor of Medicine
Director of Department of Nephrology
St. Bortolo Hospital
Vicenza, Italy
Chapter 37

Robert MacGregor Lindsay, M.D., FRCP(E), FRCP(C), FACP
Professor, Department of Medicine
The University of Western Ontario
Director of the Renal Unit
Department of Medicine
Victoria Hospital Corporation
London, Ontario, Canada
Chapter 11

Lars-Eric Lins, M.D., Ph.D.
Associate Professor, Institute of Medicine
Karolinska Institute
Senior Physician
Division of Nephrology, Department of Medicine
Karolinska Hospital
Stockholm, Sweden
Chapter 26

Robert R. Lins, M.D.
Director Nephrology Division
General Hospital Stuivenberg
Antwerp, Belgium
Chapter 38

Francisco Llach, M.D.
Professor of Medicine
University of Oklahoma Health Sciences Center
Veterans Administration Hospital
Nephrology Section
Oklahoma City, OK USA
Chapter 44

A. Peter Lundin, M.D.
Associate Professor of Medicine
State University of New York
Health Science Center at Brooklyn
Brooklyn, NY USA
Chapter 56

Michael M. Maddy, M.D.
Fellow in Nephrology
Department of Medicine
Hennepin County Medical Center
Minneapolis, MN USA
Chapter 41

John F. Maher, M.D., FACP
Professor of Medicine
Director, Nephrology Division
F. Edward Hébert School of Medicine
Uniformed Services University of the Health Sciences
Bethesda, MD USA
Chapters 1, 35, 51

Timothy H. Mathew, M.D., B.S., FRACP
Director Renal Unit
Queen Elizabeth Hospital
Adelaide, S.A., Australia
Chapter 28

Joseph H. Miller, M.D.
Associate Research Renologist
Department of Medicine
University of California at Los Angeles
Chief, Dialysis Instrumentation
Dialysis Unit, Nephrology Section
Medical Service, Wadsworth Division
West Los Angeles Veterans Administration Medical Center
Los Angeles, CA USA
Chapter 16

Charles M. Mion, M.D.
Professor of Medicine, Head Division of Nephrology
University Hospital Montpellier
Service de Néphrologie, Hôpital Saint-Charles
Montpellier, France
Chapter 24

William E. Mitch, M.D.
Professor of Medicine
Director, Renal Division
Department of Medicine
Emory University School of Medicine
Atlanta, GA USA
Chapter 53

S. Fazal Mohammad, Ph.D
Associate Professor of Pathology
University of Utah
Director, Hematology Laboratories
Institute for Biomedical Engineering
Division of Artificial Organs
Salt Lake City, UT USA
Chapter 10

John F. Moorhead, FRCP
Director
Department of Nephrology and Transplantation
The Royal Free Hospital
London, England
Chapter 36

Salim K. Mujais, M.D.
Assistant Professor of Medicine
Section of Nephrology
Northwestern University Medical School
Staff Physician
Department of Medicine, Section of Nephrology
Veterans Administration Lakeside Medical Center
Chicago, IL USA
Chapter 6

Karl D. Nolph, M.D.
Professor of Medicine
Director, Division of Nephrology
University of Missouri Health Sciences Center
Harry S. Truman Memorial Veterans Administration Hospital
Columbia, MO USA
Chapter 23

Emil Paganini, M.D., FACP
Head, Section of Dialysis and Extracorporeal Therapy
Department of Hypertension/Nephrology
The Cleveland Clinic Foundation
Cleveland, OH USA
Chapter 34

Bettine C.P. Polak, M.D.
Lecturer in Opthalmology
Erasmus University
Eye Hospital
Rotterdam, The Netherlands
Chapter 47

Manfred Pollok, M.D.
Senior Resident
Department of Nephrology
Medizinische Klinik I.
University Hospital
Cologne, FRG
Chapter 14

David S. Precious, M.D.
Chairman, Department of Oral Diagnosis and Oral Surgery
Dalhousie University
Halifax, Nova Scotia, Canada
Chapter 48

T.K. Sreepada Rao, M.D., FACP
Associate Professor of Medicine
Director of Hemodialysis
State University of New York
Brooklyn, NY USA
Chapter 43

Severin G. Ringoir, M.D.
Professor of Medicine
University of Ghent
Director, Division of Nephrology
University Hospital
Ghent, Belgium
Chapters 2, 17

Gianfranco Rizzoni M.D.
Head, Division of Nephrology and Dialysis
Department of Pediatric Research and Teaching
Ospedale Bambino Jesu
Rome, Italy
Chapter 32

Claudio Ronco, M.D.
Associate of Clinical Nephrology
Department of Nephrology
St. Bortolo Hospital
Vicenza, Italy
Chapters 15, 37

Walter Samtleben, M.D.
Privat Dozent, Nephrology Division
Medical Department I. Klinikum Grosshadern
University of Munich
München, FRG
Chapter 21

John A. Sargent, Ph.D.
Quantitative Medical Systems, Inc.
Emeryville, CA USA
Chapter 4

Ad C. Schoots, Ph.D.
Senior Researcher Analytical Biochemistry
Laboratory for Instrumental Analysis
Faculty of Chemical Engineering
Eindhoven University of Technology
Eindhoven, The Netherlands
Chapter 2

Belding H. Scribner, M.D.
Professor of Medicine
Division of Nephrology
University of Washington
Seattle, WA USA
Forewords to the First and Third Edition

Neville H. Selwood, M.D.
Deputy Director
UK Transplant Service
Southmead Hospital
Bristol, England
Chapter 31

Stanley Shaldon, M.A., M.D. (Cantab), MRCP
Professor of Nephrology
Université de Nimes
Centre Hospitalier Regional, Service de Néphrologie
Nimes, France
Chapter 12

James H. Shinaberger, M.D.
Adjunct Professor of Medicine
University of California, Los Angeles
Chief, Dialysis Program
Dialysis Unit, Nephrology Section
Medical Service, Wadsworth Division
West Los Angeles Veterans Administration Medical Center
Los Angeles, CA USA
Chapter 16

Anne M. Smith, B.Sc., M.B.Ch.B.; MRCP(UK), FRCP(C)
Clinical Assistant Professor of Medicine
The University of Western Ontario
Laboratory Hematology, and Oncology
Victoria Hospital Corporation
London Regional Cancer Centre
London, Ontario, Canada
Chapter 11

Theodore I. Steinman, M.D.
Associate Clinical Professor of Medicine
Harvard Medical School
Director Dialysis Unit
Beth Israel Hospital
Boston, MA USA
Chapter 53

William Kinnear Stewart, M.D., Ph.D., FRCP(Lond), FRCP(Edin)
Reader in Medicine
University of Dundee
Hon. Consultant Physician
General Medicine (special interest Nephrology)
Royal Infirmary
Dundee, Scotland
Chapter 8

Paul Sweny, M.D., FRCP
Senior Lecturer
Department of Nephrology and Transplantation
Royal Free Hospital Medical School
London, England
Chapter 36

Nicholas E. Tawa Jr., M.D.
Clinical Fellow in Surgery
Harvard Medical School
Resident in Surgery
Brigham and Women's Hospital
Boston, MA USA
Chapter 7

Nicholas L. Tilney, M.D.
Professor of Surgery
Director, Surgical Research Laboratories
Harvard Medical School
Director, Transplant Service
Brigham and Women's Hospital
Boston, MA USA
Chapter 9

Charles R.V. Tomson, M.B., B.S., MRCP
Medical Research Council Training Fellow
Department of Medicine
University of Newcastle upon Tyne
Royal Victoria Infirmary
Newcastle upon Tyne, England
Chapter 50

Charles Toussaint, M.D.
Professor
Department of Clinical Medicine, Nephrology
Université Libre de Bruxelles
Head, Nephrology Department
C.U.B. Hôpital Erasme
Brussels, Belgium
Chapter 39

John E. Utting, M.A. M.B., B. Chir., FFARCS
Professor of Anaesthesia
The University of Liverpool
The University Department of Anaesthesia
Royal Liverpool Hospital
Liverpool, England
Chapter 52

Albert W.J. van Doorn, Ph.D.
Scientific Consultant
Arnhem, The Netherlands
Chapter 19

Raymond Vanholder, M.D., Ph.D.
Instructor, Renal Division
University of Ghent
Associate, Renal Division
University Hospital
Ghent, Belgium
Chapters 2, 17

Zachariah Varghese, Ph.D.
Associate Director
Renal Research Unit
Royal Free Hospital
London, England
Chapter 36

Rowan G. Walker, M.D., B.S., FRACP
Director, Dialysis and Transplantation
Royal Childrens Hospital
Victoria, Australia
Chapter 27

Michael K. Ward, M.B., B.S., FRCP
Consultant Physician/Senior Lecturer in Medicine
University of Newcastle upon Tyne
Royal Victoria Infirmary
Newcastle upon Tyne, England
Chapter 50

David C. Wheeler, M.B., Ch.B., MRCP
MRC Training Fellow
Renal Research Unit
Department of Nephrology and Transplantation
The Royal Free Hospital
London, England
Chapter 36

Andrzej Wiecçek, M.D.
Department of Nephrology
Silesian School of Medicine
Katowice, Poland
Chapter 45

James F. Winchester, M.D.
Professor of Medicine
Director of Dialysis
Division of Nephrology
Georgetown University Medical Center
Washington, DC USA
Chapter 20

Robert Wineman, Ph.D.
Director of Special Projects
National Nephrology Foundation
New York, NY USA
Chapter 18

Antony J. Wing, M.A., D.M., FRCP
Consulting Physcian
St. Thomas' Hospital
London, England
Chapter 31

Celia Woffindin, B.Sc.
Scientific Officer
Renal Unit
Royal Victoria Infirmary
Newcastle upon Tyne, England
Chapter 5

INTRODUCTION

JOHN F. MAHER

'He is usually subject to constant recurrence of his symptoms; or again, almost dismissing the recollection of his ailment, he is suddenly seized with an acute attack of pericarditis, or with a still more acute attack of peritonitis, which, without any renewed warning, deprives him in eight and forty hours, of his life. Should he escape this danger likewise, other perils await him; his headaches have been observed to become more frequent; his stomach more deranged; his vision indistinct; his hearing depraved: he is suddenly seized with a convulsive fit, and becomes blind. He struggles through the attack; but again and again it returns; and before a day or a week has elapsed, worne out by convulsions, or overwhelmed by coma, the painful history of his disease is closed.'

For over a century after this classical description of end-stage renal disease by Richard Bright (1) there was virtually no change in the prognosis of these patients. In the past 30 years or so the fate of the patient with irreversible renal failure has changed dramatically, however. Adequate renal function is essential to sustain life, and in the first half of this century chronic renal failure meant an inexorably, progressively fatal course that could be delayed only a few months by rigid dietary protein restriction. The astute physician sought diligently for reversible causes of chronic renal disease such as obstructive uropathy and for such reversible complications as dehydration, infection and superimposed nephrotoxicity, but found these in less than half of the patients. Unresponsive to manipulations that sometimes restore renal function, the patient with terminal renal failure had no alternative than to face death by uremia. The physician and the relatives sat at the bedside in frustration.

Much of the mental and physical suffering that characterized renal failure as it progressed slowly to the end of life has nearly disappeared from our hospital wards. Currently it even difficult to expose our medical students to the clinical uremic syndrome and to teach them at the bedside the signs and symptoms of end-stage renal failure. The combination of gastrointestinal turmoil, twitching, lethargy, dyspnea of uncontrolled acidosis, weakness and pleuropericardial pain may not even be recognized now as uremic in origin until routine laboratory results are reported.

Today, in many parts of the world, dialysis is readily available for patients with renal failure. The patient no longers asks whether there is a chance for survival or whether treatment by dialysis is possible. Rather, the informed patient asks when dialysis will begin and how well employment and holidays can be accommodated to dialysis treatments. Can travelling, swimming, camping and skiing still be carried out? How soon can a transplantation be accomplished?

Survival rates with dialysis treatment that approach those of matched control patients with good renal function represent one of the outstanding technological achievements of the past three decades. Yet, dialysis is an imperfect substitution for renal function compared to the divine prototype. It is expensive and time consuming, indiscriminately removes solutes, fails to substitute for renal hormonal and metabolic activities and requires dietary restrictions and drug therapy to maintain the patient in suboptimal health. Obviously there is a need for much more research to improve the technology, to define more precisely the biochemical nature of uremia, to prevent the progression of renal failure and most importantly to reverse or cure the renal diseases that destroy renal function. Complacency is not warranted.

The treatment of the patient in terminal renal failure can be complicated and difficult. It requires understanding fluid and electrolyte homeostasis, and management of complications involving all the major organ systems. When dialysis first became available for a limited number of patients, a few physicians entered the field of renal replacement therapy, some of them hesitatingly, but usually attracted by the challenge of managing so complex a problem with the aid of new technology. These poineer physicians (the term 'nephrologist' came later) started more or less from scratch and saw their discipline grow rapidly. But, they could readily keep up with the modest volume of dialysis literature and learned from each other at meetings, symposia and congresses. This first generation of dialysis physicians became a family of enthusiastic, energetic physicians working in a new and fascinating field of medicine. They were viewed curiously by other colleagues, some of whom considered them gadgeteers; others were content to refer, despite skepticism, their difficult, truly terminal uremic patients, challenging them to perform 'miracles'.

This first generation is approaching, or even has already reached, the end of their careers. A second generation has taken over and a third generation of young physicians has entered the field. They face an abundant, often bewildering and widely scattered literature on dialysis and on treatment of terminal renal failure in general. Because patients are kept alive by dialysis, the opportunity has been afforded to elucidate the endocrine aspects of chronic renal failure, to study the neurological, immunological and hematological abnormalities of uremia and to identify changes in various other organ systems. New subdisciplines have developed including trace metal homeostasis and pharmacokinetics in uremia and the psychiatric aspects of life with renal substitution. It can be difficult, even frustrating, for the novice in the field to sort out amongst so much information what is important from the past, what is useful at present and what should be disregarded in between. Unless one is especially gifted with mathematical and physical knowledge, it can be a difficult, even awesome or frightening task to assimilate the information in the treatises of physics of modern dialyzers, the complicated electronics and hydraulics of modern monitoring and proportioning systems and the physics of sorbent and ion exchange regeneration systems for dialysis fluid. Therefore, a book offering an encyclopedic review of the present state of the art seemed to be useful. The contributors to this text include many of the pioneers who laid the foundation of this discipline and others who contributed importantly to its rapid growth. Those who are presently newly entering the field may find this book a useful guide to the present treatment of the patient in terminal renal failure by hemodialysis or peritoneal dialysis and they will also find descriptions of the conservative methods of treatment which necessarily accompany dialysis treatment. Others, even those first and second generation of dialysis physicians and scientists, may find the book useful as a reference guide. Accordingly, we have included detailed information and an extensive but critical review of the present concepts underlying this therapy. We have deemphasized or totally omitted, however, relatively unimportant details, outdated facts and descriptions of archaic techniques and machines, vogues and dated hypotheses.

Dialysis interposes a semi-permeable membrane between a flowing stream of blood and an appropriate rinsing solution. By convective and diffusive transport, the composition of body fluids approaches that of the dialysis solution. Simultaneous ultrafiltration decreases body fluid volumes, ordinarily toward normal. Lowering of concentrations of toxic solutes in body fluids by dialysis is ordinarily associated with clinical improvement of the uremic syndrome, while hypertension and congestive heart failure usually recede as volume excess is corrected. But, as we cannot identify precisely and understand sufficiently the toxicity of the retained solutes, we deplete indiscriminately, removing useful as well as toxic solutes in proportions dictated by membrane permeability and concentration gradients rather than according to their toxic potential. Further, we substitute poorly for the endocrine and metabolic aspects of renal regulation of body composition. Our therapy is a dramatic success compared to the natural history of progressive renal disease, but it is cumbersome, awkward and inefficient compared to the healthy kidney.

Following the initial successful dialysis for therapy of renal failure, numerous modifications in dialyzer design and technique and in other aspects of therapy soon followed, improving the efficacy of therapy. The bioengineers were able to improve flow distribution and membrane contact and to lower transport resistances. But, it now appears that additional major improvements in therapy may await increased fundamental knowledge of renal failure and the biochemistry of uremia. Empiricism may have reached its

limit. Accordingly, the complete reference work must review the basic concepts of mass transport, extracorporeal thrombogenesis, biochemical and metabolic abnormalities, organ pathophysiology and so forth to provide the fundamental basis on which new knowledge may build. Yet, the pragmatic information of why, when and how to dialyze patients must also be presented to appreciate the existing problems and to promote optimal care.

The success of dialysis and the introduction of renal biopsy are largely responsible for the development of nephrology as a clinical discipline. Yet both techniques have been harshly criticized. In the absence of morphologic understanding of the causes of end-stage renal disease and without a method to delay or avoid a fatal outcome, there was little interest in investigating chronic renal disease. These techniques changed that attitude, however. Indeed, the nephrology community and dialysis industry grew considerably. But the outsider's perception of dialysis was a 'low technology', even comparable to the 'iron lung' treatment of respiratory paralysis, diverting resources from the development of the equivalent of a poliomyelitis vaccine. Some physicians who emphasized the care of end-stage renal disease by dialysis often were lucratively rewarded monetarily but many more were slandered by their peers as pseudonephrologists. Iron lungs, however, did not provide a patient population exceeding 100,000 who presented the spectrum of abnormalities that stimulated research which clarified renal osteodystrophy, advanced immunology, developed erythropoietin, promoted development of a hepatitis vaccine, gave new insights about amyloidosis and so forth. Moreover, the funds obtained from the clinical practice of dialysis were often used to train the investigators who it is hoped can find cures to renal disease eliminating or at least decreasing the need for dialysis. The focus on that utopian goal need not belittle this remarkable technological success, however, nor ignore the immediate suffering in the quest for the long-term solution.

The science of the pathophysiology of terminal renal failure and the technology of its treatment continue to be in a state of dynamic progress. *Panta rei*: nothing is static, everything changes. Our knowledge in this field is far from petrified; it still expands and improves. Within the past decade the association of mesangial sclerosis, glomerular hyperfiltration and renal functional deterioration with a high protein intake, the clinical application of hemofiltration, of sequential filtration dialysis and of ultrashort dialysis, the initiation of continuous ambulatory peritoneal dialysis and its therapeutic variants, the availability of a hepatitis vaccine, active vitamin D metabolites and recombinant human erythropoietin, increased kinetic analysis of dialysis and of drug therapy, understanding of aluminum induced osteomalacia, improved control of hypertension, the threat of AIDS, the recognition of β_2 microglobulin related amyloidosis in long-term dialysis survivors, and cyclosporin treatment of transplant recipients have all emerged.

But technological achievements and improved diagnostic and therapeutic capability are not enough. All generations of clinical nephrologists from the first to the third and those that follow, must be aware of the enormous responsibility for the quality of treatment offered to the terminal renal failure patient who puts his life in their hands, having virtually no other choice for survival. The quality of that treatment depends on the dedication and the knowledge, the training and professional skills of the physicians, their nurses and paramedical co-workers. We should never forget that a bad treatment often means a long period of disability, of misery and of suffering if not death. We are now not only capable of saving thousands of lives, but we are also able to attain the goal of offering those patients in terminal renal failure and their families a good and enjoyable quality of life.

REFERENCE

1. Bright R: Cases and observations illustrative of renal disease accompanied with the secretion of albuminous urine. *Guys Hosp Rep* 1: 338, 1836

UREMIC TOXICITY

R. VANHOLDER, A. SCHOOTS and S. RINGOIR

INTRODUCTION

The uremic patient suffers from a syndrome that resembles poisoning by an ingested toxin. The clinical picture is well known and consists of a definite number of symptoms.

Numerous authors have tried to reproduce symptoms or demonstrate metabolic disturbances of the uremic syndrome by many *in vitro* and *in vivo* tests. Almost all these tests have been performed with uremic plasma or uremic serum. More recently fractions of uremic ultrafiltrate, obtained by gel chromatography or other separation methods, have also been evaluated in an attempt to define the substance(s) responsible for uremic toxicity.

The association of renal failure with the retention of solutes has been recognized for more than 150 years (1). It is conceivable that at least some of these solutes exert a toxic action. Firstly, the success of dialysis therapy suggests the retention of dialysable but unidentified toxins in uremia. Secondly, marked symptomatic improvement may follow the decrease of dietary protein ingestion, at least temporarily, in the predialytic stage. These proteins may function as metabolic precursors of uremic products, so that a fall in their production conceivably might result in decreased toxic effects.

Although these facts have been known for years, and tremendous efforts have been exerted to identify the specific toxin(s) that provoke the uremic syndrome, our knowledge about uremic toxin(s) has remained unsatisfactory and scattered (2), resulting in an almost purely empirical approach to treatment.

The discussion on 'the' uremic toxin is probably an oversimplification of the real problem; the entire spectrum of accumulated products may play a role, since toxicity can be due to the synergism of specific toxic effects when several components are brought together. The comparison with a 'puzzle' (the uremic puzzle) that presents its total image only after it has been completed, seems appropriate here.

It is the purpose of this chapter to review the present knowledge about uremic toxicity, with special emphasis on the methods that have been used to try to resolve this problem.

UREMIC TOXICITY

In vivo toxicity

Uremia is a clinical syndrome that in many aspects resembles systemic poisoning (3). A host of clinical symptoms have been recognized to occur when kidney function declines (4–6). Although most of these symptoms are attenuated by dialysis treatment, some may persist, even after prolonged therapy. Almost every organ system in the body is affected by uremic toxicity and the known uremic clinical symptoms and side effects are multiple (Table 1). Most striking are neurological signs and symptoms (fatigue, twitching, peripheral neuropathy), gastrointestinal problems (anorexia, hiccup, stomatitis, gastritis, parotitis, pancreatitis), cardio-vascular problems (heart failure, hypertension, pericarditis, atherosclerosis), hematological disorders of which anemia is the most important, and changes of the immunological response. Renal osteodystrophy is a specific problem as it occurs, at least in part, on a hormonal and a metabolic basis.

In spite of these multiple uremic symptoms, *in vivo* studies of uremic toxicity have rarely been performed. Essentially, four methods have been used.

A first method consists of the administration of one or more potential toxins to experimental animals. Giovanetti et al (7) used this method to demonstrate the toxicity of methylguanidine in dogs. Anemia, thrombocytopenia, weight loss, several gastrointestinal symptoms, and central and peripheral nerve dysfunction all were reported by these authors to occur after the chronic subcutaneous administration of this substance (7).

A second method is used in dialysed patients, and is characterized by attempts to counteract the elimination of one uremic solute or of a specific group of solutes, either by the addition of a substance to the dialysate (8), or by altering dialysis schedules so that only specific groups of uremic solutes are eliminated in an optimal way (9). In 1972, John-

son et al (8) developed a protocol where urea was added to dialysate to maintain blood urea concentrations at pre-fixed levels. It appeared that toxic symptoms only appeared when blood urea rose above 300 mg/dl. In a study by Lowrie et al (9), optimum elimination of small molecules like urea or of the so-called middle molecules was pursued in two separate groups; it appeared that toxic symptoms were more related to the elimination of small molecules than to that of substances with a higher molecular weight.

A third method consists of the subdivision of patient populations into a group doing well on hemodialysis, and a group showing problems or symptoms followed by a comparative study of the plasma profiles of uremic solutes in both groups (10). This approach was used by Bergström's group in 1983, resulting in the finding of a consistent elevation of the so-called 7c fraction in patients showing uremic symptoms; the concentration of this fraction was markedly less elevated in the asymptomatic patients.

A final approach is the *in vivo* evaluation in animals or in man of the influence of uremia on very specific body functions, such as parameters of autonomic nerve function (11, 12), glucose tolerance (13), or electroencephalographic and other neurophysiological abnormalities (14).

In vitro toxicity

Extensive studies by means of specific *in vitro* tests have been performed to evaluate whether one of the retained uremic solutes, or a specific group of these substances, could influence more specifically some metabolic activities in the human or the animal body. For this purpose, in most studies, uremic serum or ultrafiltrate of uremic serum was collected and studied, either as such, or after lyophylization and addition to normal serum. Uremic serum or other uremic biological fluids (e.g. pleural fluid) most currently are collected from patients in renal failure, but can also be harvested from uremic animals, e.g. rats after 5/6 nephrectomy. Some studies have been performed on normal urine, because this material is supposed to contain all solutes that are retained during uremia; it should be recognized, however, that the concentrations of many solutes in normal urine may differ substantially from those found in serum of uremic patients.

Many studies were performed following the separation of body fluids by gel chromatography (15–22). The bulk of these *in vitro* tests has been developed based on the known abnormalities occurring *in vivo* during uremia.

The *in vitro* tests of uremic toxicity can be subdivided into the following major groups (Table 2):

Studies of the immunologic system
Lamperi and Carozzi (23) evaluated T-cell growth factor activity and T-cell subset identification. The metabolic responsiveness of lymphocytes has been studied more specifically by the evaluation of ^{3}H-thymidine uptake of lymphocytes at maximal transformation (24, 25) or after stimulation (26, 27). Somewhat in parallel to the latter model, Gutman and Huang (16) directly studied bone marrow thymidine incorporation. Other currently used methods are the eval-

Table 1. Uremic clinical symptoms and side effects.

Stupor, coma	Hypogonadism
Polyneuritis	Thirst
Hiccup	Asterixis
Stomatitis	Anorexia
Parotitis	Uremic fetor
Gastritis	Motor weakness
Gastrointestinal ulcers	Malaise
Immune depression	Shortened attention span
Pericarditis	Insomnia
Anemia	Drowsiness
Bleeding	Weight loss
Pruritus	Erratic memory
Acidosis	Headache
Uremic lung	Slurred speech
Convulsions	Irritability
Fatigue	Reduced sociability
Chemical diabetes	Impotence
Vomiting, Nausea	Diminished libido
Hypertension	Dry skin
Atherosclerosis	Hypothermia
Hyperpigmentation	Restless legs
Cancer	Flapping tremor
Osteodystrophy	Cramps
Growth retardation	Tics
Hyperlipemia	Meningismus

uation of the lymphocyte immune response or proliferation or both after stimulation (22, 28, 29) and the study of E-rosette forming capacity (30). Finally, an important series of tests has evaluated granulocyte function and phagocytic response to different stimuli, either by testing granulocyte random mobility (31), granulocyte adherence (32) or direct phagocytic capacity. For the latter type of studies, polymorphonuclear leukocyte oxidative metabolism is often tested by the evaluation of the chemiluminescence of these cells (33–35). Alternative methods are the evaluation of

Table 2. In vitro tests of uremic toxicity.

Immunologic system
T-cell growth factor
T-cell subset identification
^{3}H-thymidine uptake of lymphocytes
bone marrow thymidine incorporation
lymphocyte immune response
E-rosette forming capacity
phagocytic response:
   mobility
   adherence
   chemiluminescence
   uptake of radiolabelled particles
   skin window test
   phagocytic glucose metabolism

Metabolic processes or enzymatic activities
gluconeogenesis
sodium-potassium ATP-ase activity
lactate dehydrogenase activity
mitochondrial storage of calcium
mitochondrial activity
alkaline phosphatase activity
insulin degradation

Erythrocyte status and function
fragility of red blood cells
erythrocyte membrane fluidity
in vitro iron transport
erythropoiesis
erythrocyte osmotic fragility

Coagulation
platelet cyclo-oxygenase activity
platelet aggregation
platelet glycolysis

Nerve function
isolated sural nerve conductivity

Heart cell function
beating rate of heart cells
heart cell survival
cardiovascular reflexes
effect of adenylate cyclase stimulation
beta-adrenoceptor density and affinity

Glucose metabolism
glucose utilization
insulin receptors

Drug protein binding

phagocytosis of radiolabelled particles (e.g. candida albicans) (36), of phagocytotic capacity by the skin window test (37), and of glucose metabolism by phagocytes before and after stimulation (15, 17).

Studies of metabolic processes or enzymatic activities

Numerous enzymes or other metabolic systems have been studied over the years within the context of the evaluation of uremic toxicity. By preference, these studies have been performed on tissue slices of liver, kidney, brain or muscle. Some of the systems that have been subjected to study are the gluconeogenesis of kidney cortex or liver slices (38), sodium-potassium ATP-ase activity of brain (39) or intestinal cells (40), activity of lactate dehydrogenase of kidney homogenates (20) or of rabbit muscle and beef heart (41), the mitochondrial storage of calcium (42), liver mitochondrial activity (43) and the activity of neutrophil alkaline phosphatase isoenzymes (44). Finally insulin degradation by isolated liver and muscle has also been studied (45).

Studies of erythrocyte status and function.
Studies have been conducted on fragility of red blood-cells (18), erythrocyte membrane fluidity (46), in vitro iron transport (47), erythropoiesis (48–50), and erythrocyte osmotic resistance (51, 52).

Studies of the coagulation system
Platelet cyclo-oxygenase activity has extensively been evaluated in dialysis patients by Tanaka et al and Remuzzi et al (53–55).
   Other studies have more specifically evaluated platelet aggregation (21), and platelet glycolysis (56).

Studies of nerve function
To our knowledge, in vitro studies on nerve function have only rarely been performed. One study was conducted by Funck-Brentano and his coworkers (57) in this setting, on isolated sural nerve conductivity.

Heart cell function
The beating rate and the survival of isolated heart cells was the subject of a study by Bogin et al (58). Another very recent study by Mann et al (59) focused on the chronotropic response of the heart by the evaluation of cardiovascular reflexes, of the effect of adenylate cyclase stimulation, and of beta-adrenoceptor density and affinity.

Glucose metabolism
Glucose metabolism and the response to insulin has also been the subject of extensive evaluation. Abnormal glucose utilization has been demonstrated in uremic patients (60). In vitro evaluations were mainly based on the study of glucose utilization in various tissues: striated muscle, kidney cortex, brain, liver slices, fat cells etc. (61, 62). Other studies have focused on the number of insulin receptors in chronic renal failure (63).

Changes in drug protein binding

Drug protein binding abnormalities may be considered an epiphenomenon of uremic solute retention. Although not directly toxic, these alterations may induce changes in concentration of free active drug, thereby inducing toxic side effects. Protein binding may be decreased or increased, leading to either undertreatment or drug intoxication.

Phenytoin has been the subject of repeated extensive evaluations (64–73). The protein binding characteristics of many drugs that are currently used in renal failure patients remain undetermined, however.

Comments

In vivo studies are scarce and have always been difficult to design. *In vitro* studies, on the other hand, most often evaluate only one aspect of uremic toxicity. The concentrations used do not always correspond to those encountered in the blood of uremic patients. Furthermore, these experiments only reflect acute toxicity and are not always relevant for chronic intoxication.

If samples are submitted to gel chromatography before *in vitro* testing, some of the obtained fractions may influence biological activities due to their high electrolyte and/or osmolar content or pH, and not to the organic solutes that they contain (74).

The picture is further clouded by the fact that in many instances single substances are nontoxic, causing toxicity only when mixed with other products.

Finally, the finding of substances with an *in vitro* influence on a single biochemical function may resolve a tiny part of the uremic toxicity problem, but those findings are only partially representative to what happens *in vivo* to the whole body.

By the use of *in vitro* tests, it has not only been possible to discern substances or groups of substances with an inhibitory activity on cellular or organ function, but some uremic solutes have also been shown to have no toxic effects, at least on some selected metabolic processes.

In our hands, it appeared that no inhibition of *in vitro* phagocytosis or *in vitro* protein synthesis occurred in the presence of urea (4 g/l, 66.7 mmol/l), creatinine (15 mg/100 ml, 1.3 mmol/l), arabinitol (400 mg/l, 2.6 mmol/l) erythritol (600 mg/l, 4.9 mmol/l) and myoinositol (900 mg/l, 5.0 mmol/l) in spite of concentrations of all these substances comparable with or above those that are observed in chronic renal failure patients requiring dialysis. Understanding of the toxicity or nontoxicity of uremic solutes remains confused and to a large extent unresolved, in spite of the obvious toxicity of uremic serum as such. Further multifactorial studies are needed to obtain more definite information about this topic.

BIOCHEMICAL EVALUATION OF RETAINED SOLUTES

It is undeniable that many different solutes are retained in uremia. Elaborate reviews of this subject have been published in the literature over the years (74, 75). Some of the most currently reported uremic solutes are enumerated in Table 3. Even the most detailed review, depicting all known products, remains incomplete, as the number of unknown substances probably exceeds by far the number identified. Even nowadays, new retention products are being added to the list of known uremic solutes. As an example, recent studies have enabled us to find elevated levels of the environmental pollutant hexachlorobenzene in the blood of dialyzed and non-dialyzed uremic patients (76); the latter compound is an organochlorine pesticide and is also used as a plasticizer for polyvinylchloride. High serum bromine level have previously been detected by our group in patients with renal failure (77).

Subdivision of uremic retention products

Overall, solutes that are retained during uremia can be subdivided into four main groups. First, a number of inorganic substances, such as water and electrolytes are retained. This group with often well known effects may induce acute and life-treatening complications (e.g. hyperkalemia). Sec-

Table 3. Potential uremic toxins.

Urea
Creatinine
Guanidines
Phenols
Hippurates
Benzoates
'Polypeptides'
Beta$_2$ microglobulin
Indoles
'Middle-molecules'
Ammonia
Alkaloids
Amines
Bromine
Uric acid
Cyclic AMP
Amino acids
Myoinositol
Mannitol
Oxalate
Glucuronate
Glycols
Lysozyme
Hormones
Parathormone
Natriuretic factor
Glucagon
Growth hormone
Gastrin
Prolactin

ond, an important group of low molecular weight (MW) organic substances should be mentioned (MW<300 daltons); to this group belong well known and easily determined uremic metabolites such as urea and creatinine, but also less currently evaluated derivatives such as amines, phenols and indoles. A third group is composed by the so-called middle molecules, that classically are defined to have a molecular weight of 300 to 2,000 daltons. The composition of this heterogenous group remains ill defined, in spite of prolonged and intensive research in many laboratories.

Finally, a fourth group of larger compounds up to 50,000 daltons such as larger polypeptides, beta$_2$ microglobulin and lysozyme also accumulate in renal failure and may exert toxic effects.

Identification methods

Many of the inorganic and the low molecular weight organic substances, known to accumulate in renal failure, can easily be determined by chemical methods. The study of uremic solutes becomes more complex, if an attempt is made to find as yet unknown substances, and even more complicated, when one tries to define these products. For historical reasons, the bulk of the research for unknown uremic solutes has been concentrated on the group of so-called middle molecular weight molecules. Subsequently, most of the methods used in this setting have been chosen with the aim of searching for these middle molecules.

Gel chromatography
Gel chromatography on Sephadex gels was the first approach used to separate uremic sera or other biological fluids into different fractions, and is also by far the most frequently used technique in this setting. Different types of

gels have been used (19, 78), Sephadex G-15 being the most popular (2, 15, 20–22, 79–90). With this technique, the elution volume should relate inversely to the molecular weight of the eluted solutes, at least theoretically. Thus, the solutes with the highest molecular weight should be eluted first and vice versa. Although some degree of separation of uremic solutes is obtained with this method, its resolution is not sufficient enough to allow definite conclusions about the composition of the retained substances.

Gel chromatography combined with other techniques
In many studies, gel filtration has been used only as a first line separation method, followed by a second technique in order to allow a more accurate definition of the products under study. Within the context of this multicomponent analysis, Sephadex gel chromatography has been used in conjuction with amino acid analysis (2, 79), ion-pair extraction (2), gas chromatography (2, 78, 86), gradient elution chromatography (2), isotachophoresis (2, 86), mass spectrometry (2, 78, 86), gradient elution chromatography on DEAE A-25 Sephadex microcolumns (79–80, 84, 88), high pressure liquid chromatography (22, 86), ultraviolet spectroscopy (90) and ^{1}H–^{13}C nuclear magnetic resonance (89). In spite of this extensive approach, only three groups to our knowledge have as yet been able to separate single middle molecular components of relative purity.

Firstly, Zimmerman et al (90) found that the main component of a gel chromatographic middle molecule peak (7c) was a glucuronide of ortho-hydroxyhippuric acid with a molecular weight of 371. Secondly, Cueille et al (91) described a middle molecule designated b$_{4-2}$, the main component of which appeared to be a glucuronide of an unknown compound, with a total molecular weight of 526 (92). Further study is needed to identify a specific substance within this fraction.

Table 4. Solutes (and their molecular masses) found in adjacent gel-filtration fractions.[a]

Solute	MW	Fraction number					
		13	14	15	16	17	18
Sodium (chloride)	58	O	×	O	O		
Creatinine	113				O	×	
Urea	60					O	×
Acetate	60	O	×	O	O		
Lactate	90	O	×	O			
Glucuronate	196		×				
Aspartic acid	133		×	O			
Phosphate	98	O	×				
Serine	105		×	O			
Threonine	119		×				
Glucose	180		O	O	×		
Fructose	180			×			
Glucitol	182			×	O		
Arabinitol	152			×	O		
Erythritol	122			×	O		
Myoinositol	180		O	×			

[a] Circles indicate the presence, crosses symbolize the fraction with maximum concentration, of the indicated solute in the fraction.
MW: indicates molecular mass (daltons).

Finally, Gallice et al (89) very recently identified a middle molecular compound, that also appeared to be glucuronidated ortho-hydroxyhippuric acid. This is the same substance as the one described by Zimmerman et al (90), although the latter authors used different techniques of isolation and identification. It should be stressed that, to our knowledge, the toxicity of these compounds still remains to be evaluated more thoroughly.

Disadvantages of gel chromatography
The knowledge that has resulted from the world-wide approach to the middle-molecular problem, is disappointingly small. This might be attributed to the anomalous retention behavior of gel chromatography that has been used most often as the basic separation technique. Furthermore, some other facts suggest that one should be rather careful with the results of chromatographic studies. First, artifacts might be induced by some drugs in plasma middle molecule determinations (93). It is known that salicylic acid modifies the chromatographic pattern of the middle molecule fractions in normal subjects and uremic patients (87, 94), and more exactly, peak 7c has been shown to increase in height in serum of patients to whom salicylic acid had been administered; this is not astonishing, in view of the fact that ortho-hydroxyhippuric acid, the main component of peak 7c, is one of the known metabolites of aspirin.

Furthermore, careful analysis by combined methods of the so-called middle molecular mass region has demonstrated that this fraction contained a considerable amount of substances of low molecular weight, such as carbohydrates, organic acids, amino acids, and ultraviolet absorbing solutes (86). Table 4 indicates that several small molecular substances can be found in so-called middle molecular fractions. The presence of low-molecular weight substances in the middle molecular fractions is also suggested by the molecular weight of the only truly recognized 'middle molecule', ortho-hydroxyhippuric acid glucuronide, which is surprisingly low (371 daltons) (90). All these data mandate a careful use of gel chromatography as a basic separation method, and a careful interpretation of its results; these facts have stimulated the search for alternative techniques.

Alternative separation methods

The most frequently used alternative separation methods are isotachophoresis, gas chromatography and high performance liquid chromatography (HPLC). All these methods have been used by the authors in an attempt to obtain a better separation of uremic solutes (95–101).

High performance liquid chromatography

The HPLC-technique has several advantages compared to the other techniques as it combines some important properties: known and unknown solutes are analysed simultaneously with sufficient resolution, without the need for chemical modification as in gas chromatography.

Furthermore, the method is non-destructive, so adequate

collection of fractions facilitates further characterisation of solutes with respect to biochemical activity. Also important is the fact that exact quantitation is possible as well as automation. HPLC allows the clear cut separation of at least 30 different components, that are visualized by UV absorbance or by fluorescence (102). It should, however, be stressed that the toxicity of many of these components has not as yet been demonstrated.

There is an obvious difference between pre- and postdialysis serum HPLC patterns. The HPLC-technique enables recognition of subtle differences in intradialytic extraction ratios between different dialysis techniques (100), that could not be recognized earlier with the gel chromatography method (83). Thus, in our opinion, high performance liquid chromatography appears to be a valuable tool in the study of uremic toxicity and its treatment.

Identification of solutes with a well defined chemical structure
Apart from these rather complicated, labor-intensive and multifractional analytical methods, other studies have been characterized by the search for solutes with a well defined chemical structure. Here, the group of ninhydrin-positive peptides is most important (103–106). Few data are available about the significance of these compounds as uremic toxins, and furthermore most of the reported isolation procedures of peptides are even more complex than the ones used for other uremic compounds. An exception might be the study on these compounds by a specific high performance liquid chromatography method, as recently reported by Mabuchi and Nakahashi (107). Other peptides that have been submitted to an evaluation are plasma endorphins and lipoproteins (108).

Analysis of known biologically active substances
A final approach for analysis comprises the measurement of known biochemically active compounds. In particular, different types of hormones, such as glucagon (109), and steroid hormones (110) have been analyzed. Although not entirely defined, endogenous digitalis-like fractions have also been subjected to studies by analysis of digoxin-like immunoreactivity and sodium/potassium ATP-ase inhibitory activity (111, 112).

SUBSTANCES PLAYING A ROLE IN UREMIC TOXICITY

The general opinion of nephrologists about the toxins that eventually might be responsible for the toxic symptoms observed during renal failure, has been fluctuating over the years, and so has been the transmission of these ideas into general therapeutic practice. In the early days of dialysis, it was a generally held belief that small molecular substances were the main toxins. Sometimes, however, there was a poor correlation between toxic manifestations of uremia and small molecular concentrations in uremic plasma. Scribner (113) suggested as early as 1965 that certain membranes could achieve better solute removal than others. This suggestion was based on the clinical observation that patients on long-term peritoneal dialysis were in good condition in spite of relatively high plasma concentrations of low molecular weight substances. This finally led to the 'square meter hour' hypothesis, as originally formulated by Babb et al (114). This hypothesis stressed the pathophysiological importance of substances with a higher molecular weight than the small molecules on which focus had previously been. Subsequently, the square meter hour hypothesis was changed to the middle molecule hypothesis in 1972, and removal of middle molecules was pursued intensively (114).

This statement set into motion a world-wide research. As a consequence, the early seventies became the era of belief in middle molecules. However, as time went on, and middle molecular research resulted in rather disappointing conclusions, doubt arose about the pathophysiologic role of middle molecular weight substances. This attitude was further stimulated by studies of Lowrie et al (115) and the American National Cooperative Dialysis Study (NCDS), showing a direct relation between plasma concentrations of the small molecule urea, and overall morbidity on dialysis. Subsequently, the early eighties were characterized by some skep-

Table 5. Uremic solutes and their potential toxic side effects.

Urea
  – induction of toxic symptoms: headache, vomiting, fatigue
  – inhibition of cardiac output response
Methylguanidine
  – anorexia, vomiting, diarrhea, gastric ulceration, polyneuritis
  – inhibition of *in vitro* brain sodium-potassium ATP-ase
Indoxylsulfate
  – inhibition of drug protein binding
  – defect of cellular organic acid transport
Myoinositol
  – decrease of sciatic nerve conduction velocity
Hippuric acid
  – decrease of cortical tubular para-aminohippurate and urate transport
  – inhibition of organic substance transport
  – inhibition of drug protein binding
  – (decrease of glucose tolerance)
  – (decrease of platelet cyclo-oxygenase activity)
  – (decrease of phagocytotic activity)
Peptides
  – inhibition of erythropoiesis
  – decrease in red cell osmotic resistance
  – decrease in heart cell contractility
Parathormone
  – inhibition of erythropoiesis
  – decrease in red cell osmotic resistance
  – decrease in heart cell contractility
Beta$_2$ microglobulin
  – amyloidosis
  – bone and joint disease, carpal tunnel syndrome
Spermine, polyamines
  – inhibition of erythropoiesis
  – induction of anorexia, vomiting, ataxia, seizures, hypothermia, immune deficiency.

ticism concerning middle molecules.

It is quite remarkable, that in spite of these changing moods about the substances responsible for uremic toxicity, and in spite of the concomitant changes in dialysis strategies, the responsible toxins have hardly been recognized up to now. Although it is quite certain that uremic serum influences many biological functions (see above), it has been much more difficult to identify the responsible factors, even after the subdivision into different fractions by chromatographic techniques. One of the reasons for that failure is certainly the use of gel chromatography for fractionation, since the specificity of this fractionation technique and the purity of the obtained fractions are suboptimal. Furthermore, many of these fractions contain salt, other electrolytes, and glucose and these compounds may on their turn influence biological activities. Another difficulty is the aquisition of enough substrate for analysis in uremic patients that often are also anemic, so that only small quantities of serum can be collected per patient. Here, the collection of ultrafiltrate may be of major help, although with this method larger molecules are excluded from evaluation.

For all these reasons, the knowledge of the biological toxicity of individual uremic solutes has been deceivingly low. Nevertheless, several substances have been recognized to influence one or more biological activities (Table 5).

Urea

Urea for instance has been shown to induce such toxic symptoms as headache, vomiting and fatigue, when chronic renal failure patients are dialysed against dialysate containing high concentrations of urea (8). In high concentrations, urea also decreased the cardiac output response of isolated guinea pig hearts (116). This deleterious effect was even aggravated by the addition of creatinine, guanidino-succinate and methylguanidine to the perfusion medium, suggesting that a mixture of several substances may cause more toxic side-effects than a single solute alone.

Urea may thus be toxic, but only at high concentrations, exceeding those that are currently seen in the plasma of appropriately treated chronic renal failure patients. Urea can thus not be held responsible for the bulk of uremic symptoms, observed in uremic patients.

Methylguanidine and other guanidines

Methylguanidine, when injected to healthy dogs, caused a picture of heavy intoxication, characterized by anorexia, vomiting, diarrhea, gastric ulceration and polyneuritis (117, 118). *In vitro*, brain sodium-potassium ATP-ase of uremic rats also appeared to be inhibited by methylguanidine (39).

In general, it can, however, be accepted that methylguanidine and also the other guanidines are only toxic in concentrations that are much higher than those found in uremic patients.

Indoxyl sulfate

Indoxyl sulfate has been related to drug protein binding inhibition (73, 119), and to eventual defects of the cellular organic acid transport function (120).

Myoinositol

A decrease of sciatic nerve conduction velocity was found in rats given the carbohydrate derivative, myoinositol (121). Therefore, it could be possible that myoinositol plays a role in the development of peripheral neuropathy.

Hippuric acid

It was shown in 1975 by Boumendil-Podevin and coworkers (120) that hippuric acid interfered with the para-aminohippurate and urate transport at the cortical tubular level. These data suggested that hippuric acid might inhibit the renal tubular transport of a variety of organic substances. Moreover, it was demonstrated by Porter at al (122) that hippuric acid caused net fluid secretion in proximal straight tubules isolated from rabbit kidneys. Hippuric acid has also been shown to decrease drug protein binding (72, 73). Finally, preliminary results by Dzurik et al (61) and Tanaka et al (53, 54) indicate that hippuric acid also might interfere with glucose tolerance and platelet cyclo-oxygenase activity (61, 123). Recently the authors found an inhibition by hippuric acid of the glucose consumption and the oxygen burst during the phagocytosis of Latex or Zymosan by leukocytes (123).

Peptides

Peptides may also influence biochemical functions. Abiko et al (105) were able to isolate from the hemodialysate of a uremic patient with immunodeficiency a peptide that inhibited lymphocyte stimulation.

Parathormone

In a series of elegant studies, Bogin and coworkers were able to show that parathormone had multiple toxic side effects, inducing an inhibition of erythropoiesis (52), and a decrease in red cell osmotic resistance (51), and impaired contractility of heart cells (58).

Beta$_2$ microglobulin

Beta$_2$ microglobulin has been known for years to accumulate in dialysis patients (124). Recent data indicated that the amyloidosis, that is frequently demonstrated in patients after prolonged treatment, is mainly characterized by bone and joint involvement (125) and carpal tunnel syndrome and is caused by a local deposition of beta$_2$ microglobulin (126, 127). Elimination of beta$_2$ microglobulin has been shown to vary with different types of dialyzers (128). Retrospectively, treatment with the dialyzers with the highest elimination rates of beta$_2$ microglobulin appeared to be associated with the lowest occurrence of amyloidosis (129).

Beta$_2$ microglobulin obviously exerts it's toxic action only after a prolonged period of exposure. It is, however, not entirely clear, whether beta$_2$ microglobulin related amyloidosis should be attributed directly to the accumulation of this substance, per se. The possibility exists that complement activation plays an equally important role, since this complement activation is followed by the activation and break-down of white blood cells, and since beta$_2$ microglobulin is found in high concentrations in the wall of these white blood cells. This indicates that membranes such as cuprophane, that have both low biocompatibility and a small pore size may simultaneously be characterized by an inefficient elimination and an increased production of beta$_2$ microglobulin.

Spermine and other polyamines

Spermine is a polycationic polyamine, that is retained in renal failure, and is known to influence erythropoiesis negatively (130). Other polyamines such as spermidine, putrescine and cadaverine are also found in increased concentrations in renal failure, and these substances are known to be very sticky, i.e. they have a high affinity for body proteins and cells. Polyamines are claimed by Campbell (131) to play an important role in anorexia, vomiting, ataxia, seizures, hypothermia, and immune deficiency.

Conclusions

Overall, it can be stated that our knowledge of the responsible toxins for uremic toxicity is rough, incomplete and fragmentary. Some solutes have been shown to play a role in some biological systems. The 'uremic toxin' apparently does not exist. Our knowledge is also too scanty, at the moment, to design therapy specifically or to guide modifications informatively.

MIDDLE VERSUS LOW MOLECULAR WEIGHT TOXICITY

The question now arises whether uremic toxicity is mainly due either to substances with a low molecular weight or to those of middle molecular weight. A few years ago, middle molecular weight solutes were held responsible for a number of the toxic epiphenomena of uremia, but their importance subsequently has been the subject of substantial doubt. As stated above, some commonly measured low molecular weight substances may be toxic, but most likely only in concentrations exceeding those found in chronic renal failure patients. On the other hand, it is quite certain that some small molecules such as methylguanidine, exert a straightforward toxic action. Some of these substances may exert no toxic effect as a single product, as they may only become toxic in conjunction with other compounds.

A similar or even more vague picture arises when the toxicity of so-called 'middle molecules' is taken into consideration. From the *in vitro* experiments described above, it can hardly be denied that substances with a middle molecular behavior on chromatography, may influence metabolic, physiologic and immunologic processes in the human body. It is however more difficult to translate these findings to the clinical situation. Bergström and his group (10, 132) were able to demonstrate that a group of patients doing well on hemodialysis, had a much lower concentration in the plasma of a given substance with middle molecular behavior on chromatography (fraction 7C). On the other hand, Lowrie et al (9) could not demonstrate a relationship between middle molecular elimination and dialysis morbidity, in an *in vivo* setting where the intradialytic toxin elimination rate was designed to vary. Furthermore, Kjellstrand et al (133) found no relationship between the pre-dialysis levels of middle molecules and the development of uremic neuropathy.

The question arises to the true nature of these so-called middle molecules. It has been stated by Schoots et al (86) that chromatographic middle molecular fractions contained a considerable amount of low molecular weight compounds. It is also obvious that some uremic solutes chromatographically behave like middle molecules, although their actual molecular weight is relatively low. This might be due to a number of factors that have rarely been considered until now, such as electrostatic charges, molecular configuration and protein binding. Furthermore, one should wonder whether it can be expected that a chromatographic middle molecular behavior automatically results in an intradialytic middle molecular elimination rate.

FACTORS INFLUENCING PLASMA CONCENTRATION OF UREMIC SOLUTES

There are multiple factors that may influence the plasma concentration of uremic solutes. One of the most simple examples is urea: the concentration of this low molecular weight solute depends on protein intake, general metabolic status, residual renal function, and dialysis performance (115, 134), but protein binding of urea is practically nil, and it is essentially diluted in total body water. Most other substances follow more complex kinetics due to their multi-compartmental distribution volumes, effects of protein binding and production sources other than nutrition. An example of the latter possibility is hippuric acid; the concentration of this solute might be influenced in dialysis patients by the metabolism of benzyl alcohol, a current preservative of heparin (135); furthermore, in all uremic patients, blood hippuric acid concentration might be influenced by such diverse factors, as the intake of foods and beverages containing sodium benzoate as a preservative, the breakdown of phenylalanine or phenyl containing fatty acids with an odd number of carbon atoms, environmental contact with xylenes or toluenes or both, production by the intestinal flora, and endogenous production (123, 136–139). Elimination by pathways other than the kidney, such as excretion by the gut or liver, that are of little or no importance in persons with normal renal function, may become more important as substances accumulate in the body due to inadequate kidney function.

Therefore, it is clear that the evolution of blood concentrations of any uremic solute will follow complex determinants and the factors governing their elimination remain equally complicated.

Removability

It has always been the aim of dialysis to remove a maximum quantity of toxins, and several different methods have been developed to quantify the elimination capacity of blood purification techniques.

Clearance methods

Different indirect clearance methods have been developed, to obtain an idea about the elimination of different molecules or groups of molecules during dialysis. Over the years water soluble small molecules such as urea and creatinine have become extremely popular for this purpose. Since the introduction of the middle molecular concept, substances with a size in the range of the supposed middle molecules, such as vitamin B_{12} and inulin have also been used for clearance studies (140, 141).

However, the direct estimation of the magnitude of the intradialytic elimination of large groups of unselected molecules with different size possibly gives a more accurate idea of overall solute removal. The studies within this context should preferrably be performed *in vivo* and *in vitro*, using appropriate techniques (74).

Urea kinetics

Another currently quoted marker might be the weekly time-averaged urea concentration, as suggested by studies of the American National Cooperative Dialysis Study (NCDS) (115), showing a direct relationship between the integrated and averaged plasma urea concentrations over one week and the overall morbidity on dialysis. It should, however, be kept in mind that all these studies by the NCDS were performed using cellulosic dialyzers with a relatively low molecular mass cutoff. In the meantime, dialyzers became available, especially in Europe, with more favorable sieving characteristics (142, 143). It is difficult to state at present whether urea kinetic theories, as formulated by Lowrie et al (115) and Sargent and Gotch (144), still hold for these newer and also more biocompatible membranes. Furthermore, urea might not be ideally suited as an estimate of dialysis adequacy, since it is influenced by such extradialytic factors as protein intake and catabolism. The determination of urea kinetics is complicated, labor intensive and necessitates the computation of at least three parameters: time averaged plasma urea concentration (TAC urea), mass transfer coefficient × time/distribution volume (Kt/V) and protein catabolic rate (PCR) (145).

Finally, the use of a single pool model of urea kinetics has

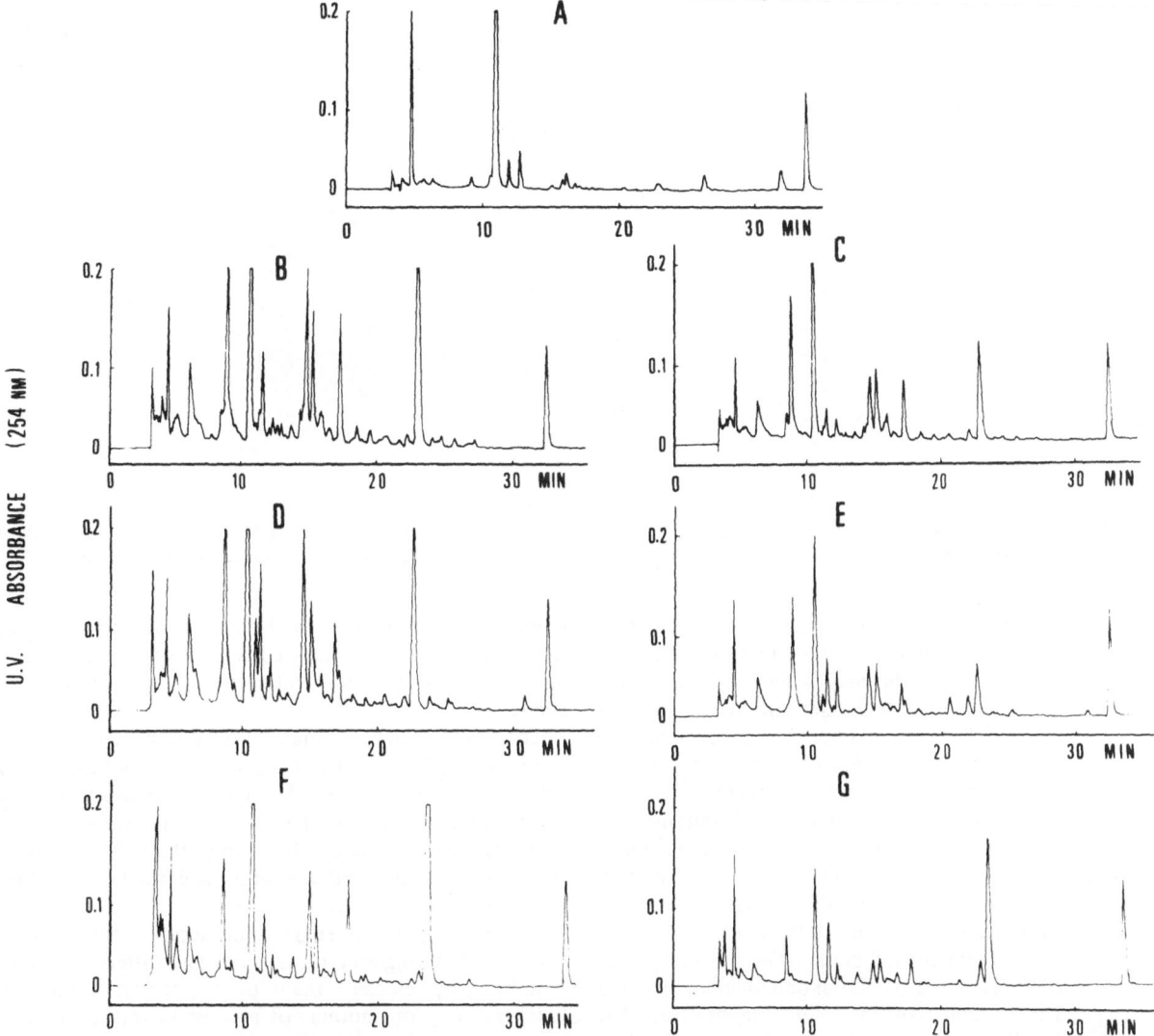

Figure 1. High performance liquid chromatogram of protein free ultrafiltrate of normal serum (A), and of uremic serum, before (B) and after conventional hemodialysis (C) (4 h), before (D) and after treatment with the two chamber technique (E) (3 h), and before (F) and after high efficiency hemodiafiltration (G) (4 h). Results are similar for 4 h conventional dialysis and 3 h two chamber technique. Results of high efficiency hemodiafiltration are better than for the two other techniques, and the post-treatment HPLC-pattern resembles most that of normal serum.

recently been criticized, because it would lead to an incorrect estimation of urea distribution volume and of protein catabolic rate (146–148).

For all these reasons, in our opinion, there should be an ongoing search for alternative markers of uremic toxicity, expecially those representing substances that are poorly removable for reasons of molecular dimension, protein binding, charge, polarity or compartmental distribution or a combination thereof.

HPLC-Studies

During the last few years the cooperative Ghent-Eindhoven group has been evaluating the elimination of multiple sol-

utes by the calculation of their dialysis ratio and their extraction. The dialysis ratio can be defined as the relation of pre- versus post-dialysis concentration, whereas extraction is the relation of the difference of pre- minus post-dialysis concentration, divided by the pre-dialysis concentration; the concentration pre- and post-dialysis and the characterization of the different solutes is performed by the HPLC-method (100, 101). These studies have resulted in a better insight into overall solute removal with different blood purification techniques and enabled us to compare different dialysis strategies to each other. For example, in a recent study, a comparison was made between three different therapeutic options: conventional hemodialysis, the two chamber technique (a combination of hemodialysis and hemofiltration

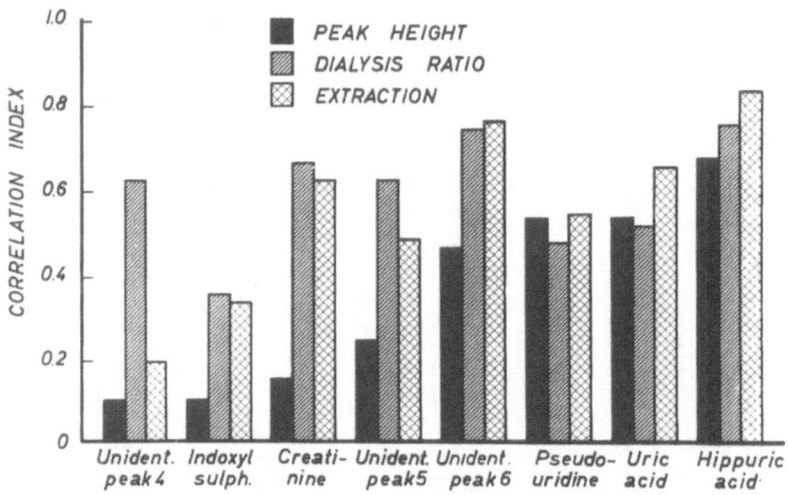

Figure 2. Correlation indices of several individual substances versus total UV absorbance for 90 hemodialysis sessions: ■ peak height, ▨ dialysis ratio, ⊠ extraction. For each of the parameters under study, the highest correlation index was found for hippuric acid.

with two dialyzers in series), and high efficiency hemodiafiltration. It appeared from these studies that with regard to solute elimination, high efficiency hemodiafiltration was superior to the two chamber technique and to conventional dialysis (Figure 1, Table 6). Although the two chamber technique was performed over 3 h, and conventional dialysis over 4 h, virtually similar results were obtained.

Within this context it is important to draw the attention to the parameter of total UV-absorbance, which is the cumulative and integrated peak height of all UV-absorbing HPLC-peaks together. In these studies, this parameter was evaluated as such, but we also studied the relative evolution before versus after dialysis, to obtain a dialysis ratio and an extraction value as well (123). It is our opinion that this value gives a good assessment of overall solute retention, and that its elimination is also a good parameter of overall solute

elimination. Preliminary studies have shown that this total UV-absorbance is inversely correlated with renal function and directly with overall retention of fluorescent uremic solutes.

The peak height of the major individual peaks was further evaluated and correlated to total UV-absorbance, in an attempt to define which individual compounds would give the most suitable reflection of overall solute retention. Similarly, dialysis ratio, and extraction of the individual peaks were also correlated with the ratio and extraction calculated for total UV-absorbance.

In brief, these data suggest the accumulation of many compounds during uremia, each having a different intradialytic behavior. Because many of these products might be toxic one way or another, or at least might be indirectly representative for overall toxicity and accumulation, they

Table 6. Dialysis efficiencies (*in vivo*) of conventional hemodialysis (CH), the two chamber technique (TCT) and high efficiency hemodiafiltration (HEH).

Peak	CH (4 h)		TCT (3 h)		HEH (4 h)	
	Ratio[b]	Extraction[b]	Ratio	Extraction	Ratio	Extraction
Creatinine	2.35 ± 0.38	0.57 ± 0.06	2.47 ± 0.28	0.60 ± 0.06	3.14 ± 0.61^c	0.67 ± 0.06^c
Pseudo-uridine	1.82 ± 0.27	0.45 ± 0.07	1.91 ± 0.26	0.49 ± 0.06	2.66 ± 0.35^c	0.65 ± 0.10^c
Uric acid	2.90 ± 0.43	0.66 ± 0.05	2.90 ± 0.37	$0.65 \pm 0\ 04$	4.18 ± 0.76^c	0.75 ± 0.04^c
Peak 4[a]	2.85 ± 0.66	0.63 ± 0.09	2.41 ± 0.98	0.59 ± 0.17	4.66 ± 0.75^c	0.77 ± 0.42^c
Peak 5[a]	1.85 ± 0.33	0.46 ± 0.08	2.01 ± 0.44	0.51 ± 0.11	2.42 ± 0.42^c	0.58 ± 0.08^c
P-OH hippuric acid	2.71 ± 0.44	0.62 ± 0.06	2.67 ± 0.38	0.62 ± 0.06	4.81 ± 1.32^c	0.78 ± 0.06^c
Hippuric acid	2.85 ± 0.53	0.64 ± 0.07	3.04 ± 0.54	0.66 ± 0.06	3.53 ± 0.88^c	0.71 ± 0.08^c
Overall UV absorption	2.48 ± 0.41	0.58 ± 0.07	2.49 ± 0.48	0.57 ± 0.06	3.20 ± 0.61^c	0.68 ± 0.06^c

[a] Peaks 4 and 5 are unidentified.

[b] Ratio: pre/post; Extraction: (pre-post)/pre.

[c] $p < 0.01$ vs CH and TCT.

might prove to be useful parameters for assessing overall elimination of toxins and adequacy of dialysis. Of all compounds that we considered, the best correlations with total UV-absorbance with regard to peak height, dialysis ratio and extraction were found for hippuric acid, as illustrated in Figure 2.

Finally, individual peak height was also correlated with residual renal function, both in non-dialyzed and dialyzed patients. To assess residual function four substances have been studied up to now: urea, creatinine, the unidentified peak 6 and hippuric acid. From these data, the hippuric acid concentration in plasma again appeared to be most suitable as an indicator of residual renal function.

CONCLUSIONS

More and more sophisticated methods have become available for the study of uremic toxicity. Nevertheless, our knowledge of the biological effects of uremic toxins and of the responsible substances remains fragmentary and a source of debate. Many of the available techniques are complicated and expensive, and have only a limited distinctive capacity. The HPLC-method is at the moment probably one of the more refined techniques, allows a clear distinction between a number of components and is not overly labor intensive.

Moreover, these is a remarkable difference between the HPLC-pattern pre- and post-dialysis. Therefore, the HPLC-method appears to us to be a valuable technique for the further study of uremic toxicity. Possibly, the performance will still be improved if this technique is combined with other separation methods.

It is not possible at the moment, to define each of the recognized products as uremic 'toxins'. The aim should be to eliminate retention products as much as possible by dialysis, in a way that the postdialysis HPLC-pattern resembles normal serum. Together with this strategy, the search for reliable markers of adequate dialysis should be continued.

ACKNOWLEDGEMENT

Table 4 is reproduced with permission, from Schoots AC et al *Clin Chem* 28: 45, 1982.

REFERENCES

1. Prevost JL, Dumas JA: Examen du sang et de son action dans les divers phénomènes de la vie. (Examination of the blood and its action in the different phenomena of life.) *Ann Chim Phys* 23: 90, 1921
2. Gordon A, Bergström J, Fürst F, Zimmerman L: Separation and characterization of uremic metabolites in biologic fluids: a screening approach to the definition of uremic toxins. *Kidney Int* 7 (Suppl 2): S45, 1975
3. Knochel JP: Pathogenesis of the uremic syndrome. *Postgraduate Med* 64: 88, 1978
4. Merrill JP, Hampers CL: Uremia. *N Engl J Med* 282: 953, 1970
5. Giovannetti S, Berlyne GM: An outline of the uremic syndrome. *Nephron* 14: 119, 1975
6. Teschan PE: The presentation of the patient with chronic renal failure, in *End-Stage Renal Disease*, edited by Stone WJ, Rabin PL, New York, Academic Press 1983, p 31
7. Giovannetti S, Biagini M, Balestri PL, Navalesi R, Giagnoni P, De Matteis A, Ferro-milone P, Perfetti C.: Uraemia-like syndrome in dogs chronically intoxicated with methylguanidine and creatinine. *Clin Sci* 36: 445, 1969
8. Johnson WJ, Hagge WW, Wagoner RD, Dinapoli RP, Rosevear JW: Effects of urea loading in patients with far-advanced renal failure. *Mayo Clin Proc* 47: 21, 1972
9. Lowrie EG, Steinberg SM, Galen MA, Gagneux SA, Lazarus JM, Gottlieb MN, Merrill JP: Factors in the dialysis regimen which contribute to alterations in the abnormalities of uremia. *Kidney Int* 10: 409, 1976
10. Asaba H, Alvestrand A, Fürst P, Bergström J: Clinical implications of uremic middle molecules in regular hemodialysis patients. *Clin Nephrol* 19: 179, 1983
11. Rockel A, Henneman H, Richwien D, Heidland A: Tyraminstimulierbares Puppillenerweiterungsvermögen – ein Parameter der autonomen Insuffizienz bei Urämie. (Pupillary reaction on tyramine – a parameter of uremic autonomic neuropathy.) *Klin Wschr* 54: 479, 1976
12. Solders G, Persson A, Wilczek H: Autonomic system dysfunction and polyneuropathy in nondiabetic uremia. *Transplantation* 41: 616, 1986
13. Briggs JD, Buchanan KD, Luke RC, Mac Kiddie MTM: Role of insulin in glucose intolerance in uraemia. *Lancet* 1: 462, 1967
14. Teschan PE: Electroencephalographic and other neurophysiological abnormalities in uremia. *Kidney Int* 7 (Suppl 2): S210, 1975
15. Ringoir S, Van Landschoot N, De Smet R: Inhibition of phagocytosis by a middle molecular fraction from uremic ultrafiltrate. *Opusc Med Techn Lundensia* 21: 13, 1979
16. Gutman RA, Huang AT: Inhibitor of marrow thymidine incorporation from sera of patients with uremia. *Kidney Int* 18: 715, 1980
17. Ringoir SMG, Van Landschoot N, De Smet R: Inhibition of phagocytosis by a middle molecular fraction from ultrafiltrate. *Clin Nephrol* 13: 109, 1980
18. Ota K, Sanaka T, Agishi T, Nakajima O: Influence of uremic middle molecules on blood cells. *Artif Organs* 4: 113, 1980
19. Dzurik R, Spustova V, Cernacek P: Inhibitor of renal gluconeogenesis (IGN): additional physiological modulator in *Biochemical Aspects of Renal Function*, edited by Rose BD, Guder WG, Oxford, Pergamon Press, 1980, p 103
20. De Smet R, Van Landschoot N, Van Der Stiggel G, Ringoir S: Isotachophoretic pattern of LDH inhibiting fractions obtained from uremic ultrafiltrate by gel chromatography. *Int J Artif Organs* 6: 67, 1983
21. Bazilinski N, Shaykh M, Dunea G, Mamdani B, Patel A, Ahmed S: Inhibition of platelet function by uremic middle molecules. *Nephron* 40: 423, 1985
22. Navarro J, Grossetete MC, DeFrosne A, Touraine JL, Traeger J: Isolation of an immunosuppressive fraction in ultrafiltrate from uremic sera. *Nephron* 40: 396, 1985
23. Lamperi S, Carozzi S: T lymphocytes, monocytes and erythropoiesis disorders in chronic renal failure. *Nephron* 39: 211, 1985
24. Korz R, Naber A, Brunner H, Buschsieweke U, Essers U:

Lymphozytentransformation und Autohämolyse unter Einwirkung höhermolekularer Urinmetabolite als potentielle Urämietoxine. (Effect of higher molecular weight urinary metabolites on lymphocyte transformation and autohemolysis.) *Klin Wschr* 53: 761, 1975

25. Korz R, Naber A, Essers U: Spontane Lymphocytentransformation bei chronischer Niereninsuffizienz. (Spontaneous lymphocyte transformation in chronic renal insufficiency.) *Klin Wschr* 53: 21, 1975

26. Del Carmen Samaniego M, Nesse A, Arrizurieta De Muchnik E: Toxinas uremicas. (Uremic toxins.) *Medicina (Buenos Aires)* 44: 252, 1984

27. Newberry WM, Sanford JP: Defective cellular immunity in renal failure: depression of reactivity of lymphocytes to phytohemagglutin by renal failure serum. *J Clin Invest* 50: 1262, 1971

28. Birkeland SA: Uremia as a state of imune defiency. *Scand J Immunol* 5: 107, 1976

29. Kurz P, Kohler H, Meuer S, Hutteroth T, Meyer Zum Buschenfelde KH: Impaired cellular immune responses in chronic renal failure: evidence for a T-cell defect. *Kidney Int* 29: 1209, 1986

30. Abiko T, Sekino H: Effects of two synthetic serum thymic factor analogues and four thymic factor fragments on the low E-rosette forming cells in patients with chronic renal failure. *Chem Pharm Bull* 30: 4448, 1982

31. Henderson LW, Miller ME, Hamilton RW, Norman ME: Hemodialysis leukopenia and polymorph random mobility – a possible correlation. *J Lab Clin Med* 85: 191, 1975

32. Lespier-Dexter LE, Guerra C, Ojeda W, Martinez-Maldonado M: Granulocyte adherence in uremia and hemodialysis. *Nephron* 24: 64, 1979

33. Ritchey EE, Wallin JD, Sham SV: Chemiluminescence and superoxide anion production by leucocytes from chronic hemodialysis patients. *Kidney Int* 19: 349, 1981

34. Nguyen AT, Lethias C, Zingraff J, Herbelin A, Naret C, Descamps-Latscha B: Hemodialysis membrane-induced activation of phagocyte oxidative metabolism detected in vivo and in vitro within microamounts of whole blood. *Kidney Int* 28: 158, 1985

35. Rhee MS, Mac Goldrick MD, Meuwissen HJ: Serum factor from patients with chronic renal failure enhances polymorphonuclear oxidative metabolism. *Nephron* 42: 6, 1986

36. Jorstad S, Smeby LC, Widerøe TE, Berg KJ: Transport of uremic toxins through conventional hemodialysis membranes. *Clin Nephrol* 12: 168, 1979

37. Ringoir S, Van Looy L, Van De Heyning P, Leroux-Roels G: Impairment of phagocytic activity of macrophages as studied by the skin window test in patients on regular hemodialysis treatment. *Clin Nephrol* 4: 234, 1975

38. Lamberts B, Brunnen H, Ochs HG, Spellerberg P, Heintz R: Effect of urine metabolites from healthy and uremic subjects on gluconeogenesis in slices of rat kidney cortex and liver. *Clin Nephrol* 6: 465, 1976

39. Minkoff L, Gaertner G, Darab M, Mercier C, Levin ML: Inhibition of brain sodium-potassium ATPase in uremic rats. *J Lab Clin Med* 80: 71, 1972

40. Kramer HJ, Backer A, Kruck F: Inhibition of intestinal ($Na^+–K^+$)-ATPase in experimental uremia. *Clin Chim Acta* 50: 13, 1974

41. Wilkinson JH, Fujimoto Y, Senesky D, Ludwig GD: Nature of the inhibitors of lactate dehydrogenase in uremic dialysates. *J Lab Clin Med* 75: 109, 1970

42. Fournier N, Gallice P, Crevat A, Murisasco A, Ducet G,

Elsen R: Action on mitochondrial calcium metabolism of an ionophorous compound isolated from uremic plasma or normal urine. *Artif Organs 9:* 22, 1985

43. Martinelli R, Rodrigues LEA, Machado AEC, Rocha M: The effect of acute uremia on liver mitochondrial activity. *Nephron* 17: 155, 1976

44. Vergnes HA, Grozdea JD: A study of the selective inhibition by urea of neutrophil alkaline phosphatase isoenzymes. *Enzyme* 34: 45, 1985

45. Rabkin R, Unterhalter SA, Duckworth WC: Effect of prolonged uremia on insulin metabolism by isolated liver and muscle. *Kidney Int* 16: 433, 1979

46. Komidori K, Kamada T, Yamashita T, Harada R, Otsuji Y, Hashimoto S, Chuman Y, Otsuji S: Erythrocyte membrane fluidity decreased in uremic hemodialyzed patients. *Nephron* 40: 185, 1985

47. Wallner SF, Vautrin RM: The anemia of chronic renal failure. Studies of iron transport in vitro. *J Lab Clin Med* 96: 67, 1980

48. Wallner SF, Vautrin RM: The anemia of chronic renal failure: studies of the effect of organic solvent extraction of serum. *J Lab Clin Med* 92: 363, 1978

49. Meytes D, Bogin E, Ma A, Dukex PP, Massry SG: Effect of parathyroid hormone on erythropoiesis. *J Clin Invest* 67: 1263, 1981

50. Delwiche F, Segal GM, Eschbach JW, Adamson JW: Hematopoietic inhibitors in chronic renal failure: lack of in vitro specificity. *Kidney Int* 29: 641, 1986

51. Bogin E, Massry SG, Levi J, Djaldetti M, Bristol G, Smith J: Effect of parathyroid hormone on osmotic fragility of human erythrocytes. *J Clin Invest* 69: 1017, 1982

52. Malachi T, Bogin E, Gafter U, Levi J: Parathyroid hormone effect on the fragility of human young and old red blood cells in uremia. *Nephron* 42: 52, 1986

53. Tanaka H, Umimoto K, Izumi N, Maekawa T, Kishimoto T, Maekawa M: Can hemodialysis remove the factor that suppresses platelet cyclo-oxygenase activity in uremic patients? *Trans Am Soc Artif Intern Organs* 31: 552, 1985

54. Tanaka H, Umimoto K, Izumi N, Maekawa T, Kishimoto T, Maekawa M: Platelet cyclo-oxygenase in haemodialysis patients: what suppresses its activity? *Proc Eur Dial Transplant Assoc Eur Ren Assoc* 22: 250, 1985

55. Remuzzi G, Benigni A, Dodesini R, Schieppati A, Livio M, De Gaetano G, Day JS, Smith WL, Pinca E, Patrignani P, Patrono C: Reduced platelet thromboxane formation in uremia. Evidence for a functional cyclo-oxygenase defect. *J Clin Invest* 71: 762, 1983

56. Tison P, Cernacek P, Silvanova E, Dzurik R: Uremic 'toxins' and blood platelet carbohydrate metabolism. *Nephron* 28: 192, 1981

57. Funck-Brentano JL, Boudet J, Sausse A, Cueille G, Man NK: In vitro sural nerve test for the evaluation of middle molecule neurotoxicity in uraemia. in *Technical Aspects of Renal Dialysis,* edited by Frost TH, Tunbridge Wells, UK, Pitman Medical, 1978, p 256

58. Bogin E, Massry SG, Harary I: Effect of parathyroid hormone on rat heart cells. *J Clin Invest* 67: 1215, 1981

59. Mann JFE, Jakobs KH, Riedel J, Ritz E: Reduced chronotropic responsiveness of the heart in experimental uremia. *Am J Physiol* 250: H846, 1986

60. Defronzo RA, Smith D, Alvestrand A: Insulin action in uremia. *Kidney Int* 24 (Suppl 16): S102, 1983

61. Dzurik R, Spustova V, Gerykova M: Pathogenesis and consequences of the alteration of glucose metabolism in renal insufficiency. in *Uremic Toxins,* edited by Ringoir S, Vanholder

R, Massry S, New York, Plenum Publ Co, 1987, p 105

62. Lockwood DH: The insulin resistance inducing factor. in *Uremic Toxins*, edited by Ringoir S, Vanholder R, Massry S, New York, Plenum Publ Co, 1987, p 97

63. Gambhir KK, Archer JA, Nerurkar SG, Cruz IA, Sanders M: Erythrocyte insulin receptors in chronic renal failure. *Nephron* 28: 4, 1981

64. Reidenberg MM, Odar-Cederlöf I, Van Bahr C, Borga O, Sjoqvist F: Protein binding of diphenylhydantoin and desmethylimipramine in plasma from patients with poor renal function. *N Engl J Med* 285: 264, 1971

65. Schoeman DW, Azarnoff DL: The alteration of plasma proteins in uremia as reflected in their ability to bind digitoxin and diphenylhydantoin. *Pharmacology* 7: 169, 1972

66. Olsen GD, Bennett WM, Porter GA: Morphine and phenytoin binding to plasma proteins in renal and hepatic failure. *Clin Pharmacol Ther* 17: 677, 1975

67. Depner TA, Gulyassy PF: Plasma protein binding in uremia: extraction and characterisation of an inhibitor. *Kidney Int* 18: 86, 1980

68. Depner TA, Stanfel LA, Jarrard EA, Gulyassy PF: Impaired plasma phenytoin binding in uremia. *Nephron* 25: 231, 1980

69. Kinniburgh DW, Boyd ND: Isolation of peptides from uremic plasma that inhibit phenytoin binding to normal plasma proteins. *Clin Pharmacol Ther* 30: 276, 1981

70. Depner TA: Suppression of tubular anion transport by an inhibitor of serum protein binding in uremia. *Kidney Int* 20: 511, 1981

71. Grossman SH, Davis D, Kitchell BB, Shand DG, Routledge PA: Diazepam and lidocaine plasma protein binding in renal disease. *Clin Pharmacol Ther* 31: 350, 1982

72. Gulyassy PF, Bottini AT, Stanfel LA, Jarrard EA, Depner TA: Isolation and chemical identification of inhibitors of plasma ligand binding. *Kidney Int* 30: 391, 1986

73. MacNamara PJ, Lalka D, Gibaldi M: Endogenous accumulation products and serum protein binding in uremia. *J Lab Clin Med* 98: 730, 1981

74. Schoots A, Mikkers F, Cramers C, De Smet R, Ringoir S: Uremic toxins and the elusive middle molecules. *Nephron* 38: 1, 1984

75. Contreras P, Later R, Navarro J, Touraine JL, Freyria AM, Traeger J: Molecules in the middle molecular weight range. *Nephron* 32: 193, 1982

76. Rutten G, Schoots A, Vanholder R, Cramers C, Ringoir S: Organochloride pesticides of serum of dialyzed and non-dialyzed uremic patients. *Nephron* 48: 217, 1988

77. Cornelis R, Ringoir S, Lameire N, Mees L, Hoste J: Blood bromine in uremic patients. *Miner Electrolyte Metab* 2: 186, 1979

78. Bultitude FW, Newham SJ: Identification of some abnormal metabolites in plasma from uremic subjects. *Clin Chem* 21: 1329, 1975

79. Fürst P, Bergström J, Gordon A, Johnson E, Zimmerman L: Separation of peptides of 'middle' molecular weight from biological fluids of patients with uremia. *Kidney Int* 7 (Suppl 2): S 272, 1975

80. Fürst P, Zimmerman L, Bergström J: Determination of endogenous middle molecules in normal and uremic body fluids. *Clin Nephrol* 5: 178, 1976

81. Oules R, Asaba H, Neuhauser M, Yahiel V, Gunnarson B, Bergström J: The removal of uremic small and middle molecules and free amino acids by carbon hemoperfusion. *Trans Am Soc Artif Intern Organs* 23: 583, 1977

82. Ringoir S, De Smet R, Becaus I: Serum middle molecules in two different strategies (PAN-open and closed) of hemodialysis. *Kidney Int* 12: 152, 1977

83. Ringoir S, De Smet R, Becaus I: Serum middle molecules in different dialysis strategies. in *Aktuelle Probleme der Dialyseverfahren und der Niereninsuffizienz,* edited by von Dittrich P, Kopp K, Friedburg, Verlag Bindernagel, 1977, p 128

84. Oules R, Asaba H, Neuhauser M, Yahiel V, Baehrendtz S, Gunnarson B, Bergström J., Fürst P: Hemoperfusion and removal of endogenous uremic middle molecules in *Artificial Kidney, Artifical Liver and Artificial Cells,* edited by Chang TMS, New York, Plenum Publ Co 1978, p 153

85. Ringoir S, De Smet R: Serum chromatographic pattern in different dialysis strategies. *Int J Artif Organs* 1: 218, 1978

86. Schoots AC, Mikkers FEP, Claessens HA, De Smet R, Van Landschoot N, Ringoir S: Characterization of uremic 'middle molecular' fractions by gas chromatography, mass spectrometry, isotachophoresis and liquid chromatography. *Clin Chem* 28: 45, 1982

87. Faguer P, Man NK, Cueille G, Funck-Brentano JL: Drug interaction in middle molecule analysis, with special reference to acetylsalicylic acid. *Artif Organs* 8: 226, 1984

88. Faguer P, Man NK, Pierrat D, Funck-Brentano JL: Semi-automated determination of the uremic toxin 'b4–2'. *Clin Chem* 30: 797, 1984

89. Gallice P, Monti JP, Crevat A, Durand C, Murisasco A: A compound from uremic plasma and from normal urine isolated by liquid chromatography and identified by nuclear magnetic resonance. *Clin Chem* 31:30, 1985

90. Zimmerman L, Fürst P, Bergström J, Jornvall H: A new glycine containing compound with a blocked amino group from uremic body fluids. *Clin Nephrol* 14: 109, 1980

91. Cueille G: Mise en évidence et évaluation des 'moyennes molécules' de la taille de la vitamine B$_{12}$ présents dans les liquides biologiques de sujets normaux et de patients urémiques. (Determination of middle molecules presenting vitamin B$_{12}$ molecular size in normal and uremic body fluids.) *J Chromatogr* 146: 55, 1978

92. Cueille G, Man NK, Farges JP, Funck-Brentano JL: Characterization of sub-peak b4.2 middle molecule. *Artif Organs* 4: 28, 1980

93. Chapman GV, Ward RA, Farrell PC: Separation and quantification of the 'middle molecules' in uremia. *Kidney Int* 17: 82, 1980

94. Asaba H, Zimmerman L, Bergström J: On drug artifacts in middle molecule analysis. *Nephron* 39: 73, 1985

95. Schoots AC, Mikkers FEP, Cramers CAMG, Ringoir S: Profiling of uremic serum by high-resolution gas chromatography-electron-impact, chemical ionization mass spectrometry. *J Chromatogr* 164: 1, 1979

96. Mikkers F, Ringoir S, De Smet R: Analytical isotachophoresis of uremic blood samples. *J Chromatogr* 162: 341, 1979

97. Mikkers F, Verheggen T, Ringoir S: Isotachophoresis of uremic metabolites. in *Protides of Biological Fluids,* edited by Peeters H, Oxford, Pergamon Press, 1979, p 727

98. Mikkers F, Ringoir S: Isotachophoresis of uremic metabolites. in *Biochemical and Biological Applications of Isotachophoresis,* edited by Adam A, Schots C, Amsterdam, Elsevier Scientific, 1980, p 127

99. Schoots A, Homan H, De Smet R, Cramers C, Vanholder R, Ringoir S: Evaluation of in vivo dialysis efficiency in hemodialysis and hemodiafiltration by reversed-phase liquid chromatography. in *First International Symposium on Single-Needle Dialysis,* edited by Ringoir S, Vanholder R, Ivanovich P, Cleveland, ISAO Press, 1984, p 151

100. Schoots AC, Homan HR, Gladdines MM, Cramers C, De Smet R, Ringoir S: Screening of UV-absorbing solutes in uremic serum by reversed phase HPLC – change of blood levels in different therapies. *Clin Chim Acta* 146: 37, 1985

101. Schoots A, Vanholder R, De Smet R, Cramers C, Ringoir S: Hippurate and an unknown compound as indicators of residual renal function in dialysed patients. in *Immune and Metabolic Aspects of Therapeutic Blood Purification Systems*, edited by Smeby LC, Jorstad S, Widerøe TE, Basel, Karger, 1986, p 240

102. Schoots A, Vanholder R, De Smet R, Cramers C, Ringoir S: Markers of uremic studied by high performance liquid chromatography (HPLC). *Abstracts Am Soc Artif Intern Organs* 15: 59, 1986

103. Abiko T, Kumikawa M, Higuchi H, Sekino H: Identification and synthesis of a heptapeptide in uremia fluid. *Biochem Biophys Res Commun* 84: 184, 1978

104. Abiko T, Onodera I, Sekino H: Isolation, structure and biological activity of the TRP-containing pentapeptide from uremic fluid. *Biochem Biophys Res Commun* 89: 813, 1979

105. Abiko T, Onodera T, Sekino HA: A peptide isolated from the hemodialysate of a uremic patient with immunodeficiency inhibits lymphocyte stimulation. *J Appl Biochem* 3: 562, 1981

106. Klein A, Sarnecka-Keller M, Hanicki Z: Middle-sized ninhydrin-positive molecules in uraemic patients treated by repeated haemodialysis. II. Chief peptide constituents of the fraction. *Clin Chim Acta* 90: 7, 1978

107. Mabuchi H, Nakahashi H: Medium-sized peptides in the blood of patients with uremia. *Nephron* 33: 232, 1983

108. Elias AN, Vaziri ND, Maksy M: Plasma beta-endorphin and beta-lipotropin in patients with end-stage renal disease – Effects of hemodialysis. *Nephron* 43: 173, 1986

109. Flanagran RWJ, Murphy RF, Buchanan KD: Circulating forms of glucagon and related peptides in normal subjects and uraemic patients. *Biochem Soc Trans* 8: 426, 1980

110. Ludwig H, Spiteller G, Matthaei D, Scheler F: Profile bei chronischen Erkrankungen. I. Steroid-Profiluntersuchungen bei Urämie. (Profile of chronic disease. I. Investigation of steroid profile in uremia.) *J Chromatogr* 146: 381, 1978

111. Greenway DC, Nanji AA: Digoxin-like immunoreactive substance in renal failure: a reappraisal. *Nephron* 41: 108, 1986

112. Kelly RA, O'Hara DS, Mitch WE, Steinman TI, Goldzer RV, Solomon HS, Smith TW: Endogenous digitalis-like factors in hypertension and chronic renal insufficiency. *Kidney Int* 30: 723, 1986

113. Scribner BH: Discussion. *Trans Am Soc Artif Intern Organs* 11: 29, 1965

114. Babb A, Farrell P, Uvelli D, Scribner B: Hemodialyzer evaluation by examination of solute molecular spectra. *Trans Am Soc Artif Intern Organs* 18: 98, 1972

115. Lowrie EG, Laird NM, Parker TF, Sargent JA: Effect of the hemodialysis prescription on patient morbidity. *N Engl J Med* 305: 1176, 1980

116. Scheuer J, Stezoski SW: The effects of uremic compounds on cardiac function and metabolism. *J Mol Cell Cardiol* 5: 287, 1973

117. Giovannetti S, Balestri PL, Barsotti G: Methylguanidine in uremia. *Arch Intern Med* 131: 709, 1973

118. Giovannetti S, Barsotti G: Uremic intoxication. *Nephron* 14: 123, 1975

119. Lindup WE, Bischop KA, Collier R: Drug binding defect of uraemic plasma: contribution of endogenous binding inhibitors. in *Protein Binding and Drug Transport*, edited by Tillement JP, Lindenlaub E, Stuttgart, Schattauer Verlag, 1986, p 397

120. Boumendil-Podevin EF, Podevin RA, Richet G: Uricosuric agents in uremic sera. Identification of indoxyl sulfate and hippuric acid. *J Clin Invest* 55: 1142, 1975

121. Clements RS, De Jesus PV, Winegrad AT: Raised plasma myoinositol levels in uraemia and experimental neuropathy. *Lancet* 1: 1137, 1973

122. Porter RD, Cathcart-Rake WF, Suk Han Wan, Whittier FC, Grantham JJ: Secretory activity and aryl acid content of serum, urine, and cerebrospinal fluid in normal and uremic man. *J Lab Clin Med* 85: 723, 1975

123. Vanholder R, Schoots A, Cramers C, De Smet R, Van Landschoot N, Wizeman V, Botella J, Ringoir S: Hippuric acid as a marker. in *Uremic Toxins*, edited by Ringoir S, Vanholder R, Massry S, New York, Plenum Publ Co, 1987, p 59

124. Vincent C, Revillard JP, Galland M, Traeger J: Serum beta 2 – microglobulin in hemodialyzed patients. *Nephron* 21: 260, 1978

125. DiRaimondo CR, Casey TT, DiRaimondo CV, Stone WJ: Pathologic fractures associated with idiopathic amyloidosis of bone in chronic hemodialysis patients. *Nephron* 43: 22, 1986

126. Shirahama T, Skinner M, Cohen AS, Gejyo F, Arakawa M, Suzuki M, Hirasawa Y: Histochemical and immunohistochemical characterization of amyloid associated with chronic hemodialysis as beta 2-microglobulin. *Lab Invest* 53: 705, 1985

127. Gejyo F, Odani S, Yamada T, Honma N, Saito H, Suzuki Y, Nakagawa Y, Kobayashi H, Maruyama Y, Hirasawa Y, Suzuki M, Arakawa M: Beta 2-microglobulin: a new form of amyloid protein associated with chronic hemodialysis. *Kidney Int* 30: 385, 1986

128. Hauglustaine D, Waer M, Michielsen P, Goebels J, Vandeputte M: Haemodialysis membranes, serum beta 2-microglobulin, and dialysis amyloidosis. *Lancet* 1: 1211, 1986

129. Vandenbroucke JM, Jadoul M, Maldague B, Juaux JP, Noel H, Van Ypersele de Strihou C: Possible role of dialysis membrane characteristics in amyloid osteo-arthropathy. *Lancet* 1: 1210, 1986

130. Radtke HW, Rege AB, La Marche MB, Bartos D, Bartos F, Campbell RA, Fischer JW: Identification of spermine as an inhibitor of erythropoiesis in patients with chronic renal failure. *J Clin Invest* 67: 1623, 1981

131. Campbell RA: Polyamines. in *Uremic Toxins*, edited by Ringoir S, Vanholder R, Massry S, New York, Plenum Publ Co, 1987, p 47

132. Bergström J., Fürst P, Zimmerman L: Uremic middle molecules exist and are biologically active. *Clin Nephrol* 11: 229, 1979

133. Kjellstrand CM, Petersen RJ, Evans RL, Shideman B, Von Hartitzsch B, Buselmeier TJ: Considerations on the middle molecule hypothesis II: neuropathy in nephrectomized patients. *Trans Am Soc Artif Intern Organs* 19: 325, 1973

134. Kopple JD, Coburn JW: Evaluation of chronic uremia. *JAMA* 227: 41, 1974

135. Farrell PC, Gotch FA, Peters JH, Berridge BJ, Lam M: Binding of hippurate in normal plasma and in uremic plasma pre- and postdialysis. *Nephron* 20: 40, 1978

136. Armstrong MD, Chao FC, Parker VJ, Wall PE: Endogenous formation of hippuric acid. *Proc Soc Exp Biol Med* 90: 675, 1955

137. Bodel PT, Cotran R, Kass EH: Cranberry juice and the antibacterial action of hippuric acid. *J Lab Clin Med* 54: 881, 1959

138. Bourke E, Frindt G, Preuss H, Rose E, Weksler M, Schreiner GE: Studies with uraemic serum on the renal transport of hippurates and tetraethylammonium in the rabbit and rat:

effects of oral neomycin. *Clin Sci* 38: 41, 1970

139. Suk Han Wan, Riegelman S: Renal contribution to overall metabolism of drugs I: Conversion of benzoic acid to hippuric acid. *J Pharm Sci* 61: 1278, 1972

140. Brown EA, Kliger AS, Finkelstein FO: Peritoneal dialysis clearances. *Nephron 21*: 310, 1978

141. Man NK, Terlain B, Paris J, Werner G, Sausse A, Funck-Brentano JL: An approach to 'middle molecules' identification in artificial kidney dialysate, with reference to neuropathy prevention. *Trans Am Soc Artif Intern Organs* 19: 320, 1973

142. Leypoldt JK, Frigon RP, Henderson LW: Dextran sieving coefficients of hemofiltration membranes. *Trans Am Soc Artif Intern Organs* 29: 678, 1983

143. Rocker A, Hertel J, Fiegel P, Abdelhamid S, Panitz N, Rockel A: Permeability and secondary membrane formation of a high flux polysulfone hemofilter. *Kidney Int* 30: 429, 1986

144. Sargent JA, Gotch FA: Mathematic modeling of dialysis therapy. *Kidney Int* 18: 2, 1980

145. Gotch FA, Sargent JA: A mechanistic analysis of the national cooperative dialysis study (NCDS). *Kidney Int* 28: 526, 1985

146. Aebischer P, Schorderet D, Juillerat A, Wauters JP, Fellay G: Comparison of urea kinetics and direct dialysis quantification in hemodialysis patients. *Trans Am Soc Artif Organs* 31: 338, 1985

147. Ilstrup K, Hanson G, Shapiro W, Keshaviah P: Examining the foundations of urea kinetics. *Trans Am Soc Artif Intern Organs* 31: 164, 1985

148. Tsang HK, Leonard EF, Le Favour GS, Cortell S: Urea dynamics during and immediately after dialysis. *asaio J* 8: 251, 1985

3

HAEMODIALYSIS: A HISTORICAL REVIEW

WILLIAM DRUKKER

THE INVENTION OF DIALYSIS (1861)

If somebody should be called the father of modern dialysis, the honour should go to a Scotsman, Thomas Graham (Figure 1), who lived from 1805–1869. He was appointed Professor of Chemistry at Anderson's University, Glasgow, in 1830 at the age of 25 (1), moving to the Chair of Chemistry at University College, London, in 1837 and was finally appointed Warden and Master Worker of the Mint, London, in 1855. Graham, an extraordinary genius, laid not only the foundation of what later became colloid chemistry, but also invented a method for separating gases by diffusion, which in later years was used for separating uranium 235 from the 238 isotope.

He demonstrated that vegetable parchment acted as a semipermeable membrane. After coating parchment with albumen to close defects, he stretched it over a wooden or guttapercha hoop, which he floated on water (Figure 2 [2]). Into this he placed, as on a seive, a fluid containing crystalloids and colloids and found that only the crystalloid material diffused through the parchment into the water. For this phenomenon Graham coined the name *dialysis*. In another experiment he used 0.5 l of urine and again demonstrated that crystalloid matter from the urine passed into the water which, after evaporation on a water bath, yielded a white crystalloid mass which appeared to be mainly urea. Graham predicted that some of his findings, particularly those on osmosis, reported in 1854, might be applied to medicine.

THE FIRST 'ARTIFICIAL KIDNEY' (1913)

Graham's experiments conclusively demonstrated that this new dialysis procedure could remove solutes from fluids containing colloids and crystalloids. However, being a chemist, he did not proceed into the field of medicine and physiology. The next step, removing solutes through a semipermeable membrane from the blood of an animal, did not take place for another fifty years and came from the United States. In 1913, John J. Abel (Figure 3) and his colleagues, Rowntree and Turner (3) of the Pharmacology Laboratory of the Johns Hopkins Medical School in Baltimore, described a method

> ... 'by which the blood of a living animal may be submitted to dialysis outside the body, and again returned to the natural circulation without exposure to air, infection by micro-organisms or any alteration which would necessarily be prejudicial to life' ...

After making the animal's blood incoagulable with hirudin, they passed it from an arterial cannula through a series of tubes made of celloidin contained in a glass jacket filled with saline or artificial serum, returning the blood through another cannula into a vein of the animal.

Their dialyser, for which they coined the name *artificial kidney*, had a series of celloidin tubes of 8 mm diameter and 40 cm long fastened by tying with a string to a system of glass manifolds, branching dichotomously. Thus, the flow of blood took place horizontally, twice in each direction through eight tubes in parallel (Figure 4). Abel and his co-workers soon became aware that only their most efficient apparatus (with 32 celloidin tubes) was suitable for larger animals of more than 20 kg weight. They suggested that flattening the tubes might improve the efficiency, more or less anticipating the flat tubing in today's coil dialysers. They mentioned also that ... 'very small tubes would undoubtedly prove valuable when the necessary time and trouble are not prohibitive' ... more or less predicting the hollow fiber type of dialysers in use today. With their apparatus, they removed from the dog either endogenous substances or foreign substances whose presence in excessive amounts endangered life. Subsequently, the investigators published in a series of articles (4–6) the results of dialysing nephrectomised dogs with their new '*vividiffusion*' apparatus, demonstrating that with a dialysing surface area of $0.32 \, m^2$ substantial quantities of non-protein nitrogen could be removed from the animals. However, the capacity of their dialyser was limited and insufficient for human application. The fragile and delicate celloidin tubes were also difficult to

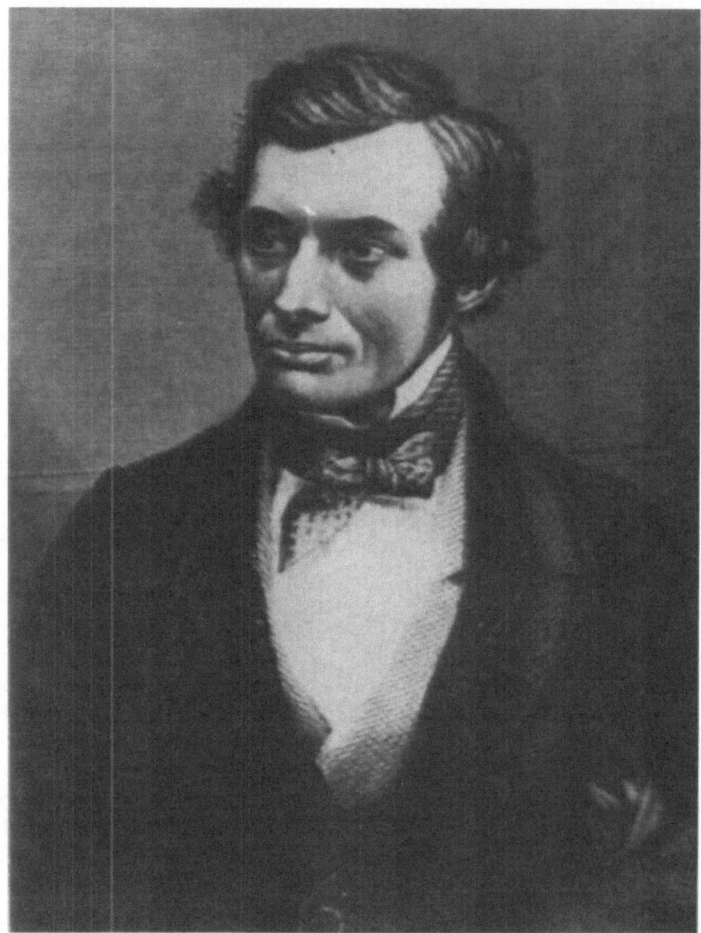

Figure 1. Thomas Graham (1805–1869), inventor of dialysis. (Engraving by C. Cook after a photograph by Claudet). From: J.S. Muspratt: *Chemistry theoretical, practical and analytical as applied and relating to the arts and manufactures,* vol. 1, Mackenzie 1853–1861.

make and handle. The also encountered difficulties with clotting of blood since heparin was not available at that time. Hirudin, which they obtained by grinding up heads of leeches in solution (... 'commercial preparations being too expensive'...), was also too toxic for human beings and was difficult to handle. However Abel and his associates developed a simple method of preparing a non-toxic hirudin solution (4) and they constructed several large surface area 'vividiffusion' devices, basically similar to their original apparatus but with 32 celloidin tubes instead of 16 and even with 192 tubes. The latter certainly must have had enough dialysing capacity for use in human patients (4).

Actually Abel was anxious to try his new invention in patients, as appears from the introductory paragraph of one of his papers, published in 1913 (4):

... 'There are numerous toxic states in which the eliminating organs of the body, more especially the kidneys, are incapable of removing from the body, at an adequate rate, the autochthonous or the foreign substances whose presence in excessive amount is detrimental to life processes. In the hope of providing a substitute in such emergencies, which might tide over a dangerous crisis... we devised a method by which the blood... may be submitted to dialysis outside the body'...

More than 10 years later Abel wrote in a letter to Heinrich Necheles at Hamburg, Germany, dated March 4, 1924:

... 'I personally also started out, quite contrary apparently to your conception of my purpose, with the view of relieving the kidney of human beings in certain pathological conditions'...

In a letter, dated December 16, 1930 to his previous co-worker Dr. Leonard Rowntree (then at the Mayo Clinic in Rochester, Minnesota) Abel refers to a paper published by Georg Haas of Gieszen, Germany, in Abderhalden's Handbuch (17, [see next section]):

... 'You will see that he [*i.e. Haas*] has modified our method. He uses venous blood and circulates this blood in a dialysing apparatus and then returns it to the vein,

Hoop Dialyser

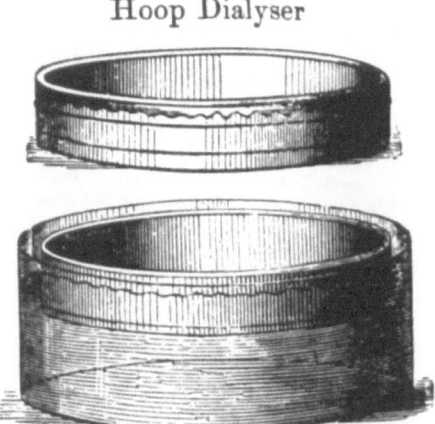

Figure 2. Hoop dialyser of Thomas Graham, with a 'dialytic septum' of parchment paper (1861 [2]).

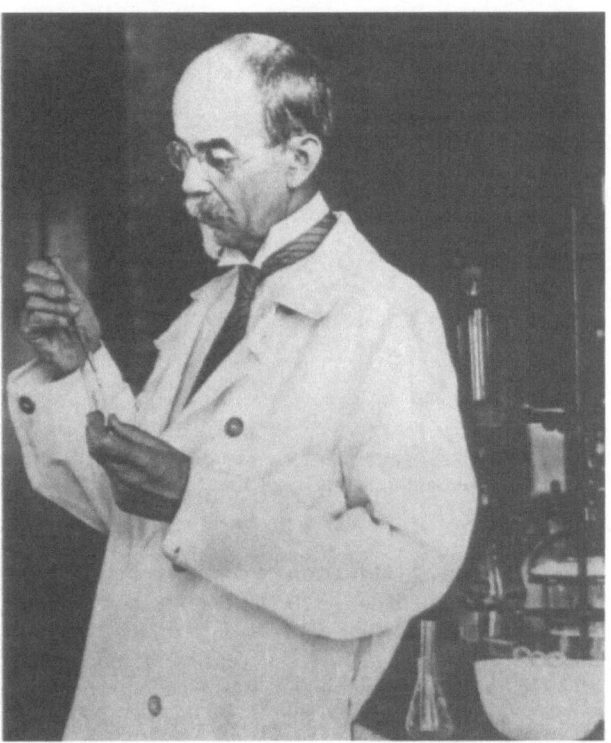

Figure 3. John Jacob Abel 1857–1938) 'a method has been devised by which the blood . . . may be submitted to dialysis outside the body . . .' (3).

taking about 3500 ccs at a time from a human being' . . .
In his letter to Necheles Abel writes (in 1924):
. . . 'My assistants and I had always hoped to try our apparatus on an appropriate case of kidney disease of mecurial *[sic]* poisoning and this was always in the backgrounds of our minds during the scientific work, which is represented in the paper reprints of which I am sending you. When the Great War came it was no longer possible for us to get leeches as these anilids ("Hirudo medici-, nalis") were imported by us in quantities of 1500 or more from Hungary. Shortly after the outbreak of the war indeed I had a consignment of 1500 leeches lieing *[sic]* at Copenhagen. The English Foreign Office ruled that this consignment was of "enemy origin" and the leeches were left to die at Copenhagen" . . .
As appears, however, from a letter, dated July 1, 1916 from the British Foreign Office, Abel could have had his leeches if he had applied to the British Government through the State Department at Washington for a transportation permit. He did not; however the unavoidable delay and the red tape would have resulted in death of the leeches anyway . . .
On the other hand, according to a footnote in the second article of Abel and his co-workers they could have obtained . . . 'good medicinal leeches from France . . . in lots of 100 or more from cupping barbers at the rate of $6 a hundred' . . ., which was rather cheap. According to the footnote there was also an American firm who hoped to be able to furnish the best leeches at 20–$25 a thousand. It remains unclear why Abel did not try to get leeches from 'non enemy origin' to continue his investigations.
In 1914 Abel stopped his work, because of the leeches problem, so never applied the 'vividiffusion apparatus' to a human being.
Even more than 15 years later Abel was still disappointed. In his letter to Rowntree (December 1930) he continues:
. . . 'As I read over the paper *[of Haas]* today I could not help thinking how unfortunate it was that our work was

stopped by the World War when we were unable to obtain the supply of leeches. . . . How would it be if a hospital such as yours would take up this whole subject again and train a special group of assistants and technicians to apply this venous method to chronic nephritics who are in the terminal stage of the disease and thus improve their condition and possibly prolong their life. I have always had the belief, and as I recall you agree with me, that something could be done by this method in cases of acute mercurial poisoning. If the blood could be washed every day, or every other day, in these cases at the time they become stuperous and unconscious, they might possibly recover. The kidney as I understood from the pathologists, has a great regenerative ability' . . .
It would be another 15 years until Abel's prediction became true: the first survivor from acute renal failure whose life was saved by an artificial kidney was dialysed by Kolff on the 3rd September 1945.
Interestingly, Dr. Leonard Rowntree witnessed one of the first clinical haemodialyses undertaken for acute poisoning about 25 years after Abel's letter at Georgetown, University Hospital in Washington, D.C.
Abel, Rowntree and Turner first demonstrated vividiffusion to their colleagues in Baltimore, on the 10th November 1912 and also demonstrated their invention in the summer of

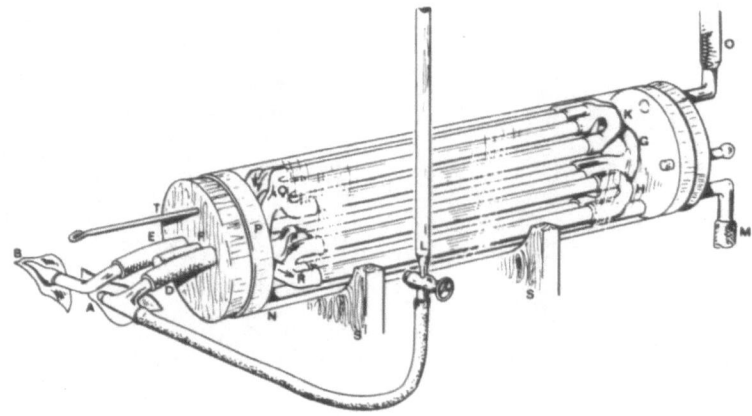

Figure 4. Vividiffusion apparatus of Abel, Rowntree and Turner with 16 celloidin tubes (1913 [4]). (A) Arterial cannula; (B) Venous cannula; (L) Burette with hirudin solution; (M) Drain; (Q) and (R) Quadruple branch points; (O) Air outlet; (T) Thermometer.

1913 in London and at the Congress of Physiology in Groningen, The Netherlands. By coincidence a young Dutch doctor named Pim Kolff, working in the Department of Medicine at the University Hospital also in Groningen started 25 years later his experiments, which led to the construction of an artificial kidney that was suitable for practical human application.

Various investigators attracted by the work from the Baltimore trio began using the new dialyser for experimental work. The two main problems, anticoagulation and a suitable membrane, remained major obstacles, however. In 1914 von Hess and McGuigan (7) used Abel's vividiffusion method in a series of experiments on the dog. They improved the apparatus by creating a pulsatile bloodflow through the celloidin tubes, which apparently helped inhibit clotting. They also enhanced the procedure by mixing the dialysis fluid at short intervals or continuously, preventing formation of a stagnant layer of fluid around the dialysing tubes. This principle of turbulent dialysis fluid flow was rediscovered some 50 years later and has found application in modern dialysers.

Several investigators on both sides of the Atlantic started preparing dialysis membranes from animal origin for dialysis purposes. Love (8) from Chicago used chicken intestines (1920). Necheles (9, 10) from Hamburg used semipermeable

conical tubes made from visceral animal peritoneum (gold-beater's skin). These tubes were compressed between metal lattice screens in order to keep the blood volume small in relation to the dialysing surface area (1923). Necheles combined a number of his 'gold-beater's skin' tubes in series and was able to dialyse bilaterally nephrectomised uraemic dogs for several hours, using hirudin (Figures 5a and 5b). He noticed a striking improvement in their condition. Later working together with Lim (11) at the Peking Union Medical College in China, he continued his experiments with dogs, using heparin for the first time.

THE FIRST HUMAN DIALYSIS (1924)

The credit for the first human dialysis must go to Georg Haas (Figure 6) from Gieszen, Germany, who lived from 1886–1971 (12–17).

In 1911 Haas started working in Hofmeisters laboratory in Strassburg, Germany on amino acid synthesis *in vivo*; he wondered whether dialysis would help him in his so far negative experimental results, by separation of intermediate metabolic products from the blood. Therefore, he circulated

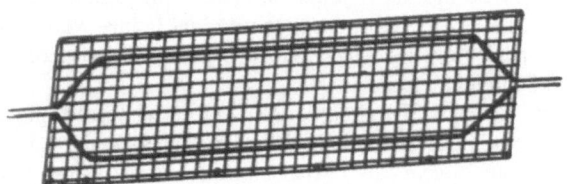

Figure 5a. Semipermeable conical tube prepared by Heinrich Necheles in 1925 from animal peritoneum, compressed between metal wire grids (9, 10).

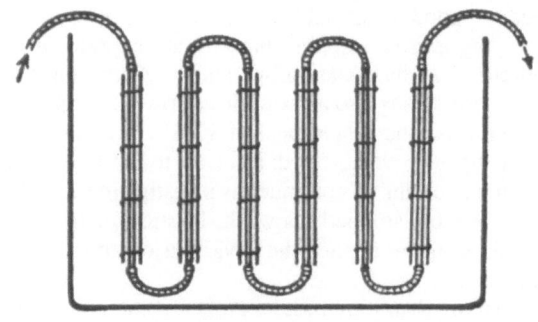

Figure 5b. Dialyser consisting of battery of 'gold-beater's skin' tubes in series constructed by Necheles (9, 10).

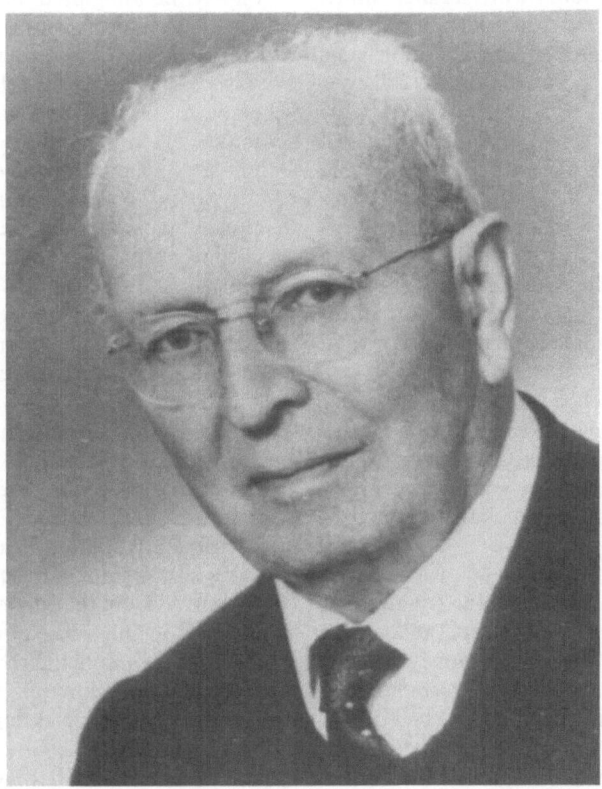

Figure 6. Georg Haas (1886–1971), who carried out the first human dialysis in 1924: '... because uraemia was a condition against which the doctor stands otherwise powerless ...' (15). Picture taken in 1968, at the age of 82.

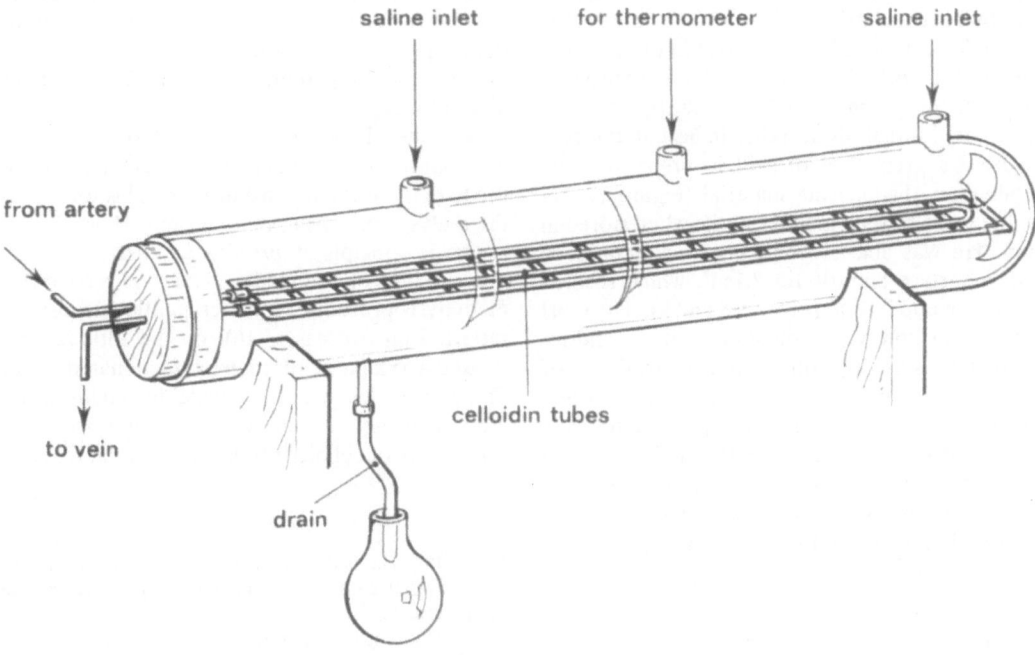

Figure 7. Glass container with pair of celloidin tubes, made by Georg Haas (1923 [17]).

blood from his animals through tubular membranes, which were prepared from reed stalks, by a procedure described in 1902 by Philippson (18), who also worked in Hofmeisters laboratory. These membranes apparently worked as dialysis membranes.

Because of World War I Haas had to return to clinical work in 1914. Working in the Department of Medicine of the University Hospital at Gieszen and the local Military Hospital he was confronted with many cases of trench nephritis some of them with rapid progression to fatal uraemia and Haas considered again a form of dialysis similar to his earlier animal experiments, instead of the customary procedures for uraemia like blood lettings, forced sweating sessions and dietary protein restriction.

... 'von der Annahme ausgehend, dass es sich bei der Urämie um der Retention von harnfähigen Stoffen handelt und dieselben wohl auch dialysabel seien, zog ich das dialysatorische Abtrennungsverfahren, das ich bei meinen intermediären Stofwechselstudien vorhatte durchzuführen, in Erwägung' ... (16).*

Having no access to the literature which was published in the Allied countries during the war, Haas remained unaware of the work of the Baltimore trio which was published in 1913 shortly before the outbreak of World War I. He resumed his experimental work but soon encountered unsurmountable difficulties: trying again different membranes prepared from reed stalks, paper and animal peritoneum, which all proved unsuitable and having no other anticoagulants than crude and toxic hirudin, Haas abondoned the project in 1917 when he was sent to Rumania to combat epidemic typhus fever. Returning in 1919 to civil medical work in post war impoverished Germany, Haas had initially no facilities to resume his experimental work. However, the work on dialysis of uraemic dogs by his compatriot Heinrich Necheles (9, 10), published in 1923, rearoused Haas' interest in dialysis. He became aware of the work of an Austrian, Franz Pregl (19), who used celloidin tubes, similar to those made by Abel and his fellow workers, for dialysis purposes in his laboratory.

Haas acquired a great deal of skill in preparing long (1.20 m) tubes from this delicate material (Figure 7). He discovered that these tubes remained sterile when stored in 60% ethanol. He was able to construct a celloidin tube dialyser with a surface area of 1.5–2.1 m², which seemed suitable for human application (Figures 8 and 9). The most serious obstacle was however to obtain a nontoxic and reliable anticoagulant, since heparin was not yet available for human application. He finally found a reasonably purified hirudin preparation of low toxicity. Using potassium iodide as a dialysable test substance, Haas performed a series of dialyses on the dog, most of them lasting 3/4–1 hour. They were well tolerated and in an hour of dialysis complete removal of the iodide from the blood was apparently achieved.

Finally, he attempted dialysis in a patient with terminal uraemia: ... 'because this was a condition against which the doctor stands otherwise powerless' ... (13).

Assisted by a surgical colleague named von der Hütten, Haas performed the first human dialysis, according to Benedum (20, 21) in the autumn of 1924. This dialysis lasted 15 minutes. No complications occurred:

... 'Somit konnte zum ersten Mal gezeigt werden, dass eine Blutauswaschung durch Dialyse am Menschen möglich und ohne jede Schädigung für den Patienten durchführbar ist' ... (13).*

No further details of this dialysis have been recorded in literature, neither is a picture available.

The second dialysis occurred on the 18th of February 1925: Haas dialysed a youthful patient in the terminal stage of uraemia, using hirudin and a continuous circulation technique. The dialysis lasted 35 min and apart from a febrile reaction, the procedure was well tolerated, but of course had no therapeutic effect (Figure 10).

Subsequently, during 1926 Haas performed another four dialyses lasting from 30 to 60 min ([15, 21] Figure 11). Bleeding occurred from the surgical cannulation wounds and the gums, presumably caused by the anticoagulant.

Once a glass container had to be replaced because of rupture of a celloidin tube, which only took 2 min (21).

Some confusion has occurred from a personal statement of Haas in 1936 (17):

... 'Ohne Kenntnis der Abelschen Arbeiten versuchte ich aus therapeutischen Gesichtspunkten im Jahre 1915 zum ersten Mal die Blutwaschung am Lebenden mit Hilfe der Dialyse durchzuführen, und zwar beim Nierenkranken' ...**

However neither case reports nor other particulars or results have been recorded in the literature. According to Benedum (21) no practical attempt of a human dialysis was done in 1915; Haas apparently only *considered* such a procedure at that time.

Obviously Haas' dialysis procedures lasted too short for any significant therapeutic effect. The main drawback was the toxicity of the impure hirudin. This forced him to limit the dialysis sessions to 30 to 60 min; Haas always observed the basic principle of *'primum nil nocere'*.

Some time elapsed before Haas again tried the new haemodialysis procedure for therapeutic purposes: in 1928 he reported on two cases (16): on the 13th January 1928 he treated a 55 kg uraemic man by fractionated dialysis, for the first time using a newly available, highly purified preparation of heparin and a dialyser of 1.5 m², consisting of three pairs of celloidin tubes with a total length of 756 cm.

---

* ... 'considering the hypothesis that uraemia is caused by retention of products which should be excreted in the urine and presumably can be removed by dialysis, I reconsidered by dialysis experiments from my previous metabolic studies' ...

* ... 'This demonstrated for the first time that a purification of the blood by dialysis in a human being was possible without damaging the patient' ...

** ... 'Without knowing of the work of Abel and collaborators I tried because of therapeutic considerations in 1915 for the first time a cleansing of the blood by means of dialysis in living individuals with kidney disease' ...

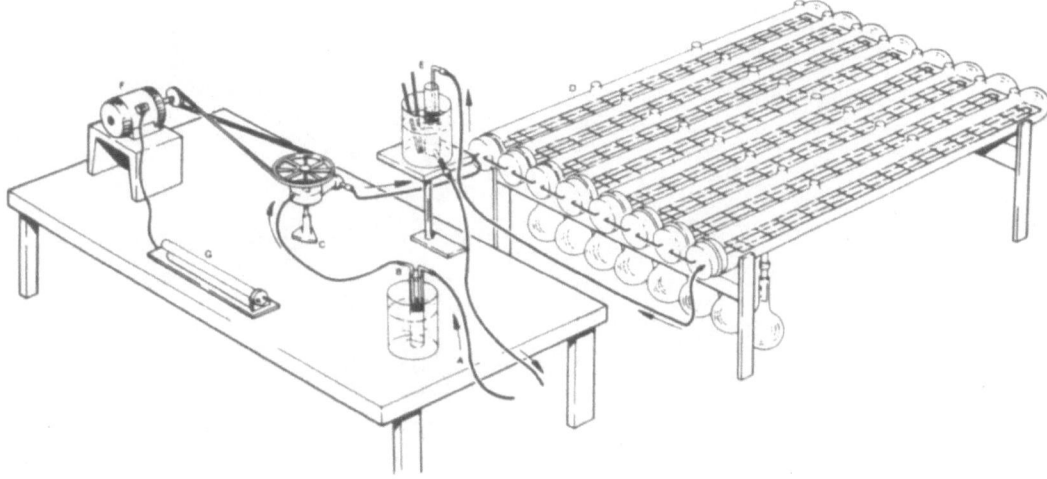

Figure 8. Battery of eight glass containers each with two celloidin dialysis tubes, used by Georg Haas in dog experiments (17). (A) Arterial bloodline; (B) Arterial blood container; (C) Blood pump; (D) Battery of dialysers with celloidin tubes; (E) venous blood collector.

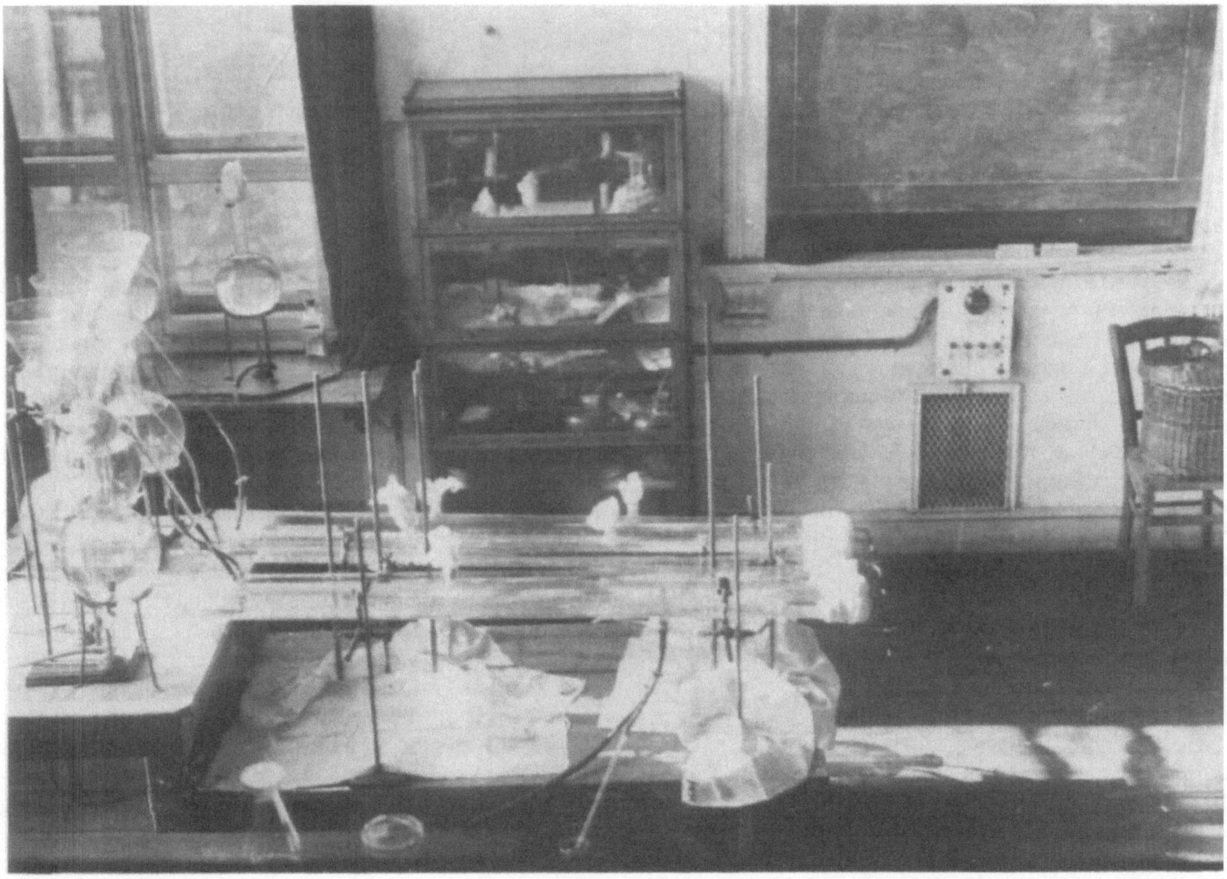

Figure 9. Battery of four glass containers with two celloidin dialysing tubes each, ready for use in a patient. Surface area appr. 2 m^2 (1926).

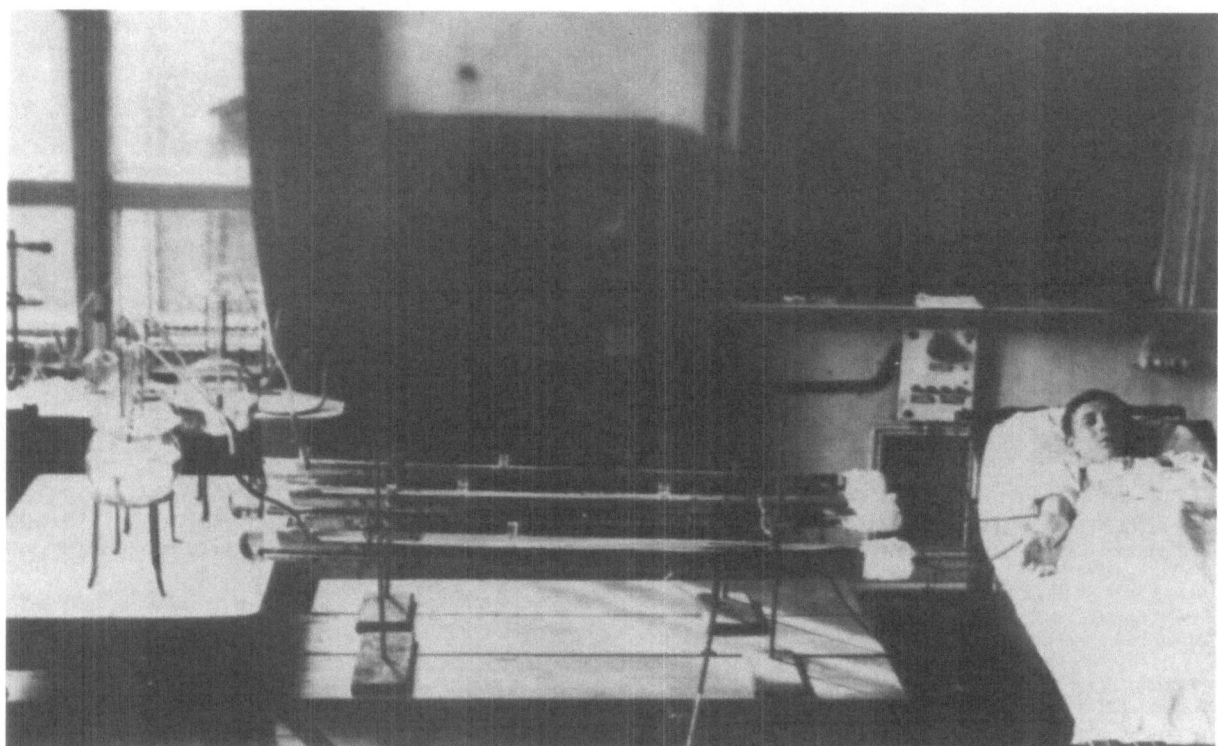

Figure 10. February 18, 1925: dialysis of a uraemic boy by Georg Haas in Giessen with three glass containers each with two celloidin tubes. This was actually the second human dialysis recorded in literature (12–17, 21).

Approximately 0.4 l of blood was taken, heparinised and circulated for half an hour through the dialyser, which was perfused with Ringer solution. The blood was reinfused into the same vein by means of a small funnel. The procedure was repeated nine times. The total removal of non-protein nitrogen was somewhat disappointing according to Haas; nevertheless the patient's clinical improvement was both subjectively and objectively impressive, lasting 6 days.

The second case was dialysed in a similar way on the 29th March 1928, the procedure being repeated after 5 weeks on 4th May 1928. After dialysing 500 ml of blood through a 2.1 m² celloidin dialyser, 2.5 g of nonprotein nitrogen was removed with a gratifying symptomatic improvement. Blood pressure decreased from 205/100 to 145/95 mm Hg.

Haas, who was obviously an astute observer, noted a temporary decrease in urine volume from 1,000 to 1,200 ml/24 h to 500 ml on the day after treatment. He offered several explanations for this phenomenon.

He also noted a decrease in the volume of the blood during the extracorporeal circulation. Actually, a loss of 100 ml from the 500 ml aliquot occurred during 30 min of dialysis. Haas discusses in his paper the explanation of this phenomenon, which actually was caused by ultrafiltration from positive pressure, not by osmotic fluid removal, because the dialysate was isotonic Ringer solution. He wondered whether this phenomenon could be of therapeutic

value in cases of nephrotic oedema . . . a cautious prophecy which later became true (22, 23).

At the end of one of his articles Haas, summarising his results, called them promising, but warned against over-optimism. His experience was only limited to a small number of experimental dialyses and Haas cautiously warned: 'one swallow does not make a summer'. His article published in 1928 (16) is a real classic in the field of dialysis.

Then follows a 9 year interval of silence on the subject during which period two important advances were made: firstly purified heparin became readily available for human application and secondly a new cellulose product named cellophane was marketed, mainly for commercial use. In 1937, a short communication was published by William Thalhimer from New York (24), who had seen a demonstration of Abel's artificial kidney when he was a medical student at Johns Hopkins University. He initially did experimental work on the treatment of uraemia with exchange transfusions and then tried to use an artificial kidney for this purpose. He constructed a dialyser replacing Abel's celloidin tubes with cellophane sausage-tube made by Visking Casing Corporation in the United States, and dialysed nephrectomised dogs, using heparin as an anticoagulant. He was, however, not very successful because the active surface of his dialyser was too small. Finally he turned again to exchange transfusions.

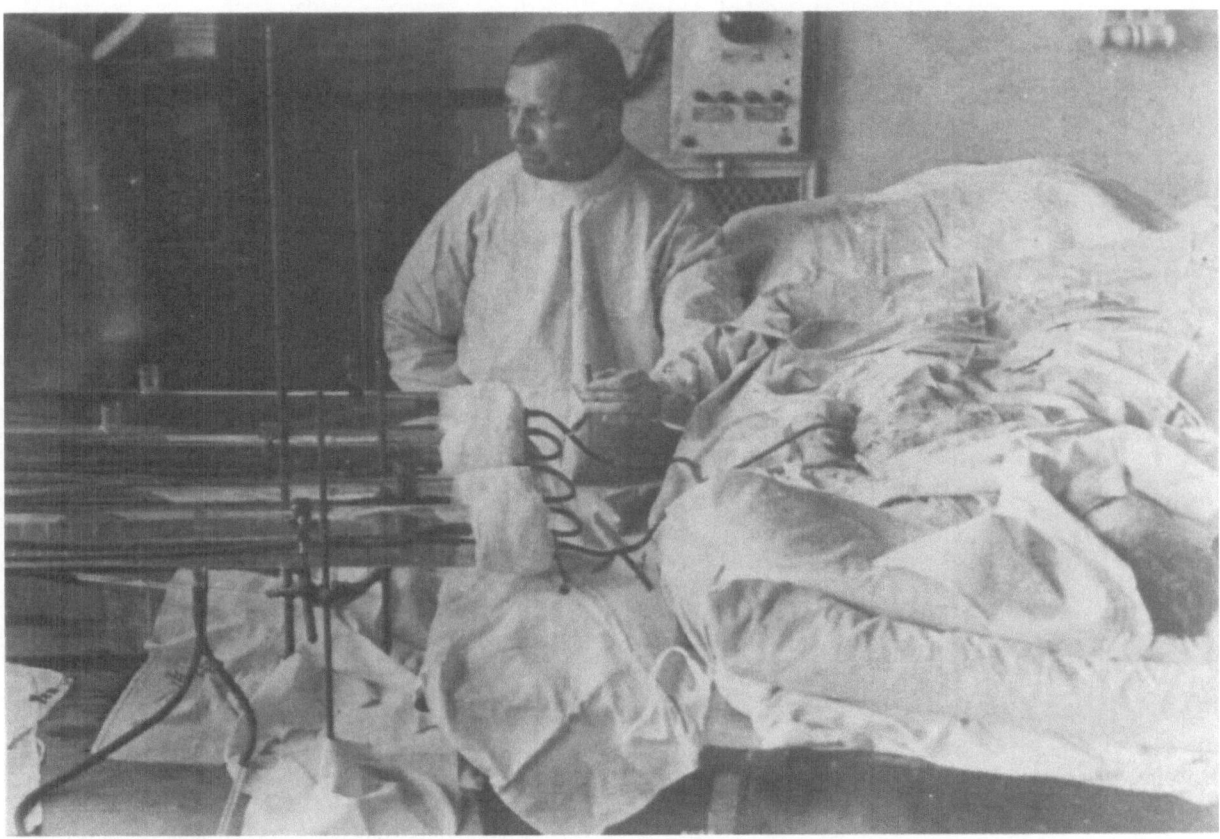

Figure 11. Georg Haas dialysing a uraemic girl. The apparatus consisted of four glass containers each provided with two celloidin dialysing tubes (1926). These experimental dialyses were performed in the lecture theatre of the Department of Medicine in Giessen, Germany.

THE ROTATING DRUM DIALYSER, CONSTRUCTED BY KOLFF AND BERK (1943)

In the late 1930's, a young doctor named Willem ('Pim') Johan Kolff (Figure 12), entered the Department of Medicine at the Groningen University Hospital in the north of The Netherlands at the age of 27. What later could be called a definite break-through was a matter of chance and coincidence. It so happened that the young doctor Kolff had to treat Jan Bruning, a uraemic 22-year-old farmer's son, who died during Kolff's early training. His death made medical history. Kolff later described his feelings of frustration as a young and inexperienced physician. Feeling helpless and depressed by the terrible suffering of his patient, just as happened to Georg Haas years before, Kolff also began to think about an apparatus that could replace renal function and thereby save patients from death by uraemia (25). Unaware of previous publications, he met Dr. Brinkman, who was a professor of biochemistry at Groningen University. He soon became young Kolff's stimulating adviser and showed him the 'wonders of cellophane'. At that time seamless cellophane tubing, used as sausage skin, had become commercially available and seemed to be an excellent material for dialysis. In order to determine how much cellophane was needed to construct an efficient artificial kidney for human use, Kolff took a 45 cm long piece of cellophane tubing, tied one end and filled it with 25 ml of water containing 0.1 g (1.7 mmol) of urea. The other end was also tied and the piece of tubing, fixed on a small wooden board, was rocked in saline (Figure 13). In 15 min all the urea had passed into the saline. Kolff repeated this experiment with 25 ml of blood, adding 400 mg (6.7 mmol) of urea and obtained similar results. By calculation, he deduced that at least 10 m of cellphane tubing were required to remove 2 g (33 mmol) of urea from 500 ml of blood in 15 min. Several types of apparatus were built, but not one appeared to be satisfactory.

On 10th May 1940, Hitler's armies invaded The Netherlands. Kolff's professor of medicine and his wife, who were Jews, committed suicide and a Dutch Nazi was appointed to the chair of medicine in Groningen. Kolff made an immediate decision. He left and found a job in the local hospital of the small town of Kampen. After settling in Kampen, Kolff started again to work on an artificial kidney. Eventually, he constructed, assisted by Hendrik Berk, who was an engineer and a managing director of Kampen's enamel factory (Fig-

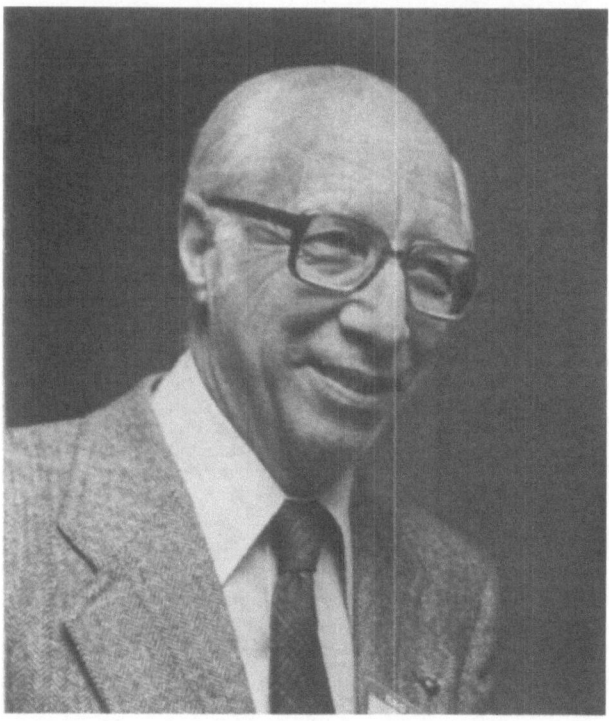

Figure 12. Willem ('Pim') Johan Kolff M.D., Ph.D. (1979).

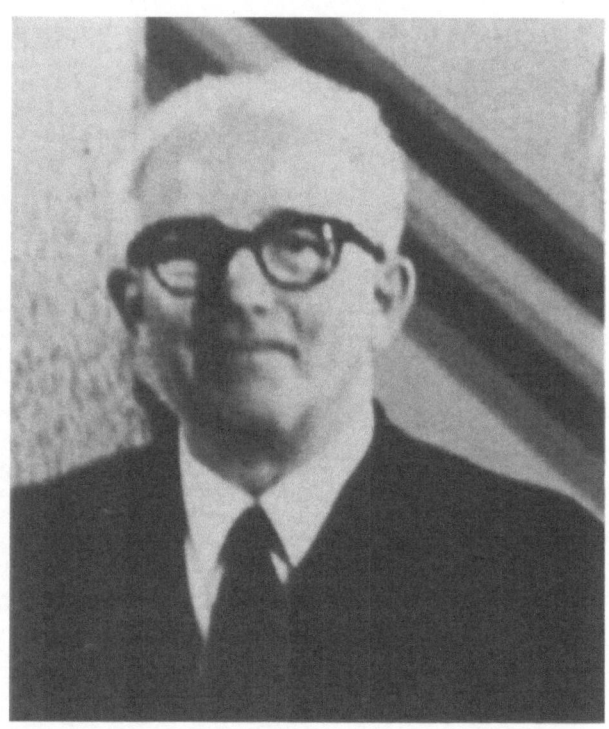

Figure 14. H.Th.J. (Hendrik) Berk, who together with Kolff designed and constructed the rotating artificial kidney in Kampen in 1942–'43 (25–30). (Picture taken in 1968, at the age of 69).

ure 14), a 'dialyser with a large surface area'. The apparatus consisted of a cylindrical drum (Figure 15a), originally made from an aluminium framework (Figure 15b). Later, drums were made from wooden laths as aluminium could no longer be obtained during the war (26–30). A 30 to 40 m length of $2^1/_2$ cm wide cellophane sausage tubing was wound on the cylinder to be perfused with the patient's blood through a rotating coupling which, according to Kolff, was copied from a Ford automobile waterpump (Figure 16). The lower half of the rotating drum was immersed in a stationary tank containing 70 l (later 100 l) of dialysis fluid.

It was actually Berk who suggested placing the drum horizontally instead of vertically, thereby making it possible to propel the blood along the cellophane tubing by rotation of the drum, eliminating the use of a bloodpump.

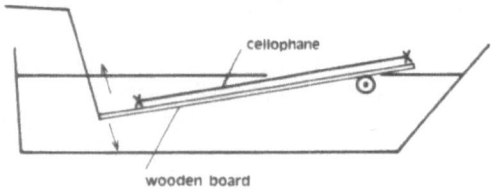

Figure 13. Kolff's first dialysis experiment: a piece of cellophane tubing filled with 'uraemic' blood and tied on a wooden board, rocken in saline (1938).

Meanwhile, purified heparin had become available and in February 1943 Kolff decided to dialyse the blood of an old gentlemen with endstage uraemia, caused by prostatic hypertrophy. He took 50 ml of blood from a vein, which was circulated through the rotating drum kidney machine and returned to a burette. By raising the burette the dialysed blood was reinfused in the patient through the same needle. When this was tolerated the procedure was repeated several times with increasing volumes of blood. No clinical effect was noted: the patient remained unconscious and died soon after the procedure (31).

Kolff's next patient, Janny Schrijver, was a 29-year-old housemaid with contracted kidneys and malignant hypertension (26–30). Upon admission she had terminal uraemia and cardiac failure. Her blood pressure was 245/150 mm Hg. Initially fractionated dialysis was performed, beginning with dialysis of 50 ml of blood. The first day, actually the 17th March 1943, 0.5 l of blood was dialysed and during subsequent days, 1.5, 3.5, 4.5 and 5.5 l per day were dialysed. Six fractionated dialyses were performed and after each treatment Janny's condition improved remarkably. With the 7th treatment, Kolff changed to continuous dialysis, taking the blood from a femoral artery by needle puncture, circulating it through the kidney machine and reinfusing the 'washed' blood by puncture of a peripheral vein. Subsequently, he had to use a radial artery and surgical cut-downs

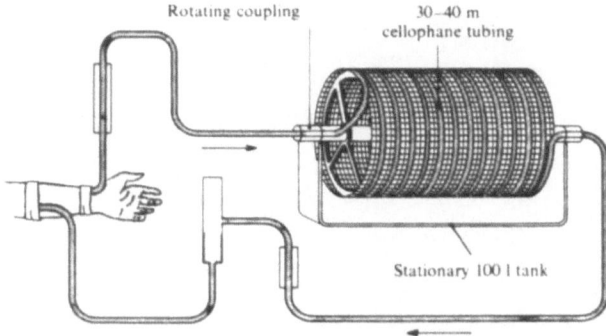

Figure 15a. Flow diagram of Kolff's rotating artificial kidney (25–30).

into the vessels became necessary for access to the circulation. This frequently caused bleeding during heparinisation. Finally Kolff and his team experienced increasing difficulties with obtaining access to the circulation and when the 11th and 12th dialysis failed because no further arteriotomies and venesections were possible, further dialysis had to be abandoned. The patient died on the 26th day of treatment.

MISFORTUNES, PROBLEMS AND UNEXPECTED SUPPORT (1943–1945)

Fate had it that the Kolff team had to struggle with a multitude of technical difficulties and problems such as membrane leaks, haemolysis, bloodline disconnections, haemorrhages and all kinds of other misfortunes. After this initial experience, they were not discouraged, however, and were resolute to continue their efforts. Kolff's tenacious character and his perseverance determined the further course of events. However, Kolff's initial ideal, the treatment of uraemic patients with irreverssible chronic renal failure by repeated dialysis, seemed still far away. Obviously, the major obstacle was achieving repeated access to the bloodstream, a problem which had to wait for another 20 years before a new approach was made. In 1946, Kolff wrote in his thesis:

> ... 'in cases of chronic (irreversible) uraemia there is in general no indication for treatment with the artificial kidney. However temporary aggravation of chronic uraemia caused by intercurrent infection, diarrhoea or surgery could benefit from a dialysis to tide the patient over the critical period' ...

Kolff tried, after these initial experiences, to limit his dialysis efforts to patients with reversible (acute) renal failure. Between the 17th March 1943 and the 27th July 1944, 15 patients were treated. Only one survived, a man treated with a sulpha drug for lobar pneumonia, who became anuric (a common complication of sulphonamide therapy in those days). One dialysis reduced his blood urea from 220 to

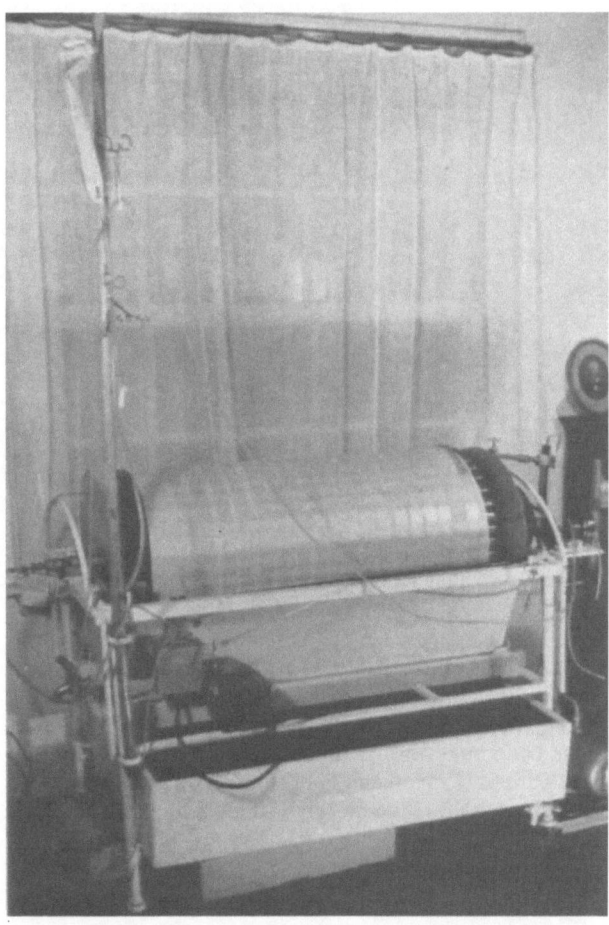

Figure 15b. Kolff's original rotating artificial kidney, used for dialysing his first patient at Kampen, The Netherlands (1943).

102 mg/dl (37 to 17 mmol/l). The next day his ureters were unblocked and cleared from sulphonamide crystals. Kolff wrote later:

> 'I never thought nor said that this man's life was saved by the artificial kidney, he might have survived without dialysis when the unblocking procedure had been done first' ...

Interestingly Kolff got quite unexpected assistance for his clinical investigations with his new device. Located at Kampen was a state chemistry laboratory which did investigations for the Government in the new land reclaimed from the Zuiderzee. All important of course were sodium (and chloride) analysis of the soil drained from seawater. Sodium at that time was chemically analysed, a laborious and time consuming procedure with uranylacetate as major test substance. During World War II this compound soon became unavailable because uranium was precious war material both in Nazi Germany and in the Allied countries.

At that time Zeiss, the well-known optical firm in Germany, had constructed a flame emission photometer, which

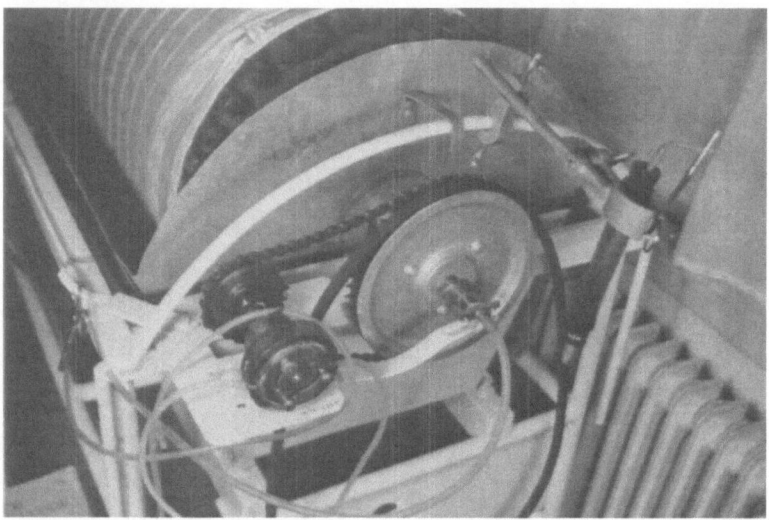

Figure 16. Rotating joint of the first rotating drum dialyser, copied from a Ford automobile waterpump (1943).

however was only suitable for potassium analysis.

The director of the soil laboratory was an agricultural Ph.D. named W.R. Domingo (Figure 17). Domingo designed and built his own flame photometer which was suitable both for sodium and potassium analysis (32).

Kolff and Domingo met by coincidence at a house of a

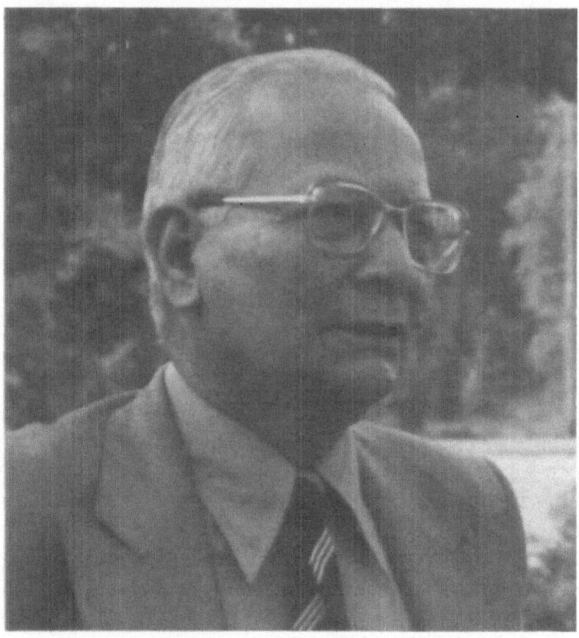

Figure 17. W.R. (Ruud) Domingo, who constructed the first flame photometer suitable for both sodium and potassium analysis (32) and who assisted Kolff with electrolyte chemistry.

Domingo relative and started talking about their mutual fields of interest and electrolyte problems. Domingo offered to help Kolff with fast and accurate sodium and potassium analyses for his dialysis patients.

After the liberation of The Netherlands by the Allied armies Domingo constructed sodium/potassium flame photometers for the Hammersmith Hospital in London, England, the Queen Wilhelmina Hospital in Amsterdam, The Netherlands and several other hospitals.

During these war years, Kolff and his team had to fight an increasing number of other problems and misfortunes; as plastic tubing was not yet available, they had to use and to reuse rubber tubing over and over again, because it was often difficult or impossible to obtain fresh supplies. Pieces had to be put together by glass tubes (where clotting often started!), heparinisation was still a problem, penicillin had become available in the Allied armies but not in the occupied countries. New venipuncture needles were not available: the old ones had to be reused and resharpened, but they became rusty on the inside and clotted easily.

Finally, conditions in the Netherlands became increasingly difficult and transportation of seriously ill patients became virtually impossible so that suitable patients for dialysis treatment could no longer be sent to Kampen, a town too small to provide an adequate number of patients locally. Kolff himself, however, was convinced that his machine was a workable device and that one day or another its value would be recognised. In later years, Kolff wondered what would have happened to his project had he not been working in occupied Holland under grim war conditions, but under more normal peaceful conditions after having treated 15 patients without a single definite therapeutic success. His coworkers and his nursing team were also convinced that one day or another the success would come and were prepared to work day and night to help Kolff with his efforts.

Undoubtedly, the war and occupation made the Dutch extremely motivated to help each other and to save their sick compatriots.

During the last year of the war, conditions became critical. Aggressiveness of the Nazis against the Dutch population sharply increased and made further use of the artificial kidney impossible. Kolff had to interrupt his dialysis programme and had to wait for another suitable case to prove that his rotating dialyser could be life saving until a few months after the liberation of The Netherlands by the Allied armies.

KOLFF's FIRST SURVIVOR (1945)

Patient no. 17 was a 67-year-old female Nazi collaborator, who was after the liberation of The Netherlands imprisoned in the military barracks of the city of Kampen. She was admitted as an acute patient to the Kampen Hospital on 3rd September 1945, suffering from acute cholecystitis with jaundice and acute renal failure with anuria, presumably caused by the treatment with a sulphonamide drug. Her condition worsened, blood urea increased from 200 to 400 mg/dl (33–67 mmol/l) and finally the patient was transferred to Kolff's 'kidney room'. At that time she was unconscious and apparently in end-stage uraemia. She was dialysed for 11 h, regained consciousness and improved dramatically. Diuresis started within a week and the patient made a good recovery. She was the first patient who owed her life to treatment with an artificial kidney (30). She died 6 years later at the age of 73 from an unrelated disease.

After the liberation of The Netherlands, Kolff went to the office of the British Information Service at The Hague and asked the medical officer if he knew of an artificial kidney developed during the war in the free world. Apparently the man did not know and Kolff concluded that none had been constructed. Actually, he was wrong since Haas in Germany had already constructed a dialyser and used it clinically in 1924 (13–17) and at the Toronto General Hospital in Canada Murray, Delorme and Thomas (33), unaware of Kolff's work, constructed during World War II a coil type artificial kidney, incorporating small bore cellophane tubing, wound around a vertical, stationary drum. This dialyser was successfully used for patients at the end of 1946.

The dialysis equipments constructed in the pre-Kolff years by the Baltimore team, by Georg Haas, Heinrich Necheles and by Thalhimer should be considered as precious relics of a period of experimental dialysis. It was Georg Haas who performed the first human dialysis, but it should be emphasised that Kolff's rotating dialyser was the first model that in practice was suitable for human application and it was in particular Kolff who made clinicians and experimentalists interested in the treatment of uraemia.

During the last year of World War II, when Kolff and his team had to interrupt their experimental work and had to put their machine temporarily out of use, they used their forced sparetime to make more artificial kidneys, receiving help from Dutch patriots wherever it was possible and even from Dutch Government officials who welcomed the opportunity to dodge or to circumvent the regulations and the supervision of the Nazi occupiers (25).

CONTRIBUTIONS OF OTHER INVESTIGATORS (1948–1949)

When the war was over Kolff gave these machines away to several hospitals to make people familiar with the technology of dialysis.

One machine went to the Royal Postgraduate Medical School at Hammersmith Hospital, London. It was promptly used, but with limited success (34).

Another machine was donated to Dr. Snapper at the Mount Sinai Hospital in New York City.

Dr. Snapper, who was a compatriot of Kolff and was previously professor of medicine at the University of Amsterdam, had left the Netherlands shortly before the World War II. His coworkers Kroop, Fishman et al started a dialysis programme in New York and performed the first human dialysis in the USA on January 26, 1948 (35).

One machine was sent to the Royal Victoria Hospital in Montreal and observations made with this dialyser were reported by De Leeuw and Blaustein (36).

Another machine was donated to professor Borst in Amsterdam, but was never used. Borst taught students that he never needed an artificial kidney machine and that the one he had was stored in the loft of his department in a somewhat rusty condition ...

Another rotating artificial kidney was sent to Poland. It went finally to the Department of Urology at the Jagiellonian University of Cracow, but was never extensively used for technical reasons and lack of trained personnel (Tadeusz Orlowski, personal communication to the author, 1977).

Others built their own machines, often with modifications and improvements. Darmady (37) a pathologist at Portsmouth and in the Isle of Wight built a rotating artificial kidney in 1946. He emphasised that it was important that the amount of blood which entered and left the machine should be controlled and provided his machine with synchronised inflow and outflow pumps. The system produced a certain amount of agitation and he pointed to the importance of turbulence which enhanced dialysis efficiency. This was later confirmed by several clinical investigators. His machine however was too bulky; therefore Darmady also constructed a machine of simpler design by passing a cellophane tube through a series of plates, 1/16th inch (1,6 mm) apart. This provided a large dialysing surface and the flow of dialysing fluid passed along a number of small grooves in the plates, which allowed the dialysing fluid to flow from the centre outwards in either direction. Unfortunately, this machine for several reasons, did not produce as satisfactory dialysis as his rotating design.

Perhaps the most successful modification of the original rotating machine was that constructed in Boston, the Kolff-Brigham machine (Figure 18 [38]). It popularised dialysis in the United States and undoubtedly reduced mortality in

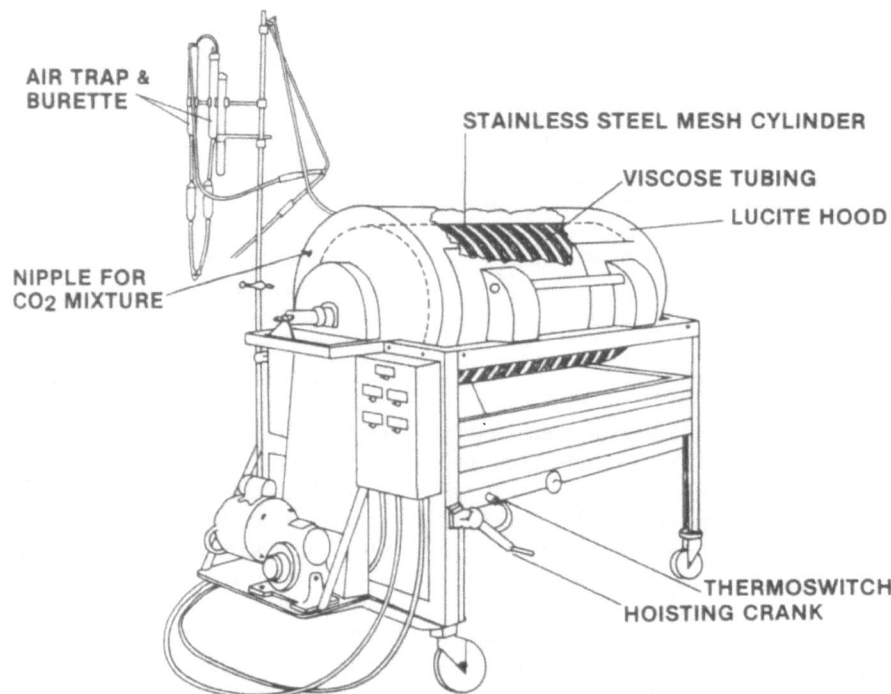

Figure 18. The Brigham modified and improved design of Kolff's rotating artificial kidney constructed by Walter, Thorn and Merrill (1948, [38, 48]). (From Alwall N: Perspective on the Development of Artificial Organs, 1985, with permission from Gambro AB, Lund, Sweden).

acute renal failure during the Korean war. Above all it brought together teams of surgeons and physicians interested both in conservative and active methods of treating patients with acute reversible types of renal failure. Gradually, as experience grew, the complete natural history of the syndrome was established.

The Kolff-Brigham machine was improved by the French firm Usifroid for the Necker Hospital in Paris and was adopted by several other hospitals in Europe, in the Middle East and even for the USSR. The team at the General Infirmary at Leeds, England increased its dialysing surface area to 3.2 m² (the Usifroid Model B) and used it occasionally even in recent years for hypercatabolic patients with acute renal failure particularly in those with potential bleeding problems, for the blood is transported through the machine by friction, thereby preventing deposition of formed elements in the blood. Regional heparinisation is rarely required when the rotating model is used. (F.M. Parsons: personal communication).

CRITICISM AND THE INFLUENCE OF BULL AND COWORKERS IN ENGLAND AND BORST IN THE NETHERLANDS (1948–1950)

Interest in the new way of treating uraemia slowly increased. But others, like Bull and co-workers (39) at the Hammersmith Hospital in London, who were acquainted with Kolff's

dialysis technique, had other views: believing that dialysis treatment had to be avoided they preferred conservative treatment by feeding the patient a high calorie, protein free diet, with peanut oil and dextrose, given by stomach tube. On the continent, Borst (40) started from the same basic principles, feeding his uraemic patients sugar and butter balls and a gruel of custard powder, sugar, butter and water. Both groups claimed satisfactory results:

> . . . 'both starvation . . . (and) injury of the erythrocytes by dialysis in the artificial kidney may be harmful' . . . (40).
> . . . 'Dialysis methods have their dangers and we believe that where this (peanut and oil regimen) is started, early dialysis should not be undertaken' . . . (39).

Both Borst and Bull were in their time and in their countries powerful and influential men. Both, at a time when pacemakers, respirators and artificial organs were still unknown, disliked medical machines and strongly opposed Kolff's 'gadgeteering'. Kolff received in Europe and in his native country little support and appreciation, but got more attention and interest in America during a tour in 1947.

He finally left the Netherlands in 1950, settling in the Cleveland Clinic in Cleveland, Ohio. But other pioneers initiated modest dialysis programmes defying the current opinion on the conservative treatment of ureaemia and the authoritative concepts of Borst and Bull.

In Hammersmith Hospital in London the early, modest dialysis programme, initiated by Bywaters and Joekes and colleagues in the late 1940's, was soon suspended because of discouraging high mortality.

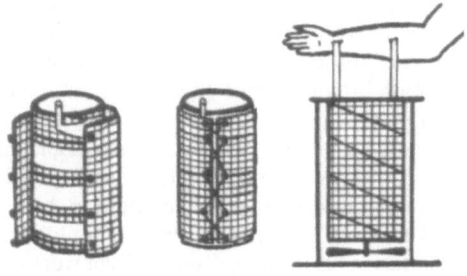

Figure 19. First Alwall dialyser (1946–1947): 10–11 m cellophane wrapped around a metal screen surrounded by a 'corset' (42).

The approach of Graham Bull (39), who was working in the same hospital, was favoured: the conservative regimen appealed to many physicians and surgeons dealing with acute renal failure cases. It became routine management in Britain between 1948 and 1956, like the more or less identical Borst treatment (40) in other European countries.

OTHER PIONEERS. THE FIRST DIALYSER WITH CONTROLLABLE ULTRA-FILTRATION (1946–1947)

Nevertheless other pioneers stimulated by the work of Kolff (41) and his first successes, continued their efforts. An interesting design was constructed by Nils Alwall in Lund, Sweden (1946–47 [42–44]): he used also cellophane tubing which was wrapped round a stationary, vertical drum made of a metal screen.

The drum and the membrane were surrounded by a second screen, as a corset fitted around the body (Figure 19). The dialyser was placed in a glass reservoir with dialysis fluid. In a later model the 'corset' was replaced by a tight fitting metal screen outer jacket: the space between the two cylinders was so calculated that the cellophane tubing could only contain a thin layer of blood (44), also causing a high resistance to blood flow and a blood pump was necessary. Both cylinders were placed in a reservoir with dialysis fluid (Figure 20), which could be closed with a tight fitting cover (not shown in the figure).

Negative pressure could be applied to the dialysis fluid reservoir. Actually this was the first dialyser which made controlled ultrafiltration possible.

The system was marketed by a Swedish firm and came into use in some 50 dialysis units in Europe and elsewhere in the 1950's, to be replaced by the twin coil artificial kidney (see further).

Alwall (45–48) like Kolff and other pioneers having misfortunes and also a high mortality in his first series of patients, was criticised in a similar way, not only in his own hospital. His colleagues invented a new term: when a terminally ill uraemic patient died despite dialysis and came to autopsy his critics talked about dialysis treatment as being 'Alwalled'... (personal communication of Mrs. Alwall to the author, 1976).

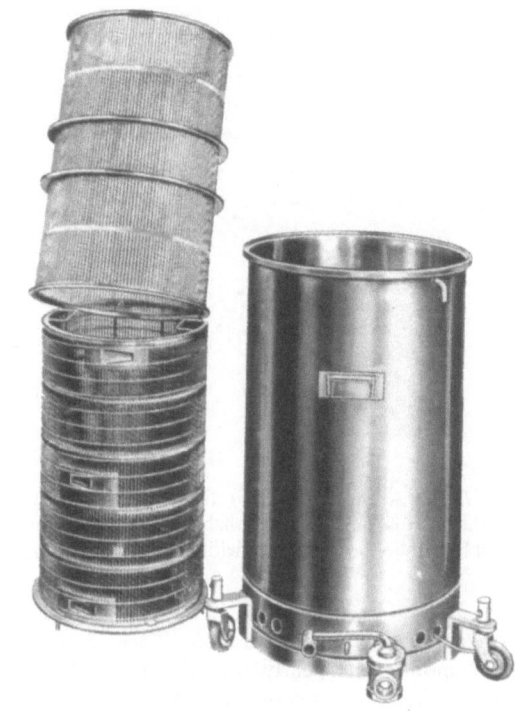

Figure 20. The first dialyser with controllable ultrafiltration, designed by Alwall (1947, 43–48).

PIONEERS IN THE UNITED KINGDOM (1955–1957)

In Leeds, UK, it fell to Dr. Frank Parsons to treat all patients with acute renal failure (49). He soon found that the dietary regimen was excellent in 'clean', non catabolic cases, but that dialysis was essential when renal failure was accompanied by severe catabolism, such as infection or following major trauma (50, 51).

During a stay in the USA, Parsons spent 3 months with Dr. John Merrill in Boston MA, to be instructed in the use of the Kolff-Brigham rotating drum dialysis machine (see Figure 18) and how to dialyse patients with acute renal failure.

After his return Parsons convinced his professor of medicine L.N. Pyrah and the Board of Governors of the hospital to buy a Kolff-Brigham rotating drum dialyser, which Parsons was keen to install against the opinion of British experts. When the machine was half way across the Atlantic Parsons was summoned to the British Medical Research Council. There he was greeted by 'Our advisers say there is no place for an artificial kidney in British medicine...'.

In a 2 h meeting Parsons recounted his experience with dialysis in Boston and the secretary of the MRC, Sir Harold Himsworth, listened intently. Parsons was finely dismissed with: 'Parsons, try it but remember that the country is against you...'.

The machine was installed in the Leeds' General Infirmary (Figure 22) and the first artificial kidney unit in the UK

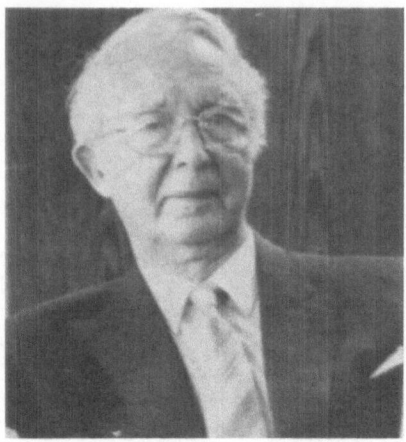

Figure 21. Nils Alwall (1904–1986), the Swedish pioneer who designed the first dialyser with controllable ultrafiltration and the first disposable parallel flow dialyser (with Messrs. Gambro AB, Sweden).

was opened on September 30, 1956.

A few months later, early in 1957, Mr. Ralph Shackman installed a French version of the Kolff-Brigham machine in the Hammersmith Hospital in London and revived the early interest in dialysis at Hammersmith some 10 years after Bywaters and Joekes ended their dialysis efforts at the same hospital.

For a while there were only two dialysis units in the UK with a roughly North/South split in referred pattern (52). The success of the Leeds unit and soon also in the unit at Hammersmith brought nephrologists to Leeds and London to train in the use of the machine and by the end of 1957 many teaching hospitals were planning to install a machine. Many others, however, took no interest and it took several years until dialysis was generally accepted in the UK.

Soon after Kolff's (41) first series of publications improved models of his rotating drum dialyser were constructed such as the Kolff-Brigham model in the USA, described above and the Usifroid model (made in France), which was adopted by the Necker Hospital in Paris and several other hospitals in Europe and even in the USSR.

THE COIL TYPE OF ARTIFICIAL KIDNEYS (1946–1955)

Perhaps one of the most important aspects of Alwall's stationary coil type of dialyser is that it foreshadowed the construction of a new generation of coil type artificial kidneys.

During World War II, Murray, Delorme and Thomas in Toronto, Canada (33, 53, see above) apparently unaware of the work of Kolff and Alwall, constructed independently a static coil type artificial kidney which resembled the Alwall system but included a very small bore cellophane tubing and started, after many efforts and a considerable period of experimenting, dialysing nephrectomised dogs and finally

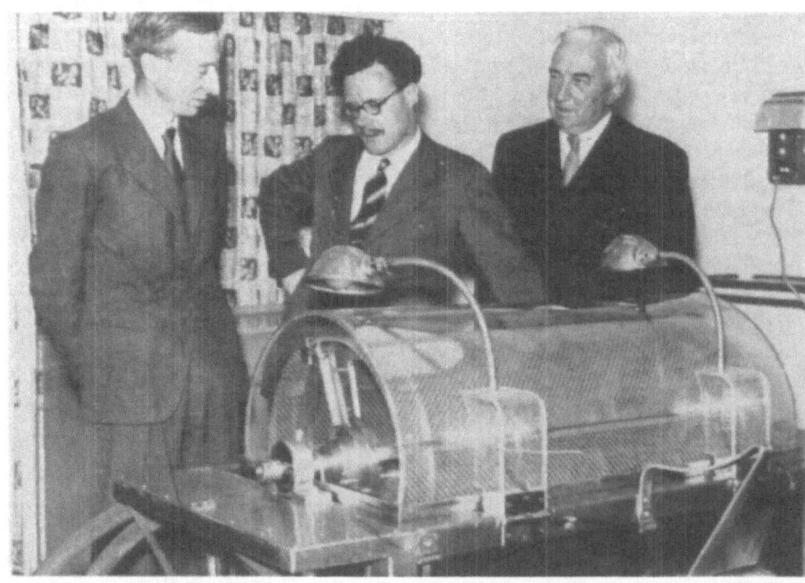

Figure 22. The first artificial kidney unit in the UK, opened September 30, 1956 at the General Infirmary at Leeds. Left Sir Harold Himsworth, secretary of the British Medical Research Council, right Sir George W. Martin, chairman of the Board of the hospital. Centre Dr. F.M. Parsons.

'Advisers say there is no place for an artificial kidney in British medicine . . . Remember, Dr. Parsons, that the country is against you . . .' (1956).

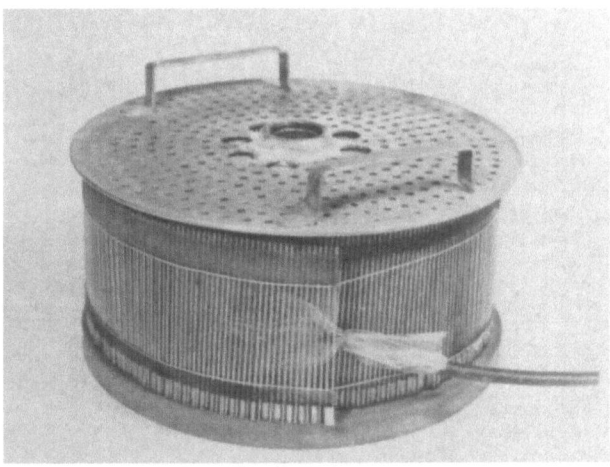

Figure 23. Stationary coil dialyser with cellophane tubing wrapped between a long strip with vertical stainless steel rods, constructed by Bodo von Garrelts, Stockholm, Sweden in 1947 (54). The surface area was later enlarged to 1.92 m²; blood volume 675 ml (50). This device was a precursor of the pressure cooker dialyser constructed by Inouye and Engelberg in 1953 (56 [Figure 24]).

used their apparatus in human patients (1946), using a specially designed, atraumatic pulsatile blood pump. In 1947 they reported details of their first successfully treated patient with acute renal failure, who was dialysed three times and recovered fully. Interestingly, they attached the patient to their machine by passing a catheter through a saphenous vein into the inferior vena cava and another cather into the opposite femoral vein, a method which is still frequently used for access to the circulation in patients with acute renal failure (53).

In Sweden Von Garrelts (54, 55) constructed a rather compact coil dialyser by wrapping cellophane tubing together with a separating device like a rope-ladder with multiple vertical metal rods, not only supporting the membrane but also allowing the dialyser to be perfused by the dialysate solution (Figure 23). This dialyser was more or less a precursor of the *coil type* of artificial kidney constructed in 1953 by Inouye and Engelberg in Philadelphia, PA (56, 57 [Figure 24]). These investigators developed a coil type of artificial kidney, using cellophane tubing wound into a helix round a stainless steel core together with a strip of plastic mesh, acting as a spacer. The coil, with a surface area of 0.9 m² was placed in a common pressure cooker through which dialysis fluid was recirculated from a 50 l tank. The blood could be circulated either with or without a blood pump and ultrafiltration could be regulated by controlling the rate at which dialysing fluid was drawn into the dialyser by a waterpump. This coil dialyser acted as a model for the 'twin coil kidney' of Kolff and Watschinger (58, 59). This 'pressure cooker' design was also a precursor of Michielsen's (60) Recirculating Single Pass (RSP) coil unit, developed about 10 years later.

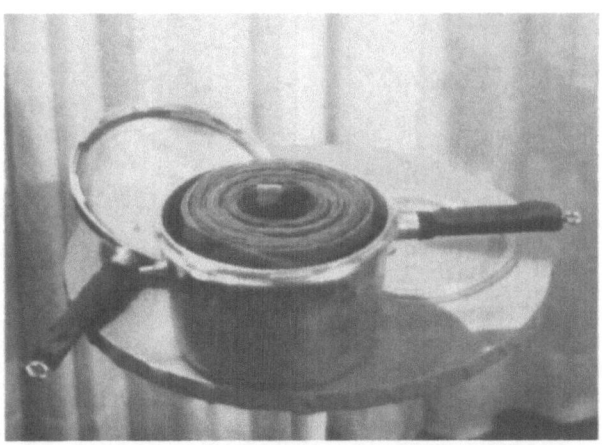

Figure 24. 'Pressure cooker' dialyser, developed by Inouye and Engelberg (56) in 1952–1953. This coil dialyser acted as a model for the 'twin coil kidney' of Kolff and Watschinger.

At that time, basically two types of artificial kidneys had been constructed: the rotating type with the cellophane tubing wrapped around a rotating drum and the stationary models like the Alwall design, the Murray dialyser and the Inouye and Engelberg coil dialyser.

PARALLEL FLOW DIALYSERS (1947–1959)

Meanwhile, another type of stationary dialyser was developed. MacNeill and colleagues from Buffalo, N.Y. (61–63) constructed in 1947 a dialyser built from short lengths of flattened cellophane tubes, 28 of which were stacked together separated by special screens, made from nylon mesh. The appearance of the MacNeill dialyser (Figure 22) had much in common with the multiple layer Gambro dialyser, marketed 20 years later. The MacNeill dialyser was portable but not disposable and had to be rebuilt and sterilised for every dialysis procedure. In fact it was the prototype of a new generation of dialysers: *the parallel flow type*.

In 1948, Skeggs and Leonards of Western Reserve University, Cleveland, Ohio (64, 65) described a different type of parallel flow dialyser,

> . . . 'consisting of a variable number of units, connected in parallel, each consisting of a single sheet of cellophane and two rubber pads (appr. 30 × 45 × 0.6 cm), the inner surfaces of which were finely grooved' . . .

Later, they used two sheets of cellophane between the rubber pads, the blood flowing between the two cellophane membranes and the grooves in the pads carrying the dialysis fluid in the opposite direction on the outer surface of the cellophane. This was the first use of the *counter current principle*. As many units as desired could easily be stacked one above the other and clamped with a holder made of two flat steel plates. The dialyser could be steam sterilised and could be perfused by arterial pressure without the aid of a

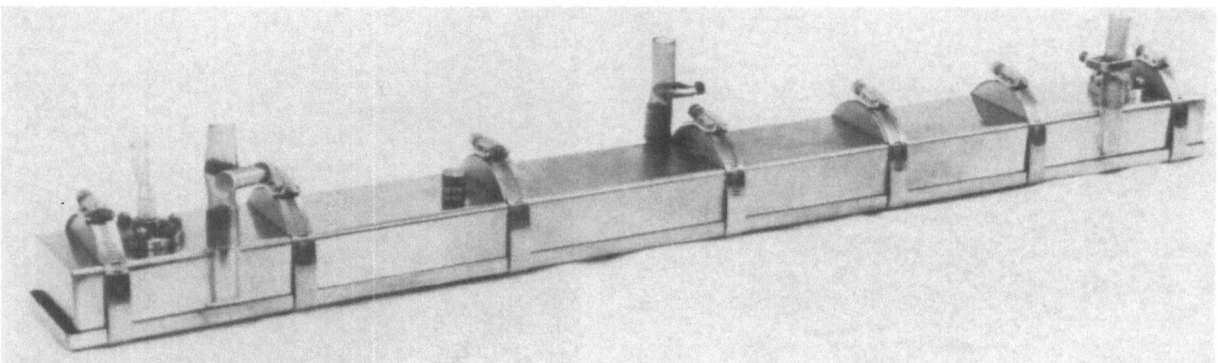

Figure 25. Plate dialyser constructed in 1947 by McNeill and associates, Buffalo NY (61–63). This dialyser was the prototype of a new generation parallel flow dialysers (see text).

blood pump. The blood volume of the dialyser was relatively small compared with the dialysing surface area.

Claus Brun built in Copenhagen a 4 m² Skeggs-Leonard's machine which must have been the largest in the world. It was theoretically 4 m² but probably channelling gave a smaller effective area.

THE 'TWIN COIL' DIALYSER (1955)

In 1955, haemodialysis was still only available in a limited number of hospitals and was applied only in exceptional cases. Many considered the procedure as experimental, laborious, expensive and dangerous. Many doubted its value.

At the first meeting of the American Society for Artificial Internal Organs on the 5th of June 1955, Watschinger and Kolff (58, 59) reported on further development of the artificial kidney of Inouye and Engelberg. To reduce the resistance in this coil dialyser, they used two cellophane tubes in parallel, each 10 m in length, giving a surface area of 1.8 m². Nevertheless, a bloodpump was necessary to obtain a blood flow of 200 ml/min from the radial artery. Both cellophane tubes and fibre glass screen with spacers were wound together around a metal core. During the initial experiments, several core sizes were tried: a beer can, a citrus can and a gallon can. The fruit juice can gave the most satisfactory results and the best pressure/flow relationship.

The urea clearance of this 'twin coil kidney' was 140 ml/min and considerable ultrafiltration took place. The amount of donor blood required to fill the two loops of cellophane tubing was about 750 ml. The dialyser itself was compact and could be presterilised by steam or by ethylene oxide. It was disposable, relatively cheap and could be mass produced. For actual dialysis the coil was placed within a small open cannister in a 100 l dialysis fluid tank with the rinsing fluid pumped crosswise through the mesh of the fibre glass screening at 30 l/min overflowing back into the dialysis fluid tank (see Figure 26a). The system was commercially produced by Travenol Laboratories in the United States (Figure 26b) and rapidly gained popularity. Kidney centres which were opened in the early post war years, changed rapidly to the twin coil artificial kidney and new centres using the machine sprang up both in Europe and in America. Nephrologists and internists became familiar with the twin coil dialysis system and the treatment of acute renal failure: more or less a breakthrough in haemodialysis occurred. The decade after 1956, the year of the introduction of the twin coil kidney, may be called '*the period of acute renal failure*'.

However, several disadvantages of the twin coil kidney soon became apparent (66). It required a blood pump and had a high blood pressure in the extracorporeal circuit which carried the hazard of membrane ruptures. Operation of the twin coil machine was not easy and required experience and skill. In those early years of clinical dialysis some considered it a 'monster to time' (52). The necessity of priming the coil with several units of donor blood exposed the patient to the risks of blood transfusion and made the system also less suitable for repetitive dialysis as is required for chronic renal failure. In addition the bacterial contamination of the open tank system was high.

Nevertheless Maher, Schreiner and Waters (67) reported in April 1961 on five patients with acute renal failure and prolonged oliguria exceeding 60 days. They survived with multiple dialyses with the twin coil system for periods between 66 and 181 days.

Their longest survivor was maintained for 181 days. He received 11 haemodialyses which required multiple arterial and venous cut downs.

ACCESS TO THE CIRCULATION (1960)

A new and original approach to the latter problem came from the studies of Alwall et al (1949 [45]), who during their experimental dialyses of anuric rabbits created an arteriovenous shunt between the carotid artery and jugular vein by siliconised glass tubes, which were joined together between treatments by a narrow glass capillary. Blood flow through the shunt was approximately 1 l/h. Heparin had to be injected every 4 to 6 h. Usually the device clotted after a week

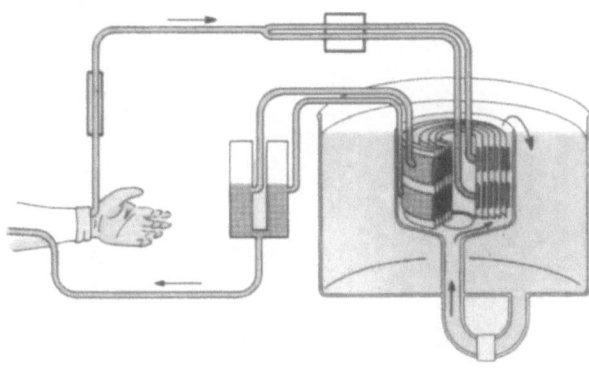

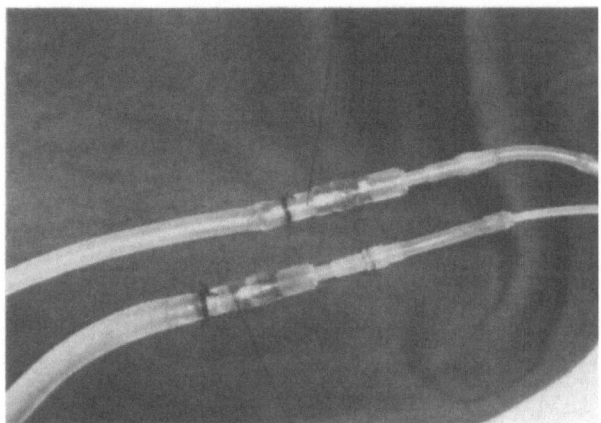

Figure 26a. 'Twin coil' artificial kidney (1955–1956 [58–59]). Flow diagram.

a

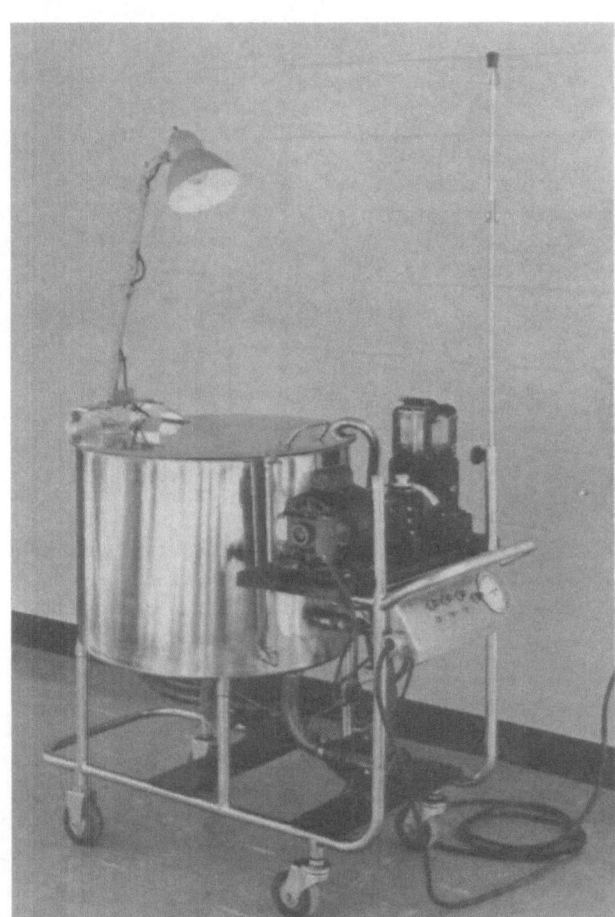

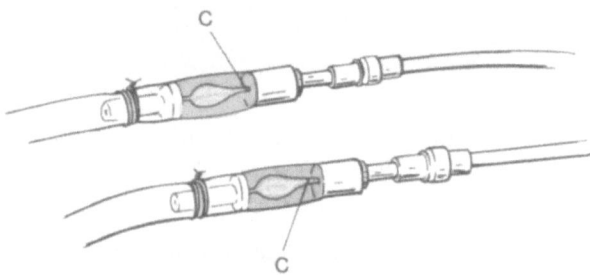

b

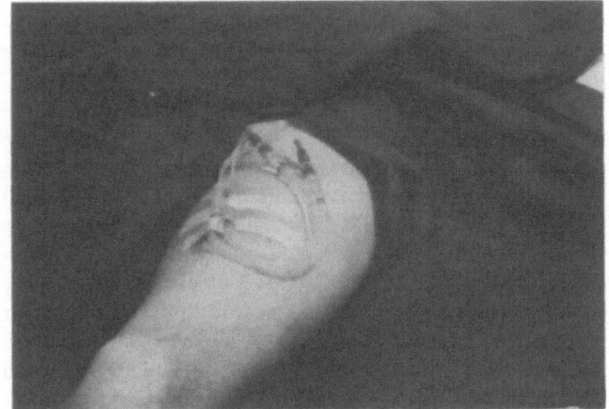

c

Figure 27a and 27b. Silastic heparin infusors connected to indwelling Teflon vena cava catheters used by Giovannetti and coworkers (1963 [68]) and Shaldon (69 [1964]). The Silastic tubing was closed at one end and filled with diluted heparin solution. This slowly perfused the catheters through the connectors which were provided with a capillary lumen (c).

Figure 26b. 'Twin coil' artificial kidney developed by Kolff, Watschinger and Travenol Laboratories.

Figure 27c. Silastic heparin infusors in situ, fixed on upper leg.

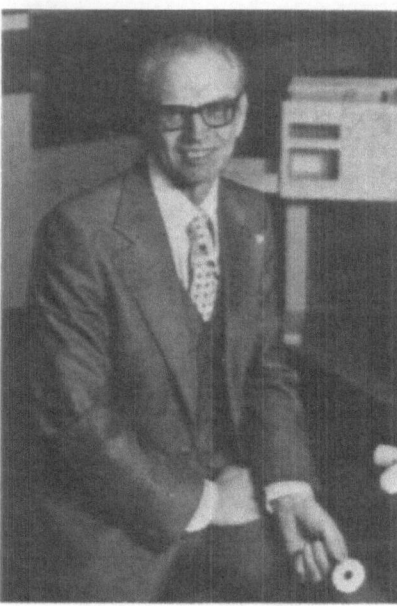

Figure 28. Wayne Quinton, who made the Teflon 'Scribner shunt', with Swageloks and the armplate (Figure 30).

or so, but the concept of an arterio-venous cannula system for repeated haemodialysis was born. The application in humans was soon abandoned however, because of frequent clotting and local infection (47).

Several reports describing various techniques and devices, allowing repeated access to the circulation, appeared between 1950 and 1960. Some of them were simple, like cannulation of the iliac veins or the inferior vena cava with single or double lumen plastic catheters introduced by percutaneous puncture of a femoral vein. Others were quite ingenious like the indwelling 'permanent' vein cannulae described in 1963 by Giovannetti and his co-workers from Pisa, Italy (68), somewhat modified by Shaldon and Rosen (69) in 1964 (Figures 27a, 27b and 27c). Obstacles such as local infection, septicaemia, recurrent clottings, clot-formations at the tip of the catheter even causing pulmonary emboli, made these devices dangerous and unsuitable for prolonged application.

Somewhat earlier, on 10th April 1960, Quinton, Dillard and Scribner ([70], Figures 28 and 29) reported at the Chicago meeting of the American Society for Artificial Internal Organs on an exteriorised bypass device made of Teflon which made the application of repeated haemodialysis for irreversible chronic renal failure a possibility. Their invention caused a major break-through and was a landmark in the history of dialysis. Two cannulae made from thin walled Teflon tubing with tapered ends were inserted, one in the radial artery and the other in the cephalic vein near the wrist of the patient, both cannulae being bent into a 180° turn beneath the skin. The external ends were connected to a curved Teflon bypass tube by means of two Swagelok cou-

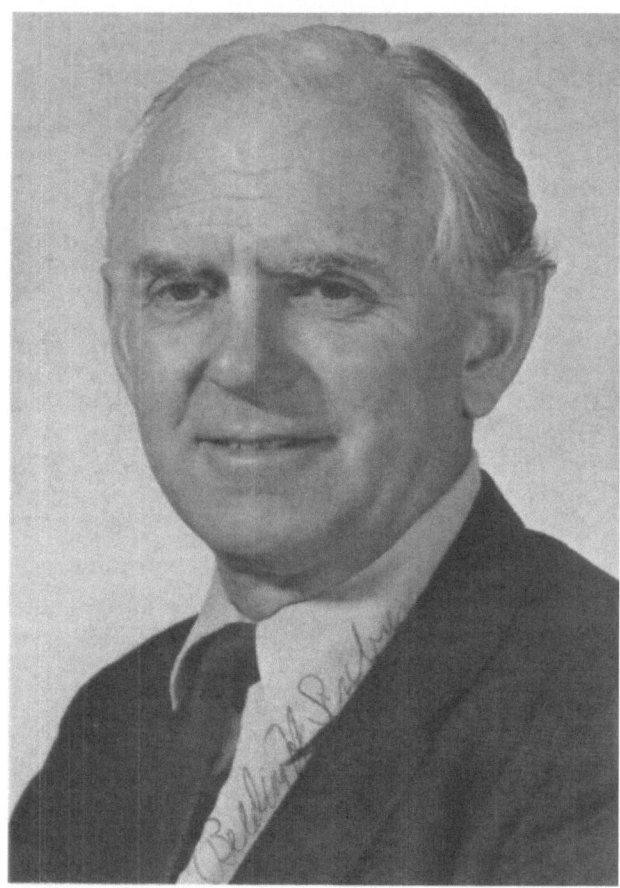

Figure 29. Belding H. Scribner, M.D. (1974).

plings, which were fixed on a stainless steel armplate (Figure 30).

Shortly thereafter, a slightly different arteriovenous shunt also made from Teflon was constructed in Edinburgh, Scotland by Sinclair, Henderson and Simpson (71) (and publish-

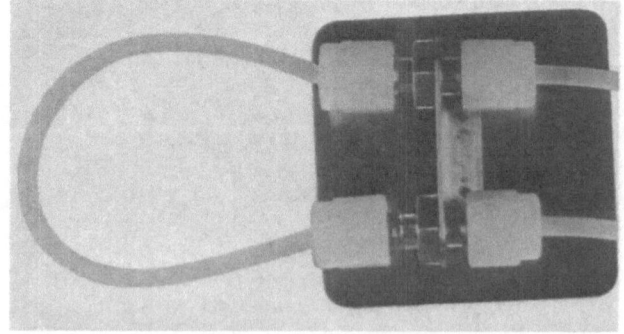

Figure 30. Prototype arterio-venous cannula system made from rigid Teflon with stainless steel armplate (Quinton, Dillard and Scribner, 1960 [70]) (Appr. actual size).

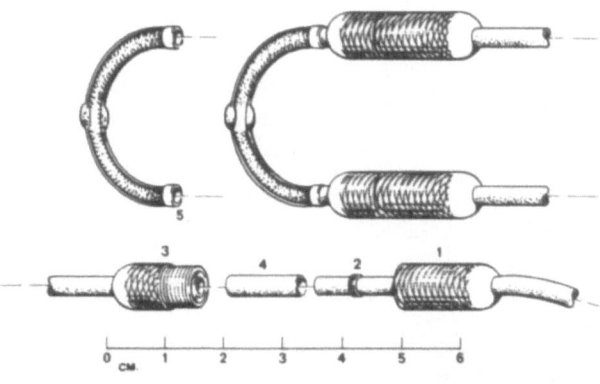

Figure 31. Edinburgh Teflon arterio-venous cannula system constructed by Sinclair, Henderson and Simpson (1961 [71]). (1) female end-piece; (2) metal collar; (3) male end-piece; (4) sleeve size-9 Teflon; (5) metal sleeve to protect U-shaped connecting segment.

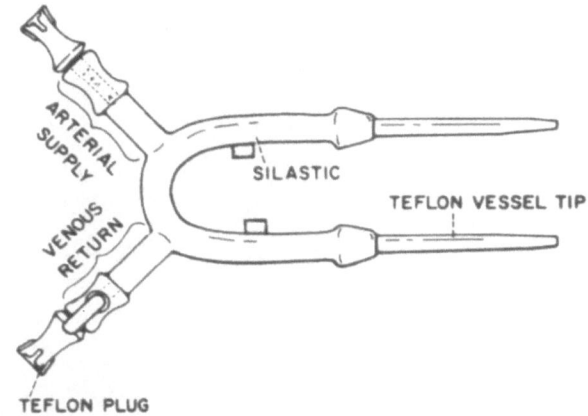

Figure 33. Buselmeier shunt (76 [1972]).

ed as a new invention in the Lancet of the 19th August 1961 [Figure 31]). The credit for the first major step towards long term replacement of renal function by regular dialysis goes, however, to Scribner and his co-workers.

The first model with rigid Teflon cannulae had only a short life expectancy, which was attributed to either mechanical damage to the Teflon tubes or to the vascular wall. The Teflon tubing also had to be shaped while heated to fit the patient's needs. Therefore special preshaped cannulae made from flexible Silastic tubing were designed with vessel tips and extension tubes made from Teflon. The armplate was omitted and the parts were secured by special metal rings (72 [1961]). Further modifications and improvements were made in the next few years, resulting in an all Silastic shunt system with a single break, a short single Teflon connector and Teflon vessel tips (73, 74). Those parts of the Teflon in contact with silicone rubber were etched to make safe connections without the use of metal rings (Figure 32).

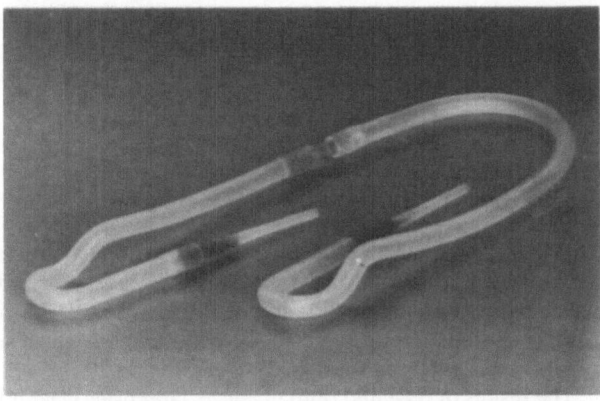

Figure 32. **All Silastic, single break 'Scribner shunt' without metal parts. Teflon parts are etched to provide safe connections (1964, 1967).**

Several commercial firms made complete sets of various shaped cannulae systems available with different sizes of vessel tips and so called reverse and straight 'winged in line' cannulae, which were easier to declot (75). A new, small, somewhat different arteriovenous shunt was designed by Buselmeier and co-workers from Minneapolis (76), which has certain advantages in particular in paediatric patients (Figure 33). The clotting problems, however and the frequency of infection, which already became apparent in 1961 (72), were not solved and still remain. Nevertheless, the 'Scribner shunt' and its modifications found wide application all over the world in every dialysis centre (77), and is still often used in acutely ill patients.

THE SEATTLE DIALYSIS SYSTEM; THE KIIL DIALYSER (1960)

At the same time Scribner (Figure 29) and co-workers presented a fresh and more sophisticated approach to haemodialysis technique. Their original aim was to perform continuous, low flow dialysis in cases of acute renal failure, using an efficient, low resistance dialyser, which made a blood pump unnecessary (78). They started originally with a deep-freeze tank containing a relatively large amount of dialysis fluid to make prolonged dialysis possible without changing the dialysis fluid. The dialysis fluid was cooled in order to reduce bacterial growth (Figures 34a, 34b, 34c). Initially the MacNeill-Collins dialyser (61–63) was tried (see Figure 25), which had a low resistance, but clotted repeatedly. Subsequently a six layer Skeggs-Leonards dialyser (64, 65) was tested. Clotting was less of a problem, but assembly was difficult. Either leaks occurred or compression of the rubber pads had to be excessive, resulting in poor flow characteristics. Finally, Scribner and his group changed to the Kiil dialyser, which was originally described in 1960 by Frederik Kiil from Oslo, Norway (79, 80 [Figures 35a, 35b and 35c]). The original four layer Kiil dialyser was modified into a two layer system and the flow path of the dialysis fluid was

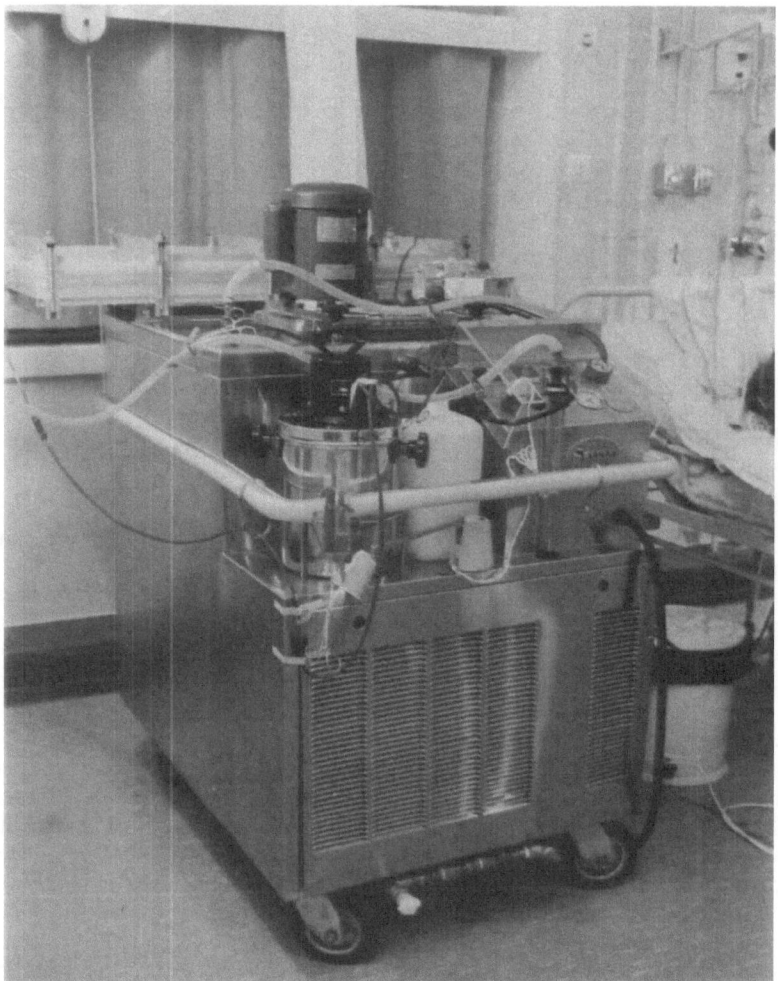

Figure 34a. The Seattle 'pumpless' haemodialysis system: 'Scribner tank' with modified two layer Kiil dialyser on top.

somewhat changed, maintaining however the counter current principle which was adopted by Kiil. An important improvement was the adoption of Cuprophane, a very thin membrane, more permeable than the original Viscose cellophane. The modified Kiil dialyser had a low volume of the blood compartment, which made priming with donor blood unnecessary. The patient's blood was washed back, using saline at the conclusion of the dialysis procedure. In addition the flow resistance of the blood compartment was low and when an arterio-venous cannulae system was used a blood pump was unnecessary: the bloodflow through the dialyser could be maintained by the arterial pressure of the patient.

Despite numerous initial problems and difficulties, the new 'low temperature continuous flow dialysis system' finally worked satisfactorily, simplifying the technique of haemodialysis considerably.

The new technique for circulatory access by (semi-)permanent arterio-venous cannulation made it basically possible to perform an unlimited number of dialyses in a single patient and Scribner decided to study the application of his dialysis system in *chronic irreversible terminal renal failure patients*.

THE FIRST SUCCESSFUL CHRONIC PATIENTS (1960)

On 9th March, 1960, a Teflon arterio-venous cannula system was inserted in the arm of Clyde Shields, a 39-year-old machinist in terminal renal failure (Figure 36) and on 23rd March, another pair of cannulae was placed in the right arm of Harvey Gentry, a 23-year-old shoe salesman.

The results of repeated (initially once, later twice weekly) haemodialyses in these first two patients were surprisingly good: both became successfully rehabilitated chronic dialysis patients. Clyde Shields lived for more than 11 years on intermittent dialysis and died in 1971 at the age of 50 from a

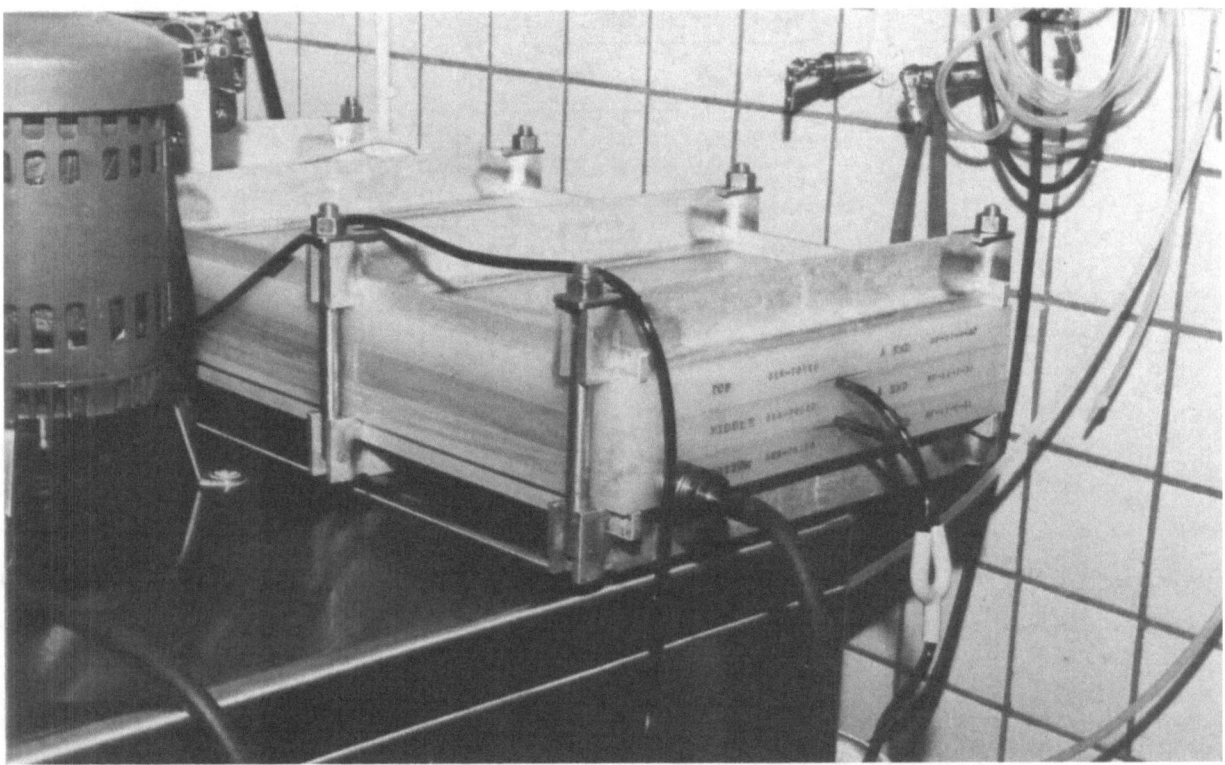

Figure 34b. Modified two layer Kiil dialyser during haemodialysis (1964).

myocardial infarction. Harvey Gentry received a successful transplant from his mother in 1968 and died suddenly in 1987 after 27 years of treatment (see Foreword). The Seattle dialysis system appeared to be so safe and reliable that patients with chronic uraemia could be haemodialysed entirely by nurses (81–83). In April, 1962, the Seattle group reported on eight patients who were on the treatment programme for periods between 4 months and 2 years (84–86). Only one death occurred after 12 months of treatment.

Others, using different techniques, had more limited success (87, 88), but it soon became apparent that successful replacement of renal function and rehabilitation by regular haemodialysis in cases of irreversible, terminal renal failure had become a reality (87, 88). In the Swedish Hospital in Seattle, an outpatient treatment centre was organised and activated early in 1962 (86, 90).

Obviously, cooling of the dialysis fluid, rewarming of the blood returning from the dialyser and performing dialysis at 20° C had been designed to avoid excessive bacterial growth in the recirculating tank system (91), but had certain disadvantages. The recirculating tank system was therefore changed into a single pass circuit. Dialysis fluid was pumped from the tank, heated to 37° C and discarded after a single passage through the dialyser (92). This increased dialysis efficiency and appeared to be a significant improvement, while bacterial counts in the system remained low (Figure 37).

INTRODUCTION OF A CENTRAL SUPPLY SYSTEM OF DIALYSIS FLUID (1963)

The introduction of the single pass technique was actually the first step in the development of a centralised dialysis fluid supply system. The second step was the substitution of acetate for bicarbonate in the dialysis fluid (93), which was based on the discovery of Mudge, Manning and Gilman (94) in 1949, that sodium acetate could act as a source of fixed base. To realise a central multipatient dialysate supply system, a concentrated solution of salts and dextrose had to be diluted with (pretreated) tapwater by means of an accurate proportioning system to obtain a continuous supply of dialysis fluid. Sodium bicarbonate solution unlike sodium acetate cannot be mixed with concentrated solutions of calcium and magnesium salts without adjusting pH to 7.4 or less.

A central system for simultaneous supply of dialysis fluid for 10 to 15 patients was designed by Dr. Albert L. Babb and his coworkers Scribner, Grimsrud, Cole and Lehman (95, 96). Dr. Babb was a faculty member of the Department of Chemical Engineering at the University of Washington at Seattle. A prototype was built with three variable speed proportioning pumps, one for 35 times normal strength salt-dextrose solution and one for water, providing dialysis fluid, on line for a 10 bed dialysis unit by mixing one part of concentrate with 34 parts of water (Figure 38). The system

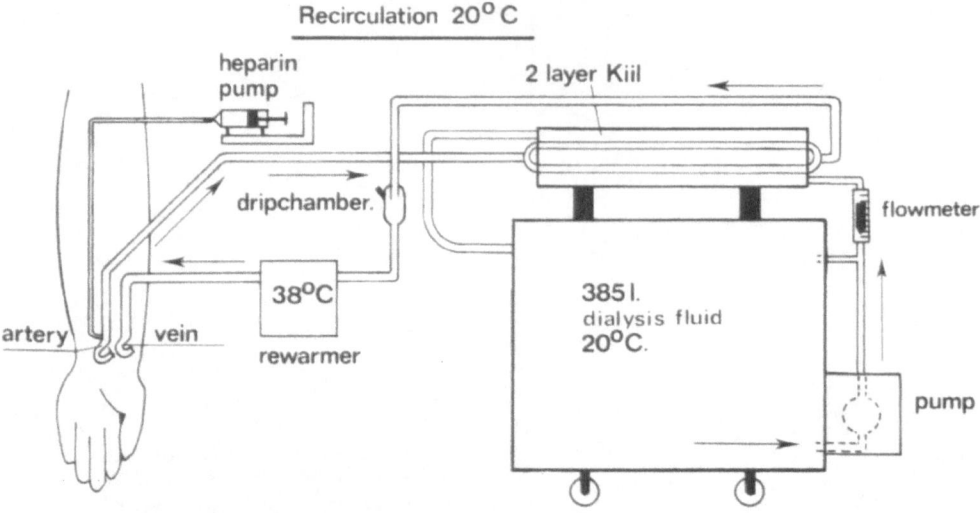

Figure 34c. Flow diagram of the original Seattle 'pumpless' haemodialysis system. The dialysis fluid was cooled and recirculated through the dialyser (1960 [78, 82, 83]).

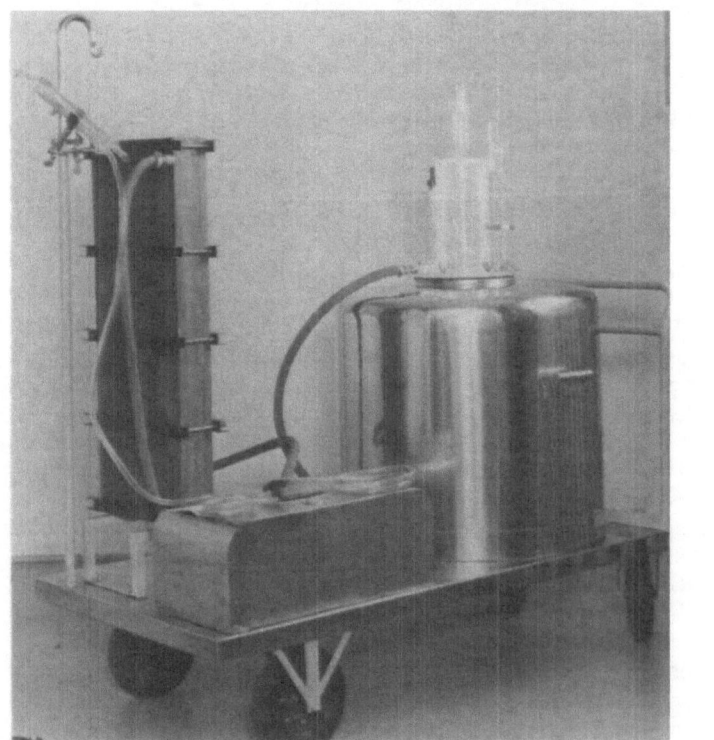

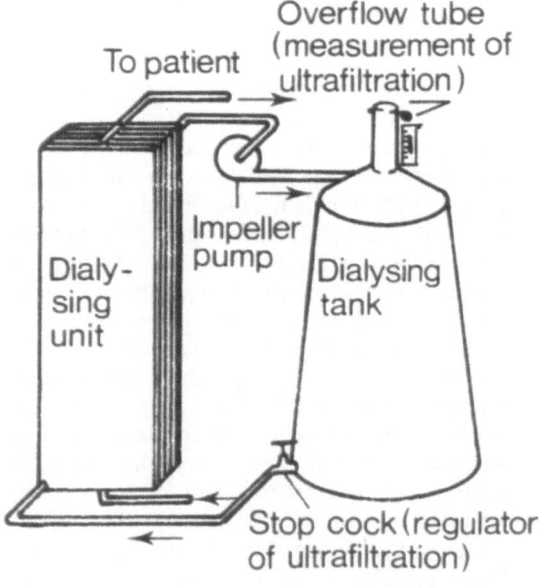

Figure 35a. Original Kiil dialyser (in vertical position) with stainless steel tank containing 300 l dialysis fluid and equipped with a open narrow overflow chimney, facilitating collection and measurement of ultrafiltrate (1960 [79, 80]).

Figure 35b. Flow diagram of the original Kiil dialysis system (79, 80).

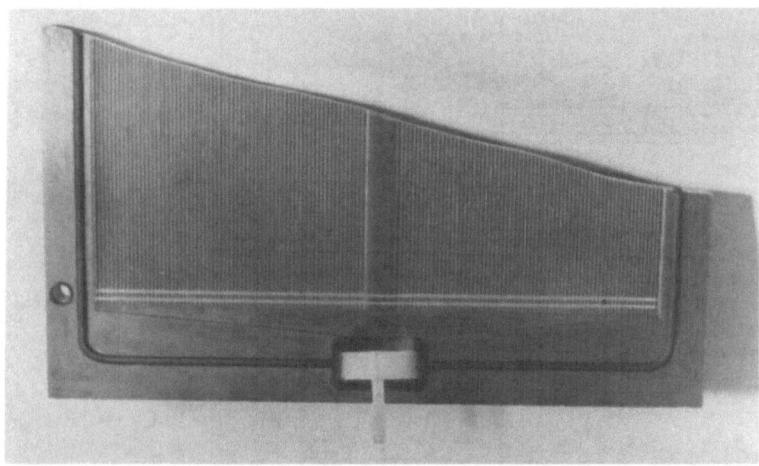

Figure 35c. End section of grooved plastic board of Kiil dialyser (made from Araldit, an epoxyresin compound [79, 80]).

had a third proportioning pump, which was envisioned for sodium bicarbonate solution, but appeared to be redundant: the investigations of Mion et al (93) had made it clear that sodium acetate was an acceptable substitute for sodium bicarbonate and could be readily mixed in the concentrate with the other salts and dextrose in the appropriate concentration. The proportioning system (called 'the monster' by the patients) was put into use in 1963 and functioned without

failure until 1967, when it was put out of use, as the dialysis unit moved to another hospital.

In terms of 1963 dollars it was estimated that the proportioning system reduced the annual cost of treatment of one patient to approximately $15,000 rather than $30,000 for thrice weekly treatment because of reduction of personnel requirement.

Surprisingly, an impressive reduction in bacterial contamination of the dialysis fluid was noted. This was explained by self sterilising properties of the concentrated bath solution (97), which, however, from later investigations (98) and the author's own experience appeared to be non existent.

The use of concentrated solutions, containing acetate, for the preparation of dialysis fluid rapidly gained wide application, both for automatic proportioning systems and also for manual preparation of dialysis fluid.

ANOTHER MILESTONE: THE START OF REGULAR DIALYSIS TREATMENT OF TERMINAL IRREVERSIBLE RENAL FAILURE (1960)

Until the early 1960's dialysis activities were limited to the treatment of acute renal failure. A few early attempts to treat patients with chronic renal failure by regularly repeated dialyses failed until the Scribner shunt became available. Then, the number of treatment centres and hence patients began to increase, but because of lack of equipment and of nephrologists and internists, who were acquainted with dialysis techniques the increase was slow; in August 1965, however, 40 centres in Europe had started treating patients with chronic renal failure and some 160 patients were on treatment (99).

Soon, the number of chronic patients requiring treatment outnumbered the available facilities, both in Europe and in the United States. But many hospitals intending to start dialysis treatment and existing dialysis centres were ham-

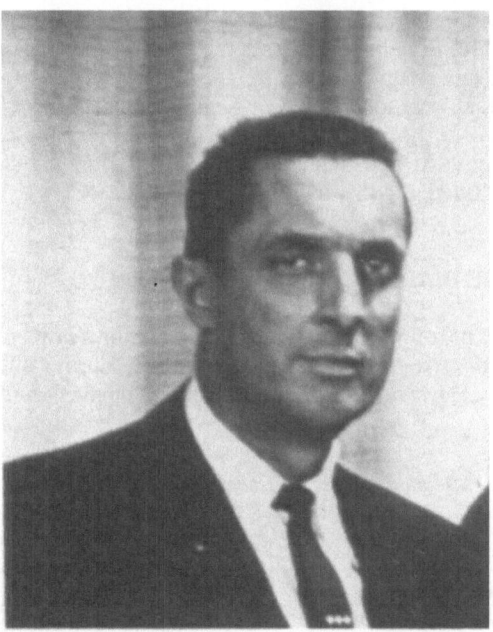

Figure 36. Mr. Clyde Shields (1921–1971), the first successful chronic dialysis patient. Picture taken in 1966 after 5 years of dialysis treatment.

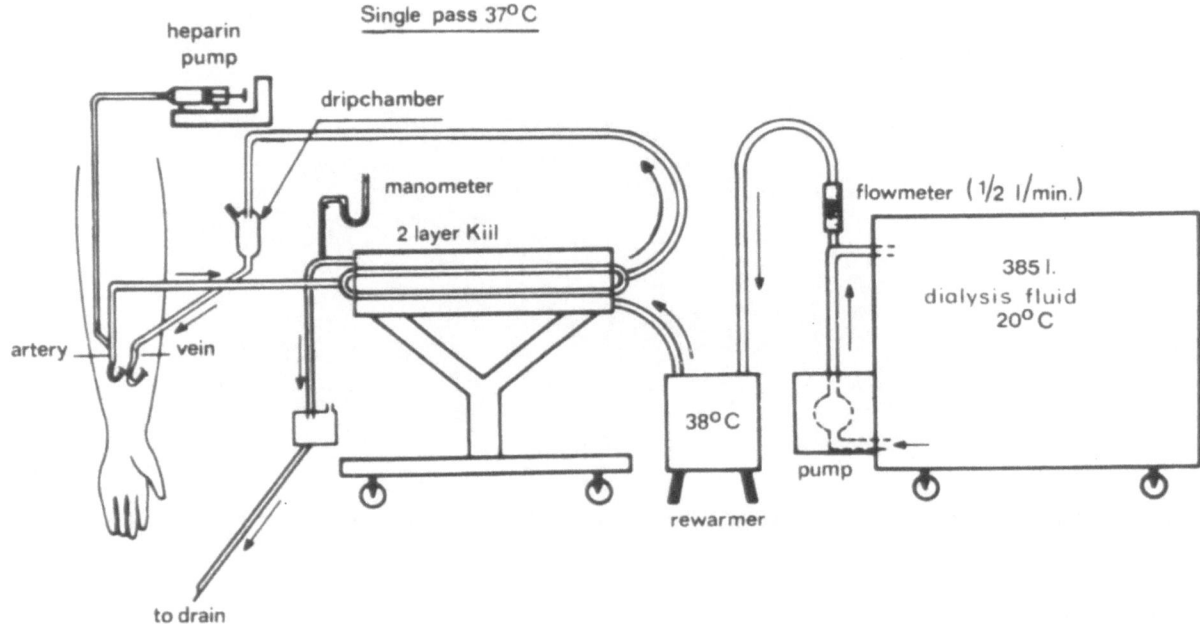

Figure 37. Flow diagram of the Seattle 'pumpless' haemodialysis system modified into a single pass system. The dialysis fluid was pumped from the tank, heated to 37°C and discarded after a single passage through the dialyser (1964 [92]). See text.

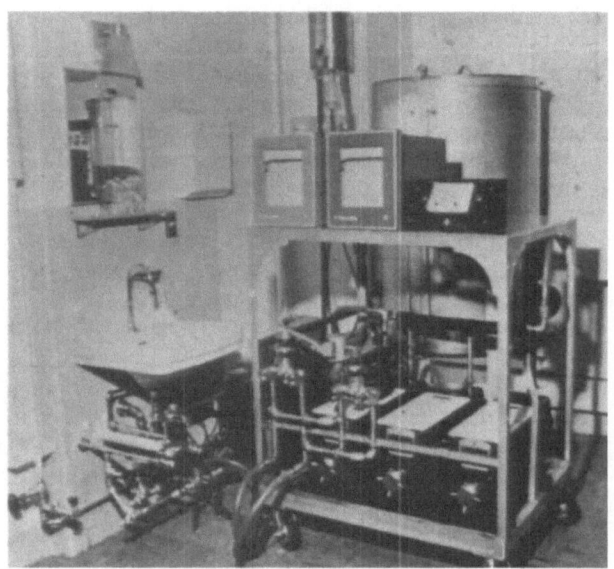

Figure 38. The original central proportioning system, called 'the Monster' by the patients, designed by A.L. Babb PhD and coworkers. The third proportioning pump (on the right) was installed for bicarbonate solution but was never used, because bicarbonate was substituted by acetate. The system functioned without any failure from 1963–1967 for 10 to 15 patients at the dialysis unit of the University Hospital at Seattle, WA.

pered at this stage by lack of money, equipment and trained personnel (99).

In Seattle, a much critisised patient selection procedure was instituted by means of a double committee (86, 90). Elsewhere however, patients were accommodated as well as possible, usually on a first come, first served basis for all medically acceptable patients.

Initially the only solution seemed to be to increase the number of hospital treatment centres and expand existing facilities. At that time, renal transplantation was still less established as a therapeutic procedure.

HOME DIALYSIS (1964) (See chapter 30)

In the next few years, a gradual increase of treatment facilities occurred both in America and in Europe (Table 1 [100]). However, enormous problems of financing and train-

Table 1. Regular dialysis treatment in Europe 1965–1968.

	1965	1966	1967	1968
No of centres	43	54	81	114
No of accepted patients	277	612	1163	2633
Alive and on regular dialysis	160	295	621	1281

(From Drukker et al (100), with permission of Excerpta Medica, Amsterdam)

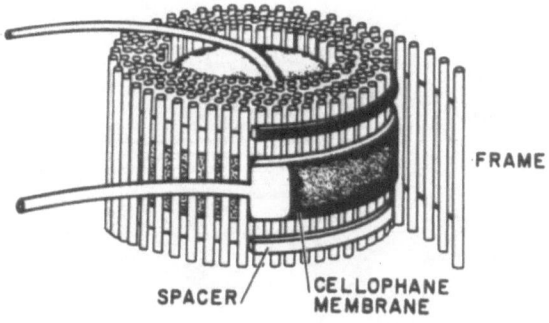

Figure 39a. Japanese coil dialyser used for home dialysis: 7 m cellophane sausage wound with a frame of plastic tubes laced with cords held on equal distance by spacers (Nosé, 1961 [105]). Surface area 0.63 m^2. This dialyser shows a striking similarity with the coil dialyser constructed by Bobo von Garrelts in Sweden in 1947 (see Figure 23).

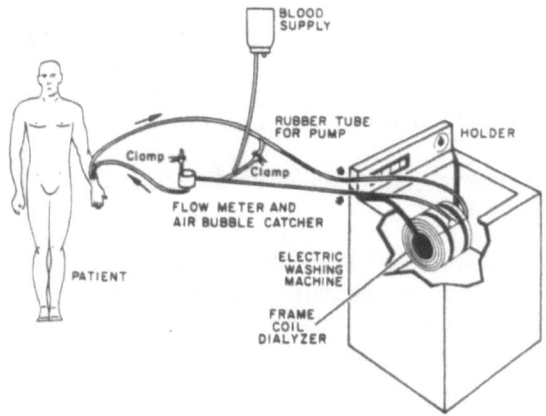

Figure 39b. Japanese home dialysis system with coil dialyser in ordinary domestic washing machine (1961 [105]).

Table 2. Europe.

Home haemodialysis % of total haemodialysis patients

year	%	
1972	17.2	
1973	18.5	
1974	18.8	
1975	19.2	
1976	19.0	
1977	15.0	
1978	14.6	← introduction of CAPD
1979	13,0	
1980	11.6	
1981	10.1	
1982	10.1	
1983	11.2	
1984	9.8	
1985	8.9	

Table 3. United Kingdom.

Home haemodialysis % of total haemodialysis patients

year	%	
1972	58.8	
1973	61.6	
1974	64.8	
1975	64.9	
1976	66.5	
1977	66.3	
1978	65.7	← introduction of CAPD
1979	64.1	
1980	62.0	
1981	61.3	
1982	60.0	
1983	59.0	
1984	56.0	
1985	51.0	

ing of doctors and nurses had to be faced and in an effort to achieve at least a partial solution of the dilemma Shaldon and co-workers of the Royal Free Hospital in London, U.K. (101–104) introduced the concept of self dialysis in September 1963. From self dialysis in the hospital to home dialysis was the next step. This step had already been made by the Japanese in 1961, according to Nosé (105 [see Figure 30a and 30b]). In America, Merrill's group (106) in Boston had already initiated home dialysis in July 1964 and satisfactory results in three patients were soon reported.

The Seattle group started their home programme in September 1964 (107). The Royal Free team began home dialysis two months later (108) their first patient being a registered nurse. Her husband, an engineer, made the Kiil dialyser and the additional dialysis equipment himself.

Merrill and colleagues (106, 109) used the disposable twin coil dialyser with recirculating dialysate, a system which was popular in America at that time. The patient's own blood was stored and used for priming the dialyser for the next dialysis. Curtis and coworkers (107) and Baillod et al. (108) used the non-disposable modified Kiil dialyser either with a 300 l static tank for dialysis fluid preparation or an automatic dialysis fluid supply system, based on the concept of the central supply machine constructed in Seattle. These single patient proportioning systems were marketed at that time both in the United States and in England.

Home dialysis soon attracted both considerable interest and criticism. It took Scribner (110) several years 'to convince both patients and colleagues that home dialysis was the only way to go'. It soon became apparent that in the home more frequent dialysis was possible with better rehabilitation. Cost was considerably less compared to hospital dialysis (110). The self sufficiency and independence were considered more than adequate compensation for the extra burden on the patient and his family (107).

In little more than 10 years approximately 16%, or more

than 10,000 patients, worldwide, practiced self dialysis in the home (111, 112).

In the mid-seventies interest in home haemodialysis, however, began to decline: in 1985 only 8.9% of all haemodialysis patients treated themselves at home (Table 2). In the U.K. the health authorities have traditionally been in favour of home dialysis. By the end of 1978 more than 65% of the total haemodialysis population in that country dialysed at home (111, 112). But thereafter the number also declined (Table 3): CAPD (continuous ambulatory peritoneal dialysis) (see chapters 22 and 25) became increasingly popular after its introduction in 1978 and was often preferred both by the doctors and the patients.

FURTHER DEVELOPMENT OF PROPORTIONING MACHINES

The multipatient proportioning system constructed by Babb and coworkers in 1962/1963 stood as a model for smaller single patient machines, designed and developed by the industry.

The construction of reliable proportioning machines has doubtless not only contributed to the safety of hospital dialysis, but in particular to the safety of self dialysis in the home setting.

Systems with motor driven piston pumps

Different systems have been developed. The simplest construction had motor driven pumps with a fixed dilution ratio (Figure 40).

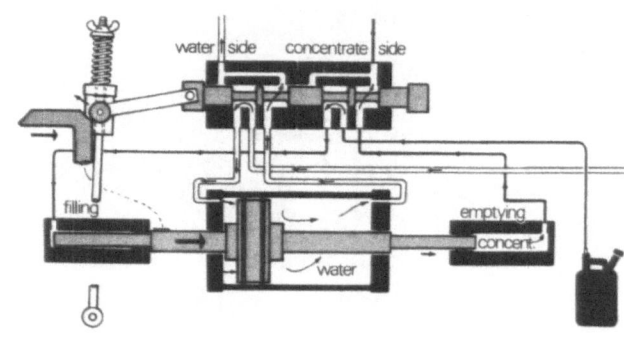

Figure 41. Proportioning device with water-driven pump system (carboy on bottom right contains concentrate). Two upper outlets, water and concentrate sides, unite in a mixing chamber. The open ended tube above the carboy is connected to the water supply. This system has also a fixed proportioning ratio.

Proportioning devices with water driven pump systems

In other systems a water driven proportioning device is used also with a fixed dilution ratio (Figure 41).

Proportioning systems with motor driven pumps with variable ratio

In still other systems, also with motor driven proportioning pump systems, the proportioning ratio can be varied between certain limits to adapt the dialysate sodium concentration to the individual requirements of the patients (Figure 42).

Systems with servo controlled electronically steered pumps

Later conductivity feed back proportioning systems were constructed. They also have the advantage of a variable proportioning ratio (Figure 43).

The presently marketed proportioning machines are com-

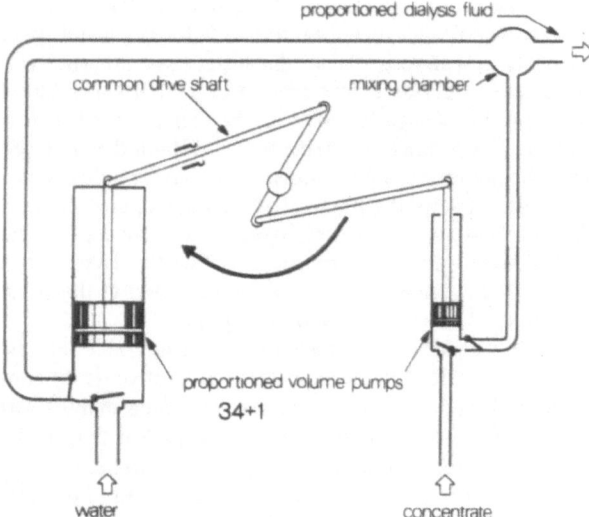

Figure 40. Motor driven piston pumps proportioning device with a fixed dilution ratio.

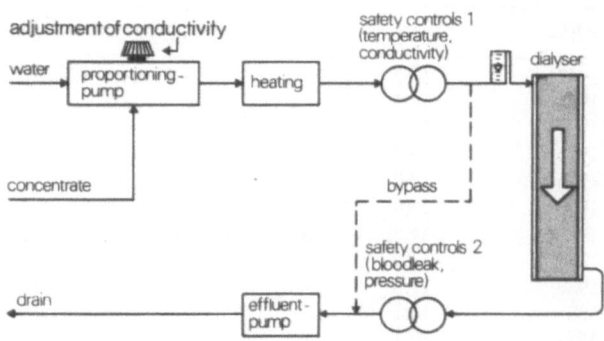

Figure 42. Proportioning system with motor driven pump. The proportioning ratio can be varied between certain limits to adapt dialysis fluid to individual requirement of the patient.

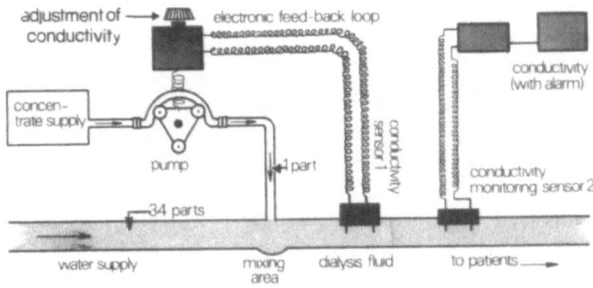

Figure 43. Proportioning system, with servo controlled speed of concentrate pump (so called electronic feed-back proportioning system) with variable proportioning ratio.

bined with highly sophisticated monitoring systems and are often technical jewels with a high degree of reliability and operating comfort.

THE ARTERIOVENOUS FISTULA (1966)

It became obvious that the arterio-venous shunt was the Achilles heel of chronic dialysis. Patients, doctors and nurses were plagued by episodes of clotting, infections and subsequent loss of shunts.

In 1966, a surgically created arterio-venous (A–V) fistula was introduced for access to the circulation by Brescia, Cimino, Appel and Hurwich from New York (113): another landmark in the history of dialysis. In the same issue of the New England Journal of Medicine a now historical editorial comment was published (114):

... 'Whether or not this new internal shunt technic can be adapted for home use remains to be determined. Although such an adaptation seems to pose some formidable problems' ...

The problems appeared to be neither insurmountable nor formidable. Shaldon (115) successfully began training patients to use the internal A–V fistula for overnight dialysis in the home and taught the patients self-needling (October 1967). The internal fistula became increasingly popular, soon dominating regular dialysis both in the home and in the hospital.

In 1975 approximately 83% of all hospital and 88% of home dialysed patients in Europe had a subcutaneous vascular access (Cimino fistula, grafts and PTFE combined) (111).

In 1978 internal access was used for 93.6% of the patients, compared to 88.4% in 1975.

The proportion of patients with external (Scribner type) shunts dropped in 1978 to 5.9% from 10.4% in 1975 (112).

THE ROLE OF THE ASAIO AND THE EDTA–ERA (1955, 1964)

In the last 25 years, haemodialysis has been the subject of intensive investigations involving bio-engineering, membrane research, biochemistry, biophysics, immunology and evaluation of clinical experience (116, 117). In America, much of this research was initially supported by the John A. Hartford Foundation, and later by the Artificial Kidney-Chronic Uremia Program of the National Institutes of Health, directed by Dr. Benjamin Burton. In the period of initial turbulence, probably nothing has been more helpful to coordinate studies and to inform investigators and clinicians than the annual meetings of the American Society for Artificial Internal Organs (ASAIO) and its Transactions. The idea of founding an American Society for Artificial Organs came from the late Dr. Peter F. Salisbury from Los Angeles, in August 1954. The new Society had 47 founding members and held its first annual meeting in Atlantic City, on the 4th and 5th June 1955, in conjunction with the American Medical Association (118).

Salisbury (119) wrote in a chronicle on the occasion of the 5th anniversary of the Society, quoting the Holy Bible 'ever since Daniel described scientific meetings with the famous words ... "many shall run to and fro and knowledge shall be increased" ...' (120).

In the first 15 years of its existence, the Society held its annual meetings in conjunction with the Federation of American Societies for Experimental Biology, usually on the east coast, in Atlantic City, sometimes in Chicago or Philadelphia. Then, they started to run to and fro, having their venues on the east and west coasts or in the midwest, and knowledge was increased immensely indeed ... In less than 20 years the membership exceeded 1000.

A similar role was played in Europe by the European Dialysis and Transplant Associaton (EDTA), which was founded in Amsterdam on 24th September 1964 (121, 122). Like the ASAIO, the EDTA has acted for many years as a forum where people could meet and could present and discuss the results of their investigations and clinical experience. Its annual statistical reports, which in 1986 included data on 110,300 patients alive and treated by dialysis and transplantation (123), became highlights and derive data from voluntary cooperation of 82 to 95% of all European centres.

In 1986 2065 centres reported to the EDTA Registry, about 82% of all known European centres. In 1986 23,320 new patients started treatment in Europe (123).

In 1982 the EDTA widened its spectrum of interest to include nephrology and a second name: 'European Renal Association (ERA) was added.

FURTHER DEVELOPMENTS; THE ROLE OF THE INDUSTRY

The initial goal of the early investigators to develop methodology by which they could keep patients in terminal chronic renal failure alive was achieved before 1965. Further refinements included increasing dialysis efficiency, shortening of dialysis time, increasing safety and comfort, miniaturisation of equipment and economising.

Other investigations were directed to prevent and to heal

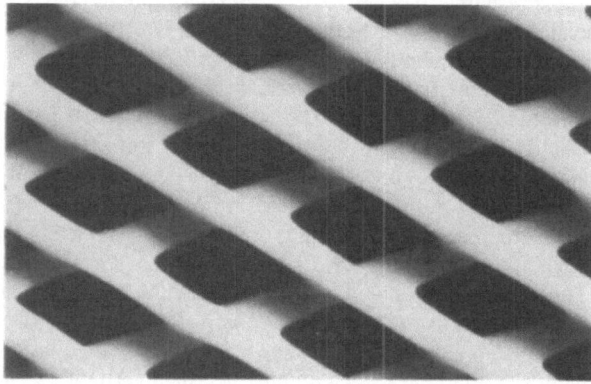

Figure 44. Hoeltzenbein mesh support used in coil dialysers (129). (See also chapter 5).

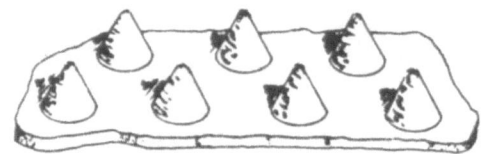

Figure 45. Multipoint membrane support (127). (See also chapter 5).

complications and to improve the health rehabilitation and quality of life of chronic dialysis patients.

On the other hand, basic research focused on haemodynamics, kinetics of solute removal and development of new membranes with better permeability characteristics, in particular for so called middle molecules (see below) and higher degrees of biocompatibility. After 1965, industry became increasingly interested in dialysis and a growing number of proportioning machines, monitoring equipment, blood pumps and ancillary equipment was constructed and introduced. A plethora of different types of dialysers was made available, both disposable (coils or parallel flow dialysers) and nondisposable such as the standard two layer Kiil and its modification with multipoint membrane support (124–128, [see also chapter 5]).

Initially basic research directed to improving the performance of dialysers came, however, primarily from outside of the industry.

The efficiency of the coil dialyser was much improved by a new mesh support designed by Hoeltzenbein (129) in 1966. It was made from polyethylene and its geometry was derived from a certain type of fishing net or from the upholstering of a Volkswagen. This membrane support (see Figure 44) eliminated spacers and increased turbulence of dialysate, decreasing the dialysing resistance of the stagnant film of dialysis fluid in direct contact with the membrane. In addition the Hoeltzenbein mesh improved the dialysis efficiency of the coil type dialyser by increasing the effective surface area of the membrane through reduced membrane contact.

The performance of coil dialysers was further improved by replacement of the cellophane membrane by thin Cuprophan, which had been used in Kiil type dialysers for several years.

The multicone membrane support was originally designed by investigators from New York, (E.F. Leonard) and from Philadelphia, (L.W. Bluemle Jr. and others) and was described in 1960 (124–128 [Figure 45, see also chapter 5]). It serves the same purpose in parallel flow dialysers as the Hoeltzenbein mesh in coils. The pyramid membrane support improved the dialyser efficiency not only by increasing the effective membrane surface area (through reduced membrane support contact) but also through improved dialysis fluid distribution (128). The advantages of the multiple cone support are particularly appreciable in situations with a low dialysate flow rate or (and) with a high transmembrane pressure for high ultrafiltration.

The multiple pyramid membrane support is employed in the non-disposable Meltec modification of the Kiil dialyser, which was used in the United Kingdom and in a number of disposable flat plate dialysers (the reader is referred to chapter 5 for more detailed information).

Around 1965, when preferences were divided between Kiil and coil dialysers (130, 131) a new design, the hollow fiber artificial kidney, or capillary dialyser was introduced (132, 133). With a short length of the blood path, a thin blood film, a highly effective membrane surface area and excellent diffusive and convective capabilities this compact dialyser could control uraemia very well. Simultaneously, in Europe, the first disposable parallel flow dialyser was introduced by Alwall (134), soon to be followed by improved models produced in Sweden by Gambro Inc.

DIFFERENT TYPES OF DIALYSERS AND MEMBRANES

The Kiil dialyser and its multipoint variant – the work horses of the 1960's – are presently obsolete. Interested nephrologists may study these historical dialysers by visiting collections of antique dialysis equipment, which are kept in a few hospitals or in the International Center of Artificial Organs and Transplantation in Cleveland, Ohio.* Coil dialysers were in the early 1980's still used in a few East European centres (in only 4% of all European dialysis patients).

Parallel flow disposable dialysers are presently used in slightly more than a quarter of all European dialysis patients; the majority of the patients (68%) dialyse with capillary hollow fibre dialysers and this proportion is still increasing.

The vast majority of the European patients dialyse with dialysers provided with Cuprophane or regenerated cellulose membranes. Presently both are considered the least

---

* Address: 8937 Euclid Ave, Cleveland, Ohio 44106, USA

biocompatible membranes (with the highest degree of complement activation [135, 136]).

The more permeable and much more biocompatible polyacrylo-nitrile membrane was used in 1984 in only 4% of the European patients. The cellulose acetate membrane with a biocomptability in between these two was used in slightly less than 4%. Other synthetic membranes with interesting characteristics are presently marketed and incorporated in capillary dialysers by several firms.

The multitude of available dialysers with different flow characteristics and different membranes including the plethora of (often non standardised) data supplied by the manufacturers is confusing to junior doctors and others who enter the field of dialysis. Confusion has been furthered by new hypotheses which have been derived from reconsiderations of old questions, i.e. what is toxic, what should be considered uraemic toxins, what should be removed?

In addition there is increasing evidence that dialysis treatment at least in a number of patients should be individualised by careful selection of the dialyser, its surface area, the type of membrane and the length of dialysis (the 'square metre/hour' concept).

THE SQUARE METRE/HOUR AND MIDDLE MOLECULE HYPOTHESES (1971)

In the early years of regular peritoneal dialysis for chronic renal failure, Scribner (137) noted that patients on chronic peritoneal dialysis, which controls traditional plasma chemistries of urea and creatinine less than haemodialysis does, often felt better (1965). Despite a certain amount of 'under-dialysis' with chronic peritoneal dialysis, peripheral neuropathy either did not occur or did not progress. Scribner presented the hypothesis that the peritoneum was more permeable and that peritoneal dialysis removed substances of higher molecular weight more efficiently than haemodialysis. Suspicion arose that the so called middle molecules played an important role in the toxicity of uraemia. Because of their size, it was suggested that they were very slowly removed compared to urea. The cellulosic membranes used in haemodialysis (e.g. cellulose acetate and cuprophane) have according to Scribner's hypothesis a rather high diffusion resistance for these species of molecules.

This speculation correlated with the hypothesis that using a given membrane, prevention of peripheral neuropathy depends on a minimum number of hours of dialysis per week, rather than on maintaining specific levels of blood urea and creatinine. Further, it was suggested that larger toxic solutes permeated the peritoneum better than cellulose membranes. These considerations led to the square metre/hour hypothesis (138, 139) and to its modification, the middle molecule hypothesis (140). Both theories suggest that inadequate removal of the middle molecules (molecular weight between 300 and 2,000) causes complications such as peripheral neuropathy, pericarditis and perhaps others.

Since the removal rate of middle molecules through a conventional haemodialysis membrane is slow, the diffusion gradient remains high throughout haemodialysis, unlike that of urea. Thus, the net removal rate of middle molecules remains rather constant during protracted dialysis and net removal is proportional to the total number of haemodialysis hours/week unlike urea which has a flow dependent removal which decreases with the decreasing plasma concentration as dialysis proceeds. Increasing the length of each dialysis may, therefore, arrest neuropathy. The Seattle group and others (139–145) presented indirect evidence that the so called middle molecules are the primary toxins causing uraemic neuropathy and other uraemic manifestations.

Until actual and accurate measurement of toxic plasma middle molecules and removal rates by dialysis are achieved, however, this index is not likely to be generally accepted and dialysis protocols will remain largely empirical. These studies may serve, however, as a warning against indiscriminate shortening of dialysis time in chronic patients on the one hand and against 'over-dialysis' on the other. *Over-dialysis,* previously considered as virtually nonexistent, may result from excessive duration of dialysis or too frequent dialysis and may affect the patient's well being adversely, possibly also causing post dialysis hangover. *Insufficient dialysis* may allow persistent hyperphosphataemia, acidaemia and abnormalities of mono- and bivalent ions and excessive concentrations of urea, creatinine, uric acid and methylguanidine, which can contribute to signs and symptoms of the uraemic syndrome.

THE SEATTLE DIALYSIS INDEX (1975)

Babb and associates (146) introduced in 1975 the concept of the 'dialysis index', a theoretical number based on several parameters, i.e. the body surface and the residual creatinine clearance of the patient, the vitamin B12 clearance of the dialyser, the membrane used and the ultrafiltration rate. This dialysis index is considered as an estimate of adequate dialysis for an individual stable chronic dialysis patient.

Nomograms have been designed for easy estimation of dialysis indices and dialysis prescriptions for stable patients (147).

DIALYSIS STRATEGIES

Short and ultra short schedules (1974–?)

The square metre/hour and middle molecule hypotheses have profoundly influenced dialysis strategies, resulting in a confusing and conflicting array of various dialysis protocols (148–150). That does not alter the fact that isolation, identification and the toxicology of so called middle molecules are still in a process of research. Several groups of investigators have been active in this slippery field full of mantraps (151, see also chapter 2).

Nevertheless in many dialysis centres, protocols were changed according to the new theories, resulting in short dialysis schedules either with large surface area dialysers or with the same type of dialyser and increased frequency, but usually with less dialysis hours per week. Experimentally short dialysis has been performed with three hollow fibre artificial kidneys in series (152) with two 1.0 m² parallel flow dialysers in series (153) or with so called large surface area dialysers, which became commercially available in the early seventies (see chapter 5). Other clinical investigators simply shortened each dialysis, decreasing substantially total weekly hours of dialysis, without increasing surface area or membrane permeability (154). Sophisticated modifications of dialysis protocols made use of a special membrane with high clearances for molecules in the critical range of 300 to 2,000 daltons (144, 145), but so far only few other special membranes have found limited practical application for dialysis (155–158).

Many early evaluations of short dialysis schedules did not take into account the fact that residual renal function contributes to removal of middle molecules (159, 160). Likewise the effect of ultrafiltration on convective removal of middle molecules (161) has been often overlooked. Residual kidney function in haemodialysis patients should be measured (162) and considered in evaluating short dialysis schedules.

Several analytical models, based on the square metre/hour, the Seattle Dialysis Index, and the middle molecule hypotheses have been introduced as guidelines for quantitation of dialysis treatment (163). In practice these models and guidelines found only limited application and the majority of dialysis protocols are still empirically determined.

With a ever increasing load of patients, dialysis time per week in hospital programs seemed only poorly adjusted to the individual patient's requirements; organisational factors apparently determined the time schedules (112).

Not only the increasing number of patients, but also economic incentives to lowering personnel costs and shortening dialysis times played a role. And of course haemodialysis patients themselves have a universal and unremitting preferences for shorter dialysis sessions (164).

In the early years of chronic dialysis, sessions with the modified two layer Kiil dialyser lasted 10 to 12 h (initially twice, later thrice weekly) with a twin coil and a Meltec multipoint modification of the Kiil slightly less.

In the 1970's when not only the need for dialysis facilities considerably increased but also with new dialysers and other dialysis equipment efficiency improved, dialysis protocols were changed, more or less according to the new theories. This resulted in shorter dialysis schedules, either with larger surface area dialysers or two or three dialysers in parallel or in serial configuration (153, 154, 163, 165, 166).

In 1977 60% of the hospital patients dialysed between 12 and 15 h per week. Most home patients dialysed longer and a substantial number of home patients were on thrice weekly schedules, dialysing 24 h per week or longer.

In the recent decade gradually a decrease occurred and presently dialysis schedules have been standardized on three times weekly for 4 h each.

In the home some patients dialyse somewhat longer; short dialysis of the 1970's has become standard dialysis in 1980: in a period of 10 years (1968–1978) average dialysis treatment time was decreased more than 50% (147).

Nevertheless efforts of further shortening of dialysis time have continued and several investigators tried to approach the limits of so called ultra-short dialysis (166–172). Daugirdas and associates (167) connected two 2.5 m² hollow fibre dialysers in series perfusing them thrice weekly with 500 ml bicarbonate-acetate dialysis fluid each for 2 h using special ultrafiltration controllers.

Rotellar and coworkers (168–170) used two 2.5 m² dialysers in parallel: blood flow was maintained at 500 ml/min. Bicarbonate containing dialysis fluid with 5 to 10 g/l dextrose was used, perfusing the dialysers with 1,000 ml/min. With these high dextrose concentrations hyperglycaemia was achieved, preventing a sudden decrease of plasma osmolality and also preventing dialysis desequilibrium and other undesired side effects (method described in 1965 [171]).

Others (173–175) performed ultra short treatment with haemodiafiltration (a combination of dialysis and haemofiltration [173, 174]). Manji et al (175) used two 1.8 m² hollow fibre dialysers in series. In the first dialyser a high transmembrane pressure was maintained resulting in a substantial convective flow.

A Japanese group (176) combined haemoperfusion and haemodialysis with a 1.3 m² hollow fibre dialyser and obtained a substantial increase of clearances of small molecules and most likely an efficient adsorbance of middle molecules by the coated charcoal, permitting reduced treatment sessions of 3 h three times weekly. Results during a treatment period of 10 months in two patients were good. It is clear that short, shorter and ultra-short dialysis has been and still is an attractive goal for clinical investigators so far resulting in an often confusing array of dialysis protocols and technologies.

Criticism

More than a decade ago, in 1974, at a symposium about new dialysis strategies, three groups presented their clinical results of short dialysis, each of them using a different mode of treatment. The then president of the meeting Prof. Jørn Hess Thaysen from Copenhagen, Denmark stood up and said:

'Well we have three gentlemen here, one gentleman uses very short dialysis with a standard dialyser. The concentration of small molecules is high and the concentration of the middle molecules is presumably also high. His results are very good. The next gentleman uses two 1 m² dialysers in series, thus obtaining a large surface area. The level of small molecules is low and the level of middle molecules is presumably low. His results are excellent. Then we have a third gentleman. He uses a dialyser with very permeable membranes to middle molecules and a small-volume recirculating dialysate system. The concentration of small molecules is high and the concentration of middle molecules is presumably low. His results are excellent too. Well gentlemen – this is very strange . . .' (177).

In the 1981 EDTA report on regular dialysis in Europe (178) it was noted, that death due to myocardial infarction was more frequent with short dialysis in elderly males and that the death rate on short dialysis was higher than on long dialysis, in particular in the Fed. Republic of Germany, both in females and elderly males.

Laurent and associates (179) from Tassin near Lyon, France reported a few years ago (1983) excellent results with long dialysis. Actually this group did not change their dialysis protocol since 1961, dialysing 24 h/week with Kiil dialysers. Excellent long-term survival figures were reported and the number of intra- and interdialytic side effects (hypotension, muscle cramps, vomiting) was surprisingly low compared with a large control group from the French registry.

The majority of the patients was dialysed during the night, a strict non transfusion policy was adhered to and blood pressure control was optimal with less than 1% of the patients on hypotensive drugs . . .

Recently Wizemann and colleagues (180) reported on their experience with a decade of short dialysis (3 × 2 to 3 h/week); after 5 years the dialysis sessions were gradually prolonged to 3 × 4 h/week. The results of the short and long dialysis protocols were compared. During the long protocol blood pressure control was significantly better and antihypertensive drugs could be discontinued in more than half the patients; the number of hypotensive episodes was significantly lower during long dialysis. Hypertrophic cardiomyopathy (documented by left sided heart catheterisation) was a common finding and could according to the authors be responsible for the high incidence of sudden death in the short dialysis population. Raja et al (181) reporting on a 10-year follow-up of a group of short treated patients (9 to 15 h/week with 'large surface area' dialysers). They noted a 10 year survival of only 30%. Laurent et al (179) reported a 10 year survival of 50% in a high risk group treated with long dialysis and in their low risk group 84% survived after 7 years and 80% after 10 years of long dialysis.

When studying the literature, doubtless the number of 'favourable' reports on short dialysis strikingly predominates over less favourable or unfavourable reports. But investigators are naturally biased to publish favourable results, studies presenting unfavourable data being unattractive to publish.

Shortcomings

Many early evaluations of short dialysis schedules did not take into account residual renal function which contributes to the removal of middle molecules (159, 160); likewise the effect of convective removal of middle molecules has been often overlooked (182).

Residual renal function should be measured (183) and considered in evaluating short dialysis schedules. Obviously the active surface area of the dialyser, blood flow, dialysis fluid flow, diet and body mass of the patient should be integrated in the protocols. An appropriate control group is essential. Obviously many, even the majority of clinical investigations on short versus long dialysis do not meet these criteria and the issue: is short (and ultrashort) dialysis a safe treatment and is it acceptable for long term regular dialysis treatment, is still undecided.

ANOTHER INDEX OF DIALYSIS (1985)

Keshaviah and Collins (164) reported recently in a well documented and well designed study on short dialysis, using the KT/V index as a parameter of dialysis adequacy.

This index, introduced in 1985 by Gotch and Sargent (184) is calculated as the product of the urea clearance (K, ml/min) of the dialyser and duration of the dialysis session (T, min), divided by the distribution volume of urea (V ml). Gotch and Sargent analysed the data of the large scale National Cooperative Dialysis Study (NCDS) in the US and determined that a KT/V value of 0.9–1.0 constitutes adequate dialysis therapy.

Values less than 0.8 are associated with a high probability of therapy failure. Keshaviah and Collins (164) also demonstrated that short and rapid dialysis treatment is well tolerated when acetate is replaced by bicarbonate and is not associated with increased mortality and morbidity if therapy is prescribed keeping KT/V greater than 1.

MORE STUDIES REQUIRED

More long term, well designed studies of short and ultra short dialysis protocols may be helpful to give the answer to the question:

'Short dialysis schedules – Finally ready to become a routine?' (Cambi, 1974 [154])

ANOTHER WARNING

But another warning sounds. Presently, after more than 20 years of chronic dialysis a new uraemic toxin (β_2-Microglobulin and a new syndrome have emerged, the β_2-M dialysis associated amyloid syndrome (185, 186; see also page 60 and 61). Practical prevention or therapy or both are yet hypothetical: high permeability membranes and prolonged dialysis or haemofiltration therapy to remove the 11,800 dalton β_2-M may be required, making the question short dialysis obsolete or controversial with a definite answer . . .

URAEMIC TOXINS; EFFORTS TO IDENTIFY MIDDLE MOLECULES (1974-?)

The symptomatology and pathophysiology of the uraemic syndrome are complex and multifactorial and not dependent on one or more specific uraemic toxins (189). Traditionally byproducts of the metabolism of nitrogen containing nutrients: proteins, polypeptides and amino acids are incriminated as responsible for uraemic toxicology. In contrast with the end-products of fat and carbohydrate metabolism (water and carbon dioxide) which can be totally eliminated by lungs and skin, the elimination of compounds derived from protein and other nitrogen containing nutrients depends on the kidneys. However, not only does the retention of toxic compounds make the renal failure patient sick finally causing death, but also progressive impairment of a multitude of hormonal and regulatory functions occurs, leading to progressive failure of multiple organ systems. In addition malfunction of one system may lead in turn to disorder and malfunction of another (Trade off hypothesis, Bricker 1972 [188]).

Nevertheless the search for and the efforts to identify uraemic toxins has been going on for a long time (151, 189).

Many simple substances may act as 'uraemic toxins' when present in the organism in excessive amounts or in abnormal concentrations because of failure of renal functions: for example water, sodium, potassium, hydrogen ions and inorganic phosphate (177). Other established compounds which may act as uraemic toxins are of a more complex nature, like parathormone (190–194), natriuretic hormone, renin and others (177, 194).

Many other substances simple or complex, have been suspected, incriminated or even listed as uraemic toxins: urea, creatinine, uric acid, the guanidines and countless others (177, 194–197). The true nature of many suspected uraemic toxins has, however, remained obscure and their pathogenicity also remained hypothetical, or, at least, doubtful and unproven (177, 194, 195).

The search for uraemic toxins gained additional impetus in recent years because of the assumption that substances with a molecular mass between 500 and 5,000 daltons were particularly toxic and the observation that these 'middle molecules' passed poorly through the cellulosic membranes commonly used in dialysers (137, 198–200). Suspicion arose that the accumulation of these more or less mysterious 'middle' molecules was not only responsible for a part of the symptomatology of uraemia but also for certain disabling and severe complications as peripheral neuropathy and pericarditis. The impact of the middle molecule hypothesis of Babb and associates (138–141) found response in a number of European research centres and a 'gold rush' started to isolate and identify middle molecules, in particular during the 1970's and early 1980's.

Most of these studies have been based on separation techniques using gel-chromatography, but later new methods for separation and quantitation of the elusive middle molecules became available.

Dzúrik and associates (201, 202) from Bratislava, Czechoslovakia using high voltage paper electrophoresis and Sephadex gel filtration demonstrated in uraemic sera peptides of 300 to 1,500 daltons, which were not detectable in normal sera.

Dall'Aglio et al (203) and Migone and coworkers (204) from Parma, Italy were able to confirm these findings and identified peptides in spent dialysate.

Other groups in Europe and also in Japan were very active in this field.

In Paris the Necker group (Funck Brentano and associates [144, 145; 205–208]) using a new polyacrylonitrile dialysis membrane (PAN), which is highly permeable and has a middle molecule clearance twice that of Cuprophan, demonstrated that severe uraemic neuropathy could be reversed with this new membrane.

These investigators identified in spent dialysate from a dialyser with a PAN membrane a chromatographic pattern similar to a pattern obtained with normal urine, observing an identical middle molecule peak in both.

With fibroblast cultures, which are sensitive to the toxic effects of middle molecules in the 300–1,500 daltons range, a high degree of toxic activity could be demonstrated with spent dialysate obtained with a polyacrylonitrile dialyser in patients with uraemic polyneuropathy and only a low degree when a Cuprophane dialyser was used.

In Stockholm, Sweden, Bergström, Fürst and coworkers (200, 209–214) using gelchromatography plus special analytical techniques (ion-exchange chromatography and iso-tachophoresis) found abnormal UV absorption 'peaks' in uraemic plasma and spent dialysis fluid from uraemic patients. Similar peaks were detected in normal urine.

These peaks became measurable in plasma when plasma creatinine concentration exceeded 400 μmol/l (4.5 mg/dl) or when the creatinine clearance was below 12 ml/min.

Ten or more different peaks were observed; peak number 7 was present only in uraemic plasma and corresponded to a molecular weight range of 1,000 to 2,000 (187).

Peak 7 material, isolated with the gel filtration procedure, could be subdivided in seven to nine subfractions by gradient elution chromatograpy on DEAE Sephadex columns. The subpeaks 7f and 7g were present in normal plasma, the other peaks were only detected in uraemic plasma.

In plasma of patients on dialysis with uraemic complications (neuropathy; pericarditis) subpeaks were especially high, in particular peak 7c. It was shown that peak 7c contained glycine and a β-glucuronidated conjugate of orthohydroxybenzoic acid (151, 211, 213).

So far the results of recent studies of middle molecules and their toxicity have been mostly based on initial separation by gel chromatography and although tremendous efforts have been invested and progress was made with interesting results, Bergström and Fürst, pioneering in this field full of booby traps and barbed wire, heaved a sigh in both previous editions of this book:

'It is to-day not possible to evaluate the exact role of the manifold compounds which accumulate in renal failure in causing or contributing to the various symptoms and biochemical abnormalities of uraemia'. (First edition in 1978 [214]).

In the second edition, in 1983 the same authors added:

'Four years later this still holds true. The new information gathered in these years has shed further light on the complexity of the problem but has not led to a breakthrough in our understanding of the nature of uraemic toxicity' (194). This opinion was shared by others (215). Nevertheless, recently applying a different chemical approach some sofar unsuspected substances have been shown to play a role in uraemic toxicity one way or another and could be considered uraemic toxins. One of these compounds is hippuric acid. In spite of its rather small molecular size of only 179 daltons it behaves like a middle molecule.

With high performance liquid chromatography hippuric acid was identified as a valuable marker for uraemic solute retention and elimination and its concentration correlated significantly with the total UV absorbance of uraemic serum, with the residual renal function and with dialytic solute extraction (216)

This correlation was substantially better than that of the classical markers such as urea and creatinine.

Other studies have already demonstrated that hippuric acid interferes with the transport of organic substances at the cellular level (217) and with drug-protein binding (218–220).

Interesting and unexpected news came from France. Assenat and colleagues (185) reported in 1980 on a syndrome observed in long-term dialysis patients, characterised by the carpal tunnel syndrome, shoulder pain and stiffness. Amyloid appeared to be deposited in carpal tunnel tissues removed at operation. Subsequently amyloid deposits were found in the synovial membranes and capsules of many other joints, and in subchrondral bone causing radiolucencies, predominantly in the wrists, hips, in the femoral neck, and in vertebral discs.

The syndrome develops slowly in patients treated by regular dialysis for at least 5 years or longer (196, 221–223). The lesions are progressive and the destructive arthropathies, spondylarthritis and even spontaneous fractures are potential factors which limit the continuation of regular dialysis treatment (222, 224).

It has been predicted that 100% of dialysis patients will be affected by the syndrome by their 20th year of treatment (225). Recently several investigators presented evidence that dialysis associated amyloidosis is caused by a new type of amyloid with an unusual and characteristic structure.

Both by amino acid sequence analysis and with immuno-histochemistry it was demonstrated that the amyloid fibrils consisted of β_2-microglobulin, a relatively small protein (molecular mass 11,800 D) normally present in plasma and excreted by glomerular filtration and catabolised after reabsorption by the renal tubular epithelium. Normal removal rate is approximately 150 mg/day (136, 186, 221, 222, 226).

In patients dialysed with classical cellulosic membranes such as Cuprophane progressive accumulation of β_2-microglobulin occurs (225–228), which is on the long term laid down forming the major constituent of the fibrils of dialysis associated amyloid that is responsible for the progressively incapacitating syndrome, briefly outlined above. β_2-microglobulin has to be considered a new uraemic toxin in long-term dialysis patients.

DIALYSIS MEMBRANES

Conventional (cellulosic) membranes

Cellophane, a polysaccharide membrane, structured by β dextrose molecules, originally marketed for packing purposes, appeared, when wetted, to be semipermeable and suitable for human dialysis (24, 25, 30).

It was used by Kolff in his rotating drum dialyser in the 1940's (25–30, see p. 28–33) and in the twin coil dialyser (58, 59, see p. 37–39) but was replaced by Scribner and coworkers (81–84) by a thinner and more permeable cellulosic membrane called Cuprophane (Cuprophan in the USA) by the manufacturers (Enka AG, Wuppertal, FRG, generic name cuprammonium rayon). Originally also marketed as

Table 4. Europe.

Year	Population (10^6)	New patients on renal replacement Rx	New patients/10^6 population	Patients on dialysis				Total on dialysis	Funct. graft	Funct. graft/10^6 population	Total on renal replacement Rx	Total/10^6 population
				Hosp. HD	Home HD	IPD	CAPD					
1972	433.6	5,481	12.6	8,502	1,819	175	–	10,321	2,752	6.3	13,248	30.5
1973	489.5	6,640	13.6	11,387	2,558	196	–	14,171	3,477	7.1	17,648	36.0
1974	486.4	7,931	16.3	14,357	3,302	268	–	19,927	4,378	9.0	22,305	45.9
1975	491.4	9,481	16.7	18,116	4,305	336	–	22,757	5,094	10.3	27,851	56.7
1976*	495.0	9,440	18.2	21,177	5,166	436	–	27,343	6,307	12.7	34,215	69.1
1977	541.0	10,166	18.7	25,344	5,953	545	–	31,842	7,402	13.6	39,735	73.5
1978**	556.8	10,523	22.1	28,438	6,563	839	–	35,546	9,074	16.3	44,914	80.7
1979	551.7	12,258	22.2	33,537	7,108	804	779	35,840	10,287	18.6	54,550	98.9
1980	573.0	14,084	24.6	40,570	7,838	910	1,839	48,408	12,394	21.6	67,412	117.6
1981***	574.2	15,889	22.7	44,777	7,981	951	3,002	52,758	14,249	24.8	80,775	140.7
1982	574.2	13,508	23.5	46,576	7,298	824	3,607	58,305	13,859	24.1	72,164	126.0
1983	574.2	19,668	34.3	62,138	8,707	984	5,563	70,845	16,489	28.7	85,188	146.0
1984	578.5	20,815	36.0	63,044	7,787	968	6,450	78,999	22,833	39.5	101,832	176.0
1985	620.2	21,004	33.9	67,328	7,441	985	7,529	82,283	25,238	40.7	108,521	175.0
1986	624.4	23,320	37.4	76,446	6,762	869	8,491	92,568	32,002	51.3	124,570	200.0

* Introduction of automatic RO PD machines.
** Introduction of CAPD.
*** Introduction of CCPD.
Data derived from the annual statistical reports of the EDTA-ERA.

flat sheets for packing purposes, they were sucessfully used as dialysis membranes in the Kiil dialyser and its modifications. Later it appeared a suitable raw material for modelling into hollow fibres, incorporated by Cordis Dow in the USA in small but efficient disposable dialysers (132, 133).

The original cellulosic membranes were successfully used for haemodialysis for several decades and Cuprophane remained the membrane of choice in the vast majority of the countless disposable dialysers both with the hollow fiber and the flat sheet configuration (see chapter 6) marketed by numerous firms. The original Cuprophane hollow fibers were later replaced by Cordis Dow by cellulose acetate (Cellulate). These cellulosic membranes are cheap and relatively easy to model into hollow fibers with different diameters and wall thicknesses. They can be readily sterilised with formaldehyde and ethylene oxide and are suitable for repeated reuse.

The world wide increase of dialysis patients (see for European figures Table 4) and limitations of available budgets in many countries urged the creation of more dialysis facilities and lower cost per treatment; the concept of short and ultra-short dialysis was born (150, 153, 154, see p. 51–53) and, not surprisingly, became rapidly popular with patients, doctors and hospital administrators. The pro's and con's of this concept have been reviewed and discussed earlier. Short dialysis required larger surface area dialysers or dialysers with more porous membranes with increased permeability for the so called middle molecules or both.

Many new membranes have been synthesised (229) but few appeared suitable for practical application and could be mass produced.

They became available for clinical evaluation in the mid-seventies (230–233 [see Table 5]). The principles of preparation, sieving and filtration properties of these membranes were reviewed by Göhl and coworkers in 1982 (234).

Filters provided with these membranes have been marketed for haemofiltration and haemodiafiltration. Because of the high hydraulic permeability (and therefore high ultrafiltration capacity) their use for haemodialysis may only be safely undertaken with modified dialysis systems permitting adaequate control of ultrafiltration (235).

This requirement and the relatively high price of these synthetic membranes have so far limited the use of these filters mainly to haemofiltration and haemodiafiltration. This, however, is presently in a process of changing.

Complement activation by cellulosic membranes and neutropenia

The majority of regular dialysis patients is dialysed with cellulosic membranes: Cuprophane, regenerated cellulose or cellulose acetate (Cellulate).

Cellulosic membranes cause profound granulocytopenia during the first 15 min of haemodialysis – a phenomenon already observed several decades ago (236–244).

More recently it became clear that cellulose, being a polysaccharide, is a potent activator of the complement cascade.

Each time dialysis is started with a new cellulosic membrane the cascade of complement activation occurs, lasting from 10 min to one hour (135, 236–248) and resulting from sequestration of neutrophils in the pulmonary vascular capillaries. This is followed by a decrease of PaO_2 and by pulmonary hypertension; interstitial pulmonary oedema may occur.

The pulmonary distress syndrome or first use syndrome

In sensitive patients a cardiopulmonary distress syndrome may develop ('dialysis lungs', 'first use syndrome' [135, 136, 245, 246]). It should be mentioned, however, that several investigators hold different views, explaining dialysis associated hypoxaemia by hypoventilation from hypocapnia caused by loss of carbon dioxide through the dialyser (249–255). Probably both mechanisms play a role (252).

Complement activation may be largely prevented with dialysers fitted with synthetic membranes which are substantially more biocompatible than cellulosic membranes (256, 257). So far complement activation (and induction of dialysis associated leucopenia) with polyacrylonitrile, polysulfone and polymethylmethacrylate (PMMA) membranes is much less or even minute (135, 248, 258–262). Probably

Table 5. Cellulosic and highly permeable membranes (229–235).

Material	Manufacturer	Marketer
Cellulose (Cuprophane)	Enka (West Germany)	Enka (West Germany)
Cellulose acetate (Cellulate)	Cordis Dow (USA, Sartorius (West Germany), Daicel (Japan)	Cordis Dow and other manufacturers
Polyacrylonitrile (PAN; AN69 or 69S)	Rhône Poulenc (France)	Hospal (Switzerland)
Polymethylmethacrylate (PMMA)	Toray (Japan)	–
Polysulfone	Amicon (USA)	Fresenius (W. Germany)
Polyamide	Gambro (Sweden)	Gambro (Sweden)
Polycarbonate	Gambro (Sweden)	Gambro (Sweden)

From Göhl et al (234) with permission.

the synthetic polyamide membrane (marketed by Gambro Corp., Sweden) is also biocompatible (253, 261).

Complement activation by acetylated cellulose membranes (such as Cellulate, the cellulose acetate incorporated in Cordis-Dow dialysers) is some 50% less compared to Cuprophane (135, 243); cellulose acetate membranes are apparently less bioincompatible than Cuprophane.

Reused or chemically modified Cuprophane (MC or Hemophan) with improved biocompatibility

Interestingly, when Cuprophane is reused biocompatibility is substantially enhanced, probably because binding sites for complement (fragment C_3) are greatly reduced by protein coating (248, 250). Complement activation of reused Cuprophane is only about 12 to 13% of the activation by new Cuprophane (248, 250).

Recently membrane specialists of ENKA Ltd, Wuppertal, West Germany (the manufacturer of Cuprophane)* presented evidence that minor chemical modifications of Cuprophane substantially improved biocompatibility of this cellulosic membrane (256). This was soon confirmed by other investigators (262, 263).

Complement activation of the modified Cuprophane membrane (preliminary called MC membrane or Hemophan) appeared to be only 1/5–1/3 of the activation by unmodified Cuprophane, as measured by the generation of the C_{3a} complement fraction. In addition dialysis efficiency and middle molecule clearances appeared to be improved (264).

Choice of membrane

From a practical point of view patients sensitive to the complement activation syndrome or the first use syndrome should not be dialysed with new Cuprophane dialysers but with dialysers either fitted with cellulose acetate or preferably with one of the synthetic membranes. These synthetic membranes are, however, expensive and require special equipment for control of ultrafiltration.

Alternatively dialyser reuse may be considered or a dialyser with the new modified Cuprophane should be used.

Dialysis with highly permeable membranes in long term patients

As discussed above the carpal-tunnel syndrome is a local manifestation of the dialysis associated amyloid syndrome which is presently recognised with increasing frequency as a painful and disabling complication in patients dialysed with Cuprophane membranes for 10 years or longer (185, 186, 221–223). It has been suggested that this syndrome will become an important, disabling complicating condition in numerous long term (>5 years) dialysis patients treated with cellulosic (Cuprophane) membranes and may affect all patients treated this way after 20 years (225).

---

* Baurmeister U, Vienken J, ENKA AG, Product Group Membrana, Wuppertal, DBR, personal communication to the author.

REMOVAL OF LOW MOLECULAR WEIGHT PROTEINS

During the previous decade it was convincingly demonstrated that the kidneys play an important role in the metabolism of low molecular weight proteins (136, 222–224, 226). Depending on molecular weight, configuration and electrical charge plasma proteins with a molecular weight of less than 65,000 are removed by glomerular filtration, reabsorbed in the proximal tubule and catabolised in the tubular epithelial cells (224, 226, 265–269). One of these proteins is β_2-microglobulin (β_2M) (molecular weight 11,800) which is normally present on the surface of mammalian cells (222, 269) and in low concentrations in human plasma (0.6 to 1.8 mg/l [50 to 150 μmol/l], 270). Other low molecular weight plasma proteins rise with increasing impairment of renal function (222, 224, 226), and a positive correlation has been found between serum β_2-M and serum creatinine levels (271). With increasing plasma and tissue levels β_2-microglobulin is laid down in fibre configuration as amyloid in synovial tissues of joints and tendons, in bones and other tissues (see p. 53, 60, 61).

It has been reported that β_2-M is removed from plasma with 'high flux', highly permeable membranes (polyacrylonitrile, polyamide and polysulfone), in contrast with cellulosic membranes, which are impermeable for small proteins (224, 228, 272–275).

Interesting results were reported by Floege and associates (275). Using the polysulfone membrane they obtained a total removal of β_2-M of 70.9 mg ($\pm$26.4) during a 3 h haemodialysis session and of 167 $\pm$ 50.9 mg during a similar haemofiltration session with the same membrane. The β_2-M blood clearance at 30 min was 54.4 $\pm$ 17.9 ml/min with haemodialysis and 87.6 $\pm$ 19.1 ml/min with haemofiltration.

Favourable results have been reported from haemodialysis with polysulfone membranes (270), which reduced β_2-M levels approximately 60% during a 6 h dialysis with a progressive reduction in pre-dialysis serum levels and remarkable improvement in shoulder pain. It has been suggested that long term dialysis patients (treated 5 years or longer) should be dialysed with one of the synthetic highly permeable membranes or alternatively treated with haemofiltration.

Interestingly so far no cases of dialysis associated amyloidosis have been reported complicating CAPD or intermittent peritoneal dialysis. Is this because the peritoneal membrane is sufficiently permeable to β_2-M or simply because peritoneal dialysis patients don't stay on this mode of treatment long enough to become symptomatic with this new syndrome?

Other, so far unanswered, questions arise. Will removal of low molecular weight proteins (and other substances with a molecular size of 65,000 D or less) be tolerated by these patients on the long term?

Is there a risk of protein malnutrition? On the other hand when dialysis with cellulosic membranes is continued, would there be a risk of other complications by accumulation of other low molecular weight proteins, normally removed and catabolised by the kidneys? We may have to wait for the answers for several, perhaps for even many years.

FURTHER PROGRESS IN ACCESS TO THE CIRCULATION (see also chapter 9)

Circulatory access, *the conditio sine qua non* for successful dialysis, also can offer problems. Sometimes access difficulties still endanger the continuation of dialysis treatment (277), but many improvements and refinements have been achieved. The classical external Scribner-Quinton arteriovenous shunt, once called the Achilles heel of chronic dialysis, has undergone many beneficial modifications, as have the surgical implantation techniques (278, 279).

Modified A-V cannulae systems

Introduction of the straight 'winged' in line cannula by Ramirez and co-workers (280) in 1966 made a straight external shunt possible, which was easy to declot. Notwithstanding such improvements, the life span of external shunts remained limited to an average of 7 to 10 months (278).

The 'large vessel applique', introduced by Thomas (281) in 1969, consists of straight Silastic cannulae with a Dacron skirt attached. In the present model, the Dacron patches are sutured to the anterior wall of the superficial femoral artery and directly to the femoral vein at the origin of the long saphenous vein which is locally excised. The obvious advantage is that the cannulae do not interrupt the blood stream in both main vessels. Originally an unacceptably high percentage of infections occurred (279) often requiring shunt removal and occasionally causing loss of a leg or even death. However, these problems decreased with the improved model, introduced in 1973 (282). Presently, the life span of the Thomas shunt seems to be much longer.

Another ingenious device is the Buselmeier shunt (283, 284) introduced in 1973). This shunt consists essentially of a small U-shaped Silastic segment with two Teflon plugged outlets (see Figure 33, p. 41). Implantation is done with standard vessel tips and the U-shaped portion is either partially or totally buried in the subcutaneous tissue, with the outlets remaining extracutaneous. The Buselmeier shunt is often preferred in paediatric dialysis.

Modified A-V fistulae

Although a well created arteriovenous fistula functions for years some patients have recurrent problems leading to obliteration of access vasculature. For these patients, other types of arteriovenous fistulas have been introduced. May and co-workers (285) introduced saphenous vein autographs as a bridge between an artery and a vein (1969). The saphenous vein can be fashioned as a loop in the forearm or as a straight bridge from the brachial artery to a distal vein. Several other modifications are possible. Chinitz and colleagues (286, 287) created bridged arteriovenous fistulae with bovine heterografts. Several others adopted this type of bridged fistula (288, 289). Others created bridged arteriove-

nous fistulae with mandril grown autografts (290) or with synthetic self sealing prosthetic material (291–293). The expanded polytetrafluoroethylene (PTFE) (Gore-Tex or Impra) self sealing conduit is an acceptable material for creating an alternative for the classical Brescia-Cimino type of A-V fistula (294).

Human umbilical cord allograft seems to be less satisfactory material for this purpose (295, 296). In special circumstances these techniques are useful but none has proved to be as satisfactory as a well created classical Brescia-Cimino type of arteriovenous fistula.

In 1978 vascular access was reevaluated in a large group of European patients (297) and compared with the year 1975; vascular access with external Scribner shunts dropped from 10.4% in 1975 to 5.9% in 1978. Internal fistula types of access (Cimino, grafts and PTFE combined) increased from 88.4% to 93.6% at the same time.

Button or no needle access

A relatively new method of access has been described as 'button' or 'no needle' method of dialysis in 1980 (298) and 1981 (299).

The 'carbon transcutaneous access device' (CTAD, Bentley Laboratories, USA), also called Dia Tab, is an access port made from vitreous carbon and is sealed with a polyethylene plug; a PTFE tubing is attached to the port.

A more or less similar device, called Hemasite (marketed by Renal Systems, USA) is constructed from titanium; the attached PTFE graft is like the CTAD access port implanted between an artery and a vein, usually at the medical site of the upper arm.

The Hemasite is provided with a resealable silicone septum with preformed slits punctured for blood access with a blunt tipped double needle access set. The slits provide haemostasis by automatic closure when the double needle set is removed. The device is expensive.

The CTAD is simpler; access is obtained by removal of the conical plug and insertion of a connector with in- and outflow tubing. The use of a 'single needle' device (see below) is essential. Both devices have been evaluated by several investigators during recent years (300–302).

Although both the Hemasite and the Dia Tab are covered with Dacron velour to promote tissue ingrowth to provide stabilisation and inhibit bacterial entry, both infection and thrombosis (and/or clotting) were of major concern (299–302), as had to be expected with implant devices interfacing with living tissues. Several cases of fatal insidious sepsis have been reported with the Hemasite device (300) and access survival with this device was in one report only 60% at one year and 30% at 2 years (302).

Also the steal syndrome and stenosis of the arterialised efferent vein have been observed with the Dia Tab button (302).

Nevertheless it has been suggested that these devices are 'promising tools and even reliable devices' for providing durable vascular access (301, 302).

Femoral or subclavian vein catheterisation

A relatively old technique which is useful in acute renal failure patients and in chronic patients temporarily lacking a standard vascular access is femoral vein catheterisation using the Seldinger method (see pages 38 and 39) either introducing two vena cava (68, 69) catheters or only one with a single needle device.

A more recent method has been introduced by Uldall and coworkers (303–305) in 1979. A single or double lumen catheter is introduced into a subclavian vein (preferably at the right side) also with the Seldinger technique and is left in place in the superior vena cava. It can stay in for 3 or 4 weeks or longer, even up to several months, with daily injection of heparin.

Insertion is technically simple and may be performed at the bedside. If the catheter (some prefer the Hickman type) is left in situ, a weekly change of the cannula is advised by some investigators (304).

A single needle device has to be used, unless a recently developed double lumen catheter is used which became commercially available in 1980 (305).

Infection of the skin exit site and of the catheter tip occurs sometimes with infection of the blood stream (304), but is much less of a problem than with the button type of access, described above.

Single needle dialysis

Haemodialysis with a single needle or catheter introduced in the early 1970's (306) has advantages in paediatric dialysis and in dialysis with percutaneous catheterisation of a femoral or subclavian vein with a single catheter (307). Several methods have been described, but probably the safest and most reliable system consists of a pump with two occluding roller heads, alternatively driven by a single motor and pressure monitored.

An expansion chamber inserted in the 'arterial' blood line is necessary, when hollow fibre dialysers, which have a low compliance, are used (307–309).

The double pump system allows excellent ultrafiltration control and permits a rather high dialyser blood flow (exceeding 250 ml/min (309). A certain amount of recirculation reduces small molecule clearances but the system's performance seems comparable to that of two needle dialysis.

This system has been used successfully not only in conventional haemodialysis but also in other extracorporeal blood purification techniques like haemofiltration, haemodiafiltration, membrane plasmapheresis and haemoperfusion (309).

SEQUENTIAL ULTRAFILTRATION AND DIALYSIS

Removal of fluid during haemodialysis by ultrafiltration, usually accomplished by negative pressure in the dialysis fluid compartment (or by positive pressure in the blood commpartment) often causes arterial hypotension or muscle cramps or both, in particular when relatively large amounts

of fluid have to be removed rapidly.

Bergström and coworkers (310) observed (in 1976) by chance that rapid ultrafiltration was much better tolerated when negative pressure was applied without dialysis fluid passing through the dialyser, plasma osmolality remaining practically constant. During recirculation dialysis with a polyacrylonitrile dialyser only a small decrease of plasma osmolality occurred and under these conditions substantial ultrafiltration was also well tolerated.

But with single-pass dialysis a rapid fall in plasma osmolality occurs, which interferes with blood pressure regulation and may cause hypotension because of a fluid shift from the plasma to the interstitial and intracellular spaces.

This fluid shift further contracts the plasma volume, which is already reduced by ultrafiltration and any additional decrease of the circulating volume may cause arterial hypotension.

They successfully introduced a dialysis protocol of sequential ultrafiltration and dialysis; in this way even large amounts of fluid could be removed without discomfort to the patient and without a fall in blood pressure. The observations of Bergström's group were confirmed by Shaldon (311) and by others (312, 313). Many dialysis machines are presently equiped to provide isolated ultrafiltration with dialysis fluid bypassing the dialyser.

REUSE OF DIALYSIS FLUID

As a rule haemodialysis requires large amounts of tap water, which must be pretreated with special equipment. Water and drain connections are required. Haemodialysis systems therefore, are in practice not portable and immobilise patients for their thrice weekly treatments. In addition in many areas in the world, city water is expensive and in short supply. To overcome these disadvantages, reuse of dialysis fluid has been tried, for example by activated carbon regeneration (314–317). Activated carbon, *per se*, has no effect on electrolytes, however, and only a limited absorption capacity for urea.

Adapting a spaceflight technological approach, Gordon et al (318–320) developed a system to regenerate a small volume of dialysis fluid (originally 5.5 l, later 6 l) by continuous recirculation through a multilayer disposable cartridge, containing urease, zirconium compounds and activated carbon. A production model of this 'Redy' system (Redy stands for Recirculating Dialysis system) was constructed by CCI-Marquardt Corporation in Van Nuys, California (later taken over by the Dutch company Organon Teknika Inc.) and marketed in 1972 (321).

The apparatus does not need fixed water- and drain connections and is semi-portable, making travelling for holiday and business purposes possible for chronic haemodialysis patients (322, 323 [see chapter 19]). Other portable and even wearable haemodialysis systems have been designed and constructed (324–328). They all had, however, certain drawbacks and found only limited practical application.

Transportable haemodialysis systems have in addition the disadvantage of a voluminous and heavy amount of accessories, like dialysers, bags with sterile saline, regeneration cartridges etc., causing transportation problems.

The Redy system underwent during the past decade several modifications and improvements and is still in practical use, both in the US, Europe and areas where water usable for dialysis is not available or in short supply.

For many patients who prefer mobile dialysis, for instance for travelling, the Redy system is presently superseded by continuous ambulatory peritoneal dialysis (CAPD) (see chapter 25).

BICARBONATE VERSUS ACETATE DIALYSIS

With the construction of an on-line dialysate proportioning system by Babb and coworkers (95) in 1964, a concentrate was prepared with sodium acetate instead of sodium bicarbonate, which was the original alkalinising anion in dialysis fluid in the early years of haemodialysis (93). This was necessary to prevent precipitation of calcium carbonate.

In recent years suspicion arose that in acute, sick patients because of a reduced rate of conversion into bicarbonate, acetate could accumulate in the blood and tissues, leading to acetate toxicity with vascular instability and hypotension (329, 330). It was also suspected that undesirable side effects of acetate could occur in stable chronic dialysis patients during dialysis with large surface area dialysers, in particular in patients who were 'slow acetate metabolisers' (331). Rapid acetate infusion, exceeding maximum utilisation, could, under these circumstances, cause rising acetate levels, leading to discomfort of the patient and to 'dialysis hangover'. Stimultaneous loss of bicarbonate from the blood through the dialyser may obviously contribute to these undesirable side effects.

The use of bicarbonate containing dialysis fluid increased between 1982 and 1985 in Europe, and in 1985 10% of all haemodialysis patients in Europe were treated by bicarbonate dialysis. Currently bicarbonate haemodialysis is used in selected patients with cardiovascular instability, in rapid, (ultra-)short (so called high efficiency) dialysis (164–170) and in sick patients in acute renal failure.

Doubtless bicarbonate dialysis is preferable even for routine dialysis, but its use instead of acetate is still not yet widespread, because of greater cost and greater technical complexity. These problems and the drawbacks have been recently summarised by Keshaviah and Collins (164), who also described the basic lay-out of a bicarbonate proportioning system.

Several single patient proportioning machines have been marketed with facilities for delivering bicarbonate dialysis fluid (332), but a number of these bicarbonate systems consist of 'add on' modules to existing acetate delivery machines, resulting in more frequent break downs and increased maintenance costs (164).

HAEMOPERFUSION

The principle of using sorbents in purification of blood dates back to 1948, when Muirhead and Reid (333) discovered that urea was adsorbed from animal blood by passing it through an ion exchange column. Sixteen years later, in 1964, Yatzidis from Athens, Greece (334) reported at the founding meeting of the European Dialysis and Transplant Association on the results of his attempts to treat uraemia by perfusing the blood of a heparinised patient over a column of activated charcoal.

It soon became apparent that activated charcoal is an effective sorbent for several 'uraemic' metabolites, e.g. creatinine and uric acid, but not for urea.

An urea sorbent

Recently a urea binding sorbent has been introduced which, however, is not yet commercially available (335, 336). In addition charcoal perfusion does not correct water and electrolyte abnormalities. It also became apparent that activated charcoal has to be coated or micro-encapsulated to prevent charcoal particles from entering the blood stream (337) and to eliminate other side-effects such as pyrogenic reactions, platelet depletion and activation of complement (as occurs with cellulosic dialysis membranes) (338).

Haemoperfusion has been experimentally used as an adjunct to dialysis treatment of chronic uraemia (339–341) without much practical success. Recently a preliminary study reported on elimination of β_2 M a low molecular weight protein, which is responsible for the dialysis associated amyloid syndrome (see page 53 and 61).

Removal of β_2-microglobulin by haemoperfusion

Beta-2 M is badly removed through cellulosic membranes, such as cellulose acetate and Cuprophane, much better by polysulfone and polyacrylonitrile membranes, but, surprisingly, seems to be badly removed by peritoneal dialysis (CAPD [342]). Haemoperfusion with specially prepared cartridges may be helpful (343).

Haemoperfusion in non renal conditions

Haemoperfusion has been experimentally tried by several groups in fulminant hepatitits with encephalopathy. After some encouraging initial results, this, however, could later not be confirmed (344–346).

The major therapeutic field of haemoperfusion is drug removal in accidental and intentional poisoning. Drugs that are water soluble are more readily removed by haemodialysis, whereas drugs that are lipid soluble are more readily removed by haemoperfusion (338), most efficiently with the nonionic resin XADL4, while other drugs (listed in several publications [338, 346] are better removed by devices containing coated charcoal.

It should be kept in mind, however, that the mainstay of treatment in the vast majority of exogenic intoxication depends on intensive supportive care ('The Scandinavian method').

Dialysis or haemoperfusion is only indicated when supportive care will be failing in patients with stage IV coma from hypnotic or (and) sedative agents (see for full information chapter 20).

HAEMOFILTRATION

Haemofiltration is a form of replacement of renal function, introduced by Henderson and co-workers (347) in 1967, originally dating back to 1928 (Brull [348]).

It is presently an alternative to conventional dialysis (i.e. removal of solutes by diffusion) and has the advantage of removal of solutes by convection which mimics the performance of the human kidney better: small and large molecules are removed at the same rate (see table 6). The birth of the middle molecule hypothesis in the early seventies (137–140, 144–147, 189, 200, 212) stimulated practical application of haemofiltration and in several centres clinical trials were initiated (350–357) in the 1970s.

Available filters

Different filters with different membranes are used: polysulfone (Amicon, USA; Fresenius, West Germany), polyamide (Berghof, West Germany; Gambro, Sweden), triacetate (Sartorius, West Germany) and polyacrylonitrile (Hospal, Switzerland) (see also p. 56 and chapter 14).

The pore diameters of these synthetic membranes are considerably larger than of the common cellulosic haemodialysis membranes, the cut off masses ranging between 15,000 and 50,000 daltons approaching the cut off mass of the natural kidney (50,000 daltons). To obtain adequate efficiency large amounts of ultrafiltrate have to be removed (20 to 30 l per session, three times weekly).

Table 6. Characteristics of different modes of blood cleansing (Reproduced from Manis and Friedman [349] slightly modified).

	Haemo-dialysis	Haemo-filtration	Haemo-perfusion (activated charcoal)
Fluid removal	Ultrafiltration	Ultrafiltration	None
Solute removal	Diffusion	Convection	Adsorption
Clearance of small molecules	High	Moderate to good	Variable
Clearance of 'middle' molecules (300–5000 D)	Low	High	High
Current use	Uraemia (Drug overdose)	Uraemia	Drug overdose Hepatic failure (Uraemia, adjunct therapy)

Predilution and postdilution

Approximately equal amounts (minus the amount of ingested and metabolically produced water) of replacement fluid have to be added, either before ('predilution mode' [351, 352]) or after the ultrafilter ('postdilution mode' [353, 354]). This is obviously one of the disadvantages of the method.

Haemofiltration was the method of choice in more than 2,500 chronic patients in Europe in 1985 and some 1,800 European patients were regularly treated by haemodiafiltration (123).

Prevention of hypotension

Both methods are considerably more effective than haemodialysis with cellulosic membranes in removing substances of higher molecular mass ('middle molecules') and are much less likely to provoke symptomatic hypotension which of course is particularly important in patients who regularly present themselves with a substantial fluid overload.

Removal of β_2-microglobulin

Recently it was demonstrated that haemofiltration effectively removes β_2-microglobulin, which is the matrix of dialysis associated amyloidosis in long term dialysis patients with the amyloid syndrome (see p. 53 and p. 60 [227, 273, 275, 276]).

It may be predicted that haemofiltration will be the treatment of choice in the future in long term haemodialysis patients to prevent or to treat the dialysis associated amyloidosis syndrome.

CAVH (continuous arterio-venous haemofiltration)

Continuous arterio-venous haemofiltration (CAVH), introduced by Kramer and associates in 1977 (358) is based on a modification designed to haemofilter an overhydrated or an acute renal failure patient by catheters introduced in a femoral artery and vein, inserting a haemofilter in between.

A spontaneous blood flow of 100 ml/min is usually obtained with a spontaneous production of 200 to 600 ml of ultrafiltrate per hour, or more with application of vacuum suction (359) or lowering the ultrafiltrate collecting bag.

CAVH is presently in many renal units the method of choice in patients with acute renal failure, sometimes in combination with intermittent haemodialysis.

PLASMA EXCHANGE

A method of 'plasmaphaeresis' had been devised by Abel and colleagues (4, 360) as early as in 1914 with the purpose of using this method for the relief of toxemia and to treat uraemia. It soon was deemed that plasmapheresis was an inefficient approach to uraemia treatment and the experiments were abandoned. Several decades later plasmapheresis found practical application in returning erythrocytes when harvesting plasma from blood donors and in 1960 Schwab and Fahey (361) reported dramatic transient improvement in two patients with hyperviscosity syndrome due to Waldenström's macroglobulinaemia.

Similar beneficial results were obtained by removal of myeloma protein from patients with hyperviscosity syndrome (362).

Techniques of plasma separation; centrifugation, membrane plasma separation

In the early 1960's efficient and repeated plasmapheresis became feasible with continuous flow centrifuges; some 20 years later suitable membranes became available making membrane plasma separation possible, which soon became the technique of choice (363, 364). Plasma separation has been introduced as standard terminology, referring to *any technique* for separation of blood into plasma and cells.

Plasmapheresis

Plasmapheresis refers to removal of plasma and its replacement with crystalloid.

Plasma exchange

Plasma exchange is the term used when plasma is separated and replaced by a protein containing solution.

Selected removal of plasma constituents

Technical improvements facilitating centrifugal apheresis and cytapheresis and the development of new membranes with different pore diameters (365) offered promising modifications and refinements of apheresis techniques.

In addition rapid development of extracorporeal dialysis technology and different methods of vascular access opened the field of apheresis to clinical investigators, in particular to immunologists and nephrologists who were interested in kidney diseases, transplantation and a number of divergent diseases, several of them having a so called 'auto-immune' pathogenesis (366–369).

Until recently the nonselectivity of the plasma constituents that are removed with plasmapheresis was felt as a drawback (370). However, attempts to increase selectivity have resulted in improved ingenious techniques.

Cascade membrane filtration

In cascade membrane filtration plasma is separated from whole blood by a first filter and then led through a second filter with smaller pores of selected diameter: specific larger molecules are removed and the filtrate, after being mixed with the cell rich residue from the first filter is returned to the patient (368, 370).

Filters with different pore diameters are presently available and a second filter with the appropriate pore size can be selected (365, 371).

Cryopheresis

Another approach to selectivity is temperature manipulation: by cooling of the plasma and the secundary filter to 0–4°C, cryoprecipitation occurs and the precipitated material can be separated from the plasma. This technique has been applied to patients with rheumatoid arthritis as an experimental therapeutic procedure with promising results (372).

Therapeutic applications

Plasmapheresis has been therapeutically applied during recent decades for a number of immunologically mediated diseases, often with concurrent immunosuppressive therapy (with corticosteroids, azathioprine or cyclosporine).

Good, even excellent results have been reported in anti-basement membrane antibody disease (Goodpasture's syndrome), combined with immunosuppression (373, 374).

Other conditions which have been treated are rapidly progressive glomerulonephritis with crescent formation, cryoglobulinaemia, systemic lupus, polyarteritis, thrombotic thrombocytopenic purpura, Wegener's disease, the hyperviscosity syndrome in myeloma and Waldenström's disease.

In a number of 'auto-immune' diseases without renal involvement (e.g. myasthenia gravis, Guillain Barré syndrome, exophthalmic Graves disease) plasma exchange has a definite therapeutic place (362).

Acute renal allograft rejection has been treated with plasmapheresis, but this gets presently little support.

Criticism

The vast and still growing literature does not present a solid perspective on the therapeutic use of plasma exchange; most case reports are anecdotal and often uncritical.

On the other hand it should be acknowledged that the type of auto-immune diseases for which plasmapheresis could be therapeutically beneficial is not suitable for controlled trials (362).

In certain diseases the immuno-pathogenetic abnormality is missing and therefore the exact nature of what should be removed is obviously lacking.

As the wide spread practice of random therapeutic use of plasma exchange continues ('hit and miss trials'), the development of objective criteria for therapeutic application of plasma exchange will remain utopian for a long time.

Unwanted side effects and risks

In this context one should be aware that the safety of plasma exchange has been a burning issue and unwanted side effects have not been rare, even in healthy donors (375).

A critical approach to therapeutic application and a perfect technology are of course mandatory.

LIPID ABNORMALITIES

High and premature mortality from cardio- and cerebro-vascular complications

In 1974, Lindner and co-workers (376) shocked the dialysis world by reporting an abnormally high premature mortality and morbidity due to atherosclerotic cardiovascular complications in Seattle dialysis patients. The incidence was much higher than for normal and hypertensive groups of comparable age. Although the group studied was rather small the data supported the figures recorded in early and more recent European statistics (99, 111, 112). Recent European statistics based on very large numbers of patients indicate that the proportion of deaths due to cardiovascular and cerebrovascular causes both in the chronic hospital haemodialysis setting and in all patients on renal replacement therapy is approximately 46%. Several studies have clarified certain pertinent metabolic lipid abnormalities in dialysis patients.

Bagdade, Porte and Bierman (377) in 1968 showed a high incidence of plasma lipid abnormalities involving mainly the triglyceride rich very-low density lipoproteins in patients with chronic renal failure, whether treated by dialysis or not.

Delayed catabolism of VLD lipoproteins and impaired triglyceride removal

Bagdade and coworkers (378) and Savdie and associates (379) demonstrated that the persistent hypertriglyceridaemia is attributable to a delay of peripheral catabolism of very-low-density lipoproteins and impaired triglyceride removal, due to a functional defect in lipoprotein lipase (380). This apparently results from the accumulation of certain uraemic toxins.

Interestingly abnormalities of lipoprotein metabolism have been demonstrated in relatively early stages of chronic renal failure, when serum creatinine was still 4 mg/dl (350 μmol/l) (381). At this stage total cholesterol and triglycerides were still unchanged.

The cause-effect relationship between lipid abnormalities (hypertriglyceridaemia) and accelerated atherosclerosis in chronic dialysis patients is presently under discussion.

Other risk factors

Doubtless risk factors preexistent prior to dialysis treatment will shorten survival because of premature atherosclerosis. On the other hand other risk factors like cigarette smoking, uncorrected or suboptimally corrected hypertension also play an important role (380, 382).

Presently hypertriglyceridaemia is considered less of a risk factor than for instance persistent hypertension. Finally it should be mentioned that hyperglyceridaemia is enhanced by dextrose in the dialysis fluid and by acetate (383, 384).

NEPHROGENIC OSTEODYSTROPHY AND VITAMIN D

Substitution of renal function by dialysis not only opened up a new field of therapeutic potentialities, but also an enormous and still continuing area of research. Many studies, related to dialysis and uraemia, had their impact in much broader fields of nephrology and renal physiology.

The mystery of renal rickets

For example, renal osteodystrophy, once infrequent, soon became a serious problem in many regular dialysis patients (385). Originally described as 'renal rickets' a series of observations brought new and exciting knowledge, clarifying vitamin D and calcium metabolism.

In 1935, Pappenheimer and Wilens (386, 387) noted parathyroid enlargement in cases of renal failure with bone disease. They could reproduce this syndrome by partial renal ablation in animals. A few years later, Liu and Chu (388) demonstrated calcium malabsorption in cases of nephrogenic osteodystrophy, which was resistant to vitamin D. However, renal osteodystrophy could be improved with unusually large doses of vitamin D or its derivative dihydrotachysterol (387). The observation of Bauer, Carlsson and Lindquist (390) that vitamin D also increased bone resorption, the demonstration of a long delay between intravenous administration of vitamin D in the rat and its physiological effects (391) and the ineffectiveness of the vitamin on resorption of bone *in vitro*, raised several questions. Although multiple interactions were apparent between the kidneys, the parathyroids, the skeleton and vitamin D, their interrelationship remained a mystery.

The liver and hydroxylation of vitamin D at the C_{25} position

An important key to the understanding of the puzzle came from the studies of DeLuca and colleagues (391) who demonstrated that vitamin D had to be hydroxylated before any physiological effects could occur. The lag period of 10 to 12 h could be cut to approximately 3 to 4 h by administration of 25-hydroxyvitamin D_3 ($25[OH]D_3$) and the 25-hydroxy-derivative appeared to be active *in vitro* on cultures of bone (392).

The liver microsomes were shown to be the site of 25-hydroxylation of vitamin D_3, which was demonstrated to be a biofeedback regulated process (393, 394). It soon became evident that $25[OH]D_3$ was not the final product in the metabolic chain of vitamin D: it had to be metabolised further before reaching full potency.

The kidneys and the hydroxylation of vitamin D at the C_1 position

The next important key to the puzzle came when Fraser and Kodicek (395, 396) revealed that the kidney was the unique source of a very potent hormone, that stimulated intestinal calcium absorption and calcium resorption from bone. DeLuca and colleagues (397) then isolated from chickens given radioactive vitamin D_3, a highly active metabolite which was identified as 1,25-dihydroxy-vitamin D_3 (398).

The implications of these findings both for the renal patient and for further research and clarification of the metabolism of calcium, vitamin D and the skeleton have been enormous. Nephrogenic bone disease became a dilemma with prolongation of life of the uraemic patient by regular dialysis. This doubtless was an impetus for the research which led to the disentanglement of the mysteries of vitamin D metabolism:

... 'the unravelling of the interrelationships between vitamin D and its metabolites is one of the triumphs of recent medical research' ... (J. Reeve]399]).

For the independent observer the completion of the jig-saw puzzle of vitamin D and its metabolites, the liver, the kidneys, the parathyroids and the skeleton by physiologists, clinical investigators and other scientists is highly impressive, even moving. Treatment of renal osteodystrophy and several other disorders with synthetic vitamin D metabolites and analogues is now available.

Nomenclature

Calcitriol, alfacalcidol, calcifedol

Calcitriol or 1,25-[OH]$_2$D$_3$ or 1a-[OH]D$_3$ (approved name alfacalcidol) which is easier to synthesise and which is converted in the liver to calcitriol by hydroxylation on the 25 position, usually provide a satisfactory response (399). Calcifedol, which is 25[OH]D$_3$ and which is the circulating form of vitamin D, is also effective but the effect may be less consistent because its full potency depends on the hydroxylation at the 1 position by the tubular cells of the kidney.

Vitamin D resistant osteomalacia

Nevertheless, recent observations which became possible after the introduction of methods for measuring 1,25-[OH]$_2$D$_3$ levels in plasma and results of long-term therapeutic trials with the new vitamin D derivatives have cast some doubt on the pathogenesis and therapy of osteomalacia either from renal or non-renal origin. With growing experience discrepancies have been observed: in some patients with osteomalacia blood levels of 1,25-[OH]$_2$D$_3$ were normal or even increased and, conversely, some patients with chronic renal failure had decreased or undetectable levels of 1,25-[OH]$_2$D$_3$ but no evidence of osteomalacia.

Also it turned out that the therapeutic results with the new vitamin D$_3$ derivatives in some patients with renal and non-renal osteomalacia were inexplicably disappointing (400). It has been suggested that the pathogenesis of nephrogenic osteomalacia is multifactorial. Recently this hypothesis gained support from observations from Newcastle upon Tyne, England, that under certain circumstances aluminium accumulation may occur in patients with chronic renal failure, the main source of aluminium uptake being the city water used for preparation of dialysis fluid (401, 402). Deposition of aluminium in bone prevents calcification and is responsible for cases of osteomalacia resistant to therapeutic doses of vitamin D$_3$ derivatives (see below and chapter 50).

ALUMINIUM TOXICITY IN DIALYSIS PATIENTS (1972)

In 1972 Alfrey and associates (403) described a new and initially poorly understood clinical entity in a group of five patients, haemodialysed in Denver, Colorado, for 3 or more years. They developed a syndrome of dyspraxia, speech abnormalities, myoclonus, seizures, personality changes and disordered encephalograms. Without exception the disease progressed to death in 3 to 7 months (403). All patients received dialysis with dialysis fluid prepared with untreated Denver city water. Trace element analysis was performed on brain tissue for a wide spectrum of elements; compared with uraemic patients who died without signs of encephalopathy and normals there were no impressive differences: rubidium and potassium concentrations in brain tissue were somewhat reduced (25–30%), in comparison with normal controls; tin (normally non detectable or less than 2 ppm [<1.7 nmol/100 g]) was the only element which was consistently increased in uraemic brain tissue, both in patients with and without the encephalopathy syndrome. The aluminium content was initially not analysed, probably because aluminium intoxication was considered highly unlikely.

Interestingly a syndrome of loss of memory, tremor, jerking movements and impaired coordination was described half a century before. In addition the relevant patient was also suffering from chronic constipation, incontinence of urine and persistent vomiting (Spofforth, 1921 [404]).

The patient was a metalworker of 46 who had been dipping red-hot metal articles contained in an aluminium holder into concentrated nitric acid. His urine was analysed and reportedly contained a large amount of aluminium.

No data were reported on renal function and on the analytical technique of aluminium determination in the urine sample, which obviously must have been rather crude in that time.

Dialysis encephalopathy and aluminium

Between 1971 and 1976, 14 more cases in the Denver regular dialysis population (405) were observed. Suspicion rose that aluminium, which is toxic for the nervous system, was responsible for the dialysis encephalopathy syndrome. This hypothesis gained support by tissue aluminium studies in brain, bone and muscle: brain tissue aluminium values were four times higher than in dialysis patients who died from other causes and ten times control values in non dialysed subjects. It appeared that the aluminium was predominantly localised in the gray matter of the brain. Aluminium concentrations in muscle and bone were also significantly higher than in controls (405).

Meanwhile similar cases were reported from Newcastle upon Tyne, England and from Ottawa, Canada. The tap water in these cities has a high aluminium content, an aluminium precipitation method being used to remove undesired colour from the water (406). In Eindhoven, The Netherlands six cases were observed and at post mortem tissue analysis very high aluminium concentrations were found in brain, bone and other tissues. The aluminium contamination was brought into the water used for preparation of the dialysis fluid by aluminium electrodes in a heating tank (407, 408). In the west of Scotland in regions with a high aluminium content of tap water (mean 420 μg/l [16 μmol/l]) the dialysis encephalopathy syndrome occurred in 14 home dialysis patients, but no cases were observed in Glasgow itself, where the city water aluminium is less than 30 μg/l (1.1 μmol/l) (409). Obviously dialysis encephalopathy had a geographical distribution, related to the aluminium content of raw or inadequately treated city water, used for dialysis fluid preparation (410–412).

Other symptoms of chronic aluminium toxicity are vitamin D resistant osteomalacia, proximal muscle weakness (414), hypochromic microcytic anaemia (413, see chapter 50).

Aluminium kinetics in dialysis patients are complex: aluminium entering the blood is eagerly bound to plasma protein and uptake from the dialysate may continue even when total plasma aluminium exceeds the dialysate aluminium concentration (415). Even when plasma has been saturated, tissue deposition is likely to continue (in brain grey matter, skeleton and muscles).

The main source of aluminium intoxication is doubtless aluminium containing city water used for preparation of dialysis fluid, either untreated or inadequately treated.

Transfer of aluminium into the patient is highly promoted by alkalinity of the dialysis fluid, either caused by high pH of the incoming raw water or by the use of bicarbonate instead of acetate in the dialysis fluid (416). A low pH (<6.5) has a similar effect (see also chapter 50).

So far dialysate pH has been routinely neglected; in this context it seems indicated to include pH monitoring and pH control of dialysis fluid in the parameters which are routinely checked.

Oral aluminium (phosphate binders)

Oral aluminium containing phosphate binders, routinely administered to dialysis patients, also may contribute to the aluminium loading of the patients. The safety of these compounds is considered as being at least questionable (415, 417–419). Dewberry and associates (420) reported on 14 patients with dialysis associated encephalopathy; 13 were dialysed with virtually aluminium free dialysis fluid, the only potential source of aluminium being oral aluminium containing phosphate binders.

Aluminium free phosphate binders

Bournerias et al (421) observed a substantial decrease of serum aluminium concentrations in 23 chronic dialysis patients, 3 having manifested Al morbidity (fracturing osteopathy and encephalopathy) after discontinuing Al containing phosphate binders, replacing them by calcium carbonate. Mean serum Al decreased from 70 to 76 μg/l (2.63 to 2.85 μmol/l) to 32 μg/l (1.2 μmol/l).

On the other hand according to data of Graf et al (422)

most of the intestinally absorbed aluminium is removed by dialysis if a dialysis fluid with a very low aluminium content (0.1–0.3 μmol/l) is used.

Nevertheless efficient aluminium free (and preferably also magnesium free) phosphate binders should replace aluminium hydroxide. Calcium carbonate recommended (423) as an alternative, is not a very efficient phosphate binder and may cause hypercalcaemia (424).

A nontoxic and very efficient phosphate binder has been developed by German investigators. Schneider and coworkers (425) demonstrated a very effective phosphate binding effect of a calcium loaded polymer (a heteropolyuromide), which belongs to a group of nontoxic, licensed food additives, and has no side effects. Another efficient nontoxic phosphate binder has been developed*, but is still not yet commercially available.

It is still unknown if the practice of cooking food in aluminium utensils and wrapping food in aluminium foil contributes to the aluminium load of renal failure patients (426–428).

Dialysis encephalopathy may be precipitated in patients who have been dialysed with aluminium containing dialysis fluid and have accumulated toxic amounts of aluminium by catabolic events like surgery (also transplantation), immobilisation and corticosteroid administration (429). This may be explained by mobilisation of aluminium from the skeleton and other depots.

Aluminium induced osteomalacia; diagnosis

Vitamin D resistant osteomalacia, presently also called aluminium osteopathy, is observed with increasing frequency. According to Cournot-Witmer (430) aluminium concentrates in bone at the mineralising layer of the osteoid. That is the site where the bone mineral is normally first deposited by an active cell-mediated proces. Sophisticated histological observations (electron microscopy, Xray microanalysis, ion microscopy) suggest that Al present in the mitochondria of the osteoblasts gradually intoxicates the cell, inducing the mineralisationdefect. In addition Al has a direct toxic effect on the parathyroid glands, resulting in low iPTH levels in patients with Al induced osteomalacia.

The diagnosis of Al induced osteopathy is based on the clinical signs and symptoms, the Xray abnormalities and demonstration of normal or decreased iPTH, normal or slightly raised alkaline phosphatase and elevated serum aluminium (and elevated aluminium in the dialysis fluid).

The diagnosis has to be confirmed by bone biopsy, which is characterised by an increased osteoid volume an increased number of osteoid lamellae, and a reduced calcification front with little osteoblastic activity. Usually there is little evidence of osteitis fibrosa. A positive aluminium stain (aurine-tricarboxylic acid) confirms the diagnosis which may also be supported by bone scintigraphy with ^{99m}Tc diphosphonate (431, 432) and a positive deferoxamine test.

---

* Organon Teknika, Turnhout, Belgium

Prevention of aluminium intoxication

The aluminium toxicity syndrome can be prevented by keeping the aluminium load of dialysis patients as low as possible by avoiding aluminium containing drugs and careful treatment of (city) water used for the preparation of the dialysis fluid. The maximum permissable aluminium concentration in the water is limited to 15 μg/l (0.56 μmol/l) in the UK or to 10 μg/l (0.38 μmol/l) in the USA.

According to Graf and coworkers (422) dialysis fluid aluminium concentration should be below 5.4 μg/l (0.2 μmol/l). Both water Al and serum levels should be below 20 μg/l (0.74 μmol/l) and preferably in the range of normal subjects (10 to 15 μg/l [0.37 to 0.56 μmol/l]), which, however, is extremely difficult to achieve. Levels should be monitored 4 to 6 times per year (422).

Therapy of aluminium intoxication

Aluminium removal has been achieved with aluminium poor dialysis fluid (less than 14 μg/l [0.5 μmol/l]) (433) and successful therapeutic results have been achieved with intravenous administration of desferrioxamine. (For further information the reader is referred to chapter 50).

DIALYSIS ASSOCIATED ANAEMIA

Pathogenesis

The anaemia of chronic dialysis patients is multifactorial: regular blood loss in the dialyser, accidental blood loss by membrane rupture, occasionally clotting of blood in the dialyser, accidental disconnection of blood lines or fistula needles and periodical iatrogenic blood loss for laboratory tests; all of these causes may lead to iron deficiency and decreased erythropoiesis. Other causes are chronic or acute haemolysis, gastrointestinal bleeding and aluminium toxicity (434, 435).

Erythropoietin defect

The major pathogenetic factor of the anaemia in chronic renal failure and chronic dialysis patients is the defect of the kidneys to produce erythropoietin (436).

Treatment with recombinant erythropoietin (1986–1988)

So far the quantities of erythropoietin derived from normal kidney tissue or plasma were minimal and insufficient for any therapeutic application. Recently however, recombinant human erythropoietin became available for clinical investigation, prepared by Ortho, Cilaq and Amgen Corp., and clinical trials both in England, France and the US (435–438) have fully confirmed that recombinant erythropoietin can increase the haemoglobin concentration, the haematocrit and also the well being of patients on haemodialysis. The production of human erythropoietin derived from recombinant DNA should be considered as another landmark in the treatment of chronic renal disease.

'Another new and important therapeutic agent has been made available through the wizardry of molecular biology.' (Erslev, 1987 [436]).

VIRAL HEPATITIS (1964–1965) (see also chapter 42)

Hepatitis B, Australia antigen

Chronic dialysis undoubtedly contributed indirectly to a totally different field of research: viral hepatitis. In 1964, Blumberg, Alter and Visnich (439) found in the serum of a multitransfused haemophiliac (an Australian aborigine), an unusual new antigen which they named Australia antigen. The significance of the new antigen was obscure until a case of mild hepatitis was correlated with transient appearance of the Australia antigen in blood (440). With the recognition that Australia antigen was found in the sera of about 10% of patients with viral hepatitis, notably those with serum hepatitis, a new era in hepatitis research began (441–444).

Outbreaks

About 1965, it became evident that serum hepatitis was a danger in dialysis units, which at that time were rapidly proliferating. Serious hepatitis outbreaks occurred not only in several European centres (Manchester, Liverpool, London, Edinburgh, Stockholm) but also in the United States (100, 442, 443). These hepatitis outbreaks were only the beginning; the major part of the iceberg was still under the surface. In the 1966 annual EDTA Report, Drukker et al (440) identified 40 cases of viral hepatitis in 19 centres out of a total of 54 reporting, i.e. 35%. In 1965/1966, 14 cases with 4 deaths occurred in patients and there were 4 deaths out of 26 cases in dialysis personnel.

In 1968 107 cases in 45 European centres were reported in patients (with seven deaths) and 70 cases in staff, luckily without fatalities (100). Subsequently, an ever increasing incidence of hepatitis in patients and staff was reported annually. Further investigations showed that after mild hepatitis B infection, persistent Australia antigenaemia (HB$_s$Ag) may develop in individuals with a diminished immune response such as patients on maintenance dialysis (444). It became evident that those with persistent Australia antigenaemia could potentially infect others (445), endangering patients and staff of dialysis units. By 1971 there were 12 major outbreaks of hepatitis resulting in 357 cases with 18 (5%) deaths. In 1975, 870 of 927 dialysis centres in Europe (93%) reported on the incidence of hepatitis amongst their staff (99). The total number of infected members of staff was 748 with 8 deaths (1.1%). The tragedy was not yet coming to an end. In 1980 2,234 new cases of hepatitis were recorded in Europe in dialysis patients: 1,800 hepatitis B, 52 A, 382 non A non B (*vide infra*) and 566 in dialysis staff, with 11 deaths (1.9%, [446]).

Hepatitis non-A non-B

Suspicion grew however that yet another type of viral hepatitis which was serologically HB$_s$Ag and HB$_s$Ab negative was responsible both for cases of post-transfusion hepatitis and dialysis associated hepatitis. This hypothesis was confirmed by Feinstone and Alter and associates (1975 [447, 448]). They observed eight hepatitis cases in a series of multiply-transfused open heart surgery patients, who were serologically not due to viral hepatitis A or B.

The aetiology of non-A, non-B hepatitis (NANB) remained initially obscure but soon it became apparent that the agent was transmissible from man to chimpanzee (449, 450) and Vitviski and co-workers (451) demonstrated a new antigen-antibody system distinct from HB$_s$Ag, which appeared specific for non-A, non-B acute hepatitis. The NANB antigen was also demonstrated in liver extract from patients with chronic NANB hepatitis.

The virus reservoir for NANB rests like the hepatitis B virus (HBV) in the so called carriers and according to the expectation NANB hepatitis is, like hepatitis B, a potential source for outbreaks in haemodialysis units.

The 1968–1970 outbreak of HB$_s$Ag negative acute hepatitis in the dialysis unit of the Fulham Hospital in London, appeared serologically unrelated to hepatitis A infection. In retrospection, 9 years later, it was concluded that this epidemic had to be classified into the category of non-A, non-B hepatitis (452).

It is both of epidemiological and clinical importance that a significant number of affected dialysis patients remain NANB carriers and that 28% of the infected Fulham patients developed chronic liver disease (452).

Detection of NANB hepatitis became possible with specific serological tests, detecting the specific non-A, non-B antigen, called hepatitis C antigen (453).

Prophylaxis

Prevention of cross infection (1970–1975)

A series of committee recommendations among others in England and the Netherlands for prophylaxis (454, 455) were partly successful. But hepatitis continued to be a serious problem in dialysis communities in the majority of countries with dialysis facilities.

Further research on hepatitis continued. Subtypes of HB$_s$Ag have been discovered (456, 457) and in 1972 Magnius and Espmark (458) discovered a new antigen called the *e* determinant. The *e* antigen has been found exclusively in HB$_s$Ag-positive sera and apparently correlates with active liver disease and infectivity. Anti *e* antibodies occur in HB$_s$Ag-positive sera and in some anti-HB$_s$ (HB$_s$Ab) containing sera. This discovery is of considerable practical importance in dialysis units.

Recently Italian investigators identified a new hepatitis agent named delta (δ), which is invariably associated with progressive liver injury in human carriers.

The agent is obligatory associated with the hepatitis B virus and apparently cannot replicate without the help of HBV.

So far δ-Ag and its antibody anti-δ seems to be common (only simultaneously with HBV markers [HB$_s$Ag and anti-HB$_s$]) in addicts who take drugs parenterally (459, 460).

One of the structural forms bearing HB$_s$Ag consists of spherical double layered ultrastructures discovered by Dane, Camerone and Briggs (461) in 1970. The so called Dane particles represent the intact virus (462, 463).

In contrast with the hepatitis B virus, the virus of hepatitis A has a short life and no carrier state has been defined (464); transmission can only occur during the acute phase of the disease. The reservoir of hepatitis B virus rests, however, in carriers. After the introduction of reliable serological tests for hepatitis B infection it became evident that with the exception of a rather small number of hepatitis cases caused by cytomegalovirus, the Epstein-Barr virus, yellow fever virus and drugs, dialysis associated hepatitis is predominantly caused by the hepatitis B virus.

Passive immunisation with gamma globulin is of temporary benefit for the prevention of hepatitis A in contacts with patients with viral hepatitis A and in subjects exposed to poor sanitary conditions (e.g. when travelling). The administration should be repeated at 4 to 6 months intervals (464, 465).

Vaccination (1980–1981)

Hyperimmune, anti-HB$_s$ gammaglobulin gives protection when administered within 48 h of infection with HBV (e.g. needlestick injury with contaminated needle) and is efficacious in protection of new patients entering dialysis units with HB$_s$Ag positive patients. Routine use is however very expensive (464, 466); obviously there still was an urgent need for active vaccination (467).

Attempts to prepare vaccines against HBV began in the early and mid 1970's (468, 469) and gave promising results.

From France, where the incidence of hepatitis B infection in dialysis units has been persistently high (470), the results of a two year study of a hepatitis B vaccine were published in 1978 by Maupas and co-workers (470, 471) and in 1981 Crosnier and colleagues reported on the results of a placebo controlled trial of a vaccine prepared at the Institut Pasteur at Paris. Both groups reported satisfactory results (472).

In 1980 Szmuness and colleagues (473) published the results of a double blind trial of an American hepatitis B vaccine in a large group of homosexual men in New York. The vaccine prepared in the Merck Institute for Therapeutic Research from HB$_s$Ag virus particles by formalin inactivation appeared highly effective over a period of at least 8 to 18 months (474). It seemed from the American study that the active immunisation even gives some protection after infection with the hepatitis B virus has occurred i.e. during the incubation period of the disease. The vaccine however induces a rather slow immune response and two booster injections (at 1 and 6 months) are required so that satisfactory immunisation is obtained.

In 1981 Szmuness and colleagues (475) presented evidence that simultaneous administration of hepatitis B immunoglobulin and hepatitis B vaccine offered immediate protection. The passively acquired antibody did not interfere with the immuno-genicity of the vaccine and did not prevent development of antibody to the vaccine.

This opened not only possibilities for post exposure prophylaxis (475) but also offered immediate protection for susceptible persons (lacking detectable hepatitis B surface antigen and antibody to HB$_s$Ag) working in (or entering) a HB$_s$Ag positive dialysis unit.

A reduced immune response to the vaccine has been noted both by the French and the American investigators in patients with naturally or artificially impaired immune response, e.g. in patients with advanced chronic renal failure and during immunosuppressive therapy (472, 475).

Results of prophylaxis and vaccination

Practical application of vaccination against hepatitis B was introduced in 1980 and the results in European dialysis units have been presented in the annual reports of the Registry of the European Dialysis and Transplant Association-European Renal Association (112, 123, 178, 446, 476–479).

The number of new cases of hepatitis B diagnosed in the years 1980–1985 in members of the staff, expressed per 1,000 patients on hospital haemodialysis, decreased rapidly in the first 2 years and continues to decline somewhat slower each year, the number of fatalities approaching zero.

The number of new cases in patients declined also rapidly from 44 per 1,000 in 1980 to 24 per 1,000 in 1982, but subsequently remained stable. (See Figure 46 and Table 7).

Large variations in the frequency of hepatitis are still found between different countries.

The number of cases of hepatitis A and non-A non-B (NANB) in staff remained stable in the years 1980–1985 if expressed per 1,000 hospital haemodialysis patients. The absolute number of NANB cases in patients, however, increased.

In patients the effect of introduction of anti-B vaccination

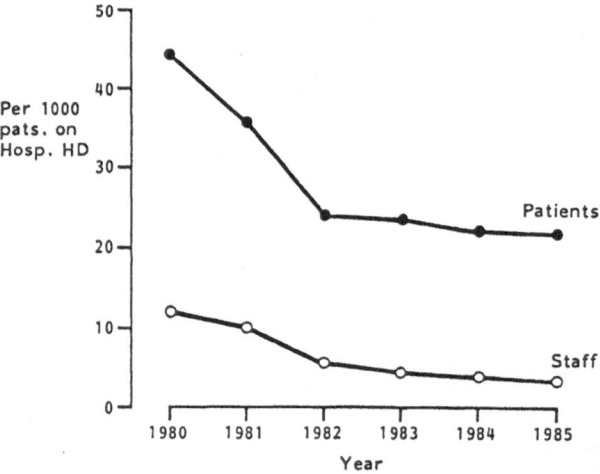

Figure 46. Presents the number of new cases of hepatitis B in Europe, diagnosed in patients and staff in each of the years 1980–1985, expressed per thousand patients on hospital haemodialysis at the end of each year. (Reproduced from the 1985 EDTA-ERA Registry report, with permission of the Registry of the EDTA-ERA).

has been somewhat disappointing, probably because antibody response in these patients is somewhat less than in healthy individuals.

In addition current hepatitis B vaccines are prepared from plasma of human hepatitis B carriers and are effective and safe (480), but for various reasons, including scarcity, cost and fear of unknown contaminants from human plasma have made acceptance, even in high risk groups, less than total (481).

Recently recombinant hepatitis B vaccine prepared from antigen expressed in yeast has been prepared in research laboratories of Merck, Sharp and Dohme, USA, with immunogenicity being comparable with the plasma derived American vaccine (480–483). This vaccine is perfectly safe

Table 7. New hepatitis cases in European dialysis units* 1980–1985.

Year	Patients					Staff				
	Hep B	Hep B/1000 Hosp. H.D.	Hep A	Hep NANB	Hep NANB/ 1000 Hosp. H.D.	Hep B	Hep B/1000 Hosp. H.D.	Hep A	Hep NANB	Deaths
1980	1801	44	52	382	9.4	493	12.2	22	51	11
1981	1614	40	63	541	12.0	460	11.5	23	41	18
1982	1360	23	71	566	12.1	315	5.6	12	52	5
1983	1473	27	85	728	11.7	275	4.9	29	24	0
1984	1402	25	41	731	11.6	251	4.4	13	96	1
1985	1384	21	54	744	11.1	236	3.6	11	38	?
1986	1338	18	?	?	?	235	3.2	?	?	?

* Data from EDTA-ERA Registry Reports. (112, 123, 178, 446, 476–479) with permission.

(484) and there is obviously no risk of unknown contaminants. This may facilitate acceptance and improve anti-B vacccination status in dialysis units.

Notwithstanding diagnostic tests for non-A, non-B hepatitis became available (451–453) a vaccine has not yet been developed.

So far, the incidence of non-A, non-B hepatitis in dialysis units seems less than of hepatitis B, but in the Netherlands, Sweden and the United Kingdom in 1979 more cases of non-A, non-B were reported than of hepatitis B.

In addition this form of hepatitis seems to be related to a high frequency of persistent hepatic dysfunction: 8 out of the 29 patients from the 1968–1970 outbreak at the Fulham renal unit in London reportedly had persistently elevated serum amino transferase activity (28%). Liver biopsy revealed chronic aggressive hepatitis in three and chronic persistent hepatitis in two (463).

Effective vaccination is urgently needed before the non-A, non-B type of hepatitis starts spreading in dialysis units.

In areas with a high frequency of primary hepatocellular carcinoma (e.g. Sub-Saharan Africa, Asia, Oceania and others) there is a close association between hepatitis B virus infection on one hand and postnecrotic cirrhosis of the liver and primary hepatocellular carcinoma on the other; primary liver carcinoma – in these areas responsible for 60% of the carcinoma deaths – commonly develops in livers with postnecrotic cirrhosis. In these areas hepatitis B virus carriers are also common.

This association supports the hypothesis that persistent hepatitis B virus infection is required for the development of most cases of primary hepatocellular carcinoma (485).

The next step in testing this hypothesis is by decreasing the frequency of hepatitis B infection by large scale vaccination, which should decrease the frequency of primary liver carcinoma in these affected areas (Blumberg and London [1981, 485]).

This may become a reality when large quantities of recombinant anti-B vaccine can be produced at relatively low cost. This would be another dialysis associated landmark in medical history.

AIDS (1981)

In Western communities human immuno deficiency virus (HIV) is predominantly sexually transmitted both homosexually and (increasingly) heterosexually.

Specific risk groups

At the time of writing (May, 1987) the infection is still virtually confined to specific risk groups: homo- and bisexual men (in particular, those who have multiple partners), past recipients of blood and blood products and drug abusers, in particular those who prostitute themselves to the money they need for their addiction (486).

Homosexual practices are still the most frequent way to transmit HIV, but heterosexual transmittance is increasing and obviously the risk of encountering (and transmitting) HIV is a high degree of promiscuity: and the risk increases with the number of different sexual partners, whatever the individual's sexual orientation (487).

Spreading of the infection continues and is still increasing, although intensive educational campaigns on 'safe sex' have started already in several countries and are on the point to be started in many others.

What about the risk that a chronic dialysis (or transplant) patient is positive for anti HIV and possibly harbours the virus? (488).

What are the risks for other dialysis patients, for the health care staff (doctors, nurses) and – indirectly – for the laboratory staff?

Some figures

According to WHO statistics the figures are staggering (489).

Early in 1987 some 100 nations are struck and 5 to 10 million people worldwide carry the virus. An estimated 100 million will be infected between 1987 and 1997.

Presently in the US some 30,000 AIDS cases have been reported and some 1.5 to 2 million people are thought to be carriers.

As predicted by the Centre for Disease Control in Atlanta, GA the total number of cases in the US will reach 270,000 between 1987 and 1992 and the total number of deaths will increase to 179,000.

The cost of treatment in 1986–1987 is already estimated to exceed a billion US$ a year and will be in 1991 an estimated US$ 14 billion annually.

Available figures from Europe seem less alarming, but this may be only temporarily because Europe is simply lagging behind in comparison with the US; by the end of January 1987 in the UK (population 56 million) 365 had died from AIDS and 686 had the disease. The number of seropositive individuals has not been mentioned in the most recent statistics (490).

In the Netherlands (population 14 million) as of December 1986 128 patients died and 72 were suffering from the disease. An estimated 10,000–20,000 were seropositive on antibodies. If 20,000 people in this country are seropositive (1 on 700) the population on replacement of renal function – 2,500 patients – must hold some 3 to 4 positive patients and among some 700 new patients, annually accepted for renal replacement therapy, there must be (at the time of writing) at least 1 seropositive patient.

There is no reason to be optimistic concerning the outlook for Europe (neither for the US or other territories). Hopefully the educational campaigns and sex instructions will produce effect; the production of an effective vaccine (or vaccines) seems still to be far away; the antiviral drug Azidothymidine (AZT) appears to be temporarily effective in decreasing mortality and morbidity in some patients with AIDS and AIDS related complex but bone marrow toxicity can be severe, requiring recurrent transfusions or even interruption of therapy, because of granulocytopenia or thrombocytopenia (491, 492). Tolerance seems to be divergent in different patients.

Results of long term trials have to be awaited.

A related drug, dideoxycytidine (DDC) is presently under trial and seems to be less toxic and more promising (489).

Guidelines for dialysis and transplant units: how to handle HIV positive patients

So far no general instructions or guidelines have been published or issued for dialysis (and transplant) units concerning handling of HIV positive patients.

Questions

Several questions arise:

1. Should all patients be tested for anti-HIV and if positive for the virus?
2. Should the patient be informed of the outcome?
3. Should all patients be tested regularly (e.g., every 3 to 6 months)?
4. Should antibody positive patients be dialysed with a personal (single patient) dialysis machine?
5. Should antibody positive patients be dialysed in an isolation area?

Obviously all precautions introduced years ago to prevent cross infection with the hepatitis B virus (493) are equally valid for the HI virus in a similar way and should strictly be adhered to, see also chapter 42.

The answers; precautions

Regarding the answers to the questions raised above it should be kept in mind that apart from blood transfusion the infection with HIV is introduced by sexual contact (486, 487) and although the epidemiology of HIV infection shows some similarities with the hepatitis B virus, HIV seems less infectious. So far only very few health professionals have developed antibodies to HIV after needlestick injuries (494). The risk of infection by contaminated needle-stick injury is small because HIV is less communicable than the hepatitis B virus. Possibly the infective dose of HIV is greater than of the hepatitis B virus. As many as 10^{13} hepatitis B virus particles are present in 1 ml of infected blood compared with only 10^4 for HIV (494).

Nevertheless seroconversion after needle-stick injury or skin contamination with HIV infected blood does occur (495, 496).

Apart from all precautions to prevent hepatitis B cross infection like incineration of used syringes, needles, dialysers, blood lines etc., the blood line puncture sites (for blood test samples) should be protected by a semicircular plastic shield and dialysis staff and laboratory workers should be carefully instructed (and supervised) (454, 493).

It is obviously important that all samples of seropositive patients are labeled with brightly colored biohazard stickers like those used for samples of hepatitis B patients or carriers

Risks for the health care staff

In 1986 the EDTA-ERA Registry committee made an inquiry of European dialysis centres on testing for HIV. Some 76% of the centres replied revealing that almost 50% tested all or most patients. More than 25,000 patients were tested: 225 (that is less than 1%) were anti HIV positive and 10 patients had died from AIDS (123).

The risk for the health care staff in Europe is very small.

Protection of patients

A non transfusion policy is important (179).

But on the other hand one should be aware that during a 4 h dialysis 10 times the total volume of blood of each patient is subjected to extracorporeal circulation, to be sure in a closed circuit. However, in exceptional situations a technical catastrophe may occur with spilling of infected blood all over the dialysis ward, as happened in a British dialysis unit many years ago (497) with unexpected consequences and cross infection of several patients in the area. This was an exceptional incident but a similar catastrophe is even presently not impossible. Therefore it should be recommended to take blood tests on anti HIV of all dialysis patients and all new patients before starting dialysis treatment. Positive patients should be dialysed in an isolation area, like hepatitis B carriers: the risk of cross infection with HIV is small, but even a minimal risk should be avoided.

The answer to the five questions, which have been put forward above, should be affirmative.

DIALYSIS TREATMENT OF NON-RENAL CONDITIONS (1960; 1977–'78)

Some 10 years ago psychiatrists, dermatologists, neurologists and dialysis physicians became interested in dialysis treatment of certain non-renal conditions.

Schizophrenia

The idea of dialysis treatment of mental disorders (schizophrenia) and myasthenia gravis originated from Switzerland and dates back to 1960 (498). Interest was renewed by Cade and Wagemaker (499–501) in 1977/78. Cade started dialysing a schizophrenic patient with hypertension and kidney disease in 1971 on her own request and described remarkable improvement of her mental condition (500). Endorphin, identified as β-leucine-5-endorphin, was isolated from the dialysing fluid of several schizophrenic patients (502–504). This however was not confirmed by others. Ever since, a number of investigators reported both negative and positive results in schizophrenic patients: the issue remained undecided. Interest however has been fading away.

Psoriasis, other conditions

Other non-renal conditions experimentally treated with dialysis are psoriasis (504–507) and myasthenia gravis (499,

504, 508, 509). Other methods of blood purification (haemofiltration, haemoperfusion and plasma exchange) have become the methods of choice for treatment of these conditions. For detailed information see chapter 49 of the 2nd edition of this book.

SOME SOCIO-ECONOMIC CONSIDERATIONS

Start and growth of replacement of renal function (1960)

For a few years after 1960 when treatment of end stage renal disease (ESRD) with dialysis began in Seattle, a closeted and anonymous committee decided which medically suitable patients would receive maintenance haemodialysis treatment; there were only a few machines and an overwhelming number of patients.

The costs were prohibitively high ($40,000 per patient/year) and financing of even a limited chronic dialysis programme raised insolvable dilemmas.

Nevertheless some 7,000 American patients received regular dialysis treatment before legislation was passed in the American Congress in 1972 under which the Federal Government would pay for the cost of dialysis treatment. In the years that the new law has been effective, the number of patients on regular dialysis treatment in the USA showed a staggering growth to approximately 85,000 in 1985 (370 per million population). Since 1972 the mean annual increase of new dialysis patients in the USA has been 5,000 to 7,000 patients per year (510, 511).

The new legislation stimulated in the U.S. a great expansion of dialysis facilities and created a big dialysis industry: approximately 36% of the total number of dialysis patients are treated in 'for profit units' (512).

In addition the new law had several unexpected side-effects: the percentage of home dialysis patients in the US decreased from 40% in 1972 to between 10 and 12% in 1979, because the new law provided economically much more attractive facilities for hospital dialysis, although home dialysis is much cheaper and survival rates and the rehabilitation figures are substantially better than with hospital dialysis (298). To reverse this highly undesirable side effect the law was altered in 1980.

Home dialysis (see also p. 47), some additional data

Home haemodialysis

Nevertheless the percentage of home haemodialysis patients decreased further to 4.7% in 1985: the introduction of continuous ambulatory peritoneal dialysis (CAPD) in the late 1970's has changed the scene.

CAPD and CCPD

CAPD (see chapter 25) and continuous cyclic peritoneal dialysis (CCPD) are essentially self treatment at home and became rapidly popular, both in the US and in Europe (see for European figures Table 4).

In the US the number of CAPD and CCPD patients had increased in 1985 to more than 12,000 patients, 14.4 percent of the total dialysis population in that country (513). In Europe CAPD grew less rapidly; in 1985 slightly more than 7,500 patients or 9% of the total dialysis population was on CAPD; home haemodialysis became less popular as in the US), the percentage decreasing from 15 to 19% in 1976–1977 to 8,9% in 1985 (see Table 2).

Geographical discrepancies

A remarkable variation of the number of regular dialysis patients in the US from state to state has been reported (512, 514), which can be only partly explained by the fact that patients in the US are sometimes dialysed in a centre across the border of the state where they are living.

The considerable differences in the dialysis rate in different states remain unexplained. Remarkable geographical differences have also been observed in the percentage of home (haemo-)dialysis patients both in the US and in Europe (123, 512, 515) and also in transplantation activities. In Europe the number of grafts varied in 1985 in different countries from 0 to 41 per million population (123, 516).

Transplantation rate in the US, expressed per million population, is twice as high as in Europe (Table 8).

Renal replacement therapy and GNP

Interestingly there is a significant correlation between the total number of patients alive on renal replacement therapy and the per capita gross national product (GNP) expressed in US dollars (516).

Some western countries with relatively high GNP, however, support fewer patients than might have been expected and others treat substantially more (516).

It is obvious that both in the US and in Europe important social, cultural and economic factors influence the numbers of patients offered treatment (517, 518). Other factors such as geographical differences in the prevalence of terminal uraemia may play a (probably minor) role.

The total number of patients on dialysis treatment was in the US (population 237 million) in 1985 84,797, i.e., 358 per

Table 8. Transplant activity.

Year	USA (pop.: 237 million)		Europe + adjacent countries (pop.: 620 million)	
	grafts	grafts/10^6 pop.	grafts	grafts/10^6 pop.
1981	4885	20,6	4556	7,8
1982	5358	22,6	5591	9,7
1983	6112	25,7	6869	12,0
1984	6968	29,4	7724	13,4
1985	7695	32,5	8201	13,2

Sources: EDTA-ERA Annual Statistical Reports; Dial Transplantation (513).

million (513). In Europe (including some adjacent countries, population 620 million) 88,243 patients were on dialysis (including haemofiltration and haemodiafiltration), i.e. 142 per million.

Some figures and cost

The annual increase of the dialysis population in Europe is presently 34 patients per million population, which is slightly higher than the annual acceptance rate in the US (between 21 and 30 per million population).

The cost of the American ESRD programme rose between 1974 and 1980 five fold from US$ 228.5 million to 1252.3 million and between 1980 and 1985 to US$ 1875.6 million (513).

In the climate of budget cutting of the present American administration the promotion of less expensive CAPD treatment and reduction of reimbursements (519) both for hospital dialysis and nonhospital dialysis (in so called free standing units) the payment for treatment of end stage renal disease decreased for the first time in 1985 from $ 1963.5 million in 1984 to $ 1875.6 million.

Figures from Europe are not readily available.

In the Netherlands (population 14 million) in 1981 some 2,000 patients were treated with regular dialysis. The annual increase of the dialysis population in this country is 450.

The cost of this national dialysis programme in 1981 was approximately $ 73 million (even with a substantial number of patients dialysed twice weekly) and is expected to increase to more than $ 390 million (for 8,000 patients [520]) by the end of the century without correction for inflation.

In the United Kingdom hospital haemodialysis has been limited by tight budgetary control and the majority (62%) of the patients practise home haemodialysis or peritoneal dialysis at home, which is cheaper.

On the other hand the group of transplanted patients in the UK continues to grow more rapidly which also helps in limiting the cost.

Nevertheless Manis and Friedman (349) were right with their statement that 'maintenance dialysis stands as an effective, costly – and incompletely understood – life sustaining regimen'. When economical retrenchments continue we should anticipate a further curtailment of dialysis facilities and ESRD programmes even in the 'rich' countries.

Hopefully it will not become necessary to turn the clock back to the early 1960's and to 'life committees' . . .

A FINAL WORD

So far the difficulties in establishing an all embracing dialysis system have been described. From Haas' faltering footsteps more than half a century ago progress has been meteoric, particularly during the past 25 years. The 'uraemic syndrome' is now a rarity having been replaced by a surprisingly good quality of life. That this has been achieved with an inanimate material such as cellophane or Cuprophane or other, synthetic membranes is almost incomprehensible, for we still have incomplete knowledge as to the nature and

biological importance of substances that pass or should pass through the membrane. It is also difficult to apportion effects on the patient between dialyses and the aftermath of physiopathological problems arising from a direct result of loss of normally functioning renal tissue.

As a result a new series of clinical and pathological problems became manifest as the life of patients with end stage renal disease was usefully extended more and more.

We were, and still are, hampered by our incomplete knowledge about the functions of normal kidneys, so it is not surprising that we are uncertain of the priorities required to build the most efficient type of artificial kidney.

Nevertheless progress is made, often slowly, sometimes unexpectedly. Treatment of patients one or more decades hence will rely not only on our knowledge and experience but also on future discoveries.

In a quarter of a century important progress was made and major problems as membrane design, vascular access, nephrogenic bone disease and disordered calcium metabolism, treatment of nephrogenic anaemia, aluminium toxicity, prevention of viral hepatitis to mention a few, have been satisfactorily solved or improved.

They are, or will be, things of the past, only to be replaced, it is anticipated, by more sophisticated or more (complex problems, for example the problem of deposition of β_2-M as dialysis associated amyloid in long-term patients whose numbers presently are rapidly increasing.

It is, however, extremely doubtful that the speculation from some clinical investigators, dating from 1979 (349), that 'innovations in the conservative treatment of uraemia may, within a decade, rival haemodialysis in both effectiveness and cost' will be confirmed.

It may take at least several decades from now to approach this ideal. We have to wait and to recall the statement of Robert Goddard: 'it is difficult to say what is impossible . . .'

In concluding this review it seems appropriate to repeat the question: 'Dialysis petrified or progressive?', which was the title of a round table discussion at the annual EDTA Congress in Tel-Aviv, Israel in 1974 (521). Considering the continuing progress made since the publication of the first and second editions of this book (August 1978 and June 1983) the answer is still obvious.

ACKNOWLEDGMENTS

The author gratefully acknowledges the courtesy of Mrs. E. Frame, The Library, University of Strathclyde, Scotland for *Photograph 1*.

Figure 2 is reproduced with kind permission from the Editor of the Philosophical Transactions of the Royal Society of London.

Photograph 3 (John Jacob Abel) was kindly supplied by Mrs Doris Thibodeau, librarian, the Johns Hopkins University Institute of the History of Medicine, Baltimore MD, USA.

Figure 4 is redrawn from a figure in the Journal of Pharmacology and Experimental Therapy with permission from the Editor and Publishers.

A number of letters of John Jacob Abel and other historical material, which is kept at the Welch Medical Library of the Johns Hopkins University, Monument Street, Baltimore, MD, USA, were photocopied and made available to the author by Mr. David

Hamilton, PhD, FRCS, consultant surgeon at the Western Infirmary, University of Glasgow, Scotland,

Photograph 6 was kindly supplied by Prof. J. Benedum, Gieszen (DBR) (20, 21).

Figures 7 and 8 are redrawn from figures originally published in Abderhalden's Handbuch der biologischen Arbeitsmethoden, with permission from the Publishers. Figure 7 has been redrawn according to figure 6 (p. 7) in Patrick McBride's book Genesis of the Artificial Kidney (published by Travenol Laboratories Inc., 1979), for the sake of clearness.

The author gratefully acknowledges the courtesy of Prof. Jost Benedum, Gieszen (DBR), for the photographs which are reproduced in *Figures 9, 10 and 11*. These figures are reproduced from originals kindley supplied by Dr. Med. Willi Haas, Erlensee/Krs. Hanau (DBR), who is a nephew of the late Dr. Georg Haas.

Figures 6, 9, 10 and 11 are reproduced with kind permission from the Editors and Publishers of the Medizin historisches Journal, Gustav Fischer Verlag, Stuttgart, New York.

Figure 13 is reproduced from Dr. Kolff's MD thesis, with permission.

Photographs 15b and 16 are by courtesy of the Municipal Museum of the City of Amsterdam.

Figure 18 is reproduced from a monograph, The Genesis of the Artificial Kidney, by Patrick McBride, Deerfield, Illinois, with permission.

Figure 19 is reproduced from the Acta Medica Scandinavia with permission from the Author and the Publishers.

Figure 20 is reproduced from a paper by Prof. Nils Alwall (48) with permission of Gambro AB, Lund, Sweden.

Figure 22 is reproduced from a photograph kindly supplied by Dr. F.M. Parsons, Leeds UK which was originally published in the Yorkshire Post in the UK.

Figure 23 was kindly supplied by Prof. Bodo von Garrelts, Stockholm, Sweden and is reproduced with his permission.

Photographs 24 and 25 were kindly supplied by Mr. Patrick T. McBride, author of Genesis of the Artificial Kidney (published by Travenol Laboratories Inc., Deerfield IL, USA, 1979), who's collection of antique dialysers and other material is permanently displayed at the International Center for Artificial Organs and Transplantation, 8937 Euclid Avenue, Cleveland OH 44106, USA.

Photograph 26b by courtesy of Baxter-Travenol Laboratories Inc., Morton Grove IL, USA.

Figure 28 is reproduced from Palmer RA, *Peritoneal Dial Bull* 2:16, 1982 (with permission).

Figure 31 was reproduced from the Lancet by kind permission from the Authors and the Editor of the Lancet.

Photographs 35a and 35c have been reproduced from original photographs kindly supplied by Dr. Frederik Kiil from Oslo, Norway.

Figure 35b is taken from a paper by Dr. Frederik Kiil in the Trans Am Soc Artif Intern Organs with permission from the Author and Editor (79, 80)

Figure 36 is reproduced from a photograph kindly supplied by Dr. Belding H. Scribner from Seattle, WA, USA.

Figure 38 was kindly supplied by Dr. Albert L. Babb PhD, Dept. of Chemical Engineering, University of Washington, Seattle WA, US.

Figures 39a and 39b are reproduced from a comment on a paper presented at an ASAIO meeting in 1965 by Dr. Y. Nosé (96) with permission from Dr. Nosé and the Editor of the Trans Am Soc Artif Intern Organs.

Figures 40–43 are (slightly modified) reproduced from Chapter 15 (written by Dr. Shaldon and Mr. Larson) in the 1st edition of this book.

Figure 45 is redrawn (slightly modified) from a diagram in a paper by Muldoon and Leonard in the Trans Am Soc Artif Intern Organs (128). With permission from the Authors and the Editor.

Figure 46 is taken from the EDTA 1985 Annual Report on Regular Dialysis and Transplantation in Europe, XVI (with permission).

REFERENCES

1. Munro AC: Thomas Graham (1805–1869). *Phil J* (*Glasgow*) 8: 30, 1971

2. Graham T: Liquid diffusion applied to analysis. *Phil Trans Roy Soc* London 151: 183, 1861

3. Abel JJ, Rowntree LC, Turner BB: On the removal of diffusible substances from the circulating blood by means of dialysis. *Trans Assoc Am Physicians* 28: 51, 1913

4. Abel JJ, Rowntree LG, Turner BB: On the removal of diffusable substances from the circulating blood of living animals by dialysis. *J Pharmacol Exp Ther* 5: 275, 1913–1914

5. Abel JJ, Rowntree LG, Turner BB: Some constituents of the blood. *J Pharmacol Exp Ther* 5: 611, 1913–1914

6. Abel JJ, Rowntree LG, Turner BB: Plasma removal with return of corpuscles (plasmaphaeresis). *J Pharmacol Exp Ther* 5: 625, 1913–1914

7. Hess CL von, McGuigan H: The condition of sugar in the blood. *J Pharmacol Exp Ther* 6: 45, 1914–1915

8. Love GH: Vividiffusion with intestinal membranes. *Med Rec* (*NY*) 98: 649, 1920

9. Necheles H: Ueber dialysieren des strömenden Blutes am Lebenden (On dialysis of the circulating blood in vivo). *Klin Wochenschr* 2: 1257, 1923 (in German)

10. Necheles H: Erwiderung zu vorstehenden Bemerkungen (Comment on the previous remarks). *Klin Wochenschr* 2: 1888, 1923 (in German)

11. Lim RKS, Necheles H: Demonstration of a gastric secretory excitant in circulating blood by vividialysis. *Proc Soc Exp Biol Med* 24: 197, 1926

12. Haas G: Dialysieren des strömenden Blutes am Lebenden (Dialysis of the circulating blood in vivo). *Klin Wochenschr* 2: 1888, 1923 (in German)

13. Haas G: Versuche der Blutauswaschung am Lebenden mit Hilfe der Dialyse (Experiments on cleansing of blood in vivo by means of dialysis). *Klin Wochenschr* 4: 13, 1925 (in German)

14. Haas G: Ueber Versuche der Blutauswaschung am Lebenden mit Hilfe der Dialyse (On experimental cleansing of blood in vivo with dialysis). *Naunyn Schmiedebergs Arch Pharmacol* 116: 158, 1926 (in German)

15. Haas G: Ueber Versuche mit Blutwaschung am Lebenden mit Hilfe der Dialyse (On experimental cleansing of blood in vivo with dialysis). *Naunyn Schmiedebergs Arch Pharmacol* 120: 371, 1927 (in German)

16. Haas G: Ueber Blutwaschung (On cleansing of blood). *Klin Wochenschr* 7: 1356, 1928 (in German)

17. Haas G: Die Methoden der Blutauswaschung (Methods of cleansing of blood). *Abderhalden's Handb Biol Arbeitsmethoden V* 8: 717, 1935 (in German)

18. Philipsson P: Ueber die Verwendbarkeit der Schilfschläuche zur Dialyse (The application of reed stalks to dialysis). *Beitr Chem Phys Path* 1: 80, 1902 (in German)

19. Pregl F: Beitrage zur Methodik des Dialysierverfahrens von E. Abderhalden (Contribution to the methodology of the dialysis procedure of E. Abderhalden) *Ferm Forsch* 1: 7, 1914 (in German)

20. Benedum J, Weise M: Georg Haas (1886–1971): Sein Beitrag zur Frühgeschichte der künstlichen Niere (Georg Haas: His contribution to the early history of the artificial kidney). *Dtsch Med Wochenschr* 103: 1674, 1978 (in German)

21. Benedum J: Georg Haas (1886–1971): Pionier der Hämodialyse (Georg Haas: Pioneer of haemodialysis). *Med Hist J* 14: 196, 1979 (in German)

22. Asaba H, Bergström J, Fürst P, Shaldon S, Wilkund S: Treatment of diuretic resistent fluid retention with ultrafiltration. *Acta Med Scand* 204: 145, 1978

23. Verbanck J, Schelstraete J, De Paepe M, Hoenich N, Ringoir S: Pure ultrafiltration by repeated puncture of a peripheral armvein as treatment of refractory edema. *Int J Artif Organs* 3: 342, 1980

24. Thalhimer W: Experimental exchange transfusion for reducing azotemia. Use of the artificial kidney for this purpose. *Proc Soc Exp Biol Med* 37: 641, 1937

25. Kolff WJ: First clinical experience with the artificial kidney. *Ann Intern Med* 62: 608, 1965

26. Kolff WJ, Berk HThJ: De kunstmatige nier: een dialysator met groot oppervlak (The artificial kidney: a dialyser with large surface area). *Ned Tijdschr Geneeskd* 87: 1684, 1943 (in Dutch)

27. Kolff WJ, Berk HThJ, ter Welle M, van der Ley AJW, van Dijk EC, van Noordwijk J: De kunstmatige nier: een dialysator met groot oppervlak (The artificial kidney: a dialyser with large surface area. *Geneesk Gids* 21: 409, 1943 (in Dutch)

28. Kolff WJ, Berk HThJ, ter Welle M, van der Ley AJW, van Dijk EC, van Noordwijk J: The artificial kidney, a dialyzer with a great area. *Acta Med Scand* 117: 121, 1944

29. Kolff WJ: Le rein artificiel: un dialyseur à grande surface (The artificial kidney: a dialyser with large surface area). *Presse Méd* 52: 103, 1944 (in French)

30. Kolff WJ: *De Kunstmatige Nier* (The artificial kidney), MD Thesis, University of Groningen, The Netherlands, Kampen, JH Kok NV, 1946 (in Dutch)

31. Thorwald J: *Die Patienten* (The Patients). München-Zürich, Droemer-Knauer Verlag 1975, p 99 (in German)

32. Domingo WR, Klijne W: A photoelectric flame photometer. *Biochem J* 45: 400, 1949

33. Murray G, Delorme E, Thomas N: Development of an artificial kidney. *Arch Surg* 55: 505, 1947

34. Bywaters EGL, Joekes BM: The artificial kidney: its clinical application in the treatment of traumatic anuria. *Proc R Soc Med* 41: 411 and 420, 1948

35. Fishman AP, Kroop JG, Leiter HE, Hyman A: Experiences with the Kolff artificial kidney. *Am J Med* 7: 15, 1949

36. De Leeuw NKM, Blaustein A: Studies of blood passed through an artificial kidney. *Blood* 4: 653, 1949

37. Darmady EM: Dialysis of blood for the treatment of uraemia. *Proc R Soc Med* 41: 410 and 418, 1948

38. Merrill JP: Dialysis in acute renal failure. In: *Replacement of Renal Function by Dialysis*, chapter 17, Edited by Drukker W, Parsons FM, Maher JF, Martinus Nijhoff, Medical Division, The Hague, Boston MA, London, 1st edition 1978, p 322

39. Bull GM, Joekes AM, Lowe KG: Conservative treatment of anuric uraemia. *Lancet* 2: 229, 1949

40. Borst JGG: Protein katabolism in uraemia. Effects of protein-free diet, infections and blood transfusions. *Lancet* 1: 824, 1948

41. Kolff WJ: Dialysis in treatment of uremia. Arch Intern Med 94: 142, 1954

42. Alwall N: On the artificial kidney. I. Apparatus for dialysis of blood in vivo. *Acta Med Scand* 128: 317, 1947

43. Alwall N, Norviit L: On the artificial kidney. II. The effectivity of the apparatus. *Acta Med Scand (Suppl)* 196: 250, 1947

44. Alwall N: *Therapeutic and Diagnostic Problems in Severe Renal Failure,* Copenhagen, Munksgaard; Stockholm, Svenska Bokförlaget; Oslo and Bergen, Universitetsforlaget, 1963 p 2

45. Alwall N, Bergsten BWB, Gedda PO, Norviit L, Steins AM: On the artificial kidney. IV. The technique in animal experiments. *Acta Med Scand* 132: 392, 1949

46. Alwall N: Experiences with treatment of uremia by dialysis of the blood in vivo ('artificial kidney') *Twenty-third meeting of the Northern Surgical Association* held in Stockholm June 26–28, 1947. Copenhagen, Munksgaard, 1948, p 418

47. Alwall N, Norviit L, Steins AM: On the artificial kidney. VII. Clinical experiences of dialytic treatment of uremia. *Acta Med Scand* 132: 587, 1949

48. Alwall N: *Historical Perspective on the Development of Artificial Organs,* Lund (Sweden) Gambro AB, 1985

49. Hamilton DNH: Developing the artificial kidney in Britain: Frank Maudsley Parsons at Leeds. In: *The University of Leeds Review,* edited by Felsenstein F, vol. 27 1984/85, University Printing Service, p 89

50. Parsons F: Historical aspects of dialysis. In *10th Ann Symposium on Renal Technology,* edited by Lawrence AE Siviter AG, Br Assoc of Renal Technicians, 1986

51. Parsons FM: Indications for haemodialysis in acute renal failure. In *Acute Renal Failure*, a Symposium, edited by Shaldon S, Cook GC, Oxford UK, Blackwell Scientific Publications 1964, p 139

52. Kerr DNS: Twenty five years of haemodialysis, a tribute to the pioneer work of the Belfast renal unit. *Ulster Med J* 54 (Suppl): 586, 1985

53. Murray G, Delorme E, Thomas N: Artificial kidney. *JAMA* 137: 1596, 1948

54. Von Garrelts B: *Twenty-third meeting of the Northern Surgical Association* held in Stockholm June 26–28, 1947, Copenhagen, Munksgaard, 1948, p 422

55. Von Garrelts B: A blood dialyzer for use in vivo. *Acta Med Scand* 155: 87, 1956

56. Inouye WY, Engelberg J: A simplified artificial dialyzer and ultrafilter. *Surg Forum* 4: 438, 1953

57. Kolff WJ: The artificial kidney – past and future. *Circulation* 15: 285, 1957

58. Watschinger B, Kolff WJ: Further development of the artificial kidney of Inouye and Engelberg. *Trans Am Soc Artif Intern Organs* 1: 37, 1955

59. Kolff WJ, Watschinger B: Further development of a coil kidney. *J Lab Clin Med* 47: 969, 1956

60. Michielsen P: A single pass system with recirculation for the twin coil kidney. *Proc Eur Dial Transplant Assoc* 2: 267, 1965

61. MacNeill AE, Doyle JE, Anthone R, Anthone S: Technic with a parallel flow straight tube blood dialyzer. *NY State J Med* 59: 4137, 1959

62. Doyle JE, Anthone R, Anthone S, MacNeill AE: Treatment of renal failure with a parallel flow, straight tubing blood dialyzer. *NY State J Med* 59: 4149, 1959

63. Doyle JE: *Extracorporeal Hemodialysis Therapy in Blood Chemistry Disorders.* Am Lecture Series no. 453, Springfield, IL, Charles C. Thomas, 1962, p 18

64. Skeggs LT Jr, Leonards JR: Studies on an artificial kidney. I. Preliminary results with a new type of continuous dialyzer. *Science* 108: 212, 1948

65. Skeggs LT Jr, Leonards JR, Heisler CR: Artificial Kidney. II. Construction and operation of an improved continuous dialyz-

er. *Proc Soc Exp Biol Med* 72: 539, 1949

66. Muehrcke RC: *Acute Renal Failure.* St Louis, The CV Mosby Company 1969, p 277

67. Maher JF, Schreiner GE, Waters TJ: Successful intermittent hemodialysis – longest reported maintenance of life in true oliguria (181 days). *Trans Am Soc Artif Intern Organs* 6: 123, 1960

68. Giovannetti S, Bigalli A, Cioni L, Della Santa M, Ballestri P: Permanent vein cannulation for repeated hemodialysis. *Acta Med Scand* 173: 1, 1963

69. Shaldon S, Rosen SM: Technique of refrigerated coil preservation haemodialysis with femoral venous catheterization. *Br Med J* 2: 411, 1964

70. Quinton W, Dillard D, Scribner BH: Cannulation of blood vessels for prolonged hemodialysis. *Trans Am Soc Artif Intern Organs* 6: 104, 1960

71. Sinclair ISR, Henderson MA, Simpson DC: Fluon arteriovenous shunt for repeated haemodialysis. *Lancet* 2: 410, 1961

72. Quinton WE, Dillard D, Cole JJ, Scribner BH: Possible improvement in the technique of long-term cannulation of blood vessels. *Trans Am Soc Artif Intern Organs* 7: 60, 1961

73. Sevitt L, Comty C, Rottka H, Shaldon S: The single break silastic teflon shunt. *Proc Eur Dial Transplant Assoc* 1: 271, 1964

74. Shaldon S: *Proc Working Conf on Chron Dialysis,* Seattle (University of Washington), December 3–5, 1967, p 16

75. Ramirez O, Swartz C, Onesti G, Mailloux L, Brest AN: The winged in-line shunt. *Trans Am Soc Artif Intern Organs* 12: 220, 1966

76. Buselmeier TJ, Kjellstrand CM, Ratazzi CC, Simmons RL, • Najarian JS: A new subcutaneous prosthetic A-V shunt: advantageous over the standard Quinton-Scribner shunt and A-V fistula. *Proc Clin Dial Transplant Forum* 2: 67, 1972

77. Wetzels E: Hämodialyse und Peritonealdialyse (Hemodialysis and Peritoneal dialysis). Berlin, Heidelberg, New York, Springer-Verlag 1969, p 127 (in German)

78. Scribner BH, Caner JEZ, Buri R, Quinton WE: The technique of continuous hemodialysis. *Trans Am Soc Artif Intern Organs* 6: 88, 1960

79. Kiil F, (Amundsen B): Development of a parallel flow artificial kidney in plastics. *Acta Chir Scand (Suppl)* 253: 142, 1960

80. Kiil F, Glover JF Jr: Parallel flow plastic hemodialyzer as a membrane oxygenator. *Trans Am Soc Artif Intern Organs* 8: 43, 1962

81. Scribner BH, Buri R, Caner JEZ, Hegstrom R, Burnell JM: The treatment of chronic uremia by means of intermittent dialysis: a preliminary report. *Trans Am Soc Artif Intern Organs* 6: 114, 1960

82. Pendras JP, Cole JJ, Tu TH, Scribner BH: Improved technique of continuous flow hemodialysis. *Trans Am Soc Artif Intern Organs* 7: 27, 1961

83. Cole JJ, Quinton WE, Williams C, Murray JS, Sherris JC: The pumpless low temperature hemodialysis system. *Trans Am Soc Artif Intern Organs* 8: 209, 1962

84. Hegstrom RM, Murray JS, Pendras JP, Burnell JM, Scribner BH: Hemodialysis in the treatment of chronic uremia. *Trans Am Soc Artif Intern Organs* 7: 136, 1961

85. Hegstrom RM, Murray JS, Pendras JP, Burnell JM, Scribner BH: Two years experience with periodical hemodialysis in the treatment of chronic uremia. *Trans Am Soc Artif Intern Organs* 8: 266, 1962

86. Murray JS, Tu WH, Alberts JB, Burnell JM, Scribner BH: A community hemodialysis center for the treatment of chronic uremia. *Trans Am Soc Artif Intern Organs* 8: 315, 1962

87. Brown HW, Maher JF, Lapierre L, Bledsoe FH, Schreiner GE: Clinical problems related to the prolonged artificial maintenance of life by hemodialysis in chronic renal failure. *Trans Am Soc Artif Intern Organs* 8: 281, 1962

88. Gonzalez FM, Pabico RL, Brown HW, Maher JF, Schreiner GE: Further experience with the use of routine intermittent hemodialysis in chronic renal failure. *Trans Am Soc Artif Intern Organs* 9: 11, 1963

89. Kolff WJ, Nakamoto S, Scudder JP: Experiences with long-term intermittent dialysis. *Trans Am Soc Artif Intern Organs* 8: 292, 1962

90. Lindholm DD, Burnell JM, Murray JS: Experience in the treatment of chronic uremia in an outpatient community hemodialysis center. *Trans Am Soc Artif Intern Organs* 9: 3, 1963

91. Sherris JC, Cole JJ, Scribner BH: Bacteriology of continuous flow hemodialysis. *Trans Am Soc Artif Intern Organs* 7: 37, 1961

92. Fry DL, Hoover PL: Single pass dialysate flow for the Seattle pumpless hemodialysis system. *Trans Am Soc Artif Intern Organs* 10: 98, 1964

93. Mion CM, Hegstrom RM, Boen ST, Scribner BH: Substitution of sodium acetate for bicarbonate in the bath fluid for hemodialysis. *Trans Am Soc Artif Intern Organs* 10: 110, 1964

94. Mudge GH, Manning JA, Gilman A: Sodium acetate as a source of fixed base. *Proc Soc Exp Biol Med* 71: 136, 1949

95. Grimsrud L, Cole JJ, Lehman GA, Babb AL, Scribner BH: A central system for the continuous preparation and distribution of hemodialysis fluid. *Trans Am Soc Artif Intern Organs* 10: 107, 1964

96. Scribner BH, Babb AL: Chronic hemodialysis in Seattle 1960–1966, part II. *Dial Transplant* 11: 324, 1982

97. Bower JD, Belle CH, Hench ME: Bactericidal properties of the concentrated artificial kidney bath solution. *Appl Microbiol* 14: 45, 1966

98. Gutch GF, Swanson JR, Ogden DA: Failure of dialysis concentrate as a bactericidal agent. *Proc Clin Dial Transplant Forum* 4: 234, 1974

99. Alberts C, Drukker W: Report on regular dialysis treatment in Europe. *Proc Eur Dial Transplant Assoc* 2: 82, 1965

100. Drukker W, Schouten WAG, Alberts C: Report on regular dialysis treatment in Europe, IV, 1968. *Proc Eur Dial Transplant Assoc* 5: 3, 1969

101. Shaldon S, Baillod RA, Comty C, Oakley J, Sevitt L: 18 Months experience with a nurse-patient operated chronic dialysis unit. *Proc Eur Dial Transplant Assoc* 1: 233, 1964

102. Shaldon S, Rae AI, Rosen SM, Silva H, Oakley J: Refrigerated femoral venous-venous haemodialysis with coil preservation for rehabilitation of terminal uraemic patients. *Br Med J* 1: 1716, 1963

103. Leading article (anonymous): New developments with artificial kidney. *Br Med J* 1: 1685, 1963

104. Shaldon S: The self service approach. *Dial Transplant* 15: 19, 1986

105. Nose Y: Discussion. *Trans Am Soc Artif Intern Organs* 11: 15, 1965

106. Merrill JP, Schupak E, Cameron E, Hampers CL: Hemodialysis in the home. *JAMA* 190: 466, 1964

107. Curtis FK, Cole JJ, Fellows HJ, Tyler LL, Scribner BH: Hemodialysis in the home. *Trans Am Soc Artif Intern Organs* 11: 7, 1965

108. Baillod RA, Comty C, Ilahi M, Konotey-Ahulu FID, Sevitt L, Shaldon S: Overnight haemodialysis in the home. *Proc Eur Dial Transplant Assoc* 2: 99, 1965

109. Hampers CL, Merrill JP, Cameron E: Hemodialysis in the

home – a family affair. *Trans Am Soc Artif Intern Organs* 11: 3, 1965

110. Scribner BH: Maintenance hemodialysis in perspective – 1969. *Proc 4th Congr Nephrol Stockholm* 3: 110, edited by Alwall N, Berglund F, Josephson BS: Basel, München, New York, Karger 1970

111. Gurland HJ, Brunner FP, Chantler C, Jacobs C, Schärer K, Selwood NH, Spies G, Wing AJ: Combined report on regular dialysis and transplantation in Europe, VI. *Proc Eur Dial Transplant Assoc* 13: 3, 1976

112. Brynger H, Brunner FP, Chantler C, Donckerwolcke RA, Jacobs C, Kramer P, Selwood NH, Wing AJ: Combined report on regular dialysis and transplantation in Europe, X, 1979, part I. *Proc Eur Dial Transplant Assoc* 17: 2, 1980

113. Brescia MJ, Cimino JE, Appel K, Hurwich BJ: Chronic hemodialysis using venapuncture and a surgically created arteriovenous fistula. *N Engl J Med* 275: 1089, 1966

114. Editorial (anonymous): Hemodialysis using an arteriovenous fistula. *N Engl J Med* 275: 1134, 1966

115. Shaldon S: The use of the arteriovenous fistula in home haemodialysis. *Proc Eur Dial Transplant Assoc* 6: 94, 1969

116. Gutch CG: Artificial kidneys: problems and approaches. *Annu Rev Biophys Bioeng* 4: 405, 1975

117. Del Greco F, Ivanovich P, Krumlovsky FA (editors): Advances in Dialysis. *Kidney Int* 18 (Suppl 10): 1980

118. Kolff WJ: The artificial kidney – past, present and future. *Trans Am Soc Artif Intern Organs* 1: 1, 1955

119. Salisbury PF: History of The American Society for Artificial Internal Organs. *Trans Am Soc Artif Intern Organs* 6: II, 1960

120. The Book of Daniel 12:4. *The Holy Bible*. Cleveland, New York, World Publishing Company (year of original publication unknown) (cited in ref. 119)

121. Drukker W: Annual Business Meeting. *Proc Eur Dial Transplant Assoc* 2: 346, 1965

122. Drukker W: The birth of the EDTA revisited. *Nieren und Hochdruckkrankheiten* 15: 309, 1986

123. Geerlings W, Tufveson G, Broyer M, Brunner FP, Brynger H, Fassbinder W, Rizzoni G, Selwood NH, Wing AJ: Combined report on regular dialysis and transplantation in Europe, XVII, 1986. (Available from Ms Sheila R Dykes, Administrator of the *EDTA-ERA Registration Committee,* St. Thomas' Hospital, Lambeth Palace Road, London SE1 7EH, UK).

124. Edson H, Keen M, Gotch F: Comparative solute transport and therapeutic effectiveness of multiple point support and standard Kiil hemodialyzers. *Trans Am Soc Artif Intern Organs* 18: 113, 1972

125. Von Hartitzsch B, Hoenich NA, Peterson RJ, Buselmeier TJ, Kerr DNS, Kjellstrand CM: Middle molecule clearance in current dialysers. *Proc Eur Dial Transplant Assoc* 10: 522, 1973

126. Leonard EF, Bluemle LW Jr: The permeability concept as applied to dialysis. *Trans Am Soc Artif Intern Organs* 6: 33, 1960

127. Bluemle LW Jr, Dickson JG Jr, Mitchell J, Podolnick MS: Permeability and hydrodynamic studies on the MacNeill-Collins dialyzer using conventional and modified membrane supports. *Trans Am Soc Artif Intern Organs* 6: 38, 1960

128. Muldoon JF, Leonard EF: Measurement of dialyzing solution film permeability under idealized conditions. *Trans Am Soc Artif Intern Organs* 6: 44, 1960

129. Hoeltzenbein J: Discussion. *Trans Am Soc Artif Intern Organs* 12: 368, 1966

130. Drukker W, Jungerius NA, Alberts C: Report on regular dialysis treatment in Europe III. *Proc Eur Dial Transplant Assoc* 4: 5, 1967

131. Anderson WW, Mann JB: Kiil versus coil dialysis – a comparative clinical study. In: *Hemodialysis, Principles and Practice.* Edited by Bailey GL, New York and London, Academic Press, 1972, p 373

132. Stewart RD, Lipps BJ, Baretta ED, Piering WR, Roth DA, Sargent JA: Short-term hemodialysis with the capillary kidney. *Trans Am Soc Artif Intern Organs* 14: 121, 1968

133. Gotch F, Lipps BJ, Weaver J Jr, Brandes J, Rosin J, Sargent JA, Oja P: Chronic dialysis with the hollow fiber artificial kidney (HFAK). *Trans Am Soc Artif Intern Organs* 15: 87, 1969

134. Alwall N: A new disposable artificial kidney: experimental and clinical experience. *Proc Eur Dial Transplant Assoc* 5: 18, 1968

135. Drukker W: Which membrane? *Dial Transplant Int* 14: 12B, 142A, 1985

136. Vanherweghem J-L, Drukker W, Schwarz A: Clinical significance of blood-device interaction in hemodialysis. A review. *Int J Artif Organs* 10: 219, 1987

137. Scribner BH: Discussion. *Trans Am Soc Artif Intern Organs* 11: 29, 1965

138. Babb AL, Popovich RP, Christopher TG, Scribner BH: The genesis of the square meter-hour hypothesis. *Trans Am Soc Artif Intern Organs* 17: 81, 1971

139. Christopher TG, Cambi V, Harker LA, Hurst PE, Popovich RP, Babb AL, Scribner BH: A study of hemodialysis with lowered dialysate flow rate. *Trans Am Soc Artif Intern Organs* 17: 92, 1971

140. Babb AL, Farrell PC, Uvelli DA, Scribner BH: Hemodialyzer evaluation by examination of solute molecular spectra. *Trans Am Soc Artif Intern Organs* 18: 98, 1972

141. Milutinovic J, Halar EM, Harker LA, Babb AL, Scribner BH: Further experience with hemodialysis at 100 ml/min dialysate flow. *Proc Clin Dial Transplant Forum* 1: 48, 1971

142. Ginn HE, Bugel HJ, James L, Hopkins P: Clinical experience with small surface area dialyzers (SSAD). *Proc Clin Dial Transplant Forum* 1: 53, 1971

143. Rosenzweig J, Babb AL, Vizzo JF, Ginn HE: Large surface area hemodialysis. *Proc Clin Dial Transplant Forum* 1: 56, 1971

144. Funck-Brentano JL: Experience with a new 'open membrane'. *Proc Clin Dial Transplant Forum* 1: 80, 1971

145. Funck-Brentano JL, Sausse A, Man NK, Granger A, Rondon-Nucete M, Zingraff J, Jungers P: Une nouvelle méthode d'hémodialyse associant une membrane à haute perméabilité pour les moyennes molécules et un bain de dialyse en circuit fermé (A new method of haemodialysis with a membrane highly permeable for middle molecules and a closed dialysis fluid circuit). *Proc Eur Dial Transplant Assoc* 9: 55, 1972 (in French)

146. Babb AL, Strand MJ, Uvelli DA, Milutinovic J, Scribner BH: Quantitative description of dialysis treatment: a dialysis index. *Kidney Int* 7 (*Suppl 2*): S23, 1975

147. Babb AL, Strand MJ, Uvelli DA, Scribner BH: The dialysis index. A practical guide to dialysis treatment. *Dial Transplant* 6(9): 9, 1977

148. Von Hartitzsch B, Hoenich NA, Peterson RJ, Buselmeier TJ, Kerr DNS, Kjellstrand CM: Middle molecule clearance in current dialysers. *Proc Eur Dial Transplant Assoc* 10: 522, 1973

149. Kjellstrand CM, Evans RI, Petersen RJ, Rust LW, Shideman J, Buselmeier TJ, Rozelle LT: Considerations of the middle

molecule hypothesis. *Proc Clin Dial Transplant Forum* 2: 127, 1972

150. Shaldon S, Florence P, Fontanier C, Polito C, Mion C: Comparison of two strategies for short dialysis using 1 m² and 2 m² surface area dialysers. *Proc Eur Dial Transplant Assoc* 12: 596, 1975

151. Middle Molecules in Uremia and Other Diseases. Proceedings of the Symposium on Present Status and Future Orientation of Middle Molecules in Uremia and Other Diseases, Avignon, France, November 28–29, 1980. *Artif Organs* 4, Suppl 1981

152. Rosenzweig J, Babb AL, Vizzo JF, Ginn HE: Large surface area hemodialysis. *Proc Clin Dial Transplant Forum* 1: 56, 1971

153. Mirahmadi KS, Kay JH, Miller JH, Gorman JT, Rosen SM: Clinical evaluation of patients dialysed with double Gambro 4 hours, 3 times per week. *Proc Eur Dial Transplant Assoc* 11: 121, 1974

154. Cambi V, Savazzi G, Arisi L, Bignardi L, Bruschi L, Rossi E, Migone L: Short dialysis schedules (SDS) – Finally ready to become routine? *Proc Eur Dial Transplant Assoc* 11: 112, 1974

155. *Proceedings of the Conference on Natural and Synthetic Membranes*, Edited by Saravis C, Gershenkorn K, Brown ME. DHEW (NIH) publ 1967

156. Leonard EF, Colton CK, Craig LD, Gessler RM, Klein E, Lontz JF, Lyman DJ, Mason RG, Nossel HL: Evaluation of membranes for hemodialyzers. *Report of the Membrane Evaluation Study Group for the Artif Kidney-Chronic Uremia Program of NIAMDD* 1974, DHEW publ no (NIH) 74: 605

157. Barbour BH, Bernstein M, Cantor PA, Fischer BS, Stone W Jr: Clinical use of NISR 440 polycarbonate membrane for hemodialysis. *Trans Am Soc Artif Intern Organs* 21: 144, 1975

158. Langlois R, Kaye M: Two year clinical trial of polycarbonate membranes for hemodialysis. *Dial Transplant* 8: 1111, 1979

159. Babb AL, Farrell PC, Strand MJ, Uvelli DA, Milutinovic J, Scribner BH: Residual renal function and chronic hemodialysis therapy. *Proc Clin Dial Transplant Forum* 2: 142, 1972

160. Von Hartitzsch B: The middle molecule in present day hemodialysis. *Proc Clin Dial Transplant Forum* 2: 149, 1972

161. Reiger J, Quellhorst E. Lowitz HD, Kong RG, Scheler F: Ultrafiltration for middle molecules in uraemia. *Proc Eur Dial Transplant Assoc* 11: 158, 1974

162. Milutinovic J, Cutler RE, Hoover P, Meysen B, Scribner BH: Measurement of residual glomerular filtration rate in the patient receiving repetitive hemodialysis. *Kidney Int* 8: 185, 1975

163. Widerøe TE, Grimsrud L, Berg KJ, Godal A, Jansen R, Jörstad S: A mathematical single-pool model for short time haemodialysis. *Proc Eur Dial Transplant Assoc* 11: 136, 1974

164. Keshaviah P, Collins A: Rapid high-efficiency bicarbonate hemodialysis. *Trans Am Soc Artif Intern Organs* 32: 17, 1986

165. Maiorca R, Castellani A, Migozzi G, Panzetta GO, Usberti M: Short time personalised dialysis: good results in spite of high levels of small and middle molecules. *Proc Eur Dial Transplant Assoc* 11: 146, 1974

166. Cambi V, Garini G, Savazzi G, Arisi L, David S, Zanelli P, Bono F, Gardini F: Short dialysis. *Proc Eur Dial Transplant Assoc-Eur Ren Assoc* 20: 111, 1983

167. Daugirdas JT, Ing TS, Humayn HH, Weber DS, Chen WT, Gandhi VC, Reid HH, Hano JE: Two-hour high-surface-area-hemodialysis: a feasibility study. *Int J Artif Organs* 4: 13, 1981

168. Rotellar E, Martinez ME, Plans A, Ferragut A: Haemodialysis: only six hours once a week. *Proc Eur Dial Transplant Assoc-Eur Ren Assoc* 22: 312, 1985

169. Rotellar E, Martinez E, Samsó JM, Barrios J, Simó R, Mulero JF, Perez MD, Bandrés S, Piñol J: Large surface hemodialysis. *Artif Organs* 10: 387, 1986

170. Rotellar E, Martinez E, Samsó JM, Barrios J, Simó R, Mulero JF, Perez D, Bandrés S, Piñol J: Why dialyze more than 6 hours a week? *Trans Am Soc Artif Intern Organs* 31: 538, 1985

171. Drukker W, Alberts Chr, Jungerius NA: Dialysate glucose concentration and plasma osmolality during haemodialysis in acute renal failure. *Proc Eur Dial Transplant Assoc* 2: 7, 1965

172. Cambi V, Buzio C, Arisi L, Calderini C, David S, Manari A, Bono F, Zanelli P: Vascular stability and middle molecules removal in hypertonic haemodiafiltration. *Proc Eur Dial Transplant Assoc* 18: 681, 1981

173. Von Albertini B, Miller JH, Gardner PW. Shinaberger JH: High-flux hemodiafiltration: under six hours/week treatment. *Trans Am Soc Artif Intern Organs* 30: 227, 1984

174. Miller JH, Von Albertini B, Gardner PW, Shinaberger JH: Technical aspects of high-flux hemodiafiltration for adequate short (under 2 hours) treatment. *Trans Am Soc Artif Intern Organs* 30: 377, 1984

175. Manji T, Maeda K, Kawaguchi S, Kobayashi K, Ohta K, Saito A, Amano I, Shimoji T, Fujisaki J: Short time dialysis with 2 m² hollow fibre kidney. *Proc Eur Dial Transplant Assoc* 11: 153, 1974

176. Odaka M, Tabata Y, Kobayashi H, Nomura Y, Soma M, Hirasawa H, Sato H, Suenaga E, Nabeta K: Three-hour maintenance dialysis combining direct haemoperfusion and haemodialysis. *Proc Eur Dial Transplant Assoc* 13: 257, 1976

177. Bergström: Citing Hess Thaysen in Uraemic Toxins. *Proc Eur Dial Transplant Assoc* 12: 579, 1975 (page 584)

178. Kramer P, Broyer M, Brunner FP, Brynger H, Donckerwolcke RA, Jacobs C, Selwood NH, Wing AJ: Combined report on regular dialysis and transplantation in Europe, XII, 1981. *Proc Eur Dial Transplant Assoc* 19: 4, 1982

179. Laurent G, Calemard E, Charra B: Long dialysis: a review of fifteen years experience in one centre (1968–1983). *Proc Eur Dial Transplant Assoc-Eur Ren Assoc* 20: 122, 1983

180. Wizemann V, Mueller K, Kramer W, Schütterle G: Ten years experience with short dialysis: A decade of cardiovascular complications. *Nephrol Dial Transplant* 1: 100, 1986 (Abstract)

181. Raja R, Kramer M, Goldstein S, Caruana R, Lerner A: Short hemodialysis – 10-year follow-up. *Trans Am Soc Artif Intern Organs* 32: 374, 1986

182. Reiger J, Quellhorst E, Lowitz HD, Kong RG, Scheler F: Ultrafiltration for middle molecules in uraemia. *Proc Eur Dial Transplant Assoc* 11: 158, 1974

183. Milutinovic J, Cutler RE, Hoover P, Meysen B, Scribner BH: Measurement of residual glomerular filtration rate in the patient receiving repetitive hemodialysis. *Kidney Int* 8: 185, 1975

184. Gotch F, Sargent JA: A mechanistic analysis of the National Cooperative Dialysis Study (NCDS). *Kidney Int.* 28: 526, 1985

185. Assenat H, Calemard E, Charra B, Laurent G, Terrat JC, Vanel T: Hémodialyse, syndrome du canal carpien et substance amyloide (Haemodialysis, carpal tunnel syndrome and amyloid material). *Nouv Presse Méd* 9: 1715, 1980 (in French)

186. Gejyo F, Yamada T, Odani S, Magakawa Y, Kunitomo T, Kataoka H, Suzuki M, Hirasawa Y, Shirahama T, Cohen AS, Schmid K: A new form of amyloid protein associated with hemodialysis was identified as β_2-microglobulin. *Biochem Biophys Res Comm* 129: 701, 1985

187. Gotch FA: A quantitative evaluation of small and middle molecule toxicity in therapy of uremia. *Dial Transplant* 9: 183, 1980

78   *William Drukker*

188. Bricker NS: On the pathogenesis of the uremic state. An exposition of the 'trade of hypothesis'. *N Engl J Med* 286: 1093, 1972

189. Bergström J, Fürst P: Uremic middle molecules. *Clin Nephrol* 5: 143, 1976

190. Massry SG, Goldstein DA: Role of parathyroid hormone in uremic toxicity. *Kidney Int* 13 (Suppl 8): S39, 1978

191. Massry SG, Goldstein DA: The search for uremic toxin(s) 'X', 'X' = PTH. *Clin Nephrol* 11: 181, 1979

192. Bogin E, Massry SG, Levi J, Djaldetti M, Bristol G, Smith J: Effect of parathyroid hormone on osmotic fragility of human erythrocytes. *J Clin Invest* 69: 1017, 1982

193. Bogin E, Massry SG, Harary I: Effect of parathyroid hormone on rat heart cells. *J Clin Invest* 67: 1215, 1981

194. Bergström J, Fürst P: Uraemic toxins. In: *Replacement of Renal Function by Dialysis,* edited by Drukker W, Parsons FM, Maher JF, 2nd edition, Dordrecht, Boston, Lancaster, Martinus Nijhoff Publ., 1983, p 354

195. Giovannetti S, Biagini M, Cione L: Evidence that methylguanidine is retained in chronic renal failure. *Experientia* 24: 341, 1968

196. Giovannetti S, Barsotti G: Dialysis of methyl guanidine. *Kidney Int* 6: 177, 1974

197. Balestri PL, Barsotti G, Camici M, Giovannetti S: High plasma fibrinogen levels and reduced fibrinolytic activity in dogs intoxicated with methyl guanidine. *Clin Nephrol* 2: 81, 1974

198. Fürst P, Asaba M, Gordon A, Zimmerman L, Bergström J: Middle molecules in uraemia. *Proc Eur Dial Transplant Assoc* 11: 417, 1974

199. Kersting F, Brass H: The effects of uraemic compounds on oxygen consumptions and mechanical activity of isolated guinea pig hearts. *Proc Eur Dial Transplant Assoc* 13: 472, 1976

200. Asaba H, Bergström J, Fürst P, Oulès R, Zimmerman L: Accumulation and excretion of middle molecules. *Proc Eur Dial Transplant Assoc* 13: 481, 1976

201. Dzúrik R, Adam J, Valončová E, Reznìček J, Zvara V: The effect of haemodialysis on blood peptide levels. *Proc Eur Dial Transplant Assoc* 8: 167, 1971

202. Dzúrik R, Božek P, Řezníček J, Oborníková A: Blood level of middle molecular substances during uraemia and haemodialysis. *Proc Eur Dial Transplant Assoc* 10: 263, 1973

203. Dall'Aglio P, Buzio C, Cambi V, Arisi L, Migone L: La rétention de moyennes molecules dans le sérum urémique (Retention of middle molecules in uraemic serum). *Proc Eur Dial Transplant Assoc* 9: 409, 1972 (in French)

204. Migone L, Dall'Aglio P, Buzio C: Middle molecules in uremic serum, urine and dialysis fluid. *Clin Nephrol* 3: 82, 1975

205. Funck-Brentano JL, Man NK, Sausse A: Effect of more porous dialysis membranes on neuropathic toxins. *Kidney Int* 7 (Suppl 2): S52, 1975

206. Man NK, Ferlain B, Paris J, Werner G, Sause A, Funck-Brentano JL: An approach to 'middle molecules: identification in artificial kidney dialysate, with reference to neuropathy prevention. *Trans Am Soc Artif Intern Organs* 19: 320, 1973

207. Man NK, Granger A, Rondon-Nucete M, Zingraff J, Jungers P, Sausse A, Funck-Brentano JL: One year follow-up of short dialysis with a membrane highly permeable to middle molecules. *Proc Eur Dial Transplant Assoc* 10: 236, 1973

208. Man NK, Cueuille G, Zingraff J, Drüeke T, Jungers P, Sausse A, Billon JP, Funck-Brentano JL: Investigations on clinico-chemical correlations in uraemic polyneuritis. *Proc Eur Dial Transplant Assoc* 11: 214, 1974

209. Bergström J, Gordon A, Fürst P, Ryhage R: A study of uremic toxicology. *Proc 7th Annu Contractors Conf Artif Kidney – Chronic Uremia Program of NIAMDD,* edited by Krueger KK, DHEW publ no (NIH) 75: 248, 1974, p 19

210. Bergström J: Uraemic toxicity. *Proc Eur Dial Transplant Assoc* 12: 579, 1975

211. Fürst P, Zimmerman L, Bergström J: Determination of endogenous middle molecules in normal and uremic body fluids. *Clin Nephrol* 5: 178, 1976

212. Bergström J, Fürst P, Zimmerman L: Uremic middle molecules exist and are biologically active. *Clin Nephrol* 11: 229, 1979

213. Zimmerman L, Baldesten A, Bergström J, Fürst P: Isotachophoretic separation of middle molecule peptides in uremic body fluids. *Clin Nephrol* 13: 183, 1980

214. Bergström J, Fürst P: Uraemic toxins. in: *Replacement of Renal Function by Dialysis,* edited by Drukker W, Parsons FM, Maher JF, 1st edition, The Hague, Boston, London, Martinus Nijhoff, 1978, p 334

215. Schoots A, Mikkers F, Cramers C, De Smet R, Ringoir S: Uremic toxins and the elusive middle molecules. *Nephron* 38: 1, 1984

216. Vanholder R, Schoots A, Cramers C, De Smet R, van Landschoot N, Wizemann V, Botella J, Ringoir S: Hippuric acid as a marker. In: *Uremic Toxins,* edited by Ringoir S, Vanholder R, Massry S, New York, Plenum Press, 1987

217. Boumendil-Podevin EF, Podevin RA, Richet G: Uricosuric agents in uremic sera. Identification of indoxyl-sulfate and hippuric acid. *J Clin Invest* 55: 1142, 1975

218. MacNamara PJ, Lalka D, Gibaldi M: Endogenous accumulation products and serum protein binding in uremia. *J Lab Clin Med* 98: 730, 1981

219. Gulyassy PF,, Bottini AT, Stanfel LA, Jarrard EA, Depner TA: Isolation and chemical identification of inhibitors of plasma ligand binding. *Kidney Int.* 30: 391, 1986

220. Vanholder P, Van Landschoot N, De Smet R, Ringoir S: Inhibition of drug protein binding during chronic renal failure. *Kidney Int.* 31: 221, 1987 (Abstract)

221. Charra B, Calemard E, Uzen M, Terrat JC, Laurent G: Carpal tunnel syndrome, shoulder pain and amyloid deposits in longterm haemodialysis patients. *Proc Eur Dial Transplant Assoc-Eur Ren Assoc* 21: 291, 1984

222. Bardin T, Kuntz D, Zingraff J, Noël JH, Droz D, Drüeke T, Funck Brentano JL, Vantelon J, Hiernaux P, Barbanel C, Lucas P: Synovial amyloidosis and beta-2 microglobulin in longterm hemodialysis patients. *Arthritis Rheum* 29: 453, 1986

223. Shirahama T, Cohen AS, Skinner M: Hemodialysis-associated amyloid of β$_2$-microglobulin nature. In: *Amyloidosis,* edited by Makkink J, van Rijswijk MH, Dordrecht, Boston, Lancaster, Martinus Nijhoff 1986, p 83

224. Bardin T, Zingraff J, Kuntz D, Drüeke T: Dialysis-related amyloidosis. *Nephrol Dial Transplant* 1: 151, 1986

225. Jadoul M, Maldague B, Vandenbroucke JM, van Ypersele de Strihou C: The natural history of dialysis-associated amyloid osteoarthropathy. The role of the dialysis membranes. *Nephrol Dial Transplant* 1: 105, 1986 (Abstract)

226. Karlsson FA, Wibell L, Evrin PE: β$_2$-microglobulin in clinical medicine. *Scand J Clin Lab Invest* 40 (Suppl 154): 40, 1980

227. Vandenbroucke JM, Van Ypersele de Strihou C: Relationship between membrane characteristics and dialysis induced changes in β$_2$-microglobulin levels. *Nephrol Dial Transplant* 1: 105, 1986

228. Bergström J, Wehle B: No change in corrected β$_2$-microglobulin concentration after Cuprophane haemodialysis. *Lancet* 1: 628, 1987

229. Lyman D: Membranes. in: *Replacement of Renal Function by Dialysis,* edited by Drukker W, Parsons FM, Maher JF, 2nd edition, Dordrecht, Boston, Lancaster, Martinus Nijhoff, 1983, p 97

230. Ota K, Okazawa T, Kumagaya E, Fujii Y, Kinura M, Nagras Y, Tsukamoto H, Tanzawa H, Sakai Y: Polymethylmethacrylate capillary kidney highly permeable to middle molecules. *Proc Eur Dial Transplant Assoc* 12: 559, 1975

231. Man N-K, Granger A, Rondon-Nucete M, Zingraff J, Jungers P, Sausse A, Funck-Brentano JL: One year follow-up of short dialysis with a membrane highly permeable to middle molecules. *Proc Eur Dial Transplant Assoc* 10: 236, 1973

232. Funck-Brentano JL, Man N-K, Sausse A: Effect of more porous dialysis membrane on neuropathic toxins. *Kidney Int* 7: 52, 1974

233. Funck-Brentano JL, Man N-K: The polyacrylonitrile membrane; use in dialysis with the Rhodial system. Use in haemofiltration. in: *Replacement of Renal Function by Dialysis,* edited by Drukker W, Parsons FM, Maher JF, 2nd edition, Dordrecht, Boston, Lancaster, Martinus Nijhoff, 1983, p 275

234. Göhl H, Konstatin P, Gullberg CA: Hemofiltration membranes. *Contrib Nephrol* 32: 20, 1982

235. Hoenich NA, Kerr DNS: Dialysers. in: *Replacement of Renal function by Dialysis,* edited by Drukker W, Parsons FM, Maher JF, 2nd edition, Dordrecht, Boston, Lancaster, Martinus Nijhoff, 1983 p 118

236. Pizziconi VB, Dorson WJ Jr, Breillat J, Hyde GM, Aniuk LM, Walsh SA, Bland LA, Brady RL: Factors affecting complement activation and neutropenia during dialysis using Cuprophane membranes. *asaio J* 7: 64, 1984

237. Mito M, Niskimura S, Kawai M, Nosé Y, Kawamura T, Yoshimoto C: On extracorporeal circulation of membrane organs (liver, kidney). *Sogoigaku* 17: 538, 1960 (cited in reference 242)

238. Kaplow LS, Goffinet JA: Profound neutropenia during the early phase of hemodialysis. *JAMA* 203: 1135, 1968

239. Papadimitriou M, Baker LRI, Seitanidis B, Sevitt LH, Kulatilake AE: White blood count in patients on regular haemodialysis. *Br Med J* 4: 67, 1969

240. Smith EKM, Jobbins K: Observations on neutropenia associated with haemodialysis. *Br Med J* 4: 70, 1969

241. Gral Th, Schroth Ph, DePalma JR, Gordon A: Leukocyte dynamics with three types of hemodialyzers. *Trans Am Soc Artif Intern Organs* 15: 45, 1969

242. Toren M, Goffinet JA, Kaplow LS: Pulmonary bed sequestration of neutrophils during hemodialysis. *Blood* 36: 337, 1970

243. Brubaker LH, Nolph KD: Mechanisms of recovery from neutropenia induced by hemodialysis. *Blood* 38: 623, 1971

244. Brubaker LH, Jensen D, Johnson L, Nothum R, Nolph K: Kinetics of stagnated-induced neutropenia during hemodialysis. *Trans Am Soc Artif Intern Organs* 18; 305, 1972

245. Craddock PR, Fehr J, Dalmasso AP, Brigham KL, Jacobs HS: Hemodialysis leukopenia: Pulmonary vascular leukostasis resulting from complement activation by dialyzer cellophane membranes. *J Clin Invest* 59: 879, 1977

246. Craddock PR, Fehr J, Brigham KL, Kronenberg RS, Jacobs HS: Complement and leukocyte-mediated pulmonary dysfunction in hemodialysis. *N Engl J Med* 296: 769, 1977

247. Craddock PR, Hammerschmidt DE: Complement mediated granulocyte activation and down-regulation during hemodialysis. *asaio J* 7: 50, 1984

248. Chenoweth DE: Biocompatibility of hemodialysis membranes. Evaluation with C_{3a} anaphylatoxin radioimmunoassays. *asaio J* 7: 44, 1984

249. Sherlock JJ, Ledwith JW, Letteri J: Hypoventilation and hypoxemia during hemodialysis: reflex response to removal of CO_2 across the dialyzer. *Trans Am Soc Artif Intern Organs* 23: 406, 1977

250. Aurigemma NM, Feldman NT, Gotlieb M, Ingram RH, Lazarus JM, Lowrie EG: Arterial oxygenation during hemodialysis. *N Engl J Med* 297: 871, 1977

251. Patterson RW, Nissenson AR, Miller J, Smith RT, Narins RG, Sullivan SP: Hypoxemia and pulmonary gas exchange during hemodialysis. *J Appl Physiol Respir Environ Exercise Physiol* 50: 259, 1981

252. Xabte B, Carter R, Shamebo M, Veicht J, Boulton Jones JM: Dialysis induced hypoxemia. *Clin Nephrol* 18: 120, 1982

253. Schaefer K, von Herrath D, Hüfler M: Stable PO_2 during hemofiltration in spite of a drop in leukocytes. *Nephron* 32: 377, 1982 (Letter to the editor)

254. Romaldini H, Rodriguez-Roisin R, Lopez FA, Ziegler TW, Bencowitz HZ, Wagner PD: The mechanisms of arterial hypoxemia during hemodialysis. *Annu Rev Respir Dis* 129: 780, 1984

255. Dolan MJ, Whipp BJ, Davidson WD, Weitzman RE, Wasserman K: Hypopnea associated with acetate hemodialysis: carbon dioxide flow dependent ventilation. *N Engl J Med* 305: 72, 1981

256. Klinkmann H: Biocomptability. *Proc Eur Dial Transplant Assoc-Eur Ren Assoc* 22: 223, 1985

257. Ringoir S, Vanholder R: An introduction to biocomptability. *Artif Organs* 10: 20, 1986

258. Knudsen F, Nielsen AH, Pedersen JO, Jersild C: Haemodialysis induced activation of complement, relates also to individual responsiveness. *Int J Artif Organs* 8: 233, 1985

259. Wegmüller E, Montandon A, Nydegger A, Descoeudres C: Biocomptability of different hemodialysis membranes: activation of complement and leukopenia. *Int J Artif Org* 9: 85, 1986

260. Levett DL, Woffinden C, Bird AG, Hoenich NA, Ward MK, Kerr DNS: Complement activation in haemodialysis: a comparison of new and re-used dialysers. *Int J Artif Organs* 9: 97, 1986

261. Göhl H, Schaefer K, Gullberg CA: Hemofiltration with different type of membranes. *Proc Eur Soc Artif Organs* 6: 180, 1979

262. Hörl WH, Schaefer RM, Heidland A: Effect of different dialysers on proteinases and proteinase inhibitors during hemodialysis. *Am J Nephrol* 5: 320, 1985

263. Bosch Th, Schmidt B, Spencer PC, Samtleben W, Pelger M, Baurmeister U, Gurland J: Ex vivo biocomptability evaluation of a new modified cellulose membrane. *Proc Int Soc Artif Organs* 1985 (in press)

264. Falkenhagen D, Zinner G, Falkenhagen U, Ahrenholz P, Holtz M, Behm E, Klinkmann H: A modified cellulose membrane (MC) with reduced complement activation. *Kidney Int* 28: 331, 1985 (Abstract)

265. Peterson PA, Evrin PE, Berggard L: Differentiation of glomerular, tubular and normal proteinuria. Determinations of urinary excretion of β_2 microglobulin, albumin and total protein. *J Clin Invest* 48: 1189, 1969

266. Bienenstock J, Poortman J: Renal clearance of 15 proteins in renal disease. *J Lab Clin Med* 75: 297, 1970

267. Maack TH: Renal handling of low molecular weight proteins. *Am J Med* 58: 57, 1975

268. Röckel A, Gilge U, Ohl B, Liewald A, Heidland A: *Contr Nephrol* 32: 40, 1982

269. Messner RP: β_2-microglobulin: an old molecule assumes a new look. *J Lab Clin Med* 104: 141, 1984

270. Gejyo F, Homma N, Suzuki Y, Arakawa M: Serum levels of β_2-microglobulin as a new form of amyloid protein in patients undergoing long-term hemodialysis. *N Engl J Med* 314–585, 1986

271. Vincent C, Révillard JP, Galland M, Traeger J: Serum beta-2 microglobilin in hemodialyzed patients. *Nephron* 21: 260, 1978

272. Forêt M, Milongo R, Meftahi H, Dechelette E, Hachache T, Kuentz F, Renversez JC, Cordonnier D: Plasma levels of $\beta_2$microglobulin in a population of 151 patients on haemodialysis. *Nephrol Dial Transplant* 1: 105, 1986 (Abstract)

273. Bommer J, Seelig HP, Seelig R, Ritz E: $\beta_2$microglobulin (β_2m) levels in haemodialysed patients. *Nephrol Dial Transplant* 1: 106, 1986

274. Chanard J, Lavaud S, Toupance O, Melin JP, Gillery P: β_2-microglobulin – associated amyloidosis in chronic haemodialysis patients. *Lancet* 1: 1212, 1986

275. Floege J, Granolleras C, Deschodt G, Branger B, Oulès R, Shaldon S, Koch KM: β_2-microglobulin kinetics during haemodialysis and haemofiltration. *Nephrol Dial Transplant* 1: 107, 1986 (Abstract)

276. Ackrill P, Robinson EL, Hill K, McClure JC: Removal of β_2-microglobulin in the relief of shoulder pain in long-term haemodialysis patients. *Nephrol Dial Transplant* 1: 58, 1986 (Abstract)

277. Higgins MR, Grace M, Bettcher KB, Silverberg DS, Dossetor JB: Blood access in hemodialysis. *Clin Nephrol* 6: 473, 1976

278. Bell PRF, Calman KC: *Surgical Aspects of Haemodialysis.* Edinburgh, London, Churchill Livingstone, 1974

279. Foran RF, Shore E, Levin PM, Freiman RL: Vascular access for hemodialysis. in: *Clinical Aspects of Uremia and Dialysis,* edited by Massry SG, Sellers AL, Springfield IL, Charles C. Thomas, 1976, p 504

280. Ramirez O, Swartz C, Onesti G, Mailloux L, Brest AN: The winged in line shunt. *Trans Am Soc Artif Intern Organs* 12: 220, 1966

281. Thomas GI: A large-vessel applique A-V shunt for hemodialysis. *Trans Am Soc Artif Intern Organs* 15: 288, 1969

282. Thomas GI: The femoral shunt to-day. *Dial Transplant* 2(1): 23, 1973

283. Buselmeier TJ, Kjellstrand CM, Simmons RL, Duncan DA, Von Hartitzsch B, Rattazzi LC, Leonard AS; Najarian JS: A totally new subcutaneous prosthetic arteriovenous shunt. *Trans Am Soc Artif Intern Organs* 19: 25, 1973

284. Buselmeier TJ, Kjellstrand CM, Quinton WE, Von Hartitzsch B, Meyer RM, Shideman JR, Bosl BM, Toledo LH, Spanos PK, McCosh TM, Simmons RL, Najarian JS: The Buselmeier shunt. *Dial Transplant* 3(1): 30, 1974

285. May J, Tiller D, Johnson J, Stewart J, Sheil AGR: Saphenous vein arteriovenous fistula in regular dialysis treatment. *N Engl J Med* 280: 770, 1969

286. Chinitz JL, Yokoyama T, Bower R, Swartz C: Self-sealing prosthesis for arteriovenous fistula in man. *Trans Am Soc Artif Intern Organs* 18: 452, 1972

287. Chinitz J, Bower R, Yokoyama T, Del Guercio E, Kim K, Swartz C: Further experience with a self-sealing prosthesis for A-V fistula. *Abstracts Am Soc Artif Intern Organs* 2: 12, 1973

288. Richie RE, Johnson K, Walker PJ, Staab EV, Ginn HE: Use of bovine xenograft for problems in vascular access. *Abstracts Am Soc Artif Intern Organs* 2: 54, 1973

289. VanderWerff BA, Rattazzi LC, Katzman HA, Schild AF: Three year experience with bovine graft arteriovenous (A-V) fistulas in 100 patients. *Trans Am Soc Artif Intern Organs* 21: 296, 1975

290. Beemer RK, Hayes JF: Hemodialysis using a mandril grown graft. *Trans Am Soc Artif Intern Organs* 19: 43, 1973

291. Flores L, Dunn I, Frumkin E, Forte R, Requena R, Ryan J, Knopf M, Kirschner·J, Levowitz BS: Dacron arteriovenous shunts for vascular access in hemodialysis. *Trans Am Soc Artif Intern Organs* 19: 33, 1973

292. Baker LD Jr, Johnson JM, Goldfarb D: Expanded polytetra-fluoroethylene (PTFE) subcutaneous arteriovenous conduit: an improved vascular access for chronic hemodialysis. *Trans Am Soc Artif Intern Organs* 22: 382, 1976

293. Kaplan MS, Mirahmadi KS, Winer RL, Gorman JT, Dabirvaziri N, Rosen SM: Comparison of 'PTFE' and bovine grafts for blood access in dialysis patients. *Trans Am Soc Artif Intern Organs* 22: 388, 1976

294. Buselmeier TJ, Rynasiewicz JJ, Sutherland DER, Howard KJ, David TD, Mauer SM, Simmons RL, Najarian JS, Kjellstrand CM: A prosthesis for blood access in patients with thrombosis of peripheral vasculature. *Dial Transplant* 6 (8): 48, 1977

295. Mindich BP, Silverman MJ, Elguezabal A, Levowitz BS: Umbilical cord vein fistula for vascular access in hemodialysis. *Trans Am Soc Artif Intern Organs* 21: 273, 1975

296. Kester RC: Vascular access for the problem patient. In *Dialysis Review,* edited by Davison AM, Tunbridge Wells, Kent, UK, Pitman Medical Publishing Co Ltd, 1978, p 106

297. Brunner FP, Brynger H, Chantler C, Donkerwolcke RA, Hathway RA, Selwood NH, Wing AJ: Combined report on regular dialysis and transplantation in Europe IX. *Proc Eur Dial Transplant Assoc* 16: 3, 1979

298. Golding AL, Nissenson AR, Higgins R, Raible D: Carbon transcutaneous access device (CTAD). *Trans Am Soc Artif Intern Organs* 26: 105, 1980

299. Martinez FJ, Cosentino LC: Blood access without skin puncture. *Trans Am Soc Artif Intern Organs* 27: 308, 1981

300. Reed WP, Light PD, Sadler JH, Ramos E: Alternative vascular access in patients lacking veins for standard arteriovenous fistulae. *Proc Eur Dial Transplant Assoc-Eur Ren Assoc* 21: 257, 1984

301. Bonalumi U, Simoni GA, Friedman D, Borzone E, Griffanti-Bartoli F: Initial experience with Hemasite vascular access device for maintenance haemodialysis. *Proc Eur Dial Transplant Assoc-Eur Ren Assoc* 21: 262, 1984

302. Smits PJH, Slooff MJH, Lichtendahl DHE, VanderHem GK: The Biocarbon® vascular access device (DiaTAB®) for haemodialysis. *Proc Eur Dial Transplant Assoc-Eur Ren Assoc* 21: 267, 1984

303. Uldall PR, Dyck RF, Woods F, Merchant N, Martin GS, Cardella CT, Sutton D, deVeber GA: A subclavian cannula for temporary vascular access of hemodialysis or plasmapheresis. *Dial Transplant* 8: 963, 1979

304. Uldall PR, Woods F, Merchant N, Bird M, Chrichton E: Two years experience with the subclavian cannula for temporary vascular access for hemodialysis and plasmapheresis. *Proc Clin Dial Transplant Forum* 9: 32, 1979

305. Uldall PR, Woods F, Merchant N, Chrichton E, Carter H: A double-lumen subclavian cannula (DLSC) for temporary hemodialysis access. *Trans Am Soc Artif Intern Organs* 26: 91, 1980

306. Kopp KF, Gutch CF, Kolff WJ: Single needle dialysis. *Trans Am Soc Artif Intern Organs* 18: 75, 1972

307. Keshaviah PR, Shaldon S: Haemodialysis monitors and monitoring. in: *Replacement of Renal Function by Dialysis,* edited by Drukker W, Parsons FM, Maher JF, 2nd edition Dordrecht, Boston, Lancaster, Martinus Nijhoff, 1983, p 223

308. Ringoir S, de Broe M, Cardon M, van Waelighem JP, Boone L: New pump system for one needle hemodialysis. *Eur Dial Transplant Assoc* (Abstract) 10: 200, 1973

309. Vanholder R, Hoenich N, Piron M, Billiouw JM, Ringoir S: Haemodialysis in a single and two needle vascular access system: a comparative review. *Proc Eur Dial Transplant Assoc-Eur Renal Assoc* 20: 176, 1983

310. Bergström J, Asaba H, Fürst P, Oulès R: Dialysis, ultrafiltration and blood pressure. *Proc Eur Dial Transplant Assoc* 13: 293, 1976

311. Shaldon S: Discussion *Proc Eur Dial Transplant Assoc* 13: 300, 1976

312. Jones EO, Ward MK, Hoenich NA, Kerr DNS: Separation of dialysis and ultrafiltration – Does it really help? *Proc Eur Dial Transpl Assoc* 14: 160, 1977

313. Ivanovich P, Huang C, Stefanovic N, Del Greco F: A useful adjunct to dialysis. *Proc Eur Dial Transplant Assoc* 14: 605, 1977

314. Blaney TL, Lindan O, Sparks RE: Adsorption: a step toward a wearable artificial kidney. *Trans Am Soc Artif Intern Organs* 12: 7, 1966

315. Jützler GA, Keller HE, Klein J, Carius J, Floss K, Dijckmans J, Fürsattel L, Leppla W: Physico-chemical investigations in regeneration of dialysis fluid. *Proc Eur Dial Transplant Assoc* 3: 265, 1966

316. Twiss EE, Paulssen MMP: Dialysis-system incorporating the use of activated charcoal. *Proc Eur Dial Transplant Assoc* 3: 262, 1966

317. Van Leer E: *Hemodialyse met Koolstofadsorptie* (Haemodialysis with charcoal adsorption). MD Thesis 1970 Univ. of Rotterdam, Drukkerij Bronder-Offset NV (in Dutch)

318. Gordon A, Greenbaum MA, Marantz LB, McArthur MJ, Maxwell MH: A sorbent-based low volume recirculating dialysate system. *Trans Am Soc Artif Intern Organs* 15: 347, 1969

319. Gordon A, Gral T, DePalma JR, Greenbaum MA, Marantz LB, McArthur MJ, Maxwell MH: A sorbent-based low volume dialysate system: preliminary studies in human subjects. *Proc Eur Dial Transplant Assoc* 7: 63, 1970

320. Gordon A, Better OS, Greenbaum MA, Marantz LB, Gral T, Maxwell MH: Clinical maintenance hemodialysis with a sorbent-based low volume dialysate regeneration system. *Trans Am Soc Artif Intern Organs* 17: 253, 1971

321. Greenbaum MA, Gordon A: A regenerative dialysis supply system. *Dial Transplant* 1 (1): 18, 1972

322. Drukker W: Introduction to the Redy system. Two long-term patients. *Nieren- u Hochdruckkrankheiten 5, (Suppl)*: 3, 1976

323. Drukker W, Parsons FM, Gordon A: Practical application of dialysate regeneration: the Redy system. in: *Replacement of Renal Function by Dialysis*, edited by Drukker W, Parsons FM, Maher JF, 2nd edition The Hague, Boston, London, Martinus Nijhoff, 1978, p 244

324. Briefel GR, Hutchisson JT, Galonsky RS, Hessert RL, Friedman EA: Compact travel hemodialysis system. *Proc Clin Dial Transplant Forum* 5: 61, 1975

325. Jacobsen SC, Stephen RL, Bulloch EC, Luntz RD, Kolff WJ: A wearable artificial kidney: functional description of hardware and clinical results. *Proc Clin Dial Transplant Forum* 5: 65, 1975

326. Stephen RL, Jacobsen SC, Atkin Thor E, Kolff WJ: Portable wearable artificial kidney (WAK) – initial evaluation. *Proc Eur Dial Transplant Assoc* 12: 511, 1975

327. Delano B, Friedman EA: Regular dialysis treatment. The portable suitcase kidney. in: *Replacement of Renal Function by Dialysis*, edited by Drukker W, Parsons FM, Maher JF, 1st edition, The Hague, Boston, London, Martinus Nijhoff, 1978, p 431

328. Kolff WJ: The future of dialysis. The WAK. in: *Replacement of Renal Function by Dialysis*, chapter 42, edited by Drukker W, Parsons FM, Maher JF, 1st edition, The Hague, Boston, London, Martinus Nijhoff, 1978, p 708

329. Scribner BH: Substitution of bicarbonate for acetate in the dialysate for the care of a critically ill patient. *Dial Transplant* 6(3): 26, 1977

330. Samar RE: Bicarbonate and acetate hemodialysis. *Contemp Dial*, August 1981, p 10

331. Tolchin DO: Acetate metabolism and high efficiency hemodialysis. *Int J Artif Organs* 2: 1, 1979

332. Gotch FA, Sargent JA, Keen M, Lam M, Prowitt M: The solute kinetics of intermittent dialysis therapy. *Proc 11th Annu Contractor's Conf Artif Kidney Program of NIAMDD*, edited by Mackey BB. DHEW publication no (NIH) 79–144, 1978, p 110

333. Muirhead EE, Reid AF: A resin artificial kidney. *J Lab Clin Med* 33: 841, 1948

334. Yatzidis H: A convenient haemoperfusion micro-apparatus over charcoal for the treatment of endogenous and exogenous intoxications, its use as an active artificial kidney. *Proc Eur Dial Transplant Assoc* 1: 83, 1964

335. Smakman R, Van Doorn AWJ, van Berlo A: Promising in-vitro results with a new urea sorbent. *Life Support Systems* (Suppl 2): 264, 1986

336. Smakman R, Van Doorn AWJ: Urea removal by means of direct binding. *Clin Nephrol* 26 Suppl. 1: S58, 1986

337. Chang TMS: Micro capsule artificial kidney in replacement of renal function: with emphasis on adsorbent hemoperfusion. in: *Replacement of Renal Function by Dialysis*, edited by Drukker W, Parsons FM, Maher JM 1st edition The Hague, Boston, London, Martinus Nijhoff, 1978, p 217

338. Winchester J: Evolution of artificial organs: Extracorporeal removal of drugs. *Artif Organs* 10: 316, 1986

339. Winchester JF, Apiliga MT, Mackay JM, Kennedy AC: Haemodialysis with charcoal haemoperfusion. *Proc Eur Dial Transplant Assoc* 12: 526, 1975

340. Winchester JF, Apiliga MT, Kennedy AC: Short term evaluation of charcoal hemoperfusion combined with dialysis in uremic patients. *Kidney Int* 10 (Suppl 7): S315, 1976

341. Winchester JF: Symposium on sorbents in uremia: Part 4. Comparison of charcoal hemoperfusion with hemodialysis. *Dial Transplant* 6(9): 46, 1977

342. Ballardie FW, Kerr DNS, Tennent G, Pepys MB: Haemodialysis versus CAPD: equal disposition to amyloidosis? *Lancet* 1: 795, 1986 (Letter to the Editor)

343. Kanwashi N, Tsuchiya T, Sugiyama M, Nishiki M, Ochi K: Elimination of low molecular weight proteins during hemoperfusion of dialysis patients using a urethane sheet embedded with powdered charcoal. *Trans Am Soc Artif Intern Organs* 32: 425, 1986

344. Chang TMS: Haemoperfusion over micro-encapsulated adsorbent in a patient with hepatic coma. *Lancet* 2: 1371, 1972

345. Williams R: Approaches to the development of artificial liver support. in: *Artificial Organs*, edited by Kennedy RM, Courtney JM, Gaylor JDS, Gilchrist T, London and Basingstoke, Macmillan Press, 1977, p 403

346. Winchester JF: Hemoperfusion. in: *Replacement of Renal Function by Dialysis*, edited by Drukker W, Parsons FM, Maher JF, 2nd edition, Dordrecht, Boston MA, Lancaster, Martinus Nijhoff, 1983, p 316

347. Henderson LW, Besarab A, Michaels A, Bluemle LW Jr:

Blood purification by ultrafiltration and fluid replacement (diafiltration). *Trans Am Soc Artif Intern Organs* 12: 216, 1967

348. Brull L: L'ultrafiltration in vivo (Ultrafiltration in vivo). *C R Soc Biol* (Paris) 99: 1607, 1928 (in French)

349. Manis T, Friedman EA: Dialytic therapy for irreversible uremia. *N Engl J Med* 301: 1254, 1321, 1979

350. Hamilton R, Ford C, Colton C, Cross R, Steinmuller S, Henderson L: Blood cleansing by diafiltration in uremic dog and man. *Trans Am Soc Artif Intern Organs* 17: 259, 1971

351. Henderson LW, Livoti LG, Ford CA, Kelly AB, Lysaght MJ: Clinical experience with intermittent hemodiafiltration. *Trans Am Soc Artif Intern Organs* 19: 119, 1973

352. Henderson LW, Colton CK, Ford C: Kinetics of hemodiafiltration. II Clinical characterization of a new blood cleansing modality. *J Lab Clin Med* 85: 372, 1975

353. Quellhorst E, Rieger J, Doht B, Beckmann H, Jacob I, Kraft B, Mietzsch G, Scheler F: Treatment of chronic uraemia by an ultrafiltration kidney. First clinical experience. *Proc Eur Dial Transplant Assoc* 13: 314, 1976

354. Quellhorst EA: Ultrafiltration and haemofiltration, practical applications. in: *Replacement of Renal Function by Dialysis*, edited by Drukker W, Parsons FM, Maher JF, 2nd edition, Dordrecht, Boston, Lancaster, Martinus Nijhoff, 1983, p 265

355. Henderson LW, Ford C, Bluemle LW, Bixler HJ: Uremic blood cleansing by diafiltration using a hollow fiber ultrafilter. *Trans Am Soc Artif Intern Organs* 16: 107, 1970

356. Baldamus CA, Schoeppe W, Koch KM: Comparison of haemodialysis (HD) and post dilution haemofiltration (HF) on an unselected dialysis population. *Proc Eur Dial Transplant Assoc* 15: 228, 1978

357. Shaldon S, Beau MC, Claret G, Deschodt G, Oulès R, Ramperez P, Mion H, Mion C: Haemofiltration with sorbent regeneration of ultrafiltrate: first clinical experience in end stage renal disease. *Proc Eur Dial Transplant Assoc* 15: 220, 1978

358. Kramer P, Wigger W, Matthaei D, Scheler F: Arteriovenous hemofiltration. A new and simple method for overhydrated patients resistant to diuretics. *Klin Wochenschrift* 55: 1121, 1977

359. Kaplan AE: Clinical trials with predilution and vacuum suction. Enhancing the efficiency of the CAVH treatment. *Trans Am Soc Artif Organs* 32: 49, 1986

360. Major RH: *A History of Medicine II*, Springfield, IL, Charles C. Thomas, 1954, p 916

361. Schwab PJ, Fahey JL: Treatment of Waldenström macroglobulinemia by plasmapheresis. *N Engl J Med* 263: 574, 1960

362. Rees AJ: Plasma exchange: principles and practice. in: *Replacement of Renal Function by Dialysis*, edited by Drukker W, Parsons FM, Maher JF, 2nd edition, Dordrecht, Boston, Lancaster, Martinus Nijhoff, 1983, p 872

363. Samtleben W, Blumenstein M, Gurland HJ: Membrane plasma separation: advantages and hazards. *Eur Dial Transplant Assoc* Abstracts XVIIth Congress, Prague 1980, p 84

364. Sprenger K, Franz HE: Membrane plasma separation (MPS): procedural recommendations. *Proc Eur Dial Transplant Assoc* 17: 353, 1980

365. Omokawa S, Malchesky PS, Sakamoto H, Flynn A, Lofters MA, Nosé Y: Changes in interleukin-1 during membrane plasmapheresis. *Trans Am Soc Intern Artif Organs* 32: 392, 1986

366. Peters DK, Rees AJ, Lockwood CM: Plasma exchange in glomerular and related auto-allergic diseases. *Proc Eur Dial Transplant Assoc* 14: 409, 1977

367. Houwert DK, Kater L, Hené RJ, Struyvenberg A: Plasma exchange in immune complex disease. *Proc Eur Dial Transplant Assoc* 16: 520, 1979

368. Ota K, Amemiya H, Sugino N, Abe M, Ono T, Kowai S, Yamana T: Double filtration plasmapheresis. *Trans Am Soc Artif Intern Organs* 26: 406, 1980

369. International symposium on plasma exchange, abstracts. *Nieren u Hochdruckkrankheiten* 9: 136, 1980

370. Balow JE: Plasmapheresis and application in treatment of renal disorders. *Artif Organs* 10: 324, 1986

371. Lysaght MJ, Samtleben W, Schmidt B, Gurland HJ: Closed loop plasmapheresis. In: *Therapeutic Hemapheresis*, edited by MacPherson JL, Kaspirin DO, Boca Raton, FL, CCR Press, 1985, p 138

372. Smit JW, Kayashima K, Kutsume C, Abe Y, Matsubara A, Malchesky PS, Krakauer RS, Nosé Y: Cryopheresis: immunochemical modulation and clinical response in auto-immune disease. *Trans Am Soc Intern Artif Organs* 28: 391, 1982

373. Lockwood CM, Rees AJ, Peason TA, Evans D, Peters DK: Immunosuppression and plasma exchange in the treatment of Goodpasture's syndrome. *Lancet* 1: 711, 1976

374. Pusey CD, Lockwood CM, Peters DK: Plasma exchange and immunopressive drugs in the treatment of glomerulonephritis due to antibodies to the glomerular basement membrane. *Int J Artif Organs* 6: 15, 1983

375. Anonymous: Hazards of apheresis. *Lancet* 2: 1025, 1982 (Editorial)

376. Lindner A, Charra B, Sherrard DJ, Scribner BH: Accelerated atherosclerosis in prolonged maintenance hemodialysis. *N Engl J Med* 290: 697, 1974

377. Bagdade JD, Porte D Jr, Bierman EL: Hypertriglyceridemia: a metabolic consequence of chronic renal failure. *N Engl J Med* 279: 181, 1968

378. Bagdade JD, Shafrir E, Wilson DE: Mechanism(s) of hyperlipidemia in chronic uremia. *Trans Am Soc Artif Intern Organs* 22: 42, 1976

379. Savdie E, Gibson JC, Crawford GA, Simons LA, Mahony JF: Impaired plasma triglyceride clearance as a feature of both uremic and posttransplant triglyceridemia. *Kidney Int* 18: 774, 1980

380. Bagdade JD: Hyperlipidemia and atherosclerosis in chronic dialysis patients. in: *Replacement of Renal Function by Dialysis*, 2nd edition edited by Drukker W, Parsons FM, Maher JF, Dordrecht, Boston, Lancaster, Martinus Nijhoff, 1983, p 588

381. Gnasso A, Haberbosch W, Augustin J, Ritz E: Abnormal lipoprotein metabolism in incipient renal failure. *Proc Eur Dial Transplant Assoc-Eur Renal Assoc* 22: 1129, 1985

382. Heuck LCh, Ritz E: Hyperlipoproteinemia in renal insufficiency. *Nephron* 25: 1, 1980

383. Swamy AP, Cestero RVM, Campbell RG, Freeman RB: Long term effect of dialysate glucose on the lipid levels of maintenance hemodialysis patients. *Trans Am Soc Artif Intern Organs* 22: 54, 1976

384. Gonzalez FM, Pearson JE, Garbus SB, Holbert RD: On the effects of acetate during hemodialysis. *Trans Am Soc Artif Intern Organs* 20a: 169, 1974

385. Boyle IT: Vitamin D and the kidney. *Proc Eur Dial Transplant Assoc* 12: 113, 1975

386. Pappenheimer AM, Wilens SL: Enlargement of parathyroid glands in renal disease. *Am J Pathol* 11: 73, 1935

387. Pappenheimer AM: Effect of reduction of kidney substance upon parathyroid glands and skeletal tissue. *J Exp Med* 64: 965, 1936

388. Liu SH, Chu HI: Studies of calcium and phosphorus metabolism with special reference to pathogenesis and effects of

dihydrotachysterol (AT10) and iron. *Medicine (Baltimore)* 22: 103, 1943

389. Nicolaysen R: Studies upon the mode of action of vitamin D_3. III The influence of vitamin D on the absorption of calcium and phosphorus in the rat. *Biochem J* 31: 122, 1937

390. Bauer GCH, Carlsson A, Lindquist B: Evaluation of accretion, resorption and exchange reactions in the skeleton. *Kungliga Fysiografiska, Sallskapet I Lund Forhandlinger* 25: 3, 1955

391. Lund J, DeLuca HF: Biologically active metabolite of vitamin D_3 from bone, liver and blood serum. *J Lipid Res* 7: 739, 1966

392. Trummel GL, Raisz LG, Blunt JW: 25-Hydroxycholecalciferol: stimulation of bone resorption on tissue culture. *Science* 163: 1450, 1969

393. DeLuca HF: The kidney as an endocrine organ for the production of 1,25-hydroxyvitamin D_3, a calcium-mobilizing hormone. *N Engl J Med* 298: 359, 1973

394. Bhattacharyya MH, DeLuca HF: The regulation of rat calciferol 25-hydroxylase. *J Biol Chem* 248: 2969, 1973

395. Fraser DR, Kodicek E: Unique biosynthesis by kidney of a biologically active vitamin D metabolite. *Nature* 228: 764, 1970

396. Kodicek E: Recent advances in vitamin D metabolism. 1,25-dihydroxycholecalciferol, a kidney hormone controlling calcium metabolism. *Clinics in Endocrinology and Metabolism* 1 no. 1 edited by McIntyre I, London, Philadelphia, Toronto, Saunders Comp Ltd, 1972, p 305.

397. Holick MF, Schnoes HK, DeLuca HF: Identification of 1,25-dihydroxycholecalciferol; a form of vitamin D_3 metabolically active in the intestine. *Proc Natl Acad Sci USA* 68: 803, 1971

398. Holick MF, Schnoes HK, DeLuca HF: Identification of 1,25-dihydroxycholecalciferol: a metabolite of vitamin D active in intestine. *Biochemistry* 10: 2799, 1971

399. Reeve J: Therapeutic applications of vitamin D analogues. *Br Med J* 2: 888, 1979

400. Velentzas C, Oreopoulos DG: 1,25-dihydroxyvitamin D_3 and osteomalacia: some unanswered questions. *Int J Artif Organs* 3: 313, 1980

401. Ward MK, Feest TG, Ellis HA, Parkinson IS, Kerr DNS, Herrington J, Goode GL: Osteomalacic dialysis osteodystrophy: evidence for a water borne aetiological agent, probably aluminium. *Lancet* 1: 84, 1978

402. Marsden SNE, Parkinson IS, Ward MK, Ellis HA, Kerr DNS: Evidence for aluminium accumulation in renal failure. *Proc Eur Dial Transplant Assoc* 16: 588, 1979

403. Alfrey AC, Miskell JM, Burks J, Contiguglia SR, Rudolph H, Lewin E, Holmes JH: Syndrome of dispraxia and multifocal seizures associated with chronic hemodialysis. *Trans Am Soc Artif Intern Organs* 18: 257, 1972

404. Spofforth J: Case of aluminium poisoning. *Lancet* 1: 1301, 1921

405. Alfrey AC, LeGendre GR, Kaehny WD: The dialysis encephalopathy syndrome. Possible aluminum intoxication. *N Engl J Med* 294: 184, 1976

406. Parkinson IS, Beckett A, Ward MK, Feest TG, Hoenich N, Strong A, Kerr DNS: Aluminium removal from water supplies. *Proc Eur Dial Transplant Assoc* 15: 586, 1978

407. Flendrig JA, Kruis H, Das AH: Aliminium intoxication: the cause of dialysis dementia? *Proc Eur Dial Transplant Assoc* 13: 355, 1976

408. Flendrig JA, Kruis H, Das AH: Aliminium and dialysis dementia. *Lancet* 1: 1235, 1976

409. Elliott HL, Macdougall AI: Aluminium studies in dialysis encephalopathy. *Proc Eur Dial Transplant Assoc* 15: 157, 1978

410. Platts MM, Goode GC, Hislop JS: Composition of the domestic water supply and the incidence of fractures and encephalopathy in patients on home dialysis. *Br Med J* 2: 657, 1977

411. Davison AM, Giles GR: The effect of transplantation on dialysis encephalopathy. *Proc Eur Dial Transplant Assoc* 16: 407, 1979

412. Wing AJ, Brunner FP, Brynger H, Chantler C, Donckerwolcke RA, Gurland HJ, Jacobs C, Kramer P, Selwood H: Dialysis dementia in Europe (Report of the Registration Committee of the European Dialysis and Transplant Association). *Lancet* 2: 190, 1980

413. Pierides AM, Edwards JWG, Cullum UX Jr, McCale JT, Ellis HA: Hemodialysis encephalopathy with osteomalacic fractures and muscle weakness. *Kidney Int* 18: 115, 1980

414. Short AIK, Winney RJ, Robson JS: Reversible microcytic hypochromic anaemia in dialysis patients due to aluminium intoxication. *Proc Eur Dial Transplant Assoc* 17: 226, 1980

415. Kaehny WD, Alfrey AC, Holman RE, Shorr WJ: Aluminum transfer during hemodialysis. *Kidney Int* 12: 361, 1977

416. Gacek EM, Babb AL, Uvelli DA, Fry DL, Scribner BH: Dialysis dementia: the role of dialysate pH in altering the dialyzability of aluminum. *Trans Am Soc Artif Intern Organs* 25: 409, 1979

417. Berlyne GM, Ben-Ari J, Pest D, Weinberger J, Stern M, Gilmore GR, Levine R: Hyperaluminaemia from aluminium resins in renal failure. *Lancet* 2: 494, 1970

418. Berlyne GM: Aluminum toxicity in renal failure. *Int J Artif Organs* 3: 60, 1980

419. Ulmer DD: Toxicity from aluminum antacids (Editorial). *N Engl J Med* 294: 184, 1976

420. Dewberry FL, McKinney PD, Stone WJ: The dialysis dementia syndrome: report of fourteen cases and review of the literature. *asaio J* 3: 102, 1980

421. Bournerias F, Monnier N, Reveillaud RJ: Risk of orally administered aluminium hydroxide and results of withdrawal. *Proc Eur Dial Transplant Assoc-Eur Ren Assoc* 20: 207, 1983

422. Graf H, Stumvoll HK, Meisinger V, Kovarik J, Woll A, Pinggera WF: Aluminum removal by hemodialysis. *Kidney Int* 19: 587, 1981

423. Slatopolsky F, Weerts C, Lopez-Hilker S, Norwood K, Zink M, Windus D, Delmez J: Calcium carbonate as a phosphate binder in patients with chronic renal failure undergoing dialysis. *N Engl J Med* 315: 157, 1986

424. Raine AEG, Oliver DO: Management of hyperphosphataemia in renal dialysis patients. *Lancet* 1: 633, 1987

425. Schneider H, Kulbe KD, Weber H, Streicher E: High effective aluminium free phosphate binder. In vitro and in vivo studies. *Proc Eur Dial Transplant Assoc-Eur Ren Assoc* 20: 725, 1983

426. Levick SE: Dementia from aluminum pots? (Letter to the editor). *N Engl J Med* 303: 164, 1980

427. Trapp GA, Cannon JB: Aluminum pots as a source of dietary aluminum (Letter to the editor). *N Engl J Med* 304: 172, 1981

428. Koning JH: Aluminum pots as a source of dietary aluminum (Letter to the editor). *N Engl J Med* 304: 172, 1981

429. Platts MM, Anastassiades E: Dialysis encephalopathy: precipitating factors and improvement in prognosis. *Clin Nephrol* 15: 223, 1981

430. Cournot-Witmer G: Aluminum osteopathy. *Contr Nephrol* 38: 59, 1984

431. Botella J, Callego JL, Fernandez-Fernandez J, Sans-Guajardo D, de Miguel A, Ramos J, Franco P, Enriques R, Sanz-Moreno C: The bone scan in patients with aluminium-associated bone disease. *Proc Eur Dial Transplant Assoc-Eur Ren*

Assoc 21: 403, 1984

432. Vanherweghem J-L, Schoutens A, Bergman P, Dhaene M, Goldman M, Fuss M, Kinnaert P: Usefulness of ^{99m}Tc pyrophosphate bone scintigraphy in the survey of dialysis osteodystrophy. *Proc Eur Dial Transplant Assoc-Eur Ren Assoc* 21: 431, 1984

433. Hodge KC, Day JP, O'Hara M, Ackrill P, Ralson AJ: Critical concentrations of aluminium in water used for dialysis. *Lancet* 2: 802, 1981

434. Eschbach JW: Hematologic problems of dialysis patients. in: *Replacement of Renal Function by Dialysis,* edited by Drukker W, Parsons FM, Maher JF, 2nd edition, Dordrecht, Boston MA, Lancaster, Martinus Nijhoff, 1983, p 630

435. Zins B, Drüeke T, Zingraff J, Bererhi L, Kreis H, Naret C, Dilons S, Castaigne JP, Peterlongo F, Casadevall N, Varet B: Erythropoietin treatment in anaemic patients on haemodialysis. *Lancet* 2: 1329, 1986

436. Erslev A: Erythropoietin coming of age. *N Engl J Med* 316: 101, 1987 (Editorial)

437. Winnearls CG, Oliver DO, Pippard MJ, Reid C, Downing MR, Cotes PM: Effects of human erythropoietin derived from recombinant DNA on the anaemia of patients maintained by chronic haemodialysis. *Lancet* 2: 1175, 1986

438. Eschbach JW, Egrie JC, Downing MR, Boowne JK, Adamson JW: Correction of the anemia of end-stage renal disease with recombinant human erythropoietin: results of a combined phase I and II clinical trial. *N Engl J Med* 316: 73, 1987

439. Blumberg BS, Alter HJ, Visnich S: A 'new' antigen in leukemia sera. *JAMA* 191: 541, 1965

440. Blumberg BS: Australia antigen, hepatitis and leukaemia. *Tokyo J Med Sci* 76: 1, 1968 (cited in ref. 296)

441. Drukker W, Alberts C, Odé A, Roozendaal KH, Wilmink J: Report on regular dialysis treatment in Europe, II, 1966. *Proc Eur Dial Transplant Assoc* 2: 90, 1966

442. Blumberg BS, Gerstley BJS, Hungerford DA, London WT, Sutnick AI: A serum antigen (Australia antigen) in Down's syndrome, leukemia and hepatitis. *Ann Intern Med* 66: 924, 1967

443. London WT, DiFiglia M, Sutnick AI, Blumberg BS: Hepatitis in hemodialysis unit: Australia antigen and host response. *N Engl J Med* 281: 571, 1969

444. Sutnick AI, Millman I, London WT, Blumberg BS: The role of Australia antigen in viral hepatitis and other diseases. *Annu Rev Med* 23: 161, 1972

445. Grob PJ, Bishof B, Naeff F: A cluster of hepatitis B transmitted by a physician. *Lancet* 2: 1218, 1981

446. Jacobs C, Broyer M, Brunner FP, Brynger H, Donckerwolcke RA, Kramer P, Selwood NH, Wing AJ, Blake PH: Combined report on regular dialysis and transplantation in Europe, XI, 1980. *Proc Eur Dial Transplant Assoc* 18: 2, 1981

447. Feinstone SM, Kapikian AZ, Purcell RH, Alter HJ, Holland PV: Transfusion-associated hepatitis not due to viral hepatitis type A or B. *N Engl J Med* 292: 767, 1975

448. Alter HJ, Holland PV, Morrow AG, Purcell RH, Feinstone SM, Moritsugu Y: Clinical and serological analysis of transfusion-associated hepatitis. *Lancet* 2: 838, 1975

449. Alter HJ, Purcell RH, Holland PV, Popper H: Transmissible agent in non-A, non-B hepatitis. *Lancet* 1: 460, 1978

450. Tabor E, Drucker JA, Hoofnagle JH, Apryl M, Gerety RJ, Sieff LB, Jackson DR, Barker LF, Pineda-Tamondong G: Transmission of non-A, non-B hepatitis from man to chimpanzee. *Lancet* 1: 463, 1978

451. Vitviski L, Prince AM, Trepo C, Brotman B: Detection of virus-associated antigen in serum and liver of patients with non-A, non-B hepatitis. *Lancet* 2: 1263, 1979

452. Galbraith RM, Dienstag JL, Purcell RH, Gower PH, Zuckerman AJ, Williams R: Non-A, non-B hepatitis associated with chronic liver disease in a haemodialysis unit. *Lancet* 1: 951, 1979

453. Shirachi R, Shiraishi H, Tateda A, Kikuchi K, Ishida N: Hepatitis C antigen in non-A, non-B post transfusion hepatitis. *Lancet* 2: 853, 1978

454. *Hepatitis and the Treatment of Chronic Renal Failure.* Report of the Advisory Group 1970–1972, chairman: Lord Rosenheim, Dept of Health and Social Security, Scottish Home and Health Dept, Welsh Office

455. *Advies inzake de Logistieke Consequenties van het Rapport van de Gezondheidsraad betreffende Maatregelen ter Profylaxe van Serumhepatitis.* (Recommendations concerning the logistic consequences from the report of the Dutch Health Council relating to the prophylaxis of serum hepatitis). Centrale Raad voor de Volksgezondheid, Rijswijk 1975 (in Dutch)

456. Zuckerman AJ: *Hepatitis Associated Antigen and Viruses* Amsterdam, London, North-Holland Publishing Co, 1972, p 12

457. Le Bouvier GL: The heterogeneity of Australia antigen. *J Infect Dis* 123: 671, 1971

458. Magnius LO, Espmark JA: New specifities in Australia antigen positive sera distinct from the Le Bouvier determinants. *J Immunol* 109: 1017, 1972

459. Raimondo G, Smedile A, Gallo L, Babbo A, Ponzetto A, Rizetto M: Multicentre study of HBV-associated delta infection and liver disease in drug addicts. *Lancet* 1: 249, 1982

460. Editorial (anonymous): Delta agent – a virus in disguise? *Lancet* 1: 259, 1982

461. Leading article (anonymous): High-titre hepatitis B immune globulin. *Br Med J* 1: 241, 1976

462. Robinson WS, Lutwick LI: The virus of hepatitis, type B, (Part I) *N Engl J Med* 295: 1168, 1976

463. Robinson WS, Lutwick LI: The virus of hepatitis type B Part II. *N Engl J Med* 295: 1232, 1976

464. Kiernan TW, Ramgopal M: Viral hepatitis: progress and problems. *Med Clin North Am* 63: 611, 1979

465. Wands JR, Kolff R, Isselbacher KJ: Acute viral hepatitis. in: Harrison's *Principles of Internal Medicine,* 9th edn International Students Edition, edited by Isselbacher KJ, Adams RD, Braunwald E, Petersdorf RG, Wilson JD, New York, McGraw-Hill Book Company, 1980, p 1466

466. Prince AM, Szmuness W, Mann MK: Hepatitis B immune globulin: Final report of a controlled, multicenter trial of efficacy in prevention of dialysis associated hepatitis. *J Infect Dis* 137: 131, 1978

467. Zuckerman AJ: Why the world needs a hepatitis vaccine. *New Scientist* 88: 167, 1980

468. Krugman S, Giles JP, Hammond J: Viral hepatitis, type B (MS-2 strain) studies on active immunization. *JAMA* 217: 41, 1971

469. Purcell RH, Gerin JL: Hepatitis B subunit vaccine. A preliminary report of safety and efficacy tests in chimpanzees. *Am J Med Sci* 270: 395, 1975

470. Maupas P, Goudeau A, Coursaget P, Drucker J, Bagros P: Hepatitis B vaccine: efficacy in high-risk settings, a two year study. *Intervirology* 10: 196, 1978

471. Maupas P, Goudeau A, Coursaget P, Drucker J, Barin F, André M: Immunization against hepatitis B in man: a pilot study of two years duration. in: *Viral Hepatitis,* edited by Vyas GN, Cohen SN, Schmidt R, Philadelphia, Franklin Institute Press, 1978, p 539

472. Crosnier J, Jungers P, Couroucé AM, Laplanche A, Benhamou E, Degos F, Lacour B, Prunet P, Cerisier Y, Guesry P: Randomised placebo-controlled trial of hepatitis B surface antigen vaccine in French haemodialysis units: I medical staff, II, haemodialysis patients. *Lancet* 1: 455 and 797, 1981

473. Szmuness W, Stevens CE, Harley EJ, Zano EA, Oleszko WR, William DC, Sadovsky R, Morrison JM, Kellner A: Hepatitis B vaccine: demonstration of efficacy in a controlled clinical trial in a high-risk population in the United States. *N Engl J Med* 303: 833, 1980

474. Dienstag JL: Toward control of hepatitis B (editorial). *N Engl J Med* 303: 874, 1980

475. Szmuness W, Stevens CE, Oleszko WR, Goodman A: Passive-active immunisation against hepatitis B: immunogenicity studies in adult Americans. *Lancet* 1: 575, 1981

476. Leading article (anonymous): Immunisation against hepatitis B. *Br Med J* 281: 1585, 1980

477. Wing AJ, Broyer M, Brunner FP, Brynger H, Challah S, Donckerwolcke RA, Gretz N, Jacobs C, Kramer P, Selwood NH: Combined report on regular dialysis and transplantation in Europe, XIII, 1982. *Proc Eur Dial Transplant Assoc-Eur Ren Assoc* 20: 61, 1983

478. Kramer P, Broyer M, Brunner FP, Brynger H, Challah S, Oulès R, Rizzoni G, Selwood NH, Wing AJ, Balás E: Combined report on regular dialysis and transplantation in Europe XIV, 1983. *Proc Eur Dial Transplant Assoc-Eur Ren Assoc* 21: 51, 1984

479. Brunner FP, Broyer M, Brynger H, Challah S, Fassbinder W, Oulès R, Rizzoni G, Selwood NH, Wing AJ: Combined report on regular dialysis and transplantation in Europe XV, 1984. *Proc Eur Dial Transplant Assoc-Eur Ren Assoc* 22: 5, 1985

480. Jilg W, Schmidt M, Zoulek G, Lorbeer B, Wilske B, Deinhardt F: Clinical evaluation of a recombinant hepatitis B vaccine. *Lancet* 2: 1174, 1984

481. Ambrosch F, Kremsner P, Wiederman G, Thisch-Niggemeyer W, Kunz C, André FE, Safary A: Boosting properties of recombinant DNA hepatitis B vaccine. *Lancet* 1: 1101, 1986

482. Valenzuela P, Gray P, Quiroga M, Zaldmar J, Goodman HM, Rutten WJ: Micleotide sequence of the gene coding for the major protein of hepatitis B surface antigen. *Nature* 280: 815, 1979

483. Valenzuela P, Medina A, Rutten WJ, Ammerer G, Hall BD: Synthesis and assembly of hepatitis B virus surface antigen particles in yeast. *Nature* 298: 347, 1982

484. Anonymous: Recombinant hepatitis B vaccine. *Med Letter* 28: 117, 1986

485. Blumberg BS, London WT: Hepatitis B virus and the prevention of primary hepatocellular carcinoma. *N Engl J Med* 304: 782, 1981 (Editorial)

486. Bradbeer C: HIV and lifestyle. *Br Med J* 294: 5, 1987

487. Kingsley LA, Kaslow R, Rinaldo Jr CR, Detre K, Odaka N, VanRaden M, Detels R, Polk BV, Chmiel J, Kelsey SF, Ostrow D, Visscher B: Risk factors for seroconversion to human immunodeficiency virus among male homosexuals. *Lancet* 1: 345, 1987

488. Smith T: Aids: a doctor's duty. *Br Med J* 294: 6, 1987

489. Wallis C, Thompon D: 'You haven't heard anything yet'. Health officials wrestle with onslaught of history's newest epidemic. *Time Magazine* 129, no. 7: 30, 1987

490. Dept. of Health and Social security: Latest figures in AIDS in the UK. *Lancet* 1: 400, 1987

491. Yarchoan R, Weinhold KJ, Lyerly HK, Gelmann E, Blum RM, Shearer GM, Mitsuya H, Collins JM, Meyers CE, Kleck-

er RW, Markham PD, Durack DT, Lehrman SN, Barry DW, Fischl MA, Gallo RC, Bolognesi DP, Broder S: Administration of 3′Azido-3′deoxythymidine, an inhibitor of HTLV-III/LAV replication to patients with AIDS or AIDS related complex. *Lancet* 1: 575, 1986

492. Anonymous: Azidothymidine for AIDS. *Med Letter* 28: 107, 1986

493. Polakoff S: Dialysis associated hepatitis. in: *Replacement of Renal Function by Dialysis*, edited by Drukker W, Parsons FM, Maher JF, 2nd edition, Dordrecht, Boston, Lancaster, Martinus Nijhoff, 1983, p 659

494. Geddes AM: Risk of AIDS to health care workers. *Br Med J* 292: 711, 1986 (Leading article)

495. Sande MA: Transmission of AIDS. The case against casual contagion. *N Engl J Med* 314: 380, 1986

496. Incidence and risk of transmission of HTLV3 infection to staff at a London hospital 1982–'85. *J Hosp Infect* 6 (Suppl. C): 15, 1985

497. Almeida JD, Kulatilake AE, Mackay DH, Shackman R, Chisholm GD, MacGregor AB, O'Donoghue EPN, Waterson AP: Possible airborne spread of serum-hepatitis virus within a haemodialysis unit. *Lancet* 2: 849, 1971

498. Thölen VH, Stricker E, Feer H, Massini MA, Staub H: Über die Anwendung der künstlichen Niere bei Schizophrenie und Myasthenia gravis (The application of the artificial kidney in cases of schizophrenia and myasthenia gravis). *Dtsch Med Wochenschr* 85: 1012, 1960 (in German)

499. Wagemaker H, Cade R: The use of hemodialysis in chronic schizophrenia. *Am J Psychiatry* 134: 6, 1977

500. Cade R, Wagemaker H: Hemodialysis as treatment for chronic schizophrenia. *Abstracts Am Soc Artif Intern Organs* 7: 7, 1978

501. Wagemaker H, Cade R: The use of hemodialysis in fourteen chronic schizophrenics. *Abstracts Am Soc Artif Intern Organs* 7: 62, 1978

502. Palmour RM, Ervin FR, Wagemaker H, Cade R: Characterization of a peptide derived from the serum of psychiatric patients. *Abstracts Ann Meeting Soc Neuroscience*, 1977

503. Kolff WJ: Dialysis of schizophrenics. Weird and novel applications of dialysis, hemofiltration, hemoperfusion and peritoneal dialysis: witchcraft? *Artif Organs* 2: 277, 1978

504. Gurland HJ: Combination of hemodialysis and hemoperfusion used in conventional dialyser format in the treatment of uremia. *Proc 12th Annu Contractor's Conf Artif Kidney – Chronic Uremia Program of NIAMDD*, edited by Mackey BB, DHEW Publication nr. (NIH) 81–1979, 1979, p 279

505. Twardowski ZJ: Abatement of psoriasis and repeated dialysis. *Ann Intern Med* 86: 510, 1977

506. Buselmeier TJ, Dahl MV, Kjellstrand CM, Goltz RW: Dialysis therapy for psoriasis. *JAMA* 240: 1270, 1978

507. Kramer P: Dialysis for psoriatic patients. *Proc 11th Ann Contractor's Conf Artif Kidney Program NIAMDD*, edited by Mackey BB, DHEW Publication no. (NIH) 79–1442, 1978, p 217

508. Korz R, Klein H, Genth E: Myasthenia gravis und Lupus erythematosus Nephritis (Myasthenia gravis and lupus erythematosus nephritis). *Dtsch Med Wochenschr* 103: 1485, 1978 (in German)

509. Gurland HJ: Is blood purification suitable for an effective cure of psoriasis? *Paper presented at the 2nd symposium on chronic renal failure*, Prague, March 1979

510. Burton BT, Kirschman GH: Demographic analysis: end stage renal disease and its treatment in the United States. *Clin Nephrol* 11: 47, 1979

511. Waterfall WK: Dialysis and transplantation. *Br Med J* 281: 726, 1980

512. Relman AS, Rennie D: Treatment of end stage renal disease. Free but not equal (Editorial). *N Engl J Med* 303: 996, 1980

513. Anonymous: Health care Financing Administration, Dept. of Health and Human Services: Medicare and non/medicare patients receiving dialysis treatments as of December 31, 1985. *Dial Transplant* 15: 544, 1986

514. Drukker W: Haemodialysis: a historical review. in: *Replacement of Renal Function by Dialysis,* edited by Drukker W, Parsons FM, Maher JF, 2nd edition, Dordrecht, Boston, Lancaster, Martinus Nijhoff, 1983, p 41

515. Editorial (anonymous): Ethics and the nephrologist. *Lancet* 1: 594, 1981

516. Wing AJ, Brunner FP, Brynger HOA, Jacobs C, Kramer P: Comparative review between dialysis and transplantation. in: *Replacement of Renal Function by Dialysis,* edited by Drukker W, Parsons FM, Maher JF, 2nd edition, Dordrecht, Boston, Lancaster, Martinus Nijhoff, 1983, p 851

517. Evans RW, Blagg CR: Treatment of end-stage renal disease (Letter to the editor). *N Engl J Med* 304: 357, 1981

518. Relman AS, Rennie D: Treatment of end-stage renal disease (Reply). *N Engl J Med* 304: 357, 1981

519. Iglehart K: Funding the endstage renal-disease program. *N Engl J Med* 306: 492, 1982

520. Parsons FM, Brunner FP, Burck HC, Gräser W, Gurland HJ, Härlen H, Schärer K, Spies GW: Statistical report. *Proc Eur Dial Transplant Assoc* 11: 3, 1974

521. Carmody M, Cattell WR, Cambi V, Koch KM, Baillod RA: Dialysis – petrified or progressive? *Proc Eur Dial Transplant Assoc* 11: 537, 1974

PRINCIPLES AND BIOPHYSICS OF DIALYSIS

JOHN A. SARGENT and FRANK A. GOTCH

INTRODUCTION

Intermittent dialysis therapy is used in chronic uremia to re-establish body water solute concentrations that cannot be achieved by the natural organ. In this sense, the dialyzer becomes an artificial kidney and it is through the transport of substances by this device that chemical and biophysical control consistent with continued survival is achieved. This chapter is organized as shown in Figure 1 and consists of two basic lines of development:

1. Consideration of the dialyzer and its operating principles.
2. Application of mass balance principles to various solute systems and the effect of dialyzer use on solute control during intermittent dialysis therapy.

Biophysical treatment of hemodialysis requires quantitative description of the interacting variables involved in this therapy; such a description, to be unambiguous, must use mathematical relationships. Certain fundamental relationships, because of their central role, have been developed in detail, such as clearance measurements and single pool solute ki-

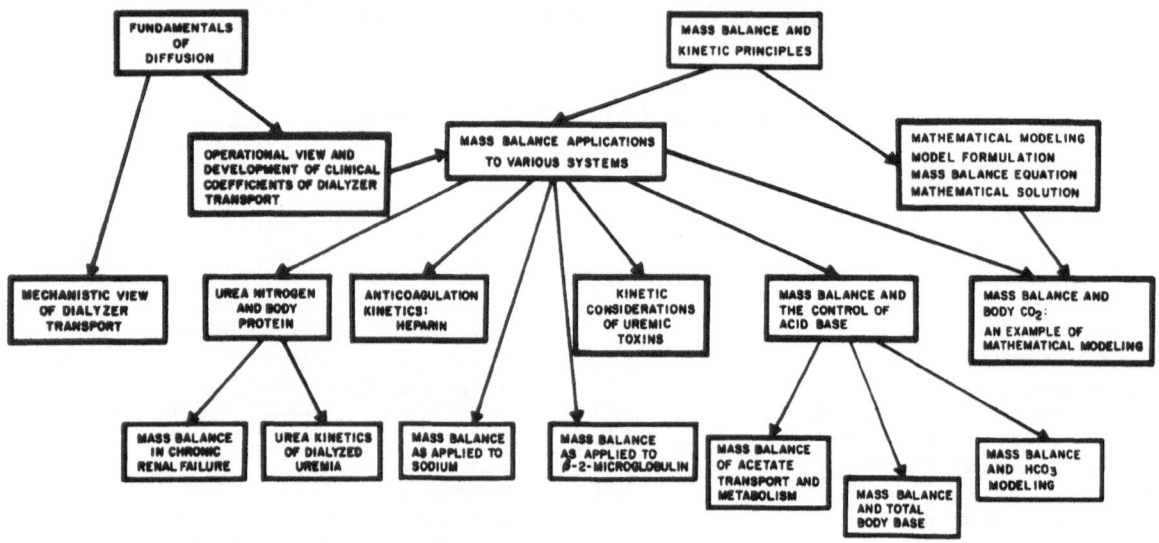

Figure 1. Diagrammatic outline of chapter organization.

netics. For solution techniques of equations and relationships that are mainly descriptive, such as double pool kinetics of larger molecules, the reader is either referred to the Appendix or to specific texts on applied mathematics. The Appendix discusses independent and dependent variables, as well as the quantitative use of relational (linear) analysis. In most cases symbols are defined in the text. For reader convenience, however, a list of symbols used appears under Nomenclature at the end of the chapter text.

The dialyzer will be considered initially, starting with a brief discussion of the fundamentals of diffusion embodied in Fick's law. The practical application of these concepts to dialyzer development or clinical use, however, requires the definition of several coefficients that can aid in either the design of dialyzers or their use in the clinic; these two aspects will be discussed in turn. The mechanistic view of transport is intended to describe what influences dialyzer properties; the discussion of the operational aspects of a dialyzer, which concerns itself with the development of relationships for dialysance and clearance, will be of value in the second part of the chapter when mass balance is considered with respect to the patient-dialyzer system.

The section which considers the mass balance of intermittent dialysis therapy begins with the fundamentals of conservation of matter and from them develops kinetic and steady state relationships that govern concentration control in dialyzed patients; these concepts are then applied to several solute systems.

FUNDAMENTALS OF MASS TRANSPORT

To remove a substance from the blood with a dialyzer, the species must move out of the blood across a membrane and into the dialysate by diffusion which is governed by Fick's Law:

$$J = -DA\frac{dc}{dx} = -DA\frac{\Delta c}{\Delta x}. \quad [1]$$

This expression states that the flux, J, of a material over a short distance, dx, is proportional to its concentration difference, dc, over this distance and the area of the diffusion front, A. The phenomological constant of proportionality resulting in equality of the above statements is the diffusivity, **D**, which has units of cm^2/sec and will be a unique property of the solute-solvent at a specific temperature. Finally, the sign convention is adopted that diffusion will be in the positive direction; material moves from the region of higher to that of lower activity so that concentration will be decreasing ($dc/dx < 0$) in the direction of flux; mathematically, therefore, the right hand side of the equation must carry a negative sign.

Equation 1 is the fundamental relationship for unidimensional diffusive movement of material and is the mass transfer analog to Fourier's Law which governs heat conduction. For practical use in the study of the operation of dialyzers, however, it is necessary to put equation 1 in less general form so that the mechanisms of transport of specific devices can be evaluated. This mechanistic approach is generally taken by engineers who desire to improve the operating characteristics and efficiency of a dialyzer. It can also be helpful to physicians in understanding the anticipated effects of different operational conditions on dialyzer performance. Typical changes in operational conditions would be dialyzer clotting, variable ultrafiltration, and non-standard flow rates. This approach also can give increased insight into what to expect from changes in the components of a dialyzer, such as the use of a different dialysis membrane.

MECHANISMS OF TRANSPORT

If the value of Δx in equation 1 is relatively constant in any one dialyzer design, the major variables that determine flux for the dialyzer will be concentration difference and area, **D** being a constant at any particular temperature for a specific chemical species. This being the case, equation 1 can be written as:

$$J = - K_o A \, \Delta C. \qquad [2a]$$

Here ΔC is an appropriately defined concentration difference. In equation 2a a new proportionality constant, the overall mass transfer coefficient, k_o, has appeared and is defined as:

$$K_o = \frac{\dfrac{J}{A}}{-\Delta C} = \frac{\text{unit flux}}{\text{driving force}} \qquad [2b]$$

K_o has units of cm/min and is independent of ΔC in the concentration range experienced in dialysis. Comparison of equations 1 and 2a shows that K_o is proportional to the diffusivity of the solute being transfered and inversely proportional to the diffusion distances characteristic of the dialyzer; this transport coefficient can be calculated from basic transport values if blood and dialysate flow rates are known as will be shown below (1–3). If equation 2a is further rewritten, the flux per unit area can be described as:

$$\text{unit flux} = \frac{J}{A} = \frac{-\Delta C}{1/K_o} = \frac{-\Delta C}{R_o}. \qquad [2c]$$

If $1/K_o$ is viewed as a resistance to transport (R_o), equation 2c can be written as:

$$\frac{\text{Mass transfer}}{\text{per unit area}} = \frac{\text{Driving force}}{\text{Resistance to transport}}. \qquad [3]$$

Equation 3 is a quantatitive statement of a fundamental physical principle which applies throughout the physical sciences. It states that there will be a flux of material proportional to the driving force and that that flux will be opposed by (or is inversely proportional to) certain resistances. This is the same form as Ohm's law of electric current flow, it is the same law that is applied to conductive heat flow, and it is in the same form as the relationship that is used to calculate peripheral resistance in circulation physiology (4).

Specifically, equation 3 shows that mass transfer is the result of the driving force relative to the resistance to transfer and is useful in that it demonstrates that flux per unit area can be improved only by increasing the driving force or decreasing the resistance. The overall resistance is an index of the difficulty in getting from the center of the blood stream to the center of the dialysate stream and is the sum of all the resistances of which it is composed (see Figure 2):

$$R_o = R_B + R_M + R_D \qquad [4]$$

where R_B = blood side resistance
where R_M = membrane resistance
$\quad\quad\ R_D$ = dialysate side resistance

In this way, the diffusion path is divided into three segments representing the three fundamental elements of a dialyzer.

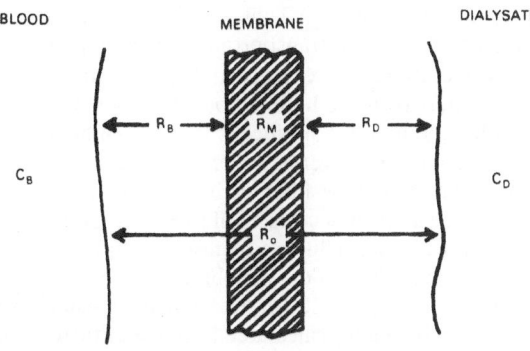

Figure 2. Schematic representation of resistances to transport in a dialyzer.

K_o was defined above as proportional to $D/\Delta x$ so that R_o, being proportional to $1/K_o$, is proportional to $\Delta x/D$. In the three segments described above, R will be:

$$R_B = \frac{\Delta x_B}{D_B}$$

$$R_M = \frac{\Delta x_M}{k D_M} = \frac{\Delta x_M}{D_M{}^*}$$

$$R_D = \frac{\Delta x_D}{D_D}$$

Where k is the solute distribution coefficient between the membrane material and the solution.

For any particular solute, the diffusivity in blood (D_B) and dialysate (D_D) of a given composition will be constant. Moreover, it should have the same value irrespective of the dialyzer, being a solution constant at operational temperatures. As a consequence, the R_B and R_D in a specific dialyzer will be governed by the Δx_B and Δx_D terms; these terms are the effective diffusion distances from the main stream to and from the membrane. To the extent that blood flows are swift and fluid channels are small, the value of Δx for both blood and dialysate will be small as will the values for R_B and R_D. The membrane resistance R_M still depends on Δx_M (the thickness of the membrane) but in addition, will be sensitive to the effective diffusivity in the membrane ($D_M{}^*$) which can vary considerably as a result of its chemical composition. In this context, a thin (small Δx_M) permeable (large $D_M{}^*$) membrane would have a small value for R_M. It should be noted, however, that the resistances are additive so that while a dialyzer with a highly permeable membrane will have low values for R_M, R_o may be high due to large values for R_B and R_D. Dialyzer efficiency can be best increased, therefore, by reducing the value of the largest resistance in equation 4. The relative values for the above resistances in four dialyzer-membrane combinations which were in common use in the early days of dialysis serves to illustrate the importance of the various resistances (see Table 1). The improvement in dialyzer design that occurred in the 1970's was spurred by the desire to reduce the overall resistance shown in Table 1.

It becomes evident from Table 1 that for urea, the predominant resistances to transport in the prototype parallel plate, Kiil dialyzer, were R_B and R_D (i.e. in the fluid streams) whereas in the hollow fiber devices with narrow fluid paths, the major resistance is in the membrane. The overall resistance, however, is lower in the latter explaining why, in general, hollow fiber dialyzers have better urea transport. For large molecules all of these dialyzers, except the one with the noncellulosic membrane, have over two thirds of the resistance in the membrane.

The overall resistance, R_o (or overall mass transfer coefficient, K_o) can be readily calculated from the diffusive dialysance, D, and knowledge of blood and dialysate flow rates (see below for discussion of diffusive dialysance). Conversely, if R_o or K_o is known the expected diffusive dialysance under specific clinical conditions of flow can be calculated (see below).

CONCENTRATION DIFFERENCE, THE DRIVING FORCE

Equation 2a states that with a specific dialyzer ($K_o A$ a constant) the removal of solute will depend directly on the concentration difference, ΔC. It is important to develop this variable further so that it can be used in computations to follow.

Logarithmic mean concentration difference

There will be a linear change in concentrations of the blood and dialysis solution as solute transfers from one to the other (shown diagrammatically in Figure 3). This figure is for counter-current flows and shows solute levels in the blood decreasing from its entry into the dialyzer at the right while

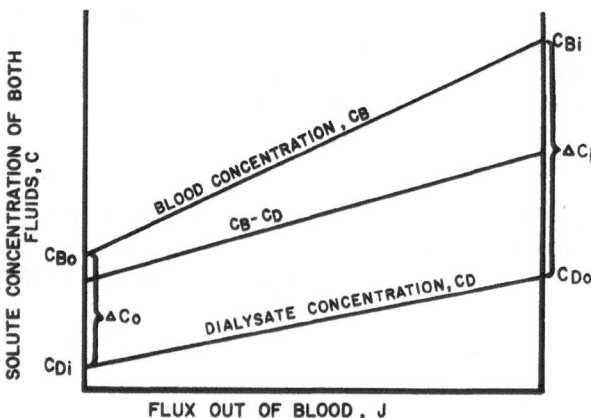

Figure 3. Graphical representation of blood and dialysate concentration as a function of flux between the two fluid streams.

concentrations in the dialysis fluid increase from its entry into the dialyzer at the left. The concentration difference at any point in the dialyzer is represented by the difference between these two lines (see the intermediate line) and it is this concentration that will determine the local flux (see equation 2a). A similar figure can be constructed for co-current flow and the analytical results to be developed below will apply equally to this case. In Figure 3 the slope of the concentration difference line will be:

$$\text{slope} = \frac{d(\Delta C)}{dJ} = \frac{\Delta C_i - \Delta C_o}{J}. \qquad [5]$$

If equation 2a is differentiated and evaluated for the very small transport area, dA, then substituted into equation 5 for dJ:

Table 1. Mass transfer resistances for various dialyzer-solute combinations.

Dialyzer and membrane	Membrane m^2	Solute	K_B^* ml/min	R_B^{**} ml/min	R_M min/cm	R_D^{**} min/cm	R_O min/cm	$\frac{R_B + R_D}{R_O}$	$\frac{R_M}{R_O}$	Ref.
Parallel ridge	1.0	Urea	80	24	19	16	59	0.68	0.32	5
Kiil-Cuprophane		Vitamin B_{12}	18	101	362	45	508	0.29	0.71	5
Parallel ridge	1.0	Urea	110	24	14	16	54	0.74	0.26	6
Kiil-polycarbonate Cordis-Dow		Vitamin B_{12}	37	101	90	45	236	0.62	0.38	6
Model 4 Hollow fiber regenerated	1.3	Urea	160	4	21	7	32	0.34	0.66	7
cellulose Cordis-Dow		Vitamin B_{12}	23	17	–	20	519	0.07	0.93	7
Model 5 Hollow fiber regenerated	2.5	Urea	185	5	21	9	35	0.40	0.60	7
cellulose		Vitamin B_{12}	40	21	–	25	536	0.09	0.91	7

* Clearances based on $Q_B = 200$ ml/min, Q_D 500 ml/min and 37° C vitamin B_{12} *in vitro*

** The value of R_B and R_D have been established from $\dfrac{\text{R urea, hollow fiber kidney}}{\text{R urea Kiil}}$

(R vitamin B_{12}, Kiil) = R vitamin B_{12}, hollow fiber kidney.

$$\frac{d(\Delta C)}{- K_0 \, dA \, \Delta C} = \frac{\Delta C_i - \Delta C_0}{J}.$$

Rearrangement yields:

$$\frac{d(\Delta C)}{\Delta C} = \frac{- K_o(\Delta C_i - \Delta C_0) \, dA}{J}.$$

Integration and solving the resulting expression for flux yields:

$$J = K_o \, A \left[\frac{\Delta C_i - \Delta C_0}{\text{Ln} \, (\Delta C_i / \Delta C_0)} \right]. \qquad [6]$$

The expression in parentheses in equation 6 is the logarithmic mean concentration difference which can be expanded as:

$$\Delta C \,(\text{Log-mean}) = \frac{(C_{Bi} - C_{Do}) - (C_{Bo} - C_{Di})}{\text{Ln} \,[(C_{Bi} - C_{Bo})/(C_{Bo} - C_{Di})]}. \qquad [7]$$

The log-mean concentration difference as represented in equation 7 is an operationally exact statement of the integrated concentration driving force in a dialyzer being operated in either counter-current or co-current mode. Equation 7, however, contains both inlet and outlet blood and dialysate concentrations which in the clinical operation of a dialyzer are tedious to obtain.

It is considerably more convenient to define a surrogate concentration driving force, $(C_{Bi} - C_{Di})$ in the clinical setting. This concentration difference can be shown to be directly proportional to the log-mean concentration difference and is clinically more convenient than equation 7 because it uses undialyzed blood and inlet dialysis fluid as reference levels to evaluate and calculate dialyzer performance. This measurement of concentration difference also adapts well to system modeling because it is possible to determine fluxes from patient's systemic concentrations alone.

OPERATIONAL CHARACTERISTICS OF THE DIALYZER

During dialysis treatment the dialyzer is the point at which mass transfer takes place either from the patient (e.g. potassium and protein catabolites) or to the patient (e.g. calcium or acetate). There is also a transfer of water from the patient to the dialysate for volume control. The two mechanisms of transport are different and are effected by virtue of dissimilar driving forces: concentration differences for the various chemical constituents and a pressure difference in the case of water. To describe the operational characteristics of a dialyzer for clinical use, it is desirable to define operational coefficients which are the analog of K_o in equation 2b and which result in a linear proportionality relating flux and driving force. The two coefficients for dialyzer water and solute flux are the ultrafiltration coefficient (K_{UF}) and dialysance (D); clearance (K) is a special case of dialysance as will be discussed below.

Ultrafiltration coefficient

Ultrafiltration Coefficient [K_{UF} (ml/min/mm Hg)] =

$$= \frac{\text{water flux}}{\text{transmembrane pressure}} = \frac{Q_F}{P_B - P_D}. \qquad [8]$$

The water flux is referred to as the ultrafiltration rate (Q_F ml/min) and the driving force is the difference in mean pressures from the blood side (P_B) to the dialysate side (P_D).

Mass transport and solute flux

Consideration of flow rates

A dialyzer is operated by manipulation of blood and dialysate flow rates. It is, therefore, appropriate to define the basis for these flows.

Because dialysate and ultrafiltrate are homogeneous aqueous fluids, their flow rates are unambiguous and represent those flows which would be calculated if a timed volumetric collection were done. Blood, in contrast, is a heterogeneous fluid which contains proteins and cellular elements. Its bulk flow rate will always exceed its water flow rate; indeed at times its non-cellular water flow rate (or plasma water) is a more relevant flow, as in the case of inulin transport; the non-cellular flow adjusted for cellular water participation is more appropriate when considering materials such as bicarbonate which readily enters cells but is in much lower cellular concentration due to Donnan effects (8–10). Bulk blood flow (Q_B), however, is routinely measured clinically and throughout the evolution of the dialysis field this quantity has been used.

In the development of the expressions to follow, Q_B will be used as the flow rate of the portion of the blood appropriate to the solute being discussed. Consequently, the quantity, $Q_B \, C_B$, will represent the mass of material in the flowing stream and Q_B will take its units from C_B (e.g. if C_B for bicarbonate is in milliequivalents per liter of blood water adjusted for red cell water and Donnan effects then Q_B will be in units of liters per minute of effective blood water flow). It should be recognized, however, that much dialysis literature and product information (such as dialyzer performance data) use the clinically measurable values of Q_B so that if other flow rates are desired they must be computed from the bulk flow and blood constants.

Protein binding

Many substances bind to plasma and body proteins (11). The relevant solute concentration with regard to dialyzer transport will be the free concentration in plasma water. However, the bound material will be in equilibrium with bound solutes to the extent of the particular solute system's solute-protein binding coefficient (11). The practical effect of solute-protein binding will be that solute analyses of plasma will yield the sum of the bound and free concentrations and will overstate the concentration driving force present. Secondly, as free solute is removed there will be un-binding of solute with the effect of supporting the free concentrations.

Consequently, depending on the kinetics of binding/unbinding – the free concentration in inlet blood, relative to dialysate concentrations, will understate the concentration driving force present during the transit of a dialyzer by the plasma.

Dialysance and clearance

Consider the dialyzer under single pass conditions as shown in Figure 4. Once flows have stabilized after the start of dialysis, the system will be nominally at steady state under which condition the mass balance will be:

$$Q_{Bi} C_{Bi} + Q_{Di} C_{Di} = (Q_{Bi} - Q_F) C_{Bo} + (Q_{Di} + Q_F) C_{Do}.$$

Rearrangement of this expression yields:

$$Q_{Bi} (C_{Bi} - C_{Bo}) + Q_F C_{Bo} = Q_{Di} (C_{Do} - C_{Di}) + Q_F C_{Do}. \qquad [9]$$

The first term on each side of equation 9 can be viewed as the diffusive component of flux whereas the second term shows the deviation from the purely diffusive case when there is a convective contribution. Both sides of the equation are expressions of solute flux during the transit of the dialyzer: The left hand side represents the solute leaving the blood; the right hand side is the solute appearing in the dialysate.

We now define a term called diffusive dialysance (D) (12), which will be a constant for a dialyzer at any specific blood and dialysis fluid flow rate.*

$$D = \frac{\text{Change in solute content of incoming blood}}{\text{Concentration Driving Force}}$$

Dialysance is the magnitude of flux to be expected per unit of concentration driving force. The next step in the mathematical development is to divide equation 9 by the concentration driving force from the blood to the dialysate. Using the inlet concentrations as discussed above the generalized inlet concentration driving force will be: $C_{Bi} - C_{Di}$. The term α, is a 'Donnan factor' defined as the ratio of ionic concentrations in dialysate and blood at equilibrium and is relevant to diffusive transport of ions.

$$\alpha = \frac{\text{Equilibrium ion concentration in dialysate}}{\text{Equilibrium ion concentration in plasma water}}.$$

$$D = \frac{Q_{Bi} (C_{Bi} - C_{Bo})}{\alpha C_{Bi} - C_{Di}} = \frac{Q_{Di} (C_{Do} - C_{Di})}{\alpha C_{Bi} - C_{Di}}. \qquad [10]$$

When non-charged solutes are being considered, $\alpha = 1$ and equation 10 becomes:

$$D = \frac{Q_{Bi} (C_{Bi} - C_{Bo})}{C_{Bi} - C_{Di}} = \frac{Q_{Di} (C_{Do} - C_{Di})}{C_{Bi} - C_{Di}}. \qquad [11]$$

Dividing equation 9 by the concentration driving force, $C_{Bi} - C_{Di}$, yields:

---

* It should be noted that this is the special case of dialysance (which will appear later) and that in this unique case, ultrafiltration, Q_F, is zero.

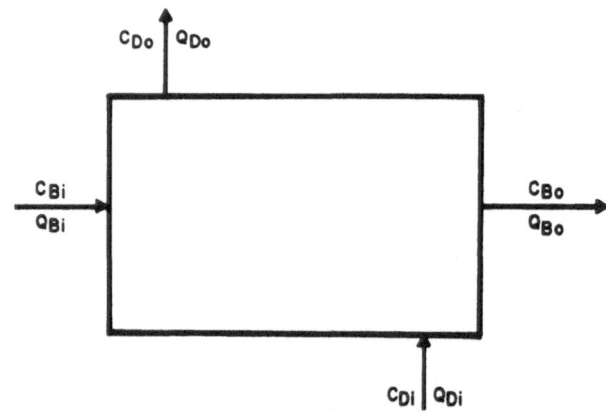

Figure 4. Schematic representation of flows and concentrations for a dialyzer operated with counter-current flows.

$$\frac{Q_{Bi} (C_{Bi} - C_{Bo})}{C_{Bi} - C_{Di}} + \frac{Q_F C_{Bo}}{C_{Bi} - C_{Di}} = \frac{Q_{Di} (C_{Do} - C_{Di})}{C_{Bi} - C_{Di}} +$$

$$\frac{Q_F C_{Do}}{C_{Bi} - C_{Di}} \qquad [12]$$

The left hand side of equation 12 becomes:

$$\frac{J}{C_{Bi} - C_{Di}} = D + \frac{Q_F C_{Bo}}{C_{Bi} - C_{Di}} = D'. \qquad [13a]$$

Where D' is the total dialysance (12). The flux out of the blood compartment is then:

$$J = D(C_{Bi} - C_{Di}) + Q_F C_{Bo}. \qquad [13b]$$

If $Q_F \ll Q_B$, equation 11 can be considered to represent the approximate relationship of blood inlet and outlet concentrations. In such a case, which is generally true during hemodialysis equation 11 can be solved for C_{Bo}. If this rearrangement is substituted into the above expression:

$$J = D(C_{Bi} - C_{Di}) + Q_F \left[C_{Bi} - \frac{D}{Q_{Bi}} (C_{Bi} - C_{Di}) \right].$$

And expanding and rearranging:

$$J = \left[D \left(1 - \frac{Q_F}{Q_{Bi}} \right) + Q_F \right] C_{Bi} - D \left(1 - \frac{Q_F}{Q_{Bi}} \right) C_{Di}. \qquad [14]$$

Equation 14 when solved for D yields:

$$D = \frac{\dfrac{J}{C_{Bi} - C_{Di}} - \dfrac{Q_F C_{Bi}}{C_{Bi} - C_{Di}}}{1 - Q_F/Q_{Bi}}. \qquad [15]$$

The flux in equation 15 can either be measured by the amount of solute lost from the blood or the amount appearing in the dialysate. Equation 9 indicates that by using the left hand side as the value for J, an expression for dialysance based on the blood side results, D_B. Analogous steps and using the right hand side of equation 9 will result in D_D.

An important special case of these expressions is when C_{Di}

= 0 which is the case with most single pass dialyzers and metabolic wastes. In this case, equation 11 becomes the definition of diffusive clearance K, which is the analog of the physiological concept (13):

$$K = \frac{Q_{Bi}(C_{Bi} - C_{Bo})}{C_{Bi}} \qquad [16]$$

and equations 13a and 15 become:

$$\frac{J}{C_{Bi}} = K + Q_F \frac{C_{Bo}}{C_{Bi}} = K' \qquad [17a]$$

$$K = \frac{\dfrac{J}{C_{Bi}} - Q_F}{1 - \dfrac{Q_F}{Q_{Bi}}}. \qquad [17b]$$

Rearrangement of this expression, or alternatively, simplification of equation 14 when $C_{Di} = 0$ yields:

$$J = [K(1 - Q_F/Q_{Bi}) + Q_F] C_{Bi} = K' C_{Bi}. \qquad [18]$$

Here K' is the total clearance and is defined as the total flux divided by the inlet blood concentration. Equations 13 and 17a mathematically combine diffusive and convective components of transport into a single first order term D' or K'.*

Because these linear coefficients relate flux to the concentration driving force, they are very useful in the kinetic description of dialysis. It should be pointed out, however, that these terms are no longer constant for a given set of blood and dialysis fluid flow rates because of their dependence on the ultrafiltration rate, Q_F.

The appearance of a diffusive and a convective term in equations 14 and 18 should not be taken as identifying the mechanism of convective transport but as a description of the net contribution that ultrafiltration will make to flux and corresponding dialysance and clearance. It is seen in equations 14 and 18 that clearance and dialysance will increase with ultrafiltration to the extent of the actual concentration present in the outflow blood.

That these equations mathematically (as opposed to physically) describe net transport is illustrated by considering equation 13a for a cation such as K^+. In such a case, the cation will be retained as plasma is ultrafiltered due to Donnan effects and $C_{Bo} > C_{Bi}$. In fact it is possible to conceive of cases where the increased dialysance above the diffusive value, due to Q_F, may be greater than the ultrafiltration flux itself as a result of the second term of equation 13a $- C_{Bo}/(\alpha C_{Bi} - C_{Di}) > 1$.

Potassium presents an illustrative case. If D(potassium (= 0.100 l/min, $C_{Bi} = 4$ mmol/l, $C_{Di} = 2$ mmol/l and $\alpha = 0.95$ (Gotch FA, Falkenhagen D, Sargent JA: Unpublished data); C_{Bo} will be approximately 3 mmol/l, and $C_{Bo}/(\alpha C_{Bi} - C_{Di}) = 1.67$, and there would be an increase of more than 3 ml/min in dialysance for each 2 ml/min of ultrafiltration.

*These expressions are those generally used in defining clearance and dialysance and also appear in Chapters 6 and 13.

Measurement of dialysance and clearance

In the context of equation 12 dialysance and clearance values should be identified as flux measured from blood or dialysis fluid and the selection of the location for sampling would appear to be based on the convenience of sampling and the analytical sensitivity of the assays used. While this is true in vitro, in vivo measurements are complicated by the complexity of blood. The unstated assumption of Figure 4 and equation 12 is that the blood flow rate, Q_B, is that of a homogeneous fluid at concentration C_B. *In vivo* conditions are at variance with this assumption: 1) Blood is heterogenous because of suspended red cells which will result in transmural solute disequilibrium for large materials and rapid transits through the dialyzer, 2) Blood is composed of certain non-aqueous constituents so that water flow (the distribution space for dissolved unbound solutes) equals the product of blood flow and the aqueous fraction.

In light of these difficulties, using dialysate values allows direct measurement of fluxes without the complexities described above. It is prudent, however, to obtain both blood and dialysate side values as a check on methods and analysis. In general, dialysance and clearance measurements used throughout this chapter, will be specified in terms of the dialysate side (K_D).

It should be noted that there are perferred methods of measuring the values in equation 9. Operationally Q_{Do} and C_{Do} can be determined from a timed aliquot of outflow dialysate; historically the preferred method of determining Q_B has been from bubble time measurement (14). The bubble time method has always been clinically tedious and this is particularly true with the advent of more rapid blood flow. An alternate method is to time blood pump revolutions (Sargent JA unpublished data). The sequence of blood and dialysate samples should be C_{Bo} and C_{Do} then C_{Bi} and C_{Di} so that sampling does not upset flow patterns. Q_F is determined from the product of ultrafiltration coefficient (K_{UF}) and the blood-dialysate pressure drop ($P_B - P_D$): a rearrangement of equation 8.

$$Q_F = K_{UF}(P_B - P_D). \qquad [19]$$

Effective blood water flow for various solutes

Blood water is the solvent for most materials, diffusively transported by the dialyzer. In general, blood water can be considered to be divided into extracellular or plasma water and intercellular or red cell water. If the hematocrit (HCT), plasma, and red cell water fractions (F_P, F_R) are known the portion of blood water flow of each can be estimated.

$$\text{Plasma water flow rate} = Q_B \left(1 - \frac{HCT}{100}\right) F_P$$

$$\text{Red cell water flow rate} = Q_B \frac{HCT}{100} F_R$$

and total blood water flow rate will be:

$$Q_{BW} = Q_B \left[F_P - \frac{HCT}{100}(F_P - F_R)\right]. \qquad [20]$$

Some substances resist somewhat transport out of the red blood cell and the contribution of the red blood cell to overall mass transfer can be modified by a coefficient γ which represents the fraction of red blood cell water that participates in the transfer during a transit of the dialyzer. That is, if during a transit of the dialyzer the plasma concentration is dropped to half its inlet value while the red blood cell concentration is reduced by only 25% γ would be 0.5. For a material for which the red blood cell membrane is essentially transparent, γ will = 1.0. For charged particles the Donnan ratio (R_D) must also be added to equation 20, where:

$$R_D = \frac{\text{anion concentration in red cells}}{\text{anion concentration in plasma water}} =$$

$$\frac{1}{\alpha} \text{ (red cell to plasma)}.$$

Substituting these factors into equation 20, the general expression for effective blood flow rate (Q_E) is:

$$Q_E = Q_B \left[F_P - \frac{HCT}{100} (F_P - F_R \gamma R_D) \right]. \qquad [21]$$

Effective blood flow rate for bicarbonate

The bicarbonate ion is a charged particle for which the red cell membrane is very permeable (8), and $\gamma = 1.0$.

Because of its charge, bicarbonate concentration in red cell water will be lower than in plasma water (i.e. $R_D < 1.0$). For bicarbonate equation 21 becomes:

$$Q_E = Q_B \left(F_P - \frac{HCT}{100} (F_P - F_R R_D) \right). \qquad [22]$$

For values of: $F_P = 0.94$, $F_R = 0.72$, and $R_D = 0.69$, equation 22 reduces to (10):

$$Q_E = Q_B \ 0.94 - 0.443 \ \frac{Hct}{100}. \qquad [22]$$

The effective flow, Q_E, can then be used in place of Q_B in the foregoing expressions and those to be developed relating D, Q_D, and Q_B to $K_O A$.

The effect of increasing hematocrit on transport

With the anticipated introduction of recombinant human erythropoetin (15, 16) the long sought ability to correct the anemia seen in most dialysis patients may become a reality. However considering equation 21, this advance would be expected to be accompanied by a reduction in effective blood flow and lower dialyzer performance at the same blood flows. The effect of doubling hematocrit on Q_E for three hypothetical substances is shown in Table 2 as calculated using equation 21. The first substance represents a small solute evenly distributed in blood water (urea would be an example). For this substance effective blood flow would decrease slightly and a 5% increase in blood flow rate would be required to compensate. The effect has been merely to add more protein (in the form of red blood cells) to the blood. The second case is a substance such as potassium that either does not distribute in red cell water, or is large enough (or metabolically retained in the red cell) that it does not appreciably move out of red cells during transit through the dialyzer. In this case the effective blood flow rate equals the plasma water flow rate and will be reduced accordingly. An increase of 33% in blood water flow rate will be required in this case to keep effective blood flow (plasma flow) rate constant. The final case is for a charged material which is easily transported out of red cells (e.g. bicarbonate). In this case the Donnan effect keeps its concentration low in cells relative to plasma and as HCT increases, the effective blood flow decreases by about 10%. An increase in blood flow of 12% would be required to keep the effective blood flow constant in this case. The effect of intermediate cases (i.e. $0 < \gamma < 1$) can be estimated from Table 2 or can be calculated using equation 21.

The values in Table 2 show the increases in blood flow rate required to keep solute fluxes constant for substances with a range of plasma – red cell distribution characteristics. It is also clear that different substances will require different adjustments so that compensation for flux rate changes for all materials will not be possible by increases in blood flow alone.

Reduced fluxes can also be compensated for by changes in dialysis fluid composition. To keep flux rates of a substance constant the right side of equation 14 must be constant when the individual variables change. With increased hematocrit the dialysate concentrations C_{Di} will have to change (from C_{D1} to C_{D2}) to account for reduction in Q_E (from Q_{E1} to Q_{E2}) which will also cause D to decrease (from D_1 to D_2 – see below).

If the left side of equation 14 remains the same, equating the right side at different hematocrits, the dialysate concen-

Table 2. Effective blood flow at different hematocrits for various substances (see Equation 21). Calculations assume blood flow of 250 ml/min, $F_P = 0.94$, and $F_R = 0.72$.

HCT	γ	R_D	Q_E	Q_B to keep Q_E const	% increase Q_B
20	1	1	224	–	
40	1	1	213	263	5%
20	0	1	188	–	
40	0	1	141	333	33%
20	1	0.69	213	–	
40	1	0.69	191	279	12%

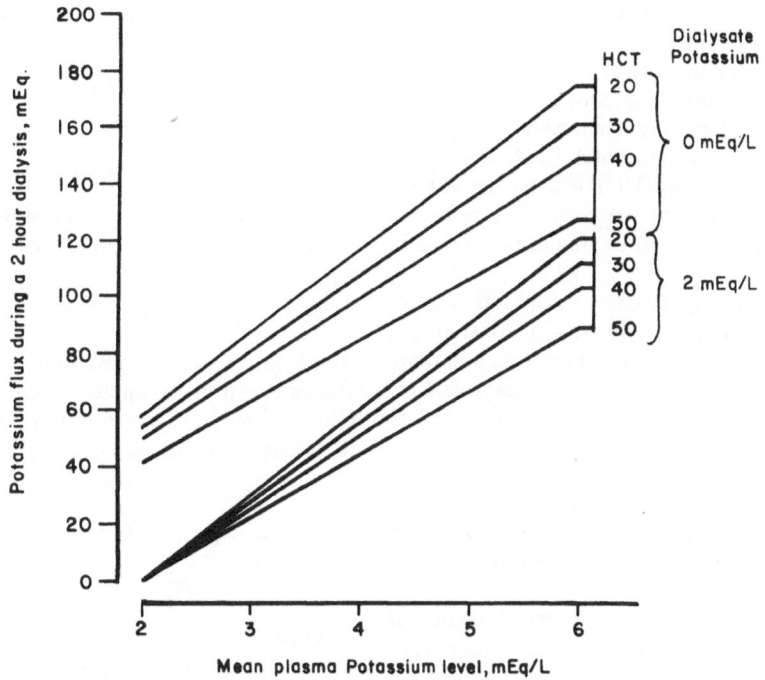

Figure 5. The effect of hematocrit on potassium transport during dialysis.

tration required to keep flux of a substance constant will be:

$$C_{D2} = \frac{D_1 C_{D1} \left(1 - \dfrac{Q_F}{Q_{E1}}\right) - C_B \left[D_1\left(1 - \dfrac{Q_F}{Q_{E1}}\right) - D_2 \left(1 - \dfrac{Q_f}{Q_{E2}}\right)\right]}{D_2 \left(1 - \dfrac{Q_F}{Q_{E2}}\right)} \quad [24]$$

Consider the case of bicarbonate with hematocrit increasing from 20% to 40% with C_{D1} = 35 mEq/l at average plasma levels of 25 mEq/l. Effective blood flows (Q_{E1} and Q_{E2}) can be read from Table 2 as 0.213 l/min and 0.191 l/min respectively. As will be discussed below, D_2 will be lower than D_1 because of the reduced effective blood flow (10). If D_1 = 0.150 l/min, D_2 = 0.142 l/min at Q_f = 0.01 l/min, equation 24 indicates that C_{D2} will have to be 35.62 mEq/l to keep bicarbonate flux constant.

Similar manipulation of equation 14 can determine what new plasma levels would result if dialysis fluid concentrations are not (or cannot) be changed (Figures 5 and 6).

For the majority of patients required dialysis fluid potassium levels can be computed with the help of equation 24. There could be a problem, however, with patients who are poorly compliant with respect to dietary K^+ restriction and have normal or high plasma K^+ level with low HCT controlled by use of zero potassium dialysis solution. Consider a patient with short dialysis (Dialysis time − td = 2 h), plasma K^+ of 5.0 mEq/l with HCT = 20. Figure 5 shows that K^+ removal in 2 h with $C_D K$ = 0 is approximately 148 mEq and that if HCT increased to 40 the CpK would have to rise to 6.0 to remove the same amount of potassium. In this case seri-

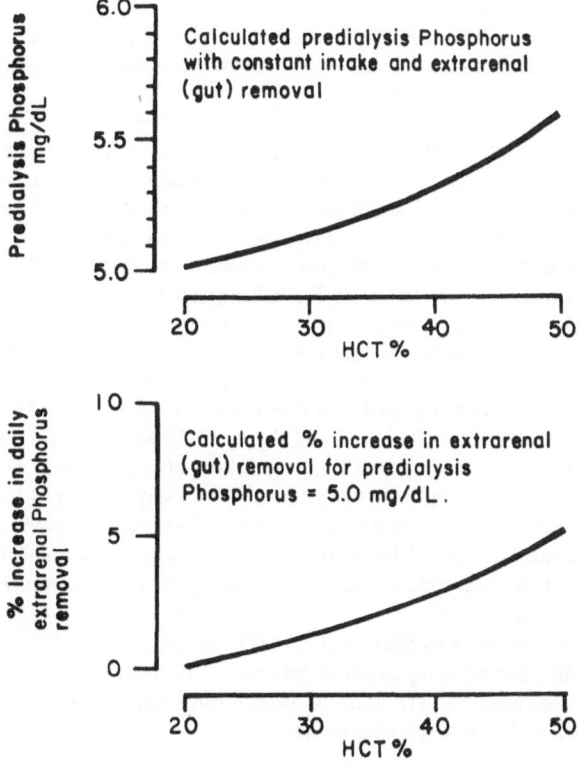

Figure 6. Expected phosphorus levels and extrarenal removal requirements with increasing hematocrit.

ous predialysis hyperkalemia could result.

The effect of decreasing inorganic phosphate (iP) dialysance (DiP) on phosphate removal is complicated because of the double pool nature of phosphate. Moreover, the bulk of phosphate removal is through the gut and mediated by binders. However, estimates of the effect of decreased phosphorus dialysance due to increased HCT can be made by a double pool analysis shown in the Appendix. The results of this analysis for a short (td = 2 h) treatment are shown in Figure 6.

The rise in predialysis phosphorus levels required to maintain zero iP balance as dialysance drops with constant gut removal was computed and is shown in Figure 6a as a function of HCT. It is apparent that as HCT increases from 20% to 40% the rise in pretreatment phosphorus would be less than 0.5 mg/dl, a modest increase.

The increase in iP binder mediated gut removal required to maintain predialysis levels constant at 5 mg/dl with decreasing DiP was also computed with results shown in Figure 6b. A 3% increase in iP binders would be required as HCT increases from 20% to 40%.

It can be concluded from the above that efficiency of dialyzer removal of the major low molecular solutes analyzed will not be seriously compromised by normalization of HCT with erythropoietin therapy. It would appear that normal HCTs will not jeopardize the current interest in the use of high flux dialyzers with short treatment times in the range of 2 h.

The interrelationship of operational constants, D, Q_B, and Q_D and the overall mass transfer coefficient – membrane area product

It is useful to determine the relationship between the operational clinical constant, diffusive dialysance, and the overall mass transfer coefficient. Equation 6 shows that for a given dialyzer K_o wil be a constant and flux will be determined solely by the magnitude of blood and dialysate concentrations; the value of K_o will not change as flows or concentrations change. Inspection of equations 10 and 11 shows that this is not true for diffusive dialysance and that the value of this constant depends directly on the flow rate. Hence, under any particular flow conditions there should be a relationship between D and K_o (or K_oA) which would be useful in determining the value of the dialyzer constant K_o from a set of clinical chemistries. Conversely, it should be possible to determine what clinical performance a dialyzer should have when blood or dialysate flow rates change or when dialyzer membrane is compromised such as in the case of clotting.

It is possible to relate K_oA and D by equating solute flux in a dialyzer using equation 14 (when $Q_F = 0$), the definition of D (see equation 11), and equations 6 and 7. Such a combination and rearrangement yields:

$$D (C_{Bi} - C_{Di}) = K_oA \frac{(C_{Bi} - C_{Do}) - (C_{Bo} - C_{Di})}{\text{Log} \frac{C_{Bi} - C_{Do}}{C_{Bo} - C_{Di}}}.$$

Manipulation of equation 11 yields the inlet and outlet concentration differences:

$$C_{Bi} - C_{Do} = (C_{Bi} - C_{Di}) (1 - D/Q_D)$$

and

$$C_{Bo} - C_{Di} = (C_{Bi} - C_{Di}) (1 - D/Q_B).$$

Substitution of these concentration terms into the equation above and rearrangement yields:

$$K_oA = \frac{Q_B}{1 - Q_B/Q_D} \text{Log} \frac{1 - D/Q_D}{1 - D/Q_B}. \qquad [25]$$

This is the expression describing K_oA and how this dialyzer constant can be computed from diffusive dialysance and clinical flows. This relationship can be rearranged to yield dialysance as a function of K_oA and flow rates:

$$D = \frac{e^{-\frac{K_oA(1-Q_B/Q_D)}{Q_B}} - 1}{\frac{e^{-\frac{K_oA(1-Q_B/Q_D)}{Q_B}}}{Q_B} - \frac{1}{Q_D}} \qquad [26]$$

Equation 25 is extremely useful in predicting the dialysance (or clearance) of a particular solute under known flow conditions if the overall mass transfer coefficient – membrane area product (K_oA) is known. Quite often a family of dialyzers will have the same design and therefore similar transport resistances. In such cases, the clinical performance of other dialyzers of same type can be accurately estimated merely by scaling the value of K_oA by the differing membrane areas in the various devices.

Equations 25 and 26 are for counter current flow. Similar expressions can be developed for co-current flow for K_oA:

$$K_oA = \frac{Q_B}{1 + Q_B/Q_D} \text{Log} \frac{Q_B}{Q_B - D(1 + Q_B/Q_D)}. \qquad [27]$$

and upon rearrangement for D:

$$D = Q_B \frac{1 - e^{-\frac{K_oA(1+Q_B/Q_D)}{Q_B}}}{1 + Q_B/Q_D}. \qquad [28]$$

Effective clearance of larger solutes with ultrafiltration

It is generally recognized that convective transport (ultrafiltration) augments solute transport (17,18). Equation 18 indicates that with smaller solutes and high clearances values (K), the effective clearance (K′) will not be greatly influenced by ultrafiltration. This is not the case, however, with larger substances where K may be of the same order of magnitude as Q_F. The effect of ultrafiltration on mass transport of solutes of different size can be illustrated using urea and a hypothetical, large molecular weight, substance which is poorly removed by diffusive transport (see Table 3). The data in Table 3 confirm that ultrafiltration plays an extremely limited role in the case of a highly cleared solute as urea (adding only 2% at high rates of ultrafiltration) but can be a major means of transport of material with limited diffusive transport potentially augmenting clearance by as much as 45%.

Transport determined by kinetic methods

The measurement of dialyzer transport by single pass methods is straight forward and accurate as long as transport rates are high so that concentration differences are sizable. In this case, values for Q_{Do}, C_{Do}, Q_F, and C_{Bi} when substituted into equation 17b will yield reliable K_d values. However, with a poorly diffusing solute where C_{Do} values may be small as will the drop in blood values, a closed loop method will yield more accurate results. With this procedure either the blood circuit or the dialysate circuit is recycled through a reservoir, and the rate of solute accumulation can be used to measure accurately transport properties (see Figure 7). Consider the system's mass balance:

Accumulation in Blood Reservoir = Flux in − Flux out

There is no flux in and substitution of equation 14 into this expression yields:

$$\frac{d(VC_B)}{dt} = D\left(1 - \frac{Q_F}{Q_{Bi}}\right)C_{Di} - \left[D\left(1 - \frac{Q_F}{Q_{Bi}}\right) + Q_F\right]C_B. \quad [29]$$

The term $d(VC_B)/dt$ indicates the rate of change of the reservoir contents. In Figure 7 where the blood loop is recycled, solute will be lost from the reservoir so that accumulation will be negative. Note that the second term of equation 29 is analogous to the one that appeared in equation 18 as the $K'C_{Bi}$ term (the product of the apparent clearance and blood inlet concentration) and accounts for the convective transport.

The solution of this expression depends on the conditions of measurement; when $Q_F = 0$, V is constant, the Q_F/Q_B terms drop out and the left hand side becomes $V(dC/dt)$ which is easily solved and yields:

$$C_B = C_{Bo}\,e^{-Dt/v} + C_{Di}(1 - e^{-Dt/v}). \quad [30a]$$

Rearranging and solving for D:

$$D = \frac{v}{t}\,Log\frac{C_{Bo} - C_{Di}}{C_{Bt} - C_{Di}}. \quad [30b]$$

Note that if the reservoir of Figure 7 is placed on the dialysate side, an equivalent expression to equation 29 results which when solved yields analogous solutions where the 'B' and 'D' sub-scripts are reversed. If Q_F is not zero, equation 29 must be solved and yields a more complicated expression which is the analog to equation 30a. (This case is solved in the Appendix).

Using the closed loop method for clearance determina-

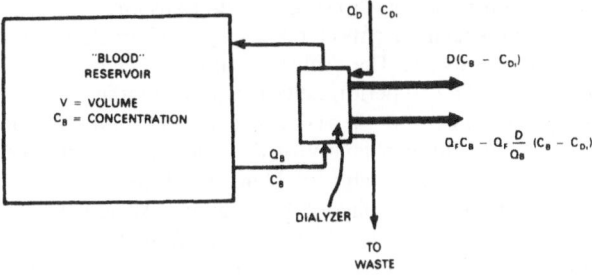

Figure 7. Schematic representation of recycle circuit for transport evaluation including flow rates and removal rates.

tion, one of the streams is recycled through a reservoir and the reservoir concentration is sampled at two times, t minutes apart. The first concentration becomes C_{Bo} (or C_{Do}), the second C_{Bt} (or C_{Dt}). The dialysance can then be calculated from equation 30b. Another method using this recycle technique and equation 30b is to take serial reservoir samples and to plot the logarithm term as a function of time. The slope of the resulting straight line will then be D/V from which the value of D can be obtained, V being known.

This technique is most suitable for materials that are poorly transported by the dialyzer so that the reservoir concentration does not change rapidly. The model shown in Figure 7 assumes that all of the material in the system is in the reservoir which is well mixed. In actuality, a significant fraction of the recycle loop can be outside (i.e. the dialyzer volume and tubing) so that this assumption is not strictly true. If D is small and V is large, however, this non-ideality becomes negligible.

The use of marker solutes

It is common practice to describe a dialyzer or membrane by the transport properties of a series of marker substances such as those listed in Table 4 (19–23). These materials when

Table 3. The effect of ultrafiltration on solute clearance for materials easily and poorly cleared by the dialyzer.

Solute	K_d	$Q_F = 5\,ml/min$		$Q_F = 10\,ml/min$	
		$Q_F = 0$ $\quad$ K_d'	K_d'/K_d	K_d'	K_d'/K_d
Urea	150	151.25	1.01	152.5	1.02
Solute 'X'	20	24.5	1.23	29.0	1.45

Table 4. Commonly used solute markers for transport studies.

Solute	Molecular weight	Ref.
NaCl	58	2
Urea	60	2
Creatinine	113	2
Uric acid	168	2
Dextrose	180	2
Sucrose	342	2
Raffinose	594	2
Bromsulfophthalein (BSP)	838	19
Cyclohepta-amylose or β Schardinger or Cyclo-dextrin	1,152	2, 21
Vitamin B_{12}	1,355	2, 19
Bacitracin	1,411	2, 19
Inulin	5,200	2, 19
Cytochrom C	13,400	2, 19

used in controlled *in vitro* studies yield transport as a function of molecular weight relationships that characterize the particular dialyzer. The difficulty with such characterizations is that *in vivo* performance cannot be predicted accurately from *in vitro* transport data because of the presence of proteins and the probability of their interaction with the membrane, the possibility of Donnan effects, and other phenomena unique to physiologic solutions. An added complication is that less than half of the listed materials (predominantly those of lower molecular weight) can be used *in vivo* so that the relationship between *in vitro* and *in vivo* values cannot be obtained easily. Finally, results of transport studies with higher molecular mass substances should be used circumspectly; membrane permeability depends on factors other than molecular mass such as molecular conformation (2, 19, 20) so that a substance of 1355 daltons (the mass of vitamin B_{12}), for example, may have transport properties far different *in vivo* from those observed for vitamin B_{12} *in vitro*.

MASS BALANCE PRINCIPLES APPLIED TO INTER-MITTENT DIALYSIS: SOLUTE KINETIC MODELING

Uremia results from the body's loss of control over its internal chemistry through the diminished capacity of the chemical regulating organ, the kidney. The fundamental assumption of dialysis treatment is that some uremic abnormalities depend on the concentration of ingested or metabolically produced toxic materials which are normally excreted by the natural kidney. The ability to keep the uremic patient alive by hemodialysis and peritoneal dialysis emphasizes that if some degree of chemical control can be restored, however imperfect, the results of uremia (particularly the predictable and imminent mortality) can be, in part, reversed. It is clear, therefore, that the passive transport of water, solutes and electrolytes which is the sole capability of dialysis, is sufficient to control the chemical imbalances which result from kidney failure.

In dialysis treatment a large number of materials, many of unknown composition (24–36) and toxicity are being removed, at unequal rates. To 'control' dialysis treatment, therefore, one might hope to select a key compound which would provide an index of treatment. To date there is no such compound although there have been numerous attempts to define one in order to develop an index of adequate treatment (5, 37–38). In reality, although control of toxic substances may be the goal of dialysis treatment, levels of a limited number of solutes, balance of fluid and electrolytes, and control of acid-base constitute the basis of current treatment adequacy on a day-to-day basis. It is with regard to the measurement and control of such substances that the concept of mass balance and solute kinetics can provide powerful tools and insights to guide treatment.

Dialysis was first mathematically modeled over three decades ago (12) with similar analysis continuing until the present time (22, 37–49). Clinical dialysis, however, has not kept pace with these advances in the quantitative understanding and ability to describe and monitor treatment. The reasons for this vary. Not all physicians consider the task of clinical management of the dialysis patient as a completely quantifiable one, a view that is at least partially justified because of the multifactorial nature of most medical problems. In addition, much of the information required by some models is unavailable to the practicing physician in the time span required for his treatment decisions. These restrictions notwithstanding the ability to describe quantitatively biochemical and physiologic processes and the abnormalities that exist in uremic patients make the process of modeling an important one for greater understanding of the disease state and better management of subsequent therapy.

Mathematical modeling of dialysis therapy represents the structured application of the principles of conservation of matter to the patient undergoing dialysis. There are many advantages to this structured approach:

1. It can describe a specific biochemical system and thereby monitor or investigate various physiologic processes, such as net rates of protein catabolism (50–52).
2. It enables one to prescribe the appropriate dialysis treatment to achieve a desired therapeutic goal, or to investigate the predictable results of altered treatment (42, 43, 53, 54).
3. It increases understanding of the controlling physiologic-biochemical mechanisms from the type of model required to describe the kinetics of a particular substance (10, 47, 55).
4. It allows determination of the controlling factors in any solute system through evaluation of the order of magnitude of various routes of input and output in a quantitatively defined system (10).
5. It allows discrimination of the causes of clinical observations and problems such as hypertension caused by sodium flux or hypoxia during acetate dialysis (10, 47).

Mathematical modeling can be viewed as 'quantified intuition' in that it mathematically relates events that are known to take place. Two aspects of mathematical modeling that should be stressed are:

1. An individual who has a thorough basic understanding of the physiologic system being modeled is best able to construct and benefit from the model (i.e. the physician who deals with specific clinical problems).
2. Putting the qualitative relationship in a mathematical context increases its value and the usefulness of information by vastly extending its range of application and the value of analyzed data (see discussion of mathematical elements in the appendix).

The basic steps of modeling are shown in Figure 8 and consist of: formulating the system description (step one) which usually involves a diagramatic representation of the system; writing the mass balance equation (step two) using the diagram; and solving the mass balance equation (step three). It should be noted that only step three requires any degree of advanced mathematical skills.

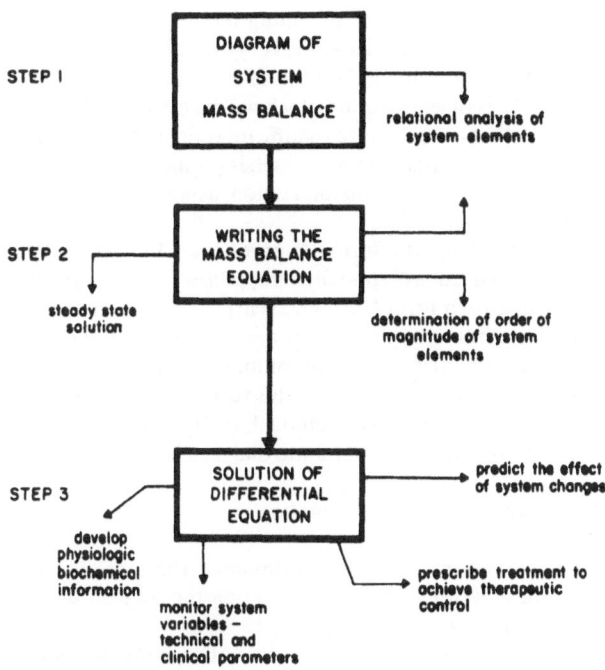

STEP 1 — DIAGRAM OF SYSTEM MASS BALANCE — relational analysis of system elements

STEP 2 — WRITING THE MASS BALANCE EQUATION — steady state solution — determination of order of magnitude of system elements

STEP 3 — SOLUTION OF DIFFERENTIAL EQUATION — predict the effect of system changes — develop physiologic biochemical information — monitor system variables – technical and clinical parameters — prescribe treatment to achieve therapeutic control

Figure 8. Diagram illustrating the steps in formulating and representing a mathematical model. Figure includes indications of uses of each stage of formulation.

MASS BALANCE CONSIDERATIONS AS APPLIED TO QUANTIFICATION OF INTERMITTENT DIALYSIS TREATMENT

The concept of conservation of matter or mass balance appears to be obvious; it is in the application of this law to a physical system, however, that it becomes an increasingly complex but an extremely powerful analytical and conceptual tool.

The Law of Conservation of Mass can be restated in the word equation:

$$\begin{matrix} \text{Accumulation} & & \text{input} & & \text{output} \\ \text{(increase in} & = & \text{to} & - & \text{from} \\ \text{system content)} & & \text{system} & & \text{system} \end{matrix} \quad [31]$$

Equation 31 forms the basis for a substantial portion of this chapter in that most relationships to follow are either applications or solutions of it.

Formulation of a model: elements of the mass balance diagram

While the application of mass balance principles to a specific system would appear not to pose any great problem, in practice it is the most difficult aspect of modeling. The difficulty lies in the need to understand fully and isolate quantitatively the specific system being modeled. It should be stressed that once the model is formulated the mathematical description of the system is predetermined, so that a deliberate attempt to represent the system accurately and quantitatively will assure the validity of subsequent steps. It is helpful if the model is formulated by use of a structured diagram. Such a diagram consists of boxes for the system and arrows for inputs and outputs.

In the following systems the model is shown as a box with arrows going into and out of it; these figures exemplify the two formal elements of this approach. The box describes the system content (generally in units of mass), such as the product of volume and concentration. Inputs add to the system content, and outputs decrease it. The manner (if any) that the inputs or outputs relate to the system content or concentration is indicated with respect to the appropriate arrows. In the case of a single box (the vast amount of figures shown in this chapter), the system is 'single pool' or one well-mixed compartment.

The system content is the total mass present at any instant. It can be contained in any physical space, such as the vascular space, the red blood cell, or the amount of dialysate recirculating through a dialyzer. The system content is the product of the compartment volume and the concentration in that space. Alternatively it can be the total system mass (irrespective of its distribution space) or simply the effect of the total mass such as in the case of heparin (56).

The quantitative description of system inputs and outputs must be consistent with the description of system content. In general, there are two common types of input/outputs: those that depend on the amount of material present in the system (first-order processes) and those that are constant (zero-order processes). The clearance of a dialyzer (K_D) is a first-order process, because material is removed as a product of K_D and concentration (see equation 18). In contrast, an effectively saturated metabolic process (such as acetate metabolism in most dialyzed patients) (55) is a constant output, or zero-order process.

The process of model formulation is best illustrated with an example.

Carbon dioxide transport in dialyzed patients

The transport of CO_2 in dialysis patients attracted considerable attention during the 1970s (57–61) and represents a good illustration of modeling techniques. The first step is to define what is meant by the CO_2 system. One must decide what forms of CO_2 are to be included, (e.g. should bicarbonate be considered part of the system?) so that all elements of the model are consistent. For this analysis we will let the CO_2 system be the total dissolved CO_2 gas in body water and let it also include the hydrated form of CO_2 (carbonic acid), but not bicarbonate. We can then draw a box such as Figure 9, that will represent the total body content of CO_2 gas at any time shown as the product of body water and CO_2 concentration (10).

Once the system is identified it is necessary to define how CO_2 is added to, and leaves the system. There are two major means of CO_2 production. The first is the oxidative metabolism of carbon containing substrates which is the ultimate origin of all body CO_2. The other is the neutralization of acid (H^+) by body bicarbonate (see reaction R-2).

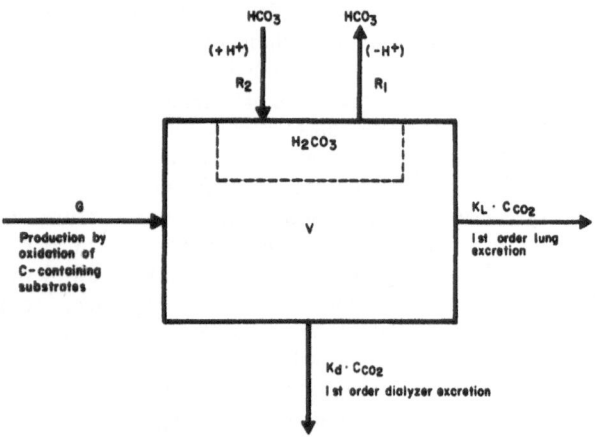

Figure 9. Model describing the CO_2 system in the dialyzed patient. (Reprinted from Kidney International, with permission.)

$$CO_2 + H_2O \rightleftarrows H_2CO_3 \rightleftarrows H^+ + HCO_3 \quad \begin{array}{l}[R\text{-}1]\\ [R\text{-}2]\end{array}$$

Carbon dioxide readily reacts with water to form carbonic acid, which will dissociate to yield H^+ and bicarbonate by reaction R-1. This system of reactions is reversible and moves to the left by reaction R-2, which represents the neutralization of acid (H^+) by bicarbonate to form H_2CO_3 and generation of CO_2. In fact, both of these reactions continue and to the extent that they are unbalanced there is net generation or consumption of CO_2.

There are two major means by which CO_2 is removed from the body water in the non-dialyzed patient. It is apparent that if reaction R-1 predominates CO_2 is removed from the system. The other route of removal is by exhalation in the lungs which will be a first order process and which will depend on the CO_2 concentration (C_{CO_2}) of the system with the lungs representing a first order excretion route which can be viewed as a lung clearance, K_L. The amount of CO_2 removed by the lungs therefore is $K_L C_{CO_2}$. In the patient not on dialysis this completely defines the system. In the dialyzed patient, however, the dialyzer will also have a CO_2 clearance (K_D) and flux by this route is $K_D C_{CO_2}$.

It is important, at this point to re-emphasize the need for an unambiguous, structured, and quantitative approach to the formulation of this model. The CO_2 system has been isolated and is the one being modeled. As such the transport of bicarbonate by the dialyzer is not relevant to the analysis; the flux of bicarbonate in the dialyzer will only affect the CO_2 through the balance of reactions R-1 and R-2 which have already been considered.

Note that the units of K_D and C_{CO_2} must be consistent and their product equal the dialyzer flux of dissolved gaseous CO_2. Clearances will most conveniently be expressed in liters per minute because CO_2 concentrations are most commonly in units of grams or milimoles per liter. This is important, because many investigators have been impressed that the dialyzer totally 'clears' incoming blood of CO_2 having CO_2 clearances equalling or exceeding blood flow (10, 60,

61). The CO_2 content of incoming blood, however, when expressed in appropriate units is very low (about 1.1 mmol/l) so that the CO_2 removed by the dialyzer is very small (10, 47). Analysis of the system (which will be completed below) will show that a much more significant route of CO_2 removal during dialysis is reaction R-1 which is promoted by bicarbonate loss and body re-alkalinization using acetate during treatment.

This completes the formulation of the CO_2 model. The CO_2 system itself is carbon dioxide, present as dissolved gas and its hydrated form (carbonic acid). CO_2 is generated by metabolic processes and the production of carbonic acid when acids are neutralized by combining with bicarbonate. It is removed by the reversal of this reaction (dissociation of H_2CO_3) and the first order removal, (CO_2 clearance) represented by the lungs (K_L) and the dialyzer (K_D).

Writing the mass balance equation

Once the systems has been formulated the mass balance equation is written. This is basically a mechanical step of substituting terms into equation 31.

The accumulation, or change in system content, will be the rate of change of the system content with time (first derivative with respect to time of the system content: d(content)/dt). It should be noted that although this term gives the intimidating appearance of 'higher mathematics' it is merely a quantitative symbol of the time dependent change of system content (i.e. accumulation). The only aspect that will change from one system to another is the representation of 'content'. In the current example, total dissolved CO_2 'content' will be the product of total body water and CO_2 concentration (not PCO_2):

$$CO_2 \text{ CONTENT} = V\,C_{CO_2}$$

$$\text{CHANGE IN SYSTEM CONTENT} = \frac{d(V\,C_{CO_2})}{dt}.$$

The input and output are taken directly from the system diagram (Figure 9) and will be the algebraic sum of all the arrows in the diagram. The zero order terms will be constants and the first order terms will be the product of first order constants (clearances) and the system concentration. Substitution of all of these terms in equation 31 yields:

$$\frac{d(V\,C_{CO_2})}{dt} = G + R_2 - R_1 - K_L C_{CO_2} - K_D C_{CO_2}. \quad [32]$$

Equation 32 is the mass balance equation for body CO_2 and, as has been stated, is a strictly mechanical reduction of the elements of the formulation, shown in Figure 9, to a mathematical form.

Use of the mass balance equation

One may be inclined to solve the above expression immediately to obtain the body CO_2 content as a function of time. For this substance this is not a very productive approach. The most useful mathematical relationship in this case, and a valuable one generally, is the mass balance equation itself.

It is instructive to consider all the terms in the specific equation to determine their relative magnitude and relation to one another. Common values for the terms listed are shown in Table 5.

Consider first the accumulation term on the left hand side of the equation 32. Computation of body CO_2 content using the values in Table 5 (i.e. $V = 40l$; $C_{CO_2} = 1.05$ mmol/l) show body CO_2 content is about 42 mmol. This is an interesting value from two standpoints. First, it should be appreciated that the entire body content of CO_2 represents only 4 min of body CO_2 production. Stated differently, there is very little 'CO_2 storage' in the body. The physiological impact of this, as is widely appreciated, is that ventilation can have a pronounced second to second effect on CO_2 levels which is extremely important in pH control through respiratory compensation in response to an acid/base insult. The second point is that a P_{CO_2} change of 10 mm Hg over a 4 h dialysis represents an average rate of change in body CO_2 content of: $d(V_{CO_2})/dt = (40) (10) (0.03)/240 = 0.05$ mmol/min or less than 0.5% of the rate of body production. It becomes clear that the change in body CO_2 content represents a small difference between two very large numbers (the rate of production at the rate of removal) and that in fact the body is effectively in steady state with respect to CO_2 content. Intuitively it would be difficult to conclude otherwise.

The system being at steady state, all the terms on the right hand side of equation 32 must add to zero. Between dialyses equation 32 reduces to: $G = K_L C_{CO_2}$; the generated CO_2 is exhaled. During dialysis the situation is more complicated. The generation of CO_2 would be expected to remain relatively constant, which from the standpoint of energetics is reasonable. During acetate dialysis reaction R1 will predominate and R2 will equal zero. Bicarbonate loss in itself will not affect this model. Usually, however, the HCO_3 lost in the dialyzer is almost quantitatively replaced by reaction R1. If plasma bicarbonate levels are 18 mEq/l approximately

Table 5. Typical values in a 70 kg patient undergoing acetate dialysis.

Inter dialytic	Intra dialytic	Ref.
V = 40l	40l	–
C = 1.05 mmol/l	1.05 mmol/l	10
(P_{CO_2} = 35 mm Hg)		
G = 11 mmol/min	11 mmol/min	60, 61
R_1 = –	2.3 mmol/min	–
R_2 = –	0	10
K_L = 10.5 l/min	8.1 l/min	10, 60
K_D = 0	0.20 l/min	10
dC = –	0.3 mmol	
	(10 mm Hg)	–
$\dfrac{d(VC)}{dt}$ = –	0.05 mm/min	–
$K_L C_{CO_2}$ = 11 mmol	8.5 mmol	–
$K_D C_{CO_2}$ = 0	0.21 mmol	–
R_2 = –	2.29 mmol	–

2.3 mEq/min will be lost and replaced by reaction R1.

Examination of the three routes of removal indicates that the effect of dialyzer CO_2 transport is vanishingly small (2%, see Table 5) and can be neglected with respect to its effect on P_{CO_2}. This fact has not been widely appreciated (60, 61).

At steady state rearrangement of equation 32 yields:

$$G - R1 - K_D C_{CO_2} = K_L C_{CO_2}.$$

Solving for K_L

$$K_L = G/C_{CO_2} - R1/C_{CO_2} - K_D. \qquad [33]$$

The 'normal' steady state relationship (in the non-dialyzed patient) of, G, K_L (K_{Ln}, and C_{CO_2} is:

$$K_{Ln} = G/C_{CO_2} \qquad [34]$$

If equation 33 is divided by equation 34 the relative value of K_L will be

$$\frac{K_L}{K_{Ln}} = 1 - R1/G - K_D/K_{Ln}. \qquad [35]$$

Substituting values into this expression from Table 5 lung clearance would be expected to drop to 77% of its normal value.

Adjustments of CO_2 levels to control pH is part of respiratory feed back in the normal individual (8, 62) although this may be complicated by hypoxia particularly at low P_{CO_2} values. During dialysis P_{CO_2} remains relatively stable (59), and equation 35 indicates that this must reflect a reduction in K_L (which is directly related to respiratory rate) to approximately three quarters of non-dialysis values in order to adjust for extra-pulmonary CO_2 excretion. It is important, therefore, that the reduced ventilation predicted by equation 35 be explained when the observed dialysis hypoxia is analyzed (58–61).

Solution of the mass balance equation

Most kinetic models (and all those to be considered) are in the form of a first order linear differential equation for which solutions and solution techniques by classical methods of applied mathematics are well known (63, 64). The solutions describe the system concentration (or system content) as function of time. Essentially the expression can then be used to predict the effect of treatment changes on a particular solute being modeled and to monitor various system parameters. This aspect of modeling has been most extensively developed for urea as described below. In the case of the CO_2 model the system is essentially at steady state (as discussed above). Consequently, third step will not be taken for this system.

These are the key steps of modeling. It is well to emphasize again that the actual mathematical steps of writing the mass balance equation and solving it (steps two and three in Figure 8) are mechanical operations which totally depend upon the model formulation (step one). Consequently, the entire validity of the solutions depend on the correct and rigorous formulation of the model itself.

MASS BALANCE AS APPLIED TO VARIOUS SOLUTE SYSTEMS

Urea nitrogen mass balance

Urea is of interest because it is the major product of protein catabolism so it can be used as an index of the patient's catabolic status and, by extension, nutritional state. Furthermore, development of the uremic syndrome depends to a large extent on protein catabolism (65–69) for which urea* generation provides a quantitative measure (see Equation A-16 in the Appendix).

Although urea is not considered highly toxic, its presence in high blood concentrations may accompany increased morbidity in dialysis patients (70–73). It has been demonstrated in a large well controlled cooperative study that elevation of BUN in the presence of adequate protein intake is associated with increased rates of hospitalization (74–78). In addition, some nitrogenous compounds that are commonly found in the dialysis patient may be stoichiometrically related to the rate of protein catabolism and consequently, to the rate of urea production.

Urea distribution and metabolism can be described quantitatively as shown in Figure 10. This figure considers urea nitrogen to be distributed in a single pool (physically approximating total body water) (79) with one route of net entry (or net generation) and one route of removal by first order processes.

Urea will enter the pool of body water as amino acids are oxidized (80, 81). As such its minute rate of net generation (absolute synthesis – absolute degradation) will not, in fact, be constant. The urea content of the body, however, is a thermodynamic property (its value being path independent) and will increase in a quasi-linear manner between dialyses. As a result the assumption that net urea generation is zero-order (constant) is considered to have practical validity.

Routes of removal are considered to be entirely first order (i.e. proportional to concentration) and accounted for solely by the residual kidney and the dialyzer. Urea diffuses into the gut where its nitrogen is converted into ammonia which is reabsorbed by the portal circulation (82, 83). Because this path is internal to the model no net gut contribution to urea removal from total body water is considered.

The analysis of this model then proceeds by writing the mass balance relationship:

Accumulation = Input − Output

$$\frac{d\,(VC)}{dt} = G - (K_R + K_D)\,C. \qquad [36]$$

Further expansion of equation 36 yields:

$$V\frac{dC}{dt} + C\frac{dV}{dt} = G - (K_R + K_D)\,C. \qquad [37]$$

---

* Because it is the nitrogen component of urea that is derived from protein, urea nitrogen is the expression used in quantitative considerations herein, but the solute itself is referred to as urea.

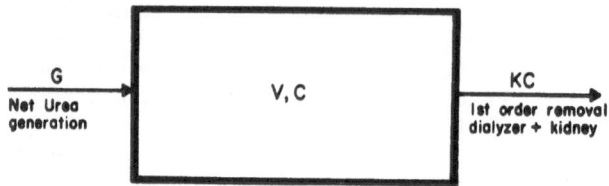

Figure 10. Model of urea nitrogen in the dialyzed patient. (Reprinted from Kidney International, with permission.)

Consideration of steady state: chronic renal failure

Before considering the solution of equation 37 it is appropriate to contemplate the mass balance equation itself with respect to the special, but more usual case of steady state when dC/dt and dV/dt are both negligible. These two quantities will always have some value, but when dialysis is not required there will be no net accumulation of body urea or water and these terms can be neglected. With respect to body solutes steady state is commonly called 'homeostasis' and in this physiological situation the left hand side of equation 37 is zero (steady state with respect to body protein is usually called zero nitrogen or protein balance). Considering equation 37 steady state for urea nitrogen can be represented as:

$$G = K_R C. \qquad [38a]$$

There are two other forms of this expression

$$K_R = G/C \qquad [38b]$$

and

$$C = G/K_R. \qquad [38c]$$

Figure 11 interrelates the three parameters shown in equations 38. The figure shows BUN as a function of time at two different levels of protein intake as renal function (urea clearance) declines. The K_R as a linear function of time is shown in a secondary K-time plot in the same figure (lower left). This figure makes use of net rate of urea nitrogen production resulting from a known quantity of protein catabolism. As is discussed further in the Appendix this accurately relates the net amount of urea that will be generated for net protein catabolic rates (PCR) from 20 g to 350 g/day in uremic and normal individuals (50, 81, 84, 85). The two forms of this relationship are (with G expressed in mg/min):

$$G = \frac{PCR - 0.294\,V}{9.35} \qquad [39a]$$

which when rearranged yields

$$PCR = 9.35G + 0.294V. \qquad [39b]$$

Figure 11 represents a progression of steady states as renal function declines. In this figure there is no change in generation. As 70 g of protein is ingested and a like amount catabolized a net quantity of 6.23 mg/min of urea nitrogen or 13.4 mg/min of urea, (i.e. 233 μmol/min) is produced, both

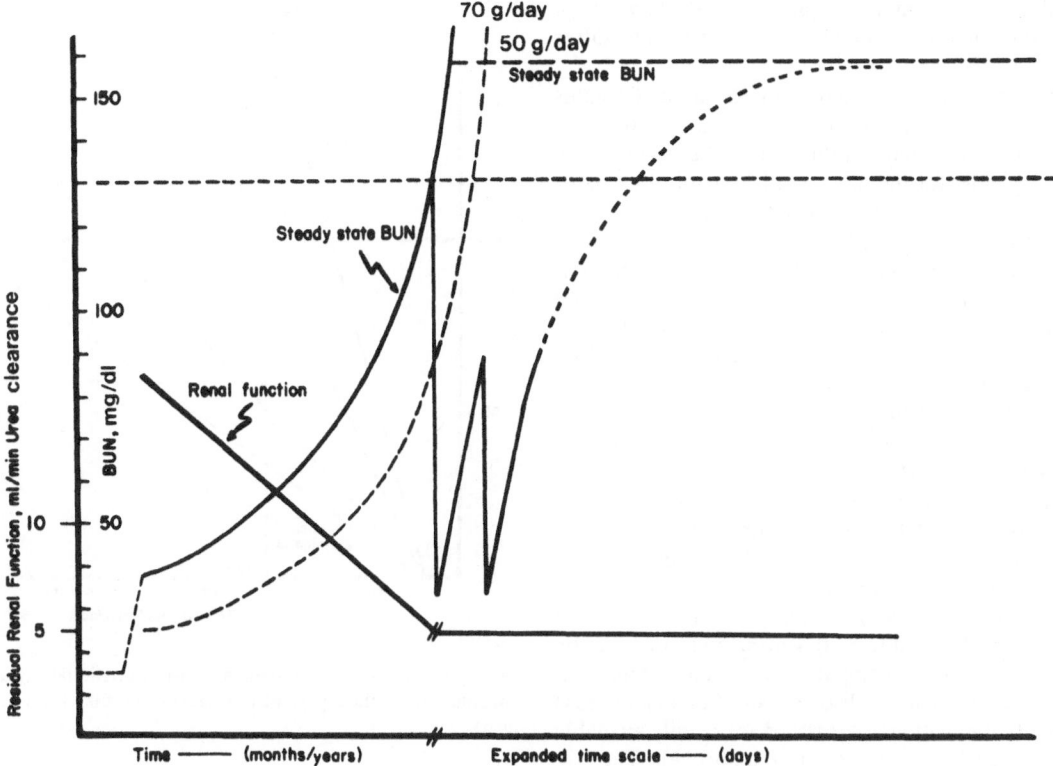

Figure 11. Blood urea nitrogen in a patient with chronic renal failure with decreasing renal function (see superimposed plot in bottom left of figure). Relationship is shown for two levels of protein intake (and net catabolism) up to the point where dialysis is instituted.

in the uremic patient with 10 ml/min of renal function, and in a normal individual. This same amount is excreted in both cases. The difference between the two is that because the flux is equal to the product of K_R and C (equation 38a) the BUN must be far higher in the uremic patient which is obviously the case.

There will be some BUN level above which every physician will consider dialysis appropriate. For this discussion 100 mg/dl (214 mg/dl of urea or 35.7 mmol/l) has been chosen as this value, to illustrate the use of steady state expressions shown in equations 38.

When K_R drops to 6 ml/min, BUN will be slightly above 100 mg/dl (35.7 mmol/l of urea) (see equation 38c). At this point the clinical decision may be to start dialysis. As seen from the figure, however, a reduction in protein intake to 50 g/day would decrease the BUN to below 70 mg/dl (25 mmol/l) and delay dialysis for an extended period. This has been the historic approach of the management of uremia (65, 86, 87). This, in fact is the spontaneous physiologic result of uremia and anorectic feed back. With an intake of 50 g/day (G = 4.09 mg/min) the BUN wil reach 100 mg/dl (35.7 mmol/l) when K_R is approximately 4 ml/min (see equation 38c). Once again the intake may be reduced.

At some point, however, dialysis will be initiated to allow a tolerable intake with acceptable BUN. It is important to realize however, that a steady state concentration still exists,

a mathematical value that may never really be attained. For an intake of 70 g/day with a K_R of 2 ml/min steady state BUN it would be 312 mg/dl (111.4 mmol/l) for example. The patient undergoes dialysis to keep BUN below this level. But at the end of a dialysis, BUN starts to increase towards this level and only the next dialysis interrupts it. The build up of BUN to a steady state value post dialysis is curvilinear because as BUN increases the remnant kidney removes more material and blunts the rate of rise (see right hand side of equation 38a and Figure 11). It is also important to recognize that as long as there is some kidney function there is mathematically a steady state BUN, which will change as K_R does. In some cases K_R will improve slightly; in such cases a re-evaluation of intake and treatment is appropriate (88).

Establishing a level of K_R

In Figure 11 the level of renal function is the major parameter to which all others must adjust. In steady state its value is shown by equation 38b which can be expanded to yield:

$$K_R = \frac{G}{C} = \frac{\text{EXCRETION RATE}}{C} = \frac{V_{ur} C_{ur}}{T_{ur}} \frac{1}{C_B}. \quad [40]$$

This expression is a general form of the classical formula for clearance: $K_R = UV/P$, where U = urine concentration (C_{ur}), V = the volume of a 24 h urine collection divided by

1440 min/day (V_{ur}/T_{ur}) and P = plasma solute level (C_B). Equation 40 recognizes that collection intervals may differ from an exact 24 h.

The right hand side of equation 40 is general for all solutes and does not rely on the presence of steady state. In this case C_B will be the average blood value during the urine collection (see Appendix for the mathematical determination of this quantity during dialysis). What is required is a urine collection of known volume, V_{ur}, and analysis of the solute concentration in that urine volume, C_{ur}, (urea nitrogen, creatinine, etc.) the duration of the collection, T_{ur}, and the average prevailing blood level of that solute C_B. In the case described above (see Figure 11), typical values for a 1500 ml 24 h collection with urine urea nitrogen (C_{ur}) 600 mg/dl (214 mmol/l) and creatinine 92 mg/dl (8.1 mmol/l) respectively would yield excretory rates (and generation for the steady state) of 9 g/day (6.25 mg/min) for urea nitrogen and 1380 mg/day (0.96 mg/min) for creatinine. For BUN and creatinine levels of 104 mg/dl (37.1 mmol/l) and 8 mg/dl (708 μmol/l) respectively, clearances will be K_R urea = 6 ml/min; K_R creatinine = 12 ml/min.

This information is useful in several ways. The net rate of urea generation obtained from this urine collection can be used in equation 39b to compute net protein catabolism. Such data are useful in many disease states (not just uremia) to assess protein nutritional status and are readily available from urine collections analyzed for urea nitrogen. The rate of creatinine generation is useful as a nutritional parameter (89). Creatinine generation rate is also a convenient check on the accuracy of the urine collection; its value is relatively stable because it is produced at a reasonably constant rate from muscle tissue. Consequently, variability of this parameter suggests inaccuracy in urine collection (either V_{ur} or T_{ur}) or analysis (C_{ur}).

The ratio of K_R urea to K_R creatinine is also a useful parameter because in chronic renal failure the ratio of these two clearances tends to remain relatively constant and can be used to estimate K_R urea from K_R creatinine values (90, 91). Once K_R urea is known, it is possible using equation 38a both to determine the level of protein intake required to keep BUN below a desired value, and the actual protein intake when a patient presents with an elevated BUN (90).

This approach is shown graphically in Figure 12 where BUN is plotted as a function of PCR for various levels of residual urea clearance. It illustrates that if K_R is known in nutritionally stable (zero nitrogen balance) patients, PCR (intake) can be accurately prescribed and determined from BUN measurements. Once clearance values have been measured a great deal of information is available from routine blood values alone. From the initial clearance determination levels of G (creatinine) and the ratio of K_R urea to K_R creatinine (K_R ratio) are known. Consequently, from subsequent values of BUN and plasma creatinine concentrations the following can be calculated:

K_R creatinine – from plasma creatinine concentration,
     G (creatinine)
     and equation 38b

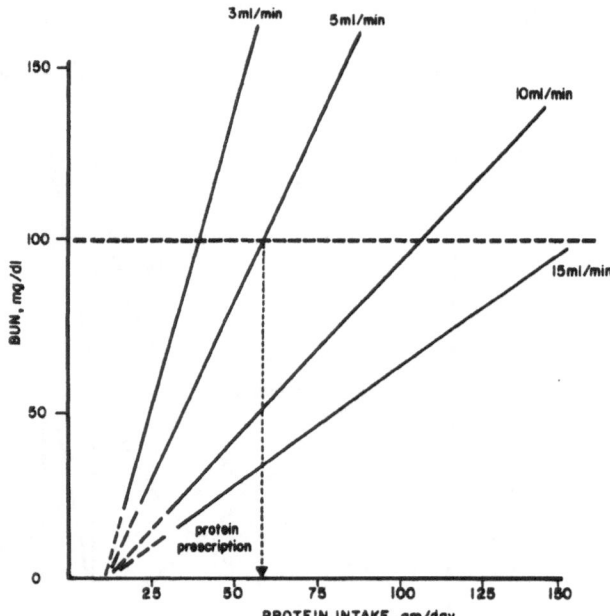

Figure 12. Blood urea nitrogen in the nutritionally stable adult chronic renal failure patient in relation to intake (and net catabolism).

K_R urea	– from K_R creatinine and the K_R ratio
G urea	– from K_R urea, BUN and equation 38a
PCR	– from equation 39b.

It is apparent that with these data available from BUN and serum creatinine levels, reducing them to a ratio of BUN/plasma creatinine concentration as has been suggested, decreases their value as analytical and nutritional parameters (92).

The technique of evaluating net protein catabolic rate using K_R ratio and G (creatinine) is useful in non-dialyzed patients and has been successfully applied to acute ill patients (91). In unpublished studies of 84 posttransplant patients, burn trauma patients, geriatric patients and normal subjects the average deviation of estimated PCR relative to those computed from 24 h urine collections was less than 10%. The value of this technique is that it permits the monitoring of catabolism in the patient who is undergoing nutritional support as well as the monitoring of renal status and nutrition in the patient with chronic renal failure.

Equation 38c shows the general determinants of BUN and creatinine levels in the undialyzed (not necessarily uremic) patient. The solute levels relate directly to net rates of generation and inversely to clearances. The widespread use of the reciprocal of plasma creatinine concentration as an index of renal function (93) and the tendency to view elevated BUNs as indicators of renal failure should be examined in the context of equation 38c. Plasma creatinine levels reflect renal function only when creatinine generation is constant. When wasting occurs simultaneously with decreasing renal function, creatinine concentration may remain relatively stable because G creatinine and K_r creatinine are decreasing at the same rate. Similarly, elevated BUN reflects the net rate of generation relative to clearance. Consequently, a high BUN may reflect a high rate of catabolism or intake (84) or reduced renal function or both. Appropriate clinical and nutritional management require that the determinants of mass balance as represented by equation 38c be evaluated individually.

Urea nitrogen kinetics in the dialyzed patient

At the point in Figure 11 when dialysis is instituted, solute concentration will oscillate at a point below steady state and the object of dialysis is to keep it within a tolerable range. Equation 37 must, therefore, be considered in its entirety.

When there is no significant change in the system volume the second term on the left of equation 37 can be dropped (dV/dT = 0) and:

$$V\frac{dC}{dt} = C - (K_R + K_D) C \qquad [41a]$$

$$\frac{dC}{dt} = \frac{G}{V} - \frac{K_R + K_D}{V} C. \qquad [41b]$$

It should be pointed out that in the steady state analysis concentration was insensitive to the system volume because there was no solute accumulation. Once dialysis is needed, however, body water serves as a container that stores solutes between treatments. Equation 41b describes this, and shows that V will significantly influence the rate of concentration increase, dC/dt, and by extension the corresponding treatment required.

The more general case, however, in the uremic patient is for V to change due to fluid retention between treatments and ultrafiltration during dialysis. In this case V as a function of time is represented as:

$$V = V_0 + \beta t. \qquad [42a]$$

And

$$\frac{dV}{dt} = \beta. \qquad [42b]$$

Where β is the rate of weight gain. Combining equations 37, 42a, and 42b and letting $K = K_R + K_D$, yields:

$$\frac{dC}{G - (K + \beta) C} = \frac{dt}{V_0 + \beta}. \qquad [43]$$

Solution of equations 41a and 43 by classical techniques (63, 64) yields analogous expression for concentration as a function of time:

$$C = C_0 e^{-Kt/V} + \frac{G}{K} [1 - e^{-Kt/V}] \qquad [44a]$$

$$C = C_0 \left(\frac{V_0 + \beta t}{V_0}\right)^{\frac{-K+\beta}{\beta}} +$$

$$+ \frac{G}{K + \beta} \left[1 - \left(\frac{V_0 + \beta t}{V_0}\right)^{\frac{-K+\beta}{\beta}}\right]. \qquad [44b]$$

Manipulations of Equation 44a for the guidance of dialysis therapy have been discussed elsewhere (42). Analogous rearrangements of equation 44b (94) provide for the same monitoring and guidance of treatment in the more general case in renal failure where volumes are changing due to expanding and contracting quantities of body water during different intervals of the therapy.

Equations 44 are used to predict the BUN concentration that will result from a specific set of therapy (t, K, and schedule) and patient (V_0, G, and β) parameters.

Although equation 44b is the more general solution of equation 37 examination of equation 44a can give some insight into the nature of these expressions. Reference to equation 38c shows that the coefficient of the second term on the right side of equation 44a is the steady state concentration if dialysis was performed indefinitely. Equation 44a can then be written as:

$$C = C_0 - e^{-Kt/V} + C_{SS} [1 - e^{-Kt/V}] \qquad [45]$$

The term, $e^{-Kt/V}$ is one that describes the rate of concentration decay in a first order system of volume V where material is being cleared at a rate K. It represents the reciprocal of $e^{+Kt/V}$ and, therefore, becomes small, approaching zero, as t becomes large. The second term is that for a system approaching steady state with constant input and first order removal. Consequently, equation 45 represents the combination of 1st order removal of material originally present in the system (1st term) plus the build up of additional material (2nd term).

By definition, any number, including e, raised to the power 0 will equal 1, so that when t = 0, equation 45 reduces to the trivial expression $C_B = C_{B0}$ which is the case by definition at t = 0. Conversely, as t becomes large C_B approaches C_{SS}.

If the patient is dialyzed for an infinite period of time, the exponential terms will approach zero, as mentioned above. The rate at which this happens will depend on the relative values of $(K_R + K_D)$ and V. If the numerator of the exponent $(K_R + K_D)$ is large compared to V, then the exponent will disappear rapidly; if the converse is true, it will remain a significant factor for long intervals. When the exponential is no longer significant, equation 45 reduces to the steady state (i.e. when the concentration has ceased to change) and the rate of material entering equals the rate of material leaving and there is no accumulation. Rarely is the patient actually dialyzed to steady state although it is important to note that even if long dialyses are used, the lowest possible concentration is that described by the ratio G/K (which is the analogue of Equation 38c).

A similar analysis of equation 44b will not lead to the same relationships. This is because the analysis that led to equation 44b is based on volume changing at a constant rate over time and at large values of t the inescapable, and impossible, result is that during very long treatments V could become negative (i.e. $- Q_F t$ be larger than V_0, β being Q_F during dialysis – see equation 42a).

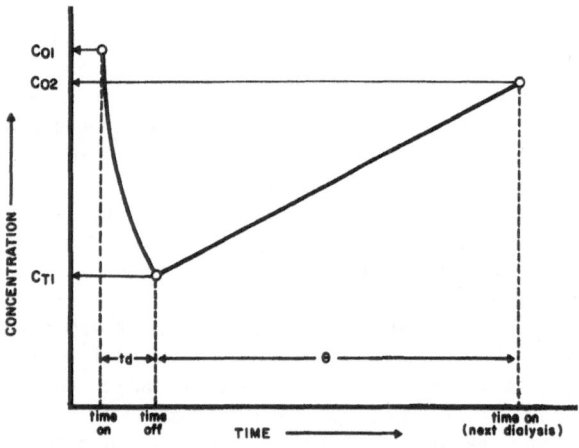

Figure 13. Blood urea nitrogen in the dialyzed patient during one dialysis cycle.

Use of mass balance equation solution

Equation 44b is used in two ways: to establish patient parameters (V and G) from clinical data (42, 94) and to predict the effect of therapy changes and prescribe dialysis treatment to achieve clinical goals (42, 43, 58, 94–96).

It is clear from equation 44b that desired BUN concentration can be achieved by manipulation of K_D and T_D (the two direct therapy parameters). Dialysis frequency is also a treatment parameter which will determine the interval over which BUN is allowed to increase between treatments (96). The use of equation 44b for predictive and prescriptive computations, however, presupposes knowledge of the patient parameters V and G. Initially values for these parameters must be developed from clinical data for the specific patient for whom the model is to be used. If the patient's level of renal function is known, examination of equation 44b shows that with BUN concentrations at the start and end of an interval as well as weight changes and treatment variables the only remaining undefined parameters in these expressions are patient volume, V_o, and urea nitrogen generation rate, G. Taking each of these constants separately, if one of them were known the other could be calculated directly from a single interval. It follows that both can be computed if the treatment parameters and BUN concentrations are known over two intervals, such as a dialysis and an inter-dialytic period (see Figure 13). The computations to obtain V and G as well as the predictive use of these solutions have been discussed elsewhere (42, 43, 47, 94).

Deviation of urea from single pool behavior

It is important to appreciate the nature of the assumption of a single well mixed compartment, i.e. a single pool model. The body has virtually an infinite number of physical compartments. Modeling attempts simplification by viewing the body as a system that acts as a single unit (single pool) or as a

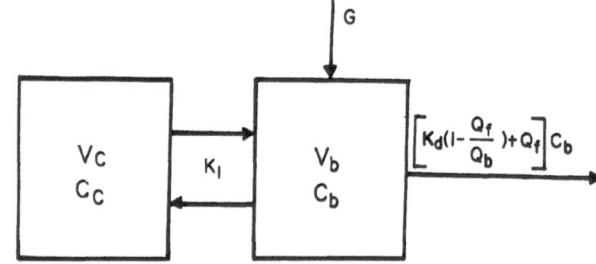

Figure 14. Two pool model for urea nitrogen in the dialyzed patient.

few discrete volumes which interconnect (multipool). For a multipool model there is mass transport between the compartments and to the extent that some of these compartments behave similarly they can be lumped as a modeled volume. Consequently, it is common to consider intracellular water as a discrete space when, in fact, it is composed of a large number of individual cells; other 'compartments' are treated similarly. Single pool modeling assumes that the body acts as a single well mixed container and relies not only on the high permeability of cells to the material being modeled, but also on the transport of the material throughout the body (i.e. the mixing) by rapidly flowing blood through a totally perfused body. Consequently, a patient in shock would tend to deviate from these assumptions, not because of any lack of permeability of cells, but because there is an upset in the normally well mixed nature of the system.

The simplifying assumption of a single pool for urea during dialysis has general validity as long as the movement of urea into and out of cells (a nonperfused compartment) from an extracellular 'compartment' is more rapid than movement of material out of this extracellular space (as happens during dialysis). When the urea transport constants from nonperfused to perfused spaces are of the same order as that of dialysis, urea will exhibit behavior that increasingly deviates from that of single pool kinetics.

With the trend toward increased dialyzer efficiency and 'rapid dialysis' (97, 98) an examination of the validity of single pool modeling of urea and other materials is important. The double pool model for urea in the dialyzed patient is shown in Figure 14. This model shows urea generation into a perfused compartment which is often considered as extracellular space (V_B, C_B). This site of urea production is considered reasonable because urea is produced in the liver and enters body water from the portal circulation. The perfused compartment is shown to communicate with the nonperfused compartment (V_C, C_C) along a concentration gradient with an intercompartmental transfer coefficient, K_1. It is important to repeat that this constant K_1 will be a combination of cell permeability and the rates of tissue perfusion. The term K_1 which combines these effects has been evaluated in dialysis patients by several investigators and has been determined to have a value of 760 – 1000 ml/min (39, 44, 99). Urea clearance with highly efficient dialyzers and rapid blood and dialysis fluid flow rates now approaches 1/4 to 1/3 of theses values of K_1.

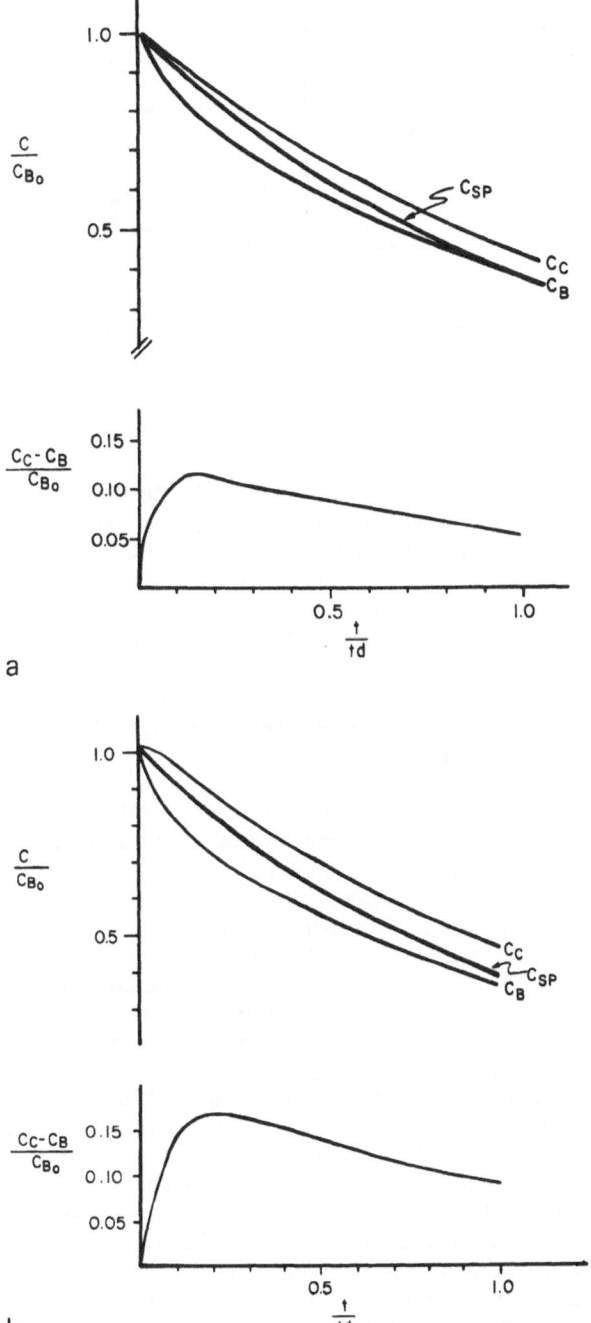

Figure 15. Urea levels (C) during dialysis computed from Two Pool Model for different dialysis times and dialyzer clearances: (A) Four hours with Kd = 175 ml/min; (B) 2.5 hours with Kd = 280 ml/min.

To determine the effect of normal and elevated urea clearances on the use of the single pool urea model discussed above, the model in Figure 14 was solved and the urea concentrations in the two compartments during treatment were computed with a 'normal' dialysis (4 h with dialyzer

urea clearance of 175 ml/min) and a 'rapid' dialysis (2.5 h with dialyzer urea clearance of 280 ml/min). The mass balance equations for this system and their solution appear in the Appendix. The hypothetical patient used for these computations was a 72 kg male undergoing dialysis, eating 1.0 g protein/kg-day, with compartment volumes of 14 l (perfused, V_B) and 28 l (nonperfused, V_C).

The urea concentrations for both compartments are shown in Figure 15A and B for the first dialysis of the week (assuming thrice weekly treatment). The total body urea concentration that would be expected if the body acted as a single pool is also shown and is intermediate between the two other curves in the upper half of those figures. The urea concentration difference between the two compartments is shown in the lower part of these figures.

As is anticipated the greater the clearance the greater is the difference in concentrations between the two pools and the greater the deviation from single pool behavior. The concentration in the non-perfused compartment tends to lag that in the perfused compartment and the difference between the two tends to peak about 30 min into the treatment. Subsequently, the non-perfused compartment concentration drops more rapidly and the concentration, C_C tends to 'catch up'.

To determine the effect of modeling this system as a single pool the double pool concentrations were considered to be the actual values during the treatments shown. The BUNs that would be measured before and after dialysis, (i.e. those in the perfused pool C_B) were then used in equation 44a–44b to estimate body water volume (the combined volumes of the perfused and non-perfused compartments). Table 6 shows that if sampling were done 'early' in dialysis equation 44b would under-estimate the combined volumes by up to 15% (almost 25% in the case of a 1 h sample for a rapid treatment). If pre- and post-treatment samples are taken, however, the under-estimation is less than 3%. Urea generation rates are over-estimated by approximately 5%.

If the patient parameters computed using equation 44b are used to determine what treatment would be required to produce a desired BUN and the actual urea level achieved in the perfused compartment is calculated using these treatment factors and the double pool model the actual BUNs exceed those expected by 2 to 4%.

Multi-compartmental models, while more mathematically elegant, present at least two difficulties: first, more physiological/anatomical parameters are needed for a complete

Table 6. Calculation of urea volume and net generation rates from urea concentrations in the perfused pool during different dialysis (see Figure 14).

	Dialysis time	1 h	2/3 T_D	T_D
V_{SP}/	Normal treatment	0.85	0.94	0.99
$V_B + V_C$	Rapid treatment	0.77	0.90	0.97
G_{SP}/	Normal treatment	1.01	1.03	1.04
G	Rapid treatment	1.01	1.04	1.06

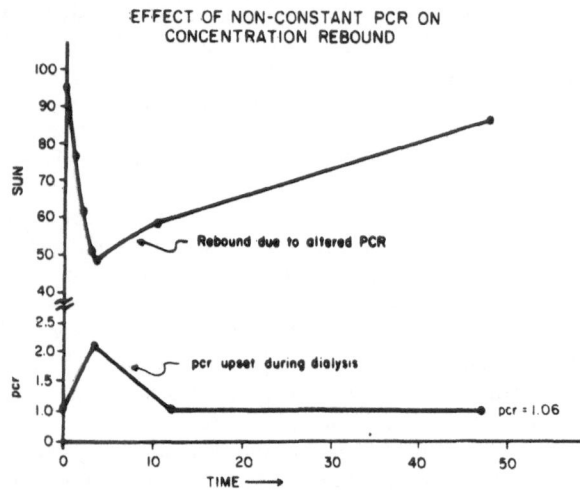

EFFECT OF NON-CONSTANT PCR ON
CONCENTRATION REBOUND

Figure 16. Illustration of the BUN (SUN) during and post dialysis in the case of non-constant net protein catabolism showing an apparent urea rebound due to increased net urea generation during and immediately post dialysis. (Reprinted from Uremia: Pathobiology of Patients Treated for 10 Years or More. edited by Giordano C, Friedman EA, Milan, Wichtig Editore, 1981, with permission.)

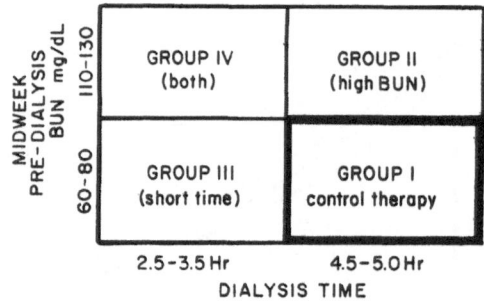

Protein Nutrition: 0.8 < dietary intake < 1.4 gm/kg/day
Weight gain: 3.5 kg/treatment

Figure 17. The design of the National Cooperative Dialysis Study.

modeling definition of the patient and second, the model may be deceptive because of the need to define the internal metabolic mechanisms in greater detail. In most multi-compartment models (45) the magnitude of many patient parameters are taken to be those published (44, 99) so that actual values are not calculated. This approach predetermines certain parameters. Thus, the model does not actually describe the specific patient and no truly individual treatment can be achieved. The assumption of parameter values, however, is required in complex models because actual calculation of patient values would require a large amount of clinical data such as interdialytic as well as pre-post solute levels. This approach makes modeling for clinical treatment inordinately complex. In contrast, a single pool model requires only pre-post concentrations for parameter calculation (42). It is this simplicity that makes a single pool model so attractive and clinically usable for the individualization of treatment (43, 53, 94).

Postulation of a multi-compartmental model presumes knowledge of internal metabolic events in some detail and in this regard may be misleading. For example, the two pool model describes the well-known rebound effect of solutes following dialysis (39) while the single pool does not. In so doing it attributes the rebound to concentration differences at the end of treatment between the two pools. There is ample evidence, however, to indicate that much of the urea rebound is due to change in rates of protein catabolism following treatment (50, 100–103). Figure 16 shows the type of rebound curve that would result from a doubling of net protein catabolic rates postdialysis, returning to predialysis levels in 8 to 10 h. Thus, although a two pool model can describe a rebound curve, it may mask some of the actual determinants of these solute levels ascribing them to concen-

tration differences in compartments rather than a pertubation of metabolic rates. In contrast the simpler model may be more clinically significant because it is less tightly defined. It allows more flexible interpretation of data which can result in greater physiological or nutritional insights because of its generality (41, 51, 90, 104).

The National Cooperative Dialysis Study (NCDS):
The clinical application of urea kinetics and operational relationships

The NCDS was conducted in the United States between 1976 and 1981. It was designed as shown in Figure 17 (76) and represents a unique example of quantitatively prescribed solute levels using a mathematical model and implementation of the dialyzer operating constants as described in this chapter to achieve them (49, 95).

There were four groups of patients in the experimental phase of the NCDS representing the combinations of the two independent variables of mid week pre-dialysis BUN and dialysis time (see Figure 17). The study was designed to hold BUN at nominal values of 70 mg/dl (25 mmol/l) and 120 mg/dl (42.9 mmol/l) mid week during dialyses of 4.5 to 5.0 h (long) and 2.5 to 3.5 h (short dialysis). All patients were initialy treated in the control phase with 'long' dialysis times and 'low' BUN treatment. After successful completion of 3 months of control therapy they were randomly assigned to the four groups shown in Figure 17.

Because dialysis time was reasonable fixed for the protocol (see Figure 17) dialyzer clearance was the main treatment parameter that was adjusted. The dialyzer clearance required to maintain each patient initially in the control group and eventually in the specific experimental group was determined from equation 44b (and mathematical rearrangements thereof) (94). With knowledge of residual kidney urea clearance present the value of 'K' in equation 44b was used to determine the dialyzer clearance required for a specific patient (i.e. for specific values of V_0, G, and β). Equations 26 and 28 were then used to determine what blood and dialysate flows (Q_B and Q_D) were needed to produce this urea clearance for the dialyzer in use (K_oA).

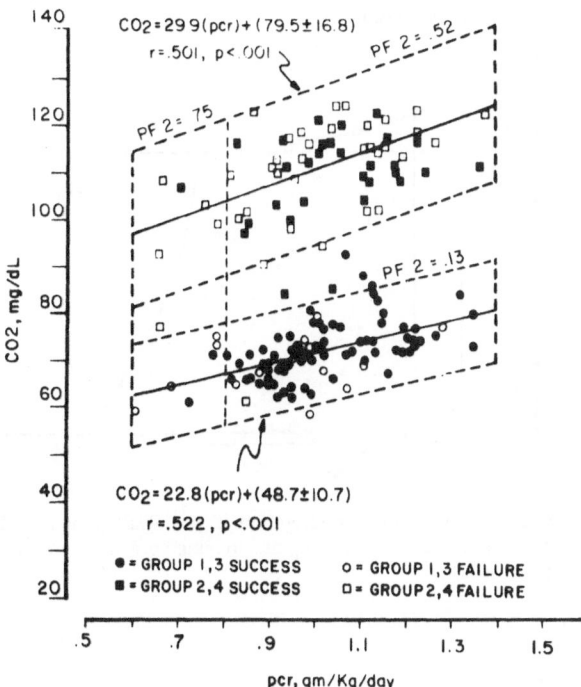

$CO_2 = 29.9(pcr) + (79.5 \pm 16.8)$
$r = .501, \, p < .001$

PF 2 = .52

PF 2 = .75

PF 2 = .13

$CO_2 = 22.8(pcr) + (48.7 \pm 10.7)$
$r = .522, \, p < .001$

● = GROUP 1,3 SUCCESS   O = GROUP 1,3 FAILURE
■ = GROUP 2,4 SUCCESS   □ = GROUP 2,4 FAILURE

pcr, gm/Kg/day

Figure 18. The locus of all patients in the National Cooperative Dialysis Study mapped by average mid-week predialysis BUN (CO_2, mg/dl) and PCR (gm/kg/day). Symbols are: O, group 1,3 success; O, group 1,3 failures; [ ], group 2,4 success; [ ], group 2,4 failure. (Reprinted from Kidney International, with permission.)

Clearances that were possible to achieve in the NCDS protocol using dialyzers and clinical blood and dialysate flows in use at that time ranged from approximately 90 ml/min with all dialyzers to a maximum of approximately 200 to 250 ml/min (the former value was for the smaller dialyzers used; the latter was for dialyzers with nominal 2.5 m² membrane area) (94).

A graphical representation of the NCDS results is shown in Figure 18 (78) as a map relating average mid week predialysis BUN (C 0_2: C = BUN; 0 = pre-dialysis at T = 0; 2 = second dialysis) to protein catabolic rate pcr – g/kg/day. Protein catabolic rate for patients in nutritional steady state (such as those in the NCDS) will be equivalent to protein intake (105).

The two regions that are blocked off by parallelograms signify the BUN regions explored in the study with the upper region representing the patients with high BUNs (groups 2 and 4 of Figure 17) and the lower region representing those patients with low BUNs (groups 1 and 3 in Figure 17). Figure 18 shows that by using the operational relationships developed in this chapter (i.e. Equations 25–28 which relate K_oA, Q_B and Q_D to desired K_D) and the urea kinetics model, a carefully controlled multicenter, clinical study protocol, such as that described in Figure 17, can be successfully implemented.

Modeling the anticoagulation activity of heparin

Heparin is the usual anticoagulant for hemodialysis. The need to model this material stems from the fact, which has generally been ignored in the pharmacology literature, that biological sensitivity and elimination of heparin varies widely (56). In formulating this model, a slightly different approach is followed. The characteristic of interest with heparin is its anticoagulant effect, measured as the clotting time prolongation (56) rather than concentration. Consequently, it is this response to heparin that is the appropriate parameter to model. In this analysis, therefore, the anticoagulation response (R) or clotting time prolongation relative to baseline levels resulting from systemic heparinization, will be considered a direct measure of the system content (see Figure 19).

Input to the system, after initial heparin loading, is a zero order infusion rate, I_r, quantified as units/hour. A coefficient is required to convert the infusion rate to increased clotting time response, so input is I_rS. This coefficient, S, (clotting time prolongation per unit) is the 'sensitivity' of the clotting system to added heparin. This response is found to be linear and insensitive to dose level for therapeutic quantities of this drug (56). Output or deactivation of anticoagulation in response to heparin is first order (116–118) and described as the product of the response and an elimination constant, K. This completes the model formulation.

Mass balance is then written:

$$\frac{dR}{dt} = I_rS - KR. \qquad [46a]$$

At steady state the right side of equation 46a will equal zero and the steady state infusion rate necessary for the required response will be:

$$I_r = \frac{KR}{S}. \qquad [46b]$$

Solution of equation 46a yields:

$$Rt = R_oe^{-Kt} + \frac{I_RS}{K}(1 - e^{-Kt}) \qquad [47]$$

Both S and K are individual patient constants and must be determined for each individual. The sensitivity, S, is evaluated by measurement of the change in clotting response to a step change in heparin as represented by bolus dose:

$$S = \frac{R - R_o}{dose}. \qquad [48]$$

It is apparent from equation 47 that the elimination or deactivation constant, K, can be calculated from the decrease clotting response with time once heparin infusion has stopped from

$$K = -\frac{1}{T} \, Ln \, \frac{R_T}{R_o}.$$

The technique of having to discontinue heparin administration in order to determine a value for K, however, is

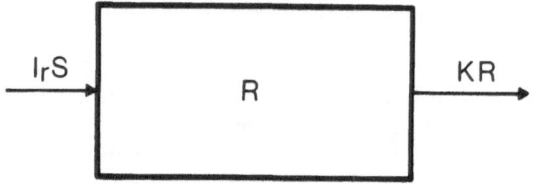

Figure 19. Model of heparin.

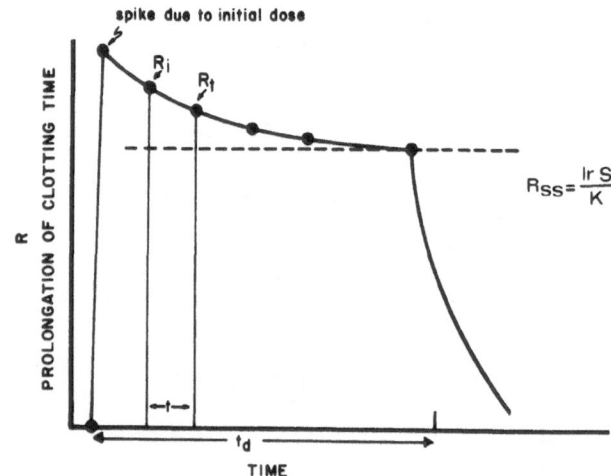

Figure 20. Clotting time prolongation in a dialysis patient with systemic heparinization consisting of a loading dose and a constant infusion thereafter.

inconvenient because it may require a patient to remain after the dialysis is discontinued or be at risk of unacceptable clotting levels during treatment. Recognizing this, a method was developed to calculate the heparin elimination constant from serial clotting times for a dialysis patient receiving a constant heparin infusion. Examination of equation 48 shows that K appears both in the I_rS/K term as well as the exponent, and as such this expression cannot be directly solved for K although there will be a unique value for this metabolic constant for any specific value of R_T, R_o, I_r, and S. A specific rearrangement of equation 48 which avoids the use of logarithms, common in analagous urea kinetic solutions (42) is shown in equation 49.

$$K = \frac{I_rS\,(1 - e^{Kt})}{R_I - R_Te^{Kt}}.$$ [49]

Equation 49 is used when the infusion rate, I_r, is known and the sensitivity, S, has been calculated for clotting time response values after the start of dialysis as shown in Figure 20. Both R_i and R_t are measured by standard techniques (although some form of the whole blood partial thromboplastin time is preferred because of its speed and reproducibility). The computation requires that equation 49 be 'primed' with a 'starting' value of K. This value is then used to compute the right-hand-side of equation 49, which will yield a 'closer' value for K (the left-hand-side of the equation). This new K value is then used to recompute another value of K until this system of calculations converges to a unique value.

Acid base control in dialysis patients

The maintenance of body pH is a fundamental aspect of normal homeostasis ultimately controlled through net acid excretion by the kidneys. As with other solutes, impairment of renal function results in loss of homeostatic control over H^+. This upset must be considered as one of the most severe complications of renal failure, particularly because of the highly reactive nature of acids and bases and the narrow range of pH consistent with life (approximately 6.8 to 7.8 in man). The entire metabolic structure of the body relies on the maintenance of optimal pH; the clinical signs of lowered pH in acidosis are well known: hyperventilation due to respiratory compensation, K^+ elevation due to cellular neutralization of H^+, low bicarbonate from H^+ neutralization, and eventual bone deterioration from long term H^+ buffering. Perhaps one of the most critical aspects of this problem is that acid must be buffered immediately upon generation.

Unlike other solutes where body water acts as a 'storage vessel' between treatments, the body has a very low capacitance for H^+ and the bulk of H^+ storage must be accomplished by the body buffer system which then must be realkalinized during dialysis treatment.

Acid generation from metabolic processes

Metabolism of various substrates will have a net acid (H^+ producing) or basic (H^+ consuming) effect depending on their composition. Christensen (109, 110) pointed out that to determine the acidic or basic effect of a biochemical reaction it is most convenient to consider the overall reaction (substrate to products) from the standpoint of a charge balance, and to add H^+ as a product or reactant to accomplish this overall adjustment of charge. In this manner acid producing reactions yield products that are more negative than their reactants and generate H^+. Conversely, reactions whose products have a more positive electrical charge than the reactants, have consumed H^+ and have a basic effect. Consideration of NH_4Cl, which is a typical material to produce experimental acidosis, illustrates Christensen's point

$$NH_4Cl\ (+CO_2) \rightarrow urea + H_2O + Cl^-.$$ [R-3]

The complete catabolism of ammonium chloride will yield urea and water from the oxidation of nitrogen and will strand Cl^- in body water. The net effect is the same as adding equivalent amounts of HCl. To balance the reactions with respect to charge H^+ must be added to the right hand side of the reaction

$$2\ NH_4Cl\ (+CO_2) = urea + H_2O + 2(Cl^- + H^+).$$ [R-4]

Metabolism of an organic anion will have the reverse effect as can be illustrated with the acetate anion whose products are neutral CO_2 and water:

Organic anion + H⁺ = H₂O + CO₂   [R-5a]

$$\text{Organic anion} + H^+ = H_2O + CO_2 \qquad [R\text{-}5a]$$

$$\text{acetate} + (H^+) = 2H_2O + 2CO_2. \qquad [R\text{-}5b]$$

Writing this expression in traditional biochemical form tends to confuse this point.

$$\text{ATP} \longrightarrow \text{AMP} + \text{PP}$$

$$\text{Acetate} \longrightarrow \text{Acetyl-S-CoA} + H_2O. \qquad [R\text{-}6]$$

$$\text{HSCoA}$$

Chemical balance shows, however, that as written there is one more hydrogen in the products than in the reactants.

Reactions R-5 and R-6 illustrate that the popular concept that acetate produces bicarbonate is figurative at best (60, 61), the alkalanizing effect of acetate being through its consumption of H⁺ as it is metabolized. Bicarbonate is produced by the unique reaction of carbonic acid dissociation (see reaction R-1 above). The only connection between these two reactions is that one consumes hydrogen ion (acetate metabolism) whereas the other produces it (dissociation of carbonic acid).

This method of considering metabolic reactions would then predict that ingested citric acid, formic acid (even nitric acid) would have no net effect on body acid base status because these compounds are electrically neutral on ingestion and will produce only neutral products. Although pH will decrease transiently, metabolism of the anion (base equivalent) will eventually reverse the response.

Net acid generation as related to protein catabolism and intake

Catabolism of protein should have a predictable acidic effect. This is because of the two sulfur containing amino acids – cystine and methionine – which when metabolized will abandon their sulfur as a negatively charged sulfate ion.

$$\begin{array}{ccc} H & HHH & \\ \text{H-C-S-C-C-C-COO}^- & \rightarrow H_2O + CO_2 + \text{Urea} \\ H & HHN & + SO_4^= (2H^+) \qquad [R\text{-}7] \\ & + H_3^+ & \end{array}$$

(methionine)

In addition to its direct acidic effect protein is a good index of general intake of various substances (49, 111). Analysis of metabolically and clinically controlled studies where both H⁺ and nitrogen balances were done (Figure 21) shows that net rates of protein catabolism can be used to obtain good estimates of the net quantity of acid being produced (0.77 mEq/g of protein catabolized (122–126).

Acetate metabolism

Appreciation of the alkalinizing effect of acetate metabolism, shown in reaction R-5, led Mion and coworkers in 1965 to substitute this anion for the more commonly used bicarbonate (117). This opened the way for the development of single concentrate dialysis proportioning systems (118). The

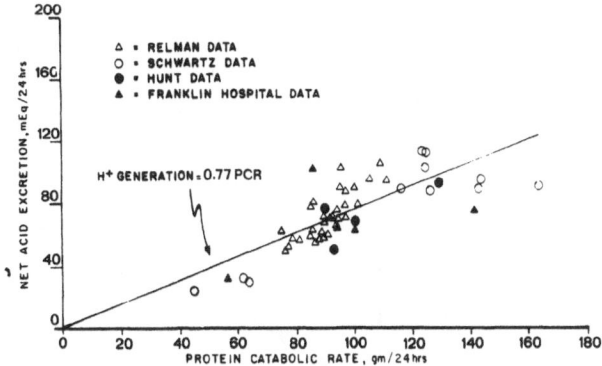

Figure 21. Hydrogen ion (acid) generation as a function of net rates of protein catabolism.

disadvantages of using bicarbonate in dialysate solutions are its poor solubility, its instability, and the requirement of high concentrations of dissolved CO₂ to keep pH in the range where magnesium and calcium will remain soluble (119). The advantages of acetate are its high solubility and perceived rapid rate of metabolism (120, 121).

Model formulation of acetate metabolism presents a major problem. Once again a single pool is sought (see Figure 22). Input to the system is uncomplicated being diffusive transport from dialysate to blood in the dialyzer, as described in equation 14. The output from the system presents some difficulty, however. A typical acetate concentration profile during and immediately after dialysis is shown in Figure 23 and is the one that is commonly found in dialysis patients (55, 122). Examination of this figure reveals an asymmetry between the concentration build-up, which may take as long as 2 to 3 h during dialysis and the rapid reduction of acetate to low plasma levels in less than an hour after dialysis. These kinetics are not consistent with a first order metabolic process.

Many metabolic systems show non-linear behavior as described by Michaelis-Menten type kinetics and shown in Figure 24. The type of system shown indicates first order metabolism at low substrate levels (e.g. a doubling of metabolic rate for a doubling of substrate); as substrate builds up, however, there is less of an increase in metabolic rate approaching saturation levels. If acetate metabolism were in the shaded region of the figure its conversion to acetyl C₀A shown in reaction R-6 would show very little sensitivity to

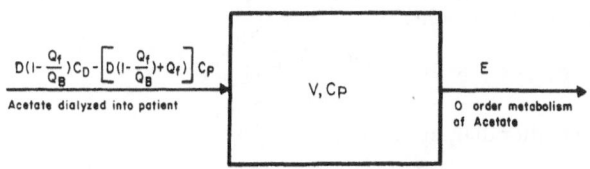

Figure 22. Model of acetate transport and metabolism in dialyzed patients.

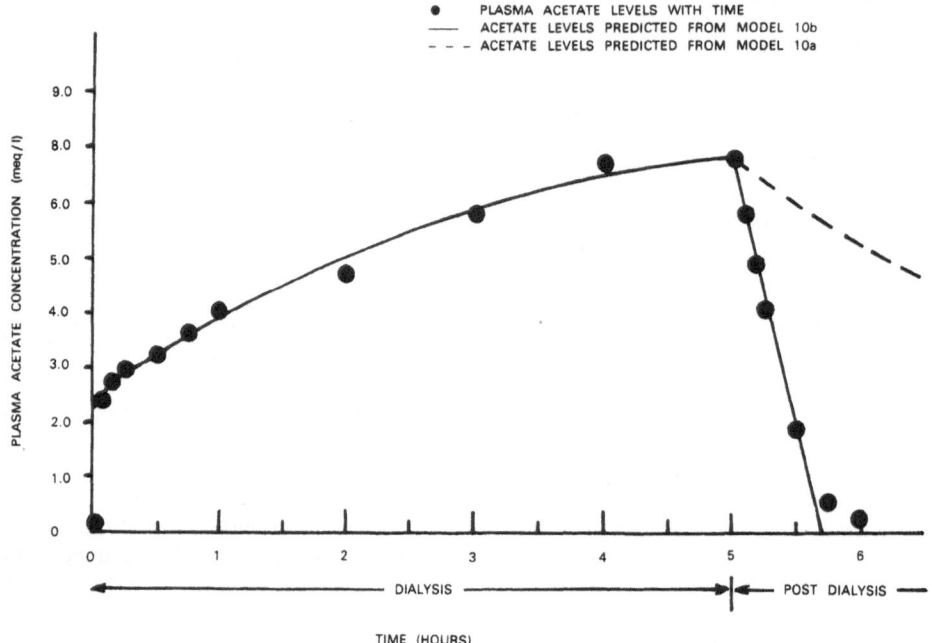

Figure 23. Acetate concentration with time in a typical dialysis patient during and shortly after a 5 h treatment.

changing acetate levels and would be effectively constant (or zero order). When this output is used, the model in Figure 22 results. This yields the mass balance expression:

$$\frac{d(VC_P)}{dt} = D\left(1 - \frac{Q_F}{Q_B}\right)C_D - \left[D\left(1 - \frac{Q_F}{Q_B}\right) + Q_F\right]C_P - E. \quad [50a]$$

If ultrafiltration can be neglected (i.e. Q_F and dV/dt approach zero) then Equation 50a becomes:

$$V\frac{d(C_P)}{dt} = D(C_{Di} - C_P) - E. \quad [50b]$$

Using the assumption of constant ultrafiltration (see equations 42a and b) and solving for acetate concentration during dialysis yields:

$$C_P = C_{Po}\left(\frac{V_0 - Q_F t}{V_0}\right)^{D(1/Q_F - 1/Q_B)} + \left[D\left(1 - \frac{Q_F}{Q_B}\right) - E\right]$$

$$\left[1 - \left(\frac{V_0 - Q_F t}{V_0}\right)^{D(1/Q_F - 1/Q_B)}\right]. \quad [51a]$$

And when extracellular volume can be considered constant (dV/dt and Q_F are negligible see Equation 50b) an analogous expression results:

$$C_P = C_{Po}\, e^{-Dt/V} + \frac{DC_{Di} - E}{D}(1 - e^{-Dt/v}) \quad [51b]$$

and after dialysis in both cases:

$$C_P = C_{Pt} - \frac{E}{V}t. \quad [52]$$

From Figure 23 it is clear that acetate metabolism slows when acetate concentration is below 2 mEq/l post dialysis. Reference to Figure 24 would indicate that below these acetate levels the metabolic reaction is below the shaded region and in the linear range (the reaction is now first order).

It is seen that equation 51b is of the same form as equation 45 and that $(D\,C_{Di} - E)/D$ will be the steady state plasma level (C_{Pss}) at large values of t (i.e. when $e^{-Dt/V}$ is very small). It is clear that if steady state concentrations are known or

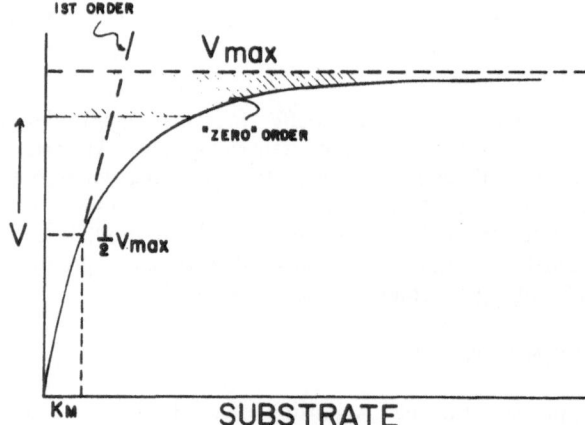

Figure 24. Velocity of a metabolic reaction (V, mEq/min) as a function of substrate levels (mEq/l) which would result from Michaelis-Menten kinetics.

can be approximated and D is known then the value of E can be estimated from

$$E = D(C_{Di} - C_{Pss}) \qquad [53]$$

rearrangement of equation 51b allows another computation of E:

$$E = D \left(C_{Di} - \frac{C_P - C_{Po}\, e^{-Dt/V}}{1 - e^{-Dt/V}} \right) \qquad [54]$$

where V is assumed to be extracellular water and is taken as 1/3 of total body water (or V urea from the urea kinetic calculations). Values of E computed by both methods for the data shown in Figure 24 are shown in Table 7 and agree very closely.

Body base

Because of the critical nature of acid base control it is important to describe quantitatively the elements of H^+ and buffer base in the patient.

Acid-base kinetics are conceptually complex because of the labile nature of the solute, H^+, for which mass balance equations must be written. In addition, although several hundred milliequivalents of H^+ may be generated and removed during a complete dialysis cycle, the free concentration in body water remains vanishingly small (0.000030 – 0.000045 mEq/l) because of instantaneous reactions between H^+ and the large buffer pool in the body.

$$H^+ + buffer^- = buffer\, H. \qquad [R\text{-}8]$$

Table 7. Acetate concentration in a patient dialyzed with 39 mmol/l in the dialysis fluid for 5 h. D acetate = 0.120 l/min.

Time: t-relative to the start of dialysis, 0-relative to its end (min)	Plasma concentration (mmol/l)	E (from equation 54)	E (from equation 53)
0	0	–	–
60	4.0	3.63	–
120	4.7	3.87	–
180	5.8	3.74	–
240	6.7	3.66	–
300	6.8	3.73	–
		3.73	3.74

Table 8. Magnitude of elements in H^+ balances over one dialysis cycle.

Hydrogen generation (from dietary sources)	100–200 mEq
Bicarbonate loss during acetate dialysis	500 mEq
Acetate uptake	600–800 mEq
Organic acid production	0–200 mEq
Organic anion loss (net H^+ production)	0–100 mEq
Body H^+ content	0.0017 mEq

This can be more fully appreciated by reference to Table 8 which shows the various elements of H^+ balance in a 70 Kg dialysis patient ingesting from 0.8 to 1.6 g protein/Kg/day dialyzed with acetate dialysate using a 1.3 m^2 regenerated cellulose dialyzer.

Ironically, from a strict mass balance sense, the modeled species (H^+) can be ignored because it is present in negligible quantities. In fact, H^+ balance is so treated, and the difference between H^+ production and elimination is taken as equal to the degree of buffer depletion (i.e. R-8 goes to completion and $d(H^+)/dt = 0$). In the discussion to follow, the model is of the body content of basic equivalents, and their increase or decrease in content can be considered as the negative of H^+ balance. In this context body buffer (i.e. adding basic equivalents) is 'negative H^+ balance', and acidification of body buffer (i.e. removing basic equivalents) is 'positive H^+ balance'.

Body base model formulation requires an in depth consideration of all elements that affect acid base status and consequently becomes quite complex. Step 1 of Figure 8 indicates that it is first necessary to define the system. However, consideration of the bicarbonate system is appropriate before the body base system is defined.

Bicarbonate modeling

Bicarbonate is traditionally and superficially treated pharmokinetically as distributed in a single pool volume (generally estimated to be 40% body weight) (114, 115, 123). If a general model of bicarbonate is formulated for dialysis with dialytic uptake of HCO_3^- and its removal by H^+ generation (gH^+) Figure 26a results. If a fixed distribution volume is assumed the mass balance equation becomes:

$$V\frac{dC_P}{dt} = D(C_{Di} - C_{Pi}) - gH^+. \qquad [55a]$$

Solution of this expression yields:

$$C_P = C_{Po}\, e^{-Dt/V} + \left(C_{Di} - \frac{gH^+}{D} \right)(1 - e^{-Dt/V}). \qquad [55b]$$

Rearrangement of equation 55b yields an expression for V:

$$V = Dt\, Log\, \frac{C_{Po} - (C_{Di} - gH^+/D)}{C_{Pt} - (C_{Di} - gH^+/D)}. \qquad [55c]$$

From the change in plasma concentration under known dialysis conditions of D and C_{Di} during bicarbonate dialysis, V can be calculated (where gH^+/D is considered negligible).

Values calculated using this equation occasionally show large and variable bicarbonate volumes (124). A similar variation of bicarbonate space depending on the level of acidosis has been reported (125).

Re-evaluation of the model shows that the fault may lie with the use of traditional pharmacokinetic techniques as embodied in Figure 25a and Equation 55c. Such methods are normally applied to a specific solute which occupies a unique physical volume. This may be modified in the case of protein binding because an additional storage capacity for

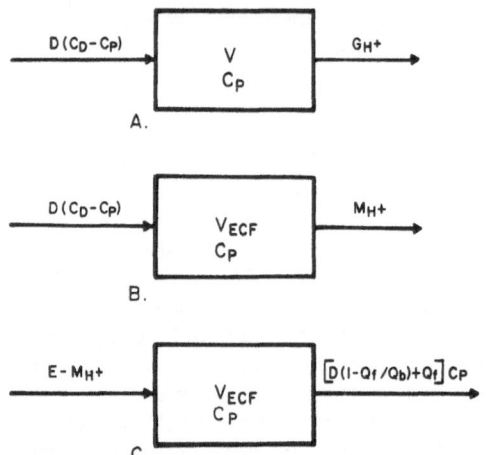

Figure 25. Models of the bicarbonate system during bicarbonate dialysis showing two versions of the model: a) using apparent bicarbonate space, b) using a fixed volume approximating extracellular volume and a mobilization constant, and c) during acetate dialysis.

the substance is present and V is correspondingly larger (i.e. 'distribution volume' for a bound substance will be larger than its physical distribution space). Bicarbonate, however, because of its interrelation with H+ and through it the other buffer systems, represents a highly labile material which may disappear from extracellular space either by diffusion into cells or by neutralization of H+ released from other buffers (123).

It does not seem unreasonable to consider that during the interdialytic period, generated H+ will progressively deplete buffer stores and that during dialysis the infused bicarbonate will have to restore these buffers. The extent of restoration may vary depending on the state of depletion which will reflect the magnitude of interdialytic H+ generation. A constant term like g_{H^+} must then be retained but its definition will differ as it will not be the generation of H+ but the apparent movement of HCO_3^- out of extracellular space. The disappearance of bicarbonate from this space can be described in terms of m_{H^+} or 'hydrogen ion mobilization' which is intended to include diffusive movement of HCO_3^- out of the extracellular volume. The V term in the equation then becomes constant whose value is known or can be determined. Rearrangement of the mass balance equation for the model shown in Figure 25b yields:

$$V_{ecf} \frac{dC_P}{dt} = D(C_D - C_P) - m_{H^+} \qquad [56a]$$

$$m_{H^+} = D\left[(C_D - C_{Po}) - \frac{(C_{Bt} - C_{Bo})}{1 - e^{-Dt/v}}\right]. \qquad [56b]$$

Note in this expression C_{Po} represents bicarbonate concentration at the start of dialysis. Equation 56b shows that m_{H^+} is the difference of two terms, the initial rate of diffusive flux into extracellular space, and a term that contains the amount

of rise of bicarbonate in that space. The second term accounts for the fact that HCO_3^- content of extracellular space is increasing. Examination of this expression shows what intuition would suggest, that the greater the rise in bicarbonate ($C_{Bt} > C_{Bo}$) during a treatment the smaller the alkalinization of other buffers will be. The lack of equivalence of this increased content with the flux from the dialyzer is accounted for by basic equivalents that have moved into other anatomical areas. Consequently, using typical intradialytic values for C_D, C_{Po}, C_{Pt}, V, D, and t, the extent of titration of buffers can be calculated. Thus if $C_D = 35\,mEq/l$, $C_{Po} = 20\,mEq/l$, $C_{Pt} = 23\,mEq/l$ over a 1 h period and V = 13 l, D = 0.100 l/min, the bicarbonate is disappearing (mH^+) at a rate of 0.69 mmol/min during this interval. The average flux into the patient $D(C_D - C_B)$ would be approximately 0.1 (35 − 21.5) or 1.35 mmol/min of which 49% would contribute to a rise in extracellular bicarbonate concentration. These illustrative data demonstrate an analytical technique that can estimate the H+ balance during the process of acid-based correction with dialysis treatment. The adoption of model b in Figure 25 should increase understanding of what is actually occurring in the body, whereas a 'distribution space' for bicarbonate tends to blur the fact that the kinetics of this substance are interrelated both to the movement of H+ and the status of body buffers.

Expected bicarbonate levels during acetate dialysis

The model shown in Figure 25c depicts bicarbonate mass balance during acetate dialysis. This model is the reverse of models 25a and 25b, which described bicarbonate dialysis. In this case bicarbonate is being dialyzed out of extracellular space; this model also incorporates volume changes during treatment. There will be some addition of HCO_3^- to the system resulting from the alkalinizing effect of acetate metabolism and the consumption of H+, some of which will come from reaction R-1. The rate of HCO_3^- production is shown as the rate of alkalinization by metabolic conversion of acetate to acetyl-co-a (E) modified to account for the fact that only part of the H+ consumed by this reaction will come from H_2CO_3 (see R-1). This modification is indicated as the acetate conversion rate less the hydrogen ion mobilization term (E − mH^+). Because of the relatively small contribution of gH^+ and the difficulty of separating it from the mH^+ term it is included in this term for the purposes of this model.

The mass balance equation becomes:

$$\frac{d(V_{ecf}C_P)}{dt} = V_{ecf}\frac{dC_P}{dt} + C_P\frac{dV_{ecf}}{dt} =$$

$$(E - mH^+) - \left[D\left(1 - \frac{Q_F}{Q_B}\right) + Q_F\right]C_P. \qquad [57a]$$

If most of the intradialytic volume change comes from changes in extracellular water volume, equations 42a and 42b can be used to define the change in this space. With this substitution solution of equation 57a yields:

$$C_P = C_{Po} \left(\frac{V_0 - Q_F t}{V_0}\right)^{D(1/Q_F - 1/Q_B)} + \frac{E - m_{H^+}}{D(1 - Q_F/Q_B)}$$

$$\left[1 - \left(\frac{V_0 - Q_F t}{V_0}\right)^{D(1/Q_F - 1/Q_B)}\right] \qquad [57b]$$

Equations 51a and 57b can be used to calculate the expected end dialysis plasma acetate and bicarbonate levels that would result with increasing dialyzer flux rates of these materials. The following patient and dialyzer parameters were used to examine these relationships: urea volume 36 l; $V_{ecf}(end) = 12 l$; $V_{ecf}(start) = 14.5 l$; $E = 3.8 \, mEq/min$; $C_P HCO_3(start) = 20 \, mEq/l$; with treatment delivered during a dialysis designed to provide total urea clearance equal to urea volume (i.e. KT/V urea = 1.0) but conducted over differing intervals. Under these conditions dialyzer clearances will increase as dialysis time is shortened. Bicarbonate and acetate dialysance values were taken to be 83% and 70% of the required urea clearance respectively; C_D(acetate) = 37 mEq/l; mH+ (the alkalinization required to restore body base equivalents depleted between treatments) is 123 mEq divided by the length of dialysis in minutes. Dialysis times were varied from 4 to 2 h.

The end dialysis bicarbonate and acetate levels expected to result from these treatment conditions are shown in Figure 26. It can be seen that acetate levels are near zero at the end of a 4 h treatment but steadily increase as treatment becomes more rapid reaching a level of 15 mEq/l at the end of a 2 h treatment. This curve reflects acetate flux increasing beyond the acetate metabolic rate with more rapid dialysis.

Bicarbonate levels at the end of treatment decrease as dialysis becomes more rapid due to increasing net dialyzer bicarbonate loss which exceeds the rate of alkalinization from acetate metabolism and its contribution to the H_2CO_3 neutralization reaction (see R-1). At the end of a 2 h dialysis the blood acetate level is 15 mEq/l and higher than blood bicarbonate which is 13 mEq/l. The analysis indicates that acute metabolic acidosis and striking acetatemia would result if high flux 2 h dialysis was performed using dialysis fluid buffered with acetate. It cannot be concluded that net correction of acidosis would be inadequate since the large extracellular acetate inventory will be rapidly metabolized over 30 to 45 min after dialysis and will result in rapid bicarbonate generation. The magnitude of post dialysis acetate metabolism can be estimated from the patient parameters used for this analysis. The acetate inventory in V_{ecf} can be calculated from this volume and end dialysis acetate concentrations = 12(15) = 180 mEq. Thus 180 mEq H+ will be consumed and result in some combination of cell buffer alkalinization and bicarbonate production. Since in this analysis it was assumed that m_{H^+} during dialysis resulted in full alkalinization of cell buffers during dialysis (which is not likely to be strictly correct), the rise in bicarbonate post dialysis could be estimated as 180/12 = 15.0 mEq/l and the plasma bicarbonate 30 to 40 min after dialysis would be 13 + 15 = 28 mEq/l. In fact, it would be expected that a similar percentage of the alkalinizing potential of the conversion of acetate to acetyl-co-A would go to alkalinize other buffers

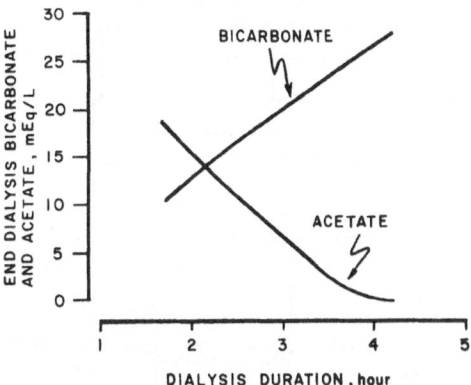

Figure 26. End dialysis bicarbonate and acetate levels during different length treatments where normalized treatment (KT/V) remains the same.

and a smaller rise in ultimate plasma HCO_3^- would be expected.

The curves in Figure 25b demonstrate that acetate will not be a suitable dialysate buffer for correction of metabolic acidosis as dialysis times are shortened and as dialyzer flux rates increase. The point at which it is necessary to change from acetate to bicarbonate for an individual patient will clearly depend on his parameters as shown in equations 51a and 57b (particularily the value of E). In any event, as bicarbonate flux rates progressively exceed acetate metabolic rates progessive acetatemia and metabolic acidosis will be induced during dialysis followed by very rapid postdialysis alkalinization from acetate metabolism.

The body base model

The model shown in Figure 25b represents only the bicarbonate portion of the overall base content of the body. Figure 27 shows its incorporation into the overall model of body base equivalents. It is included as the bottom half of the inner box which is the bicarbonate portion of buffer base equivalents, that are capable of interacting with other body buffers. The inner box represents the body base equivalents and is separated into three sections. Base equivalents in extracellular water are illustrated as including the HCO_3^-, just discussed, as well as the non-buffer materials in extracellular water (top right) such as lactate, acetate, and other organic anions (see R-5). The top left section of this box represents the non-extracellular buffers in basic form. The size of the space belies its extent which is actually greater than half of the total buffer base capacity of the body (123). Communication between these three compartments is indicated. As was discussed, addition of HCO_3 to the extracellular pool will not quantitatively increase the extracellular bicarbonate content because there will be 'mobilization' of bicarbonate (or transfer of base equivalents) to other buffer systems. Similarly, when the buffers are acidified the buffer load will distribute among bicarbonate and other buffer systems as shown by the H+ accumulation term A_{H^+}

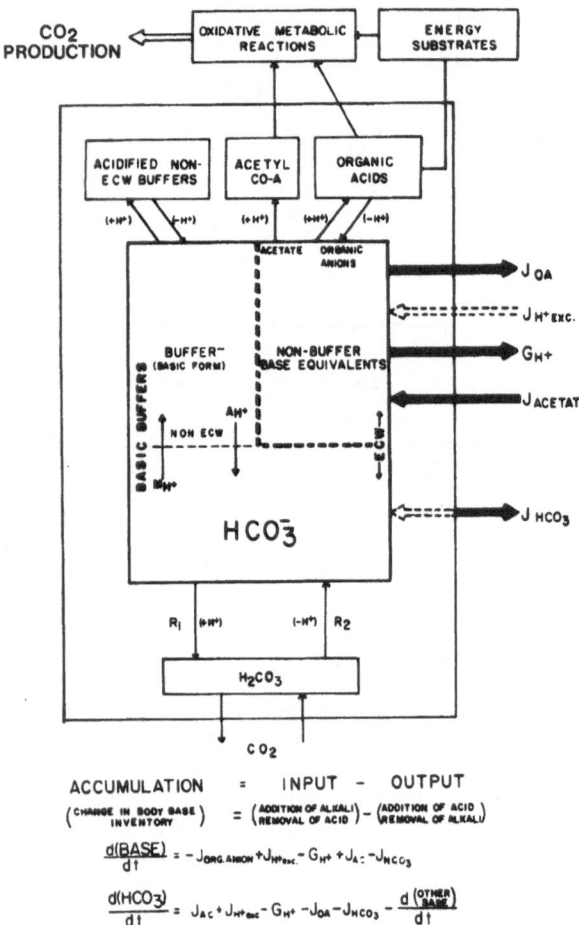

ACCUMULATION = INPUT − OUTPUT

$$\left(\begin{array}{c}\text{CHANGE IN BODY BASE}\\\text{INVENTORY}\end{array}\right) = \left(\begin{array}{c}\text{ADDITION OF ALKALI}\\\text{REMOVAL OF ACID}\end{array}\right) - \left(\begin{array}{c}\text{ADDITION OF ACID}\\\text{REMOVAL OF ALKALI}\end{array}\right)$$

$$\frac{d(\text{BASE})}{dt} = -J_{\text{ORG.ANION}} + J_{\text{H}^+\text{Exc}} - G_{\text{H}^+} + J_{\text{AC}} - J_{\text{HCO}_3}$$

$$\frac{d(\text{HCO}_3)}{dt} = J_{\text{AC}} + J_{\text{H}^+\text{exc}} - G_{\text{H}^+} - J_{\text{OA}} - J_{\text{HCO}_3} - \frac{d(\text{OTHER BASE})}{dt}$$

Figure 27. Model of body base equivalents.

which indicates that as the extracellular compartment sustains an acid load, base equivalents will move into that compartment to restore partially the bicarbonate level (i.e. non extracellular buffers will neutralize some of the added H^+). In Figure 27 the outer box encloses the system but also contains internal sources capable of producing buffer base if alkalinized, such as carbonic acid, organic acids, and acidified non extracellular buffers.

Consider the example of lactic acid production by anaerobic metabolism:

$$\text{glucose} = \text{lactate-} + (\text{H}^+). \qquad [\text{R-9}]$$

Glucose (an energy substrate – upper right) has produced lactic acid (an organic acid). Both lactate and H^+ are added to the internal box of the figure. H^+, however, will combine with a buffer base, HCO_3^- for example, and produce H_2CO_3, which may in turn be exhaled in its anhydrous form CO_2. These reactions, however, will have no effect on the total base content because the decrease in HCO_3^- has been matched by the addition of lactate, a base equivalent (i.e. a substance capable of removing H^+ from the system when it is metabolized see R-5a).

It should be emphasized that carbon dioxide interaction with the body base system will have no net effect on the base content, for it is a neutral substance, although it can profoundly effect the system pH through its relation with the carbonic acid-bicarbonate system. The net excretion or retention of carbon dioxide, however, will not effect the body base content.

With reference to Figure 27 only the bold arrows represent net inputs and outputs for the system. All other arrows represent the transfer of neutral materials which have no net effect on the overall acid base status.

Consider first the inputs of the system: The ways that the body buffer system content can increase. A total of three inputs are considered. Renal excretion of acids (j_{H^+}Exc), will effect a net increase because net removal of hydrogen ion will cause a net movement of base equivalents from one of the internal buffer systems (e.g. alkalinization of non-extracellular buffers or dissociation of H_2CO_3 by reaction R-1). Body base can be increased directly by flux of acetate into the patient (direct addition of base equivalents).

Alternatively, bicarbonate (if used in the dialysis fluid) can be a pathway to increase base content of the system. Note that once in the system, the acetate to acetyl-CoA conversion will be coupled to one of the other internal systems alkalinizing a non-extracellular buffer or net dissociation of H_2CO_3. In this light it is apparent that non-stoichiometric appearance of bicarbonate during acetate metabolism (60, 61) should, in fact, be predicted because of the variety of substances capable of providing the hydrogen ion consumed in the acetate metabolic reaction.

Routes of output or ways in which base equivalents will be removed from the system will be: by removal of organic anions which are themselves base equivalents (e.g. lactate); by acid generation g_{H^+}, or by bicarbonate loss during acetate dialysis. These outputs (and inputs) are totally general. If the diet is low in protein and high in alkaline material (sodium citrate for example) g_{H^+} will be negative and there will be a net base increase. Also if bicarbonate is given by mouth or some other unbalanced organic anion such as monosodium glutamate is ingested this contribution can be dealt with by incorporating the flux of these substances in J_{HCO_3} or J_{OA} terms and appropriate adjustment of algebraic sign.

Referring to the section 'Formulation of a model' and Figure 8 it will be apparent that the model in Figure 27 has not been completely specified. The normal step would be to relate the inputs and outputs to the system content. In this case 'body base' consists of a collection of substances which may interrelate in a manner that cannot be defined on the basis of current research. These difficulties of specifying this model further will be discussed below.

Writing the mass balance equation yields

$$\frac{d(\text{Base})}{dt} = -J_{\text{OA}} + J_{\text{H}^+}\text{Exc} - g_{\text{H}^+} + J_{\text{AC}} - J_{\text{HCO}_3}. \quad [57]$$

This expression is totally general and not restricted to dialysis or even uremia. Consider the stable individual not on dialysis (i.e. Jac = 0), presumably in steady state (d(base)/dt = 0)

$$j_{H+}Exc = g_{H+} + J_{OA} + J_{HCO_3}. \qquad [58]$$

This indicates that H^+ excretion will balance H^+ generation plus the loss of organic anions and bicarbonate. Acid base upsets can also be described by Figure 27 and equations 57 and 58. Consider, for example, ketoacidosis in diabetes mellitus. When fat is a major energy substrate, there is generation and neutralization of organic acids represented by their dissociation into the buffer pool. The immediate effect will be neutralization of H^+ by some other buffer, which the organic anion will replace as a body base equivalent, the body base content staying constant. The elevated levels of organic anions, however, will result in urinary excretion of these materials (J_{OA}). If $j_{H+}Exc$ can increase to accommodate the buffer loss (see equation 58), there will be no net acidification of the system. If not base content will be reduced (see equation 57).

If body base is separated into bicarbonate and other buffers, equation 57 can be rewritten and solved for the HCO_3^- terms:

$$\frac{d(HCO_3^-)}{dt} + J_{HCO_3^-} =$$

$$J_{AC} - g_{H+} - J_{OA} - \frac{d(other\ base)}{dt} + J_{H+}Exc. \qquad [59]$$

Equation 59 indicates that HCO_3^- removal from the system plus the increase in HCO_3^- content will equal the combination of the five terms on the right side. It should, once again, be noted that for acetate flux and metabolism to be equal to HCO_3^- mass balance as has been anticipated by some (60, 61) the algebraic sum of the last four terms must be zero an improbable result during such a metabolically disruptive event as dialysis. Consequently, the non-equivalence of acetate uptake and bicarbonate appearance described by others (60, 61) should not be surprising.

Control of acid base: solution of the model

The goal of acid base control during dialysis treatment is to minimize the depletion of body buffers between dialyses and the non-extra-cellular buffers (bone) long term, and to restore adequately the basic buffer forms during treatment.

As alluded to above there is very little therapeutic control of interdialytic base depletion, that primarily results from acid forming foods in the diet and appears in the forgoing relationships as g_{H+}. In addition, intake of fluid, which will not have an overall effect on body buffers, causes movement of base equivalents into the extra-cellular compartment to supply buffer to this space as it expands (dilutional acidosis) (125). Hence, while Figure 27 represents a useful model it cannot yet be adequately formulated.

The system content as represented by the internal box in Figure 27 cannot be accurately specified. More information about the composition and interrelation of buffers as implied by the terms aH^+ and mH^+ is required. Because HCO_3^- is the measureable component of body buffer and the one to which output and input relate knowledge of how HCO_3^- and other buffers interact is required. Also of interest is the location of the acetate alkalinization step and whether it has its effect directly on extracellular buffers or through non-extracellular buffers. The dashed lines shown in Figure 27 may have certain resistances associated with them so that the addition of HCO_3^- to the extracellular fluid may have a different effect than equivalent alkalinization using acetate and indications of this possibility have been observed. The alkalinizing effect of acetate may also depend on transport of a co-ion, e.g. sodium, and therefore complete specification of the model will rely on another solute system which is changing during dialysis. For these reasons the model as described in Figure 27 must be considered as partially specified, for which the mass balance equation (equations 57–59) are an accurate representation, but for which insufficient information is available for complete formulation for the purposes of guiding treatment.

The effect of fluid retention and removal

A few comments are appropriate with respect to the marginal ability to correct acid base during dialysis. The acidification of the system between treatments was discussed primarily with respect to protein and acid generation. In addition, as fluid is consumed and retained in body water some dilutional acidosis occurs (i.e. base equivalents move into extracellular fluid acidifying cell buffers in the process, to sustain extracellular buffer levels). Although this will not change total body base equivalents, intracellular buffers will be depleted. The need to remove the retained fluid during dialysis, however, markedly blunts the ability to alkalinize the patient. Equation 14 shows that with Q_F of zero and 15 ml/min under the same bicarbonate conditions discussed above (see bicarbonate model) flux would be 1.35 mEq/min versus 0.91 mEq/min or a 31% drop when $Q_F = 15$ ml/min (900 ml/h).

Creatinine

Creatinine is traditionally grouped with urea as a major uremic catabolite, the concentration of which, should be controlled (126–128). That plasma creatinine concentration provides valuable nutritional information through its relationship to body muscle mass is well established (89). In this regard, it can be more accurate to view creatinine, or at least its production rate, as an outcome measure of dialysis therapy rather than control variable.

Plasma creatinine concentration is widely used in the predialysis patient as a rough inverse correlate to kidney function (93), although there is evidence that creatinine production drops in chronic uremia disproportionately to the decrease in lean body mass (129–131). Nevertheless, the relative constancy of creatinine production from the spontaneous and non-enzymatic dehydration of creatine phosphate has made it useful as an endogenous marker in progressive renal failure. Through its utility as a marker of renal function it has become associated with other catabolites and has assumed as importance that is unwarranted for its role as a metabolic product. It does not represent the end product of a major metabolic pathway, although it is associated with the energy pathway in muscle tissue through its connection with the creatine – phosphocreatine system. It can be shown that creatinine follows single pool kinetics (127) although not as closely as urea (128).

Sodium

There continues to be significant intradialytic morbidity associated with regular dialysis therapy. This morbidity comprises multiple symptoms including headache, nausea and vomiting, fatigue, hypotension and severe muscle cramps. The most frequent and objective symptoms are hypotension and muscle cramps which require medical intervention and occur in 15 to 40% of treatments in different centers.

Several studies have shown that increasing the dialysis fluid concentration of Na (C_{DNa}) reduces morbidity during dialysis (132–134). This therapeutic maneuver has been effective but can cause excessive body Na content and volume overload. Consequently a model would seem highly desirable for quantitative assessment of interdialytic Na and volume loading and intradialytic Na and volume removal.

Hemofiltration has been widely reported to reduce morbidity compared to hemodialysis (135–146). In view of the strong dependence of treatment morbidity during dialysis on dialysate sodium concentration an evaluation of comparative hemofiltration morbidity should include assessment of Na flux in the compared therapies.

Measurement of sodium concentration and activity

Until recently blood and dialysate inlet Na concentrations (C_B, C_D) have been routinely measured by the flame photometer (F) in clinical practice. The Na diffusion gradient or driving force for diffusive Na flux (J) across the dialyzer, however, is a function of the Na activity in the blood and dialysate streams which is correctly measured with an ion selective electrode (ISE). The flame photometer correctly measures Na concentration of the two streams but does not provide a correct measure of the Na activity; the ion selective electrode does.

The reason for these differences is that the electrode measures the ionized Na concentration in the aqueous phase of each stream but does not include Na ionically complexed with anions, particularly protein (147), bicarbonate (148) and acetate. The flame method measures total Na content per unit volume irrespective of ionization state and sample water fraction. These differences between measurement methods indicate that the Na diffusion gradient across the dialyzer should be measured by ion selective electrode and Na flux should be measured by flame photometry.

These relationships have been verified in *in vitro* and *in vivo* studies (148). These studies also showed that the osmotic distribution of Na in the blood stream is equal to the total water content of red cells plus plasma since Na mass balance between the blood and dialysate streams was achieved when QB was defined by the aqueous phase flow rate. Thus Qe for sodium equals the total blood water flow rate.

Relationships between measurement methods for blood and dialysate

The flame and electrode measurements of Na agree fairly closely in blood under usual conditions (149–151). In dialysate they differ substantially with electrode values typically being lower than flame values due to the high concentrations of acetate or bicarbonate. A predictable relationship has been reported between electrode and flame methods for both blood and dialysate in the presence of acetate or bicarbonate anions (Ca), as shown in Table 9.

The impact of measurement methods on clinical practice

There are important clinical consequences of the relationships in equation 60 (see Table 9). In order to achieve a zero Na diffusive gradient across the dialyzer, the Na activity in blood and dialysate must be equal and from the above considerations it follows that $1.01\,C_PF = 0.965\,C_DF$ or $C_DF = 1.05\,C_PF$. Thus if $C_PF = 140$, for a zero diffusion gradient C_DF must be 147 mEq/l or about 7 mEq/l higher than blood Na.

These relationships have resulted in some controversy in recent years between dialysate manufacturers and consumers. Many clinical laboratories now use electrode measurements because of its technical simplicity compared to flame measurements. Consequently, dialysate concentrate which is prepared to provide a Na content (determined correctly by F) of 140 mEq/l with standard 35:1 dilution will show Na concentration measured by electrode of only 135 mEq/l. When the consumer finds a dialysate electrode Na value of 135 mEq/l he is likely to conclude the concentrate is 4% low while the manufacturers data shows the actual Na content is 140 mEq/l. Both measurements are correct but confusion results because the parameters being measured (concentration or activity) are not widely understood by most clinicians.

Equivalency of Na flux in hemodialysis and hemodiltration studies

The relationships between flame and electrode measurement of Na shown in Table 9 also have significant implications with respect to comparative Na flux in hemodialysis (J_{HD}) and postdilution hemofiltration (J_{HF}). Sodium flux into

Table 9. The relationship of ion selective electrode and flame photometer determination of sodium concentrations in blood and dialysate samples

Fluid	Relationship	Reference	Equation
Blood plasma	$C_PE/C_PF = 1.01$	139–141	[60a]
Dialysate	$C_DE/C_{DF} = 0.99e^{-0.00063Ca}$	139	[60b]

Solution of the dialysate equation in Table 9 for typical dialysate acetate or bicarbonate concentration of 40 mEq/l shows that $C_DE/C_DF = 0.965$.

the patient during hemodialysis is described by a version of equation 14:

$$J_{HD} = D \ (1 - Q_F/Q_E) \ C_D - [D(1 - Q_F/Q_E) + Q_F] \ C_P \quad [61a]$$

where D is Na dialysance, Q_F is ultrafiltration rate, Q_E is blood water flow rate, C_D is inlet dialysate Na concentration, and C_P is inlet plasma Na concentration. The values for C_D and C_P represent the Na activity se when C_D and C_P are measured by flame photometer, the effective concentrations are:

$$J_{HD} = D(1 - Q_F/Q_E) \ (0.965 \ C_D F) -$$
$$[D(1 - Q_F/Q_E) + Q_F] \ (1.01 \ C_P F) \quad [61b]$$

In the case of postdilution hemofiltration Na flux can be described by:

$$J_{HF} = (Q_{HF} - Q_F) \ C_S - Q_{HF} \ (C_F) \quad [62]$$

where J_{HF} is Na flux into the patient, Q_{HF} is an analogue of D and represents the total hemofiltration rate, Q_F is net fluid removal rate, $(Q_{HF} - Q_F)$ is substitution fluid infusion rate, C_S is substitution fluid Na concentration, C_F is hemofiltrate Na concentration.

When C_S and C_F are measured by flame photometer, the effective Na concentrations will be:

$$J_{HF} = (Q_{HF} - Q_F) \ C_S F - Q_{HF} \ (0.985 \ C_P F). \quad [63]$$

There is no correction for $C_S F$ because it is infused directly into the blood stream. The coefficient 0.985 is applied to the term $C_P F$ based on several reports indicating the mean ratio $C_F F/C_P F = 0.985$ (152–154).

The $C_D F$ value relative to $C_S F$ required for $J_{HD} = J_{HF}$ can be calculated by combining equations 61b and 63 and solving for $C_D F$ as follows:

$$C_D F = \left(\frac{1}{0.965 \ D \ (1 - Q_F/Q_E)} \right)$$
$$[Q_{HF} \ (C_S F - 0.985 C_P F) - Q_F(C_S F - 1.01 \ C_P F)$$
$$+ \ [D(1 - Q_F/Q_E) \ 1.01 \ C_P F] \quad [64]$$

Equation 64 can be evaluated for the following set of typical treatment parameters: $D = Q_{HF} = 0.160 \, l/min$; $Q_F = 0.010 \, l/min$; $Q_E = 0.200 \, l/min$; $C_P F = C_S F = 140 \, mEq/l$. Solution of Equation 64 for these data results in $C_D F = 149 \, mEq/l$ when $C_S F = 140 \, mEq/l$ and $J_{HD} = J_{HF}$.

There has been considerable controversy regarding the ratio of $C_F F/C_P F$ (14, 155, 156). If it is assumed that this ratio is 1.00 (i.e. the first two terms in the numerator of equation 64 are neglected), solution of the above data shows $C_D F = 147$ when $C_S F = 140 \, mEq/l$ and $J_{HD} = J_{HF}$.

This analysis of the effective Na concentrations in hemodialysis and hemofiltration indicates that dialysate Na concentrations must be 7 to 9 mEq/l higher than substitution fluid Na concentration for equal Na flux with both therapies. Dialysate Na concentration is known to influence strongly treatment morbidity which in hemofiltration has been reported to be lower than for hemodialysis when $C_D F = C_S F$. Consideration of the effective Na concentrations with these two therapies indicates that reduced morbidity with hemo-

filtration may be due to lower Na removal in hemofiltration when $C_D F = C_S F$.

The difference between these two treatments under the same initial dialysis conditions can be illustrated further by computing the difference in sodium flux resulting from both therapies. Substituting the initial parameters used in the above computation into Equations 61b and 62 assuming that $C_D F = 140 \, mEq/l$ and computing the flux difference yields J_{HD}, J_{HF}, and $J_{HD} - J_{HF}$ of $- 2.37 \, mEq/min - 1.06$, $- 1.31$ mEq/min. The instantaneous effect of this difference on the vascular compartment would be to move $1.31/140 = 0.0094 \, l/min$ (9.4 ml/min) out of the extracellular compartment which would have the same effect early in dialysis of nearly doubling the ultrafiltration rate (i.e. 10 ml/min ultrafiltration plus 9.4 ml/min osmotically drawn into cells).

Sodium distribution volume

It has long been known that osmotic equilibrium exists throughout body water (157). Although there are multiple small anatomical subdivisions of total body water (V), (158), with respect to osmotic equilibrium it can be described as a two compartment system comprised of extracellular and intracellular water (V_E and V_C) as diagrammed in Figure 28. Osmotic equilibrium exists between compartments because of the high hydraulic permeability of cell membranes; any change in the osmotically active solute content of V_C or V_E selectively results in net water flux until the concentration of solute in both compartments is again equal.

Owing to the passive nature of water flux between V_E and V_C due only to the osmotic driving force, it follows that the volume of each compartment will be determined by the relative contents of osmotically active solute in each compartment and the total amount of water distributed between the compartments. Although there are multiple solutes present in body water, the bulk of osmolality in V_E is contributed by sodium salts and in V_C it is contributed by potassium salts. The asymmetric distribution of Na and K is achieved by active transport mechanisms in cell membranes resulting in high transcellular concentration gradients for Na and K. It has been shown by isotope dilution studies that plasma Na (C_{Na}) over a wide concentration range linearly depends on the rapidly exchangeable body sodium and potassium content (Na_{Ex}, K_{Ex}) and total body water, V.

The relationship found was (159):

$$C_{Na} = \frac{Na_{Ex} + K_{Ex}}{V}. \quad [65]$$

The rapidly exchangeable quantities, $Na_{Ex} + K_{Ex}$, were postulated to be measures of the osmotically active Na and K salts in V_E and V_C respectively. The relationship in Equation 65 provided confirmation of this postulate and demonstrated that the effective osmotic driving force controlling body water distribution between V_E and V_C was determined by Na and K salts in the two compartments respectively. The sum of Na_{Ex} and K_{Ex} can be considered equal to the total osmotically active cation (C^+) in body water and Equation 65 can then be written.

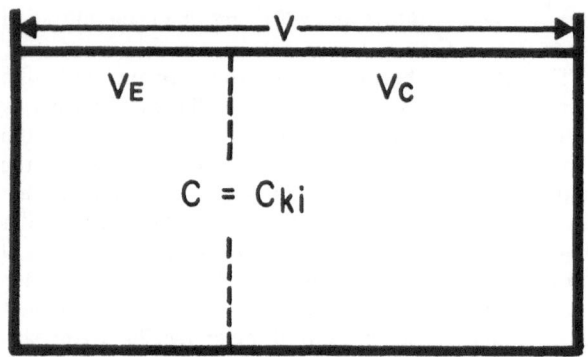

Figure 28. Two compartment distribution of osmotically active sodium and potassium in body water.

$$C_{Na} = \frac{C^+}{V} \tag{66}$$

Equation 66 is a powerful physiologic statement showing that C^+ can readily be calculated from the product $C_{Na}V$. Serial change in C^+ can be computed from serial changes in C_{Na} if V is either constant or undergoes a quantified change, ΔV. This can be illustrated as follows: Consider initial composition to be represented by C_{Na_1}, V_1 and C^+_1; assume that C_{Na_2} is measured after a known ΔV and unknown change in C^+ due to changes in body water content of Na and K, ΔNa and ΔK. The serial composition relationships will be:

$$C_{Na_1} = \frac{C^+_1}{V_1} \tag{67a}$$

$$C_{Na_2} = \frac{C^+_1 + \Delta Na + \Delta K}{V_1 + \Delta V}. \tag{67b}$$

The change in C^+, which is by definition $\Delta Na + \Delta K$, can be determined by subtraction of equation 67a from 67b and rearrangement:

$$(\Delta Na + \Delta K) = (C_{Na_2} - C_{Na_1}) V_1 + (C_{Na_2}) (\Delta V). \tag{67c}$$

Assuming all quantities on the right hand side of equation 67c can be measured, the relationships in equation 67c provide a simple method to calculate ΔC^+ or $\Delta Na + \Delta K$.

The clinical material used to establish the relationships in equation 65 was comprised of a spectrum of patients with chronic illness with C_{Na} ranging from hyponatremic to modest hypernatremic levels (159). In the hyponatremia of chronic illness, depletion of cellular K^+ often was the major compositional change present causing H_2O to move out of cells diluting Na^+ in extracellular fluid.

In the dialysis patient there are regular small oscillations in body water K^+ content with interdialytic loading of excess K^+ followed after 2 or 3 days by dialytic removal of the excess. Thus the body K^+ content, in the absence of an associated severe K^+ depleting chronic illness, oscillates between mild excess and normal.

Because of normal K^+ sequestration in cells, potassium loads should result in small changes in plasma K^+ levels, (156, 160, 161). Studies in dialysis patients, however, in-

dicate that K^+ loading and removal can be accurately estimated by considering changes in potassium levels to extend over total body water. That is, a 3 mEq/l reduction in K^+ in a patient with 40 l of total body water will reflect 120 mEq of potassium removal. The reasons behind this apparent contradiction of asymmetric potassium distribution are not clear. It may relate to the small changes in potassium which makes this approximation usable. Thus ΔK is negligible and equation 67b can be rewritten as:

$$\Delta Na = C_{Na_2}(V_1 + \Delta V) - (C_{Na_1}) (V_1). \tag{68}$$

It is apparent from equation 68 that although anatomically Na is confined to V_E, its osmotic distribution is V, and a single pool equal to total body water can be used to model sodium in steady state. It should be emphasized that the magnitude of change in the Na^+ content of body water can be computed from equation 68 only if there are no unusual asymmetrically distributed solutes which are loaded or removed from body water during the dialysis cycle. Consequently, if solutes such as dextrose or mannitol are present equation 68 should not be used to calculate the change in body Na content. Both of these materials can accumulate in V_E. Consequently in the diabetic patient with substantial changes in blood sugar during dialysis or in the mannitol treated patient, equation 68 would be invalid due to unaccounted for changes in osmotically active solute in V_E resulting in net transcompartmental water flux independent of ΔNa.

A third solute which can have a significant impact on these relationships is urea. At steady state there is concentration equilibrium between V_E and V_C for urea and thus urea will not influence water distribution between these components. During dialysis a urea concentration gradient develops between the two compartments (i.e. cellular urea concentration will be higher than extracellular concentration – see Figure 15) which will transiently pull water into cells. This urea disequilibrium then introduces another osmotic effect in addition to that of Na and as in the case of mannitol and dextrose equation 68 should be used with caution.

Calculation of Δ_{Na} and Δ_V over the dialysis treatment cycle

A flow diagram of body compositional relationships over the dialysis treatment cycle is shown in Figure 29. In order to calculate values for interdialytic dietary Na loading and subsequent intradialytic sodium removal from serial values of C_{Na} it is necessary to determine V and ΔV. Total body water is coextensive with the urea distribution volume (79) so that the variable volume urea kinetic model described earlier can be used to determine end-dialysis volume (V_t). Over short 2 to 3 day interdialytic intervals, change in body weight is traditionally used as a measure of change in V (volume loading, V_L). Similarly, change in body weight from pre- to postdialysis is used to measure the volume of fluid removal, V_R.

The magnitude of sodium removal is equal to $C^+_{o2} - C^+_{t1}$ (see Figure 29) and described by:

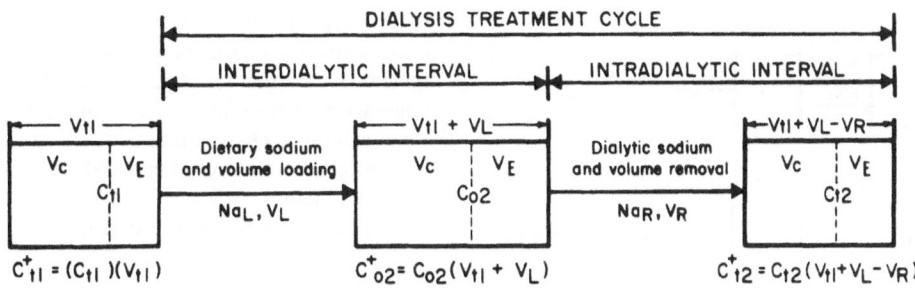

Figure 29. Flow diagram of interdialytic Na and volume loading and intradialytic Na and volume removal.

sodium loading $= C_{o2} (V_{t1} + V_L) - (C_{t1}) (V_{t1}).$ [69]

The magnitude of sodium removal is equal to $C^+_{o2} - C^+_{t2}$ and described by:

sodium removal $= C_{o2} (V_{t1} + V_L)$
$$- C_{t2} (V_{t1} + V_L - V_R). \qquad [70]$$

Sodium balance $\Delta(C_{Na}V)$ over the treatment cycle by definition equals sodium loading less sodium removal and can be determined by subtracting equation 70 from 69 resulting in:

$$\Delta C_{Na}V = (C_{t2} - C_{t1}) V_{t1} + C_{t2} (V_L - V_R). \qquad [71]$$

Equations 69 to 71 provide a simple method to quantify Na loading, removal and balance over the treatment cycle from several measured values of C_{Na} and use of urea kinetics to determine V_t and changes in weight to determine V_L and V_R.

The usual therapeutic goal for each treatment cycle is to achieve zero Na and V balance; that is, to remove during dialysis exactly the quantity of dietary sodium and water loaded since the previous dialysis. Inspection of equation 71 shows that to achieve this, the end dialysis sodium concentration must always be returned to the same value ($C_{t2} = C_{t1}$) and the net fluid removed during dialysis must equal the interdialytic weight gain ($V_L = V_R$). The first term on the right side of equation 71 can be viewed as being controlled by the diffusive Na concentration gradient between blood and dialysate; the second term can be viewed as being controlled by the magnitude of ultrafiltration. Current state of the art dialysis therapy provides reasonable assurance that $V_R = V_L$ by matching the ultrafiltration to the interdialytic weight gain but does not assure that $C_{t2} = C_{t1}$ since there is no attempt to individualize the diffusive Na gradient for each treatment. This would require measurement of C_{o2} and use of a model to individualize dialysis fluid Na^+ concentration as will be discussed.

The relative impact on Na^+ balance resulting from mismatch of diffusive gradient and ultrafiltration can be shown by consideration of equation 71. Assume average values of $V_t = 38.01$ and $C_{t2} = 140 \, mmol/l$. For a 1.0 mmol/l difference between C_{t2} and C_{t1} there will be a 38 mmol change in Na balance and for each 0.11 mismatch between V_L and V_R

there will be a difference of 14 mmol. It is apparent that both diffusion and ultrafiltration must be individualized for each treatment if no change in Na balance is to result.

Modeling extracellular water and osmotic interactions

The preceding discussion provides the theoretical basis for a single pool Na distribution model as well as methods to compute change in Na and water balance over the interdialytic and intradialytic intervals. Sodium and volume loading between dialyses will depend entirely on dietary Na and water intake and can be quite variable. In order to achieve zero Na balance over each dialysis cycle reliably, it is necessary to target a constant end-dialysis Na concentration irrespective of predialysis concentration as shown by equation 71. Sodium concentration, however, depends on the amount of Na present as well as the volume of extracellular water which will change during dialysis depending on ultrafiltration and on osmotic factors.

In addition, extracellular water is the system of interest because its content will directly influence hypotension and intradialytic patient morbidity. Extracellular water will be influenced, however, by two major factors: The ultrafiltration rate across the dialyzer induced by a blood-dialysate pressure difference (the analogue of convective transport of a solute); and the osmotic movement of water due to changes in osmotically active solutes (the analogue of diffusive transport of a solute). The model for this system, therefore, involves other systems in a similar manner as did the body base model.

There are three interacting systems that will influence extracellular water content and these systems are shown in Figure 30. They are: 1. The body water system (Figure 30a); 2. The sodium system (Figure 30b); and 3. The system designated as that for 'other osmotically active solutes' (Figure 30c). This latter system is general and will be seen to be the same as Figure 14 for urea if 'I' is equated to urea generation rate (G) and if Q_F is set to zero. This model, however, can also be used to describe such osmotic agents as mannitol with 'I' as an infusion rate and with K_I approaching zero (effectively confining mannitol to extracellular water).

Each of these models will be considered in turn. Although extracellular water is the system of interest it is actually part of total body water as described in Figure 30a. This system is

---

* The subscripts o2 and t1 relate to the start (time = 0) and end (time = t) of the first dialysis (number 1) or second dialysis (number 2).

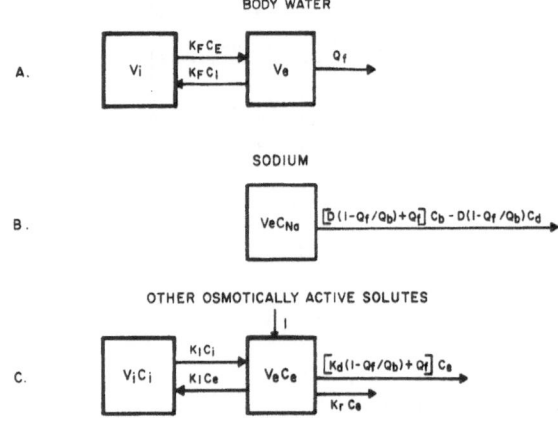

Figure 30. Model for body water and osmotically active solutes during dialysis.

considered as consisting of two compartments – intracellular and extracellular water. Movement of water out of the extracellular space occurs by ultrafiltration (Q_F) across the dialyzer and depends on the hydraulic permeability of the dialyzer (its ultrafiltration coefficient) and the mean transmembrane pressure (see equation 19). For purposes of this model the ultrafiltration rate is considered constant which is generally the case during dialysis. Movement of water between intra- and extracellular compartments depends on the relative concentration of osmotically active solutes in these compartments (CI and CE). Higher concentrations in extracellular water (CE) cause movement of water into this compartment. Conversely, higher concentrations in intracellular water (CI) cause water to move from the extracellular space into cells. In general, therefore, it is desirable for (CE – CI) to be positive or zero so that there will be refilling of the extracellular volume or at least no volume change. If (CE – CI) is negative, water will move out of the extracellular space both across the dialyzer and into cells in which case hypotension and some degree of vascular collapse is likely.

Osmotically active solutes (CI and CE above) will consist of electrolytes (predominantly sodium as discussed above) and nonelectrolytes (such as urea). The model for sodium is shown in Figure 30b. It is a single pool model and its content will be influenced, during dialysis, by diffusive and convective transport as described in Equation 14.

Figure 30c describes other osmotically active solutes (nonelectrolytes) examples of which are urea and exogenous materials. A specific case of this model for urea was presented in Figure 14. In this system the intracellular pool is basically passive with the only route of solute entry being diffusion from the extracellular space. Material enters the extracellular space either through generation (urea: I = G) or by constant infusion (in the case of exogenous solutes). The second route by which material is added to the extracel-

lular space is by diffusion from the intracellular space down a concentration gradient controlled by an intercompartmental transfer coefficient of K_L. Material is removed from this compartment by dialysis (see equation 14) or continuing renal clearance (K_R) of this material or both.

Considering each of these systems separately the mass balance equations will be:

Body water system (Figure 30a):

$$\frac{d(V_i)}{dt} = K_F \, (CI - CE) \qquad [72a]$$

$$\frac{d(V_e)}{dt} = -Q_F - K_F \, (CI - CE) \qquad [72b]$$

Sodium system (Figure 30b):

$$\frac{d(V_e C_{Na})}{dt} = -\left[D \left(1 - \frac{Q_F}{Q_B} \right) + Q_F \right] C_{Na}$$

$$+ D \left(1 - \frac{Q_F}{Q_B} \right) C_d. \qquad [73]$$

Other osmotically active solutes (Figure 30c):

$$\frac{d(V_i C_i)}{dt} = -K_1 \, (C_i - C_e) \qquad [74a]$$

$$\frac{d(V_e C_e)}{dt} = K_1 \, (C_i - C_e) + I$$

$$- \left[K_D \left(1 - \frac{Q_F}{Q_B} \right) + Q_F \right] C_e - K_R C_e \qquad [74b]$$

A model similar to the one shown in Figures 30 has been used to obtain *in vivo* measurements of the whole-body cell ultrafiltration (K_F) and urea mass transfer (K_1) coefficients (99). In these studies the Q_F and $C_D Na$ were manipulated to remove either 1.01 of Na free water or 130 mEq Na without water removal over 30 min of dialysis (99). Frequent measurements of blood Na and urea during the 30 min of dialysis and a following 30 min period of equilibration were used to calculate K_F and K_1 values from numerical solution of the mass balance expressions (equations 72 to 74).

These studies yielded mean values of K_1 of 760 ml/min which agrees with other reported values (22, 39). Contrary to common intuition, that water transport into and out of cells is 'rapid', values of K_F were 0.2 ml/min/mm Hg (i.e. the entire body cell diffusion area is less permeable to water than most dialyzers). The transcapillary ultrafiltration coefficient is considerably higher and of the order of 5 ml/min/mm Hg (162).

It is clear from Figure 30 that extracellular volume with potential impact on intradialytic morbidity requires a complex and a multi-system model. In contrast however, to the body base system, most of the interrelationships between the water, sodium, and urea systems can be quantitatively defined. What is also clear is that intradialytic hypotension is far more complicated than has perhaps been appreciated and depends on more factors than strictly ultrafiltration rates for its control.

Clinical applications of the extracellular water model

A major goal of each dialysis is removal of dietary Na^+ and water that has accumulated since the previous treatment with minimal risk of intradialytic morbidity such as symptomatic hypotension and muscle cramps. At present there are not clear guidelines for optimizing Na^+ and H_2O removal. A number of empirically developed dialysate Na^+ profiles have been reported to reduce morbidity associated with ultrafiltration (163) but a consensus has not been reached regarding their value. It would seem probable that clinical optimization of ultrafiltration will require quantification of the relationships between several different systems including various body fluid compartments and definition of circulatory hemodynamics. Unfortunately such information is not yet available.

Decreasing intradialytic morbidity can be viewed as a problem of selecting the best means of removing the interdialytic Na^+ and water load during dialysis. The means of accomplishing this removal remains ultrafiltration and the selecting of an appropriate dialysis solution Na^+ concentration. However, with the current designs of dialysis fluid delivery equipment it is increasingly possible to have both of these parameters change during the course of dialysis. This evolution in dialytic control makes it possible to investigate if variable, or even individualized, prescriptions for Na^+ and water removal may provide more optimal treatment.

Current understanding of water 'kinetics' as described above provides the basis for considering possible optimization of Na^+ and water removal. For balance over the treatment cycle the interdialytic Na^+ load should be removed during the subsequent treatment. The ultrafiltration rate, Q_F, may be variable but the integrated product of ultrafiltration rate and dialysis time over the course of a treatment should equal the patient's interdialytic weight gain. Examination of Figure 30b and Equation 73 indicates that the dialysis fluid Na^+ concentration required to produce a specific rate of change in the extracellular Na^+ is:

$$C_d = \frac{d(V_eC_{Na})/dt + [D(1 + Q_F/Q_B) + Q_F]C_{Na}}{D(1 + Q_F/Q_B)} \quad [75]$$

It may be useful to select the desired value for $d(V_eC_{Na})/dt$ (either constant or variable) during the course of a treatment. An illustration of possible methods of removing accumulated Na^+ is shown in Figure 31. In each case the pre- and postdialysis extracellular Na^+ content are the same, but the rate of change is different. The top line indicates the major decrease in Na^+ content is toward the end of the treatment. This might be the case if there were concern that large urea flux combined with Na^+ removal would contract extracellular volume (V_e) too rapidly and Na^+ removal would be delayed until much of the urea load had been removed (see Figure 15 above). The lower line is the opposite case where there is accelerated removal of sodium early in dialysis. This case is more of a logical contrast to the previous case and may have limited clinical use because of the rapid decrease in extracellular volume that would be intuitively expected if this option were used. The intermediate (straight) line in-

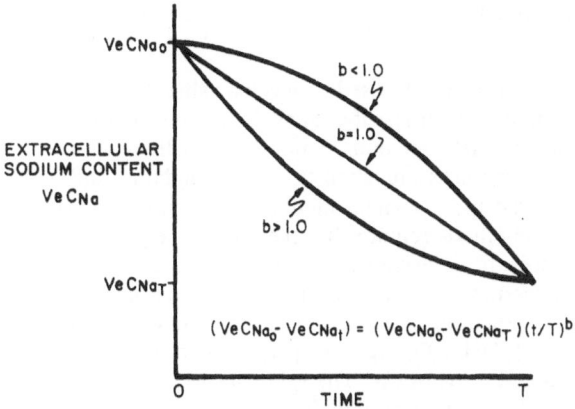

Figure 31. Possible means of decreasing extracellular sodium content during dialysis.

dicates a constant decrease in extracellular Na^+ during the treatment.

It should be noted that the term $d(V_eC_{Na})/dt$ indicates the slope of the line in Figure 31. For the straight line, where the slope is constant, this term will be constant and negative. For the upper line this term will change with time and will be increasingly negative during the treatment; for the bottom line this term will also be a function of time and will be increasingly positive (i.e. will be less negative) throughout the dialysis.

It should also be stressed that the relationships shown in Figure 31 do not directly show what is happening to either Na^+ concentration (C_{Na}) or extracellular volume (V_e) but their product. Consequently, the upper line could be produced by a rapid initial decrease in extracellular volume and a rise in sodium concentration as well as a relatively constant or increasing extracellular volume and more rapidly decreasing Na^+ concentrations. Consequently, a prescription of the Na^+ removal rate may also require some control of the rate of change of either extracellular volume or Na^+ concentrations. In fact further investigation may indicate that either of these rates may be the parameter that should be controlled during dialysis rather than their product recognizing that $d(V_eC_{Na})/dt = V_e(dC_{Na}/dt) + C_{Na}(dV_e/dt)$.

Nonetheless a prescriptive expression for curves such as those shown in Figure 31 can be expressed as:

Total change in sodium content at any time	=	Total change in sodium content during the course of the treatment	$\left(\dfrac{t}{T}\right)^b$

$$V_eC_{Na_0} - V_eC_{Na_t}) = (V_eC_{Na_0} - V_eC_{Na_T})\left(\frac{t}{T}\right)^b$$

and,

$$V_eC_{Na_t} = V_eC_{Na_0} - (V_eC_{Na_0} - V_eC_{Na_T})\left(\frac{t}{T}\right)^b. \quad [76a]$$

Differentiation of equation 76a yields:

$$\frac{d(V_e C_{Na})}{dt} = -b(V_e C_{Na_0} - V_e C_{Na_T})\left(\frac{t}{T}\right)^{b-1}. \qquad [76b]$$

Equation 76b can be used to develop values for $d(V_e C_{Na})/dt$ in equation 75 at specific times during the treatment. It is apparent that equation 75 now defines the dialysate N_a^+ concentration as a function of both C_{Na} and time and should be solved using general methods for non-linear systems. These methods require that the terms in equation 75, for example, be determined over very short intervals of time to produce new system values for recomputation. For example, in equation 75 if intervals of a minute were chosen the value of $[D(1 + Q_F/Q_B) + Q_F]C_{Na}$ would be computed using the initial value of C_{Na}. The value of $(d/V_e C_{Na})/dt$ would be computed from equation 76b at mid-interval (i.e.: $t = 0.5$ min) and C_{DNa} could be computed for the first minute of dialysis. The value of V_e Would then be computed from the multisystem model described above. This value would then be used in either equation 73 and equation 76b to determine C_{Na} after one minute. This value would then be used to compute C_{dNa} during the second minute, etc.

It should be apparent from examination of equations 72 to 74 that a substantial number of physiologic parameters must be estimated and historic data must assumed to represent current patient values for implemention of the extracellular water model described above. These requirements may limit the clinical accuracy of the model and a clinical data base will be required to evaluate its precision in actual use.

Use of the extracellular water – sodium model to counter the intradialytic urea gradient

It should also be possible to use the above model to determine a dialysate N_a^+ profile to counter balance the transcellular osmotic urea gradient ($C_i U - C_e U$) with an osmotic cation gradient ($C_e - C_i$) and thus prevent any water movement into cells during dialysis. This application may be particularly useful in dialysis of patients with acute renal failure or during the initial dialyses of patients with chronic renal failure and high BUNs.

The goal of this therapeutic maneuver is to determine the dialysate N_a^+ profile, as defined by $d(V_e C_{Na})/dt$, to exactly counter the urea gradient in order to solve equation 75 for the dialysate N_a^+ concentration throughout the treatment.

The desired extracellular sodium profile will be:

$$\frac{dC_e}{dt} = \frac{dC_{Na}}{dt} = \frac{d(C_i U - C_e U)}{dt} = \frac{dC_i U}{dt} - \frac{dC_e U}{dt}. \qquad [77]$$

The rate of change in extracellular N_a^+ shown in Equation 75 can be described as:

$$\frac{d(V_e C_e)}{dt} = V_e \frac{dC_e}{dt} + C_e \frac{dV_e}{dt}.$$

If intracellular volume is to remain constant, ultrafiltration will be exclusively from the extracellular fluid (i.e. $V_e = V_{eo} - Q_F t$) and:

$$\frac{d(V_e C_e)}{dt} = (V_{eo} - Q_F t)\frac{dC_e}{dt} - C_e Q_F \qquad [78]$$

Combining equations 77 and 78:

$$\frac{d(V_e C_{Na})}{dt} = (V_{eo} - Q_F t)\left(\frac{dC_i U}{dt} - \frac{dC_e U}{dt}\right) - C_{Na} Q_F. \qquad [79a]$$

Because of the constraints of the treatment (i.e. holding intracellular volume constant) $d(C_i U)/dt$ and $d(C_e U)/dt$ can be determined by use of equations 74a and 74b:

$$\frac{dC_i U}{dt} = -\frac{K_1}{V_i}(C_i U - C_e U) \qquad [79b]$$

and

$$\frac{dC_e U}{dt} = \frac{1}{V_{eo} - Q_F t}\left[K_1(C_i U - C_e U) + G\right.$$
$$\left. - K_D(1 - Q_F/Q_B)C_e U - K_R C_e U\right]. \qquad [79c]$$

Equation 79a is used with equation 75 as equation 76b was above over short intervals to compute the desired dialysis solution N_a^+ concentration during dialysis. In this case the value of $d(V_e C_{Na})/dt$ is computed from equation 79a using equations 79b and 79c to compute values for $dC_i U/dt$ and $dC_e U/dt$. These expressions use values of $C_e U$ and $C_i U$ which are calculated from equations 74a and 74b (adapted for urea).

The use of osmotically active solutes to counter urea disequilibrium

Another approach to balancing the urea gradient and associated water movement in acute or high BUN dialysis is to use an exogenous osmotically active solute such as mannitol. If the intracellular volume can be kept constant (as in the previous case) this case is computationally somewhat easier because equation 74b (adapted for mannitol i.e. $K_1 = 0$) can be solved in same manner as the single pool variable volume urea model. If this is done, and the impact of renal excretion of mannitol during dialysis is considered negligible (i.e. $K_R = 0$), the expression for mannitol concentration at any time will be:

$$C_M = C_{Mo}\left(\frac{V_{eo} - Q_F t}{V_{eo}}\right)^{K(1/Q_F - 1/Q_B)} +$$
$$\frac{I}{K(1 - Q_F/Q_B)}\left[1 - \left(\frac{V_{eo} - Q_F t}{V_{eo}}\right)^{K(1/Q_F - 1/Q_B)}\right]. \qquad [80]$$

Equation 80 can then be rearranged to yield the infusion rate necessary to keep the mannitol at the desired concentration which in this case will be the difference between urea concentrations in the two modeled compartments ($C_i U - C_e U$).

For intracellular volume to be constant N_a^+ must be controlled to assure that there is no intercompartmental water movement due to unbalanced cation concentrations. If N_a^+ is not controlled the assumptions of $dV_i/dt = 0$ and

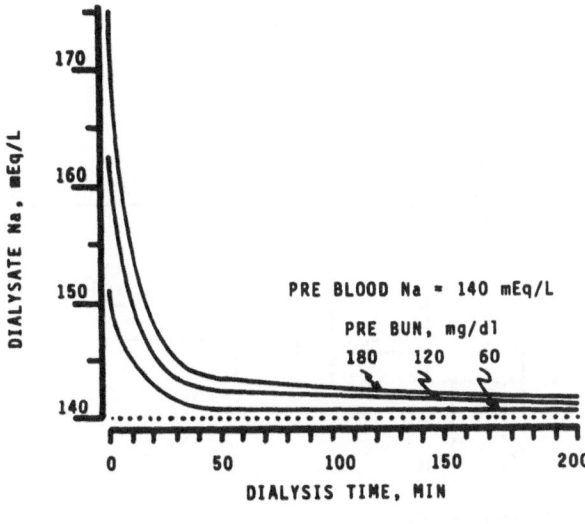

DIALYSATE Na PROFILE TO HOLD Vi CONSTANT

Figure 32. Dialysate sodium concentration required during dialysis to counteract urea gradient.

$V_e = V_{eo} - Q_F$ t may not be valid and mannitol concentration will not be an analytical function of time as shown in equation 80. If the volumes V_i and V_e are not controlled this system must be solved in the manner as the previous two cases – by step-wise calculations using small increments of time to determine the mannitol infusion rate with time.

If the assumptions of constant intracellular volume and ultrafiltration from the extracellular compartment alone are valid then this system of equations may be solved analytically. That is, the concentrations in the extracellular and intercellular compartments (presuming that these coincide with the perfused and nonperfused compartments described above for urea) are distinct functions of time. Consequently, it is possible to describe the infusion rate of mannitol to counter this urea disequilibrium as an analytical function, i.e. iterative methods should not be needed.

It should be noted that consistent with the discussion of modeling compartments above, it is important to appreciate that the models shown in Figure 30 may not be the same physiological spaces. That is, the 'nonperfused' urea compartment may not be coincident with the intracellular compartment. To the extent that this is the case the methods described to control urea induced water movement may be inexact. For example, the mean whole body K_l of 760 ml/min may represent some combination of cell membrane resistance to urea transport and nonideality of cell perfusion. In this case a therapeutically induced increase in osmotically active materials (i.e. Na^+ or mannitol) extracellularly could result in local regions of cell dehydration transiently.

The transcellular urea gradient and total osmolar drop in BUN have been discussed above and indicate that greater problems with urea induced water movement should be encountered at high urea removal rates. Reports to date have generally indicated less intradialytic morbidity with

high flux dialysis times in the range of 2 h (164). However, these short treatment times have generally been accompanied by conversion from acetate to bicarbonate dialysis, the use of volumetric ultrafiltration control systems and more biocompatible membranes all of which very likely contributed heavily to decreased morbidity. There is still significant morbidity in the range of 10% with optimized high flux dialysis which could in part be due to the increased transcellular urea gradient.

Intradialytic morbidity studies using mannitol infusions have been designed to evaluate symptoms with infusion rates high enough to counterbalance the total osmolar drop in BUN during dialysis (165–167). These designs will result in infused mannitol doses that are four or five times those required to prevent cell swelling, and should cause cell dehydration, expansion of extracellular volume and high plasma mannitol levels at the end of dialysis. If the purpose of mannitol is to prevent osmotically driven cell swelling due to the transcellular urea gradient, much smaller infusions during the first half hour of dialysis adequate to counterbalance the transcellular urea osmotic gradient should be administered.

The computations described above to counter urea gradients with extracellular sodium were performed to calculate the C_{DNa} profile which would be required to hold V_i constant with results shown in Figure 32. Average physiologic parameters were used and the rate of dialysis was such that t = 220 min for Kt/V urea = 1.0. It can be seen that the initial C_{DNa} would have to be 10 to 35 mEq/l greater than CeNa. The profiles for high flux dialysis would be very similar since although the initial transcellular urea osmotic gradient is higher, the dialysance of Na^+ is much higher so the dialysate to blood Na^+ gradient would not be appreciably different.

The multisystems model for extracellular water shown in Figure 30, as with the body base model, is very flexible. It can be used to guide the ultrafiltration aspect of normal dialysis when deliberate removal of both water and N_a^+ is required, particularly in the presence of a possible urea gradient which can 'pull' water into cells. It can be used to guide a wider range of 'nonroutine' treatments when efficient removal of water, electrolytes, and solutes are required, such as described as above. At this time the extent of application of this model has not been extensively evaluated. Nevertheless it has the potential for greatly enhanced control of dialysis treatment with the goal of reducing intradialytic patient morbidity.

The single pool interdialytic and double pool intradialytic models of Na^+, urea and water flux can be used to write dialysis prescriptions which will achieve targeted changes in Na^+ balance and intracellular and extracellular compartment volume during dialysis. At present there is not an adequate clinical data base to assess the utility of this model in reducing intradialytic morbidity in routine chronic dialysis.

We have had preliminary experience using the double pool Na^+ model to prescribe either a dialysate Na^+ profile or a mannitol infusion to hold V_i constant during the initial dialyses in four patients with acute renal failure and predialysis BUN ranging from 110 to 200 mg/dl. In each instance a full treatment was provided in the first dialysis of these patients resulting in a 60 to 70% drop in BUN over 3 to 4 h. The modeled therapy was highly successful in these patients who did not manifest dialysis disequilibrium.

Beta₂ microglobulin

Over the past several years evidence has accumulated linking beta₂ microglobulin (b₂m) to long term complications in dialysis patients (168, 169). The toxicity of b₂m results from its possible polymerization reactions which produce amyloid material (168–171) which preferentially deposits in synovia and bone (168) (where it may result in tumoral masses and pathological fractures) but also in skin (172) and many viscera (173).

The function of b₂m is not known. It is structurally associated with the general class of globulins involved with the immune system. However, little is known about this substance such as the regulation of its production and what may affect it; if it is a degradation product of some other process; or if it is a primary material produced to fill some, yet unknown, physiologic role.

Blood levels of b₂m are 20 to 50 times normal in dialysis patients. This has led to speculation that the rate of amyloid formation in these patients is in some way b₂m concentration dependent and that lowering blood levels through enhanced removal by dialysis might reduce amyloid formation.

It is reasonably well established that b₂m distributes as an unbound monomer (174) in two body water compartments, plasma (V_p) and interstitial fluid (V_{is}) (175, 176) as depicted in Figure 33a. As in other double pool models there will be concentration dependent transfer between compartments as described by a first order intercompartmental transfer coefficient (K_1).

Figure 33a shows generation of b₂m into V_{is} and removal from V_P primarily by renal clearance in normal subjects. It is not known if production of b₂m in a specific individual is constant or whether there is some degree of feedback control over its production or product inhibition. Other aspects of b₂m production will be discussed below.

The model indicates that removal (in the absence of dialysis) will be by renal clearance and metabolic routes (K_m and Γ). Monomeric b₂m is readily filtered at the glomerulus and reabsorbed into the proximal tubule where it is quantitatively catabolized (177). Thus plasma clearance is proportional to glomerular filtration rate (GFR).

The relationship between b₂m clearance and inulin clearance (K_i) has been studied by Vincent et al (175) at low levels of renal function (inulin clearances from 0 to 10 ml/min). From these studies the clearance of b₂m appears to follow the relationship: $K_{b2m} = 0.6k_i + 1.9$. This relationship would seem to indicate that renal clearance of b₂m is approximately 60% of GFR.

The above clearance relationship also indicates that there is some degree of b₂m catabolism or a metabolic clearance (K_m) which is approximately 2 ml/min. This term is shown in

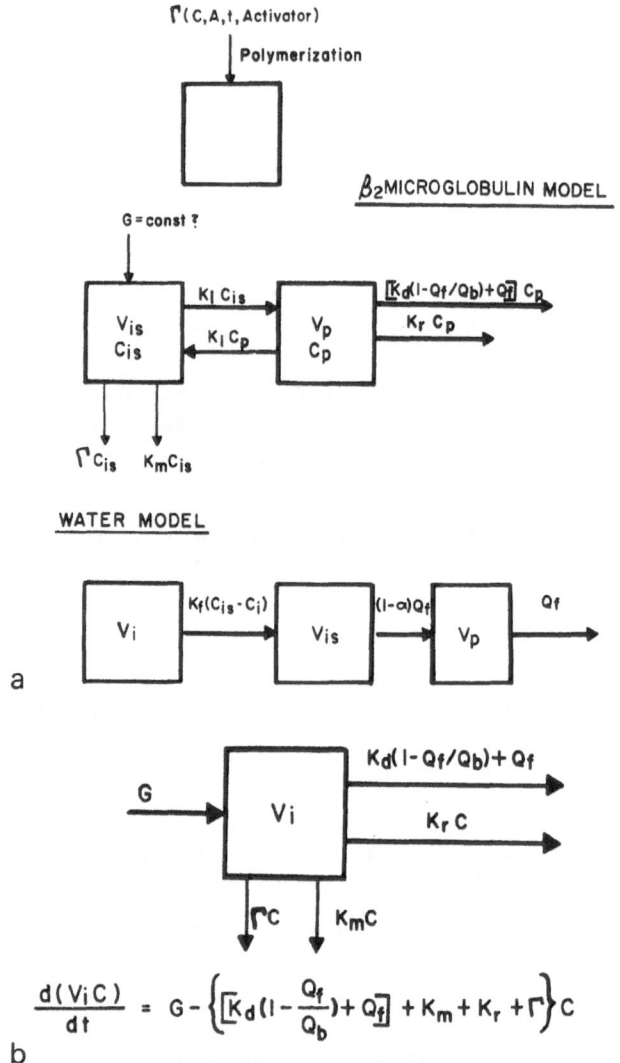

Figure 33. Model for Beta-2-microglobulin and body water: (A) considering Beta-2-microglobulin as distributed in two pools; (B) Treating Beta-2- microglobulin as distributed in a single pool.

Figure 33a as b₂m removal from interstitial water at the rate of K_mC. The model also indicates the possibility of b₂m serving as a substrate for biochemical reactions such as the postulated polymerization to amyloid at a rate ΓC_{is}. If this reaction exists, its rate of reaction (expressed as a clearance, Γ) may be variable and may depend on other factors not shown in this strictly concentration model.

The turnover of b₂m on lymphocyte cell membranes has been studied in tissue culture and found to be quite variable with $T_{1/2}$ ranging from 1.5 to 11.7 h (178). A large portion of the turnover in these studies appears to be via shedding of b₂m from the cell surface.

Whole body production of b₂m is substantially increased in such diseases as lymphoproliferative diseases, rheumatoid arthritis, Crohn's disease, chronic hepatitis, sarcoidoses, vasculitis, AIDS, Hodgkin's disease, leukemia and multiple myeloma (174, 179, 186). However, there appears to be marked variability in b_2m appearance even in the absence of these disorders.

In patients with renal insufficiency ($K_{Rb_2m} < 40\,ml/min$) b_2m appearance rates seem to range from 0.04 to 0.25 mg/min. At more normal levels of renal function ($K_{Rb_2m} > 70\,ml/min$) appearance rates range from 0.12 to 0.25 mg/min. It is apparent from these estimates that b_2m appearance is highly variable and some degree of product inhibition may be present (i.e. there was some decrease in b_2m appearance at high concentrations and low clearances). This observation, however, cannot be established at a statistically significant level. Recent studies suggest that as b_2m levels are reduced in renal failure patients treated with highly permeable membrane therapy, b_2m levels do not drop which would indicate the possibility that production or appearance rates increase as b_2m concentrations decrease.

Finally, there is considerable controversy concerning the effect of dialysis, per se, on b_2m appearance. It has been repeatedly observed that plasma b_2m rises during dialysis with cuprophan membranes which has led to the speculation that membranes with poor biocompatibility resulting in complement activation may cause increased shedding of b_2m. It is known that b_2m is not cleared by cuprophan membranes, moreover, the volume of distribution for b_2m ($V_p + V_i$ in the model) is relatively small and may be reduced as much as 20% to 30% by ultrafiltration during dialysis so that a substantial rise in plasma b_2m could be expected simply from concentration of the b_2m present.

Bergström and co-workers (181) have reported that plasma b_2m is unchanged after cuprophan dialysis when the level is corrected for ultrafiltration. Shaldon et al (182) reported that there is no change in plasma b_2m with sham dialysis but a substantial rise occurs with isovolemic dialysis with cuprophan. This has been interpreted to reflect increased cell shedding of b_2m due to 'cell swelling, resulting from the fall in osmolality because of urea removal. The effect of osmolality has been studied by Mahiout et al (183) who correlated the change in plasma b_2m with change in plasma osmolality during dialysis with dialysate Na^+ of 140 and 155 mEq/l. However, it is very likely that this correlation is due entirely to large changes in extracellular fluid volume related to dialysate Na^+.

The model shown in Figure 33a ignores the role of biocompatability in b_2m appearance (if present) and shows b_2m addition to the interstitial compartment only. If blood-membrane interactions are important an appearance term should also be associated with the plasma compartment.

The model shows dialytic removal of b_2m as described in equation 14. Cellulose and cellulose acetate membranes that have historically been used in chronic hemodialysis are virtually impermeable to b_2m. In this case Kd is zero and this term drops out of the model. More recently dialysis membranes of materials such as polysulfone and polyacrylonitrile have been developed that have increased permeability to materials in this size range.

The mass balance equation for the models shown are:

Beta$_2$ microglobulin model:

$$\frac{d(V_{is}C_{is})}{dt} = G - K_1(C_{is} - C_P) - K_MC_{is} - \Gamma C_{is} \quad [81a]$$

$$\frac{d(V_pC_P)}{dt} = K_1(C_{is} - C_P)$$

$$- \left[K_D\left(1 - \frac{Q_F}{Q_B}\right) + Q_F\right]C_P - K_RC_P \quad [81b]$$

Water model:

$$\frac{dV_i}{dt} = -K_F(C_{is} - C_i) \quad [81c]$$

$$\frac{dV_{is}}{dt} = K_F(C_{is} - C_i) - (1 - a)Q_F \quad [81d]$$

$$\frac{dV_P}{dt} = (1 - a)\,Q_F - Q_F = -aQ_F. \quad [81e]$$

It should be apparent that some of the terms in the above relationships are unknown such as Γ. In addition, some may be variable and depend on factors other than concentration or time such as G and Γ. As such it will be difficult to solve these relationships in an unequivocal manner.

Consider initially the situation of steady state with traditional dialyzers. In this case b_2m dialyzer clearance can be considered negligible and $K_D = 0$. In the absence of kidney function equation 81b shows that b_2m content will remain reasonably stable in the plasma compartment with the concentration increasing as V_P decreases (due to ultrafiltration) and content will change somewhat if plasma volume changes cause differences in C_P and C_{is}. In fact, the plasma concentration will basically reflect what is occurring in the interstitial compartment.

If the system is truly in steady state (i.e. content of both compartments is not changing) then it is clear that b_2m appearance will be off-set by removal: $G = K_MC_{is} - \Gamma C_{is}$. If, as expected ΓC_{is} is very small with respect to K_MC_{is} it can be neglected and: $C_{is} = G/K_m$. It is apparent from this steady state expression that with K_m being small and G varying considerably (0.04 to 0.24 mg/min) a wide range of C_{is} can be expected. The above relationship would predict C_P values ranging from 20 to 120 mg/l which, in fact, are seen in clinical reports. This wide range in C_P, however, may not be entirely due to variation in b_2m appearance since small variations in K_m would also result in wide dispersion of C_P steady state values.

Until recently conventional dialyzers were virtually impermeable to substances of the size of b_2m (both diffusively and convectively). With newer membranes such as polyacrylonitrile and polysulfone it is now possible to achieve clearance for b_2m in the range of 40 to 90 ml/min and by using such devices it should be possible to lower concentrations of this material.

The impact of using dialyzers that are highly permeable to b_2m can be investigated using the model shown in Figure 33a and equations 81a to e. For calculation purposes the postulated conversion of b_2m to amyloid (ΓC_{is}) can be ignored because such a pathway (while important if present) is small from a mass flow standpoint. Consequently, this term can be dropped from equation 81a. Even with this simplification solution of the equations shown should be used with caution. Much of the information shown in Figure 34a is based on estimates (V_P, V_{is}, K_1, K_m, a, etc). In addition, G may be variable and increase with b_2m removal.

Preliminary, unpublished studies suggest that despite high flux dialysis predialysis b_2m concentrations are not reduced. The conclusion generally drawn from these observations is that as b_2m is removed with more permeable dialyzer membranes its appearance rate increases so that the original predialyzer levels are restored. However, it must be pointed out that b_2m mass balance measurement has not been attempted in these studies and would be required to establish this conclusion. For example, the b_2m concentrations (both before and after dialysis) depend strongly on extracellular volume which may vary up to 30% and, if not accounted for, could result in considerable scatter in predialysis concentrations. Further, the magnitude of removal has generally not been documented carefully. The large molecular mass of b_2m (12 kilodaltons) places this solute in the region where membrane permeability is decreasing rapidly as a function of molecular size. The variability in a commercial membrane permeability to b_2m *in vivo* has not been carefully studied nor has the effect of various cleaning agents on membrane b_2m permeability been studied. Consequently, the level of *in vivo* b_2m clearance provided may have been poorly controlled.

The solution of equations 81 a to e is complex generally requiring a computer and iterative solution. An alternative approach is to simplify the model shown in Figure 33a (see Figure 33b) to a single pool model. As long as the dialyzer clearances remain at values approximately $0.5 K_1$ or less the single pool model will reasonably estimate b_2m concentrations to be expected using dialytic and filtration therapy. Calculation using V_P/V_{is} of 3/121 and K_D of 90 ml/min (the highest clearance now available) indicate that calculated posttreatment concentrations are underestimated by approximately 20%. When clearance is 40 ml/min calculated posttreatment b_2m levels are underestimated by 5%.

The use of the models shown in Figure 33 (a and b) will be along the lines of other models such as the urea model: That is, to determine what b_2m concentrations will result from a given level of therapy; to estimate b_2m production rates; or to evaluate how much treatment (clearance and time) is needed for a specific patient to control b_2m levels.

At this time it is not known what adequate treatment is regarding b_2m. It should be remembered that its toxicity is inferred from the presence of identical material in excised amyloid and the assumption that production of amyloid is caused by the higher than normal levels of b_2m present in dialysis patients. Although this is a reasonable hypothesis, the mechanism by which b_2m may result in amyloid production is not clear. Concentrations of b_2m are high shortly after the initiation of chronic hemodialysis (184) while amyloid formation, is either delayed almost a decade despite virtually constant b_2m concentrations or this length of time may be required to recognize its formation. There is some indirect evidence suggesting that aluminum may augment the rate of amyloid appearance since there is a correlation between excess body burden of aluminum and the clinical appearance of amyloid (168, 171, 180). Another mystery is why there is a predilection for amyloid deposition in synovia and bone and not other anatomical regions.

Kinetic consideration of uremic toxins

The concept of a uremic toxin is an old one. It is normal to consider that as other regulated substances accumulate in the absence of excretory capacity, so do certain substances that are systemic toxins. This concept is in part supported by the unresponsiveness of some lesions to the regulation of the commonly measured materials by dialysis. Toxic substances have been generally presumed to be certain peptides which are normally excreted. This presumption has been supported by detection of various substances in normal urine (185) which are found in uremic plasma but are absent in uremic urine (29, 31). Peptide production can be pictured by the hypothetical scheme shown in Figure 34.

In this scheme are shown a protein and substance γ; the protein is initially cleaved to A and B, and these two peptide fragments subsequently break down into various intermediate peptides until the final products G, H, I, and L result which are normally excreted in the urine. Substance γ is some other material that undergoes various metabolic steps which result in Z; Z may or may not be excreted by the kidney. It is only reasonable to presume in this scheme that the impaired removal of these hypothetical catabolic products will cause disruptions, perhaps toxic in nature. There has been the feeling that one or more of such substances are toxins and that their accumulation results in various uremic lesions (18, 33, 37, 38, 186).

This concept was pursued in the early 1970s by attempting to accelerate 'toxin' removal using different dialysis protocols (5, 187, 188) and more permeable dialysis membranes; in addition, certain quantifications and indices of therapy, partially based on these materials, were proposed (5, 37, 38). The rationale behind these studies was that the materials to be removed vary in size so that during dialysis they would be removed at different rates, the smaller ones being removed more rapidly than the larger ones (i.e. during dialysis the rates of elimination, V_{e1}, V_{e2}, V_{e3}, and V_{e4}, which might be similar in the natural organ, are different and depend on the size of the individual solute and the dialyzer characteristics). Consequently, the larger materials or 'middle molecules' (32, 186) would accumulate to a greater extent than the smaller catabolites and if toxic, would aggravate a given uremic lesion, the neurological system being one of the target areas (189).

In this regard, it has been suggested that the peritoneum is a far more permeable membrane than those used in hemodialyzers and that removal of 'middle molecules' is more efficient with peritoneal dialysis (5). Observation of patients undergoing this therapy supports this hypothesis by the less frequent occurrence of neuropathy (190) a lesion thought to result from middle molecule accumulation (5, 21). More

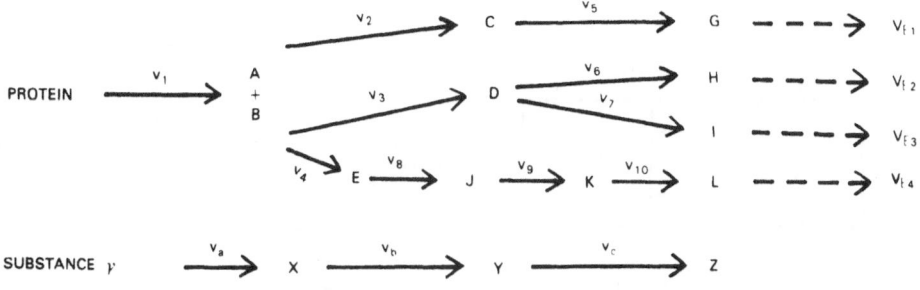

Figure 34. Hypothetical metabolic scheme involving catabolism of a protein and the biochemical pathways for some other substance γ.

recent analysis of peritoneal dialysis questions this contention (191). Other analyses of patients undergoing peritoneal dialysis, however, suggests that there may be a lower rate of some catabolic reactions (protein catabolism and urea generation) than in hemodialysis patients (17); this would lower correspondingly the level of several of the hypothetical catabolic materials discussed above but because this is caused by lower overall catabolic rates some level of undernutrition should be expected in such cases.

Nevertheless, the presence of several catabolic materials G, H, I and L in high concentrations and the possible toxicity of one or more of these substances is certainly valid. The analysis becomes immediately more complex, however, due to the size of the materials involved and the heterogenicity of the body. Kinetic analysis of such solute systems requires multicompartmental models in order that the levels of these unknown catabolites which will result from different types of dialysis therapy can be estimated and the effects of different dialyzers and protocols can be evaluated.

The steps of model formulation are similar to those discussed above with the exception that it is now necessary to abandon the simplicity of a single well mixed system. Two basic models are shown in Figure 35 (a and b), the difference between the two being the site of solute generation. Figure 35a indicates that material is generated into the perfused pool which would be the case if the solute in question were produced in the liver so that it had to traverse the extracellular system to reach cells. Figure 35b represents the case where the material is produced in cells. In either case there is a resistance to movement between the two compartments. The transport constant in this case is the intercompartmental transport coefficient (K_1) which has units of flow. Note that the model shown in Figure 35a was used to model urea and is the same as that in Figures 14 and 30c.

These models have been discussed at length by others (22, 45) but it is instructive to consider briefly the basic differences between them. In 'case A' the peripheral pool acts as a capacitance, and the perfused compartment will go through large swings, the concentration being low immediately post-dialysis and building up to levels higher than the peripheral compartment as the interdialytic period progresses. There will be solute movement alternately out of and into the peripheral pool during the dialysis cycle.

In contrast, 'case B' shows that the peripheral pool connects the site of generation and the site of excretion. As such the peripheral pool concentration will be elevated, because it is only through a high concentration difference that material can be transported into the perfused pool. Ironically, in 'case B' the uremic levels are closer to normal (relatively) because the same transport situation exists in health i.e. large concentration gradients being required for transport out of cells. This may be seen more clearly if steady state mass balance is examined in the two pools of model 35b:

$$G = K_1(C_{C_{Ss}} - C_{B_{Ss}})$$ [82a]

$$K_1(C_{C_{Ss}} - C_{B_{Ss}}) = K_R C_{B_{Ss}}.$$ [82b]

Solution of these equations for the steady state concentration in pool C yields:

$$C_{C_{Ss}} = \frac{G}{K_R} \left[1 + \frac{K_R}{K_1} \right].$$ [83]

Equation 83 shows that for peripheral generation the concentration will approach G/K_R when K_1 becomes large but will be higher with decreasing values of K_1 (e.g. for $K_1 = 5$ ml/min and K_R (normal) of 125 ml/min, the K_R/K_1 term results in normal steady state concentrations in the peripheral pool 26 times G/K_R). Thus, a minimal toxic effect of decreased transport out of extracellular space with model 35b would be expected if the effector site was situated in pool C because of the high normal levels in this pool.

In models such as Figure 35a and 35b mass balance expressions are written for each pool and the resulting differential equations are then solved simultaneously. Solutions for each of these cases are shown in the Appendix.

The case with metabolic interactions

The foregoing discussion of middle molecules in a multicompartmental setting is entirely hypothetical; such analyses point up the difficulties to be encountered when 'toxic' substances are not measured and their site of action is not known. In addition, the complexity of the kinetic system requiring knowledge of production rates and rates of transport between compartments coupled with the paucity of knowledge of these fundamental parameters makes this area of research a very demanding one.

Attempts to date to demonstrate a cause and effect rela-

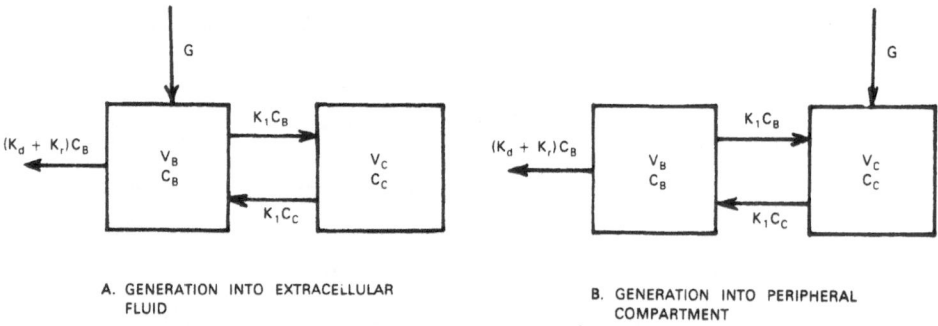

Figure 35. Two versions of a two compartment model for large molecular weight substances. Model a shows generation of material into the perfused (extracellular) compartment; model b shows generation into the perpherial (cellular) compartment.

tionship with respect to lowering levels of middle molecular weight toxins have been somewhat ambiguous (33, 192). There have been reports of improved blood pressure control (193) and decreased neuropathy (194) with similar high permeability protocols.

The two pool analysis of uremic toxins views the metabolic network shown in Figure 34 as a series of independent reactions that will depend on the removal rate alone for their level in the body. Reconsidering this figure shows that while this approach may be attractive, it is probably overly simplistic.

Consider the path for the protein to fragment B and the three pathways resulting in end products H, I, and L. If the clearances of L, H, and I are restricted, these substances will build up uniformly. However, if L is removed more rapidly than H and I, as would be the case during dialysis with urea (L) and large molecules, then the levels of H and I would be much higher relative to normal than the level of L would be; this interrelationship of catabolites has been the basis of the preceding discussion.

It is instructive, however, to consider the case where the paths are not independent. Let reaction V_4 be much faster than V_3 so that comparatively small amounts of H and I are formed with respect to L. At steady state, i.e. with the natural kidney still functioning, V_4, V_8, V_9, V_{10}, and V_{e4} will all be equal because none of the intermediates E, J, or K are accumulating. This will also be true of the chain of reactions resulting in H and I, i.e. $V_3 = V_6 + V_7 = V_{e2} + V_{e3}$. In this system, the complete blockage of pathways V_6 and V_7 will not significantly increase production of E because the predominant reaction is already in this direction. Reduction of V_{e4}, however, would cause reaction V_{10}, V_9 and V_8 to slow which would increase B and the rates of reactions V_3, V_6, and V_7. If L is a common catabolite, such as urea, then its elevation in the steady state case would cause corresponding elevation of the levels of K, J, E, and B. Urea's immediate precursor arginine has, in fact, been shown to be higher than normal in uremic patients (195). In addition, if pathway V_3 existed, higher levels of D, H, and I would be expected. In fact, H and I would increase more than L even if they were cleared at the same rate because V_3 has been increased with respect to V_4. In the dialysis patient where V_{e2} and V_{e3} would

possibly be less than V_{e4}, levels of H and I would be that much higher.

Up to this point, we have considered the ultimate products of these hypothetical biochemical reactions to be the potentially toxic materials. It is quite possible that intermediate substances C, D, E, J, or K might be metabolically active materials. As such, the elevated concentrations existing when the described pathways are blocked might reach toxic levels, or one of these materials (D, for example) might inhibit reaction Vb in another metabolic pathway. This in turn might result in either toxic levels of X in the metabolic reaction series in which D does not itself participate, or the creation of some lesion because of the abnormally low levels of substance Z.

The above discussion has viewed the series of reactions with regard to what may occur at different steady state levels. In the dialysis patient, however, the levels of G, H, I and L will be continually changing, which will cause the levels of intermediates to change with lags appropriate to the kinetics of the individual reactions. This would then cause a system of metabolic perturbations to exist in the dialysis patient and would be a new syndrome not found in nondialyzed patients and the perturbations themselves might cause toxic effects that would not be the result of any specific compound.

That the above discussion describes some catabolites is indicated by the kinetic behavior of various 'middle molecular' weight compounds (36) (see Figure 36). Two 'typical' curves shown in this figure demonstrate markedly different behavior. Figure 36a shows classical double pool behavior (39) for compounds 7f and 7g of Asaba et al (36). The modest concentration rebound and short transient times indicate that there is only slight multipool behavior. The short rebound transient also indicates that K_1 values are probably large relative to the dialyzer clearance so that re-equilibration takes place rapidly. The behavior shown by these materials is not much different than that of urea, creatinine, or uric acid (39, 126, 127).

Figure 36b shows a totally different and confusing concentration pattern, particularly post dialysis. It is clear from this curve (which is a composite of peptides 7a, 7b, and 7c of Asaba and coworkers [36]) that both models shown in Fig-

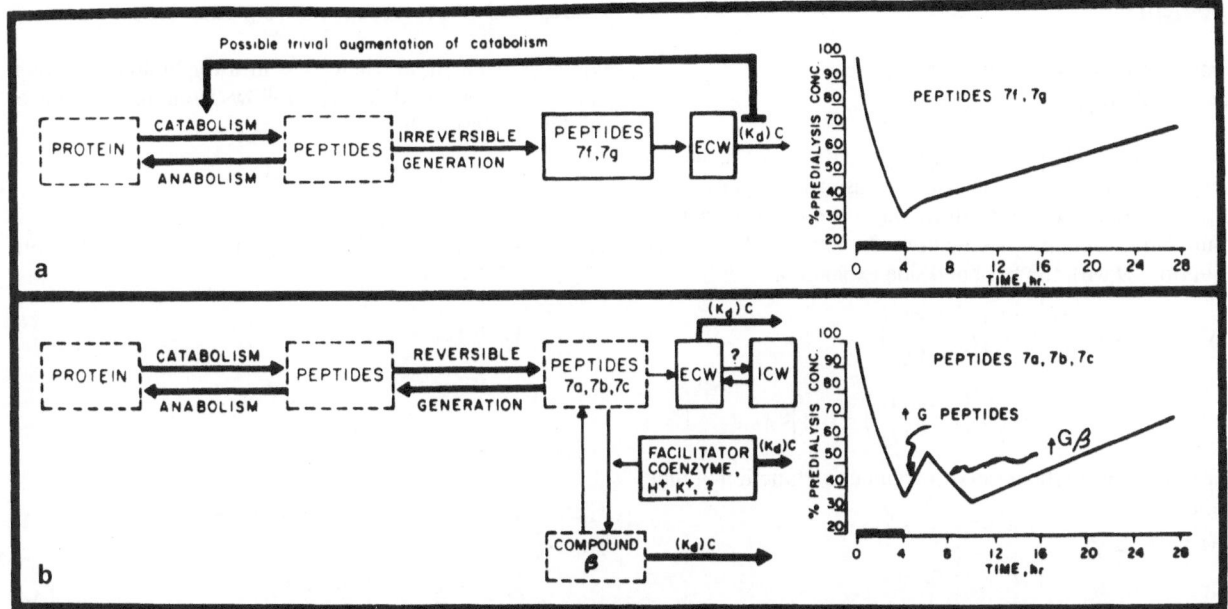

Figure 36. Concentration/time behavior or two types of peptides reported by Asaba et al (36) showing possible explanations for the kinetics of these materials. Reprinted by permission from Middle Molecules in Uremia and other diseases. (Supplement to Volume 4, Artificial Organs), Copyright © 1981 by the International Society for Artificial Organs.

ure 35 are inadequate. What is most disturbing about these compounds is the rapid rise post treatment followed by a drop even below post dialysis levels. The model in Figure 37b should be viewed as a specific but hypothetical example of the general diagram shown in Figure 34 and constructed to represent a possible explanation of the concentration behavior of the peptide shown.

Consider that these peptides are metabolic intermediates and are ultimately catabolized to compound beta. Both the peptides and beta are dialyzable and will accumulate in the uremic patient after dialysis. Further, the metabolic reaction of the peptide to beta requires a facilitator, co-enzyme, or cofactor (be it an electrolyte, optimal pH, etc.). Consider what, under these specific conditions, would happen as a result of dialysis. During dialysis all of these materials – the peptide, the facilitator, and beta – decrease in concentration. Immediately at the end of treatment there is a marked increase in peptide levels both because of re-equilibration between intracellular and extracellular water and the increased production of this material from the precursor peptide. In addition, because the facilitator has been dialyzed to low concentrations, the degradation of 7a, b and c to beta is temporarily blocked. The combination of increased production of these peptides into a 'dead-ended' system will result in a rapid rise in their concentration post dialysis.

The facilitator is gradually repleted post dialysis to the point where the catabolism of the peptide to beta can proceed and there is a rapid decrease of peptide levels as beta (which was also removed during treatment) increases. Once this reaction scheme is back to 'normal' the concentration of the peptides gradually rises as levels of beta increase, dependent on the reaction constant for the peptide/beta reaction. Note also, that the final slope of peptide build-up is more gradual than that immediately post dialysis because the same amount of peptide generation is both accumulating and supplying substrate for the 'beta reaction'.

This reaction scheme, while entirely hypothetical, is a possible explanation of curves such as the one shown in Figure 36b. Moreover what this figure shows is not a traditional 'toxin' but a very labile compound which appears and is degraded by multiple pathways, and depends on the level of reactants and products for its kinetic behavior, and which may require cofactors and certain optimum biochemical conditions for normal reactions to take place. In short, it is a typical biochemical compound in a uremic setting. Curves such as that in Figure 36b serve to remind us that uremia, particularly dialyzed uremia, where homeostasis no longer exists, is a very disruptive metabolic state. And it is very likely that there is a high degree of 'toxicity' associated with such metabolic chaos.

APPENDIX

Dialyzer transport measurements: the case with ultrafiltration

The use of recycle methods of dialyzer transport measurement were described above for the case where there is no ultrafiltration. When ultrafiltration is present ($Q_F \neq 0$) a solution different from equations 30 results. Reconsider Equation 29 with the left hand side expanded:

$$V \frac{dC_B}{dt} + C_B \frac{dV}{dt} = D \left(1 - \frac{Q_F}{Q_B}\right) C_{Di}$$
$$- \left[D \left(1 - \frac{Q_F}{Q_B}\right) + Q_F\right] C_B \qquad [A1]$$

The size of the 'blood' reservoir volume as a function of time will be:

$$V = V_0 - Q_F t$$

and

$$\frac{dV}{dt} = -Q_F.$$

Substitution of these relationships into equation A1 rearrangement and solution yield:

$$C_{Bt} = C_{Di} + (C_{Bo} - C_{Di}) \left[(V_0 - Q_F t)/V_0\right]^{D(1/Q_F - 1/Q_B)}. \qquad [A2]$$

Solving for D:

$$D = \frac{Q_F}{1 - Q_F/Q_B} \frac{\mathrm{Log} \dfrac{(C_{Bt} - C_{Di})}{(C_{Bo} - C_{Di})}}{\mathrm{Log} \dfrac{(V_0 - Q_F t)}{V_0}}. \qquad [A3]$$

Appropriate reservoir sampling for equation variables will yield dialysance values (see text).

Average blood concentration during urine collection

Figure A1 shows that when concentration build up between dialyses is considered linear, it follows from the principle of similarity (196) that:

$$\frac{C_0 - C_t}{\theta_t} = \frac{C_{01} - C_t}{\theta_1} = \frac{C_{02} - C_t}{\theta_2}$$

The value of starting and ending collection concentrations (C_{o1} and C_{o2}) will be:

$$C_{01} = C_t + (C_0 - C_t) \frac{\theta_1}{\theta_2}$$

and

$$C_{02} = C_t + (C_0 - C_t) \frac{\theta_2}{\theta_t}.$$

The average collection concentration will be the average of C_{o1} and C_{o2} or:

$$\tilde{C}_B = C_t + \frac{(C_0 - C_t)(\theta_1 + \theta_2)}{2\theta_t}. \qquad [A4]$$

Two pool analysis of 'middle molecule' kinetics

The model in Figure 35 assumes distribution in two well mixed spaces: Compartment B, a perfused space and Compartment C, a non-perfused space. Between these two compartments there is transport by first order mechanism K_1. Two variations of the model are considered: (A) with generation into the perfused space and (B) with generation into the non-perfused space.

The removal of 'middle molecules' from the system is by first order elimination from compartment B by the dialyzer and natural organ if present. Note for simplicity both models assume constant pool volumes i.e.:

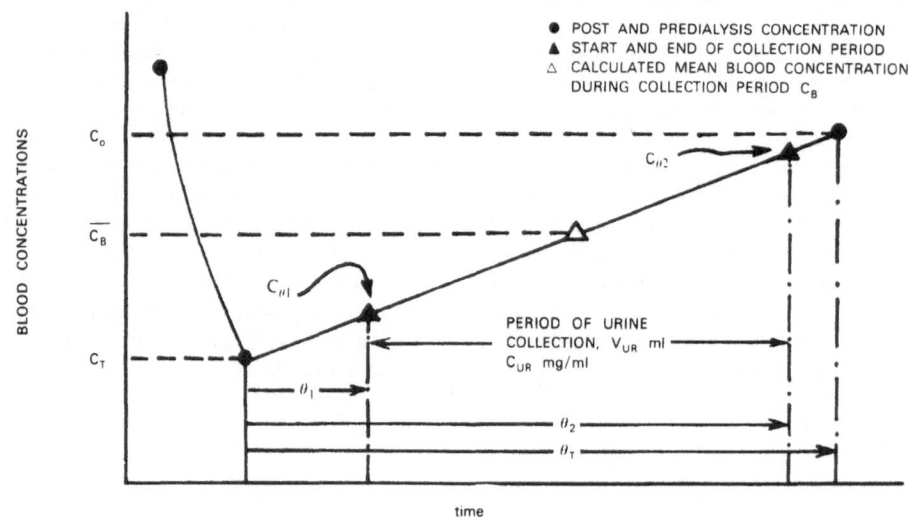

Figure A-1. Blood concentration and time values post dialysis required to calculate residual kidney clearance in the dialyzed patient.

$$\frac{dV_C}{d_c} = \frac{dV_B}{d_c} = 0.$$

As has been discussed, this assumption is not entirely valid in dialysis where fluid volume increases between dialysis and where a major treatment consideration is its decrease during a treatment session. As was considered during the analysis of extracellular volume, the manner of changes in both C_B and C_C will depend on ultrafiltration rates and transport of osmotically active solutes. However, it is felt that for general consideration of middle molecules assuming constant volumes will permit more useful mathematical expressions while not compromising the analysis significantly.

Model A represents the case where the solute is generated into the perfused space, for example if such substances were synthesized in the liver during protein catabolism. The defining equations for this model during all phases of dialysis are:

$$V_B \frac{dC_B}{dt} = G - K_1(C_B - C_C) - (K_R + K_D)\, C_B \quad [A5]$$

(compartment B)

$$V_C \frac{dC_C}{dt} = K_1(C_B - C_C) \quad [A6]$$

(compartment C)

The method of solution employed has been to put both equations A5 and A6 into Laplace transform space and alternately solve them simultaneously for the transformed concentration in each space. These expressions are then easily inverted by standard techniques to yield (63, 64):

$$C_B = \left[\frac{C_{C0}\,K_1}{V_B} + \frac{C_{B0}\,K_1}{V_C} + \frac{G}{V_B} - \frac{G\,K_1}{V_B V_C}\frac{1}{\beta}\right.$$
$$\left. - C_{B0}\right]\beta\ \frac{e^{-\beta c}}{\alpha - \beta} \quad [A7]$$
$$- \frac{C_{C0}\,K_1}{V_B} + \frac{C_{B0}\,K_1}{V_C} + \frac{G}{V_B} - \frac{GK_L}{V_B V_C}\frac{1}{\alpha}$$
$$- C_{B0}\,\alpha \bigg]\frac{e^{-\alpha t}}{\alpha - \beta} + \frac{G\,K_1}{V_B V_{C\alpha\beta}}$$

$$C_C = \left[\frac{C_{B0}\,K_1}{V_C} + \frac{C_{C0}(K_1 + K_R + K_D)}{V_B}\right.$$
$$- \frac{G\,K_1}{V_B V_C}\frac{1}{\beta} - C_{C0}\,\beta \bigg]\frac{e^{-\beta t}}{\alpha - \beta} \quad [A8]$$
$$- \left[\frac{C_{B0}\,K_1}{V_C} + \frac{C_{C0}\,(K_1 + K_R + K_D)}{V_B} - \frac{G\,K_1}{V_B V_C}\frac{1}{\alpha}\right.$$
$$- C_{C0}\,\alpha \bigg]\frac{e^{-\alpha t}}{\alpha - \beta} + \frac{G\,K_1}{V_B V_C \alpha\beta}.$$

Where α and β are defined by:

$$\alpha \text{ and } \beta = \frac{1}{2}\left[\frac{K_1}{V_C} + \frac{K_1 + K_R + K_D}{V_C}\right.$$

$$\pm \left(\frac{K_1}{V_C} + \frac{K_1 + K_R + K_D}{V_B}\right)^2 - 4\,\frac{K_1(K_R + K_D)}{V_B\,V_C}.$$

Off dialysis these equations still hold except in the case of the anephric patient; this special case can be approximated by letting K_R approach zero (i.e., by letting K_R have a very small value). C_{B0} and C0 will be the initial values for the particular interval being considered; predialysis for the dialytic period, end-dialysis values for the period between treatments.

Model B represents the case where the solute is generated into the peripheral space in a manner similar to creatinine. The defining equations for this model during all phases of dialysis are:

$$V_B\frac{dC_B}{dt} = -K_1(C_B - C_C) - (K_R + K_D)C_B \quad [A9]$$

$$V_C\frac{dC_C}{dt} = G + K_1(C_B - C_C). \quad [A10]$$

The same solution method described above was used to solve equations A9 and A10 and results in:

$$C_B = \left[\frac{C_{C0}\,K_1}{V_B} + \frac{C_{B0}\,K_1}{V_C}\right.$$
$$- \frac{GK_1}{V_B V_C}\frac{1}{\beta} - C_{B0}\,\beta\bigg]\frac{e^{-\beta t}}{\alpha - \beta} \quad [A11]$$
$$- \left[\frac{C_{C0}\,K_1}{V_B} + \frac{C_{B0}\,K_1}{V_C}\right.$$
$$- \frac{GK_1}{V_B V_C}\frac{1}{\alpha} - C_{B0}\,\alpha\bigg]\frac{e^{-\alpha t}}{\alpha - \beta} + \frac{GK_1}{V_B V_C\,\alpha\beta}$$

$$C_C = \left[\frac{C_{B0}\,K_1}{V_C} + \frac{C_{C0}(K_1 + K_R + K_D)}{V_B} + \frac{G}{V_B}\right.$$
$$- \frac{G(K_1 + K_R + K_D)}{V_C V_B}\frac{1}{\beta} - C_{C0}\,\beta\bigg]\frac{e^{\beta t}}{\alpha - \beta} \quad [A12]$$
$$- \left[\frac{C_{B0}\,K_1}{V_C} + \frac{C_{C0}(K_1 + K_R + K_D)}{V_B} + \frac{G}{V_B}\right.$$
$$- \frac{G(K_1 + K_R + K_D)}{V_C V_B}\frac{1}{\alpha} - C_{C0}\,\alpha\bigg]\frac{e^{-\alpha t}}{\alpha - \beta}$$
$$+ \frac{G(K_1 + K_R + K_D)}{V_B V_C\,\alpha\beta}$$

The value of α and β will be the same for the two models. Inspection of equations A11 and A12 shows that a steady state (i.e. $e^{-\alpha t}$ and $e^{-\beta t}$ equal zero) the concentration is represented by the constant term which is different for two compartments B and C. In the non-dialysis case, C_B will be less than C_C because the residual clearance, K_R, appears in the numerator of the constant term for equation A12 but not in the corresponding one in equation A11. What is indicated is that in the normal patient where K_R may exceed 100 ml/min, there will be a profound intercompartmental concentration difference in the case of model B which was discussed previously.

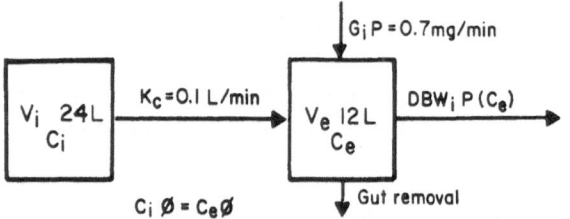

Figure A-2. Model for phosphorus mass balance in dialyzed patients.

Inorganic phorphorus balance in dialysis patients

A two pool model for analysis of inorganic phosphorus balance during dialysis is shown in Figure A2. Input is via dietary phosphorus intake, in the gut into the extracellular pool (V_e). There is phosphorus distribution into the intracellular pool (V_i) but this pool remains passive much as model A discussed above. Transfer between compartments is described by the intracompartmental transfer coefficient (K_C). Removal of phosphorus is by dialysis D_{BWiP} (C_e) and gut removal using phosphorus binders.

Mass balance equations for the system shown in Figure A2 are:

$$\frac{d(V_i\, C_i)}{dt} = -\, K_C(C_i - C_e) \qquad\qquad [A13a]$$

$$\frac{d(V_e\, C_e)}{dt} = K_C(C_i - C_e)$$
$$+ \, G_iP - D_{BWiP}\,(C_e) - \text{gut}. \qquad [A13b]$$

Solution of these relationships are analogous to those shown in equations A7 and A8. Using this model and the following system parameters phosphorus removal during 2 h, thrice weekly dialysis was computed:

Table A-1. Typical parameters for phosphorus model.

V_i:	24 l
V_e:	12 l
K_C:	0.100 l/min
G_iP:	100 mg/day
$C_{oi}P$:	5.0 mg/dl
K_pA_iP:	0.62 l/min
Q_B:	0.40 l/min
Q_D:	0.80 l/min
Q_F:	0.021 l/min
H_{ct}:	20 to 40%
gamma:	0

Removal through the gut using phosphorus binders was computed as the difference in intake and removal during dialysis. The results of this dialysis have been discussed and are shown in Figure 6.

Mathematical concepts and relational analysis

Independent and dependent variables and linear regressions

Medical science and clinical practice are characterized by, among other things, the vast amounts of data and information both available and obtained for patients. It is important to consider such clinical data in a structured manner particularly if relationships between variables are to be investigated.

A broad distinction can be made between those parameters that cause other effects, or in terms of which other effects are measured (such as time) and the effects themselves. Those that are the cause or reference parameters are generally referred to as *independent variables* and their effects or results are *dependent variables*. Thus, as will be discussed below, when protein is catabolized, urea is generated. The protein being catabolized will cause the urea to be generated (not the other way around) so that the amount of protein being catabolized is considered to be the independent variable. The amount of urea produced is considered to be the dependent variable.

This independent/dependent variable relationship in many biological systems is linked. For example, protein catabolism will also produce acid (H^+), another dependent variable; the production of acid, however, will lower plasma bicarbonate concentration which will neutralize the generated acid and in this context H^+ generation will be an independent variable and HCO_3 will be a dependent variable. Bicarbonate will be an independent variable in the buffer reactions which will cause respiratory changes (as quantitatively described by the Henderson-Hasselbalch equation). These examples of related physiological variables illustrates that the examination of clinical data can be much more meaningful when the concept of independent and dependent variables is kept in mind.

This is clearly the case when relationships and correlations between variables are investigated using linear analysis. Analyses for linear correlations is an attempt to obtain a direct relationship between two variables. Most commonly when such a relationship is found the analysis is considered complete when in fact it has only begun.

This is the starting point for in depth analysis because a non-trivial relationship between variables allows a fundamental property of that variable system to be described in an unequivocal mathematical form of a straight line. In addition, analysis of composite data will often reveal a fundamental relationship that is more accurate than any of the points that make it up. An example of this is the determination of bicarbonate dialysance values from the slope of a plot of flux as a function of concentration driving force $J = f(C_{Bi} - C_{Di})$ rather than by direct computation using equation 10 (10).

The relationship that results from a linear regression analysis is:

$$Y = aX + b. \qquad\qquad [A14]$$

The presence of an expression, in this exact form, on a linear regression plot, i.e. the use of y rather than the actual variables being related, however, belies a reluctance to take the next step. In addition, it should be noted that this general mathematical form indicates that the dependent variable should be plotted on the vertical axis (ordinate) as a function of the independent variable on the horizontal axis (abscissa) so that equation A13 shows what can be expected to happen to Y (a dependent variable) when X (an independent variable) changes.

Consider, for example, the data of Borah and colleagues (50, 51, 197) relating net urea generation rate and net rates of protein catabolism (see Figure A3) the dependent variable will be the net urea generation because it is caused by protein catabolism and oxidation of amino acids; the net rate of protein catabolism will be the independent variable. The linear regression is shown in Figure A3 and results in the relationship:

$$G = 0.154 \, PCR - 1.7 \quad (\text{not } Y = 0.154 \, X - 1.7). \quad [A15a]$$

This relationship can now be used in various ways. First, it can be used to estimate what the rate of urea generation will be at various levels of intake, e.g. 400 g/day protein intake such as the patient of Richards and Brown (84). Second, it is important to consider the equation constants, specifically the coefficient of PCR and the intercept.

The slope indicates that for each 10 g of protein catabolized, 1.54 g of urea nitrogen will be generated. This is 96% of the nitrogen content of protein and indicates that there may be some other non-urea catabolites that will be produced in a linear manner when protein is catabolized. A slight dependence of creatinine generation on protein generation has been found (198) and there may be other trace catabolites whose net production increases as the net amount of protein catabolism does.

The intercept (-1.7) should also be considered. There are two intercepts that should be evaluated (when G = 0 and when PCR = 0). When PCR = 0, i.e. when there is no net catabolism, extrapolation of the relationship would indicate that there will be negative generation (or that urea will be consumed). Physically what this would mean is that urea would be consumed to produce the other nitrogen base materials that are produced and excreted at a fixed rate (see below). It appears that this conclusion is more a result of the mathematics than actual physiology, and would not be expected to occur under normal circumstances; the relationship will become discontinuous at some point before G = 0. In this context it is important to emphasize that one should be cautious in extrapolating relationships into domains outside the range of the data used. Extrapolation into ranges where discontinuity would be expected (very low levels of protein catabolism in the present case) should be attempted with caution. Evaluation of the PCR intercept (where G = 0) gives other information:

$$0 = 0.154 \, PCR - 1.7$$

$$PCR = 1.7/0.154 = 11.04 \quad [A15b]$$

The PCR intercept indicates that in the patients Borah and

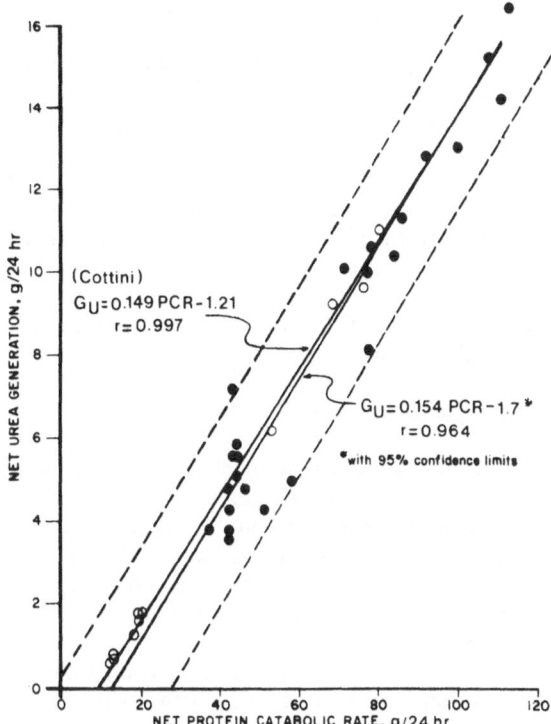

Figure A-3. Relationship between net protein catabolic rate and net urea nitrogen generation in uremic subjects. Data shown are those from two populations: Cottini (197) and Borah (50). Reprinted by permission, Dialysis & Transplantation 10: 314, 1981.

coworkers (50) studied there is an obligatory rate of catabolism (i.e. not linearly related to PCR) of 11 g/day. This obligatory catabolic rate includes creatinine production and nitrogen excretion in stool. If, as is likely, this rate of obligatory nitrogen loss is a function of body size then the Borah relationship can be generalized by adjusting this intercept value relative to body size by keeping the same slope, i.e. the same linear relation of G to PCR. In this case when the intercept is scaled by the volume of total body water (in Borah's patients 37.6 liters) the relationship when solved for the PCR becomes

$$PCR = 6.49 \, G + 0.294 \, V \quad [A16a]$$

or if G is in mg/min:

$$PCR = 9.35 \, G + 0.294 \, V. \quad [A16b]$$

Graphically, this adaption to body size shifts the G/PCR line to the left (for smaller individuals) and to the right (for larger ones) with the slope remaining the same. Such a modification has been shown to be valid for estimation of PCR in pediatric patients (81, 198). Similarly, if obligatory or fixed losses are known to be different, i.e. as they would be in peritoneal dialysis, a similar shift in the relation of Figure A3 would be appropriate. Data from Blumnkrantz et al (85) from CAPD patients shows such a shift, although the analysis did not follow the lines described above.

This example, while fundamental to the urea nitrogen discussion in this chapter, is meant to illustrate the logical progression and extensive use that can be made of linear relational analysis.

It is critical to add that if there is a linear relationship between variables, an extended evaluation of the elements of that relationship is important. If such analysis (examination of slopes and intercepts) does not result in useful information then it is likely that the key, or fundamental, variables are not being related.

Therapeutic extension of clinical information through mathematical reduction of data

Nutritional management of acute dialysis:

Linear reduction of data reduces clinical information to quantitative form, increasing its therapeutic use as has been discussed above. It can also extend these collective data to broader areas of therapy and treatment decision. The relation of net rates of catabolism as a function of energy and protein intake in the acute dialysis patient provides a pertinent example (51, 199, 200).

Often in the acute dialysis patient undergoing total parenteral nutrition a relation will exist between the rate of energy input to the patient and the net rate of protein catabolism (see Figure A4 [51, 201]). Such relationships have been found by many investigators and (202–206) clinical observations are commonly made of negative nitrogen balance in patients with large energy demands that are not met, e.g. protein-calorie malnutrition.

This clinical 'understanding' of the interaction of net protein catabolism and energy intake, however, can be further extended and made into a powerful therapeutic tool if it is reduced to quantitative form. The relationship shown in Figure A4 is a PCR-energy relationship for an acute dialysis patient receiving total parenteral nutrition (energy in the form of 70% dextrose). In this figure energy is the independent variable because, as is shown, the change in the energy level is the factor influencing the net rate of protein catabolism. It should be noted that the metabolic interrelationships in the acute dialysis patient are clearly complex, but in terms of Figure A4 it is the change in energy that is shown to influence the PCR. For this particular patient during this specific illness the relation was:

$$PCR = 59 - 0.007 \, Kcal. \qquad [A17]$$

Equation A17 indicates that for each 1000 Kcal (4,200 KJ) of additional dextrose energy given the PCR will be reduced by 7 g/day. When no exogenous dextrose is given the PCR will be 59 g/day. It should be stressed that Figure A4 is specific for the patient-illness for which it was determined. A different patient will have a different relation; moreover the effect of dextrose input would be expected to be different for the same patient during another illness.

This expression which reduces the multiple PCR/energy observations to a mathematical relation can then be used to determine the probable effect of giving more or less energy

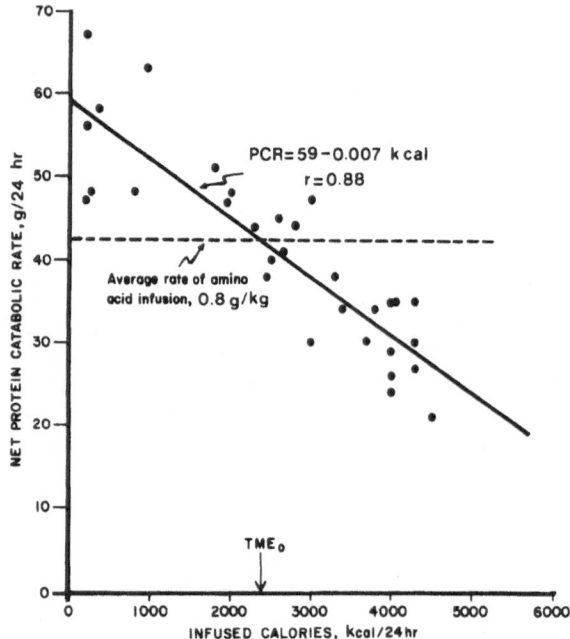

Figure A-4. Net protein catabolic rate as a function of glucose calorie infusion in a 73 year old male with acute renal failure. PCR = 59 − 0.007 Kcal. Reprinted by permission, Dialysis & Transplantation 10(4): 314, 1981.

in the form of dextrose, much the way that the G/PCR relation (see Figure A3) was used to determine the effect of increased catabolism on BUN or to determine the PCR from computed G values. The analysis, however, should not stop here.

In addition to the problems of catabolite accumulation in acute dialysis patients, there is the problem of volume control. As more protein and dextrose are administered there is an obligatory addition of water. This added volume load using an energy 'stock solution' with C_e Kcal/ml 'energy concentration' and an amino acid stock solution of C_{aa} mg amino acids/ml, however, can be accurately estimated and can be shown to be:

$$V = \frac{PPI}{(1000 - E/C_e) \, C_{aa}} + V_a. \qquad [A18]$$

In this expression PPI is the 'effective parenteral protein intake' and V_a is the additional volume required to supply the desired electrolytes to the intravenous solution. For 70% dextrose monohydrate C_e will be 2.38 Kcal/ml; C_{aa} will be 0.085 g amino acids/ml for standard amino acid solutions.

The amount of protein administered for a specific energy input, E, and volume of solution, V, will be:

$$PPI = (1000 - E/C_e) \, C_{aa}(V - V_a). \qquad [A19]$$

For the degree of nitrogen balance $PPI - PCR = dP/dt$, equations A17 (in general form) and A19 can be combined (see graphical representation Figure A5) to yield:

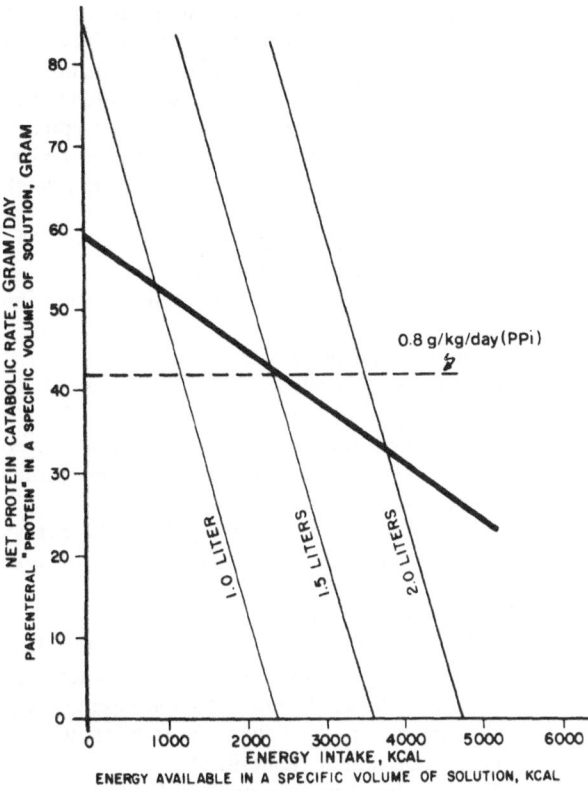

Figure A-5. The energy-catabolism-volume relationships in the acute renal failure patient. Isovolumic lines for total volumes of 1, 1.5, and 2 liters are shown superimposed on the PCR/Energy relation of Figure A-3. The figure shows the nutrient constraints of parenteral fluid mixing as well as the therapeutic constraints of treating such a patient. Reprinted by permission, Dialysis & Transplantation 10(4): 314, 1981.

$$dP/dt = (1000 - E/C_e)\, C_{aa}(V - V_a)$$
$$- (PCR_o - bE) \qquad [A20]$$

In equation A20 PCR_0 is the PCR when no energy is given (the PCR intercept) and b is the slope of the PCR/E relation (see Figure A4). Equation A20 presents the treatment/nutritional problem in unequivocal form. The three clinical factors that have to be considered, and how they interrelate, are shown:

1. dP/dt: The degree of protein balance (positive, negative, or zero)
2. E: The amount of energy to be administered.
3. Vf: The amount of fluid to be administered.

The choice of independent variable now rests with the physician. Volume may be controlling and dP/dt and E will then have to adjust to the need for control of fluid. Or the status of protein balance (dP/dt) may be the primary clinical consideration.

The effect of amino acid administration

It is common when a patient is found to be protein depleted or in negative nitrogen balance, to supply intravenous amino acids. The methods of prescribing amino acid administration and the degree of evaluation of this therapy has been found to be somewhat arbitrary (91).

Administration of amino acids will increase protein catabolism because on an intuitive basis it is highly unlikely that additional protein (irrespective of its 'quality') will be quantitively anabolized. Consequently, it would be useful to evaluate PCR as a function of PPI. If this were done and the slope of this analysis proved equal to 1.0, one could conclude that the administrattion of amino acids was having little effect on the catabolic state of the patient. If, however, the slope was less than 1.0, this would indicate an anabolic effect and the magnitude of that effect could be determined.

It should be noted that energy and protein will have counteracting effects on PCR (energy lowers it, protein increases it). Consequently, the common practice of modifying nutritional support by increasing or decreasing the quantity of solutions (containing both energy and amino acids) administered, may show no effect on PCR (91).

Summary

The essential point to be drawn from the forgoing development is that there is information contained in clinical data that remains untapped, even when such information is analyzed by elegant statistical techniques. The need is generally not for more data or more sophisticated analysis; it is for a more structured analysis of the information available to provide greater understanding.

The initial step, as in the process of modeling, is a conceptual one: which variables are controlling (the independent variables), and which ones respond (the dependent variables). The independent-dependent variable statistical analysis will yield certain direct (or linear) relationships. The question must be asked: Do they make sense? An important means to answer this question is by examination of the slope and intercept values of the specific linear relationship. If these show physically or physiologically impossible situations there is reason to re-examine the original data. If these basic parameters seem devoid of any physical meaning it is likely that a different presentation of the data will yield more important information.

Finally, once a linear relation has been discovered and found to be relevant it represents a precise analytical and clinical tool. The tool should be examined, 'fashioned', and used to predict clinical behavior and estimate the magnitude of metabolic events. Such a tool, which represents the quantitative distillation of physiological properties and behavior in man, provides a unique means to use clinical information and an opportunity to greatly expand the domain of clinical investigation and medical understanding.

NOMENCLATURE

A   Area: cm^2; dA: differential area

α   Donnan factor; fraction of ultrafiltration from plasma volume

aH^+ Addition of H^+ to extracellular water from intracellular water; this term is the reverse of mH^+; mEq/min

b   Exponent of expression for control of extracellular sodium content during dialysis

C   Concentration; mg/ml, mEq/l; C_{aa}: amino acid concentration in stock solution for parenteral nutrition; C_B: blood concentration; C_C: concentration in pool C in a two pool model; C_{CO_2}: concentration of gaseous CO_2; $\overline{C_D}$: dialysate concentration; C_e: energy concentration of glucose stock solution for parenteral nutrition; C_F: concentration in hemofiltrate; C_0: initial concentration – pre-dialysis; C_t: end-dialysis concentration; C_{UR}: urine concentration: C_{SS}, C_{BSS}, C_{CSS}: steady state concentration; C_{01}, C_{02}: C_0 for two sequential dialyses; C_{Bi}, C_{Di}: inlet concentrations; C_{Na}: sodium concentration; C_P: plasma concentrations – C_{Po}, C_{PT}, and C_{PSS} represent initial, end dialysis, and steady state values; C_{PR}: concentration of proteins in plasma: $\overline{C_B}$: mean concentration: ΔC: concentration difference in flux expressions dc/dx: change of concentration with distance – indicates a concentration gradient $\Delta c/\Delta x$: gradient over the fixed distance Δx; C(Log-mean): concentration driving force in a dialyzer; dC/dt: time rate of change in concentration

C^+ Total osmotically active cation, $Na_{ex} + K_{ex}$; mEq

D   Diffusive dialysance; ml/min, l/min; D': apparent dialysance

d   ( )/dt Rate of change of ( ) with respect to time

D   Diffusivity, cm^2/sec; **Db**: diffusivity in blood; **Dd**: diffisivity in dialysate; **Dm**: diffusivity in the membrane; **Dm***: effective diffusivity in the membrane

E   Zero order enzymatic conversion rate of acetate to acetyl-C_oA: mEq/min; glucose energy infused as part of parenteral nutrition: Kcal

F   Fraction; FF: filtration fraction in hemofiltration; F_p: water fraction in plasma; F_R: water fraction of the red cell

G   Generation rate: mg/min, mM/min, mEq/min; in the case of urea G: the net rate of urea nitrogen generation from net protein catabolism; g_{H+}: rate of hydrogen ion production

Γ   Rate of beta-2-microglobulin removal from interstitial water to form amyloid, expressed as a clearance, ml/min

HCT   hematocrit, per cent

Ir   Infusion rate of heparin: units/h

J   Flux; mass/time, mg/min, mEq/min; Jac: flux of acetate into a patient: $J_{H+ Exc}$: flux of H^+ out of patient by renal excretion; J_{HCO_3}: flux of bicarbonate out of a patient; J_{OA}: flux of organic anions

K   Diffusive clearance or transport constant; K_o: overall mass transfer coefficient, cm/min; K: clearance, ml/min, l/min; K_B: clearance based on blood side flux; K_D: clearance based on dialysate side flux; K_L: lung clearance (of CO_2); K_{Ln}: normal lung clearance: K_R: residual renal clearance; K': apparent clearance; K_1: intercompartmental transport coefficient in a two pool model; K_{UF}: ultrafiltration coefficient, ml/min/mm Hg

k   Solute distribution coefficient

K_{ex} Total exchangeable potassium: mEq

mH^+ Mobilization of H^+ out of extracellular water into other buffers: mEq/min

Na_{ex} Total exchangeable sodium: mEq

P   Pressure: mm Hg; Pb: blood side pressure; Pd: dialysate side pressure; P: average pressure

P   Tissue protein content of the body: g; dP/dt: rate of change of tissue protein content with time – protein balance

PCR   Net rate of protein catabolism: g/day; PCR: net rate of protein catabolism relative to normal body weight

PPI   Parenteral protein intake; g/day

Q   Flow rate; ml/min, l/min; Q_B: blood flow; Q_D: dialysate flow; Q_E: effective blood water flow rate: Q_F ultrafiltrate flow; Q_F: ultrafiltration rate; Q_{Bi}, Q_{Di}: inlet flow rates to the dialyze; Q_S: rate of addition of substitution fluid in hemofiltration

R   Mass transfer resistance, min/cm; R_B: mass transfer resistance in blood phase; R_D: mass transfer resistance in dialysate phase; R_m: mass transfer resistance in the membrane; R_o. over all mass transfer resistance

R   Response of body clotting mechanism to a heparin load; prolongation of clotting time: sec; R_i: R at the start of an interval; R_o: initial value of R – baseline value; R_t: R at the end of an interval

S   Sensitivity of an individual to heparin: response/unit; sec clotting prolongation/unit of heparin

T(t)   Time: minutes; t_d: duration of dialysis; T_{ur}: length of a urine collection

V   Volume: ml, l; volume of distribution of specific species; volume of parenteral solutions given to a patient; V_a: volume of electrolytes added to parenteral solutions; V_B: volume of compartment b in a two pool model; V_C: volume of compartment c in a two compartment model; V_{ecf}: volume of extra-cellular fluid; V_f: amount of fluid to be administered to the patient receiving total parenteral nutrition; V_L: inter-dialytic volume loading; V_R: intra-dialytic volume removal; V_0: initial volume; V_{ur}: volume of a urine collection; dV/dt: time rate of change in volume

X(x)   Distance, cm; dx: differential distance; Δx: diffusion distance; Δ_B: thickness of blood film; Δx_D: thickness of dialysate film; Δx_M: membrane thickness

α, β   Exponent in two pool analysis, min -1

β   Rate of weight gain: g/min, kg/day

θ   Inter-dialytic interval; minutes

REFERENCES

1. Michaels AS: Operating parameters and performance criteria for hemodialyzers and other membrane-separation devices. *Trans Am Soc Artif Intern Organs* 12: 387, 1966
2. Gotch FA, Autian J, Colton CK, Ginn HE, Lipps BJ, Lowrie EG: *The Evaluation of Hemodialyzers*, DHEW publication No (NIH) 72–103, 1971–1972
3. Klein E, Autian J, Bower JD, Buffaloe G, Centella L, Colton CK, Darby TD, Farrell PC, Holland FF, Kennedy RS, Lipps B Jr, Mason R, Nolph KD, Villarroel F, Wathen RL: *Evaluation of Hemodialyzers and Dialysis Membranes*. DHEW Publication No (NIH) 77–1294, 1977
4. Guyton AC: *Textbook of Medical Physiology*. Philadelphia, WB Saunders, 6th edition, 1981, p 208
5. Babb AL, Popovich RP, Christopher TG, Scribner BH: The genesis of the square meter-hour hypothesis. *Trans Am Soc Artif Intern Organs* 17: 81, 1971
6. Klein E: Membranes and materials evaluation. *Proc 7th Annu Contractors' Conf Artif Kidney-Chronic Uremia Program* NIAMDD edited by Krueger KK, DHEW publ no (NIH) 75–248: 85, 1974
7. Gotch FA, Sargent JA, Keen ML, Seid MA, Foster R: Comparative treatment time with Kiil, Gambro and Cordis-Dow Kidneys. *Proc Clin Dial Transplant Forum* 3: 217, 1973
8. Comroe JH: *Physiology of Respiration*. Chicago, Year Book Medical Publishers, 2nd edition, 1975, p 60
9. Pitts RF: *Physiology of the Kidney and Body Fluids*. Chicago, Year Book Medical Publishers, 2nd edition, 1968, p 29
10. Sargent JA, Gotch FA: Bicarbonate and carbon dioxide transport during dialysis therapy. *asaio J* 2: 61, 1979
11. Farrell PC, Grib NL, Fry DL, Popovich RP, Broviac JW, Babb AL: A comparison of in vitro and in vivo solutes – protein binding interactions in normal and uremic subjects. *Trans Am Soc Artif Intern Organs* 18: 268, 1972
12. Wolf AV, Remp DG, Killey JE, Currie GD: Artificial kidney function: Kinetics of hemodialysis. *J Clin Invest* 30: 1062, 1951
13. Smith HW: *The Kidney: Structure and Function in Health and Disease*. New York, Oxford University Press, 1951, p 39
14. Gotch FA: Hemodialysis: Technique and kinetic considerations. in *The Kidney*, edited by Brenner BM, Rector FC Jr, Philadelphia, WB Saunders Company, 1976, p 1673
15. Eschbach JW, Egrie JC, Downing MR, Browne JK, Adamson JW: Correction of the anemia of end-stage renal disease with recombinant human erythropoietin: results of a combined phase I and phase II clinical trial. *N Engl J Med* 316: 73, 1987.
16. Erslev A: Erythropoietin coming of age. *N Engl J Med* 316: 101, 1987
17. Nolph KD, Nothum RJ, Maher JF: Effects of ultrafiltration on dialysance in commercially available coils. *Kidney Int* 2: 293, 1972
18. Nolph KD, Nothum RJ, Maher JF: Ultrafiltration: A mechanism for removal of intermediate molecular weight substances in coil dialyzers. *Kidney Int* 6: 55, 1974
19. Farrell PC, Babb AL: Estimation of the permeability of cellulosic membranes from solute dimensions and diffusivities. *J Biomed Mater Res* 7: 25, 1973
20. Bottomley S, Parsons FM, Broughton PMG: The dialysis of non-electrolytes through regenerated cellulose (Cuprophane). I. The effect of molecular size: *J Appl Polym Sci* 16: 2115, 1972
21. Babb AL, Farrell PC, Uvelli DA, Scribner BH: Hemodialyzer evaluation by examination of solute molelcular spectra.

Trans Am Soc Artif Intern Organs 18: 98, 1972
22. Popovich RP, Hlavinka DJ, Bomar JB, Monerief JW, Dechard JF: The consequences of physiological resistances on metabolic removal from the patient – artificial kidney system. *Trans Am Soc Artif Intern Organs* 21: 108, 1975
23. French D: The Schardinger dextrins. *Adv Carbohydrate Chem* 12: 189, 1957
24. Schreiner GE: The search for the uremic toxin(s). *Kidney Int* 7 (Suppl 3): S270, 1975
25. Horowitz HI: Uremic toxins and platelet function. *Arch Intern Med* 127: 823, 1970
26. Cohen BD: Guanidinosuccinic acid in uremia. *Arch Intern Med* 126: 846, 1970
27. Giovannetti S, Biagini M, Cioni L: Evidence that methyl guanidine is retained in chronic renal failure. *Experientia* 24: 341, 1968
28. Schmidt EG, McElvian NS, Bowen JJ: Plasma amino acids and the ether soluble phenols in uremia. *Am J Clin Path* 20: 253, 1950
29. Gordon A, Bergström J, Fürst P, Zimmerman L: Separation and characterization of uremic metabolites in biologic fluids: A screening approach to the definition of uremic toxins. *Kidney Int* 7(Suppl 3): S45, 1975
30. Giovanetti S, Barsotti G: Dialysis of methylguanidine. *Kidney Int* 6: 177, 1974
31. Fürst P, Bergström J, Gordon A, Johnsson E, Zimmerman L: Separation of peptides of 'middle' molecular weight from biological fluids of patients with uremia. *Kidney Int* 7(Suppl 3): S272, 1975
32. Funck-Brentano J, Man NK, Sausse A, Zingraff J, Boudet J, Becker A, Cueiile GF: Characterization of a 1100–1300 MW uremic neurotoxin. *Trans Am Soc Artif Intern Organs* 22: 163, 1976
33. Bergström J, Fürst P, Zimmerman L: Uremic middle molecules exist and are biologically active. *Clin Nephrol* 11: 229, 1979
34. Bergström J, Fürst P: Uremic toxins. *Kidney Int* 12(Suppl 8): S9, 1978
35. Asaba H, Bergström J, Fürst P, Oules R, Zimmerman L: Accumulation and excretion of middle molecules. *Proc Eur Dial Transplant Assoc* 13: 481, 1976
36. Asaba H, Fürst P, Oules R, Ward M, Yahiel V, Zimmerman L, Bergström J: The effect of hemodialysis on endogenous middle molecules in uremic patients. *Clin Nephrol* 11: 257, 1979
37. Babb AL, Strand MJ, Uvelli DA, Milutinovic J, Scribner BH: Quantitiative description of dialysis treatment: A dialysis index. *Kidney Int* 7(Suppl 2): S23, 1975
38. Babb AL, Strand MJ, Uvelli DA, Scribner BH: The dialysis index: A practical guide to dialysis treatment. *Dial Transplant* 6: 9, 1977
39. Bell RL, Curtis FK, Babb AL: Analog simulation of the patient- artificial kidney system. *Trans Am Soc Artif Intern Organs* 11: 183, 1965
40. King PH, Baker WR, Ginn HE, Frost AB: Computer optimization of hemodialysis. *Trans Am Soc Artif Intern Organs* 14: 389, 1968
41. Dedrick RL: Pharmacodynamic considerations for chronic hemodialysis. *Kidney Int* 7(Suppl 2): S-7, 1975
42. Sargent JA, Gotch FA: The analysis of concentration dependence of uremic lesions in clinical studies. *Kidney Int* 7(Suppl 2): S35, 1975
43. Gotch FA, Sargent JA, Keen MI, Lee M: Individualized quantified dialysis therapy of uremia. *Proc Clin Dial Trans-*

plant Forum 4: 27, 1974

44. Gotch FA, Farrell PC and Sargent JA: Theoretical considerations of molecular transport in dialysis and sorbent therapy for uremia. *J Dial* 1: 105, 1976

45. Frost TH, Kerr DNS: Kinetics of hemodialysis: A theoretical study of the removal of solutes in chronic renal failure compared to normal health. *Kidney Int* 12: 41, 1977

46. Sargent JA: Kinetic modeling in the guidance of dialysis therapy Dial Transplant 8: 1101, 1979

47. Sargent JA, Gotch FA: Mathematical modelling of dialysis therapy. Kidney Int 18(Suppl 10): S-2, 1980

48. Sargent JA: Which mathematical model to guide clinical dialysis? in *Uremia – Pathobiology of Patients Treated for Ten Years Or More* Giordano C, Friedman EA, Milan, Wichtig Editore, 1980, p 209, Milano

49. Sargent JA, Lowrie EG: Which mathematical model to study uremic toxicity? *Clin Nephrol* 17: 303, 1982

50. Borah MF, Schoenfeld PY, Gotch FA, Sargent JA, Wolfson M, Humphreys MH: Nitrogen balance during intermittent dialysis therapy of uremia. *Kidney Int* 14: 491, 1978

51. Sargent JA, Gotch FA, Borah M, Piercy L, Spinozzi N, Schoenfeld P, Humphreys M: Urea kinetics: A guide to nutritional management of renal failure. *Am J Clin Nutr* 31: 1696, 1978

52. Cogan MG, Sargent JA, Yarbrough SG, Vincenti F, Amend WJ: Prevention of prednisone-induced negative nitrogen balance. *Ann Intern Med* 95: 158, 1981

53. Gotch FA, Sargent JA, Keen ML, Lam M, Prowitt M, Grady M: Clinical results of intermittent dialysis therapy (IDT) guided by ongoing kinetic analysis or urea metabolism. *Trans Am Soc Artif Intern Organs* 22: 175, 1976

54. Sargent JA: Urea kinetics: A quantitative guide to nutrition and treatment in renal disease. *Dial Transplant* 10: 275, 1981

55. Sargent JA: *The Role of Acetate in Acid Base Corrections during Hemodialysis Treatment,* Doctoral dissertation, University of California, Berkeley, 1976.

56. Gotch FA, Keen ML: Precise control of minimal heparinization for high bleeding risk hemodialysis. *Trans Am Soc Artif Intern Organs* 23: 168, 1977

57. Sherlock JE, Yoon Y, Ledwith JW, Letteri JM: Respiratory gas exchange during hemodialysis. *Proc Clin Dial Transplant Forum* 2: 171, 1972

58. Sherlock JE, Ledwith JW, Letteri JM: Hypoventilation and hypoxemia during hemodialysis: reflex response to removal of CO_2 across the dialyzer. *Trans Am Soc Artif Intern Organs* 23: 406, 1977

59. Aurigemma NM, Feldman NT, Gottlieb M, Ingram RH, Lazarus JM, Lowrie EG: Arterial oxygenation during hemodialysis. *N Engl J Med* 297: 871, 1977

60. Tolchin N, Rogers JL, Hayashi J, Lewis EJ: Metabolic consequences of high mass-transfer hemodialysis. *Kidney Int* 11: 366, 1977

61. Tolchin N, Roberts JL, Lewis EJ: Respiratory gas exchange by high efficiency hemodialysis. *Nephron* 21: 137, 1978

62. Guyton AC: *Textbook of Medical Physiology.* Philadelphia WB Saunders, 6th edition, 1981, p 518

63. Kreyszig E: *Advanced Engineering Mathematics,* New York, John Wiley and Sons, 1972, p 24, 147

64. Sokolnikoff IS, Redheffer RM: *Mathematics of Physics and Modern Engineering.* New York, McGraw Hill, 1958, p 23, 756

65. Giovanetti S, Maggiore Q: A low nitrogen diet with proteins of high biological value for severe chronic uremia. *Lancet* 1: 1000, 1964

66. Shaw AB, Bazzard FJ, Booth EM, Nilwarangkur S, Berlyne GM: The treatment of chronic renal failure by modified Giovannetti diet. *Q J Med* 34: 237, 1965

67. Kerr DNR, Robson A, Elliott RW, Ashcroft R: Diet in chronic renal failure. *Proc Roy Soc Med* 60: 115, 1967

68. Franklin SS, Gordon A, Kleeman CR, Maxwell MH: Use of a balanced low-protein diet in chronic renal failure. *JAMA* 202: 477, 1967

69. Kopple JD, Sorensen MK, Coburn JW, Gordon A, Rubini ME: Controlled comparison of 20 g and 40 g protein diets in the treatment of chronic uremia. *Am J Clin Nutr* 21: 553, 1968

70. Hewlett AW, Gilbert QO, Wickett AD: The toxic effects of urea on normal individuals. *Arch Intern Med* 18: 636, 1916

71. Grollman EF, Grollman A: Toxicity of urea and its role in the pathogenesis of uremia. *J Clin Invest* 38: 749, 1959

72. Cohen BD, Handelsman DG, Narayan Pai B: Toxicity arising from the urea cycle. *Kidney Int* 7 (Suppl 3): S285, 1975

73. Johnson WJ, Hagge WW, Wagoner RD, Dinapoli RP, Rosevear JW: Toxicity arising from urea. *Kidney Int* 7(Suppl 3): S288, 1975

74. Lowrie EG, Laird NM, Parker TF, Sargent JA: Effect of the Hemodialysis prescription on patient morbidity: Report from the national cooperative dialysis study. *N Engl J Med* 305: 1176, 1981

75. Luke RG: Uremia and the BUN. *N Engl J Med* 305: 1213, 1981

76. Lowrie EG, Laird NM, Henry RP: Protocol for the national cooperative dialysis study, Kidney Int 23(Suppl 13): S11, 1983

77. Laird NM, Berkey CS, Lowrie EG: Modeling success or failure of dialysis therapy: The national cooperative dialysis study. *Kidney Int* 23(Suppl 13): S101, 1983

78. Gotch FA, Sargent JA: A Mechanistic analysis of the national cooperative dialysis study (NCDS). *Kidney Int* 28: 526, 1985

79. Steffenson KA: Some determinations of the total body water in man by means of intravenous injections of urea. *Acta Physiol Scand* 13: 282, 1947

80. Lehnnger AL: *Biochemistry,* New York, Worth Publishers, 1970, p 433

81. Sargent JA, Gotch FA: Is urea generation adaptive? *Controv Nephrol* 1: 451, 1979

82. Walser M, Bodenlos LJ: Urea metabolism in man. *J Clin Invest* 38: 1617, 1959

83. Wolpert E, Phillips SF, Summerskill WHJ: Transport or urea and ammonia production in the human colon. *Lancet* 2: 1387, 1971

84. Richards P, Brown CL: Urea metabolism in an azotemic woman with normal renal function. *Lancet* 2: 207, 1975

85. Blumenkrantz MJ, Kopple JD, Moran JK, Grodstein GP, Coburn JW: Nitrogen and urea metabolism during continuous ambulatory peritoneal dialysis. *Kidney Int* 20: 78, 1981

86. Berlyne GM, Shaw AB, Nilwaramgkur S: Dietary treatment of chronic renal failure. Experience with a modified Giovanetti diet. *Nephron* 2: 129, 1965

87. Walser M: The conservative management of the uremic patient. in *The Kidney* edited by Brenner BM, Rector FC, Philadelphia, WB Saunders Co, 1976, p 1613

88. Bennett N: Urea kinetics: A dietitian's clinical tool in the nutritional management of patients with end stage renal disease. *Dial Transplant* 10: 332, 1981

89. Forbes G, Bruining GJ: Urinary creatinine excretion and lean body mass. *Am J Clin Nutr* 29: 1359, 1976

90. Sargent JA, Gotch FA: Mass balance: A quantitative guide to clinical nutritional therapy I: The predialysis renal disease patient. *J Am Dietetic Assoc* 75, 547, 1979

91. Sargent JA: Assessing the utility and improving the effectiveness of nutritional support. *Nutr Clin Prac* 1: 29, 1986

92. Kopple JD, Coburn JW: Evaluation of chronic uremia. Importance of serum urea nitrogen, serum creatinine, and their ratio. *JAMA* 227: 41, 1974

93. Rutherford WE, Blondin J, Miller JP, Greenwalt AS, Vavra JD: Chronic progressive renal disease: Rate of change of serum creatinine concentration. *Kidney Int* 11: 62, 1977

94. Sargent JA: Control of dialysis by a single-pool urea model; the national cooperative dialysis study. *Kidney Int* 23(Suppl 13): S2, 1983

95. Cestero RVM, Thunberg B, Jain VK: Diagnostic value of modeled therapy: nutritional status and technical problems of treatment. *Dial Transplant* 10: 302, 1981

96. Acchiardo SR, Moore LW: Urea kinetics: The possibility of selectively reduced treatment frequency. *Dial Transplant* 10: 295, 1981

97. Collins A, Keshaviah P, Berkseth R, Ilstrup K, McMichael C, Ebben J: Short efficient hemodialysis with reduced symptoms. *Kidney Int* 27: 158, 1985

98. Keshaviah P, Collins A: Rapid high-efficiency bicarbonate hemodialysis. *Trans Am Soc Artif Intern Organs* 32: 17, 1986

99. Heineken FG, Evans MC, Keen ML, Gotch FA: Intercompartmental fluid shifts in hemodialysis patients. *Biotechnol Progr* 3: 2, 1987

100. Shackman R, Chisholm GD, Holden AJ, Pigott RW: Urea distribution in the body after haemodialysis. *Br Med J* 2: 355, 1962

101. Wathen R, Keshaviah P, Hommeyer R, Cadwell K, Comty C: Role of dialysate glucose in preventing gluconeogenesis during hemodialysis. *Trans Am Soc Artif Intern Organs* 23: 393, 1977

102. Wathen RL, Keshaviah P, Hommeyer P, Cadwell K, Comty CM: The metabolic effects of hemodialysis with and without glucose in the dialysate. *Am J Clin Nutr* 31: 1870, 1978

103. Farrell PC, Hone PW: Dialysis induced catabolism. *Am J Clin Nutr* 33: 1417, 1980

104. Wineman RJ, Sargent JA, Piercy L: Nutritional implications of renal disease, II. The dietitian's key role in studies of dialysis therapy. *J Am Diet Assoc* 70: 483, 1977

105. Sargent JA, Gotch FA, Henry RA, Bennett N: Mass balance: a quantitative guide to clinical nutritional therapy. *J Am Diet Assoc* 75: 551, 1979

106. Olsson P, Lagergen H, Er S: The elimination from plasma of intravenous heparin. *Acta Med Scand* 173: 619, 1963

107. Eiber HB, Danishefsky I, Borelli JJ: Studies with radioactive heparin in humans. Angiology 2: 40, 1960

108. Estes JW: The kinetics of heparin. *Ann N Y Acad Sci* 179: 187, 1971

109. Christensen HN: General concepts of neutrality regulation. *Am J Surg* 103: 286, 1962

110. Christensen HN: *Diagnostic Biochemistry: Quantitative Distribution of Body Constituents and their Physiological Interpretation*. New York, Oxford University Press, 1959, p 122

111. Isaksson B: Urinary nitrogen output as a validity test in dietary surveys. *Am J Clin Nutr* 33: 4, 1980

112. Gotch FA, Sargent JA: Measurement of H+ balance during acetete and biocarbonate dialysis therapy. *Kidney Int* 16: 887, 1979

113. Relman AS, Schwartz WB: The effects of DOCA on electrolyte balance in normal man and its relation to sodium chloride intake. *Yale J Biol Med* 24: 540, 1952

114. Schwartz WB, Jenson RL, Relman AS: The disposition of acid administered to sodium – depleted subjects: the renal response and the role of the whole body buffers. *J Clin Invest* 33: 587, 1954

115. Schwartz WB, Orning KJ, Porter R: The internal distribution of hydrogen ions with varying degrees of metabolic acidosis. *J Clin Invest* 36: 373, 1957

116. Hunt JH: The influence of dietary sulfur on the urinary output of acid in man. *Clin Sci* 5: 119, 1956

117. Mion CM, Hegstrom RM, Boen ST, Scribner BH: Substitution of sodium acetate for sodium bicarbonate in the bath fluid for hemodialysis. *Trans Am Soc Artif Intern Organs* 10: 110, 1964

118. Grimsrud L, Cole JJ, Lehman GA, Babb AL, Scribner BH: A central system for the continuous preparation and distribution of hemodialysis fluid. *Trans Am Soc Artif Intern Organs*, 10: 107, 1964

119. Sargent JA, Gotch FA, Lam MA, Prowitt M, Keen ML: Technical aspects of on line proportioning of bicarbonate dialysate, *Proc Clin Dial Transplant Forum* 7: 109, 1977

120. Krebs HA: The biochemical lesions in ketosis. *Arch Intern Med* 107: 119, 1961

121. Lundquist F: Production and utilization of free acetate in man. *Nature* 193: 579, 1962

122. Kaiser BA, Potter DE, Bryant RE, Vreman HJ, Weiner MW: Acid-base changes and acetate metabolism during routine and high-efficiency hemodialysis in children. *Kidney Int* 19: 70, 1981

123. Swan RC, Pitts RF: Neutralization of infused acid by nephrectomized dogs. *J Clin Invest* 34: 205, 1955

124. Gotch FA, Borah MF, Keen ML, Lam MA, Provitt M, Sargent JA: The solute kinetics of intermittent dialysis therapy. *Third Annual Report of Artificial Kidney Chronic Uremia Program NIAMDD* 1977, p 48

125. Garella S, Dana CL, Chazan JA: Severity of metabolic acidosis as a determinant of bicarbonate requirements. *N Engl J Med* 289: 121, 1973

126. Dombec DH, Klein E, Wendt RP: Evaluation of two pool model for predicting serum creatinine levels during intra and interdialytic periods. *Trans Am Soc Artif Intern Organs* 21: 117, 1975

127. Sanfelippo ML, Hall DA, Walker WE, Swenson RS: Quantitative evaluation of hemodialysis therapy using a simple mathematical model and a programmable pocket calculator. *Trans Am Soc Artif Intern Organs*, 21: 125, 1975

128. Katz MA, Hull AR: Transcellular creatinine disequilibrium and its significance in hemodialysis. *Nephron* 12: 171, 1974

129. Jones JD, Burnett PC: Implication of creatinine and gut flora in the uremic syndrome: Induction of 'creatinine' in colon contents of the rat by dietary creatinine. *Clin Chem* 18: 280, 1972

130. Jones JD, Burnett PC: Creatinine metabolism in humans with decreased renal function: creatinine deficit. *Clin Chem* 20: 1204, 1974

134. Mitch WE, Walser M: A proposed mechanism for reduced creatinine excretion in severe chronic renal failure. *Nephron* 21: 248, 1978

132. Wehle B, Asaba H, Castenfors J, Fürst P, Grahn A, Gunnarson B, Shaldon S, Berström J: The influence of dialysis fluid composition on the blood pressure response during dialysis. *Clin Nephrol* 10: 62, 1978

133. Ogden DA: A double crossover comparison of high and low sodium dialysis. *Proc Clin Dial Transplant Forum* 8: 157, 1978

134. Van Stone JC, Cook J: Decreased postdialysis fatigue with increased dialysate sodium concentration. *Proc Clin Dial Transplant Forum*, 8: 152, 1978

135. Quellhorst D, Reiger J, Doht B, Beckman H, Jacob I, Kraft B, Mietzsch G, Scheler F: Treatment of chronic uraemia by an ultrafiltration kidney – first clinical experience. *Proc Eur Dial Transplant Assoc* 13: 314, 1976

136. Maekawa M, Kishimoto T, Ohyama T, Tanaka H: Present status of hemofiltration and hemodiafiltration in Japan. *Artif Organs* 4: 85, 1980

137. Kakagwa S: Multifactorial evaluation of hemofiltration therapy in comparison with conventional hemodialysis. *Artif Organs* 4: 94, 1980

138. Streicher E, Schneider H: Clinical experience in hemofiltration. *Int J Artif Organs* 3: 221, 1980

139. Schneider H, Streicher D, Hachmann H, Chmiel H, von Mylius U: Clinical experience with haemofiltration. *Proc Eur Dial Transplant Assoc* 14: 136, 1977

140. Baldamus CA, Knobloch M, Schoeppe W, Koch KM: Hemodialysis/hemofiltration. A report of a controlled cross-over study. *Int J Artif Organs* 3: 211, 1980

141. Shaldon S, Beau MC, Claret G, Deschodt G, Oules R, Ramperez P, Mion H, Mion C: Haemofiltration with sorbent regeneration of ultrafiltrate: first clinical experience in end stage renal disease. *Proc Eur Dial Transplant Assoc* 15: 220, 1978

142. Shaldon, Deschodt G, Beau MC, Claret G, Mion H, Mion C: Vascular stability during high flux haemofiltration (HF). *Proc Eur Dial Transplant Assoc* 16: 695, 1979

143 Shaldon S, Beau MC, Deschodt G, Ramperez P, Mion C: Vascular stability during hemofiltration. *Trans Am Soc Artif Intern Organs* 26: 391, 1980

144. Baldamus CA, Ernst W, Fassbinder W, Koch KM: Differing haemodynamic stability due to differing sympathetic response: comparison of ultrafiltration, haemodialysis and haemofiltration. *Proc Eur Dial Transplant Assoc* 17: 205, 1980

145. Shaldon S, Beau MC, Deschodt G, Flavier JL, Gullberg CA, Ramperez P, Mion C: Two years clinical experience with short hour high efficiency haemofiltration (HF). *Abstracts Clin Dial Transplant Forum* p. 52, 1980

146. Quellhorst E. Schuenemann B, Hildebrand U, Falda Z: Response of the vascular system to different modification of haemofiltration and haemodialysis. *Proc Eur Dial Transplant Assoc* 17: 197, 1980

147. Ladenson JH: Direct potentiometric analysis of sodium and potassium in human plasma: Evidence for electrolyte interaction with a non protein, protein-associated substance (S). *J Lab Clin Med* 90: 654, 1977

148. Shyr C, Young CC: Effect of sample protein concentration on results of analysis for sodium and potassium in serum. *Clin Chem* 26: 1517, 1980

149. Coleman RL: Differences in electrolyte results as measured by direct potentiometry (ISE) and flame photometry. Bulletin from Nova Biomedical, Newton, MA

150. Gotch FA, Evans MC, Keen ML: Measurement of the effective dialyzer Na diffusion gradient in vitro and in vivo. *Trans Am Soc Artif Intern Organs* 31: 354, 1985

151. Flannery JM: Differences in electrolyte results as measured by direct potentiometry (ion selective electrode) and flame photometry. Bulletin from Nova Biomedical, Newton, MA

152. Bijster P, Vader HL, Vink CLJ: An evaluation of the Corning 902 direct potentiometric sodium/potassium analyzer. *J Automatic Chem* 4: 125, 1982

153. Aluer A, Belledonne M, Saciaggi A, Glabman S, Bosch J: Sodium fluxes during hemodialysis. *Trans Am Soc Artif Intern Organs* 29: 684, 1983

154. Nolph KD, Stoltz ML, Carter CB, Fox M, Maher JF: Factors affecting the composition of ultrafiltrate from hemodialysis coils. *Trans Am Soc Artif Intern Organs* 16: 495, 1970

155. Shinaberger JH, Brautbar N, Miller JH, Gardner PN: Successful application of sequential hemofiltration followed by diffusion dialysis with standard dialysis equipment. *Trans Am Soc Artif Intern Organs* 24: 677, 1978

156. Flear CTG, Bhattacharya SS, Sung CM: Solute and water exchanges between cells and extracellular fluids in health and disturbances after trauma. *J Pen J Parenter Enteral Nutr* 4: 98, 1980

157. Maffly RH: The body fluids: Volume, composition, and physical chemistry. in *The Kidney* edited by Brenner BM, Rector FC, Philadelphia, WB Saunders Co, 1976, p 65

158. Edelman IS, Leibman J: Anatomy of body water and electrolytes. *Am J Med* 27: 256, 1959

159. Edelman IS, Leibman J, O'Meara MP, Birkenfeld LW: Interrelations between serum sodium concentration, serum osmolarity and total exchangeable sodium, total exchangeable potassium and total body water. *J Clin Invest* 37: 1236, 1958

160. Feig PU, Shook A, Sterns RH: Effect of potassium removal during hemodialysis on the plasma potassium concentration. *Nephron* 27: 25–30, 1981

161. Feig PU, Pring M, Guzzo J, Singer I: Disposition of intravenous potassium in anuric man: A kinetic analysis. Kidney Int. 15: 651–660, 1979

162. Landis EM, Pappenheimer JR: Exchange of substances through the capillary walls *Handbook of Physiology*, Section II, Circulation, Volume 22, Washington DC, Am Physiol Soc, 1963, p 961

163. Maeda K, Saito A, Kawaguchi S: Hemodiafiltration with sodium concentration-controlled dialysate. *Artif Organs* 4: 121, 1980

164. Keen M, Evans M, Gotch FA: Comparison of morbidity in high flux dialysis (HFD) and conventional dialysis (CD). *Kidney Int* 31: 235, 1987

165. Acchiardo S, Burk L, Bannister D: High-flux (HF) hemodialysis (HD). *Kidney Int* 31: 226, 1987

166. Kjellstrand CM, Rosa AA, Shideman JR: Hypotension during hemodialysis: osmolality fall is an important pathogenetic factor. *asaio J* 3: 11, 1980

167. Heinrich EL, Woodard TD, Blackley JD, Gomez-Sanchez C, Pettinger W, Cronin RE: Role of osmolality in blood pressure stability after dialysis and ultrafiltration. *Kidney Int* 18: 480, 1980

168. DiRaimondo C, Stone W: AB$_2$M amyoidosis. *Int J Artif Organs* 10: 281, 1987

169. Sethi D, Gower P: Synocial fluid B$_2$-M levels in dialysis arthropathy. *New Engl J Med* 315: 1419, 1986

170. Gejyo F, Odani S, Yamada R, Honma N, Saito H, Suzuki Y, Nakagawa Y, Kobayashi H, Maruyama Y, Hirasawa Y, Suzuki M, Arakawa M: B$_2$-microglobulin: a new form of amyloid protein associated with chronic hemodialysis. *Kidney Int* 30: 385, 1986

171. Gorevic P, Munoz P, Casey T: Polymerization of intact B$_2$/microglobulin in tissue cases amuloidosis in patients on chronic hemodialysis. *Proc Natl Acad Sci USA* 83: 7908, 1986

172. Kachel H, Altmeyer P, Baldamus C, Koch K: Deposition of amyloid-like substance as a possible complication of regular dialysis treatment. *Contrib Nephrol* 36: 127, 1983

173. Ogawa H, Saito A, Hirabayashi N, Hara K: Amyloid deposition in systemic organs in long-term hemodialysis patients. *Clin Nephrol* 28: 199, 1987

174. Messmer RP, B$_2$-microglobulin: an old molecule assumes a new look. *J Lab Clin Med* 104: 141, 1984

175. Vincent C, Pozet N, Revillard J: Plasma B$_2$-microglobulin turnover in renal insufficiency. *Acta Clin Belg* 35(Suppl 10): 1, 1980

176. Karlsson F, Groth T, Sege K, Wibell L, Peterson P: Turnover in humans of B$_2$-microgolulin: The constant chain of HLA-antigens. *Eur J Clin Invest* 10: 293, 1980

177. Schardijn G, Statius Van Eps L: B$_2$-microglobulin: Its significance in the evaluation of renal function. *Kidney Int* 32: 635, 1987

178. Cresswell P, Springer T, Strominger JL, Turner MJ, Grey HM, Kubo RT: Immunological identity of the small subunit of HLA antigens and B$_2$-microglobulin and its turnover on the cell membrane. *Proc Nat Acid Sci USA* 71: 2123, 1974

179. Statius Van Eps L, Schardijn G: B$_2$-microglobulin and the renal tubule, in *Non- Invasive Diagnosis of Kidney Disease*, edited by Lubec G, Basel, Karger, 1983, p 103

180. Bhalla R, Safai B, Mertelsmann R, Schwartz MK: Abnormally high concentrations of B$_2$-M in acquired immunodeficiency syndrome (AIDS) patients. *Clin Chem* 29: 1560, 1983

181. Bergström J, Wehle B: No change in corrected B$_2$-M concentration after cuprophane hemodialysis. Lancet 1: 628, 1987

182. Shaldon S, Koch KM, Dinarello CA, Colton CK, Knudsen PJ, Floege J, Granolleras C: B$_2$-microglobulin and haemodialysis. Lancet 1: 925, 1987

193. Mahiout A, Ludat K, Schultze G: Alteration of blood osmolality induces a shift of B$_2$-M plasma levels in patients undergoing hemodialysis. *Nephrol Dial Transplant* 2: 448, 1987

194. Geiyo F, Homma N, Suziki Y, Arakawa M: Serum levels of Beta-2-microglobulin as a new form of amyloid protein in patients undergoing long-term hemodialysis. *N Engl J Med* 314: 585, 1986

185. Burzynski SR: Biologically active peptides in human urine: I. Isolation of a group of medium size peptides. *Physiol Chem Physics* 5: 437, 1973

186. Scribner BH, Babb AL: Evidence for toxins of middle molecular weight. *Kidney Int* 7(Suppl 3): S349, 1975

187. Shinaberger JH, Miller JH, Rosenblatt MG, Gardner PW, Carpenter GW, Martin FE: Clinical studies of 'low flow' dialysis with membranes highly permeable to middle weight molecules. *Trans Am Soc Artif Intern Organs* 18: 82, 1972

188. Rattazzi T, Wathen R, Comty C, Raij L, Leonard A, Shapiro F: The comparison of low flow (Qd200) to regular flow (Qd500) dialysis. *Trans Am Soc Artif Intern Organs*, 20: 402, 1974

189. Ginn HE, Teschan PE, Walker PJ, Bourne JR, Macalyne F, Ward JW, McLain LW, Johnson HB, Hamel B: Neurotoxicity in uremia. *Kidney Int* 7 (suppl 3): S357, 1975

190. Tenckhoff H, Curtis FK: Experience with maintenance peritoneal dialysis in the home. *Trans Am Soc Artif Intern Organs* 16: 90, 1970

191. Gotch FA: A quantitative evaluation of small and middle molecule toxicity in therapy of uremia. *Dial Transplant* 9: 183, 1980

192. Gotch FA, Sargent JA, Modelling of middle molecules in clinical studies. Symposium on present status and future orientation of middle molecules in uremia and other diseases. *Artif Organs* 4: 133, 1980

193. Henderson LW, Stone RA, Ford CA, Lysagth MJ: Blood pressure control with hemodiafiltration. *Proc 10th Annu Contractors: Conf Artif Kidney* – Chronic Uremia Program NIAMDD, DHEW Publication No. (NIH) 77-1442, 1977, p 110

194. Funck-Brentano JL, Man NK, Sausse A, Cueille G, Zingraff J, Drueke T, Jungers P, Billon JP: Neuropathy and 'middle' molecule toxins. *Kidney Int* 7(Suppl 3): S352, 1975

195. Gulyassy PRF, Peters JH, Lin SC, Ryan PM: Hemodialysis and plasma amino acid composition in chronic renal failure. *Am J Clin Nutr* 21: 565, 1968

196. Bartsch HJ: *Handbook of Mathematical Formulas*. Translated by Liebscher H, New York, Academic Press, 1974, p 139

197. Cottini ERP, Gallina DK, Dominguez JE: Urea excretion in adult humans with varying degrees of kidney malfunction fed milk, egg or an amino acid mixture: Assessment of nitrogen balance. *J Nutr* 103: 11, 1973

198. Bleiler RE, Schedl HP: Creatinine excretion: variability in relationship to diet and body size. *J Lab Clin Med* 59: 945, 1962

199. Harmon WE, Spinozzi N, Meyer A, Grupe WE: Use of protein catabolic rate to monitor pediatric hemodialysis. *Dial Transplant* 10: 324, 1981

200. Sargent JA, Gotch FA: Nutrition and treatment of the acutely ill patient using urea kinetics. *Dial Transplant* 10: 314, 1981

201. Sargent JA: Urea mass balance: Nutrition and treatment of the acutely ill patient. *Nutr Support Services* 2: 2, 1982

202. Cuthbertson DP: The metabolic response to injury and its nutritional implications: retrospect and prospect. *JPET J Parenter Enteral Nutr* 3: 1078, 1979

203. Long JM, Wilmore DW, Mason AD: Effect of carbohydrate and fat intake on nitrogen excretion during total intravenous feeding. *Ann Surg* 185: 417, 1977

204. Clowes GHA Jr, O'Donnell TF Jr, Blackburn GL, et al: Energy metabolism and proteolysis in traumatized and septic man. *Surg Clin North Am* 56: 1169, 1976

206. Clowes GHA Jr, O'Donnell TF Jr, Ryan NT: Energy metabolism in sepsis: treatment based on different patterns in shock and high output stage. Ann Surg 179: 684, 1974

206. Wolfe BM, Culebras JM, Sim AJW, Ball MR, Moore FD: Substrate interaction in intravenous feeding: comparative effects of carbohydrate and fat on amino acid ultilization in fasting man. Ann Surg 186: 518, 1977

5

DIALYSERS

NICHOLAS A. HOENICH, CELIA WOFFINDIN and MICHAEL K. WARD

INTRODUCTION

From a historical view point, the treatment of renal failure by artificial support has been synonymous with haemodialysis. The past decade has, however, seen the evolution and clinical application of a number of new modalities of treatment which retain their reliance on a device containing an artificial membrane. The techniques are summarised in Table 1.

Despite the advent of these new techniques and associated devices, haemodialysis remains the most widely used mode of treatment for renal failure.

THE IDEAL HAEMODIALYSER

Before surveying existing devices, the requirements of an ideal haemodialyser need to be considered (Table 2). Many requirements interrelate while others are mutually exclusive. The extent to which current designs conform to this ideal may vary considerably since each design represents the manufacturer's solution to the conflicting demands of the ideal.

The choice of haemodialyser or device with which the patient is treated becomes a compromise. On the one hand it may be governed by the philosophy of treatment, on the

Table 1. Modalities of treatment of renal failure by artificial organs.

Technique	Description of technique	Device used
Haemodialysis	Diffusive transport of molecules across a membrane with convective transport	Haemodialyser
Sequential Ultrafiltration/Dialysis	Convective transport of molecules across a membrane followed by diffusive transport	Haemodialyser
Haemofiltration	A process in which uremic whole blood is cleansed by convective transport (ultrafiltration) after dilution of the blood with a physiological solution	Haemofilter
Haemodiafiltration	Simultaneous haemodialysis and haemofiltration	Haemofilter
Biofiltration		Haemodialyser
Continuous Arterio Venous Haemofiltration (CAVH)	A process in which uraemic whole blood is cleansed by convective transport (ultrafiltration) without a blood pump	Haemofilter
Plasma Separation	Separation of plasma components in whole blood across a membrane by filtration	Plasmafilter

other financial considerations may play an important part, and in consequence it may not be possible to select a dialyser whose performance characteristics totally meet the needs of the patient. Fortunately, patients tolerate not only the wide range of strategies employed but also the wide range of functional performances produced by the devices.

CLASSIFICATION AND USE OF DEVICE TYPE

Haemodialysers in clinical use may be classified as designed

Table 2. Requirements of an ideal haemodialyser.

High clearance of small and middle molecular weight solutes
Negligible loss of vital solutes across the semipermeable membrane
Adequate range of ultrafiltration
Low residual blood volume and good washback characteristics
High reliability
Nontoxic construction
Low cost
Re-use potential

for multiple use or for single use. Multiple use dialysers are available in parallel plate configuration, while those designed for single use may be of parallel plate, coil or hollow fibre configuration. Of these, the parallel plate and hollow fibre variants may also be used for the newer modalities of treatment such as haemofiltration and haemodiafiltration.

Up to 1968, four fifths of European dialyses were undertaken using either the multiple use flat plate (Kiil) or single use twin coil designs (1). The early 1970's saw the introduction of single use parallel plate and this was followed by a period of rapid technical development, which improved functional performance. This led to the growth and availability of disposable designs not only in the parallel plate and coil, but later of hollow fibre designs, a trend which has persisted to date (Table 3).

The proportion of European patients using the principal categories of dialyser during the period 1975–1984 has been monitored by the European Dialysis and Transplant Association – European Renal Association (EDTA-ERA) and is shown in Table 4. The proportion of patients routinely using

Table 3. Numbers of different types of dialyser manufactured from 1976–1985.

Year	Non disposable	Disposable				Total
	Flat plate	Flat plate	Coil	Hollow fibre	Haemofilter	
1976	7	19	32	8	–	56
1977	8	22	38	16	6	90
1978	8	31	40	21	6	106
1979	8	34	42	35	11	130
1980	9	56	44	72	16	197
1981	9	66	37	96	18	226
1982	10	81	34	141	23	289
1983	10	86	28	158	29	311
1984	10	87	28	197	30	352
1985	10	92	28	258	34	422

haemofiltration is also shown. Individual countries, however, differ in their utilization of devices and for comparison, the United Kingdom utilization is shown (Table 5).

CLASSIFICATION OF MEMBRANES

The first dialyser developed by Abel, Rowntree and Turner, used tubular membranes made from nitro cellulose (2). The rotating drum kidney described by Kolff and Berk (3), a successor to this early device, used regenerated cellulose membranes in the form of tubing (originally produced for sausage casings). Although advances in the technology of dialysers were made over the next two decades, the membrane used remained regenerated cellulose (although during this period it became available in not only tubular, but also flat sheet and hollow fibre form). The development of a number of manufacturing processes to produce this mem-

brane has resulted in its availability under a variety of trade names (Table 6).

The advent of the middle molecular hypothesis (4) highlighted a failing of these widely used membranes. Development of synthetic membranes and modification of cellulose based membranes to overcome their inability to remove middle molecular weight solutes followed and such membranes have seen a limited clinical application. Although these membranes were originally developed to improve middle molecular clearance, their biocompatibility compared to cellulose based membranes has resulted in a more widespread clinical interest and their use is growing, as demonstrated by data from the EDTA-ERA registry survey (Figure 1). The success of membrane based therapy in the treatment of renal failure led to the use of similar techniques for the separation of plasma from whole blood and the development of membranes specifically for this purpose.

Table 4. The proportion (as a per cent) of patients using the four main types of haemodialyser in Europe during the period 1975–1985.

Year	Non disposable	Disposable			
	Flat plate	Flat plate	Coil	Hollow fibre	Haemofilter
1975	13.7	40.2	35.2	10.4	
1976	11.0	42.2	35.8	10.4	
1977	8.7	43.2	31.4	14.6	
1978	6.4	46.0	27.7	19.8	
1979	4.7	44.7	22.3	28.3	
1980	3.1	45.7	16.6	34.6	1.2
1981	2.1	41.1	11.1	43.8	1.7
1982	1.3	37.1	7.0	52.6	2.1
1983	0.8	31.2	5.3	60.6	2.1
1984	0.5	27.2	4.0	66.3	2.0
1985	0.4	25.4	2.7	69.4	2.0

Results based on responses to the EDTA-ERA patient questionnaire which asked for the dialyser most commonly used during a particular year.

Table 5. The proportion (as a per cent) of patients using the four main types of haemodialyser in the United Kingdom during the period 1975–1985.

Year	Non disposable	Disposable			
	Flat plate	Flat plate	Coil	Hollow fibre	Haemofilter
1975	70	8.9	13.1	10.9	
1976	61.6	13.3	13.4	11.6	
1977	56	16.8	12.1	22.2	
1978	41.6	22.8	10.7	19.6	
1979	38.5	28.6	8.7	23.9	
1980	31.4	30.7	8.7	29	
1981	20.5	36.5	7.8	35	
1982	9.7	41.4	6.8	41.9	0.2
1983	6.4	42.6	2.5	48.3	0.1
1984	2.0	41.7	4.1	52.1	0.1
1985	1.3	31.3	1.7	65.7	0.2

Results based on responses to the EDTA-ERA patient questionnaire which asked for the dialyser most commonly used during a particular year.

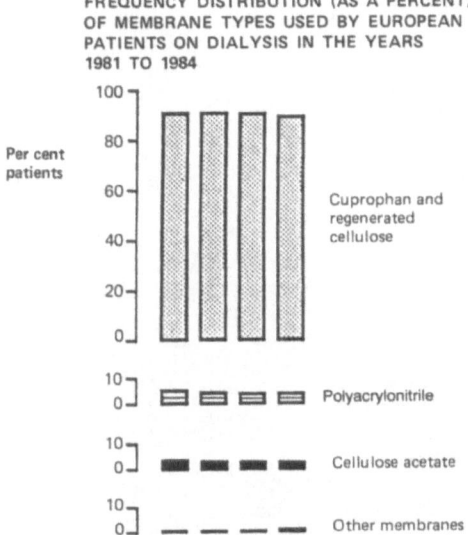

FREQUENCY DISTRIBUTION (AS A PERCENT) OF MEMBRANE TYPES USED BY EUROPEAN PATIENTS ON DIALYSIS IN THE YEARS 1981 TO 1984

Figure 1.

as well as middle molecules due to the reduction in obstructed membrane area as well as improved mixing of the dialysate during its passage through the device. This was achieved by cross cutting of the longitudinal grooves, a concept based on the pioneering work of Bluemle and colleagues (5). These devices were introduced commercially in the United States by the Western Gear Company (6). The United Kingdom variant of this design was manufactured by Meltec Ltd (7). Although this company is no longer in existence, a number of their dialysers remain in clinical use today, together with a modified variant (M3 Micropoint) in which the depth of the cross cut has been reduced and the blood manifold modified.

The use of this type of dialyser declined over recent years for a number of reasons. Firstly, they have to be built either weekly or for each dialysis and sterilized before use. Some patients and staff find the boards used bulky and difficult to handle, while successful leak free operation depends upon the skill of the person building the device. The dialyser is sterilised by formaldehyde which is toxic (8–10), has an unpleasant smell and prolonged handling and exposure may give rise to allergic skin and respiratory tract reactions (8, 9). Formaldehyde is difficult to eliminate totally from the dialyser (11–13), and monitoring formadehyde exposure in a clinical setting has proved difficult and time consuming (14,15). The formation of anti-N-antibodies in patients who dialyse with devices sterilised with formaldehyde has given rise to significant clinical problems (16–18). Its presence in dialysers has also been implicated in causing haemolysis (19) and anaphylactic shock (20).

DEVICES IN CURRENT CLINICAL USE

Haemodialysers

Multiple use parallel plate designs

The earlier parallel plate type dialysers, based on a design by Kiil were, by the 1970's, largely replaced by multipoint variants. Such devices were manufactured widely and while retaining the basic features of the Kiil design, offered substantial improvement in their ability to remove small solutes

Single use parallel plate designs

Early variants of such dialysers were a compromise between current designs and the previously described multiple use devices in as much as they contained a disposable membrane

Table 6. Classification of membranes used in the treatment of renal failure.

Membrane		Trade name	Use
Cellulose Based	Regenerated cellulose	Cuprophan®	HD, HF
		Cellophane	HD
		Cuprammonium Rayon	HD
	Modified cellulose	Hemophan	HD
	Cellulose acetate[1]	Cellulate®	HD, HF
	Cellulose hydrate		HD, HF
	Cellulose triacetate		HF
	Saponified cellulose ester	SCE	HD
Synthetic	Polyacrylonitrile	PAN 15	HD, HF, HDF
		AN 69	
	Polysulfone		HF, HD, HDF
	Polycarbonate	Gambrane®	HD
	Polymethylmethacrylate	PMMA	HD, HF
	Polyethylene vinyl alcohol	EVAL	HD, HF
	Polypropylene		PS
	Polyamide		HF

[1] Trade name refers to material produced by CD Medical.

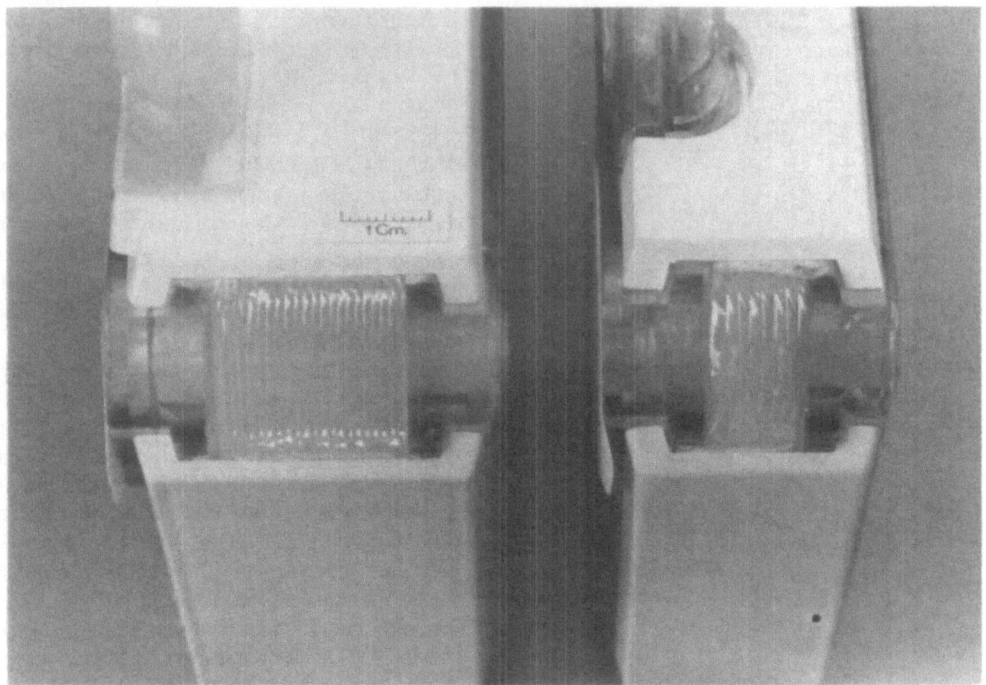

Figure 2. Multiple layer configuration used in current disposable haemodialyser.

insert in a solid clamping frame (21). The first commercially produced single use parallel plate design was the Gambro-Alwall dialyser (22,23). Current designs are smaller and more compact than their predecessors. They are pre-sterilized and offer a high degree of convenience compared with the multiple use designs. The reduction in size has been achieved by a multiple layer configuration (Figure 2) which requires a high precision during manufacture and assembly to ensure an even distribution through the blood and dialysate pathways.

These stringent requirements during manufacture were not easily attained leading to variability in the functional performance of early designs. They have largely been eliminated as manufacturing technology has improved and current performance characteristics are comparable or superior to those of multiple use designs.

The search for improved performance by incorporation of thinner blood and dialysate fluid pathways and the need to reduce manufacturing costs led to a move away from moulded plastic plates. Alternative forms of support structure such as non-woven polypropylene mesh were tried. Their use allowed a further reduction in the size of the device (Figure 3). The effectiveness of such devices may, however, be compromised by inadequately degassed dialysis fluid due to the adherence of bubbles to the mesh structure with consequent reduction in effective surface area of the device (24).

Single use parallel plate designs retain the advantages of their rebuildable counterparts. Being fully disposable and presterilized they avoid the use of formaldehyde and are rarely associated with pyrogen reactions. As shown in Table 3, a number of different designs are available from major artificial organ manufacturers. The use of this variant of haemodialyser in the early 1970's accounted for nearly half of the European dialysers, but more recently their market share has declined in favour of hollow fibre devices.

Coil designs

The coil haemodialyser was the first single use device constructed. In its early form it utilized a tubular membrane supported by a fibre glass mesh wound around a central core (Figure 4). This original design, together with the rebuildable plate design described above, accounted for up to four fifths of haemodialyses in Europe in the late 1960's.

The original design manufactured by Travenol Laboratories had a high blood compartment volume and compliance under normal operating conditions resulting from the poor support given by the mesh. It required priming by blood, and had a low and unpredictable performance due to variable blood film thickness and the difficulty in maintaining a constant flow of dialysis fluid across the coil while in its holding container. This latter defect was initially overcome by enclosing the device in an inflatable plastic cuff which in later versions was replaced by a solid outer casing (Figure 5) and the fibre glass mesh by the Hoeltzenbein mesh (25). In one current design the mesh has been replaced by an extruded multipoint support sheet bearing a series of truncated pyramids.

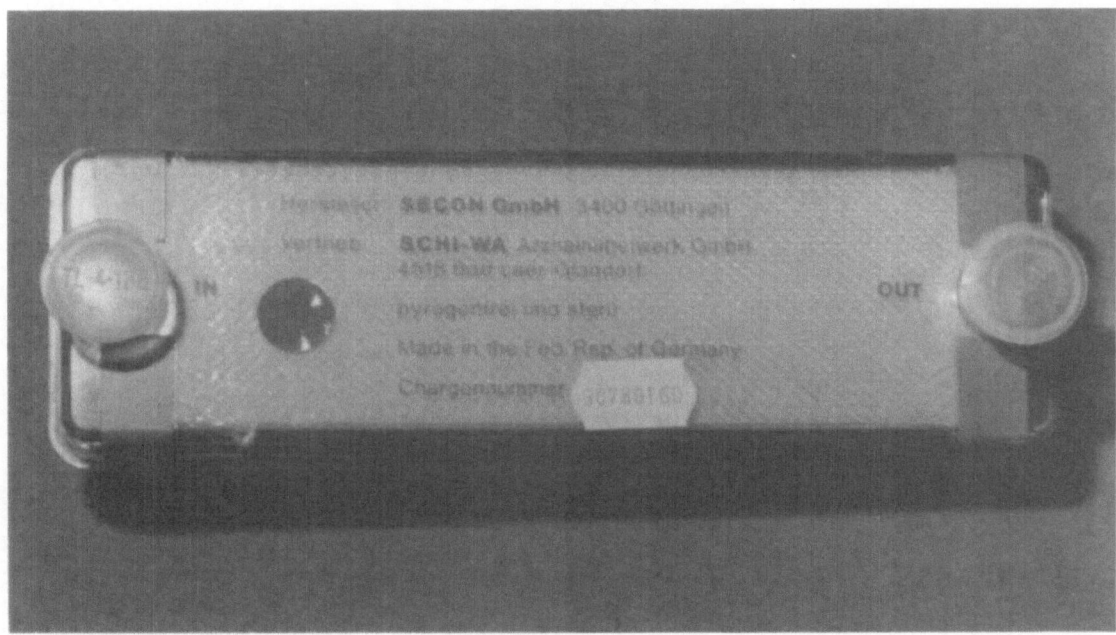

Figure 3. Miniature multiple layer disposable haemodialyser utilising a non-woven polypropylene mesh membrane support.

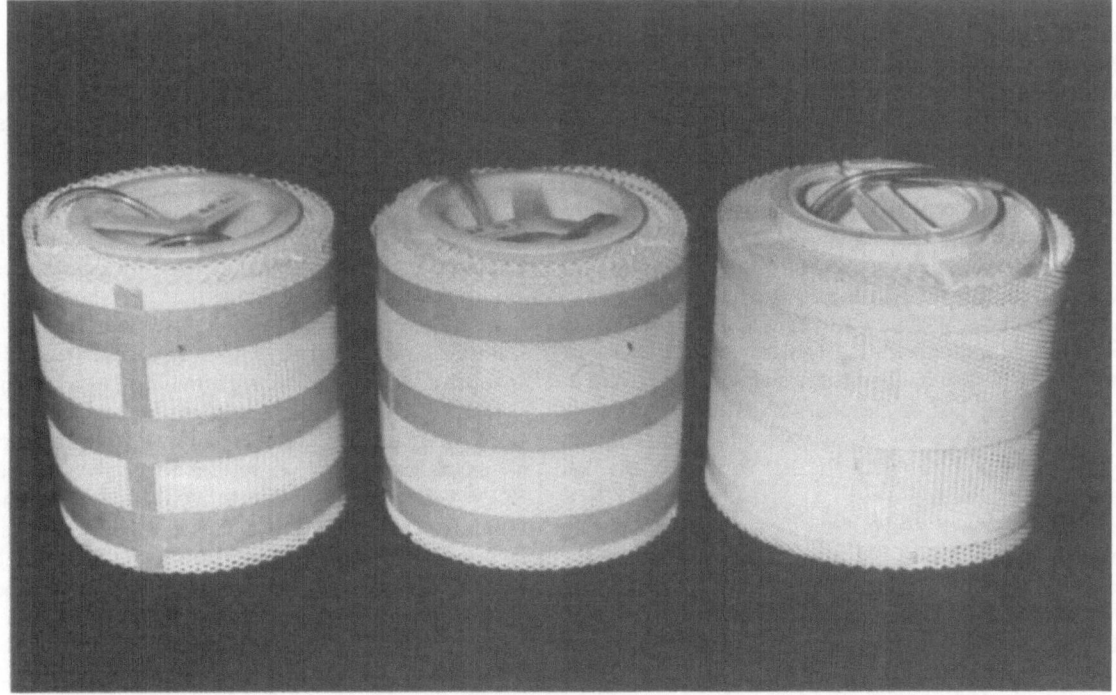

Figure 4. Early coil haemodialyser.

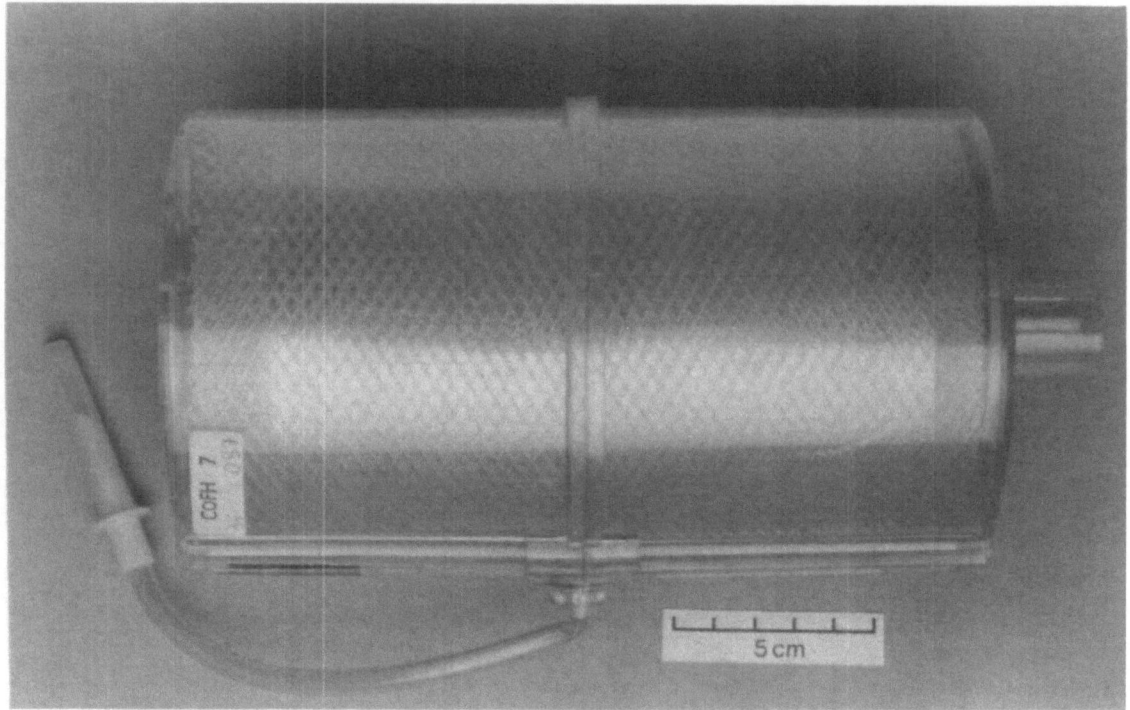

Figure 5. Current clinically used coil haemodialyser.

Current clinically used designs owe their origins to these developments which have been further refined by the use of a wider tubular membrane and the replacement of the traditional folding of the membrane at the inlet and outlet manifolds where the membrane joins the blood tubing by distribution manifolds which ensure a more even flow across the width of the membrane and eliminate the stagnant areas within the folds.

Coil devices use a high dialysate flow rate (25 to 30 l/min) obtained by the recirculation of dialysate through the device by a high speed pump with flow at right angles to that of the blood. Such flow configuration enhances solute transport across the membrane but limits coil dialyser use to recirculating or recirculating single pass (RSP) dialysate supply systems. To enable the devices to be used with conventional dialysate supply systems fully encased variants of the coil have been produced.

Coil dialysers have a high blood flow resistance, due to their construction, which is further influenced by the patient's haematocrit which leads during clinical use to a high and variable ultrafiltration rate which is difficult to control. Coil dialysers are inexpensive compared to other single use devices and may be used with less sophisticated dialysate supply systems. Their use has declined in the past decade in favour of other single use devices and currently accounts for less than 3% of European dialysers.

Hollow fibre designs

Abel, Rowntree and Turner (2) demonstrated the feasibility of removing metabolites from the blood of animals by the use of nitro-cellulose tubes bathed in saline and thus created the first hollow fibre dialyser.

The present designs of hollow fibre haemodialysers may be traced to the experimental design produced by the Dow Chemical Company in the late 1960's which utilised cellulose hollow fibres originally designed for de-salination purposes. This experimental design was subsequently manufactured commercially by Dow's Medical Division (Cordis-Dow) in a range of sizes using formalin as a sterilizing agent.

Until 1975 regenerated cellulose fibres manufactured by Cordis were the only commercially available fibres for use in haemodialysers. In 1975 the monopoly was broken, and Enka Ag complemented their production of flat sheet and tubular membranes with a range of hollow fibres manufactured by the cuprammonium process. The availability of an alternative source of membrane, together with the development of mathematical theory for the capillary artificial kidney allowing for optimization of solute transport characteristics, (26) led a large number of manufacturers to extend their production range of dialysers to include hollow fibres.

Many of the designs produced were copies of the classical design described by Stewart and colleagues (27) and consist-

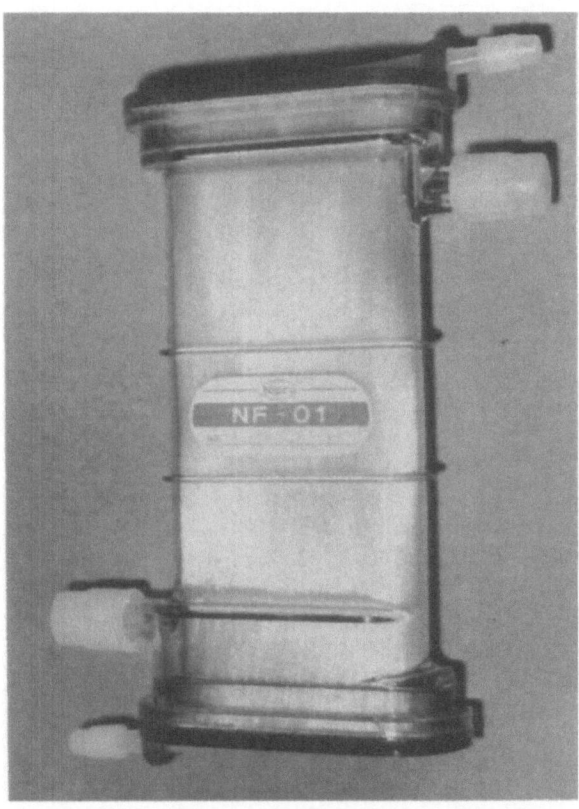

Figure 6. Rectangular block arrangement of hollow fibres designed to minimise flow maldistribution in the dialysate pathway of the haemodialyser.

ed of a bundle of fibres encased in a perspex tubular housing, the choice for this configuration being governed by the fact that it is comparatively easy to obtain a tight seal between the header and housing. Blood entered and left the device via manifolds, which were designed in such a way that the blood velocity and pressure drops were the same for all the fibres in the bundle thereby ensuring an even distribution of the blood though the fibre lumens. Dialysate flowed in a counter-current direction through the fibre bundle. Such designs, while theoretically efficient, were nevertheless subject to problems related to their design, e.g., chanelling or preferential flow through the fibres which resulted in a lowered efficiency. Early manifold designs were associated with extensive thrombus formation and clotted fibres, due to the presence of stagnant areas in the manifold. Distortion of the fibres by the potting and cutting process produced irregular blood flow distribution (28).

A variety of design solutions were used to eliminate these problems. Nakagawa and colleagues (29) arranged the fibres in a rectangular block (Figure 6), while Lee and Taylor (30) developed a triple bundle configuration in which the dialysate flow paths are interconnected in series while the blood compartments are connected in parallel. Cobe Laboratories, in a now discontinued series of designs, used a

baffled crossflow dialysate flow. Sorin, on the other hand, spirally wound the fibres around a central core, a concept used by several other manufacturers. In more recent variants of such dialysers, the central core has been omitted.

Many hollow fibre designs incorporate knitted fibres (Figure 7). Fibre knitting is associated with a number of disadvantages, namely higher cost, low fibre packing density in the bundle and a degree of fibre-strangulation by the warp yarn (31).

Stagnation in the blood inlet and outlet manifolds has been overcome by a design described by Sigdell (26) in which the blood enters the header manifold tangentially to the orientation of the fibres (Figure 8). This creates a circular and turbulent flow pattern in the manifold eliminating the stagnant areas. This optimized design has seen clinical introduction and is used in the Erika and Fresenius series of dialysers. All these design solutions, while theoretically efficient, are expensive to sustain in volume production.

In hollow fibre designs the membrane surface area may be changed by altering the number of fibres, the fibre length or the fibre diameter. The availability of thinner fibres has resulted in smaller, more compact designs (Figure 9). The development of injection moulding, and the use of newly developed plastic materials, allowed the design of smaller header manifolds optimised for better blood flow distribution. The problem of uneven dialysate flow distribution or channelling, a feature of earlier designs, has been solved by the use of deflector baffles at the dialysate entry and exit ports.

Paediatric designs

The use of haemodialysis to treat end-stage renal failure in children is well recognised and accepted (32,33). Although alternative treatments such as continuous ambulatory peritoneal dialysis (CAPD) (34, 35) and continuous cyclic peritoneal dialysis (CCPD) (35) are available and the use of high permeability membranes for haemodiafiltration and haemofiltration have been tried (36,37), conventional haemodialysis remains the mainstay of treatment for the uraemic child unable or unwilling to receive a transplant. The techniques of dialysis are comparable to those used in adults but adaptations to both the equipment and treatment schedules are necessary to meet paediatric needs (38) (see also Chapter 28).

A fundamental requirement of paediatric dialysis is the maintenance of the extracorporeal circuit volume (blood lines and dialyser) below 10% of the child's total blood volume (38). Larger extracorporeal volumes may lead to hypotension during treatment and fluid overload at the termination of treatment.

In choosing a dialyser for paediatric use, a nomogram of the type shown in Figure 10 may be useful and allows the appropriate size of device to be selected for the child in question. Further points to bear in mind when selecting a device for paediatric use is that too efficient dialysis results in a rapid fall in extracellular osmolality leading to dialysis disequilibrium. For the choice of the correct dialyser size, the use of the relationship

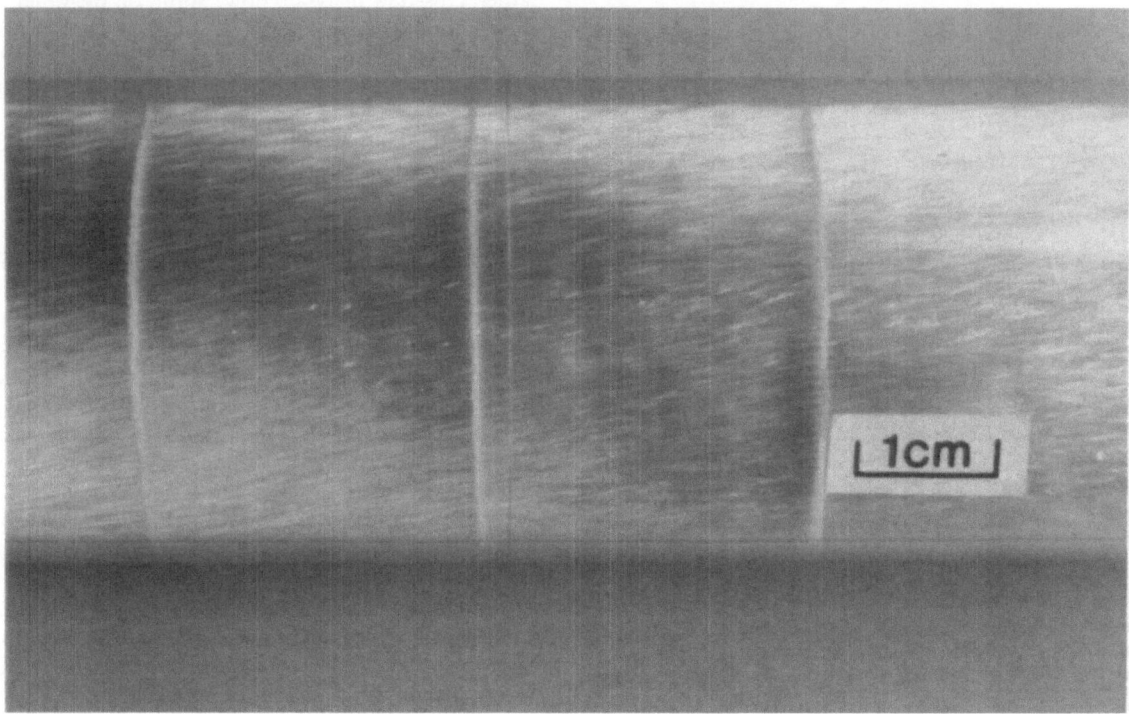

Figure 7. Warp yarn knitting of hollow fibres.

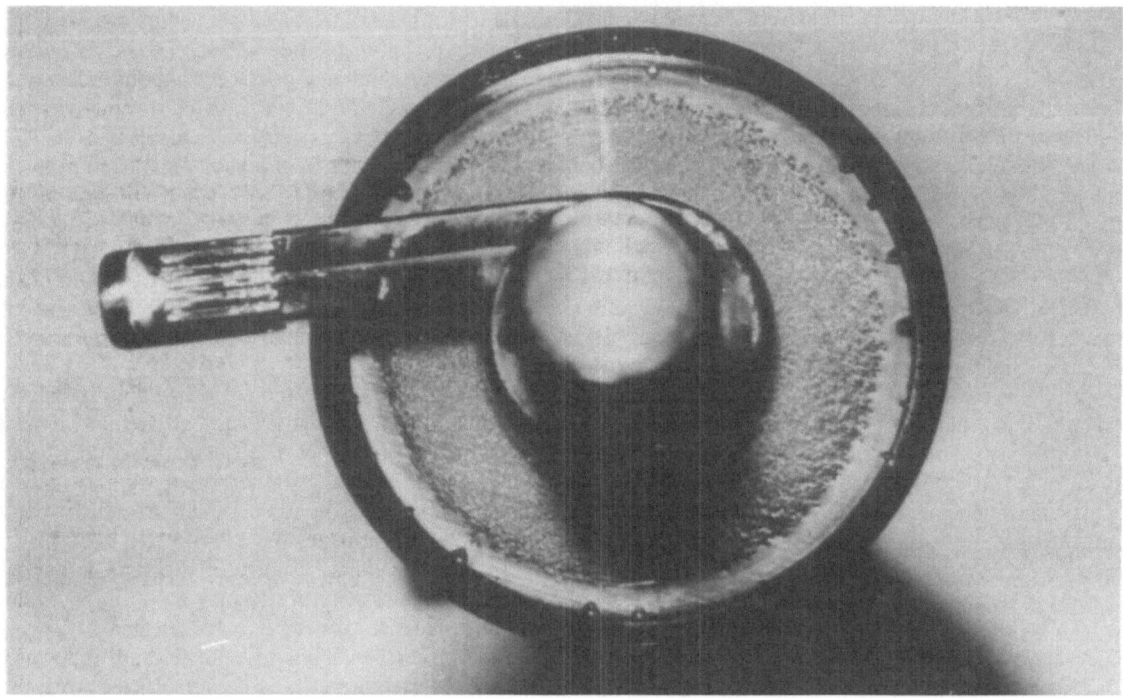

Figure 8. Optimised blood manifold used in hollow fibre dialysers designed to eliminate the clotting of peripheral fibres.

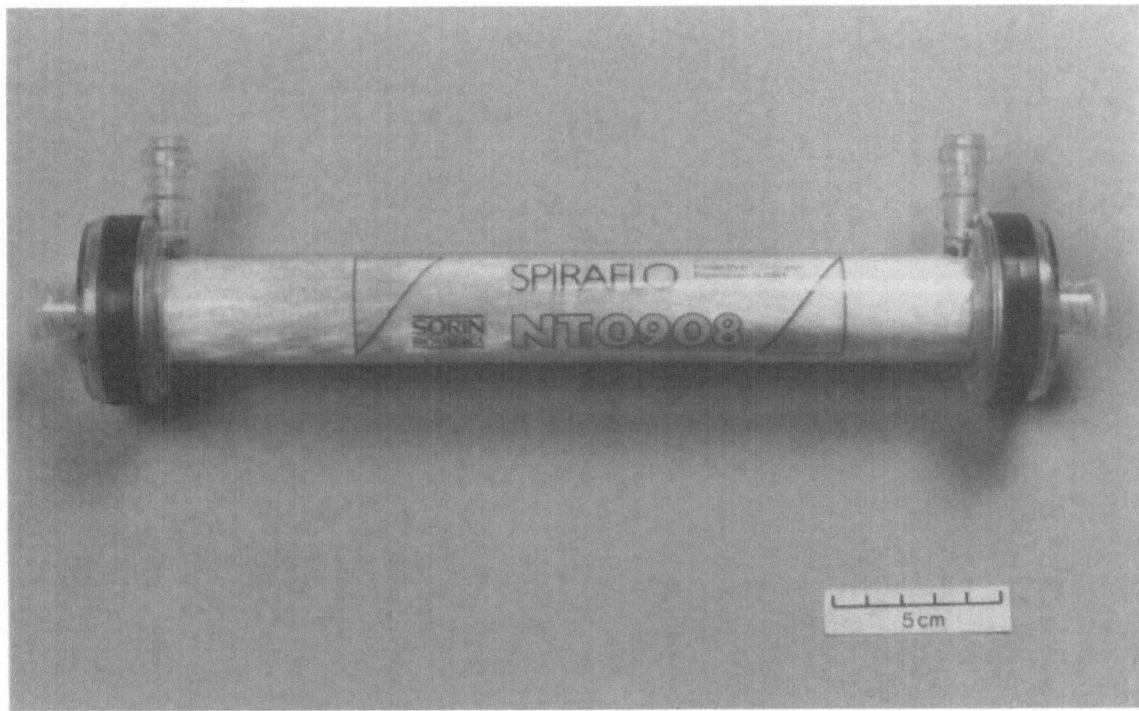

Figure 9. Current clinically used hollow fibre haemodialyser.

$$\frac{\text{Dialyser Surface Area}}{\text{Patient Surface Area}} = 0.75$$

has been proposed (38). Dialysis induced disequilibrium may be avoided by maintaining urea clearance below 4 ml/min/kg. Ultrafiltration needs to be less than 5% of the total body weight to avoid side effects such as vomiting and muscle cramps.

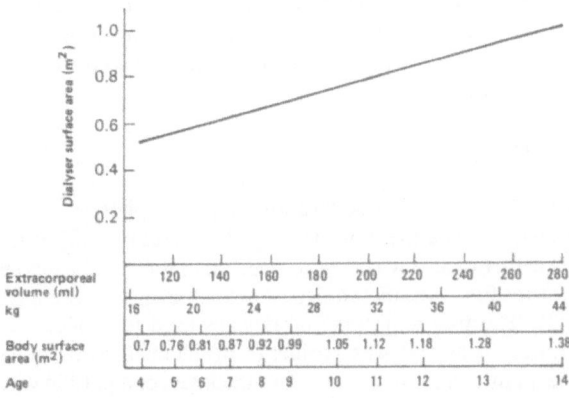

Figure 10. Nomogram for the selection of paediatric haemodialyser.

The high calorie, protein and fluid intake requirement of children necessitates more dialysis in relation to body weight compared with adults. Ideally, paediatric dialysis schedules should be more frequent than those for adults. However, this is often impractical, necessitating the need for longer treatments which may increase the incidence of dialysis related complications.

Haemofilters and high flux dialysers

During conventional haemodialysis, water and solutes are removed by diffusion and filtration. The use of ultrafiltration across synthetic membranes to obtain plasma water samples dates back to the late 1800's. In 1967, Henderson and co-workers published a new method of blood purification in which ultrafiltrate extracted from blood by the application of a hydrostatic pressure gradient across a highly permeable membrane was replaced by a solution of comparable composition to that of extracellular fluid (39). This technique, initially called diafiltration, was subsequently renamed haemofiltration (40).

The clinical application of this technique, which resembles the filtration process of the human kidney, became possible in the 1960's with the availability of an isotropic synthetic polymeric membrane with a high hydraulic permeability and controlled pore size (39). The latter part of the 1970's saw the development of flat plate and hollow fibre devices for use in haemofiltration.

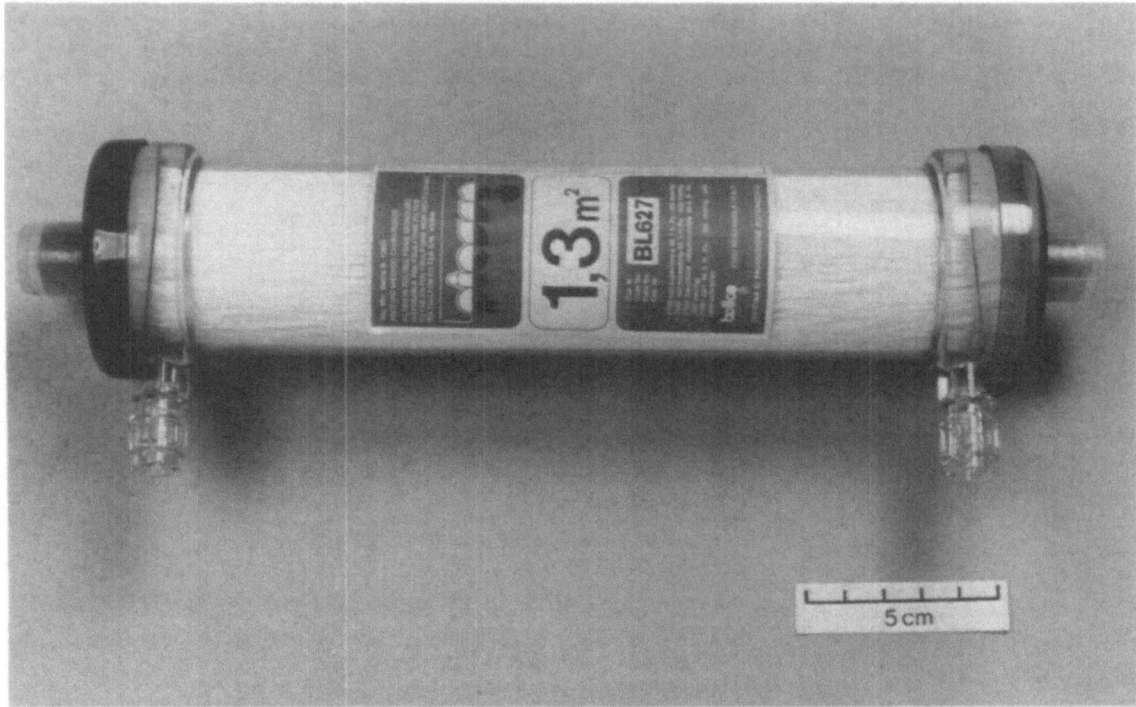

Figure 11. Hollow fibre haemodialyser, utilising high permeability polysulfone membranes suitable for haemofiltration and haemodiafiltration.

Hollow fibre haemofilters

Hollow fibre haemofilters in current production consist largely of conventional tubular bundle designs (Figure 11). The membranes used allow various types of sterilisation methods but most devices are ethylene oxide sterilised.

Variants of hollow fibre designs are those intended for use in continuous arterio-venous haemofiltration (CAVH). This modality of treatment is used widely for the treatment of acute renal failure (41–43) and relies on the patient's blood pressure to provide the flow in the extracorporeal circuit and, in consequence, such devices must possess a low flow resistance and thus tend to be smaller than those intended for conventional haemofiltration (Figure 12).

Parallel plate haemofilters

Whereas hollow fibre haemofilters have similar configurations, flat plate haemofilters, like haemodialysers, allow variations in the blood flow distribution and membrane support configuration.

The first flat plate haemofilters were flat plate haemodialysers such as the Rhone Poulenc RP6, containing polyacrylonitrile (AN 69S) membranes, or the Gambro Lundia Major haemodialyser, containing Cuprophan HDF membranes. Current variants of the dialysers continue to use the same membranes. A device manufactured by Sartorius

GmbH utilises a disc configuration in which the membrane layers and support plates are sealed at the edges. Blood enters at the centre of the disc and is directed radially to the outside. To maintain an even blood film thickness through the multiple pathways the disc is clamped in a holder during use.

For optimum filtration performance and prevention of concentration polarization at the membrane surface during use, a high shear rate needs to be maintained in the device (44). Vortex mixing produced by pulsatile pumping causes the blood to flow in circular streamlines and reduces concentration polarization (Figure 13). Laboratory studies with such a device demonstrated increases in filtration rate of 30% compared with the same membrane in a conventional device (45).

Plasma separators

Therapeutic plasma separation or plasmapheresis may be used in the treatment of a variety of diseases (46–48). Initially, centrifugal devices were used; membrane plasma separators first became clinically available in the late 1970's (49). The first experimental devices used flat sheet membranes. Their use was subject to problems associated with the maintenance of a blood film thickness compatible with a high shear rate across the membrane, a prerequisite for the maintenance of flux across the membrane (50). Subsequent

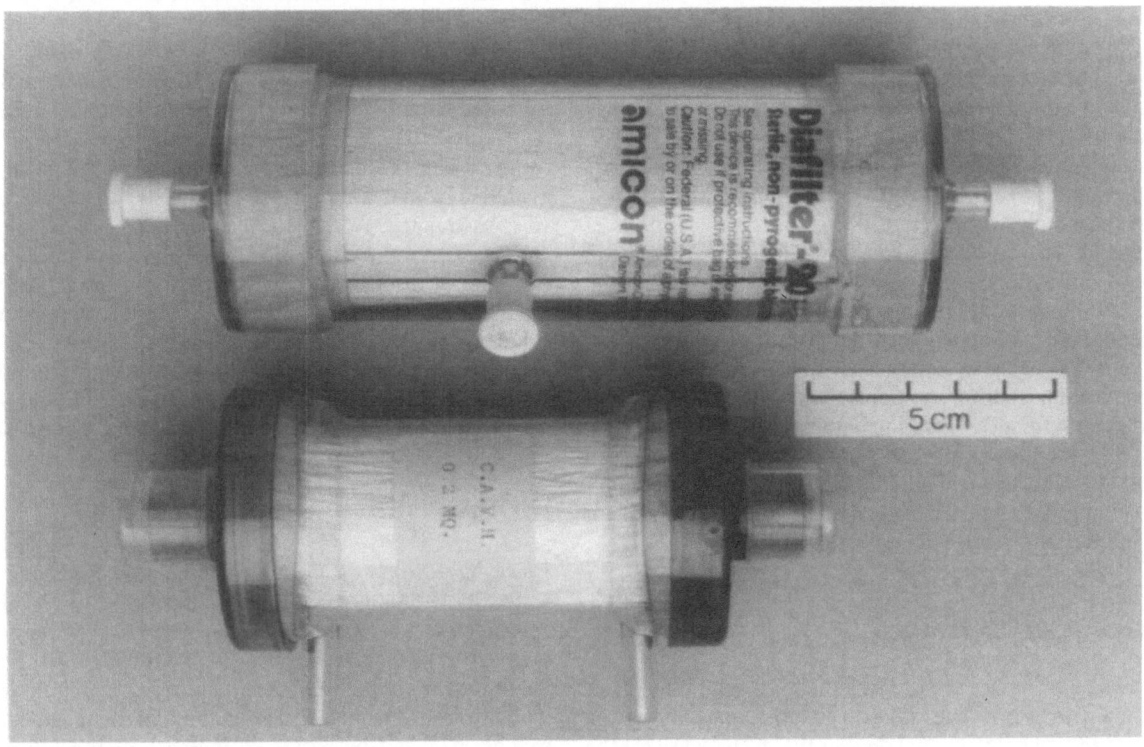

Figure 12. Hollow fibre devices suitable for use in continuous arteriovenous haemofiltration (CAVH).

clinically used devices have opted for a hollow fibre config-uration similar to those used in haemodialysers and haemo-filters. The therapeutic plasma exchange (TPE) system pro-duced by Cobe Laboratories retains the flat sheet config-uration and overcomes the above problem by a special fluid cycler consisting of a microprocessor controlled hydraulic clamp which compresses or releases the filter stack and varies the blood film thickness for the prevailing blood flow

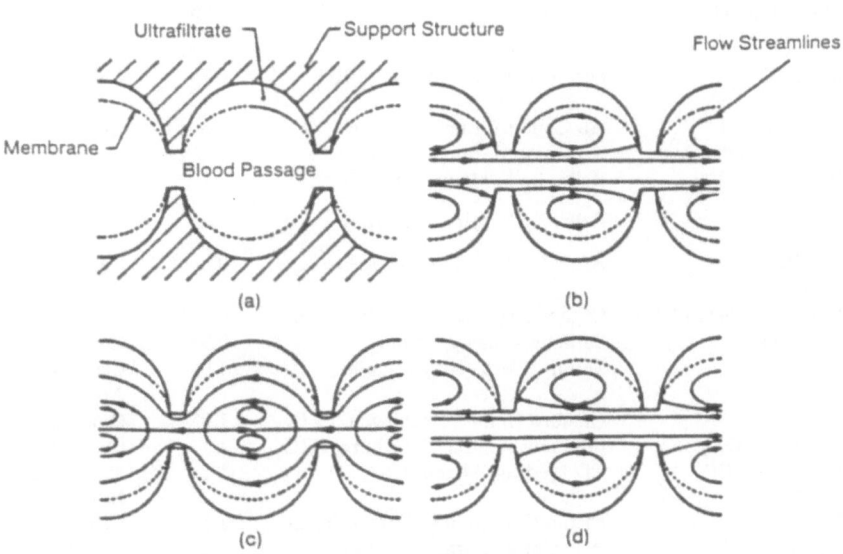

Figure 13. Vortex mixing in a parallel plate haemofilter produced by the use of oscillatory flows.

and haematocrit to achieve optimal plasma filtration rate.

Device performance is governed not only by geometry and fluid dynamic factors, but also by membrane properties. The membranes used in such devices have pore sizes ranging from 0.1 to 0.6 microns in size and allow the separation of solutes of several million dalton molecular weight from cellular elements. In contrast to conventional haemodialysers or haemofilters, they operate at lower transmembrane pressures since high transmembrane pressures can lead to haemolysis, deterioration of plasma flux and molecular removal (51). In consequence, the use of a given membrane material defines the operating conditions for a device. Thus, a given device must be operated according to the specified conditions for that particular module, with considerations of the blood's cellular and macromolecular solute concentrations which also influence operating parameters (52).

Use of membrane plasma separators may be achieved with haemodialysis equipment. However, integrated control systems have been produced to allow safer, convenient and more cost effective use of such devices.

DEVICE PERFORMANCE

The choice of device for the treatment of renal failure has continued to grow. The clinician is faced not only with a wide variety of conventional devices that he may use for the treatment of renal insufficiency, but also with a choice of therapeutic techniques.

This section is not intended to provide the reader with a catalogue of device performance. Such information may be obtained from manufacturers or from our own studies undertaken on behalf of the Department of Health and Social Security in the United Kingdom, details regarding which are available from the authors, or in published reviews (53,54). In consequence, we have selected devices whose physical characteristics are summarised in Tables 7–9 for comparison, and to use for the description of the fundamentals of device performance of clinical importance, as well as the principles involving their measurement, together with their influencing factors. This should allow the clinician to make rational choices and can be used to analyse the reasons for the differences between devices, should he wish to undertake his own comparative studies.

Blood flow

Blood flow in artificial organs influences functional performance in a number of ways. In haemodialysis it influences the clearance of small molecules and ultrafiltration particularly in designs that have a high pathway resistance. In haemofiltration the influence of concentration polarization may be diminished by increasing the wall shear rate and this can be achieved by either an increase of the blood flow

Table 7. Standard haemodialysers – physical characteristics.

Dialyser type	Name	Manufacturer	Surface area (m²)	Membrane Type	Micron thickness
Non disposable Flat Plate	M3 Multipoint		1.03	Cuprophan	11
Disposable Flat Plate	MTL 133	Secon GmbH, Gottingen, FRG	0.75	Cellulose Hydrate	20
	Lundia 10-3N	Ab Gambro, Lund, Sweden	0.8	Cuprophan	10
	Lundia PRO5	Ab Gambro, Lund, Sweden	1.1	Gambrane	16
	BL 501 BRAVO	Bellco SpA, Mirandola, Italy	1.1	Cuprophan	16
Disposable Coil	Vita 2HP	Bellco SpA, Mirandola, Italy	1.2	Cuprophan	18
Disposable Hollow Fibre	AM 100M	Asahi Medical, Tokyo, Japan	0.8	Cuprammonium Rayon	11
	Nephross Allegro HF	Organon Teknika, Oss, Netherlands	0.9	Cuprophan	6.5
	NT 10.11	Sorin SpA, Saluggia, Italy	0.96	Cuprophan	11
	TAF 10	Terumo Corp, Tokyo, Japan	1.0	Cellulose Acetate	12
	FP 100	Gambro GmbH, Hechingen, FRG	1.05	Gambrane	15
	Hemoflow D2	Fresenius Ag, Bad Homburg, FRG	1.1	Cuprophan	10
	CDAK 90 SCE	CD Medical, Miami, USA	1.1	Saponified Cellulose Ester	30
	FB 110T	Nissho Corporation, Tokyo, Japan	1.1	Cellulose Acetate	15
	BL 612M	Bellco SpA, Mirandola, Italy	1.2	Cuprophan	11
	GF 120M	Gambro GmbH, Hechingen, FRG	1.2	Cuprophan	11

Plasma separation in membrane devices is also governed by flow dynamics through the device. Accurate knowledge of the blood flow is of critical importance in obtaining optimal performance; despite this, it is often neglected by investigators undertaking measurements on device performance. *In vitro* measurement of simulated blood flow can be easily accomplished by a timed collection at the outflow of the device. The measured flow rate must, where applicable, be corrected for the ultrafiltration rate which may be measured directly or calculated from a previously constructed graph relating transmembrane pressure to flow rate. *In vivo* or when there is only a limited volume of simulated blood available, the measurement of flow rate is more difficult. A commonly used method is by the use of calibrated blood pumps, the calibration being performed either at the beginning or the end of the study and based upon the presumption that the flow generated by a roller pump is the product of the rotational speed of the rollers and the stroke volume. Many currently used blood pumps measure the rotating speed of the rollers by a tachometer and multiply this reading by a constant stroke volume to display the volumetric flow rate. This method, while acceptable for routine clinical use during trouble free haemodialysis, is subject to serious error of clinical significance due to variations in the internal diameter of the pump insert. Inadequate occlusion between the roller and the pump insert leads to back flow. In the presence of high inlet negative pressures incomplete filling of the pump insert occurs. The actual flow rate may be substantially less than that calculated and displayed or pre-set on the blood pump.

Incomplete occlusion of the blood pump segment and variations in the flow due to the varying pressures downstream of the pump may be minimised by selection of the blood pump. Punctilious attention to detail and the appropriate selection of blood tubing sets are important when undertaking research studies. Recalibration at the end of each *in vivo* study should be performed.

Table 8. High flux devices – physical characteristics.

Dialyser type	Name	Manufacturer	Surface area (m²)	Membrane Type	Micron thickness	Clinical use
Disposable Flat plate	Biospal 2400S	Hospal, Lyons, France	1.0	AN69S	22	HD, HF, HDF
Disposable Hollow Fibre	HF 060	Sorin SpA, Saluggia, Italy	0.7	Polysulfone	40	HF
	PAN 150	Asahi Medical, Tokyo, Japan	1.1	Polyacrylonitrile	55	HD, HF, HDF
	AN 69HF	Hospal, Lyons, France	1.15	AN 69HF	45	HD, HF, HDF
	F 60	Fresenius Ag, Bad Homburg, FRG	1.25	Polysulfone	40	HF, HDF
	B1-100	Toray Medical, Tokyo, Japan	1.36	PMMA	40	HF
	CD Duoflux	CD Medical, Miami, USA	1.4	Cellulate	30	HD, HF

Table 9. Devices suitable for paediatric use.

Device	Name	Manufacturer	Surface area (m²)	Clearance Urea	Clearance Creat	Blood compt. Vol. (ml)	UF coeff. ml/hr/mm Hg	Ref.
Disposable Flat plate	Mini Mini Minor	Ab Gambro, Lund, Sweden	0.1	19[a]	8[a]	15[c]	0.37	193
	Mini Minor	Ab Gambro, Lund, Sweden	0.23	48	33	20[c]	0.5	193
	Lundia 10-1N[b]	Ab Gambro, Lund, Sweden	0.40	103	74	46[c]	1.5	
	Lundia 10-2N[b]	Ab Gambro, Lund, Sweden	0.70	133	103	60[c]	3.1	
Hollow Fibre	FB 50T	Nissho Co, Tokyo, Japan	0.50	108	81	38	2.7	
	Hemoflow D1	Fresenius Ag, Bad, Homburg, FRG	0.60	148	111	49	3.4	
	SF 06	Sorin Spa, Saluggia, Italy	0.60	128	92	55	1.9	
	Nephross Lento HF	Organon Teknika, Oss, Netherlands	0.70	141	110	51	2.4	

[a] At a blood flow of 100 ml/min.

[b] Also available in low (L) and high (H). Ultrafiltration versions.

[c] At a transmembrane pressure of 100 mm Hg.

[d] Where no reference is quoted in this and subsequent tables the data are those obtained at Newcastle upon Tyne.

Pressures at the inlet side of the blood pump during clinical use vary considerably. Our unpublished observations (H. Tanboga, N. Hoenich, 1977) showed that all roller pumps respond to a low inflow pressure by producing a decreased flow at a given setting and the fall off begins before most circuits collapse upstream of the pump. This source of error can be avoided by monitoring the pressure in the arterial line upstream of the pump or by the incorporation of a thin walled collapsible sac (mouse) in the extracorporeal circuit before the pump that detects the fall in pressure more readily than the thicker walled tubing.

Other methods of *in vivo* monitoring of blood flow include electromagnetic and ultrasonic devices and inexpensive in line flow meters which utilise a small float or a 'pressure head' of blood in a twin chamber consisting of a measuring chamber above the venous drip chamber interconnected by means of a small orifice. A quadratic scale is incorporated into the wall of the chamber allowing visual estimation of the blood flow. Such in line flow meters are unable to provide accuracy at low flow rates sufficient for research purposes, while at clinical flow rates their reading may be vitiated by the presence of froth. These devices faded from clinical use.

Electromagnetic flow meters use probes which are incorporated into the blood lines necessitating sterilisation between uses which shortens the life of the probe. They are expensive and with the risk of transmission of hepatitis, confining their use to laboratory and animal experiments.

Ultrasonic flow meters use clip on probes which are sensitive to changes in blood tubing dimensions and rely upon the attainment of an acoustic contact between the blood tubing and the probe which cannot be checked after the experiment. The accuracy of ultrasonic and electromagnetic flow meters ranges between ± 5 and $\pm 15\%$ (55).

Bubble transit techniques are an accurate and inexpensive method of *in vivo* blood flow measurement. In this method a small bubble of air is injected into the arterial segment of the extracorporeal circuit and the time of its passage between two marks a fixed distance apart ('race track') is measured. This method of measurement is used routinely in our experimental studies and the factors affecting the transit time have been studied. An accuracy of $\pm 3\%$ over the clinical range of blood flows can be achieved routinely provided the undermentioned conditions are maintained and procedures followed.

1. An adequate length of 'race track' is used. Many blood lines already incorporate 50 cm segments suitable for bubble transit measurements. Such lengths are too short, since with a 5 mm internal diameter, the transit times over the clinical range of blood flows lie between 2 and 8 seconds. To improve accuracy in measurement we routinely use a 200 cm 'race track' which ensures that the transit time lies between 8 and 30 seconds for such flows.

2. The 'race tracks' should be kept horizontal to avoid errors introduced by the lower density of air compared with the blood.

3. The length of 'race track' should be measured prior to the commencement of dialysis to minimize stretching. Commercial PVC tubing is sufficiently constant to give an accuracy of $\pm 3\%$ provided it is not stretched during track measurement.

4. The 'race track' should be calibrated with bank blood whose haematocrit is of the same range as the patients since bubble speed is influenced by fluid viscosity. *In vitro* studies have shown that the variation introduced within the haematocrit range 27 to 40% is 5% (56).

5. A single air bubble (0.5 ml) is injected. Its passage is measured in triplicate at each flow rate with a stop watch measuring to 0.1 sec. If the air bubble fragments after injection, the observation is discarded.

6. The internal diameter of the tubing should be sufficiently constant. Variations in this parameter have the same effect on calculated blood flow as discussed above for pump segments. Our experience has shown that this parameter is sufficiently constant thereby not necessitating recalibration at each experiment. However, it is a wise precaution to recheck calibration from time to time during a series of experiments.

Such a technique is suitable for conventional two needle treatments or when access is by a double lumen catheter. Single needle access using single pump or double pump systems generates a cyclic tidal flow pattern in the extracorporeal circuit. Consequently not only do blood flow rates differ in the different parts of the extracorporeal circuit but high blood flows occur transiently during the aspiration (inflow) and return phases (See Chapter 17). A number of the current clinically used systems provide a direct read out of the flows achieved based on the principles described above for single pump systems which are subject to the same limitations. To overcome these and to measure the blood flow in such systems we developed a technique based upon the fact that when using such systems the blood flow in the extracorporeal circuit between the dialyser venous outlet and the venous drip chamber (in the case of single pump tidal flow systems and the venous compliance chamber in double pump tidal flow systems) is largely independent of the cyclic variations induced by the blood pump since they are damped by the dialyser allowing the blood flow to be measured by bubble transit techniques.

We have used two alternative techniques – in our early studies we maintained a 200 cm race track but increased the number of measurements at each blood flow. This has the same effect as lengthening the 'race track' but avoids the problems of excessive extracorporeal volumes. Currently, we use a 400 cm 'race track' inserted into the venous segment of the extracorporeal circuit between the dialyser venous outlet and the venous drip expansion chamber and measure the transit time of five bubbles. This adds marginally to the extracorporeal volume but produces an error comparable with that for two needle measurements provided the flow interruption in switching from the aspiration to return phase does not exceed 1 second.

Measurement of bubble transit time involves the repeated insertion of a needle into an injection site. Careful instruction in the use of the technique is necessary to prevent the risk of accidental needle injury to fingers which may be further minimised by the use of injection sites that incorporate a protective guard on the underside of the site. Because of this risk and the possibility of aerosol generation when puncturing an injection site under positive pressure, it is our view that such techniques should not be used with patients who are HB_sAg positive or HIV positive.

The use of bubble transit time in CAVH is impractical; Bosch (57) has described a method of blood flow measurement for use in CAVH which relies on the measurement of the ultrafiltration rate, and the blood haematocrit at both the inlet and outlet to the filter and allows the blood flow to be calculated from

$$Q_{Bi} = \frac{(Q_F \, HCT_o)}{(HCT_i - HCT_o)}$$

plasma flow may be calculated from

$$Q_{Pi} = [Q_{Bi} - \text{erythrocyte mass}]$$

where erythrocyte mass (ml/min) at the inlet = $(Q_{Bi} \times HCT_i)/100$.

PERFORMANCE PARAMETERS

The performance parameters of any device may be categorised into those that relate to its physical properties, mass transfer properties and its physiological effects.

PERFORMANCE PARAMETERS RELATED TO PHYSICAL PROPERTIES

Blood compartment volume

Construction features of any device govern properties such as ease of handling, packaging, size, ease of preparation and setting up as well as the volume contained within the device's blood or dialysate pathways.

The blood compartment volume of any device is of importance not only to the clinician, but also to the design engineer. In the clinical setting it is an important contributory component of the extracorporeal circuit volume while in engineering terms, it is normally expressed as blood film thickness obtained by dividing the blood compartment volume by the device surface area. It is an important factor governing the exchange of molecular species between the blood and the boundary wall or membrane.

Historically, blood compartment volume was important. Early devices were so large as to require priming with donor blood. Since 1960, there has been a steady reduction in this parameter (with a concomitant increase in performance) such that currently the volume contained in many devices is exceeded by the volume contained by the blood lines with which it is used (Tables 10,11).

Blood compartments of devices utilising compliant flat sheet or tubular membranes change with increasing transmembrane pressure, this increase being referred to as compliance and is a function of not only the applied pressure, but also of the membrane thickness, grain orientation and support geometry. Blood compartment volumes of devices incorporating hollow fibre membranes remain constant over a wide pressure range.

The volume of the blood compartment may be expressed in terms of blood path geometry. For flat plate or coil devices it is given by:

$$\bar{L} \, W \, h_B \, N$$

while for hollow fibres it is given by:

$$\frac{\pi \, d^2 \bar{L} N}{4}$$

Table 10. Standard haemodialysers blood compartment volume (ml).

	Transmembrane pressure (mm Hg)	
	100	*200*
M3 Micropoint	151	+16
MTL 133	37	+ 9
Lundia 10-3N	85	+ 8
Lundia PRO5	65	+15
BL 501 Bravo	109	+25
Vita 2HP	238	+47
AM 100M	63[a]	
Nephross Allegro HF	49	
NT 10-11	79	
TAF 10	73	
FD 100	84	
Hemoflow D2	83	
CDAK 90 SCE	77	
FB 110T	72	
BL 612M Prima	73	
GF 120 M	83	

[a] All hollow fibre measurements made by air evacuation of fibres after priming.

Table 11. High flux devices blood compartment volume (ml).

	Transmembrane pressure (mm Hg)	
	100	*200*
Biospal 2400S (194)	79[a]	–
HF 060	35[b]	
PAN 150	56	
AN 69 HF	77	
F 60 (195)	75	
B1-100	83	
CD Duoflux	–	

[a] At a transmembrane pressure of 70 mm Hg.
[b] All measurements from Newcastle made by air evacuation of fibres after priming.

Calculation of the blood compartment volume by the above formula in the case of hollow fibre devices uses the dry fibre dimensions. When the fibres are primed with saline, fluid is absorbed into the fibre walls and the fibre swells with consequent changes in both fibre internal diameter and wall thickness causing an increase in blood compartment volume. This increase has been expressed mathematically by Sigdell (58). In practical terms these changes are small but may influence the device's mass transport characteristics.

Blood compartment volumes and compliance may be measured by filling the compartment with a fluid such as vegetable oil or kerosene in vitro. In our own studies we combined measurement of this parameter with the measurement of ultrafiltration characteristics by using a solution to which the membrane is permeable. For devices containing highly permeable membranes we use a non permeable fluid (vegetable or corn oil).

Flow resistance

Blood pathway

For haemodialysers, the resistance to flow in the blood pathway is governed by the pathway geometry. For flat plate devices with a large width to height ratio, the relationship between flow rate and flow resistance is given by:

$$\triangle P_B = \frac{12 \mu \bar{L}}{W h^3 N} Q_B$$

while for circular passages the expression is:

$$\triangle P_B = \frac{128 \mu \bar{L}}{\pi N d^4} Q_B.$$

The above relationships measure pressure drop in dynes/cm^2 and also hold for haemofilters. To convert these pressure drops to the more commonly used mm Hg, the equations shown should be multiplied by 7.5×10^{-4} (mm Hg/dyne/cm^2).

These equations show that $\triangle P_B$ is linearly related to Q_B provided the blood pathway geometry and fluid viscosity are constant.

Blood exhibits an anomalous viscosity which increases with increasing haematocrit. It tends to decrease in small passages such as capillary tubes with an internal diameter of less than 100 microns and increase with decreasing shear rate (59,60).

Deviations from linearity due to changes in blood pathway geometry may be a consequence of dimensional variations in this parameter, resulting from inappropriate support of the membrane or variations that may be introduced during manufacture.

Blood flow resistance can be measured *in vitro* using blood or an aqueous solution, or *in vivo*. It is most commonly measured in vitro using an aqueous solution. To estimate the *in vivo* pressure drop a conversion factor may be used if direct measurement is unavailable. To establish this conversion factor we have measured the pressure drop directly with blood of haematocrit of 20%, and combined the results

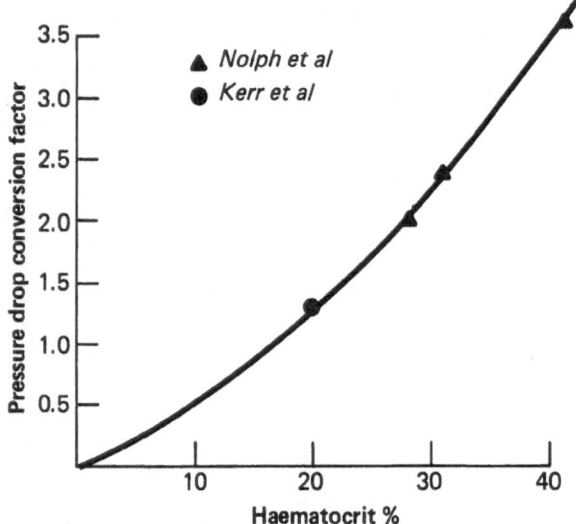

Figure 14. Conversion factor for blood compartment pressure drop from aqueous solution measurement to blood of varying haematocrit.

with those of Nolph and colleagues (61) for haematocrit values of 26, 31 and 41% (Figure 14).

Care should be exercised when using such a conversion factor since there is a considerable scatter in the relationship between blood viscosity and haematocrit.

Dialysate pathway

The equations governing dialysate pathway resistance and flow rate are comparable with those given for the blood pathway. The value of this parameter is of importance in haemodialysers since they operate in conjunction with a negative pressure in the dialysate pathway. Excessive pressure drops may limit the use of the device to certain delivery systems while variations in this parameter can lead to unpredictability in the solute and water removal characteristics of the device.

Flow distribution

Flow non-idealities may occur in either the blood or dialysate pathways due to random dimensional variations in the path geometry introduced during manufacture or due to design defects.

The uniformity of flow distribution is important in as much as variability influences solute transport characteristics, and causes flow stagnation leading to increased thrombus formation and blood loss.

Flow visualisation studies may be performed by dye or tracer isotopes (62) injected into the pathway and linking the pathway outflow to a suitable flow-through analyser. This technique may be extended to the analysis of the mean residence time and the variance of distribution to provide a more detailed fluid dynamic analysis of the results.

Blood loss

Blood loss during haemodialysis and other extracorporeal circulation procedures is due to a number of causes that include sampling for biochemical control, bleeding from the access site at the start or termination of the procedure and technical causes such as accidental rupture of the membrane, clotting episodes during therapy and loss at the termination of treatment. The cumulative total from all these sources has been studied and been shown to be as high as 5 1/annum (63,64). The wider availability of microanalytical laboratory methods has reduced the volume of samples required for biochemical analysis but iatrogenic loss remains the largest component of the total blood loss during extracorporeal circulation procedures.

Large amounts of blood may be lost through membrane rupture or leak. These problems may be traced to membrane defects, shipment, storage and handling prior to and during use as well as defects in manufacture. Current devices are pressure tested during manufacture and these problems have largely disappeared. This has not always been the case (65). In the case of nondisposable devices the leak rate depends upon the skill and care of the persons building it.

Leak rates are difficult to assess since multiple centre studies extending over several thousand treatments are required, even for devices with a relatively high (>5%) leak rate.

Blood loss at the termination of treatment may be effectively assessed during clinical use. However, the magnitude of this loss is subject not only to the device itself, but the technique of extracorporeal circuit rinsing as well as the degree of anticoagulation achieved during use. All currently used devices are sufficiently thrombogenic to require the administration of an anticoagulant. The mechanism of thrombus formation in an artificial organ such as a haemodialyser or haemofilter is complex and a consequence of the patient's thrombus generating potential, the surface properties of the material in contact with blood and the local fluid dynamic and mass transfer conditions (66–68). A reduction in the thrombus formation during clinical use by the administration of antiplatelet drugs such as prostacyclin (69) has been explored but due to the high cost of the drugs, has not seen widespread clinical use and heparin remains the most widely used method of anticoagulation during extracorporeal circulation. The technique of heparin administration and the assessment of the adequacy of anticoagulation resulting from such administration is discussed elsewhere in this book (Chapter 11).

The blood remaining in the extracorporeal circuit at the termination of therapy consists of two distinct components. First, the fluid blood component which is related to the design of the device, the volume of the rinse back solution and the technique of washback. The second component is the clotted residue formed despite adequate heparinisation which is trapped and cannot be removed either by increasing the volume of rinseback or by altering the washback technique short of dislodging the clot.

Measurement of the two components differs. Fluid residue retained in the extracorporeal circuit may be measured colorimetrically whereby the haemoglobin content of the patient's blood taken immediately prior to the termination of treatment is compared with the haemoglobin content of the fluid retained in the circuit. A number of methods for this purpose have been described (70–72). In our own studies after the termination of washback, the contents of the extracorporeal circuit are recirculated under minimal ultrafiltration conditions through one litre of ammoniated water (0.04% NH_3). Haemoglobin content of the patient's blood and the ammoniated water is measured spectrophotometrically using a technique described by Cripps (73) and the blood retained calculated from the formula:

$$RBV = \frac{U\ (1000 + \text{Extracorporeal circuit volume})}{200\,S}$$

where

U = haemoglobin concentration of residual fluid
S = haemoglobin concentration of arterial sample taken prior to the termination of treatment diluted 1 : 200 in 0.04% NH_3.

The measurement of circuit volume is determined separately or by the draining of the contents of the circuit into a measuring cylinder. Both these methods are subject to inaccuracies but their influence on the final result is small, unless the extracorporeal circuit volume is excessively large.

Although the accuracy of such an estimation has been questioned (74) it remains widely used in clinical practice.

Clotted blood residue may be assessed visually. However, such assessment is likely to underestimate the residue. It is most readily measured by the labelling of the patient's red cells with a radioactive tracer and comparing the tracer concentration in the device at the termination of treatment with a sample of the patient's blood taken prior to the termination of treatment which is diluted in a geometry of similar dimensions to the device under test and counting them both in either a bulk sample counter, whole body counter or by a gamma camera. Radioisotope markers that may be used for this purpose include Technetium-99M, Iron-59 and Chromium-51 – of these ^{51}Cr and ^{99}Tc are preferable since they may be used immediately whereas some 2 weeks must be allowed for the incorporation of the ^{59}Fe into the red cells.

These procedures use small amounts of activity (approximately 50 uCi) and the resulting body burdens are low. Their use, however, has not been wide due to ethical considerations.

A comparison of blood loss is given in Table 12. These results refer to haemodialysers only. They show a wide scatter but the mean loss is small in comparison with losses from other sources. No such comparative data are available for haemofilters, possibly due to their limited use compared with haemodialysers. Gohl and Konstantin (75) have commented that provided proper rinseback procedures are used, residual blood loss is comparable with that for dialysers.

Table 12. Standard haemodialysers blood loss (ml).

	Fluid blood retained (ml)		Saline Rinse volume (ml)	Rinse volume[a] / Circuit volume
	Mean	Range		
M3 Micropoint	5.3	2.2 – 10.9	600	1.64
MTL 133	2.3	1.0 – 4.1	500	1.87
Lundia 10-3N	0.9	0 – 1.0	600	2.53
Lundia PRO 5	3.8	1.8 – 7.0	600	1.46
BL 501 Bravo	3.3	1.3 – 5.1	600	2.04
Vita 2 HP	2.0	0.3 – 3.9	800	0.60
AM 100M				
Nephross Allegro HF				
NT 10-11				
TAF 10	2.9	1.6 – 5.1	600	1.49
FD 100				
Hemoflow D2				
CDAK 90 SCE	4.4	1.3 – 16.3	600	1.69
FB 110T	1.6	0.7 – 4.8	600	1.44
BL 612M Prima	2.0	0.8 – 3.2	600	1.68
GF 120M	1.0	0.4 – 1.5	600	1.80

Washout characteristics

Currently practised short dialysis schedules with small high efficiency haemodialysers have resulted in the desirability of minimising fluid given to the patient at the termination of treatment without incurring unacceptably high blood losses. To permit this to be achieved, a measure of the haemodialyser's washout characteristics is required. Such a technique not only allows optimisation of the fluid required, but also enables various rinseback techniques to be studied.

Theoretical and experimental work relating to this subject has been described by a number of authors (76,77). Our own studies have involved a non invasive technique using ^{51}Cr labelled red cells by which blood recovery curves for any dialyser may be established and related to the ratio of washback volume/circuit volume (78) (Figure 15). Although this method is suitable for both *in vitro* and *in vivo* measurements, the need to expose the patient to radiation and the special equipment required limits its use. *In vitro* data may be more readily established by on line spectrophotometric monitoring of a non dialysable tracer. The extrapolation of data obtained by such a technique to *in vivo* is not without difficulty since during clinical use the membrane may be distorted or the device partially clotted. Consequently, the visual observation of the venous bubble chamber may prove a sufficiently simple and acceptable clinical guide to dialyser washout characteristics.

SOLUTE TRANSPORT CHARACTERISTICS

Clearance and dialysance

Analogous to the clearance concept from renal physiology the overall solute transport characteristics may be expressed in terms of clearance or dialysance. Clearance is the operational parameter of the device that focuses on the removal of solute from the patient and is the most meaningful parameter clinically since it describes the device as part of the circulatory system. Clearance is defined as the amount of solute removed from the blood per unit of time, divided by the incoming blood concentration and represents the volumetric rate of removal. Dialysance is used by engineers in the comparison of the overall solute removal at a given blood flow for different haemodialyser designs. It is defined as the amount of solute removed from the blood per unit of time divided by the concentration difference between incoming blood and dialysate.

By consideration of the mass balance across the device the above definitions may be expressed in terms of concentration gradients and flow rates such that:

$$K_B = \frac{(C_{Bi} - C_{Bo})\ Q_{Bi}}{C_{Bi}} + \frac{Q_F\ C_{Bo}}{C_{Bi}}$$

for the blood side of the dialyser, and

$$K_D = \frac{(C_{Do} - C_{Di})Q_{Di}}{C_{Bi}} + \frac{Q_F\ C_{Do}}{C_{Bi}}$$

for the dialysate side of the dialyser.

Equivalent expressions for dialysance are:

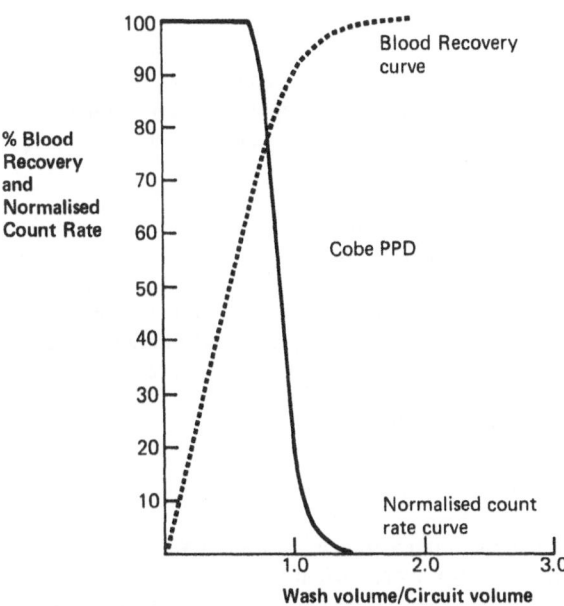

Figure 15. Normalised count rate curve and its derived blood recovery curve for a parallel plate haemodialyser.

$$D_B = \frac{(C_{Bi} - C_{Bo})Q_{Bi}}{(C_{Bi} - C_{Di})} + \frac{Q_F C_{Bo}}{(C_{Bi} - C_{Di})}$$

and

$$D_D = \frac{(C_{Do} - C_{Di})Q_{Di}}{(C_{Bi} - C_{Di})} + \frac{Q_F C_{Do}}{(C_{Bi} - C_{Di})}$$

For negligible ultrafiltration $(Q_F \rightarrow 0)$ the above expressions reduce to the more commonly used relationships.

$$K_B = \frac{(C_{Bi} - C_{Bo})}{C_{Bi}} Q_B$$

$$K_D = \frac{(C_{Do} - C_{Di})}{C_{Bi}} Q_D$$

$$D_B = \frac{(C_{Bi} - C_{Bo})}{(C_{Bi} - C_{Di})} Q_B$$

$$D_D = \frac{(C_{Do} - C_{Di})}{(C_{Bi} - C_{Di})} Q_D$$

From the above formulae the relationship between clearance and dialysance may be established. It is given by

$$K_B = \frac{(C_{Bi} - C_{Di})}{C_{Bi}} D_B$$

The two expressions are only equal when $C_{Di} = 0$, i.e. single pass dialysis. In all other cases, clearance is less than dialysance, an important point to bear in mind when considering a comparison of devices whose construction demands different dialysate supply systems, for example, coil dialysers used with rapidly recirculated dialysate and dialysers used in single pass systems. In the former, the clearance is equal to the dialysance in the initial minutes of treatment and decreases throughout treatment as the solute concentration increases in the tank, whereas for single pass systems it remains the same throughout treatment.

There are instances where the relationship between clearance and dialysance is more complex. The first of these is when a coil type dialyser is being used with a recirculating single pass system (RSP) rather than a pure recirculating system. In recirculating single pass a small volume of dialysate (5 to 10 l) is recirculated through the dialyser at a flow rate corresponding to that which would be used in pure recirculation systems. Simultaneously, dialysate is drawn from the system to waste and fresh dialysis fluid is added at the same rate as the withdrawal. For such systems, an expression relating clearance to dialysance has been derived by von Hartitzsch (79) and is given by

$$K_B = \frac{D_B}{1 + D_B/Q_B}.$$

This relationship permits the comparison of coil dialysers with parallel plate or hollow fibre types without giving an erroneous impression of relative efficiency. Since it is only valid in the case of well mixed dialysate, it should not be used during the first hour of dialysis when rapid changes in the solute reservoir concentration may be present.

A second case in which the clearance is modified is in single needle systems where recirculation, or the mixing of fresh blood with that which has already been through the haemodialyser occurs. The modified relationship under these circumstances has been derived by Gotch (56) and is given by

$$K_R = \frac{(1 - R')}{1 - R' \ (1 - K/Q_B)}.$$

The above relationships all relate to whole blood clearance, in haemofiltration in contrast to haemodialysis, the solute removal is by convection rather than diffusion as the solute is cleared from the blood by removal of plasma water. This necessitates knowledge of the precise distribution of the solute. To allow the equivalent calculations to those used in haemodialysis to be made, it is necessary to introduce the concept of sieving coefficient, defined as the ratio of solute concentration in the ultrafiltrate and the concentration in bulk plasma water such that

$$S = \frac{C_F}{C_W} = \frac{2 \ C_F}{C_{Wi} + C_{Wo}}.$$

If the concentration of solutes is equal in the blood and filtrate then $S = 1$, on the other hand if the membrane is impermeable to the solute $S = 0$.

Bulk plasma water concentration is related to whole blood concentration and plasma concentration such that

$$\frac{C_P}{C_W} = 1 - \varphi$$

φ = volume fraction of the hydrated protein and

$$\frac{C_B}{C_P} = 1 - H + Hk.$$

The relationships for the calculation of whole blood clearances for specified operating conditions during haemofiltration have been described in detail by Colton et al (80) and Henderson et al (81) and are given below.

for pre-dilution

$$K_B = Q_B \frac{(1 - H)}{(1 - H + Hk)}$$

$$\left\{ 1 - \left[\frac{(1 - \varphi)(1 - H) + Q_D/Q_B \ (1 - Q_F/Q_D)}{(1 - \varphi)(1 - H) + Q_D/Q_B} \right]^S \right\}$$

for post-dilution

$$K_B = Q_B \frac{(1 - H)}{(1 - H + Hk)}$$

$$\left\{ 1 - \left[\frac{(1 - \varphi)(1 - H + Q_F/Q_B)}{(1 - \varphi)(1 - H)} \right]^S \right\}.$$

Plasma clearance may be calculated from

$$K_P = \frac{Q_F C_F}{C_{Pi}}.$$

In the case of solute removed by ultrafiltration alone, such as during CAVH, whole blood clearance is equivalent to the plasma clearance such that

$$K_B = \frac{Q_F C_F}{C_{Bi}}.$$

If the effects of the exclusion volume of the hydrated proteins and the exclusion of larger molecular weight solutes are neglected the relationship simplifies to

$$K_B = Q_F S.$$

During haemodiafiltration, solute removal is principally by diffusion but the removal of large molecular weight solutes is augmented by convection. Gupta and Jaffrin (82) showed that the overall clearance is less than the clearance of each process occurring separately due to the interaction between convection and diffusion and may be expressed as

$$K_{HFD} = K_B + \frac{Q_F}{2}.$$

Overall mass transfer coefficient

Measurement of clearance is normally sufficient for clinical purposes. However, such measurements offer no insight into the mass exchange phenomena occurring within the device and for an effective interdisciplinary approach, the overall mass transfer coefficient which is the reciprocal of the overall mass transfer resistance (R_T) needs to be used if such insight is required.

In the absence of significant ultrafiltration, the relationships between overall mass transfer resistance and dialysance have been derived and may be used to analyse the phenomena occurring in a haemodialyser in any of the clinically used flow configurations (Table 13).

Table 13. Relationship of dialysance to total mass transfer resistance.

Flow geometry	Dialysance (D)	Total mass transfer resistance (R_T)
Co-Parallel	$Q_B \left[\dfrac{1 - \left[\exp - J\left(1 + \dfrac{Q_B}{Q_D}\right) \right]}{1 + \dfrac{Q_B}{Q_D}} \right]$	$\dfrac{S(Q_B + Q_D)}{Q_B Q_D \ln\left[\dfrac{1}{1 - \dfrac{D}{Q_B} - \dfrac{D}{Q_D}} \right]}$
Contra-Parallel	$Q_B \left[\dfrac{1 - \left[\exp - J\left(1 - \dfrac{Q_B}{Q_D}\right) \right]}{1 - \dfrac{Q_B}{Q_D} \exp\left[- J\left(1 - \dfrac{Q_B}{Q_D}\right) \right]} \right]$	$\dfrac{S(Q_B - Q_D)}{Q_B Q_D \ln\left[\dfrac{1 - \dfrac{D}{Q_B}}{1 - \dfrac{D}{Q_D}} \right]}$
Cross-Flow*	$\dfrac{Q_B}{2} \left[\left[\dfrac{1 - \exp\left[- J\left(1 + \dfrac{Q_B}{Q_D}\right) \right]}{1 + \dfrac{Q_B}{Q_D}} \right] + \left[\dfrac{1 - \exp\left[- J\left(1 - \dfrac{Q_B}{Q_D}\right) \right]}{1 - \dfrac{Q_B}{Q_D} \exp\left[- J\left(1 - \dfrac{Q_B}{Q_D}\right) \right]} \right] \right]$	$\dfrac{S}{2Q_B Q_D} \left[\ln\left[\dfrac{Q_B + Q_D}{1 - \dfrac{D}{Q_B} - \dfrac{D}{Q_D}} \right] + \dfrac{Q_B - Q_D}{\ln\left[\dfrac{1 - \dfrac{D}{Q_B}}{1 - \dfrac{D}{Q_D}} \right]} \right]$

Where $J = \dfrac{S}{R_T Q_B}$

* Approximate equation only. For exact equations refer to Kays and London, Compact Heat Exchangers, 2nd ed. New York, McGraw Hill, 1964.

Table 14. Compounds suitable for solute transport characterization.

Compound	Molecular mass (daltons)	
Sodium chloride	58	small molecules
Urea	60	
Creatinine	113	
Phosphate	136	
Uric acid	168	
Dextrose	180	
Sucrose	342	middle molecules
EDTA	380	
Raffinose	504	
Vitamin B$_{12}$	1,355	
Inulin	5,200	
Cytochrome C	13,400	large molecules
Haemoglobin	68,000	
Albumin	69,000	

Assessment of solute transport characteristics

Prior to 1968, publications dealing with haemodialyser performance included only information relating to the clearance of small molecular weight solutes namely urea and creatinine.

Following the advent of the 'middle molecular hypothesis' (4) coupled with the increased utilisation of high permeability membranes for alternative therapies, it is common practice to describe device or membrane solute transport by the use of marker solutes, such as those shown in Table 14. Although these compounds describe *in vitro* solute transport characteristics, their use in vivo or the extrapolation of *in vitro* data to *in vivo*, is subject to constraints resulting from phenomena unique to physiological solutions such as whole blood, and their interaction with the membrane.

For conventional haemodialysers solute transport is related to blood flow (Figure 16). The shape of the relationship is governed by constraints imposed by the blood flow and the product of device surface area and overall mass transfer coefficient. This relationship is the same for all designs and solutes and allows experimental data to be fitted to a curve of a standard shape given by:

$$K_B = \frac{Q_B}{a + b \ Q_B}$$

where a and b are constants.

This may be transformed into a linear relationship by a simple arithmetic manipulation allowing linear regression analysis of the data. A typical analysis using this technique for a specimen dialyser is shown in Figure 17. The bars above and below the line at standard blood flow rates indicate the 95% confidence limits of the estimate while the probability limits of the data are represented by dashed lines. In such analyses the confidence limits may be made as narrow as desired by increasing the number of observations. Increasing the number of observations does not influence the probability limit since this represents the variability in observations caused by the experimental technique and dialyser variability. Provided gross inaccuracies from a single dialyser are excluded this parameter may be used as a measure of consistency.

Table 15 summarises mean *in vivo* clearance data of haemodialysers for small molecules established for patients whose mean haematocrit was 24%. Clearance of middle molecular weight solutes for standard haemodialysers is summarised in Table 16, and high flux devices in Table 17.

Table 15. Standard haemodialysers. *In vivo* clearance of small molecules at a blood flow of 200 ml/min.

	Urea clearance (ml/min)	Range	Creatinine clearance (ml/min)	Range
M3 Micropoint	147 ± 1.1	141–156	118 ± 0.7	111–123
MTL 133				
Lundia 10-3N	147 ± 3.2	137–156	112 ± 3.8	98–130
Lundia PRO 5	161 ± 2.6	149–172	145 ± 4.2	130–161
BL 501 Bravo	135 ± 0.9	128–145	108 ± 1.7	97–119
Vita 2 HP	122 ± 2.2	114–129	98 ± 1.0	93–105
AM 100M	133 ± 3.6	115–159	102 ± 3.7	85–128
Nephross Allegro HF	159 ± 2.5	152–167	139 ± 3.9	127–152
NT 10-11	149 ± 3.4	137–167	125 ± 4.0	111–145
TAF 10	152 ± 2.3	143–164	122 ± 4.5	103–147
FD 100	154 ± 4.7	135–179	137 ± 4.6	115–167
Hemoflow D2	167 ± 4.1	145–196	132 ± 6.0	102–182
CDAK 90 SCE	156 ± 1.2	149–164	118 ± 2.1	108–132
FB 110T	167 ± 1.4	159–172	143 ± 2.0	135–154
BL 612M Prima	159 ± 2.5	147–169	132 ± 2.6	119–149
GF 120 M	154 ± 1.2	147–161	130 ± 1.7	119–141

Dialysate flow 500 to 530 ml/min, Temperature 38° C.

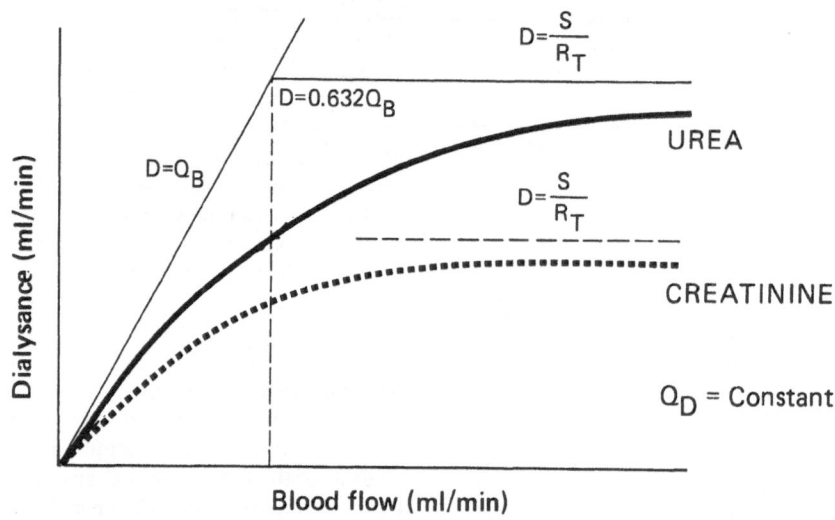

Figure 16. The relationship between dialysance and blood flow. This relationship is applicable to any device. The curves are limited by the constraints shown which intercept at a point given by $0.632 \, Q_B$.

Table 16. Standard Haemodialysers. *In vitro* clearance of small and middle molecular weight solutes at a blood flow of 200 ml/min.

	Urea (60)	Creatinine (113)	PO₄ (138)	Vitamin B₁₂ (1355)
M3 Micropoint	152	122	–	42.8
MTL 133	133	101	–	27.0
Lundia 10-3N	142	109	–	26.3
Lundia PRO 5	155	134	98	59.1
BL 501 Bravo	139	108	–	32.0
Vita 2 HP	123	91	–	30.8
AM 100M	139	113	94	30.3
Nephross Allegro HF	164	141	123	39.1
NT 10-11	157	129	106	22.3
TAF 10	161	134	–	62.8
FD 100	158	141	111	70.3
Hemoflow D2	178	145	–	40.8
CDAK 90 SCE	153	121	–	23.0
FB 110T	166	138	113	43.1
BL 612M Prima	163	137	–	34.0
GF 120M	168	132	–	32.6

Dialysate flow 500 to 530 ml/min, Temperature 38° C. Figures in parentheses refer to molecular weight. Mean results extrapolated to zero ultrafiltration shown.

Table 17. High flux devices. *In vivo* clearance of small and middle molecular weight solutes at a blood flow of 200 ml/min.

	Urea (60)	Creatinine (113)	PO₄ (138)	Vitamin B₁₂ (1355)	Ref.
Biospal 2400S[a]	165	136	121	69	194
HF 060	151	137	126	80.2	
PAN 150	158	144	135	83.7	
AN 69 HF	164	151	131	78.2	
F60	190	182	176	125	195
B1-100	151	127	102	49.5	
CD Duoflux	158	137	120	72.2	

Dialysate flow 500 to 530 ml/min, Temperature 38° C. Figures in parentheses refer to molecular weight.
[a] Manufacturers' results at an ultrafiltration rate of 10 ml/min. Mean results extrapolated to zero ultrafiltration shown.

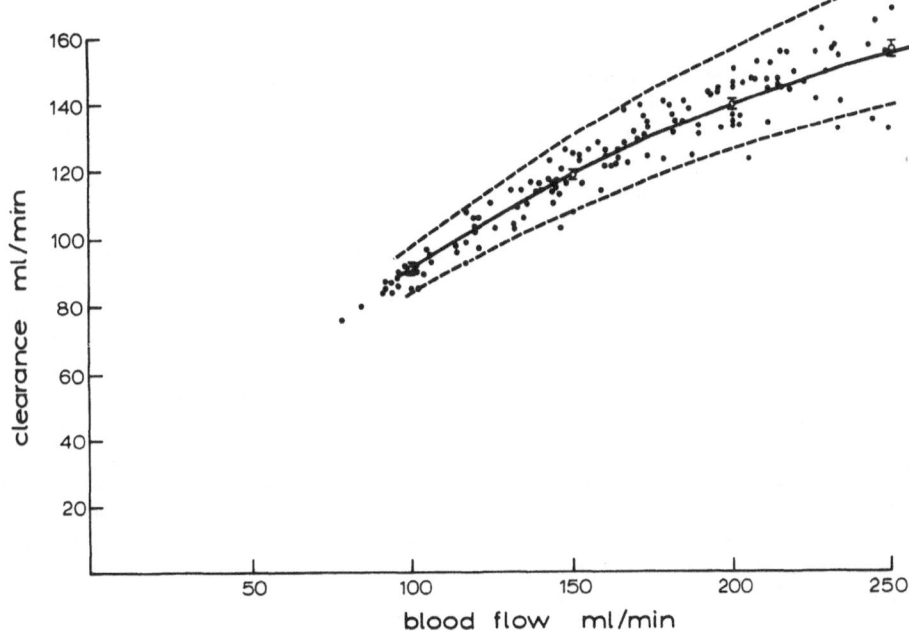

Figure 17. Experimental data for a haemodialyser showing 95% confidence and probability limits.

Factors influencing solute transport

Ultrafiltration (convective mass transfer)

In conventional haemodialysis the effects of ultrafiltration on the clearance of small molecules are in the order of 3% provided the ultrafiltration rate is less than 5 ml/min (83).

The effects of ultrafiltration on the clearance characteristics of haemodialysers have been studied by Nolph et al (84–86). Their studies demonstrate an increase in clearance due to the contribution of convective mass transport which in the case of devices with compliant pathways may be associated with a decrease in diffusive clearance due to expansion of the blood pathway or increased draping of the membrane over the membrane support.

Red cell and protein concentration effects

In vitro measurements are normally performed using aqueous solutions. *In vivo* studies involve a complex heterogenous solution in which the solute diffusion rates may be reduced due to the movement of solutes around or through the formed elements (87) as well as protein binding (88–90).

The effect of haematocrit on clearance of small molecules has been studied by Woffindin (91) who demonstrated a negligible effect on urea clearance but a measurable effect on creatinine clearance, findings that suggest disequilibrium between the red cell and plasma creatinine levels. Mass transport may also be influenced by solute charge and the adsorption of proteins on to the surface of the membrane.

These effects have been studied for haemodialysis by Grossman, Kopp and Frey (92) who showed that the difference between in vitro and in vivo clearance for urea is of the order of 3% for the haematocrit range 20 to 30% over the clinical range of blood flows.

Temperature

The determination of solute transport properties and clinical therapy are undertaken at a constant temperature (37 ± 1°C). The removal of macromolecules in plasma separation may be performed at a reduced temperature (cryofiltration). Such a reduction in temperature will reduce solute transport compared to that obtained at higher temperatures for a given membrane (50).

Flow rate

The relationship between solute removal and blood flow is shown in Figure 16. The relationship between solute transport rate and dialysate flow rate is a similar shape. The role of dialysate flow rate on solute transport has been studied by Sigdell and Tersteegen (93) who defined a practically feasible upper limit for dialysate flow rate as being twice the blood flow, while for specific instances where clearance of middle weight solutes is of interest, they suggested that a dialysate flow rate equivalent to the blood flow may be sufficient since the removal of large molecular weight solutes is less dependent on dialysate flow rate. Low flow rate dialysis has seen a limited clinical application (94,95) but it is not utilised widely and a flow rate of 500 ml/min remains the standard.

Dialysate degassing

Adequate dialysate degassing is now achieved by the majority of proportionating systems by the use of negative pressure and heat exchangers. The use of bicarbonate based dialysis fluid as well as dialysate regeneration may, however, continue to pose problems due to the excess of CO_2 in the dialysis fluid. This may lead to the accumulation of gas in the dialysate pathway, loss of surface area due to membrane masking and a decrease in solute removal with time (96).

Membrane characteristics

The membrane is the principal barrier to diffusion for large and middle molecular weight solutes. It is less important for low molecular weight solutes where the principal barrier to diffusion lies in the fluid films surrounding the membrane rather than the membrane itself. The hydrophilicity or hydrophobicity of the membrane material as well as its surface charge play a major role in adsorption of proteins on to membrane surfaces which, in turn, influence the transport properties of the membrane (97–99).

WATER TRANSPORT CHARACTERISTICS

During haemodialysis and haemofiltration, whole blood – a complex mixture of water, proteins and cells – is filtered, resulting in the removal of both water and solutes, whereas in membrane plasmapheresis all blood components except cells are filtered.

The fluid removed during extracorporeal therapy has two components, one due to the hydrostatic transmembrane pressure gradient ($Q_{F(h)}$) the other due to the osmotic transmembrane pressure gradient ($Q_{F(osm)}$) such that

$$Q_F = Q_{F(h)} + Q_{F(osm)}.$$

The osmotic transmembrane pressure gradient is the algebraic sum of the osmotic gradients for each of the molecular species present on either side of the membrane. During haemodialysis, the overall molarity of the dialysis fluid is comparable to that of the blood and the influence of this component is small, unless solutes such as dextrose are added. A special case of osmotic pressure gradient is that due to the proteins in the plasma, since the membranes are impermeable to protein and the dialysate is protein free; these molecules exert their full osmotic force which is referred to as plasma protein concentration or colloid osmotic pressure. At normal plasma protein concentrations this pressure is about 25 mm Hg and modifies hydrostatic pressure such that it may be written algebraically as

$$[\Delta P_{M(h)} - \Delta P_{osm}].$$

The relative importance of this correction is small in haemodialysis or haemofiltration where the hydraulic pressure gradient dominates as the principal force in water removal. CAVH on the other hand functions at low pressures and colloid osmotic pressure has a significant effect on the filtration rate.

In haemodialysis, water transport characteristics may be quantified in terms of membrane surface area, hydraulic permeability and hydrostatic pressure gradient such that

$$Q_F = L_h \; A \; \Delta P_{M(h)}$$

the mean hydrostatic pressure given by

$$P_{M(h)} = \frac{(P_{Bi} + P_{Bo})}{2} - \frac{(P_{Di} + P_{Do})}{2}.$$

In practice the relationship between mean hydrostatic or transmembrane pressure and ultrafiltration rate may most readily be studied *in vitro* where if the studies are performed under conditions of balanced osmolality a straight line relationship is obtained, the slope of the line representing the ultrafiltration coefficient of the device. If the appropriate correction for plasma oncotic pressures is made then it is possible to predict *in vivo* ultrafiltration based on *in vitro* measurements. During *in vitro* studies pressures at all entry and exit points of the device are monitored. Such comprehensive monitoring is not always available during clinical use. However as

$$P_B = P_{Bi} - P_{Bo}$$

by definition, and

$$P_D = P_{Di} - P_{Do}$$

so the mean hydrostatic pressure may be expressed in terms of measured pressures by algebraic substition provided the pressure drops in the blood and dialysate pathways are small. Under such circumstance $P_{M(h)}$ approximates to the arithmetic sum of the two normally measured pressures (P_{Bo} and P_{Do}). The pressure drop across the pathways may be affected by thrombus formation, the variable relationship between haematocrit and viscosity, and lead to difficulties in predicting the *in vivo* ultrafiltration from *in vitro* measurements.

A modification to the above approximation needs to be made when using devices in conjunction with pressure-pressure controlled single needle systems using two pumps. In such systems the dialyser is isolated by the pumps in the extracorporeal circuit and the pressure across the dialyser varies continuously since the blood outlet pressure is used to switch the cycle. The assumption that the pressure drop in the blood pathway is negligible cannot be made in these circumstances and a correction factor derived from considering the blood pathway pressures at the maximum and minimum pressures during a cycle needs to be added to the arithmetic sum of the two most commonly measured pressures during dialysis (P_{Bo} and P_{Do}) such that

$$P_{M(h)SN} = P_{Bo} - P_{Do} + \frac{\Delta P_{Bmax} + \Delta P_{Bmin}}{4}$$

where ΔP_{Bmin} and ΔP_{Bmax} represent the minimum and maximum blood pathway pressure drops during each cycle. If such a correction is made, it is possible to use the ultrafiltration coefficients when the device is used in single needle mode.

In haemofiltration, the filtrate flux is less dependent upon the mean hydrostatic pressure and is governed by the haemodynamic conditions. Theoretical relationships using the concentration polarization model have been derived. These relationships are summarised elsewhere (75) and describe the ultrafiltration flux for both flat sheet and hollow fibre devices in terms of geometric dimensions, mean flow rate through the device and wall shear rate.

Table 18 summarises the *in vitro* and *in vivo* ultrafiltration characteristics of standard haemodialysers. *In vitro* results for devices incorporating high flux membranes suitable for haemofiltration or haemodiafiltration are shown in Table 19.

Ideally, *in vitro* and *in vivo* ultrafiltration characteristics for haemodialysers, but not for haemofilters, should be comparable. Experimental studies for haemodialysers from our group show a wider variation between *in vitro* and *in vivo* results than those reported by Keshaviah et al (100), whose studies' differences ranged between 1 and 10% when correcting for plasma oncotic pressure and is a consequence

of membrane fouling by proteins and blood components, a factor that increases in importance for haemofiltration. On the rare occasions that *in vivo* data exceed *in vitro data* at the same transmembrane pressure, it is probably the consequence of interdevice variability.

Taking all factors that contribute to the inter device variability the prediction of the *in vivo* ultrafiltration rate has shown the greatest variability. This variability is of clinical significance in that it is probably responsible for many hypotensive episodes during treatment. This is likely to be of less clinical significance in the future as the use of the newer generation of proportionating systems incorporating ultrafiltration control and monitoring become more widespread.

In accord with ultrafiltration monitoring studies, extrapolation of *in vitro* aqueous data to *in vivo* is not possible due to considerable differences between patients of plasma protein composition and significant variations in membrane permeability.

Factors influencing water transport

Water transport in haemodialysis and haemofiltration depends upon a variety of factors some of which are interlinked and related to the characteristics of the membrane, operating conditions, device geometry, blood composition and temperature.

Table 18. Standard haemodialysers. Ultrafiltration coefficient (ml/hr/mm Hg) measured at a blood flow of 200 ml/min.

	In vitro	*In vivo*
M3 Micropoint	4.4	–
MTL 133	6.1	3.6
Lundia 10-3N	3.9	2.4
Lundia PRO 5	6.8	6.8
BL 501 Bravo	4.4	2.9
Vita 2 HP	4.9	4.6
AM 100M	3.4	2.4
Nephross Allegro HF	5.2	4.9
NT 10.11	3.2	2.7
TAF 10	5.1	4.4
FD 100	5.7	7.1
Hemoflow D2	5.9	4.9
CDAK 90 SCE	2.9	2.6
FB 110T	5.8	5.5
BL 612M Prima	4.4	3.9
GF 120M	3.6	2.9

Dialysate flow 500 to 530 ml/min. Temperature 38° C.

Table 19. High flux devices. Ultrafiltration coefficient (ml/hr/mm Hg) at a blood flow of 200 ml/min.

	In vitro
Biospal 2400	42
HF 060	–
PAN 150	–
AN 69 HF	37.6
F 60	–
B1-100	11.8
CF Duoflux	25.4

Membrane characteristics

Membranes used in artificial organs are batch produced and as such are subject to inter-batch variations.

Ultrafiltration may also be influenced by storage conditions, temperature and humidity, factors which have been studied by Sato and Kidaka (101), who as a result of their experimental studies postulated that in the amorphous region of cellulose, adsorbed molecules of water in the presence of high levels of humidity served as molecular cross links through hydrogen bonding and this reduces the size of the fine pores causing a decrease in ultrafiltration. Other membrane characteristics that have been studied in this context are membrane charge and wettability in haemofilters (99).

Takesawa et al (102) studied the effects of methods of sterilisation on the structure and permeability of regenerated cellulose membranes and demonstrated that both gamma irradiation and autoclave sterilisation influenced hydraulic permeability. These changes being a consequence of pore shrinkage induced by the sterilisation technique.

Membrane porosity may also be affected by strain, particularly in the case of flat sheet membranes where an increase in membrane permeability can occur due to stretching of the membrane over the support structure, although in practice, part of this increase may be cancelled by the draping of the membrane over the support structure (103). Because storage conditions can influence device performance, the manufacturers' recommendations should be followed.

Blood composition

The influence of plasma protein concentration on ultrafiltration rates used in conventional haemodialysis is small. At ultrafiltration rates associated with haemofiltration, its role becomes more significant. In the clinical setting, differences in ultrafiltration rate at equivalent blood flow rates and haematocrits have been noted for different patients using the same filter, while no quantitative studies have been made these differences are thought to be a consequence of differences in protein composition especially lipoproteins.

Haematocrit also influences filtration flux in both conventional and continuous arterio-venous haemofiltration. In the latter the haemoconcentration causes an increase in haematocrit and protein concentration, as well as viscosity, which in turn, increases the flow path pressure drop causing a decrease in blood flow and filtration flux. In conventional haemofiltration, the role of haematocrit has been studied by Okazaki and Yoshida (104) who found a complicated dependence in which variations from normal haematocrit led to variations in the flux.

Fluid dynamic conditions

The role of fluid dynamic conditions in determining ultrafiltration rate is complex, and is related to the device geometry. Its role is particularly important in haemofilters where the filtration flux depends upon the shear rate or the velocity gradient at the membrane surface. Shear rate influences the concentration polarization. However, whereas a high shear rate is desirable in clinical practice, the attainment of such an ideal is limited by the available blood flow and the inability to reduce the blood film thickness below a certain limit due to its influence on pathway resistance.

Temperature

During haemodialysis, temperature differences between the blood and dialysate may exist which influence the ultrafiltration rate (105). Temperature also influences ultrafiltrate flux, and a linear relationship between temperature and ultrafiltration exists over the clinical range of temperatures (61, 106). In haemofiltration values at 37° C being some 34% higher than those established at room temperature (44).

PLASMA FILTRATION

In plasmapheresis or plasma separation, the plasma proteins pass through the membrane which retains formed elements including red cells.

The flow pressure relationship in plasma separation is similar to that seen in haemofiltration in as much as filtration initially rises with increasing transmembrane pressure but then reaches a plateau where further increases in transmembrane pressure do not result in an increase in plasma flux. The point of transition depends on the flow rate through the device and represents the occurrence of haemolysis or cell damage.

In common with haemofiltration, mathematical theories explaining such behaviour have been developed and have been reviewed by Malchesky (51).

Factors influencing plasma filtration

In common with haemofiltration and ultrafiltration, major factors influencing the separation of plasma from whole blood include characteristics of the membrane, operating conditions, device geometry and blood composition (50).

PHYSIOLOGICAL EFFECTS

In describing physiological effects resulting from use of a device, discussion will be confined to effects for which the device is directly responsible. Kinetic considerations, as a consequence of solute removal, are considered in Chapter 4.

REACTIONS MEDIATED BY DEVICES

Blood membrane interactions

Thrombus formation

When non coagulated blood comes into contact with a foreign surface, protein adsorption occurs almost instantaneously and is followed by platelet adhesion and activation of the intrinsic coagulation pathway. To prevent such thrombosis, heparin is used as an anticoagulant.

Dialysis may trigger coagulation or thrombus formation, not only by membrane contact but also by contact with other components of the extracorporeal circuit. The underlying mechanisms for thrombus formation are complex and are probably related to the affinity of a given surface for proteins (98, 99), although factors such as fluid dynamic conditions within the device (107, 108) and patient response to the anticoagulant (109, 110) also play a part.

Heparin requirements during therapy may be assessed by kinetic modelling techniques (111, 112). Patients vary in their requirements while the optimal dose is unknown (113, 114). Too little heparin results in fibrin formation and platelet adhesion, while too much heparin leads to a risk of haemorrhage. In addition, long term high doses of heparin during extracorporeal therapy may lead to osteoporosis (115).

Alternative methods of anticoagulation during extracorporeal therapy have included the use of prostacyclin (69, 116), low molecular weight heparin (117, 118) and hypertonic trisodium citrate (119–121) but heparin remains the most widely used anticoagulant. Requirements during maintenance haemodialysis are established by kinetic methods; such techniques also may be applied to other forms of extracorporeal therapy provided corrections for the elimination of heparin are made.

In addition to contributing to the blood loss at the termination of therapy, foreign surface induced thrombus formation may also be implicated in the formation and subsequent release into the patient's circulation of microemboli (122).

Damage to blood components

During extracorporeal circulation, damage to blood components occurs. The cause of this damage may be mechanical, such as haemolysis induced by blood pumps (123) or the consequence of shear at the membrane surface which may result in not only red cell damage but also platelet damage (124).

The damage incurred during haemodialysis has been studied, and in the case of platelets, Lindsay et al (125) demonstrated a link between platelet damage and clot formation.

The influence of shear rates on red cells has been studied by Blackshear and Patankar (126) who concluded that under laminar flow conditions the damage to erythrocytes was not significant. The role of shear on red and white cell damage during haemofiltration and plasma separation is complex and relates not only to the critical haemolytic point, the transmembrane pressure at which lysis occurs which itself, may be membrane dependent, but also to various other factors including cell diameter, cell membrane tension, membrane pore diameter and cell pore residence time (44,51).

Leucopenia

In the early stages of extracorporeal therapy, a drop in leucocytes occurs which is reversed by the end of the first hour of therapy (Figure 18). The cause of this drop is sequestration of leucocytes in the lung vasculature (127–130) secondary to the activation of complement.

Many studies have shown that the type of membrane plays a major role in the extent of leucopenia and complement activation. Cellulosic membranes produce a profound leucopenia (131–134) but the magnitude of the changes may be influenced by the chemical processes the cellulose undergoes during manufacture (134, 135). Synthetic materials such as those used for haemofiltration (polyacrylonitrile, polysulfone) cause little or no leucopenia (131–134, 136).

White cell activation by complement and/or surface contact is now thought to play a part in the cause of acute cardiorespiratory problems in patients with reduced cardiorespiratory reserve and contribute to the morbidity associated with long term therapy (135).

The differences between membranes have stimulated substantial scientific interest and manufacturers of cellulose based membranes are modifying their production techniques to adjust the bioincompatibility of cellulose membranes to that of synthetic membranes (137). Licencing authorities in discussions set international standards of bioincompatibility and are pressing for such measurements as white cell count changes, and complement activation to be made available when submitting applications for new devices.

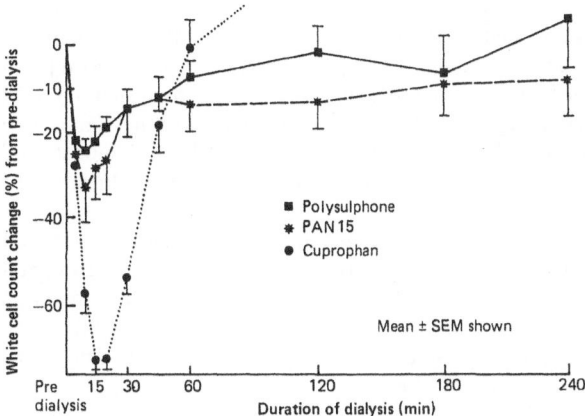

Figure 18. Haemodialysis membrane induced leucopenia.

Eosinophilia

Eosinophilia has been described by a number of investigators as a haemodialysis associated phenomenon (138–140). Its occurrence may express an allergic response to a treatment specific antigen exposition, as eosinophils are considered to modulate local immediate hypersensitivity reactions. On the other hand, it has also been suggested that it may be uraemia related (141).

Complement activation

Activation of the complement system occurs during extracorporeal circulation manifested by a fall in the total complement activity of serum or by falls in complement factors such as C3 or Factor B. More recently, interest has focused on the activated complement components, C3a and C5a.

The activation is a direct consequence of blood membrane contact during therapy (128–130). In common with leucopenia, complement activation by different membranes has received extensive study (131–133, 142–144) but like leucopenia, it remains an interesting laboratory phenomenon without definite clinical implications although Hakim (145) has linked the level of C3 activation with the occurrence of hypersensitivity reactions.

Hypoxia

Patients receiving dialysis treatment experience a fall in arterial oxygen tension (PaO$_2$), which occurs over the same time span as the leucopenia and ranges between 5 and 25%.

The cause of hypoxia, observed during dialysis has been widely studied and the subject of a number of reviews (146–148). Despite extensive study the subject remains inadequately explained and its cause is attributed to both membrane dependent and membrane independent factors. The former involve complement activation induced neutropenia, leading to lung sequestration; membrane independent causes include CO_2 loss to acetate containing dialysate (149), microemboli (150), increased oxygen consumption due to acetate metabolism (149, 151) and treatment induced pH changes. Studies with synthetic membranes (135, 152) and bicarbonate based dialysate (153) have demonstrated decreased complement activation and the amelioration of hypoxia.

In common with leucopenia and complement activation it is uncertain whether its repeated occurrence is detrimental to long term patient survival. The possibility that repeated exposure to activated leucocytes may be associated with irreversible pathological changes is speculative, but merits further investigation.

Haemodialysis related amyloidosis

Amyloid deposits derived from β_2 microglobulin have been identified in the synovium and carpal tunnel tissue of patients treated by long term dialysis (154). The epidemiology of dialysis related amyloidosis is ill defined but it appears to relate to duration of therapy and is rarely seen before the eighth year on dialysis. It affects 50% of patients at 10 years, and 100% at 15 years (155). With the recognition of this long term complication, interest has focused on the mechanisms of production and rate of removal during therapy (155–159).

However, at present it is not clear to what extent the elevated levels observed are a consequence of inadequate removal during therapy, particularly with Cuprophan membranes, or of membrane bioincompatibility with release into the extracellular fluid resulting from the generation of β_2 microglobulin by contact between blood and the membrane (160, 161).

Elution of toxic substances

The manufacture of devices is controlled by Good Manufacturing Practices (GMP) regulations.

Materials used in the construction of devices may be toxic despite their compliance with toxicity standards drawn up for quite different purposes, the toxicity being cumulative since patients on long term renal replacement therapy have a life expectancy beyond two decades.

Membranes contain small amounts of trace metals which may be released during therapy (162, 163).

Acute anaphylactoid reactions using haemodialysers (164, 165), haemofilters (164) and membrane plasma separators (164) have been described in the literature. Such reactions occur within minutes of start of treatment with new devices sterilised with ethylene oxide.

Although a number of authors have described the occurrence of these reactions in their patient populations (164, 166) the only large scale study to assess the incidence of the reactions has been undertaken by Villarroel and Ciarkowski (167) who, on the basis of a 2 year survey of the United States' haemodialysis population, calculated the incidence of reactions as 3.3 reactions per 1,000 patients per annum for hollow fibre dialysers and 0.3 reactions per year per 1,000 patients using flat plate dialysers.

An added complication is the likelihood that there are two types of reactions. The first starts immediately on initiation of treatment, although it may be delayed up to 30 min or more into treatment. Its symptoms are severe and require the administration of antihistamines, epinephrine or steroids and the termination of treatment. The second category of somewhat milder reactions also takes place early during treatment, the most predominant symptoms being chest or back pain but usually it is not necessary to discontinue treatment.

The factors responsible for the reactions are unknown, the most commonly suggested potential cause has been allergic reactions against ethylene oxide used to sterilise the devices (168–171). Since the production of hollow fibres involves the use of a number of toxic substances such as isopropyl myristrate, methanol and freon, their inadequate removal either during manufacture or preparation for use may also be responsible (172). This latter cause remains a distinct possibility as in a number of cases inadequate rinsing of new dialysers prior to use has been identified as a predisposing factor (164).

Rubber components in connectors, tubing and 'O' rings are used widely in haemodialysis equipment, and allergic reactions to these components may occur (173).

Plasticisers and other compounds may leach out of blood lines and bags used in intravenous infusion (174–176). Spallation of particles from blood pump inserts (177, 178) may lead to accumulation of silicone in haemodialysis patients which in turn leads to foreign body reaction with granuloma formation and can be associated with hypercalcemia (179). The migration of acetylated hemicellulose from capillary dialysers leading to scleritis or iritis has also been reported (180).

All new devices contain particulate debris similar to that described in intravenous fluids (181). Although no reactions have been specifically attributed to such particles, Ogden (182) showed that the total particulate weight in filtered blood compartment effluent was 1.2 to 2.2 mg and 0.8 to 1.1 mg in the first and second litre of effluent; some, but probably not all, particles would be removed during priming.

The repeated exposure of dialysis patients to hazards such as these renders them vulnerable, but hard evidence of harm is scant, although eluates from tubing sets and dialysers have been shown to produce cardiac arrythmias (183).

Pyrogen and endotoxin reactions

Pyrogen reactions occur as a complication of extracorporeal therapy. The cause of these reactions in many cases remains a mystery, particularly as the intact dialyser membrane provides an effective barrier against endotoxin from the dialysate (184, 185).

When nondisposable or rebuildable dialysers were used widely, pyrogen reactions were frequently encountered. Manual assembly, soaking of the membranes and chemical sterilisation provided opportunities for the contamination of the blood circuit.

The epidemiology of febrile reactions with disposable dialysers has been the subject of two studies in which the reported incidence of reactions differed significantly. Whereas Kolmos and Moller (186) reported an incidence of 11% in a study of 2,000 dialysers, Schaefer et al (187) in a larger and more recent study, reported an incidence of 4.84%. Both studies agree that the principal cause of the reactions was a result of endogenous factors such as infection, rather than exogenous factors such as dialysate bacteria and pyrogens. The incidence of such reactions during haemofiltration was given by Schaefer et al (187) as 0.81%, while Frei and Koch (188) in a retrospective questionnaire based study of centres practising haemofiltration and haemodiafiltration, elicited a fever incidence of 0.19% in 135,000 treatments.

COST

The membrane separation device constitutes the most expensive disposable component of the extracorporeal circuit.

The cost of devices can vary substantially from country to country, or even centre to centre as many manufacturers offer bulk purchase discounts, particularly for haemodialysers.

In general, devices for haemodialysis utilising cellulose based membranes are less expensive than those using synthetic membranes. For haemodialysers there has been a recent trend towards lower prices in the presence of over capacity in production. The costs of devices for haemofiltration, haemodiafiltration and plasma separation are substantially higher reflecting the increased cost of the membranes used in such devices, as well as their less widespread use and smaller market.

SPECIAL APPLICATIONS OF DEVICES

All devices may be considered as simple mass exchangers and as such, suitable for other potential applications (Table 20).

Table 20. Special applications of renal replacement therapy devices.

Application	Suitable device	Ref.
Heat exchange for hypothermia	Haemodialyser	
Partial respiratory support	Haemodialyser	196
Isolated ultrafiltration for congestive heart failure or fluid overload	Haemodialyser Haemofilter	197
Ascites filtration and reinfusion	Haemofilter Haemodialyser	198–200
Treatment of combined hepatic and renal failure	Haemodialyser	201, 202
Treatment of hepatic failure	Haemofilter Haemodialyser Plasma separator	203–206

CHOICE OF DEVICE

The choice of device for routine use in renal replacement therapy is a complex decision involving not only the functional performance of the device, but also the equipment available as well as the philosophy of treatment.

In haemodialysis, a wide range of devices are available which, coupled with the ability to model mathematically the physiological processes, allows a degree of individualisation of therapy. In practice, however, such individualisation is often limited by practical considerations.

Devices utilising Cuprophan or other cellulose based membranes, remain most widely used in the context of renal replacement therapy. Use of devices utilising synthetic membranes are at present confined to patients being treated by haemofiltration, CAVH or haemodiafiltration, and in conventional haemodialysis for those patients in whom hypersensitivity or allergic reactions to cellulose based membranes have been experienced. Long term therapy has been associated with polyarthropathy thought to be due to production of and failure to remove β_2 microglobulin by cellulose based membranes. It seems likely that bioincompatibility and associated long term morbidity will influence future choices of haemodialysers.

FUTURE TRENDS IN DEVICE DESIGN

Haemodialysers

The relationship between dialyser design parameters and functional performance characteristics is shown in Table 21. Of these, surface area, geometry of blood and dialysate pathways (30,31) and the minimisation of boundary layers at the membrane surface have all received attention (45) and have led to improved performance. Further improvements are likely from the use of the recently developed 5 micron Cuprophan membranes, which allow a reduction in device surface area without change in functional performance, as measured by urea clearance and ultrafiltration (189), such an approach will also help to minimise bioincompatibility (190, 191). If long term mortality and morbidity can be attributed to bioincompatibility then more biocompatible devices will be developed though cost will be a major factor in their implementation into clinical practice.

Haemofilters and high flux devices

The primary purpose of haemofilters and high flux devices, like haemodialysers, is solute removal which is achieved by filtration rather than diffusion. In such devices the maintenance of high flux across the membrane throughout treatment is of critical importance. Flux is governed by concentration polarization of proteins at the membrane surface and relates to the geometric dimensions of the device and the shear rate. Shear rate in turn is governed by clinical parameters such as blood flow, haematocrit and protein composition. These parameters vary between patients, making opti-

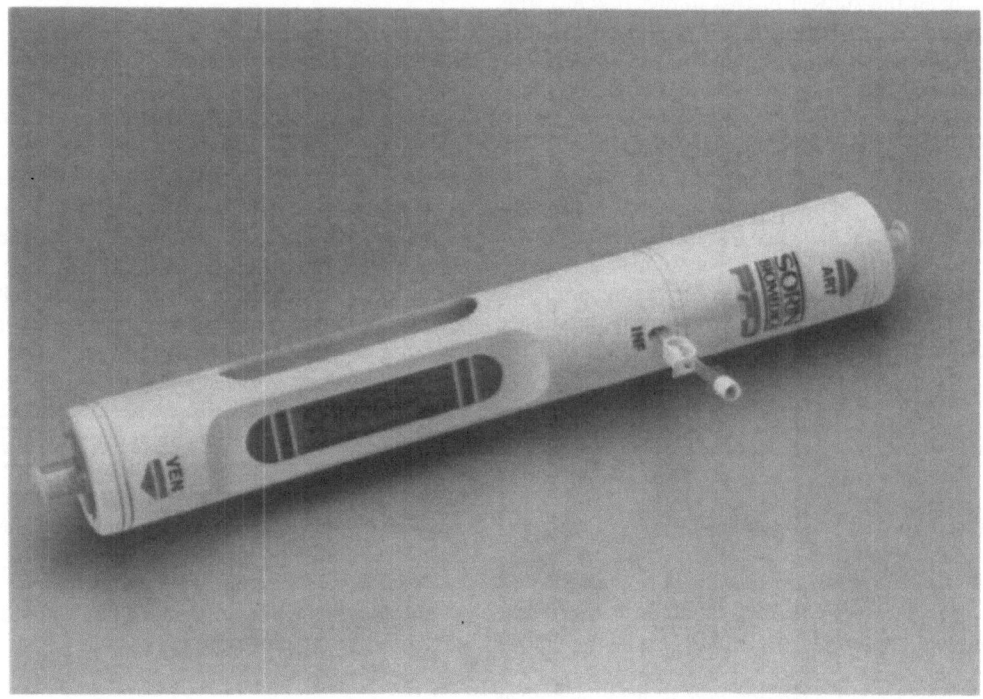

Figure 19. Combined haemodialyser and haemofilter.

misation of shear rate at present difficult. Future designs by monitoring clinical parameters may allow this ideal to be attained. An alternative approach is by the use of vortex mixing in which the boundary layers at the membrane surface are broken up (Figure 13).

Solute transport through high flux membranes is exclusively by convective mass transfer and whereas it is effective for the removal of middle molecular weight solutes, it is less effective for low molecular weight solutes. Haemodiafiltration combines haemodialysis and haemofiltration, but the combined solute total removal rate is less than the sum of the removal rates by diffusion and convection (82). Improvement of solute transport may be achieved by the combination of a haemodialyser and haemofilter into a single unit (Figure 19) (192).

Table 21. Optimization of device design. Influence of design variables on clinical parameters.

Design variable	Clinical parameter					
	Solute removal		Fluid removal	Flow resistance	Blood compartment volume	Blood loss
	Small molecules	Middle molecules				
Device						
Surface area	+	+	+	−	+	+
Blood pathway geometry	++	+	+	+	+	++
Dialysate pathway geometry	+	−	+	+	−	−
Membrane						
Permeability	+	++	++	−	−	−
Geometry	−	+	+	+	−	+

++ Positive influence.
+ Marginal effect.
− No effect.

Plasma filters

The next step in the advancement of plasma separation is likely to focus on the improvement of specificity of the technique that will allow a single toxic substance from the plasma to be removed.

Many of the above developments critically depend upon developments in membrane technology and monitoring equipment. The future radical developments in device design will not only depend upon the availability of new membranes, but also upon the positive identification of the toxins required to be removed.

NOMENCLATURE

C	Concentration
D	Dialysance
HCT or H	Haematocrit
K	Clearance
L	Permeability
$\bar{L}$	Length
N	Integer
P	Pressure
Q	Volumetric flow rate
R	Mass transfer resistance
R'	Recirculation
S	Surface area
S	Sieving coefficient
W	Width
φ	Volume fraction of hydrated proteins
π	Constant
d	Diameter
h	Pathway height
k	Equilibrium solute distribution (partition coefficient) between red cells and plasma
s	Integer
u	Viscosity

Subscripts

B	Blood
D	Dialysate
F	Flux
HFD	Haemodiafiltration
M	Membrane
P	Plasma
R	Recirculation
SN	Single needle
T	Total
W	Water
h	Hydraulic
i	Inlet
max	Maximum
min	Minimum
o	Outlet
Osm	Osmotic

References

1. Drukker W, Haagsma-Schouten WAG, Alberts Chr. Spoek MG: Report on regular dialysis treatment in Europe V, 1969. *Proc Eur Dial Transplant Assoc* 6: 99, 1969
2. Abel JJ, Rowntree LG, Turner BB: On the removal of diffusible substances from the circulating blood of living animals by dialysis. *J Pharmacol Exp Ther* 5: 275, 1913–1914
3. Kolff WJ, Berk HTJ, ter Welle M, van der Ley AJW, van Dijk EC, van Noordwijk J: De kunstmatige nier, een dialysator met groot oppervlak (The artificial kidney, a dialyser with a large surface area). *Geneesk Gids* 21: 409, 1943 (in Dutch)
4. Babb AL, Farrell PC, Uvelli DA, Scribner BH: Hemodialyzer evaluation by examination of solute molecular spectra. *Trans Am Soc Artif Intern Organs* 18: 98, 1972
5. Bluemle LW, Dickson JG, Mitchell J, Podolnick MS: Permeability and hydrodynamic studies on the MacNeil Collins dialyzer using conventional and modified membrane supports. *Trans Am Soc Artif Intern Organs* 6: 38, 1960
6. Edson H, Keen M, Gotch F: Comparative solute transport and therapeutic effectiveness of multiple point support and standard Kiil hemodialyzers. *Trans Am Soc Artif Intern Organs* 18; 113, 1972
7. von Hartitzsch B, Hoenich NA: Meltec Multipoint haemodialyser. *Br Med J* 1: 237, 1972
8. Sakula A: Formalin asthma in hospital laboratory staff. *Lancet* 2: 816, 1975
9. Porter JAH: Acute respiratory distress following formalin inhalation. *Lancet* 2: 603, 1975
10. Hendrick DJ, Lane DJ: Formalin asthma in hospital staff. *Br Med J* 1: 607, 1975
11. Lewis KJ, Dewar PJ, Ward MK, Kerr DNS: Formation of anti-N-like antibodies in dialysis patients: effect of different methods of dialyzer rinsing to remove formaldehyde. *Clin Nephrol* 15: 39, 1981
12. Gotch FA, Keen ML: Formaldehyde kinetics in reused dialyzers. *Trans Am Soc Artif Intern Organs* 29: 396, 1983
13. Hakim RM, Friedrich RA, Lowrie EG, Mantilla JM, Lee C: Formaldehyde kinetics and bacteriology in dialyzers. *Kidney Int* 28: 936, 1985
14. Woffindin C, Hoenich NA: Some aspects of residual formaldehyde testing when reusing hemodialyzers. *Int J Artif Organs* 8: 313, 1985
15. Stragier A, Wenderickx D: Increased sensitivity of residual formaldehyde testing in reused dialysers. *Int J Artif Organs* 9: 277, 1986
16. Howell ED, Perkins HA: Anti-N-like antibodies in the sera of patients undergoing chronic hemodialysis. *Vox Sang* 23: 291, 1972
17. Crosson JT, Moulds J, Comty CM, Polesky HF: A clinical study of anti-N_{DP} in the sera of patients in a large repetitive hemodialysis program. *Kidney Int* 10: 463, 1976
18. Fassbinder W, Seidl S, Koch KM: The role of formaldehyde in the formation of haemodialysis-associated Anti-N-like antibodies. *Vox Sang* 35: 41, 1978
19. Orringer EP, Mattern WD: Formaldehyde-induced hemolysis during chronic hemodialysis. *N Engl J Med* 294: 1416, 1976
20. Maurice F, Rivory JP, Larsson PH, Johansson SGO, Bousquet J: Anaphylactic shock caused by formaldehyde in a patient undergoing long-term hemodialysis. *J Allergy Clin Immunol* 77: 594, 1986
21. McDonald HP, Merrill JP: A disposable parallel flow unit for the MacNeill-Collins artificial kidney – Description and evaluation. *Trans Am Soc Artif Intern Organs* 6: 7, 1960

22. Malchesky PS, Mrava GL, Nose Y: A totally disposable presterilized dialyzer. *Arch Intern Med* 127: 278, 1971

23. Alwall N: A new disposable artificial kidney: experimental and clinical experience. *Proc Eur Dial Transplant Assoc* 5: 18, 1968

24. Hoenich NA, White T, Luno J, Liano F, Kerr DNS: Disposable dialysers-current trends and experiences. In *Technical Aspects of Renal Dialysis,* edited by Frost TH, Tunbridge Wells, Pitman Medical, 1977, p 38

25. Hoeltzenbein J: Efficient and inexpensive, no-prime, no blood-loss haemodialysis system. *Proc Eur Dial Transplant Assoc* 5: 316, 1969

26. Sigdell JE: *A Mathematical Theory for the Capillary Artificial Kidney.* Stuttgart, Hippokrates Verlag, 1974

27. Stewart RD, Cerny JC, Mahon HI: The capillary 'Kidney'. Preliminary report. *Univ Michigan Med Center J* 30: 116, 1964

28. Agishi T, Ota K, Nose Y: Is hollow fibre occlusion due to maldistribution of blood? *Proc Eur Dial Transplant Assoc* 12: 519, 1975

29. Nakagawa S, Koshikawa S, Ishida Y, Uematsu M, Ishibashi K: Development of flat type hollow fibre dialyser (NF-01): achievement of better performance than cylinder type with same membrane area. in: *Technical Aspects of Renal Dialysis* edited by Frost TH, Tunbridge Wells, Pitman Medical, 1977, p 29

30. Lee KH, Taylor JA: Multi-chambered dialyzers and their efficiencies. *Artif Organs* 3: 137, 1979

31. Sigdell JE: New hollow-fiber dialyzers. *Artif Organs* 9: 205, 1985

32. Broyer M, Brunner FP, Brynger H, Fassbinder W, Guillou PJ, Oules R: Demography of dialysis and transplantation in children in Europe, 1984. *Nephrol Dial Transplant* 1: 9, 1986

33. Trachtman H, Hackney P, Tejani A: Pediatric hemodialysis: A decade's (1974–1984) perspective. *Kidney Int* 30: S15, 1986

34. Baluarte HJ, Morgenstern BZ, Kaiser BA, Polinsky MS, Perlman SA, Gruskin AB: Clinical aspects of continuous ambulatory peritoneal dialysis in children. *Dial Transplant* 14: 18, 1985

35. Leichter HE, Salusky IB, Alliapoulos JC, Hall T, Jordan SC, Ettenger RB, Fine RN: CAPD and CCPD in children: an experience of three and a half years. *Dial Transplant* 13: 382, 1984

36. Fischbach M, Tarral E, Koehl C, Coumaros G, Geisert J: High permeable membranes in children: HD or HDF for an optimal blood purification? *Nieren und Hochdruckkrankh* 14: 162, 1985

37. Muller-Wiefel DE, Rauh W, Wingen AM, Mehls O, Scharer K: Hemofiltration in children. *Contr Nephrol* 32: 128, 1982

38. Gardiner AOP, Sawyer AN, Donckerwolcke RA, Haycock GB, Murphy A, Ogg CS, Winder EA, Chantler C: Assessment of dialysis requirement for children on regular hemodialysis. *Dial Transplant* 11: 754, 1982

39. Henderson LW: The beginning of hemofiltration. *Contr Nephrol* 32: 1, 1982

40. Henderson LW, Besarab A, Michaels A, Bluemle LW Jr: Blood purification by ultrafiltration and fluid replacement (diafiltration). *Trans Am Soc Artif Int Organs* 13: 216, 1967

41. Golper TA: Continuous arteriovenous hemofiltration in acute renal failure. *Am J Kidney Dis* 6: 373, 1985

42. Kaplan AA, Longnecker RE, Folkert VW: Continuous arteriovenous hemofiltration. *Ann Intern Med* 100: 358, 1984

43. Dodd NJ, O'Donovan RM, Bennett-Jones DN, Rylance PB, Bewick M, Parsons V, Weston MJ: Arteriovenous haemofiltration: a recent advance in the management of renal failure. *Br Med J* 287: 1008, 1983

44. Ofsthun NJ, Colton CK, Lysaght MJ: Determinants of fluid and solute removal rates during hemofiltration. in: *Hemofiltration,* edited by Henderson LW, Quellhorst EA, Baldamus CA, Lysaght MJ, Berlin, Heidelberg, Springer-Verlag, 1986, p 18

45. Jeffree MA, Peacock J, Sobey IJ, Bellhouse BJ, Increased maximum haemofiltration rates in a vortex mixing haemofilter. *Proc Eur Soc Artif Organs* 8: 150, 1981

46. Vangelista A, Frasca GM, Bonomini V: Parameters for indication of plasmapheresis and the interpretation of results. *Clin Nephrol* 26: S64, 1986

47. Freeman JG, Matthewson K, Record CO: Plasmapheresis in acute liver failure. *Int J Artif Organs* 9: 433, 1986

48. Smith JW, Malchesky PS, Nose Y: Membrane plasmapheresis and the developing technology of plasma therapy. *Cleve Clin Q* 51: 135, 1984

49. Gurland HJ, Samtleben W, Blumenstein M, Randerson DH, Schmidt B: Clinical applications of macromolecular separations. *Trans Am Soc Artif Int Organs* 27: 356, 1981

50. Malchesky PS, Wojcicki J, Horiuchi T, Lee JM, Nose Y: Membrane separation processes for macromolecule removal. in: *Plasmapheresis,* edited by Nose Y, Malchesky PS, Smith JW, Cleveland, ISAO Press, 1983, p 51

51. Malchesky PS: Membrane plasma separation: critical issues. in: *Therapeutic Apheresis: A Critical Look,* edited by Nose Y, Malchesky PS, Smith JW, Cleveland, ISAO Press, 1984 p 93

52. Sueoka A, Malchesky PS, Nose Y: Effects of blood composition in membrane plasma separation. in: *Plasmapheresis,* edited by Nose Y, Malchesky PS, Smith JW, Cleveland, ISAO Press, 1983, p 93

53. Sigdell JE: New hollow-fiber dialyzers. *Artif Organs* 9: 69, 1985

54. Sigdell JE: New hollow-fiber dialyzers on the market. *Artif Organs* 8: 365, 1984

55. Lunt MJ, Powell RJ, Cattell WR: Evaluation of an ultrasonic doppler flowmeter for measurement of extracorporeal blood flow during renal dialysis. in: *Technical Aspects of Renal Dialysis,* edited by Frost TH, Tunbridge Wells, Pitman Medical, 1977, p 210

56. Gotch FA: Hemodialysis: technical and kinetic considerations. in *The Kidney,* edited by Brenner BM, Rector FC Jr, Philadelphia, London, Toronto, Sydney, WB Saunders Co, 1976, p 1672

57. Bosch JP: Continuous arteriovenous hemofiltration. in *Hemofiltration,* edited by Henderson LW, Quellhorst EA, Baldamus CA, Lysaght MJ, Berlin, Heidelberg, Springer-Verlag, 1986, p 234

58. Sigdell JE: Comparison of hollow fiber dialyzers. *Artif Organs,* 5: 401, 1981

59. Pirofsky, B: The determination of blood viscosity in man by a method based on Poiseuille's Law. *J Clin Invest* 32: 292, 1953

60. Lowrie EG, Hampers CL, Merrill JP: Physical principles in hemodialysis. in *Haemodialysis: Principles and Practice,* edited by Bailey GL, New York, Academic Press, 1972, p 195

61. Nolph KD, Fox M, Maher JF: Factors affecting the ultrafiltration rate from standard dialysis coils. *Trans Am Soc Artif Intern Organs* 16: 487, 1970

62. Gunnarsson B, Asaba H, Bergström J, Kiibus A, Soderborg B: Application of gamma camera technique for hemodynamic study of parallel flow dialyzers. *Artif Organs* 4: 201, 1980

63. Longnecker RE, Goffinet JA, Hendler ED: Blood loss during maintenance hemodialysis. *Trans Am Soc Artif Intern Organs* 20: 135, 1974

64. Ireland R, Lutkin J, Evans R, Sharpstone P, Trafford A:

Blood losses from patients on chronic hemodialysis. *Dial Transplant* 11: 782, 1982

65. Stewart WK, Fleming LW: The rupture problem with haemodialysers. *Br J Hosp Med (Equip Suppl)* May 1974, p 47

66. Butruille YA, Leonard EF, Litwak RS: Platelet-platelet interactions and non-adhesive encounters on biomaterials. *Trans Am Soc Intern Organs* 21: 609, 1975

67. Schultz JS, Lindenauer SM, Penner JA, Barenberg S: Determinants of thrombus formation on surfaces. *Trans Am Soc Artif Intern Organs* 26: 279, 1980

68. Petschek H, Adamis D, Kantrowitz AR: Stagnation flow thrombus formation. *Trans Am Soc Artif Intern Organs* 14: 256, 1969

69. Rylance PB, Gordge MP, Ireland H, Lane DA, Weston MJ: Haemodialysis with prostacylin (Epoprostenol) alone. *Proc Eur Dial Transplant Assoc* 21: 281, 1984

70. Lindsay RM, Burton JA, Edward N, Dargie HJ, Prentice CRM, Kennedy AC: Dialyzer blood loss. *Clin Nephrol* 1: 29, 1973

71. Miller JH, Shinaberger JH, Gardner PW: Comparison of new hemodialyzers: 1974–1975. *Dial Transplant* 4: 40, 1975

72. Gorgels J, Tan BH: An evaluation of the performance of current dialyzers in routine use and in vitro. *Dial Transplant* 5: 68, 1976

73. Cripps CM: Rapid method for the estimation of plasma haemoglobin levels. *J Clin Pathol* 21: 110, 1968

74. Lindsay RM, Burton JA, King P, Davidson JF, Boddy K, Kennedy AC: The measurement of dialyzer blood loss. *Clin Nephrol* 1: 24, 1973

75. Gohl H, Konstantin P: Membranes and filters for hemofiltration. in: *Hemofiltration*, edited by Henderson LW, Quellhorst EA, Baldamus CA, Lysaght MJ, Berlin, Heidelberg, Springer-Verlag, 1986, p 42

76. Frost TH, Petrie CJS, Saleh TAM: Hydrodynamics of purging blood filled extra-corporeal circuits. *Institute of Mathematics and its Applications*. August/September: 205, 1978

77. Tello R, March R, Lowrie EG: A model of the reinfusion process at termination of hemodialysis. *Dial Transplant* 12: 444, 1983

78. Clayton CB, Hoenich NA, Keir MJ: The measurement of dialyser washout characteristics. in: *Technical Aspects of Renal Dialysis*, edited by Frost TH, Tunbridge Wells, Pitman Medical 1977, p 65

79. von Hartitzsch B, Hoenich NA, Samson P, Erickson J, Ashcroft RA, Kerr DNS: A clinical evaluation of the new dialysers. *Kidney Int* 3: 35, 1973

80. Colton CK, Henderson LW, Ford CA, Lysaght MJ: Kinetics of hemodiafiltration. I. In vitro transport characteristics of a hollow-fiber blood ultrafilter. *J Lab Clin Med* 85: 355, 1975

81. Henderson LW, Colton CK, Ford CA: Kinetics of hemodiafiltration. II. Clinical characterization of a new blood cleansing modality. *J Lab Clin Med* 85: 372, 1975

82. Gupta BB, Jaffrin MY: In vitro study of combined convection-diffusion mass transfer in hemodialysers. *Int J Artif Organs* 7: 263, 1984

83. Kramer P, Tonnis HJ, Eichelberg B, Kattermann R, Scheler F: Distortion of dialysance by ultrafiltration, and its correction by means of a simple method. *Proc Eur Dial Transplant Assoc* 8: 460, 1971

84. Nolph KD, Nothum RJ, Maher JF: Effects of ultrafiltration on dialysance in commercially available coils. *Kidney Int* 2: 293, 1972

85. Nolph KD, Hopkins C, Van Stone J: Effects of ultrafiltration on solute clearances in parallel plate dialyzers. *Clin Nephrol* 8: 453, 1977

86. Nolph KD, Twardowski ZJ, Hopkins CA, Rubin J, Van Stone JC: Effects of ultrafiltration on solute clearances in Cuprophan and cellulose hollow fiber dialysers: in vitro and clinical studies. *J Lab Clin Med* 91: 998, 1978

87. Colton CK, Smith KA, Merrill EW, Reece JM: Diffusion of organic solutes in stagnant plasma and red cell suspensions. *Chem Eng Progress Symp Series* 66: 85, 1970

88. Farrell PC, Ward RA, Hone PW: Uric acid: binding levels of urate ions in normal and uraemic plasma, and in human serum albumin. *Biochem Pharmacol* 24: 1885, 1975

89. Farrell PC, Grib NL, Fry DL, Popovich RP, Broviac JW, Babb AL: A comparison of in vitro and in vivo solute-protein binding interactions in normal and uremic subjects. *Trans Am Soc Artif Intern Organs* 18: 268, 1972

90. Skalsky M, Schindhelm K, Farrell PC: Creatinine transfer between red cells and plasma: a comparison between normal and uremic subjects. *Nephron* 22: 514, 1978

91. Woffindin C, Hoenich NA, Kerr DNS: The effect of hematocrit on the clearance of small molecules during hemodialysis. *Int J Artif Organs* 6: 127, 1983

92. Grossman NDF, Kopp KF, Frey J: Transport of urea by erythrocytes during haemodialysis. *Proc Eur Dial Transplant Assoc* 4: 250, 1967

93. Sigdell JE, Tersteegen B: Clearance of a dialyzer under varying operating conditions. *Artif Organs* 10: 219, 1986

94. Christopher TG, Cambi V, Harker LA, Hurst PE, Popovich RP, Babb AL, Scribner BH: A study of hemodialysis with lowered dialysate flow rate. *Trans Am Soc Artif Intern Organs* 17: 92, 1971

95. Shinaberger JH, Miller JH, Rosenblatt MG, Gardner PW, Carpenter GW, Martin FE: Clinical studies of 'low flow' dialysis with membranes highly permeable to middle weight molecules. *Trans Am Soc Artif Intern Organs* 18: 82, 1972

96. Hoenich NA, White T, Conceicao S, Luno J, Liano F, Kerr DNS: High efficiency dialysers, miniature and cuprophan hollow fibre. *Proc Eur Dial Transplant Assoc* 14: 601, 1977

97. Rubin JE, Fani K, Friedman EA, Berlyne GM: Use of fluorescent antisera (FAS) to identify blood components deposited on dialyzer membranes. *Trans Am Soc Artif Intern Organs*, 24: 471, 1978

98. Fumero R, Muttoni M, Scuri S, Tanzi MC, Cairo G: Blood-membrane interactions during hemodialysis: the influence of fluid-dynamics, membrane structure and manufacturing process. *Proc Eur Soc Artif Organs*, 13: 301, 1986

99. Lehmann HD, Biesinger U, Bergkvist G, Goehl H, Weber H, Krauth E, Kulbe KD: Haemofilter efficiency as a result of membrane charge and wettability. in: *Biomaterials in Artificial Organs*, edited by Paul JP, Gaylor JDS, Courtney JM, Gilchrist T, London, Basingstoke, Macmillan Press Ltd, 1984, p 238

100. Keshaviah PR, Constantini EG, Luehmann DA, Shapiro FL: Dialyzer ultrafiltration coefficients: comparison between in vitro and in vivo values. *Artif Organs* 6: 23, 1982

101. Sato H, Kidaka T: Effect of moisture on and kinetic features of the ultrafiltration rate of dialysis membrane. *Artif Organs* 5: 286, 1981

102. Takesawa S, Ohmi S, Konno Y, Sekiguchi M, Shitaokoshi S, Takahashi T, Hidai H, Sakai, K: Varying methods of sterilisation, and their effects on the structure and permeability of dialysis membranes. *Nephrol Dial Transplant* 1: 254, 1987

103. Potter LJ, Frost TH: The effect of strain and pre-tension on the permeability of cellulose membranes and on the performance of flat bed dialysers. in: *Technical Aspects of Renal Dialysis*, edited by Frost TH, Tunbridge Wells, Pitman Press, 1977, p 112

104. Okazaki M, Yoshida F: Ultrafiltration of blood: effect of hematocrit on ultrafiltration rate. *Ann Biomed Eng* 4: 138, 1976

105. Grossmann DF, Kopp KF: Thermo-osmotic effect and ultrafiltration in the artificial kidney. Experience with the 'coil kidney'. *Proc Eur Dial Transplant Assoc* 3: 299, 1966

106. Nolph KD, Groshong TD, Maher JF: Estimation of weight loss during coil dialysis. Kidney Int 1: 182, 1972

107. Blackshear PL Jr, Forstrom RJ: Fluid dynamics of blood cells and applications to hemodialysis. *Proc 10th Annu Contractors Conf Artif Kidney program NIAMDD* edited by Mackey BB, DHEW Publ No (NIH) 77–1442, 1977, p 58

108. Blackshear PL Jr, Forstrom RJ: Fluid dynamics of blood cells and applications to hemodialysis. *Proc 8th Annu Contractors' Conf Artif Kidney Program NIAMDD,* edited by Mackey BB, DHEW Publ No (NIH) 75–248, 1975, p 59

109. Wilhelmsson S, Lins LE: Heparin elimination and hemostasis in hemodialysis. *Clin Nephrol* 22: 303, 1984

110. Lindsay RM: Variable heparin requirements during hemodialysis – Why? *asaio J* 3: 81, 1980

111. Gotch FA, Keen ML: Precise control of minimal heparinization for high bleeding risk hemodialysis. *Trans Am Soc Artif Intern Organs* 23: 168, 1977

112. Khazine F, Simons O: Pharmacokinetics monitoring of heparin therapy for regular hemodialysis. *Artif Organs* 9: 59, 1985

113. Cipolle RJ, Seifert RD, Neilan BA, Zaske DE, Haus E: Heparin kinetics: Variables related to disposition and dosage. *Clin Pharmacol Ther* 29: 387, 1981

114. Talstad I, Kjelby K: Analysis of heparinization methods during hemodialysis. *Am J Clin Pathol* 84: 317, 1985

115. Griffiths GC, Nichols G, Asher JD, Flanagan B: Heparin osteoporosis. *JAMA* 193: 85, 1965

116. Camici M, Evangelisti L: Prostacyclin and heparin during haemodialysis: Comparative effects. *Life Support Systems* 4: 205, 1986

117. Lane DA, Ireland H, Flynn A, Anastassiades E, Curtis JR: Haemodialysis with low MW heparin: Dosage requirements for the elimination of extracorporeal fibrin formation. *Nephrol Dial Transplant* 1: 179, 1986

118. Renaud H, Moriniere P, Dieval J, Abdull-Massih Z, Dkhissi H, Toutlemonde F, Delobel J, Fournier A: Low molecular weight heparin in haemodialysis and haemofiltration – comparison with unfractioned heparin. *Proc Eur Dial Transplant Assoc* 21: 276, 1984

119. von Brecht JH, Flanigan MJ, Freeman RM, Lim VS: Regional anticoagulation: Hemodialysis with hypertonic trisodium citrate. *Am J Kidney Dis* 8: 196, 1986

120. Flanigan MJ, von Brecht J, Freeman RM, Lim VS: Reducing the hemorrhagic complications of hemodialysis: A controlled comparison of low-dose heparin and citrate anticoagulation. *Am J Kidney Dis* 9: 147, 1987

121. Kelleher SP, Schulman G: Severe metabolic alkalosis complicating regional citrate hemodialysis. *Am J Kidney Dis* 9: 235, 1987

122. Bischel MD, Scoles BG, Mohler JG: Evidence for pulmonary microembolization during hemodialysis. *Chest* 67: 335, 1975

123. Veitch P, Hawkins F, Frost TH, Jolly D, Kerr DNS: Factors affecting haemolysis in extracorporeal dialysis circuits. in: *Technical Aspects of Renal Dialysis,* edited by Frost TH, Tunbridge Wells, Pitman Medical, 1977, p 218

124. Leonard EF: Biocompatibility issues in single-needle dialysis. in: *1st Int Symposium on Single-Needle Dialysis,* edited by Ringoir S, Vanholder R, Ivanovich P, Cleveland, ISAO Press, 1984, p 203

125. Lindsay RM, Prentice CRM, Davidson JF, Burton JA. McNicol GP: Haemostatic changes during dialysis associated with thrombus formation on dialysis membranes. *Br Med J* 4: 454, 1972

126. Blackshear PL Jr, Patankar SV: Fluid dynamics of blood cells and applications to hemodialysis. *Proc 11th Annu Contractors' Conf Artif Kidney Program NIAMDD,* edited by Mackey BB, DHEW Publ No (NIH) 79–1442, 1978, p 97

127. Toren M, Goffinet JA, Kaplow LS: Pulmonary bed sequestration of neutrophils during hemodialysis. *Blood* 36: 337, 1970

128. Craddock PR, Hammerschmidt D, White JG, Dalmasso AP, Jacob HS: Complement (C5a)-induced granulocyte aggregation in vitro. *J Clin Invest* 60: 260, 1977

129. Craddock PR, Fehr J, Brigham KL, Kronenberg RS, Jacob HS: Complement and leukocyte-mediated pulmonary dysfunction in hemodialysis. *N Engl J Med* 296: 769, 1977

130. Craddock PR, Fehr J, Dalmasso AP, Brigham KL, Jacob HS: Hemodialysis leukopenia. Pulmonary vascular leukostasis resulting from complement activation by dialyzer cellophane membranes. *J Clin Invest* 59: 879, 1977

131. Amadori A, Candi P, Sasdelli M, Massai G, Favilla S, Passaleva A, Ricci M: Hemodialysis leukopenia and complement function with different dialyzers. *Kidney Int* 24: 775, 1983

132. Jacob AI, Gavellas G, Zarco R, Perez G, Bourgoignie JJ: Leukopenia, hypoxia, and complement function with different hemodialysis membranes. *Kidney Int* 18: 505, 1980

133. Wegmuller E, Montandon A, Nydegger U, Descoeudres C: Biocompatibility of different hemodialysis membranes: activation of complement and leukopenia. *Int J Artif Organs* 9: 85, 1986

134. Woffindin C, Johnston SRD, Hoenich NA, Quereshi M, Kerr DNS: Membrane-induced neutropenia. In: *Biomaterials in Artificial Organs,* edited by Paul JP, Gaylor JDS, Courtney JM, Gilchrist T, London, Basingstoke, Macmillan Press Ltd, 1984, p 64

135. Ivanovich P, Chenoweth DE, Schmidt R, Klinkmann H, Boxer LA, Jacob HS, Hammerschmidt DE: Cellulose acetate hemodialysis membranes are better tolerated than Cuprophan. *Contr Nephrol* 37: 78, 1984

136. Fawcett S, Hoenich NA, Woffindin C, Ward MK: Influence of high permeability synthetic membranes on gas exchange and lung function during hemodialysis. *Contr Nephrol* 46: 83, 1985

137. Bosch T, Schmidt B, Samtleben W, Gurland HJ: Biocompatibility and clinical performance of a new modified cellulose membrane. *Clin Nephrol* 26: S22, 1986

138. Scheuermann EH, Fassbinder W, Frei U, Koch KM, Baldamus CA: Eosinophilia in hemodialysis. *Contr Nephrol* 36: 133, 1983

139. Novello AC, Port FK: Hemodialysis eosinophilia. *Int J Artif Organs* 5: 5, 1982

140. Bodner G, Peer G, Zakuth V, Spirer ZH, Aviram A: Dialysis-induced eosinophilia. *Nephron* 32: 63, 1982

141. Backenroth R, Spinowitz BS, Galler M, Golden RA, Rascoff JH, Charytan C: Comparison of eosinophilia in patients undergoing peritoneal dialysis and hemodialysis. *Am J Kidney Dis* 8: 186, 1986

142. Cheung AK, Henderson LW: Effects of complement activation by hemodialysis membranes. *Am J Nephrol* 6: 81, 1986

143. Levett DL, Woffindin C, Bird AG, Hoenich NA, Ward MK, Kerr DNS: Complement activation in haemodialysis: a comparison of new and re-used dialysers. *Int J Artif Organs* 9: 97, 1986

144. Levett DL, Woffindin C, Bird AG, Hoenich NA, Ward MK,

Kerr DNS: Haemodialysis-induced activation of complement. *Blood Purif* 4: 185, 1986

145. Hakim RM: Clinical sequelae of complement activation in hemodialysis. *Clin Nephrol* 26: S9, 1986

146. Eiser AR: Pulmonary gas exchange during hemodialysis and peritoneal dialysis: Interaction between respiration and metabolism. *Am J Kidney Disease* 6: 131, 1985

147. Francos GC, Besarab A, Burke JF, Peters J, Tahamont MV, Gee MH, Flynn JT, Gzesh D: Dialysis-induced hypoxemia: Membrane dependent and membrane independent causes. *Am J Kidney Disease* 5: 191, 1985

148. Nissenson AR, Kraut JA, Shinaberger JH: Dialysis-associated hypoxemia: Pathogenesis and prevention. *asaio J* 7: 1, 1984

149. Sherlock J, Ledwith J, Letteri J: Hypoventilation and hypoxemia during hemodialysis. Reflex response to removal of CO_2 across the dialyzer. *Trans Am Soc Artif Intern Organs* 23: 406, 1977

150. Bischel MD, Scoles BG, Mohler JG: Evidence for pulmonary microembolization during hemodialysis. *Chest* 67: 335, 1975

151. Patterson RW, Nissenson AR, Miller J, Smith RT, Narins RG, Sullivan SF: Hypoxemia and pulmonary gas exchange during hemodialysis. *J Appl Physiol* 50: 259, 1981

152. Hakim RM, Lowrie EG: Hemodialysis-associated neutropenia and hypoxemia: the effect of dialyzer membrane materials. *Nephron* 32: 32, 1982

153. Nissenson AR: Prevention of dialysis-induced hypoxemia by bicarbonate dialysis. *Trans Am Soc Artif Intern Organs* 26: 339, 1980

154. Bardin T, Zingraff J, Kuntz D, Drüeke T: Dialysis – related amyloidosis. *Nephrol Dial Transpl* 1: 151, 1986

155. Floege J, Granolleras C, Bingel M, Deschodt G, Branger B, Oules R, Koch KM, Shaldon S: B_2-microglobulin kinetics during haemodialysis and haemofiltration. *Nephrol Dial Transpl* 1: 223, 1987

156. Rockel A, Hertel J, Fiegel P, Abdelhamid S, Panitz N, Walb D: Permeability and secondary membrane formation of a high flux polysulfone hemofilter. *Kidney Int* 30: 429, 1986

157. Shaldon S, Koch KM, Dinarello CA, Colton CK, Knudsen PJ, Floege J, Granolleras C: B_2-microglobulin and haemodialysis. *Lancet* 1: 925, 1987

158. Bonal J, Pastor MC, Romero R, Corominas A, Caralps A: B_2-microglobulin and haemodialysis. *Lancet* 1: 926, 1987

159. Mayer G, Thum J, Woloszczuk W, Graf H: B_2-microglobulin and haemodialysis. *Lancet* 1: 927, 1987

160. Hauglustaine D, Waer M, Michielsen P, Goebels J, Vandeputte M: Haemodialysis membranes, serum B_2-microglobulin, and dialysis amyloidosis. *Lancet*, 1: 1211, 1986

161. Bergström J, Wehle B: No change in corrected B_2-microglobulin concentration after Cuprophane haemodialysis. *Lancet* 1: 628, 1987

162. Zazgornik J, Schmidt P: Effects of zinc-containing dialysis membranes on zinc metabolism in patients on RDT. *Proc Eur Dial Transplant Assoc* 9: 548, 1972

163. Barbour BH, Bischel M, Abrams DE: Copper accumulation in patients undergoing chronic hemodialysis. The role of Cuprophan. *Nephron* 8: 455, 1971

164. Nicholls AJ, Platts MM: Anaphylactoid reactions due to haemodialysis, haemofiltration, or membrane plasma separation. *Br Med J* 285: 1607, 1982

165. Daugirdas JT, Ing TS, Roxe DM, Ivanovich PT, Krumlovsky F, Popli S, McLaughlin MM: Severe anaphylactoid reactions to Cuprammonium cellulose hemodialyzers. *Arch Intern Med* 145: 489, 1985

166. Foret M, Kuentz F, Hachache T, Christollet M, Milongo R, Meftahi H, Dechelette E, Cordonnier DJ: Hypersensitivity reactions during haemodialysis in France. *Proc Eur Dial Transplant Assoc Eur Ren Assoc* 22: 181, 1985

167. Villarroel F, Ciarkowski AA: A survey on hypersensitivity reactions in hemodialysis. *Artif Organs* 9: 231, 1985

168. Pearson F, Bruszer G, Lee W, Sagona M, Sargent H, Woods E, Dolovich J, Caruana R: Ethylene oxide sensitivity in hemodialysis patients. *Artif Organs*, 11: 100, 1987

169. Bommer J, Ritz E: Ethylene oxide (ETO) as a major cause of anaphylactoid reactions in dialysis (A Review). *Artif Organs* 11: 111, 1987

170. Marshall CP, Pearson FC, Sagona MA, Lee W, Wathen RL, Ward RA, Dolovich J: Reactions during hemodialysis caused by allergy to ethylene oxide gas sterilization. *J Allergy Clin Immunol* 75: 563, 1985

171. Lemke HD, Kuentz F, Foret M: Mechanisms of hypersensitivity reactions during hemodialysis. *Trans Am Soc Artif Intern Organs* 31: 149, 1985

172. Keshaviah P, Luekmann D, Shapiro F, Comty CM: Investigation of the risks and hazards associated with hemodialysis devices. *FDA Medical Device Standards Publication, Technical Report*, DHEW publication, contract no 223-78-5046, US Govt Printing Office, 1980

173. Buxton PK, Going SM, Hunter JAA, Winney RJ: Allergic reaction to rubber chemicals in haemodialysis equipment. *Br Med J* 287: 1513, 1983

174. Ljunggren L: Plasticizer migration from blood lines in hemodialysis. *Artif Organs* 8: 99, 1984

175. Bommer J, Von Sonntag C, Buchler N, Ritz E: Diethylhexyl phthalate leakage from dialysis tubing. *Proc Int Soc Artif Organs* 1: 504, 1983

176. Kevy S, Jacobson M: Hepatic effects of the leaching of phthalate ester plasticizer and silicon. *Contr Nephrol* 36: 82, 1983

177. Barron D, Harbottle S, Hoenich NA, Morley AR, Appleton D, McCabe JF: Particle spallation induced by blood pumps in hemodialysis tubing sets. *Artif Organs* 10: 226, 1986

178. Leong ASY, Disney APS, Gove DW: Spallation and migration of silicone from blood-pump tubing in patients in hemodialysis. *N Engl J Med* 306: 135, 1982

179. Altmann P, Dodd S, Williams A, Marsh F, Cunningham J: Silicone-induced hypercalcaemia in haemodialysis patients. *Nephrol Dial Transpl* 2: 26, 1987

180. Oba T, Tsuji K, Nakamura A, Shintani H, Mizumachi S, Kikuchi H, Kaniwa M, Kojima S, Kanohta K, Kawasaki Y, Furuya T, Matsumoto K, Tobe M: Migration of acetylated hemicellulose from capillary hemodialyzer to blood, causing scleritis and/or iritis. *Artif Organs* 8: 429, 1984

181. Marshall L, Lloyd G: Intravenous fluid filtration. *Care of the Critically Ill* 3 (1): 10, 1987

182. Ogden DA: Clinical responses to new and reprocessed hemodialyzers. in *Guide to Reprocessing of Hemodialyzers*, edited by Deane N, Wineman RJ, Bemis JA, The Hague, Martinus Nijhoff, 1986, p 87

183. Autian J, Lawrence WH, Dillingham EO, Beyer SA, Bigelow CL, Kleiman A: Detection of toxicity of extracted constituents from dialyzers and components. *Proc 10th Annu Contractors Conf Artif Kidney Program NIAMDD*, edited by Mackey BB, DHEW publ No (NIH) 77-1442, 1977, p 71

184. Port FK, Bernick JJ: Pyrogen and endotoxin reactions during hemodialysis. *Contr Nephrol* 36: 100, 1983

185. Bernick JJ, Port FK, Favero MS: In vivo studies of dialysis-related endotoxemia and bacteremia. *Nephron* 27: 307, 1981

186. Kolmos HJ, Moller S: The epidemiology of febrile reactions in

haemodialysis. *Acta Med Scand* 203: 345, 1978

187. Schaefer K, von Herrath D, Hufler M, Pauls A: The occurrence of fever during hemodialysis and hemofiltration. A comparative study. *Int J Artif Organs,* 9: 247, 1986

188. Frei U, Koch KM: Fever and shock during haemofiltration. *Contr Nephrol* 36: 107, 1983

189. Van der Steen A: Research on dialyzers with improved biocompatibility. *Clin Nephrol* 26: S39, 1986

190. Schaefer RM, Rautenberg W, Neumann S, Heidland A, Horl WH: Improvement of dialyzer compatibility by reduction of membrane surface area. *Clin Nephrol* 26: S35, 1986

191. Mahiout A, Meinhold H, Kessel M, Schulze H, Baurmeister U: Dialyzer membranes: effect of surface area and chemical modification of cellulose on complement and platelet activation. *Artif Organs* 11: 149, 1987

192. Botella J, Ghezzi PM, Zucchelli P, Koutsikos D, Sanz-Moreno C, Nigrelli S, Santoro A, Spongano M, Cento G: Two-chamber technique: Adequate philosophy for blood purification. *Nephrol Dial Transpl* 1: 101, 1986

193. Anonymous: Manufacturers' Technical Information, Ab Gambro, Lund, Sweden

194. Anonymous: Manufacturers' Technical Information, Hospal, Lyons, France

195. Anonymous: Manufacturers' Technical Information, Fresenius Ag, Bad Homburg, FRG

196. Kostopoulos C, Rassidakis A, Johios J, Rokas S, Kontoleon P, Ziroyannis P, Moulopoulos S: Cuprophan and cellulose acetate hemodialyzers for partial respiratory support. *Proc Eur Soc Artif Organs* 13: 279, 1986

197. Verbanck J, Schelstraete J, De Paepe M, Hoenich N, Lameire N, Ringoir S: Pure ultrafiltration by repeated puncture of a peripheral arm-vein as treatment of refractory edema. *Int J Artif Organs* 3: 342, 1980

198. Epstein M, Perez GO, Bedoya LA, Molina R: Continuous arterio-venous ultrafiltration in cirrhotic patients with ascites or renal failure. *Int J Artif Organs* 9: 253, 1986

199. Landini S, Coli U, Fracasso A, Morachiello P, Righetto F, Scanferia F, Gallenda F, Bazzato G: Spontaneous ascites filtration and reinfusion (SAFR) as ambulatory chronic treatment for hepatorenal syndrome. *Trans Am Soc Artif Intern Organs* 31: 439, 1985

200. Landini S, Coli U, Fracasso A, Morachiello P, Righetto F, Scanferla F, Genchi R, Bazzato G: Spontaneous ascites filtration and reinfusion (SAFR) in cirrhotic patients. *Int J Artif Organs* 8: 277, 1985

201. Adler AJ, Feldman J, Friedman EA, Berlyne GM: Use of extracorporeal ascites dialysis in combined hepatic and renal failure. *Nephron* 30: 31, 1982

202. Strand V, Mayor G, Ristow G, Greenbaum D, Mayle J, Rosenbaum R: Concomitant renal and hepatic failure treated by polyacrylonitrile membrane hemodialysis. *Int J Artif Organs* 4: 136, 1981

203. Denis J, Guerin J-M, Opolon P, Huguet C, Levy V-G, Poupon R: Hemofiltration with a high permeability membrane in the treatment of fulminant or end stage Wilson's disease. *asaio J* 6: 36, 1983

204. Matsushita M, Nose Y: Artificial liver. *Artif Organs* 10: 378, 1986

205. Wilkinson SP, Weston MJ, Parsons V, Williams R. Dialysis in the treatment of renal failure in patients with liver disease. *Clin Nephrol* 8: 287, 1977

206. Al Mardini H, Hoenich N, Bartlett K, Record CO: Comparative value of different dialysis membranes, including a carbon coated membrane for removal of noxious substances in hepatic coma. *Int J Artif Organs* 2: 290, 1979

MEMBRANES FOR EXTRACORPOREAL THERAPY

SALIM K. MUJAIS and PETER IVANOVICH

INTRODUCTION

The maintenance of a stable internal milieu by the kidney involves an intricate array of functions, and calls into play a variety of mechanisms including hydraulic forces, selective permeability barriers, specialized transport systems and exactingly regulated synthetic machinery. Replacement of renal function artificially is a formidable task in view of the need to balance intended goals and available technologies. The elegant apparent simplicity of the hemodialysis concept contrasts sharply with the acknowledged complexity of renal mechanisms. It is a tribute to the imaginative approach of hemodialysis pioneers to attempt a formidable task with simple means. With time, however, the ostensible simplicity of dialysis has been shown to mask cardinal sophistication and an underlying complexity.

The central component of the hemodialysis process is the membrane which is the ultimate determinant of the success of therapy. Early membranes were, like other components of the procedure, technologically primitive. While modernization of the other components of the procedure is reaching a plateau, improvements in membrane quality, efficiency, and safety are, and need to be, continuously improving. The approach that we will follow in this chapter will be first to put the present state and future of membrane qualities in perspective by defining the characteristics of the ideal dialysis membrane; and second, to present a comparative overview of available membranes as a guide for dialysis prescription and patient safety.

Membranes are traditionally perceived as *diffusive-convective structures*. Information emerging from new studies, however, suggests a more complex role. Membranes have now to be viewed in reference to their capacity to activate plasma proteins and enzymatic cascades of the coagulation and complement pathways, hence they can be conceived of as *activator or interactive structures*. Additionally, membranes are capable of binding plasma components, hence their new aspect as *adsorptive structures*.

CHARACTERISTICS OF AN IDEAL MEMBRANE

What wishes would we request from this modern genie encased in a sealed dialyser? As the legendary Aladdin did we shall choose three, but with more cunning, will define these wishes in categories rather than items. An ideal membrane would need to be ideal in three areas: diffusive, reactive and adsorptive properties.

Diffusive-convective properties

Ideal *diffusive-convective* properties would include high diffusion for small solutes, particularly phosphate; selective permeability to specific toxic molecules of medium to large molecular weight (middle molecules and β_2-microglobulin); and a water permeability that allows easy and controllable ultrafiltration.

Reactive properties

Ideal *reactive* properties will intuitively lie in the negative zone. An ideal membrane is expected to be inert with no interaction with blood components: no activation of complement or coagulation pathways; no interaction with nucleated blood cells and the ensuing release of monokines and enzymes; no trapping of, or damage to, cellular blood constituents.

Adsorptive properties

Ideal *adsorptive* properties need to be qualified depending on the use for the membrane. In membranes used for regular dialysis, indiscriminate protein and drug binding should be viewed as a negative property. Adsorption leads to interference with plasma constituents and depletion of drug stores, thereby necessitating adjustements of drug doses intermittently to parallel the intermittent nature of the therapy. Protein binding can also limit the therapeutic usefulness of a membrane by limiting its diffusive capacity. This becomes particularly important with the advent of the new high flux membranes (1). Some selective adsorptive properties can, however, be viewed as positive, such as binding of pathologic proteins, a term we use to characterize those proteins that accumulate in abnormal quantities in dialysis patients and lead to pathology, such as β_2-microglobulin implicated in the pathogenesis of localized amyloidosis and carpal tunnel syndrome (2–4). Removal of specific abnormal proteins in nonuremic conditions is also a desirable characteristic, and work along those lines is progressing (5, 6). Indeed, it will not be long before membrane-immobilized monoclonal antibodies (5) or hormones (6), become routine therapy.

Physical characteristics

The ideal membrane will also need to have physical characteristics that will insure its operative usefulness such as physical integrity (no predisposition to rupture or particle release, stability under variant pressure gradients) and limited compliance and distensibility. Finally, it should be remembered that the membrane is an integral part of a system and that those properties that are deemed ideal for the membrane need to be complemented by the properties of the entire operative system.

CHARACTERISTICS OF AVAILABLE MEMBRANES

Membranes made from a wide variety of material have been evaluated and used for extracorporeal therapy (Table 1). These can be divided conveniently into those of cellulosic origin and those of synthetic origin. This large number of chemicals reflects the continuing search for membranes with better characteristics either by alteration in the chemical constitution of available membranes or by synthesis of new membranes. In both of these processes a great deal of ingenuity has been manifested, particularly in the former. The fortuitous choice of cellulose by dialysis pioneers could not have been more appropriate in view of the amenability of the polymer to useful manipulations.

Physico-chemical characteristics

The chemical diversity of membranes is reflected in differing physico-chemical characteristics, transport properties, and interactive behavior. Two physico-chemical characteristics of clinical relevance are the hydrophilicity of membranes and their charge since both play a role in influencing adsorption of the solute to membrane surface and thereby affect the transport characteristics of the membrane.

Hydrophilicity

Hydrophilicity is a measure of wettability and is due to the interaction of terminal groups, such as carboxyl, amino or hydroxyl groups, with water by hydrogen bonding (7). Cellulose and cellulose based membranes and polyethylene-polyvinyl alcohol copolymer have high hydrophilicity, whereas polyacrylonitrile, polyamide and polymethyl methacrylate have low hydrophilicity (7). The lower the hydrophilicity of a membrane, the greater the adsorption of protein during use. In addition to differences in hydrophilicity, membranes can differ in the response to wetting. Cuprophan membranes for example double in thickness when wetted, cellulose acetate has minimal increase in thickness whereas synthetic membranes do not swell (8, 9).

Charge

Membrane surface charge is created by dissociation of groups into ions when immersed in water. Negative charges are created by dissociating acidic groups such as carboxyl ($COOH \rightarrow COO^- + H^+$) or sulfonyl groups whereas positive charge by quarternation of amino compounds ($NH_3 + H^+ \rightarrow NH_4^+$) (7). The net charge on a membrane surface depends on the balance of various dissociating groups. It is also altered by the adsorption of proteins (10). Basic membrane charge, and its alteration by the adsorbing protein, are likely insignificant for small solutes, but may affect the sieving of large molecular weight substances (10).

Symmetry

Membranes can have a *symmetric* structure whereby both sides of the membrane are similar, either because a skin is present on both sides or because the membrane is uniform throughout. Alternatively, they can be asymmetric with the

Table 1. Chemicals used as membranes for extracorporeal therapy.

Cellulosic membranes
Regenerated cellulose
Cuprophan (Cuprammonium rayon and derivatives)
Cellulose acetate, diacetate, and triacetate
Saponified cellulose ester

Synthetic polymers
By linear polycondensation
Polysulfone and sulfonated polysulfone
Polyamide (aromatic and aliphatic-aromatic)
Polyether-sulfone
Polycarbonate
By linear addition
Ethylene-vinylalcohol copolymer
Polymethyl methacrylate
Polyacrilonitrile
Polyacrylonitrile-Na methallyl sulfonate
Polyethylene-polyvinyl alcohol
Polyelectrolytes

Modified from (7).

skin on one side, usually that which interfaces with blood, with the remaining part of the membrane more porous and serving a supportive function. These two structural forms are produced by varying the process of manufacture. Asymmetric membranes are produced by rapid precipitation (see below for detail on membrane manufacturing). Symmetric membranes are obtained by slow precipitation. In asymmetric membranes, the skin is responsible for the permeability properties of the membrane. Asymmetry allows for very high diffusive permeability and asymmetric membranes are therefore commonly used in hemofiltration. Polyamide and polysulfone membranes in clinical use, are examples of asymmetric membranes. The symmetry or asymmetry of a membrane is independent of the chemical nature of the membrane, and depends almost exclusively on the precipitation step because symmetric and asymmetric membranes have been produced from the same chemical such as polyacrylonitrile (7).

Thickness

The diffusive flux or permeability accross a membrane is the result of the ratio of diffusion coefficient to membrane *thickness*. The diffusion coefficient depends on the pore structure of the membrane and the interaction of the solute with the polymer. This characteristic is set by the preparation process of the membrane and is independent of membrane thickness. It follows that reduction of membrane thickness for the same diffusion coefficient leads to higher diffusive permeability. The historical trend in membrane manufacture, particularly for cuprophan, is for decreasing thickness allowing for greater diffusion and permitting reduction in membrane surface area. For a preset clearance of urea of 150 ml/min, reduction of membrane thickness from $16\,\mu M$ to $5\,\mu M$, allows reduction of surface area from 1.6 to $0.5\,m^2$. The latter change can be expected to reduce further problems with biocompatibility as well as lower priming volume. The effect of reduction in membrane thickness for cuprophan hollow fiber dialysers can be gleaned from inspection of Table 2. For the product of every manufacturer, a thinner membrane leads to a substantial increase in ultrafiltration coefficient. For the listed hollow fibers, reduction of membrane thickness from $11\,\mu M$ to 8 or $9\,\mu M$ results in an increase in ultrafiltration coefficient from 3.9 ± 0.1 to 5.35 ± 0.2 ml/h/mm Hg, an increment in vitamin B_{12} clearance from $37.4 \pm$ to 47.2 ± 2.1 ml/min, and a modest improvement in urea clearance from 162.8 ± 2.2 to 169.4 ± 2.6 ml/min. Table 3 lists representative thickness of currently used membranes. It is noted that synthetic highly permeable membranes are thicker than less permeable cellulosic membranes. This apparent paradox is resolved by the greater diffusion coefficient of synthetic membranes.

Membrane chemistry and manufacturing

An examination of the chemical basis of membranes and the

Table 2. Characteristics of cuprophan hollow fiber dialysers of $1\,m^2$ surface area.

Manufacturer	Fiber wall (μM)	Kf ml/min/ mm Hg	Clearance (ml/min)	
			urea	vitamin B_{12}
Bellco (BL611L)	11	3.3	154	33
COBE (HF100)	11	4.2	165	33
ERIKA (C-10)	10	5.2	175	50
FRESENIUS (C1,0)	11	4.0	169	36
FRESENIUS (D2)	10	6.3	180	50
GAMBRO (120M)	11	4.4	167	44
GAMBRO (120H)	8	6.1	171	55
HOSPAL (110)	11	4.0	170	34
Idemsa (10N)	11	3.7	164	39
Inphardial (3)	8	5.3	173	47
Renak (E-10L)	16	2.9	147	32
Renak (E-10M)	11	4.3	165	42
Renak (E10-H)	9	5.4	170	52
I-Flow (100)	16	2.7	153	53
Niprizer (C-110)	11	4.4	163	43
Niprizer (D-110)	16	3.2	155	34
Niprizer (F-110)	8	6.1	176	51
Nephross (andante)	11	4.2	165	33
SECON (119)	11	3.1	155	30
SECON (120)	8	3.9	157	35
SMAD (GL10)	9	4.6	160	40
SORIN (NT1108)	8	5.3	163	45
SORIN (SF1.0)	11	3.3	145	33
TERUMO (TE10)	11	3.7	160	41
TRAVENOL (CF.15.11)	11	4.1	175	46

changes in properties that follow chemical alterations of basic molecules is very instructive. Cellulose was the first membrane material used in hemodialysis and, with its derivatives, remains by far the most used membrane in the field. Cellulose is a naturally occuring linear condensation D-glucose polymer obtained from cotton linters with cellobiose (dimer of glucose) as the fundamental structural unit. Cuprophan and cellulose acetates are derived from cellulose. Most other types are of synthetic origin.

Although the chemical details may differ, most membranes are formed along the following general scheme: 1) formation of the soluble polymer; 2) controlled precipitation of the solid polymer; and 3) final geometric finishing and manufacture. The first two steps are referred to as *phase inversion* since the alternation from solvent to nonsolvent solutions induces a change in membrane state from a liquid phase to a solid phase. Manipulation of membrane characteristics can be done at any and all of these steps. The relative composition and chemical nature can be altered in step 1. Partial evaporation of the solvent can be used to create a skin on the membrane and induce the asymmetric state. Membrane symmetry can be produced by passing the polymer material through a gelling medium that gradually transfers the membrane into a solid phase. This is controlled during step 2. Masking of membrane surface is feasible in step 3. Illustrative examples of these interventions follow for some of the membranes.

Cellulosic membranes

Regenerated cellulose is produced by initially dissolving the cellulose in sodium hydroxide. The material is then aged, treated with carbon disulfide, and excess sodium hydroxide is added. The cellulose is then regenerated and the membrane formed by extruding this solution into an acid bath. Membrane properties can be altered by changing the condition during this operation and rigid control of all the steps is

Table 3. Thickness of currently used membranes.

Membrane type	Dry thickness (μM)
Cellulosic	
Cuprophan	7 to 17*
Cuprophan HDF	8 to 20*
Regenerated cellulose	8 to 13*
Modified regenerated cellulose	26*
Saponified cellulose ester	18 to 30
Cellulose acetate	15 to 16*
Cellulose triacetate	85
Synthetic	
Ethylene-vinylalcohol copolymer	32
Polymethyl methacrylate	25 to 40
Polycarbonate	20 to 60
Polyacrilonitrile	20 to 55
Polysulfone	40 to 70
Polyamide	50

* Wet thickness greater than dry.

required to insure a membrane of consistent quality. Cuprophan is developed by a slightly different method. The cellulose is dissolved in an ammonium solution of copper hydroxide rather than in sodium hydroxide. A copper-ammonia-cellulose complex is formed which when extruded into an acid bath yields a cellulosic membrane with the cuprammonium radical incorporated in its structure. This gives the membrane better diffusion and ultrafiltration properties than ordinary regenerated cellulose. The amount of residual copper is small. Unlike non-cellulosic membranes with high glycerin content (polyacrylonitrile 50%), the glycerin content of cuprophan is low (5%), yet sufficient to prevent the formation of cellulose bonds between the cellulose fibrils and allows maintenance of the basic pore structure even when the membrane is dry. Increasing glycerin content of cuprophan allows achieving a higher flux and higher solute transport characteristics and makes the membrane suitable for hemodiafiltration (11). A further modification of cuprophan is performed by introducing tertiary amino groups into some cellubiosis units of the cellulose molecule by means of stable ether bonds and minimal modification of hydroxyl groups. This new membrane (Hemophan) retains all the physical properties of cuprophan and its low thrombogenicity, but has less of a neutropenic effect and less complement activation (7, 12).

For cellulose acetate the acetylation is performed before membrane formation in acid. Acetylation in various degrees increases solute permeability and ultrafiltration (7). These cellulose esters have the advantage of being soluble in a wide range of solvents which facilitates variations in membrane properties and allows different manufacturing processes. This advantage is balanced, however, by poor strength and poor chemical resistance requiring relatively high membrane thickness (Table 3). Furthermore, cellulose acetates are more thrombogenic than cuprophan is (13).

All of these cellulosic membranes have free hydroxyl groups on their surface that may be responsible for the complement activation observed when these membranes are used (14). Elimination of direct contact between blood and the active hydroxyl groups would, theoretically, reduce complement activation. Japanese investigators have developed a new cellulosic membrane by masking the membrane surface during the finishing process with a synthetic polymer (14). The masking layer was formed of a nearly monomolecular thickness with the masking polymer strongly bound to OH and COOH groups of the membrane surface. This treatment expectedly decreased the hydrophilicity of the membrane which is dependent on OH and COOH groups, and created a positive surface charge because of the cationic amino groups of the polymer. The increased hydrophobicity of the membrane favors protein adsorption and may further prevent interaction between OH groups and complement. These changes significantly altered the complement activating ability of the membrane and its neutropenic effects to levels comparable with synthetic polymers (14). This masking by polymer had no significant effect on the permeability and diffusion characteristics of the membrane (14).

Synthetic polymers

Synthetic polymers are rapidly becoming popular membranes for various forms of extracorporeal therapy. These polymers are commercially available thermoplastics and are widely used in apparel and appliances. Many are not biomaterials specially synthesized for extracorporeal application. Nevertheless, most of these polymers lack the labile nucleophiles required for recognition by the complement system. The resulting lower complement activation is an important advantage.

Polyamides offer the advantage of possessing extremely asymmetric structure and high filtration rates (15). Their high mechanical strength and flexibility allow the fabrication of thin and pressure resistant fibers and increase their usefulness in hemofiltration (15). A draw back to some polyamides is protein binding which can impair filtration.

The polycarbonate-polyether copolymer has been introduced into extracorporeal therapy because of several useful properties including good mechanical characteristics, low thrombogenicity, and the ease of modification of the basic aromatic polycarbonate backbone to alter membrane properties chemically and select for favorable final characteristics (8, 9). The copolymer is formed by polycondensation of two polymers (bisphenol A = polycarbonate and polyethylene glycol = polyether) that are initially dissolved together (8). The membrane that is formed with phase inversion is asymmetric and, unlike cellulosic membranes, does not swell when wetted (8, 9). Finally, polycarbonate membranes appear to have biocompatibility characteristics that are intermediate between cuprophan and polyacrylonitrile (16). The latter polymer is characterized by good wettability that leads to high filtration rates combined with high diffusive permeability.

Polysulfone membranes present the interesting situation of a uniform, symmetrical membrane with very high permeability, the latter a characteristic usually associated with asymmetric membranes. At the luminal side, the membrane is evenly covered by pores of identical size. The inner and outer sides of the membrane merge into the porous foam structure of the entire membrane without any compact boundary layers to impede transport (17). Use of this membrane, as other highly permeable membranes, leads to equal solute clearances across therapeutic modalities (18) and negates the superiority of filtration procedures over hemodialysis when this membrane is used (17).

Biocompatibility profile

The last decade has witnessed a tremendous increase in attention to the issue of membrane biocompatibility. New indices of blood-membrane interactions are introduced in parallel with advances in molecular medicine (Table 4). The availability of assays for monokines has allowed exploration of this new avenue of interaction between the membrane and nucleated blood cells. It is now recognized that increased production of monokines, particularly interleukin 1 (30) and tumor necrosis factor (31) occurs during dialysis. It is postulated that these compounds may be responsible for some of the consequences of dialytic therapy that were heretofore unexplained. Interleukin-1 may be invoked to explain the rise in body temperature observed with dialysis (32). Tumor necrosis factor is a catabolic monokine with the ability to induce hemodynamic changes (32). It may play a role in both the vascular instability in a few patients and the more universal catabolism observed during the procedure. The detailed aspects of biocompatibility are more appropriately explored in other chapters with a more comprehensive evaluation of the contribution of the various components of the extracorporeal system. The role of membranes will be briefly discussed presently to highlight some important comparative aspects. Table 4 represents a qualitative summary of a few of the many comparative studies available, and is meant to illustrate first, the propensity of cuprophan membranes to be the most frequently associated with the least biocompatible behavior as judged by multiple parameters. This propensity, however, has been successfully reduced by either chemical alteration of cuprophan (Hemophan) or by masking of surface OH groups with polymers. Second, for some parameters, notably the coagulation profile, the chem-

Table 4. Overview of comparative biocompatibility.

Parameter	Relative order	Ref.
Coagulation profile		
Heparin consumption	CU> PS = PMMA	19
Fibrinogen half-life	CU = CH = CA = PC = PAN	20
FDP generation	CU = CH = CA = PC = PAN	20, 21
Factor VIII antigen	CU = CH = CA = PC = PAN	20, 21
β-thromboglobulin generation	CU = PC> EVAL> PAN	21, 22
Complement activation	CU> CA> PC> PS> PAN	16, 23, 24
Nucleated cell activation		
Granulocyte adherence	CU> EVAL> PAN = PS	25
Leukopenia	CU> CA> PC> PAN = PS = PMMA	23, 24, 26, 27
Granulocyte elastase	CH> CU = PMMA> EVAL = PS = PAN	26–29

CU = cuprophan; CH = cellulose hydrate; CA = cellulose acetate; PC = polycarbonate; PS = polysulfone; PAN = polyacrylonitrile; PMMA = Polymethyl methacrylate; EVAL = ethelenevinyl alcohol; FDP = fibrin degeneration products.

ical nature of the membrane is of little consequence i.e. all membranes are equally interactive in vivo. This finding contrasts with in vitro differences in thrombogenicity (13) and suggests equalization of risk because of major patient- or procedure-related factors. Thirdly, while as a group synthetic membranes are better than cellulosic membranes, they display intragroup differences.

Membrane biocompatibility is closely related to the issue of membrane-induced pathology. Although the non-ideal biocompatible behavior of available membranes is responsible for induction of pathology, it should be reiterated that membranes are integral parts of a therapeutic system, and that other constituents of the system may contribute significantly to observed pathology. Identified culprit components of the system include particulate release from tubing, potting material and residuals of sterilization procedures.

Adsorptive profile

Binding of circulating compounds can have both salutory and detrimental effects. $\beta2$-microglobulin binding has recently been hailed as a beneficial effect under the presumption that this protein is responsible for the development of amyloidosis in patients on long-term hemodialysis and specifically that responsible for carpal tunnel syndrome. The relative adsorption of this protein differs for the various types of membranes depending on their degree of hydrophobicity (PMMA 20 to 30 mg/m^2; PAN 49 mg/m^2; Polyamide 30 to 80 mg/m^2) (2–4). In all cases, however, the removal remains less that the generation rate of the protein, the alteration in blood levels is variable, and the therapeutic benefit is still unproven. While it can be argued that binding and removal of a pathologic protein in beneficial, the property may not be selective and binding or activation of other proteins may accompany the salutary effect. Furthermore, adsorption of proteins may interfere with the permeability characteristics of the membrane. In vitro studies have shown that exposure to plasma greatly reduced hydraulic permeability of polysulfone and polyacrylonitrile membranes without affecting solute permeability (1). Other studies, however, have shown a decrease in the sieving coefficient for inulin on exposure of hemofilter membranes to plasma (Table 5). Membranes may differ not only in the amount of protein adsorbed, but also in the type adsorbed (33). It should be noted that many adsorbed proteins can not be easily desorbed and may affect membrane reuse.

In addition to proteins, membranes are capable of adsorbing drugs such as gentamicin (34) and thus interfere with the circulating levels of medications and necessitate adjustment of dosages to maintain desired therapeutic levels.

MEMBRANE CHOICES FOR SPECIFIC APPLICATIONS

A few years ago, it would have been possible to divide membranes into specific groups, each serving a specific therapeutic category. Cellulosic membranes would have been assigned exclusively to hemodialysis and synthetic polymers to hemofiltration. Unfortunately for writers, but fortunately for the art of extracorporeal therapy, such a classification can no more be made unabashedly. Newly developed cellulosic membranes readily overlap several therapeutic categories in their usefulness. Furthermore, the recognition that the high diffusive and convective properties of synthetic polymers can be exploited for better hemodialysis when ultrafiltration is controllable (high flux dialysis), has brought forth a most interesting situation. With some qualifications, it can be argued that among presently available membranes, there are several that can be succesfully used for multiple therapeutic modalities. An illustration of this is in the new polysulfone membrane that has been used with equally remarkable success in hemodialysis, hemofiltration and hemodiafiltration (17, 18). Nephrologists have *l'embarras du choix,* and the variations in dialysis requirements can be met with a richer armamentarium. The enthusiasm for membrane versatility has to be tempered, however, because of the need for better clinical evaluations and for practical and financial considerations. In addition, it can still be argued that there are best membranes for every particular therapy, and that the ideal versatile membrane is not yet at hand (7). The use of the same membrane in multiple therapeutic modalities relegates the burden of defining the characteristics of the modality to the other components of the extracorporeal system. Thus with a membrane of very high permeability, the avoidance of backfiltration when the membrane is used for hemodialysis must rest in attention to the pressure gradient between the dialysate and the venous end of the dialyser (35). In most clinical conditions, however, filtration of a significant degree is utilized to remove excess fluid in a short duration. The negative dialysate pressure utilized may be sufficient to keep the gradient in favor of

Table 5. Effect of protein adsorption on inulin sieving coefficient.

Membrane	Sieving coefficient		
	In saline	*In blood*	*% change*
Polysulfone	0.99	0.52	47.5
Polyacrylonitrile	0.87	0.33	62
Cellulose triacetate	0.99	0.78	21
Cuprophan HDF	0.80	0.75	6.25

Modified from (7).

filtration and no backfiltration would occur (17). Finally, the availability of these versatile membranes is influencing the design of extracorporeal systems and encouraging the development of multipurpose systems adequate for multiple therapeutic modalities depending on dialysis prescription (36).

The limited, but encouraging versatility of available membranes is illustrated in Table 6. This versatility is expected to increase with the present trend in extracorporeal therapy to utilize high flux short dialysis. The physician's choice of the appropriate tool for a particular modality is no more membrane restricted, but rather determined by considerations of availability, cost and overall properties of dialysers. These are covered in other chapters in this book.

FUTURE DIRECTIONS IN MEMBRANES

Extracorporeal therapy is rapidly becoming a broad and diverse discipline playing an important role in the treatment of many diseases. New applications are necessitating new technologies and the latter are successfully used to ameliorate established modalities of treatment. The future of membranes lies in balancing functional gains with increased patient safety. Future membranes will need to move close towards criteria defined by renal scientists. These criteria need to be continuously updated as our understanding of pathophysiology improves. We have brought the genie out of Aladdin's lamp and the range of wishes is unlimited. Membranes can now be manipulated to play a more intricate and a more useful role than simple barriers. One can consider the possibility of membrane-bound heparin or other anticoagulants to avoid systemic anticoagulation in patients with bleeding disorders. Membranes with specific catalytic functions, such as sites for specific adsorption of compounds, can be developed for substance-specific removal. Alternatively, this task may be achieved by combining membranes with other systems, such as columns equipped with binders for specific compounds, or with substrates for specific biochemical reactions. Use of multiple membranes simultaneously in series is an avenue worthy of exploration. From the vantage point of membranes, the future of extracorporeal therapy appears very promising.

Table 6. Versatility of available membranes.

Membrane	Reported uses
Cellulose, regenerated	HD, HDF
Cellulose acetates	HD, HDF, HF
Cuprophan and derivatives	HD, HDF
Polysulfone	HD, HDF, HF, CAVH
Polyacrylonitrile	HD, HDF, HF, CAVH
Polyamide	HF, CAVH
Polycarbonate-polyether	HD, HDF, HF
Polyethelene-polyvinyl	HD, HDF, HF

HD = hemodialysis; HDF = hemodiafiltration; HF = hemofiltration; CAVH = continuous arteriovenous hemofiltration.

REFERENCES

1. Bosch T, Schmidt B, Samtleben W, Gurland HJ: Effect of protein adsorption on diffusive and convective transport through polysulfone membranes. *Contr Nephrol* 46: 14, 1985
2. Ono T, Kataoka H, Kunimoto T: Quantitative analysis on the removal of β2-microglobulin from chronic dialysis patients. *Blood Purif* 4: 212, 1986
3. Goldmann M, Thayse C, Dhaene M, Lagmiche M, Amraoui Z, Lambert P, Vanherweghem JL: Adsorption of β2-microglobulin on dialysis membranes: a quantitative study. *Blood Purif* 5 (1987) in press
4. Kaiser J, Gohl H, von Herrath D, Schaefer K: Very effective removal of β2-microglobulin with a modified polyamide membrane. *Blood Purif* 5 (1987) in press
5. McManus D, Randerson DH: A membrane immobilized monoclonal antibody immunoadsorption system. *Trans Am Soc Artif Intern Organs* 32: 81, 1986
6. Singh P, Goldman J, Jackson CE: Preparation and in vitro evaluation of a new extracorporeal dialyser with immobilized insulin. *Artif Organs* 6: 145, 1982
7. Gohl H, Konstantin P: Membranes and filters for hemofiltration. in *Hemofiltration*, edited by Henderson LW, Quellhorst EA, Baldamus CA, Lysaght MJ, Berlin, Springer-Verlag, 1986, p 41
8. Konstantin P, Bailey RM: Polycarbonate-Polyether (PC-PE) flat sheet membrane: manufacture, structure and performance. *Blood Purif* 4: 6, 1985
9. Gohl H, Raff M, Harttig H, Deppisch R: PC-PE hollow fiber membrane. Structure, performance characteristics and manufacturing. *Blood Purif* 4: 23, 1985
10. Leypoldt JK, Frigon RP, Henderson LW: Macromolecular charge affects hemofilter solute sieving. *Trans Am Soc Artif Intern Organs* 32: 384, 1986
11. Henne W, Duenweg G, Bandel W: A new cellulose membrane generation for hemodialysis and hemofiltration. *Artif Organs* 3: 466, 1979
12. Mahiout A, Jorres A, Meinhold H, Kessel M: Prostaglandin production and extracorporeal complement activation by dialyser membranes. *Trans Am Soc Artif Intern Organs* 32: 88, 1986
13. Lontz J: Membranes and other material. *Proc 6th Annu Contractors Conf Artif Kidney Program of NIAMDD*, edited by Krueger KK, DHEW publ no (NIH) 74–248 1973
14. Akizawa T, Kitaoka T, Koshikawa S, Watanabe T, Imamura K, Tsurumi T, Suma Y, Eiga S: Development of a regenerated cellulose non-complement activating membrane for hemodialysis. *Trans Am Soc Artif Intern Organs* 32: 76, 1986
15. Streicher E, Schneider H: Asymmetric polyamide hollow fiber filters in the hemofiltration system. *J Dial* 1: 727, 1977
16. Henderson LW, Chenoweth DE, Shinaberger JH, Miller J, Konstantin P: Preliminary report on complement activating potential of polycarbonate membrane. *Blood Purif* 4: 74, 1986
17. Streicher E, Schneider H: The development of a polysulfone membrane. *Contr Nephrol* 46: 1, 1985
18. Streicher E, Schneider H: Polysulfone membrane mimicking human glomerular basement membrane. *Lancet* 2: 1136, 1983
19. Hildebrand U, Quellhorst E: Influence of various membranes on the coagulation system during dialysis. *Contr Nephrol* 46: 92, 1985
20. Gasparotto ML, Bertoli M, Vertolli U, Ruffatti A, Stoppa ML, Di Landro D, Romagnoli GF: Biocompatibility of various dialysis membranes as assessed by coagulation assay. *Contr Nephrol* 37: 96, 1984

21. Notohamiprodjo M, Andrassy K, Bommer J, Ritz E: Dialysis membranes and coagulation system. *Blood Purif* 4: 130, 1985

22. Martin-Malo A, Velasco F, Castillo D, Perez R, Andres P, Torres A, Aljama P: Factors affecting the plasma beta-thromboglobulin levels during dialysis. in *Immune and Metabolic Aspects of Therapeutic Blood Purification Systems*, Basel, Karger, 1986, p 18

23. Henderson LW, Chenoweth D: Biocompatibility of artificial organs: An overview. *Blood Purif* 5: 100, 1987

24. Aljama P, Martin-Malo A, Castillo D, Velasco F, Torres A, Perez R, Castro M: Anaphylotoxin C5a generation and dialysis-induced leukopenia with different hemodialyzer membranes. *Blood Purif* 4: 88, 1986

25. Aljama P, Martin-Malo A, Perez R, Castillo D, Torres A, Velasco F: Granulocyte adherence during hemodialysis. *Contr Nephrol* 46: 75, 1985

26. Schaefer RM, Heidland A, Horl WH: Release of leukocyte elastase during hemodialysis. Effect of different dialysis membranes. *Contr Nephrol* 46: 109, 1985

27. Fawcett S, Hoenich NA, Woffindin C, Ward MK: Influence of high permeability synthetic membranes on gas exchange and lung function during hemodialysis. *Contr Nephrol* 46: 83, 1985

28. Horl WH, Steinhauer HB, Schollmeyer P: Plasma levels of granulocyte elastase during hemodialysis: effect of different dialyzer membranes. *Kidney Int* 28: 791, 1985

29. Horl WH, Schafer RM, Heidland A: Effect of different dialysers on proteinases and proteinase inhibitors during hemodialysis. *Am J Nephrol* 5: 320, 1985

30. Yamagami S, Yoshihara H, Kishimoto T, Sugimura T, Niwa M, Maekawa M: Cuprophan membrane induces interleukin-1 activity. *Trans Am Soc Artif Intern Organs* 32: 98, 1986

31. Lonnemann G, van der Meer JWM, Cannon JG, Dinarello CA: Induction of tumor necrosis factor during extracorporeal blood purification. *N Engl J Med* 317: 963, 1987

32. Dinarello CA, Mier JW: Lymphokines. *N Engl J Med* 317: 940, 1987

33. Barozzi C, Cairo G, Fumero R, Scuri S, Tanzi MC, Tieghi G: Protein-membrane interactions during hemodialysis. in *Immune and Metabolic Aspects of Therapeutic Blood Purification Systems*, Basel, Karger, 1986, p 1

34. Rumpf KW, Reiger J, Ansorg R, Doht B, Scheler F: Binding of antibiotics by dialysis membranes and its clinical relevance. *Proc Eur Dial Transplant Assoc* 607, 1977

35. Stiller S, Mann H, Brunner H: Backfiltration in hemodialysis with highly permeable membranes. *Contr Nephrol* 46: 23, 1985

36. Canaud B, N'Guyen QV, Lagarde C, Stec F, Polaschegg HD, Mion C: Clinical evaluation a multipurpose dialysis system adequate for hemodialysis or for post dilution hemofiltration/ hemodiafiltration with online preparation of substitution fluid from dialysate. *Contr Nephrol* 46: 184, 1985

PRETREATMENT AND PREPARATION OF CITY WATER FOR HEMODIALYSIS

PRAKASH R. KESHAVIAH

INTRODUCTION

During the early years of hemodialysis, the need for water purification was not widely recognized, in part because patient survival on dialysis was short. However, the increased survival of the dialysis patient has brought a growing recognition of the need to treat city water supplies for hemodialysis.

The need for water treatment for hemodialysis

While regulated municipal supplies may be safe for drinking purposes, very few are suitable for hemodialysis without some form of treatment. Drinking water regulations (1) are based on a weekly exposure of about 14 l, whereas the patient on hemodialysis is exposed to between 300 and 400 l/week. These patients have diminished renal function and, hence, compromised urinary excretion of toxins. Further, unlike gastrointestinal absorption, diffusion across the dialysis membrane is non-selective. Toxic substances may, therefore, directly diffuse into the patient's blood stream. If these toxins bind to plasma proteins, even a small gradient for diffusion from dialysate to blood can result in substantial toxic loads (2) because of the sustained gradient for diffusion. The requirements for water used in hemodialysis are, therefore, much more stringent than those for drinking water, necessitating additional treatment.

Contaminants with documented toxicity

The substances that have been documented as toxic in the hemodialysis setting are listed in Table 1 along with the toxic effects that have resulted from exposure to them. It is of interest that most of these toxic substances are not regulated by drinking water standards. Water that is safe for drinking may, therefore, be hazardous for the patient on hemodialysis underscoring the need to treat city water for hemodialysis.

Aluminium sulfate (alum) is used as a flocculant in municipal water treatment. In the absence of appropriate water treatment, high levels of aluminium in the water supply have been associated with fatal dialysis encephalopathy (3–6) and renal bone disease (7, 8).

Many municipal water supplies are hard due to the presence of calcium and magnesium. Excessive levels of calcium and magnesium in the resulting dialysate have resulted in the hard water syndrome (9–11) characterized by nausea, vomiting, muscular weakness, skin flushing and hyper- or hypotension.

Chloramines are widely used as bactericidal agents in municipal water treatment. Chloramines denature hemoglobin by direct oxidation as well as by inhibition of the hexose monophosphate shunt. Hemolysis, Heinz body hemolytic anemias and methemoglobinemias have resulted from chloramine exposure (12–14).

High levels of naturally occurring copper as well as leaching of copper from the distribution system and from the dialysis machine by acidic water have resulted in nausea, chills, headaches, liver damage and fatal hemolysis (15–17).

Municipal water supplies are fluoridated to prevent dental caries. Even at the recommended level of 1 mg/l (53 μmol/l) continued exposure of the dialysis patient to fluoride can lead to osteomalacia, osteoporosis and other bone diseases (18–20). Accidental over-fluoridation of the water supply during municipal treatment was associated with symptoms in eight dialysis patients and one death (21).

Bacterial contamination and the use of fertilizers may result in a high level of nitrate in the water supply. Nitrate levels above 10 mg/l (161 μmol/l) can cause methemoglobinemia with cyanosis, hypotension and nausea (22).

Table 1. Water contaminants and the lowest concentrations associated with toxicity in the hemodialysis setting.

Contaminant	Toxic effects	Lowest toxic level (mg/l)
Aluminium	Dialysis encephalopathy, renal bone disease	0.06
Calcium/Magnesium	Hard water syndrome: nausea, vomiting, muscular weakness, flushed feeling, hypertension, hypotension	88 (Ca^{++})
Chloramines	Hemolysis, anemia, methemoglobinemia	0.25
Copper	Nausea, chills, headache, liver damage, fatal hemolysis	0.49
Fluoride	Osteomalacia, osteoporosis, other bone diseases	1.0
Nitrate	Methemoglobinemia with cyanosis, hypotension, nausea	21 (as N)
Sodium	Hypertension, pulmonary edema, confusion, vomiting, headache, tachycardia, shortness of breath, seizures, coma, death	300
Sulfate	Nausea, vomiting, metabolic acidosis	200
Zinc	Anemia, nausea, vomiting, fever	0.2
Microbial	Pyrexial reactions: chills, fever, nausea, hypotension, cyanosis	–

Hypernatremia and death have resulted from high sodium levels in the water supply (23, 24). One such episode (23) resulted from water softener malfunction during home dialysis.

Sulfate concentrations above 200 mg/l (2.1 μmol/l) increase the amount of lead leached from pipes. High concentrations of sulfate have been associated with nausea, vomiting and metabolic acidosis (25). The use of galvanized iron in the water treatment and distribution system has led to high levels of zinc in the water used for dialysis fluid with the development of a syndrome characterized by anemia, nausea, vomiting and fever (26).

Trace metals such as cadmium, manganese, strontium and tin have accumulated in the tissues of dialysis patients (27). The clinical consequences of such accumulation are not well understood.

Asellus aquaticus, a fresh water louse, thrives in water mains giving the water an unpleasant odor and taste. To overcome this problem, pyrethrins are used in concentrations of approximately 0.001 mg/l. No untoward effects of pyrethrin exposure have been noted in the dialysis setting. Outbreaks of pyrogen reactions have been described in several dialysis programs (28–30). These outbreaks are often associated with microbial and endotoxin contamination of the dialysate. Such contamination is usually a consequence of inadequate cleaning and disinfection of the water treatment system and dialysis equipment.

WATER TREATMENT OPTIONS – ADVANTAGES, DISADVANTAGES AND CONSIDERATIONS IN THEIR CHOICE

Along with the growing cognizance of the hazards of untreated water, there has been increased awareness of the options suitable for treating water used for hemodialysis. The water treatment options available today to the dialysis practitioner are listed in Table 2.

We will now consider each of these options, examine the advantages and disadvantages of the water treatment option and the considerations that go into choosing a particular water treatment strategy.

Sediment filtration

Sediment filtration is used to remove large particulates from the water supply. Particulate removal is necessary to protect the dialysis equipment downstream of the filter. Ultrafiltration devices, reverse osmosis devices and hemodialysis machines are all susceptible to pluggage by particulate matter with clinical consequences that vary depending on the mode of equipment failure. Sediment filters afford protection to these devices and, hence, safeguard patients from the consequences of particulate pluggage. In a sediment filter, filtration of particulate material is accomplished by size exclusion as the water percolates through screens, meshes, closely packed fibers or a porous matrix. A schematic representation of a sediment filter is shown in Figure 1. Sediment filters are rated by nominal pore size for particulate exclusion as well as by the maximum flow rate at which they may be operated. Once filter capacity is exceeded, particulates may break through into the effluent stream. The continued operational efficacy of a sediment filter is monitored by measuring the pressure drop across the filter. Once the pressure drop exceeds the value specified by the manufacturer, the filter must be replaced.

A problem associated with sediment filters is proliferation of microbial organisms on the filter medium with subsequent contamination of the equipment downstream. Patient consequences of such contamination include pyrogen reactions, bacteremias and sepsis. Disinfection of the water treatment system at regular intervals and timely replacement of filters will minimize this problem. Another problem associated with such filters is sloughing of filter media into

Table 2. Water treatment options.

Sediment filtration
Softening
Activated carbon filtration
Deionization
Reverse osmosis
Ultrafiltration
Distillation

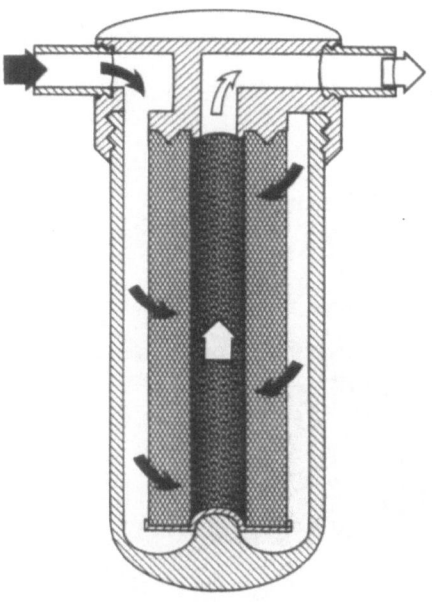

Figure 1. Schematic representation of a sediment filter. (Reprinted from the F.D.A. report 'Investigation of the Risks and Hazards Associated with Hemodialysis Devices', Prakash Keshaviah, Principal Investigator.)

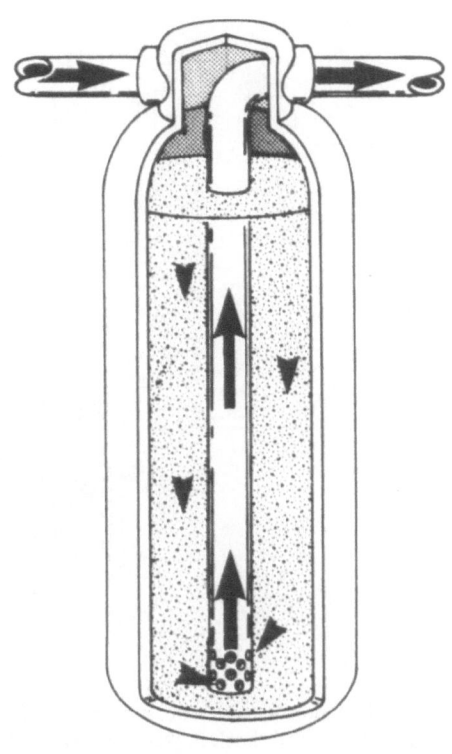

Figure 2. Schematic representation of a water softener. (Reprinted from the F.D.A. report 'Investigation of the Risks and Hazards Associated with Hemodialysis Devices', Prakash Keshaviah, Principal Investigator.)

the effluent stream. Also, toxic residues from the filter medium may be released into the water supply. It has been reported that a filter made of cotton fibers held together by thermosetting polymers allowed the leaching of formaldehyde into the effluent water causing an outbreak of hemolytic anemia in 12 patients (31). Sediment filters may be used at several points in the water treatment system: for prefiltration of the city water supply, downstream of carbon filters that are susceptible to the release of carbon fines and at the inlet of the hemodialysis delivery system.

Water softeners

Water softeners (Figure 2) are ion exchangers containing a cationic resin that exchanges sodium ions for calcium, magnesium and other polyvalent cations. When all of the sodium ions on the resin have been exchanged, the resin is said to be exhausted and the softener has to be regenerated. A concentrated solution of sodium chloride is used for regeneration with reversal of the ion exchange process, sodium ions being restored on the resin matrix. Water softeners have to be sized according to the hardness of the water supply, the rate of water consumption and the ion exchange capacity of the resin. The effectiveness of softening is monitored by measuring the hardness of the effluent water with suitable kits. Water softening is required, not only to prevent the hard water syndrome, but also to pretreat water for reverse osmosis (RO) devices to protect the RO membrane from scale build up and subsequent failure.

If water softeners are regenerated on site, they must be

equipped with bypass valves to ensure that regeneration does not occur during dialysis. In a reported case, accidental power interruption to the water softener caused a mistiming of the generation cycle so that regeneration occured during dialysis with patient symptoms of hypernatremia including thirst, vomiting, back pain, headache and disorientation (23). If the water softener is provided with an automatic bypass valve, supply water will bypass the resin during regeneration, thereby, preventing hypernatremia. Another problem with softeners, as with sediment filters, is that of microbial proliferation. This can be minimized with back washing of the resin during regeneration. If the resin of the softener is regenerated at a commercial facility, care must be taken to ensure that the resin from the dialysis center is not admixed with resins from other non-medical users to prevent microbial and toxic contamination of the resin. Cross contamination of resin between urban and rural users with heavy microbial contamination of the urban users' resin has been described (32). Microbial proliferation in the water softener depends to some extent on the design of the resin bed. The problem is exacerbated if the flow path incorporates areas of stagnation and dead ends. Rigorous disinfection and periodic surveillance of the effluent can control this problem. If the water softener is followed by a membrane process such as ultrafiltration or reverse osmosis, bacterial removal is effectively accomplished.

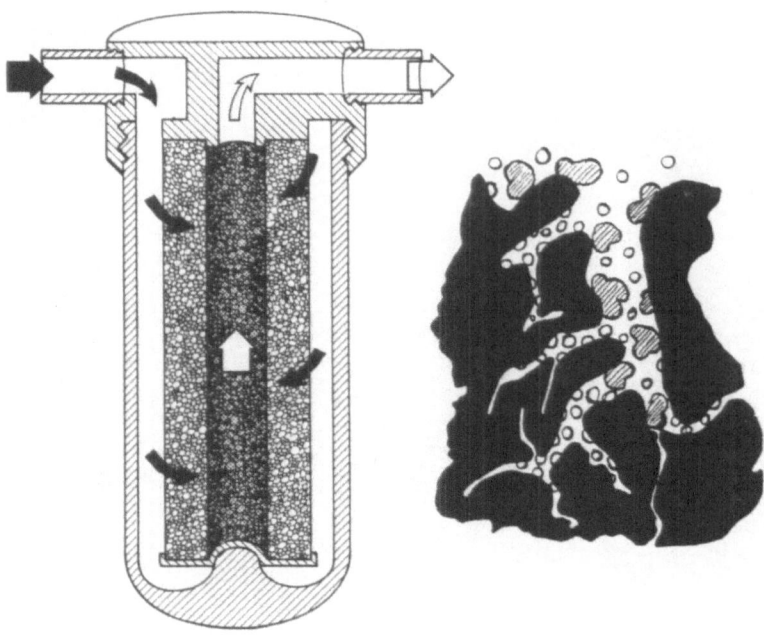

Figure 3. Representation of an activated carbon filter. (Reprinted from the F.D.A. report 'Investigation of the Risks and Hazards Associated with Hemodialysis Devices', Prakash Keshaviah, Principal Investigator.)

Activated carbon filtration

Activated carbon filters remove chlorine, chloramines and dissolved organics (60 to 300 daltons) by the process of adsorption. As shown in the schematic (Figure 3), activated carbon has a microporous structure with a very large surface area to weight ratio to facilitate adsorption of chlorine, chloramines and smaller organic contaminants. In choosing a carbon filter and sizing it for a water supply, it is important to recognize that the adsorption capacity and the rate of removal depend upon the source of carbon (coal, petroleum derivatives, pecan shells, wood, bone, etc.) and the nature of the activation process. Activation of carbon is achieved by heating and exposure to steam to create the fine pore structure of the medium. When the adsorptive capacity of the carbon filter is exhausted, adsorbed substances will spill over into the effluent. Measuring the effluent concentration of chlorine or chloramine is, hence, a convenient method for monitoring the efficacy of a carbon filter. Carbon filters cannot be regenerated effectively and must be replaced when exhausted. Carbon filters, because of their microporous structure, tend to release carbon particles called fines. Sediment filters must, therefore, be used downstream of carbon filters to trap these fines and prevent them from plugging equipment downstream.

Some types of reverse osmosis membranes are susceptible to damage by chlorine. Carbon filtration must, therefore, be used as a pretreatment when such RO membranes are used. Carbon filters effectively remove smaller organic contaminants while RO membranes are very effective in the removal of larger organics. The combination of carbon filtration and reverse osmosis is, therefore, ideal when the water supply has a high concentration of organics. Carbon filtration may also be necessary as pretreatment for deionizers which are incapable of removing chlorine and organics such as chloramine.

Because of the porosity of activated carbon and its affinity for organics, carbon filters are susceptible to microbial contamination and proliferation. Chlorine and chloramine which normally retard bacterial growth are removed by the carbon filter and organic nutrients are adsorbed, thereby exacerbating the proliferation of bacteria in the efferent portions of the carbon bed and downstream of the carbon filter. Appropriate disinfection of water treatment devices downstream of a carbon filter is important to limit the bacterial contamination of the treated water.

Chloramines are being used increasingly as a substitute for chlorine in municipal water treatment because chlorine reacts with naturally occurring organic compounds in the water supply to form trihalomethanes which have been shown to be carcinogenic (33). The United States Environmental Protection Agency (EPA) has promulgated a maximum level of 0.1 mg/l for total trihalomethanes in drinking water necessitating the use of chloramines in municipal water treatment. Chloramines in concentrations as low as 0.25 mg/l can cause hemolysis, anemia and methemoglobinemia in dialysis patients (12–14). The improper sizing of a carbon filter or the absence of appropriate monitoring of effluent concentrations can, therefore, create an extremely hazardous situation when chloramines are used as bactericidal agents.

Deionization

Deionizers, as the name implies, are used for the removal of dissolved inorganic ions in the water supply. They are, like softeners, based on the principle of ion exchange. Two types of ion exchange resins are used – cationic and anionic. Cationic resins exchange hydrogen ions for cations and anionic resins exchange hydroxyl ions for anions. In a mixed bed deionizer, the cationic and anionic resins are mixed, the exchanged hydrogen and hydroxyl ions combining to form neutral water. Mixed bed deionizers can produce water of a very high quality. The efficacy of the deionizer is measured in terms of the resistivity of the effluent water. Mixed bed deionizers can produce an effluent with a resistivity in excess of 1 megohm/cm. Dual bed deionizers, with the cationic and anionic resins in separate beds, produce water of a lower quality than mixed bed deionizers but are less expensive to operate. Dual bed systems are, therefore, sometimes used as a pretreatment for mixed bed deionizers.

As with softeners, when the ion exchange capacity of the cationic and anionic resins is exhausted, regeneration is necessary. Cationic resins are regenerated using strong acids and anionic resins are regenerated using strong alkalis. Deionizer efficacy is monitored by measuring the resistivity of the effluent. When the resistivity falls below a preset value, usually 1 megohm/cm, regeneration is necessary. When a deionizer is exhausted, previously adsorbed ions may be eluted into the effluent depending on the affinity of the ions for the resin. With cationic resins, the affinities are as below:

$$Ca^{++} > Mg^{++} > K^+ > Na^+ > H^+.$$

With anions, the affinities are ordered:

$$NO_3^- > SO_4^{--} > NO_2^- > Cl^- > HCO_3^- > OH^- > F^-.$$

In a reported episode a defective resistivity monitor resulted in the deionizer being used beyond the point of exhaustion with very high levels of fluoride in the effluent (34). The patient developed severe osteomalacia, bone resorption and decreased bone formation. When a deionizer is nearing exhaustion, another potential risk exists, namely, imbalance between cationic and anionic exchange capacities. An acidic effluent usually results because the ion exchange capacity favors the cationic resin. Two types of hazards are described as a result of acidic effluents from deionizers. In one episode, copper was leached from the piping and dialysis machine components with consequent copper induced toxicity manifested as hemolytic anemia, nausea, vomiting, chills and anorexia (17). In the other episode, acidic dialysate resulted in heparin inactivation with subsequent clotting in dialyzers (35). Resistivity monitors used for deionizers must be temperature compensated for appropriate monitoring of deionizer efficacy. Resistivity varies with temperature and if the monitor is not temperature compensated, exhaustion may go undetected in situations where the inlet water temperature varies widely.

During commercial regeneration of deionizer resins, it must be ensured that resins from dialysis centers are not admixed with resins of non-medical users. Deionizers are used industrially for recovery of plating metals such as chromium and silver. If admixture of resins takes place, traces of such toxic metals may remain bound to the resin and may be eluted into the water used for dialysis, with toxic consequences. Also, the chemicals used for regenerating the resins must not contain high levels of toxic impurities and adequate rinsing of these chemicals must be ensured before the deionizer is suitable for dialysis water treatment. As with softeners and carbon filters, deionizers are also susceptible to microbial contamination and proliferation. However, if regeneration is performed at reasonable intervals, bacterial quality of the effluent may be controllable. With certain municipal supplies, effluents from deionizers have been found to contain nitrosodimethylamine, a suspected carcinogen (36). In such situations, carbon filters must be used to pretreat the water before deionization. As with carbon filters, deionizer resins may slough particles, requiring the use of sediment filters downstream of the deionizer.

Reverse osmosis

Reverse osmosis is a membrane based process that rejects 90 to 98% of monovalent ions and 95 to 99% of divalent ions by molecular sieving (>200 daltons) and ionic exclusion. This form of water treatment is effective for removal of dissolved inorganics, dissolved organics, bacteria, pyrogens and particulates. When two solutions of different ionic concentrations are separated by a semipermeable membrane, flow of solvent takes place from the less concentrated to the more concentrated side. This phenomenon is called osmosis. Osmotic pressure is the pressure that must be applied to the concentrated solution side of the membrane to prevent this flow. When this applied pressure exceeds the osmotic pressure, there is reversal of flow, solvent flowing from the more concentrated to the less concentrated side. This is called reverse osmosis and is the basis for the water treatment process. Several types of membranes have been used for reverse osmosis, e.g. cellulosic, aromatic polyamides, polyimides, polyfuranes and thin film composite membranes. Geometrical configurations include plate and frame, tubular, helical tube, spiral wound and hollow fiber configurations.

The spiral wound and hollow fiber configurations are most frequently used in water treatment for hemodialysis and are shown schematically in Figures 4 and 5 respectively. The performance of reverse osmosis devices is monitored by measuring the resistivity of the feed water and product water and calculating the percent rejection from these measurements. In some cases, the effluent may also be analyzed for specific contaminants to confirm the rejection measured by resistivity. Reverse osmosis membranes are susceptible to fouling if the feed water is not appropriately pretreated. Calcium, magnesium, iron and manganese, if present in high concentrations, can form scales on RO membranes with loss of efficacy and failure of the membranes. Some

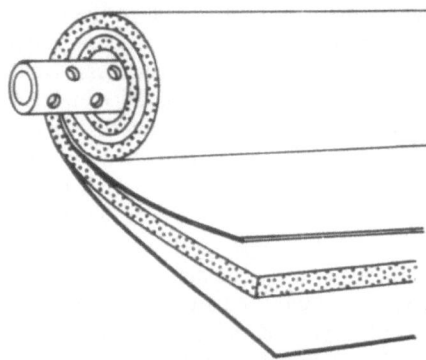

Figure 4. A spiral wound reverse osmosis module. (Reprinted from the F.D.A. report 'Investigation of the Risks and Hazards Associated with Hemodialysis Devices', Prakash Keshaviah, Principal Investigator.)

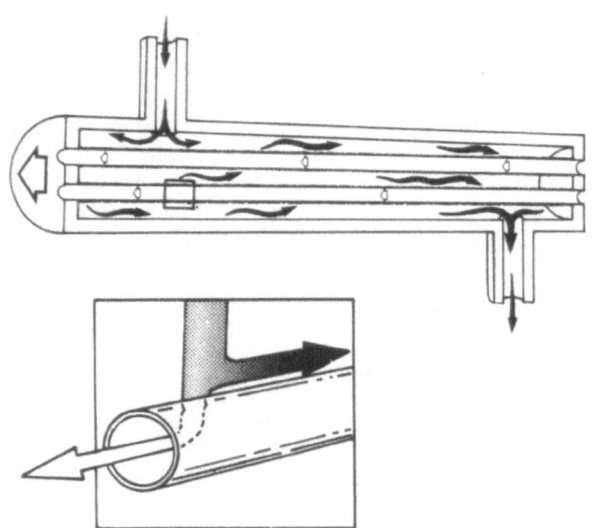

Figure 5. Hollow fiber reverse osmosis module showing the product water flow through a wall of a single fiber and the reject flow tangential to the fiber. (Reprinted from the F.D.A. report 'Investigation of the Risks and Hazards Associated with Hemodialysis Devices', Prakash Keshaviah, Principal Investigator.)

membranes are also susceptible to damage by chlorine and chloramines. Cellulosic membranes are vulnerable to pH values above 8 and are also susceptible to bacterial degradation. Reverse osmosis modules are expensive and once damaged, the ability to regenerate the membrane is limited. However, beyond the initial capital cost, water treatment by reverse osmosis is relatively inexpensive and is a mode of treatment that effectively removes all four types of contaminants, i.e. organic, inorganic, particulate and microbial. While reverse osmosis is effective for removal of bacteria, viruses and pyrogens, microbial infestation of the module can occur, with microorganisms and pyrogens penetrating small defects in the membrane or leaky seals. Bacterial contamination of the product water can, therefore, occur and disinfection of reverse osmosis modules must be performed according to an appropriate schedule. With high levels of contaminants such as fluoride and nitrate in the feed water, reverse osmosis alone may not be an adequate form of treatment. A deionizer may be required to polish the product water of the reverse osmosis module. Such a scheme can create a problem with microbial contamination and a downstream ultrafilter may be required to limit such contamination.

Ultrafiltration

Ultrafiltration, like reverse osmosis, is a membrane process, but the pores of ultrafiltration membranes are much larger than those of reverse osmosis membranes. Ionic exclusion is, therefore, not accomplished with ultrafiltration membranes, but ultrafiltration membranes can remove bacteria, viruses, pyrogen and particulates. Thin polymeric membranes are used in ultrafilters in a sheet or tubular configuration. Different nominal pore sizes and flow capacities are available. The effectiveness of the ultrafilter is monitored by measuring the pressure drop across the filter, as with sediment filters. Ultrafilters may be used as pretreatment for reverse osmosis modules to prevent bacterial contamination of the RO modules and fouling by colloids and particulates.

Ultrafilters may be regenerated by chemicals and, with certain ultrafilter designs, by back flushing. Some ultrafilters are disposable and replaced when pressure drops exceed manufacturer's specifications. Ultrafilters are also used as the last stage of water treatment to control bacterial contamination in the product water when upstream devices introduce such contamination. There has been limited use of ultrafilters for water treatment in hemodialysis but increased use of these filters is anticipated as they are relatively inexpensive and easy to use.

Distillation

Distillation is a process that is effective for the removal of non-volatile organic and inorganic substances, particulates, colloids, microorganisms and pyrogens. It is an effective but expensive form of water treatment and is not commonly used for hemodialysis. Water is converted to the vapor phase with subsequent condensation of the vapor back to the liquid phase by cooling. This form of water treatment often requires the use of storage tanks and distribution pumps. The system may, therefore, be susceptible to bacterial proliferation even though the treatment process, itself, is effective in the removal of bacteria and pyrogens. Distillation is not effective for volatile contaminants because they are carried over in the vapor. Distillation systems are continuously reusable but maintenance requirements are stringent. Monitoring of efficacy is accomplished by resistivity measurements of the product water or by measuring the concentration of relevant species in the product water.

Water purification systems

The water purification system consists of combinations of the various water treatment options described above, as well as other components such as piping, valves, tanks, pumps and other devices needed for the transport, handling and purification of water. The materials of construction should be such that the chemical quality of the water is unaffected by contact with these materials. Polyvinylchloride, polypropylene and nylon are considered sufficiently inert materials for such use. Metals such as copper, brass, zinc and stainless steel should be avoided because of the potential for leaching of toxic materials into the water supply. The water system should be designed to avoid dead ends and areas of stagnation which promote bacterial proliferation. Bacterial proliferation can also be minimized by avoiding oversized pipes, holding tanks and pressure vessels, whenever possible. The system should also be designed for convenient cleaning and disinfection and it should be ensured that adequate contact with the disinfectant occurs and that rinse out of disinfectant is facilitated. The specifics of a water purification system depend on several factors that include the capacity of the system, the nature of the incoming water supply, seasonal variations in quality and the final quality of the product water. It is, therefore, not practical to specify a standard configuration that all hemodialysis units must have in order to meet a product water standard. Water treatment systems have to be individualized for the particular application and it is the responsibility of the supplier of the system as well as the user to ensure that the final product quality meets water quality standards, taking into consideration the worst case, with seasonal variations of incoming water quality.

WATER QUALITY STANDARDS FOR HEMODIALYSIS

Standards organizations of various countries have proposed water quality standards. In the United States, the Association for the Advancement of Medical Instrumentation (AAMI) has developed a comprehensive water quality standard that has since become an American National Standard (37). Many of the recommendations of the Food and Drug Administration (FDA) sponsored study on the risks and

Table 3. Water quality standard for substances documented as toxic in hemodialysis.

Substance	Maximum concentration (mg/l)	Rationale
Aluminium	0.01	Based on lowest toxic
Chloramines	0.10	levels reported in the
Copper	0.10	dialysis literature
Fluoride	0.20	with appropriate
Nitrate	2.0	margin of safety
Sulfate	100	
Zinc	0.10	

hazards of hemodialysis systems (38) were adopted by AAMI and incorporated into their standard. We will consider water quality standards for inorganic substances, organic and radioactive substances and for the microbiological quality of the water used for hemodialysis.

Inorganic substances

Inorganic substances may be divided into three categories – non-toxic substances normally included in dialysate, toxic substances described in the dialysis literature and toxic substances regulated by the EPA drinking water standards which have not yet been implicated as toxic in the dialysis setting. Maximum recommended concentrations for these three classes of substances are listed in Tables 3, 4 and 5 along with the rationale used for establishing these maximums. For substances regulated by drinking water standards (Table 5), one should ideally set the level at the no transfer level, the level at which no transfer occurs from dialysate to blood. No transfer levels have been established for some of these substances (2). However, these no transfer levels were established using radioisotopes of these substances and the levels are sometimes below the detection limit of standard analytical methods established by the EPA (39). One could also set limits for these substances based on the fact that the dialysis patient is exposed to 25 times the drinking water exposure. However, a 25 fold reduction in the concentration of these substances may be difficult to achieve in the practical setting of dialysis. The standard sets the concentration of these substances at 10% of the EPA drinking water standard based on the pragmatic consid-

Table 4. Water quality standard for non-toxic substances normally included in dialysate.

Substance	Maximum concentration (mg/l)	Rationale
Calcium	2 (0.1 mEq/l)	Based on allowable
Magnesium	4 (0.3 mEq/l)	margin for error in
Potassium	8 (0.2 mEq/l)	final dialysate
Sodium	70 (3.0 mEq/l)	

Table 5. Water quality standard for toxic substances regulated in the EPA drinking water standards.

Substance	Maximum concentration (mg/l)	Rationale
Arsenic	0.005	10% of EPA level or
Barium	0.01	'no-transer' level,
Cadmium	0.001	whichever is higher
Chromium	0.014	
Lead	0.005	
Mercury	0.0002	
Selenium	0.09	
Silver	0.005	

eration that reverse osmosis devices, which are frequently used for water treatment in dialysis, remove more than 90% of total dissolved inorganic solids in the feed water. In addition to the above recommendations, the AAMI standard also sets a maximum level of 0.5 mg/l for chlorine because of its potential toxicity.

Organic and radioactive substances

The EPA drinking water standards include chlorinated hydrocarbons (pesticides), chlorophenoxys (herbicides) and man-made nuclides emitting alpha, beta and photon radioactivity. At this time, not enough information is available to set maximum contaminant levels for these substances in the water used for hemodialysis. Hence, no water standard recommendations are possible. However, one should note that the combination of activated carbon filtration and reverse osmosis is very effective in removing a wide range of organic materials. Activated carbon filters will remove organics with a molecular weight between 60 and 300 daltons, while reverse osmosis membranes will remove organics with a molecular weight greater than 200 daltons. Radioactive isotopes will be removed by mechanisms similar to those that eliminate their non-radioactive counterparts.

Microbiology

Based on the studies of the Centers for Disease Control (30, 40), the AAMI limit for microbiological contamination has been set at a maximum total viable count of 200 cfu/ml for the water used to prepare dialysate. Further, a maximum of 2,000 cfu/ml has been established for effluent dialysate at the end of the dialysis procedure. No standard has been established for the endotoxin contamination of the water used to prepare dialysis solution; however, for water used for reprocessing dialyzers for multiple use, a maximum limit of 1 ng/ml of bacterial lipopolysaccharide (measured by the limulus amebocyte assay) has been established by the AAMI standard for reuse of hemodialyzers (41). If the water treatment system for dialysis fluid is also used to prepare the water for reuse, care should be taken to ensure that both the dialysis solution water quality standard and the reuse water quality standard are met by the system.

WATER QUALITY MONITORING

Water quality monitoring ensures the proper performance of the water treatment equipment and also ensures patient safety. When a water treatment system is first installed, it is essential to ensure that all components of the system, as well as the final product, meet the specifications of the system supplier and the final water quality standard. Such testing should take into consideration seasonal variations of the incoming water quality. After the system has been validated, regular monitoring of water quality ensures appropriate operation of the system and patient safety related to water quality. Frequency of monitoring is an important

consideration, but one for which no simple guidelines can be established that apply to all dialysis programs. The quality of the incoming water supply is variable and the performance of the water treatment equipment may change with time. The ideal of very frequent monitoring has to be tempered by the pragmatic reality of cost. State and local agencies must be consulted regarding seasonal water quality variations, as well as variations in the municipal treatment methods, before an adequate monitoring schedule is established. The nature and configuration of the water treatment system is also an important determinant of the frequency of monitoring. The manufacturer of the system should advise the dialysis program regarding schedules of regeneration and replacement of various components. However, monitoring of water quality is the responsibility of the dialysis unit. AAMI has established some guidelines concerning the frequency of monitoring but these should be viewed cautiously in light of the above remarks. The AAMI recommendation is that chemical contaminants in the product water should be analyzed every 12 months if reverse osmosis and/or deionizers are used. For other types of treatment devices, a frequency of 3 months is recommended with additional monitoring at times of expected high concentrations in the incoming supply. AAMI also recommends that the microbiological quality of the product water should be checked monthly and also when warranted by pyrogen reactions or bacteremias in the dialysis unit. The AAMI standard acknowledges that such frequent monitoring may not be suited to the home dialysis setting. AAMI also recommends that initially, when the water treatment system is first installed, monthly testing should be performed and a data record maintained of such testing. Once an historical record has been developed, testing can be done less frequently.

In monitoring the quality of the final product water to ensure compliance with product water standards, the various contaminant concentrations have to be individually analyzed. The American Public Health Association references the analytical methods in their publication 'Standard Methods For the Examination of Water and Waste Water' (42). The EPA in the United States also has a publication, 'Methods for Chemical Analysis for Water and Wastes' (39). It is recommended that these analytical methods be used for monitoring the quality of the final product water. For microbiological quality of the product water, the 1.0 ml calibrated loop technique is inadequate. Pour or spread plate techniques or a membrane filter technique should be used. Samples must be assayed within 30 min of collection, or if stored at 5°C, within 24 h. Standard methods agar, blood agar or tryptic soy agar may be used as a culture medium and the colonies should be counted after incubation at 37°C for 48 h. These methods may have to be modified if contamination with mycobacteria is suspected (43). Also if bicarbonate dialysis is being used, the microbiology of dialysate should be assayed using a salt supplemented agar such as tryptic soy agar rather than standard methods agar. The use of standard methods agar for bicarbonate dialysate results in an underestimation of the actual level of bacterial contamination (44).

While the final product water is analyzed for all contaminants specified in the water quality standard on an annual basis, it should be kept in mind that more frequent monitoring of individual components of the water treatment system takes place with the use of appropriate monitors at each water treatment device. For instance, the performance of a reverse osmosis module can be checked continuously with measurements of resistivity and percent rejection determined from such resistivity measurements. Similarly, the product water of deionizers is checked continuously using a resistivity monitor. Carbon filters need to be checked fairly frequently for free chlorine in the effluent of the carbon filter in order to ensure that the carbon has not been exhausted. Free chlorine levels in feed water to the reverse osmosis unit may also need to be measured frequently when membranes sensitive to chlorine are being used. If reverse osmosis membranes are sensitive to pH, the pH of the feed water to the reverse osmosis unit needs to be checked often, especially in situations where season variations are encountered. Chloramines in the final product water also need to be monitored frequently. Bacterial monitoring on a monthly basis may be adequate when the system is well designed and is frequently disinfected. However, in many systems, weekly cultures may be necessary to safeguard against extensive proliferation of bacteria over the period of a month. The efficacy of the water softener should also be checked periodically depending on the capacity of the system and the degree of hardness of the feed water. Test kits are available for frequent monitoring at a fairly low cost. Just as system design has to be individualized to meet the needs of a particular dialysis program, the monitoring schedule should also be individualized to meet those needs. It is difficult to make specific recommendations that apply universally.

RESPONSIBILITY OF THE SUPPLIERS AND USERS OF WATER TREATMENT EQUIPMENT

In the United States, water treatment equipment has been classified by the FDA as medical devices. The Good Manufacturing Practices act (45), therefore, applies to the manufacture of such equipment. In addition to these responsibilities, the manufacturer has additional responsibilities in supplying a water treatment system to meet water quality standards. Before a system is installed, the supplier should obtain a certified laboratory analysis of the feed water from the dialysis center, local water authorities or EPA certified laboratories. This analysis should be used in deciding on the type and capacity of the system and a disclosure document should be prepared by the supplier indicating expected concentrations at various points of the treatment system. In addition, the manufacturer should provide details such as inlet water temperatures, pressures, flow rates, generic nature of materials contacting water, chemicals that are not compatible with materials of construction and non-toxicity of chemicals such as flocculants required for the water treatment system. Upon installing the system, the manufacturer should validate the system for a time duration adequate to determine appropriate performance of all components of the system. The manufacturer should also specify the schedules for replacement or regeneration of various devices in the system. Methods of disinfection, maintenance schedules and guidelines, troubleshooting procedures and spare parts lists should also be provided. Beyond the initial installation, testing and validation of the system, its maintenance and safe operation thereafter, become the responsibility of the dialysis unit. These responsibilities include frequent monitoring of water quality, periodic cleaning and disinfection, and maintenance of various components of the system. Any untoward consequences that result from inadequate water quality are the responsibility of the dialysis practitioner. It should not be forgotten that the patient on dialysis is exposed in 3 years to an amount of water that is consumed by the normal individual in a lifetime. Only a thin non-selective membrane separates the blood of the dialysis patient from the various contaminants in the water used for dialysate preparation. Every year more than 2,000 new chemicals are being introduced, all of which can potentially enter water supplies and are potentially toxic. It is not an exaggeration to state that inadequate water treatment is one of the gravest risks posed to the health of the patient on dialysis.

REFERENCES

1. Environmental Protection Agency, Office of Water Supply. National Interim Primary Drinking Water Regulations, U.S. Government Printing Office, Washington, D.C., 1978
2. NIH Report – Trace Metal Protein Binding, Gulf South Research Institute, 1979
3. Alfrey AC, Mishell M, Burks SR, Contiguglia P, Rudolph H, Lewin E, Holmes JH: Syndrome of dyspraxia and multifocal seizures associated with chronic hemodialysis. *Trans Am Soc Artif Intern Organs* 18: 257, 1972
4. Platts MM, Moorhead PJ, Grech P: Dialysis dementia. *Lancet* 2: 159, 1973
5. Alfrey AC: Dialysis encephalopathy syndrome. *Annu Rev Med* 29: 93, 1978
6. Dunea G, Mahurkar SD, Mamdani B, Smith EC: Role of aluminum in dialysis dementia. *Ann Intern Med* 88: 502, 1978
7. Platts MM, Goode GC, Hislop JS: Composition of the domestic water supply and the incidence of fractures and encephalopathy in patients on home dialysis. *Br Med J* 2: 657, 1977
8. Ward MK, Ellis HA, Feest TG, Parkinson IS, Kerr DNS, Herrington J, Goode GL: Osteomalacic dialysis osteodystrophy: Evidence for a water-borne aetiological agent, probably aluminum. *Lancet* 1: 841, 1978
9. Freeman RM, Lawton RL, Chamberlain MA: Hard-water syndrome. *N Engl J Med* 276: 1113, 1967
10. Evans DB, Slapak M: Pancreatitis in the hard water syndrome. *Br Med J* 3: 748, 1975
11. Drukker W: The hard water syndrome: A potential hazard during hemodialysis. *Proc Eur Dial Transplant Assoc* 5: 284, 1968
12. Yawata Y, Kjellstrand C, Buselmeier T, Howe R, Jacob H: Hemolysis in dialyzed patients: Tap water-induced red blood cell metabolic deficiency. *Trans Am Soc Artif Intern Organs* 18: 301, 1972
13. Botella J, Traver JA, Sanz-Guajardo D, Torres MT, Sanjuan I,

Zabala P: Chloramines, an aggravating factor in the anaemia of patients on regular dialysis treatment. *Proc Eur Dial Transplant Assoc* 14: 192, 1977

14. Neilan BA, Ehlers SM, Kolpin CF, Eaton JW: Prevention of chloramine-induced hemolysis in dialyzed patients. *Clin Nephrol* 10: 105, 1978

15. Ivanovich P, Manzler A, Drake R: Acute hemolysis following hemodialysis. *Trans Am Soc Artif Intern Organs* 15: 316, 1969

16. Manzler AD, Schreiner AW: Copper-induced acute hemolytic anemia. A new complication of hemodialysis. *Ann Intern Med* 73: 409, 1970

17. Natter BJ, Pederson J, Psimenos G, Lindeman RD: Lethal copper intoxication in hemodialysis. *Trans Am Soc Artif Intern Organs* 15: 309, 1969

18. Siddiqui JY, Simpson SW, Ellis HE, Kerr DNS, Appleton DR, Robinson BH, Hawkins JB, Robertson PW, Taves DR: Fluoride and bone disease in patients on regular hemodialysis. *Proc Eur Dial Transplant Assoc* 8: 149, 1971

19. Jowsey J, Johnson WJ, Taves DR, Kelly PJ: Effects of dialysate calcium and fluoride on bone disease during regular hemodialysis. *J Lab Clin Med* 79: 204, 1972

20. Lough J, Noonan R, Gagnon R, Kaye M: Effects of fluoride on bone in chronic renal failure. *Arch Pathol* 99: 484, 1975

21. Anderson R, Beard JH, Sorley D: Fluoride intoxication in a dialysis unit – Maryland. MMWR 29: 134, 1980

22. Carlson DJ, Shaprio FL: Methemoglobinemia from well water nitrates: A complication of home dialysis. *Ann Intern Med* 73: 757, 1970

23. Nickey WA, Chinitz VL, Kim KE, Onesti G, Swartz C: Hypernatremia from water softener and malfunction during home dialysis. *JAMA* 214: 915, 1970

24. Robson M: Dialysate sodium concentration, hypertension, and pulmonary edema in hemodialysis patients. *Dial Transplant* 7: 678, 1978

25. Comty C, Luehmann D, Wathen R, Shapiro F: Prescription water for chronic hemodialysis. *Trans Am Soc Artif Intern Organs* 20: 189, 1974

26. Gallery EDM, Blomfield J, Dixon SR: Acute zinc toxicity in haemodialysis. *Br Med J* 4: 331, 1973

27. Alfrey AC, LeGendre GR, Kaehny WD: The dialysis encephalopathy syndrome: possible aluminum intoxication. *N Engl J Med* 294: 184, 1976

28. Robinson PJA, Rosen SM: Pyrexial reactions during haemodialysis. *Br Med J* 1: 528, 1971

29. Raij L, Shapiro FL, Michael AF: Endotoxemia in febrile reactions during hemodialysis. *Kidney Int* 4: 57, 1973

30. Favero MS, Petersen NJ, Boyer KM, Carson LA, Bond WW: Microbial contamination of renal dialysis systems and associated health risks. *Trans Am Soc Artif Intern Organs* 20: 175, 1974

31. Orringer EP, Mattern WD: Formaldehyde-induced hemolysis during chronic hemodialysis. *N Engl J Med* 294: 1416, 1976

32. Stamm JM, Engelhard WE, Parsons JE: Microbiological study of water-softener resins. *Appl Microbiol* 18: 376, 1969

33. Wilkins JR, Reches NA, Kruse CW: Organic chemical contaminants in drinking water. *Am J Epidemiol* 10: 420, 1979

34. Johnson WJ, Taves DR: Exposure to excessive fluoride during hemodialysis. *Kidney Int* 5: 451, 1974

35. Schwarzbeck A, Wagner L, Squarr HU, Strauch M: pH-dependent heparin inactivation during hemodialysis. *Dial Transplant* 7: 740, 1978

36. Kirkwood R, Dunn S, Thomasson L, Simenhoff ML: Generation of the precarcinogen dimethyl nitrosamine (DMNA) in dialysate water. *Trans Am Soc Artif Intern Organs* 27: 168, 1981

37. Association for the Advancement of Medical Instrumentation: American National Standard for Hemodialysis Systems. Arlington, Virginia, AAMI, 1982

38. Keshaviah P, Luehmann D, Shapiro F, Comty CM: *Investigation of the Risks and Hazards associated with Hemodialysis Devices* Technical Report, Contract 223–78–5046, Silver Spring, MD, US Dept Health Education and Welfare, Food and Drug Administration, Bureau of Medical Devices, 1980

39. U.S. Environmental Protection Agency, Research and Development. Methods for Chemical Analysis of Water and Wastes, March 1979

40. Favero MS, Petersen NJ: Microbiological guidelines for hemodialysis systems. *Dial Transplant* 6: 34, 1977

41. Association for the Advancement of Medical Instrumentation: Recommended Practice for Reuse of Hemodialyzers. Arlington, Virginia, 1986

42. American Public Health Association: Standard Methods for the Examination of Water and Waste Water, 15th edition, APHA, AWWA, WPCF, Washington D.C., 1980

43. Bolan G, Reingold AL, Carson LA, Silcox VA, Woodley CL, Hayes PS, Hightower AW, McFarland L, Brown J, Petersen NJ, Favero MS, Good RC, Broome CF: Infections th mycobacterium chelonei in patients receiving dialysis and using processed dialyzers. *J Infect Dis* 152: 1013, 1985

44. Ebben J, Hirsch D, Luehmann D, Collins A, Keshaviah P: Microbiological contamination of liquid bicarbonate concentrate (LBC) for hemodialysis (HD). *Trans Am Soc Artif Intern Organs* 33: 269, 1987

45. U.S. Dept. of Health & Human Services, Food & Drug Administration: Device Good Manufacturing Practices Manual, 3rd edition, November 1984

THE COMPOSITION OF DIALYSIS FLUID

WILLIAM K. STEWART

HISTORICAL

Kolff (1) anticipated most of the problems that have been encountered in formulating a suitable dialysis fluid for haemodialysis. After many trials he advocated a low sodium, high potassium fluid (Table 1). The major problem was the high pH of the solution and the presence of bicarbonate which affected the solubility of calcium salts. Kolff attempted to adjust pH by bubbling CO_2 into the dialysis fluid. He finally used tap water containing calcium 1.0 mmol/l and gave calcium gluconate intravenously post-dialysis. To avoid haemolysis, dextrose monohydrate was added.

For early coil-type dialysers immersed in a fixed volume tank of dialysis fluid (e.g. Kolff-Travenol Tank) it was essential to remove the dialysate and renew the dialysis fluid every 2 h in order to achieve higher clearances (6). With these systems each 'bath' of dialysis fluid was adjusted to near pH 7.4 with lactic acid and bubbled CO_2, following which the calcium chloride was added. Any citrated and heparinised blood used for 'priming' the extracorporeal cir-

Table 1. Composition of extracellular fluid and of former and contemporary haemodialysis fluids (references in parenthesis).

	Serum (2)	Serum water (2)	Interstitial (2)	Earliest dialysis fluid (1)	1960's dialysis fluid (3–5)		1986 dialysis fluid** Extreme range majority	
Sodium mmol/l	142	152.7	145	126.5	130–135		109–148	128–140
Potassium mmol/l	4.0	4.3	4.0	5.4	0–1.5		0–4.0	1.0–2.0
Calcium mmol/l	2.5	1.5	1.5	1.0	1.25		0–1.75	1.5–1.75
Magnesium mmol/l	0.8	0.5	0.5	not stated	0.5		0–1.5	0.5–0.85
Chloride mmol/l	101	108.5	114	10	100.5		87–117	95–109
Bicarbonate mmol/l	27B	29.3B	31B	23.9B	35–40A		0–46.7A	35–40A
					1961 (3)	*1965 (4)*		
Glucose mmol/l	5.0	–	–	83–111 or 166*	111	11	0–30	11
g/dl	0.09	–	–	1.5–2.0 or 3.0*	2.0	0.2	0–0.54	0.2X

* = for fluid removal
B = bicarbonate; A = acetate
** = Courtesy of Macarthys Medical Ltd.
X = 78% at 0.2 ± 0.02, 16% at nil.

cuit was dialysed against the adjusted bath fluid before being connected to the patient so as to avoid hypocalcaemic effects (7).

The concentration of the principal electrolytes in extracellular fluid is given in Table 1 (2). Empirically, the composition of dialysis fluid should probably be similar to that of normal interstitial fluid appropriately corrected for the small protein component of the latter. In practice considerable variation has been advocated in both cation and anion concentrations. The common composition of dialysis fluid used in the early 1960's is listed (Table 1). The content of dextrose was reduced in later years, once ultrafiltration by pump-generated hydrostatic pressure had been shown to be superior to the earlier transmembrane osmolar gradient method of achieving water shift (3). Concentrations of other components have changed considerably since. The wide range of concentrations currently commercially-available (late 1980s) reflects disparate fluids used for particular clinical circumstances.

Since a main aim of haemodialysis is to restore physiological amounts and concentrations of univalent and divalent ions in the patient's intracellular and extracellular fluids as a result of diffusional transfers between dialysis fluid and blood plasma, the level of individual ions in dialysis fluid might be set arbitrarily at the mean levels found in plasma water. In this way sub- or hyper-normal concentrations in patients would tend to be corrected given time by equilibration along the concentration gradient. Accordingly, dialysis fluid sodium and potassium levels might be set at the respective median values for these cations in plasma water, while calcium and magnesium could likewise be set at the median levels for the diffusable fraction in plasma water of each divalent cation. This simplistic ideal is departed from in particular circumstances, such as acute renal failure, after parathyroid surgery and when the degree of urgency of an individual electrolyte abnormality calls for rapid correction.

Before 1975 the popularity of centralised dialysis fluid delivery systems, each linked to up to 30 dialysis positions and using commercially-manufactured dialysis fluid concentrate, led to more standardisation of dialysis fluid composition. A typical example of the dialysis fluid used for all 30 patients in such units might be Na 140, K 1.5, Ca 1.87, Mg 0.5 (all mmol/l). Departures from such dialysis fluid formulations are increasingly adopted now to meet individual patient needs. Individualised prescribing of dialysis content has become possible now that bedside (single patient) proportionating pump-monitors are widely available. Using these single-patient machines, the proportion of diluent water to concentrate can be varied within certain limits and, additionally, selected single components can be added to the concentrate prior to dilution provided that adequate care is taken to ensure complete mixing with the concentrate before dilution and use. In this way the level in dialysis fluid of sodium, potassium, calcium and magnesium can be individually increased according to need. Conversely, an increase of the dilution factor (conventionally 1:35 by volume) can decrease all concentrations if necessary.

When the stratagem of adding concentrated individual

electrolyte solutions is employed, it is essential that the content of the solutions so added is carefully calculated, prepared in advance and distinctively labelled. The act of addition to the concentrate and mixing must be properly witnessed and confirmed by formal labelling of the concentrate container. Unless these additions are made with established formality there is a serious risk of confusion or worse through unintentional double additions. Since the resultant composition cannot be easily checked analytically before use in clinical circumstances, it is vital that all the calculations, pharmaceutical preparation and labelling are undertaken with deliberation and in circumstances where double-checking is possible. These additives, for example high concentration potassium salt solution, are probably best stored in separate locked cupboards.

The role of the final concentration of each electrolyte and dextrose will be examined in detail.

INDIVIDUAL CONCENTRATIONS OF ELECTROLYTES AND DEXTROSE

Sodium

In dialysis fluid, as in extracellular fluid, sodium is the major determinant of osmolality. The early 1970's saw moves away from the hitherto unquestioned dialysis fluid with a low sodium concentration relative to plasma and especially to plasma water (Table 1) (8–10). The use of dialysis fluid with sodium as low as 115 mmol/l and as high as 155 mmol/l (11, 12) has been described, but the extremes are infrequently used. In 1976 most United Kingdom and continental European dialysis centres still chose a sodium concentration of less than 135 mmol/l, with a mean level of 130 mmol/l (13). The low sodium concentration in maintenance haemodialysis was carried forward from the earlier requirement (14) for a sodium gradient of about 20 mmol/l between dialysis fluid and plasma water. The rate of removal of sodium from the patient with early non-convective techniques was determined by the concentration difference across the dialysis membrane. Extraction of water in early haemodialysers was effected by osmotically-induced ultrafiltration, osmolality of dialysis fluid being increased relative to blood plasma by using unphysiologically-high concentrations of dextrose (>1.5 g/dl) which more than out-weighed the otherwise low dialysis fluid osmolarity due to low sodium concentrations.

Current haemodialysers are much more robust than earlier models and rupture of membranes is uncommon. Such dialysers are capable of withstanding higher hydrostatic pressures within the blood compartment. With these physical changes in dialyser characteristics, ultrafiltration nowadays is brought about predominantly by a hydrostatic pressure difference across the dialysis membrane. Ultrafiltration is capable of inducing net convective shifts of water, sodium and other micromolecular solutes from plasma to dialysate even in the absence of those concentrations gradients necessary for passive diffusion-induced transfers. Hydrostatically-effected movement of water, and accompanying solute by solvent-drag, has the great merit of easy control because transmembrane pressure can be adjusted according to clinical circumstances. In consequence there has been a marked trend upwards in transmembrane pressures. Concomitantly, dialysis fluid sodium concentrations have increased and glucose concentrations have decreased (13). The ultrafiltration of 2 kg of plasma water will remove about 260 mmol of sodium (as well as other solutes), an amount approximately equal to that ingested by the average patient during 3 days. Thus accumulated dietary sodium can be removed by hydrostatic ultrafiltration alone (15) and the original justification for a sodium concentration gradient across the dialyser has gone.

Dialysis centres imposing severe restrictions of salt and water intake for their patients may avoid the need for much ultrafiltration (e.g. >2.0 l in 5 h). Such centres continue to emphasise the need for minimal interdialytic weight gain by the patient and prefer the use of hyponatric dialysis fluid, possibly because its use appears to minimise thirst, spontaneous water intake and occasionally hypertension in the patients. However, there have always been some patients who, despite adequate dialysis and removal of sodium with a concentration of sodium in dialysis fluid at 130 mmol/l, remained hypertensive (16). Recently low sodium dialysis fluid (circa 130 mmol/l) has been shown to result in recurrent cerebral water intoxication (17).

Current usage

Figure 1 illustrates the current range of dialysis fluid sodium concentrations for the majority of United Kingdom users. Only 5% of solutions supplied have sodium concentrations less than 130 mmol/l and the vast majority lie between 130 and 136 mmol/l. Ten per cent have sodium concentrations above 136 mmol/l.

It should be recognised, however, that concentrate supplied by the manufacturer is not always a reliable indicator of the final dialysis concentrations used. Not all dilute X35. Some dialysis units underdilute the concentrate, or use water-softening devices which may increase the final sodium concentration by up to 6 mmol/l.

The 1980 figures show a clear trend upwards in the sodium concentration used compared with 1974 (12). The change is particularly noticeable compared with the figures for 1967, when 80% of European dialysis centres were using sodium concentrations of 130 mmol/l (18). This dropped to 28% for United Kingdom centres in 1980. Since 1980 there has been no further trend upwards in sodium concentrations. Boquin and colleagues in 1977 (19) surveyed the concentration of sodium in the dialysis fluid obtained from concentrate supplied by the three main manufacturers in the United States (covering 75% of the market) and found that 35% had a sodium concentration of 130 to 133 mmol/l, 61% had 134 to 136 mmol/l, but only 4% were in the 137 to 140 mmol/l range.

Relationship to intra-dialytic upset and osmolal change

The role of sodium concentration in dialysis fluid was seen originally in terms of 'dialysis dysequilibrium syndrome' (DDS) alone. The core symptomatology of DDS included headache, nausea, vomiting and muscle cramps with other less frequent components such as hypotension, hypoxaemia, acidosis and anterior chest pain. Unfortunately for the clinician it is now apparent that hypotension, the commonest side-effect of haemodialysis, can result from hypovolaemia, vasomotor instability, and probably other factors in addition to DDS. There appear to exist several overlapping intra-dialytic upsets of which DDS is only one.

DDS was formerly largely equated with dialysis-induced change in extracellular fluid osmolality and resultant movements of water between body compartments. Every dialysis treatment, with concentration-induced diffusional changes of non-sodium solutes such as phosphate and bicarbonate across the dialyser membrane, necessarily involves a drop in plasma osmolality. Ultrafiltration does not produce significant change in osmolality.

During dialysis with dialysis fluid sodium of 130 mmol/l or less, the blood returning to the patient will be hyponatraemic. Consequently the general plasma sodium concentration will decrease progressively over the course of the dialysis session. This reduction in extracellular sodium concentration, as well as the concomitant lowering of plasma urea concentrations, will produce a situation where the intracellular fluid is relatively hyperosmolar to extracellular fluid and there will be a consequent movement of water from the extracellular space to the intracellular space. In the case of low sodium dialysis the decrease in extracellular osmolality is of the order of 30 mOsm/kg plasma water, from about 310 mOsm/kg plasma water pre-dialysis to 280 mOsm/kg plasma water post-dialysis. Clinically these osmolality-related changes are expressed mainly by nausea and vomiting, muscle cramps, hypotension and heachaches (20). Cerebral overhydration is also thought to play a part (17).

It has to be recognised that maintenance dialysis treatment cannot be undertaken without the extraction of osmotically-active substances from the patient. On a priori grounds the therapeutic aim must be to minimise both the extent and rate of osmolal changes. The concentration of sodium in dialysis fluid should be chosen with these desiderata in mind. Sodium concentration is the variable which can most easily be manipulated so as to reduce the extent of osmolal change. It follows that no single sodium concentration is ideal for everyone. The concentration selected will vary on the one hand according to the haemodialysis technique employed (particularly the extent of ultrafiltration used and the temporal inter-relation between ultrafiltration and dialysis) and on the other hand according to dietary restrictions and patient compliance, especially related to water and salt intakes.

The use of an increased sodium concentration in dialysis fluid has been the main approach adopted so as to reduce the extent of change in the osmolality of body fluids during the dialysis session. Other strategies include (a) sequential dialysis, i.e. ultrafiltration (convective transfer) followed by dialysis (diffusion transfer) to separate in time solute from water removal (21, 22), (b) infusions of mannitol to counteract the reduction in plasma osmolality as urea is dialysed out of the extracellular fluid (23, 24), (c) high concentrations of dextrose in dialysis fluid (23, 25), (d) glycerol in dialysis fluid (26), and (e) hypertonic saline infusions (27). Other investigators have advocated the use of haemofiltration (diafiltration or haemodiafiltration) in which replacement fluids are infused either before (pre-dialyser) or after the ultrafiltration process (post-dialyser) (28–30) and have claimed a marked reduction in the symptoms of disequilibrium which so often accompany low sodium dialysis. Cambi and colleagues (31) have recommended ultrashort dialysis (2 h) with recirculation of 20 to 40 l dialysate in a closed system, using sodium concentrations of 132 mmol/l or 140 mmol/l.

Coincidental with the observations that higher rates of ultrafiltration could be tolerated as long as sodium concentrations in dialysis fluid were higher (10, 12, 19, 32, 33), Bergström and his co-workers (21) recommended the temporal separation of the ultrafiltration process from the dialysis process. When the dialysis phase, which followed ultrafiltration, was carried out with sodium concentrations of 145 mmol/l, patient tolerance was better than when the sodium concentration was only 133 mmol/l. Reduction in blood volume has been shown to be less during dialysis with 145 mmol/l of sodium compared with 130 mmol/l (34). Liebau and colleagues (11) recommended increasing the sodium concentration of dialysis fluid to as high as 155 mmol/l to promote better control of blood pressure in patients with uncontrollable hypertension at lower sodium concentrations. Locatelli and colleagues (12) also showed that sodium concentrations in dialysis fluid as high as 155 mmol/l enabled toleration of high ultrafiltration rates (3 l/h) with concurrent dialysis. Schuenemann and colleagues (35) have pointed out that the body is more sensitive to concentration changes than to volume changes. It was once believed that the reduction in plasma volume during the course of a haemodialysis treatment session was responsible for much dialysis-related upset but it has gradually become apparent that diffusion-produced changes in individual plasma electrolyte and solute concentrations and in osmolality seem to mediate much of the trouble (12, 20, 23).

Recent studies continue to confirm the benefits obtained with higher dialysis fluid sodium concentrations (36, 37). 'Redy machine' dialysis is also better tolerated, especially for children, with a sodium concentration of 140 mmol/l compared with 130 mmol/l (38). Murisasco et al (39) advocate the use of individualised sequential sodium dialysis, and suggest that patients tend to divide into two groups. In one group plasma sodium changes are predictable and dialysis fluid sodium level can be chosen to minimise change so that pre- and post-dialysis plasma sodium concentrations are alike. In the other group a uniform plasma sodium concentration maintained by using a single individually-selected dialysis fluid sodium is not possible and intermittent alternating phases (30 to 90 min) of hypertonic and hypotonic dialysis fluid is required throughout each dialysis. The patients in this group have either excess sodium concentration or excess water load post-dialysis. One of the inherent difficulties in matching dialysis fluid sodium individually to each patient lies in the limited accuracy of the measuring and diluting devices used (40, 41). This inaccuracy applies both to the commercial dialysis fluid concentrates and to the dilutional adjustments made by proportionating systems at the bedside. Accuracy in the product dialysis fluid of the order of better than ± 2% is ordinarily unobtainable, e.g. 140 mmol Na per litre ± 2.8. Similarly serum sodium measurement is liable to imprecision.

Limitations of increased sodium dialysis and reduced osmolal change

Even with higher sodium concentrations in dialysis fluid, acetate-based dialysis can induce changes which produce symptoms, electroencephalogram (EEG) alterations and vasomotor instability which could be regarded as typical of DDS (42). Some authors have found that higher sodium concentrations, although reducing DDS, have given rise to problems of thirst and unacceptable inter-dialysis weight-gains (43, 33). Redaelli and colleagues (45) have shown that truly isonatric dialysis, with sodium concentrations in dialysis fluid matched to that in the patient's plasma water, actually causes a small sodium gain. A movement of water from extracellular to intracellular space is probably responsible for an increase of around 3 mmol/l in plasma water sodium concentrations during dialysis with isonatric dialysis fluid. Locatelli and colleagues (46) have pointed out that any particular sodium concentration in dialysis fluid (e.g. 140 mmol/l) is not inherently 'high' or 'low' in itself, but should be related to the individual patient's plasma water sodium. A sodium in dialysis fluid of 140 mmol/l could be high for a hypoproteinaemic hyponatraemic patient, and low for a sodium-overloaded patient. It should be recognised that as far as extra-cellular fluid is concerned minimising sodium concentration change and minimising osmolal change are mutually exclusive. A dialysis fluid sodium which maintains unchanged plasma sodium concentrations will mean reduction in plasma osmolality, due mainly to urea concentration decreases. A dialysis fluid which would minimise induced changes in plasma osmolality would require to have a hypernatraemic sodium concentration in order that the increase in plasma sodium during dialysis would counteract the osmolar effect of the inevitable fall in plasma urea. This could have disadvantages in the long term.

The contribution to osmolal change from diffusion of constituents such as creatinine and phosphate is minimal relative to urea and sodium. Other methods aimed at reducing plasma osmolality changes to the unavoidable minimum necessitated by urea diffusion have various disadvantages. Mannitol, being possibly toxic in prolonged usage, is seldom used (47). The use of glyercol has been criticised by Van Stone and colleagues (48) who consider sodium or dextrose to be more physiological. Haemofiltration has its advocates (29, 49) but is relatively expensive.

Sodium modelling and future trends

Redaelli and colleagues (45) recommended matching sodium concentrations in dialysis fluid to that in the plasma of the individual patient, to counteract ultrafiltration-produced increases in plasma water sodium. In practical terms, this means a sodium concentration in dialysis fluid several mmol/l lower than the patient's plasma water sodium. In their experience this turned out to be, on average, a sodium concentration of 142 mmol/l (termed by them 'adequate' sodium in dialysis fluid).

Individual matching of dialysis fluid concentration to patient needs has not proved practical in most dialysis units, though the principle has much to recommend it. The advent of variable-dilution proportioning machines has made this ideal approach attainable in some centres. The ultimate form of such individual 'optimisation' is 'sodium modelling'. This involves selecting dialysis fluid sodium concentrations for each patient on the basis of previous observations on his (her) pre- and post-dialysis plasma sodium levels (39). Some programmes involve changing dialysis fluid sodium during dialysis in accordance with computer-calculated predictions derived from the patients' intradialytic sodium and water-loading characteristics (50). Ultrafiltration can be similarly programmed on an individual patient's recent characteristics. All such predictions are based on computer simulation models with one or more constituent compartments. They remain experimental and problematic but their success to date in reducing dialysis-related patient upset points to the critical role of dialysis fluid sodium concentration, and its variation and interrelationship to ultrafiltration, during each haemodialysis.

The future trend may well be to vary sodium in dialysis fluid throughout an individual dialysis (51–53). This approach avoids the loss of valuable diffusional dialysis time which occurs when using pure ultrafiltration (as in sequential ultrafiltration/dialysis), a factor especially important in the face of the trend towards shorter dialysis treatment times. Locatelli and colleagues (54) believe that the use of higher dialysis fluid sodium concentration with concurrent ultrafiltration is better than sequential ultrafiltration and dialysis in all but the heavily water-overloaded patient. Patients with cellular overhydration have responded well to gradual reduction of dialysis fluid sodium throughout a dialysis period, combined with replacement fluid at 140 mmol/l sodium concentration (52). Chen and colleagues (53) found that, compared with standard dialysis at 130 mmol/l, an extra litre of fluid could be removed with a continuously decreasing sodium concentration in dialysis fluid from 150 to 133 mmol/l, before arterial blood pressure was affected. Dumler and colleagues (51) dialysed patients against a sodium concentration of 150 mmol/l for 3 h and then at 130 mmol/l for 1 h and found fewer symptoms of 'disequilibrium' compared to using sodium concentrations of 140 mmol/l throughout a dialysis. The aim of these strategies was to counteract the osmolality fall accompanying urea removal by allowing sodium influx during the first hours of dialysis and thereafter to remove sodium during the later part of the dialysis treatment session. This approach may prove useful in those few refractory patients who have excessive thirst and weight gain when treated with a higher sodium concentration in dialysis fluid and, paradoxically, hypotension and cramps when treated with a lower sodium concentration.

Potassium

Potassium homeostasis is considerably affected in both acute and chronic renal failure. The dialysis solutions suitable for acute and chronic renal failure will be discussed separately.

Acute renal failure

Control of hyperkalaemia during the early oliguric phase is important, being particularly difficult in patients with a hypermetabolic response when the initial rise in the level of potassium in the plasma frequently exceeds other biochemical markers of uraemia. If internal bleeding has been an additional complication the rapid release of potassium from lysis of red blood cells leads to an increased hazard. Hyperkalaemia in early days was most readily corrected by withholding potassium from the dialysis fluid (55) for the first 60 min of dialysis unless the patient was receiving digitalis or similar drugs. When release of intracellular potassium is excessive (i.e. from large haematomas or haemolysis) a deliberate attempt to produce a partial depletion of total body potassium (TBK) using a zero or relatively low potassium concentration in dialysis fluid for a longer period of time can delay the recurrence of hyperkalaemia. In contrast, during prolonged diarrhoea and vomiting, the development of hypokalaemia should be prevented by adding potassium to the dialysis fluid.

With modern flow-to-waste proportioning systems, control of plasma potassium in acute renal failure requires care. A wide range of dialysis fluid concentrates, each with a different potassium level, is to be avoided. A single dialysis concentrate giving on dilution 1.5 mmol/l potassium can be used with locally-prepared or commercial potassium chloride additives. Such additives must be rigorously controlled in use (i.e. stock holding, act of mixing, labelling of container). Ideally the potassium concentration in the resultant dialysis fluid should be checked directly by a potassium-measuring electrode system before dialysis is commenced. While low potassium dialysis fluid (e.g. 1.5 mmol/l) is useful early in the course of acute renal failure it is an error to continue with that concentration when the patient is dialysed daily and may eat poorly and/or have potassium losses by other routes. Accordingly, it is often convenient to dialyse with a fluid containing 4 mmol/l of potassium to prevent inadvertent depletion.

Chronic renal failure

For potassium (and also magnesium) there are ranges of plasma values beyond the normal reference range which are not associated with adverse clinical effects. This is fortunate, for some accumulation of total body potassium is inevitable between dialyses when the oliguric patient on maintenance dialysis is eating normal food. Considerable flexibility is automatically included in a maintenance dialysis regimen, because the quantity of each cation removed, assuming a fixed concentration in the dialysis fluid, increases as the plasma value rises and, conversely, decreases as that in the plasma falls. Reverse movement of potassium down a concentration gradient into the patient can occur in potassium-depleted individuals, and can be arranged if needed. Thus small changes in daily dietary intake are acceptable. The concentration of potassium used in the dialysis fluid must depend on dietary intake, type of dialyser used and the duration and frequency of dialysis (56) so that there is no single ideal value applicable to all clinical conditions. Intracellular potassium is also dependent on the acid-base balance so that the relative levels of sodium, chloride and acetate (likewise bicarbonate) in dialysis fluid are also important determinants of potassium balance. Unfortunately all those factors which affect potassium homeostasis in patients treated by regular dialysis have not been stated in the majority of reported investigations so that it becomes difficult, if not impossible, to make an accurate assessment (57). Currently used fluids have potassium concentrations ranging from 0 to 4 mmol/l, with most between 1 and 2 mmol/l.

The plasma concentration of potassium is not a reliable guide to total body content though most would agree that persistently low values, particularly before dialysis, are indicative of a total body deficit. Red cell concentrations (58) may give a better indication of total body potassium (TBK). As a result, investigations to ascertain the optimum concentration of potassium in dialysis fluid have been mainly directed towards measurement of either TBK or potassium content of muscle obtained by biopsy. Exchangeable potassium values using ^{42}K or ^{43}K (76) underestimate TBK in renal failure possibly due to their slow distribution. Using ^{40}K techniques several investigators (59–61) found no evidence of potassium depletion in patients taking a moderately restricted potassium diet and dialysed against usual dialysis fluid potassium concentrations. When the potassium intake was low or the level in the dialysis fluid was less than 1.5 mmol/l (or both) (56) then TBK was below normal. Some caution is necessary in the interpretation of these data. For instance, an attempt was made to correct the acidosis resulting from the use of one of the dialysis fluids (shown previously to give normal values of TBK [60]) by elevating the acetate in the dialysis fluid by 5 mmol/l at the expense of chloride (62). Profound symptomatic hypokalaemia developed in all patients which was corrected by temporarily raising the potassium concentration in dialysis fluid to 5 mmol/l. As no other changes had been introduced potassium appeared to have moved intracellularly in response to correction of metabolic acidosis. Thus TBK, as measured by ^{40}K is not always an infallible guide to the state of potassium balance or the dialysis fluid potassium required, but is a non-invasive investigation allowing measurements to be made repeatedly over an indefinite period of time. It must

also be remembered that some reduction in TBK should be expected because most patients with renal failure have a reduced red cell mass (56).

The other main method used for estimating potassium content of the body has been by analysis of muscle biopsies (57, 63). Intracellular potassium appears to be low in chronic renal failure but returns to normal after institution of dialysis, provided dialysis fluid potassium is not too low (57). Whether this improvement in potassium content after starting intermittent dialysis is due to improved dietary intake, decreased intracellular water or correction of acidosis is not clear.

On the available evidence a free dietary intake of 60 to 80 mmol potassium per day with a thrice weekly dialysis schedule, each dialysis lasting 4 to 5 h, seems to give an acceptable potassium balance when the dialysis fluid contains about 1.5 mmol/l. There will inevitably be some minor asymptomatic hyperkalaemia before dialysis and hypokalaemia immediately after dialysis. With shorter dialysis times and larger (1.5 m²) dialysers (64) potassium balance seemed to remain unaltered. If the concentration of potassium in the dialysis fluid is greater than 1.5 mmol/l or dialysis is undertaken only twice per week some dietary restriction of potassium is probably required, since hyperkalaemia is still a major cause of death in patients treated by regular dialysis (65), particularly following treatment interruptions.

If dietary intake is temporarily reduced (e.g. during intercurrent illness), oral supplementation of potassium or an increased level in the dialysis fluid (e.g. raised to 3.5 mmol/l by additives) may be necessary. Should the time interval between dialyses be temporarily lengthened (e.g. in case of difficulties with vascular access) plasma potassium must be measured frequently and any tendency for the development of hyperkalaemia corrected by using an orally administered calcium cation-exchange resin (66).

Quintanilla and Weffer (67) have pointed out that one large meal could contain sufficient potassium to raise plasma potassium dangerously high in renal patients, were it not for the ability of the tissues to 'soak up' potassium rapidly. Patients on dialysis are critically dependent on this tissue storage and on colonic epithelial excretion of potassium (68) between dialyses. The effect of uraemia on aldosterone metabolism can significantly interfere with potassium adaptability (67). Diabetic patients are particularly at risk of hyperkalaemia, due to hyperglycaemia. Heparin has also been implicated as a possible factor in the development of hyperkalaemia (69). All these influences must be borne in mind when choosing the dialysis fluid potassium for a unit or when interpreting anomalous levels for an individual patient.

Calcium

In the past, account had to be taken of the calcium content of the water supply used to dilute the concentrate as this could add up to 0.2 or 0.4 mmol/l (0.7 to 1.5 mg/dl) of calcium. Most units now use reverse osmosis of the mains water used for dialysis and allowing for water calcium content has become irrelevant. Units which allowed for untreated mains water calcium should remember to make the necessary upward adjustment in concentrate calcium when reverse osmosis is installed. For occasional use with individual patients it is possible to increase calcium in dialysis fluid by adding a calculated amount of calcium chloride dihydrate in solution to a known quantity of concentrate and mixing well.

The diffusible fraction of calcium in the plasma of patients with renal failure was reported to be higher than in normal subjects, values ranging from 57.6 to 64.3% (70) of the total plasma calcium value, so that the minimum amount of calcium in dialysis fluid to achieve a zero or slightly positive balance to the patients was found to be about 1.5 to 1.55 mmol/l (6 to 6.2 mg/dl) (70). Early studies on mineralisation of bone indicated that calcium was lost from the skeleton when calcium fell below 1.5 mmol/l (6 mg/dl) in dialysis fluid (71). Increasing the concentration to 1.75 mmol/l (7 mg/dl) prevented a fall in the metacarpal bone index and a further increase to 2.0 mmol/l (8 mg/dl) resulted in an increase in total body calcium in patients with osteomalacia (72). Discussion on adequacy of calcium concentration in dialysis fluid has been focused on the range 1.5 to 2.0 mmol/l (6 to 8 mg/dl).

Some treatment techniques such as ultrafiltration and haemofiltration, lead to convective loss of calcium from plasma to dialysate. During ultrafiltration for example, diffusible but not protein-bound calcium will be removed pari passu with water and sodium.

Manipulation of calcium concentration in dialysis fluid can be used readily to augment the delivery of calcium to the patient during haemodialysis. The calcium concentration in dialysis fluid and the concomitant levels of plasma inorganic phosphate have been shown to be the two major influences controlling the flux of calcium across the dialyser during haemodialysis (73). Calcium transfers from dialysis fluid to patient of 8 to 43 mmol/weekly can be effected with single-pass systems by varying dialysis fluid calcium and can be used to correct evident calcium deficits. In recirculating systems 'reverse dialysis' of calcium (i.e. into the patient) is difficult to control due to the progressive decrease in calcium in the recirculated dialysis fluid.

During the last 15 years the traditional level of 1.25 to 1.5 mmol/l (5 to 6 mg/dl) calcium in dialysis fluid has been increased in several units in the hope of normalising overall calcium balance (74) and perhaps obviating hyperparathyroidism and osteodystrophy. The majority of current dialysis fluids have between 1.5 and 1.75 mmol/l (6 to 7 mg/dl) of calcium (Figure 1). Levels as high as 2.0 mmol/l (8 mg/dl) of calcium in dialysis fluid have been recommended (73). Overt post-dialytic hypercalcaemia has been reported as uncommon when using 1.75 mmol/l (7 mg/dl) of calcium in dialysis fluid (75). Even transient dialysis-related hypercalcaemia readily provokes unpleasant nausea, vomiting and hypertension (76) and should be avoided. Moreover, covert soft tissue calcification is widespread in dialysed patients, and of obscure causation (77). A positive calcium-balance and an intermittent rapid influx of extraneous calcium cannot be assumed to be entirely beneficial, indeed it may be

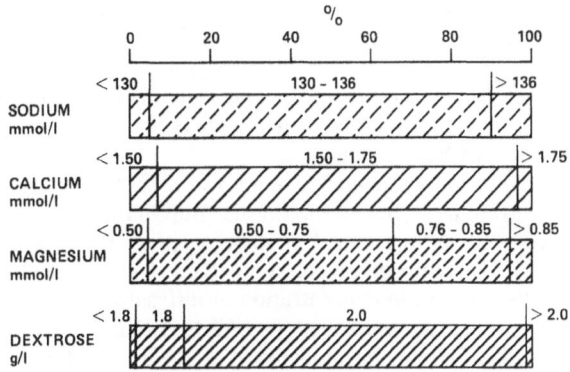

Figure 1. Current (1987) range of sodium, calcium, magnesium and dextrose concentrations of haemodialysis fluids supplied to the U.K. (courtesy of Macarthy Medical).

harmful. Divalent ions may influence blood pressure by altering vascular tone (78). The inward movement of calcium in particular during dialysis can increase cardiac contractility (79), especially as it occurs at a time of plasma potassium reduction (80). Furthermore, increased divalent ions in skin have been related to the common problem of pruritus in dialysed patients (81).

Despite the trend to higher calcium concentration in dialysis fluid some advocate, and many continue to use, traditional lower and possibly safer levels between 1.5 to 1.6 mmol/l (6 to 6.4 mg/dl). Effective treatment with active vitamin D sterols may be affected by calcium concentrations in dialysis fluid (82). Dialysis fluid calcium concentrations above 1.75 mmol/l (7 mg/dl) suppress parathyroid hormone (PTH) secretion in some short-term studies (83) but not in others (84). Effects of intermittent dialysis on parathyroid function or bone status are not necessarily persistent and may be less potent than the effects produced by pharmacologic doses of vitamin D_3 metabolites (85).

The recent urge to increase calcium concentrations in dialysis fluid should be tempered by realisation that the effect of active vitamin D metabolites and analogues such as 1,25-dihydroxyvitamin D_3 ($1,25(OH)_2D_3$) or 1 α hydroxyvitamin D_3 ($1\alpha(OH)D_3$) is additional to the effect of high calcium in dialysis fluid (82). The pharmacological use of sterols which influence intestinal calcium absorption is also inherently more constant, controllable and physiological than the adoption of high calcium concentrations in dialysis fluids. These sterols suppress parathyroid overactivity but long established parathyroid hyperplasia only regresses slowly (86).

There are both advantages and disadvantages in the two approaches to the correction of negative calcium balance in patients on intermittent dialysis, i.e. 'reverse dialysis' of calcium and vitamin D analogues. An increased calcium concentration in the dialysis fluid presents practical difficulties in preparing appropriate concentrates and ensuring that the correct one is used for individual patients. Furthermore, it will have a short-lived effect in suppressing parathyroid overactivity. Use of calcitriol or equivalent vitamin D sterol certainly increases absorption of dietary calcium and can seemingly balance any tendency to calcium loss when a low calcium concentration in dialysis fluid (1.375 mmol/l [5.5 mg/dl]) is used. Nevertheless, careful monitoring of plasma calcium levels and drug dosage is required to avoid unwanted hypercalcaemia.

Contemporary attempts to optimise dialysis fluid calcium concentrations seem over-optimistic. Bulk-purchased commercial concentrate aimed at some arbitrary level, is unlikely to be appropriate for more than a few individual patients. The mean concentration of diffusable calcium in blood plasma is approximately 1.60 to 1.65 mmol/l (6.4–6.6 mg/dl). Patients haemodialysed at 1.625 mmol/l gained on average only 3.0 mmol calcium during one dialysis but the variation in the group of patients ranged from −16.4 to +18 mmol (−650 to +720 mg) (87). It should be remembered that ultrafiltration of 2.0 l of fluid will remove circa 3.5 mmol (140 mg) calcium from the patient each dialysis. Patients subjected to high ultrafiltration will lose proportionately more calcium and be in more negative calcium balance than those with low ultrafiltration at any given dialysis fluid concentration. It would therefore make sense to increase dialysis fluid calcium to compensate in units applying high ultrafiltration, such as those using higher (isonatric) dialysis fluid sodium concentrations. While in maintenance haemodialysis conditions it is not possible to match each patients with an appropriate dialysis fluid, the adoption of around 1.63 mmol calcium/l (6.5 mg/dl) will probably minimise calcium transfers. As a policy the concentration of calcium in dialysis fluid should be just high enough to avoid the development of a negative calcium balance across the dialyser. It is recognised that this alone will not stabilise bone metabolism.

Magnesium

Magnesium is predominantly intracellular, but the physiological plasma concentration is stabilised within the range 0.70 to 1.10 mmol/l (1.7 to 2.7 mg/dl), approximately 25% being protein-bound, and the rest diffusible (0.52 to 0.82 mmol/l, 1.3 to 2.0 mg/dl), mostly in the ionised form (88). Absorption of dietary magnesium in renal failure appears to be normal (89) and continues unaltered despite the development of hypermagnesaemia or tissue excess (88) so that in renal failure care must be taken whenever magnesium-containing medication is used.

The kidney is the main regulator of extracellular magnesium concentration. As renal failure progresses with reduced glomerular filtration, hypermagnesaemia is inevitable if dietary intake is normal. Magnesium excess has been associated with cardiac abnormalities (at plasma concentrations approaching 5 mmol/l, 12 mg/dl) and with effects on the nervous system, such as loss of deep tendon reflexes, at plasma concentrations above 3 mmol/l (7.3 mg/dl) (88). Magnesium deficiency also affects the nervous system, causing neuromuscular disturbances and tremor.

The relationships between magnesium, PTH and bone metabolism, both in the presence and absence of renal fail-ure, are complex. Investigations have been beset by problems of PTH assay and have often been inconsistent (90). Although some have indicated that acute hypermagnesaemia tends to reduce PTH production (88) more recent studies have shown no change in PTH status with varying dialysis fluid magnesium concentrations (91). Lower dialysis fluid magnesium can decrease bone magnesium without any alteration in PTH levels (91). Others have shown that increased magnesium concentrations can suppress the release of PTH, but do not alter the rate of synthesis (92). In chronic renal failure, the effect of magnesium is subservient to the overriding effect of calcium on PTH production, hypocalcaemia being a far more potent stimulus than varying magnesium concentrations (88).

A survey of dialysis fluid concentrates for the United Kingdom market in 1980 found magnesium concentrations in dialysis fluid ranging from 0 to 1.0 mmol/l (2.4 mg/dl) with 80% of fluids between 0.50 and 0.80 mmol/l (1.2–1.95 mg/dl). In the early days of maintenance haemodialysis a dialysis fluid magnesium of 0.5 to 0.7 mmol/l was usual so practice did not change markedly over two decades. The position in 1987 is unchanged. Despite the recommendations (91) that dialysis fluid magnesium should be 0.25 mmol/l (0.6 mg/dl) or less and continued reports on the benefits of low magnesium dialysis (93), 90% of currently supplied dialysis fluids in the United Kingdom (Figure 1) have magnesium concentrations ranging from 0.5 to 0.85 mmol/l (1.2 to 2.1 mg/dl) and only 5% use less than 0.5 mmol/l. Magnesium-free dialysis fluid has been advocated for patients given magnesium-containing antacids to control phosphate absorption (94, 95), but there is a strong body of opinion against using magnesium-containing drugs in patients with renal failure, dialysed or not (94, 96). Drüeke (95) considers 0.4 to 0.6 mmol/l (1 to 1.5 mg/dl) of magnesium to be appropriate for dialysis fluid if oral magnesium drugs are avoided. Magnesium concentrations of 0.25 mmol/l (0.6 mg/dl) are recommended for peritoneal dialysis fluid (97). The aim should be to normalise extracellular magnesium as much as possible and avoid either prolonged hypermagnesaemia or hypomagnesaemia. Overall, prolonged hypermagnesaemia appears to carry more dangers than temporary hypomagnesaemia under established maintenance haemodialysis conditions. Low magnesium concentrations in dialysis fluid (0.2 mmol/l [0.5 mg/dl]) (98–100) result in normal to high normal predialysis plasma magnesium concentrations, decreasing to mildly low concentrations post-dialysis which return to normal a few hours later. Thus plasma magnesium can be made to fluctuate across the normal range. Low plasma magnesium is always associated with low plasma potassium, but hypokalaemia can exist without hypomagnesaemia (96).

Lowering magnesium in dialysis fluid to between 0 to 0.2 mmol/l (0.5 mg/dl) has resulted in improved nerve conduction velocities (93, 100), erythrocyte magnesium concentrations nearer normal (99), less pruritus (101) and improvements of renal osteodystrophy (102), though some of these claims have been disputed (103).

It is accepted that magnesium retention, rather than depletion, is the main problem in renal failure and excess magnesium may be a factor in both renal bone disease (94, 104) and soft tissue calcification (80, 90, 105). In contrast, it has recently been suggested (106) that hypermagnesaemia protects against soft tissue calcification. Erythrocyte and tissue magnesium concentrations appear to remain high even with the long term use of low magnesium dialysis fluid (99, 103). Although the overt effects of acutely high plasma magnesium concentrations are seldom seen in patients on intermittent dialysis, the avoidance of even moderate hypermagnesaemia would seem a desirable goal. This aim is even more relevant today when more units are attempting to use magnesium-containing rather than aluminium-containing drugs to reduce phosphate absorption. Nevertheless the majority of dialysis units, however, accept moderate hypermagnesaemia as a matter of course, with pre-dialysis values in the 1.5 to 2.0 mmol/l (3.7 to 4.9 mg/dl) range using a dialysis fluid magnesium concentration of 0.5 to 0.7 mmol/l (1.2 to 1.7 mg/dl) (103).

Future trends in dialysis fluid magnesium concentrations will probably be downwards, to a possible mean between 0.2 and 0.3 mmol/l (0.5 to 0.7 mg/dl) which, on present evidence, would appear to be the most acceptable level. As dialysis times become shorter, magnesium retention may be increased, and it would seem sensible to lower magnesium in dialysis fluids accordingly, in order to keep plasma magnesium within the reference range as much as possible. On the other hand if dietary intake of magnesium decreases for any reason (e.g. anorexia or diarrhoea), it would be wise to monitor plasma magnesium concentrations and supplement by oral, parenteral or higher dialysis fluid concentrations when sub-normal pre-dialysis values are found. Magnesium has an important role in the regulation of intracellular protein synthesis (107). It is also worth remembering that the administration of aminoglycoside antibiotics can produce magnesium, calcium and potassium wasting (96). In the absence of magnesium-containing oral drugs, magnesium-free dialysis fluid is contraindicated (108) since symptomatic magnesium depletion with PTH suppression can develop in some patients. Lack of magnesium may also play a role in the development of dialysis-related cramps (108).

Hard-water syndrome

Dialysis fluid calcium levels of 3.6 mmol/l (14.4 mg/dl) and magnesium levels of 1.5 mmol/l (3.7 mg/dl) have been reported after failure of mains water treatment systems (109, 110), causing acute symptoms of hypertension, sweating, warmth, nausea and vomiting, with progressing lethargy and weakness. These were isolated instances, but dialysis staff should be aware of the possibility of malfunctions in the dialysis fluid delivery systems if rapidly developing clinical symptoms occur during a dialysis session.

Acetate and bicarbonate

In the 1960's acetate replaced bicarbonate as the buffer substrate in haemodialysis fluid to ensure adequate solubility of the calcium and magnesium salts. This change was considered to be a major advance in formulation. It enabled concentrates to be prepared commercially and bought in bulk. The amount of acetate diffusing into the circulation during a routine haemodialysis of that time was estimated at about 90 mmol/h. The recommended concentration of acetate in dialysis fluid (5) was determined at 35 mmol/l and values close to this concentration are still used.

Acetate was almost universally adopted and it is surprising that only in relatively recent years has its metabolism been studied in patients with renal failure and its use questioned. It took more than a decade before it was realised (111) that critically-ill often-septic patients in acute renal failure were especially intolerant of acetate in dialysis fluid. In particular, ultrafiltration was relatively poorly tolerated in such patients.

Present day dialysers are relatively more efficient and frequently have larger surface areas. A further gain in clearance rates and enhanced transfer of acetate to the patient followed the replacement of the Scribner shunt with the arterio-venous fistula, which allows a much greater flow rate of blood through the dialyser. Many investigators have found that the larger dialysing areas and enhanced blood flow rates allow more than 300 mmol/h of acetate to be transferred to the patient during dialysis (112). This can cause some biochemical disturbances. A rise in the anion gap develops and plasma bicarbonate decreases as acetate rises, thereby indicating that bicarbonate regeneration is not as rapid as the bicarbonate loss. In contrast when using bicarbonate in dialysis fluid there is a progressive fall in anion gap as the bicarbonate concentration rises and waste-metabolite anions are removed (113). After dialysis any accumulated acetate is rapidly metabolised to bicarbonate (114). In maintenance haemodialysis the majority of individuals exposed regularly to acetate develop a degree of tolerance, although there may be a subset who are slow disposers of acetate (115).

The 1980's have seen a marked increase in the number of papers recommending bicarbonate dialysis (116). There is no doubt that bicarbonate dialysis is the treatment of choice in acute renal failure (117, 118) and for elderly or diabetic patients, or those with cardiovascular instability, on maintenance haemodialysis. Central nervous system symptoms and tolerance of ultrafiltration are improved by bicarbonate haemodialysis (113, 119, 120) though muscle cramps appear to be an exception (121). A high (isonatric) sodium concentration is needed to reduce muscle cramps (8). Also use of a high sodium dialysis fluid will reduce the need for bicarbonate dialysis fluid, since the high sodium leads to better blood pressure control, better tolerance of ultrafiltration and fewer symptoms irrespective of whether the fluid is acetate or bicarbonate based (122, 123).

Most recent reports agree that bicarbonate dialysis prevents haemodynamic instability during haemodialysis and minimises blood pressure changes (115, 124–126). Acetate dialysis leads to an increase in cardiac output while vascular resistance and myocardial O_2 supply decrease (127) and when O_2 demand exceeds the supply the myocardium becomes hypoperfused. There is less change in left ventricular function with bicarbonate dialysis (126). Although acetate may be incorporated into lipids (128) lipid balance does not differ appreciably, comparing bicarbonate and acetate dialysis (129), nor do some of the metabolic parameters affecting blood pressure, such as plasma renin activity and kininogen which increase during dialysis irrespective of acetate or bicarbonate (130). The improved blood pressure control on bicarbonate is therefore attributed to improvements in vascular resistance (127) and to less change in plasma volume (125).

Acid-base balance and the degree of hypoxaemia both fluctuate less on bicarbonate dialysis (115, 120, 131) but hypoxaemia does still occur in bicarbonate dialysis (129). With acetate dialysis hypoxaemia is aggravated by CO_2 loss (132, 133), which leads to hypoventilation. The type of dialyser membrane used however, can have a marked effect on this aspect of haemodialysis (133–137). Recent studies have shown that PaO_2 and leucocyte counts are more stable using polyacrylonitrile (PAN) membranes, irrespective of dialysate buffer, and that PaO_2 and leucocytes both decrease using cuprophane membranes (135, 138). The decrease in PaO_2, caused by CO_2 loss and hypoventilation during acetate dialysis, is less with PAN membranes (133). Francos et al (136) have distinguished between the two components of hypoxaemia – one component membrane-dependent (i.e. absent with PAN membranes, present with cuprophane membranes and aggravated by acetate dialysis) and the other component independent of the membrane used and due to the CO_2 loss caused by acetate dialysis. On both counts bicarbonate is to be preferred to acetate. Vaziri et al (137), however, have shown that a change from single pass to recirculation with cellulose membranes can reduce the hypoxaemia and CO_2 loss during acetate dialysis.

Acetate may interfere with buffering mechanisms not only in extracellular fluid but also in bone. Calcium phosphate and calcium carbonate crystals from bone can dissolve releasing these respective anions which then act as buffering agents. Gotch and colleagues (139) have suggested that in the long-term, an accumulated base deficit occurs as bone buffers are used to correct acidosis. This can be reduced with bicarbonate dialysis.

Bicarbonate 'biofiltration' (replacement of excess ultrafiltrate with a solution of high bicarbonate concentration post-dialyser) during acetate haemodialysis has been recommended by Panzetta et al (140) and might be an alternative though expensive approach which would avoid the technical problems associated with bicarbonate dialysis fluid delivery, such as calcium precipitation (141) (see below).

Relevance to rapid dialysis

High efficiency dialysis of short duration (2 to 3 h), 'rapid dialysis', as advocated increasingly over the past 10 years (142), is more tolerable with bicarbonate-based fluid since the rapid infusion of acetate exacerbates nearly all the problems apparent with longer duration acetate haemodialysis (143).

It has also been recommended (144) that the bicarbonate

fluid should be isonatric. If haemodiafiltration is used with rapid dialysis, the replacement solution should be hypertonic, that is hypernatric (144). Some have used pre-dialysis intravenous boluses or infusions of hypertonic saline or bicarbonate during rapid dialysis (145). In contrast, Rubin and Berlyne (146) have suggested that if dialysis fluid sodium concentration is high enough (e.g. 145 mmol/l) rapid dialysis can be both effective and without any increased symptoms even with acetate as the buffer.

The high efficiency non-cellulose membranes are more biologically inert and therefore of themselves of benefit in reducing acute leucopenia during haemodialysis, but this desirable effect is also evident during standard length dialysis of 4 to 5 h. The adequacy of rapid dialysis over the long-term has also been questioned (147), but recent evidence indicates that changes in morbidity and mortality are related to the plasma urea level maintained overall in the patient, rather than to the finite length of a dialysis session (148).

Production of bicarbonate-containing dialysis fluid

Bicarbonate-based dialysis generally involves a special three-stream, two-pump proportionating monitor with attendant increase in complexity and cost. If this increased technical requirement was not involved, bicarbonate dialysis would probably be universally adopted for both chronic and acute dialysis since it is clearly more 'physiological'.

Instability of the bicarbonate anion in aqueous solution at physiological pH and especially in the presence of calcium and magnesium cations is usually circumvented by separating the bicarbonate-containing and divalent cation-containing dialysis fluid concentrates into separate compartments. Perforce, bicarbonate-containing dialysis fluids are usually constituted immediately prior to use by the admixture with heated and degassed water of two concentrates, formulated as a matching pair, one bicarbonate-containing and the other calcium-containing. The calcium-containing concentrate is diluted with water and this diluted solution is then used to dilute the bicarbonate-containing solution to produce the fully diluted dialysis fluid close to the point of use in the dialyser. In practice four or five different bicarbonate concentrations can be chosen within a fairly limited range, each determining a different sodium concentration. Dextrose, if used, can be in either the calcium-containing or the bicarbonate-containing concentrate.

Underlying all such systems is the principle that when diluted solutions containing divalent cations (calcium and magnesium) meet sodium bicarbonate, residence time in the fluid-flow pathway is momentary before entering the dialyser (the 'last minute' mixing principle). The water solubility limit of calcium carbonate is in fact exceeded but metastability of the carbonate usually delays precipitation sufficiently to obviate any significant deposition and obstruction. Traces of other contaminant carbonates or particulate materials in the bicarbonate concentrate will promote precipitation of calcium carbonate. Included in the calcium-containing concentrate is a small quantity of usually acetic acid which in combination with the 'excess' bicarbonate in the other solution helps prevent the precipitation of calcium carbonate. The use of bicarbonate-containing dialysis fluid requires careful and regular maintenance of the fluid pathway. During maintenance the flowpath must be irrigated with a decalcifying solution (20% citric acid in water rinse) to remove trace deposits of calcium carbonate.

Certain pharmaceutical properties of the 'parent' concentrates and the product dialysis fluid should be remembered. The bicarbonate concentrate is not stable over long periods. Loss of CO_2 from solution, as for example through poorly secured closure of the container, may lead to precipitation, especially of trace calcium carbonate (141). Storage should be minimal and in cool conditions. Bicarbonate concentrate having a high salt concentration should inhibit bacterial growth during storage but contamination with microorganisms such as *Pseudomonas paucimobilis* and *Bacillus sps.* occurred in this unit and in others (140, 150). Bacterial contamination means that toxic products including pyrogens (endotoxins) are present in the fluid which can add to the ill effects of dialysis. The calcium-containing concentrate is acidic and does not support bacterial growth.

Attempts have been made to supply more stable liquid bicarbonate concentrates (151, 152) with storage times of up to 2 years but the ingredient used to maintain stability (a non-dialysable sequesterant) is undisclosed (152). Pre-packaged bicarbonate powder must be dissolved immediately prior to use, but prolonged and vigorous agitation is usually required and dangers arise if solution is incomplete. Variations on these approaches may prove in the end to provide the answer to the technological difficulties of bicarbonate dialysis fluid production and delivery.

Acetate and chloride

The chloride content of dialysis fluid is predetermined by the limiting electrochemical relationship wherein total anion charges must equal total cation charges. Thus:

Total cations (in mEq/l) = acetate + chloride (in mEq/l).

In this context it should be remembered that it is the equivalent concentrations that must be equal, not the molar concentrations. Potassium, calcium and magnesium salts are usually present in the concentrate as the chlorides, the mEq contribution of chloride from these salts being relatively small (2.5 to 6.0 mEq/l in total). Sodium, being the major cation, is provided by both sodium acetate and sodium chloride, and the relative amounts of each can be varied. The usual practice is to decide the acetate level required and to make up the balance with the chloride salt. One cannot lower the acetate content without increasing the chloride content and vice-versa. Similarly the total sodium content, which can range as discussed earlier from 130 to 145 mEq/l, will determine the chloride concentration if the acetate component has been fixed. Relative to acetate (or bicarbonate) the chloride concentration in dialysis fluid seems to have little or no effect per se. The range in current use varies between 92 and 111 mEq/l. Rather empirically, the acetate (or bicarbonate) concentration in haemodialysis fluid has come to be about 40 mEq/l. Lower concentrations of acetate in dialysis fluid are associated with some acidosis under maintenance haemodialysis conditions (153) presumably because of a relative hyperchloraemia or underprovision of fixed base.

In general terms, in stable dialysis patients the concentrations of acetate and chloride in dialysis fluid should be chosen to give a normal post-dialysis concentration of plasma bicarbonate. This results usually in a sodium:chloride ratio in the dialysis fluid around 3:2.

Dextrose

The efficacy of hydraulic ultrafiltration and the ability to control it by adjustment of transmembrane pressure with modern pump-monitors, has made dextrose-mediated osmotic extraction of water unnecessary. High dextrose-containing dialysis fluid (>100 mmol/l) (>1.8 g/dl), as employed in the past (3) could effect quite marked symptomatic reactive hypoglycaemia and hyponatraemia shortly after the dialysis treatment was completed. Such high concentrations of dextrose in dialysis fluid have no recommendation nowadays.

Contemporary dialysis fluids are dextrose-free, isoglycemic or slightly above (5.5 to 11 mmol/l [100 to 200 mg/dl]). Most patients tolerate regular haemodialysis treatment with dextrose-free fluid without evident ill-effect despite a loss of about 25 g of glucose across the dialyser (154, 155) and minor reductions in plasma glucose and insulin (155). Dextrose-free dialysis fluid has been advocated (156) mostly on the theoretical grounds that the avoidance of this extraneous glucose infusion will lessen ultimate serum cholesterol and triglyceride levels, and thereby reduce the long-term complications of atherosclerosis. Recent studies (156) suggest that all patients on haemodialysis have hypertriglyceridaemia and mild hyper-cholesterolaemia irrespective of 'high' (11 mmol/l [200 mg/dl]) or 'low' (5.5 mmol/l [100 mg/dl]) dialysis fluid glucose, and that the lipidaemia is accounted for predominantly by normal low-density and high very-low-density lipoproteins. The higher insulin and growth hormone levels associated with higher glucose in dialysis fluid did not appear to influence the lipid status of the patients (157) or haemodynamic parameters. There may be a gradual decrease in triglyceride and cholesterol concentrations with increasing duration of dialysis (156). The use of dextrose-free fluid may involve a recurrent metabolic stress to the patient with aggravated intradialytic change in serum osmolality, concomitant EEG changes (158) and stimulation of gluconeogenesis (159). The presence of dextrose minimises some of the disturbances of acetate-based haemodialysis (160).

While dextrose-free dialysis fluid does not always produce hypoglycaemia when in routine use, spontaneous symptomatic hypoglycaemia to the point of coma is a recognised though rare complication of maintenance haemodialysis (161). Such hypoglycaemic episodes may occur in diabetic or in non-diabetic patients and have been associated with concurrent propranolol (162) or aspirin therapy (163).

The effect of omitting dextrose on gluconeogenesis is probably of importance. Blood pyruvate (154, 164) fell and acetoacetate and β-hydroxy-butyrate markedly increased (154) during dextrose-free dialysis in the fasting state. In the presence of dextrose there was little change in all three substances. Using dextrose-free dialysis fluid there was up to 60% reduction in whole blood alanine concentration (164). An increased protein catabolic rate was observed during dialysis with both dextrose-free and dextrose-containing dialysis fluid.

Despite the findings that modest amounts of dextrose may be beneficial many nephrologists use dextrose-free dialysis fluids which seem to cause few, if any, clinical abnormalities. It has also been suggested that there is less need for dextrose in bicarbonate based dialysis (160). Absence of dextrose could be advantageous in discouraging growth of contaminating bacteria.

On current evidence, as first principles might suggest, there seems to be some advantage in dialysis fluid which has a dextrose concentration approximately isomolar with fasting plasma glucose (approximately 5 mmol/l [90 mg/dl]), but few units in the UK appear to be using such fluid (Figure 1). The majority (78%) are using 10 to 12 mmol/l (180 to 220 mg/dl).

Fluoride

Although fluoride is known to accumulate in haemodialysed patients, especially where the tap water is fluoridinated (165), recognisable ill effects are infrequent or absent. Such accumulation can be appreciable before haemodialysis treatment begins (166) and is reflected in raised bone and serum levels of the element. While an isolated anecdotal example of cardiotoxicity from dialysis fluid fluoride has been claimed (167), there is no unequivocal evidence that the undoubtedly increased body burden of fluoride is harmful. The increased bone content may be a factor mitigating in some measure against dialysis osteodystrophy (166) by rendering bone more resistant to excess parathyroid hormone (168).

The role of inadvertent fluoride accumulation in the haemodialysed patient remains conjectural. It is perhaps fortunate that reverse osmosis treatment of water for haemodialysis virtually eliminates fluoride from the diluent water and may progressively reduce the plasma level of diet-derived fluoride (169). Deionisers, where still used, must be well-serviced since, in the near-exhausted phase, excessive quantities of fluoride may be eluted before divalent ion saturation is noticed (170).

CONTAMINANTS AND OTHER SUBSTANCES

Although haemodialysis began using dialysis fluid prepared with untreated tap water, instances of both chemical and bacterial contamination have led to the widespread adoption of water treatment prior to use in haemodialysis. Harmful chemicals still present in tap water which is safe for drinking must be removed before the water enters a dialysis system. Frequently water authorities add substances such as aluminium sulphate (alum) or ferrous sulphate at irregular or seasonal intervals to raw water, which may cause problems in conventional dialysis systems. Rarely, unexpected material such as zinc or copper may inadvertently be introduced into water supplies near to the point of delivery. Most authorities maintain high standards of purification in water supplied to domestic establishments (particular attention being paid to bacterial contamination) but these standards vary throughout the world and it is advisable for each dialysis centre to make appropriate enquiries for there may be potential hazards peculiar to certain areas. It is now mandatory to check water quality in any new home-dialysis unit location before initiating treatment. Particular care is needed in isolated rural areas. Liaison with the water supply company chemist is often helpful. Standards for concentrate quality and advice on water quality have been established by both the Association for Advancement of Medical Instrumentation (AAMI) in the USA (171) and by the British Pharmacopoeia (172). The recommendations for water are not mandatory in the UK since the British Pharmacopoeia has no jurisdiction over British Water Boards.

Particulate

Particulate contamination can arise with sedimentary material from filter beds and iron oxides from the distribution pipework or from acid concentrates in the bicarbonate system (173). While inapparent in a small volume, the large quantities involved in haemodialysis (circa 500 ml per minute) make such particulates important in relation to the later stages of water treatment (i.e. deionisation and reverse osmosis in the clinical unit). Filters of woven polypropylene with an exclusion limit of >30 microns are effective as a main unit filter to protect the final individual pump-monitor filters (often carbon-based) which should be seen as indicators of failure more proximally, rather than filters for particulates in their own right. A block of the final machine filter results in hydrostatic pressure reduction within the pump-monitor and interference with ongoing dialysis treatment.

Chemical

Chemical contamination from aluminium has received increasing attention in recent years due to the occurrence of dialysis-related encephalopathy and fracturing osteomalacia. Since 1974, the inadvertent aluminium content of dialysis fluid has been shown to be capable of delivering toxic even lethal amounts across the dialyser membrane into the patient (174). Tap water used for dilution of concentrate was the usual source of that aluminium. Although purification treatment of water for haemodialysis is now mandatory and aluminium levels <10 μg/l (0.37 μmol/l) are achieved, the dialysis fluid concentrates still contain some aluminium.

Accordingly it is necessary to monitor the diluted dialysis fluid for aluminium. A satisfactory low concentration of aluminium in dialysis fluid would be <30 μg/l (1.1 μmol/l). The EEC Directive for 1986 stipulates <30 μg/l for both diluted dialysis fluid and water to come into force on 1 January 1989 (175). The AAMI limit is currently 10 μg/l (0.37 μmol/l) (171, 174).

Bacterial

Bacterial contamination, which can introduce a variety of pyrogens (176), must be minimised. The liability of poorly maintained intramural water distribution systems to bacterial/algal contamination is such that expensive constant- or pulsed-flow systems have been advocated (177). The dialysist, however, has little or no control over the water employed by the pharmaceutical manufacturer in the preparation of dialysis concentrate. While severe endotoxin-mediated febrile reactions during haemodialysis are now rare, especially since the widespread adoption of disposable dialysers and lines, it is possible that less flagrant endotoxin-induced dialysis 'reactions' (nausea, vomiting, hypotension, heachache, fever) are still occurring. These may be mediated by a mechanism involving interleukin-1 release (178). The increasing use of dialysers with highly permeable membranes for high-flux dialysis, brings an enhanced potential for the passage of dialysis fluid-borne endotoxin into the blood compartment. Such passage, a feature of high porosity membranes even when structurally intact, results from both diffusive and convective (back-filtration) mechanisms (179). The risk of entry of pyogenic derivatives into the patient is less with conventional membranes and in this respect plate dialysers are preferable to capillary configurations (179).

Virtually all water supplies require further processing immediately upstream from the dialysis equipment. At a minimum this entails filtration to abstract suspended sediments, sometimes water-softening, and carbon filtration followed by reverse osmosis (RO). Periodic replacement of these in-line sediment filters at short intervals and of the RO membrane at longer intervals is essential to avoid build-up of particulates on both items of equipment with eventual pressure/flow difficulties or even progressive bacterial or (and) algal contamination. RO membranes reject a very high percentage of inorganic ions (Table 2) and organic

substances greater than 200 daltons. It is to be noted that RO units work on a percentage rejection basis and not to any given absolute value in the product water and it is essential for all dialysis centres to analyse their product water at regular intervals. Such measurement also gives warning of a partial breakdown of an RO unit. Table 2 shows that fluoride has a relatively low rejection ratio (and, though not shown, a similar value is found for bicarbonate). The rejection of fluoride (and bicarbonate) is affected by the pH of the feed water. Units practising dialyser re-use need to check for residual formaldehyde.

The water component of haemodialysis fluid cannot be assumed to be inherently innocuous. More work on the purity of concentrate solutions and evidence about manufacturers' quality control seems indicated.

Other substances

Although dialysis removes certain essential substances, such as water-soluble vitamins and amino-acids, these are not added to dialysis fluid on account of expense and can usually be replaced by an adequate diet and some supplements.

CONSTITUTION OF DIALYSIS FLUID

Proportionating machines

Tank systems have now been totally superceded by proportionating systems. While the recirculation of 'one batch' dialysis fluid still has its advocates (137) most centres use single-pass run-to-waste dialysis fluid to avoid bacterial complications. Recirculation during acetate dialysis with a cellulose membrane greatly reduced hypoxaemia and dialyser CO_2 loss compared with single pass use (137). This illustrates that the delivery system can affect patient well-being, all other factors being equal.

The multiple stream proportionating pump-monitors used for bicarbonate-containing dialysis fluid production (e.g. Gambro BCN-10-1; Cobe Centry 2) have complex feedback control-loops using the conductivity of the mixture at successive levels in the product stream to control the pumps delivering each of the two concentrates. It is important that the pair of salt concentrates used is compatible with the particular three-stream machine being employed (see previous section). While centralised bulk-supply systems are available for bicarbonate dialysis fluid, single-patient multiple-stream proportionating pump-monitors at each bedside are currently more usual and are preferable due to the less bacteriostatic nature of bicarbonate dialysis fluid. Nevertheless, Thayse et al (180) used a central proportionating system for bicarbonate dialysis distributed to up to 30 dialysis patients without evidence of bacterial build-up.

Use of special paired concentrates for bicarbonate dialysis raises some safety considerations. Each concentrate alone is unsuitable for use in single-stream proportionators. Reports have appeared describing the inadvertent use of the acid (calcium-containing) concentrate of a pair for bicarbonate

Table 2. Average rejection rates of a reverse osmosis unit.

Substance	% Rejection
Calcium	96–98
Magnesium	96–98
Sodium	85–95
Potassium	85–95
Aluminium	98–99
Sulphate	95–98
Chloride	85–95
Nitrate	60–85
Fluoride	86–95

dialysis instead of conventional acetate-containing dialysis fluid concentrate (181). This misuse caused severe acidosis. Most manufacturers of three-stream machines incorporate some safeguard against inadvertent swap-over of the paired concentrates or use of conventional acetate-based concentrate instead of the acid concentrate of the matched pair. The safeguards include variously pH checks, special connectors and coloured containers or built-in limited-range conductivity acceptance on the part of the machine's metering devices. The best safeguard is trained staff well aware of the special potential for trouble and explicit labelling.

Temperature control

Untested a priori reasoning led to the adoption of 'body temperature', taken as 37°C, for the optimum temperature of dialysis fluid. Conventional pump-monitoring equipment heats the concentrate/tapwater mixture to 37°C ± 0.5 (range). Overheating through failure of the surveillance devices may lead to gross haemolysis in the dialyser blood compartment with, depending on severity, a clinical syndrome involving vomiting, dyspnoea, chest pain and collapse (182) and the theoretical possibility of hypercalcaemia with cardiac arrest. By contrast, chilling, through a failure of the heat exchanger, may produce shivering in the patient. These two extremes aside, a case has been made for the adoption of 35° or 35.8°C for dialysis fluid, that is, 1° to 2° less than is usual with contemporary dialysis, as a new standard. This is justified by the idea that limb arterio-venous fistula blood is normally 1°C less than body core temperature and a controlled trial with dialysis fluid at 35.8°C showed a moderate benefit in terms of arterial blood pressure stability during dialysis as well as less intradialytic heat gain (183). A reduced incidence of hypotension without any significant differences in hypoxaemia parameters occurred using 35°C (184).

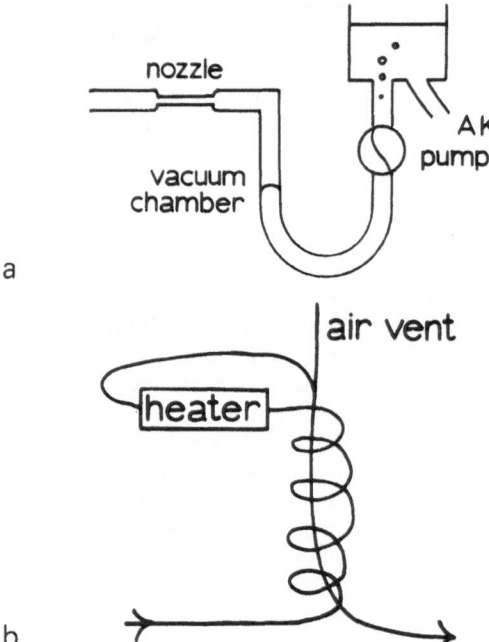

a

b

Figure 2. De-aeration methods (a) negative pressure (b) heat exchanger.

De-aeration of dialysis fluid

Since the solubility of air in water decreases as temperature is increased or as pressure in water is decreased, there is a marked liability for dissolved air to appear as bubbles when dialysis fluid is heated to 37°C and subatmospheric (negative) pressures are applied (Table 3). Such bubbles can interfere with conductivity measurement and solute transfers across dialyser membranes. The concomitant supersaturated phase (with high pO_2 levels), antecedent to bubble formation, may effect some gas transfer across the dialyser membrane into the blood compartment, with resultant increase in air trapping and blood foaming in the bubble trap of the extracorporeal circuit (185, 186).

The disadvantages of such bubble formation in dialysis fluid during use makes de-aeration mandatory in all pump-monitors which employ negative pressure ultrafiltration. The de-aeration devices (Figure 2) subject the mains water, or the dialysis fluid as finally constituted, to either negative pressure with venting off of gas or less commonly, transient heating of the mains water to 'pasteurisation-temperatures' at circa 70°C.

In conclusion, familiarity with dialysis fluid should never engender a casual attitude in dialysis staff. There is no ideal for all patients. It should be remembered that dialysis fluid carries the potential for unexpected ill-effects.

Table 3. Approximate solubility of air in water at varying temperatures and pressures.

Temperature of town mains °C	Saturated air content at 760 mm Hg ml/l	Quantity to be removed on heating to 37°C at 760 mm Hg* ml/l
5	25.5	11.5
10	23.0	9.0
15	20.5	6.5
20	18.5	4.5
25	17.0	3.0
30	15.5	1.5
35	14.5	0.5
37	14.0	–

* Plus an additional 4.0 ml/l if pressure reduced to 560 mm Hg (i.e. – 200 mm Hg).

ACKNOWLEDGEMENTS

Thanks are due to Macarthy Medical Ltd., Romford, UK

for supplying the information for Figure 1, and to Culligan, High Wycombe, UK for the data given in Table 2.

Figure 2a is reproduced from Proc Eur Dial Transplant Assoc 5: 1968 by kind permission of the Editors and Excerpta Medica Foundation.

REFERENCES

1. Kolff WJ: *New Ways of Treating Uraemia.* London, J & A Churchill, 1947
2. Diem K, Lentner C (Editors): *Documenta Geigy Scientific Tables* 7th Edn Basle, JR Geigy, 1970, p 523
3. Scribner BH, Hegstrom RM, Buri R: Treatment of chronic uremia by means of hemodialysis: a progress report. in *Proc 1st Int Congr Nephrol,* Basel, New York, S Karger, 1961, p 616
4. Cole JJ, Fritzen JR, Vizzo JE, van Paasschen WH, Grimsrud L: One year's experience with a central dialysate supply system in a hospital. *Trans Am Soc Artif Intern Organs* 11: 22, 1965
5. Mion CM, Hegstrom RM, Boen SI, Scribner BH: Substitution of sodium acetate for sodium bicarbonate in the bath fluid for hemodialysis. *Trans Am Soc Artif Intern Organs* 10: 110, 1964
6. Wolf AV, Remp DG, Kiley JE, Currie GD: Artificial kidney function: kinetics of hemodialysis. *J Clin Invest* 30: 1062, 1951
7. Parsons FM, McCracken BH: The use and function of the artificial kidney. *Br J Urol* 30: 463, 1958
8. Stewart WK, Fleming LW, Manuel MA: Benefits obtained by the use of high sodium dialysate during maintenance haemodialysis. *Proc Eur Dial Transplant Assoc* 9: 111, 1972
9. Port FK, Johnson WJ, Klass DW: Prevention of dialysis disequilibrium syndrome by use of high sodium concentration in the dialysate. *Kidney Int* 3: 327, 1973
10. Stewart WK, Fleming LW: Blood pressure control during maintenance haemodialysis with isonatric (high sodium) dialysate. *Postgrad Med J* 50: 260, 1974
11. Liebau H, Eisenbach GM, Mariss P, Hilfenhaus M: Role of sodium and water in hypertensive patients on maintenance hemodialysis. *Contrib Nephrol* 8: 126, 1977
12. Locatelli F, Costanzo R, Di Filippo S, Pedrini L, Marai P, Pozzi C, Ponti R, Sforzini S, Redaelli B: Ultrafiltration and high sodium concentration dialysis: pathophysiological correlation. *Proc Eur Dial Transplant Assoc* 15: 253, 1978
13. Stewart WK, Fleming LW, McLean S: Is hyponatric dialysis appropriate? a survey of dialysate sodium concentration in the United Kingdom. *Dial Transplant* 6: 9, 1977
14. Moriarty MV, Parsons FM: Hypernatraemia during peritoneal dialysis. *Proc Eur Dial Transplant Assoc* 3: 359, 1966
15. Nolph KD, Hopkins CA, New D, Antwiler GD, Popovich RP: Differences in solute sieving with osmotic vs. hydrostatic ultrafiltration. *Trans Am Soc Artif Intern Organs* 22: 618, 1976
16. Haruyama T, Shitomi K, Kaneda H, Takeuchi M, Murata T: Development of malignant hypertension as a result of negative sodium balance. *Nippon Jinzo Gakkai Shi* 19: 441, 1977
17. Winney RJ, Kean DM, Best JKK, Smith MA: Changes in brain water with haemodialysis. *Lancet* 2: 1107, 1986
18. Drukker W, Jungerius NA, Alberts C: Report on regular dialysis treatment in Europe III. 1967. *Proc Eur Dial Transplant Assoc* 4: 3, 1967
19. Boquin E, Parnell S, Grondin G, Wollard C, Leonard D, Michaels R, Levin NW: Crossover study of the effect of different dialysate sodium concentrations in large surface area

short-term dialysis. *Proc Clin Dial Transplant Forum* 7: 48, 1977
20. Gordon A, Maxwell MH: Water, electrolyte, and acid-base disorders associated with acute and chronic dialysis. in *Clinical Disorders of Fluid and Electrolyte Metabolism,* 3rd edn, edited by Maxwell MH, Kleeman CR, New York, McGraw-Hill, 1980, p 827
21. Bergström J: Ultrafiltration without dialysis for removal of fluid and solutes in uremia. *Clin Nephrol* 9: 156, 1978
22. Wehle B, Asaba H, Castenfors J, Fürst P, Gunnarsson B, Shaldon S, Bergström J: Hemodynamic changes during sequential ultrafiltration and dialysis. *Kidney Int* 15: 411, 1979
23. Rodrigo F, Shideman J, McHugh R, Buselmeier T, Kjellstrand C: Osmolality changes during hemodialysis: natural history, clinical correlations, and influence of dialysate glucose and intravenous mannitol. *Ann Intern Med* 86: 554, 1977
24. Henrich WL, Woodard TD, Blachley JD, Gomez-Sanchez C, Pettinger W, Cronin RE: Role of osmolality in blood pressure stability after dialysis and ultrafiltration. *Kidney Int* 18: 480, 1980
25. Leski M, Niethammer T, Wyss T: Glucose-enriched dialysate and tolerance to maintenance hemodialysis. *Nephron* 24: 271, 1979
26. Arieff AI, Lazarowitz VC, Guisado R: Experimental dialysis disequilibrium syndrome: prevention with glycerol. *Kidney Int* 14: 270, 1978
27. Jenkins PG, Dreher WH: Dialysis-induced muscle cramps: treatment with hypertonic saline and theory as to etiology. *Trans Am Soc Artif Intern Organs* 21: 479, 1975
28. Kohnle W, Heimsch E, Schmidt-Wiederkehr P, Franz HE: Acid base status during treatment of chronic uremia with diafiltration. *J Dial* 1: 419, 1977
29. Henderson LW: Pre vs. post dilution hemofiltration. *Clin Nephrol* 11: 120, 1979
30. Kishimoto T, Yamagami S, Tanaka H, Ohyama T, Yamamoto T, Yamakawa M, Nishino M, Yoshimoto S, Maekawa M: Superiority of hemofiltration to hemodialysis for treatment of chronic renal failure: comparative studies between hemofiltration and hemodialysis on dialysis disequilibrium syndrome. *Artif Organs* 4: 86, 1980
31. Cambi V, Arisi L, Bignardi L, Garini G, Rossi E, Savazzi G, Migone L: Critical appraisal of hemofiltration and ultrafiltration. The development of ultra-short dialysis: preliminary results. *J Dial* 2: 143, 1978
32. Levine T, Falk B, Henriquez M, Raja RM, Kramer MS, Rosenbaum JL: Effects of varying dialysate sodium using large surface area dialyzers. *Trans Am Soc Artif Intern Organs* 24: 139, 1978
33. Man NK, Pils P, Di Guilio D, Zingraff J, Drüeke T, Jungers P, Funck-Brentano JL: Tolerance to high ultrafiltration rates during closed batch hemodialysis. *Artif Organs* 2: 154, 1978
34. Funck-Brentano JL: Ultrafiltration and diffusion techniques with the polyacrylonitrile membrane dialyzer. *Proc Renal Physicians Assoc* 2: 9, 1978
35. Schuenemann B, Borghardt J, Falda Z, Jacob I, Kramer P, Kraft B, Quellhorst E: Reactions of blood pressure and body spaces to hemofiltration treatment. *Trans Am Soc Artif Intern Organs* 24: 687, 1978
36. Cybulsky AVE, Matni A, Hollomby DJ: Effects of high sodium dialysate during maintenance hemodialysis. *Nephron* 41: 57, 1985
37. Bosch J, Ponti R, Glabman S, Lauer A: Sodium fluxes during hemodialysis. *Nephron* 45: 86, 1987
38. Eaves JA, Beare JE: The advantages of high sodium dialysate

for children less than 24 kilogrammes. in *Proceedings 7th British Symposium on Renal Technology,* Warwick, edited by Deller A, Aldridge C, Kilvington M, Gambro, 1982, p 124

39. Murisasco A, France G, Leblond G, Durand C, El Mehdi M, Crevat A, Elsen R, Boobes Y, Baz M: Sequential sodium therapy allows correction of sodium-volume balance and reduces morbidity. *Clin Nephrol.* 24: 201, 1985

40. Dadson IP: Conductivity and its relationship to dialysate composition. *Am Assoc Nephrol Nurses Technicians J* 9: 19, 1982

41. Ragon A, Reynier JP, Murisasco A, Elsen R, Leblond G: Dialysate sodium control during modeling in hemodialysis. *Artif Organs* 9: 63, 1985

42. Hampl H, Klopp HW, Michels N, Mahiout A, Schilling HP, Wolfgruber M, Schiller R, Hanefield F, Kessel M: Electroencephalogram investigations of the disequilibrium syndrome during bicarbonate and acetate dialysis. *Proc Eur Dial Transplant Assoc* 19: 351, 1982

43. Wilkinson R, Barber SG, Robson V: Cramps, thirst and hypertension in hemodialysis patients – the influence of dialysate sodium concentration. *Clin Nephrol* 7: 101, 1977

44. Robson M, Oren A, Ravid M: Dialysate sodium concentration, hypertension and pulmonary edema in hemodialysis patients. *Dial Transplant* 7: 678, 1978

45. Redaelli B, Sforzini S, Bondoldi G, Dadone C, Di Filippo S, Filoramo F, Limido D, Mimmo R, Pincella G, Vigano MR: Hemodialysis with 'adequate' sodium concentration in dialysate. *Int J Artif Organs* 2: 133, 1979

46. Locatelli F, Costanzo R, Di Filippo S: High sodium dialysate. *Int J Artif Organs* 2: 171, 1979

47. Swamy AP, Cestero RVM: Mannitol and maintenance hemodialysis. *Artif Organs* 3: 116, 1979

48. Van Stone JC, Meyer R, Murrin C, Cook J: Hemodialysis with glycerol dialysate. *Trans Am Soc Artif Intern Organs* 25: 354, 1979

49. Quellhorst EA, Schuenemann B, Mietzsch G: Long-term hemofiltration in 'poor-risk' patients. *Trans Am Soc Artif Intern Organs* 33: 758, 1987

50. Funck-Brentano J-L, Man NK: Optimization of Na content in dialysis fluid. *Nephron* 36: 197, 1984

51. Dumler F, Grondin G, Levin NW: Sequential high/low sodium hemodialysis: an alternative to ultrafiltration. *Trans Am Soc Artif Intern Organs* 25: 351, 1979

52. Maeda K, Saito A, Kawaguchi S, Asada A, Niwa T, Ohta K, Kobayashi K: Hemodiafiltration with sodium concentration-controlled dialysate. *Artif Organs* 4: 121, 1980

53. Chen W-T, Ing TS, Daugirdas JT, Humayun HM, Brescia DJ, Gandhi VC, Hano JE, Kheirbek AO: Hydrostatic ultrafiltration during hemodialysis using decreasing sodium dialysate. *Artif Organs* 4: 187, 1980

54. Locatelli F, Costanzo R, De Filippo S, Pedrini L, Marai P, Pozzi C, Ponti R, Sforzini S, Redaelli B: Controlled sequential ultrafiltration dialysis, iso-osmotic dialysis, isonatric dialysis: pathophysiological and clinical evaluations. *Dial Transplant* 8: 622, 1979

55. Merrill JP: *The Treatment of Renal Failure.* New York, Grune and Stratton Inc 1955, p 185

56. Oh MS, Levison SP, Carroll HJ: Content and distribution of water and electrolytes in maintenance hemodialysis. *Nephron* 14: 421, 1975

57. Butkus DE, Alfrey AC, Miller NL: Tissue potassium in chronic dialysis patients. *Nephron* 13: 314, 1974

58. Hagemann I, Schilling E, Krocker B, Precht K, Buchali K, Kruse I, Pietsch R, Eichhorst E, Seewald R: Untersuchungen des Elektrolytgehaltes in Erythrozyten im chronischen Hamo-

dialyse-Programm bei Anwendung unterschiedlicher Spullosungen. (The electrolyte content in erythrocytes in the long-term dialysis programme during use of different irrigating solutions). *Z Urol Neprhol* 66: 255, 1974 (In German)

59. Boddy K, King PC, Lindsay RM, Briggs JD, Winchester JF, Kennedy AC: Total body potassium in non-dialysed and dialysed patients with chronic renal failure. *Br Med J* 1: 771, 1972

60. Morgan AG, Burkinshaw L, Robinson PJA, Rosen SM: Potassium balance and acid-base changes in patients undergoing regular haemodialysis therapy. *Br Med J* 1: 779, 1970

61. Cohn SH, Cinque TJ, Dombroski CS, Letteri JM: Determination of body composition by neutron activation analysis in patient with renal failure. *J Lab Clin Med* 79: 97, 1972

62. Atkinson PJ, Hancock DA, Acharya VN, Parsons FM, Proctor EA, Reed GW: Changes in skeletal mineral in patients on prolonged maintenance dialysis. *Br Med J* 4: 519, 1973

63. Maschio G, Bazzato G, Bertaglia E, Sardini D, Mioni G, D'Angelo A, Marzo A: Intracellular pH and electrolyte content of skeletal muscle in patients with chronic renal acidosis. *Nephron* 7: 481, 1970

64. Martin AM, Oduro-Dominah A, Gibbins JK, Devapal D, Mitchell DC: Regular short haemodialysis in end-stage renal failure. *Br Med J* 3: 758, 1975

65. Brynger H, Brunner FP, Chantler C, Donckerwolcke RA, Jacobs C, Kramer P, Selwood NH, Wing AJ: Combined report on regular dialysis and transplantation in Europe, X, 1979. *Proc Eur Dial Transplant Assoc* 17: 4, 1980

66. Berlyne GM, Janabi K, Shaw AB, Hocken AG: Treatment of hyperkalaemia with a calcium-resin. *Lancet* 1: 169, 1966

67. Quintanilla AP, Wefer MI: Hyperkalemia in the patient on chronic dialysis. *Int J Artif Organs* 10: 17, 1987

68. Sandle GI, Gaiger S, Tapster S, Goodship THJ: Evidence for large intestinal control of potassium homeostasis in uraemic patients undergoing long-term haemodialysis. *Clin Sci* 73: 247, 1987

69. Edes TE, Sunderrajan EV: Heparin-induced hyperkalemia. *Arch Intern Med* 145: 1070, 1985

70. Wing AJ: Optimum calcium concentration of dialysis fluid for maintenance haemodialysis. *Br Med J* 4: 145, 1968

71. Bone JM, Davison AM, Robson JS: Role of dialysate calcium concentration in osteoporosis in patients on haemodialysis. *Lancet* 1: 1047, 1972

72. Denney JD, Sherrard DJ, Nelp WB, Chesnut CH, Baylink DJ, Murano RI, Hinn G: Total body calcium and long-term calcium balance in chronic renal disease. *J Lab Clin Med* 82: 226, 1973

73. Goldsmith RS, Furszyfer J, Johnson WJ, Beeler GW Jr, Taylor WF: Calcium flux during hemodialysis. *Nephron* 20: 132, 1978

74. Ritz E: Azotemic osteodystrophy – indications for intervention. *Prog Biochem Pharmacol* 17: 251, 1980

75. Johnson WJ: Persistent severe hypercalcemia during maintenance hemodialysis. *Ann Intern Med* 93: 272, 1980

76. Zawada ET Jr, Bennett EP, Stinson JB, Ramirez G: Serum calcium in blood pressure regulation during hemodialysis. *Arch Intern Med* 141: 657, 1981

77. Kuzela DC, Huffer WE, Conger JD, Winter SD, Hammond WS: Soft tissue calcification in chronic dialysis patients. *Am J Pathol* 86: 403, 1977

78. Zawada ET, Simmons J, Sica D: The importance of divalent ions to blood pressure regulation during hemodialysis. *Int J Artif Organs* 7: 245, 1984

79. Henrich WL, Hunt JM, Nixon JV: Increased ionized calcium and left ventricular contractility during hemodialysis. *N Engl J Med* 310: 19, 1984

80. Haddy FJ, Scott JB, Emerson TE, Overbeck HW, Daugherty RM: Effects of generalized changes in plasma electrolyte concentration and osmolarity on blood pressure in the anesthetized dog. *Circ Res (Suppl)* 24: I.59, 1969

81. Blachley JD, Blankenship DM, Menter A, Parker TF, Knochel JP: Uremic pruritus: skin divalent ion content and response to ultraviolet phototherapy. *Am J Kidney Dis* 5: 237, 1985

82. Winney RJ, Bone JM, Anderson TJ, Robson JS: Treatment of renal osteodystrophy with 1 alpha-hydroxycholecalciferol (1 alpha-OH-D₃) in conjunction with a high dialysate calcium. *Calcif Tissue Res* 22 (Suppl): 94, 1977

83. Goldsmith RS, Furszyfer J, Johnson WJ, Fournier AE, Sizemore GW, Arnaud CD: Etiology of hyperparathyroidism and bone disease during chronic hemodialysis III. Evaluation of parathyroid suppressibility. *J Clin Invest* 52: 173, 1973

84. Drüeke T, Bordier PJ, Man NK, Jungers P, Marie P: Effects of high dialysate calcium concentration on bone remodelling, serum bio-chemistry, and parathyroid hormone in patients with renal osteo-dystrophy. *Kidney Int* 11: 267, 1977

85. Bouillon R, Verberckmoes R, de Moor P: Influence of dialysate calcium concentration and vitamin D on serum parathyroid hormone during repetitive dialysis. *Kidney Int* 7: 422, 1975

86. Cundy T, Kanis JA, Earnshaw M, Woods CG: Comparative effects of alphacalcidol and parathyroidectomy with vitamin D in hyperparathyroid renal bone disease. *Q J Med* 60: 659, 1986

87. Carney SL, Gillies AHG: Effect of an optimum dialysis fluid calcium concentration on calcium mass transfer during maintenance hemodialysis. *Clin Nephrol* 24: 28, 1985

88. Massry SG: The clinical pathophysiology of magnesium: *Contrib Nephrol* 14: 64, 1978

89. Schmidt P, Kotzaurek R, Zazgornik J, Hysek H: Magnesium metabolism in patients on regular dialysis treatment. *Clin Sci* 41: 131, 1971

90. Brautbar N, Kleeman CR: Disordered divalent ion metabolism in kidney disease: comments on pathogenesis and treatment. *Adv Nephrol* 8: 179, 1979

91. Gonella M: Plasma and tissue levels of magnesium in chronically hemodialyzed patients: effects of dialysate magnesium levels. *Nephron* 34: 141, 1983

92. Heidland A, Wetzels E: Discussion: magnesium metabolism. *Contrib Nephrol* 38: 203, 1984

93. Ahmad R: Magnesium induced neuropathy in patient undergoing haemodialysis. *Br Med J* 288: 1654, 1984 (unreviewed report)

94. Brunner FP, Thiel G: The use of magnesium-containing phosphate binders in patients with end-stage renal disease on maintenance haemodialysis [letter]. *Nephron* 32: 266, 1982

95. Drüeke T: Does Mg excess play a role in renal osteodystrophy. *Contrib Nephrol* 38: 195, 1984

96. Massry SG: Magnesium homeostasis in patients with renal failure. *Contrib Nephrol* 38: 175, 1984

97. Mandelbaum JM, Heistand ML, Schardin KE: Six months' experience with PD-2 solution. *Dial Transplant* 12: 259, 1983

98. Johny KV, Lawrence JR, O'Halloran MW, Weilby ML: Effect of haemodialysis on erythrocyte and plasma potassium, magnesium, sodium and calcium. *Nephron* 8: 81, 1971

99. Stewart WK, Fleming LW: The effect of dialysate magnesium on plasma and erythrocyte magnesium and potassium concentrations during maintenance haemodialysis. *Nephron* 10: 222, 1973

100. Fleming LW, Lenman JAR, Stewart WK: Effect of magnesi-
um on nerve conduction velocity during regular dialysis treatment. *J Neurol Neurosurg Psychiatry* 35: 342, 1972

101. Graf H, Kovarik J, Stummvoll HK, Wolf A: Disappearance of uraemic pruritus after lowering dialysate magnesium concentration. *Br Med J* 2: 1478, 1979

102. Burnell JM, Teubner E: Effects of decreasing dialysate magnesium in patients with chronic renal failure. *Proc Clin Dial Transplant Forum* 5: 191, 1976

103. Catto GRD, Reid IW, MacLeod M: The effect of low magnesium dialysate on plasma, ultrafiltrable, erythrocyte and bone magnesium concentrations from patients on maintenance haemodialysis. *Nephron* 13: 372, 1974

104. Alfrey AC, Miller NL: Bone magnesium pools in uraemia. *J Clin Invest* 52: 3019, 1973

105. Posner AS, Betts F, Blumenthal NC: Role of ATP and Mg in the stabilization of biological and synthetic amorphous calcium phosphates. *Calcif Tissue Res* 22 (Suppl): 208, 1977

106. Meema HE, Oreopoulos DG, Rapoport A: Serum magnesium level and arterial calcification in end-stage renal disease. *Kidney Int* 32: 388, 1987

107. Terasaki M, Rubin H: Evidence that intracellular magnesium is present in cells at a regulatory concentration for protein synthesis. *Proc Nat Acad Sci USA* 82: 7324, 1985

108. Kenny MA, Casillas E, Ahmad S: Magnesium, calcium and PTH relationships in dialysis patients after magnesium repletion. *Nephron* 46: 199, 1987

109. Freeman RM, Lawton RL: The hard-water syndrome. *Med Instrum* 8: 201, 1974

110. Drukker W: The hard water syndrome: a potential hazard during regular dialysis treatment. *Proc Eur Dial Transplant Assoc* 5: 284, 1968

111. Novello A, Kelsch RC, Easterling RE: Acetate intolerance during hemodialysis. *Clin Nephrol* 5: 29, 1976

112. Kaiser BA, Potter DE, Bryant RE, Vreman HJ, Weiner MW: Acid-base changes and acetate metabolism during routine and high-efficiency hemodialysis in children. *Kidney Int* 19: 70, 1981

113. Van Stone JC, Cook J: The effect of bicarbonate dialysate in stable chronic hemodialysis patients. *Dial Transplant* 8: 703, 1979

114. Kveim M, Nesbakken R: Utilization of exogenous acetate during hemodialysis. *Trans Am Soc Artif Intern Organs* 21: 138, 1975

115. Hakim RM, Pontzer MA, Tilton D, Lazarus JM, Gottlieb MN: Effects of acetate and bicarbonate dialysate in stable chronic dialysis patients. *Kidney Int* 28: 535, 1985

116. Mastrangelo F: Bicarbonate dialysis – pro. *Int J Artif Organs* 10: 145, 1987

117. Huyghebaert MF, Dhainaut J-F, Monsallier JF, Schlemmer B: Bicarbonate hemodialysis of patients with acute renal failure and severe sepsis. *Critical Care Med* 13; 840, 1985

118. Leunissen KML, Hoorntje SJ, Fiers HA, Dekkers WT, Mulder AW: Acetate versus bicarbonate hemodialysis in critically ill patients. *Nephron* 42: 146, 1986

119. Mastrangelo F, Rizzelli S, Corliano C, Montinaro AM, De Blasi V, Alfonso L, Aprile M, Napoli M, Laforgia R: Benefits of bicarbonate dialysis. *Kidney Int* 28 (Suppl 17): S188, 1985

120. Schilling H, Lehmann H, Hampl H: Studies on circulatory stability during bicarbonate hemodialysis with constant dialysate sodium versus acetate hemodialysis with sequential dialysate sodium. *Artif Organs* 9: 17, 1985

121. Uldall PR, Kennedy I, Craske H, Porrett E, Aid J, Woods F, Levine D: A double-blind controlled trial of acetate versus bicarbonate dialysate. *Proc Clin Dial Transplant Forum* 10: 220, 1980

216   *William K. Stewart*

122. Bijaphala S, Bell AJ, Bennett CA, Evans SM, Dawborn JK: Comparison of high and low sodium bicarbonate and acetate dialysis in stable chronic hemodialysis patients. *Clin Nephrol* 23: 179, 1985

123. Maggiore Q, Enia G, Catalano C, Polimeni RM: Bicarbonate dialysis – con. *Int J Artif Organs* 10: 151, 1987

124. Graefe U, Milutinovich J, Follette WC, Vizzo JE, Babb AL, Scribner BH: Less dialysis-induced morbidity and vascular instability with bicarbonate in dialysate. *Ann Intern Med* 88: 332, 1978

125. Hsu CH, Swartz RD, Somermeyer MG, Raj A: Bicarbonate hemodialysis: Influence on plasma refilling and hemodynamic stability. *Nephron* 38: 202, 1984

126. Leenen FHH, Buda AJ, Smith DL, Farrel S, Levine DZ, Uldall PR: Hemodynamic changes during acetate and bicarbonate dialysis. *Artif Organs* 8: 411, 1984

127. Wolff J, Pedersen T, Rossen M, Cleemann-Rasmussen K: Effects of acetate and bicarbonate dialysis on cardiac performance, transmural myocardial perfusion and acid-base balance. *Int J Artif Organs* 9: 105, 1986

128. Rorke SJ, Davidson WD, Guo SS, Morin RJ: Metabolic fate of ^{14}C-acetate during dialysis. *Proc Eur Dial Transplant Assoc* 13: 394, 1976

129. Duarte R: Blood pressure, ventilation and lipid imbalance during hemodialysis: effect of dialysate composition. *Blood Purif* 3: 199, 1985

130. Ksiazek A, Solski J, Sokolowska G: Sympathetic activity, plasma renin activity (PRA) and kininogen levels in patients haemodialysed with acetate and bicarbonate. *Int Urol Nephrol* 16: 337, 1984

131. Nissenson AR: Prevention of dialysis-induced hypoxemia by bicarbonate dialysis. *Trans Am Soc Artif Intern Organs* 26: 339, 1980

132. Dolan MJ, Whipp EJ, Davidson WD, Weitzman RE, Wasserman K: Hypopnea associated with acetate hemodialysis: carbon dioxide-flow-dependent ventilation. *N Engl J Med* 305: 72, 1981

133. Igarashi H, Kioi S, Gejyo F, Arakawa M: Physiologic approach to dialysis-induced hypoxemia. *Nephron* 41: 62, 1985

134. Raja R, Kramer M, Rosenbaum JL, Bollisay C, Krug M: Dialysis hypoxemia with varying dialyzers and dialysate – role of acetate in etiology. *Abstracts Am Soc Artif Intern Organs* 9: 60, 1980

135. De Backer WA, Verpooten GA, Borgonjon DJ, Vermeire PA, Lins RR, De Broe ME: Hypoxemia during hemodialysis: Effects of different membranes and dialysate compositions. *Kidney Int* 23: 738, 1983

136. Francos GC, Besarab A, Burke JF, Peters J, Tahamont MV, Gee MH, Flynn JT, Gzesh D: Dialysis-induced hypoxemia: Membrane dependent and membrane independent causes. *Am J Kidney Dis* 5: 191, 1985

137. Vaziri ND, Wilson A, Mukai D, Darwish R, Rutz A, Hyatt J, Moreno C: Dialysis hypoxemia – role of dialyser membrane and dialysate delivery system. *Am J Med* 77: 828, 1984

138. Craddock PR, Fehr J, Brigham KL, Kronenberg RS, Jacob HS: Complement and leucocyte-mediated pulmonary dysfunction in hemodialysis. *N Engl J Med* 296, 769, 1977

139. Gotch FA, Sargent JA, Keen M, Lam M, Prowitt MH: The solute kinetics of intermittent dialysis therapy. *Proc 11th Annu Contractor's Conf Artif Kidney Program of NIAMDD,* Edited by Mackey BB, DHEW publ no (NIH) 79, 1442, 1978, p 110

140. Panzetta G, Tessitore N, Valvo E, Lupo A, Loschiavo C, Fabris A, Oldrizzi L, Gammaro L, Rugiu C, Bellotti Z, Maschio G: Biofiltration in the treatment of patients with acetate

dialysis intolerance. *Clin Nephrol* 26: 33, 1986

141. Klein E, Ward RA, Harding GB: Calcium carbonate precipitation in bicarbonate hemodialysis. *Artif Organs* 10: 248, 1986

142. Keshaviah PR: Rapid dialysis therapy. *Artif Organs* 10: 173, 1986

143. Collins A, Ilstrup K, Hanson G, Berkseth R, Keshaviah P: Rapid-high-efficiency hemodialysis. *Artif Organs* 10: 185, 1986

144. Ghezzi PM, Sanz-Moreno C, Gervasio R, Migrelli S, Botella J: Technical requirements for rapid high efficiency therapy in uremic patients. *Trans Am Soc Artif Intern Organs* 33: 546, 1987

145. Manohar NL, Gorfien PC, Namba T, Louis BM, Lipner HI: Rapid improvement of uremic neuropathy on short high-efficiency hemodialysis with special reference to middle molecules. *Trans Am Soc Artif Intern Organs* 33: 274, 1987

146. Rubin JE, Berlyne GM: Long-term follow-up of patients on short-time dialysis. *Trans Am Soc Artif Intern Organs* 33: 540, 1987

147. Teschan PE: Clinical estimates of treatment adequacy. *Artif Organs* 10: 201, 1986

148. Raja RM, Kramer MS, Goldstein SJ, Mendez M, Kobrin SM: Factors affecting morbidity and mortality during long-term short dialysis. *Trans Am Soc Artif Intern Organs* 33: 538, 1987

149. Ebben JP, Hirsch DN, Luchmann DA, Collins AJ, Keshaviah PR: Microbiologic contamination of liquid bicarbonate concentrate for hemodialysis. *Trans Am Soc Artif Intern Organs* 33: 269, 1987

150. Bland LA, Ridgeway MR, Aguero SM, Carson LA, Favero MS: Potential bacteriologic and endotoxin hazards associated with liquid bicarbonate concentrate. *Trans Am Soc Artif Intern Organs* 33: 542, 1987

151. von Brecht JH: Liquid bicarbonate dialysate: interdialytic and storage characteristics. *Dial Transplant* 14: 75, 1985

152. Nissenson AR, Ackerman RA, Meyers SA, Bridsall SK: Stable liquid bicarbonate hemodialysate (LBD). *Dial Transplant* 14: 78, 1985

153. Bjaeldager PAL, Christiansen E, Jensen HA, Pauley PK: Improved effect of hemodialysis on acidemic patients from an acetate concentration of 38 mmol/l. *Nephron* 27: 142, 1981

154. Wathen R, Keshaviah P, Hommeyer P, Caldwell K, Comty C: Role of dialysate glucose in preventing gluconeogenesis during hemodialysis. *Trans Am Soc Artif Intern Organs* 23: 393, 1977

155. Wathen RL, Keshaviah P, Hommeyer P, Caldwell K, Comty CM: The metabolic effects of hemodialysis with and without glucose in the dialysate. *Am J Clin Nutr* 31: 1870, 1978

156. Swamy AP, Cestero RVM, Campbell RG, Freeman RB: Long-term effect of dialysate glucose on the lipid levels of maintenance hemodialysis patients. *Trans Am Soc Artif Intern Organs* 22: 54, 1976

157. Ramirez G, Butcher DE, Morrison AD: Glucose concentration in the dialysate and lipid abnormalities in chronic hemodialysis patients. *Int J Artif Organs* 10: 31, 1987

158. Ramirez G, Bercaw BL, Butcher DE, Mathis HL, Brueggemeyer C, Newton JL: The role of glucose in hemodialysis: the effects of glucose-free dialysate. *Am J Kidney Dis* 7: 413, 1986

159. Ward RA, Shirlow MJ, Hayes JM, Chapman GV, Farrell PC: Protein-catabolism during hemodialysis. *Am J Clin Nutr* 32: 2443, 1979

160. Ward RA, Wathen RL, Williams TE, Harding GB: Hemodialysate composition and intradialytic metabolic, acid-base and potassium changes. *Kidney Int* 32: 129, 1987

161. Anonymous: Uraemic hypoglycaemia (Editorial). *Lancet* 1: 660, 1986

162. Grajower MM, Walter L, Albin J: Hypoglycemia in chronic hemodialysis patients: associated with propranolol use. *Nephron* 26: 126, 1980

163. Fassett RG, Oliver JR, Mathew TH: Hypoglycemia in end-stage renal disease. *Dial Transplant* 12: 543, 1983

164. Ganda OP, Aoki TT, Soldner JS, Morrison RS, Cahill GF Jr: Hormone-fuel concentrations in anephric subjects. *J Clin Invest* 57: 1403, 1976

165. Oreopoulos DG, Taves DR, Rabinovich S, Meema HE, Murray T, Fenton SS, deVeber GA: Fluoride and dialysis osteodystrophy: results of a double-blind study. *Trans Am Soc Artif Intern Organs* 20: 203, 1974

166. Erben J, Hajakova B, Pantucek M, Kubes L: Fluoride metabolism and renal osteodystrophy in regular dialysis treatment. *Proc Eur Dial Transplant Assoc* 21: 421, 1984

167. McIvor M, Baltazar RF, Beltram J, Mower MM, Wenk R, Lustgarten J, Solomon J: Hyperkalemia and cardiac arrest from fluoride exposure during hemodialysis. *Am J Cardiol* 51: 901, 1983

168. Parsons V, Davies C, Ogg CS, Siddiqui JY, Goode GC: The ionic composition of bone from patients with chronic renal failure and on RDT, with special reference to fluoride and aluminium. *Proc Eur Dial Transplant Assoc* 8: 139, 1971

169. Chaleil D, Simon P, Tessier B, Cartier F, Allain P: Blood plasma fluoride in haemodialysed patients. *Clin Chim Acta* 156: 105, 1986

170. Johnson WJ, Taves DR: Exposure to excessive fluoride during hemodialysis. *Kidney Int* 5: 451, 1974

171. D'Amico G, Petrella E: Standardization of hemodialysis materials. *Kidney Int* 28 (Suppl 7): S105, 1985

172. British Pharmacopoeia 1980, Addendum 1983, p 295, and Appendix XVIIIE, (6/84) pA58

173. Stephens D: The origin and control of rust-coloured precipitates in bicarbonate dialysate lines. *Dial Transplant* 15: 250, 1986

174. Alfrey AC: Aluminium metabolism. *Kidney Int* 29 (Suppl 18): S8, 1986

175. European Economic Community Resolution 86/C 184.04 *Official J Eur Comm* C184. 16 July 1986

176. Kolmos HJ: Hygienic problems in dialysis. *Danish Med Bull* 32: 338, 1985

177. Bommer K, Ritz E: Water quality – a neglected problem in hemodialysis. *Nephron* 46: 1, 1987

178. Shaldon S, Deschodt G, Branger B, Granolleras C, Baldamus CA, Koch KM, Lysaght MJ, Dinarello CA: Haemodialysis hypotension: the interleukin hypothesis re-stated. *Proc Eur Dial Transplant Assoc* 22: 229, 1985

179. Schmidt M, Baldamus CA, Schoeppe W: Back filtration in hemodialysis with highly permeable membranes. *Blood Purif* 2: 108, 1984

180. Thayse C, Vanherweghem J-L, Verbanck P, Walleman P, Durieux A: Description of a central proportioning and delivery system for bicarbonate dialysis. *Nephron* 29: 198, 1981

181. Brueggemeyer CD, Ramirez G: Dialysate concentrate: A potential source for lethal complications. *Nephron* 46: 397, 1987

182. Berkes SL, Kahn SI, Chazan JA, Garella S: Prolonged hemolysis from overheated dialysate. *Ann Intern Med* 83: 363, 1975

183. Lindholm T, Thysell H, Yamamoto Y, Forsberg B, Gullberg CÅ: Temperature and vascular stability in hemodialysis. *Nephron* 39: 130, 1985

184. Marcen R, Quereda C, Lamas S, Orofono L, Teruel JL, Ortuno J: Hypoxemia and dialysate temperature. *Nephron* 45: 74, 1987

185. Von Hartitzsch B, Hoenich NA, Johnson J, Brewis RAL, Kerr DNS: The problem of de-aeration – cause, consequence, cure. *Proc Eur Dial Transplant Assoc* 9: 605, 1972

186. Drukker W, v d Werff B, Meinsma K: De-aeration of dialysis fluid. *Dial Transplant* 3: 33, 1974

ANGIOACCESS IN THE RENAL FAILURE PATIENT

NICHOLAS E. TAWA JR and NICHOLAS L. TILNEY

INTRODUCTION

The introduction of extracorporeal dialysis of blood by Kolff et al (1) in 1943 provided a means whereby patients with end stage renal failure could be sustained for prolonged periods. Intermittent catheterization of distal arteries and veins using glass or metal cannulae was performed originally, with the vessels ligated following each procedure. Chronic dialysis was not feasible until the introduction of the external arteriovenous shunt by Quinton, Dillard and Scribner in 1960 (2) and the endogenous fistula by Brescia, Cimino and colleagues in 1966 (3), approaches that afforded routine intermittent access to the circulation. The increased availability of synthetic vascular prostheses has allowed a greater procedural choice, particularly in chronic dialysis patients who have exhausted peripheral venous sites. In recent years placement of external shunts has diminished coincident with the greater popularity of permanent subcutaneous vascular grafts for long-term use or percutaneous catheters for acute use. In this chapter we review general techniques of placement, care, revision and repair, as well as expectations for long term patency of vascular access procedures for dialysis.

TECHNIQUES FOR TEMPORARY ACCESS

Urgent vascular access is often required for treatment of acute renal failure or during the maturation period of recently created or revised permanent arteriovenous fistulae. Such maturation is mandatory for endogenous fistulae since the non-arterialized recipient vein cannot withstand repeated venipuncture. In addition, various investigators have described tunnel hematomas in as many as 75% of synthetic grafts punctured within several days of implantation (4).

External devices such as the Quinton-Scribner, Allen-Brown, or Thomas shunts, are effective for high flow dialy-sis in individuals in whom cannulation of the femoral or subclavian veins is difficult or contraindicated, or those in whom coagulopathy precludes venipuncture with large bore cannulae (2). However, such accesses have been associated with poor patency rates and a high incidence of sepsis, particularly (in the femoral triangle) with the Thomas shunt (5). In addition, important distal vessels are sacrificed by their use. Today, the percutaneous transvenous catheter, placed intermittently for dialysis or left in place for relatively brief periods, has obviated many of these problems and has become the procedure of choice for temporary access.

External shunts

The Scribner shunt is comprised of two Silastic tubes that can be fitted with tapered Teflon tips of various sizes to enter a given vessel. The tubes are joined by a Teflon connector when the shunt is not in use; for dialysis, it can be disconnected and the tubing joined directly to the machine. Once a tip of appropriate size has been chosen, it is important to moisten it and insert its base a short distance into the Silastic tubing; as kinking or creasing of the Teflon may cause thrombosis, a damaged tip should be replaced. The Ramiriz wing tip modification, which is designed to prevent extrusion or dislodgement, also makes the shunt more difficult to remove and is not recommended.

As the procedure can be performed under local anesthesia, it is particularly helpful in intensive care unit patients with acute renal failure which is expected to reverse itself. If available, the distal radial artery and cephalic vein are cannulated; the large basilic vein in the posterior aspect of the forearm may also be used if necessary. The cannula tip should not cross a joint or be placed in a potentially ischemic extremity. The appropriate vessels are isolated via small skin incisions, encircled with ligatures proximally and distally, and the distal ends ligated (Figure 1). A small trans-

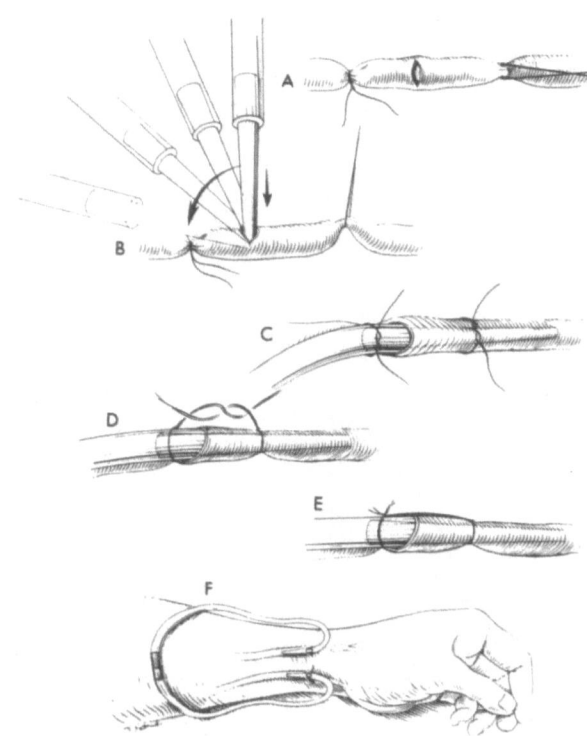

Figure 1. A. The radial artery and an adjacent vein are isolated and ligated distally. B. The largest convenient Teflon cannulae is inserted into the vessels via a transverse incision. C. The tip and Silastic tubing are tied in place proximally and distally. D. These ligatures are then tied together to prevent extrusion of the tip. E. The tip should lie so as not to angulate or kink the vessel. F. The completed Scribner shunt lies conveniently along the forearm. (Reprinted with permission of WB Saunders Co.)

verse arteriotomy or venotomy is made and the proximal vessel dilated to accept the largest tip possible, avoiding intimal cracking or dissection. Small arterial tips should be chosen in diabetic patients, as the intima may roll up ahead of the advancing Teflon if the tip is too large. The tip is advanced to a point where the Silastic tubing abuts the opening into the vessel and is tied in place with the proximal ligature. The Silastic tubing is secured with the distal ligature and both proximal and distal ends tied together to prevent extrusion of the cannula. A subcutaneous pocket is made to hold the U-shaped Silastic tubing, the distal ends of which exit from the skin through separate stab wounds on the proximal forearm. After adequate flow is assured by heparinized saline flushing, the external limbs of the shunt are connected with a Teflon connector. The shunt is protected by wrapping the forearm loosely with an elastic bandage.

Care of these shunts is minimal; the skin and exiting Silastic tubing should be cleaned daily. Thrombosis can occur if the tubing kinks or with low flow and hypotension. The shunt should not be used as a route for intravenous medication or for monitoring of arterial pressure; during

other surgical procedures, blood pressure measurements should never be taken in the access arm. A thrombosed shunt can occasionally be cleared using a #3 Fogarty catheter; alternatively, streptokinase injected into the clotted shunt will often lyse small thrombi at the tip. More often, a thrombosed or poorly flowing shunt will have to be replaced or the tips moved more proximally in the same vessels.

Most series have reported patency rates for external shunts ranging from 2 to 15 months (6, 7). Thrombosis, infection, kinking of the tubing or fibrous intimal hyperplasia of the native vessel at the level of the tip all contribute to failure. Chronic administration of low dose aspirin may help to insure patency (8, 9). Thus, although an effective access can be created quickly using a Scribner shunt, the relatively high incidence of thrombosis and infection, the potential for dislodgement and hemorrhage, and the elimination of important sites for an endogenous fistula are all disadvantages of the method.

Percutaneous transvenous catheterization

Percutaneous catheterization of the femoral vein for dialysis was first described by Shaldon et al in 1961 (10–13). Either a single lumen or double lumen coaxial catheter may be used. The former suffers from diminished clearance because of significant dead space and recirculation requiring increased duration and frequency of dialysis; the double lumen coaxial catheter allows continuous and effective venous return.

After groin skin preparation, the femoral vein immediately below the inguinal ligament is catheterized with a 16 gauge cannula. A spring guidewire is then passed into the proximal iliac vein, the cannula withdrawn, and a Teflon catheter inserted over the guidewire. The guidewire is then removed and the dialysis tubing fixed to a Luer-lock at the end of the venous catheter. Complications happen infrequently but include ileofemoral venous thrombosis, local infection at the catheter site, retroperitoneal hemorrhage secondary to venous perforation, and arteriovenous fistula (14, 15). As most of these complications occur during insertion, the catheter is usually left indwelling; the patient remains hospitalized during its use but may ambulate. These catheters may be maintained up to 2 weeks with meticulous skin care. Heparinized saline (1000 units in 500 ml) is infused continuously at 5 ml/h for patency. The catheter may also be flushed with 1,500 units of heparin every 12 h and capped.

Placement of a temporary catheter in the subclavian vein is technically more difficult than in the femoral region but preferable to it. The incidence of infection is lower, the catheter may remain in place for prolonged periods with scrupulous skin care, and the mobility of the patient is not affected; all of these factors allow the individual to remain at home. The catheter is flushed with heparin as previously described. This short catheter may be introduced either using the infraclavicular or supraclavicular route (16–18). The patient lies supine with the bed in Trendelenburg position to increase venous distension. A rolled towel is placed between the shoulder blades and the head is turned to the side opposite the insertion site. After prepping and draping, the sternal notch and clavicular joint are palpated. A site midway along the clavicle is anesthetized and a 16 gauge cannula is passed directly beneath the clavicle, aiming at the sternal notch. Slight continuous suction on the syringe is kept; a flash back of blood into the syringe shows that the vessel has been entered. The syringe is detached and a guidewire inserted through the cannula, which is then removed. The dialysis catheter is passed over the wire into the vein. The patient is then sent for an upright chest film to rule out pneumothorax and check catheter position. Placement is adequate if the tip lies in the superior vena cava or the junction of the superior vena cava and right atrium.

A modification of this technique is operative placement of a double lumen Silastic catheter into the central venous system via the internal jugular vein (Quinton-Hickman catheter). Proper positioning is confirmed by fluoroscopy. The catheter is then tunneled subcutaneously to a remote exit site on the anterior chest. A proximal Dacron cuff provides a barrier to infection. These catheters may be expected to have a lower incidence of septic complications and other percutaneous devices and are useful for patients in whom dialysis may be terminated within 3 to 6 months (19), or in those in whom more permanent access is planned.

TECHNIQUES FOR CHRONIC ACCESS

General principles

Arteriovenous fistulae are of endogenous vein or prosthetic material. They are optimally placed just deep to the dermis to prevent erosion through the skin while permitting easy puncture. Provided a vein of adequate size is easily visible, the endogenous (Cimino) fistula at the wrist or at the antecubital space is preferred as a first procedure because of long-term patency and a low incidence of infection. Such fistulae are impractical for patients whose cephalic veins are sclerosed or thrombosed because of continued use, or in post-menopausal women with small, fragile veins lying deep in the subcutaneous fat. Cimino fistulae, particularly at the wrist, are often unsuccessful in the diabetic patient because of inadequate arterial inflow. Preoperative planning includes adequate hydration, prevention of hypotension and vasoconstriction, and perioperative antibiotics, particularly for placement of prosthetic materials. Repeated venipuncture in the arm to be used for access is an anathema.

In selecting a fistula site (20, 21), the upper extremity is preferred because the incidence of infection is lower and development of arterial steal syndrome less critical than in the leg (Figure 2). These considerations are especially important in patients at greater risk for atherosclerosis and ischemia, such as elderly or diabetic persons. Similarly, the saphenous vein should be spared when possible for future arterial reconstruction. The most distal site available should be used to keep maximal vessel length for future revision. Finally, the non-dominant arm is preferred for ease of venipuncture by the patient and to keep the dominant arm free during dialysis.

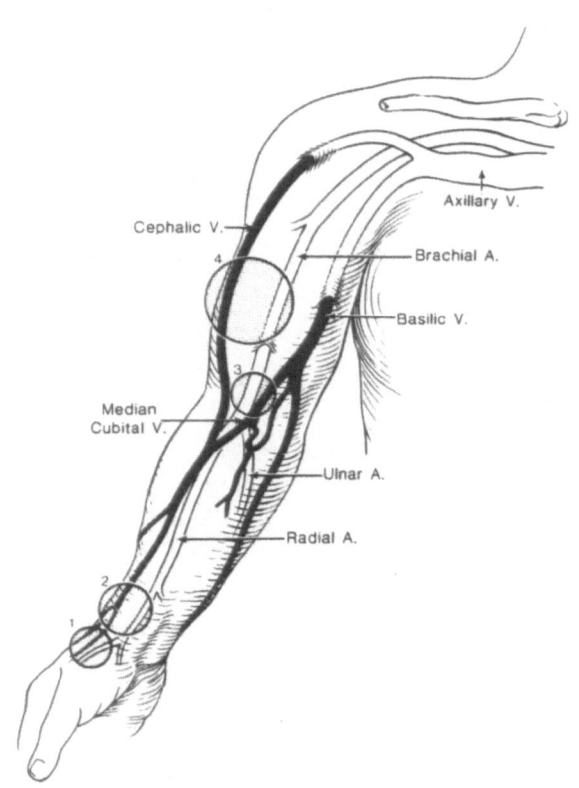

Figure 2. The most widely used sites for creation of arteriovenous fistula are circled. (Reprinted with permission of WB Saunders Co.)

Endogenous fistulae

The radial artery and cephalic vein at the wrist are preferred for initial creation of a Cimino fistula, although other upper extremity sites can be used. Unlike the side-to-side anastomosis first described for wrist fistulae, an end-vein to side-artery anastomosis with preservation of the distal radial artery should be performed, as it results in a reduced incidence of arterial steal and distal venous hypertension (22–24). Furthermore, patency rates for the two approaches are equal (24).

An outpatient procedure performed under local anesthesia, the fistula is constructed exposing radial artery and distal cephalic vein via a transverse incision (Figure 3). A smaller catheter is passed up the vein to dilate it, and the vein is irrigated to ensure patency. The end-to-side anastomosis is then performed with continuous 6–0 monofilament suture. If possible, the confluence of two major venous tributaries is fashioned as an onlay patch after each distal branch has been ligated and divided a few millimeters from their junction. The vein proximal to the anastomosis should be isolated for 2 to 3 cm to ensure maximal dilation for arterial flow. On completion of the anastomosis and release of the occlusive vessel loops, a thrill should be palpable over the proximal vein. Absence of a thrill, and a bounding pulse, suggest venous outflow obstruction.

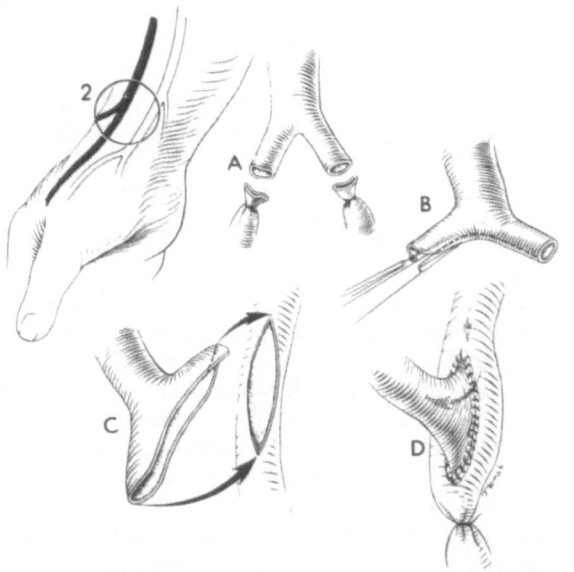

Figure 3. A Cimino fistula is made most commonly at the wrist (Area 2). A. The cephalic vein is isolated at its bifurcation and the distal branches ligated. B. This is opened. C. The widened area is then shaped for a patch graft. D. An end-to-side anastomosis is created using fine suture. The distal artery can be ligated if desired. (Reprinted with permission of WB Saunders Co.)

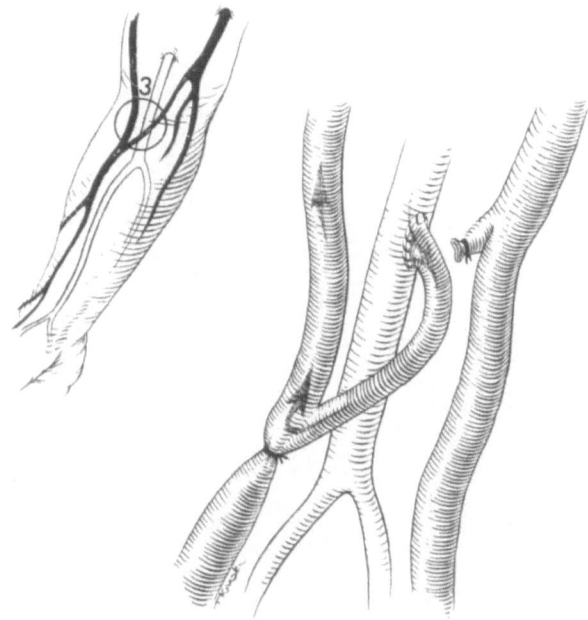

Figure 4. The median cubital vein may be anastomosed to the brachial artery for an upper arm Cimino fistula (Area 3). (Reprinted with permission of WB Saunders Co.)

Upper arm fistulae are satisfactory if vessels at the wrist are inadequate, in individuals with obvious proximal cephalic or antecubital veins, or in those with a previous failed distal Cimino fistula which produced proximal venous dilatation. Using the end-to-side technique, the median cubital vein is isolated from its junction with the basilic system above the elbow and anastomosed to the proximal brachial artery (Figure 4), or the cephalic vein is divided, mobilized, and anastomosed to the artery above or below the antecubital crease (Figure 5). Extra length may be achieved by isolating a large venous branch proximally into the forearm.

When the venous anatomy of the arm precludes an endogenous fistula, a saphenous vein segment may be used as an autograft through a looped or curved tunnel between an adequate upper extremity artery and vein (23, 25, 26). The technique is occasionally useful in those individuals who seem to be allergic to Teflon. The incidence of infection in such grafts is less than with prosthetic ones, but the long-term occurrence of diffuse stenosis is higher (27). In individuals whose upper extremity sites have been exhausted, the saphenous vein may be used in-situ as a loop fistula in the thigh. It is isolated through a series of longitudinal incisions to the level of the knee (Figure 6). Branches are carefully ligated. The saphenofemoral junction is kept intact and the vein passed in a U-shaped tunnel to the common femoral artery where it is anastomosed end-to-side. Although used as a last resort, the technique is effective in some difficult long-term patients, particularly those few who seem to react adversely to Teflon with sterile inflammation.

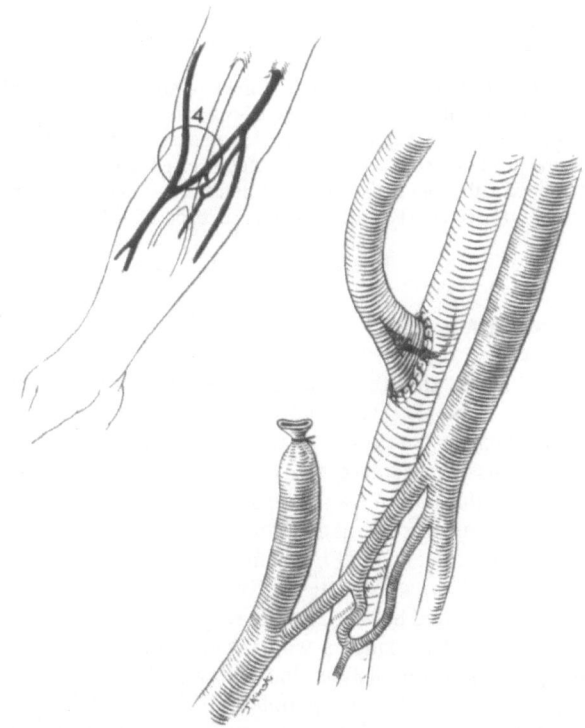

Figure 5. The cephalic vein can be anastomosed to the brachial artery for an upper arm Cimino fistula (Area 4). (Reprinted with permission of WB Saunders Co.)

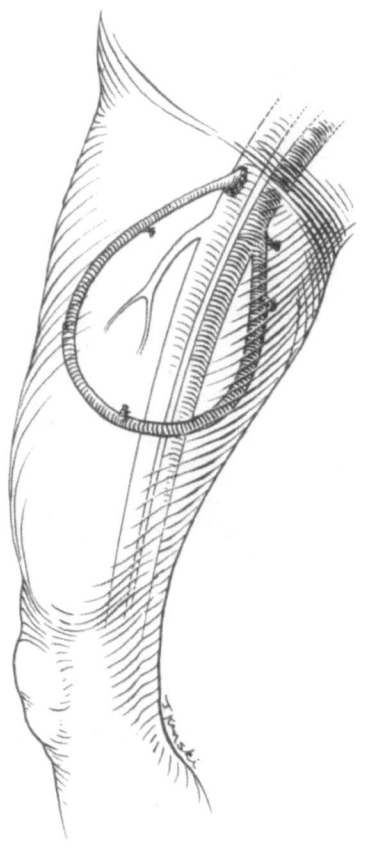

Figure 6. An autogenous saphenous vein loop fistula can be created in the groin when upper arm sites have been exhausted. The saphenous vein is isolated carefully from below the knee to the saphenofemoral junction. All branches are carefully ligated. The vein is then positioned in the superficial tunnel and its distal end anastomosed to the femoral artery. (Reprinted with permission of WB Saunders Co.)

Synthetic grafts

For permanent endogenous access, use of the patient's own vein is desirable despite a relatively high initial failure rate. When veins are inadequate or unavailable, however, prosthetic grafts become necessary even though the rate of infection and thrombosis may be higher. Prosthetic grafts have been more satisfactory than biological ones. Expanded polytetra-fluorethylene (PTFE), is the most popular vascular prosthesis; it has patency rates between 58% and 95% at one year and 36% and 86% at 2 years, surprisingly higher than those reported in patients with Cimino fistulae (27–29). Adequate flow for dialysis and a low incidence of high output cardiac failure or peripheral steal syndrome are achieved with 6 mm PTFE, the most common diameter used. Grafts bearing a spiral external support are useful if joint lines must be crossed.

For PTFE grafts as with endogenous fistulae, the most distal site available on the upper extremity is used first. A loop configuration has a significantly higher patency rate than straight PTFE (30) and is preferred. A loop graft lying on the ventral aspect of the forearm may be created using the distal brachial artery as inflow and the largest available vein, either the basilic or cephalic and usually proximal to the antecubital crease, as outflow (Figure 7). In patients in whom a previous forearm graft was removed due to infection, a new forearm loop graft may be made using more proximal vessels following healing. If necessary the proximal basilic vein in the mid or upper arm, the axillary vein in the axillary fossa, or the subclavian vein in the infraclavicular position may be used (Figure 8). In the upper arm, the graft should run on the lateral aspect of the biceps as it is not only difficult to cannulate on the medial aspect but uncomfortable for the patient to hold the arm in external rotation during dialysis.

Techniques in placement of access prostheses are the same as those used in standard peripheral vascular surgery. After isolating appropriate vessels at a chosen site, a shallow subcutaneous tunnel is created using a curved tunneler and the graft placed within it (31). Such tunnelers should be the same diameter as the graft to prevent seroma formation. Kinking or twisting of the graft is to be avoided. After the vessels are occluded with loops, the graft is beveled obliquely and placed end-to-side to the vessel using continuous 5–0 or 6–0 monofilament suture. Upon completion of the first anastomosis, heparinized saline is placed in the vessel, the graft clamped and the second anastomosis constructed. Systemic heparinization is rarely necessary. As in the Cimino fistula, it is helpful to isolate a short segment of vein proximal to the anastomosis to allow dilatation with arterial flow. A venous thrill should be palpable after this maneuver. As a bounding pulse in the absence of a thrill suggests venous obstruction, on table arteriography may be helpful. The extremity is elevated for 48 to 72 h after operation to diminish swelling which represents expression of a plasma ultrafiltrate across the initially porous PTFE graft. New grafts should not be used for at least 3 weeks to allow tissue incorporation and thus to avoid hematoma or pseudoaneurysm formation due to premature puncture, which may be a potential source of infection.

In difficult patients with multiple previous failures, vessels of the lower extremity may be used as a last resort. Prosthetic fistulae may be positioned between the distal superficial femoral or popliteal artery and the proximal saphenous or femoral vein, or a femoro-femoral loop constructed over the anterior medial aspect of the upper thigh between the common or proximal superficial femoral artery and saphenous or femoral vein (32). Some have advocated axillary-axillary or brachial-internal jugular grafts in such patients although such grafts running across the neck or sternum are disfiguring (33). Grafts in the lower extremity should be avoided in diabetic or older individuals with peripheral vascular compromise.

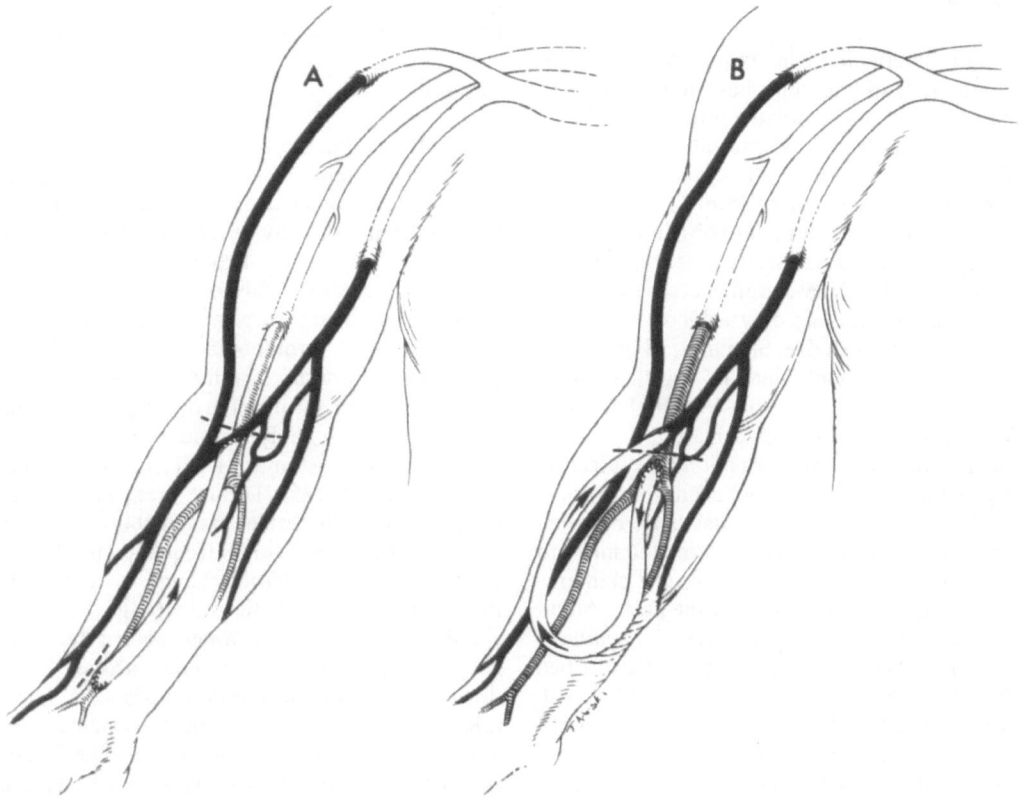

Figure 7. Prosthetic material is used commonly for dialysis access in the forearm. A. A straight graft can run between distal radial artery and a convenient venous channel at the antecubital space. B. A forearm loop prosthesis is placed in a U configuration between brachial artery and a convenient vein at the antecubital space. (Reprinted with permission of WB Saunders Co.)

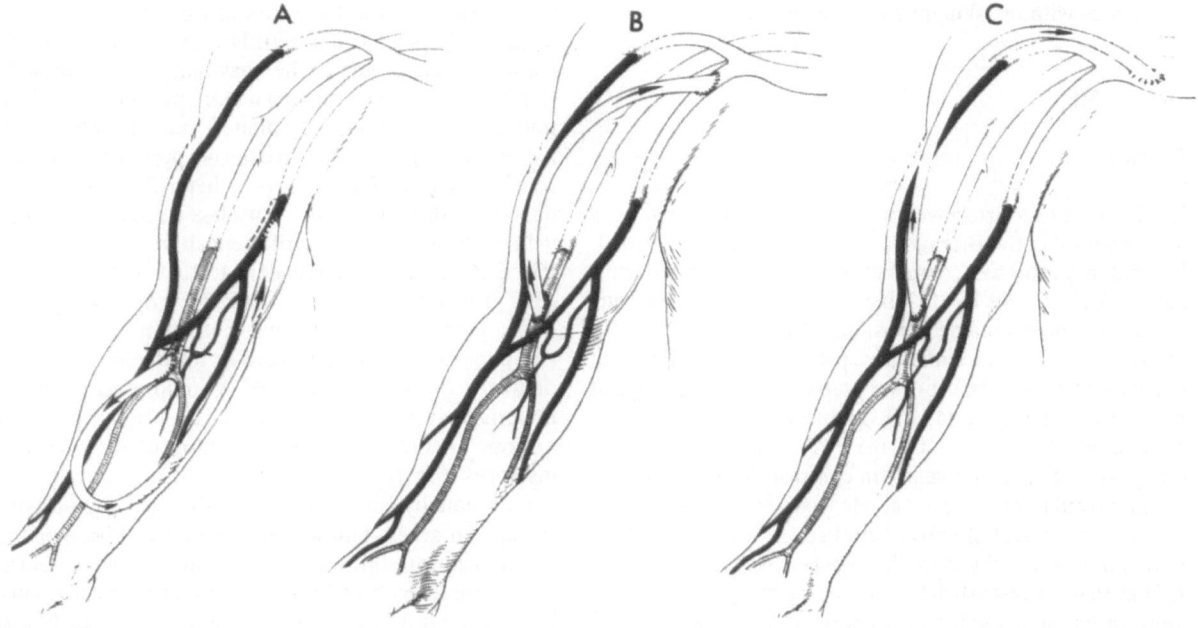

Figure 8. When more proximal veins have all been used, the venous limb of the prosthesis can be anastomosed more proximally to the basilic vein. B. A new prosthetic graft may be placed between the brachial artery and the proximal brachial vein in the axilla. C. The venous end can also be anastomosed to the subclavian vein. (Reprinted with permission of WB Saunders Co.)

Alternative devices

Although no graft material has been thoroughly satisfactory, biological materials in particular have not lived up to their potential and seem inappropriate for dialysis patients. Bovine grafts, prepared from cow carotid artery treated with aldehyde and alcohol, show a one year cumulative patency rate in several series ranging from 33% and 95%; however, at 2 years, patency rates fall to 6% and 24% (27, 34–37). Stenosis at the venous anastomosis is common and the rate of infection high. If these grafts become infected, they rapidly degenerate, leaving only a blood-filled subcutaneous tunnel lined with sludge. Similarly, while human umbilical vein has been available since 1974, little enthusiasm has been shown for its use (38, 39). We feel that use of such grafts for dialysis access are contra-indicated.

A low incidence of hematoma formation and infection following early (within 72 h of operation) needle puncture of PTFE and bovine carotid heterografts has been reported when very superficial and constrictive subdermal tunnels are used (4). However, this technique may promote skin erosion and pseudoaneurysm formation over the graft. An alternative approach allowing immediate use of a synthetic graft is a self-sealing dialysis prosthesis. It consists of two coaxial PTFE tubes, the space between them filled with silicone rubber sealant. Excellent results have been shown in a canine model (40). Recently, a hemasite-incorporated graft has been described which obviates needle puncture at the time of dialysis; this potentially allows early use while reducing the risk of graft infection, pseudoaneurysm formation, and thrombosis. In a limited series of 11 patients, the cumulative patency rate at one year was 70% (41). However, infection arising at the junction of the metallic hemasite device with the skin may be problematic.

OUTCOME

Patency rates

In a review of 324 arteriovenous conduits constructed over a 4 year period at the Brigham and Women's Hospital, excellent patency rates were demonstrated for both Cimino fistulae and PTFE grafts by life table analysis (29). These results confirmed those obtained previously by others (25, 28, 30, 46) and suggested the cumulative patency rates for PTFE in particular to exceed most other grafts, particularly those of biological origin (27, 44, 47). In the Brigham series, the cumulative patency rates for 163 PTFE grafts were 83% at one year and 70% at 2 years. In contrast, 64% of over 150 Cimino fistulae were patent at one year and 50% at 2 years. The lower survival of native vein fistulae was the result of early failures, usually in the first post-operative month. Although in most cases such failure was secondary to the use of veins of marginal quality noted at operation, it was elected to proceed in the hope that a synthetic graft could be avoided. There was no difference in patency of Cimino fistulae created at the wrist and in the antecubital fossa. Important-

ly, when the earlier failures were not considered, PTFE grafts and endogenous fistulae had equivalent survival.

Thrombosis

Thrombosis is the most common cause of fistula failure. In the Brigham series (29), 50% of PTFE grafts required thrombectomy or revision to maintain their function. Although thrombosis may be induced by external pressure on the fistula, dehydration, hypotension or hypovolemia (usually associated with dialysis), or a hypercoaguable state often occurring after surgery, outflow stenosis is at fault in the majority of thrombosed PTFE and Cimino fistulae. Stenosis usually occurs near the venous anastomosis because of fibrotic valves, through the development of fibrous intimal hyperplasia probably secondary to turbulence and high flow, or at the anastomosis itself from localized ingrowth of endothelial cells (25). Diffuse areas of stenosis may also develop within the fistula, presumably due to accumulation of organized laminar clot at frequently used puncture sites. In addition, atherosclerotic changes have been described in the neointima of synthetic grafts (48).

Although usually performed soon after thrombosis to keep within the dialysis schedule, successful restoration of thrombosed fistulae can be accomplished as long as 2 weeks following the event. As initial treatment, thrombectomy under local anesthesia is undertaken. The fistula is opened surgically through a small transverse incision placed near the anastomosis of Cimino fistulae or near the venous anastomosis for synthetic grafts. Clot is removed using an appropriate Fogarty balloon-tipped catheter. If fistula thrombosis is due to mechanical obstruction, the underlying cause must be corrected; for example, in Cimino fistulae, a short stenotic segment found in the vein itself can be repaired locally using a vein patch (Figure 9). However, when stenosis of a Cimino fistula occurs at the anastomotic site, a new fistula should be created by making a more proximal arterial anastomosis using the already dilated vein. Rarely, a Cimino fistula will clot secondary to external pressure. These can be reopened using a fine Fogarty catheter. If thrombophlebitis develops, thrombectomy is useless because the inflamed vein reclots. Correction of stenosis results in prolonged PTFE graft survival equivalent to that of unrevised grafts (29). It is noteworthy that for PTFE grafts, a significantly higher cumulative patency was noted if an outflow stenosis was bypassed as compared either to simple thrombectomy or to the use of a patch (29). A jump graft of prosthetic material may easily be run between the original prosthesis to a more proximal uninvolved portion of the vein in such instances (Figure 10).

Occasionally percutaneous transluminal angioplasty may salvage an access failing from a venous stenosis, although experience with this technique is limited. In a recent study (49), local injection of streptokinase and percutaneous balloon angioplasty were used in conjunction to restore shunt patency after thrombosis. Seventeen (52%) of the 33 shunts in this series were restored to function without surgical intervention; 21% had restoration of flow but required sur-

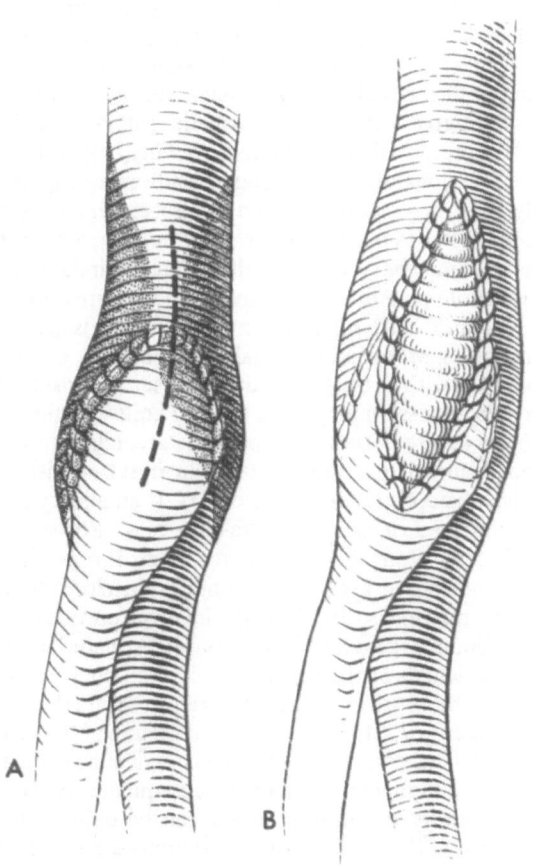

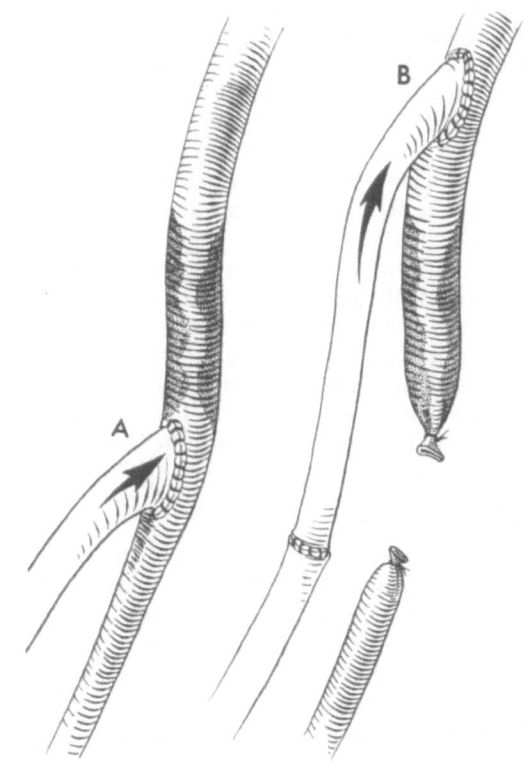

Figure 10. Lengthy stenoses proximal to the graft-venous anastomosis can be bypassed using a jump graft anastomosed to a normal proximal segment of vein. (Reprinted with permission of WB Saunders Co.)

Figure 9. A stenosis at or near the graft venous anastomosis can be patched using native vein or prosthetic material. (Reprinted with permission of WB Saunders Co.)

gical correction of an underlying problem such as a pseudoaneurysm or a stenosis that resisted balloon angioplasty. Nine (27%) showed no improvement. Further follow-up of these patients is needed to determine the long-term efficacy of this approach.

Aneurysmal complications of arteriovenous fistulae are unusual, but these may be an additional cause for thrombosis. True aneurysms of Cimino fistulae occur primarily at the anastomotic site and along areas of the vein where venipunctures are made repeatedly. The majority remain asymptomatic although occasionally the overlying skin may become thin and erode, or the aneurysm can thrombose or become infected. If symptomatic, posing a cosmetic problem, or bothersome to the patient when renal function is regained after successful transplantation, the normal vessels immediately adjacent to the dilatation can be ligated, the aneurysm excised and a new fistula constructed more proximally if desired. Thrombosis can occur from progressive layering of laminar clot both in sacular aneurysms and in large fusiform aneurysms involving much of the venous limb. Although it is sometimes possible to remove such a clot with a Fogarty catheter or by expressing the thrombus from the aneurysm

by direct pressure via a venotomy, one usually has to open immediately into the sac to remove the clot. Most Cimino fistulae with thrombosed aneurysms cannot be repaired and have to be established elsewhere.

In PTFE grafts, pseudoaneurysms result from unsealed needle puncture sites anywhere along their course. By producing areas of reduced flow, they contribute to graft thrombosis. Like true aneurysms, they may become locally symptomatic or cosmetically undesirable. Overall, pseudoaneurysm formation in PTFE accounts for only 2% of malfunctions (29); treatment is by local excision and restoration of continuity with an interposition graft.

Ischemia

Ischemic symptoms of the hand or forearm distal to a well-functioning fistula are not common but may be difficult to resolve. Both arterial insufficiency and venous hypertension contribute to the low flow state. Poor arterial inflow to the hand results from direct shunting to the proximal fistula and from a vascular steal phenomenon, in which blood flows retrograde from the palmar arches through the radial artery into the fistula. For example, when thumb blood pressure was used as an index of perfusion, occlusion of the radial artery distal to a Cimino fistula resulted in a significant increase in pressure in 88% of patients studied, only a small proportion of whom had ischemic symptoms (50). In one series (51), 42% of patients with side-to-side radiocephalic fistulae and 16% of those with end-to-side fistulae had intermittent hand claudication with exercise. A cool, bluish, and painful hand with rest pain is often relieved by placing the hand in a dependent position. This condition is more common in diabetic patients.

As the majority of ischemic symptoms improve within several weeks following fistula placement, a period of temporization is essential. Occasionally, symptoms are severe enough to demand surgical recourse; this entails narrowing the fistula by banding it with a ligature or by use of a tapered interposition graft. Reduced fistula flow, at least theoretically, drives more arterial blood distally into the hand. Although this maneuver is occasionally effective, it is hardly a panacea, and a few individuals retain permanent hand weakness.

In contrast, when a patient presents with venous hypertension, the situation may be different. A proximal venous occlusion or stenosis of a major vein may sometimes be demonstrated on arteriogram, with major collateralization around it, often with significant retrograde venous flow into the distal venous system. Such occlusion may be bypassed, or if extensive or very proximal, a new access must be made.

Cardiac failure

A rare problem associated with arteriovenous fistulae is high output cardiac failure (52). Patients with this complication are characterized by cardiac disease pre-existing before the angioaccess procedure, including congestive heart failure of any cause, prolonged hypertension, or coronary artery disease. Excessive flow through the fistula, usually between 20 to 50% of the cardiac output, with a concomitant rise in venous return, causes a deleterious rise in cardiac preload. By reducing fistula flow with simple ligation, banding, or interposition of a tapered synthetic segment, cardiac performance may be increased significantly.

Infection

A common cause of prosthetic access failure is infection; for example, at Brigham and Women's Hospital, graft sepsis accounted for 19% of PTFE graft complications (29). By contrast, infection of Cimino fistulae is rare, usually localized to a needle site and often treated effectively by antibiotics and local care. In prosthetic grafts, infection appears to correlate with the completeness of the neointimal lining and time following graft insertion (27, 53, 54). Staphylococcus aureus, Staphylococcus epidermidis, other gram positive cocci, and a variety of gram negative organisms are causative agents, in descending order of frequency. Bacteria may be inoculated during graft puncture for dialysis; the presence of a peri-graft hematoma or aneurysm with associated thrombus increases the risk of infection (55, 56). This risk is also heightened during thrombectomy or reconstructive procedures on the access. Therefore, strict aseptic technique during dialysis and perioperative antibiotics at operation are mandatory (25, 54). In inner city populations, direct injection of ilicit street drugs into the access is a surprisingly common source of infection. Prosthetic graft infection has a variable presentation. Although swelling, erythema, or fluid collections around the superficially placed graft are easily identified, graft infection is also extremely subtle, with few obvious manifestations; occasionally, the interior of the graft may be colonized without external inflammation in the febrile patient with positive blood cultures. In addition, human T-cell lymphotropic virus infection is becoming an increasing problem in the dialysis population, especially in patients with a history of drug abuse. The associated immunosuppression may mask signs of graft infection.

With a severe abscess or septicemia secondary to an infected Cimino fistula, the infected vein must be excised and the subcutaneous tunnel drained (53). If an aneurysm becomes infected, incision and drainage may also be necessary. In 50% of infected PTFE prostheses, it is possible to bypass a localized area with a jump graft, close the new incisions, then excise and drain the involved portion (29). If the infection is generalized and purulent material tracks along the length of the prosthesis, or if an anastomosis is involved, the entire graft should be removed and the tunnel packed open (29, 54, 57). Although resection of the venous and arterial anastomoses has been recommended in the face of extensive tunnel infection (54), subsequent repair of the involved artery to ensure patency can be quite difficult, particularly if the edges of the arteriotomy are friable or if the patient is a diabetic. Recently it was shown that a 2 to 3 mm oversewn cuff of PTFE may be safely left at the arterial anastomosis if the remainder of the graft, including the venous anastomosis, is excised and the entire tunnel tract debrided and irrigated with antibiotics. This method is recommended if progressive, severe infection stops short of the anastomotic site (57). The healed extremity may be used again for another graft, using more proximal vessels.

The type and location of the access also influences rates of infection and treatment. As noted, the incidence of infection in biological grafts is higher than in native vessels; once infected, such grafts dissolve (58). Furthermore, the incidence of bacteremic episodes in individuals with prosthetic grafts is twice that of those with endogenous fistulae and three times higher for patients with fistulae placed in the groin regardless of the material used (59). Infections in the femoral triangle are especially difficult to control. In one large series, 27 out of 161 patients (17%) with groin fistulae developed infection (60). Bacteremia from a septic focus may produce serious complications, including septic pulmonary emboli, myocardial abscess, endocarditis, empyema, meningitis, osteomyelitis, or infection of joint prostheses. However, in the aforementioned study, most patients with infected abscesses were treated appropriately for 4 to 6 weeks beginning within 48 h of discovery; 71% of these became afebrile within 3 days (58). Nine cases of endocarditis, usually of the aortic valve (2.7% of those on chronic hemodialysis), were found in another study; the diagnosis was difficult, although the development of murmurs, central nervous system abnormalities of varying degrees of seriousness, and occasional peripheral emboli were described (61).

DIABETES

The patient with diabetes mellitus and end-stage kidney failure often poses the most difficult problems for the surgeon. The most common causes for hospitalization of such patients are the creation and revision of vascular dialysis accesses. Arteries of the upper extremity may be small with diffuse arteriosclerosis, fragility of the arterial wall, and calcification of the media, making anastomosis challenging. Arterial inflow may be unsatisfactory for well-functioning fistulae. Insertion of Scribner shunts may be difficult, as the radial artery does not dilate and the loose intima tends to push up in front of the advancing Teflon tip. The groin should not be used as an access site in these individuals because of their increased propensity for infection and because peripheral vascular involvement of the lower extremities is almost invariable. Access infections are potential hazards regardless of the type of prosthesis used (62). One series has described the necessity for 2.5 accesses per patient year in diabetic patients, a number exceeding that of the general dialysis population (63). Necrosis and painful ulceration of the finger tips has been described in diabetic patients bearing upper extremity fistulae, presumably secondary to vascular steal in conjunction with compromised microcirculation (64) and inability of the distal arterial tree to dilate.

REFERENCES

1. Graham WB: Historical aspects of hemodialysis. *Transplant Proc* 9: xlix, 1977
2. Quinton WE, Dillard DH, Scribner BH: Cannulation of blood vessels for prolonged hemodialysis. *Trans Am Soc Artif Intern Organs* 6: 104, 1960
3. Brescia MJ, Cimino JE, Appel K, Hurwich BJ: Chronic hemodialysis using venipuncture and a surgically created arteriovenous fistula. *N Engl J Med* 275: 1089, 1966
4. Taucher LA: Immediate, safe hemodialysis into arteriovenous fistulas created with a new tunneler. *Am J Surg* 150: 212, 1985
5. Corry RJ, Patel NP, West JC: Surgical management of complications of vascular access for hemodialysis. *Surg Gynecol Obstet* 151: 49, 1980
6. Ishihara AM, Myers CH: Longevity of arteriovenous shunts for dialysis. *Ann Surg* 168: 281, 1968
7. Foran RF, Golding AL, Treiman RL, DePalma JR: Quinton-Scribner cannulas for hemodialysis: Review of four years' experience. *Calif Med* 112: 8, 1970
8. Harter HR, Burch JW, Majerus PW, Stanford N, Delmez JA, Anderson CB, Weerts CA: Prevention of thrombosis in patients on hemodialysis by low dose aspirin. *N Engl J Med* 301: 577, 1979
9. Chesebro JH, Clements IP, Elveback LR, Fuster V, Smith HC, Bardsley WT, Frye RL, Holmes DR Jr, Vlietstra RE, Pluth JR, Wallace RB, Puga FJ, Orszulak TA, Piehler JM, Schaff HV,

Danielson GK: A platelet-inhibitor-drug trial in coronary-artery bypass operationss. *N Engl J Med* 307: 73, 1982
10. Shaldon S, Chiandussi L, Higgs B: Hemodialysis by percutaneous catheterization of the femoral artery and vein with regional heparinization. *Lancet* 2: 857, 1961
11. Shaldon S, Silva H, Pomeroy J, Rae AI, Rosen SM: Percutaneous femoral venous catheterization and reusable dialyzers in the treatment of acute renal failure. *Trans Am Soc Artif Intern Organs* 10: 133, 1964
12. Nidus B, Matalon R, Katz C: Hemodialysis using femoral vessel cannulation. *Nephron* 13: 416, 1974
13. Arana VA, Hodson JM, Menno AD, McMahon JJ: Percutaneous femoral vein catheterization in patients receiving hemodialysis. *J Urol* 106: 492, 1971
14. Kjellstrand CM, Merino GE, Mauer SM, Casali R, Buselmeier TJ: Complications of percutaneous femoral vein catheterization for hemodialysis. *Clin Nephrol* 4: 37, 1975
15. Fulley TJ, Mahoney JJ, Juncos LI, Hawkins RF: Arteriovenous fistula after femoral vein catheterization. *JAMA* 236: 2943, 1976
16. Defalque RJ: Subclavian puncture: A review. *Anesth Analg* 47: 677, 1968
17. Erben J, Kvanicka J, Bastecky J: Experience with routine use of subclavian vein cannulation in hemodialysis. *Proc Eur Dial Transplant Assoc* 6: 59, 1969
18. DeCubber A, DeWolt C, Lameire N: Single needle hemodialysis with the double headpump via the subclavian vein. *Proc Eur Dial Transplant Assoc* 7: 1261, 1978
19. McGonigle DJ, Schrock LG, Hickman RO: Experience using central venous access for long-term hemodialysis. A new concept. *Am J Surg* 145: 571, 1983
20. Whittemore AD: Vascular access for hemodialysis, in *Surgical Care of the Patient with Renal Failure*, edited by Tilney NL, Lazarus JM, Philadelphia, WB Saunders Co., 1982, p 49
21. Tilney NL, Whittemore AD: Dialysis access in difficult patients, in *Vascular Surgery*, edited by Bell PRF, Tilney NL, London, Butterworths, 1984, p 175
22. Bossell JA, Abbott JA, Lim RC: A radial steal syndrome with arteriovenous fistula for hemodialysis. *Ann Intern Med* 75: 387, 1971
23. May J, Tiller D, Johnson J, Stewart J, Sheil AG: Saphenous vein arteriovenous fistula in regular dialysis treatment. *N Engl J Med* 280: 770, 1969
24. Wedgwood KR, Wiggins PA, Guillou PJ: A prospective study of end-to-side vs side-to-side arteriovenous fistulas for haemodialysis. *Br J Surg* 71: 540, 1984
25. Jenkins AM, Buist TAS, Glover SD: Medium-term follow-up of forty autogenous vein and forty polytetrafluorethylene (Gortex) grafts for vascular access. *Surgery* 88: 667, 1980
26. Gerardet RE, Hackett RE, Goodwin NJ, Friedman EA: Thirteen months' experience with the saphenous vein graft arteriovenous fistula for maintenance hemodialysis. *Trans Am Soc Artif Intern Organs* 16: 285, 1970
27. Morgan AP, Dammin GJ, Lazarus JM: Failure modes in secondary vascular access for hemodialysis. *asaio J* 1: 44, 1978
28. Hammill FS, Johnson GG, Collins GM: A critical appraisal of the changing approaches to vascular access for chronic dialysis. *Proc Eur Dial Transplant Assoc* 9: 325, 1980
29. Palder SB, Kirkman RL, Whittemore AD, Hakim RM, Lazarus JM, Tilney NL: Vascular access for hemodialysis. *Ann Surg* 202: 235, 1985
30. Munda R, First MR, Alexander JW, Linneman CC Jr, Fidler JP, Kittur D: Polytetrafluoroethylene graft survival in hemodialysis. *JAMA* 249: 219, 1983

31. Salvatierra O Jr, Feduska NJ: Construction of the optimal tunnel for interposition arteriovenous hemodialysis fistulas. *Surgery* 94: 508, 1983

32. Mandel SR, McDougal EG: Popliteal artery to saphenous vein vascular access for hemodialysis. *Surg Gynecol Obstet* 160: 358, 1985

33. Haimov M: Vascular access for hemodialysis-new modifications for the difficult patient. *Surgery* 92: 109, 1982

34. Rosenthal JJ, Spigelman A, Gaspar MR, Mavius HJ: Problems with bovine heterografts for hemodialysis. *Am J Surg* 130: 182, 1975

35. Johnson JM, Kenoyer MR, Johnson KE, Potter DJ, Nickas GM, Williams T: The modified bovine heterograft in vascular access for chronic hemodialysis. *Ann Surg* 183: 62, 1976

36. Hurt AV, Batello-Cruz M, Skipper BJ, Teaf SR, Sterling WA Jr: Bovine carotid artery heterograft versus polytetrafluoroethylene grafts. *Am J Surg* 146: 844, 1983

37. Naimov M, Jacobson NJ: Experience with modified bovine arterial heterograft in peripheral reconstruction and vascular access for hemodialysis. *Ann Surg* 180: 291, 1974

38. Mindich BP, Silverman MJ, Elguezabal A, Levowitz BS: Umbilical cord vein fistula for vascular access in hemodialysis. *Trans Am Soc Artif Intern Organs* 21: 273, 1975

39. Dardik H, Ibrahim IK, Dardik I: Arteriovenous fistulas constructed with modified human umbilical cord vein graft. *Arch Surg* 111: 60, 1976

40. Schanzer H, Martinelli GP, Bock G, Pierce EC: A self-sealing dialysis prosthesis. *Ann Surg* 204: 574, 1986

41. Jain KM, Patil KD, Grochowski EC, Argyres SN: The hemasite-incorporated graft. Operative technique and early results. *Am J Surg* 148: 637, 1984

42. Ehrenfeld WK: Surgical techniques for hemodialysis access. in *Peripheral Arterial Disease*, edited by Barker WF, 2nd edition, Philadelphia, WB Saunders Co, 1975, p 462

43. Rohr MS, Browder MD, Frentz GD, McDonald JC: Arteriovenous fistula for long-term dialysis. *Arch Surg* 113: 153, 1978

44. Tellis VA, Kohlberg WI, Bhat DJ, Driscoll B, Veith FJ: Expanded polytetrafluoroethylene graft fistula for chronic hemodialysis. *Ann Surg* 189: 101, 1979

45. Sabanayagam P, Schwartz AB, Soricelli RR, Chinitz JL, Lyons P: Experience with 100 reinforced expanded PTFE grafts for angioaccess in hemodialysis. *Trans Am Soc Artif Intern Organs* 26: 582, 1980

46. Etheredge EE, Haid SD, Maeser MN, Sicard GA, Anderson CB: Salvage operations for malfunctioning polytetrafluoroethylene hemodialysis access grafts. *Surgery* 94: 464, 1983

47. Sabanayagam P, Soricelli R, Schwartz A: Experience with 225 expanded PTFE arteriovenous fistulae for chronic maintenance hemodialysis. Presented at the Annual Meeting of the European Society for Artificial Organs, Geneva, Switzerland, Sept. 29–Oct. 1, 1979

48. Selman SH, Rhodes RS, Anderson JM, DePalma RG, Clowes AW: Atheromatous changes in expanded polytetrafluorethylene grafts. *Surgery* 87: 630, 1980

49. Zeit RM, Cope C: Failed hemodialysis shunts. One year of experience with aggressive treatment. *Radiology* 154: 353, 1985

50. Duncan H, Ferguson L, Faris I: Incidence of the radial steal syndrome in patients with Brescia fistula for hemodialysis: its clinical significance. *J Vasc Surg* 4: 144, 1986

51. Kinnaert P, Strugven J, Mathieu J, Vereerstraeten P, Toussaint C, Van Geertruyden J: Intermittent claudication of the hand after creation of an arteriovenous fistula in the forearm. *Am J Surg* 139, 838, 1980

52. Anderson CB, Codd JR, Graff RA, Groce MA, Harter HR, Newton WT: Cardiac failure and upper extremity arteriovenous dialysis fistulas. Case reports and a review of the literature. *Arch Intern Med* 36: 292, 1976

53. Nsouli KA, Lazarus JM, Schoenbaum SC, Gottlieb MN, Lowrie EG, Shocair M: Bacteremic infection in hemodialysis. *Arch Intern Med* 139: 1255, 1979

54. Bhat DJ, Tellis VA, Kohlberg WI, Driscoll B, Veith FJ: Management of sepsis involving expanded polytetrafluoroethylene grafts for hemodialysis access. *Surgery* 187: 445, 1980

55. Malone JM, Moore WS, Campagna G, Bean B: Bacteremic infectability of vascular grafts: the influence of pseudointimal integrity and duration of graft function. *Surgery* 78: 211, 1975

56. Roon AJ, Malone JM, Moore WS, Bean B, Campagna G: Bacteremic infectability: a function of vascular graft material and design. *J Surg Res* 22: 489, 1977

57. Gifford RM: Management of tunnel infections of dialysis polytetrafluoroethylene grafts. *J Vasc Surg* 2: 854, 1985

58. Dobkin JF, Miller MH, Steigbigel NA: Septicemia in patients on chronic hemodialysis. *Ann Intern Med* 88: 28, 1978

59. O'Brien TF: Infection in dialysis and transplant patients. in *Surgical Care of the Patient with Renal Failure*, edited by Tilney NL, Lazarus JM, Philadelphia, WB Saunders Co, 1982, p 67

60. Morgan AP, Knight DC, Tilney NL, Lazarus JM: Femoral triangle sepsis in dialysis patients. *Ann Aurg* 191: 460, 1980

61. Leonard A, Raij L, Shapiro FL: Bacterial endocarditis in regularly dialyzed patients. *Kidney Int* 4: 407, 1973

62. Morgan AP, Lazarus JM: Vascular access for dialysis. Am J Surg 129: 432, 1975

63. Crofford OB: DHEW Publication No (NIH) 76–1018, Washington, DC 1975, p 1

64. Najarian JS, Sutherland DER, Simmons RL, Howard RJ, Kjellstrand CM, Mauer SM, Kennedy W, Ramsay R, Barbosa J, Goetz FC: Kidney transplantation for the uremic diabetic patient. *Surg Gynecol Obstet* 144: 682, 1977

EXTRACORPOREAL THROMBOGENESIS: MECHANISMS AND PREVENTION

S. FAZAL MOHAMMAD

INTRODUCTION

Blood-contacting prosthetic devices are playing an increasing role in the practice of medicine, and trends indicate that their use will continue to grow. Not only are hemodialyzers, blood oxygenators, and catheters used routinely, but the number of vascular grafts, heart valves, ventricular assist devices, and even total artificial hearts implanted in patients, grew steadily in the past decade. Through the use of these devices we have learned that thrombogenesis remains a potential problem when blood contacts an artificial surface (1, 2).

A number of diverse reactions are initiated when blood contacts with an artificial surface (3–6). Immediately following the exposure of most artificial surfaces to blood, various plasma proteins begin to adsorb to those surfaces (7). The interaction of plasma proteins with artificial surfaces can initiate the activation of the intrinsic as well as extrinsic blood coagulation, the kinin, the complement, and the fibrinolytic systems (8). Ultimately, thrombin may be formed, and this enzyme may adsorb to artificial surfaces in an active state and thus augment localized activation of previously adsorbed plasma proteins. As various proteins are being adsorbed to an artificial surface and establishing an equilibrium state, blood cells begin to adhere to the protein layer. While erythrocytes seem to adhere poorly to such a surface, platelets and leukocytes, especially neutrophils, are attracted to the adsorbed protein layer, frequently in large numbers. Adhesion of platelets and leukocytes to the artificial surface may lead to activation of the extrinsic blood coagulation system through the exposure of tissue factor-like activity which is present on the plasma membranes of the adherent cells.

Exposure of blood to an artificial surface may lead only to protein adsorption followed by adhesion of a few blood cells, or the reactions may be more intense. The series of events outlined in Figure 1 may culminate in the formation of a white mural thrombus composed of fibrin, platelets, leukocytes, and passively trapped erythrocytes (Figure 2). Numerous diverse factors influence formation of mural thrombi.

The chemical and physical nature of the polymeric surface itself appears to play an important role (9) not only in protein adsorption, but also in the subsequent adhesion and activation of platelets and leukocytes. Rheologic factors also play an important role, both in adsorption and activation of plasma proteins, as well as adhesion and activation of cells. Carefully conducted studies have demonstrated that turbulence enhances thrombus formation, while laminar flow decreases the possibility of thrombosis (10). Stasis or vortical flow, even when confined to relatively small areas, can serve as powerful initiators of thrombosis. The active states of various blood components themselves appear to play poorly understood roles in thrombus formation.

Normally, the blood coagulation sequences are maintained in a fine state of balance by the interaction of activating mechanisms with numerous inactivating or neutralizing pathways (11, 12). Enhanced activation of coagulation factors through contact of blood with artificial surfaces and adherent cells, and the possible loss of inactivating factors, either due to their adsorption to these surfaces or by denaturation, can enhance the risk of thrombus formation. Similarly, alterations in the state of reactivity of platelets and leukocytes brought about by their contact with, or proximity to artificial surfaces or by shear-stress induced changes, may enable these cells to participate actively in thrombotic processes. Formation of a mural thrombus, whether it be simply a single layer of adherent cells or whether it be a true thrombus that contains blood cells and fibrin, can lead to the formation of emboli. These thromboemboli can obstruct

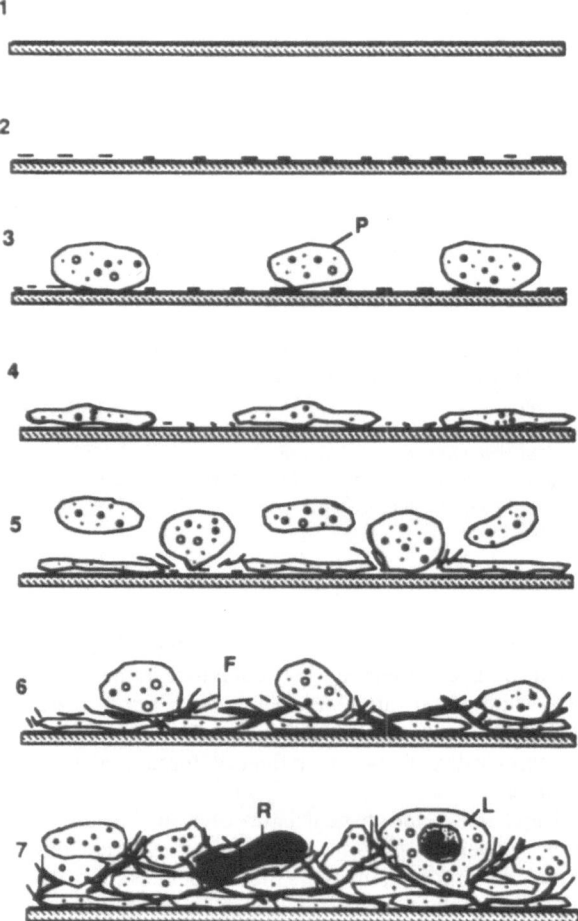

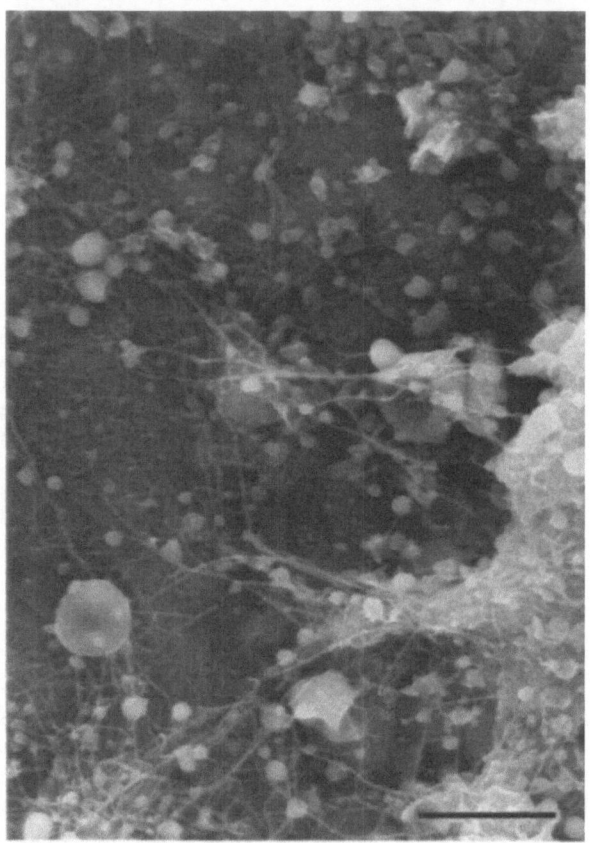

Figure 2. Scanning electron micrograph showing adherent platelets and fibrin (F) network with trapped erythrocytes (R) and leukocytes (L). This figure represents stage 7 in Figure 1.

Figure 1. Schematic illustration of sequence of reactions between blood and an artificial surface (1). Immediately upon contact with blood, plasma proteins interact with surface and certain proteins are adsorbed to the surface (2). Circulating platelets (P) are also attracted to the interface (3). These platelets adhere and undergo a series of changes that include spreading (see Figure 2) and release of ADP, thromboxane A2 and other highly reactive products from their granules (4, 5). Adsorbed plasma proteins and adherent platelets may activate coagulation (and complement) pathways resulting in the generation of thrombin and formation of fibrin (5, 6). Substances released from platelets and local generation of thrombin may escalate the above reactions thus depositing a large number of platelets enmeshed in the fibrin (F) network (6). Erythrocytes (R) and leukocytes (L) may also be trapped in the fibrin network resulting in the formation of thrombus (7) at the blood-material interface.

blood vessels distal to the point of their origin, and depending upon their size and location when lodged, can produce serious consequences. Certain pharmaceuticals, apart from the anticoagulants heparin and warfarin, can reduce the risk of thrombosis by inhibiting certain reactions in platelets and leukocytes.

Since activation of blood coagulation is a necessary component of artificial surface-induced thrombus formation, the use of anticoagulants is considered necessary during hemodialysis or during circulation of blood through other extracorporeal devices (13). Because of its immediate effect, heparin is the most commonly used anticoagulant today (14). Heparin has been used not only as a soluble anticoagulant, but also to coat artificial surfaces in efforts to improve their blood compatibility. A number of approaches have been used to incorporate heparin at the polymer interface. Efforts have been made to incorporate heparin in the polymer matrix in a manner that will obtain the slow but sustained release of the heparin (15). Alternately, heparin has been covalently bonded to the surface (16). This has been shown to diminish the formation of thrombi by processes that are poorly understood at this time. Although a potent anticoagulant, heparin has been shown to stimulate platelets (17), and in some studies with heparinized surfaces, greater adhesion of platelets has been noted (18). Therefore, to minimize adhesion and activation of platelets on heparinized surfaces, efforts have been made to incorporate an antiplatelet agent along with heparin. Surfaces coated with PGE_1-heparin have shown considerable promise, since they appear to have minimal adhesion or activation of proteins or platelets (19). The presence in blood of antiplatelet agents such as aspirin, dipyridamole, sulfinpyrazone, or prostaglandin I_2 also helps improve compatibility of blood with artificial surfaces (20).

INTERACTIONS OF BLOOD COMPONENTS WITH ARTIFICIAL SURFACES

The importance of the interactions of soluble and cellular elements of blood with artificial surfaces is obvious in the use of any extracorporeal or intracorporeal device that interfaces with blood. The following comments concerning the various mechanisms, whereby interaction of blood-soluble and cellular components with surfaces lead to thrombus formation, emphasize events that can take place during hemodialysis, or when blood contact other artificial organs and devices such as cannulas, catheters, vascular shunts, blood conduits, oxygenators, artificial heart valves, artificial blood vessels, ventricular assist devices, and total artificial hearts. In the discussions that follow, references to the literature, have been selective citing, wherever possible, pertinent review articles.

Adsorption of plasma proteins

The adsorption of plasma proteins to artificial surfaces has been studied extensively, and virtually every physical and chemical property of materials has been examined (21, 22). As pointed out earlier, carefully planned studies have documented that immediately after contact of blood with an artificial surface, plasma proteins begin to adsorb at the interface (7). Scarborough and coworkers (23) documented the adsorption of proteins by exposing a glass slide to native blood for only 5 sec and then examining thin sections of the slide by transmission electron microscopy. They observed a thin layer of plasma proteins at the interface, even after such a brief exposure to blood.

Soon after hemodialysis was introduced for treatment of patients with chronic renal failure, concern was voiced about denaturation of plasma proteins exposed to surfaces in various hemodialyzers and in other extracorporeal devices (24). These concerns still persist, and probable denaturation of plasma proteins has been shown to influence platelet function adversely (25).

Interest in the mechanism of activation of the intrinsic blood coagulation system has led to numerous studies of the interaction of certain blood coagulation factors with artificial surfaces. Activation of the intrinsic blood coagulation system by exposure of blood to artificial surfaces has been attributed to adsorption of certain of the procoagulants, and such work continues with exciting advances in our understanding of protein adsorption (26–32). Vroman and associates (33–36) devised numerous unique methods for studying the interactions of proteins with artificial surfaces, and used several ingenious techniques for visualizing these reactions. These investigators have shown that a number of plasma proteins including albumin, globulins, and fibrinogen interact with artificial surfaces in a highly complex manner. This has been confirmed by others who used similar techniques (37, 38). Oja and coworkers (39) used a different approach and studied the removal from plasma of specific blood coagulation factors following exposure of the plasma to artificial surfaces. Lyman and Brash (40–43) studied the interactions of plasma proteins with a large number of artificial surfaces, particularly hydrophobic polymers. The importance of flow effects in plasma protein adsorption to surfaces was emphasized by their work and that of others (44–46). These investigators and others (47, 48) have shown that in the early stages of blood-material interactions, adsorbed plasma proteins frequently exist in a state of equilibrium with nonadsorbed proteins. This equilibrium is influenced both by the specific surfaces tested and by the presence (and concentration) of different species of proteins in solution. It is now generally agreed that unless protein concentration is low, protein molecules are adsorbed to most artificial surfaces to form a monolayer, with relatively little distortion of the various species of molecules present. Adsorption of molecular species that take part in the activation of the intrinsic blood-coagulation system (26–31), as well as other protein species, may represent important exceptions to this statement.

Although activation of adsorbed proteins is a major concern, thrombin adsorption to artificial surfaces may be one of the most important single steps in development of thrombogenesis. Thrombin is adsorbed firmly to many artificial surfaces and in most cases it is adsorbed in an enzymatically active form. Waugh and coworkers (49, 50) were early leaders in studies of this type. Chuang and coworkers (51, 52) added new insights about thrombin interactions with artificial surfaces. The importance of thrombin adsorption, particularly as it may remain enzymatically active, suggests that this phenomenon should be given more attention and the role of adsorbed thrombin in the formation of mural thrombi studied more carefully. Artificial surfaces exposed to blood may become foci for adsorption and concentration of active thrombin molecules. Furthermore, platelets have been shown to bind thrombin (53, 54), and platelets adherent to an artificial surface could serve as points for concentration of thrombin in a localized area. It is evident that thrombin forms even in well-heparinized blood that is exposed extracorporeally to various artificial surfaces. These artificial surfaces may then act to adsorb out the activated thrombin molecules and concentrate them so that they can serve to enhance the activation of the blood-coagulation system at the interface.

Recently, *ex-vivo* studies of protein adsorption involving different types of flow chambers and various flow conditions have been reported (55–57). In some of this work, purified, radiolabelled plasma proteins have been used. Results from these studies generally support early investigations conducted with different techniques in that protein adsorption has been shown to occur rapidly. Of more interest are findings showing that protein species adsorbed initially may be replaced later by different protein species. These recent studies are of particular importance because they have been conducted with blood that is returned to living experimental animals, permitting the organism to react to surface-exposed blood in various ways. Equally exciting are reports of changes in supposedly 'immobile' polymer surface groups brought about by contact of the polymer in water, which rendered the surface less reactive with proteins. The latter studies extend the pioneering work done by Merrill and associates (5).

In summary, many workers have documented that various proteins from plasma interact in a complex manner with artificial surfaces (3–6, 23, 58–61) and these interactions are affected by the nature of the polymeric surface as well as the composition of the plasma proteins. The consequences of these interactions are numerous and diverse, but our understanding of these complex reactions is still in its infancy. In a more optimistic vein, it must be noted that several investigators have reported the formation of a passivating or blood-compatible protein layer on certain artificial surfaces exposed to blood for prolonged periods of time (62, 63). These studies deserve further attention (64).

Adhesion of platelets

During extracorporeal circulation of blood, the platelet count decreases significantly; carefully conducted studies have demonstrated that the low platelet count is generally due to hemodilution (65) and adherence to interfaces in the extracorporeal device (65, 67). Since plasma proteins adsorb at the interface immediately following the contact of blood with artificial surfaces, cell-surface interactions, particularly reactions of platelets at the interface, are believed to be mediated by these adsorbed proteins. Therefore, reactions of platelets with adsorbed plasma proteins have received attention from several investigators (68–72). In most test systems, albumin adsorbed to artificial surfaces has little effect on the subsequent adherence of platelets, but fibrinogen coating of a surface enhances platelet adherence. Interfaces coated with gamma globulin also show enhanced adhesion of platelets with concomitant increase in platelet-release reaction (73, 74). The effect of fibrinogen on platelet adhesion can be demonstrated at extremely low concentrations (68, 75, 76). However, in interpreting such experiments, it must be realized that in the absence of proteins, platelets often adhere avidly to bare (uncoated) artificial surfaces (77). In contrast to the effect of fibrinogen and gamma globulins, numerous investigators have shown that the exposure of artificial surfaces to albumin or mixed plasma proteins appreciably decreases the subsequent reaction of platelets with these surfaces (68, 73, 78–81). Purified albumin was found to be a useful coating on artificial surfaces when inhibition of platelet adhesion was desired. The effect of other plasma proteins, either alone or in combination, has been examined, but their role in platelet adhesion is not well understood (78, 79).

The mechanisms by which albumin or mixtures of plasma proteins affect platelet adhesion is also not clear. Recently, Mohammad and colleagues (77, 82, 83) have shown the presence of a naturally occurring complex of albumin and immunoglobulin G in blood. This albumin-IgG complex has been shown to inhibit markedly the adhesion of platelets to a number of artificial surfaces. Further studies are necessary to elucidate the mechanism by which albumin-IgG complex interacts with surfaces and whether such complexes play any role in circulating blood.

In addition to activation and adsorption of coagulation factors, extracorporeal circulation causes denaturation of plasma proteins (84, 85) and activation of complement proteins C3a and C5a. Decreased circulating concentrations of C1, C3, and C4 and an increase of C3a have been reported (86–88).

The surface energies of artificial surfaces that have acquired coatings of plasma proteins were found to be remarkably similar, regardless of the composition of the material (89–92). This may explain why so many different types of artificial surfaces react similarly when placed in contact with blood. However, there is general agreement that surface energy alone does not determine the degree of compatibility of a polymeric surface with blood. Other factors must influence this phenomenon. The role of the carbohydrate content of proteins in influencing platelet adhesion to artificial surfaces was studied by Lee and Kim (93). They found that platelet adhesion to adsorbed proteins paralleled the saccharide content of the proteins, which may explain why albumin, a protein that contains no carbohydrate, may not be as attractive to platelets as fibrinogen, fibronectin or gammaglobulin, each of which contain sugar moieties (94).

Treatment of heparinized surfaces with fibrinogen solutions, platelet-free plasma, or serum does not protect against subsequent platelet adhesion, whereas incubation of the heparinized surface with albumin reduces adhesion of platelets to that surface (59, 61, 95, 96). Hence, heparinization of a surface in itself does not prevent subsequent protein adsorption, but it may influence the types and amounts of proteins adsorbed, which may in turn affect the interaction of cells.

It is now generally recognized that the adsorbed plasma proteins (23, 58, 59, 97–101) and rheologic factors (102–107) play important roles in the generation of thrombi as well as embolization. Despite this, our knowledge of the composition of thrombus-generating surface coatings and of passive or protective coatings is remarkably scanty. This lack of knowledge is due largely to inadequate techniques for detecting and quantitating the various components of the adsorbed protein layers that form on surfaces of extracorporeal devices that contact blood. Not only must we come to understand the mechanisms whereby adsorbed protein layers attract platelets, but we must also develop interfaces that will discourage or prevent platelet and leukocyte adhesion. Existing polymers are being modified in a number of ways to make them more blood compatible, and new polymers are emerging that may be inherently more compatible with blood.

Recently, new insights have been gained concerning the increasingly complex ways in which platelet adhesion to protein-coated artificial surfaces can influence thrombus

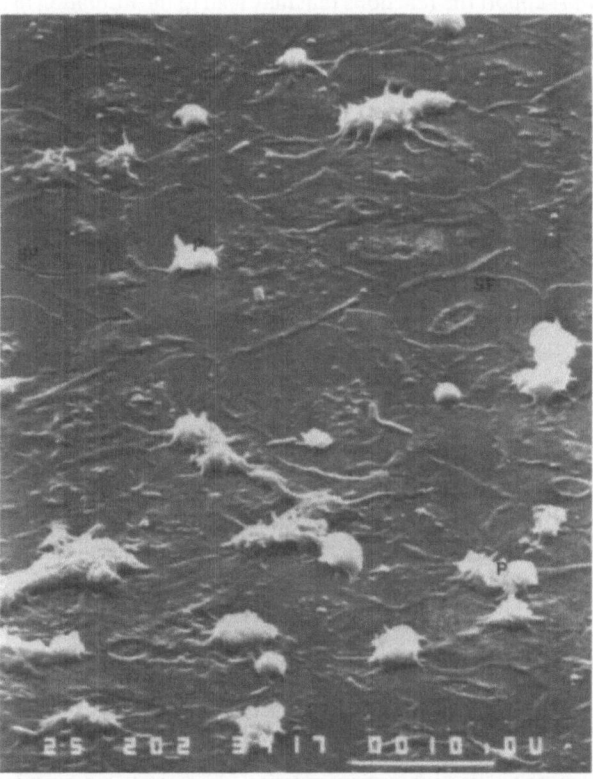

Figure 3. Scanning electron micrograph of a glass slide exposed to heparinized blood for 5 min. The slide was rinsed with 0.15 M NaCl and fixed with glutaraldehyde. Note the adherent platelets many of which have spread completely with their granules clustered generally in the center (SP). The adherent platelets have attracted other platelets (P). This micrograph represents stages 4 and 5 in Figure 1.

formation. In some cases but by no means all, adhesion stimulates platelets to undergo a complex series of reactions that enhance the platelet aggregation and activation of blood coagulation (108). Activated platelets change shape to produce pseudopods that appear to facilitate the spread of the cells on a surface (Figure 3). Shape change frequently is followed by the release reaction (109–111), generation and release of thromboxane A_2 (112), production of platelet-activating factor (113, 114), and platelet Factor 3 activity (115, 116); binding of fibrinogen (117–119), Factor Va (120, 121), and Factor Xa (122, 123) to specific 'receptors' on the outer surface of the platelet plasma membrane; and generation of Factor XIa on the plasma-membrane surface (124, 125). Release of serotonin, ADP, thromboxane A_2, and other platelet activating factors leads to aggregation of nearby nonadherent platelets (108). Release of platelet Factor 4 (PF4) from activated platelets can neutralize heparin (126, 127). Binding of fibrinogen to a platelet plasma membrane is considered an essential step for ADP-induced aggregation (128). Platelet Factor 3 activity serves as a procoagulant which may be related to the binding of activated Factors V and X on the platelet surface. Activation of Factor XI and

binding of Factors Va and Xa by platelets markedly enhances blood coagulation sequences in the neighborhood of adherent and aggregated platelets, with the ultimate formation of thrombin, an enzyme that also binds to platelets (129, 130), and converts fibrinogen to fibrin. Fibrin stabilizes platelet aggregates. Thus, appropriate stimuli, admittedly incompletely understood at present, arising from adsorbed plasma proteins, adherent cells, or artificial surfaces themselves, trigger a variety of changes at the interface that may promote adhesion and aggregation of platelets, and activate blood coagulation factors, thus enhancing the risk of thromboembolization (131–133). Along with the risk of thrombogenesis during extracorporeal circulation of blood, the risk of bleeding also increases in some patients. It has been shown that platelets circulating through extracorporeal devices become less responsive (133) to the soluble agonists mentioned above. During this circulation, besides releasing thromboxane A_2, PF4, and other substances, thrombospondin, a platelet-derived protein, appears in plasma. Plasma thrombospondin concentration is proportional to the duration of blood circulation through the extracorporeal device (133–135).

It is possible that the loss of platelet function, consumption of certain coagulation factors, or other plasma proteins and changes in the composition of blood collectively result in subnormal hemostatic processes, thus enhancing the risk of bleeding. In patients on hemodialysis, uremia is known to cause a qualitative defect in platelet function, which can also contribute to bleeding (136).

Adhesion of leukocytes

Adhesion of leukocytes to artificial surfaces has been less well studied than has the adhesion of platelets, although research in this area has accelerated recently. It was realized early that hemodialysis was associated with a precipitous but short-lasting fall in the peripheral leukocyte count (137, 138). This fall in leukocytes was followed by a gradual rise to normal or even supranormal levels (139). Various studies showed that the initial fall in leukocytes is due only in small part to adhesion of these cells to artificial surfaces that contact blood. The major part of the leukopenia that develops soon after hemodialysis is initiated relates to sequestration of leukocytes within the patient's vascular system (139). The role of activated complement components, particularly C5a, in dialysis-associated leukopenia has received considerable attention (140–143). Another active area of research involves the studies of alteration of leukocyte functions secondary to exposure of blood to artificial surfaces. The consequences of the adhesion of leukocytes to artificial surfaces are several, including potential immunologic consequences. Several investigators have suggested that adhesion of leukocytes to artificial surfaces is associated with the exposure of tissue factor activity in or on the leukocyte plasma membrane (144–146). Adherent leukocytes may also release certain factors, either stored in cytoplasmic granules or generated within these cells, that can influence blood coagulation (147–150) as well as platelet aggregation. In the latter case, it has been shown that stimulated leukocytes can release powerful platelet aggregation inducers, platelet activating factor (PAF) (151) and thromboxane A_2 (152, 153). Morphologic studies indicate that adherent leukocytes may attract platelets that subsequently adhere to them (154–159). These interactions of leukocytes and platelets deserve further investigation.

It is possible that adherent leukocytes serve as scavengers that remove adherent platelets and fibrin. This role has not yet been clarified fully, but numerous reports indicate that neutrophils and macrophages can phagocytose adherent platelets, fibrin, or denatured proteins. Despite the presence of numerous adherent platelets and leukocytes (158–162), the efficiency of reused dialysis membranes does not seem to be noticeably impaired (163, 164), although not all investigators agree with this observation (165). This raises the question of whether adhesion of leukocytes or platelets to hemodialysis membranes has any significance unless it leads to the formation of mural thrombi of emboli, or produces changes in blood that alter certain functions of circulating platelets or leukocytes.

Adhesion of erythrocytes

Although erythrocytes adhere to artificial surfaces *in vitro* (166), microscopic evaluation of hemodialysis membranes following clinical use indicates that relatively few erythrocytes adhere firmly to these surfaces (162, 165, 166). Adherent platelets and leukocytes far outnumber adherent erythrocytes unless a fibrin clot is present, which traps the red cells. Erythrocytes do adhere avidly to artificial surfaces in the absence of proteins, but when proteins are present, adhesion is markedly reduced. In a number of *in vitro* studies, erythrocytes have been shown to adhere to artificial surfaces by a small area of their plasma membrane (167). Such adherent erythrocytes can be deformed by shear stresses and the main part of the cell may be torn away from the adherent portion, leaving behind the adherent part of the cell membrane. Flow conditions play an important role in determining the extent of interaction between erythrocytes and the artificial surface, both in hemodialyzers as well as other blood-contacting prosthetic devices (168, 169). Rheologic factors associated with flow rate, turbulence, and stasis are also important in attracting erythrocytes and other blood cells to a dialysis membrane (170, 171).

The interaction of erythrocytes with artificial surfaces, including hemodialysis membranes, can enhance blood coagulation through several mechanisms. If erythrocytes are disrupted during or after their adhesion on an artificial surface, thromboplastic substances may appear on the surface of the cell or be released from the injured cells (60, 61). These thromboplastic substances can augment the activation of the blood coagulation system. Damaged or disrupted erythrocytes also release a number of substances, including ADP, that may activate the platelets and enhance the adhesion of circulating platelets to the interface or to those platelets already adherent to the hemodialysis membrane. Thus, adhesion and subsequent disruption of erythrocytes

will support the reactions that may lead to the formation of a mural thrombus.

INTERACTION OF BLOOD COMPONENTS WITH HEMODIALYSIS MEMBRANES IN CLINICAL APPLICATIONS

During hemodialysis, the blood that is exposed to dialysis membranes is heparinized. The degree to which plasma proteins adsorb to hemodialysis membranes and the degree to which platelets and leukocytes adhere to this adsorbed protein layer vary from patient to patient. This may depend on the effective level of heparin present in the blood of the patients. The dose of heparin required to achieve a certain degree of inhibition of blood coagulation also varies among patients for reasons 'that are not completely understood (172). Heparin carries a considerable negative charge, which permits it to interact with artificial surfaces, plasma proteins, and with platelets and leukocytes. The amount of heparin present appears to be highly important in determining the interaction of soluble and cellular components of the blood with hemodialysis membranes (95). As stated above, PF4 released from adherent platelets will neutralize the anticoagulant activities of heparin. Therefore, increased platelet adhesion may neutralize a significant amount of circulating heparin, necessitating larger doses of heparin to maintain effective anticoagulation. Certain basic proteins released from stimulated leukocytes also can neutralize heparin more or less in the same manner as PF4 does.

In certain hemodialysis patients, increased numbers of thromboembolic complications occur during hemodialysis compared to the experiences of other patients. These thromboembolic-prone individuals may require increased amounts of heparin to prevent thromboembolism for reasons that are not well understood. Hemodialysis patients have been shown to have circulating platelets that are altered in certain of their functional properties (131, 132). Perhaps altered rheologic states encountered within the hemodialyzers result in damage and activation of the platelets. Certain other aspects of the blood coagulation and fibrinolytic system also may be altered in these patients (136). The inclusion of certain antithrombotic or antiplatelet drugs in the patient's therapeutic regimen may decrease the propensity to thromboembolism. Finally, heparinization of surfaces in the ex-vivo blood circuit, including membrane surfaces, may decrease interactions of blood with these surfaces and permit dialysis to be performed with little or no anticoagulant added to the blood.

Recent evidence indicates that heparin may lower the circulating plasma concentration of prostaglandin I_2 (PGI_2) levels (173). PGI_2, a potent antiplatelet agent, inhibits platelet adhesion and aggregation, and prevents the release reaction. Thus, heparin, a two-edged sword, may enhance platelet-mediated reactions at the interface by activating the circulating as well as adherent platelets, while at the same time effectively inhibiting the blood coagulation pathway.

Undesirable reactions of blood with artificial surfaces

continue to be among the most challenging problems in the use of hemodialyzers. These blood-artificial surface interactions appear to be major obstacles to successful use of artificial organs that contact blood. The necessity of using heparin or other anticoagulants to overcome the thrombogenicity of artificial surfaces will be discussed in other chapters in this book. Further, the interactions between artificial surfaces and plasma proteins on one hand, and the cellular elements of blood on the other, have been discussed earlier in this chapter.

As stated above, a variety of factors appear to play important roles when blood contacts a foreign surface. Exposure of blood to an artificial surface may result in rapid contact activation of certain of the blood coagulation factors in addition to alterations (activation) of platelets and leukocytes. Moreover, rheologic conditions such as turbulence, pressure fluctuations, and shear stresses generated at the interface between the artificial surface and flowing blood, have significant impacts on thrombus formation. Further, the electrokinetic surface charge of an artificial surface may determine to some extent the degree of thrombus formation at the interface.

THE INFLUENCE OF BLOOD FLOW ON BLOOD-MATERIAL INTERACTION

Blood and plasma both exhibit non-Newtonian behavior, particularly under low rates of shear (174–177). It has been demonstrated that due to inward migration of cells in the laminar flow circulation mode, blood cells, particularly erythrocytes, tend to circulate away from the vessel or container wall. This leaves a cell-free marginal zone of plasma at the blood-vessel and wall interface (178, 179). Goldsmith (179) demonstrated that this cell-free marginal zone of plasma shrinks when circulating cell concentrations increase, as occurs at the surface of a dialysis membrane. Cellular interactions and collisions give rise to sideways or radial movements, and cells including platelets and leukocytes are occasionally pushed against the wall, thus creating flow conditions in which platelets interact with vessel or container wall (180). At higher rates of shear (15 dynes/cm^2), erythrocytes may undergo morphologic alterations. Further increases in shear rates result in leakage of potassium and hemoglobin, while even further increases ultimately can cause lysis of the cells (181–184). Leakage of various substances, particularly ADP from erythrocytes under high shear stresses, can induce the aggregation of platelets. The release of ADP from erythrocytes may be of considerable significance since lysis of even small number of cells may result in appreciable amounts of ADP. In addition to the impact of substances released from erythrocytes, it has been shown that circulating platelets are even more sensitive to high shear stress. Brown et al (102) observed that a shear stress of only 50 dynes/cm^2 liberates adenine neucleotides and serotonin from intact platelets, whereas a shear stress of 100 dynes/cm^2 lyses these cells in a rotational viscometer. These observations clearly suggest marked susceptibility of platelets to shear stress. Even slight damage to platelets can induce the release reaction, which in turn will induce further changes in nearby circulating platelets, leading to formation of mural thrombi or circulating platelet aggregates. The amount of mural thrombus formed and the size of circulating platelet or leukocyte aggregates are factors that can markedly influence flow conditions. Disturbed flow may not only increase the chances of interactions between a container wall and the cellular components of blood, it may also alter the pattern of adsorbed plasma proteins at the interface. Altered deposition of soluble components onto the surrounding container walls can greatly influence the attractiveness of the wall for cellular components, especially in areas of persistently distorted flow. Increased adsorptive deposition of various plasma proteins on container walls in an area of turbulent or vortical flow, and associated increase in adherence of platelets has been demonstrated experimentally (Copley (185, 186) suggested that in addition to fibrin deposition and aggregation of cellular elements of blood, a time-dependent progressive adsorption of certain other plasma proteins may also contribute to thrombogenesis. If this indeed is true, this latter process could be enhanced due to the newly generated electrokinetic status of a particular artificial surface. Such a surface may become thrombogenic after a certain period of time, even under laminar flow conditions. It is obvious, therefore, that thrombogenicity of artificial surfaces is a result of the interplay of a variety of factors. This complexity makes the task of elucidating the various mechanisms involved in thrombus formation exceedingly difficult. Most certainly, rheologic factors and the chemical and physical nature of the particular artificial surface in contact with flowing blood may ultimately be the determining factors in the blood-material interactions.

APPROACHES TO THE PREVENTION OF THROMBOSIS DURING HEMODIALYSIS

Practical approaches to the prevention of thrombosis during hemodialysis include the use of improved dialysis membranes, various modifications of surfaces of biomaterials, endothelialization of blood-contacting surfaces, and the use of soluble antithrombotic and antiplatelet agents. Membrane selection and the use of improved membranes may also help minimize the adverse blood-material interactions. Several new or improved membranes currently under clinical trial, and extensive research and development efforts to obtain new surfaces should, in the near future, provide surfaces that will be more compatible with blood than those presently available. Various modifications of existing blood-contacting surfaces may also help minimize or eliminate problems associated with adhesion of platelets and leukocytes, and activation of adsorbed coagulation factors (187).

Effects of soluble antithrombotic or antiplatelet agents

Two undesirable but commonly observed events that frequently follow the extracorporeal circulation of blood are deposition of fibrin, and adherence of platelets and leukocytes to the blood-contacting artificial surface. While anticoagulants such as heparin prevent the formation of fibrin, they generally have minimal inhibitory effect on platelet adherence at the concentrations commonly used clinically. Therefore, even with clinically adequate levels of circulating heparin, the ability of platelets to adhere to artificial surfaces and the possibility of formation of platelet aggregates due to altered flow conditions remain relatively unchanged or may even be enhanced (188). It may be important in this context to note a recent observation that suggests that heparin, even at low concentrations, can stimulate platelet aggregation, the platelet release reaction, and thromboxane A_2 production in the presence of subthreshold concentrations of a variety of aggregating agents (189, 190). This is of critical concern in light of suggestions summarized in the preceding paragraphs that note the possibility of shear-stress-induced release of ADP by erythrocytes or platelets (191). Since it may be difficult to avoid excessive shear stresses completely during extracorporeal circulation, release of small concentrations of substances such as ADP, serotonin, platelet activating factor, and thromboxane A_2 may not be totally avoidable. Such substances then could produce substantial platelet aggregation in the presence of heparin. Published reports suggest that in the presence of heparin, platelets release significantly more thromboxane A_2 when they are challenged by epinephrine, ADP or arachidonic acid (190).

One approach to overcoming injurious alterations of blood cells with subsequent enhancement of platelet aggregation has been the use of antiplatelet or antithrombotic drugs. Dipyridamole appears to be one of the agents of choice (192). Aspirin also has been shown to decrease the adhesion of platelets to hemodialysis membranes (193, 194), as has RA-233, an analog of dipyridamole (195). While these drugs minimize undesirable reactions in platelets, some contradictions have been reported. Mielke et al (196) found aspirin ineffective in extracorporeal circulation in oxygenators, while dipyridamole used under similar conditions markedly inhibited platelet stimulation. Gurewich and Lipinski (197) found Suloctodil, a vascular antispasmotic, to be the most effective antithrombotic agent in a predrug trial in animal models of thrombosis. In the same study, dipyridamole was shown to be more effective than aspirin. Dipyridamole also inhibits fibrin deposition in experimental animal models of thrombosis (198). This drug reduced effectively the thromboembolic complications associated with the use of prosthetic heart valves (199, 200). Sulfinpyrazone, another antiplatelet agent, also has been effective in inhibiting thrombus formation when given to patients with prosthetic heart valves (201). It has been suggested that prostaglandin E_1 (PGE_1) (202, 203) and PGI_2, a potent platelet aggregation inhibitor synthesized predominantly by endothelial cells *in vivo* (204), may be important in preventing platelet aggregation. The possibility of using PGI_2 alone or with heparin in extracorporeal circulation of blood has been investigated in several laboratories with promising results. Coppe et al (205) observed that PGI_2 prevented loss of platelets during extracorporeal circulation. Weston et al (206) and Bunting and associates (207) found that PGI_2 prevents thrombocytopenia, adhesion of platelets to dialyzer surfaces, and microembolization. They also observed that in the presence of PGI_2 it was possible to perform hemodialysis without adding anticoagulants. These reports point to the possibility of using PGI_2 or a suitable analog in extracorporeal circulation in the future. Hypotension, however, is a significant side-effect of PGI_2 administration because it is also a potent vasodilator.

It has been observed that when the use of any one antiplatelet agent fails to prevent thrombosis, a combination of two different agents often proves effective (208). Well-designed, extensive trials are in progress to test the effectiveness of a variety of antiplatelet agents in human subjects in which blood is exposed to artificial surfaces (192). Results of such trials will help establish the relative efficacies of antiplatelet drugs in preventing thromboembolism during hemodialysis. Although much attention has focused on the clinical use of oxygenators or artificial heart valves, thromboembolism associated with the use of any of the artificial devices that contact blood present a clinically significant challenge. Thus, an agent found to be effective in the prevention of mural thrombosis or a polymeric surface that shows promise in any one type of artificial organ may well prove useful in preventing thromboembolic complications in hemodialyzers or other blood-contacting prosthetic devices.

Although a number of antiplatelet agents are presently known, the effects of only a few of them have been studied carefully in patients undergoing hemodialysis. Several symposia proceedings and reviews have recently appeared, reporting the effectiveness of a number of antiplatelet drugs in prevention of thromboembolism (192, 209–212). In many cases, the effect of antiplatelet agents has been evaluated critically.

Modifications of surfaces of biomaterials that contact blood

Heparinization of surfaces

Gott and associates (213) explored the use of heparinized surfaces during the early 1960's to address the questions concerning thrombogenesis when artificial prosthetic valves were beginning to be used increasingly in open-heart surgery. In their original method, an ionic bonding took place of the negatively charged sulfate groups of the heparin molecule with a quaternary ammonium salt on a graphite polymer surface. This graphite-benzalkonium-heparin (GBH) surface showed remarkably good blood-compatibility compared to surfaces such as glass, polycarbonate, or silicone. Unfortunately, it was found later that this GBH procedure could not be applied to flexible materials such as cellophane or polyvinyl chloride. In addition, desorption of heparin from the surface was found to occur rapidly. Investigators at Battelle laboratories improved the GBH using chloromethylation of a polystyrene surface followed by quaternization with dimethylanaline (214). Heparin can be attached to such a treated surface by ionic bonding. Several polymer surfaces such as polyethylene, polyvinyl chloride, cellophane, and silicone rubber have been heparinized successfully by this technique. More recently, numerous other methods have been introduced for quaternization of polymer surfaces, with subsequent bonding of heparin by ionic forces. Yen and Rembaum (215) used a polyurethane-containing pendant amino group and quaternized this by treatment with hydrochloric acid. Merker et al (216) introduced as a heparin binder a quaternized 3-amino-propyl triethoxysilane on the silica filler present in commercially available silicone rubber. Heparin milled into a silicone rubber (Hepacone) during fabrication was used by Hufnagel et al (217), and Grode and associates (218) succeeded in quaternizing a number of different polymers by use of a bile-soluble quaternary ammonium salt, triduodecyl methyl ammonium chloride (TDMAC). The heating and cooling technique was used by Langeren and coworkers to induce penetration of a cationic surfactant into polymer surfaces (219). Heparin could then bind to the deeply deposited cationic sites. Chawla and Chung (220) used a radiation grafting method to achieve the binding of heparin to a cellulose membrane. An inorganic heparin complex system was used by Dycke (221) to prepare several nonthrombogenic polymer surfaces. Martin et al (222) have shown that quaternary ammonium salts of polymers containing tertiary amino groups such as acrylnonitrile-dimethylaminoethyl methacrylate (ANDMAEMA) could be formed by treatment of the polymer surface with acid at 50°C. Lindsay and associates (96) modified this procedure by further treatment of these membranes with ethylene oxide after heparin was bonded. A hydrophilic polymer surface which binds heparin ionically was developed by Idezuki et al (223). Cross-linking of TDMAC or cationic-bonded heparin with 1% gluteraldehyde has been used successfully to reduce the desorption of heparin. Heparin bonded to surfaces by ionic exchange reactions is unstable, however, and desorption and dissociation of heparin from polymer surfaces can occur under both *in-vivo* and *in-vitro* conditions (224). Attempts have been made to bond heparin covalently to polymer surfaces via carboxylic groups, amino groups, or hydroxyl groups of the heparin. Leininger and associates (225) modified their previous efforts by developing a one-step heparin-TDMAC complex for heparin binding. Halpern and Shibakawa (226) have shown that polystyrene can be converted into isocyanate-polystyrene, and that heparin can be coupled to this modified polystyrene by a formamide bond. A polymer with cross-linked heparin has also been prepared by Merrill et al (227). In addition, they were able to attach heparin molecules to cellulose membranes with ethylene amine (228). Schmer (229, 230) has shown that amino groups of heparin can be attached to either substituted or unsubstituted agarose by cyanogen bromide activation, as in peptide synthesis. Hoffman and coworkers (231) have shown that heparin and protein molecules can be bound covalently to radiation-grafted hydrogels using an approach similar to that of Schmer. Surfaces with covalently bonded heparin have shown great improvement over surfaces with ionically bonded heparin with respect to decreased *in-vitro* or *in-vivo* leaching of the bound heparin.

However, these surfaces still do not appear ideal since complete prevention of thrombus formation has not been achieved to date and published observations suggest that heparinized surfaces may preferentially attract circulating platelets (232).

Major problems in the early development of heparin-bonded surfaces for clinical usage were the slow leaching of heparin as well as leaching of toxic agents used in grafting and quaternizing polymer surfaces. The use of covalently bonded, heparinized surfaces has come close to solving the problem of desorption of heparin following exposure of heparinized surfaces to blood. However, in some cases these surfaces have been less effective in the prevention of thrombosis than were ionically heparinized surfaces. This is most probably due to the fact that harsher conditions are required to attach heparin to polymers covalently than in the case with ionic attachment. These harsh conditions likely caused physical damage to the surface. These changes included craze, roughness and opacification (233), but this was not totally unexpected. In addition, the heterogeneity of heparin preparations used for virtually all studies may have contributed to some of the adverse effects. For example, it was shown that several commercial preparations of heparin could contain as many as 21 different components, with molecular sizes ranging from 3,000 to 39,000. Only heparin of polymer size greater than 7,000 (66% of the total) has been shown to have desirable anticoagulant activities (234). Recently, multiple functional domains of the heparin molecule have been shown by Oosta et al (235). The conditions used to attach heparin to surfaces may cause denaturation and enhance the risk of fragmentation of heparin molecules before, during, or after bonding. Another obvious disadvantage in grafting heparin to dialyzer surfaces has been the resultant impairment of diffusion in these membranes. Further, radioautography of ^{35}S-heparin-coated surfaces has clearly shown that the surface concentration of heparin was nonhomogeneous for several polymers tested. This nonuniformity of heparin distribution at the interface may permit formation of small thrombi at specific loci deficient in bound heparin (236). Difficulties in sterilization of heparinized surfaces also have been encountered in clinical applications.

Therefore, in order to develop a heparin bonded surface that is highly thromboresistant, it is essential to understand the mechanisms by which such surfaces interact with blood. Unfortunately, these mechanisms have not been elucidated clearly to date. An attractive hypothesis states that a micro-atmosphere of heparin is created at the polymer surface (233). According to this hypothesis, the heparinized surface is simply serving as a heparin reservoir during contact with blood. However, recent progress in covalently bonding of heparin seems to refute this hypothesis, since these new surfaces have been shown to be thromboresistant under conditions in which there is little or no evidence for desorption of heparin. Recent findings suggest that plasma proteins adsorbed to heparinized surfaces may play important roles in the interaction of these surfaces with other soluble plasma components and with blood cells. Heparinized surfaces are known not to activate Factor XII (227).

The patterns of radioactively labeled plasma proteins adsorbed to heparin-bonded surfaces and to nonheparinized parent polymer surfaces are surprisingly similar (237). Preincubation of heparinized surfaces with albumin solutions resulted in some inhibition of platelet adhesion (237, 238), an effect found also with the same surfaces that had not been coated with heparin. Recently, heparin cofactors have been eluted from heparinized surfaces, and one of these has been identified as antithrombin III, an agent known to inhibit thrombin mediated effects (239, 240). However, it is highly likely that as yet unidentified proteins adsorb on heparin-bonded surfaces in minute quantities. These unidentified proteins may be responsible for the antithrombogenicity of heparinized surfaces. Highly sensitive techniques such as radioimmunoassays have been used to identify (241, 242) and quantitate plasma proteins adsorbed on artificial surfaces. These techniques may be applied also to identify and quantitate plasma proteins adsorbed to heparinized surfaces.

Other modifications of surfaces

Incorporation of prostaglandin derivatives known to inhibit platelet functions at the interface may be another approach to enhance the blood compatibility of artificial surfaces. PGI_2 has been shown to be effective in reducing thrombogenesis (243), especially when it is used in combination with heparin (244). However, the short half-life of PGI_2 in aqueous solutions (about 3.5 min) and the difficulty of conjugating PGI_2 to surfaces without reducing its potency makes the use of surface-bound PGI_2 as a nonthrombogenic surface unattractive. Heparin may decrease the effect of PGI_2 on platelets. Grode et al (245) have shown that artificial surfaces with covalently bound PGE_1 inhibit platelet adherence. A controlled release of PGE_1 from polymer matrices has been designed and tested by McRea and Kim (246). The PGE_1 was incorporated into Biomer and polyvinyl-chloride during casting and was released at a slow rate from the polymer into the soluble phase. This system will not only protect the potency of PGE_1 but will permit the antithrombogenic effect to last for an extended time. Such a system also may be applicable to labile agents such as PGI_2. On the other hand, pharmacologists have searched vigorously in the past few years for analogues of PGI_2 that possess greater stability and are of equal or better potency. Several analogues have become available as a result of these efforts (247–250). However, the biological activities of those analogues, when used *in-vivo,* or *ex-vivo* in humans, and particularly during extracorporeal circulation have not been fully examined.

Surface passivation with adsorbed plasma proteins

Passivation of dialysis membranes, or other biomaterials with whole blood or blood components, has attracted some attention in the past since no artificial surfaces have been found to be totally unattractive to plasma proteins. Surfaces precoated with albumin (43, 251), gelatin (252), or whole blood (253) have been used with varying degrees of success.

The use of platelet adhesion inhibitors (86, 116) and lipoprotein (87) as a precoating to discourage platelet interactions with artificial surfaces may also be feasible. The major task of passivation is the immobilization of the precoated substances at the interface. Although formalin or glutaraldehyde seem to be highly effective in stabilizing precoated surfaces (252, 253), the leaching of these chemicals into blood is undesirable. Furthermore, the passivated surfaces may not have a long, effective life span since new proteins or blood cellular components may be adsorbed to these stabilized coatings.

Reuse of a hemodialyzer by the same patient has been shown to produce a lesser degree of thrombosis than use of a new device. The efficacy of dialysis with reusable dialyzers surprisingly was found not to be diminished appreciably. Furthermore, with dialyzer reuse, the cost reductions can be substantial. However, because of the temporal limitations of dialyzer reuse with the same patient, the high risk of contamination with bacteria during flushing and storage, and the threat that toxic or immunologically active substances may leach from the sterilized dialyzer, this practice is not recommended by the manufacturers.

Endothelialization of materials

A radically different approach to increase the blood compatibility of materials is to cover the material's surface with a viable layer of endothelial cells (254). However, this approach remains academic because of the enormous problems concerning the growing of endothelial cells on the artificial surfaces. Furthermore, in clinical applications the endothelial cells must be obtained initially from the same patient who will use the cell-coated device. Whether an endothelial monolayer present on the hemodialysis membrane will adversely affect the efficiency of dialysis is also unknown at present. Other cell types, such as fetal fibroblasts, have been used with some success in work with nonhuman mammals. The major advantage of using endothelialized interfaces may be that this will present a dynamic interface to the circulating blood. Besides presenting a blood compatible surface, endothelial cells are capable of releasing PGI_2 and plasminogen activator in the presence of appropriate chemical stimuli. Endothelial cells may also bind heparin from circulating blood. All of these properties of endothelial cells may be useful in presenting to the blood an ultimate and compatible interface.

REFERENCES

1. Copley AL, Seaman GVF (editors): *Surface Phenomena in Hemorheology: Their Theoretical, Experimental and Clinical Aspects.* New York, N Y Acad Sci, 1983
2. Salzman EW: Interaction of blood with artificial surfaces. in *Hemostasis and Thrombosis,* edited by Colman RW, Hirsh J, Marder VJ, Salzman EW, New York, Lippincott, 1987, p 1335
3. Forbes CD, Prentice CRM: Thrombus formation and artificial surfaces. *Br Med Bull* 34: 201, 1978
4. Lindsay RM, Mason RG, Kim SW, Andrade JD, Hakim RM:

Blood surface interactions – report of ASAIO panel conference. *Trans Am Soc Artif Intern Organs* 26: 603, 1980

5. Merrill EW: Properties of material affecting the behavior of blood at their surface. *Ann NY Acad Sci* 283: 6, 1977

6. Andrade JD, Coleman DL, VanWagoner R: Perspectives and future developments in the field of blood-materials interactions. in: *Interactions of the Blood with Natural and Artificial Surfaces,* edited by Salzman E, New York, Marcel Dekker, 1981, p 201

7. Andrade JD, Nagaoka S, Cooper S, Okano T, Kim SW: Surfaces and blood compatibility: current hypotheses. *asaio J* 10: 75, 1987

8. Mason RG, Chuang HYK, Mohammad SF, Saba HI: Thrombosis and artificial surfaces. in *The Thromboembolic Disorders,* edited by Van der Loo J, Prentice CRM, Beller FK, New York, Schattauer Verlag, 1983, p 533

9. Salzman EW, Merrill EW: Interaction of blood with artificial surfaces. in *Hemostasis and Thrombosis,* edited by Colman RW, Hirsh J, Marder VJ, Salzman EW, New York, Lippincott, 1982, p 931

10. Baier RE: Key events in blood interactions. *Artif Organs* 2: 422, 1978

11. Jackson CM, Nemerson Y: Blood Coagulation. *Annu Rev Biochem* 49: 765, 1980

12. Nemerson Y, Furie B: Zymogens and cofactors of blood coagulation. *CRC Crit Rev Biochem* 9: 45, 1980

13. Edmunds LH, Addonizio VP: Extracorporeal circulation. in *Hemostasis and Thrombosis,* edited by Colman RW, Hirsh J, Marder VJ, Salzman EW, New York, Lippincott, 1987, p 901

14. Jaques LB: 40 years of heparin research – past and future. in *Heparin: Structure, Cellular Function and Clinical Applications,* edited by McDuffie NM, New York, Academic Press, 1979, p 373

15. Kim SW, Ebert CD, Lin JY, McRea JC: Non-thrombogenic polymers: pharmaceutical approach. *asaio J* 6: 76, 1983

16. Heyman P, Cho C, McRea J, Kim SW: Heparinized polyurethanes: in-vitro and in-vivo studies. *J Biomed Mat Res* 19: 419, 1985

17. Mohammad SF, Anderson WH, Smith JB, Chuang HYK, Mason RG: Effects of heparin on platelet aggregation and release and thromboxane A₂ production. *Am J Pathol* 104: 132, 1981

18. Salzman EW, Merrill EW, Binder A: Protein-platelet interaction on heparinized surfaces. *J Biomed Mater Res* 3: 69, 1969

19. Jacobs H, Okano T, Kim SW: Heparin-PGE₁ conjugate releasing polymers. *J Controlled Release* 2: 313, 1985

20. Joint Committee for Stroke Resources: Cerebral ischemia: the role of thrombosis and of antithrombotic therapy. *Stroke* 8: 150, 1977

21. Anderson JM, Koftke-Merchant K: Platelet interactions with biomaterials. *CRC Critical Reviews in Biocomposition* 1: 111, 1985

22. Sawyer PN: Surface charge and thrombosis. *Ann N Y Acad Sci* 416: 561, 1984

23. Scarborough DE, Mason RG, Dalldorf FG: Morphologic manifestations of blood-solid interfacial reactions. *Lab Invest* 20: 164, 1969

24. Lee WH Jr, Krumhaar D, Fonkalsrud EW, Scheide OA, Maloney JV Jr: Denaturation of plasma proteins as a cause of morbidity and death after intracardiac operations. *Surgery* 56: 29, 1961

25. Wallace HW, Liquoir EM, Stein TP, Brooks H: Denaturated plasma and platelet function. *Trans Am Soc Artif Intern Organs* 21: 450, 1975

26. Nossel HL: Activation of factors XII and XI in thrombogenesis. *Bull NY Acad Med* 48: 281, 1972

27. Cochrane CG, Revak SD, Wuepper KD: Activation of Hageman factor in solid and fluid phases. *J Exp Med* 138: 1564, 1973

28. Schiffman S, Lee P: Partial purification and characterization of contact activation cofactor. *J Clin Invest* 56: 1082, 1975

29. Griffin JH, Cochrane CG: Mechanisms for the involvement of high molecular weight kininogen in surface-dependent reactions of Hageman factor. *Proc Natl Acad Sci USA* 73: 2554, 1976

30. Cochrane CG, Wiggins RC, Revak SD: Activation of the contact system on a surface. in *Hemostasis, Prostaglandins, and Renal Disease,* edited by Remuzzi G, Mecca G, de Gaetano G, New York, Raven Press, 1980, p 125

31. Silverberg M, Dunn JT, Garen L, Kaplan AP: Autoactivation of human Hageman factor. *J Biol Chem* 255: 7281, 1980

32. Mannhalter C, Schiffman S: Surface adsorption of factor XI. Association of adsorption sites with the heavy chain of activated factor XI. *Thromb Haemost* 43: 124, 1980

33. Vroman L, Adams AL: Possible involvement of fibrogen and proteolysisin surface activation. *Thromb Diath Haemorrh* 18: 510, 1967

34. Vroman L, Adams AL, Klings M: Interactions among human blood proteins at interfaces. *Fed Proc* 30: 1494, 1971

35. Vroman L: What factors determine thrombogenicity? *Bull NY Acad Med* 48: 302, 1972

36. Vroman L, Adams AL, Fischer GC, Munoz PC: Interaction of high molecular weight kininogen, factor XII, and fibrinogen in plasma at interfaces. *Fed Proc* 30: 1494, 1971

37. Morrissey BW, Stromberg RR: The conformation of adsorbed blood proteins by infrared bound fraction measurements. *J Colloid Interface Sci* 56: 557, 1976

38. Morrissey BW, Stromberg RR: The conformation of adsorbed blood proteins by infrared bound fraction measurements. *J Colloid Interface Sci* 46: 152, 1976

39. Oja PD, Holmes GW: Specific coagulation factor adsorption as related to functional groups on surfaces. *J Biomed Mater Res* 3: 165, 1969

40. Lyman DJ, Brash JL, Chikin SW, Klein KG, Carini M: The effect of chemical structure and surface properties of synthetic polymers on the coagulation of blood. II. Protein and platelet interaction on polymer surfaces. *Trans Am Soc Artif Intern Organs* 14: 250, 1968

41. Brash H, Lyman DJ: Adsorption of plasma proteins in solution to uncharged, hydrophobic polymer surfaces. *J Biomed Mater Res* 3: 175, 1969

42. Lyman DJ, Klein KG, Brash JL, Fritzinger BK: The interaction of platelets with polymer surfaces. I. Uncharged hydrophobic polymer surfaces. *Thromb Diath Haemorrh* 23: 120, 1970

43. Brash JL, Lyman DJ: Adsorption of proteins and lipids to nonbiological surfaces. in *The Chemistry of Biosurfaces,* edited by Hair ML, New York, Marcel Dekker, 1971, vol 1, p 177

44. Friedman LI, Liem H, Grabowski EF, Leonard EF, McCord CW: Inconsequentiality of surface properties for initial platelet adhesion. *Trans Am Soc Artif Intern Organs* 16: 63, 1970

45. Turitto VT, Leonard EF: Platelet adhesion to a spinning surface. *Trans Am Soc Artif Organs* 18: 348, 1972

46. Eberhart RC, Lynch ME, Bilge FH, Arts HA: Effects of fluid shear and temperature on protein adsorption on Teflon surfaces. *Trans Am Soc Artif Intern Organs* 26: 185, 1980

47. Lee RG, Kim SW: Adsorption of proteins onto hydrophobic polymer surfaces: Adsorption isotherms and kinetics. *J Biomed Mater Res* 8: 251, 1974

48. Lee RG, Adamson C, Kim SW, Lyman DJ: Determination of the surface energy of proteinated polymer surfaces. *Thromb Res* 3: 87, 1973

49. Waugh DF, Baughman DJ: Thrombin adsorption and possible relations to thrombus formation. *J Biomed Mater Res* 3: 145, 1969

50. Waugh DF, Lippe JA, Freund Y: Interaction of bovine thrombin and plasma albumin with low-energy surfaces. *J Biomed Mat Res* 12: 599, 1978

51. Chuang HYK, Sharma NC, Mohammad SF, Mason RG: Adsorption of thrombin onto artificial surfaces and its detection by an immunoradiometric assay. *Artif Organs* 3 (Suppl): 226, 1979

52. Chuang HYK, Mohammad SF, Sharma NC, Mason RG: Interaction of human a-thrombin with artificial surfaces and reactivity of adsorbed a-thrombin. *J Biomed Mater Res* 14: 467, 1980

53. Shuman MA, Tollefsen DM, Majerus PW: The binding of human and bovine thrombin to human platelets. *Blood* 47: 43, 1976

54. Mohammad SF, Whitworth C, Chuang HYK, Lundblad RL, Mason RG: Multiple active forms of thrombin-binding to platelets and effects on platelet function. *Proc Natl Acad Sci USA* 73: 1660, 1976

55. Didisheim P, Stropp JQ, Borowick JH, Grabowski AF: Species differences in platelet adhesion to biomaterials: investigation by a new two-stage technique. *asaio J* 2: 124, 1979

56. Schultz JS, Lindenauer SM, Penner JA, Barenberg S: Determinants of thrombus formation on surfaces. *Trans Am Soc Artif Intern Organs* 26: 279, 1980

57. Hanson SR, Harker LA, Ratner BD, Hoffman AS: In vivo evaluation of artificial surfaces with a nonhuman primate model of arterial thrombogenesis. *J Lab Clin Med* 95: 289, 1980

58. Salzman EW: Role of platelets in blood-surface interactions. *Fed Proc* 30: 1503, 1971

59. Salzman EW: Nonthrombeogenic surfaces: critical review. *Blood* 38: 509, 1971

60. Scarborough DE: The pathogenesis of thrombosis in artificial organs and vessels. *Curr Top Pathol* 54: 95, 1971

61. Salzman EW: Surface effects in hemostasis and thrombosis. in *The Chemistry of Biosurfaces*, edited by Hair ML, New York, Marcel Dekker, 1972, vol 2, p 489

62. Mohammad SF, Olsen DB: Reduced platelet adhesion and activation of coagulation factors on polyurethane treated with albumin-IgG complex. *Trans Am Soc Artif Intern Organs* 32: 323, 1986

63. Grevelink J, Wu F, Kolff WJ, Mohammad SF: Study of platelet function in a calf with artificial ventricles attached to an ex-vivo shunt. *Trans Am Soc Artif Intern Organs* 32: 177, 1986

64. Baier RE, DePalma VA, Furuse A, Gott VL, Lucas TY, Sawyer PN, Srinivasan S, Stanczweski B: Thrombo-resistance of glass cleaned by glow discharge treatment in argon. *Abstracts Am Soc Artif Intern Organs* 2: 3, 1973

65. Edmunds LH, Ellison N, Colman RW: Niewiarowski S, Rao AK, Addonizio VP, Stephenson LW, Edie RN: Platelet function during open heart surgery: Comparison to the membrane and bubble oxygenators. *J Thor Cardiovasc Surg* 83: 805, 1982

66. Salzman EW: Measurement of platelet adhesiveness. *J Lab Clin Med* 62: 724, 1963

67. Hope AF, Heyns A du P, Lotter MG, van Reenan OR, de Kock F, Badenhorst PN, Pieters H, Kotze H, Meyer JM, Minaar PC: Kinetics and sites of sequestration of indium[111]-labeled human platelets during cardiopulmonary bypass. *J Thor Cardiovasc Surg* 81: 880, 1981

68. Packham MA, Evans G, Glynn MF, Mustard JF: Effects of plasma proteins on interaction of platelets with glass surfaces. *J Lab Clin Med* 73: 686, 1969

69. Brash JL: Hydrophobic polymer surfaces and their interactions with blood. *Ann N Y Acad Sci* 283: 356, 1977

70. Andrade JD, Hlady V: Protein adsorption and material biocompatibility. *Adv Polymer Sci* 79: 1, 1986

71. Andrade JD, Coleman JD, Didisheim P, Hanson SR, Mason RG, Merrill E: Blood-materials interactions: 20 years of frustration. *Trans Am Soc Artif Intern Organs* 27: 659, 1981

72. Colman RW: Surface-mediated defense reactions: the plasma contact activation system. *J Clin Invest* 73: 1249, 1984

73. Lyman DJ, Klein KG, Brash JJ, Fritzinger BK, Andrade JD, Bonomo FS: Platelet interaction with protein-coated surfaces: an approach to thrombo-resistant surfaces. in *Platelet Adhesion and Aggregation in Thrombosis: Countermeasures*, edited by Mammem EF, Anderson GF, Barnhard MI, Stuttgart FRG, FX Schattauer Verlag, 1970, p 109

74. Evans G, Mustard JF: Platelet-surface reaction and thrombosis. *Surgery* 64: 273, 1968

75. Zucker MB, Vroman L: Platelet adhesion induced by fibrinogen adsorbed onto glass. *Proc Soc Exp Biol Med* 131: 318, 1969

76. Mason RG, Shermer RW, Zucker WH: Effects of certain purified plasma proteins on the compatibility of glass with blood. *Am J Pathol* 73: 183, 1973

77. Sharma N, Mohammad SF, Chuang HYK, Mason RG: Inhibition of platelet adhesion to glass by certain human plasma and serum proteins. *asaio J* 3: 43, 1980

78. George JN: Direct assesment of platelet adhesion to glass: a study of the forces of interactions and the effects of plasma and serum factors, platelet function, and modification of the glass surface. *Blood* 40: 862, 1972

79. Mohammad SF, Hardison MD, Glenn CH, Morton BD, Bolan JC, Mason RG: Adhesion of human blood platelets to glass and polymer surfaces. I. Studies with platelets in plasma. *Haemostasis* 3: 257, 1974

80. Andrade JD, Kunitomo K, Van Wagenen R, Kastigir B, Gough D, Kolff WJ: Coated adsorbents for direct blood perfusion: hema/activated carbon. *Trans Am Soc Artif Intern Organs* 17: 222, 1971

81. Andrade JD: Interfacial phenomena and biomaterials. *Med Instrum* 7: 110, 1973

82. Mohammad SF, Hardison MD, Chuang HYK, Mason RG: Adhesion of human blood platelets to glass and polymer surfaces. II. Demonstration of the presence of natural platelet adhesion inhibitor in plasma and serum. *Haemostasis* 5: 96, 1976

83. Sharma NC, Mohammad SF, Chuang HYK, Mason RG: Isolation and some of the physiochemical and immunologic properties of a platelet adhesion inhibitor from human serum. *Thromb Res* 17: 683, 1980

84. Lee WH, Krumhaar D, Fonkalsrud E: Denaturation of plasma proteins as other cause of morbidity and death after intracardiac operations. *Surgery* 50: 29, 1961

85. Zapol WM, Levy RI, Kolobow T: In-vitro denaturation of plasma alpha lipoproteins in the dog. *Curr Topic Surg Res* 1: 449, 1969

86. Clark RE, Beauchamp RA, Magrath RA, Brooks JD, Ferguson TB, Weldon CS: Comparison of bubble and membrane oxygenators in short and long perfusions. *J Thor Cardiovasc Surg* 78: 655, 1979

87. Chenoweth DE, Cooper SW, Hugli TE, Stewart RW, Blackstone EH, Kirklin JW: Complement activation during cardiopulmonary bypass. *N Engl J Med* 304: 497, 1981

88. Boralessa H, Shifferli JA, Zaimi F, Watts E, Whitwam JG, Rees AJ: Perioperative changes in complement associated with cardiopulmonary bypass. *Br J Anaesth* 54: 1047, 1982

89. Leininger RI, Mirkovitch V, Beck RE, Andrus PG, Kolff WJ: The zeta potentials of some selected solids in respect to plasma and plasma fractions. *Trans Am Soc Artif Intern Organs* 10: 239, 1964

90. Baier RE, Gott VL, Feruse A: Surface chemical evaluation of thromboresistant materials before and after venous implantation. *Trans Am Soc Artif Intern Organs* 16: 50, 1970

91. Lee RG, Adamson C, Kim SW: Competetive adsorption of plasma proteins onto polymer surfaces. *Thromb Res* 4: 485, 1974

92. Kaelble DH, Moacanin J: A surface energy analysis of bioadhesion. *Polymer* 18: 475, 1977

93. Lee RG, Kim SW: The role of carbohydrate in platelet adhesion to foreign surfaces. *J Biomed Mater Res* 8: 393, 1974

94. Barber TA, Lambrecht LK, Mosher DL, Cooper SL: Influence of serum proteins on thrombosis and leukocyte adherence on polymer surfaces. *Scan Electron Microsc* 3: 881, 1979

95. Salzman EW, Merrill EW, Binder A, Wolf CFW, Ashford TP, Austen WG: Protein-platelet interaction on heparinized surfaces. *J Biomed Mater Res* 3: 69, 1969

96. Lindsay RM, Rourke J, Reid B, Friesen M, Linton AL, Courtney J, Gilchrist T: Platelets, foreign surfaces, and heparin. *Trans Am Soc Artif Intern Organs* 22: 292, 1976

97. Mason RG: The interaction of blood hemostatic elements with artificial surfaces. *Prog Hemost Thromb* 1: 141, 1972

98. Berger S, Salzman EW, Merrill EW, Wong PSL: The reaction of platelets with prosthetic surfaces. in *Platelets: Production, Function, Transfusion and Storage,* edited by Baldini MG, Ebbe S, New York, Grune and Stratton, 1974, p 299

99. Berger S, Salzman EW: Thromboembolic complications of prosthetic devices. *Prog Hemost Thromb* 2: 273, 1974

100. Mason RG, Mohammad SF, Chuang HYK, Richardson PD: The adhesion of platelets to subendothelium, collagen and artificial surfaces. *Semin Thromb Hemostas* 3: 98, 1976

101. Wethersby PK, Horbett TA, Hoffman AS: A new method for analysis of the adsorbed plasma protein layer on biomaterial surfaces. *Trans Am Soc Artif Intern Organs* 22: 242, 1976

102. Brown CH III, Lemuth RF, Hellums JD, Leverett LB, Alfrey CP: Response of human platelets to shear stress. *Trans Am Soc Artif Intern Organs* 21: 35, 1975

103. Brown CH III, Leverett LB, Lewis SW, Alfrey CP Jr, Hellums JD: Morphological, biochemical and functional changes in human platelets subjected to shear stress. *J Lab Clin Med* 86: 462, 1975

104. Johnston CG, Marzec U, Bernstein EF: Effects of surface injury and shear stress on platelet aggregation and serotonin release. *Trans Am Soc Artif Intern Organs* 21: 413, 1975

105. Roohk HV, Pick J, Hill R, Hung E, Bartlett RH: Kinetics of fibrinogen and platelet adherence to biomaterials. *Trans Am Soc Artif Intern Organs* 22: 1, 1976

106. Hung TC, Hochmuth RM, Joist JH, Sutera SP: Shear-induced aggregation and lysis of platelets. *Trans Am Soc Artif Intern Organs* 22: 285, 1976

107. Butruille YA, Leonard EF, Litwak RS: Platelet-platelet interactions and non-adhesive encounters on biomaterials. *Trans Am Soc Artif Intern Organs* 21: 609, 1975

108. Guidelines for blood-material interactions: Report of the National Heart, Lung and Blood Institute Working Group, *NIH Publication* No 85–2185, 1985, p 19

109. Whicher JS, Uniyal S, Brash JL: Platelet-foreign surface surface interactions: the release reaction from singly adherent platelets and adherent platelet aggregates. *Trans Am Soc Artif Intern Organs* 26: 268, 1980

110. Clagett GP, Russo M, Hufnagle H, Collins CJ Jr, Rich NM: Platelet serotonin changes in dogs with prosthetic aortic grafts. *J Surg Res* 28: 223, 1980

111. Malmgren R, Larson R, Olson P, Radegran K: Serotonin uptake and release by platelets adhering to polyethylene. *Haemostasis* 8: 400, 1979

112. Burch JW, Majerus PW: The role of prostaglandins in platelet function. Semin Hematol 16: 196, 1979

113. Chignard M, LeCouedic JP, Tence M, Vargaftig BB, Benveniste J: The role of platelet-activating factor in platelet aggregation. *Nature* 279: 799, 1979

114. Chap H, Mauco G, Simon MF, Benveniste J, Douste-Blazy L: Biosynthetic labelling of platelet activating factor from radioactive acetate by stimulated platelets. *Nature* 289: 312, 1981

115. Sharma NC, Mohammad SF, Chuang HYK, Mason RG: Isolation and physiochemical and immunologic characterization of human platelet factor 3. *Thromb Res* 16: 673, 1979

116. Sharma NC, Mohammad SF, Chuang HYK, Mason RG: Characterization of a platelet adhesion inhibitor from human serum and plasma as a complex of albumin with immunoglobulin G. *Fed Proc* 40: 810, 1981

117. Mustard JF, Packham MA, Kinlough-Rathbone RL, Perry DW, Regoezzi E: Fibrinogen and ADP-induced platelet aggregation. *Blood* 52: 453, 1978

118. Marguerie GA, Plow EF, Edgington TS: Human platelets possess an inducible and saturable receptor specific for fibrinogen. *J Biol Chem* 254: 5357, 1979

119. Tomikawa M, Iwamoto M, Soderman S, Blomback R: Effect of fibrinogen on ADP-induced platelet aggregation. *Thromb Res* 19: 841, 1980

120. Osterud B, Rapaport SI, Lavine KL: Factor V activity of platelets: evidence for an activated factor V molecule and for a platelet activator. *Blood* 49: 819, 1977

121. Vicic WJ, Lages B, Weiss HJ: Release of human platelet factor V activity is induced by both collagen and ADP and is inhibited by aspirin. *Blood* 56: 448, 1980

122. Miletich JP, Jackson CM, Majerus PW: Properties of the factor Xa binding site on human platelets. *Proc Natl Acad Sci USA* 74: 4033, 1977

123. Miletich JP, Jackson CM, Majerus PW: Properties of the factor Xa binding site on human platelets. *J Biol Chem* 253: 6908, 1978

124. Lipcomb MS, Walsh PN: Human platelets and factor XI. Localization in platelet membranes of factor XI like activity and its functional distinction from plasma factor XI. *J Clin Invest* 63: 1006, 1977

125. Walsh PN, Griffin JH: Contributions of human platelets to the proteolytic activation of blood coagulation factors XII and XI. *Blood* 57: 106, 1981

126. Kaplan KL, Owen J: Plasma levels of beta-thromboglobulin and platelet factor 4 as indices of platelet activation in vivo. *Blood* 57: 199, 1981

127. Kaplan KL, Owen J: Radioimmunoassay of platelet factor 4. in *Methods in Enzymology, Vol 70,* edited by Vunakis HV, Langone JJ, New York, Academic Press, 1981, p 226

128. Hawiger J: Adhesive interactions of blood cells and the vessel wall. in *Hemostasis and Thrombosis,* edited by Colman RW, Hirsh J, Marder VJ, Salzman EW, New York, Lippincott, 1987, p 182

129. McGregor JL, Clemetson KJ, James E, Luscher EF, Dechavanne M: Characterization of human blood platelet membrane proteins and glycoproteins by their isoelectric point (pI)

and apparent molecular weight using two-dimensional electrophoresis and surface-labelling techniques. *Biochim Biophys Acta* 599: 473, 1980

130. Ganguly P, Fossett NG: Inhibition of thrombin-induced platelet aggregation by a derivative of wheat germ agglutinin. Evidence for a physiologic receptor of thrombin in human platelets. *Blood* 57: 343, 1981

131. Hennessy VL Jr, Hicks RE, Niewiarowsky S, Edmunds LH Jr, Coleman RW: Function of human platelets during extracorporeal circulation. *Am J Physiol* 232: 4622, 1977

132. Clagett GP, Russo M, Hufnagel H: Platelet changes after placement of aortic prostheses in dogs. *J Lab Clin Med* 97: 345, 1981

133. Harker LA, Malpass TW, Branson HE, Hessel EA II, Slichter SJ: Mechanism of abnormal bleeding in patients undergoing cardiopulmonary bypass: acquired transient platelet dysfunction associated with selective alpha granule release. *Blood* 56: 824, 1980

134. Davies GC, Sobel M, Salzman EW: Elevated plasma fibrinopeptide A and thromboxane A$_2$ levels during cardiopulmonary bypass. *Circulation* 61: 808, 1980

135. Harker LA, Marzec UM, Ginsberg MH: Thrombospondin levels in plasma, platelets and urine in normal subjects, subjects receiving heparin, thoracotomy patients and patients undergoing cardiopulmonary bypass. *Thromb Haemost* 50: 40, 1983

136. Lindsay RM, Prentice CRM, Davidson JF, Burton JA, McNicol GP: Haemostatic changes during dialysis associated with thrombus formation on dialysis membranes. *Br Med J* 2: 454, 1972

137. Kaplow JS, Goffinet JA: Profound neutropenia during the early phase of hemodialysis. *JAMA* 203: 1335, 1968

138. Toren M, Goffinet JA, Kaplow LS: Pulmonary bed sequestration of neutrophils during hemodialysis. *Blood* 36: 337, 1970

139. Jensen DP, Brubaker LH, Nolph KD, Johnson CA, Nothum RJ: Hemodialysis coil-induced transient neutropenia and overshoot neutrophilia in normal man. *Blood* 41: 399, 1973

140. O'Flaherty J, Craddock PR, Jacob US: Altered granulocyte adhesiveness (GA) during in vivo complement (C) activation. *Blood* 48: 987, 1976

141. Wauters JP, Lambert PH: Hemodialysis induced leukopenia: role of cellophane membrane and complement activation. *Kidney Int* (Abstract) 12: 77, 1977

142. Aljama P, Bird PAE, Ward MK, Feest TG, Walker W, Tanboga H, Sussman M, Kerr DNS: Haemodialysis-induced leukopenia and activation of complement: effects of different membranes. *Proc Eur Dial Transplant Assoc* 15: 144, 1978

143. Skubitz KM, Craddock PR: Reversal of hemodialysis granulocytopenia and pulmonary leukostasis. *J Clin Invest* 67: 1383, 1981

144. Zacharski LR, McIntyre OR: Membrane-mediated synthesis of tissue factor (thromboplastin) in cultured fibroblasts. *Blood* 41: 679, 1973

145. Garg SK, Niemetz J: Tissue factor activity of normal leukemic cells. *Blood* 42: 729, 1973

146. Rickles FR, Hardin JA, Pitlick FA, Hoger LW, Conrad ME: Tissue factor activity in lymphocyte cultures from normal individuals and patients with hemophilia A. *J Clin Invest* 52: 1427, 1973

147. Rapaport SI, Hjost PF: The blood clotting properties of rabbit peritoneal leukocytes in vitro. *Thromb Diath Haemorrh* 17: 222, 1967

148. Kociba GJ, Griesemer Ra: Disseminated intravascular coagulation induced with leukocyte procoagulant. *Am J Pathol* 69: 407, 1972

149. Saba HI, Herion JC, Walker RJ, Roberts HR: Effects of lysosomal cationic proteins from polymorphonuclear leukocytes upon the fibrinogen and fibrinolysis system. *Thromb Res* 7: 543, 1975

150. Niemetz J, Muhlfelder T, Chievego ME, Troy B: Procoagulant activity of leukocytes. *Ann NY Acad Sci* 283, 208, 1977

151. Camussi G, Mencia-Huerta JM, Benveniste J: Release of platelet activating factor and histamine. I. Effect of immune complexes, complement and neutrophils on human and rabbit mastocytes and basophils. *Immunology* 33: 523, 1977

152. Morley J, Bray MA, Jones RW, Nugtenen DH, Van Dorp DA: Prostaglandin and thromboxane production by human and guinea-pig macrophages and leukocytes. *Prostaglandins* 17: 729, 1979

153. Beckman RS: Prostaglandin production by human blood monocytes and mouse peritoneal macrophages: synthesis dependent on in vivo culture conditions. *Prostaglandins* 21: 9, 1981

154. Dutton RC, Webber AJ, Johnson SA, Baier RE: Microstructure of initial thrombus formation on foreign materials. *J Biomed Mater Res* 3: 13, 1969

155. Baier RE, Dutton RC: Initial events in interactions of blood with a foreign surface. *J Biomed Mater Res* 3: 191, 1969

156. Ahearn DJ, Marshall JW, Nothum RJ, Esterly JA, Nolph KD, Maher JF: Morphologic studies of dialysis membranes – adherence of blood components to air rinsed coils. *Trans Am Soc Artif Intern Organs* 19: 435, 1973

157. Mason RG, Wolf RH, Zucker WH, Shinoda BA: Dynamics of thrombus formation upon an artificial surface in vivo: effects of antithrombotic agents. *Am J Pathol* 82: 187, 1978

158. Mason RG, Zucker WH, Bilinsky RT, Shinoda BA, Mohammad SF: Blood components deposited on used and reused dialysis membranes. *Biomater Med Devices Artif Organs* 4: 333, 1976

159. Lindsay RM, Prentice CRM, Burton JA, Ferguson D, Kennedy AC: The role of the platelet-dialysis membrane interaction in thrombus formation and blood loss during hemodialysis. *Trans Am Soc Artif Intern Organs* 19: 487, 1973

160. Bjornson J, Kierulf P, Eika C, Godal HC: Fibrin deposits in the Kiil dialyzer. *Scand J Haematol* 1: 379, 1973

161. Marshall JW, Ahearn DJ, Nothum RJ, Esterly J, Nolph KD, Maher JF: Adherence of blood components to dialyzer membranes. Morphological studies. *Nephron* 12: 157, 1974

162. Schwartz GH, Stenzel RH, Kohno I, Ast D, Miyata T, Rubin AL: Deposition of blood cells on collagen and Cuprophane membranes. J Biomed Mater Res 9: 453, 1975

163. Bilinsky RT, Morris AJ: Hemodialysis coil reuse. *JAMA* 218: 1806, 1971

164. Siemsen AW, Lumeng J, Wong EGC, Wong LMF, Ching A, Ennio JA, McGowan RF: Clinical laboratory evaluation of coil reuse. *Trans Am Soc Artif Intern Organs* 20: 585, 1974

165. Kramer P, Matthaei D, Go JG, Winckler K, Schieler F: Effect of blood factor deposits in reused dialysers on the dialysance of middle weight molecules. *Proc Eur Dial Transplant Assoc* 9: 278, 1972

166. George JN, Weed RI, Reed CF: Adhesion of human erythrocytes to glass: the nature of the interaction and the effect of serum and plasma. *J Cell Physiol* 77: 51, 1971

167. Hochmuth RM, Mohandas N, Spaeth EE, Williamson JR, Blackshear PL Jr, Johnson DW: Surface adhesion, deformation and detachment at low shear of red cells and white cells. *Trans Am Soc Artif Intern Organs* 18: 325, 1972

168. Goldsmith HL: The flow of model particles and blood cells and its relation to thrombogenesis. *Prog Hemostas Thromb* 1: 97, 1972

169. Goldsmith HL: The effects of flow and fluid mechanical stress on red cells and platelets. *Trans Am Soc Artif Intern Organs* 20: 21, 1974

170. Bartelt K, Forstrom R, Blackshear PL Jr: Blood platelet deposition onto filtering surfaces – effect of concentration polarization. *Abstracts Am Soc Artif Intern Organs* 5: 7, 1976

171. Forstrom RJ, Bartelt K, Blackshear PL Jr, Wood T: Formed element deposition onto filtering walls. *Trans Am Soc Artif Intern Organs* 21: 602, 1975

172. Wessler S, Gitel S: Control of heparin therapy. *Prog Hemost Thromb* 3: 311, 1976

173. Saba HI, Saba SR, Blackburn CA, Hartman RC, Mason RG: Heparin neutralization of PGI$_2$: effects upon platelets. *Science* 205: 499, 1979

174. Charm S, Kurland GS: Viscometry of human blood for shear rates of 0–100,000 sec^{-1}. *Nature* 206: 617, 1965

175. Copley AL, Scott-Blair GW: Hemorheological method for the study of blood systems and of processes in blood coagulation. in *Flow Properties of Blood,* edited by Copley AL, Stainsby G, London, Pergamon Press, 1960, p 412

176. Rand PW, Lacombe E, Hunt HE, Austin WH: Viscosity of normal human blood under normothermic and hypothermic conditions. *J Appl Physiol* 19: 117, 1964

177. Peric B: Viscosity of the blood at low shear rates. *Isr J Exp Med* 11: 139, 1963

178. Blackshear PL Jr, Forstrom JR, Dorman FD, Voss GO: Effect of flow on cells near walls. *Fed Proc* 30: 1600, 1971

179. Goldsmith HL: Red cell motions and wall interactions in tube flow. *Fed Proc* 30: 1578, 1971

180. Grabowski EF, Friedman LI, Leonard EF: Effects of shear rates on the diffusion and adhesion of blood platelets to a foreign surface. *Indust Eng Chem Fundam* 11: 224, 1972

181. Nevaril CG, Lynch EC, Alfrey CP Jr, Hellums JD: Erythrocyte damage and destruction induced by shear stress. *J Lab Clin Med* 71: 784, 1968

182. Bernstein EF: Certain aspects of blood interfacial phenomena – red blood cells. *Fed Proc* 30: 1510, 1971

183. MacCallum RN, O'Bannon W, Hellums JD, Alfrey CP, Lynch EC: Viscometric instruments for studies on red blood cell damage. in *Rheology of Biological Systems,* edited by Gabelnick HL, Litt M, Springfield IL, Charles C Thomas, 1973, p 70

184. Solen KA, Whiffen JD, Lightfoot EN: The effect of shear, specific surface and air interface on the developments of blood emboli and hemolysis. *J Biomed Mater Res* 12: 381, 1978

185. Copley AL: Hemorheological aspects of the endothelium-plasma interface. *Microvasc Res* 8: 192, 1974

186. Copley AL: Non-Newtonian behavior of surface layers of human plasma protein systems and a new concept of the initiation of thrombosis. *Biorheology* 10: 541, 1971

187. Hoffman AS: Blood-material interactions: An overview. in *Biomaterials, Advances in Chemistry* series no. 199, edited by Cooper SL, Peppas NA, Hoffman AS, Ratner BD, Am Chem Soc, Washington DC, 1982, p 3

188. Lindon J, Rosenberg R, Merrill E, Salzman E: Interaction of human platelets with heparinized agarose gel. *J Lab Clin Med* 91: 47, 1978

189. Anderson WH, Mohammad SF, Chuang HYK, Mason RG: Heparin potentiates synthesis of thromboxane A$_2$ in human platelets. *Adv Prostaglandin Thromboxane Res* 6: 287, 1980

190. Mohammad SF, Anderson WH, Smith JB, Chuang HYK, Mason RG: Effects of heparin on platelet aggregation, release reaction and thromboxane A$_2$ production. *Am J Pathol* 104: 132, 1981

191. Wurzinger LJ, Opitz R, Wolf M, Schmid-Schonbein H: Ultrastructural investigations on the question of mechanical activation of blood platelets. *Blut* 54: 97, 1987

192. Harker LA, Hirsh J, Gent M, Genton E: Critical evaluation of platelet inhibiting drugs in thrombotic disease. *Prog Hematol* 9: 229, 1975

193. Stewart JH, Farrell PC, Dixon M: Reduction of platelet and fibrin deposition in haemodialysers by aspirin administration. *Aust NZ J Med* 5: 117, 1975

194. Lindsay RM, Prentice CRM, Ferguson D, Burton JA, McNicol GP: Reduction of thrombus formation on dialyser membranes by aspirin and RA 233. *Lancet* 2: 1287, 1972

195. Sullivan JM, Harken DE, Gorlin R: Pharmacologic control of thromboembolic complications of cardiac valve replacement. *N Eng J Med* 284: 1391, 1971

196. Mielke CH, deLeval M, Hill JD, Macur MF, Gerbode F: Drug influence on platelet loss during extracorporeal circulation. *J Thor Cardiovasc Surg* 66: 845, 1973

197. Gurewich V, Lipinski B: Evaluation of antithrombotic properties of 'Suloctodil' in comparison with aspirin and dipyridamole. *Thromb Res* 9: 101, 1976

198. Gurewich V, Lipinski B, Wetmore R: Inhibition of intravascular fibrin deposition by dipyridamole in experimental animals. *Blood* 45: 569, 1975

199. Harker LA, Slichter SJ: Studies of platelets and fibrinogen kinetics in patients with prosthetic heart valves. *N Engl J Med* 293: 1302, 1970

200. Arrants JE, Hairston P, Lee WH Jr: Use of dipyridamole in preventing thromboembolism following valve replacement. *Chest* 58: 275, 1970

201. Welly HS, Genton E: Altered platelet function in patients with prosthetic mitral valves – effect of sulfinpyrazone therapy. *Circulation* 42: 967, 1970

202. Addonizio VP, Macarak EJ, Niewiarowski S, Colman RW, Edmunds LH: Preservation of human platelets with PGE$_1$ during in vitro cardiopulmonary bypass. *Trans Am Soc Artif Intern Organs* 23: 639, 1977

203. Addonizio VP, Strauss JF, Macavak EJ, Colman RW, Edmunds LH: Preservation of platelet number with PGE$_1$ during total cardiopulmonary bypass in rhesus monkeys. *Surgery* 83: 619, 1978

204. Mohammad SF, Mason RG, Eichwald EJ, Shively JA: Healthy and impaired vascular endothelium. in *Blood platelet function and medicinal chemistry,* edited by Lasslo L, New York, Alan R Liss, 1984, p 129

205. Coppe D, Wonders T, Snider M, Salzman EW: Preservation of platelet number and function during extracorporeal membrane oxygenation by regional infusion of prostacyclin. in *Prostacyclin,* edited by Vane JR, Bergstrom S, New York, Raven Press, 1979, p 385

206. Weston MJ, Woods HF, Ash G, Bunting S, Moncada S, Vane JR: Prostacyclin as an alternative to heparin in dogs. in *Prostacyclin,* edited by Vane JR, Bergstrom S, New York, Raven Press, 1979, p 349

207. Bunting S, Moncada S, Vane J, Woods HF, Weston MF: Prostacyclin improves hemocompatibility during charcoal hemoperfusion. in *Prostacyclin,* edited by Vane JR, Bergstrom S, New York, Raven Press, 1979, p 361

208. Harker LA: In vivo evaluation of antithrombin therapy in man. *Thromb Diath Haemorrh* 60 (suppl): 481, 1974

209. Didisheim P, Shimomoto T, Yamazaki H: Platelets, thrombosis and inhibitors. *Thromb Diath Haemorrh* 60 (suppl), 1974

210. Mason RG, Sargi K, Brinkhous KM: Antithrombotic agents – their effects on platelets and methods for their evaluation. in

Cardiovascular Drugs, edited by McMahon FG, New York, Futura, 1974, p 183

211. Hirsh J, Cade JF, Gallus AS, Schonbaum E: *Platelet, Drugs and Thrombosis.* New York, Basel, S Karger, 1975

212. Harker LA, Gent M: The use of agents that modify platelet function in the management of thrombotic disorders. in *Haemostasis and Thrombosis,* edited by Colman RW, Hirsh J, Marder VJ, Salzman EW, New York, Lippincott, 1987, p 1439

213. Gott VL: Wall-bound heparin – historical background and current clinical applications. *Adv Exp Med Biol* 52: 351, 1974

214. Leininger RI, Cooper CW, Epstein MM, Falb RD, Grode GA: Nonthrombogenic plastic surfaces. *Science* 152: 1625, 1966

215. Yen SPS, Rembaum A: Complexes of heparin with elastomeric positive polyelectrolytes. *J Biomed Mater Res* 1: 83, 1971

216. Merker RI, Elyash LJ, Mayhew SH, Wany JYC: The heparinization of silicone rubber using aminoorganosilane coupling agents. in *Artificial Heart Program Conference,* edited by Hagyeli RJ, National Heart Institute, Washington DC, 1969, p 29

217. Hufnagel CA, Conrad PW, Gillespie JF, Pifarre R, Ilano A, Yokoyama T: Comparative study of cardiac and vascular implants in relation to thrombosis. *Surgery* 61: 11, 1967

218. Grode GA, Anderson SJ, Crotte HM, Falb RD: Nonthrombogenic materials via a simple coating process. *Trans Am Soc Artif Intern Organs* 15: 1, 1969

219. Lagergren HR, Eriksson JC: Plastics with a stable surface monolayer of cross-linked heparin – preparation and evaluation. *Trans Am Soc Artif Intern Organs* 17: 10, 1971

220. Chawla AS, Chang TMS: Nonthrombogenic surface by radiation grafting of heparin – preparation, in vitro and in vivo studies. *Biomater Med Devices Artif Organs* 2: 157, 1974

221. Dycke MF: Inorganic heparin complexes for the preparation of nonthrombogenic surfaces. *J Biomed Mater Res* 6: 115, 1972

222. Martin RE, Shuey HF, Saltonstall GW Jr: Improved membranes for hemodialysis. *J Macromol Sci Chem A* 4: 635, 1970

223. Idezuki Y, Watanabe H, Hagiwara M, Kanasugi K, Mori Y, Nagaoka S, Hagio M, Yamamoto K, Tanjawa H: Mechanism of antithrombogenicity of a new heparinized hydrophilic polymer: Chronic in vivo studies and clinical application. *Trans Am Soc Artif Intern Organs* 21: 436, 1975

224. Eberle JW, Manton JR, Meals CR, Whitley DE, Rea WJ: Cross-linked heparin binding of a membrane oxygenator system. *J Biomed Mater Res* 7: 145, 1973

225. Leininger RI, Crowley JP, Falb RD, Grode GA: Three year's experience in vivo and in vitro with surfaces and devices tested by the heparin complex method. *Trans Am Soc Artif Intern Organs* 18: 312, 1972

226. Halpern BD, Shibakawa R: Heparin covalently bonded to polymer surface. *Adv Chem Ser* 87: 197, 1968

227. Merrill EW, Salzman EW, Wong PSL, Ashford TP, Brown AH, Austen WG: Polyvinyl alcohol-heparin hydrogel 'G'. *J Appl Physiol* 29: 723, 1970

228. Merrill EW, Salzman EW, Lipps BJ Jr, Gilliland ER, Austen WG, Joison E: Antithrombogenic cellulose membranes for blood dialysis. *Trans Am Soc Artif Intern Organs* 12: 139, 1966

229. Schmer G: The biological activity of covalently immobilized heparin. *Trans Am Soc Artif Intern Organs* 18: 321, 1972

230. Schmer G, Teng LNL, Cole JJ, Vizzo JE, Francisco MM, Scribner BH: Successful use of a totally heparin grafted hemodialysis system in sheep. *Trans Am Soc Artif Intern Organs* 22: 654, 1976

231. Hoffman AS, Schmer G, Harris C, Kraft WG: Covalent binding of biomolecules to radiation-grafted hydrogel on inert polymer surfaces. *Trans Am Soc Artif Intern Organs* 18: 10, 1972

232. Lansson R, Eriksson JC, Lagesgren H, Olsson P: Platelet and plasma coagulation compatibility of heparinized and sulphated surface. *Thromb Res* 15: 157, 1979

233. Falb RD, Leininger RI, Grode G, Crowley J: Surface-bound heparin. *Adv Exp Med Biol* 52: 365, 1974

234. Nader HG, McDuffe NM, Diettich CP: Heparin fractionation by electrofocusing. Presence of 21 components of different molecular weights. *Biochem Biophys Res Commun* 57: 488, 1974

235. Oosta GM, Gardner WT, Beeler DL, Rosenberg RD: Multiple functional domains of the heparin molecule. *Proc Natl Acad Sci USA,* 78, 829, 1981

236. Stewart GP, Wilkow MA: Mechanism of failure of biocompatible-treated surfaces. *J Biomed Mater Res* 10: 413, 1976

237. Falb RD, Takahashi MT, Grode GA, Leininger RI: Studies on the stability and protein adsorption characteristics of heparinized polymer surfaces by radioisotopic labeling techniques. *J Biomed Mater Res* 1: 239, 1967

238. Coleman DL, Atwood AI, Andrade JD: Platelet retention by albuminated glass and polystyrene beads. *J Bioengineering* 1: 33, 1976

239. Gentry PW, Alexander B: Specific coagulation factor adsorption to insoluble heparin. *Biochem Biophys Res Commun* 50: 500, 1973

240. Thaler E, Schmer G: A simple 2-step isolation procedure for human antithrombin II/III and its biological activity after insolubilization to agarose. *Trans Am Soc Artif Intern Organs* 20: 516, 1974

241. Chuang HYK, Crowther PE, Mohammad SF, Mason RG: Identification and quantitation of plasma proteins adsorbed to artificial surfaces by use of ^{125}I-labeled specific antibodies. *Fed Proc* 37: 444, 1978

242. Chuang HYK, Mohammad SF, Sharma NC, Mason RG: Radioimmunoassays of human fibrinogen and alpha-thrombin adsorbed to artificial surfaces. *Fed Proc* 40: 806, 1981

243. Woods HF, Ash G, Weston MH, Bunting S, Moncada S, Vane JR: Prostacyclin can replace heparin in haemodialysis in dogs. *Lancet* 2: 1075, 1978

244. Turney JH, Woods HF, Weston MJ: The use of prostacyclin in extracorporeal circuits. in *Hemostasis, Prostaglandins, and Renal Disease,* edited by Remuzzi G, Mecca G, Gaetano G, New York, Raven Press, 1981, p 353

245. Grode GA, Putman J, Crowley, Leininger RI, Falb RD: Surface-immobilized prostaglandin as a platelet protective agent. *Trans Am Soc Artif Intern Organs* 20: 38, 1974

246. McRea JC, Kim SW: Characterization of controlled release of prostaglandin from polymer matrices for thrombus prevention. *Trans Am Soc Artif Intern Organs* 24: 746, 1978

247. Van Drup DA, Van Evert WC, Van der Wolf L: 20-methylprostacyclin, a powerful unnatural platelet aggregation inhibitor. *Prostaglandins* 16: 953, 1978

248. Dembinska-Kiec A, Rucker W, Schomhofer PS, Gandolf C: Prostacyclin analogs: antiaggregatory potency and enhancement of cAMP levels in human platelet rich plasma. *Thromb Haemost* 42: 1340, 1979

249. Whittle BJR, Moncada S, Whiting F, Vane JR: Carbacyclin – a potent stable prostacyclin analogue for the inhibition of platelet aggregation. *Prostaglandins* 19: 605, 1980

250. Malmstem C, Claesson HE: Inhibition of platelet aggregation and elevation of cyclic-AMP levels in platelets by 13, 14-deydro PGI_2 methyl ester. *Prostaglandins Med* 4: 453, 1980

251. Imai Y, Tajima K, Nose Y: Biolized materials for cardiovascular prosthesis. *Trans Am Soc Artif Intern Organs* 17: 6, 1971

252. Harasaki H, Kiraly R, Murabayashi S, Pepoy M, Fields A, Kambic H, Hillegass D, Nose Y: Cross-linked gelatin as blood contacting surface. *Proc 2nd Meeting of ISAO,* 1979, p 203

253. Kambic H, Barenburg S, Harasaki H, Gibbons D, Kiraly R, Nose Y; Glutaraldehyde-protein complexes as blood compatible coatings. *Trans Am Soc Artif Intern Organs* 24: 426, 1978

254. Mansfield PB, Wechezak AR, Sauvage LR: Preventing thrombus on artificial vascular surfaces: true endothelial cell linings. *Trans Am Soc Artif Intern Organs* 21: 264, 1975

11

PRACTICAL USE OF ANTICOAGULANTS

ROBERT M. LINDSAY and ANNE M. SMITH

INTRODUCTION

To use anticoagulants optimally during dialysis it is necessary to understand hemostasis, how to evaluate it and how therapeutic agents interfere with it. Knowledge of the hemostatic defects found in uremia and the influence of dialysis upon these is necessary, as is an understanding of foreign surface induced coagulation. This chapter presents such information before providing a practical guide to anticoagulant use.

SUMMARY OF THE HEMOSTATIC SYSTEM

(This section is not extensively referenced; further details may be obtained from major coagulation texts) (1–6).

When a blood vessel is injured spontaneous arrest of bleeding occurs due to the formation of an impervious seal. This hemostatic plug is formed by three major mechanisms: 1) vessel wall contraction, 2) platelet adherence to the vessel wall and platelet aggregation and 3) formation and maintenance of fibrin clots by activation of blood coagulation. These reactions occur simultaneously and are mutually interdependent.

It is convenient to separate hemostasis into two continuous stages, primary and secondary. Primary hemostasis results from vasoconstriction, platelet adhesion and aggregation in which a platelet plug is produced. Bleeding may recur unless the friable platelet plug is reinforced by a tough fibrin mesh. Secondary hemostasis requires blood coagulation, and the production of fibrin. The hemostatic plug is maintained until healing is complete. Tissue repair then occurs and the fibrin-platelet plug is gradually dissolved by fibrinolysis and replaced by organized tissue.

Before considering the particular problems relating to hemostasis and anticoagulation in hemodialysis, it is important to understand the physiology of normal hemostasis. A brief description follows in the next few sections.

Role of the blood vessel

Vascular injury induces vasoconstriction resulting in immediate control of bleeding. The factors initiating vasoconstriction are poorly understood. Vessels with muscular walls contract but vasoconstriction occurs even in the microcirculation in vessels without smooth muscle cells. The mechanism appears to be humoral and may be due to the release of vasoconstrictor thromboxane A_2 from platelets as adhesion and aggregation occur. The stimulus to hemostatic plug formation is damage to the vascular endothelium. The endothelial cell plays an active role in hemostasis by synthesizing and secreting substances involved in the formation and localization of the hemostatic plug. Such substances are von Willebrand's factor (VIII : WF), prostacyclin and plasminogen activator. Von Willebrand's factor is part of the factor VIII molecule which also possesses VIII clotting activity. It is involved in the adhesion of platelets to subendothelium. Lack of VIII : WF will prolong bleeding. Prostacyclin (PGI_2)

is synthesized from arachidonic acid in the endothelial cells. It inhibits platelet aggregation and prevents platelet deposition on normal blood vessel endothelium. It may help localize the hemostatic plug to the site of the vascular injury. Plasminogen activator is an enzyme that converts plasminogen to plasmin, which then lyses fibrin. Release of this enzyme by damaged endothelium also helps to localize the hemostatic plug. Exposed endothelium provides a surface for adhesion and activated blood coagulation.

Primary hemostasis

Vascular injury resulting in endothelial damage exposes connective tissue (collagen, microfibrils, and basement membrane) to blood and causes platelets to undergo a sequence of responses. Within seconds of injury platelets gather at the site of vascular damage and start to adhere to the endothelial surface. Platelets have a particular affinity for collagen. Platelet adhesion at the site of vessel wall injury is followed by the appearance of a mass of aggregated platelets occluding the vessel lumen and arresting blood flow. Within a short time fibrin is seen at the periphery and in the interstices of the platelet aggregate.

The physiological stimulus to platelet aggregation appears to be exposure of the platelet membrane to collagen. Platelets undergo a shape change from a disc to a rounded form with pseudopods and undergo a secretory process (called the release reaction) analogous to endocrine gland secretion. Certain substances including ADP, ATP, serotonin, are discharged from cytoplasmic granules within the platelet. Collagen, ADP, thrombin, epinephrine, and serotonin may all induce platelet aggregation by activation of the enzyme phospholipase A_2 in the platelet membrane causing conversion of membrane phospholipid to a number of fatty acids including arachidonic acid. This is converted by the platelet enzyme cyclo-oxygenase to cyclic endoperoxides, which are further converted by the enzyme thromboxane synthetase to thromboxane A_2 (Figure 1). The latter is a powerful inducer of platelet aggregation and its production also causes the release of ADP from platelet granules which triggers further platelet aggregation. Details of platelets and platelet function are given later.

Secondary hemostasis

Hemostatic plugs are composed mainly of aggregated platelets but fibrin is necessary to stabilize the plug and bind it to the vessel wall. Fibrin is the end result of blood coagulation and its appearance in the plugs indicates local generation of thrombin.

Plasma contains at least ten proteins directly involved in blood coagulation. Two further proteins involved in the kallikrein-kinin system participate in the coagulation process. The nomenclature of the coagulation factors is shown in Table 1. Most coagulation factors are referred to by Roman numerals, except fibrinogen and prothrombin, which are usually referred to by their proper names and not as factors I and II, respectively. Most clotting factors exist in

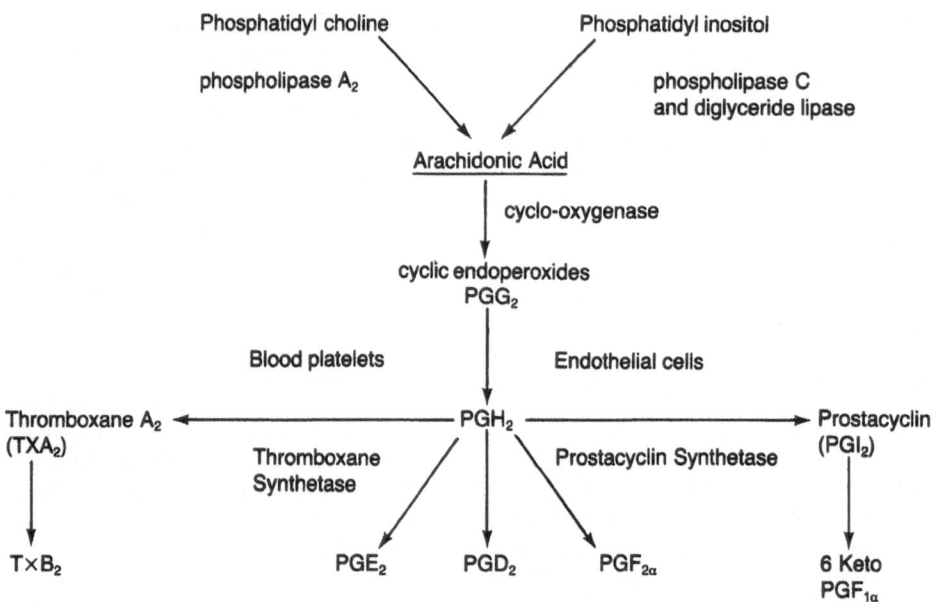

Figure 1. Prostaglandin pathway.

plasma as inert precursors and are converted to their active enzymic form during coagulation. The letter 'a' accompanying a Roman numeral (e.g. factor Xa) indicates the factor is in its activated form. Clotting factors act either as substrates which under the influence of enzymes are themselves converted into active enzymes or they act as cofactors in complexes formed by enzyme and substrate.

Blood coagulation results from the conversion of a soluble

Table 1. Coagulation factors (procoagulants).

Factor	Synonyms	Normal plasma concentration (mg/dl)
I	Fibrinogen	200–400
II	Prothrombin	10
III	Tissue thromboplastin, tissue factor	0
IV	Calcium ion	4–5
V	Proaccelerin, labile factor	1
VII	Serum prothrombin conversion accelerator, stable factor	0.05
VIII	Antihemophilic factor	1–2
IX	Christmas factor	0.3
X	Stuart-Prower factor	1
XI	Plasma thromboplastin antecedent (PTA)	0.5
XII	Hageman factor	3
XIII	Fibrin stabilising factor (FSF)	1–2
prekallikrein	Fletcher factor	5
High molecular weight kininogen	Fitzgerald factor, contact activation cofactor	6

plasma protein, fibrinogen, into insoluble fibrin and is catalysed by the enzyme thrombin. Thrombin is not normally present in the circulating blood but exists as an inert precursor prothrombin. Figure 2 illustrates a simplified view of blood coagulation.

The generation of thrombin from prothrombin results from two separate chains of reactions, the extrinsic and intrinsic pathways. The difference between the two pathways is the way in which factor X is activated. Both pathways share a common pathway after the activation of factor X. The steps leading to the formation of thrombin in both pathways consist of a series of proenzyme-enzyme conversions, each enzyme sequentially activating the proenzyme next in line, i.e. the cascade hypothesis of blood coagulation (see Figure 2).

The concept of two separate pathways is of practical value. The prothrombin time (PT) screens the extrinsic system and the partial thromboplastin time (PTT), the intrinsic system. Abnormalities in the PT help localize the problem to the extrinsic system and in the PTT, the intrinsic system. If both PT and PTT are abnormal a defect is likely in the common pathway.

Extrinsic pathway (Figure 3)

Within seconds of vascular injury, tissue thromboplastin released from damaged cells forms a complex with factor VII which activates factor X. At the same time, platelet phospholipid (platelet factor 3 [PL3]) procoagulant activity becomes available to plasma as a result of the change in platelet membrane architecture (induced by platelet adhesion). Platelet phospholipid activity provides a surface onto which activated factor X (Xa) binds to catalyse the conversion of prothrombin to thrombin. Activation of factor

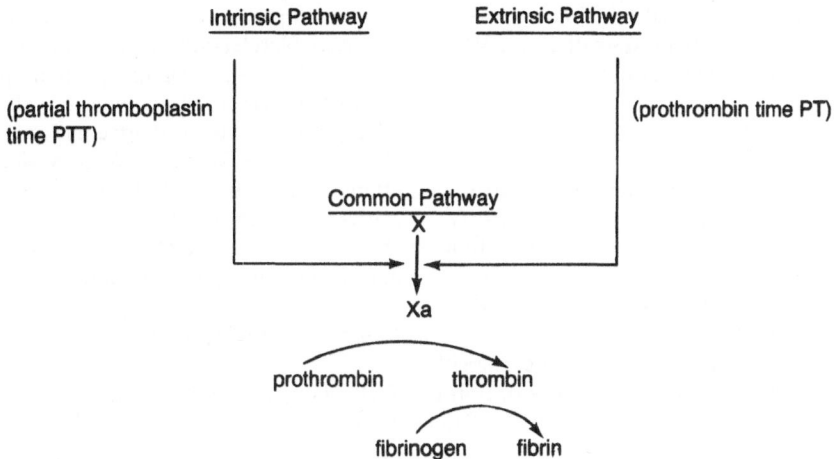

Figure 2. Simplified scheme of blood coagulation.

X, via the extrinsic pathway, results in the generation of small amounts of thrombin that initiate feedback reactions and accelerates the formation of the hemostatic plug.

Intrinsic pathway (Figure 3)

The essential features of this pathway are that factor XII is activated (XIIa) by contact with a foreign surface (e.g.

exposed collagen). The reaction is accelerated in the presence of prekallikrein (Fletcher factor). Factor XIIa activates factor XI to XIa, a reaction facilitated by either high molecular weight kininogen (HMWK) or Fletcher factor. Calcium ions are not required up to this stage of coagulation. Factor XIIa also interacts with the extrinsic pathway by converting the single chain factor VII molecule to a double chain molecule with many times more activity.

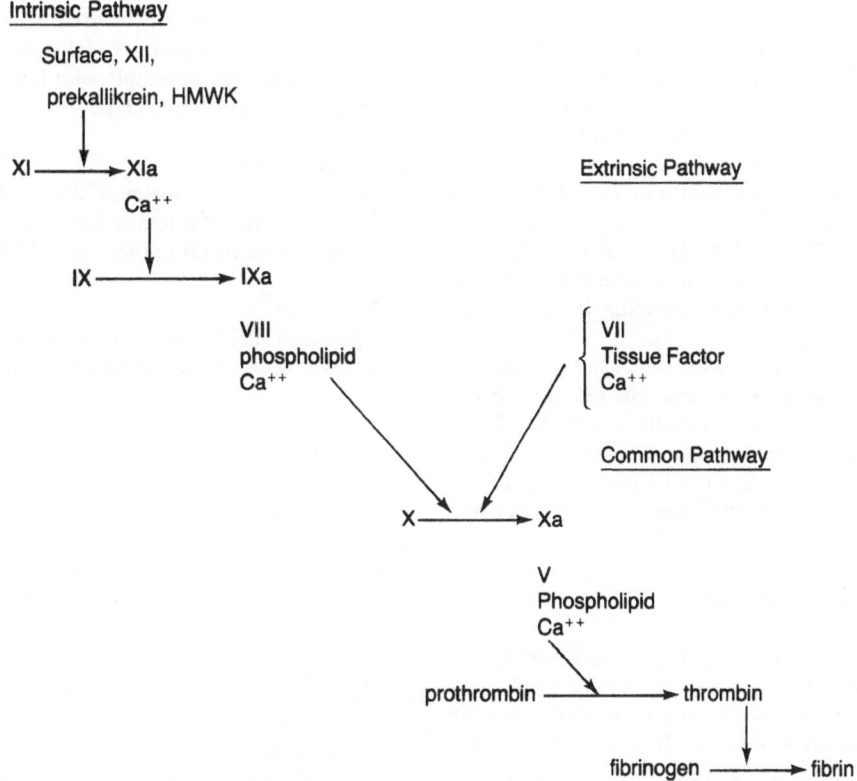

Figure 3. A scheme for blood coagulation.

Factor XIa (in the presence of calcium ions) converts factor IX to IXa which, in turn, complexes with factor VIII, Ca^{++} and phospholipid to activate factor X.

Common pathway (Figure 3)

Once factor X has been activated, whether by the extrinsic or intrinsic pathway mechanism, it complexes with factor V, Ca^{++} and phospholipid, to convert prothrombin to thrombin. The main action of thrombin is to split fibrinopeptides A and B from fibrinogen to produce fibrin monomer which then undergoes polymerization to form a visible clot.

Thrombin also activates factor XIII (in the presence of Ca^{++} which catalyses the formation of cross links of fibrin chains producing a stable clot more resistant to the lytic action of plasmin.

Links between intrinsic and extrinsic pathways

The distinction between the two independent pathways has become blurred as feedback mechanisms and interactions outside the classical schemes have been found. Activated factor XII can rapidly convert factor VII into a form that upon combination with tissue factor, has increased activity as an activator of factor X. Factor XII triggers the intrinsic pathway and appears to prime the extrinsic pathway. Similarly, Xa (whether activated via the intrinsic or extrinsic pathway) also enhances factor VIII activity. There also appears to be a direct activation of factor IX via the tissue factor-factor VII-Ca complex.

Although division of coagulation into the three pathways (intrinsic, extrinsic, and common) is, therefore, artificial, it still has a practical use. The tests used to screen for abnormalities in coagulation localize the problem to one of the three pathways, therefore, narrowing down the factors likely to be involved. The prothrombin time (PT) reflects abnormality in factor VII predominantly, whereas the partial thromboplastin time (PTT) reflects factors XII, XI, IX, and VIII. If both PT and PTT are abnormal, then the problem is mainly in the common pathway reflecting factors X, V, prothrombin or fibrinogen.

Liver disease provides a good example: here all factors synthesized in the liver may be affected, i.e. fibrinogen, prothrombin, VII, IX, X, and V, therefore, both the PT and PTT will be affected. In hemophilia A (factor VIII deficiency) on the other hand, only the PTT is affected. Hence, it remains useful clinically to subdivide the process of coagulation.

Localization of the hemostatic plug

Blood coagulation is an autocatalytic process resulting in a rapid generation of thrombin within the vascular system at the site of injury. It is obviously important that thrombin production is restricted to this site. If allowed to disperse and remain active in the circulation, diffuse intravascular clotting would occur. A number of mechanisms ensure localization of the hemostatic process. Clotting factor interac-

tions and thrombin generation occur more efficiently on the surface of platelets where phospholipid (PL3) facilitates the spatial relationships of the proteins prior to interaction. Factor V is present in platelets as well as in plasma. When released from platelets it appears to act as a receptor on the platelet surface for factor X activation. Thrombin generation tends to be confined to the region of the platelet aggregation. Activated clotting factors dispersed from the immediate area of plug formation are rapidly inactivated by naturally occurring plasma inhibitors.

Naturally occurring plasma inhibitors

Well characterized inhibitors include antithrombin III (heparin cofactor) α$_2$ macroglobulin, α$_1$ antitrypsin, α$_2$ antiplasmin, C1 inactivator (C1 esterase inhibitor) and protein C (Table 2). Concentrations of inhibitors are higher than those of coagulation factors or plasminogen. They comprise approximately 20% of the globulin fraction of human plasma and act to limit and localize thrombosis, fibrinolysis, and inflammatory reactions.

Antithrombin III (AT III)

It is an α$_2$ globulin (approximately 64,000 daltons). It is a major inhibitor of thrombin but also inhibits XIIa, XIa, Xa, IXa, prekallikrein and plasmin. Its action is greatly enhanced by heparin which is present in mast cells. Heparin binds to AT III inducing a conformational change such that arginine at the reactive site is more accessible to the active serine site of thrombin (or the other serine proteases). The physiological importance of AT III is shown by the repeated thrombotic episodes in people with hereditary AT III deficiency (<50% of normal AT III).

α$_2$ Macroglobulin

This is a large plasma protein (725,000 daltons) which also inhibits thrombin but is less active than AT III. Deficiencies do not appear to result in increased thrombosis.

α$_1$ Antitrypsin

This protein (50,000 daltons) inhibits factor XIa and plasmin; deficiency does not result in thrombosis.

Table 2. Naturally occurring plasma inhibitors.

Inhibitors	Normal plasma concentration (mg/dl)
Antithrombin III (heparin cofactor)	18–30
α$_2$-Macroglobulin	150–350
α$_1$-Antitrypsin	200–400
α$_2$-Plasmin Inhibitor (α$_2$-antiplasmin)	5.7
C1 inactivator (C1 esterase inhibitor)	15–35
Protein C	0.4

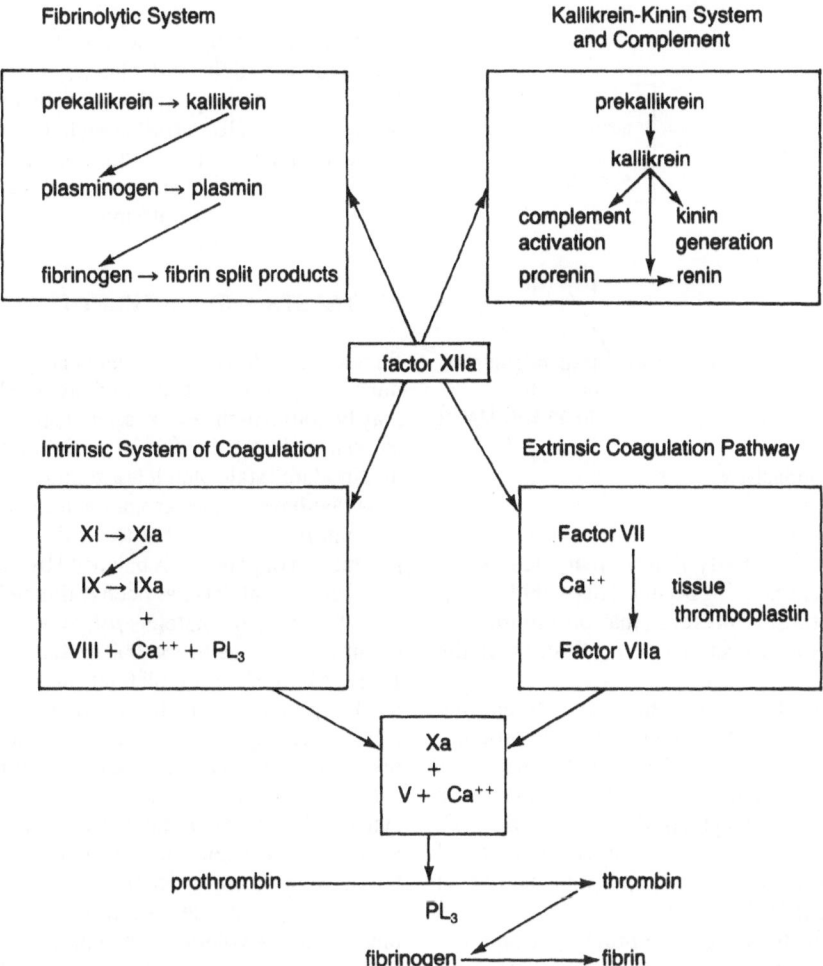

Figure 4. Activation of factor XII is pivotal in a number of physiologic processes.

α_2 Plasmin inhibitor

Interferes with binding of plasminogen to fibrin. Inherited deficiency results in severe hemorrhagic tendency.

C1 Inactivator (C1 esterase inhibitor)

This was initially identified as an inhibitor of C1 esterase in the complement system. Subsequently, it was found to inhibit plasmin, plasma kallikrein, factor XIIa and XIa. Deficiency of this inhibitor is not associated with a thrombotic tendency.

Protein C

This is a recently identified vitamin K dependent plasma protein. It is converted to its active form by thrombin helped by another vitamin K dependent factor, protein S. Activated protein C interacts with an endothelial surface cofactor, thrombomodulin, which rapidly inactivates factors V and VIII and inhibits prothrombin activation. Hereditary deficiency of protein C leads to increased thrombotic episodes.

Contact factor activation

Activation of factor XII is pivotal in a number of physiological processes. As previously mentioned, factor XIIa initiates the intrinsic pathway of coagulation by activating factor XI and activates the extrinsic pathway by converting VII to VIIa. In addition to its role in coagulation, factor XII activates the fibrinolytic, kallikrein-kinin complement and renin-angiotensin systems (Figure 4).

Although factor XII has these roles, coagulation can occur efficiently in people with factor XII deficiency. Such people tend, in fact, to have if anything a thrombotic tendency as exemplified by Mr. Hageman who, lacking factor XII, died of a pulmonary embolus.

Role of fibrinolysis in hemostasis

Fibrinolysis is the dissolution of fibrin clots (Figure 5). It is an essential host defense mechanism preventing vascular occlusion. The role of fibrinolysis in normal hemostasis is

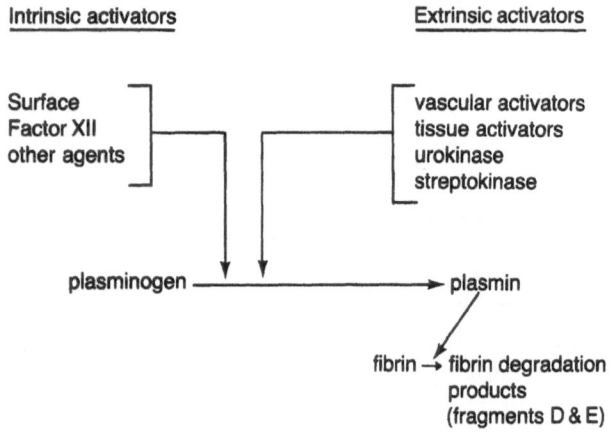

Figure 5. A scheme for fibrinolysis.

uncertain. If fibrinolytic activity is too great, hemostatic plugs break down and rebleeding occurs. This would infer it is not useful in hemostasis. However, it may be important in localizing the plug and in eventual recanalization of the injured vessel.

Fibrinolysis occurs by the action of the proteolytic enzyme plasmin, which attacks fibrin to produce a soluble product, fragment X. Further degradation of fragment X produces lower molecular weight fragments Y and D. Fragment Y is finally degraded to another fragment D plus a fragment E. One mole of fibrin produces two moles of fragment D and one mole of fragment E. These fragments are called fibrin degradation products (FDP).

Plasmin is formed by the action of a proteolytic enzyme, plasminogen activator, on an inactive β globulin precursor, plasminogen. Plasminogen activator is found in many tissues and is secreted into the blood by vascular endothelial cells. It is probably also formed in the blood from a precursor protein plasminogen proactivator, factor XIIa being involved in this conversion. The various forms of plasminogen activator in the blood and tissues are immunologically distinct. The naturally occurring inhibitor of plasmin (α_2 antiplasmin) has already been described. α_2 macroglobulin, AT III, α_1 antitrypsin and C1 inactivator, also inhibit plasmin. Inhibitors to plasminogen activators may also exist, but have not been adequately characterized.

There is recent evidence to suggest that activation of plasminogen in fibrin clots is regulated as follows. When the vascular wall is injured, tissue factor and plasminogen activator are released. Tissue factor initiates the extrinsic pathway of formation of thrombin which then forms fibrin clots. Both plasminogen and the vascular activator specifically bind to fibrin. The formation of plasmin then occurs in situ dissolving the clots. α_2 antiplasmin is also incorporated into the clots by the action of factor XIIIa to control the clot dissolution. Any plasmin escaping into the circulation is rapidly inactivated by the circulating natural inhibitors. If uncontrolled plasmin production occurs a bleeding tendency results because plasmin not only induces the dissolution of

clots but also digests factors V, VIII, and fibrinogen. The FDP's produced by the action of plasmin also inhibit the action of thrombin and platelet aggregation, which also leads to a bleeding tendency. Obviously the fibrinolytic mechanism is well controlled such that hemorrhage does not occur normally. Extra stimulation of fibrinolysis by agents such as streptokinase and urokinase can cause hemorrhage due to these effects of plasmin.

PLATELETS AND PLATELET FUNCTION

Platelets are derived from megakaryocytes which are produced by pluripotent myeloid stem cells. Megakaryocytes may be found in the extravascular space of the bone marrow as well as in the lungs and peripheral circulation. In the unstimulated state platelets are small, anuclate disc-shaped cells that have an average diameter of 2 to 3 μm and have a circulatory life-span of 9 to 12 days. In the steady state, production of platelets is balanced by destruction. The turnover rate of platelets has been estimated to be approximately 35,000 $\pm$ 4,300 platelets/μl/day with the normal platelet count in the range of 150,000 to 400,000/mm^3 (150 to 400 $\times$ 10^9/l). About $^1/_3$ of the platelets are in a splenic pool which freely exchanges with the circulation. Platelet production can increase up to approximately eight times normal when necessary. Megakaryocytopoiesis is stimulated by thrombocytopenia (decreased platelets), or suppressed by thrombocytosis (increased platelets). Therefore, a regulatory mechanism involving a hormone, thrombopoietin, has been postulated. With thrombocytopenia the marrow may accelerate production of platelets by three possible mechanisms: an increase in the volume of megakaryocytes, with an increase in the average number of nuclei per cell; an increase in the total number of megakaryocytes by an influx of cells from the stem cell pool; and a shortening of the maturation time of megakaryocytes. Platelets produced under stressed conditions are larger than normal. It is unclear whether in the unstressed state, young platelets are larger than old platelets. Platelets can disappear from the circulation through senescence, immunological destruction, or platelet consumption (non-immune destruction including coagulation) in physiological or pathological states associated with platelet activity. Any platelet destructive process is usually associated with increased thrombocytopoeisis. If platelet production keeps pace with destruction circulating platelet counts remain normal, if not, thrombocytopenia ensues.

Platelet structure

Platelets are highly evolved specialized structures. The mature platelet has unique morphological features (Figure 6) that subserve platelet function. Platelets can be activated by many substances. These can be divided into three categories: proteolytic enzymes such as thrombin, or trypsin; large molecules, such as collagen, aggregated IgG and insoluble immune complexes; and small molecules such as ADP, serotonin, arachidonic acid and epinephrine.

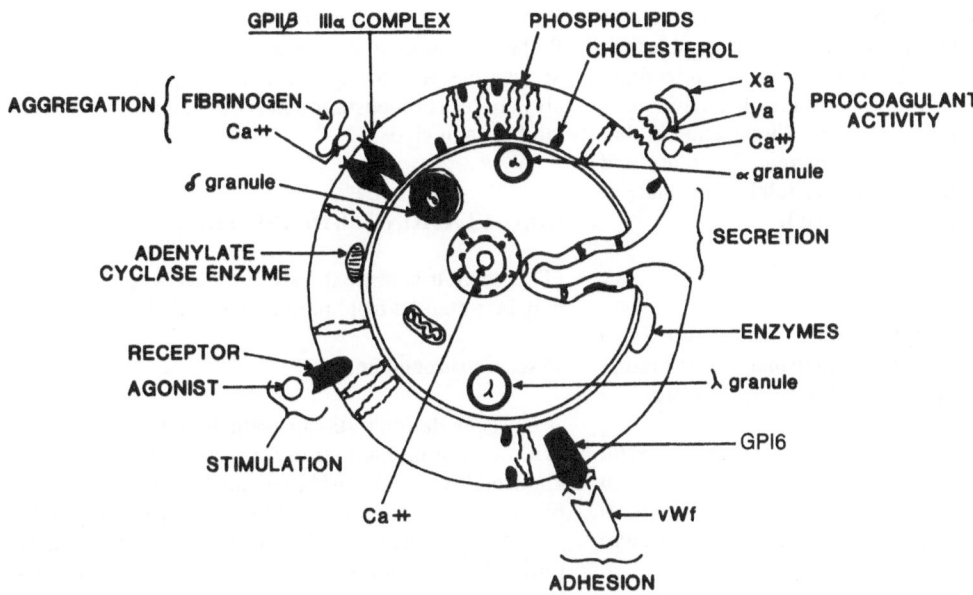

Figure 6. Schematic structure and function of the platelet (for details see text).

When platelets combine with aggregating agents under physiological conditions they rapidly lose their disc shape and become irregular spheres with multiple pseudopods. Surface contour changes are accompanied by movement of cytoplasmic granules toward the cell center where they are closely encircled by the centrally displaced circumferential band of microtubules and microfilaments. This is the so-called 'shape change' reaction. During the shape change the individual platelets become adhesive and begin to aggregate.

Platelet adhesion

The platelet membrane contains 'clothes-pin' shaped phospholipids in a bilayer 8 nm thick with polar head groups oriented to the aqueous environment and each pair of flexible fatty acid chains (wavy lines in Figure 6) oriented towards the hydrophobic middle of the bilayer. Interspersed are cholesterol (small black ellipsoids), proteins, and glycoproteins. Protruding from the surface is glycoprotein Ib (GPIb) to which von Willebrand factor binds in the process of platelet adhesion to the subendothelium. The von Willebrand factor probably has a bridging action between GPIb and subendothelium.

After adhering to the subendothelium a shape change occurs and platelets begin to release their granular contents. The mechanisms underlying both the release reaction and aggregation appear to depend on prostaglandin synthesis (Figure 1).

Platelet aggregation and the release reaction (Figure 6)

Platelet aggregation and secretion are initiated by the binding of agonists such as thrombin, epinephrine, or ADP, to specific receptors. In the presence of extracellular calcium ions, aggregation is completed by binding of fibrinogen to the glycoproteins (GPIIb and GPIIIa) in the platelet membrane. Thrombospondin (a glycoprotein) released from alpha granules contained in the platelets may act as the endogenous platelet ligand forming a complex with fibrinogen stabilizing the platelet aggregates. Prostaglandin synthesis with production of cyclic endoperoxides takes place on the membrane of the cell, the open canalicular system, and the dense tubular system (center). These synthetic reactions require enzymes such as phospholipase A_2 and cyclo-oxygenase. The release reaction requires transfer of Ca from nucleated calcium stores into the cytosol, an event that triggers secretion from the alpha granules, dense granules, and lysosomes (λ granules) (Table 3).

Thrombin can induce the platelet release reaction at a concentration lower than that required to activate phospholipase A_2 so that the release mechanism can probably proceed by an alternative pathway. Both cyclic endoperoxides and thromboxane A_2 (Figure 1) are potent inducers of release and aggregation.

Procoagulant activity of platelets

The procoagulant activity of platelets is initiated by binding factor Va to its surface receptor. Factor Va, in the presence of calcium ions, acts as the receptor for Xa thereby activating prothrombin at the cell surface. By providing specific surface features for the intrinsic and extrinsic systems of coagulation, platelets play a key role in hemostasis.

Inhibitors of platelet function

Platelet function is partially autoregulated by membrane

adenylate cyclase enzyme complex (AC); this enzyme plus cyclic AMP-dependent phosphodiesterases, determines the platelet content of cyclic AMP, an inhibitor of platelet function. Cyclic AMP blocks the production of arachidonate from platelet phospholipids (Figure 1). Circumstances that elevate cyclic AMP levels such as increased activity and decreased phosphodiesterase activity, inhibit the platelet release reaction (see antiplatelet agents).

Clot retraction

Clot retraction is mediated by platelet actomyosin (also called thrombosthenin). Platelets help to maintain the integrity of small vessels and in thrombocytopenic states red blood cells leak through vessel walls.

Vascular tissue and endothelial cells produce prostacyclin (PGI_2) which potently inhibits platelet aggregation and probably plays an important role in preventing thrombus formation. The cyclic endoperoxide PGH_2 is metabolised to

Table 3. Platelet granule contents.

α Granules
　Platelet-specific proteins (low molecular weight)
　　PF4
　　Low-affinity PF4
　β-Thromboglobulin
　　Platelet basic protein
　Mitogenic factors (platelet-derived growth factor)
　High molecular weight glycoproteins
　　Fibrinogen
　　von Willebrand factor
　　Factor VIII
　　Fibronectin
　　Thrombospondin
　　Factor V
　　HMWK
　Albumin
Dense bodies (δ granules)
　ADP
　ATP
　Calcium
　Pyrophosphate
Lysosomal enzymes (λ granules)
　Acid phosphatase
　β-N-Acetylglucosaminidase
　β-Galactosidase
　β-Glycerophosphatase
Granular proteins of uncertain location
　Cathepsins
　　Endoglucosidase
　Cyclic-3′, 5′-phosphodiesterase
　Collagenase
　Vascular permeability factors
　Proelestase and elastase
　$α_1$-Protease inhibitor
　$α_2$-Macroglobulin
　Antiplasmin
　Bactericidal protein
　Aryl sulfatase

form prostacyclin. Thromboxane A_2 is also formed from PGH_2, so compounds having opposite effects on platelets are synthesized through very similar pathways. This probably enables homeostatic control of platelet aggregation and inhibition in vivo.

COAGULATION TESTS AND THEIR USE

(This section is not extensively referenced; further details may be obtained from major coagulation texts) (1–6).

Tests of procoagulants

A few coagulation tests can evaluate procoagulant function. With a minimal number of screening tests, the hemostatic abnormality can be isolated quickly. All these tests are based on the eventual formation of fibrin strands that can be detected by either optical or electrical devices. In each case, prolongation of test time may represent an abnormally low factor concentration, the presence of a biologically inactive factor(s) or an inhibitor(s).

The partial thromboplastin time (PTT)

This tests the intrinsic system of coagulation. The time consuming reactions which take place when blood is allowed to clot in a glass tube are: first those leading to contact activation, and second, those causing platelet aggregation and availability of phospholipid (platelet factor 3, [PL3]). If these reactions are accelerated or bypassed, any delays in the clotting sequences commencing with the activation of factor IX become more obvious. Plasma is, therefore, preincubated with kaolin to activate contact factors and various types of phospholipids are added to replace platelet activity.

The PTT with kaolin is a sensitive, quick, practical way of demonstrating defects in coagulation too small to lead to prolongation of the whole blood clotting time. It will detect deficiencies of factors V, VIII, IX, X, XI, and XII, as well as the presence of circulating anticoagulants.

A PTT of 7 seconds or more longer than the control should be considered abnormal. A prolonged PTT will not determine which factor is deficient. Specific factor assays are required for precise determination of the particular factor deficiency. The normal range for PTT varies between laboratories depending on reagents and methods used but is approximately 25 to 36 sec.

Prothrombin time (PT)

The clotting time of plasma after the addition of brain extract was introduced originally for prothrombin activity (hence, its name). It is now known to measure factors V, VII, X, and prothrombin. It is also sensitive to the presence of heparin and to hypofibrinogenemia. The principle of the prothrombin time is based on a potent preparation of human or rabbit brain emulsion added to citrated plasma. The mixture is recalcified and the clotting time estimated.

The prothrombin time is a non specific indicator of the extrinsic blood coagulation system. Normal range is 8 to 12 seconds (this varies among laboratories depending on reagents and methods used).

Thrombin clotting time (TCT)

Thrombin is added to plasma and the clotting time measured. The thrombin clotting time reflects conversion of fibrinogen to fibrin. The commonest causes of an increased TCT are the presence of heparin, or fibrin degradation products (FDP) or the depletion of fibrinogen. Dysfibrinogenemia can also result in a prolonged TCT. In multiple myeloma the abnormal globulin interferes with fibrin polymerization and may result in a prolonged TCT.

Reptilase time (RT)

A purified thrombin-like snake enzyme, from the Bothrops Atrox, may be used to replace thrombin in the thrombin clotting time tests. The snake venom is not inhibited by heparin, so that a prolonged TCT and a normal RT is diagnostic of the presence of heparin in the plasma. The RT is less prolonged than TCT in the presence of FDP. Dysfibrinogenemia, however, may cause the RT to be more prolonged than the TCT.

Fibrinogen

Fibrinogen can be quantified by using optical or automated methods. Dysfibrinogenemia can be characterized by immuno-electrophoresis.

Fibrin/fibrinogen degradation products (FDPs)

There are several methods to determine the presence of fibrin or fibrinogen degradation products. Most are based on agglutination reactions in the presence of FDP's which can be quantified. A common method involves a suspension of latex particles coated with antihuman fibrinogen which is mixed with serum. Agglutination is seen in the presence of FDP.

Assay of factor XIII

Factor XIII is activated during clotting from an inactive precursor. Calcium ions and thrombin are necessary for this activation. Activated factor XIII stabilizes the fibrin clot by a transamidation process. The stable clot is insoluble in 5-molar urea, whereas clots from a plasma deficient in factor XIII are soluble. A simple quantitative assay can be done based on clot solubility in 5-molar urea.

Circulating anticoagulants

Some coagulation abnormalities are caused by inhibition of specific factors rather than the lack of a factor. If a plasma is deficient in a particular factor or factors, addition of a normal sample will correct the deficiency whereas if the deficiency is caused by an inhibitor, the latter will affect the normal sample with which it is mixed, giving a prolonged coagulation time (e.g. using the PT or the activated partial thromboplastin time, APTT [see below]).

The lupus anticoagulant

The lupus anticoagulant appears to be an antibody (IgG, or IgM) with specificity for negatively charged phospholipids resulting in a prolonged APTT. A platelet neutralization test can be done to demonstrate the lupus anticoagulant. In general, plasma containing the lupus inhibitor will demonstrate a shortened APTT with the addition of free stored platelets which provide the phospholipid.

These tests can be performed by the nephrology team and are sufficient for preliminary investigation of the renal patient with a coagulation abnormality. More specific assays of the coagulation-fibrinolytic systems should remain within the realm of the hematologist whose help may be required. The latter may offer the following in certain circumstances:

Tests of plasminogen and plasmin

Tests for measuring plasminogen and plasmin levels directly are available in some laboratories. The activation of the plasminogen-plasmin system can also be inferred from the findings of a long thrombin time, a low fibrinogen level, and a raised level of fibrin degradation products.

Euglobulin-lysis time

Another test used to measure plasminogen-plasmin activation is the euglobulin-lysis time. In this test, a variant of the clot lysis time, the inhibitors of fibrinolysis have been substantially removed so as to shorten the time required to complete the assay. The rate of lysis of clotted I^{125}-fibrinogen can also be used to assess fibrinolysis.

D-dimer test

Measurement of FDP's does not distinguish between degradation of fibrin or fibrinogen. The D-dimer only detects fibrin derivatives exposed to the action of activated factor XIII. Activated factor XIII cross links fibrin and upon doing so provides specific antigenic determinants at the D-domain. When this cross linked fibrin is subjected to plasmin's action the D-domains of fibrin yield is the D-dimer. Detection of this D-dimer in plasma utilizing a monoclonal antibody offers a more specific test for fibrinolysis in-vivo.

The D-dimers are detectible in deep venous thrombosis and pulmonary embolism and may help distinguish pulmonary embolism from other pulmonary conditions. The test is also more specific for in vivo fibrinolysis and disseminated vascular coagulation. It can monitor clot lysis more specifically when using thrombolytic therapy. The disadvantage of the test is that it does not distinguish physiological from pathological conditions. For example, the test can be elevated due to healing postsurgery and could not distinguish a deep venous thrombosis developing in this situation. False positive results may also occur due to the presence of a rheumatoid factor.

The D-dimer test may have a place in the detection of *in vivo* fibrinolysis as it is sensitive, specific, and easily done by an immunoassay by latex agglutination. The presence of heparin, streptokinase or fibrinogen, does not interfere with the test.

Fibrinopeptides A and B

These are split from fibrinogen by thrombin. Radioimmunoassays have been developed especially for fibrinopeptide A. Increased levels of fibrinopeptide A have been found in vascular occlusive disease, post operatively with patients with thrombophlebitis, pulmonary embolism, acute infections, and in some patients with cancer, burns, fractures, systemic lupus erythematosus and active nephritis. Tests can be useful in certain conditions and can be more sensitive than detection of FDP's. The D-dimer test described above may prove to be more useful.

TESTS FOR MONITORING HEMODIALYSIS ANTICOAGULATION

Whole blood clotting time

The test is carried out in new glass test tubes measuring 3″ by $^3/_8$″ (76 mm by 9.5 mm). Venous blood is collected in a plastic or siliconized glass syringe by clean venipuncture using a 19 to 21 gauge needle. One milliliter of blood is placed directly in each of four tubes at 37° C and the tubes are tilted in turn at 30 sec intervals until each tube can be inverted without spilling blood. A stop watch is started once the blood is placed in the tubes and the clotting time is recorded from this time until the blood solidifies. The clotting time of each tube is recorded separately and the average of the four tests is reported. The clotting time of normal blood usually lies between 3 and 6 min.

Dialysis heparinization used to be monitored by whole blood clotting times and with systemic use of heparin, clotting times of around 15 to 20 min were usual. The obvious difficulty with this technique is that rapid adjustments in heparin dose cannot be made due to the prolonged clotting time. Whole blood activated clotting time improves such monitoring.

Whole blood activated clotting time (WBACT)

This test differs from the whole blood clotting time in that an activator of surface contact factors is added (kaolin, earth, or ground glass) to speed up the initial stages of the coagulation cascade. Thus, a normal WBACT ranges from 90 to 140 sec. During dialysis when 'ideal' amounts of heparin are given (i.e. sufficient to prevent thrombus formation on artificial surfaces without causing bleeding) the WBACT lies

between 200 and 240 sec. This time is short enough to adjust heparin dosage rapidly, if necessary. To carry out a WBACT the following are required:
1) Dry heat block calibrated to 37° C ± 0.5
2) Automatic pipette to deliver 0.2 ml
3) Stop watch
4) 12 mm × 75 mm glass test tubes
5) Tuberculin syringes with 21 gauge needles
6) Reagent (which will vary according to the manufacturer).

Set up:
1) Preheat test tubes in the heat block for 30 min.
2) Dispense 0.2 ml of reagent in test tubes.
3) Allow 10 min for reagents to warm.

Test procedure:
1) With tuberculin needle and syringe withdraw 0.4 ml sample of blood.
2) Remove needle from syringe and immediately dispense blood into warm test tube with reagent.
3) Start stop watch.
4) Gently swirl the mixture, return to heat block.
5) At 35 sec withdraw tube with tilt so that blood spreads along half of its length.
6) Return tube to heat block.
7) Repeat steps 5 and 6 exactly every 5 sec.
8) The WBACT is when blood gels or turns into a solid clot.

Useful devices which will perform WBACT and electrically rotate the glass tube and record electronically the clotting time are the Hemochron system (International Technidyne Corporation, New Jersey, USA) and the HemoTec system (HemoTec Inc., Englewood, CO, USA). Both excellently correlate the WBACT and heparin levels; the HemoTec system is the more sensitive of the two (R.M. Lindsay, personal observations).

Whole blood activated partial thromboplastin time (WBAPTT)

This test can also monitor dialysis heparinization and is based on the same principle as the WBACT except that the activator contains a platelet lipid surrogate as well as a foreign surface. An example of such a reagent is Thrombofax (Ortho-diagnostics) which was until recently widely used in dialysis units but unfortunately is now difficult to obtain. The procedure for the WBAPTT is identical to that for the WBACT, but the clotting times are somewhat shorter.

Activated partial thromboplastin time (APTT)

This is identical to the WBAPTT save plasma, rather than whole blood, is used. For this reason it is not ideal for clinical use but is a laboratory test.

TESTS OF PLATELETS AND PLATELET FUNCTION

(This section is not extensively referenced; further details may be obtained from major coagulation texts) (1–6)

Peripheral smear evaluation and platelet count

Examination of peripheral blood smear quickly provides definitive information. On a well seen normal smear there will be approximately ten platelets per high power ($\times 1,000$ magnification) field which corresponds to a normal platelet count ranging from 150 to $400 \times 10^9/l$ or 150,000 to $400,000/\mu l$.

Bleeding time

The bleeding time is defined as the interval between the infliction of a small standard cut and the moment when bleeding stops. Although this seems simple there are many variables. It is the most difficult test of hemostasis to standardize (7). When carefully standardized it gives reproducible results and affords the most important evaluation of a patient with a bleeding tendency.

The bleeding time measures the interruption by the platelet of the defect in the blood vessel wall and the subsequent formation of the hemostatic plug. It measures the early stages of hemostasis. A long bleeding time occurs when the number of circulating platelets is decreased, the platelets are abnormal in function, or when they cannot interrupt the vascular wall defect.

There are numerous methods for performing the bleeding test. All are modified from two techniques: The Duke technique (using an ear lobe puncture) or the Ivy technique (a puncture or incision is made in the forearm while the capillaries are under increased constant pressure from an inflated blood pressure cuff on the upper arm). The most useful way of performing the test is to use a template which allows a standardized depth of incision.

The bleeding time is usually normal when platelet counts exceed $100,000/mm^3$ ($100 \times 10^9/l$) and is prolonged in an inverse linear fashion when related to lower counts. A prolonged bleeding time with a platelet count exceeding $100,000/\mu l$ indicates impaired platelet function.

Platelet aggregometry

A platelet aggregometer is a simple device that records light transmission through a suspension of platelets. When platelets aggregate, light passes through the suspension more easily. To test aggregation a scale for each sample is set up from 0% (using platelet rich plasma) to 100% (platelet free plasma). Platelet rich plasma is placed in a cuvette and gently stirred into concentrations of an appropriate aggregation agent such as ADP, collagen, or thrombin, are added. As platelets aggregate the rate of increase of light transmission can be measured and recorded on a scale thereby estimating the velocity of platelet aggregation (%/minute).

Platelet factor 4 (PF4) and beta thromboglobulin (BTG) estimation

PF4 and BTG are platelet specific proteins which are released from the alpha granules (Table 3) as part of the basic platelet release reaction. These proteins can be measured by radioimmunoassay and elevated levels indicate recent platelet activity.

ANTICOAGULANTS

Heparin

Heparin is present in most tissues but exists in highest concentration in the liver and the lungs. It is water soluble and may be precipitated by alcohol, acetone and acid. Heparin is usually prepared by extraction from animal tissue in water, alkali or potassium thiocyanate and purified by repeated precipitations with alcohol or acetone. From chemical analysis of the purest preparations, Jorpes (8) found that it was composed almost entirely of hexuronic acid, hexosamine, and ash. The ash contained 7 to 8% sulfur and the anticoagulant activity was proportional to the sulfur content. Heparin carries a strong electronegative charge; in a 2% solution the specific conductance is 85×10^{-4} mhos. Commercial heparins consist of a polydisperse mixture of polysaccharides of variable molecular weights (approximately 10,000) and other properties (9). Furthermore, heparin can be separated into fractions with active and inactive anticoagulant properties (10). Because heparins are available, a suitable chemical assay is impossible. Therefore, standardization of a sample of heparin is based on comparison *in vitro* with a known standard in a nonspecific assay of anticoagulant activity. The USP unit of heparin is the quantity that will prevent 1.0 ml of citrated sheep plasma from clotting for 1 h after the addition of 0.2 ml of 1:100 $CaCl_2$ solution. Heparin sodium USP must contain at least 120 USP units/mg and is available in sterile water for intravenous injection in concentrations of 250 to 40,000 USP units/ml (11).

The anticoagulant effect of heparin occurs because it acts on the intrinsic coagulation pathway (Figure 3). It acts by enhancing the action of antithrombin III (ATIII) by binding to its lysyl groups, inducing a conformational change which increases the inhibitory action on factors XIIa, XIa, IXa, and Xa and thrombin. The heparin and ATIII complex inhibits thrombin preferentially. When formation of the ATIII-thrombin complex has occurred heparin readily dissociates from the complex. It, therefore, acts as a catalyst of the neutralizing process. Heparin stimulates the degradation of ATIII by thrombin and results in the reduction of circulating ATIII seen in patients who receive continuous therapy with heparin. Heparin also inhibits thrombin and factor Xa by a direct effect that is due to electrostatic attraction. The inhibition involves formation of reversible complexes that interfere with the procoagulant effects of both enzymes. This action probably accounts for the known antithrombotic effect of heparin that is frequently accompanied by bleeding, one of the major side effects of heparin therapy. At low heparin concentrations, fibrinogen acts as an antithrombin apparently due to an induced change in the charge of fibrinogen by heparin.

Heparin may be given in a low dose prophylactically in the

absence of actual thrombosis, or in larger doses to prevent further thrombosis and embolism in patients who already have established thrombosis. Heparin does not cause clot lysis. It acts to prevent further thrombosis and allows the normal fibrinolytic system to reabsorb the clot and allow recanalization.

When administered in low doses, prophylactically, heparin is usually given subcutaneously. For therapeutic use it should be given intravenously preferably by continuous infusions rather than by intermittent injection. Intramuscular injection of heparin is to be avoided because of the real hazard of muscle hematoma formation.

There are two general types of assays of the action of heparin on coagulation: those determining the effect on clotting in general and those measuring the rate of specific clotting protease inactivation. Present experience suggests that neither type can, in the individual patient, predict with assurance antithrombotic efficacy or protect from hemorrhage.

As noted earlier, less heparin is required for thrombosis prophylaxis than to prevent extension of thrombosis after intravascular coagulation has occurred. When overt thrombosis is extensive, more heparin may be required than when intravascular coagulation is minimal. On this basis, heparin therapy can be divided into three categories: Low dose (10,000 to 20,000 units/day), medium dose (20,000 to 60,000 units/day), and large dose (60,000 to 100,000 units/day). Low dose heparin, usually given subcutaneously, reduces significantly the incidence of postoperative pulmonary emboli, does not produce significant bleeding and requires no monitoring (12). medium dose heparin, given by constant intravenous infusion, is probably effective and safe for established venous thromboembolism. Monitoring is not essential but can give early warning of impending hemorrhage (12). Large dose heparin for florid thromboembolism is apparently safe if limited to under 48 h, but thereafter the risk of hemorrhage is high (12). The dosages of heparin required to conduct hemodialysis safely are given subsequently.

Heparin and platelets

The interrelations between heparin and platelets are complex and are only incompletely understood. Part of the complexity results from the heterogenerity of the currently available heparin preparations. Heparin in combination with ATIII is an extremely potent inhibitor of thrombin. Since the latter is one of the most potent platelet aggregating agents there is no doubt that heparin exerts an 'empty platelet effect' when thrombin is being generated.

Heparin may also induce thrombocytopenia (13). Most reductions are modest with counts rarely dropping below 100,000/ul (100×10^9/l). The mechanism of this is not certain. It occurs between the 2nd and 15th day following full dose heparin. Platelet counts return to normal rapidly after heparin is discontinued and may do so even if therapy is

continued. A much rarer reaction, usually begins several days after heparin is started and becomes severe between the 7th and 14th day. An immunological mechanism is suggested by the interval between the onset of thrombocytopenia and the start of therapy, the rapid increase in platelet count following discontinuation of heparin and the equally rapid decline in platelets after readministering heparin. Heparin-dependent antiplatelet antibodies have been identified in most patients with severe thrombocytopenia. The antibody appears to be directed against a platelet-heparin complex, but there may be some antibody-heparin interaction as well, and these latter complexes may directly aggregate circulating platelets. This *in vivo* aggregation can, itself, produce thrombosis. The thromboses are arterial rather than venous and can be disastrous with major arterial occlusions including myocardial infarction. The use of low dose heparin does not protect against this complication.

If mild thrombocytopenia ($>50 \times 10^9$/l) occurs during heparin therapy, start oral anticoagulants and closely monitor the platelet count stopping the heparin in 2 to 3 days. If already on oral anticoagulants it is reasonable to stop the heparin.

If the thrombocytopenia is severe ($<50 \times 10^9$/l) heparin must be stopped because of the risk of major arteriothrombosis. Ancrod, a defibrinating agent, would be an alternative anticoagulant to use when an anticoagulant is vital and may be started once the platelet count is greater than $50,000/\mu$l. If a patient has had heparin-associated thrombocytopenia further thromboembolic episodes should not be treated with heparin. Ancrod would be the treatment of choice in the initial phase until oral anticoagulants can be used. Furthermore, heparin cannot be used for dialysis anticoagulation; ancrod or citrate (preferably) are used in this situation.

This immunological interaction between platelets and heparin probably explains some recorded phenomena which are of relevance to blood-foreign surface interactions and, hence, to hemodialysis. As early as 1938 Best (14) showed that heparin did not prevent 'white thrombus' formation in cellophane arteriovenous shunts in rabbits but did so in other species. When blood is passed through glass bead columns, decreased (15), increased (16, 17) and unchanged (18) retention of platelets have been reported in the presence of heparin. These disparities may reflect variation in techniques for measuring platelet retention. Thompson and his colleagues (19) clearly demonstrated that heparin in final concentrations of 3 to 4 units/ml, *in vitro* or in plasma from volunteers given the drug, caused both increased retention of platelets within a test cell lined by cuprophan dialysis membranes (20) and also potentiation of platelet aggregation by ADP and adrenaline. Neither different heparin brands nor batch variations influenced these effects. Furthermore, Lindsay and colleagues (21) showed that commercial heparin in concentrations used during hemodialysis increases the retention of platelets on foreign surfaces such as those in the dialyzer circuit.

Coumarin and indandione anticoagulants

Oral anticoagulants are widely used in the prevention of recurrent thrombosis. Their action is to reduce the levels of vitamin K-dependent clotting factors. Vitamin K catalyzes the formation of γ-carboxyglutamic acids at specific sites in procoagulant factors II, VII, IX and X, as well as in the anticoagulant factors protein C and protein S. These modified amino acids are responsible for calcium and phospholipid surface binding and, thus, are essential for the functional activity of the vitamin K dependent enzyme. Coumarin blocks the regeneration of vitamin K, and thereby indirectly blocks formation of the γ-carboxyglutanic acid residue. When the action of vitamin K is blocked, unmodified proteins called PIVKAs (protein induced by vitamin K antagonists) appear in the circulation. While PIVKA's do not appear to have any physiologically important functional activity they may affect the PT assay performed with some reagents. Several days of treatment with coumarin drugs are required to reduce clotting factor activity to the proper therapeutic range. This is dependent on the different half lives and biological removal of the factors from the circulation.

The initiation stage of coumarin drug therapy represents a period of rapid change in procoagulant and anticoagulant factor levels and, therefore, risk of both bleeding and thrombosis are increased. When circulating levels of the vitamin K dependent factors are approximately 20 to 30% of normal, the risk of further thrombosis is sufficiently reduced and there is minimal risk of bleeding.

The most commonly used test for monitoring oral anticoagulant therapy is the PT which is influenced by the functional levels of factors II, VII, and X, as well as other factors not affected by oral anticoagulants. The reproducibility and reliability of this test are important for the optimal treatment of the patient. Variations in the test are common. Therefore, a new method to standardize reporting of prothrombin times for patients on oral anticoagulants has been recommended by the World Health Organization along with the International Committee on Thrombosis and Hemostasis; the International Normalized Ratio (INR) (22, 23). The responsiveness of thromboplastin reagent towards plasma samples containing an oral anticoagulant is described by an International Sensitivity Index (ISI). The use of the INR system should make treatment of patients at risk for thrombosis safer and more effective. An internationally accepted system of standardization will facilitate a better definition of the therapeutic range. INR can enable the physician to make a direct comparison between PT values regardless of the reagent-instrument system used and make interlaboratory correlation easy. The normal therapeutic range for INR is 2 to 4. This compares to therapeutic range of the PT (when using the most widely used commercial rabbit brain thromboplastins) of 15 to 18 sec with a control range of 9 to 12 sec.

There is a relatively high incidence of adverse reactions to indandione oral anticoagulants. There are mainly hypersensitivity reactions including skin rashes, pyrexia, diarrhea, neutropenia, thrombocytopenia, hepatitis and nephropathy. Therefore, these drugs have been largely supplanted by the various coumarin derivatives, especially warfarin (Coumadin) and bishydroxy-coumarin (Dicumarol). Bleeding is the main side effect of warfarin but skin necrosis is a rare complication which can occur in patients with protein C deficiency at the start of warfarin therapy. Coumarins also cross the placenta and should not be used in pregnancy as hemorrhage of the newborn may occur; congenital defects, spontaneous abortions and stillbirths have been described.

Many commonly used drugs (Table 4) interact with the coumarin drugs. They may act on any of the various mechanisms involved in the absorption, transport, biotransformation and excretion of these anticoagulants. Barbiturates antagonize the action of coumarins leading to 'Coumarin resistance' and potential overdosage when they are withdrawn. Other drugs such as salicylates and phenobarbitone potentiate coumarin action. Broad spectrum antibiotics and nonabsorbable sulfonamides suppress vitamin K synthesis by gut flora and may potentiate the action of coumarin. The actions of phenytoin, tolbutamide and chlorpropamide may be potentiated by coumarins. The physician should be aware of the many drugs that can interact with the coumarin anticoagulants. There are many other factors which modify the effects of the coumarin drugs, especially the functional effficiency of the liver and dietary intake of vitamin K.

Anticoagulant therapy should be done smoothly without giving a loading dose. The prothrombin time becomes maximally prolonged 36 to 72 h following administration of the coumarins due to factor VII reduction. However, the antithrombotic action is not maximal until plasma levels of factors IX, X, and prothrombin are significantly depressed. This may require several days of therapy. Consequently, it is safer to give approximately 10 mg of warfarin daily until the prothrombin time is within the therapeutic range and then adjust the dose of warfarin to keep the PT at 1.5 to 1.8 x

Table 4. Drug and other interactions with warfarin.

Increased response	Decreased response
phenylbutazone	cholestyramine
sulfinpyrazone	barbiturates
clofibrate	rifampin
acetylsalicylic acid	oral contraceptives
disulfiram (antabuse)	griseofulvin
trimethoprim-sulfamethazole	carbamazepine
sulfonamides	uremia
cimetidine	hypothyroidism
alcohol	
chloramphenicol	
metronidazole	
cephalosporins (third generation)	
anabolic steroids	
allopurinol	
thyroxine	
amiodarone	
combination of antibiotics	
poor vitamin K intake	
malabsorption	

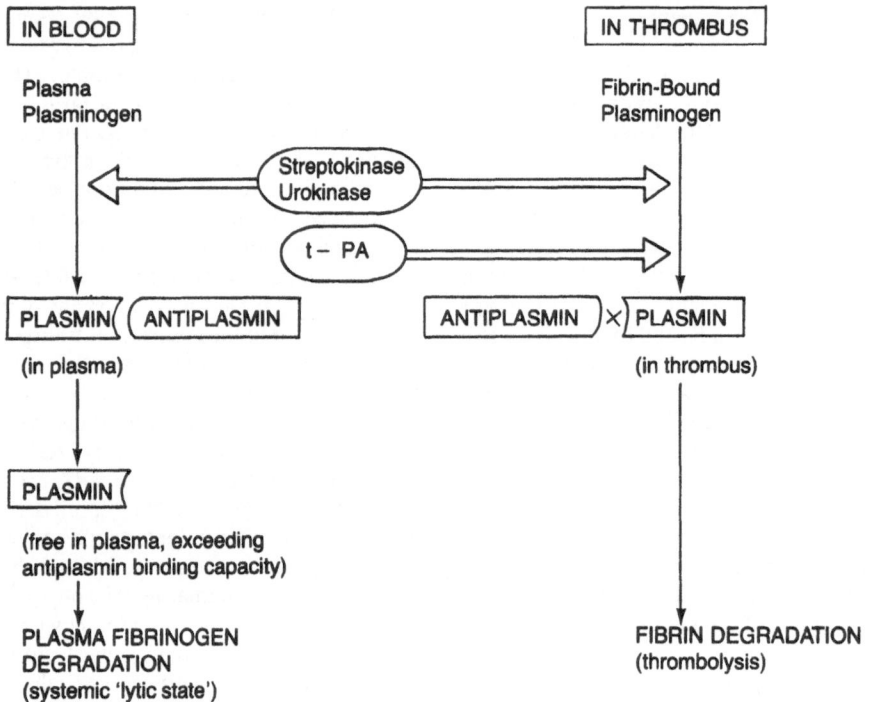

Figure 7. Schematic mechanism of action of fibrinolytic agents.

normal control (INR 2 to 4 times). It is therapeutically as effective and less dangerous than giving a large loading dose.

THROMBOLYTIC AGENTS

There are three thrombolytic agents: the commonly used streptokinase, urokinase, and the newest thrombolytic agent tissue plasminogen activator (t-PA).

Thrombolytic agents (24–26) stimulate the formation of plasmin, the active enzyme which digests the fibrin clot. Streptokinase and urokinase indiscriminantly activate both plasma plasminogen and fibrin bound plasminogen. Plasmin generated in plasma is rapidly neutralized by α_2 antiplasmin. However, when sufficient plasmin is formed to exhaust the blood antiplasmin binding capacity, free circulating plasmin can degrade plasma fibrinogen. This systemic 'lytic' state can cause bleeding as well as clot lysis. Tissue plasminogen activator preferentially activates fibrin-bound plasminogen. This generates fibrin-bound plasmin which is inaccessible to neutralization by α_2 antiplasmin. Fibrin-bound plasmin in the thrombus promotes local fibrin degradation (thrombolysis) with little or no systemic effects on circulating plasma fibrinogen. A schematic diagram of the action of thrombolytic agents is shown below in Figure 7.

Streptokinase and urokinase

These agents are utilized for a variety of thromboembolic conditions even though the exact indications are not well elucidated. Beside the question of efficacy, the major reason for reluctance in the use of thrombolytic agents is the high rate of bleeding complications in the early therapeutic trials. With proper care and avoidance of invasive procedures the rate of bleeding complications may be equivalent to the rate seen with heparin. Streptokinase is approved for use in acute pulmonary embolism, deep venous thrombosis, arterial thrombosis, acute myocardial infarction, and occlusion of vascular access shunts (e.g. for dialysis). Urokinase is only approved for acute pulmonary embolism and occlusion of vascular access shunts.

Streptokinase

Streptokinase was the first activator of the fibrinolytic system to become available. It is a protein with the electrophorectic mobility of human β-globulin and its molecular mass is about 43,000 daltons. It is produced from many forms of Streptococci from which it acquires its name, but plasminogen activator activity can be produced by many organisms including E coli, Staphylococci, Pseudomonas, and Clostridia. There is very marked species variability in the response to streptokinase; human plasminogen is more readily activated than rabbit, canine or bovine plasminogens. Streptokinase, like other streptococcal proteins, can be antigenic in man, and antibodies are detected in the normal population in varying amounts. Because it is rapidly bound by antibody, enough streptokinase must be given to bind antibody and any other non-specific inhibitors before the fibrinolytic enzyme system is affected. Thus, the effect on lysis times *in vitro* is dose dependent. The optimum concentration of streptokinase is considered to be 1,000 to 2,000 units/ml of plasma. When streptokinase is discontinued, fibrinolytic activity declines to preinfusion levels within an hour. However, a coagulation defect persists for up to 24 h because of the digestion of coagulation factors such as fibrinogen, factors V and VIII and, perhaps, some inhibition of platelet aggregation.

Urokinase

It has been known since 1885 that urine has proteolytic activity. Specific fibrinolytic activity was noted by Macfarlane and Pilling (27), and shown by Williams (28) to be due to a plasminogen activator in urine; the name urokinase was suggested by Sobel and collegues (29).

Urokinase is a colorless protein (54,000 daltons) that is highly stable over a wide pH and temperature range. It is, itself, a proteolytic enzyme which activates plasminogen according to first order kinetics likely by splitting lysine or arginine bonds or both. It seems likely that urokinase is elaborated by the kidneys. Urokinase appears to be nonantigenic and less toxic than streptokinase. Although a serum inhibitor is present, its levels are much more constant than with streptokinase so it is easier to use a fixed priming dose and a uniform maintenance dose on a body weight basis. Moreover, in *in vitro* systems containing both fibrinogen and fibrin, urokinase as compared with streptokinase, produces relatively more fibrinolysis and less break down of fibrinogen so anticoagulant effects are less likely.

Thrombolytic therapy

Thrombolytic agents should be administered in a loading dose with approximately 1,250,000 units of streptokinase over a period of 30 min or 4,400 IU/kg of urokinase over 10 min. Hydrocortisone 100 mg should be given before and every 12 to 24 h during streptokinase therapy to prevent side effects.

Following a loading dose, streptokinase is given in a maintenance dose of 100,000 Units/h for 24 h in pulmonary embolism and 42 to 72 h in deep venous thrombosis. Urokinase is given in a dose of 4,400 IU/kg/h for 12 to 24 h in pulmonary embolism and 24 to 48 h in deep venous thrombosis. Anticoagulant therapy (usually heparin) is initiated after thrombolytic drugs have been stopped and the APTT falls to approximately twice the control value. A loading dose of heparin is not necessary unless the APTT is well below the therapeutic range. Therapy is then continued for the usual period of approximately 10 days.

Thrombolytic therapy does not require close monitoring of the control value since a fixed dose is given in most situations. The only reason to monitor therapy is to ensure that at least a fibrinolytic state has been reached. A fibrinolytic state can most conveniently be determined by a thrombin time (TT) that should be obtained prior to therapy and approximately 3 to 4 h after initiation of treatment. The goal

is to achieve a significant prolongation above the baseline value which for the TT is more than 3 sec above the control value. If not achieved, a repeat loading dose should be given and its effect measured 3 h later. Patients who fail to achieve a fibrinolytic state with streptokinase should be switched to urokinase since antibody neutralization of streptokinase may be responsible.

Hemorrhage is the major complication of thrombolytic therapy as it is with all anticoagulants. Scrupulous care must be exercised to exclude patients with recent surgery or recent invasive procedures and to avoid invasive procedures during therapy. Venous phlebotomy should be reduced to a minimum and pressure dressings should be used at the venipuncture site. Contraindications to therapy must be closely observed to avoid treating patients at risk of bleeding. Minor local bleeding can be controlled locally but major bleeding requires discontinuation of therapy. Packed red cells can be given to replace blood loss and fresh frozen plasma or cryoprecipitate can be given to correct the coagulopathy. The half life of streptokinase (and urokinase) is very short (15 min) and, thus, the fibrinolytic state resolves quickly. It is very rarely needed to give an antifibrinolytic agent such as aminocaproic acid.

Streptokinase is associated with a high incidence of fever and allergic reactions and some patients experience nausea, vomiting, and flushing with treatment. These reactions can be treated with antihistamines and antipyretics such as acetaminophen or possibly prevented with hydrocortisone which, as indicated above, should be given before starting therapy and every 12 to 24 h during treatment.

Local therapy

Special mention should be given to local therapy in which direct infusion is given into peripheral vessels including dialysis access shunts which have clotted. The infusion catheter should be adjacent to or directly in the substance of the thrombus. Streptokinase should be given by continuous infusion for 24 to 72 h in a dose of 7,500 IU/h (no loading dose). In general, a systemic fibrinolytic effect is not evident but may become manifest 16 to 18 h after infusion. The thrombin time performed at 8 to 12 h intervals may help identify whether a systemic fibrinolytic effect has occurred. Monitoring the success of thrombolytic therapy is usually done by injecting contrast material locally. For local infusions urokinase is seldom used and appropriate doses have not been established. Depending upon the reason for the thrombolytic therapy, heparin may be required (e.g. femoral artery thrombosis). If given, it should be administered immediately in a standard loading dose followed by continuous infusion as done routinely.

Recombinant human tissue plasminogen activator (rt-PA)

As indicated above streptokinase and urokinase activate the fibrinolytic system by converting both circulating and fibrin bound plasminogen to plasmin and a systemic fibrinolytic state ensues. In contrast rt-PA (30–32) derived from a non-cancerous mammalian cell line through DNA technology, is a potent thrombolytic agent achieving rapid thrombolysis through a high affinity for fibrin and a low activity for circulating plasma plasminogen. Plasminogen activation by rt-PA is enhanced in the presence of fibrin and, therefore, it is relatively clot specific converting fibrin-bound plasminogen on the clot surface. Initially, it was thought that no systemic fibrinogenolysis occurred. However, rt-PA infusions do result in a systemic lytic state but much less marked than with streptokinase or urokinase and usually only after longer infusion times. Fibrin specificity is, therefore, relative because it can be overcome and fibrinogenolysis may occur.

Trials using rt-PA have shown it to be safe and effective as a thrombolytic agent. As it avoids the profound systemic fibrinogenolysis associated with the currently employed thrombolytic agents it appears likely to replace the use of both streptokinase and urokinase in the very near future.

INHIBITORS OF FIBRINOLYSIS

Epsilon aminocaproic acid (EACA)

The fibrinolysis inhibitory effects of EACA appear to be principally via inhibition of plasminogen activator substances and to a lesser degree through antiplasmin activity. The drug is absorbed rapidly following oral administration and whether administered by the oral or intravenous route a major portion of the compound is recovered and metabolized in the urine. The renal clearance of EACA is high (about 75% of the creatinine clearance); thus, the drug is excreted rapidly. After prolonged administration EACA distributes throughout the extravascular and intravascular compartments and readily penetrates human red blood cells and other tissue cells. The usual intravenous dose is 0.1 g/kg every 6 h, for severe bleeding or 1 g/h following a 5 g loading dose orally. Total daily dose should not exceed 30 g.

Tranexamic acid (AMCA)

This agent has properties similar to those of EACA but is more potent on a weight basis. It is absorbed well from the gastrointestinal tract although less completely than EACA and is widely distributed throughout body fluid compartments and excreted in the urine. The dose is 10 mg/kg intravenously or 30 to 50 mg/kg orally every 4 h for control of systemically enhanced fibrinolysis.

The therapeutic use of inhibitors of fibrinolysis is indicated for primary systemic fibrinolysis sufficient to cause hemorrhage. This situation is extremely rare. Although bleeding due to local fibrinolysis has been controlled by EACA or AMCA, side effects are often unacceptably high. For example, although bleeding from the kidney can be controlled in hemophiliac patients the high incidence of urinary tract obstruction makes their use unjustifiable. Thrombotic episodes may occur remote from the site of bleeding if these agents are given systemically. These drugs should not be used without advice of a hematologist.

ANCROD

Ancrod is an enzyme purified from the venom of the Malayan pit viper. Its use as an antithrombotic agent resulted from the observation that bites from the viper caused hypofibrinogenemia but little bleeding. The proteolytic effect of ancrod on fibrinogen differs from that of thrombin in that ancrod cleaves only fibrinopeptide A from the fibrinogen molecule. The resultant fibrin is more susceptible to fibrinolysis. Ancrod does not activate factor XIII and does not diminish factors V, VIII, IX, or X. FDPs rise during the first 36 h of treatment and then return to normal rapidly. Following cessation of therapy fibrinogen takes 2 to 3 weeks to reach normal levels. Ancrod must be given parenterally, preferably intravenously because intramuscular therapy often results in drug resistance. Doses recommended are 1 U/kg intravenously for the first 12 h followed by 0.5 U/kg every 12 h thereafter. Fibrinogen levels are used to monitor ancrod aiming for approximately 50 mg/dl (0.5 g/l). Bleeding is not a frequent complication. If it does occur, fibrinogen replacement can be given (by the use of cryoprecipitate) and an antivenom is available.

ANTIPLATELET AGENTS

Antiplatelet agents: effect on vessel wall prostacyclin production

Understanding of the use of platelet inhibitor drugs in thrombosis has to take into account the natural contribution of the vessel wall to the inhibition of thrombosis. The vessel wall may inhibit the process of thrombosis in at least two ways. One of these is in the release of plasminogen activator which can cause the localized formation of plasmin to lyse fibrin. The second mechanism is associated with formation of a prostaglandin metabolite, initially discovered by Moncada and colleagues (33) and subsequently named prostacyclin (34). This compound seems to be the main prostaglandin metabolite in vascular tissue, being most highly concentrated on the endothelium, and progressively decreasing in activity towards the adventitial surface (35, 36). Prostacyclin is a potent systemic vasodilator (37) and the most potent inhibitor of platelet aggregation yet discovered (33). It inhibits platelet adherence to damaged vessel walls (38–40) and possesses antithrombotic properties (40, 41). Prostacyclin activates platelet membrane adenyl cyclase which in turn increases platelet cyclic AMP.

Presumably, similar to the synthesis of the prostaglandin, thromboxane A_2, by the platelet, the vessel wall synthesizes prostacyclin from its own precursors; arachidonic acid is converted into cyclic endoperoxides by the cyclo-oxygenase enzyme and such endoperoxides are subsequently converted into prostacyclin by a prostacyclin synthetase enzyme. It appears, therefore, that the generation of prostacyclin is a physiologic mechanism that protects the vessel wall from platelet deposition and an imbalance between the formation of prostacyclin and thromboxane A_2 may be one of the mechanisms leading to thrombosis. If this is the case, one might expect that drugs used to inhibit platelet activation might also inhibit prostacyclin formation and hence, nullify the desired effect of preventing thrombosis in natural vessels.

Aspirin (acetylsalicylic acid)

Aspirin (42) is hydrolyzed into a salicylate and the free acetyl group released covalently binds to cyclo-oxygenase in the platelet. Acetylation of cyclo-oxygenase irreversibly inhibits the enzyme. Therefore, in platelets, incapable of re-synthesizing unacetylated cyclo-oxygenase, the inhibitory effects of aspirin persist for the life time of the platelet (7 to 10 days). Endothelial cells, however, can resynthesize cyclo-oxygenase thus regaining their capacity to produce prostaglandin PGI_2 (prostacyclin) within hours. Simultaneous inhibition of vascular PGI_2 formation would tend to negate the antithrombotic effect of aspirin in blocking platelet thromboxane synthesis causing 'the aspirin dilemma'. There is evidence that platelet cyclo-oxygenase may be more sensitive to inhibition by aspirin than vascular cyclo-oxygenase. It has been found that a single low dose of aspirin 40 to 80 mg can almost completely inhibit platelet aggregation and thromboxane synthesis while largely sparing vascular prostacyclin (PGI_2) forming capacity. It may be that aspirin should be administered on a less frequent than daily basis.

Nonsteroidal anti-inflammatory drugs and sulfinpyrazone

These drugs compete with arachidonic acid for binding to cyclo-oxygenase in a dose dependent manner. Therefore, these drugs can cause reversible inhibition of platelet cyclo-oxygenase the function of which is restored as the drugs are eliminated from the circulation (i.e. within hours). Sulfin-pyrazone is inferior to aspirin in the management of patients with transient cerebral ischemia and unstable angina and the results with secondary prevention of myocardial infarction have been inconsistent.

Dipyridamole

The mechanism of antiplatelet action of this drug is not clearly defined. It inhibits platelet cyclic AMP phosphodiesterase resulting in accumulation of cyclic AMP. In addition, dipyridamole may stimulate vascular prostacylin release, potentiate the effects of prostacyclin and inhibit thromboxane formation. Dipyridamole has been shown to normalize increased platelet turnover in patients with prosthetic heart valves, arterial grafts, arteriovenous shunts, and aortocoronary grafts. Unlike aspirin, it does not inhibit platelet aggregation or prolong the bleeding time at blood concentrations achieved with therapeutic dosage. The clinical antithrombotic efficacy of dipyridamole is primarily observed in combination with aspirin with which it may have additive effects. It is used as an adjunct to aspirin and may be effective in the secondary prevention of myocardial infarct, prosthetic heart valve embolism, and coronary artery graft occlusion.

Fish oil containing omega-3 fatty acids

The omega-3 fatty acid eicosapentaenoic acid (EPA) is similar to arachidonic acid in that it contains 20 carbons but it contains five rather than four double bonds and it competes with arachidonic acid for incorporation into membrane phospholipids (43). Phospholipase activated platelets release both EPA and arachidonic acid and these free fatty acids then compete as substrates for cyclo-oxygenase. In platelets, the predominant product of EPA metabolism is thromboxane A_3 which does not possess the potent platelet aggregatory and vasoconstrictory properties of thromboxane A_2 formed from arachidonic acid. In contrast, PGI_3 derived from EPA, released from endothelial cell membrane phospholipids in subjects taking fish oils retains the antiplatelet and vasodilatory properties of PGI_2 (prostacyclin) that is derived from arachidonic acid. The antithrombotic and antiatherogenic effects of the omega-3 fatty acids that have been recently described are unlikely to be due exclusively to their modest antiplatelet action. Effects on serum lipids, cell membrane fluidity and leukocyte function, probably also contribute to their beneficial action. In Eskimos who consume a considerable amount of fish oil the ratio of EPA to arachidonic acid in platelet membrane lipids approximates unity.

Thromboxane synthetase inhibitors

Experience so far with thromboxane synthetase inhibitors has been disappointing. Current preparations lack prolonged and complete inhibition of thromboxane formation and there are platelet agonist effects of the endoperoxides that accumulate with thromboxane synthetase inhibition.

Prostacyclin and stable analogues

These bind to specific platelet surface receptors and inhibit platelet activation by raising intracellular levels of cyclic AMP. Since prostacyclin is unstable it must be administered by continuous intravenous infusion. Recently developed stable prostacyclin analogues such as iloprost (Schering Health Care, UK) are active when used orally. Increasing clinical applications of these agents include their use in cardiopulmonary bypass and hemodialysis to prevent extracorporeal platelet activation and consumption, in peripheral vascular disease, Raynaud's phenomenon, pre-eclampsia and thrombotic thrombocytopenic purpura. Some of the efficacy of prostacyclin may be attributable not only to its antiplatelet action but also to favorable hemodynamic effects.

Ideal dose and therapeutic combinations of commonly used antiplatelet agents

Recent evidence indicates that the prescribed dose of each of the platelet inhibitor drugs may be crucial in determining the final therapeutic outcome of the patient. A recent summary of this evidence is outlined below (44).

Acetylsalicylic acid (aspirin)

A very low dosage of aspirin (40 to 325 mg/day) is sufficient in most patients to have an antithrombotic effect inhibiting platelet cyclo-oxygenase without affecting vessel wall prostacyclin synthesis.

An intermediate dosage of aspirin (0.5 to 1.5 g/day) may be potentially beneficial to some patients whereas to others the antithrombotic effect may be partially abolished by the inhibition of prostacyclin synthesis.

Larger doses of aspirin (more than 1.5 g/day), may be potentially beneficial in a few patients and it appears that only very high dosages (perhaps more than 10 g/day, might promote thrombosis.

Dipyridamole and its combination with aspirin

Most of the information regarding the ideal potential antithrombotic dose of dipyridamole has been obtained by platelet survival studies (45). The decreased platelet survival found in patients with prosthetic heart valves could be lengthened by high dosage dipyridamole therapy (100 mg four times per day). A similar correction could be produced by the combination of intermediate dosages of dipyridamole (100 mg/day) and aspirin (1 g/day) (46). Moncada and Korbut (47) examined various intravenous doses of both drugs singly and in combination in the rabbit and observed that maximal inhibition of platelet aggregation in flowing blood was obtained by combining intermediate dosages of dipyridamole (3 mg/kg) and aspirin (10 mg/kg). Such a combination has therapeutic attraction because each drug affects platelet metabolism at a different level and, therefore, might be expected to increase the probability of therapeutic effectiveness.

Sulfinpyrazone

The available evidence suggests that 400 mg of sulfinpyrazone per day has virtually no effect on platelets whereas 800 mg/day is highly effective and that this latter dosage has only a minimal effect on prostacyclin formation so it is unlikely to promote thrombus formation.

Table 5. Side effects of antiplatelet agents.

Side effect	Percentage of patients using		
	Aspirin	Sulfin-pyrazone	Dipyri-damole
Gastrointestinal upset	18	? (Negligible)	12
Bleeding	7	3	4
Headache	4	? (low)	9
Skin rash	2	?	3

Drug side effects

The most commonly used platelet inhibitor drugs (aspirin, dipyridamole, and sulfinpyrazone) are potent pharmacological agents with known side effects. This is important because when they are used as antithrombotic agents they usually are given for prolonged periods. Table 5 summarizes the most important side effects when compared with placebo; the data have been compiled by Fuster and Chesebro (44) from recent prospective studies.

Aspirin

Ingestion of 1.0 g of aspirin per day will cause gastrointestinal side effects in about 20% of patients and 7% will have a bleeding complication, most often of the gastroduodenal tract, that will necessitate medical attention. Plasma uric acid levels can increase in patients with good renal function and clinical gout can be precipitated. This latter complication is not relevant to the dialysis population. Allergy, particularly in the form of skin rashes, is uncommon.

Dipyridamole

Gastrointestinal symptoms such as epigastric discomfort and nausea occur in approximately 10% of patients taking dipyridamole. These symptoms, however, tend to subside after a few days of medication particularly if the drug is given with meals. In contrast with aspirin when dipyridamole is given alone or in combination with anticoagulants it does not seem to increase the incidence of gastritis, gastroduodenal ulcer, or the tendency to bleed. Because dipyridamole is a vasodilator headaches occur in almost 10% of patients but they become a major problem only rarely.

Sulfinpyrazone

Side effects caused by sulfinpyrazone seem to be less pronounced than those noted with aspirin or dipyridamole. In particular, there are fewer gastrointestinal side effects. As noted previously sulfinpyrazone increases the sensitivity to oral coumarin anticoagulants and prolongs the prothrombin time. Thus, modification of coumadin dosage is highly likely when the two drugs are used together. The drug is, of course, a potent uricosuric agent. In the nondialysis population the possibility of precipitation of uric acid stones must be considered. Sulfinpyrazone also increases the sensitivity of sulfonylurea hypoglycemic agents and, if prescribed, attention should be given to the blood glucose level.

THE BLEEDING TENDENCY OF UREMIA

A bleeding tendency is common in uremia; this has been known since 1907 (48). While deficiencies in factors V and VII occur in some uremic patients (49), platelet abnormalities form the major coagulation defects in such patients and these may be both quantitative and qualitative. These abnormalities, which have been reviewed by Rabiner (50) often prolong bleeding time (51, 52). However, whether the uremic individual has a prolonged bleeding time, thrombocytopenia, or qualitative platelet abnormalities either alone or in combination, platelet life span appears to be normal (51) even when the patient is maintained on dialysis (53). When arteriovenous shunts are used for vascular access, however, platelet survival is shortened (45).

Both the qualitative and quantitative platelet abnormalities can improve with dialysis. This was first noted over 20 years ago by several groups (51, 54–56), who concluded that the thrombocytopathy of uremia was due to dialyzable factors that suppressed megakaryocytes and hence decreased platelet production and, in addition, acted as circulating toxins impairing the platelet release reaction. More recent studies have confirmed this and have shown that efficient hemodialysis or peritoneal dialysis can return platelet function to normal in spite of the trauma of the extracorporeal circuit (57–61). It appears, however, that the uremic platelet defect is not entirely explained by dialyzable toxins and that there may be nondialyzable plasma factors as well. There may be decreased concentrations of factor VIII-von Willebrand activity which are not corrected by dialysis (62). This accounts for the fact that the infusion of cryoprecipitate (providing factor VIII-von Willebrand activity) and desmopresin (which stimulates release of von Willebrand factor from endothelial cells) will shorten the prolonged bleeding time in uremic subjects (63). There is also a nondialyzable heat labile factor in the plasma of uremic patients capable of inhibiting production of platelet cyclo-oxygenase and at the same time stimulating endothelial prostacyclin production (64). Both effects, of course will lead to defective platelet adhesion-aggregation. Di Minno and colleagues (65) suggest that uremic platelets have a defect in arachidonic acid production from phospholipids and a storage pool defect; the first is improved by dialysis, the second is not.

Another factor that must be taken into account in any consideration of the uremic platelet defect is the influence of the hematocrit. As early as 1910 Duke (66) noticed that in some forms of anemia the bleeding time was prolonged out of proportion to any coexisting thrombocytopenia and that reversal of anemia by blood transfusion correlates with a shortening or correction of the bleeding time. These observations have been subsequently confirmed (67, 68). These studies initially could not exclude the possibility that improvements in the bleeding time after transfusion of homologous red cells was related to hemostatic components adsorbed onto the red cell membrane and made available at the site of hemostatic plug formation. However, a very recent paper showing that the increase in autologous red cells induced by recombitant human erythropoeitin also correlated with a shortening or return to normal of the bleeding time definitely establishes a role for red cells in the pathyphysiology of the uremic hemostatic defect (69). These observations may be of relevance for good quality hemodialysis is likely to be associated with the achievement of satisfactory hemoglobin levels and that in the near future the use of recombitant human erythropoeitin may become more widespread.

The platelet defect and its ability to be improved by dialysis may influence the interaction between blood foreign surfaces and anticoagulants that occurs during hemodialysis. This interaction will now be discussed in some detail.

HEMODIALYSIS: THE PROBLEMS OF THROMBOSIS AND ANTICOAGULATION

When blood flows over a foreign surface, protein adsorption occurs immediately (70). Frequently, this is followed by platelet adhesion (71) and activation of the intrinsic coagulation pathway (72). The last two phenomena occur more or less independently (73), but in the latter stage of blood clotting on a foreign surface there is a mutual interaction between the coagulation process and the platelet reaction. When prothrombin is converted to thrombin the platelet release reaction will be stimulated enhancing platelet-adhesion-aggregation. On the other hand, during the platelet release reaction which follows platelet foreign surface contact, platelet factor III is released and augments the classical coagulation pathway. The end result is, of course, thrombus formation. The situation may also be enhanced by adherence of leukocytes since Niemetz and his colleagues (74) demonstrated that leukocytes obtained from the used membranes of an artificial kidney have enhanced procoagulant activity. The relative importance of white cell adhesion in the final common pathway (i.e. thrombus formation) is not fully determined. There is recent interest, however, in alternative pathway complement activation occurring when blood contacts the cellulose based membranes used in the artificial kidney and it is known that this is associated with a transient leukopenia and leukocyte aggregation (75). Further studies have suggested that C5a production in the complement cascade is the factor which causes both neutropenia and leukocyte aggregation (76). It is highly possible, therefore, that C5a induced leukocyte aggregation is associated with the release of leukocyte thromboxane A_2 which, in turn, may lead to *in vivo* platelet aggregation and destruction by those platelets on the foreign surface. Studies of this possible interaction are indicated.

The role of the platelet in surface induced thrombus formation appears to be well-defined. To prevent thrombosis taking place during hemodialysis, heparin is used. But, it has been pointed out that heparin has no inhibitory effect on the platelet foreign surface interaction. Indeed, it has been shown that in concentrations used during hemodialysis it actually enhances ADP induced platelet aggregation (19) and the retention of platelets on a foreign surface (21). Thus, heparin cannot be considered as an ideal anticoagulant for extracorporeal use. Thrombus formation can take place upon the membranes of the artificial kidney in spite of adequate heparinization and this may be associated with the fall in platelet count over the course of dialysis and with demonstrable retention of platelets by that membrane surface (77). The hypothesis that platelet retention by that membrane is an important step in the reaction which subsequently leads to thrombus formation has been proven by a double blind trial involving antiplatelet agents (78). Furthermore, the substitution of a dialysis membrane with low platelet retaining properties into a dialyzer known to have enhanced *in vivo* thrombus formation also reduced the amount of thrombus formed during the dialysis procedure (79). Thus, the nature of the dialysis membrane and the geometry to which that membrane conforms are important (80).

From the heparin anticoagulation point of view the patient walks a tight rope between under anticoagulation with the risk of blood clotting, and over heparinization with potential bleeding from cannulation sites and other areas such as the gut and uterus. Because of these problems more precise control of heparin anticoagulation has been recommended using a series of WBACTs (or WBAPTTs) to delineate a 'heparin profile' for the patient. From this profile an indication of the heparin loading dose required and the rate of constant infusion necessary during dialysis can be calculated (81). Details of the mathematical modelling approach to heparin therapy are given in Chapter 4. There is no doubt that with a given patient, over a short period of time, the 'heparin profile' works and trouble free dialysis anticoagulation can be achieved. However, in spite of this technique, variability in heparin requirements has been noted in dialysis patients. It appears that heparinization cannot be uniformly judged on a body weight basis and that a given patient may require different heparin dosages from time to time. It may be that currently available commercial heparin has variable potency. On the other hand, it may equally be possible that some of the variability rests with the uremic patient and his dialysis treatment; for example, efficient hemodialysis can improve platelet function in spite of extracorporeal trauma. Thus, it can be anticipated that platelet function in a given patient will be different at the commencement of renal replacement therapy from that found after 6 months of adequate dialysis. Accordingly, the patient's propensity to have platelet retention by relatively bioincompatible materials will change with improvement of uremia by dialysis treatment. Furthermore, the platelet dialysis membrane interaction is implicated in thrombus formation during hemodialysis. Platelet retention by foreign surfaces in this situation is followed by the release of platelet constituents including platelet factor 4 (PF4) which is released in parallel with serotonin (82). PF4 appears to be a substance in the molecular weight range of 7,000 to 9,000 which has heparin neutralizing activity (HNA) (83). Any demonstrable HNA in plasma is believed to be a function of PF4 released by platelets and its level, if raised, is likely to reflect recent or continuing platelet activity as might be found in arterial thrombosis (84). HNA levels have been increased in the plasma of patients with end-stage renal disease treated by hemodialysis but not in nondialyzed patients with severe chronic renal failure, patients treated by peritoneal dialysis or in those with normal renal function who have been exposed to the extracorporeal circulation of the heart lung bypass, 48 to 72 h before testing (85). It was postulated, therefore, that the trauma of extracorporeal circulation causes platelets to release PF4 which is not cleared by dialysis but is by the human kidney. The elevation of plasma

HNA, so caused, must have therapeutic implications for heparin dosage schedules during hemodialysis. For example, a 70 kg man with end-stage renal failure and hematocrit of 20% is likely to have a plasma volume of about 4,000 ml and at a plasma HNA level of 0.140 units/ml has the immediate ability to neutralize 560 units of heparin. A continuous infusion of 7,000 units of heparin over 3 h will run at 40 units/min, a common dialysis procedure. There is, therefore, the potential for complete neutralization of heparin over the first 14 min of infusion. During this period, the platelet foreign surface interaction will generate further HNA release and prolong the period of serious underdosage. If a continuous heparin infusion is contemplated it may be advisable to start this at least 15 min before dialysis commences or to use an adequate systemic loading dose. It has already been confirmed that there is a correlation between an elevated plasma HNA level and the necessity to give greater than normal heparin dosages during hemodialysis (85).

There has been interest in the use of prostacyclin (PGI_2) for dialysis anticoagulation. Woods and his colleagues (86) demonstrated that dogs could be dialyzed without heparin if a constant infusion of prostacyclin (2 μ/g/min; equivalent to 60 to 100 ng/kg/min) was used. They subsequently demonstrated that this agent can be used safely for human dialysis and that an infusion of 9 ng/kg/min has significant heparin sparing effects (87). They proposed that the sparing of heparin consumption and the enhancement of its biological activity by prostacyclin are due to the prevention of release of platelet antiheparin activity (PF4). In another study it was shown that prostacyclin could be used as a sole anticoagulant in 10 patients on long-term dialysis and in one patient undergoing dialysis for acute renal failure who had bled on three occasions when heparin was used. The authors administered prostacyclin intravenously for 10 min before starting dialysis and via the arterial line during the procedure adjusting the dosage to avoid drug induced hypotension. Each patient underwent 240 min of dialysis and received an average of only 423 ng of prostacyclin/kg of body weight. No clinically important changes in the intrinsic clotting system were noted and there was no evidence of hemorrhage or thrombosis within the dialyzers. It was concluded that prostacyclin could replace heparin safely as a sole antithrombotic agent during hemodialysis and that this agent might be advantageous if ordinary anticoagulation is contraindicated (88). More recently other authors drew very similar conclusions (89). An interesting observation made by the latter authors, however, was that the prostacyclin so used prevented platelet activation but not the elevation of fibrinopeptide A as a marker of fibrin generation. They felt that this may explain why some patients develop clot in the dialysis circuit during prostacyclin only dialysis. However, this could be abolished by using prostacyclin in combination with heparin. Whether or not widespread use of prostacyclin for dialysis will occur will depend upon the frequency of undesirable clinical side effects such as drug induced hypotension and on its availability and cost. Interestingly there have been very few publications on such use of prostacyclin in the past 5 years.

PRACTICAL USE OF ANTICOAGULANTS

With this background a practical guide to the use of the various anticoagulants agents for dialysis patients can be given. This will be presented separately as it relates to hemodialysis anticoagulation and to the prevention of clotting in blood access devices.

Hemodialysis anticoagulation

Systemic heparin anticoagulation for the majority of hemodialysis patients

It will be clear from the data presented that heparin is not an ideal anticoagulant for hemodialysis and yet is the only one generally available. Thrombus formation may take place during hemodialysis despite apparently adequate heparinization and the platelet foreign surface interaction is of major importance in its occurrence. The ability of platelets to release their contents is likely to be enhanced by the improvement in the uremic syndrome resulting from adequate dialysis and will be stimulated by the materials used in the hemodialysis circuit which are of poor biocompatibility. It is likely, therefore, that variations in heparin dosage for hemodialysis are common within the dialysis population and these cannot necessarily be judged by body weight. Taking all this into account, the following have been suggested as guidelines for the better monitoring of heparin anticoagulation for the patient on maintenance dialysis (90):

1) The patient should have heparin requirements assessed during a series of WBACT's (or WBAPTT's as described by Gotch and Keen [81]) during the first three hemodialyses the patient receives. From the information, so obtained, an indication of the heparin loading dose and the rate of constant infusion required during dialysis will be ascertained. (Details of the methodology and calculations are provided as an appendix to this chapter).

2) When the patient is established on a regular hemodialysis schedule the heparin/WBACT profile should be assessed monthly.

3) Should any untoward clotting or hemorrhagic tendencies be noted, emergency reassessment of the heparin/WBACT profile should be made.

4) If untoward clotting episodes occur in spite of apparently good heparinization techniques then ideally, the patient's platelet function should be examined with particular reference to the release of PF4 and assessment of plasma HNA levels. If enhanced platelet activity and elevated plasma HNA levels are found, it is reasonable to treat the patient with an antiplatelet agent such as acetylsalicylic acid in low dose. If such investigations are not available the antiplatelet agent should be tried empirically.

Heparinization procedures for the at risk hemodialysis patient

Frequently hemodialysis is required for an acute or chronic uremic patient with an intercurrent hemorrhagic problem (such as gastrointestinal bleeding or menorrhagia) or a situation exists when over heparinization might be dangerous, as in the patient with pericarditis or in association with recent surgery. In such situations minimal heparinization or 'regional heparinization' with neutralization of circulating heparin by protamine sulfate or even hemodialysis without anticoagulation has been employed.

Minimal heparinization

A technique of 'minimal heparinization' has been evaluated (Hood SA, Holmes L, and Lindsay RM, unpublished) which is suitable for such a high risk situation and appears to obviate successfully the need for the regional technique. The basis of the minimal heparinization technique is to reduce the total heparin dosage given to the dialysis patient by 50%. The dialyzer and lines are primed with saline in the usual way and 1,000 units of heparin are added to the system 2 min prior to the termination of (re)circulation. The patient then receives an initial bolus of heparin into the venous return cannula and after the commencement of dialysis, heparin is given at a constant infusion which is terminated 30 min before the planned cessation of dialysis. The amounts of heparin given as initial bolus and at a constant infusion are 50% of those known to be ideal according to the standard systemic heparinization schedule. The heparin dosage can be safely reduced to a mean of 2,750 units/4 h of dialysis without inducing significant thrombus formation and whilst maintaining a blood loss in the dialyzers and lines of less than 5 ml. Further reductions in heparin are possible but then the dialyzer blood loss increases and the risk of clotting the venous return system is greater. The investigators also felt there might be some advantage in using dialyzers with cellulose acetate membranes as opposed to cuprophan membranes when utilizing such a technique. Throughout the course of each dialysis it is important to conduct serial WBACTs at hourly intervals and these should be maintained at around 200 sec throughout the course of dialysis. Close monitoring of WBACT in each individual patient can allow fine adjustements, if necessary, in the rate of heparin infusion.

Regional heparinization

A constant heparin infusion with a solution of 200 units of heparin/ml in 0.9% saline is made into the inlet line of the dialyzer. Simultaneously, a constant infusion of a solution of 2 mg of protamine sulfate/ml in 0.9% saline is made into the outlet line before the blood return to the patient. At the beginning of dialysis a minimal loading dose of heparin is given i.e. 50% of that normally required, if known, or empirically 500 units plus that in the priming solution. At the commencement of dialysis both infusion pumps are started;

separate pumps being employed so that the rate of heparin or protamine can be increased or decreased. The objective is to keep the patient's WBACT between 80 and 100 sec and the extracorporeal circuit of the artificial kidney at the therapeutic level, namely, 200 to 250 sec. The good dialysis nurse becomes very adept at adjusting the infusions of heparin and protamine sulfate to regulate the desired clotting times.

A 'heparin rebound' phenomenon may occur after regional heparinization. Even with a normal WBACT at the end of dialysis a rebound state of anticoagulation may occur from 2 to 4 h after the cessation of dialysis and persist for up to 10 h, possibly causing hemorrhage. It is believed that this heparin rebound is caused by the heparin-protamine complex being broken down in the reticuloendothelial system and the anticoagulant re-entering the circulation.

In view of this rebound and the fact that protamine sulfate in large doses also has an anticoagulant action, large amounts of protamine should be avoided. In other words, the secret of good regional heparinization is to decrease the heparin infusion thereby decreasing the WBACT rather than increase the protamine.

Protamine at the termination of dialysis

However dialysis anticoagulation has been carried out in a high risk situation, should the patient's WBACT be prolonged and if it is felt that there is a significant risk of bleeding, then the intravenous administration of protamine can be given to the patient to neutralize any remaining heparin. Should it be necessary to neutralize heparin urgently, one has to accept that the potency of batches both of heparin and protamine sulfate vary, but the usually accepted dose of protamine sulfate is 1 to 1.5 mg per 100 units of heparin. By personal experience, the author considers that generally only 50% of the recommended protamine dosage should be given and no more than 50 mg in any 10 min period.

Should time permit, it is possible to have a heparin: protamine titration test carried out. Here a known volume (10 ml) of blood is taken from the patient immediately postdialysis and protamine is added by titration until a WBACT (or other test such as a thrombin time) is returned to normal. By estimating the patient's blood volume, the exact amount of protamine required to neutralize circulating heparin can be calculated. Again, we suggest that only half the recommended protamine dosage should be given and then protamine titration checked once more.

Dialysis without anticoagulation

Several groups have evaluated various techniques for hemodialysis without any anticoagulation. Glaser et al (91) were successful in performing heparin-free dialysis. Sanders et al (92) reviewed their retrospective experience predominantly in renal transplant patients and showed a high success rate in avoiding anticoagulants while achieving excellent solute clearances with hollow fiber dialyzers. They did not report any bleeding complications associated with the 'no-heparin' technique. Schwab et al (93) evaluated a protocol for hemodialysis without anticoagulation in a large number of hospitalized patients with relative contraindications to anticoagulation. They found that they were able to conduct such hemodialysis successfully in 91% of cases. Only 7% of attempts required conversion to a low dose heparin regimen because of clotting in the extracorporeal dialysis circuit and 2% of the dialysis treatments resulted in clotting sufficient to interrupt hemodialysis. The protocol used by this group was as follows: 1) Plate dialyzers only were used. 2) Immediately prior to use, parallel plates and blood lines were flushed for 10 to 15 min with 1.0 l of 0.9% sodium chloride solution containing 3,000 units of heparin. Heparin was then flushed from the dialyzer with at least a further 1 l of 0.9% saline before blood flow was initiated. 3) Blood flow rates as high as possible were aimed for. 4) Hemodynamics were optimized to maintain systolic blood pressure above 100 mm Hg. 5) The hemodialyzer was flushed with 50 to 100 ml of 0.9% saline every 15 min to detect any signs of partial clotting and to prevent hemoconcentration. If partial clotting could not be resolved with saline flushes the patient received a low dose heparin regime. 6) If more than 2 l of fluid had to be removed from the patient or if the blood pressure was unstable, minimal fluid loss was aimed for during the dialysis procedure; fluid was then subsequently removed by sequential ultrafiltration. 7) Blood transfusions were not given during 'no-heparin' hemodialysis. 8) One to one nursing is essential with such a protocol.

A very similar protocol employing intermittent saline flushes was described by Caruana (94).

Dialysis with prostacyclin infusion

The use of prostacyclin would seem very appropriate for the high risk group and its use could increase rapidly in the next few years. In many countries, certainly in North America, the drug is only available for experimental use at this time. When available, the dosage regimes previously suggested would be appropriate.

Dialysis using ancrod

Ancrod with its unique effect on fibrinogen has been used in place of heparin as an anticoagulant during dialysis and was observed to reduce the formation of fibrin on the membranes of the Kiil dialyzer (95). However, it would be impractical to use this drug routinely for dialysis as its administration is more complex than heparinization and, as it is not easily neutralized, the patient would have a hypofibrinogenemic clotting defect for sometime after dialysis which might lead to excessive blood loss from arteriovenous fistula puncture sites.

Dialysis using citrate anticoagulation

Regional citrate anticoagulation has been used for patients considered at risk for bleeding and in those with sensitivity to heparin resulting in thrombocytopenia. Various techniques have been described, e.g. those of Pinnick et al (96) and of Von Brecht et al (97). These methods use citrate as a calcium chelator, to prevent activation of the clotting cascade in the extracorporeal circuit, plus intravenous Ca infusions and multiple serum Ca measurements to prevent hypocalcemia. Complications of citrate regional anticoagulation include hypocalcemia and citrate toxicity with nausea, parasthesiae, muscle cramps, tetany and hypotension (97). Kelleher and Schulman (98) describe metabolic alkalosis as an additional complication. Despite these potential complications, Flanigan et al (99) have demonstrated that dialysis using citrate anticoagulation is a viable alternative for patients needing heparin free dialysis and there are fewer bleeding episodes with this form of anticoagulation compared with low dow systemic heparin. In the author's experience, the simplest and most efficacious method for such anticoagulation is that developed from the extensive experience of Dr. D. Ward and colleagues (University of California, San Diego) which is as follows:

1) Prepare 0.2 mol trisodium citrate (sterile); 1.5 l for a 4 h procedure.
2) Prepare 5% CaCl$_2$ (sterile); 120 ml for a 4 h procedure.
3) Prepare a single pass system dialysis machine (i.e. not a dialysate regenerating system such as the Redy), and prepare the dialysis circuit as usual and prime without heparin.
4) Use a Ca-free dialysis solution; other dialysate constituents as usual including the Mg concentration.
5) Connect the vascular access lines with 4 way stop-cocks in both arterial and venous lines as close to the patient as possible.
6) Set up the citrate and CaCl$_2$ infusions. The citrate to the arterial line and CaCl$_2$ to the venous line using IVAC (or similar) pumps.
7) Commence blood flow into the system and simultaneously start the citrate infusion at 300 ml/h.
8) As soon as blood is in the venous return line, commence the CaCl$_2$ infusion at 30 ml/h.
9) Monitor the patient as follows: a) for anticoagulation control use WBACT's (e.g. by Hemochron system; used by Ward) on blood samples drawn immediately predialyzer (i.e. between the citrate infusion and the dialyzer). These should be performed at 15 min, 30 min, then every 30 min throughout dialysis. If the WBACT is less than 250 sec, increase citrate pump to 350 ml/h. If WBACT exceeds 350 sec, decrease citrate pump to 250 ml/h. b) Ionized calcium levels should be drawn from a peripheral vein at 15 min, 1 h and hourly throughout dialysis. Normal values are 1.1 to 1.3 mmol/l. The calcium chloride infusion rate can be adjusted as necessary, e.g. if ionized calcium is below 1 mmol/l increase calcium infusion rate to 35 ml/h. It is unlikely that elevated Ca levels will occur, but if so, simply reduce the infusion rate.
10) If the blood pump stops during dialysis then stop both IVAC's immediately. This is especially vital for the citrate infusion as trisodium citrate is very sclerosing and must not back up into the arterial line.
11) The above procedure is satisfactory for blood flow rates between 150 and 350 ml/min.

Anticoagulant use with blood access devices

Prophylaxis for shunts

We have to consider how best to maintain patency of devices, such as Teflon-Silastic arteriovenous shunts and foreign material grafts, which may be implanted subcutaneously to be used as blood conduits. Both sulfinpyrazone (100) and acetylsalicylic acid (101) prolong shunt life without causing significant morbidity. Anticoagulation with coumadin, on the other hand, also prolongs shunt life (102) but increases hemorrhagic complications. As far as the dose of the antiplatelet agent required to keep the Teflon-Silastic arteriovenous shunt patent, one can theorize that this device will not endothelialize and, therefore, it is not necessary to be concerned about suppressing prostacyclin generation. Most centers prescribe aspirin in the intermediate dosage range i.e. 650 mg (3.6 mmol/day) but theoretically, the low dose (40 to 325 mg/day) is probably sufficient. Sulfinpyrazone is usually given in the dosage of 200 mg 3 or 4 times a day. Because aspirin irreversibly inhibits the cyclo-oxygenase system in the platelet, it might be thought that the drug could be given once or twice a week and still have the desired effect. However, if platelet survival is approximately 10 days (likely to be even less in a patient with an arteriovenous shunt) then 10% of a platelet population will be renewed each day by new nonaffected platelets. For this reason, aspirin should be given daily. The efficacy of dipyridamole either alone or in combination with aspirin on patency should be studied. As mentioned previously, however, there is a theoretical advantage of combining the two drugs, so it would be reasonable to prescribe a low to intermediate dosage of aspirin in combination with dipyridamole 100 mg/day.

There does not appear to be any prospective study clearly demonstrated the value of antiplatelet agents in maintaining patency of foreign material grafts. There is no doubt that platelet foreign surface interaction takes place with their use. Clagett and colleagues (103) have demonstrated shortened platelet survival after the placement of Dacron aortic prostheses in dogs. Harker et al (104) have also demonstrated that the decreased platelet survival associated with prosthetic arterial grafts will return towards normal within 9 months in humans and within 6 weeks in baboons. In the baboon it was shown that normalization of platelet survival correlated with the degree of graft endothelialization. Both aspirin and dipyridamole can prevent platelet aggregation and adherence to such vascular grafts in animal studies (105). The actuarial survival curve of PTFE (gortex) (polytetrafluoroethylene) grafts (see Chapter 9) of our hemodialysis patients revealed that 50% of the grafts are lost within the first 10 months. Thereafter, the survival curve improves dramatically. It would appear, therefore, that this might be the time when graft endothelialization takes place. If an antiplatelet agent is to be used, therefore, it would seem that the dosage of the drug is not important in the early stages, but after 10 months when endothelialization has taken place one might have to consider the potential effects on decreasing prostacyclin production. Prospective trials of antiplatelet agents in various dosages with the use of such grafts is indicated.

A policy that has been adopted by many units (including ours) which appears to be satisfactory is that antiplatelet agents are prescribed to the patient with a previous history of blood access thrombosis or after his first clotting episode. They are, however, not prescribed routinely. Coumadin anticoagulation is only employed after further thrombotic episodes in spite of the use of antiplatelet agents.

Anticoagulants in the treatment of thrombosed shunts and grafts

When a Teflon-Silastic shunt clots, it can often be declotted mechanically either by irrigation with heparinized saline and the dextrous use of suction by syringe (see also Chapter 9). If one is fortunate and restores flow through the shunt, there is a clear indication for the commencement of either antiplatelet agents or a coumadin type of anticoagulant. If the declotting procedures are not successful, surgical help is needed and replacement of the clotted tip or tips is necessary. In the past many units attempted lytic therapy and infused streptokinase (106, 107) or urokinase (108–110) to declot such shunts. None of these authors gave detailed follow up regarding the long term patency achieved by such methods and most nephrologists would now agree that the success rate of lytic therapy in this area is poor. At present there is no information on the use of rt-PA in this situation. There are no reports to suggest that lytic therapy has a place in the management of thrombosed fistulae or prosthetic grafts and the management of such problems rests with early surgical intervention.

FUTURE DEVELOPMENTS

In the future we will undoubtedly see improvements in the biocompatibility of surfaces used in the artificial kidney and in other artificial organ systems. Considerable research in pharmacological manipulations of surfaces bringing about the controlled release of bioactive agents such as heparin and prostaglandins promises to reduce significantly the surface thrombosis without upsetting the coagulation status of the patient. In addition to preparing surfaces that will release heparin, other investigators, including the Swedish group, have been examining the possibility of covalently bonding heparin to a surface where it is not released into the microenvironment yet maintains its activity. Their method has shown that a surface so treated is highly thromboresistant in terms of reduced platelet adhesion, surface catalysed adsorption and inhibition of thrombin and capacity to prevent clotting of nonanticoagulated blood (111). The topic of biocompatibility has been reviewed recently ([112] and Chapter 6).

In addition, there is considerable research at present into the understanding of the anticoagulant, antithrombotic, and hemorrhagic effects of heparin; these three effects do not necessarily relate directly to each other. Stemming from this research is the development of heparinoids which have been shown in experimental animals to be as effective in preventing thrombosis but at the same time induce less hemorrhage than heparin. At least one study has been made of a low molecular weight heparinoid derived from animal intestinal mucosal tissue in human volunteers and in hemodialysis patients. This study has shown that the heparinoid was as successful as heparin in preventing clotting of the extracorporeal circuit but had no effect upon platelets (whereas heparin stimulated ADP induced platelet aggregation and increased plasma PF4 levels) and in contrast to heparin the low molecular weight heparinoid had only a minor effect on the activated partial thromboplastin time and thrombin time while both compounds induced anti Xa activity in plasma (113). It is almost certain, therefore, that in the not too distant future such heparinoids will be available which may be ideal for hemodialysis anticoagulation.

APPENDIX

1) To use the WBACT to calculate heparin dosage for dialysis in a given patient.

Procedure:

Action	*Comments*
1. Use non-heparinized saline in priming the dialyzer.	1. This allows accurate assessment of heparin received by the patient.
2. Do a baseline whole blood activated clotting time (WBACT) (#1).	2. This is unheparinized blood.
3. Administer loading dose of 1,500 to 2,000 units of heparin to the patient.	3. Systemic heparinization is recommended before the extracorporeal circuit is attached to the patient.
4. Follow with 10 ml of normal saline.	4. To ensure that entire loading dose of heparin enters the patient's circulation.
5. Allow 3 to 5 min to pass.	5. To ensure optimal patient response.
6. Do a WBACT (#2)	6. –
7. Initiate dialysis.	7. Do *not* begin heparin pump at this time.
8. Calculate patient response to heparin.	8. Response = WBACT #2 – WBACT #1
9. Calculate patient sensitivity to heparin.	9. Sensitivity = $\dfrac{\text{response}}{\text{heparin dose}}$
10. Do a WBACT (#3) *exactly* 30 min. after bolus dose of heparin was given.	10. This will allow calculation of patient's elimination rate of heparin (K)*
11. Begin the heparin pump at the desired dosage.	11. Give bolus as well if WBACT is below 200 sec.
12. Do a WBACT on a $\frac{1}{2}$ hourly basis.	12. Hourly infusion rate = $\dfrac{(\text{desired WBACT-WBACT \#1})\,(K)}{\text{sensitivity}}$
13. Stop heparin prior to termination of dialysis according to calculations.	13. Time (hours) = $\dfrac{1}{K}\text{Log}_e\left[\dfrac{\text{desired WBACT-WBACT \#1}}{\text{lowest WBACT before take-off-WBACT \#1}}\right]$
14. Do a final WBACT just prior to finishing dialysis.	

2) To use the WBACT to monitor a given dialysis.

Procedure:

Action	*Comments*
1. Do a baseline WBACT.	1. –
2. Administer loading dose of 1,500 to 2,000 units of heparin to the patient.	2. Systemic heparinization is recommended. Loading dose of 1,500 units is based on average patient sensitivity of 0.06 sec/unit, thereby elevating WBACT to 230 to 260 sec, i.e., peaking above the ideal range.
3. Follow with 10 ml normal saline.	3. To ensure that loading dose enters patient for optimal patient response.
4. Allow 3 min to pass.	4. Follow usual procedures.
5. Do a WBACT 3 min after venous line is attached.	5. This will give patient's response to heparinized saline in dialyzer.
6. Give bolus dose as necessary.	6. For every 10 sec WBACT is below 200 sec give 250 units.
7. Do a WBACT 30 to 60 min later.	7. To check constant infusion rate.
8. Adjust infusion rate if necessary.	8. For every 10 sec WBACT is above or below 220 sec, change heparin infusion rate by 250 units. NOTE: If WBACT is below 200 sec, give bolus dose of heparin.
9. Do WBACT test at hourly intervals.	9. To check infusion rate.
10. Stop heparin infusion $\frac{1}{2}$ hour before termination of dialysis.	10. –

$$* \; K \text{ (elimination rate in hours)} = \text{Log}_e\left[\frac{\text{Response}}{\text{WBACT \#3-WBACT \#1}}\right] \times \frac{1}{\text{Time (hours)}}$$

$$= 2 \times \text{Log}_e\left[\frac{\text{Response}}{\text{WBACT \#3-WBACT \#1}}\right] \text{ (for 30 min test period.)}$$

The data will give an ideal hourly infusion rate for heparin (see 12 above) and an ideal loading dose can also be calculated as follows:

$$\text{Loading dose} = \frac{\text{Desired WBACT} - \text{WBACT\#1}}{\text{Sensitivity}}$$

11. Do a WBACT test.

11. A WBACT value at this time is most desirable to help determine the exact time for discontinuing the heparin infusion for subsequent dialysis.

12. Do a final WBACT 30 min after discontinuing infusion – just before taking the patient off.

12. For every 20 sec WBACT is above 200 sec stop heparin pump 15 min earlier next dialysis. For every 20 sec WBACT is below 200 sec, leave heparin pump on 15 min longer.

The clotting times can be graphed as shown in Figure 8.

Note the WBACT times given in this appendix are those found in the author's unit using the HemoTec (HemoTec Inc., Englewood CO) or the Hemochron (International Technidyne Corp., New Jersey) systems. Times found in other units may vary according to the reagent and system used; each unit must set up its own standards.

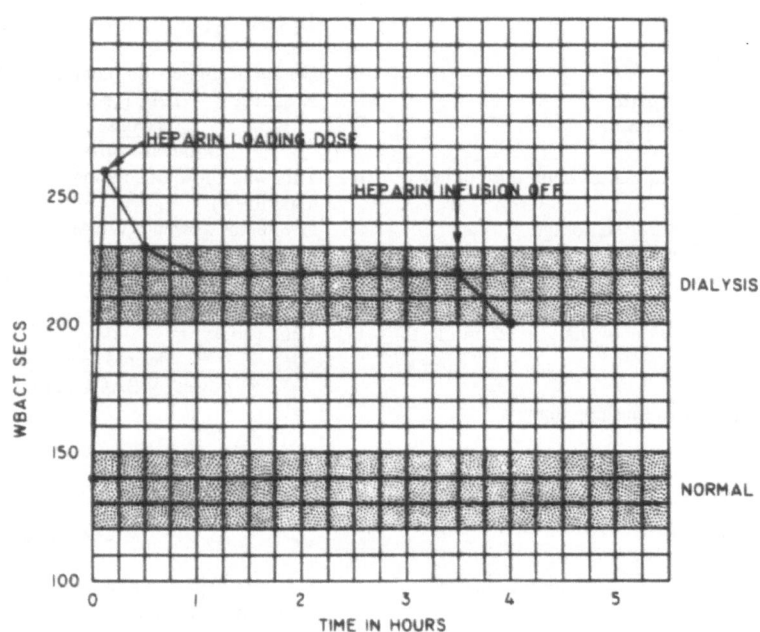

Figure 8. A typical heparin/WBACT profile for a 4 h hemodialysis. The ideal loading dose of heparin should cause a slight overshoot of desired dialysis WBACT range. If it does not, it is slightly more difficult to achieve a steady heparin infusion rate.

REFERENCES

1. Jandl JH: Blood: *Textbook of Hematology.* Boston, Toronto, Little, Brown, and Co, 1987
2. Ratnoff O, Forbes CD: *Disorders of Hemostasis.* Orlando Grune and Stratton Inc, 1984
3. Schumacher HR, Garvin DF, Triplett DA: *Introduction to Laboratory Hematology and Hematopathology.* New York, Alan R. Liss Inc, 1984
4. Dacie Sir JV, Lewis SM: *Practical Haematology.* 6th edition, Edinburgh, Churchill Livingstone, 1984
5. Hirsh J: *Venous Thromboembolism: Guide to Management.* Missisauga, Ontario, DuPont Pharmaceuticals, 1986
6. Lee GR, Boggs DR, Bithell TC, Foerster J, Athene JW, Lubene JN: *Clinical Hematology.* Philadelphia, Lea and Febiger, 1981
7. Bowie EJW, Owen CA Jr: Standardisation of the bleeding time. *Scand J Haematol* 25 (Suppl 37): 87, 1980

8. Jorpes JE: *Heparin in the Treatment of Thrombosis. An Account of its Chemistry, Physiology and Application in Medicine,* London, Oxford University Press, 1946
9. Cifonelli JA, King J: Structural studies on heparins with unusually high N-acetylglucosamine contents. *Biochim Biophys Acta* 320: 331, 1973
10. Rosenberg RD, Lam LH: Heparinized surface – a comment. *Ann NY Acad Sci* 283: 404, 1977
11. O'Reilly RA: Anticoagulant, antithrombotic and thrombolytic drugs. in *The Pharmacological Basis of Therapeutics,* edited by Gilman AG, Goodman LS, Gilman A, 6th edition, New York, MacMillan Publishing Co, 1980
12. Wessler S, Gitel S: Control of heparin therapy. *Prog Hemost Thromb* 3: 311, 1976
13. King DJ, Kelton JG: Heparin-associated thrombocytopenia. *Ann Intern Med* 100: 535, 1984
14. Best CH: Heparin and thrombosis. *Br Med J* 2: 977, 1938
15. Moolten SE, Vroman L, Vroman GMS: Role of blood plate-

lets in thromboembolism. *Arch Intern Med* 84: 667, 1949

16. O'Brien JR, Shoobridge SM, Finch WJ: Comparison of the effect of heparin and citrate on platelet aggregation. *J Clin Path* 22, 1969

17. Bowie EJW, Owen CA, Thompson JH: A test of platelet adhesiveness. *Mayo Clin Proc* 44: 306, 1969

18. Salzman EW: Measurement of platelet adhesiveness. A simple in vitro technique demonstrating an abnormality in von Willebrand's disease. *J Lab Clin Med* 62: 724, 1963

19. Thomson C, Forbes CD, Prentice CR: The potentiation of platelet aggregation by heparin in vitro and in vivo. *Clin Sci Mol Med* 45: 485, 1973

20. Lindsay RM, Prentice CRM, Ferguson D, Muir WM, McNicol GP: A method for the measurement of platelet adhesiveness by use of dialysis membranes in a test-cell. *Br J Haematol* 24: 377, 1973

21. Lindsay RM, Rourke JTB, Reid BD, Linton AL, Gilchrist T, Courtney J, Edwards RO: The role of heparin on platelet retention by acrylonitrile co-polymer dialysis membranes. *J Lab Clin Med* 89: 4, 1977

22. Loeliger EA: ICSH/ICTH recommendations for reporting prothrombin time in oral anticoagulant control. *Acta Haematol* (Basel) 72: 405, 1984

23. Barrow DA, Maynard JR: Standardisation of the prothrombin time for monitoring oral anticoagulant therapy: the international normalised ratio. *Dade Coagulation Technical Bulletin* #19, 1987

24. Sherry S, Bell WR, Duckert H, Fletcher P, Gurewich V, Marder VJ, Roberts H, Salzman EW, Sasahara A, Verstraete M: Thrombolytic therapy in thrombosis: a National Institutes of Health Consensus Development Conference. *Ann Intern Med* 93: 141, 1980

25. Bell WR, Meek AG: Guidelines for the use of thrombolytic agents. *N Engl J Med* 301: 1266, 1979

26. Marder VJ: The use of thrombolytic agents: choice of patient drug administration, laboratory monitoring. *Ann Intern Med* 90: 802, 1979

27. Macfarlane RG, Pilling J: Fibrinolytic activity of normal urine. *Nature* 159: 779, 1947

28. Williams JRB: The fibrinolytic activity of urine. *Br J Exp Pathol* 32: 530, 1951

29. Sobel GW, Mohler SR, Jones NW, Dowdy AB, Guest MM: Urokinase: an activator of plasma profibrinolysin extracted from urine. *Am J Physiol* 171: 768, 1952

30. Thorsen S, Glas-Greenwalt P, Astrup T: Differences in the binding to fibrin of urokinase and tissue plasminogen activator. *Thromb Diath Haemorrh* 28: 65, 1972

31. Risius B, Graor RA, Geisinger MA, Zelch MG, Lucas FV, Young JR, Grossbard EB: Recombinant human tissue-type plasminogen activator for thrombolysis in peripheral arteries and bypass grafts. *Radiology* 160: 183, 1986

32. Collen D, Topol EJ, Tiefenbrunn AJ, Gold HK, Weisfeldt ML, Sobel BE, Leinbach RC, Brinker JA, Ludbrook PA, Yasuda I, Bulkley BH, Robison AK, Hutter AM Jr, Bell WR, Spadaro JJ Jr, Khaw BA, Grossbard EB: Coronary thrombolysis with recombinant human tissue-type plasminogen activator: a prospective, randomized, placebo-controlled trial. *Circulation* 70: 1012, 1984

33. Moncada S, Gryglewski R, Bunting S, Vane JR: An enzyme isolated from arteries transforms prostaglandin endoperoxides to an unstable substance that inhibits platelet aggregation. *Nature* 263: 663, 1976

34. Johnson RA, Morton DR, Kinner JH, Gorman RR, McGuire JC, Sun FF, Whitaker N, Bunting S, Salman J, Moncada S, Vane JR: The chemical structure of prostaglandin × (prostacyclin). *Prostaglandins* 12: 915, 1976

35. Moncada S, Herman AG, Higgs EA, Vane JR: Differential formation of prostacyclin (PGx or PGI2) by layers of the arterial wall: An explanation for the anti-thrombotic properties of vascular endothelium. *Thromb Res* 11: 323, 1977

36. MacIntyre DE, Pearson JD, Gordon JL: Localisation and stimulation of prostacyclin production in vascular cells. *Nature* 271: 549, 1978

37. Armstrong JN, Lattimer N, Moncada S, Vane JR: Comparison of the vasodepressor effects of prostacyclin and 6-oxylprostaglandin F1 alpha with those of prostaglandin E2 in rats and rabbits. *Br J Pharmacol* 62: 125, 1978

38. Cazenave JP, Dejana E, Kinlough-Rathbone RL, Richardson M, Packham MA, Mustard JF: Prostaglandins I2 and E1 reduce rabbit and human platelet adherence without inhibiting serotonin release from adherent platelets. *Thromb Res* 15: 273, 1979

39. Higgs EA, Moncada S, Vane JR, Caen JP, Michel H, Tobelem G: Effect of prostacyclin (PGI2) and platelet adhesion to rabbit arterial subendothelium. *Prostaglandins* 16: 17, 1978

40. Weiss HJ, Turitto VT: Prostacyclin (prostaglandin I2, PGI2) inhibits platelet adhesion and thrombus formation on subendothelium. *Blood* 53: 244, 1979

41. Higgs EA, Higgs GA, Moncada S, Vane JR: Prostacyclin (PGI2) inhibits the formation of platelet thrombi in arterioles and venules of the hamster cheek pouch. *Br J Pharmacol* 63: 535, 1978

42. Aspirin and other antiplatelet drugs in the prophylaxis of thrombosis. *Blood Rev* 1: 9, 1987

43. Goodnight SH, Harris WS, Connor WE: The effects of dietary W3 fatty acids on platelet composition and function in man. A prospective controlled study. *Blood* 58: 880, 1981

44. Fuster V, Chesebro JH: Series on pharmacology in practice. 10. Anti-thrombotic therapy: role of platelet-inhibitor drugs. 11. Pharmacological effects of platelet-inhibitor drugs. *Mayo Clin Proc* 56: 185, 1981

45. Harker LA, Slichter SJ: Platelet and fibrinogen consumption in man. *N Engl J Med* 287: 999, 1972

46. Harker LA: In vivo evaluation of antithrombotic therapy in man. *Thromb Diath Haemorrh* (suppl 60): 481, 1974

47. Moncada S, Korbut R: Dipyridamole and other phosphodiesterase inhibitors act as antithrombotic agents by potentiating endogenous prostacyclin. *Lancet* 1: 1286, 1978

48. Riesman D: Hemorrhages in the course of Bright's disease with a nephrotic origin. *Am J Med Sci* 134: 709, 1907

49. Donner L, Neuwirtova: The hemostatic defect of acute and chronic uraemia. *Thromb Diath Haemorrh* 5: 319, 1960

50. Rabiner SF: Uremic bleeding. *Prog Hemost Thromb* 1: 233, 1972

51. Castaldi PA, Rosenberg MC, Stewart JH: The bleeding disorder of uraemia. *Lancet* 2: 66, 1966

52. Salzman EW, Neri LL: Adhesiveness of blood platelets in uremia. *Thromb Diath Haemorrh* 15: 84, 1966

53. George CRP, Slichter SJ, Quadracci LJ, Striker GE, Harker LA: A kinetic evaluation of hemostasis in renal disease. *N Engl J Med* 291: 1111, 1974

54. Stewart JH, Castaldi PA: Uraemic bleeding: A reversible platelet defect corrected by dialysis. *Q J Med* 36: 409, 1967

55. Rabiner SF, Hrodek O: Platelet factor 3 in normal subjects and patients with renal failure. *J Clin Invest* 47: 901, 1968

56. Joist JH, Pechan J, Schikowski U, Hubner G, Gross R: Studies on the nature and etiology of uremic thrombocytopathy. *Verh Dtsch Ges Inn Med* 75: 476, 1969

57. Lindsay RM, Moorthy AV, Koens F, Linton AL: Platelet function in dialyzed and non-dialyzed patients with chronic renal failure. *Clin Nephrol* 4: 52, 1975

58. Lindsay RM, Friesen M, Koens F, Linton AL, Oreopoulos D, DeVeber G: Platelet function in patients on long term peritoneal dialysis. *Clin Nephrol* 6: 335, 1976

59. Lindsay RM, Friesen M, Aronstam A, Andrus F, Clark WF, Linton AL: Improvement of platelet function by increased frequency of hemodialysis *Clin Nephrol* 10: 67, 1978

60. Nenci GG, Berrettini M, Agnelli G, Parise P, Buoncristiani U, Ballatori E: Effect of peritoneal dialysis, haemodialysis and kidney transplantation on blood platelet function. I. Platelet aggregation by ADP and epinephrine. *Nephron* 23: 287, 1979

61. Jorgenson KA, Ingeberg S: Platelets and platelet function in patients with chronic ureamia on maintenance hemodialysis. *Nephron* 23: 233, 1979

62. Kazatchkine M, Sultan Y, Caen JP, Bariety J: Bleeding in renal failure: a possible cause. *Br Med J* 2: 612, 1976

63. Remuzzi G, Pusineri F: Coagulation defects in uremia. *Kidney Int* 33(Suppl 24): S123, 1988

64. Remuzzi G, Livio M, Cavenaghi AE, Marchesi D, Mecca G, Donati MB, de Gaetano G: Unbalanced prostaglandin synthesis and plasma factors in uraemic bleeding a hypothesis. *Thromb Res* 13: 531, 1978

65. Di Minno G, Martinez J, McKean ML, De La Rosa J, Burke JF, Murphy S: Platelet dysfunction in uremia. Multifaceted defect partially corrected by dialysis. *Am J Med* 79: 552, 1985

66. Duke WW: The relation of blood platelets to hemorrhagic disease. *JAMA* 60: 1185, 1910

67. Livio M, Gotti E, Marchesi D, Mecca G, Remuzzi G, De Gaetano G: Uremic bleeding: role of anemia and beneficial effect of red cell transfusions. *Lancet* 2: 1013, 1982

68. Fernandez F, Goudable C, Sie P, Ton-That H, Durand D, Suc JM, Boneu B: Low hematocrit and prolonged bleeding time in uremic patients: effect of red cell transfusions. *Br J Hematol* 59: 139, 1985

69. Moia M, Vizzotto L, Cattaneo M, Mannucci PM, Cassati S, Pontichelli C: Improvement in the hemostatic defect of uremia after treatment with recombitant human erythropoeitin. *Lancet* 2: 1127, 1987

70. Brash JL, Lyman DJ: Adsorption of proteins and lipids to non-biological surfaces. in *The Chemistry of Biosurfaces,* edited by Hair ML, New York, Marcel Dekker Inc, 1971, p 177

71. Salzman EW: Role of platelets in blood-surface interactions. *Fec Proc* 30: 1503, 1971

72. Vroman L, Adams AL, Klings M: Interactions among human blood proteins at interfaces. *Fed Proc* 30: 1494, 1971

73. Feijen J: Thrombogenesis caused by blood-foreign surface interaction. in *Artificial Organs,* edited by Kenedi RM, Courtney JM, Gaylor JDS, Gilchrist T, Baltimore, Univ Park Press, 1976, p 235

74. Niemetz J, Muhlfelder T, Chierego ME, Troy B: Procoagulant activity of leukocytes. *Ann NY Acad Sci* 283: 208, 1977

75. Craddock PR, Fehr J, Brigham KL, Kronenberg RS, Jacob HS: Complement and leukocyte-mediated pulmonary dysfunction in hemodialysis. *N Engl J Med* 296: 769, 1977

76. Jacob HS, Craddock PR, Hammerschmidt DE, Moldow DF: Complement-induced granulocyte aggregation: an unsuspected mechanism of disease. *N Engl J Med* 302: 89, 1980

77. Lindsay RM, Prentice CRM, Davidson JF, Burton JA, McNicol GP: Haemostatic changes during dialysis associated with the thrombus formation on dialysis membranes. *Br Med J* 4: 454, 1972

78. Lindsay RM, Ferguson D, Prentice CRM, Burton JA, McNicol GP: Reduction of thrombus formation on dialyzer membranes by aspirin and RA233. *Lancet* 2: 1287, 1972

79. Lindsay RM, Rourke J, Reid B, Friesen M, Linton AL, Courtney J, Gilchrist T: Platelets, foreign surfaces and heparin. *Trans Am Soc Artif Intern Organs* 22: 292, 1976

80. Wilkinson R, Lindsay RM, Burton JA: The membrane support system and thrombus formation on dialysis membranes. *Proc Eur Dial Transplant Assoc* 10: 306, 1973

81. Gotch FA, Keen ML: Precise control of minimal heparinization for high bleeding risk hemodialysis. *Trans Am Soc Artif Intern Organs* 23: 168, 1977

82. Harada K, Zucker MB: Simultaneous development of PF4 activity and release of 14C-serotonin. *Thromb Diath Haemorrh* 25: 41, 1971

83. Rucinski B, Niewiarowski J, James P, Walz DA, Budzynski AZ: Antiheparin proteins secreted by human platelets: purification, characterization, and radioimmunoassay. *Blood* 53: 47, 1979

84. O'Brien JR: Antithrombin III and heparin clotting times in atherosclerosis and thrombosis. *Thromb Diath Haemorrh* 32: 116, 1974

85. Aronstam A, Dennis B, Friesen MJ, Clark WF, Linton AL, Lindsay RM: Heparin neutralizing activity in patients with renal disease on maintenance haemodialysis. *Thromb Diath Haemorrh* 35: 695, 1978

86. Woods HF, Ash G, Weston MJ, Bunting S, Moncada S, Vane JR: Prostacyclin can replace heparin in haemodialysis in dogs. *Lancet* 2: 1075, 1978

87. Turney JH, Fewell MR, Williams LC, Parsons V, Weston MH: Platelet protection and heparin sparing with prostacylin regular dialysis therapy. *Lancet* 2: 219, 1980

88. Zusman RM, Rubin RH, Cato AE, Cocchetto DM, Crow JW, Tolkoff-Rubin N: Haemodialysis using prostacyclin instead of heparin as the sole antithrombotic agent. *N Engl J Med* 304: 934, 1981

89. Rylance PB, Gordge MP, Ireland H, Lane DA, Weston MJ: Haemodialysis with prostacyclin (Epoprostenol) alone *Proc Eur Dial Transplant Assoc Eur Renal Assoc* 21: 281, 1984

90. Lindsay RM: Variable heparin requirements during hemodialysis-Why? *asaio J* 3: 81, 1980

91. Glaser P, Guedsder R, Rouby J, Eurin VB: Hemodialysis without heparin is possible. *Lancet* 1: 579, 1979

92. Sanders PW, Taylor H, Curtis J: Hemodialysis without anticoagulation. *Am J Kidney Dis* 5: 32, 1985

93. Schwab SJ, Onorato JJ, Sharar LR, Dennis PA: Hemodialysis without anticoagulation: 1 year prospective trial in hospitalized patients at risk for bleeding. *Am J Med* 83: 405, 1987

94. Caruana RJ, Raiai RM, Bush JV, Kramer MS, Goldstein SJ: Heparin free dialysis: comparative data and results in high risk patients. *Kidney Int* 31: 1351, 1987

95. Hall GH, Holman HM, Webster ADB: Anticoagulation by ancrod for haemodialysis. *Br Med J* 4: 591, 1970

96. Pinnick RV, Wiegmann TB, Diederich DA: Regional citrate anticoagulation for hemodialysis in the patient at high risk for bleeding. *N Engl J Med* 308: 258, 1983

97. von Brecht JH, Flanigan MJ, Freeman RM, Lim VS: Regional anticoagulation: hemodialysis with hypertonic trisodium citrate. *Am J Kidney Dis* 8: 196, 1986

98. Kelleher SO, Schulman G: Severe metabolic alkalosis complicated regional citrate hemodialysis. *Am J Kidney Dis* 9: 235, 1987

99. Flanigan MJ, von Brecht J, Freeman RM, Lim VS: Reducing the hemorrhagic complications of HD: a controlled compari-

son of low dose citrate anticoagulation. *Am J Kidney Dis* 9: 147, 1987

100. Kaedi A, Pinio GF, Shimizu A, Drivedi H, Hirsch J, Gent M: Arteriovenous shunt thrombosis: Prevention by sulfinpyrazone. *N Engl J Med* 290: 304, 1974

101. Harter HR, Burch JW, Majerus PW, Stanford N, Delmez JA, Anderson CB, Weerts CA: Prevention of thrombosis in patients on hemodialysis by low-dose aspirin. *N Engl J Med* 301: 577, 1979

102. Wing AJ, Curtis JR, de Wardener HE: Reduction of clotting in Scribner shunts by long-term anticoagulation. *Br Med J* 3: 143, 1976

103. Clagett GP, Russo M, Hufnagel H: Platelet changes after placement of aortic prostheses in dogs. I. Biochemical and functional alterations. *J Lab Clin Med* 97: 345, 1981

104. Harker LA, Slichter S, Sauvage LR: Platelet consumption by arterial prostheses: The effects of endothelialization and pharmocologic inhibition of platelet function. *Ann Surg* 186: 594, 1977

105. Oblath RW, Buckley FO, Green RM, Schwartz SI, DeWeese JA: Prevention of platelet aggregation and adherence to prosthetic vascular grafts by aspirin and dipyridamole. *Surgery* 84: 37, 1978

106. Clunie GJA, Martin AM, Nolan B: Intermittent haemodialysis: insertion and care of the Silastic Teflon cannula. *Br Med J* 3(Suppl July-Sept): 88, 1967

107. Anderson DC, Martin AN, Clunie GJA, Stewart WK, Robson AS: The use of streptokinase in the declotting of arteriovenous shunts. *Proc Eur Dial Transplant Assoc* 4: 55, 1967

108. Watt DL, Dun BP, Livingston WR, MacDougall AI, MacKay RKS, Obineche EN, Rennie JB: The use of urokinase in declotting arteriovenous shunts. *Proc Eur Dial Transplant Assoc* 6: 88, 1969

109. McIntosh CS, Petrie JC, MacLeod N: Maintenance of Silastic-Teflon shunts for intermittent haemodialysis. *Br Med J* 4: 717, 1969

110. Clunie GJA, Hartley L: Treatment of clotting in external-arteriovenous shunts with a fibrinolytic enzyme. *Med J Aust* 2: 463, 1969

111. Larm O, Larsson R, Olsson P: A new non-thrombogenic surface prepared by selective covalent binding of heparin via a modified reducing terminal residue. *Biomat Med Devices Artif Organs* 11: (2 and 3), 1984

112. Lindsay RM, Mason R, Kim SW, Andrade JD, Hawkin RM: Blood surface interactions. *Trans Am Soc Artif Intern Organs* 26: 603, 1980

113. ten Cate H, Henny CP, ten Cate JW, Buller HR, Mooy MC, Surachno S, Wilmink JM: Anticoagulant effects of a low molecular weight heparinoid (Org 10172) in human volunteers and dialysis patients. *Thromb Res* 39: 211, 1985

HEMODIALYSIS MONITORS AND MONITORING

PRAKASH R. KESHAVIAH and STANLEY SHALDON

INTRODUCTION

Worldwide acceptance of hemodialysis for achieving long-term survival of patients with end stage renal failure may have obscured the inherent danger of this technique to the patient. The technique evolved rapidly from the intensive care unit with continuous nurse/doctor observation of the patients in 1960 (1), to the patient's own home, where unattended overnight hemodialysis was first performed in 1964 with a passive flow system and without the use of a blood pump (2). The universal preference for the arteriovenous (A-V) fistula (3) with its implied use of a blood pump, and the use of more efficient dialyzers together with the requirement that the patient accepts more responsibility for his own treatment (4, 5), have placed even greater emphasis on the need for adequate equipment and monitoring.

It is difficult to estimate the true incidence and severity of technical mishaps in hemodialysis from a review of the scientific literature. This may, in part, be due to the reluctance of dialysis centers to publish their unfortunate accidents. It may also be a consequence of a major secondary complication obscuring the primary event. For example, infections still are a principal cause of death in dialysis patients, accounting for 20% of mortality (6). It is likely that many of them relate to a primary technical fault as opposed to reduced immune response of uremic patients. A comprehensive survey of the risks and hazards associated with hemo-

dialysis equipment was compiled in 1980 (7) under the sponsorship of the Food and Drug Administration (FDA) of the USA. The reader is also referred to Chapter 33 of this book for a survey of the acute complications associated with hemodialysis.

In striving for safety in hemodialysis, one must recognize that safety is a relative rather than an absolute concept. The addition of safety features should be considered in terms of the added cost, complexity, increased maintenance and most importantly, overall effectiveness of treatment. Equipment should be designed around the 'fail-safe' concept defined by Grimsrud et al (8) as follows: 'In the event of an excursion of the variables outside their control limits, or a breakdown of the monitoring or control equipment itself, the system will automatically return to a safe configuration'. Safe configuration refers to patient isolation, and hence protection from the malfunction and its effects but does not usually include rectification of the cause of an alarm. Such rectification usually depends on appropriate human action. It is, therefore, important to note that safety depends not only on an equipment design, but also on a properly trained operator. It is not possible to substitute one for the other.

Standards for hemodialysis equipment have been formulated by agencies in many countries including USA, UK, Canada, Japan and West Germany. In the USA, the Association for the Advancement of Medical Instrumentation (AAMI) has been active in the development of voluntary standards. The AAMI standard has been approved by the American National Standards Institute, Inc. and has become an American National Standard (9). Many of the recommendations of the FDA report on risks and hazards of hemodialysis equipment (7) have been adopted in this standard.

This chapter will focus on the monitoring of the extracorporeal blood and dialysate circuits. Equipment used in these circuits will be described and the parameters that need to be measured and monitored will be defined. Principles of measurement and the accuracy and resolution requirements of these monitors will also be defined. In addition to the monitoring requirements of the blood and dialysate circuits, ultrafiltration control systems and special dialysis schemes such as single needle dialysis, sequential ultrafiltration and diffusion and bicarbonate dialysis systems will be discussed. Monitoring of the patient during dialysis will also be considered briefly.

Preceding detailed discussion of individual monitors, certain requirements that are common to all monitors and constitute an approach to the ideal monitoring system are enumerated below:

1. The location and sensitivity of monitors should detect changes in the variable monitored before these changes can affect the patient.
2. Functional testing of alarms should be easily accomplished without special tools so that testing may be incorporated into the dialysis procedure. It should also be possible to test and calibrate each monitor independently using external standards.
3. The minimum sensitivity and maximum spread of alarm limits should be internally set with operator adjustments being possible only within this range. Operator adjustments should not disable the alarm.
4. Fail-safe design and system stability may be compromised with interdependence of monitors and their circuitry. This may also be true if control and monitoring functions have common sensors and circuitry. Hence, control and monitoring functions should be independent of each other and individual monitors should be independent. Further, the monitor should be critically sensitive to only one variable.
6. Audible and visual alarms should be provided. A muting switch, if provided, should affect *only* the audible alarm and for a limited time (e.g. 90 to 120 sec). It should be impossible to resume dialysis as long as the alarm condition exists or with the monitors inactivated. Visual alarms should be designed for clarity and readability at a distance of 2 m. Audible alarms should be rated at no less than 70 decibels ('A' scale) at 3 m.
7. In an alarm condition, patient protection should occur by passive mechanisms inherent to system design rather than by specific reactive mechanisms.
8. With isolated loss of power, the affected monitor displays should indicate either the high or low range rather than the central, normal range to prevent the operator from assuming normal operation. Loss of power to the overall system should be indicated by an alarm (audible and

visual) and patient protection schemes should activate automatically.
9. The hydraulic and electrical components within a piece of equipment should be separated, the electrical circuits being adequately isolated from liquid leaks. The outside of the equipment should be shielded from liquid spills.

THE EXTRACORPOREAL BLOOD CIRCUIT

A typical hemodialysis blood circuit is illustrated in Figure 1. With the advent of the A-V fistula, blood is pumped from the patient via the access through the dialyzer and back to the patient. The portion of the circuit from the patient to the dialyzer is commonly referred to as the arterial segment and that from the dialyzer back to the patient as the venous segment. The sites at which pressures in the blood circuit are usually measured are between the patient's access and the blood pump, at an arterial trap between the blood pump and the dialyzer and at the venous air trap located downstream of the dialyzer. The air detector is usually located on the venous air trap with the clamp that is activated by the air detector being positioned just below the air trap. Heparin, for anticoagulation, is typically infused downstream of the blood pump. Patient isolation from alarm conditions in the blood circuit is usually effected by stopping the blood pump and clamping the venous blood tubing.

Flow monitoring

The flow rate at which blood perfuses the dialyzer is an important parameter because it influences the efficiency of solute transport across the dialyzer membrane. Small solutes such as urea and creatinine are said to be flow limited because their clearances are influenced to a greater extent by the blood and dialysis fluid flow rates than by the diffusive resistance of the dialyzer membrane. On the other hand, large solutes such as vitamin B_{12} are membrane limited, their clearances being mainly influenced by the diffusive resistance of the membrane and to a much smaller extent by blood and dialysis solution flow rates. Dialyzer clearances of small solutes increase as blood and dialysis fluid flow rates increase but at a diminishing rate, a relative clearance plateau being reached beyond a certain blood or dialysis fluid flow rate.

In the early days of hemodialysis, cannulas were used for blood access, thereby allowing passive perfusion of the blood circuit by the patient's systemic blood pressure. The predominant use of the A-V fistula nowadays, necessitates the use of a blood pump for perfusion of the blood circuit, because the pressure gradient between the fistula needles is not sufficient to achieve adequate flow. Blood pumps used in hemodialysis may be free-standing or an integral part of the dialysis fluid delivery system. The type of blood pump most commonly used is the peristaltic roller pump. A compressible segment of the 'arterial' blood tubing is inserted into a curved roller track in the blood pump and the rotation of the rollers compresses the tubing, forcing blood out of the

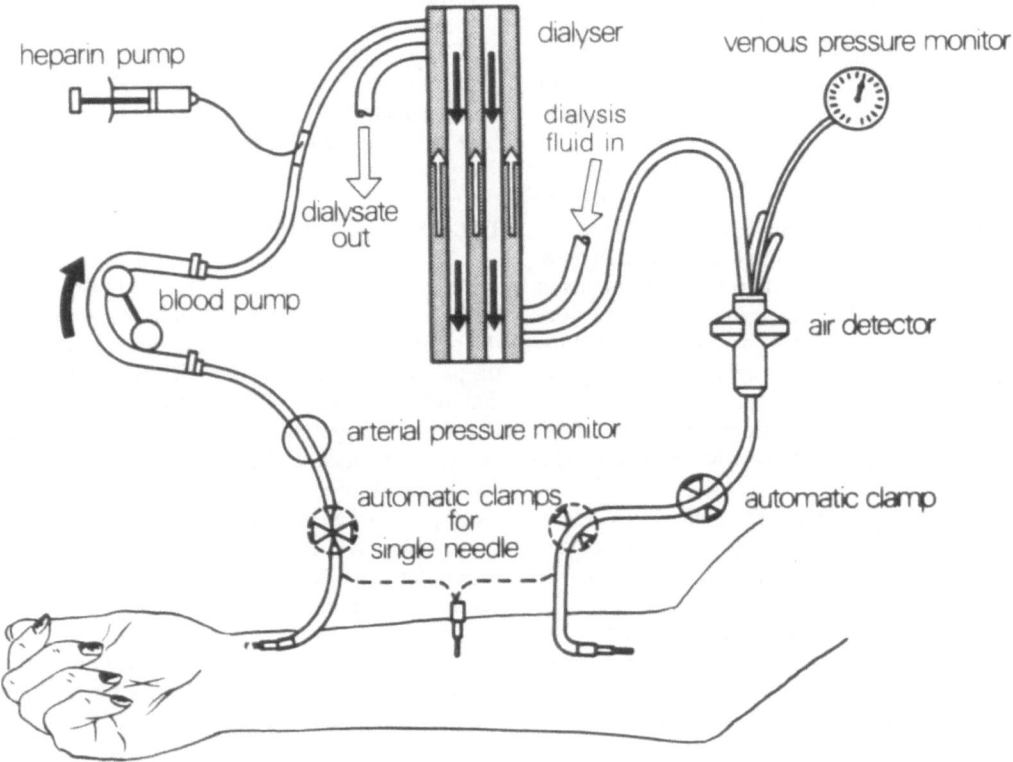

Figure 1. Typical haemodialysis blood circuit.

pump segment. After passage of the roller, the tubing resumes its original shape and blood is drawn in to refill the pump segment.

The roller pumps used in hemodialysis have between one and three rollers on the pump head, most often two. Increasing the number of rollers on the pump head increases the frequency of pulsation but decreases the pulse amplitude (pulse pressure). The occlusion of the pump segment between the roller track and the rollers is usually adjustable. Inadequate occlusion causes back flow, foaming and possibly, hemolysis. Over-occlusion can lead to tubing damage, and hence blood leaks, as well as increased hemolysis. Many blood pumps use spring loaded rollers for optimal occlusion, correcting for small variations in tubing diameter, wall thickness and hardness.

Blood pumps are usually designed to accomodate a range of tubing sizes as well as single/dual pump segments. In pumps that incorporate a direct display of blood flow rate, provisions are made to correlate choice of tubing size and number of segments to flow rate, either through the use of multiple scales on the display or through selector switches. Blood pumps are usually provided with a tool for manual operation in the event of a power failure.

Hemolysis is a problem of considerable magnitude in blood pumps used for cardiopulmonary bypass because of the high blood flow rates. In hemodialysis, however, the flow rates are much lower and studies indicate that immediate and delayed hemolysis in the extracorporeal circuit are too small to be of consequence (10, 11). Moreover, in well-dialyzed patients, red cell survival approaches normal, suggesting that there is no delayed hemolysis due to sublethal damage in the extracorporeal circulation (12).

With some blood pumps the operator is inadequately protected from the rotating parts of the pump. Either there is no safety cover or some rotating parts protrude through the cover. Some pumps have a mechanical or electrical safety shut-off feature in high torque situations. This not only protects the pumps from damage but also provides for operator safety.

It is highly desirable to have the electrical components of blood pumps shielded from liquid spills. In the absence of such shielding, a saline spill may not only damage the pump circuit but could also result in dangerous current leakage. High current leakage may also be observed in older pumps that have been subjected to salt corrosion. The use of a low voltage DC motor reduces the electrical hazard associated with a blood pump.

Calibrated blood pump

The flow output of a blood pump is the product of pump speed and stroke volume. If stroke volume is constant, flow output is directly proportional to pump speed. Many blood pumps have a meter that supposedly indicates the speed of operation and hence the flow rate. The displayed parameter is not really pump speed but armature voltage, to which pump speed is proportional. Under normal inlet voltage conditions this is valid. However, inlet voltages fluctuate by at least ± 10%. Therefore, with the same meter indication, voltage fluctuations could result in varying pump speeds. There are pumps that have a true tachometer display. This is more desirable than an armature voltage indicator. If stroke volume varies, precise measurement of pump speed will not indicate flow rates accurately. Stroke volume variations, arising from variations in the internal diameter of the pump segment, may cause flow rate errors as large as ± 20%. With extreme inlet suction pressures (subatmospheric pressures), the pump segment refills incompletely, reducing stroke volume. Depending on the thickness and durometer of the pump segment, the stroke volume may also decrease with continued pumping because of a time dependent loss of pump segment elasticity. The stroke volume is also reduced by retrograde flow when the pump outlet pressure exceeds the occlusive pressure setting of the rollers. In all of these situations, the actual flow rate is less than that indicated by pump speed.

A blood pump that displays armature voltage may be calibrated using banked blood or a fluid of similar viscosity. The calibration is, however, valid only if the pressures at the pump inlet and outlet simulate those in clinical use. As the pressures in clinical use vary considerably, the calibration may be inaccurate because of the changes in stroke volume associated with different inlet and outlet pressures.

Bubble transit time

A clinically used measure of the blood flow rate is the 'bubble transit time'. In this method an air bubble is injected into the blood circuit and the transit time of the bubble across a certain length of tubing is measured. A suitable calibration is used to convert the transit time to a flow rate. Blood tubing for hemodialysis usually incorporates a 50 cm 'race track'. The race track is merely a segment of blood tubing with two markings spaced at the required distance to allow convenient measurement of the bubble transit time. Several factors contribute to inaccuracies with this method. The race track must be horizontal during the measurement and this is often neglected in the routine clinical setting. The bubble size significantly influences the accuracy of the method. Small bubbles that travel along the axis of flow overestimate the actual flow rate because the velocity profile across the tube cross-section is parabolic, the center line velocity being twice the mean velocity. The method is more accurate when the bubble fills the entire tubing cross-section. Variations in the internal diameter of the blood tubing and hence the volume of the race track are another source of error. Inaccuracies in the time measurement also add to the error of the method. At a typical blood flow rate of 200 ml/min, a race track length of 50 cm, and an internal diamter of 0.48 cm (3/16″), the bubble transit time is as small as 2.5 sec.

The transit time is even smaller with higher flow rates and, hence, susceptible to larger measurement errors. To improve accuracy, race track lengths as large as 2 m have been used. If extending the race track increases the length of blood tubing used, the extracorporeal volume may be larger than desired. The risk of hepatitis transmission through an accidental needle stab exists with this method. The risk is minimized if there is a protective guard on the underside of the injection site. Aerosol transmission of virus particles from puncturing a tube under positive pressures does, however, exist. The risk of accidental needle stabs and aerosol transmission can be eliminated with an infusion 'T' for injecting the bubble. Despite these criticisms, under ideal conditions of measurement, it may be possible to establish a good correlation between the bubble transit time and the blood flow rate (see Chapter 5 for further details of the 'bubble transit time' method).

Electromagnetic flow devices

Electromagnetic flow devices have been employed in hemodialysis. The electromagnetic method is an invasive technique which requires that the electrodes directly contact blood. Although the method is very accurate, the need to clean and sterilize the blood contaminated transducers together with the risk of transmission of hepatitis, have largely precluded its clinical use.

Ultrasonic flow meters

Ultrasonic flow meters employ the principle that the passage of a blood cell will reflect part of the transmitted ultrasonic wave and cause a frequency change which can be detected by the 'Doppler shift' which is directly proportional to the particle speed. This value in cm/min multiplied by the inner cross-section of the blood tubing in cm^2 yields a flow rate in ml/min. Calibration of the inner diameter of the tubing is critical. In addition, the sonic contact between transducer and tubing must be adequate and requires the use of a silicone gel to improve the sonic transport. It is possible to monitor the electrical read out of blood flow with a high/low alarm contact system. In spite of the theoretical advantages, the expense and unreliability of current ultrasonic meters have prevented their use for routine clinical monitoring of blood flow rate.

Bubble trap flow indicator

Some blood tubing sets have a visual flow meter incorporated into the disposable bubble trap which is modified into two chambers separated by a disc containing a central hole through which the blood flows. A small tube allows free communication of air between the top of each chamber. As a result the height of the column of blood in the upper chamber is related to flow-rate. An appropriate scale is affixed to the upper chamber graduated from 100 to 400 ml/min.

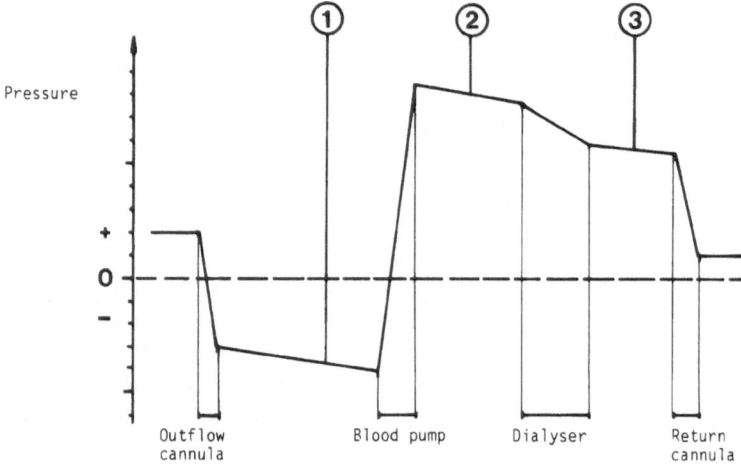

Figure 2. Pressure profile in the blood circuit. Pressure 1 is negative before the pump and pressures 2 and 3 are positive after it.

Pressure monitoring

Pressures in the blood circuit are monitored for two reasons. pressure monitoring is used to detect tubing separations as well as obstructions caused by clots, kinks or clamps. Pressures are also measured to aid in controlling fluid removal from the patient. In hemodialysis, fluid removal is achieved by applying a hydrostatic pressure differential across the dialyzer membrane, fluid being forced through membrane pores. This process is called ultrafiltration and the applied pressure differential is referred to as the transmembrane pressure (TMP). The TMP may be generated by applying positive (above-atmospheric) blood compartment pressures, negative dialysate compartment pressures, or a combination of both. The blood compartment pressure used in calculating the TMP is estimated by averaging the pressures at the inlet and outlet of the dialyzer. In routine clinical practice, as the pressure drop across the blood compartment is small, the pressure in the venous air trap is used as a reasonable approximation of the blood compartment pressure. This approximation becomes less valid as the blood flow rate and hematocrit rise. The indirect control of the ultrafiltration rate by adjusting the TMP is slowly being replaced by ultrafiltration control systems built into the newer dialysate delivery systems. These ultrafiltration control systems are capable of controlling the rate of ultrafiltration directly, the TMP becoming a dependent parameter rather than an independent controlling parameter.

The pressure profile in the blood circuit is depicted in Figure 2. Pressures that exceed atmospheric pressure are considered positive and those below atmospheric are negative. As seen in the figure, pressures upstream of the blood pump may be negative while those downstream of the pump are positive. It is the energy supplied by the pump that raises pressures from a negative to a positive level. Pressure monitoring is desirable at the locations indicated in Figure 2 for the following reasons:

The pressure before the blood pump (1 of Figure 2) is negative due to the resistance of the access site needle and tubing set. It is desirable to have as little negative pressure as possible for a given blood flow rate to avoid suction of the vessel wall into the lumen of the needle and to minimize the risk of air entry at bad joints. The length and internal bore of the fistula needle can increase the resistance by 100% if 38 mm by 1.5 mm needles are used instead of 15 mm by 2.0 mm needles (13).

The pressure between the blood pump (2 of Figure 2) and the dialyzer is always positive. As indicated earlier, its measurement permits a calculation of the transmembrane pressure when used in conjunction with the venous pressure. The 'venous' pressure, that is, the pressure after the dialyzer (3 of Figure 2), is measured in the air trap downstream of the dialyzer. Increase in resistance between the air trap and the return access site will cause a rise in pressure which may rupture the dialyzer. Reductions in blood flow as well as any disruption of the tubing between the bubble trap and the venous needle will reduce pressure and activate a low alarm. In addition, any alarm which stops the blood pump will cause the pressure at this point to drop and will usually result in a low pressure alarm.

Blood circuit pressure monitors and alarms are usually incorporated into the dialysate delivery system. There are three types of pressure monitors commonly in use.

Mechanical manometers

Mechanical manometers have mechanical, optical, or electronic contacts and depend upon a change in pressure causing a movement within bellows or Bourdon tubes which, by means of amplifying levers and gears, is then registered by a pointer. The pointer position is related to a graduated pressure scale. The mechanical alarm contacts are essentially make or break contacts which depend upon a junction between the moving pointer and the fixed alarm contact. In selecting a mechanical contact from the fail safe point of view, it is essential that the circuit be broken by the alarm

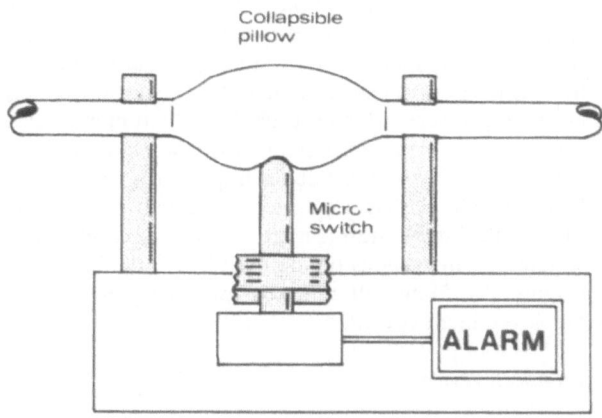

Figure 3. Collapsible 'pillow' pressure monitor.

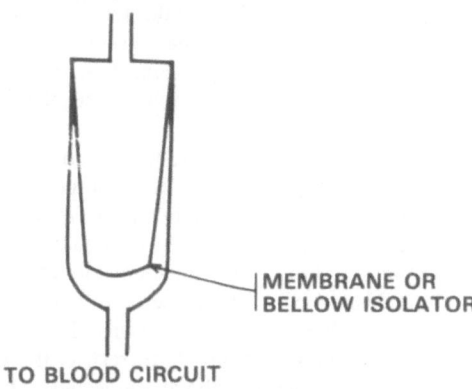

Figure 4. Blood pressure monitor isolator.

situation. It is also important that the voltage and current passing through the contact be sufficient to make the circuit. This will depend upon the surface area and the material used. Low resistance gold plating is frequently used because it resists oxidation which would cause an increase in resistance. DC circuits (12 to 24 V) are commonly employed, with high resistance components to safeguard against possible increase in resistance by oxidation of contacts. This type of alarm monitor with a range of −250 to +400 mm Hg is the oldest and perhaps the least reliable of pressure monitors.

Mechanical manometers with optical or electronic contacts are more reliable, theoretically. The contact between the moving pointer and the fixed alarm setting depends upon the pointer interrupting a light beam to a photosensitive cell. With electronic contacts the pointer changes the frequency of an oscillator circuit and thereby triggers an alarm. Although these methods involve more components and are expensive, the mechanical moving parts are reduced, resulting in greater reliability.

Electronic manometers

A pressure transducer picks up the pressure signal and converts it to an electrical signal. This value is then amplified and displayed either on a meter or as a digital read-out graduated in mm Hg. The alarm settings in the electronic system may be preset or adjustable either from the display panel or by the use of trim potentiometers inside the monitor. To visualize the alarm settings an adjustable graduated dial indicator with a fixed pressure range between high and low alarm points is sometimes provided. The indicator can be set to the pressure determined by the pointer on the meter. An alternative approach is the use of the electronic signal to record the pressure, with adjustable visible alarm contacts operated either by an optical device or by changing the frequency within an oscillator. The advantage of this system is that one has the more reliable measurement of pressure and at the same time visible adjustable alarm settings.

Enclosed pressure sack or pillow monitor

This device (Figure 3) is usually situated between the patient and the blood pump and is a crude method of detecting excessive negative pressure. The sack maintains the pressure when full and holds a microswitch in the make position; when the sack collapses the microswitch breaks and causes an alarm. The sack and the microswitch may be calibrated to alarm at a minimum given negative pressure which depends upon the thinness of the wall of the sack and the spring force of the microswitch. Even with such calibration, the pillow monitor is susceptible to frequent false alarms. It cannot be used in single needle dialysis.

Blood pressure monitor isolators

With all manometers and pressure transducers it is desirable that there is some form of isolation between the blood and the actual monitoring device. The development of isolators was necessitated originally because of the risk of transmission of hepatitis. Subsequently, protection of the monitor from blood contamination and the difficulty in cleaning it resulted in a rapid adoption of some form of disposable elastic non-permeable membrane or bellows used as a pressure monitor isolator (Figure 4). The alternative type of pressure isolator, in the form of a pore filter which closes on contact with liquids, is excellent for protecting the monitor but has a major disadvantage. After closure, no further pressure change can be recorded; thus unless the filter is changed, the monitor is rendered inoperative. Pressure isolators with hydrophobic membranes are also in use. These isolators can continue to transmit pressure even upon some wetting with liquid. However, if the isolator is filled with blood and clotting occurs, the pressure measurement will be unreliable, necessitating replacement of the isolator.

Pressure monitors should have an accuracy of ± 10 mm Hg at pressures less than 50 mm Hg and ± 10% of the indicated pressure at pressures above 50 mm Hg. The tolerance of ± 10 mm Hg is necessary to detect blood line separations occurring when blood circuit pressures are low. The tolerance of $\pm 10\%$ of the indicated pressure at pressures greater than 50 mm Hg is based on considerations of ultrafiltration control and prediction. The accuracy of the alarms should be ± 10 mm Hg relative to the indicated alarm setting.

Blood circuit pressure alarms, when activated, should shut the blood pump off and activate audible and visual signals of the alarm condition. When the cause of the alarm has been corrected, there should be a manual obligation to restart the blood pump. The maximum spread of pressure alarm limits should be internally set with operator adjustments being possible only within this range. For detection of separations, it would be desirable to restrict the low limit setting to pressures that are above atmospheric. If the low limit were set in the subatmospheric range, separations may remain undetected. This requirement may create a problem in priming the circuit before the initiation of dialysis. It is common practice to spread the alarm limits beyond the safe range during the priming procedure. A possible solution to this problem would be to incorporate a time delay of up to 60 sec inactivating the low alarm thereby enabling the pump to prime the circuit. It is undesirable to be able to bypass the low alarm setting.

Air leak monitoring

When hemodialysis is performed without a blood pump, the entire blood circuit is under positive pressure and embolism consequent to air entry into the blood circuit is extremely unlikely. However, with the predominant use of the A-V fistula pump circuit nowadays, the risk of air embolism has increased enormously as negative pressures are developed between the arterial fistula needle and the blood pump. The incidence of major air embolism has been reported as 1 per 2,000 hemodialyses (14). Foam-emboli with micro-bubbles of air mixed with blood are more common than pure air emboli and the mortality is around 25% of all reported cases. The causes of air entry include falling out of the outflow needle, leaks around any joint between the outflow needle and the blood pump, air entry from an empty intravenous glass fluid container infusion system before the blood pump, and air entry from the heparin infusion system placed before the blood pump. Reduction in the incidence of these accidents can be achieved by eliminating all joints and needle punctures before the blood pump and by infusion of heparin and saline downstream of the blood pump. Efficient degassing of the dialysis fluid will also reduce micro-bubble transport across the dialyzer membrane. However, despite minimizing these risks, air detectors remain essential. They are recommended for all hemodialysis blood circuits where subatmospheric pressure can be generated.

The ideal air detector will respond to the presence of foam or air and not to saline. It should not require bypass in order to prime the blood circuit. It should register an audible and visible alarm, fulfil the basic requirements of fail safe monitoring, be powered independently of the blood pump (and not in series with the pump's electrical supply) and in an alarm situation, must stop the blood pump. However, because of the high compliance of many disposable dialyzers, stopping of the blood pump will not prevent an air embolism, as the passive expulsion of air from an air-filled dialyzer under pressure will still reach the patient in most cases. Therefore, a solenoid clamping device which occludes the venous tube below the bubble trap is also required (see Figure 1). The air detector devices are usually placed around the venous bubble trap (Figure 5a), but some models are situated on the venous tubing itself below the bubble trap (Figure 5b). Many different physical principles have been employed in air detection.

Photocell devices

The earliest air detectors consisted of a light source which triggered a photocell situated on the opposite side of the bubble trap; the cell did not react if blood obstructed the light path. These devices were insensitive to foam and could not react if the light path was obstructed by fibrin deposits on the inner wall of the bubble trap. In addition, ambient light could reach the photocell and cause false alarms. Infrared light photocell devices have increased the sensitivity to air but are still not foolproof against obstruction to the passage of the infrared waves, or sensitive enough to be 100% reliable against foam without causing multiple false alarms.

Capacitance devices

Capacitance devices (15) are based upon the principle of change in the frequency of an oscillator circuit, which will vary with the presence of air or fluid within the range of the circuit, and with the thickness of the bubble trap wall, or an admixture of the two. By using two or more capacitor plates to surround the bubble trap, sensitive to different frequencies, changes in oscillation can predict the presence of air, foam, saline or blood in the bubble trap. Thus, theoretically, this device could fulfill all the requirements of the ideal detector. However, because of volume changes within the bubble trap associated with alterations in the venous pressure, variations in wall thickness of the bubble trap and alterations in the blood viscosity according to individual hematocrit levels, this device has proven too difficult to use. It must be calibrated for each patient and the sensitivity adjusted accordingly. In addition, it is not absolutely reliable for foam detection.

Ultrasonic devices

Ultrasonic devices (16) are based on the principle of the transmission of ultrasonic waves across the bubble trap. A voltage source to a transmitting ceramic crystal causes vibrations; ultrasonic waves then pass through the bubble trap to a ceramic crystal receiver, which vibrates on sensing the waves and creates a measurable electrical signal. Because blood or other fluids transmit sound more efficiently than air, a decrease in the intensity of the ultrasonic wave is easily

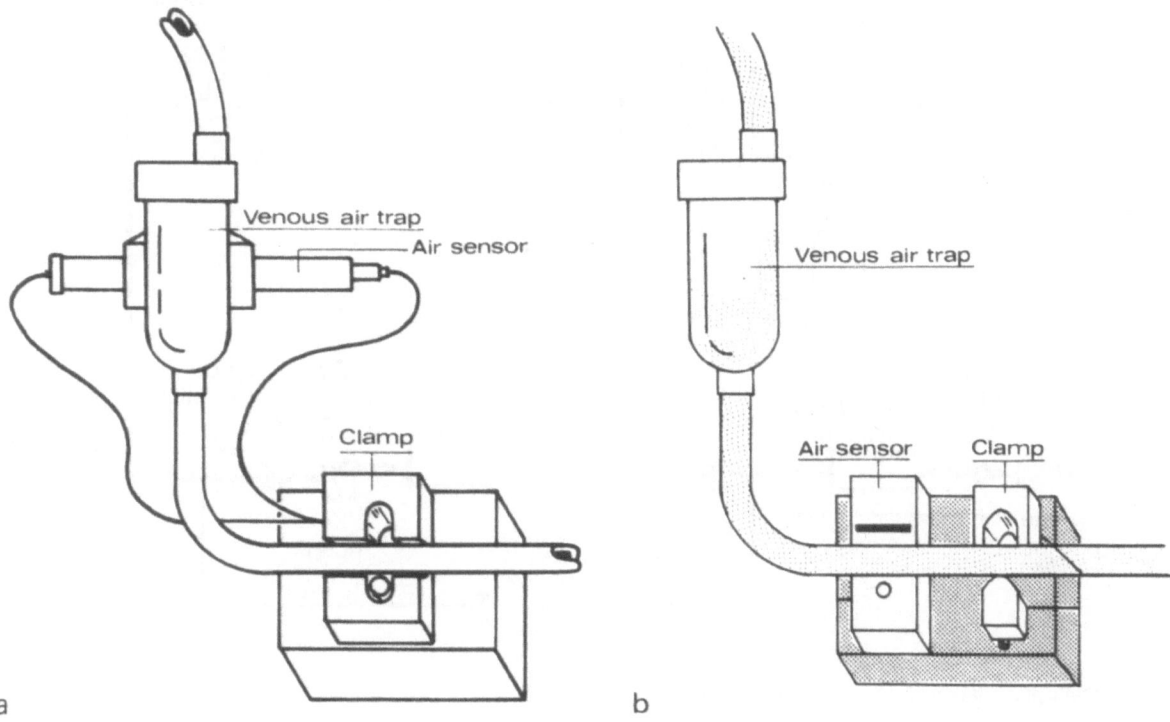

Figure 5. A. Air detector with sensor positioned on venous air trap and clamp on venous blood return line; B. Air detector with sensor and clamp positioned on venous blood return line.

detected. The major advantage of this technique is the specific damping effect on ultrasonic transmission of bubbles. Thus, this is probably the most reliable device for foam detection.

Blood line clamp

The ideal blood clamp should be occlusive against the maximal pressure generated in the blood circuit (up to 800 mm Hg) and not damage the blood tubing. In addition it should not restrict the tubing in the open position. It is usually powered by a solenoid valve with or without a mechanical spring lever working on the 'anvil' principle. For it to be fail-safe, it should close on 'break' and be held open in the 'make' position. However, in the event of electrical power failure, it becomes difficult to return the dialyzer blood content to the patient. For this reason some clamps are designed to function in the reverse sequence, which is, nevertheless, basically undesirable.

The volume of air required to cause clinical symptoms is uncertain. It has been reported that as little as 5 ml of air can be fatal (17), but it is generally accepted that volumes necessary to cause death range from 65 to 125 ml of rapidly injected air (18). Ward, et al (14) in analyzing their experiences with air embolism suggest that humans are probably sensitive to less air than 1 ml/kg/min. During hemodialysis air entering the patient may range from a massive bolus of

air to a short stream of microbubbles. Von Hartitszch and Medlock (19) report symptoms of nausea and vomiting attributed to a continuous stream of microbubbles which were 1 to 1.5 mm in diameter. Others report that no symptoms have occurred as a consequence of microbubble embolization (20). It is, therefore, difficult to specify minimum sensitivity of air detection until further research has established susceptibility limits for air occurring as large boluses, as large visible bubbles and as microbubbles or foam. If the air detector is extremely sensitive, it becomes subject to numerous false alarms and runs the risk of being inactivated by dialysis personnel.

Infusion pumps for anticoagulation

Infusion pumps are used to instill heparin, and sometimes protamine, into the blood circuit to control anticoagulation of blood. There are two types of infusion pumps used in hemodialysis, syringe pumps and peristaltic pumps. Syringe pumps are more commonly used. Infusion pumps may have fixed rates of infusion or variable rates ranging from 0.5 to 6.0 ml/h. They may either be free-standing units or incorporated into the dialysis fluid delivery system.

The site of infusion is sometimes located upstream of the blood pump which increases the risk of air embolism because of the subatmospheric pressures in this segment of the blood circuit. It is, therefore, preferable to locate the site of

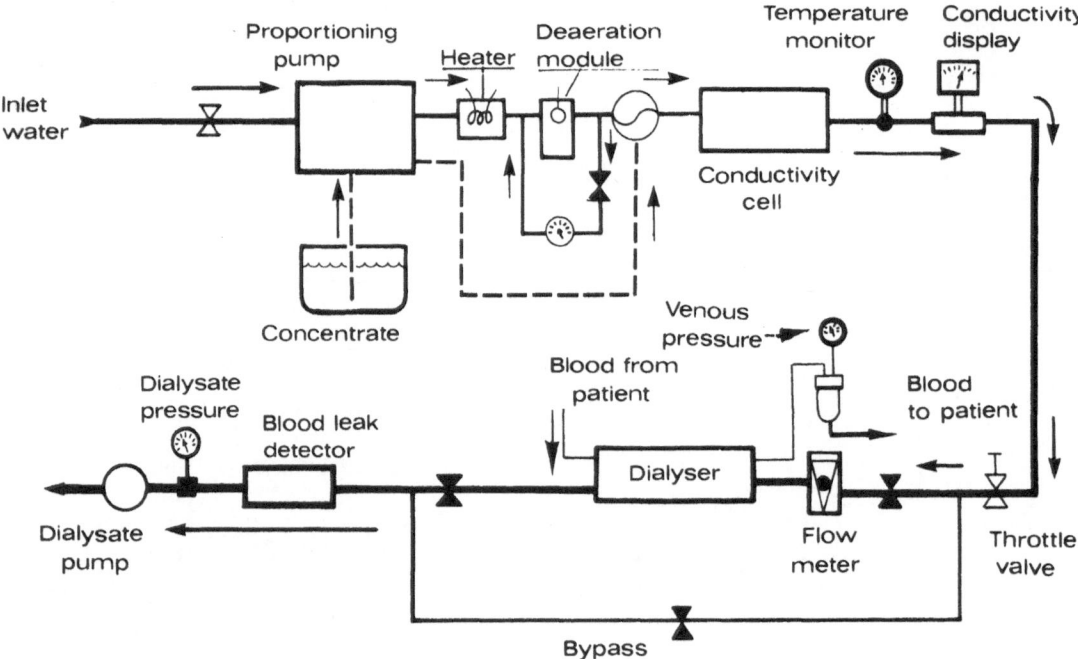

Figure 6. Schematic presentation of single pass dialysis fluid circuit.

infusion downstream of the blood pump, the venous air trap being a convenient location except for heparin. The infusion pump should be capable of accurate delivery against the pressures typically generated downstream of the blood pump. With syringe pumps, the inclusion of 'end of stroke' and 'infusion interrupted' (e.g. power failure) alarms are considered desirable. However, with adequate clinical surveillance of the dialysis, these features are not considered absolutely essential.

THE DIALYSIS FLUID CIRCUIT

The dialysate compartment of the dialyzer is perfused with dialysis fluid by the dialysate delivery system under appropriate conditions of concentration, temperature, pressure and flow. Monitors and alarms incorporated into the system monitor, and in some systems control, hydrostatic pressures applied across the dialyzer membrane for fluid removal. They also safeguard against dialyzer blood leaks and sudden changes of pressure in the blood circuit associated with separations and obstructions. In most current delivery systems, the blood pump, heparin infusion pump and air detector are built into the system with provisions for appropriate connections to, and positioning of, the blood tubing. The advantages of such an integrated system include a less cluttered treatment area, simplified operations and elimination of human errors in interconnecting free-standing devices.

Dialysate delivery systems may be single pass, recirculating single pass or recirculating systems. Each type may be further divided into single patient or multiple patient (cen-

tral) systems. In the single pass system, dialysis fluid is delivered to the dialyzer and, after a single pass, is pumped out to the drain. In the recirculating single pass system, dialysate is recirculated in the dialysate circuit with fresh dialysis solution being continuously introduced into the circuit, displacing dialysate and causing it to overflow to the drain. In the older recirculating systems, a large volume of dialysate was recirculated in the circuit with no provisions for supplying fresh dialysis fluid or overflow from the recirculating dialysate. At the treatment's beginning, the closed loop was filled with fresh dialysis solution; at the treatment's end, the spent dialysate was drained from the closed loop. In a newer version of this concept, a much smaller recirculating dialysate loop is used, with frequent replacement of the spent dialysate with fresh dialysis solution. In such a system, some loss of time and dialysis efficiency occurs with draining and filling of the recirculating loop.

Dialysis solution may be prepared as a batch process (manual or automated) or may be continuously proportioned (on-line). In single pass systems, dialysis solution is generally prepared on-line by proportioning water and concentrate. Recirculating systems are usually batch systems. Recirculating single pass systems may be batch or proportioning systems.

The composition of dialysis fluid and its preparation in recirculating and recirculating single pass systems are discussed in Chapter 8 and the clinical problems associated with incorrect formulation are discussed in Chapter 33. This chapter deals primarily with the single pass system, the system most commonly used today.

The introduction of dialysis fluid concentrate and the

principle of fluid proportioning in 1964 revolutionized hemodialysis. It eliminated the need for manual production of large quantities of dialysis solution used in batch systems, reduced the bacteriological problem and opened the way for single pass dialysis at 37° C. The basic single pass dialysate circuit used with either a central supply system and bedside monitors or an individual patient unit is illustrated in Figure 6. The continuous production of dialysis solution is achieved with a proportioning device, mixing water and concentrate. Water is heated and deaerated before being mixed with concentrate. The quality of the resulting dialysis fluid is assured by conductivity and temperature monitoring. If the quality of the fluid is outside prescribed limits, it by-passes the dialyzer. Normally, dialysate perfuses the dialyzer under conditions of controlled flow and pressure. The presence of red cells in dialysate, in case of a membrane rupture, is detected by a blood leak monitor situated after the dialyzer. The dialysate pressure is monitored by a pressure monitor and the dialysate then passes to drain via an effluent pump which creates the flow and pressure requirements of the circuit.

The dialysate delivery system consists of the proportioning device, conductivity monitoring, temperature regulation and monitoring, blood leak detection, dialysis fluid pressure and flow regulation and monitoring. In addition to these functions the dialysate delivery system also deaerates dialysate, interfaces with the air detector and blood pump and incorporates a disinfection scheme using chemicals or hot water. Typically, blood circuit pressure monitors and alarm circuitry are incorporated into the dialysate delivery system.

Conductivity monitoring

In proportioning systems, treated water and concentrate are mixed in the desired ratio, electrical conductivity being the parameter commonly used to monitor appropriate proportioning. The proportioning ratio may be fixed, adjustable to a desired value or continuously variable with servo-control based on continuous, internal conductivity monitoring.

Proportioning pumps may be motor or water driven. Motor driven pumps may be of the piston, plunger or membrane type and are usually bulky and noisy but have functioned well for over 10 years with very few problems. Water driven pumps are driven by water pressure and are generally quieter and smaller than motor driven pumps. Servo-control systems may have a peristaltic pump whose speed is servo-controlled or a venturi orifice whose opening is servo-controlled. Though separate sensors are usually used for monitoring and for control, the two conductivity cells are usually identical in design and the possibility of simultaneous failures exists. Further, crystallization of concentrate in a venturi orifice can cause problems. The advantages of the servo-controlled system are potential miniaturization and lower costs.

Fatalities have been associated with improper proportioning of dialysate (21–23). In many instances, human error and negligence were contributing factors. Easily accessible by-pass switches or a re-zeroing feature constitute poor design

practice and increase the potential for human errors. Improper proportioning can also result from clogging of the concentrate filter and other orifices and metering ports in the proportioning system. The probability of such clogging increases if the particulate contamination of concentrate is not controlled.

The principle of monitoring proportioning of concentrate and water is an indirect one, which depends upon the specific conductivity of the total ionic content of the dialysate. Temperature changes influence the measurement by about 1.7%/° C in the clinical range of operation. Conductivity is expressed in mS (milliSiemens) or mmhos/cm (milli 'mhos' per centimeter where 'mho' represents the reciprocal of ohm). Dialysate (sodium concentration 130 to 150 mEq/l) has a conductivity of approximately 13 to 15 mS. Conductivity is monitored in conductivity cells which may function by one of two methods. The resistive or impedance method is more commonly used. Two electrodes are immersed in the dialysate and an alternating current of high frequency (1 Khz) pulses through the fluid. When changes in temperature are compensated, the only variable is the electrical resistance of the dialysate which causes an alteration in the current passing between the electrodes, which may be read on a meter. Temperature compensation requires a separate circuit consisting of a thermistor which senses temperature changes in the range of 34 to 41° C and corrects the conductivity output signal accordingly. The alternative method is inductive where two electro-magnetic coils replace electrodes and the alteration in the current passing through them represents changes in the conductivity of the dialysate. Temperature compensation is again necessary. It is always mandatory, when calibrating a new conductivity cell or changing the concentrate formula, to correlate a given conductivity reading to a direct measurement of the sodium concentration in the dialysate by flame photometry, as the conductivity varies with the ratios of chloride to acetate or bicarbonate and the presence or absence of glucose.

Problems arising with conductivity measurement are usually due to coating of the electrodes with deposits from the dialysate or with air bubbles from deaeration of the dialysate. These artefacts increase the resistance resulting in a false low conductivity measurement. Design of the cell to prevent gas accumulation is important. It should have a small fluid channel pathway, and the electrodes should be made of an anticorrosive and non-toxic material. The induction coil method has the advantage that air bubbles have a smaller effect upon current changes. Design of the conductivity monitoring system is extremely important for the safety of the hemodialysis. It must follow the fail-safe basis described above. The meter design is usually of the continuous scale type where its range should not exceed the physiological limits of safety, i.e. the equivalent of 120 to 160 mEq/l sodium (approximately 12 to 16 mS). If, however, the meter is of the zero type, the percentage deviation from a precalibrated known conductivity set at zero should not exceed ± 10%. Both types should detect 1% changes easily. The alarm setpoints should not be movable beyond the safe limits of the physiological range of conductivity. The acceptable limits of the alarm setpoints vary in clinical practice, but are usually ± 3% of the desired measurement. It is essential that the monitor be independent of the system controlling proportioning and that the control system be based on a different monitoring principle. Thus, the tendency nowadays to sacrifice safety in this area for the sake of miniaturization and low cost (as in most servo-controlled systems) is regrettable. Conductivity monitors should activate automatically during the dialysis mode and it should not be possible to circumvent these monitors or their alarms when a dialyzer is connected to the delivery system. The triggering of an alarm, when there is an error in the quality of the dialysate, must stop the delivery to the dialyzer, diverting the fluid to drain, and at the same time cause an audible and visual alarm. Methods of interruption of the dialysate supply to the dialyzer during an alarm include solenoid valve bypass systems or stopping the suction pump which normally draws the fluid through the dialyzer. It is, however, usual to continue to produce and monitor dialysis solution during an alarm period in order to permit correction of the error while the machine is in the bypass or safe modality.

Temperature monitoring

Early designs of delivery systems used cold dialysate to retard bacterial growth in the recirculation reservoir with heat exchangers provided for rewarming the blood. Modern delivery systems utilize a thermostatically controlled heater to warm the incoming water which is then mixed with concentrate at room temperature, the temperature sensor being located downstream of the point of mixing. The temperature of the dialysate is maintained within the physiological range of 36°C to 42°C. Though red cell hemolysis may result only at temperatures greater than 45°C, protein denaturation can take place above 42°C (24).

Overheated dialysate can cause hemolysis and even death (25, 26). One report (26) indicates that exposure of blood to 47°C to 51°C caused a form of chronic hemolysis rather than sudden, massive hemolysis. Underheated dialysate causes patient discomfort from chilling but does not usually damage the formed elements in blood. It has, however, been reported that low temperature dialysate can activate an anti-N-like cold agglutinin precipitating extracorporeal coagulation (27).

Heat exchangers and (or) immersion heating elements are used to generate the required temperature. They should be constructed from passivated stainless steel and never from copper or aluminum, because of the risk of copper or aluminum intoxication. To reduce the risk of corrosion, it is preferable that water alone be in contact with the heating element and that dilution of the concentrate occur after the heating of the water. With a single pass (500 ml/min) delivery system, 1.5 kW is sufficient to raise cold water to the dialysing temperature. If hot water disinfection is required, a reduction in flow to 200 to 300 ml/min will permit the 1.5 kW heating source to raise the water temperature to 85°C. The 1.5 kW energy requirement enables the machine to draw its electrical supply from a standard domestic wall socket in most countries.

The heating system control may employ a mechanical thermostat with large temperature swings between the on and off settings or a precise closed loop proportioning band with continuous adjustment of the heating element current compensating for temperature fluctuations detected by the sensor. The advantage of the latter system is that the lag time between a temperature deviation and its correction is much shorter, so that the volume of the fluid dead space, necessary to damp out temperature fluctuations, can be reduced considerably. The thermostat system usually requires a reservoir of at least one liter to produce a constant temperature. This is undesirable as it constitutes a source of bacterial growth during dialysis and presents problems of cleaning and adequate sterilization, which tend to be time consuming because of the large volume.

The accuracy of temperature control and monitoring should be ± 1°C. The monitor should have at least a high alarm limit with audible and visual alarms. The accuracy of the monitor and high alarm set point should be such that dialysate temperature does not exceed 42°C, inclusive of monitor and alarm set point errors. Temperature monitors and alarms should be independent of temperature controls and adjustments should be possible only within the physiological range of 36°C to 42°C. It should not be possible to circumvent the monitor or its alarm when a dialyzer is connected to the delivery system. If hot water disinfection is used, means, such as a shunt-interlock system, should be provided to prevent dialysis during the disinfection cycle.

Pressure monitoring

As indicated earlier, the determination of transmembrane pressure for fluid removal requires measurement of the pressure in the dialysate compartment. Single pass proportioning systems are sometimes referred to as negative pressure systems because they can generate negative dialysate pressures for facilitating fluid removal. The negative pressure may be generated either by locating a constricting valve upstream of the dialyzer and a dialysate pump downstream of the dialyzer or by using two pumps, one on either side of the dialyzer, the downstream pump being operated at a faster flow setting than the upstream one. Dialysate pumps should be self-priming and capable of pumping air during the priming of the circuit.

As with the blood compartment pressure, the dialysate compartment pressure can be estimated by averaging the inlet and outlet pressures. However, as the dialysate compartment pressure drop is usually small, in most delivery systems only one of the two pressures is measured for calculating the transmembrane pressure (TMP).

Dialysate pressures are measured with mechanical or electronic manometers similar to those used for blood circuit pressures. If the manometer is located on a 'T' fitting rather than in a 'flow through' configuration, stagnant areas inaccessible to sterilant exist and there is the potential for bacterial contamination and proliferation. Dialysate pressure monitors usually include high and low limit alarms with

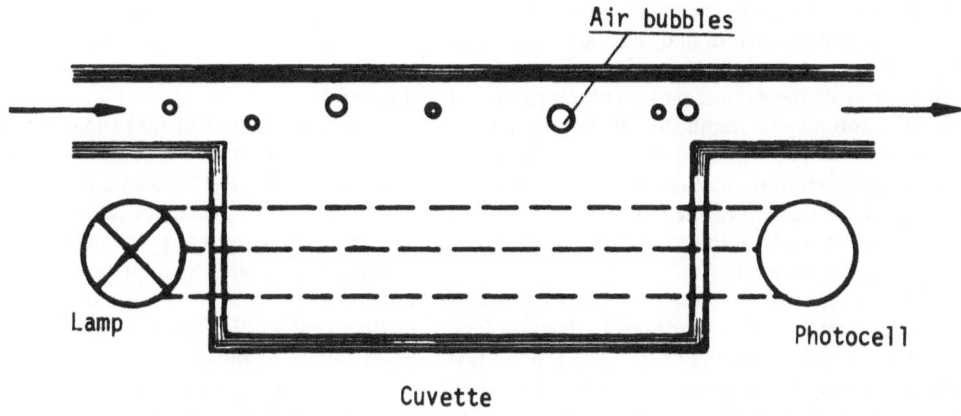

Figure 7. Bloodleak sensor with a flow-through configuration.

audible and visual indications of the alarm condition.

Some dialysate delivery systems display the TMP. The TMP is usually based on one blood compartment and one dialysate compartment pressure and is, therefore, an approximation of the true TMP. Some systems also provide servo-control of the TMP, thus maintaining a constant TMP even with changing blood compartment pressures.

Dialysate pressure monitors should have a range of -400 to $+300$ mm Hg and be accurate to ± 20 mm Hg or $\pm 10\%$ of the indicated reading, whichever is greater. The same limits on accuracy apply to the TMP display for systems that display this parameter rather than the dialysate pressure. Alarms which are adjustable should not allow settings outside the monitor's scaled range. The alarm setting accuracy should be ± 10 mm Hg or $\pm 10\%$ of the setting whichever is greater.

If positive dialysate pressures are achievable, safeguards should be provided to prevent dialysate compartment pressures from exceeding blood compartment pressures. This is necessary, because if a membrane leak develops, not only will the leak go undetected because of the pressure gradient from dialysate to blood, but the blood circuit will also be contaminated with non-sterile dialysate.

Flow monitoring

As with blood flow rates, dialyzer clearances of small solutes increase as the dialysis fluid flow rate rises but at a diminishing rate until a relative clearance plateau is reached. The dialysis fluid flow rate is, therefore, one determinant of solute transport across the dialyzer membrane. Typically, the dialysis fluid flow rate is 500 ml/min for single pass systems. At this flow rate dialyzer clearances are less sensitive to changes in dialysis fluid flow rate than to changes in the blood flow rate.

In some single pass delivery systems, the proportioning pumps deliver dialysis solution to a storage vessel from which the dialyzer is perfused by a separate pump. In other systems, the proportioning pump also functions as the dialy-

sis fluid delivery pump. Not all delivery systems display the flow rate and few systems incorporate alarms for out of range flow rates. In some systems, the dialysate flow rate is internally set and operator adjustment of flow rates is not easily accomplished. These features all relate to the non-critical nature of the flow rate in terms of patient safety. In systems that display dialysate flow rate, a calibrated flow meter is usually provided, situated either before or after the dialyzer. An accuracy of $\pm 10\%$ of indicated flow is considered quite adequate.

Blood leak monitoring

Delivery systems incorporate a sensor, usually of the photo-optical type, that can detect the presence of blood in dialysate. Some sensors use the visible light spectrum while others use the blue spectrum for improved sensitivity. In the event of a blood leak, there are audible and visual indications of the alarm condition and power to the blood pump is interrupted. In addition, in some systems, the flow of dialysate bypasses the dialyzer. The threshold of blood leak detection is adjustable in some systems, so that, with a minor blood leak, the threshold is increased and dialysis continued.

As the osmolality of dialysate is not very different from that of blood, the red cells entering dialysate, in the event of a membrane leak, do not hemolyze. Blood leak detection is, therefore, accomplished by measuring the change in optical transmission caused by the scattering of light by hemoglobin-containing red cells. Some manufacturers use hemoglobin standards for calibrating blood leak sensors. This may lead to inaccuracies of calibration, because with a membrane leak the hemoglobin is within the red cell membrane rather than in solution.

The blood leak sensor usually has a 'flow-through' configuration (Figure 7). Some sensor designs are susceptible to false alarms produced by trapping of air bubbles in the optical path. The incidence of this artefact can be minimized by efficient deaeration of dialysate and by appropriate design of the sensor. For example, if the light path is situated at the bottom of the sensor cuvette and the fluid enters and leaves at the top, buoyancy of the air bubbles will help keep the air bubbles out of the optical path. The sensitivity of blood leak detection may be diminished if the windows of the cuvette become coated with deposits from the dialysate. The cuvette should, therefore, be easily accessible for regular cleaning and it should be possible to introduce a control filter to check the sensitivity of the sensor and intactness of the electrical monitoring circuits.

In some delivery systems, the blood leak is not quantitated, and instead, a relative index of the magnitude of the leak is provided. This makes estimation of the actual blood loss difficult especially if hemoglobin standards have been used for calibration. Quantifying the detector in milliliters of blood per liter of dialysate, a detection threshold of 0.25 ml/l for nonadjustable detectors and a maximum threshold of 0.35 ml/l for adjustable detectors are recommended. Such a calibration can be achieved using a blood standard having the characteristics of uremic blood with a subnormal hematocrit. Having initially calibrated the detector with a blood standard, subsequent testing of the detector can be done by more convenient methods such as the interposition of an optical filter.

Dialysis fluid deaeration

The feed water to the delivery system usually has a considerable amount of dissolved air, especially during the cold, winter months. Dialysis solution prepared from this water has a tendency to 'degas' under conditions of negative pressure and heating to operating temperatures. The gas that comes out of solution may result in flow maldistribution in the dialyzer's dialysate compartment by 'air-locking' or obstructing flow passages. Membrane masking by air bubbles may also result. As a consequence, solute clearances may be reduced. In addition, dialysate compartment pressure drops could increase, making TMP estimation, and hence ultrafiltration prediction, unreliable. When dialysate has a high concentration of dissolved air, air may cross the dialyzer membrane into blood and contribute to foaming in the venous air trap (28, 29). Foaming is undesirable because of the potential for air embolism as well as microembolism from small clots formed at the blood-air interface.

Deaeration of dialysate in delivery systems is usually achieved by first heating incoming water to physiologic temperatures, and then subjecting it to extreme negative pressures (300 to 600 mm Hg below atmospheric) and venting air released from solution. The negative pressures are usually achieved by a constricting valve upstream from a pump that recirculates water in a closed loop which contains an air trap and vent (Figure 6). Some systems use elevated temperatures rather than negative pressure for deaeration. The incoming water is heated to temperatures around 85° C to facilitate deaeration. In such systems, a heat exchanger is used to cool the deaerated stream by heat transfer to the incoming water. Some delivery systems do not have good deaeration capabilities and merely incorporate a filter that

provides nucleation sites for air bubble formation. These small bubbles then coalesce into larger ones which are vented. This scheme does not accomplish effective removal of dissolved air.

Von Hartitzsch et al (28) suggested limiting the pO_2 of dialysate entering the dialyzer to no more than 150 mm Hg. Drukker, Werff and Meinsma (29), based on more recent experience, indicated that problems related to air in dialysate are non-existent at pO_2 values under 130 mm Hg. Inlet water temperatures and pressures greatly influence the amount of air which comes out of solution. Therefore, rather than rely on dialysate pO_2 values, the efficacy of deaeration should be quantitated. An example of such quantitation would be to assume a standard inlet water condition (e.g. 4° C at 760 mm Hg) and to then choose the lowest clinically relevant negative pressure (e.g. −500 mm Hg) at which no air comes out of solution. The volume of air at inlet conditions less the saturation volume at the chosen negative pressure is denoted as 100% removal and the actual removal expressed as a percentage of this total.

Disinfection of the dialysis fluid delivery system

The input water to the dialyzer is usually contaminated with common water bacteria unless it has been adequately pretreated. Water softeners and deionizers can contribute to bacterial proliferation because of their inherent 'dead spaces'. Dialysate at 37° C, especially if it contains glucose, supports bacterial growth. Dialysate delivery systems, therefore, require periodic disinfection to prevent excessive bacterial contamination of dialysate. Disinfection may be achieved either with hot water at 90° C to 95° C or with chemicals such as formaldehyde, sodium hypochlorite or peracetic acid.

Delivery systems usually have a mode switch that initiates the disinfection, cool-down (for hot water sterilization) and rinse cycles. The disinfection cycle should not only allow adequate contact time, but also expose all parts of the flow circuit to the disinfectant. In systems designed to introduce disinfectant in the concentrate line, the dialysate-contacting but not the water-containing parts of the flow circuit are disinfected. With hot water disinfection, cooling may be achieved by rinsing the whole circuit with cool dialysate, thereby cooling and rinsing simultaneously. Hot water disinfection may caramelize residual glucose and lead to flow obstructions and coating of blood leak detector lenses. In some delivery systems the disinfection, cool-down (for hot water disinfection) and rinse phases are automatically sequenced with adequate time for each phase.

An important requirement of the delivery system is that it prevents the operator from dialyzing a patient during the disinfection, cool or rinse cycles. Once the disinfection cycle is initiated, it should be impossible for the dialyze mode to be selected until the cycle has been completed. This can be achieved by means such as a shunt interlock switch. The shunt connector activates a microswitch that prevents initiation of dialysis. Further, the temperature and conductivity monitors are overridden during this phase. An additional safeguard would be to have no power to the blood pump during this phase. Further, in systems that proportion the disinfectant, some means should be provided that will necessitate replacing the disinfectant with concentrate before selecting the dialyze mode. This is especially important for central systems.

In systems that have dead ends, 'T-joints' and areas of reduced flow, inadequate disinfection may result with consequent contamination of the dialysate by bacteria and pyrogens. The problem is magnified because these systems are also susceptible to bacterial proliferation. Such system designs may also lead to inadequate rinse-out of disinfectant and potential toxic reactions.

The connection of the drain line of the delivery system to the drain receptacle should be such as to prevent backsiphoning and contamination due to retrograde growth of drain piping organisms. An air gap at the drain connection is one means of achieving this.

Formaldehyde is a very effective disinfectant and is widely used in dialysis for disinfecting delivery systems as well as for disinfecting dialyzers for multiple use. Formaldehyde is, however, an unpleasant toxic substance and there is, hence, the risk of patient and staff exposure to formaldehyde from spills, splashes and fumes. Inhalation of formaldehyde has been associated with asthmatic reactions (30) and contact dermatitis due to formaldehyde in clothing textiles has been reported (31). Inadequate rinsing of formaldehyde could result in formaldehyde crossing the membrane into the blood circuit. Toxic symptoms produced by formaldehyde include transitory burning sensation in the vascular region, an uneasy feeling with a smothering sensation, a drop in blood pressure and a strange taste in the mouth (32). Chronic toxicity of formaldehyde is not well documented but neurological and retinal disturbances, metabolic acidosis and hemolysis have been suspected (33). Formaldehyde may also be a potent inactivator of heparin (32) and thereby contribute to clotting and resultant blood loss. There is considerable circumstantial evidence (34–38) linking the use of formaldehyde to the formation of anti-N-like antibodies especially in the context of dialyzer disinfection with formaldehyde. The clinical significance of this relatively rare antibody is not well known but is has been implicated in renal allograft failure (39) and a shortened red cell life span (40). It has been demonstrated (40, 41) that the formaldehyde-induced alteration of red cell membranes is dose-dependent and that the formation of anti-N-like antibodies can be prevented by reducing the residual formaldehyde concentration below 10 μg/ml. (See also Chapter 18).

The Clinitest ®, which is widely used for formaldehyde detection, has been shown to be incapable of detecting concentrations under 15 μg/ml (32). The Hantzsch test has been proposed as a more sensitive screening test for residual formaldehyde (32).

Hypochlorite and peracetic acid have also been used to disinfect dialysate delivery systems. A major disadvantage of both hypochlorite and peracetic acid is their corrosive effect on metals. Hypochlorite is also considered to be a less effective disinfectant than formaldehyde or peracetic acid.

However, hypochlorite very effectively breaks up and dissolves bacterial slime or biofilm that forms on various components of the dialysate circuit.

Microbiological quality and pyrogenicity of dialysate

Sepsis, bacteremias and pyrogen reactions in patients on dialysis have been associated with contaminated dialysate (42–44). The underlying causes for contamination of the dialysate include contaminated water supplies, contaminated concentrate, inadequate system disinfection, inappropriate drain connections with back siphoning from the drain, improper system design and system failures.

Standards have been established for the microbiological quality of water used to prepare dialysis solution as well as for the effluent dialysate at the end of the dialysis session. According to the AAMI standard (9), total viable counts should not exceed 200 cfu/ml in water and 2,000 cfu/ml in effluent dialysate. Standards limiting the pyrogen concentration of dialysate have yet to be established. Concentrate standards indicate that either the concentrate should be non-pyrogenic or the water and chemicals used to manufacture the concentrate should be non-pyrogenic. The concentrate standard has been successfully met by manufacturers for acetate concentrates but problems have been encountered with aqueous and powder formulations of bicarbonate concentrate (45). Even with aqueous bicarbonate concentrates labeled as bacteristatic by the manufacturer, high microbial and endotoxin levels have been measured (45) and it has been demonstrated that these concentrates, once contaminated, support rapid proliferation of organisms with a consequent rise of endotoxin concentrations. Microbial levels of the order of 10^5 cfu/ml and pyrogen levels of 12 to 24 ng/ml have been demonstrated. Dialysate made from these concentrates will also have a high level of bacterial and endotoxin contamination with potential risks to the patient unless appropriate control measures are instituted. These include avoidance of prolonged storage of concentrate, frequent cleaning and disinfection of delivery systems and of concentrate containers, as well as frequent monitoring of dialysate quality. If microbiological and endotoxin quality of dialysate are still inadequate, ultraviolet irradiation or membrane filtration of concentrate may be necessary.

Standards limiting the endotoxin levels of dialysate need to be established. This is especially important with the use of high permeability membranes. Such membranes allow the passage of solutes of the order of 10,000 daltons and also have very high ultrafiltration coefficients necessitating the use of an ultrafiltration control system. As discussed later in this chapter, the use of these membranes with an ultrafiltration controller results in substantial rates of reverse filtration from dialysate to blood, with the potential risk of carryover into blood of reactive endotoxin fragments, 10,000 daltons in size or smaller.

Electrical safety

The potential for electric shock in dialysis patients exists because of the current transmission capability of a circuit which includes extracorporeal blood, the dialyzer membrane, and dialysate. If the equipment is appropriately grounded, this hazard does not exist. However, with restrictions on equipment current leakage, the seriousness of the hazard can be minimized when equipment grounding is absent or inappropriate.

Lefferson and Goss (46) described circumstances in which an electric current may flow through this circuit. These include broken ground wires, and dialysis machinery and other applicances not being at the same ground potential. They illustrated methods of reducing the hazards from a broken ground wire by reducing the amount of current leakage using isolation transformers or high impedance leakage current paths. The hazard of dialysis machinery and other appliances not being at the same ground potential is a particular risk for home dialysis patients; hospitals generally have equipotential ground systems.

Deller (47) has shown that the typical total impedance of the combination of dialysate, blood lines, blood, and dialyzer is about 400 kiloohms. Hence, dialysis patients have little danger of electric shock during normal conditions of no ground or insulation failures. However, when direct contact is made with the device, the protective impedance of the blood and dialysate circuit is bypassed and the potential for electric shock exists. Frize et al (48), described an experiment in which a dog was connected to a current source and ground via the cephalic vein in the left foreleg and muscles or the righ rear leg. Current at 60 Hz was applied to a level of 85 milliamperes, RMS. No pump (heart) failure or fibrillation occurred.

Proposed limits for dialysis machines range from 100 to 500 microamperes. AAMI and the American National Standards Institute, Inc (ANSI) have determined that risk current limits for dialysis machines should be set at 100 microamperes, RMS (49). We believe that this limit implies a large margin of safety.

Other electrical hazards of dialysis equipment exist in addition to those described as leakage currents or grounds at unequal potential. Electrical components of dialyzers operate in an environment in which liquid spills are common. The spills occur because of frequent intravenous fluid administration, priming of extracorporeal circuits with saline, connection of dialysate supply hoses to dialyzers, and maintenance of hydraulic components within dialysate supply devices. External switches and plugs or receptacles are especially susceptible to spills. Such spills cause violent short circuits to develop, with fire and destruction of circuitry commonly resulting.

Overview of system safety

Some manufacturers allow the user to choose the specific configuration of monitors desired. A basic system is offered, and other system monitors are optional. Although such flexibility is sometimes desirable, it may allow patient safety to be compromised in favor of low equipment cost. Relative to patient safety, a minimum system can be proposed which should have the following monitors:

1. Temperature monitor with at least a high limit alarm.
2. Conductivity monitor with high and low limit alarms.
3. At least one manometric device with high and low limit alarms for blood circuit pressure monitoring.
4. Blood leak detector with a quantifiable level of detection.
5. Provisions for interfacing with an air detector, if it is not included as part of the system.
6. At least one dialysate pressure monitor with high and low limit alarms (for delivery systems that rely on dialysate pressure control for fluid removal). The recommendations made earlier for each type of monitor also apply to the minimum system.

When free standing devices such as the air detector, blood pump and infusion pump are used in conjunction with the dialysate delivery system, suitable interfacing should be provided so that the addition of accessories does not compromise the integrity of monitoring and alarms.

As indicated earlier, functional testing of monitors and alarms should be easily accomplished without the need for special tools so that such testing may be incorporated into the dialysis procedure. Such testing should not be limited to a check of the electronic monitoring and alarm circuitry but should also include the sensors. It should be possible to test and calibrate each monitor independently using external standards.

ULTRAFILTRATION CONTROL SYSTEMS

The control of ultrafiltration by controlling the transmembrane pressure is fraught with many uncertainties. It assumes accurate measurement of four pressures (blood inlet and outlet and dialysate inlet and outlet pressures) as well as accurate knowledge of the *in vivo* ultrafiltration coefficient of the dialyzer. Further, accuracy requires a correction for the oncotic pressure of plasma proteins. In the clinical setting only two pressures are usually measured, the blood outlet pressure and either the dialysate inlet or outlet pressure depending on the type of delivery system in use. Further, the pressure measuring devices used are not located at the same horizontal fluid level. Hence, errors due to vertical fluid columns exist. The ultrafiltration coefficient of the dialyzer specified by the manufacturer is usually a nominal value with a ± 10 to 20% deviation around the mean. If the dialyzer is reprocessed for multiple use, further uncertainties regarding the ultrafiltration coefficient exist as the coefficient may change with reprocessing. In the light of all these uncertainties, the control of ultrafiltration becomes a guessing game and corrections to the transmembrane pressure may often be necessary during dialysis to achieve the desired ideal finishing weight. Consequently, the patient may be subjected to varying rates of ultrafiltration with the potential for hypovolemic hypotension or inadequate fluid removal.

The recent introduction of ultrafiltration control systems to measure and control directly the rate of ultrafiltration makes fluid removal during dialysis uniform, accurate and

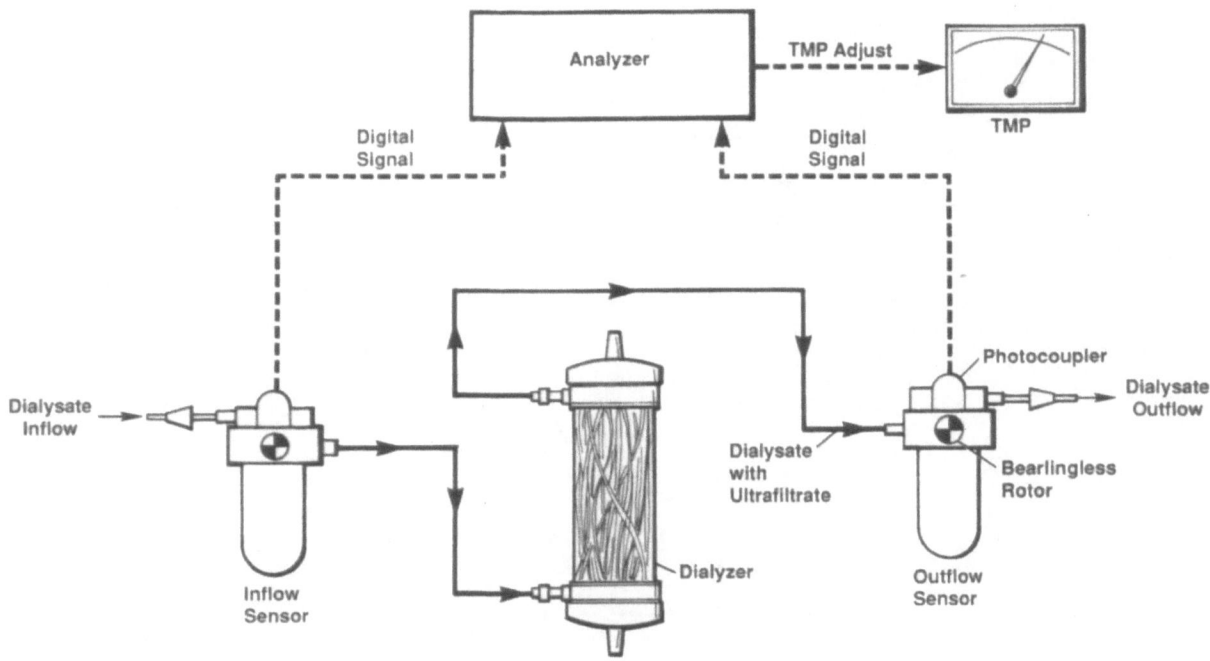

Figure 8. Schematic representation of the flow sensor scheme of ultrafiltration control.

predictable. With a fixed ultrafiltration rate, weight loss is linear and the desired finishing weight is approached predictably with a potential accuracy of ± 200 g.

There are three basic types of ultrafiltration control systems: flow sensors, balancers, and closed loops.

Flow sensor systems

This system (Figure 8) uses flow sensors in the dialysate inflow and outflow streams to measure the rate of dialysate flow to and from the dialyzer. The difference between the outflow and inflow rates is the rate of ultrafiltration. This difference is measured by digital circuitry and is fed back to the transmembrane pressure circuit. The transmembrane pressure is varied until the measured and desired rates of ultrafiltration become equal. Two types of sensors have been used. One is a bearingless rotor the speed of rotation of which is measured with an optical beam and correlated to flow rate. The other is an electromagnetic flow sensor which measures the voltage developed by the flow of a conductive solution through a magnetic field. The voltage developed is proportional to the flow rate. In the electromagnetic scheme, the inflow and outflow streams flow through a differential flow sensor so that the difference is directly measured rather than measuring each flow rate and then calculating the difference. In both the rotor and electromagnetic schemes, the flow sensors must be kept clean and free of bacterial slime and particulates for accurate determination of the flow rates. Frequent bleaching of the flow sensors is recommended to ensure cleanliness and reliable operation.

Volumetric balancing systems

The balancing system (Figure 9) uses matched pumps (usually diaphragm pumps) with appropriate valving to keep the dialysate inflow exactly equal to the dialysate outflow, thus establishing a quasi-closed loop. As shown in the schematic, two diaphragm pumps are used out of phase, to establish matched continuous flow of dialysate. A separate pump is used to remove fluid from this non-compliant quasi-closed loop at the desired rate of ultrafiltration. The fluid loop being non-compliant, ultrafiltrate flow across the dialysis membrane takes place to match the rate of fluid removal by the pump. The accuracy of this system depends on two factors, accurate calibration of the pump that withdraws fluid from the loop and accurate balancing of the dialysate inflow and outflow rates. Accurate balancing requires appropriate design and functioning of the matched pumps as well as appropriate sealing of the valves used in the balancing system. The presence of bacterial slime or particulates can compromise the valve seals with consequent inaccuracies of ultrafiltration control.

Closed loop system

The closed loop system (Figure 10) resembles in some respects the balancing system. Instead of a quasi-closed loop, an actual closed loop with recirculating dialysate flow is used. As in the balancing system, a separate pump withdraws fluid from the closed loop with a matched flow of ultrafiltrate across the dialyzer membrane. As uremic toxins

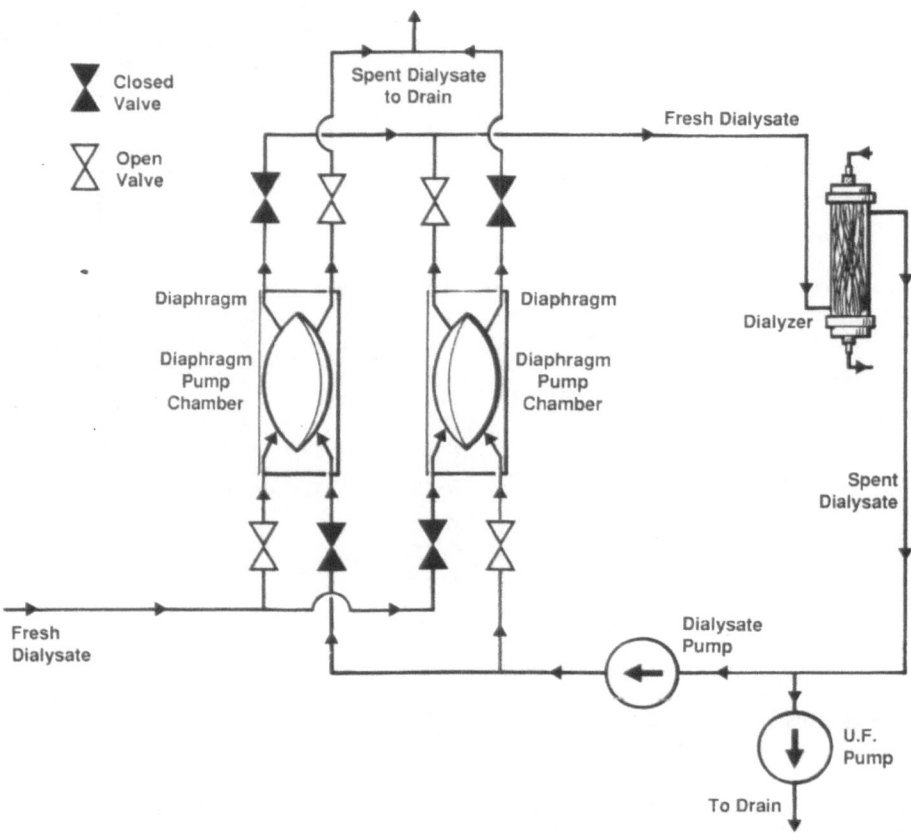

Figure 9. Ultrafiltration control based on the balancing scheme.

build up in the closed loop, the dialysate is periodically discharged to drain and fresh dialysis fluid is used to fill the closed loop. The accuracy of this type of system depends only on the accuracy of the pump used for fluid withdrawal. However, the drawbacks of the closed loop scheme include microbiological contamination of the closed loop, loss of effective dialysis time in emptying and filling the loop and some loss of dialysis efficiency as toxin concentrations build up in the closed loop decreasing the diffuse gradient across the dialyzer membrane.

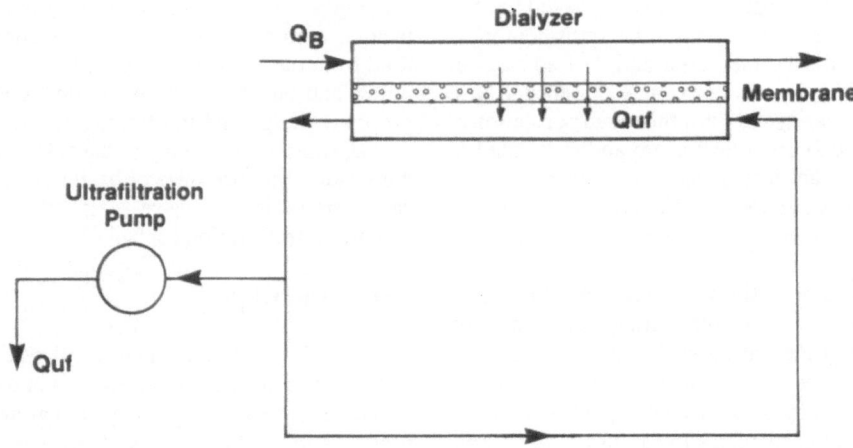

Figure 10. The closed loop ultrafiltration control system.

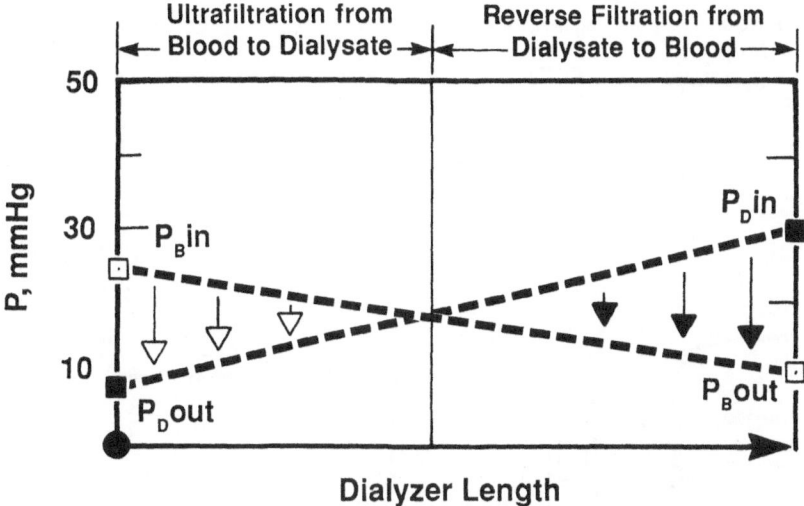

Figure 11. Blood and dialysate pressure profiles along the length of a high permeability dialyzer showing the occurrence of ultrafiltration from blood to dialysate and reverse filtration from dialysate to blood at the afferent and efferent ends respectively.

There is currently great interest in the use of highly permeable membranes for dialysis. These membranes have very high ultrafiltration coefficients (20 to 60 ml/h/mm Hg) and also allow passage of solutes as large as 10,000 to 20,000 daltons. When such membranes are used with an ultrafiltration controller, a high rate of filtration occurs from blood to dialysate in the afferent part of the dialyzer with reverse filtration from the dialysate to blood in the efferent part so that net ultrafiltration is commensurate with patient needs. This is shown schematically in Figure 11. With substantial rates of reverse filtration, the potential exists for carryover of reactive endotoxin fragments from dialysate into blood. Further, in the event of a membrane leak, there is the grave risk of undetected bacterial and endotoxin contamination of blood. Some manufacturers have tried to address this problem by instituting a TMP alarm when the TMP is less than a certain value. However, if this limit is very low, reverse filtration may still occur, and if it is set too high, it may not be possible to limit obligatory ultrafiltration with high permeability membranes, saline replacement becoming necessary. If the use of high permeability membranes for large solute removal is shown to be clinically desirable, new stringent standards for the microbiological and endotoxin quality of dialysate may be mandatory.

SPECIAL MONITORING SCHEMES

Single needle systems

The need for the single needle technique (See Chapter 17) arose on the basis that two needles were more difficult to insert than one and that one puncture gave a longer fistula life (50). The latter hypothesis has not been proven, although 7% (51) of fistula dialysis are performed with single

needle systems. The technique works poorly where it is most needed, namely in patients with poor vascular access, particularly where there is a low blood flow through the A-V fistula. However, when fistula perfusion is adequate but only a short segment of fistula is available, as in pediatric dialysis, single needle dialysis may permit satisfactory use of the fistula. The disadvantages of single needle dialysis include an increase in mechanical devices, reduction in blood flow, and an ever present risk of recirculation and inefficient dialysis. In addition, the dialyzer must be compliant or a compliant chamber used for optimal results. This may increase the extracorporeal blood volume.

The basic principle involves alternating the direction of blood flow through a single access needle joined to a Y-junction which connects the two ends of the classical blood circuit (Figure 1). The alteration of direction of flow can be achieved in different ways. One system (Figure 12) uses two clamps, one situated on the arterial and the other on the venous line as close to the Y-junction as possible. When the arterial clamp is opened, the pump draws blood out against the closed venous clamp and the situation reverses when the venous clamp is opened and the arterial clamp is closed. Pressure monitoring of the venous bubble trap with high/low-alarm contacts can be made to operate the clamps, i.e. the high pressure contact opens the venous clamp and closes the arterial clamp and vice versa. Under these conditions of pressure/pressure regulation, the blood pump never stops and this is contrary to all basic pressure monitoring considerations. An alternative is the timed opening and closing of the clamps with pressure monitoring still controlling the blood pump. Time-time systems may be hazardous because of the relative independence of the stroke volumes for the two phases with the possibility of a mismatch. The continuous operation of the blood pump even when the arterial clamp is closed leads to extreme subatmospheric pressures

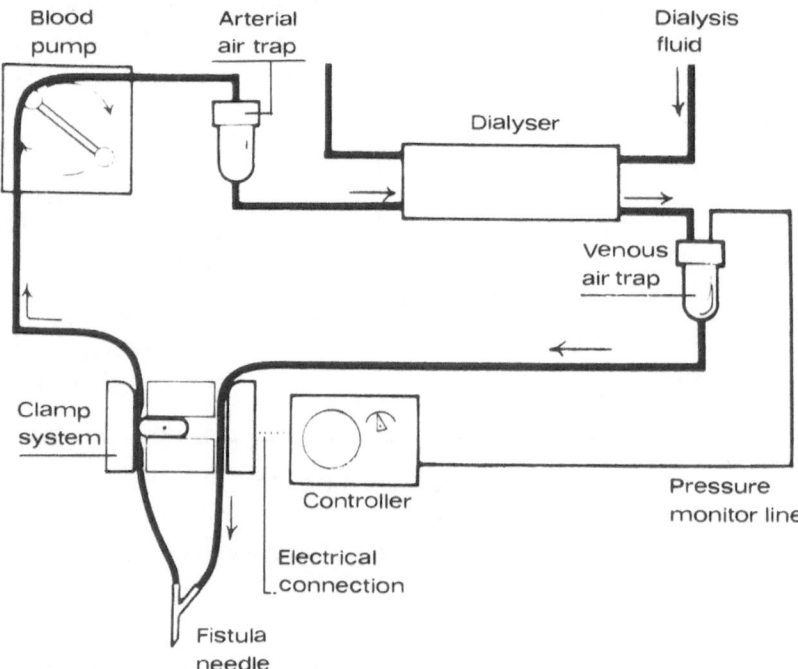

Figure 12. One type of single needle system with continuous blood pump operation and alternate activation of arterial and venous clamps.

between the angioaccess and the blood pump. This can lead to foaming from 'degassing' of blood with the potential for clotting in the dialyzer. Also the effective blood flow is reduced because of the incomplete filling of the pump segment. Further, upon the opening of the arterial clamp, the sudden exposure of the patient's access to an extreme subatmospheric pressure can be detrimental. The generation of extreme subatmospheric pressures also increases the potential for air embolism.

In another type of single needle system, there is intermittent operation of the blood pump with a single venous clamp. When the blood pump is on, the venous clamp is closed and blood is drawn out of the patient into the extracorporeal circuit. The venous air trap pressure increases as a consequence and at a pre-set high pressure limit, the pump is shut off and the clamp opened, blood being returned to the patient. This lowers the venous air trap pressure and when the low pre-set pressure limit is reached, the clamp closes and the pump is turned on to recycle the operation. This system is simpler to operate than the two clamp system but is relatively inefficient because of intermittent blood pumping. In yet another system, two blood pumps are used which operate sequentially, one situated before and the other after the dialyzer. No clamps are required as the occlusive pumps also function as clamps. The objection to this system is that an unmonitored pressure can build up between the 'venous' blood pump and the patient's access with the risk of hematoma formation and damage to the fistula. Newer versions of this system include a second pressure monitor to prevent this. In addition, two sites of sub-atmospheric pressure are developed in the blood circuit.

Single needle systems are more complex from the viewpoint of operation and safety monitoring. The efficiency of solute transport is compromised by recirculation. It is difficult to measure the 'true' blood flow with most single needle systems. The beneficial effect on fistula longevity with one instead of two punctures for each dialysis has not been established. The use of single needle dialysis as a last resort in the face of fistula problems is ill-advised when fistula perfusion is poor because of increased recirculation causing less effective treatment. In acute renal failure, the use of percutaneous catheterization (52) of a major vein (femoral or subclavian) with a single needle system reduces the 'indwelling catheter risk' (See also Chapter 9). Double lumen, single needles have been developed for hemodialysis. Newer designs eliminate some of the early problems with the double lumen concept. With a well-designed double lumen needle, the benefits of a single venipuncture may be utilized without the use of special, more complex equipment. However, not all patients tolerate the larger diameter double lumen needles.

Sequential ultrafiltration and diffusion

Sequential ultrafiltration and diffusion is a mode of therapy that requires the divorcing and sequencing of fluid and solute removal, these two processes being simultaneous during conventional hemodialysis. Isolated ultrafiltration i.e. fluid removal without simultaneous solute removal by diffusion, may precede or follow the phase of pure diffusive solute removal. The observation that isolated ultrafiltration did not produce symptomatic hypotension was first reported in 1972 (53), and confirmed in 1975 (54). In 1976 it was demonstrated that ultrafiltration alone was well tolerated but not when combined with diffusion (classical acetate dialysis) in susceptible patients (55). The potential benefit of separating diffusion and ultrafiltration sequentially during one treatment session was also shown in 1976 using the Rhone-Poulenc high flux dialyzer (RP6) when the patient lost 4 kg during 1 h without change in pulse or blood pressure and then tolerated 3 h of asymptomatic acetate dialysis without weight loss (56). However, further studies revealed a tendency for the blood pressure to drop in the absence of weight loss (57). Subsequent investigation of the hemodynamic changes indicated a compensatory increase of the peripheral resistance during isolated ultrafiltration, but a failure of the peripheral resistance to rise during acetate dialysis (58–60). This observation has been confirmed and associated with a rise in circulating catecholamines during isolated ultrafiltration but not during acetate hemodialysis with ultrafiltration (61). This difference is unexplained.

During isolated ultrafiltration, no dialysis fluid perfuses the dialyzer but the required hydrostatic pressure gradient is established across the dialyzer membrane for the desired rate of fluid removal. This can be accomplished in several ways. The simplest is to use a venous clamp on the blood tubing to generate adequate positive blood compartment pressures, the dialysate compartment being open to the atmosphere. With this scheme, the ultrafiltrate can be collected readily and the rate of fluid removal easily determined. The generation of high blood compartment pressures does, however, increase the possibility of tubing separations and membrane ruptures as in coil dialysis. Pressure monitoring of the blood compartment pressure is, therefore, important, especially as it is difficult to regulate the blood compartment pressure precisely with most venous clamps. Also, some form of blood leak detection should be used, to prevent excessive blood loss in the ultrafiltrate with membrane ruptures. Isolated ultrafiltration can also be performed using negative pressures in the dialysate compartment generated either by a suction pump, or a vacuum source. Alternatively, a conventional dialysate delivery system can generate negative pressures in the dialysate compartment during the bypass mode of operation. With the negative pressure schemes, it may be more difficult to measure the rate of ultrafiltration than with the positive pressure scheme but it is easier to control the negative pressure. If a suction pump is used, the rate of ultrafiltration can be controlled by regulating the speed of the pump. The difficulty, however, lies in the fact that the ultrafiltrate tends to 'degas' under subatmospheric pressures, resulting in a mixture of fluid and gas being pumped. To avoid this, a gas trap with provisions for venting the gas under conditions of negative pressure is required. If a vacuum source is used, a graduated collection vessel can be used for measuring the ultrafiltration rate. With the dialysate bypass scheme, the ultrafiltrate mixes with dialysate and is, therefore, not accessible for direct measurement of flow rate unless special provisions for diverting the ultrafiltrate through a flow meter are included. In all of these schemes monitoring of patient weight can also assess the fluid removal rate. The negative pressure schemes should also incorporate a blood leak detector which should be located as close to the dialyzer as possible, to prevent delays between the incidence of the rupture and the activation of the blood leak alarm.

Bicarbonate dialysis systems

The use of bicarbonate dialysis is increasing with the recognition that vascular stability during dialysis is improved with bicarbonate relative to acetate. Several studies have demonstrated (60–63) that the compensatory vasoconstrictive response to hypovolemia is inhibited when acetate is used as the buffer source in hemodialysis. The vasoconstrictive response is intact during isolated ultrafiltration, hemofiltration and bicarbonate hemodialysis (60, 64, 65). With standard treatments of 4 to 5 h, the benefits of bicarbonate over acetate are obvious in only a small percentage of the dialysis population. However, with shortened duration of treatment (2 to 3 h) the benefits of bicarbonate in maintaining vascular stability, reducing intradialytic symptoms and achieving ideal finishing weights are clear cut (66).

Until recently, bicarbonate dialysis has been utilized sparingly because of the complexity of the equipment necessary for delivering bicarbonate dialysate. Two concentrates are necessary, a bicarbonate concentrate containing sodium bicarbonate and sodium chloride and an acidified concentrate containing sodium chloride, potassium chloride, calcium chloride, magnesium chloride, dextrose and acetic acid. In order to mix appropriately these two concentrates with water, two proportioning systems with associated monitoring, control and alarms are necessary. Bicarbonate dialysis is usually accomplished with 'add-on' modules for standard acetate delivery systems. As a consequence, these modules are often not well-integrated with the rest of the system and malfunction frequently. They also require more personnel-intensive calibration, cleaning and maintenance. The potential for mix-ups between the two concentrates with adverse clinical consequences exists. For all these reasons, there has been limited utilization of bicarbonate dialysis despite its clinical advantages.

Two concentrates are required for bicarbonate dialysis because precipitation of calcium and magnesium carbonates would occur if the calcium and magnesium chlorides and sodium bicarbonate were included at the desired concentrations in a single concentrate. Acetic acid is included in the calcium and magnesium containing concentrate to achieve a slightly acidic pH when the two concentrates are mixed, thereby preventing precipitation of the calcium and magnesium salts. Acetic acid reacts with sodium bicarbonate to produce sodium acetate and carbonic acid. The carbonic acid facilitates the retention of the calcium and magnesium salts in solution. In some systems, the water and bicarbonate concentrates are proportioned first, with subsequent addition of the acidified concentrate. In other systems, the order of addition of the two concentrates is reversed. Most systems use conductivity monitoring for ensuring appropriate proportioning. Some systems also have a pH monitor whose main function is to ensure that the appropriate concentrates are being used in the two step proportioning and that no mix-ups have occurred. This is especially important with systems that use variable proportioning based on the servo-feedback scheme. In such systems, in the absence of pH monitoring, even when the two concentrates are mixed-up, the servo system will vary the proportioning ratio to bring the conductivity into the correct range. As a consequence, the final dialysate may be extremely acidic with potential risks to the patient or extremely alkaline with the potential for precipitation of the calcium and magnesium salts and subsequent malfunction of the system. If the precipitation is rapid and extensive, severe damage to the system may result. With the current state of the art, problems related to calibration drift, accuracy and reliability of pH monitors have been experienced. Manufacturers who use fixed ratio proportioning have, therefore, opted to not include pH monitors in their systems and rely only on conductivity measurements for monitoring. As long as the composition of the concentrate for which the system is calibrated remains unchanged, this may be adequate; but when concentrate formulation varies there may be safety problems in the absence of pH monitoring.

Even with appropriate system calibration and operation, problems of precipitation occur frequently with bicarbonate modules. This may be a consequence of system design. The mixing chambers for the addition of the two concentrates and the distance between them should be designed to ensure complete mixing with a homogeneous final composition; otherwise, local concentration may be high enough to trigger precipitation. Further, if pulsatile proportioning pumps are used, bolus doses of concentrate may be discharged with poor mixing and high local concentrations, thereby, triggering precipitation. Carbonate precipitation may also be due to variable feed water pH, variations in concentrate formulation, inadequate system cleaning and inadequate rinse out of an alkaline disinfectant such as bleach.

Technological improvements in the design and integration of bicarbonate modules are necessary before bicarbonate dialysis can become as easy and routine as acetate dialysis. At present, bicarbonate systems demand a much greater personnel commitment for cleaning, disinfection and maintenance than do acetate systems.

One technological innovation that has allowed large scale delivery of bicarbonate dialysis is the hybrid bicarbonate system designed by the Regional Kidney Disease Program (RKDP) in Minneapolis (67). This system is a hybrid of central proportioning of water and bicarbonate concentrate and patient station proportioning of the bicarbonated water and acidified concentrate (Figure 13). Fixed ratio proportioning with piston pumps (Modified Drake-Willock pump) is used for the centralized proportioning of water and bicarbonate concentrate in a 19:1 ratio with conductivity monitoring. The resulting bicarbonated water is delivered into a tank with level sensors. The bicarbonated water is then pumped from the tank to the individual patient stations in a recirculating loop. At the patient station, a standard 'ace-

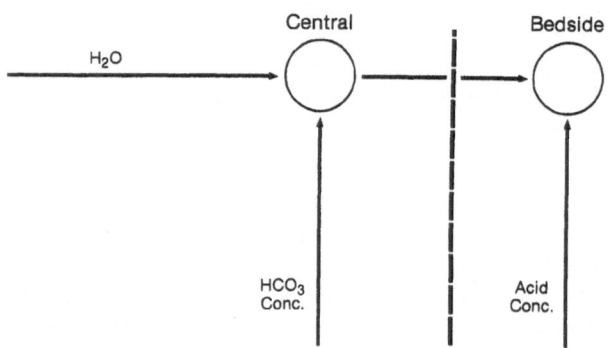

Schematic of Hybrid Bicarbonate System

Figure 13. Hybrid scheme of bicarbonate proportioning designed by the Regional Kidney Disease Program, Minneapolis. (Reprinted with permission from 'Technical Requirements for Rapid High-Efficiency Therapies', P. Keshaviah, D. Luehmann, K. Ilstrup and A. Collins, Artificial Organs 10: 189–194, 1986.)

tate' delivery system is used to proportion the bicarbonated water and acidified concentrate in a 34:1 ratio. Small (8 station) and large (35 station) hybrid systems have been built and the RKDP clinical experience with this scheme is of the order of 100,000 dialyses. The advantages of the system include simplicity, reduced hardware costs (relative to the costs of outfitting each patient station with a bicarbonate module), reduced wastage of bicarbonate concentrate, smaller potential for mix-ups of concentrates and a greatly reduced personnel component for maintenance and operation of the system. Because of the system design, the bicarbonate is well mixed in the water before the acidified concentrate is added, greatly reducing the potential for calcium and magnesium precipitation.

As stated earlier, system cleaning and disinfection is especially important with bicarbonate dialysis because of the potential for bacterial contamination of the bicarbonate concentrate and the rapidity of bacterial proliferation in this concentrate. Microbial levels of 10^5 cfu/ml and endotoxin levels of 12 to 24 ng/ml in the concentrate have been documented. If prolonged storage of the bicarbonate concentrate is avoided and if the concentrate containers are cleaned and disinfected frequently, it is possible to limit the contamination of the concentrate. However, to limit the contamination of the final dialysate, it is also necessary to clean and disinfect the delivery system frequently and to monitor the bacterial and endotoxin levels periodically. Unless such measures are adopted, the advantages of bicarbonate dialysis may be overshadowed by the potential risk of pyrogen reactions, bacteremias and sepsis.

PATIENT MONITORING

One of the most difficult parameters to measure in the dialysis patient is the dry body weight (see also Chapter 13).

Indeed, it is possible that the true dry weight is never known, as measurements of total body water and the extracellular space are related to a standard derived from a normal population (68). The observation that most dialysis patients undergo substantial diuresis and weight loss following successful transplantation suggests that these patients were overhydrated. Because of the ever-present risk of overhydration and associated volume hypertension, the monitoring of body weight and blood pressure before and after each dialysis has become traditional. The aim is to control the blood pressure by ultrafiltration (inducing weight loss) and avoid hypertension or orthostatic hypotension. To succeed, the patient must cooperate and restrict salt and water intake to avoid large swings in body weight.

Monitoring of the patient's blood pressure and heart rate during dialysis is also traditional, the frequency of the observation depending upon the unit and staff availability. Measurement of weight loss during a dialysis may not be required when using a reliable ultrafiltration control system. However, weight monitoring independently checks the accuracy and reliability of the ultrafiltration control system. With isolated ultrafiltration, direct collection and measurement of the volume of ultrafiltrate obviates the need for weight measurement during dialysis.

Long term monitoring of body weight is a difficult problem for the dialysis physician. In the absence of overt clinical signs of dehydration or overhydration, the blood pressure is often used as an index of correct hydration. However, this rule may prove fallacious and much clinical experience may be necessary to adjust the individual body weight according to circumstances. In the early months of treatment, following initial progressive weight loss with blood pressure control, the patient should gain weight at the rate of 0.5 to 1.0 kg per month if he is receiving an adequate protein and calorie intake and was malnourished initially (68). True weight gains of 5 kg are not unusual during the first year of treatment. After this, it is uncommon to see substantial weight gains in stable adult patients. It is difficult to judge this type of weight gain and a tendency to ultrafilter the patient into shock to prove whether the weight gain is dry weight gain or not is a bad practice. In the absence of overt edema, it is better to allow progressive weight gain if the blood pressure does not exceed normal limits and to ask the patient if he feels better keeping the extra weight. With patients over the age of 60 years, a mild systolic hypertension is often better tolerated than the rigorous prescription of a dry body weight designed to produce a normal blood pressure. However, some patients feel bloated when they are too heavy and will insist upon a lower weight. The monitoring of the hematocrit may be useful in judging weight changes. Weight gain associated with salt and water retention dilutes the red cell mass and may be associated with an unexplained progressive reduction of the hematocrit. Conversely, unexpected rises in the hematocrit may suggest extracellular dehydration. A frequent problem is wasting with maintenance of actual body weight. This can induce hypertension without apparent weight gain or signs of overt overhydration. The cause is usually malnutrition due to an inadequate diet or any cata-

bolic process, particularly infection. The clue is often a rise in blood pressure without weight gain associated with a reduction in the hematocrit. The treatment is more aggressive ultrafiltration together with the correction of the causative factor. Continuous monitoring of blood pressure and weight are the fundamentals by which the dry body weight of the dialysis patient is judged. It is often difficult for the patient to monitor these correctly for himself and a regular review of blood pressure and weight is necessary for all dialysis patients.

REFERENCES

1. Scribner BH, Buri R, Caner JEZ, Hegstrom R, Burnell JM: The treatment of chronic uremia by means of intermittent hemodialysis. A preliminary report. *Trans Am Soc Artif Intern Organs* 6: 114, 1960
2. Shaldon S: Experience to date with home hemodialysis. *Proc Working Conf on Chronic Dialysis*, University of Washington, Seattle, WA, 1964, p 66
3. Brescia MJ, Cimino JE, Appel K, Hurwich BJ: Chronic hemodialysis using venipuncture and surgically created arterio-venous fistula. *N Engl J Med* 275: 1089, 1966
4. Shaldon S: Independence in maintenance haemodialysis. *Lancet* 1: 520, 1968
5. Cambi V, Savazzi G, Arisi L, Bignardi L, Bruschi G, Rossi E, Migone L: Short dialysis schedules (SDS) – Finally ready to become a routine? *Proc Eur Dial Transplant Assoc* 1: 112, 1974
6. Gurland JH, Brunner FP, v Dehn H, Harlen H, Parsons FM, Schärer K: Combined report on regular dialysis and transplantation in Europe, III. 1972. *Proc Eur Dial Transplant Assoc* 10 XVII, 1973
7. Keshaviah PR, Luehmann D, Shapiro F, Comty C: Investigation of the Risks and Hazards associated with Hemodialysis Devices. Technical Report, Silver Spring, MD, US Dept. Health, Education and Welfare, Food and Drug Administration, Bureau of Medical Devices, 1980
8. Grimsrud HJ, Cole JJ, Eschbach JW, Babb AL, Scribner BH: Safety aspects of hemodialysis. *Trans Am Soc Artif Intern Organs* 20: 770, 1974
9. Association for the Advancement of Medical Instrumentation. American National Standard for hemodialysis systems, 1982. Arlington, VA
10. Bernstein EF, Indeglia RA, Shea MA, Varco RL: Sublethal damage to the red blood cell from pumping. *Circulation* 35 (Suppl 1): 226, 1967
11. Hyde SE III, Sadler JH: Red blood cell destruction in hemodialysis. *Trans Am Soc Artif Intern Organs* 15: 50, 1969
12. von Hartitzsch B, Carr D, Kjellstrand CM, Kerr DNS: Normal red cell survival in well dialyzed patients. *Trans Am Soc Artif Intern Organs* 19: 471, 1973
13. Shaldon S, Ahmed R, Oag D, Crockett RE, Opperman F, Koch KM: The use of the A-V fistula in overnight home haemodialysis in children. *Proc Eur Dial Transplant Assoc* 8: 65, 1971
14. Ward MK, Shadforth M, Hill AVL, Kerr DNS: Air embolism during haemodialysis. *Br Med J* 2: 74, 1971
15. Beullens T, Beelen R, Van Ypersele de Strihou C: Devices for air detection during dialyses. *Proc Eur Dial Transplant Assoc* 8: 412, 1971
16. Nishi RY: Ultrasonic detection of bubbles with Doppler flow transducers. *Ultrasonics* 10: 173, 1972
17. Blagg CR: Acute complications associated with hemodialysis.

in *Replacement of Renal Function by Dialysis,* first edition, edited by Drukker W, Parsons FM, Maher JF, The Hague, Martinus Nijhoff, 1978, p 486

18. Weseley SA: Air embolism during hemodialysis. *Dial Transplant* 2: 14, 1972
19. von Hartitzsch B, Medlock R: New devices to prevent air foam emboli. *Dial Transplant* 8: 515, 1979
20. De Palma JR, Shinaberger JH, Abukurah AR: Air embolism hazards in maintenance hemodialysis. *Abstracts Am Soc Artif Intern Organs* 5: 20, 1976
21. Said R, Quintanilla A, Levin N, Ivanovich P: Acute hemolysis due to profound hypo-osmolality. A complication of hemodialysis. *J Dial* : 447, 1977
22. Linder A, Moskovtchenko JF, Traeger J: Accidental mass hypernatremia during hemodialysis. *Nephron* 9: 99, 1972
23. Bluemle LW Jr: Current status of chronic hemodialysis. *Am J Med* 44: 749, 1968
24. Kachmar JF, Grant GH: Proteins and amino acids. in *Fundamentals of Clinical Chemistry,* edited by Tietz NW, Philadelphia, WB Saunders Co, 1976, p 264
25. Fortner RW, Nowakowski A, Carter CB, King LH, Knepshield JH: Death due to overheated dialysate during dialysis. *Ann Intern Med* 73: 443, 1970
26. Berkes SL, Kahn SI, Chazan JA, Garella S: Prolonged hemolysis from overheated dialysate. *Ann Intern Med* 83: 363, 1975
27. Harrison PB, Jansson K, Kronenberg H, Mahony JF, Tiller D: Cold agglutinin formation in patients undergoing haemodialysis. A possible relationship to dialyser re-use. *Aust NZ J Med* 5: 195, 1975
28. von Hartitzsch B, Hoenich NA, Johnson J, Brewis RAL, Kerr DNS: The problem of de-aeration – Cause, consequence, cure. *Proc Eur Dial Transplant Assoc* 9: 605, 1972
29. Drukker W, van der Werff B, Meinsma K: Deaeration of dialysis fluid. *Dial Transplant* 3: 33, 1974
30. Hendrick DJ, Lane DJ: Formaline asthma in hospital staff. *Br Med J* 1: 607, 1975
31. O'Quinn SE, Kennedy CB: Contact dermatitis due to formaldehyde in clothing textiles. *JAMA* 194: 123, 1965
32. Ogden DA, Myers LE, Eskelson CD, Ziegler EJ: Iatrogenic administration of formaldehyde to hemodialysis patients. *Proc Clin Dial Transplant Forum* 3: 141, 1973
33. Reveillaud RJ, Deschamps A, Aubert Ph: Risks of i.v. administration of formaldehyde to hemodialyzed patients. *Kidney Int* 1: 292, 1977
34. Howell D, Perkins HA: Anti-N-like antibodies in the sera of patients undergoing chronic hemodialysis. *Vox Sang* 23: 291, 1972
35. White WL, Miller GE, Kaehny WD: Formaldehyde in the pathogenesis of hemodialysis-related anti-N antibodies. *Transfusion* 17: 443, 1977
36. Crosson JT, Moulds J, Comty CM, Polesky F: A clinical study of anti-N_{DP} in the sera of patients in a large repetitive hemodialysis program. *Kidney Int* 10: 463, 1976
37. Shaldon S, Chevallet M, Maraoui M, Mion C: Dialysis associated auto-antibodies. *Proc Eur Dial Transplant Assoc* 13: 339, 1976
38. Fassbinder W, Pilar J, Scheuermann E, Koch M: Formaldehyde and the occurrence of anti-N-like cold agglutinins in RDT patients. *Proc Eur Dial Transplant Assoc* 13: 333, 1976
39. Belzer FO, Kountz SL, Perkins HA: Red cell cold auto-agglutinins as a cause of failure of renal allotransplantation. *Transplantation* 11: 422, 1971
40. Koch KM, Frei U, Fassbinder W: Hemolysis and anemia in anti-N-like antibody positive hemodialysis patients. *Trans Am Soc Artif Intern Organs* 24: 709, 1978

41. Lewis KJ, Dewar PJ, Ward MK, Kerr DNS: Formation of anti-N-like antibodies in dialysis patients: Effect of different methods of dialyzer rinsing to remove formaldehyde. *Clin Nephrol* 15: 39, 1981
42. Sherris JC, Cole JJ, Scribner BH: Bacteriology of continuous flow hemodialysis. *Trans Am Soc Artif Intern Organs* 7: 37, 1961
43. Favero MS, Petersen NJ, Boyer KM, Carson LA, Bond WW: Microbial contamination of renal dialysis systems and associated health risks. *Trans Am Soc Artif Intern Organs* 20: 175, 1974
44. Curtis JR, Wing AJ, Coleman JC: Bacillus cereus bacteraemia: A complication of intermittent haemodialysis. *Lancet* 1: 136, 1967
45. Ebben J, Hirsch D, Luehmann D, Collins A, Keshaviah P: Microbiological contamination of liquid bicarbonate concentrate (LBC) for hemodialysis (HD). *Trans Am Soc Artif Intern Organs* 33: 269, 1987
46. Lefferson P, Goss J: Risk current vs leakage current. *Dial Transplant* 2: 42, 1973
47. Deller AG: Electrical safety in dialysis. *J Med Eng Tech* 3: 186, 1979
48. Frize M, Scott J, Durie N, Park G: Fibrillation caused by leakage from dialysis machines – What is the danger? *Med Biol Eng Comput* 16: 124, 1978
49. Association for the Advancement of Medical Instrumentation. Safe current limits for electromedical apparatus, American National Standard, 1978, Arlington, VA
50. Kopp KF, Gutch CF, Kolff WJ: Single needle dialyses. *Trans Am Soc Artif Intern Organs* 18: 75, 1972
51. Gurland HJ, Brunner FP, Chantler C, Jacobs C, Schärer K, Selwood NH, Spies G, Wing AJ: Combined report on regular dialysis and transplantation in Europe, VI, 1976. *Proc Eur Dial Transplant Assoc* 13: 3, 1976
52. Shaldon S, Chiandusse L, Higgs B: Haemodialysis by percutaneous catheterisation of the femoral artery and vein with regional heparinization. *Lancet* 2: 857, 1961
53. Kobayashi K, Shibata M, Kato K, Kato S, Nakamura S, Kurachi K, Yasuda B, Ohta K, Maeda K, Imai T, Kawaguchi S, Shimizu K, Yamazaki T, Maji T, Nomura T: Studies on the development of a new method of controlling the amount and contents of body fluids (extracorporeal ultrafiltration method: ECUM) and the application of this method for patients receiving long term hemodialysis. *Jap J Nephrol* 14: 1, 1972
54. Ing TS, Ashbach DL, Kanter A, Oyama HJ, Armbruster KFW, Merkel FK: Fluid removal and negative-pressure hydrostatic ultrafiltration using a partial vacuum. *Nephron* 14: 451, 1975
55. Bergström J, Asaba H, Fürst P, Oules R: Dialysis ultrafiltration and blood pressure. *Proc Eur Dial Transplant Assoc* 13: 293, 1976
56. Shaldon S: Sequential ultrafiltration and dialysis. *Proc Eur Dial Transplant Assoc* 13: 300, 1976
57. Asaba H, Bergström J, Fürst P, Lindh K, Mion C, Oules R, Shaldon S: Sequential ultrafiltration and diffusion as alternative to conventional haemodialysis. *Proc Clin Dial Transplant Forum* 6: 129, 1976
58. Hampl H, Paeprer H, Unger V, Kessel M: Hemodynamic studies during hemodialysis in comparison to sequential ultrafiltration and hemofiltration. *J Dial* 3: 51, 1979
59. Wehle B, Asaba H, Castenfors J, Fürst P, Gunnarsson B, Shaldon S, Bergström J: Hemodynamic changes during sequential ultrafiltration and dialysis. *Kidney Int* 15: 411, 1979
60. Keshaviah P, Ilstrup K, Constantini E, Berkseth R, Shapiro F:

The influence of ultrafiltration (UF) and diffusion (D) on cardiovascular parameters. *Trans Am Soc Artif Intern Organs* 26: 328, 1980

61. Koch KM, Ernst W, Baldamus CA, Brecht HM, Georges J, Fassbinder W: Sympathetic activity and hemodynamics in hemodialysis ultrafiltration and hemofiltration. *Kidney Int* (abstract) 16: 891, 1979

62. Liang CS, Lowenstein JM: Metabolic control of the circulation: Effects of acetate and pyruvate. *J Clin Invest* 62: 1029, 1977

63. Keshaviah P: The role of acetate in the etiology of symptomatic hypotension. *Artif Organs* 6: 378, 1982

64. Shaldon S, Beau MC, Deschoft G, Ramperez P, Mion C: Vascular stability during hemofiltration. *Trans Am Soc Artif Intern Organs* 26: 391, 1980

65. Wehle B, Asaba H, Castenfors J, Gunnarsson B, Bergström J: Influence of dialysate composition on cardiovascular function in iso-osmotic hemodialysis. *Proc Eur Dial Transplant Assoc* 18: 153, 1981

66. Keshaviah P, Collins A: Rapid high-efficiency bicarbonate hemodialysis. *Trans Am Soc Artif Intern Organs* 32: 17, 1986

67. Luehmann D, Hirsch D, Ebben J, Collins A, Keshaviah P: Hybrid hardware scheme for bicarbonate dialysis. *Progr Artif Organs* 3: 188, 1985

68. Comty CM: Factors influencing body composition in terminal uraemics treated by regular haemodialysis. *Proc Eur Dial Transplant Assoc* 4: 216, 1967

BIOPHYSICS OF ULTRAFILTRATION AND HEMOFILTRATION

LEE W. HENDERSON

INTRODUCTION

Removal of excess body water is an important function of both the artificial kidney and peritoneal dialysis. More recently, solute removal in conjunction with ultrafiltration has been exploited as an alternative to diffusion as a means for cleaning uremic blood. This chapter deals with the practical and theoretical aspects of ultrafiltration and convective mass transfer across the artificial kidney and peritoneal mass transfer barriers.

THEORETICAL BACKGROUND

Hemodialysis

When a concentration gradient exists across a semipermeable membrane, both solute and water tend with time to move in a direction to discharge that gradient. Solute and water move in opposite directions across the membrane to achieve equilibrium. The gradient may be expressed in terms emphasizing the solute (e.g. number of milligrams per deciliter of solute on side A, minus the number on side B) or in terms emphasizing the water (e.g. number of milliosmoles on side A, minus the number on side B). Osmolality indicates the number of solute particles per kilogram of water. Alternatively, it may be conceptualized as the number of water molecules per kilogram of solution, i.e. the 'concentration of water'. While the concentration of water is not commonly spoken about by physical chemists, it may be a helpful concept to understand the intimate events in the small domain of the water filled channels in dialysis membranes. There are two ways that a concentration gradient for water may be achieved: osmotically and hydrostatically. For artificial kidney membranes both osmotic and hydrostatic (hydraulic) force may be used to achieve the concentration gradient necessary to cause ultrafiltration, i.e. the separation of plasma water from macromolecular constituents such as protein and cellular elements. For reasons that will become apparent hydrostatic force is the more effective.

An equation that relates ultrafiltration rate to these forces is frequently written

$$J_f = \frac{Q_f}{A} = L_p \, (\Delta P + \Delta \pi). \qquad [1]$$

Ultrafiltration rate per unit area of membrane = (permeability of membrane to water) × (hydrostatic force + osmotic force) where

J_f = the volume flux rate per unit membrane area across the membrane for water (ml/min/cm²),[1]

L_p = the permeability of the membrane for water, i.e. the volumetric flow rate of water per unit area of membrane per unit pressure gradient (ml/min/cm²/mm Hg).

Q_f = flow rate of ultrafiltrate (ml/min),

A = area of the membrane (cm²),

ΔP = the hydraulic pressure gradient from blood path to dialysis fluid path (mm Hg),

$\Delta \pi$ = the osmotic pressure gradient from blood path to dialysis fluid path (mm Hg);

$\Delta \pi$ is frequently expressed as mOsm/l and may be converted to mm Hg using $1.0 \, \text{mOsm} \approx 19 \, \text{mm Hg}$.

The hydrostatic and osmotic forces are summed in this equation, since with hemodialysis there is a deliberate, usually hydrostatic, gradient favoring water movement from blood to dialysate. When isotonic dialysis fluid is used, the osmotic pressure provided by the plasma proteins favors

---

[1] Because ml = cm³ the expression can be reduced to cm/min.

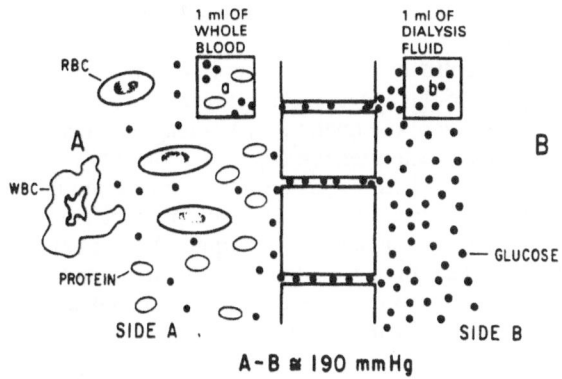

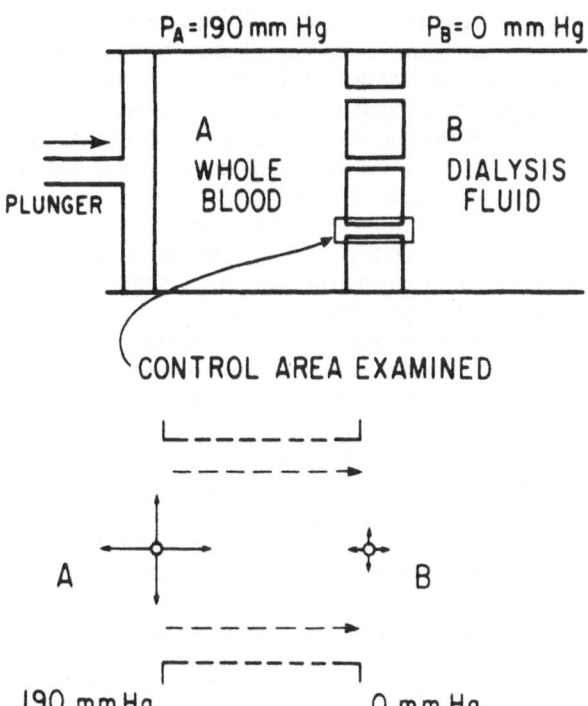

Figure 1. Diagrammatic sketch of a semipermeable membrane dividing whole blood (side A) and dialysis fluid (side B). Glucose (anhydrous) is present on side B at 280 mg/dl (15.6 mmol/l). The pores in the membrane are too small to allow passage of cell elements and protein. An osmolar gradient from A to B of approximately 190 mm Hg (5890–5700 mm Hg) is diagrammatically shown in 1 ml control volumes a and b where the amount of water per milliliter of solution is greater in a than b (see text for further discussion).

Figure 2. Diagrammatic sketch of a rigid membrane dividing whole blood (side A) and iso-osmolar dialysis fluid (side B). A piston on side A provides 190 mm Hg pressure on the whole blood. A single pore in the membrane is depicted below. An average water molecule just outside each end of the pore is depicted as an open circle (O). Vectors for the random motion of these molecules are given. The length of the vector depicts the number of water molecules moving in the direction indicated. An imbalance in the vectors within the pore is such that more water molecules are moving into the pore from side A than from side B with a resultant net flux from A to B down the length of the pore.

water movement from the dialysis solution to blood and the contribution of $\Delta\pi$ to J_f is negative. The two forces $\Delta\pi$ and ΔP may be examined conceptually for an artificial kidney membrane with the aid of Figures 1 and 2. Consider Figure 1 showing two perfectly mixed solutions (blood and dialysis fluid) separated by a membrane that contains homogeneously distributed water filled pores (drawn in cross section as right circular cylinders). Further, the membrane is perfectly semipermeable with respect to blood proteins and formed elements. That is, no cells or protein traverse the pores which have too small a diameter to accommodate these comparatively large molecules and blood cells. Figure 1 shows the events at the pore when an osmotically active solute such as glucose (as anhydrous d-glucose, mass = 180 daltons) is present in high concentration (280 mg/dl = 15.6 mmol/l) on the dialysis fluid side of the membrane (side B). As noted, the concentration of water may be considered to relate inversely to the concentration of solute. That is, for a given volume of solution the greater number of dissolved solute particles (molecules, ions) the fewer number of water molecules can be present. The osmolality of the plasma is 300 mOsm/l. Figure 1 depicts the instant after these two solutions appear on each side of the membrane. Further, there is no difference in hydrostatic pressure across the membrane (consider the membrane 'floppy', such that no hydrostatic pressure gradient can be sustained). At this instant, there is a concentration gradient for water across the pores from A to B. The magnitude of this pressure gradient is 10 mOsm/l or 190 mm Hg (1.0 mOsm/l = 19 mm Hg). Water moves very swiftly to discharge such concentration gradients. Water rarely if ever moves by single molecule diffusion[2], but rather by 'bulk' or 'plug' flow in which movement of 'blocks' of water occur much as you would consider the

movement of pure water in a pipe when an inlet to outlet pressure gradient is applied. It is apparent that in subsequent instances this rather straightforward conceptualization becomes much more complicated. To cite some of the events, glucose is small enough to move by diffusion down its concentration gradient from B to A reducing the osmotic driving force; further, the water arriving on side B dilutes the glucose concentration adjacent to the membrane lengthening the diffusion path over which the concentration gradients apply and slowing their discharge. Further, protein, a macromolecular structure present in solution on the blood side (A), cannot cross the membrane and will exert an osmotic effect (oncotic pressure) favoring water reabsorption from the dialysate. Finally, ionic charges on the solute particles and the requirement for electroneutrality across the membrane will modulate the movement of electrolytes in response to their concentration gradient. Before moving

---

[2] Tritiated water in a beaker can distribute by single molecule diffusion.

to a somewhat more rigorous description, it can be helpful to consider a comparable conceptualization for the circumstance in which an hydraulic (hydrostatic) pressure gradient exists. Figure 2 depicts a rigid membrane with blood on side A and dialysis fluid on side B. As in the previous example, the composition of electrolytes in plasma water and dialysis fluid are identical as are the measured osmolalities and this time there is no difference in glucose concentration. The plunger on side A exerts 190 mm Hg of hydrostatic pressure. A single pore in the membrane is depicted in the lower part of Figure 2. The higher hydrostatic pressure on side A is a measure of the greater number of bombardments per second of solute and solvent particles on a given surface area of the container, one surface of which is our semi-permeable membrane. An 'average' water molecule just outside the pore in the membrane is shown for each side. The average magnitude and direction of water molecule movement is given by the vector arrows. In the bulk phase of solution outside the pore such motion is random and is schematically shown in Figure 2 as four arrows of equal length reflecting the sums of all intermediate vectors for each quadrant. The greater number of bombardments of the end of the pore on side A as opposed to side B means that there is net movement of water from A to B down the pore. It should be noted that solute particles that are small enough not to be hindered by the pore, (the pore diameter being substantially larger than the hydrated radius of the solute), will move with the water because of the frictional forces between water and the solute particle. This convecting of solutes along with water through a membrane in response to a pressure gradient (osmotic or hydrostatic) is termed 'solvent drag'. When the membrane exerts no restraining force (sieving effect on the solute, i.e. the solution does not change in concentration as it traverses the membrane), then the terms 'bulk', 'plug' or 'Poiseuillian' flow describe the event. In the present example, of course, protein and cell elements are blocked from crossing the membranes by pore size and the solute concentration of plasma water does change as the ultrafiltrate is formed.

The osmotic and hydrostatic movement of water, while commonly considered to give the same result, differ in a potentially important respect. In order for a solute to exert an osmotic force it is a necessary constraint that the solute particle be of such a size that there is resistance to its movement through the channels in the membrane. The hydrated radius of the solute then must approach in size the mean radius of the pores in the membrane. For a small solute such as glucose it means that only membranes containing pores with radii near in size to that of glucose participate in the osmotically driven generation of ultrafiltrate. Treating these channels as a parallel array of right circular cylinders or pores has proven useful in simplifying the arithmetic commonly employed to describe them (but may not be an accurate description of the clinical circumstance.) In a membrane with heterogeneously dispersed pore sizes it will mean that pores with larger radii do not participate. Quite the contrary would be true for an hydrostatic driving force as water flow through a pore is directly proportional to the fourth power of the radius of that pore (Poiseuille again). As such, large pores dominate in conducting hydrostatic ultra-filtration.

Let us return now to equation 1, and a more formal description of the above events. In general, the hydraulic pressure gradient of equation 1 (ΔP) may be taken as the average blood path pressure (P_B) minus the dialysate path pressure (P_D). These values are readily measured in most artificial kidney monitors. The osmotic pressure gradient is somewhat more complicated to compute. Van't Hoff's Law of Osmotic Pressure adequately describes the osmotic pressure difference between two solutions (e.g. blood and dialysis fluid) in the absence of a membrane:

$$\Delta\pi = RT \left[\sum_{j=1}^{m} C_j^B - \sum_{j=1}^{n} C_j^D \right]$$

where B and D identify the two solutions and

$\sum_{j=1}^{m} C_j^B$ = The sum $(1 + 2 + 3 \ldots m)$ of the concentrations[3] of all solute particles in blood (B)

$\sum_{j=1}^{m} C_j^D$ = The sum of the concentrations of all solute particles in dialysis fluid (D)

= The temperature in degrees Kelvin

= The gas constant = 0.0623 when units of $\dfrac{\text{liter} \times \text{mm Hg}}{\text{mmol} \times \text{degree}}$ are used

We wish to compute the $\Delta\pi$ across a semipermeable membrane. An ideal semipermeable membrane permits permeation of one species, e.g. water, with no resistance while blocking entry to all other species, e.g. protein. Currently used cellulosic dialysis membranes may be considered to be ideally semipermeable for water and protein. In the dialysis setting, however, there are a host of other osmotically active solutes, most of which diffuse across the membrane. To assess the contribution a given solute makes to the overall transmembrane osmotic pressure gradient, it is necessary to know how readily it permeates the membranes, as compared with water in response to an applied hydraulic pressure gradient. This may be expressed as

$$\frac{N}{Q_f} = C_w (1 - \varepsilon) \qquad [3]$$

where

N = the net flux rate of solute movement across the membrane (moles/min):

Q_f = the net flux rate of water movement across the membrane (ml/min):

ε = a property of the membrane termed the 'rejection coefficient' and is a measure of the degree to which the membrane restrains movement of the solute. If the membrane pore is much larger than both the water molecule and

---

[3] Partially or completely dissociated electrolytes contribute more solute particles to the solution than their molar concentration would identify. For example, NaCl at concentrations used in dialysis fluid, dissociates almost completely into its constituent ions, providing nearly double the number of osmotically active particles that would be expected from the molality and Avogadro's number.

the solute particle, both will traverse the membrane without hindrance, and the ultrafiltrate's concentration (C_f)

$$C_f = \frac{N}{Q_f} \qquad [4]$$

is unchanged from the retentate, i.e. the concentration of the solution does not change as it crosses the membrane. In this instance

$$C_f = C_w$$

and by equation 3,

$$\varepsilon = 0 = \text{rejection coefficient.}$$

For protein, which is completely rejected by the membrane, however,

$$\varepsilon = 1.$$

The rejection coefficient, therefore, will have values that range from zero to 1, depending on the degree of stearic hindrance presented by the membrane to the hydrated solute particle. At times, it is more convenient to refer to the sieving coefficient (S) of a membrane for a given solute:

$$\varepsilon = 1 - S \qquad [5]$$

$$S = \frac{C_f}{C_w} \qquad [6]$$

The Van't Hoff equation applied across the membrane may be written using Staverman's reflection coefficient (σ), which may be considered the measure of a membrane's 'semipermeability' for a given solute and as such is closely related to, but different from the rejection coefficient (ε)[4]

$$\Delta\pi = RT\sigma_j \left[\sum_{j=1}^{m} C_j^B - \sum_{j=1}^{n} C_j^D \right]$$

or, converting concentration terms for each side of the membrane into osmolar gradients we have the more useful

$$\Delta\pi = \sum_{j=1}^{n} (\Delta\pi_j \, \sigma_j) \qquad [8]$$

$$= (\Delta\pi_1 \, \sigma_1) + (\Delta\pi_2 \, \sigma_2) + \ldots \text{ etc.} \qquad [9]$$

Equation 2 may now be written more precisely as

$$Q_f = AL_p \left(\Delta P + \sum_{j=1}^{n} \Delta\pi_1 \, \sigma_1 \right) \qquad [10]$$

The concentration of the ultrafiltrate C_f under carefully controlled conditions not only depends on σ, but, as has been shown by Spiegler and Kadem (1), varies with the

---

[4] ε is readily measured during clinical or bench experiments with ultrafiltration. It may be considered a phenomenologic parameter that will be reflective of such things as the rate of flow of the solution through the membrane, the mixing present at the membrane surface as well as the pore structure of the membrane. σ on the other hand must be computed from ε values taking into account such matters as filtration flow rate and unstirred layers at the membrane surface. As such, σ is an intrinsic property of the membrane/solute pair and remains a constant number over a wide range of operating conditions. One may analogize between ε and clearance and σ and the membrane mass transfer resistance (R_m).

volume flow rate J_f (ml/min/cm^2) of ultrafiltrate.

$$C_f = \frac{J_s}{J_f} = (1 - \varepsilon) \, C_w \qquad [11]$$

where J_s is the solute flux rate (mol/min/cm^2). ε then may be related to σ using the Spiegler equation (2):

$$\varepsilon = \sigma \, \frac{\varepsilon^\beta - 1}{\varepsilon^\beta - \sigma} \qquad [12]$$

where $\beta = J_f(1 - \sigma)/P_m$ and P_m = the permeability of the membrane for the solute considered (cm/min)

when J_f is very large ε approaches σ

when J_f is very small ε approaches $\dfrac{J_f\sigma}{P_m}$.

These relationships of ε and σ point out that the difference between σ, the intrinsic property of the membrane/solute pair, and ε the phenomenologic coefficient, may be considered as the contribution made by diffusive transport toward the observed net movement of the solute, i.e. diffusion across the filtering membrane will lessen the amount of measured rejection and ε will be less than σ.

The ultrafiltration rate in the human glomerulus and capillary beds such as that in the splanchnic circulation, interestingly, are dominated by consideration of oncotic pressure. The importance of oncotic pressure lies not in its magnitude, which is small in absolute terms (1 to 1.5 mOsm/l or 19 to 28 mm Hg), but rather because it is nearly equal to the hydraulic pressure gradient across the capillary wall. By contrast, in the artificial kidney, under usual operating conditions (where ΔP ranges from 20 to 250 mm Hg) hydraulic pressure (ΔP) almost invariably exceeds oncotic pressure. Small solutes, other than protein, present in dialysis fluid or in uremic plasma (e.g., glucose and urea) contribute substantially to the osmolality of the solution (25 to 100 mOsm/l or 475 to 1900 mm Hg), but because their reflection coefficient across cellophane is less than unity cause less water flux across the membrane than might otherwise be expected.

Peritoneal dialysis

A detailed description of the peritoneum appears in chapter 23. Concepts of the peritoneal mass transfer resistance have recently become more complex with the invoking of models that comprise capillaries uniformly 'smeared' within supporting interstitium, the so called distributed model (3,4) and the postulating of two barriers to transport configured in series (5) to explain better the functional performance of this 'membrane'. In addition, the role of the lymphatics in both water and solute transport must now be taken into account (6). To begin with, our analysis considers the peritoneal membrane as the domain that separates the bulk phase of plasma water from that of well-mixed dialysis fluid. Such a description then comprises both the anatomical structures such as the vascular endothelium and mesothelium, and in addition, all of their attendant unstirred layers. Unlike hemodialysis, ultrafiltration across the peritoneal membrane is accomplished almost exclusively by osmotic force.

The peritoneal membrane is not perfectly semipermeable (i.e. is somewhat leaky) for the solutes to be considered, making quantitation of the driving force for ultrafiltration more complicated. Glucose moves across the peritoneal membrane at a rate consonant with its rather small size (180 daltons). Even protein molecules such as albumin (69,000 daltons) traverse the peritoneal membrane to a small extent.

As noted for the artificial kidney the peritoneal membrane is not ideally semipermeable for a host of solutes and the correction factor (σ) for each solute concentration gradient ($\Delta\pi$) must be applied to adjust that gradient for the degree of the membrane's 'semipermeability' for that solute. Analogous to equation 10 for artificial membranes these concepts may be set down as follows:

$$Q_f = AL_p \ (\Delta\pi^1\sigma^1 \text{ and } \Delta\pi_2\sigma_2 + \dots \text{etc.} \qquad [13]$$

where: $\Delta\pi_1\sigma_1$ would equal to osmotic driving gradient for sodium $\Delta\pi_2\sigma_2$ would equal that for potassium, etc, until each solute present on each side of the membrane was represented. This equation was previously written for the artificial kidney (e.q. 10) with a term to express the hydrostatic driving force resulting from the blood to bath (ΔP). Because the peritoneal space under normal circumstances is free of significant quantities of fluid, we may reasonably assume that the hydrostatic and oncotic forces at play across the capillary membrane from arteriolar to venular end are in balance with lymphatic run off. To effect net accumulation of ultrafiltrate in the peritoneal space, these forces must be unbalanced by the osmotic force contributed by glucose in dialysis fluid. For a 2 l exchange added to the peritoneal space, the hydrostatic force contributed would result from the elastic recoil of the abdominal wall or the hydrostatic head of pressure generated by the 'column' of water above the dependent portion of the peritoneal membrane or both. As such, it would be expected to be small and to favor net uptake across the peritoneal membrane from 'bath to blood'. To be precise, this force must be added as a component of ΔP. Lastly, in considering this simplification there is the unlikely possibility that hypertonic dialysis fluid by some mechanism may alter the afferent/efferent resistances of the peritoneal capillary bed in such a manner as to enhance the hydrostatic pressure gradient thereby causing ultrafiltration. Solutes that were nearly equal or equal in concentration on both sides of the membrane would, of course, contribute little or no driving force for ultrafiltration. Solutes such as glucose, urea and protein, for example, which by therapeutic intent or biological circumstance will have significant concentration gradients across the membrane, may contribute significant osmotic driving force.

To understand just how much, or even relatively how much force for ultrafiltration across the peritoneal membrane would be contributed, for example, when glucose is contrasted with protein or urea, requires further exploration of the term σ and an appreciation that the larger a solute is in terms of its molecular size the less likely it is to be present in biologic solutions at a concentration that contributes much to the total osmolality.

Albumin, for example, has a reasonable high σ. That is to say albumin moves through the membrane with difficulty. It is commonly present in the plasma at a concentration of 3.5 g/dl. Taking an average molecular mass of 60,000 and assuming $\sigma = 1$, the osmolar contribution of albumin to resisting movement of plasma water into the peritoneal space is only

$$\frac{35 \text{ g/kg H}_2\text{O}}{60,000} = 0.0006 \text{ Osm/kg H}_2\text{O}$$
$$= 0.6 \text{ mOsm/kg H}_2\text{O} = 11 \text{ mm Hg}$$

Dextrose monohydrate on the other hand at a concentration of 1.5 or 4.25 g/dl in the dialysis fluid (1.36 or 3.86 g/dl of dextrose anhydrous) and 100 mg/dl in plasma would contribute a maximum potential osmolar driving gradient for ultrafiltration of either 70 mOsm (1330 mm Hg) or 209 mOsm (3987 mm Hg)[5]. This maximum is never manifest, however, because σ for dextrose across the peritoneal membrane is less than unity. Furthermore, with time, the concentration gradient deteriorates (Figure 3). There are at least two components to this discharge of the gradient. The first is diffusion of dextrose into the plasma and the second is convective water movement countercurrent to the dextrose. Clinically, the net movement of water is obtained as the difference between inflow and outflow volumes. As such, it represents an average value. Lymphatic uptake from the cavity (not commonly measured) modulates this net movement of water (6). Figure 4 shows the relationship of net water flow rate and dialysate volume with time for a solution containing 4.25% dextrose monohydrate (7) while Figure 3 relates the osmolar gradient and the dextrose concentration with time. To determine the osmotic force contributed by urea (u), with a molecular weight of 60, consider the following circumstance: for a plasma urea concentration of 300 mg/dl (50 mmol/l, BUN of 140 mg/dl) it offers a 50 mOsm (950 mm Hg) maximum potential osmolar driving gradient for water movement. Clinical wisdom identifies that 'isotonic' (1.5% dextrose containing) dialysis solutions used in a patient with a BUN concentration of 150 ± 20 mg/dl (about 54 mmol/l of blood urea) usually results in little or no net removal of excess total body water. In this circumstance for average values of π for a 60 min exchange time then $\sigma_u\pi_u \approx \sigma_g\pi_g$ where starting values for $\pi = 950$ and $\pi_g = 1482$.

Therefore, $\sigma_u < \sigma_g$ and $\dfrac{\sigma_u}{\sigma_g}$ = about 0.6. This approximation assumes the role of lymphatic uptake of fluid in the adult is quantitatively small. This value reconciles reasonably with the ratio computed for measured values of σ for urea and glucose reported in Table 1 of 0.5. With cellulose membranes for laboratory use (i.e. not Cuprophane) studied in vitro (8), the values obtained are $\sigma_u = 0.024$ and $\sigma_g = 0.20$, i.e. σ_u/σ_g = about 0.1 suggesting that this synthetic membrane is a good deal 'tighter' than the peritoneal membrane. A similar conclusion for Cuprophane was arrived at by

---

[5] Dextrose (d-glucose) is added to dialysis solution to provide an osmolar gradient for ultrafiltration. Expressed as d-glucose, H₂O (dextrose monohydrate, 198 daltons), the concentrations are 1.5 g/dl or 4.25 g/dl, whereas the concentrations of dextrose anhydrous are 1.36 or 3.86 g/dl.

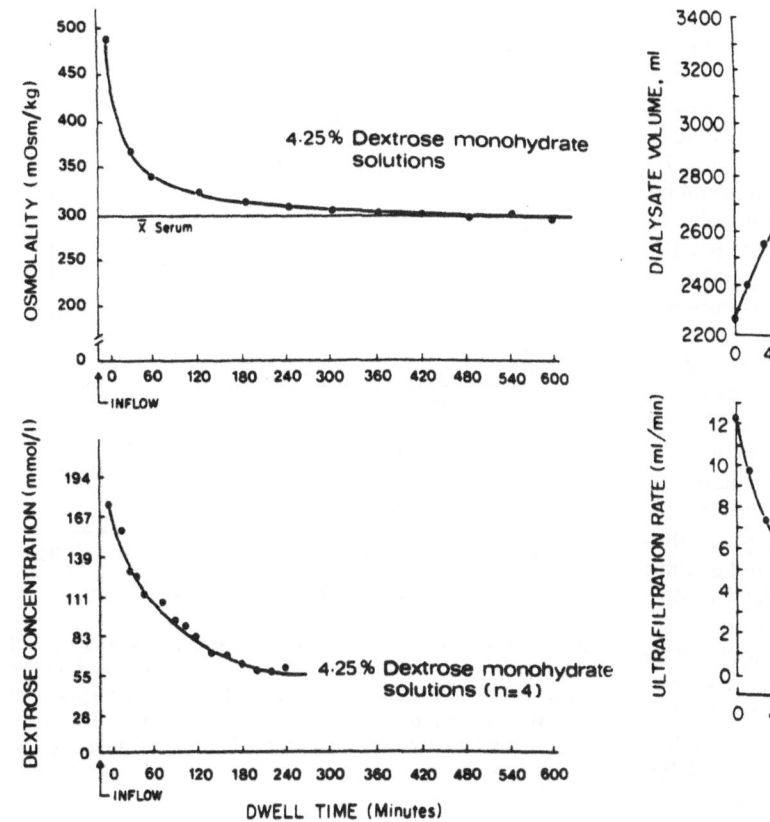

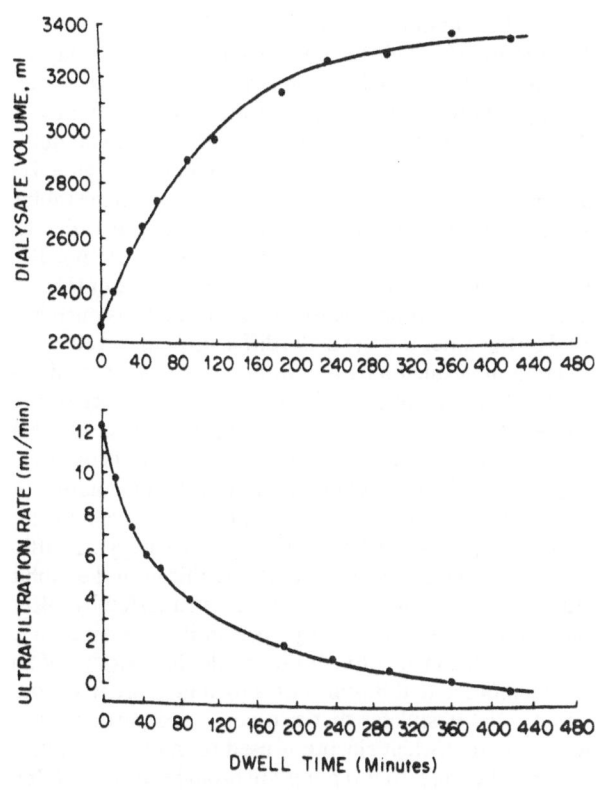

Figure 3. Change in d-glucose concentration and osmolality of a solution containing 4.25% dextrose monohydrate plotted vs dwell time.

Figure 4. Dialysate volume and the rate of ultrafiltration are plotted vs dwell time for a solution containing 4.25% dextrose monohydrate.

another line of reasoning (9). At present, there is rather limited information about σ for the peritoneal membrane and the various solutes that are present in the peritoneal dialysis system (i.e. soluble constituents of uremic plasma water and dialysis fluid) (5,10). As with hemodialysis what is usually measured clinically is the sieving coefficient(s) (eq. 6) or rejection coefficient (ε) as described in equations 5 and 6. Table 1 lists these values for several relevant solutes (10–14). To gain insight into the relationship of the rejection coefficient and Staverman's reflection coefficient for the peritoneal membrane where direct measurements are difficult to make, consider the following empirical formulation. With reference to equations 11 and 12:

When J_f is large ε approaches σ as a limit

When J_f is small ε approaches $\dfrac{J_f\sigma}{P_m}$.

Using a best guess estimate for the area of peritoneal membrane, participating in the process (we will take a small but defensible area of $0.5\,m^2$ (9) in order to err if at all on the high side when estimating the ultrafiltration flux rate for the peritoneal membrane), one would judge the J_f for peritoneal membrane to be 'small'. With reference to Figure 3 and 4 the maximum net ultrafiltrate rate measured at the onset of a

4.25% exchange when the glucose gradient is greatest, ranges from 12 to 16 ml/min (7). Adding substantial lymphatic drainage might raise the 'true' maximum ultrafiltration rate to 20 ml/min. 'True' in this instance refers to the ultrafiltration rate of fluid into the peritoneal space not the net amount usually measured as drained volume from which lymphatic drainage is lost back into the patient. For an estimated membrane area of $0.5\,m^2$, J_f computes to $8 \times 10^{-3}\,ml/min/cm^2$. Contrast this with hemodialysis where a $1.0\,m^2$ hollow fiber Cuprophane dialyzer may be expected to remove 5 l of excess total body water over a 4 h treatment period: $J_f \approx 2 \times 10^{-3}\,ml/min/cm^2$. This value for Cuprophane is of the same order of magnitude as that for peritoneal ultrafiltration and is considered 'small' (2). Hence, for a given solute moving convectively across the peritoneum it is expected that $\varepsilon \approx J_f\sigma/P_m$. This relationship has been used by us and others to compute σ values from the experimental parameters of filtration flow rate (J_f) and measured rejection coefficient (ε) (5, 10). Figure 5 plots σ vs. molecular weight in a rabbit model using neutral dextran studied in a size dispersion that corresponds in molecular size range from inulin (13 Å, 5.2 kilodaltons [kd]) to albumin (35 Å, 69 kd). Of note are the uniformly high values that are relatively independent of molecular size. This pattern points out that in the rabbit the peritoneal membrane is remarkably 'tight' when studied by ultrafiltration (5). This same surprising conclusion may be reached independently by examining Table 1 which shows that even solutes as small in size as urea and creatinine are held back by this membrane that is considered to be quite open when tested using diffusion based methods. Figure 6 is a plot of the same polydispersed neutral dextran in the rabbit but this time the experiment was conducted in order to compute the diffusive mass transfer coefficient (PA). PA has been divided by the diffusion coefficient in water (D) for the given dextran molecule to factor out the resistance imposed by the water present in the diffusion path traversed by a dextran molecule on its way from plasma water to dialysate. PA/D compares the diffusive transport rate across the barriers to mass transport that comprise the peritoneal membrane to that across a simple film of water of comparable thickness. The point of interest is the rather flat nature of the curve between 13 and 30 Å, i.e. little if any size dependence of transport through these barriers indicating very little restriction to diffusion by them. This reaffirms in the rabbit model that the peritoneal membrane when tested by diffusion behaves as if it were very open in its pore structure. There have been two efforts to reconcile this paradox of an open membrane to diffusion with a tight membrane to convection. One postulates that two pore sizes participate in such a way that when glucose is used to induce ultrafiltration, only the small (tight) pores are brought to bear. Nolph et al (15) have laid out this synthesis including considerable anatomical support for the presence of two pore sizes in the peritoneal membrane. For diffusion using this dual pore model, both small and large pores are postulated to participate making the membrane appear open to diffusion as the large pores dominate in conducting the transport. When hypertonic solutions induce osmotically driven transport only the small pores are presumed to participate as glucose can only exert an osmotic driving force on a pore for which it exhibits a reflection coefficient of greater than zero. The

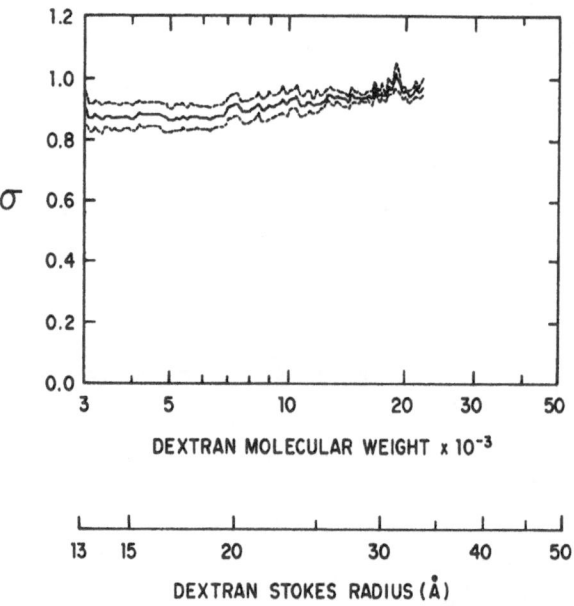

Figure 5. The values for the reflection coefficient (σ) of neutral dextran are plotted as a function of molecular weight and Stokes radius. The mean value is shown with bracketing curves at ±1 SEM. For reference inulin (5,200) daltons) in this test system has a Stokes radius of approximately 13 Å and albumin (69,000 daltons) of 35 Å.

large pore is postulated to exhibit a radius that is significantly larger than glucose for which σ = 0. The results of our recent experiments in the rabbit employing intraperitoneal vacuum as the driving force for ultrafiltration are at odds with this heteroporosity model of the peritoneal membrane (16). With vacuum driven ultrafiltration, convective transport of water and solute should primarily occur through the large pores and hence σ values should be lower than for

Table 1. Sieving and reflection coefficients measured for the human peritoneal membrane[a].

Solute	Daltons	Hydrated radius (Å)	S ± SEM[b]	1-σ (range)	Ref.
Urea	60	2.7	0.81 ± 0.03		11
			0.63 ± 0.06[c]		14
				0.82 (0.9–0.73)	10
Creatinine	113	–	0.57 ± 0.09[c]	0.67 (0.83–0.51)	14,
Uric acid	168	–	–	0.63 (0.83–0.54)	10
Chloride	35	3.86	0.78 ± 0.2	–	12
Potassium	37	3.96	0.36 ± 0.2	–	13
Dextrose	180	4.4	0.40 ± 0.04[c]	0.62 (0.82–0.57)	14,
Sodium	23	5.12	0.54 ± 0.2	–	12
			0.56 ± 0.04[c]		
Inulin	5,200	12.0	0.83 ± 0.04	0.63 (0.91–0.30)	11
			0.41 ± 0.08[c]		
Albumin	69,000	35.5	<0.02	–	a

[a] = See text for explanation.
[b] = S = sieving coefficient (± one standard error of the mean).
[c] = Sieving coefficient values for these studies were obtained using 4.25% dextrose monohydrate containing solutions, a 30 min dwell and 20 min drain time. The other values reported are for 7% solution, a 30 min dwell and 30 min drain time.

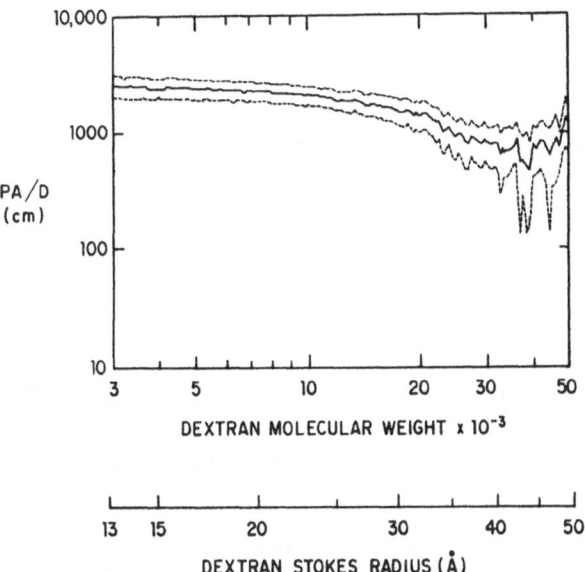

Figure 6. The overall mass transfer coefficient (PA) value for neutral dextran divided by its diffusion coefficient (D) in isotonic saline is plotted as a function of molecular weight and Stokes radius. The mean value is shown with bracketing curves at ± 1 SEM.

osmotically driven ultrafiltration. The results of these experiments do not support heteroporosity alone as an explanation for the behavior of the peritoneal transport barrier. A more complex model will likely be needed to explain all experimental observations.

A second effort at reconciliation of the paradox may be found in our rabbit work which postulates the functional equivalent of two mass transfer resistances coupled in series existing between capillary lumen and peritoneal cavity. Our anatomical candidates for these two resistances and their special characteristics are as follows: The proximal membrane would be the capillary endothelium which anatomically has been shown to be but a few microns thick (17). Its transport characteristics for diffusion would be dominated by its very thinness recognizing that membrane permeability is proportional to the diffusivity of the solute in the membrane and inversely proportional to the thickness of the membrane (length of the diffusion path within the membrane). The thinness of the capillary endothelium then would make for a high permeability. The other property of the endothelium must be that it predominantly contains pores that are 'tight'. This would serve as the dominant restraining barrier during osmotic convective transport making the peritoneal membrane appear tight. The second or distal barrier would be the interstitium and its overlying mesothelial membrane. This barrier would have two important properties, an openness to both convective and diffusive transport and a substantial thickness (50 to 100 microns). Anatomically, this thickness has been shown to be correct (17). Diffusive transport then would display the familiar size dependence commonly reported and imposed

by the length of the diffusion path. Little or no additional resistance would be imposed by this open second membrane a feature compatible with the flat PA/D curve shown in Figure 6.

Recent work by Flessner, Dedrick and colleagues (3, 4) using a rat model of peritoneal dialysis puts forward a distributed model of peritoneal transport. This model has so far been limited to its application to diffusive transport and as such will not be commented upon in detail here. The underlying concept is that for analytical purposes the capillary is 'smeared' evenly throughout the tissue considered, in this instance, the peritoneal membrane. The permeability area product employed applies to the capillary wall rather than the overall peritoneal membrane. The model shows a remarkably good degree of 'fit' with experimental data both presented by Flessner and Dedrick et al and taken from the literature (3). Further testing of the distributed model in the convective mode and comparison with the dual barrier model is indicated.

SIEVING COEFFICIENT MEASUREMENT

Hemodialysis

The clinical yield is small from measuring sieving coefficients for hemodialysis membranes such as Cuprophane which have comparatively low hydraulic permeability (approximately ten or more times less) when contrasted with hemofiltration membranes. At maximum, 5 l of excess total body water would be removed per treatment. As such, the maximum amount of urea, creatinine and other small uremic solutes to be removed would be that contained in 5 l of uremic plasma water. Furthermore, measurements by Green et al (18) show small but significant rejection of these solutes by cuprophane (Table 2).

If the traditional concern is accepted that solutes of 500 daltons or less, rather than 'middle molecules' are important for removal in uremia, then hemodialysis treatment may be considered to be dominated by the diffusive rather than the convective component of mass transfer. Transport of such small solutes by convection may be considered as quantitatively insignificant when contrasted with diffusive transport

Table 2. Comparison of hemodialysis membrane sieving coefficients.

Solute	Daltons	Å	Sieving coefficients	
			Cuprophane	AN69
Urea	60	5.1	1.00	1.00
Sucrose	342	9.2	0.79	0.98
vit. B_{12}	1,355	14.6	0.63	0.94
Inulin	5,200	22.9	0.31	0.78

AN69 = polyacrylonitrile membrane distributed in sheet plate dialyzer format by Rhône Poulenc Corporation, France, Å refers to molecular diameter.

obviating the need to know about the membrane sieving properties for them. Electrolyte transport, however, is an important exception. Sodium, for example, commonly appears in dialysis fluid in a concentration slightly lower than, but nearly equivalent to, that in plasma water. As such, the diffusive loss from plasma water to bath is markedly reduced making the relative contribution of convective loss dominate the net balance of sodium per treatment. For example, if 3.0 l of plasma water at a sodium concentration of 140 mmol/l are removed during a 4.0 h treatment and the 420 mmol of sodium lost by ultrafiltration far exceeds that lost down the modest 2 mmol/l concentration gradient (for total equilibration with bath sodium the value is 70 to 80 mmol) established when the bath sodium concentration is 138 mmol/l. Sorbent cartridge dialysis with dialysis fluid sodium concentrations that start well below and rise to supernormal levels during treatment relies in no small measure on convective sodium removal to restore sodium balance in the sodium and volume overloaded patient (19). Calcium concentrations in the dialysis fluid (6 ± 1 mg/dl, or 1.5 mmol/l) also exceed somewhat those in normal plasma water (5 mg/dl or 1.25 mmol/l). The protein bound calcium of course is not available for convective loss due to nearly complete restraint of protein by the membrane. Net negative calcium balance during therapy may result if 3.0 l of plasma water are removed, each containing 50 mg/l (1.25 mmol/l) of unbound calcium. The 150 mg (3.75 mmol) of calcium removed will exceed that moving into the plasma down the modest 1 to 2 mg/dl (0.25 to 0.5 mmol/l) bath to blood concentration gradient. As routine dialysis treatment time shortens (6 to 4 h) the potential net negative calcium balances may be even greater. In the case of potassium, convective loss augments the diffusive loss down the usual blood to bath gradient set for that ion.

It should be noted that ionic charge can affect electrolyte distribution across a dialysis membrane. There have been relatively few experiments with artificial kidney membranes to examine this phenomenon (20). The experimental design of these studies does not permit a clear judgement as to whether the influence of charge bearing protein such as albumin present on the blood side of the membrane exercises a Gibbs-Donnan like charge effect during isolated ultrafiltration through the membrane or whether sufficient diffusive interchange between the 'blood' and the ultrafiltered droplet hanging on the membrane resulted in the observed deviations from unity in the sieving coefficient. Suffice it to say that in this system the cation and anion concentration distribution are quantitatively very similar to that expected at diffusion equilibrium as described by Donnan (21). As a practical matter when the 'plasma' concentrations of cations are corrected for both the displaced volume effect of protein ('Protocrit') and for Gibbs-Donnan distribution the concentrations in the plasma water are virtually the same as those in the ultrafiltrate (20,22).

Lastly, the plasma clearance for inulin (5,200 daltons), a test 'middle molecule', across 1 m² of cuprophane is 4 ml/min by diffusion. For a 3.0 l fluid removal over a 4.0 h hemodialysis the convective clearance would be on the order of 12 ml/

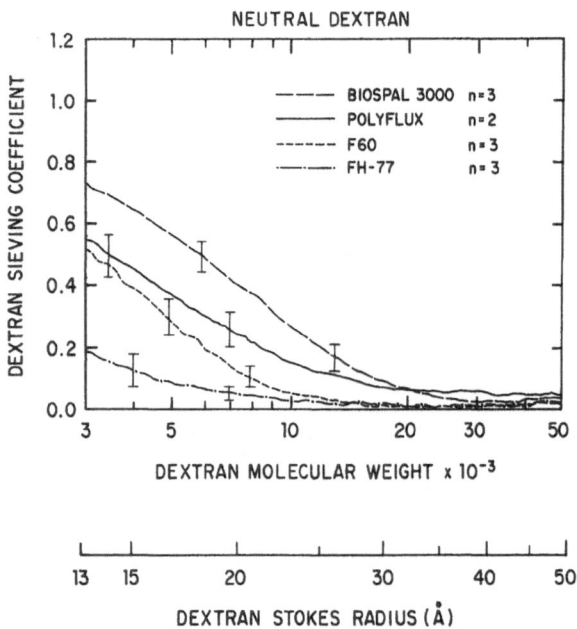

Figure 7. Sieving coefficients for polydispersed neutral dextran are plotted vs molecular weight and Stokes radius for several hollow fiber membranes used for hemofiltration. The polyacrylonitrile membrane from Hospal (Biospal 3000) is contrasted with the polysulfone membrane from Fresenius (F-60) and two polyamide membranes from Gambro (FH-77 and polyflux). Means values with error bar (± 1 SEM) are shown.

min if the membrane did not restrain the passage of the solute. Cuprophane is a relatively 'tight' membrane and the sieving coefficient for inulin is 0.3 (Table 2) reducing the purely convective clearance to 4 ml/min (18). Cuprophane is likely to be typical of the other cellulosic dialysis membranes such as cellulose acetate or cellophane for which there are no studies of sieving properties. Noncellulosic membranes used for hemodialysis such as the polyacrylonitrile membrane from Hospal (3000S) or polysulfone membrane from Fresenius (F-60) have a far higher hydraulic permeability than cuprophane as well as a more open pore structure. They require special fluid cycling equipment in order to use them for hemodialysis. They may also be used for hemofiltration and for that matter hemodiafiltration. Sieving coefficients for these membranes and for others that are exclusively used for hemofiltration are shown in Figure 7. Suffice it to say that convective transport of middle molecules can readily be accomplished with these more open membranes, even under circumstances where these membranes are presumably being used for pure hemodialysis. In this instance, because of the membrane's high hydraulic permeability, the fluid cyclers must employ a fixed volume in the dialysate circuit. This requirement coupled with the pressure drop in the blood path from inflow to outflow end sets up an internal convection loop in which ultrafiltration from blood to dialysate occurs at the inflow end of the membrane and from dialysate to blood at the outflow (Fig-

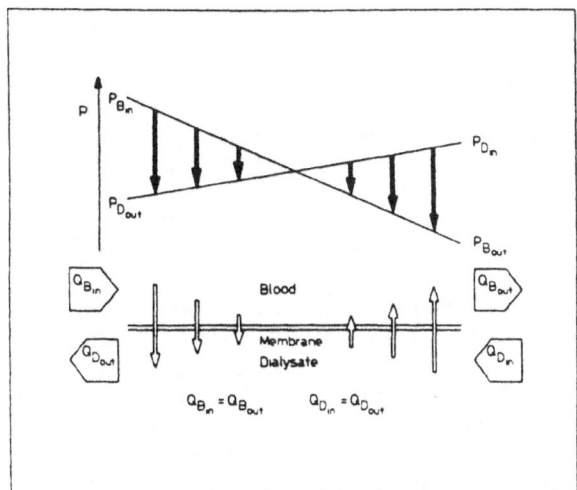

Figure 8. The pair of lines in the upper half of the figure represent the pressure (P) on the dialysis fluid and blood side of the membrane. The heavy solid arrows show the direction and magnitude (length) of the driving pressure along the length of the flow paths from inflow (in) to outflow (out). In the lower half of the figure the vertical open arrows represent the direction and magnitude of flow of ultrafiltrate over the length of the flow paths. It is clear that ultrafiltered plasma water leaves the blood path and is swept to drain with the spent dialysate. Similarly fresh dialysis fluid is ultrafiltered into the blood at the blood outflow end of the membrane. These conditions exist in certain membranes with high hydraulic permeability when operated at zero net ultrafiltration (23).

ure 8). Schmidt (23) has explored these events in a quantitative manner for a polysulfone hollow fiber membrane and concludes that convective transport accounts for some 25% of the net clearance of inulin sized molecules in this inadvertent hemodiafiltration mode.

Peritoneal dialysis

For peritoneal dialysis, past experiments to measure the sieving coefficient (S) have involved infusing hypertonic peritoneal dialysis fluid that contains the relevant solute in a concentration equal to that in plasma water. The average concentration of this solute in ultrafiltrate ($\bar{C}_f$) may be computed from the concentrations of the solute measured on inflowing and outflowing dialysis fluid. The number of milligrams of solute transported by convection into the peritoneal space is computed as the difference and factored for the time of the exchange to obtain an average rate of solute removal ($\bar{Q}_s$ = mmol/min). Similarly, the volume of dialysis fluid removed in excess of that infused provides the volume of ultrafiltrate which is also factored for the exchange time ($\bar{Q}_f$ = ml/min) as

$$C_f = \frac{J_s \text{ (mmol/min membrane area)}^6}{J_f \text{ (ml/min/membrane area)}} \quad [14]$$

$$\bar{C}_f = \frac{\bar{Q}_s}{\bar{Q}_f} \quad [15]$$

The concentration of the solute in the plasma water available from a peripheral vessel (artery or vein) is then measured and is presumed to represent the concentration of that solute on the 'blood side' of the peritoneal membrane. Peripheral blood water is usually estimated by sampling plasma concentration and applying a correction factor to convert the measured value to plasma water concentration (C_w).

$$\frac{\bar{C}_f}{C_w} = S = 1 - \varepsilon \quad [16]$$

$$C_w = \frac{C_p}{1 - \varphi}$$

where φ, the volume fraction of hydrated protein, is taken as 0.0107 times the concentration of total plasma proteins (7.4 g/dl) in normal plasma (24).

In criticism of this method the potential impact of lymphatic flow from the cavity is not addressed. Loss of volume from the peritoneal cavity to the vascular space via the lymphatics will mean, first, that the true volume of ultrafiltrate generated will be underestimated (i.e. a low $\bar{Q}_f$). Secondly, the solute flux via the ultrafiltrate will appear to be less due to loss via the lymphatics reducing mass of solute in the dialysate ($\bar{Q}_s$). It is apparent from equation 15 that the error induced by ignoring lymphatic flow may to some degree be self cancelling. This suggests that the values for S reported in Table 1 using this 'diffusion blocked' methodology may well be quite reasonable values but experimental confirmation is needed. At present the reported studies are in conflict about the means for quantitating lymph flow rate from the cavity.

The observed sieving coefficients for the electrolytes that are below unity (Table 1), should make the clinician expect hypernatremia and hyperchloridemia when substantial fluid removal occurs. As with hemodialysis, potassium is removed by diffusion in addition to convection (unlike sodium and chloride) and offers few problems. Treatment of these iatrogenic concentration increments may be accomplished either by offering sodium chloride-free water in amounts calculated to offset the sodium chloride-free water lost as ultrafiltrate, or by alternating hypotonic or isotonic fluid with hypertonic exchanges, to permit diffusion equilibrium or water reabsorption to readjust these high values toward normal. At times plasma glucose levels rise considerably above the usual values of 300 to 500 mg/dl (16.7 to 27.8 mmol/l) when dialysis fluid containing 4.25% dextrose monohydrate is used, resulting in an osmolar shift of water out of cells. This would artifactually ameliorate the hypernatremia induced by serial hypertonic exchanges. With the return to isotonic exchanges or discontinuance of the dialysis, hyperglycemia would abate and water would move intracellularly revealing the true degree of hypernatremia. At present there is no information on sieving coefficients for

---

[6] It is assumed that the area of the membrane for movement of the solute is the same as that for movement of water and hence, may be cancelled out of the ratio, a point that needs experimental demonstration.

other electrolytes. More recent experiments (5,10) employ mathematical relationships found in equation 12 to compute the values of σ rather than the diffusion blocked methodology previously employed to determine sieving coefficients. To perform these calculations and derive σ accurately, it is prerequisite to measure accurately peritoneal fluid volume and its changes with time. Methods for measuring peritoneal volume will be addressed in a subsequent section on solute transport by ultrafiltration.

CLINICAL APPLICATION OF ULTRAFILTRATION

Hemodialysis

Patients with chronic renal failure requiring treatment with the artificial kidney usually require reduction of their total body water in conjunction with their dialysis. For each dialysis a judgement must be rendered as to how much fluid should be removed during treatment. This presupposes that two pieces of information are available: 1) the extent that the patient deviates from the proper total body water content and 2) the ultrafiltration rate of the artificial kidney to be used.

The concept of 'dry' weight of a hemodialysis patient is widely accepted and usually defined as the body weight below which hypotension or symptoms such as muscle cramps, particularly in the legs or both occur. Should the patient be upright, signs and symptoms of postural hypotension may be manifest. The patient's 'dry' weight is only established after several weeks of conscious effort by the hemodialysis staff to achieve an asymptomatic minimum weight level. Implied in this definition is the absence of clinically demonstrable fluid accumulation in tissues or body cavities unexplained by local derangements, e.g. thrombophlebitis, or pericarditis. Once established, this value is the basis for the judgement of excesses of total body water requiring removal. This empirical concept is exceedingly useful clinically. Table 3 gives total body water (tritiated water space) in liters and as a percent of body weight in 16 stable end stage renal failure patients on hemodialysis treatment for at least 6 months. Whole blood volume (I^{131}-Albumin + ^{51}Cr-RBC) in liters and as a fraction of total body weight is given for the same group. The measurements were made post treatment and all were considered to be at 'dry' weight. The values given do not differ from those of normal subjects (Henderson LW, San Felippo ML, Barg AP, O'Connor DT: Unpublished observations).

At present, most dialysis membranes are used in capillary fiber format. Sheet plate devices are next most common with coil dialyzers much in the minority. The end to end pressure drop in hollow fiber dialyzers is on the order of 15 to 20 mm Hg at 200 ± 50 ml/min blood flow rates. This low figure means a near zero obligatory ultrafiltration rate as it is virtually offset by the oncotic force of the plasma proteins. Most sheet plate devices share this characteristic. In these units dialysis fluid is often pulled through the dialyzer rather than pushed and a hydrostatic pressure for ultrafiltration is achieved by the dialysis fluid pump pulling against a partially occluded (by an adjustable clamp) inflow line generating a negative dialysate side pressure or the blood pump pumping against a partially occluded return line increasing blood side hydrostatic pressure or both. Resistance to flow in the unclamped dialysate path is sufficiently low so that at satisfactory flow rates (200 to 500 ml/min) little, if any, obligatory ultrafiltration occurs. The ultrafiltration rate of the device used is usually offered by the manufacturer as a graph of the rate of fluid loss vs transmembrane pressure. Reasonable prediction of fluid loss per treatment time can be made from these graphs. In marked contrast, however, are the coils for which a significant pressure drop is noted. For unencased coils the pressure gradient may be clearly estimated by averaging the inflow and outflow pressures of the blood path. Most dialysis fluid delivery systems do not provide an inflow pressure. Estimates of the transmembrane pressure from outflow pressure measurements alone modified by experience with a given piece of equipment are, however, quite satisfactory clinically. As Nolph, Fox and Maher (25) have identified, encased coils through which dialysis fluid is pumped have a significant back pressure which reduces the transmembrane pressure as estimated from blood path pressure measurement alone. Encased coils show a somewhat lower obligatory fluid loss due to the lower intrinsic transmembrane pressure. Experience with the coil fluid delivery system combination or information from the manufacturer or both is required to predict fluid loss accurately with time.

New fluid delivery equipment for hemodialysis is now available that provides direct and accurate measurement of the flow rate of ultrafiltrate as a difference in flow rates of dialysis fluid entering and leaving the membrane package. In addition, the total volume of ultrafiltrate generated at any point in the treatment may be displayed. Lastly, this information will provide the ability to program fluid loss for a given treatment to achieve any pattern desired, e.g. 'linear' weight loss with time.

Dialysis induced symptomatic hypotension

Symptomatic hypotension is common during hemodialysis treatments, but a distinct rarity with peritoneal dialysis. A clinical pattern of dizziness, malaise, nausea, and cramps accompanied by a fall in blood pressure, requiring some therapeutic intervention occurs in approximately 25% of

Table 3. Total body water and whole blood volume in 16 stable maintenance dialysis patients at 'dry' weight.

	$\bar{X}$
Total body water (liters)	43.17 ± 1.1
Total body water/kg body wt (%)	59.81 ± 1.6
Whole blood volume (ml)	4,480 ± 283
Whole blood volume/kg body wt (%)	5.92 ± 0.37

$\bar{X}$ = mean ± 1 = standard error of the mean.

hemodialysis treatments. The common perception is that this syndrome is the result of a high rate and volume of removal of excess body water.

In removing excess total body water to achieve dry weight it is quite possible with present day membranes and equipment to remove fluid from the vascular space more swiftly than it can be retrieved from the interstitium and intracellular compartments. Rather than review the pathophysiology of the shock that attends vascular volume depletion in a setting of uremic autonomic neuropathy, activation of complement via the alternate pathway and allergic response to dialyzer membrane contaminants (26–28), I will focus on the differences between hemofiltration and hemodialysis in response to fluid removal. This comparison points out that hemofiltration is associated with some salutary properties that need to be defined further. Specifically, work by ourselves and virtually any group that has done an orderly comparison of the two techniques shows a reduction in the incidence of symptomatic hypotension by about 50% on switching from hemodialysis to hemofiltration (27). This does not appear to be simply the result of better attention paid to the sodium and volume status that attends hemofiltration. Two common observations characterize the pathophysiologic response to fluid removal with hemodialysis that are not present with hemofiltration (29–33). Total peripheral resistance in each study was shown to fall in the fourth hour of hemodialysis at a time when net fluid removal was maximal. Furthermore, and probably etiologically linked to this fall in peripheral resistance was a failure to release norepinephrine in response to the vascular volume depletion. For comparable net fluid removal in these patients with hemofiltration both of these normal physiologic responses were intact. In the Quellhorst study (33), the same membrane (polyacrylonitrile, Hospal) was used for hemodialysis and for hemofiltration. This points strongly away from bioincompatibility of the membrane as an underlying mechanism. There are at least two potential explanatory mechanisms. First, and I think most likely, is the loss by convection of a solute that is sufficiently large to have a low to negligible diffusive loss, i.e. 3 to 10 kd molecular weight. This solute would have to be a suppressor of norepinephrine release and possibly a peripheral vasodilator as well. A second mechanism would involve the presence of unsterile dialysis fluid and interaction of some noxious constituent thereof with blood elements in such a manner as to derange the normal physiologic responses to vascular volume depletion noted above. Vigorous investigation of this latter mechanism is underway but a clear link between, for example, IL-1 release from acetate or pyrogen stimulated monocytes and symptomatic hypotension has not yet surfaced. Work on the former mechanism (34) has cast doubt on a promising middle molecule (atrial natriuretic factor) which has the prerequisite ability to block norepinephrine release and reduce peripheral resistance. This study shows a fall to normal of plasma atrial natriuretic factor as volume depletion with hemodialysis occurs. This is so, not because of its elimination across the dialyzer, but rather as its stimulus for elaboration is reduced and endogenous clearance which is high (3 l/min). This clinically important area is in vital need of more study.

Peritoneal dialysis

Ultrafiltration across the peritoneal membrane must be accomplished osmotically. Glucose, sorbitol, mannitol and other osmotically active solutes have been used to create the pressure gradient. Commercially available dialysis solutions most often offer a 1.5 g/dl or a 4.25 g/dl dextrose monohydrate solution. The measured osmolality of the 1.5 g/dl solution is 350 mOsm/l, well above that for a normal plasma, but quite comparable to that of the patient with renal failure when the blood urea nitrogen concentration is 150 to 200 mg/dl (blood urea 54 to 72 mmol/l). The 4.25 g/dl dextrose monohydrate solution, however, is considerably more hypertonic than even uremic plasma and 2 l will induce about 300 to 500 ml of ultrafiltrate per 30 min exchange. There is considerable variability among patients with regard to the negative fluid balance due to ultrafiltration. An explanation may well be that the membrane involved is biological and subject to differences between patients as well as changes with time in the same patient or the rate of lymphatic drainage from the peritoneal cavity differs amongst patients. With a 30 to 70 min exchange a net ultrafiltration rate of 7 to 16 ml/min is achieved, which contrasts with rates of 0 to 35 ml/min that may be easily obtained with a standard Cuprophane dialysis membrane. As intermittent peritoneal dialysis is usually conducted over at least 12 h and not uncommonly in acute renal failure for 24 to 48 h compared to 4 to 6 h for extracorporeal hemodialysis many clinicians prefer peritoneal dialysis when large volumes (over 5.0 l) of body water must be removed. The slower removal rate permitted by the longer treatment time, means fewer symptoms related to depletion of vascular volume, since the rate of movement of fluid entering the vascular compartment from interstitial and possibly intracellular sources can compensate for the fluid removal. The rate of mobilization of extravascular fluid is specific to the individual. Fluid sequestered in body cavities such as the pleura or the pericardium usually is recruited very slowly and may take weeks or months of repeated efforts to remove, even in the absence of any identifiable cause for local fluid accumulation such as active pleuritis or pericarditis.

The important role of the lymphatics has recently emerged in studies on animals from the Missouri group (6,35). Their work and that of others previously indicate in animals lymphatic loss of fluid from the peritoneal cavity is at a relatively constant rate, is nonsize discriminatory in its transport of solutes, probably occurs predominantly via entering lacunae on the underside of the diaphragm and plays a quantitatively significant role in the net balance of fluid during peritoneal dialysis. Studies in man are sure to follow and likely to confirm many of the observations made in the animal models.

A recent preliminary report by Mistry et al (36) evaluated an alternative to dextrose monohydrate as the osmotically active solute in peritoneal dialysis fluid. The caloric load imposed by dextrose is substantial and in many cases undesirable. Their use of a 16.8 kd starch derived glucose polymer is of interest from several standpoints. First, it provides a substantially greater net ultrafiltration than dextrose monohydrate alone and as expected far less absorption resulting in 50% less caloric load. More clinical testing is clearly warranted.

SOLUTE TRANSPORT BY ULTRAFILTRATION DURING DIALYSIS

Hemodialysis

While the concept of solute rejection by the membrane is important, in order to understand why $\Delta\pi\sigma$ contributes comparatively little to the transmembrane pressure when fluid is removed from a patient during dialysis, it is vital to the understanding of convective mass transfer. From equation 3 it is apparent that the membrane property (ε) dictates the respective velocities of solute (N) and solvent (Q_f) movement across the membrane. No concentration gradient is necessary for solute transport by convection. While transport by diffusion is always size-dependent (i.e. small solutes are transported faster than large ones), convective mass transfer is not necessarily dependent on solute size. The respective contributions of convection and diffusion in conventional dialyzers has long been ignored, largely because of the comparatively low hydraulic permeability of Cuprophane. The advent of more water permeable ('high flux') membranes, however, has directed interest to this area. At present there is comparatively little information on sieving coefficients for uremic solutes across cellulosic dialysis membranes. Current fluid cycling equipment, however, permits the use for hemodialysis of membranes normally classed, because of their high hydraulic permeability, as hemofiltration membranes. In Table 2 the sieving properties of cuprophane are compared with those of the most open of the currently available dialysis membranes.

An expression for combined diffusive and convective clearance (and dialysance) may be derived from equations for clearance (and dialysance) and from consideration of mass balance across a dialyzer in which ultrafiltration is occurring:

$$Q_{Bi}C_{Bi} = Q_{Bo}C_{Bo} + Q_fC_f$$

$$\text{Clearance} = \frac{Q_{Bo}(C_{Bi} - C_{Bo})}{C_{Bi}} + Q_f \tag{17}$$

$$= \frac{Q_{Di}(C_{Do} - C_{Di})}{C_{Bi}} + \frac{Q_fC_{Do}}{C_{Bi}} \tag{18}$$

$$\text{Dialysance} = \frac{Q_{Bo}(C_{Bi} - C_{Bo}) + Q_fC_{Do}}{C_{Bi} - C_{Di}}$$

$$= \frac{Q_{Di}(C_{Do} - C_{Di}) + Q_fC_{Do}}{C_{Bi} - C_{Di}}. \tag{19}$$

These equations provide a clinically satisfactory means for describing mass transfer when both solute transport processes are ongoing. Two points of importance should be noted. *First*, equations relating dialysance and membrane

mass transfer resistances are not valid in the presence of ultrafiltration. Hence, values obtained from equations 18 and 19 should not be used to calculate the overall mass transfer resistance of a membrane/solute pair. The hydraulic permeability of Cuprophane is low so that the transmembrane pressure gradients, resulting from the blood path resistance to flow, which is intrinsic to many clinical dialyzers, results in low enough ultrafiltration rates to permit use of these equations. As previously noted, if high flux membranes are used and transmembrane pressure is regulated by adjustment of pressure on the dialysis fluid side of the membrane to block net ultrafiltration, see for example Schmidt (23), these equations again will be in error. In this situation, convective flux will continue at the inflow end of the blood path where a blood-to-dialysate pressure gradient exists. At the outflow end the pressure gradient is reversed, and, owing to the comparatively high flow rate for dialysis fluid ($Q_D \gg Q_B$), the solute concentration of the dialysis fluid re-entering the blood path is lower than the ultrafiltrate formed at the inflow end ('Starling flow'). Calculated mass transfer resistances for poorly diffusing solutes are then artifactually low. *Second*, while equations 18 and 19 are useful in deriving expected chemical benefits from treatment, they offer little insight into the interaction between convection and diffusion when both are operating in a given dialyzer (as noted in the section on ultrafiltration, σ changes with J_f).

Villarroel and colleagues (2) have developed a simplified form of the Spiegler and Kadem equation (1) that describes solute transport as the sum of a convective and diffusive term:

$$J_s = P_m\Delta C + \bar{C}(1 - \sigma) J_f \tag{20}$$

where J_f is ultrafiltrate flux and

$$\bar{C} = C_B - Z (C_B - C_D) \tag{21}$$

and (the factor)

$$Z = \frac{1}{\beta} - \frac{1}{e^\beta - 1}. \tag{22}$$

Beta is given by

$$\beta = (1 - \sigma) \frac{J_f}{P_m} \tag{23}$$

If $0<\beta<3$ then $\frac{1}{3} < Z < \frac{1}{2}$.

If $\beta>3$ then $Z = \frac{1}{\beta}$ and

$$J_s = C_B (1 - \sigma) J_f. \tag{24}$$

These relationships point out that as ultrafiltration rate, *in vitro*, increases, the overall contribution to net solute transport made by diffusion decreases to zero, an observation already made by Nolph and associates (37). The studies of Villarroel and colleagues (2) demonstrated that for dialysis membranes tested *in vitro*, equation 16 shows a reasonable degree of agreement (within 5%) with the results obtained

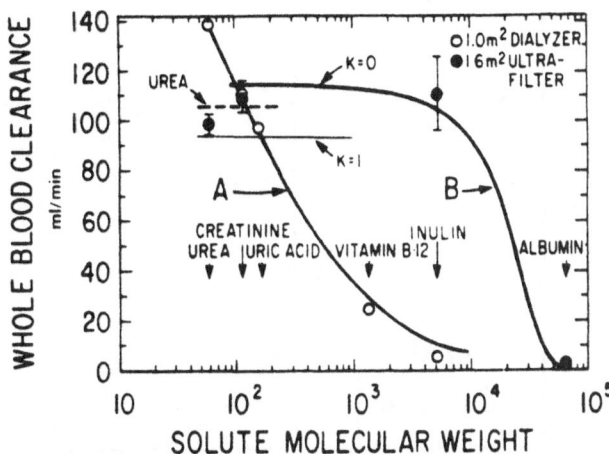

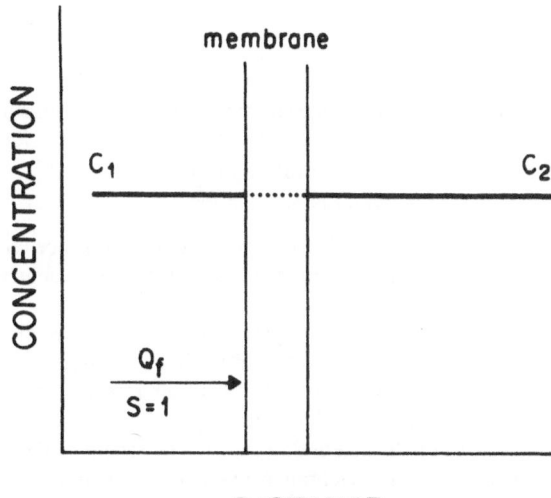

Figure 9. Whole blood clearance is plotted against the log of solute molecular weight. Curve A shows the solute clearance pattern for a 1.0 m² dialyzer operated with no ultrafiltration where solute transport is by diffusion. Curve B shows such a pattern for a 1.6 m² ultrafilter where solute transport is by convection. Normal human kidneys display a clearance pattern very similar to curve B. Small solutes (<200 molecular weight) are better cleared by diffusion. K ranges from 0 to 1 and describes the distribution of solute between plasma and the red blood cell (see text on hemofiltration for further discussion of K).

Figure 10. Concentration profile for a solute with sieving coefficient (S) = 1 during ultrafiltration across a membrane. The dialysis fluid has been made up to contain a concentration of the solute (C_2) equal to that in plasma water (C_1).

with the more rigorous and complex Spiegler equation. As can be predicted, the impact of convective mass transport is most impressive on solutes that diffuse poorly through the membrane. Figure 9 plots clearance by diffusion (curve A) and clearance by convection (curve B) against log molecular weight. It is apparent that for 'conventional' uremic solutes (less than 200 daltons) curve A shows a higher clearance than curve B (38,39). Figure 9 shows two extreme cases for comparison. Clearance is plotted vs molecular weight for diffusion using cuprophane membrane (curve A). This contrasts with curve B where clearance by pure convection is plotted. As we move toward use of more hydraulically permeable membranes where the interplay between convection and diffusion may not be externally apparent in terms of net water movement, we will see an improvement in the transport of larger molecules that is more reflective of curve B. Hemodiafiltration will be commented upon subsequently.

Peritoneal dialysis

The ability of solutes to move across the peritoneal membrane in the absence of a driving concentration gradient was demonstrated in 1966 for urea (40). Important to the understanding of the mechanisms for movement of solutes into the dialysis fluid is the role that the membrane plays in restraining or modulating such movement. The concept of membrane sieving or rejection as explored above, is central to an understanding of how solute movement occurs. Solute mass transfer and its quantitation has been dealt with in some detail elsewhere (see Chapter 4). Therefore, these comments are restricted to convective mass transfer across the peritoneum and the impact that this may have on simultaneously occurring diffusive mass transfer. The usual calculation of peritoneal clearance using the conventional relationship

$$\text{clearance} = \frac{\text{average mass removed per minute in the dialysate}}{\text{plasma concentration}}$$

will provide an average rate of plasma clearance that will not distinguish the comparative contributions of convection and diffusion, but which is perfectly satisfactory for clinical judgments relating to the rate of solute removal. Table 1 offers sieving coefficient values for urea, inulin, glucose, sodium, potassium and chloride. At present, data in humans on larger biological solutes are not yet available. Figure 5 shows sieving coefficients for neutral polydispersed dextrans over the range of sizes from inulin (5,200 daltons) to protein sized molecules in a rabbit model.

Take the case of an uncharged solute of small weight for which S = 1. Let us assume for the moment that urea fulfills these criteria. Figure 10 depicts this concentration profile across a membrane separating blood and dialysis fluid. The concentration for urea has been adjusted to be equal in plasma water and dialysis fluid. The concentration profile is drawn for the conditions existing a few moments after the onset of ultrafiltration and is linear. That is, there is no change in the concentration of the ultrafiltered plasma water as it crosses the membrane and its attendant 'unstirred' layers. In this circumstance the average convective clearance of urea will be the product of the sieving coefficient and the ultrafiltration rate.

$$S_u = \frac{\bar{C}_{f_u}}{\bar{C}_{w_u}} \quad [25]$$

$$S_u \bar{Q}_f = \frac{\bar{C}_{f_u}}{\bar{C}_{w_u}} \bar{Q}_f = \begin{array}{l} \text{Average clearance of urea from plasma} \\ \text{water by convection} \qquad [26] \end{array}$$

$$\frac{\text{Mass removed by ultrafiltration exchange/time}}{\text{Plasma water concentration}}$$

$\bar{Q}_f$ would usually be obtained as the volume difference (Inflow volume – Outflow volume) divided by the exchange time.

It is apparent that the average convective clearance for a solute with $S = 1$ is equal to the ultrafiltration rate.

The measurement of the ultrafiltration rate as usually performed clinically provides an average value. The glucose generated osmotic gradient deteriorates exponentially with time. The convective clearance described then is also an average value for the plasma cleared over the time interval of the exchange rather than an instantaneous value.

In the usual clinical situation where one may wish to quantify the convective clearance for a solute such as urea, there is no urea present in the dialysis fluid. Diffusion and convection then occur simultaneously during the exchange.

Impact of convection on diffusion

While there are theoretical treatments for the comparative contributions of diffusion and convection to overall clearance rate for the peritoneal (41,42) and hemodialysis membranes (2,43), there are only a few *in vivo* experiments to substantiate the respective contributions of these forces to net mass transfer (5,14,40–42). Reasoning from this work and from analogy with synthetic membranes *in vitro* a qualitative appreciation of the interaction between these two modes of solute transport may be developed. Figure 11 differs from Figure 10 in that there is no ultrafiltration occurring and the circumstance is presented where there is no urea in the dialysis fluid. Figure 11 depicts the concentration profile when diffusion alone occurs. The fall in concentration from bulk phase plasma to the surface of the membrane represents the 'blood side' unstirred layer that is partially depleted of solute by diffusion across the membrane into the dialysis fluid. Similarly, the 'dialysate side' unstirred layer is depicted as a continuing reduction in concentration with distance in the dialysis fluid before achieving the dialysate bulk phase concentration (which at the start will be zero). With peritoneal dialysis there is comparatively little mixing of unstirred layers of dialysate when compared with hemodialysis. This component of resistance to transport for peritoneal dialysis should then be significant. Imposing a transmembrane driving force for ultrafiltration on the conditions shown in Figure 11 results in the changes shown in Figure 12. The reduction to zero (or toward zero for a more diffusively permeable solute) of the blood side fluid film will enhance diffusion by shortening the length of the path over which the gradient for diffusion is acting (D_1 to D_2) between bulk phase blood and bulk phase dialysate. In addition, the drop in concentration within the membrane has been oblit-

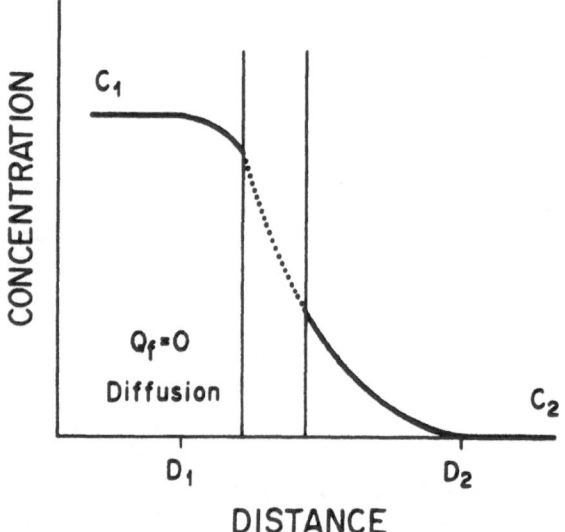

Figure 11. Concentration profile for a solute that diffuses across a membrane in the absence of any ultrafiltration. The 'steepness' of the driving gradient for diffusion is depicted by the difference in concentrations between the bulk phase of the plasma water (C_1) and that of the dialysis fluid (C_2) acting over the distance D_1 to D_2, i.e. $\dfrac{C_1 - C_2}{D_1 - D_2}$.

erated, also shortening the path over which the concentration gradient is exercised. Finally, the dialysate side film shifts away from the membrane. In the event that mechanical mixing may be somewhat better away from the membrane, there will be some enhancement of diffusion. Alternatively, if mechanical mixing is less good the diffusion path may be lengthened and diffusive transport reduced (37). This formulation assumes no changes in the membrane to alter its permeability characteristics as a result of adding an osmotic agent to the bath.

Figure 13 shows the circumstance for a larger uncharged solute where there is significant membrane restraint ($S<1$). The solute is convected to the membrane surface where the concentration builds up ('concentration polarization' or 'solute polarization') (44). The concentration within the membrane falls with distance and the dialysate side film is displaced in a manner analogous to the situation in Figure 12. Again, the overall effect is to steepen the concentration gradient enhancing the diffusive component of transport. Precise quantitation of this enhancement for the solutes routinely dealt with in uremic plasma, is not presently possible for the peritoneal membrane and may not be in view of data, that indicate that exposure to hypertonic solutions not only increase membrane permeability, but membrane area (increase in number of capillary loops perfused?) as well (11).

Finally, in considering the impact of convection on diffusion it should be apparent that solute size is important. For larger solutes with poor diffusive permeability for the membrane (referred to now without its attendant fluid films),

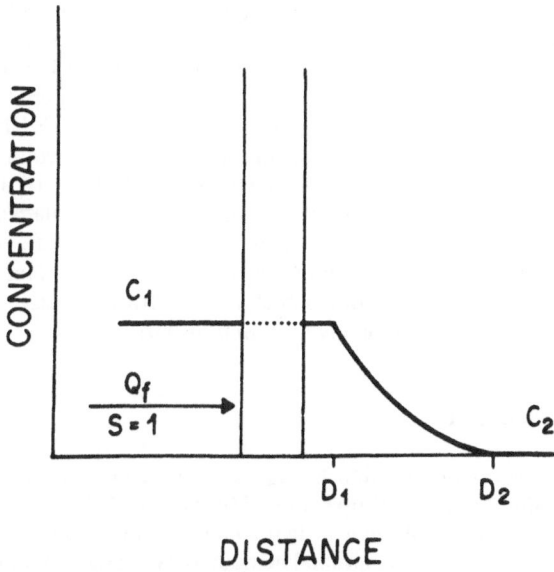

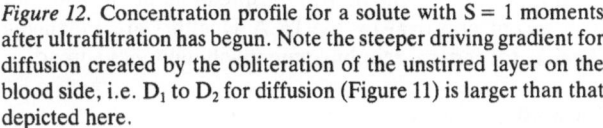

Figure 12. Concentration profile for a solute with S = 1 moments after ultrafiltration has begun. Note the steeper driving gradient for diffusion created by the obliteration of the unstirred layer on the blood side, i.e. D_1 to D_2 for diffusion (Figure 11) is larger than that depicted here.

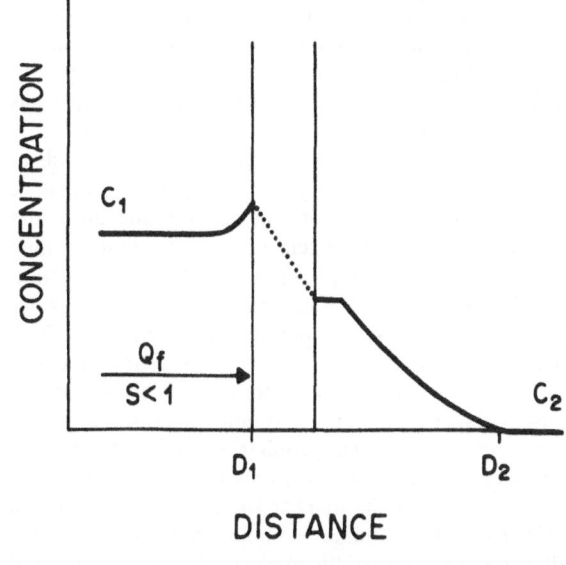

Figure 13. Concentration profile for a solute that is partially restrained by the membrane (S<1) moments after the onset of ultrafiltration. The concentration gradient is made steeper by the build-up of solute on the membrane and acts over a shorter distance than was the case for simple diffusion (as in Figure 11).

convective mass transport, if the sieving coefficient for that solute is high enough, can contribute the major portion of the total mass transported. As a corollary, the fraction of overall mass transfer resistance to diffusion contributed by unstirred fluid films becomes less as the solute considered becomes larger due to the membrane dominating the serial resistance to transport (45).

Albumin, the smallest of the traditional plasma proteins and plasma protein in general, merit special comment with respect to peritoneal dialysis. The presence of protein in the initiating exchange (i.e. the 'ascites' present) and its subsequent decline over the next few exchanges to a steady state level point out the fact that under usual circumstances there is a loss of protein from the plasma into the peritoneal space. The capillary membrane is the likely source. Albumin is the predominant protein. Table 1 lists a sieving coefficient (S) for albumin of <0.02. Glomerular restraint of albumin in animals is somewhat more complete with S≈0.003 (46). The figure given in Table 1 for the peritoneal membrane is not rigorously arrived at, as there are no experiments to determine this value so far reported. Rather, it derives from data for protein (precipitable by trichloracetic acid) loss in a series of isotonic exchanges (1.3 ± 0.1 g, n = 13) taken after washout and subtracted from losses in hypertonic solution (1.7 ± 2 g) to which no protein had been added to block diffusion. The ultrafiltrate concentration of 0.06 g/dl divided by a normal plasma albumin of 3.5 g/dl = 0.02. This figure is purely an estimate as diffusive loss is not blocked and it is assumed that only albumin is convected when, in point of fact, small amounts of other proteins are also present. This estimate of 'peritoneal membrane' restraint in man, how-

ever, approaches that for the glomerular membrane in animals. Further, the presence of protein in spent peritoneal dialysate is frequently cited as a point for the peritoneal membrane as being 'very permeable' when contrasted with hemodialysis or hemofiltration membranes. It should be noted, however, that for convective transport more than 98% of the protein is held back by this 'very permeable' membrane even under the stress of hypertonic solutions. Examination of Figure 5 also supports the 'tightness' of this membrane in the rabbit when tested with convective transport. For perspective, cuprophane PT-150 has a transmittance (T_r) value ($T_r \approx S$) for egg albumin (44,000 daltons, 46.6 Å) of 0.002 and the more permeable Rhône-Poulenc AN 69 (PA) dialysis membrane has a value of 0.04 (18). In light of its slow diffusivity, it seems likely that the predominant mechanism for protein loss across the peritoneal membrane is convective even in the presence of isotonic dialysis solutions. The presence of dialysis fluid would, of course, 'trap' by massive dilution, protein lost from the capillary that normally would, under steady state circumstances, be either returned to the vascular space via the lymphatics or less likely be convected back across the venular end of the capillary bed. It is of interest that lymphatic drainage from the peritoneal cavity accomplishes solute transport by a mechanism that is independent of solute size up to and including solute particles, e.g. red blood cells. This almost surely means by bulk flow of peritoneal fluid through open channels rather than by diffusion. The quantitative importance of this transport path is now under study. Work in rats and rabbits place its quantitative importance as significant accounting for 20 to 25% of the net water transaction taking place during an hypertonic exchange (6). As flow rate across the diaphragm is proportional to respiratory rate and this in turn is in general inversely related to body size, i.e. small size begets a high rate, it will be important to confirm this quantitative importance of animal data in adult humans as well as in the pediatric population.

An important consideration in studies of peritoneal ultrafiltration is the method used to measure the volume of peritoneal dialysate and how it changes with time during the exchange. The rigor with which this is done will determine the rigor of mass transport parameters such as the reflection coefficient (σ) for convection and the area permeability product (PA) or dialysance parameter for diffusion. This latter may be computed from either isotonic or hypertonic exchanges. Its accuracy when computed from hypertonic exchanges depends on accurate volume measurements. We have recently studied this problem by indicator dilution methodology (47,48). We as others before us noted that lymphatic uptake of the marker solute (e.g. radiolabeled albumin, Evans Blue albumin complex, red blood cells) was significant and dilution of the marker solute by ultrafiltered water resulted in a systematic error that overestimated the volume due to loss through the lymphatics. We resorted to using both the traditional method of placing an index solute in the infused dialysate at the beginning of the exchange and following its concentration serially with time and also employing a second index solute applied at intervals for an 'instantaneous' indicator dilution measure of volume. This latter technique meant repeated additions of index solute for this instantaneous assessment and gave values comparable to those obtained by simply draining the abdomen and measuring the volume with a graduated cylinder. We next formulated a model of fluid transport that included 'lymphatic'[7] run-off and from mathematical first principles derived the fact that for the most rigorous assessment of mass transport parameters, it was necessary to use both volume measurements, i.e. that from the common way of using the index solute with its systematic error and the instantaneous value (48). Further, and at least counter to my intuition, if only one of these volume methods is to be used the best (and quite reasonable) values for computed mass transfer parameters are given by the common method. Comparison of

---

[7] Methods for measuring lymphatic flow rate from the cavity entail quantitating the departure of a large index solute, e.g. radiolabeled or dye labeled albumin. Work by Flessner et al in the rat (49) and Rippe et al (50) in CAPD patients show that there is a significant departure of such index solutes from the peritoneal cavity and that at 3 to 4 h these solutes remain sequestered in the interstitial tissues. That is, they have not entered the vascular space as would be expected had they departed the peritoneal cavity via the lymphatics. As much as 50% of radiolabeled fibrinogen departing the peritoneal cavity of the rat does not return to the vascular space during the 4 h study. Our model does not assume loss of the index solute from the cavity via a lymphatic path but rather assumes the general case of its departure by any nonsize discriminatory pathway. Hence, the use of the term 'lymphatic' in quotes. The quantitative impact of true lymphatic drainage of the peritoneal cavity will await further clarification of this problem.

actual data obtained in a rabbit model confirmed this mathematical prediction (48). That is, we used both methods to compute our PA and σ values. These most rigorously computed values were then compared with values computed using one or the other indicator dilution methods alone. This work happily validates many fine studies using this volume measurement method conducted without knowledge of the systematic error it introduces. Lastly, one may speculate on why the common method provides the most accurate figure to compute PA and σ. Possibly, it is because this volume with its systematic error is somehow more truly reflective of the area of membrane involved in transport.

HEMOFILTRATION

By now, hemofiltration has moved from an experimental technique to clinical application. More efficient clearance of intermediate molecular weight solutes with hemofiltration compared with conventional hemodialysis suggests that this technique will become more widespread in the near future. The recent approval by the USA Health Care Financing Agency for federal reimbursement will help that spread.

Theoretical aspects

Solute removal by hemodialysis as a diffusion based process is size discriminatory, i.e. small molecules such as the conventionally recognized uremic solutes, (urea [60 daltons], creatinine [113], uric [168]) diffuse rapidly in water and through water filled 'pores' in membranes and are removed with commonly available dialysis equipment at clearances that are similar to those for intact human kidneys (see Table 4). It should be remembered, however, that the continuously functioning human kidney provides a net weekly clearance that dramatically exceeds even the most efficient artificial kidney applied for 12 to 15 h per week. Large solutes on the other hand that diffuse poorly are cleared slowly by hemodialysis. The process of hemofiltration in which whole blood is diluted with a physiologic solution of electrolytes either before or after it is ultrafiltered across a membrane to remove convectively undesirable solutes, is diagrammatically shown in Figure 14. Blood is introduced into the membrane package and a transmembrane pressure gradient is accomplished either by creating a negative pressure in the casing outside of the membrane or positively pressurizing the blood path by partially clamping the blood outflow line while pumping blood into the inflow port or both. The membrane used is selected for its high hydraulic permeability and retentivity characteristics. The latter should mimic those of the human glomerular basement membrane.

The ultrafiltrate formed should contain little or no macrosolutes (protein) and no cellular elements. Microsolutes, e.g. electrolytes, urea, creatinine, uric acid, glucose, phosphate and sulfate, should be present in the ultrafiltrate in the same concentration as in plasma water. Intermediate molecular weight solutes (300 up to 30,000 daltons) identified

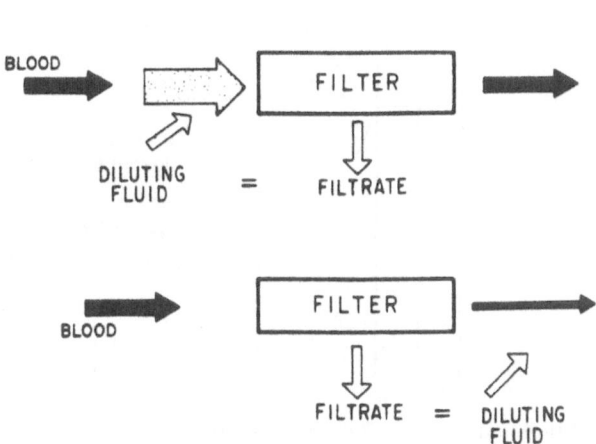

PREDILUTION / POST DILUTION

Figure 14. Diagram of hemofiltration showing two modes of replacing ultrafiltrate to the blood path.

(but not fully characterized) as present in abnormal concentrations in uremic plasma will be removed convectively along with the microsolutes. Depending on the size of the membrane pores and the solute particles, a certain percentage of these intermediate molecular weight solutes will be retained. Figure 9 shows the clearance pattern for an Amicon XM-50 ultrafilter. It is apparent that like the human kidney, inulin with a molecular weight of 5,200 is cleared at the same rate (approximately 100 ml/min) as creatinine (113 daltons) at the operating conditions of this experimental 1.6 m² device.

It is obvious that replacement of water, desirable electrolytes and glucose, simulating 'tubular reabsorption' are required to maintain a satisfactory blood volume and composition. Table 5 gives the composition of a typical replacement solution. With reference to Figure 14, diluting fluid may be introduced before (predilution) or after (postdilution) the ultrafilter.

At present there are at least four membrane formulations with high enough hydraulic permeability for hemofiltration. Most are noncellulosic, i.e. polysulfone, polyacrylonitrile and polyamide. One formulation of cellulose acetate has proven satisfactory. Some of their solute transport characteristics are depicted in Figure 7.

Factors affecting ultrafiltration flow rate

Solute mass transfer rate across the membrane is governed by the rate of ultrafiltration and the sieving coefficient of the membrane. Equation 1 gives the general form of the relationship of forces governing the ultrafiltrate flux (J_f) across membranes with relatively low hydraulic permeability. A more useful equation for membranes having a high hydraulic permeability and used to ultrafilter protein containing solutions such as plasma or blood is needed. Figure 15 shows the results of an experiment in which a sheet of high flux membrane is placed in a stirred cell and transmembrane pressure is induced. Saline flux is linearly related to transmembrane pressure. When protein is present, however, the flux rate shows a linear relationship at low transmembrane pressures but eventually reaches a plateau at which time pressure increments do not increase flux rate. An increase in protein concentration of the solution being filtered results in a lower plateau of water flux but increasing stirrer speed

Table 4. Comparison of commonly reported whole blood clearance patterns for hemofiltration, the human kidney and hollow fiber hemodialysis.

Solute	Daltons	Clearance (ml/min)		
		Hemofiltration	*Human kidney*	*Hemodialysis*
Inulin	5,200	117	218	6
Creatinine	113	108	218	120
Urea	60	101	136	140

Table 5. Diluting fluid composition.

	mmol/l		*mmol/l*
Sodium	133 (132–140)	Chloride	105 (100–110)
Potassium	2 (0–4.0)	Acetate	37 (35–40)
Calcium	1.75 (1.25–2.0)	–	–
Magnesium	0.75	–	–
	Dextrose anhydrous 0–5.6 mmol/l		

Common values given, with range in brackets. Values in milliequivalents per liter are: Calcium 3.5 (2.5–4.0) mEq/l, Magnesium 1.5 mEq/l, and in mass units Dextrose 0–100 mg/dl.

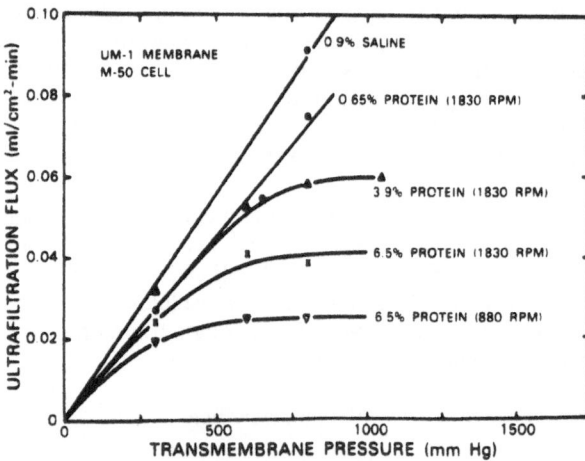

Figure 15. Ultrafiltration flux rate in a stirred cell with sheet ultrafiltration membrane is plotted against transmembrane pressure. The influence of changes in protein concentration can be seen. For saline (0% protein) the response is linear. Increasing protein concentration in the bulk solution decreases the plateau value for the flux rate of water. Increasing stirrer speed reduces the thickness of the polarized layer of protein on the membrane and increases the flux rate for water at any given protein concentration. (RPM = stirrer speed, revolutions per minute, see text).

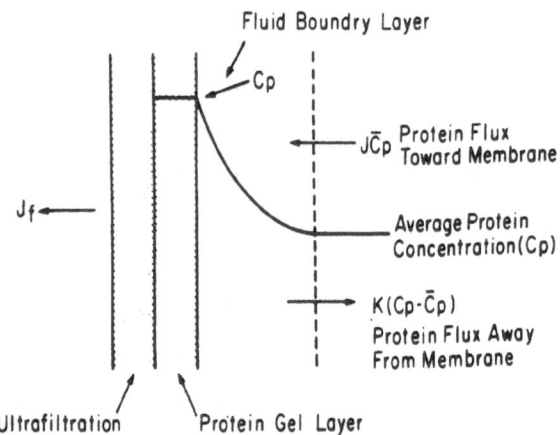

CONCENTRATION POLARIZATION

Figure 16. Diagram of the events at the membrane during ultrafiltration of a protein containing solution. Protein is moved to the membrane surface (polarized) in conjunction with the water traversing the membrane. It is moved away from the membrane by diffusion and shear forces generated by flow over the membrane. Thickness of the protein layer at steady state represents the net balance of these two processes. The concentration profile for protein is shown.

elevates this level. Experiments such as these have permitted a reasonable empirical description of the events at the membrane level (38,39,44,51,52). Figure 16 is a diagrammatic representation of such events. During the ultrafiltration of blood, protein containing solution moves to the membrane surface where water and the microsolutes continue to move unimpeded across the discriminating surface. Protein, however, is sieved out and remains behind (concentration polarization). The thickness of this polarized protein layer is determined by the amount of protein delivered to the surface (protein concentration in the bulk phase of plasma times the flow rate for water through the membrane) and the amount diffusing back from the surface (back flux). Factors that influence the back flux are the concentration gradient between the bulk phase of the solution and the polarized layer of protein at the membrane and the shear forces that 'stir' the protein layer. In the stirred cell with sheet membrane used to generate the data for Figure 15 increasing stirrer speed decreases the thickness of the polarized protein layer and increases the water flux rate. In a hollow fiber unit increasing flow rate down the fiber reduces the thickness of this layer. Previous work with hollow fiber ultrafilters using plasma permitted several useful correlations relating variables of protein concentration in the bulk phase of plasma (C_p), the slope of the velocity profile for whole blood at the fiber wall, that is the shear rate (γ_w) and the fiber length from the inlet (x):

$$J_f = 3.40 \times 10^{-5} \left[\frac{\gamma_w}{X}\right]^{1/3} \ln \frac{28.7}{C_p}. \qquad [27]$$

This semiempirical relationship states that for a hollow fiber unit J_f, the water flux rate averaged across the entire membrane falls with increase of plasma protein concentration, that the faster the end to end flow rate down the fiber the higher the flux, but the longer the fiber the lower the flux rate. The impact of introducing red blood cells, i.e. ultrafiltering whole blood as studied by Okazaki and Yoshida (51) changes these relationships as red cells augment the diffusion of protein away from the membrane, i.e. act as a stirring force. As such, there is an increasing influence of γ_w as hematocrit rises, i.e. the exponent on γ_w rises from 0.3 to 0.8 as hematocrit was changed from 0.0 to 44%. While more work needs to be done in refining these relationships into a truly predictive equation, this semiempirical relationship remains useful to help conceptualize the interaction of the forces that govern water flux rate across the membrane.

Another useful formulation relates net ultrafiltration flow rate (Q_f) to the membrane area of the device (A), the diameter of the fiber (d) and the blood flow rate entering the device:

$$Q_f \alpha (A/d)^{2/3} (Q_{Bi})^{1/3}. \qquad [28]$$

This points out that Q_f is independent of fiber length so long as (A/d) is held constant. It might be incorrectly assumed that for a given total membrane area J_f could be increased by shortening the length of the fibers and increasing their numbers holding total surface area constant. However, this is not true; if a given blood flow is directed into a greater number of fibers the shear rate in each fiber will fall and J_f will decrease as a result. Figure 17 depicts the differences in net flow of ultrafiltrate (Q_f) and ultrafiltrate flux (J_f) and their dependence on fiber length, i.e. (A/d) increasing.

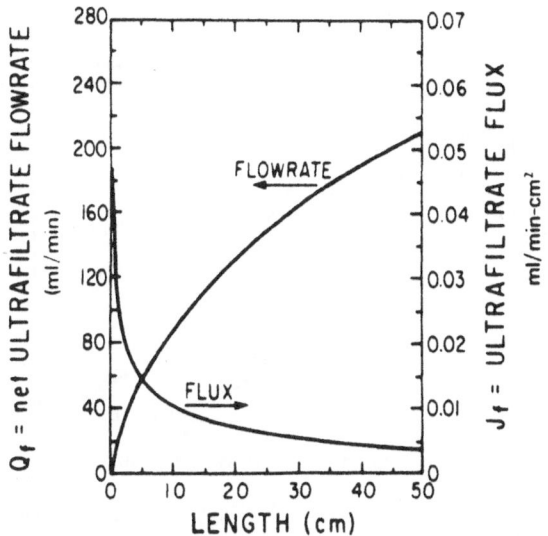

Figure 17. Net ultrafiltrate flow rate and ultrafiltrate flux are plotted against distance from the fiber inlet, for a 4,000 fiber unit with fiber internal diameter of $200 \, \mu m$ operated in the predilution mode ($Q_B = Q_f = 200 \, ml/min$). With a 20 cm length, a $1.0 \, m^2$ total transport area is present.

Factors affecting solute transport

The other factor governing clearance of a solute is, of course, the degree of openness of the membrane as measured by its sieving (S) or reflection (σ) coefficient for that solute. The relationship between the phenomenologic membrane parameter S (or ε) and the intrinsic membrane property σ has already been explored (see equations 11, 12 and supporting text). What is of importance to note here are the special circumstances that pertain to hemofiltration and how they are relevant to the relationship between S and σ. For solutes that are small in comparison with the pore diameter and are not held back, the concentration does not change as they traverse the pores in the membrane, i.e. the concentration of the solute in the ultrafiltrate (C_f) is the same as in the plasma water (C_w) and their ratio, the sieving coefficient (S), is 1.0:

$$S = \frac{C_f}{C_w} = 1. \qquad [29]$$

Equation 29 is valid locally anywhere along the fiber, but C_f and C_w vary with length. Operationally, we have access to the inflow and outflow blood of the ultrafilter as well as to the ultrafiltrate. S can be measured using the average of inflow and outflow plasma water concentration as an approximation of C_w for solutes with S<1, i.e.

$$S = \frac{2C_f}{C_{wi} + C_{wo}}. \qquad [30]$$

This approximation has been shown to be reasonably accurate (better than 1%) for flow conditions reported with hollow fiber hemofiltration (38, 39). In this instance (S = 1)

there will be no concentration gradient for the solute across the membrane to drive diffusion. As such, there is no contribution by diffusion to S and S and σ may be considered operationally equivalent. For solutes of such a size that S<1 for the membrane, we potentially have a very different situation. The build up of protein (S = 0) at the membrane surface referred to as concentration polarization has been discussed above. An analogous circumstance applies to a partially sieved solute (e.g. S = 0.5). One may envision a concentration profile that is qualitatively the same as that shown for protein in Figure 16 or as depicted for the peritoneal membrane in Figure 13. At steady state (i.e. after a minute or two of operation) there will be a significant concentration gradient for diffusive transport from blood to ultrafiltrate. That is, the concentration of the solute in the polarized layer will be higher than that in the plasma water being ultrafiltered and, by virtue of membrane restraint, the concentration in the ultrafiltrate will be lower than that in the plasma water. With reference to Figure 13 the driving gradient for diffusion between the polarized solute layer and that in the ultrafiltrate stream operates over the shortest possible distance, i.e. the thickness of only the separating synthetic membrane. The unstirred layers of fluid on both sides of the membrane that in the absence of ultrafiltration contribute to the overall mass transfer resistance to diffusive transport are swept away by the filtrate stream. Our expectation then is for values of S (or ε) to depart significantly (S>σ) from values of σ by virtue of solute added to the filtrate stream by diffusion.

Hemofiltration is usually conducted with a transmembrane pressure gradient that falls on the plateau region of the plot of ultrafiltration flux rate and transmembrane pressure (see Figure 15). For clinical hemofiltration membrane this would be approximately 200 mm Hg or above. As such, the filtrate flux rate (J_f) is at its maximum for the membrane and flow and concentration conditions present. With reference to equations 11 and 12, J_f is considered large and the relative contribution of convected to diffused solute is small, i.e. S (or ε) approaches σ.

A second point to consider is that both logic and theory would predict that if a solute with S<1 is polarized to the wall of an ultrafiltering membrane that this higher concentration will, in point of fact, perturb measured sieving coefficients such that they will be higher than would occur in the absence of such a concentration build up at the membrane. Said another way, the solution being ultrafiltered by the membrane carries a solute concentration that is higher than we are aware of by measuring concentrations in the domain that is remote from the membrane on the 'blood side'. These influences on S push in opposite directions as filtrate flux rate (J_f) is increased. That is, the diffusive component of transport drops away and S falls approaching σ whereas solute brought to and held at the membrane surface by the filtrate stream should make S rise above σ. One would expect as J_f increased to see a nadir reached for S that would be close to but still greater than σ and that with further increase in J_f, the measured S would rise in response to polarization of the test solute.

In a pragmatic check of these theoretical circumstances in the range of clinically relevant operating parameters, we conducted experiments with hemofiltration membranes that were being operated in the plateau region (53). Our test solute was polydispersed neutral dextran of sizes that ranged between full rejection by the membrane and nearly uninhibited passage. Two widely differing 'blood flows' (of plasma *in vitro*) were used (100 and 700 ml/min). We wished with our higher blood flow rate to sweep away the polarized layer of dextrans at the membrane surface and hence establish the true sieving coefficient. We were unable to show any difference in S for test solutes of any size at the two flow rates. In a second set of experiments in which 'blood flow rate' was held constant and the filtration rate per unit area of membrane (J_f) was increased, the dextran S fell in a manner consonant with the dependence of S and J_f previously described. We were unable to show a rise in S as J_f increased to its maximum for the membrane used suggesting that within practical operating limits of the hemofiltration membranes used, diffusive augmentation of S above σ are all that we need to contend with. The relationship may be rigorously stated as:

$$S = \frac{1 - \sigma}{1 - \sigma \left[-J_v \frac{(1 - \sigma)}{P_m} \right]}.$$

(Note the lack of a term implicating concentration polarization of the test solute.

It should be noted that change of charge on the solute molecule as noted for biological filtration membranes may contribute to its degree of sieving for certain membranes.

Recent work (54,55) points out that anionic dextran sulfate is preferentially rejected by the negatively charged polyacrylonitrile membrane (Biospal 3000S) but moves identically with neutral dextran of the same size across the uncharged polysulfone membrane (Fresenius F-60). Whether this is purely the effect of charge-charge interaction or whether membrane composition plays a role remains to be clarified. More work in this area of solute charge and transport is clearly needed to develop a full understanding of the intimate mechanisms involved in what clearly is a complex interaction.

The data from Table 6 and Figure 18 show that solute sieving for some membranes depends strongly on the presence of protein. An 'irreversible' (to saline rinsing) fouling of these membranes lowers sieving coefficients for solutes of all sizes (56).

Table 6. Inulin sieving coefficients for hemofiltration membranes at common clinical operating parameters.

Membrane	Inulin sieving coefficient	
	Saline	Whole blood
Amicon XP-50	0.97 ± 0.04	0.28 ± 0.08
Asahi PAN-15	0.94 ± 0.09	0.13 ± 0.05
Sartorius Hemofilter	–	0.59 ± 0.10
Rhône Poulenc RP-6	0.84 ± 0.01	0.78 ± 0.05

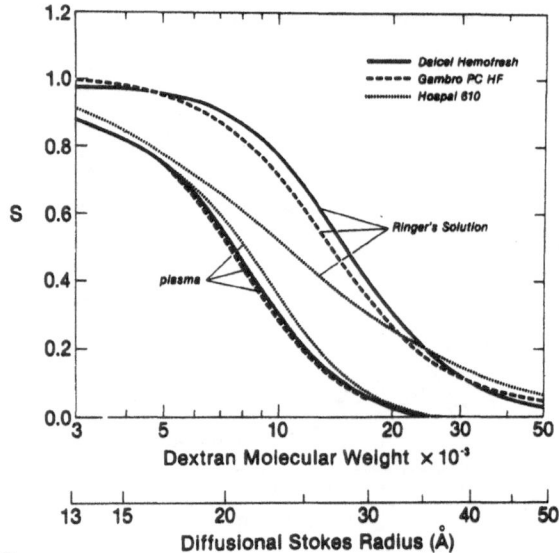

a

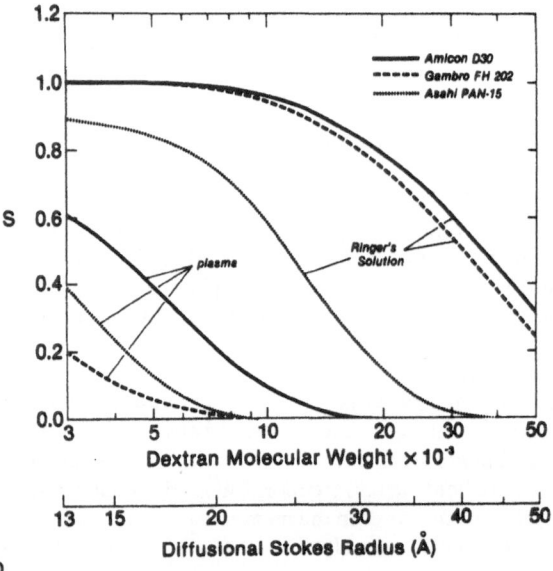

b

Figure 18. Sieving profiles for neutral polydisperse dextran vs molecular weight or Stokes radius are shown for a variety of membranes tested with Ringer's solution and then with plasma. The upper pannel shows data for sheet membranes and the lower panel those for hollow fiber membranes. Inulin (5,200 daltons) in this test system has a 13 to 14 Å and albumin (69,000) a 35 Å Stokes radius.

Solute concentration in plasma water (C_w) is related to the measured concentration of that solute (in the absence of protein binding) by:

$$\frac{C_p}{C_w} = 1 - \varphi \qquad [31]$$

where φ (the volume fraction of plasma proteins- the 'protocrit') may be calculated as the product of 0.0107 and the

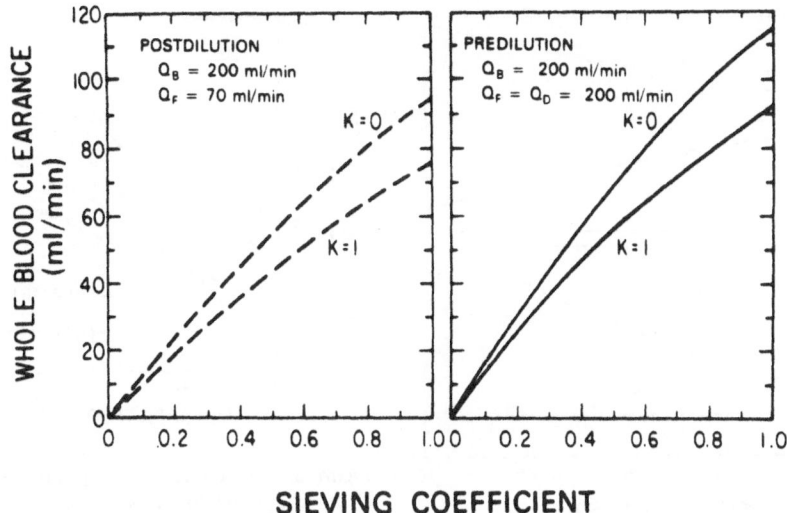

SIEVING COEFFICIENT

Figure 19. Whole blood clearance is plotted against sieving coefficient with pre- and postdilution for the range of K from 0 to 1 for 200 ml/min blood flow. Predilution results in a higher clearance.

total concentration of plasma proteins in g/dl (24). Whole blood concentration (C_B) is related to plasma concentration as

$$\frac{C_B}{C_p} = 1 - H + HK \qquad [32]$$

where H is the hematocrit, expressed as a decimal, and K is the distribution coefficient between red cells and plasma. For a solute entirely excluded from the red cell such as inulin, K = 0 whereas if there is no difference in concentration across the red cell membrane then K = 1. The high hemoglobin concentration precludes K ever reaching 1.0 for passively distributed solutes. Typical K values (38,39) for some solutes are

Inulin = 0.00
Urea = 0.86
Creatinine = 0.73.

Clearance

We may now express solute clearance in terms of flow rates and the sieving coefficient for that solute. By definition clearance is the mass of solute removed divided by the concentration of that solute in the whole blood or plasma. The mass removed in the ultrafiltrate (C_fQ_f) is easily determined.

$$\text{Plasma clearance} = \frac{C_f Q_f}{C_w} = Q_f S. \qquad [33]$$

For certain solutes where a significant plasma blank may be present, e.g. for inulin, a form of the clearance equation may be useful if balanced operation pertains (i.e. the flow rates for diluting fluid and ultrafiltrate are equal).

$$\text{Whole blood clearance} = Q_B \frac{C_{pi} - C_{po}}{C_{pi}}. \qquad [34]$$

Concentration corrections of K and H cancel out of the fraction as do the blank values. In predilution mode, C_{pi} should be sampled before dilution. In postdilution mode, C_{po} should be sampled after dilution.

Measurements of solute concentration and flow on the blood side of the membrane make it possible to compute a mass balance:

$$C_{bi}Q_i - C_{Bo}Q_{ho} = Q_f C_f. \qquad [35]$$

The mass lost from blood should appear in the ultrafiltrate. This calculation may also be used to assess adsorption of solute by the membrane but it is a relatively insensitive index in that the mass remaining is measured rather than that adsorbed and the latter quantity is likely to fall within the error of measurement of the former. Figure 19 illustrates the impact of sieving coefficient on whole blood clearance rate for the range of K from 0 to 1 and compares pre- and postdilution modes of operation for a fixed set of flow conditions (38,39,52). It should be noted that for a given clearance rate the requirement for diluting fluid in the postdilution mode is roughly half that for predilution. Further, for a given sieving coefficient. clearance is higher in the predilution mode. Figure 20 shows the impact of the hematocrit on whole blood clearance for the range of K from 0 to 1 at the same flow conditions as in Figure 19. The sieving coefficient was held at 1.0. Finally Figure 21 shows the impact of ultrafiltration flow rate on whole blood clearance. It should be noted that for the post dilution mode there is a limit placed on the ultrafiltration flow rate by the concentration of plasma protein and red cells. The filtration fraction (glomerular filtration rate/renal plasma flow rate) achieved by the human glomerulus is 0.20 ± 0.05. Higher values occur in congestive heart failure or other abnormal circumstances. What

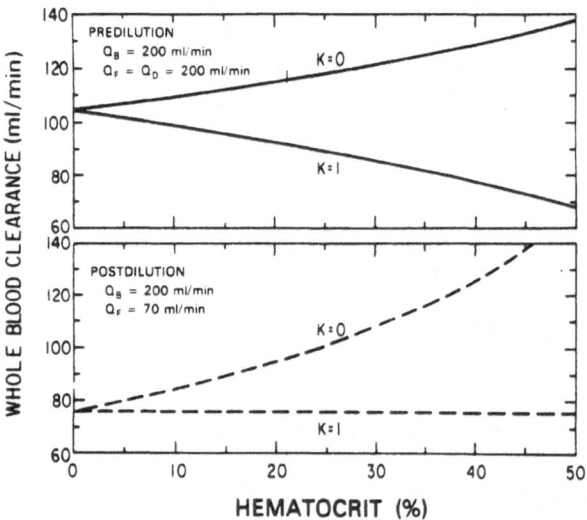

Figure 20. Effect of hematocrit on whole blood clearance by hemofiltration for the range of solute distributions (K = 0 to 1) in pre- and postdilution mode. For an intracellular solute in ready equilibrium with plasma water (K = 1) there is no change in clearance with hematocrit in the postdilution mode.

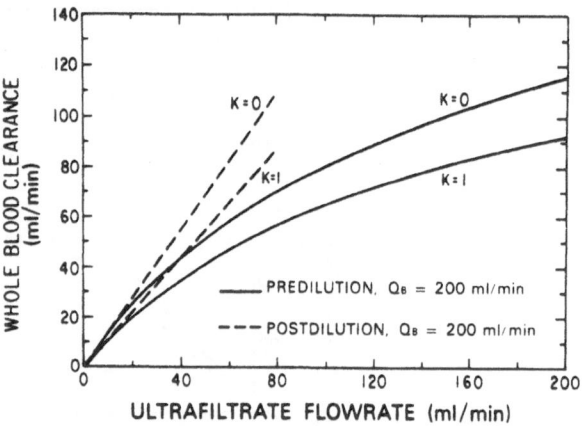

Figure 21. The effect of ultrafiltration flow rate on whole blood clearance, plotted for pre- and postdilution mode. The postdilution mode curves are terminated at a filtration fraction of 0.5 (see text).

filtration fraction is permissible in ultrafiltration from the standpoint of protein denaturation, red cell damage and plugging of the ultrafilter from overly viscous 'blood' is not yet clear. The curves for post dilution are plotted up to a filtration fraction of 0.5. This likely reflects an upper limit.

For clearance calculations with hemofiltration, it is important to identify the space distribution of the solute in whole blood. Clearance is commonly expressed for either plasma or whole blood depending on the solute concentration. If a solute is distributed exclusively in the plasma water then:

$$C_{Bi} < C_{pi} < C_{wi}. \qquad [36]$$

Continuity requires that

$$Q_{Bi}(C_{Bi} - C_{Bo}) = Q_{pi}(C_{pi} - C_{po})$$
$$= Q_{wi}(C_{wi} - C_{wo}) \qquad [37]$$

and it follows that clearance from whole blood >plasma >plasma water.

Methodologically, it is not consistent to calculate clearance of whole blood from plasma solute concentrations (C_p) and whole blood flow rate (Q_B). That calculation assumes that blood is homogeneous from a concentration standpoint, i.e. that the concentration of solutes inside and outside the cell are the same. This clearly does not apply for electrolytes which distribute either by Donnan equilibrium or are actively kept inside or outside the cells. Furthermore, each non-electrolyte solute can be expected to have a unique space of distribution in whole blood. For example, inulin appears to be distributed in the plasma water alone, whereas urea also has an intracellular distribution.

A second problem is closely linked to the first and relates to the rate at which solutes move across the blood cell

membrane in response to a concentration driving force. Each solute can be expected to have a unique flux rate depending on such factors as size, charge and lipid solubility.

The solute available for removal in the plasma water will depend on whether there is a significant solute distribution within the blood cell and on its flux rate from cell to plasma water.

Studies on urea movement out of the cell in response to the concentration gradient established by 50% dilution of whole blood in predilution mode hemofiltration indicate swift equilibration between red cell and plasma water (57).

This likely will not be the case for other larger solutes or those bearing a charge. Frost et al (58) summarize much of the information, scant as it is, on the mass transfer resistances imposed by the cell wall. For solutes that are small, i.e. 200 daltons or less, the mass transfer coefficient across the cell wall exceeds that across the dialyzer membrane. For larger solutes the reverse is true. More data on this subject will be important to obtain as treatment time is shortened and transport of solutes from extravascular locations will come to dominate resistances to solute removal.

DERIVATIVE TECHNIQUES

Continuous arteriovenous hemofiltration

The clinical and technical aspects of this variant of hemofiltration may be found in Chapter 15. This section describes important underlying differences in water and solute transport with continuous arteriovenous hemofiltration (CAVH) when contrasted with those for conventional hemofiltration.

With respect to fluid transport rates, the water movement stems from arterial pressure which generates a lower pressure gradient that that which drives hemofiltration, i.e. transmembrane pressure is commonly less than 100 mm Hg in CAVH. This means that the filter is operated well below the plateau region noted in Figure 15 where filtration rate is plotted against transmembrane pressure. Said another way, concentration polarization of protein does not limit the water flux rate (J_f). This has important implications for filter design as it means that membrane hydraulic permeability is the important determinant of the filtration flow rate during clinical operation of CAVH filters (59). This contrasts with routine hemofiltration where the polarized protein layer, not the membrane hydraulic permeability governs J_f. Return of the control of this important governing parameter for clearance to the hands of the design engineer has not as yet been translated into membranes with hydraulic permeability that exceed those routinely used for hemofiltration. Hydraulic permeability for these latter membranes has not been systematically examined at driving pressures relevant to CAVH. It seems likely that a new set of filters designed to operate at 150 mm Hg or less will be forthcoming and permit better clearance at lower pressures than currently are available which are constructed using hemofiltration membrane scaled down in size for use in CAVH.

As is predictable from prior considerations (equations 5, 11 and 12) when a CAVH filter is operated at these low flows there is a significant diffusive component to the clearance, i.e. S is larger than σ. Figure 22 plots the dependence of neutral dextran sieving coefficients on ultrafiltration flow rate (53) over the range 10 to 97 ml/min for a constant blood flow rate using a commonly available CAVH filter (Amicon D-30). At the lower molecular weight end there is a sharp difference in sieving with low flow rates increasing S by more than a factor of two (0.39 to 0.82). Again, a design constraint is present indicating that increasing clearance is best achieved by providing sufficient membrane area so that flow rate of filtrate per unit area of membrane (J_f) is kept low and yet overall filtration rate (Q_f) remains high as does the net solute transport rate that has its convective component augmented by diffusion.

The principle identified in the above paragraph is carried to its logical fruition by providing a concentration gradient even for solutes that pass the membrane with a sieving coefficient of unity. This is readily achieved by circulating dialysis fluid through the casing of the filter at a slow (10 to 15 ml/min) rate, i.e. continuous arteriovenous hemodiafiltration (CAVHD) (60). Again, a design constraint for optimizing such a filter may be identified; namely that the membrane selected for these derivative techniques should be both very open to water flow and the convection of solute but also that it be thin. This thinness would provide a short diffusion path from blood to 'dialysate' and thus high diffusive permeability. Most asymmetric membranes used for hemofiltration are thick and spongy (50 to 70 microns) when contrasted with cuprophane (15 to 20 microns when wet). Again, deliberate exploitation by industry of this potential advantage is expected.

It is apparent that optimizing membranes for CAVH and CAVHD is a different matter than for HF.

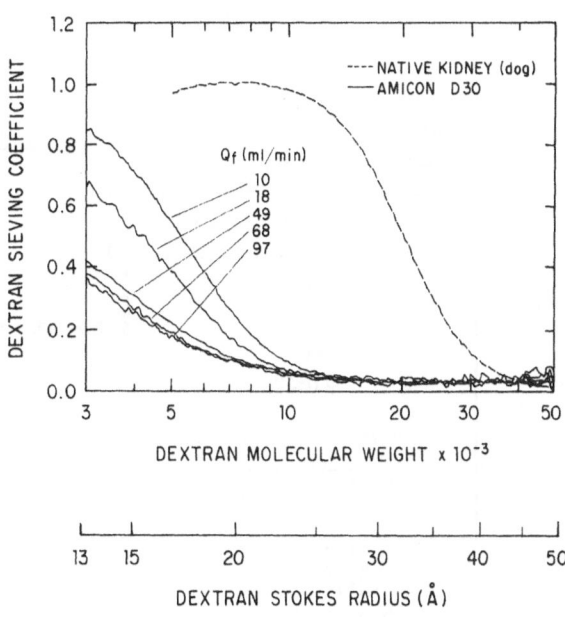

Figure 22. The sieving profile for an Amicon D-30 CAVH filter is compared with that for dog glomerular membrane over the range of dextran sizes from 13 to 50 Å. At increasing ultrafiltration rate the D-30 membrane shows a fall in sieving coefficient. Clearance (Q_f × S) however rises as ultrafiltration rate increases.

Hemodiafiltration

This combination of hemodialysis and hemofiltration was first exploited by Leber et al (61), with the deliberate aim of capturing the best features of both techniques, namely, the high clearance of conventional small solutes by diffusion coupled with the high clearances of middle molecules by convection. A recent resurgence in this very logical approach has occurred in conjunction with the interest in shortening treatment time. Figure 23 is taken from our work using two filtration membrane modules in series. This bench study was undertaken to determine the feasibility of this approach. von Albertini et al (62,63) have shown it to be applicable *in vivo*. At higher than conventional flow rates for blood (500 ml/min) and dialysis fluid (1000 ml/min) and using two ultrafilters in series they have achieved a technically satisfactory 2 h treatment that by computation against standards of adequacy put forward by the National Cooperative Dialysis Study is more than satisfactory. A very important element in shortening treatment time is the preservation of cardiovascular stability. Vascular refilling rate and urea disequilibrium between intracellular and extracellular space is made materially worse by compressing 4 h changes into 2 h. The need to preserve the beneficial effects that attend convective transport then will be crucial. Limited clinical experience reported by Shinaberger in Chapter 16 supports this preservation.

HEMODIAFILTRATION HYBRID SYSTEM

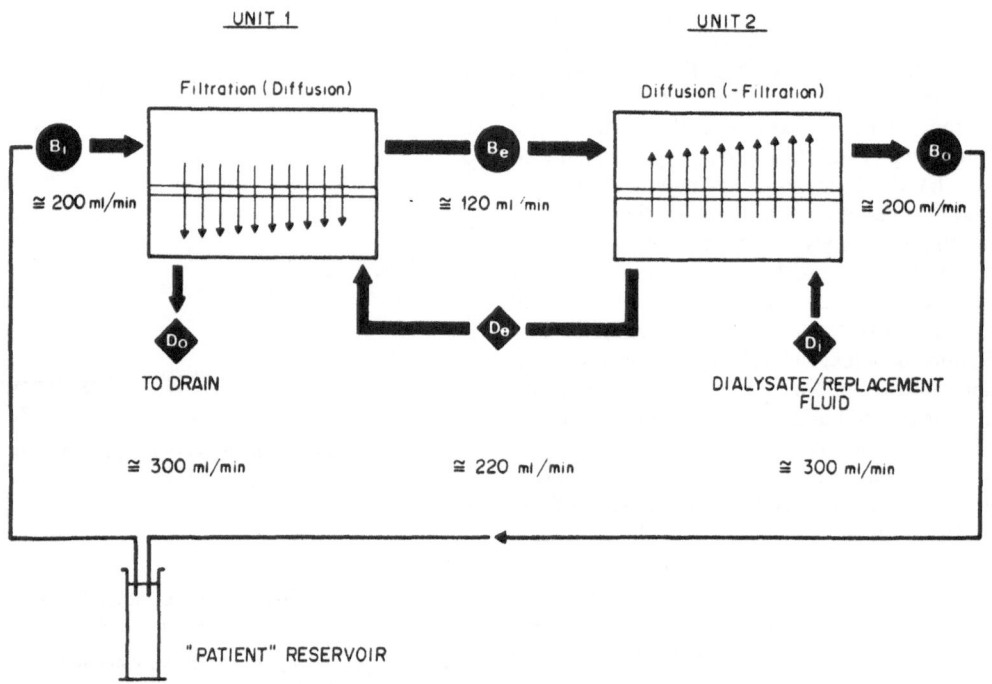

Figure 23. The hybrid system depicted here extends the principle noted in Figure 8. The hemofiltration membrane of unit 1 acts primarily to remove uremic plasma water which is swept to drain (D$_o$) by the dialysate flowing in the casing. Diffusional loss of uremic solutes also occurs in unit 1. Unit 2 acts to filter 'dialysate' into the blood path and maintain patient fluid balance. Diffusional solute loss across the membrane in unit 2 also occurs.

With respect to solute transport, it should be noted that sifting out the respective contributions of diffusion and convection to overall mass transport in a system as complex as that present when hemodiafiltration is performed has yet to be accomplished. Overall transport is well represented by clearance calculations of the sort presented in equations 18 and 19.

REFERENCES

1. Spiegler KS, Kadem O: Transport coefficients and salt rejection in uncharged hyperfiltration membranes. *Desalination* 1: 311, 1966
2. Villarroel F, Klein E, Holland F: Solute flux in hemodialysis and hemofiltration membranes. *Trans Am Soc Artif Intern Organs* 23: 225, 1977
3. Dedrick RL, Flessner MF, Collins JM, Schultz JS: Commentary: Is the peritoneum a membrane? *asaio J* 5: 1, 1982
4. Flessner MF, Dedrick RL, Schultz JS: A distributed model of peritoneal – plasma transport: Theoretical considerations. *Am J Physiol* 246: R597, 1984
5. Leypoldt JK, Parker HR, Frigon RP, Henderson LW: Molecular size dependence of peritoneal transport. *J Lab Clin Med* 110: 207, 1987
6. Nolph KD, Mactier R, Khanna R, Twardowski ZJ, Moore H, McGary T: The kinetics of ultrafiltration during peritoneal dialysis: The role of the lymphatics. *Kidney Int* 32: 219, 1987
7. Rubin J, Nolph KD, Popovich RP, Moncrief JW, Prowant B: Drainage volume during continuous ambulatory peritoneal dialysis. *asaio J* 2: 54, 1979
8. Durbin RP: Osmotic flow of water across permeable cellulose membranes. *J Gen Physiol* 44: 315, 1960
9. Henderson LW: The problem of peritoneal membrane area and permeability. *Kidney Int* 3: 409, 1973
10. Pyle WK, Moncrief JW, Popovich RP: Peritoneal transport evaluation in CAPD. in *CAPD Update; Continuous Ambulatory Peritoneal Dialysis,* edited by Moncrief JW, Popovich RP, New York, Masson Publ USA Inc, 1981, p 35
11. Henderson LW, Nolph KD: Altered permeability of the peritoneal membrane after using hypertonic peritoneal fluid. *J Clin Invest* 48: 922, 1969
12. Nolph KD, Hano JE, Teschan PE: Peritoneal sodium transport during hypertonic peritoneal dialysis. *Ann Intern Med* 70: 931, 1969
13. Brown ST, Ahearn DJ, Nolph KD: Potassium removal with peritoneal dialysis. *Kidney Int* 4: 67, 1973
14. Rubin J, Klein E, Bower JD: Investigation of the net sieving coefficient of the peritoneal membrane during peritoneal dialysis. *asaio J* 5: 9, 1982
15. Nolph KD, Miller FN, Pyle WK, Popovich RP, Sorkin MI: An hypothesis to explain the ultrafiltration characteristics of peritoneal dialysis. *Kidney Int* 20: 543, 1981

16. Bell JL, Leypoldt JK, Frigon RP, Henderson LW: Hetero-porosity model of peritoneal transport is not supported by hydraulically-driven convective transport. *Kidney Int* 33: 243, 1988

17. Nolph KD, Twardowski ZJ: The peritoneal dialysis system. in *Peritoneal Dialysis*, 2nd edition, edited by Nolph KD, Martinus Nijhoff, The Hague, 1985, p 23

18. Green DM, Antwiler GD, Moncrief JW, Decherd JF, Popovich RP: Measurement of the transmittance coefficient spectrum of Cuprophan and RP 69 membranes: Applications to middle molecule removal via ultrafiltration. *Trans Am Soc Artif Intern Organs* 22: 627, 1976

19. Henderson LW: Redy or not. *asaio J* 2: 49, 1979

20. Nolph KD, Stoltz ML, Carter CB, Fox M, Maher JF: Factors affecting the composition of ultrafiltrate from hemodialysis coils. *Trans Am Soc Artif Intern Organs* 16: 495, 1970

21. Donnan FG: Theory of membrane equilibria. *Chem Reviews* 1: 73, 1924–25

22. Ramenofsky JA, Prestidge H, Ford C, Sanfelippo ML, Henderson LW: Novel applications for hemofiltration membranes. *Trans Am Soc Artif Intern Organs* 27: 613, 1981

23. Schmidt M, Baldamus CA, Schoeppe W: Back filtration in hemodialyzers with highly permeable membranes. *Blood Purif* 2: 108, 1984

24. Colton CK, Smith KA, Merrill EW, Friedman S: Diffusion of urea in flowing blood. *Am Inst Chem Engineering J* 17: 800, 1971

25. Nolph KD, Fox M, Maher JF: Factors affecting the ultrafiltration rate from standard dialysis coils. *Trans Am Soc Artif Intern Organs* 16: 487, 1970

26. Henderson LW: Symptomatic hypotension during hemodialysis. *Kidney Int* 17: 571, 1980

27. Henderson LW: Heterogeneity of cardiovascular response to hemofiltration. *Kidney Int* 29: 901, 1986

28. Henderson LW, Chenoweth D: Biocompatibility of artificial organs: An overview. *Blood Purif* 5: 100, 1987

29. Shaldon S, Baldamus CA, Koch KM, Lysaght MJ: Of sodium, symptomatology and syllogism. *Blood Purif* 1: 16, 1983

30. Wehle B, Asaba H, Castenfors J, Fürst P, Gunnarson B, Shaldon S, Bergström J: Hemodynamic changes during sequential ultrafiltration and dialysis. *Kidney Int* 15: 411, 1979

31. Hampl H, Paeprer H, Unger V, Kessel M: Hemodynamic studies during hemodialysis in comparison to sequential ultrafiltration and hemofiltration. *J Dial* 3: 51, 1979

32. Chen WT, Chaignon M, Omvik P, Tarazi RC, Bravo EL, Nakamoto S: Hemodynamic studies in chronic hemodialysis patients with hemofiltration/ultrafiltration. *Trans Am Soc Artif Intern Organs* 24: 662, 1978

33. Quellhorst E, Schuenemann B, Hildebrand U, Falda Z: Response of the vascular system to different modifications of haemofiltration and haemodialysis. *Proc Eur Dial Transplant Assoc* 17: 197, 1980

34. Saxenhofer H, Gnadinger MP, Weidmann P, Shaw S, Schohn D, Hess C, Uehlinger DE, Jahn H: Plasma levels and dialysance of atrial natriuretic peptide in terminal renal failure. *Kidney Int* 32: 554, 1987

35. Mactier RA, Khanna R, Twardowski ZJ, Nolph KD: Role of the peritoneal cavity lymphatic absorption in peritoneal dialysis. Editorial review, *Kidney Int* 32: 165, 1987

36. Mistry CD, Mallick NP, Gokal R: Ultrafiltration with an isosmotic solution during long peritoneal dialysis exchanges. *Lancet* 2: 178: 1987

37. Husted FC, Nolph KD, Vitale FC, Maher JF: Detrimental effects of ultrafiltration on diffusion in coils. *J Lab Clin Med* 87: 435, 1976

38. Colton CK, Henderson LW, Ford CA, Lysaght MJ: Kinetics of hemodiafiltration. I. In vitro transport characteristics of a hollow fiber blood ultrafilter. *J Lab Clin Med* 85: 355, 1975

39. Henderson LW, Colton CK, Ford C: Kinetics of hemodiafiltration. II. Clinical characterization of a new blood cleansing modality. *J Lab Clin Med* 85: 372, 1975

40. Henderson LW: Peritoneal ultrafiltration dialysis: enhanced urea transfer using hypertonic peritoneal dialysis fluid. *J Clin Invest* 45: 950, 1966

41. Babb AL, Johansen PJ, Strand MJ, Tenckhoff H, Scribner BH: Bidirectional permeability of the human peritoneum to middle molecules. *Proc Eur Dial Transpl Assoc* 10: 247, 1973

42. Randerson DH, Farrell PC: Mass transfer properties of the human peritoneum. *asaio J* 3: 140, 1980

43. Andreoli TE, Schafer JA, Troutman SL: Coupling of solute and solvent flows in porous lipid bilayer membranes. *J Gen Physiol* 57: 479, 1971

44. Blatt WF, Dravid A, Michaels AS, Nelson L: Solute polarization and cake formation in membrane ultrafiltration: Causes, consequences and control techniques. in *Membrane Science and Technology*, edited by Flinn JE, New York, Plenum Corporation, 1970, p 47

45. Colton CK: *Permeability and transport studies in batch and flow dialyzers with application to hemodialysis. Ph.D. Thesis*, Massachusetts Institute of Technology, Cambridge, MA, 1969

46. Carone FA, Banks DB, Post RS: Micropuncture study of albumin excretion in the normal rat. *Am J Physiol* 55: 19A, 1969

47. Pust AH, Leypoldt JK, Frigon RP, Henderson LW: Peritoneal dialysate volume determined by indicator dilution measurements. *Kidney Int* 33: 64, 1988

48. Leypoldt JK, Pust AH, Frigon RP, Henderson LW: Dialysate volume measurements required for determining peritoneal solute transport. *Kidney Int* 34: 254, 1988

49. Flessner MF, Parker RJ, Sieber SM: Peritoneal lymphatic uptake of fibrinogen and erythrocytes in the rat. *Am J Physiol* 244: H89, 1983

50. Rippe B, Stelin G, Ahlem J: Lymph flow from the peritoneal cavity in CAPD patients. in *Frontiers in Peritoneal Dialysis*, edited by Maher JF, Winchester JF, New York, Field, Rich and Assoc, 1986, p 24

51. Okazaki M, Yoshida F: Ultrafiltration of blood: Effect of hematocrit on ultrafiltration rate. *Ann Biomed Eng* 4: 138, 1976

52. Lysaght MJ, Ford CA, Colton CK, Stone RA, Henderson LW: Mass transfer in clinical blood ultrafiltration devices – a review. in *Technical Aspects of Renal Dialysis*, edited by Frost TH, Tunbridge Wells, UK, Pitman Medical Publ Co, 1978, p 81

53. Henderson LW, Leypoldt JK, Frigon RP: The impact of membrane area on solute clearance in continuous arteriovenous hemofiltration. in *Proc Int Symp on Continuous Arteriovenous Hemofiltration,* edited by La Greca G, Fabris A, Ronco C, Milan, Wichtig Editore, 1986, p 37

54. Leypoldt JK, Frigon RP, Henderson LW: Macromolecular charge effects hemofilter solute sieving. *Trans Am Soc Artif Intern Organs* 32: 384, 1986

55. Leypoldt JK, Frigon RP, Okamoto S, Henderson LW: Macrosolute charge independent of sign decreases sieving coefficient. Abstract 5th Annu Mtg Int Soc Blood Purification. *Blood Purif* (in press) 1988

56. Frigon RP, Leypoldt JK, Alford MF, Uyeji S, Henderson LW: Hemofilter solute sieving is not governed by dynamically polarized protein. *Trans Am Soc Artif Intern Organs* 30: 486, 1984

57. Cheung AK, Alford MF, Wilson MM, Leypoldt JK, Henderson LW: Urea movement across erythrocyte membrane during artificial kidney treatment. *Kidney Int* 23: 866, 1983

58. Frost TH, Kerr DNS: Kinetics of hemodialysis: A theoretical study of the removal of solutes in chronic renal failure compared to normal health. *Kidney Int* 12: 41, 1977

59. Lysaght MJ, Schmidt B, Gurland HJ: Filtration rates and pressure driving forces in AV filtration. *Blood Purif* 1: 178, 1983

60. Schneider NS, Geronemus RP: Continuous arteriovenous hemodialysis. *Kidney Int* 33 (Suppl 24): S 159, 1988

61. Leber HW, Wizemann V, Goubeaud G, Rawer P, Schutterle G: Simultaneous hemofiltration/hemodialysis: An effective alternative to hemofiltration and conventional hemodialysis in the treatment of uremic patients. *Clin Nephrol* 9: 115, 1978

62. von Albertini B, Miller JH, Gardner PW, Shinaberger JH: High flux hemodiafiltration: Under six hours per week treatment. *Trans Am Soc Artif Intern Organs* 30: 227, 1984

63. Miller JH, von Albertini B, Gardner BW, Shinaberger JH: Technical aspects of high flux hemodiafiltration for adequate short [under two hours] treatment. *Trans Am Soc Artif Intern Organs* 30: 377, 1984.

ULTRAFILTRATION AND HEMOFILTRATION: PRACTICAL APPLICATIONS

CONRAD A. BALDAMUS and MANFRED POLLOK

HISTORICAL BACKGROUND

The modern era of hemofiltration began with its clinical application in 1976. Before that, Henderson and colleagues (1, 2), Quellhorst and associates (3–6), and Dorson and Markowitz (7, 8) had contributed to the physical principles (9, 10), reported first clinical results (6) and recycled purified ultrafiltrate (11). This work would have been inconceivable without the membrane technology developed by industrial firms, such as Amicon (9) and Sartorius (3). The dialysis community became curious about the new technology when in 1976 the first workshop on hemofiltration was held in Braunlage (Table 1) initiated by the German group of Quellhorst. At this meeting a variety of clinical benefits were reported (12) including improvement of anemia, neuropathy, lipid metabolism, hypertension control, hyperparathyroidism and symptomatology. This impressive list of advantages recommended hemofiltration as the panacea in end-stage renal disease (ESRD) treatment. Thereafter industry developed automatic balancing equipment (13) on a volumetric or gravimetric basis and different membranes for flat sheet or hollow fiber filters; simultaneously the complicated dynamics of fluid and solute transfer (9, 10) were elucidated. In time more thoroughly controlled clinical studies refuted many of the benefits attributed to hemofiltration. However improved intratreatment symptomatology and hemodynamic stability remained advantages of hemofiltration (14). Since the late 1970s hemofiltration, especially by the postdilution technique, established itself as a recognized method of extracorporeal blood purification (15), though the high expense of sterile, pyrogen-free substitution fluid impeded the propagation of this procedure. In Europe at present about 3% of the ESRD population is treated by hemofiltration (16).

ESTABLISHED CLINICAL ADVANTAGES

Improved hemodynamics

One of the earliest clinical findings was an improved posttreatment symptomatology with hemofiltration (6). Less fatigue, less washed out feeling and a more stable posttreatment blood pressure were reported uniformly, so that interest focussed directly on hemodynamic differences between hemodialysis and hemofiltration. Quellhorst and associates (6) and Henderson and colleagues (17) independently reported a more stable blood pressure during hemofiltration compared with that during hemodialysis. Subsequently many investigators confirmed these phenomena and revealed the underlying pathophysiologic mechanisms (Table 2).

In a controlled cross-over study Baldamus et al (34) described the relations between the intratreatment blood pressure, changes in peripheral resistance and serum levels of norepinephrine, an indicator for sympathetic tone (Figures 1–3). With a constant ultrafiltration rate during hemofiltration or isolated ultrafiltration, blood pressure remained stable while during bicarbonate hemodialysis (and even more so with acetate hemodialysis) blood pressure decreased. Concomitantly the pulse rate remained constant with ultrafiltration and hemofiltration, whereas it rose steeply during acetate hemodialysis. Bicarbonate caused a moderate increase in pulse rate. Cardiac output, measured invasively, fell significantly during ultrafiltration and hemofiltration but remained unchanged during acetate and bicarbonate hemodialysis. The total peripheral resistance increased during hemofiltration and ultrafiltration but remained constant with bicarbonate hemodialysis and fell during acetate hemodialysis. Sympathetic tone, as indicated by the plasma norepinephrine concentration, increased significantly during ultrafiltration and hemofiltration but remained nearly un-

Table 1. Program of the Braunlage Workshop on Hemofiltration. September 25, 1976.

Introduction	F. Scheler, Göttingen
Principles of hemofiltration in comparison to hemodialysis	E. Quellhorst, Hannoversch-Muenden
Construction and special features of hemofiltration systems	J. Rieger, Göttingen: B. Doht, Hannoversch-Muenden
Predilution hemofiltration	H. Mann, Aachen
Variations in negative pressure during hemofiltration	M. Hueffler, D.v. Herrath, G. Asmus, K. Schaeffer, Berlin
Hemofiltration with hollow fibers	E. Streicher, H. Schneider, Stuttgart
Application of convective transport to artificial kidneys by means of hemofiltration	N.K. Man, A. Sausse, Paris
Hollow-fiber membranes	U. Mylius, Tuchingen
Cellulose-nitrate membranes	H. Perl, Göttingen
Lactate or acetate substitution fluid buffer	C-D. Seufert, H.D. Soling, Göttingen
Calcium balance in hemofiltration	Ch. Fuchs, Göttingen
Loss of amino acids in hemofiltration	H. Mann, Aachen
Role of clotting factors during hemofiltration	H. Koestering, Göttingen
Kinetics of leukocyte and colony-forming units in the blood of uremic patients on hemofiltration and hemodialysis	H.L. Franz, U/M
Clinical results of hemofiltration	B. Doht, Hannoversch-Muenden; D.v. Herrath, M. Hueffler, G. Asmos, K. Schaeffer, Berlin; H. Schneider, E. Streicher, Stuttgart
Control of dialysis-resistant hypertension with hemofiltration	B. Schunemann, Hannoversch-Muenden; J. Girndt, Göttingen
Changes in nerve-conduction velocities with long-term hemofiltration	H. Beckemen, Hannoversch-Muenden
Comparison of lipid changes in hemodialysis and hemofiltration	H. Henning, Göttingen
Elimination of drugs during hemofiltration	P. Kramer, K.W. Rumpf, Göttingen
Excursions in PTH, vitamin D, and digoxin during chronic hemofiltration	K. Schaeffer, G. Offerman, D.v. Herrath, G. Asmus, M. Hueffler, Berlin

Table 2. Hemodynamic changes during various extracorporeal treatments for uremia (14).

First author	Reference	Year	Treatment	Pre-/post-treatment change				
				BP	HR	CO	TPR	PNA
Bergström	18	1976	HD·A	−	+			
			UF	c	c			
Graefe	19	1977	UF	c				
			HD·A, Na 133	− −				
			HD·B, Na 133	−				
Brecht	20	1978	HD·A					c
Bergström	21, 22	1978	UF/HD·A	c/−		−/+	+/−	
			HD·A/UF	−/c		+/−	−/+	
Pogglitsch	23	1978	UF/HD·A	−/−		c/+	+/−	
			HD·A	−		c	−	
Zucchelli	24, 25	1978	HD·A				c	
Canella	26	1978	UF	c				+
			HD·A	−				c
Baldamus	27	1978	HD·A	−	+			
			HF·A	c	(+)			
Shaldon	28	1979	HD·A	−	+	+	c	
			HF·A	c	c	−	+	
Quellhorst	29, 30	1979	HD·A	−				
			HF·A	c				
Hampl	31, 32	1979	HD·A	−	+	(−)	c	
		1980	UF/HD·A	c/−	c/+	−/c	+/c	
			HF·L	c	c	−	+	
Baldamus	33	1980	HF·A	c	(+)	−	+	+
	34	1982	UF	c	(+)	−	+	+
			HD·A	−	+	+	−	c

Table 2. (Continued).

First author	Reference	Year	Treatment	BP	HR	CO	TPR	PNA
					Pre-/post-treatment change			
HD·B	—	(+)	+	c	c			
Quellhorst	35	1980	HD·L	−	+	+	c	c
			HF·L	c	+	−	+	+
Shaldon	36	1980	HD·A	− −	+		−	
			HD·B	−	+		c	
			HF·A	c	(+)		+	
			HF·B	c	c		+	
Keshaviah	37	1980	HD·A	−	+	−	c	
			UF/HD·A	c/−	+/c	−/c	+/−	
Henrich	38	1980	HD·A	−	+			c
			UF	c	−			+
			HD+Man	c	c			c
Wehle	39	1981	HD·A, Na140+U	−		+	−	
	51	1979	HD·B, Na140+U	−		+	−	
			HD·B, Na133+U	− −		c	−	
Aljama	40	1982	HD·A	−		c	−	
			HD·B	c		−	c	
			HF·A	c		−	+	
			UF	c		−	+	
Cini	41	1982	UF/HD·A	c/c	c/+	−/+	+/−	
			HD·A/UF	c/c	+/c	+/−	c/+	
Hampl	42	1982	HD·A	−	+	c	c	
			HD·B	c	c	−	+	
Kishimoto	43	1982	HD·A	−		c	−	
			UF	c		−	+	
Vincent	44	1982	HD·A	−	+	−	c	
			HD·B	c	c	−	(+)	
Schick	45	1983	HD·A	−	+	c	−	c
			HD·B	c	+	c	c	c
Frewin	46	1984	HD·A	−				−
Leenen	47	1984	HD·A	−	++	+	−	
			HD·B	c	c	c	c	
Freyschuss	48	1984	UF	c	c	−	+	
			HD·A	c	++	(+)	−	
Zucchelli	49	1984	HD·A	−	+		c	c
			HF·A	c	c		+	+
Schneider	50	1985	HFD·A	−	+	−	c	+
			HFD·B	c	+	+	c	(−)
			HDF·A	c	+	−	+	+
			HDF·B	c	+	+	−	−
			HF·A	c	+	−	+	+
			HF·B	c	(+)	+	−	c

UF ultrafiltration; HF, hemofiltration; HD, hemodialysis; UF/HD, HD/UF, sequential therapy, UF followed by HD or vice versa; HDF, hemodiafiltration; HFD, high-flux hemodialysis; ·A, acetate dialysate/replacement fluid; ·B, bicarbonate dialysate/replacement fluid; ·L, lactate dialysate/replacement fluid; Na 140, Na 133, sodium concentration in dialysate; +U, urea-containing dialysate; + Man, mannitol containing dialysate; BP, blood pressure; HR, heart rate; CO, cardiac output; TPR, total peripheral vascular resistance; PNA, plasma noradrenaline concentration; c, pre- and post-treatment are comparable; −, decrease, (−) weak, − − strong; +, increase, (+) weak, ++ strong.

changed during acetate and bicarbonate dialysis. Similar observations were reported by other investigators (Table 2) showing that the uremic patient on regular hemodialysis treatment is able to react physiologically at least qualitatively to volume removal. During hemofiltration this physiologic response is maintained. In contrast during hemodialysis the same patient fails to react appropriately to fluid withdrawal, decreasing rather than increasing vascular resistance. The reasons for these different hemodynamic reactions are still unknown, though they are probably related to blunting of sympathetic tone during hemodialysis. The suspected factors are listed in Table 3 and will be discussed in detail.

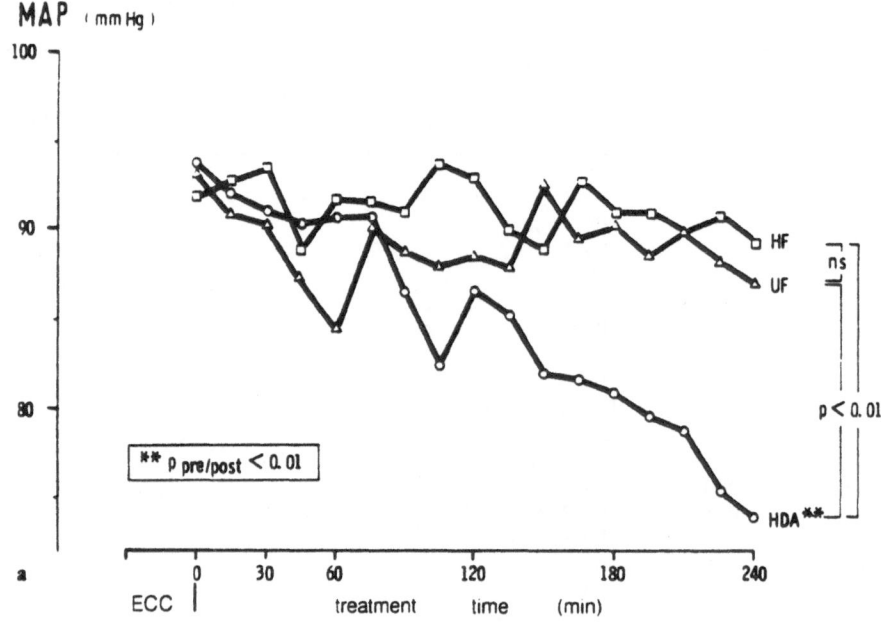

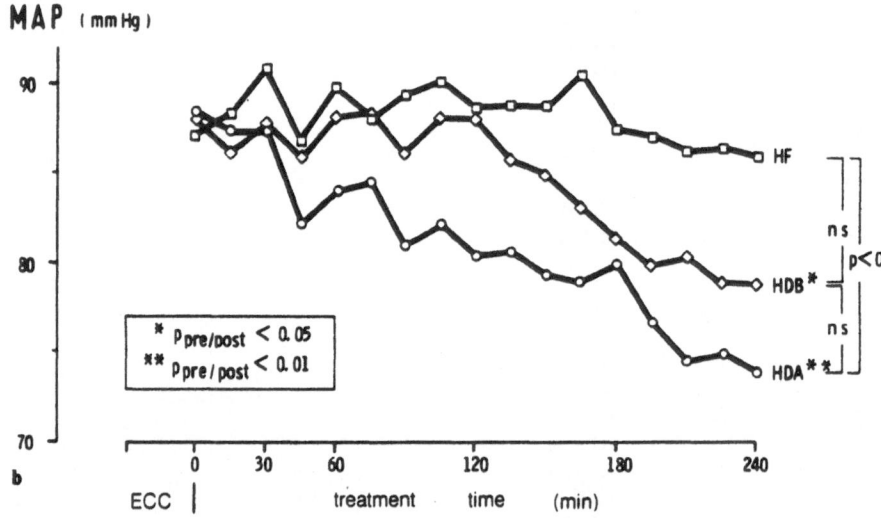

Figure 1. Mean arterial blood pressure (MAP) during ultrafiltration (UF), hemofiltration (HF), acetate (HDA) and bicarbonate hemodialysis (HDB) EEC: extracorporeal circulation.

Mechanisms involved

Ultrafiltration, mandatory in ESRD treatment, results in intravascular *hypovolemia* and correspondingly in an increase in plasma colloid osmotic pressure, initiating a volume shift from the interstitial to the intravascular space. Hypotension occurs if ultrafiltration exceeds vascular refilling and when other mechanisms, e.g. increase in vascular tone or heart rate fail to compensate adequately. The vascular refilling rate in dialysis patients exceeds that of normal patients after hemorrhage and has been measured to be in the range of 300 ml/h (52–54). Systemic hypotension starts to occur at a blood volume of 50 ml/kg body weight (53). Hemodynamic consequences of hypovolemia do not depend on the absolute blood volume only, but on the mobilisation of blood from venous, mainly pulmonary, capacitance vessels (55) and also on total peripheral resistance. During hemodialysis (54) the compliance of these venous capacitance vessels, regulated by sympathetic venous tone, may not adjust adequately to the hemodynamic demands in hypovolemia. This poor response is attributed mainly to autonomic neuropathy. Little is known about sympathetic regulation of

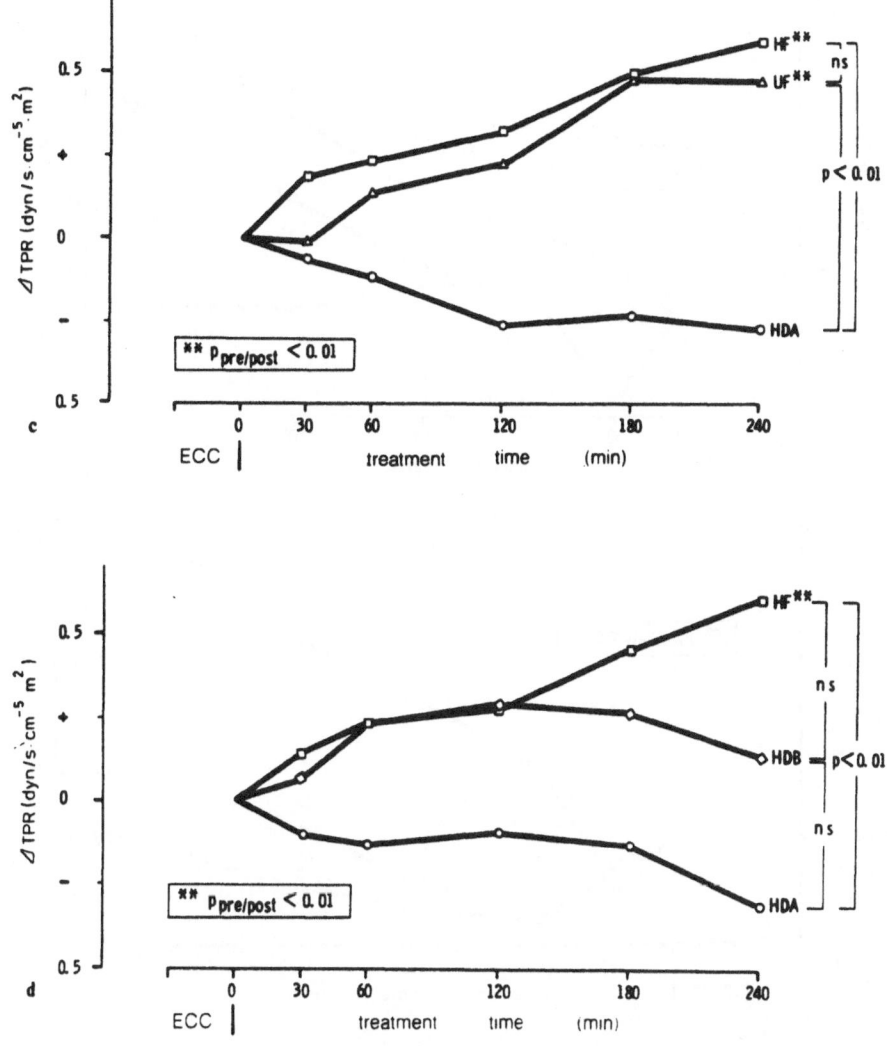

Figure 2. Change of total peripheral resistance (Δ TPR) during ultrafiltration (UF), hemofiltration (HF), acetate (HDA) and bicarbonate hemodialysis (HDB) EEC: extracorporeal circulation.

Table 3. Mechanisms which possibly interfere with blood pressure regulation during hemofiltration and hemodialysis (14).

Pathogenetic factors	Mediators	Pathophysiologic factors	Underlying pathology
Ultrafiltration	Hypovolemia	Myocardial contractility	Heart disease
Solute removal	Electrolyte imbalance	Heart rate	Vascular disease
Solute uptake	Acid-base changes	Vascular volume	Autonomic neuropathy
Membrane/blood interaction	Prostaglandins	TPR	Medication
	Complement activation		
	White blood cell products		
	Platelet products		
	Antidiuretic hormone (ADH)		
	Atrial natriuretic factor		
	Interleukin-1		
	Catecholamines		

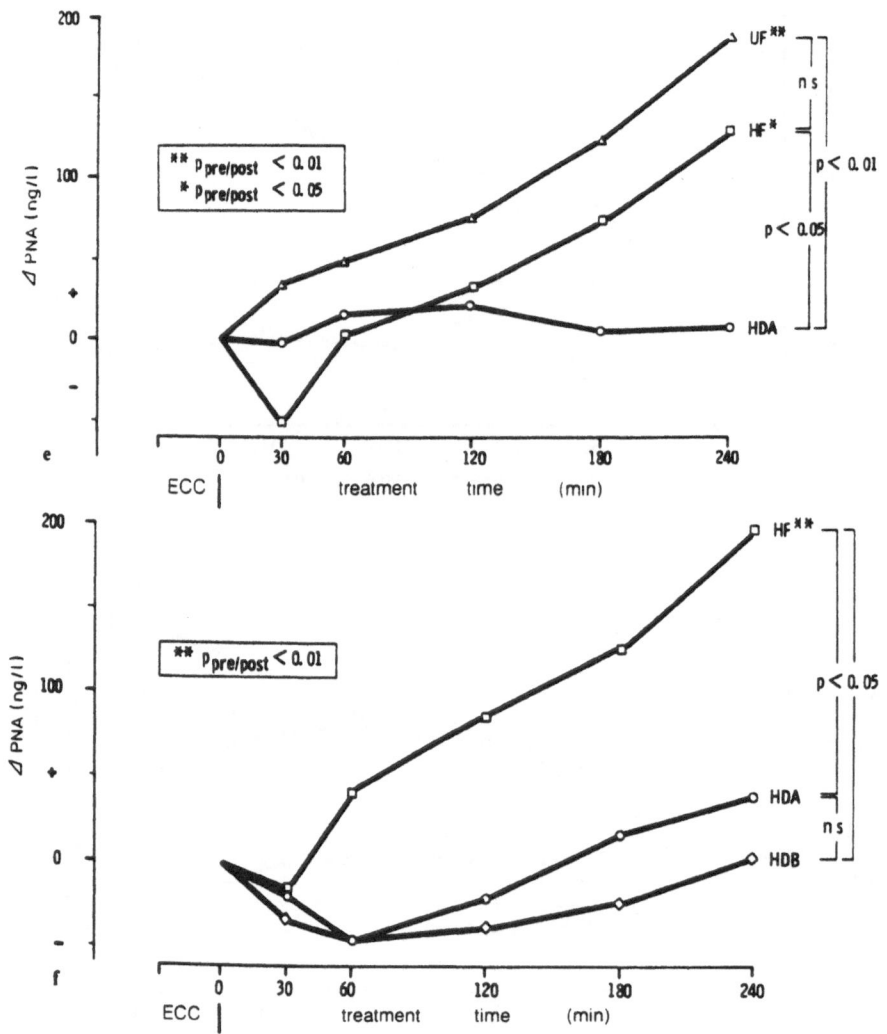

Figure 3. Change of plasma norepinephrine (Δ PNA) during ultrafiltration (UF), hemofiltration (HF), acetate (HDA) and bicarbonate hemodialysis (HDB).

intrathoracic blood volume with respect to ultrafiltration in uremic patients. Hypovolemia culminates in circulatory shock with all the deleterious consequences when circulation no longer complies with the vital needs of organ perfusion.

The better hemodynamic stability during isolated ultrafiltration hemofiltration has been attributed to the absence of or smaller *osmotic changes* in contrast to hemodialysis (5, 30, 39). Based on a well designed cross over study with high and low efficiency dialysis, Shaldon et al (56) demonstrated that the absolute change in osmolality with hemodialysis was not the major contributing factor to hypotension. Hemodynamic stability in ESRD treatment does not depend on the absolute change in osmolality but on changes in concentrations of those solutes that cannot equilibrate immediately between extracellular and intracellular space (Figure 4). The main variant in regard to these 'oncotic solutes' during

dialysis is sodium. Interstitial sodium concentration varies with changes of its concentration in dialysis solution or substitution fluid. Gotch et al (57) focussed on the role of sodium with respect to differences between hemodialysis and hemofiltration. They explained the better hemodynamic stability during hemofiltration by an increased sodium load. In patients undergoing hemodialysis and hemofiltration at comparable starting points Baldamus et al (58) correlated the individual sodium loss with the change of blood pressure and total peripheral resistance (Figure 5). Irrespective of sodium loss, blood pressure remained stable during hemofiltration but dropped with increasing sodium loss during hemodialysis. The blood pressure during hemofiltration was stabilized by an increasing total peripheral resistance parallel to the sodium loss. In contrast patients undergoing hemodialysis were not able to increase total peripheral resistance as sodium loss increased.

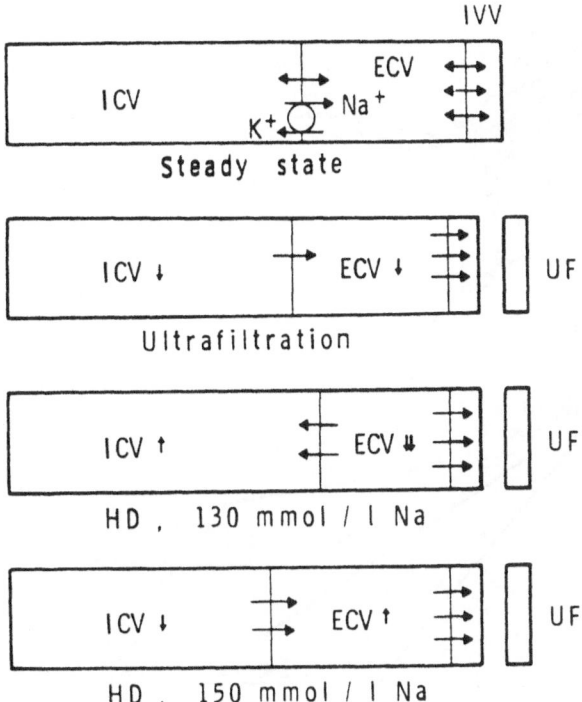

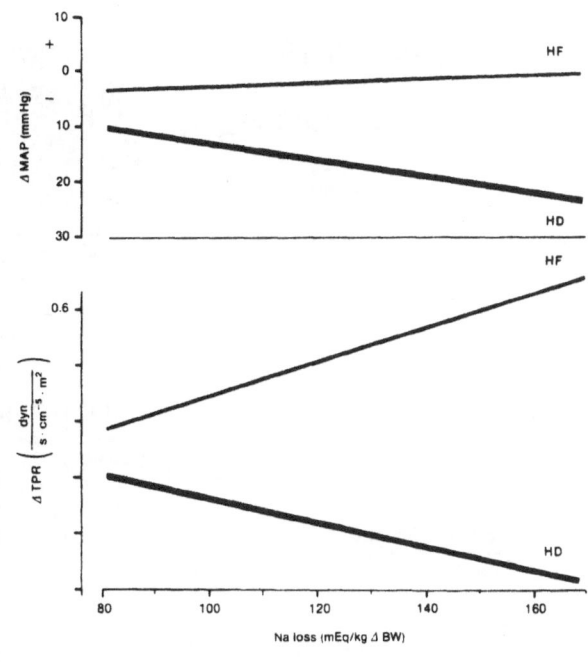

Figure 4. Volume shifts during hemodialysis (HD). In the steady-state body compartments are constant. Intravascular volume (IV) is maintained mainly by the colloid oncotic pressure of proteins. Equilibrium of intracellular (ICV) and extracellular (ECV) volume is regulated mainly by the sodium-potassium pump, and by the passive permeability of the cell membrane. Ultrafiltration (UF) leads to redistribution: ICV, ECV, and IVV decrease. During hemodialysis with low sodium concentration in the dialysate, the interstitial sodium concentration decreases. This leads to a volume flux from the ECV to the ICV and aggravates intravascular hypovolemia caused by UF. In contrast, during high-sodium dialysis, interstitial sodium concentration rises, which causes a volume flux from ICV to ECV and improves vascular refilling.

Figure 5. Correlation of change in mean arterial blood pressure (Δ MAP) and total peripheral vascular resistance (Δ TRP) with individual sodium loss, given as mEq/kg weight loss per treatment. The same patients underwent hemodialysis (HD) and hemofiltration (HF) at standardized working conditions: 3 kg linear weight loss and identical small-solute clearances and treatment time. Even at high sodium loss, i.e., a decrease in interstitial sodium concentration, blood pressure is maintained in HF by an increased TPR. In contrast, in HD TPR even decreases with increasing sodium loss and as a result of this blood pressure falls.

Among the *electrolyte changes* sodium plays a triple role in regulating intratreatment hemodynamics. As discussed above, sodium causes a transcellular volume shift. An increase in extracellular sodium concentration stimulates vasopressin secretion and thereby increases total peripheral vascular resistance. Furthermore, a falling serum sodium concentration increases renin release resulting in a rise of blood pressure (59).

During treatment of ESRD potassium is removed whereas calcium is supplied. Both electrolytes influence hemodynamics. A decrease in extracellular potassium concentration causes vasoconstriction (60) most likely due to its action on the sarcolemmal (Na-K)-ATPase. A rise in ionized calcium increases total peripheral resistance (61) and improves cardiac contractility (62). Acidosis blunts this response. Differences in hemodynamics might be due to variations in electrolyte balances; however, controlled studies examining these influences are lacking.

Differences in hemodynamics have been attributed to the buffer substrate in dialysate. Therefore, it is interesting to review the studies comparing acetate and bicarbonate hemodialysis with acetate and bicarbonate hemofiltration (34, 36, 50). Doubtless, acetate at relevant plasma concentrations lowers total peripheral vascular resistance which must be compensated for by a higher cardiac output (63). Most authors report a decrease in vascular resistance during acetate dialysis and little or no increase during bicarbonate dialysis (34, 36, 40, 44, 45). In contrast, total peripheral resistance increases adequately during hemofiltration regardless of whether acetate or bicarbonate is used as buffer in the replacement fluid. Provided that urea clearance and acetate concentration in dialysis fluid and in hemofiltration substitution fluid are identical, the acetate load in hemofiltration exceeds that in hemodialysis (14).

Vasoactive hormones have been claimed to contribute to the hemodynamic stability during hemofiltration. Theoretically, substances interfering with sympathetic activity might be generated during hemodialysis but not during hemofiltration. Removal of these substances during hemofiltration is another possible explanation for the different responses. Despite a higher clearance of norepinephrine during hemofiltration at comparable urea clearances elevated plasma

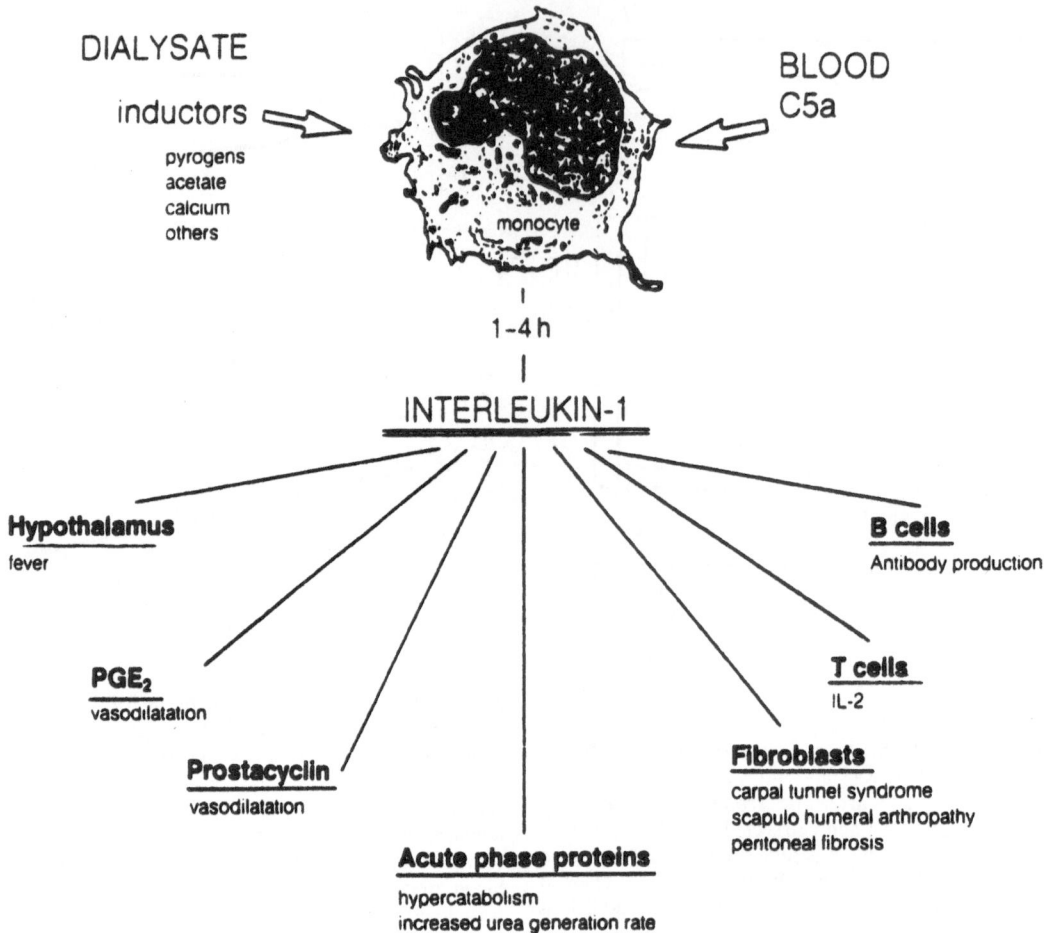

Figure 6. Possible consequences of dialysis-associated IL-1 production by activated monocytes.

norepinephrine levels were found during hemofiltration compared with those during hemodialysis. Vasopressin, a powerful vasoconstrictor, is released either by an increase in extracellular osmolality, e.g. an increased plasma sodium concentration or by stimulation of the renin angiotensin system in hypovolemia. Whether there are differences between hemodialysis and hemofiltration in vasopressin release remains unknown.

The atrial natriuretic factor (ANF) is a potent vasodilating hormone released by volume loading and subsequent atrial dilatation. At the end of the interdialytic period ANF is generally increased but secretion tapers with intratreatment weight reduction (64, 65). Since the atrial natriuretic factor (3,000 daltons) is removed effectively during hemofiltration but not during hemodialysis, its vasodilating effect might become noticeable during hemodialysis.

Maggiore et al (66) were the first to describe improved hemodynamic stability when extracorporeal blood was returned at low *temperature*. They were able to show that the hemodynamic differences between hemodialysis and hemofiltration diminished with low temperature treatment (67,

68). However the maximal drop in blood pressure during warm hemofiltration was less than during warm hemodialysis. In similar experiments Schäfer et al (69) and others (70) found no significant difference in hemodynamic stability if the temperature of the replacement fluid was varied within a range that did not inconvenience the patient.

Blood device interaction is unavoidable in extracorporeal treatment. Blood contacts dialyzer or filter, blood lines, connections and other items directly. Residues of the manufacturing or sterilizing process diffuse into the plasma to bind to its lipophilic constituents. The most thoroughly investigated blood device interaction is complement activation by cellulosic membranes occuring immediately after blood contacts the membrane (71–73). While complement is activated in the very first minutes of dialysis, hypotension occurs late in treatment. Complement activation may influence hemodynamics by interleukin 1 (IL 1) production (74). The interleukin 1 hypothesis was presented first by Henderson et al (75) and later promoted by Shaldon et al (76). Based on clinical observations in chronic dialysis patients, such as rise of temperature during treatment, low plasma zinc concentration and increased plasma levels of acute phase proteins, they postulated the activation of IL 1 during dialysis (Figure 6). The complement component C5A binds to macrophages and induces IL 1 production with a time lag of 1 to 4 h. This coincides with the peak incidence of hypotensive episodes during hemodialysis. Endotoxin (77–79) in dialysate stimulates IL 1 liberation. Pyrogens adsorb extensively to dialysis membranes and may penetrate the membrane to gain access to the blood stream. Circulating or membrane-bound pyrogens stimulate adherent monocytes to produce IL 1 as supported by experimental data. Principal differences in membrane transport may be responsible for differences in IL 1 production between hemodialysis and hemofiltration (76). Because IL 1 stimulation decreases blood pressure (80), it can explain the hemodynamic differences seen between hemodialysis and hemofiltration.

Autonomic neuropathy, frequently found in uremic patients (81, 82), predisposes to intratreatment hypotension. Treatment-specific differences especially in baroreceptor responses could not be demonstrated between hemodialysis and hemofiltration (83). Patients with 'uremic cardiomyopathy' or other forms of cardiac impairment are especially sensitive to volume removal resulting in intratreatment hypotension. Hemofiltration is of particular benefit for these patients. Because of their high sensitivity further studies especially in these patients might help to clarify specific pathogenetic aspects of hemodialysis associated hypotension.

Improved solute removal

Originally hemofiltration was introduced because the middle molecule hypothesis attributed medical benefits to better removal of solutes with a higher molecular weight. The initially reported clinical advantages of hemofiltration such as improvement of uremic neuropathy (6) seemed to confirm this hypothesis. When the middle molecule hypothesis could not be proven removal of higher molecular weight solutes by hemofiltration became a neglected field of interest. Only recently when dialysis associated β_2 microglobulin-associated amyloidosis (84–86) was recognized as a late complication of dialysis treatment, the removal of higher molecular weight solutes again became an important promoter for hemofiltration.

During the late 1970s and early 1980s amyloidosis was recognized as a late complication in long term hemodialysis patients (87). With growing time on dialysis patients increasingly suffered from carpal tunnel syndrome, shoulder-arm-pain, and bone cysts all of which were shown to be preferred sites of amyloid deposition (87). In 1985 and 1986

Table 4. Characteristics of filters frequently used for hemofiltration.

Manufacturer	Type of filter	Membrane material	Membrane area (m²)	Inner diameter (µm)	Fiber length (mm)	Blood volume (ml)	UF at QB (ml/min) 100 at TMP (mmHg) 60	200 500	400 500	Sieving coeff. f. B2-Microglobulin	B2M-absorption
Amicon	D 20	polysulfone	0,25	200	130	20	5–15	–	–		
	D 30	polysulfone	0,6	200	215	40	10–25	–	–		?
	D 40	polysulfone	1,10	200		75	–	70– 90	90–120		
ASAHI	PAN 150	polyacrylo-	1,10	210	215	75	–	80– 90	–		
	PAN 200	nitrile	1,40	210	240	100	–	80–100	110–130	<0,2	0
	PAN 250		2,00	210	240	140	–	80–100	120–150		
Cordis Dow	Duoflux	cell. acetate	1,80	200	250	135	–	60– 80	80–100		?
Fresenius	AU 600	polysulfone	1,35	220	255	90	30–35	–	–		
	HF 60		1,25	200	255	75	–	90–100	110–130	0,6	0
	HF 80		1,90	200	255	120	–	110–120	180–200		
Gambro	FH 66	polyamide	0,60	215	140	43	15–20	–	–		
	FH 77		1,40	215	250	90	–	75– 95	110–150	>0,2	
	FH 88		2,00	215	250	137	–	75– 95	140–180	+	
	Polyflux 130		1,30	220	210	85	–	80– 90	130–160	0,6	
Hospal	Multiflow	AN 69	0,6	240	135	49	15–17	–	–		
	Filtral 12	polyacrylo-	1,2	240	200	90	–	100–110		0,6	
	Filtral 16	nitrile	1,7	240	260	122	–	130			+
Sartorius	SM 400 42	cellulose	0,6	flat sheet			–	85–115	110–150		
	SM 400 43	triacetate	1,0	flat sheet				100–120	130–180	<0,7	0
Toray	B1-L	PMMA	2,10	240	230	155	–	70– 80	80–100	?	?

these amyloid deposits were identified as beta$_2$ microglobulin amyloid fibrils (85). Although beta$_2$ microglobulin amyloidosis occurs in all forms of renal replacement therapy patients on hemofiltration might benefit from removal of this small protein by the treatment. Whether amyloidosis can be prevented by hemofiltration is still unclear because very few patients have been treated exclusively by hemofiltration continuously for more than 8 years. Furthermore, the hemofilters applied in the early days of hemofiltration had a rather low sieving coefficient for beta$_2$ microglobulin (B2M) (Table 4). Using recently developed hemofilters with high sieving coefficients for B2M it has been shown that pretreatment B2M levels can be reduced by high-efficient hemofiltration or hemodiafiltration (88). Whether hemofiltration also influences formation of beta$_2$ microglobulin remains to be tested.

It has been claimed that long-term treatment with highly permeable membranes used in a dialysis mode (89) leads to B2M amyloidosis less frequently than treatment with cuprophane hemodialysis does. Biocompatibility preventing the induction of acute phase proteins might be the major factor accounting for this difference. Cuprophane dialysis induces complement activation in contrast to polyacrylonitrile. In addition convective transport in high flux cellulosic hemodialysis (76) might lead to immediate removal of activated complement components or IL 1 generated from membrane adherent macrophages (79).

Removal of higher molecular weight peptides (6,000 to 50,000 daltons) might become a major benefit of hemofiltration in contrast to diffusive transport modes, especially in connection with removal of hormones and such immunological modifiers as tumor necrosis factor (90), IL 1 (79), IL 2, IL 2 receptors (91), complement and others. Treatment of iron overload or aluminum intoxication or both by deferoxamine became another domain of hemofiltration. The water soluble Fe- or Al-deferoxamine (DFO) complex with a size of about 700 daltons easily passes the hemofilter with a clearance equal to urea clearance (92). In contrast DFO clearance by hemodialysis is restricted to less than 70% of the urea clearance.

Quantification of therapy

Assessment of treatment quality of hemofiltration is very simple. Interruptions of therapy or changes in filter quality do not influence the efficiency of treatment as long as the ultrafiltration volume remains constant. Kinetics and mass balances can easily be performed by measuring appropriate parameters in plasma and in total ultrafiltrate (93).

HEMOFILTRATION TECHNIQUE

Procedures

Clinical hemofiltration can be performed with substitution fluid administered either as pre-dilution, post-dilution or if two filters are used, as mid-dilution alone or as a mixture of pre-, mid- and post-dilution. In clinical settings usually the post-dilution mode is applied because substitution fluid is expensive. A plasma filtration fraction of about 50% can be achieved. Intracellular solutes within erythrocytes cannot be cleared by post-dilution hemofiltration. Therefore, small solutes with high mass transfer rates across cell membranes such as urea can never be cleared as efficiently as in hemodialysis. However, comparably high mass transfer rates are possible in the pre- and mid-dilution mode. Here intracellular solutes diffuse along a concentration gradient created by the infused fluid and depending on the dilution ratio (94).

Hardware

The extracorporeal circuit must be monitored during hemofiltration in a similar way as during regular hemodialysis. Instead of preparation of dialysis solution and its conductivity control, hemofiltration equipment balances the filtered volume with the infused volume. This can either be achieved gravimetrically, volumetrically or by flow cells (13). Since large volumes are exchanged in a short treatment time, the accurate control of fluid balance is critical. Imbalance can rapidly lead to life-threatening volume depletion or hyperhydration of the patient. Volumetric balancing is technically difficult to achieve, mainly because substitution fluid is delivered under positive pressure whereas the ultrafiltrate is generated under negative pressure. Air bubbles develop in the bicarbonate containing ultrafiltrate. This interferes with volumetric control of the ultrafiltrate. Therefore the ultrafiltrate has to be degassed in an additional step. Because of this technical complexity volumetric hemofiltration systems have been abandoned.

Gravimetric control of ultrafiltrate and substitution fluid has become the most widely used monitoring system in hemofiltration. Usually two scales are balanced by a microprocessor which is also able to integrate a continuous weight loss. Single scale systems measuring the combined weight of ultrafiltrate and substitution fluid require a monitor indicating the effectiveness of the hemofiltration process. In early days of hemofiltration mechanical scales were used with adequate fluid balance. They have been replaced by electronic scales. Balancing ultrafiltrate and substitution fluid by flow cells has not reached clinical application, however modern dialysis equipment may be used for this purpose if sterile and pyrogen-free dialysate is produced (95).

Filters

Filters are designed as flat plate or hollow fiber filters and are equipped with cellulosic or synthetic membranes. Polyacrylonitrile (AN69) and cellulose acetate membranes are widely used in flat sheet devices. Hollow fibers consist of either polyamide, polysulfone, polyacrylonitrile, or polymethylmethacrylate membrane material. Sieving coefficients *in vivo* for inulin (5,200 daltons) vary between 0.3 and 0.8. Those for beta$_2$ microglobulin (molecular weight 11,800) range from less than 0.1 to 0.6. Sieving coefficients determined in aqueous solution are reduced *in vivo* by pro-

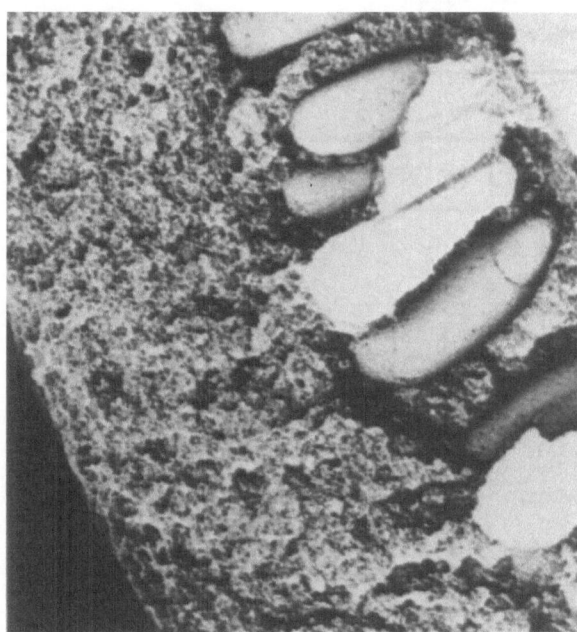

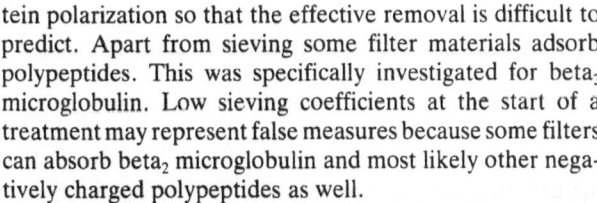

Figure 7. Cross section through the wall of a polyacrylonitrile hollow fiber (PAN 200), wall thickness 50 um.

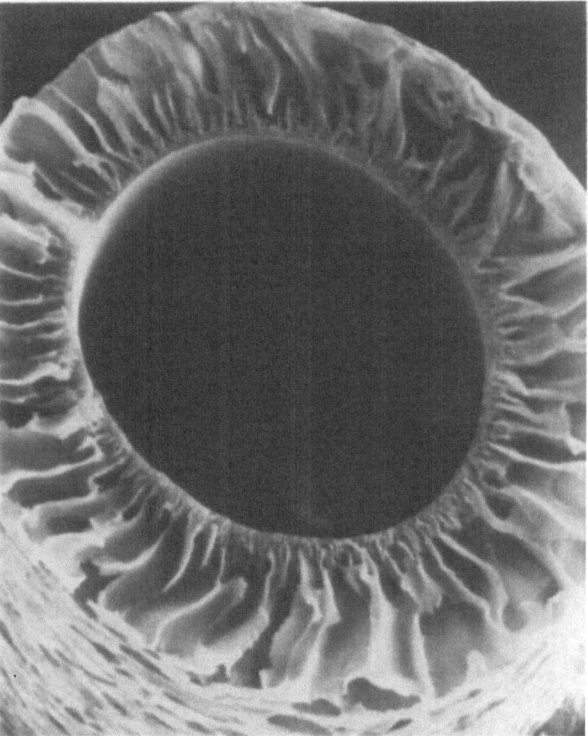

Figure 8. Cross section of an asymmetric skinned polysulfone hollow fiber.

tein polarization so that the effective removal is difficult to predict. Apart from sieving some filter materials adsorb polypeptides. This was specifically investigated for beta$_2$ microglobulin. Low sieving coefficients at the start of a treatment may represent false measures because some filters can absorb beta$_2$ microglobulin and most likely other negatively charged polypeptides as well.

Table 4 depicts the sieving and absorption characteristics of various filters. An ideal hemofilter mimics the normal glomerulus. Membrane structure must permit a high plasma water flux but also that of molecules up to the size of albumin. All filter membranes consist of a skinned surface in contact with blood and of a sponge- or fingerlike supporting structure (Figures 7, 8).

Membranes can be divided in three groups (Figure 9): fluid membranes, finely porous membranes, and microporous (coarse) membranes. For filtration only finely porous membranes are used and they are subdivided into gel and heteroporous membranes (96).

Substitution fluid

During hemofiltration the amount of ultrafiltrate minus the desired weight loss is replaced by sterile, pyrogen free substitution fluid. It is usually infused at a rate between 100 and 180 ml/min. In no other clinical setting are these high infusion rates established for a time of more than 2 h amounting to a parenteral infusion of 25 to 35 l. Therefore, a high standard in regard to fluid quality, e.g. sterility, absence of pyrogens and other foreign material is mandatory. Severe

complications and casualties due to contaminated substitution fluid occurred in the early days of hemofiltration (97). Commercially available hemofiltration fluid is packed in 4.5 to 5 l bags and sterility of these great volumes demands additional technical efforts. After the manufacturer's quality control, the handling, shipping and storing of these bags can lead to contamination. Wrapping of the fluid containing bag in a second sterile plastic envelope has eliminated this problem. In view of these high quality standards the costs of sterile substitution fluid became a factor limiting the widespread application of hemofiltration and in particular of the pre- or mid-dilution mode. The way to solve this financial problem is the on-site production of sterile and pyrogen-free substitution fluid. This had already been performed in the very early days of hemofiltration (98), but was not used extensively. Recently it became commercially available (95). From an electrolyte concentrate and reverse osmosis water, a proportioning system manufactures substitution fluid of the desired composition. After the passage through bacteria- and pyrogen-filters this substitution fluid is infused directly (on line) or is stored for minutes or hours before its consumption (batch) (Figure 10). Regular dialysis machines with additional safety devices for maintaining sterility are now being clinically tested. They are equipped with volumetric or flow cell balancing systems. Electively the physician can perform hemodialysis, hemodiafiltration, and he-

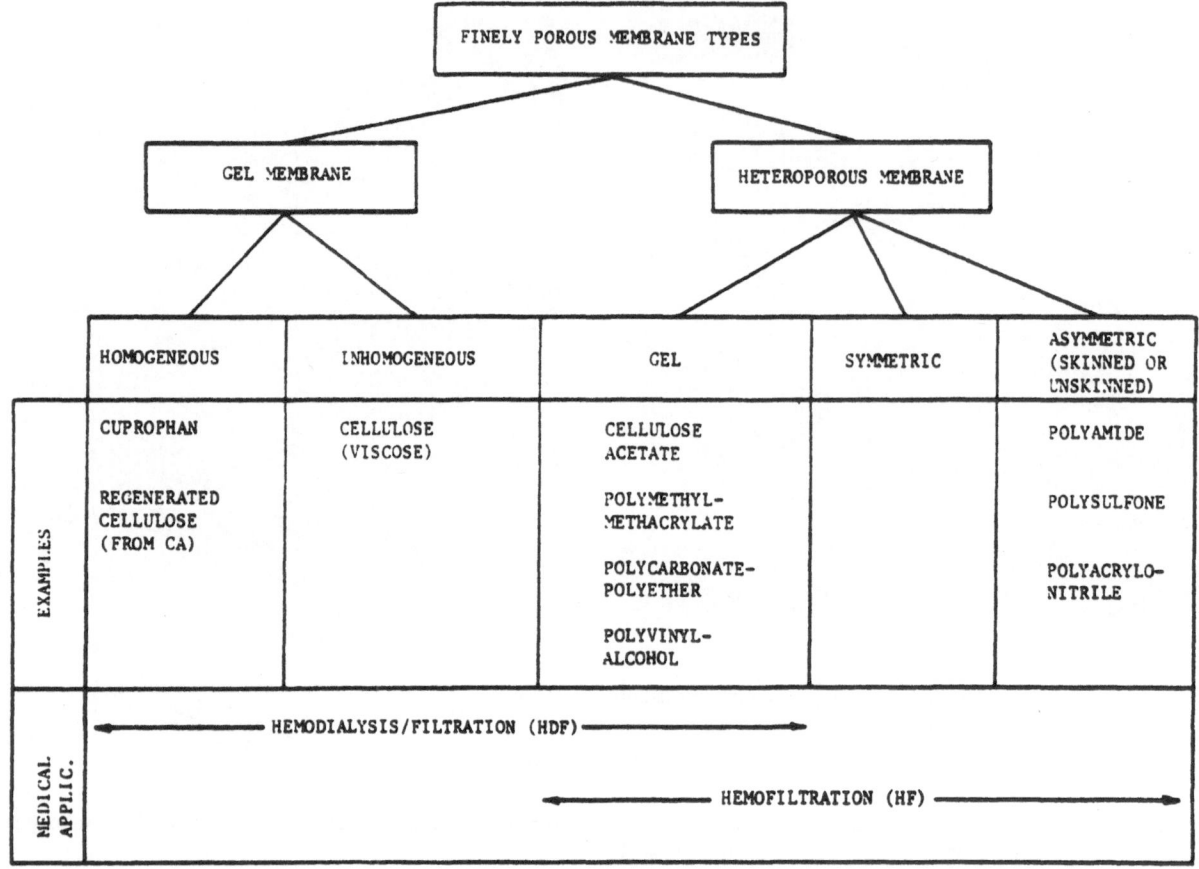

Figure 9. Classification of finely porous membrane types.

mofiltration with the same machine. This kind of hybrid dialysis equipment (Figure 11) may become the hardware of choice for the last decade of this century. The use of sterile, pyrogen-free dialysis fluid may improve biocompatibility (99).

The replacement fluid usually contains: sodium 140, potassium 2,0, calcium 2,0, magnesium 0,75, chloride 102,5 and lactate 45 mmol/l, summing up to an osmolarity of 292 mmol/l. Some manufacturers add glucose to this solution. According to individual necessities potassium free solution is available and calcium and sodium content vary. In some solutions lactate is replaced by acetate. Bicarbonate buffered replacement fluid can be produced on site only with the above mentioned proportioning systems.

CLINICAL CONSIDERATIONS

On theoretical grounds a high blood flow is required to achieve adequate filtration rates of 120 to 180 ml/min. This requires extracorporeal blood flows of 350 to 500 ml/min. Hemofiltration requires optimal arteriovenous fistulas to achieve such flow rates. Hemodynamic impairment from high shunt volume leading eventually to congestive heart

failure, is a danger especially for patients with impaired cardiac function, a group who might benefit from hemofiltration therapy most. On the other hand these patients suffer from progressive arteriosclerosis, and it can become difficult to achieve adequate flow rates through subcutaneous arteriovenous fistulas in such a population. If hemofiltration has to be performed at low blood flow rates, it is necessary either to prolong treatment time or to perform hemofiltration in a pre-dilution mode.

Inadequate blood flow may also be due to high flow resistance of small bore needles. Short (20 mm) needles with an internal diameter between 1.8 and 2 mm should be used for hemofiltration. The venous needles should have similar dimensions. Short, wide bore needles prevent a falsely high venous pressure.

Because of the necessity for high fistula blood flow rates, saphenous loops, brachial arteriovenous fistulas, heterografts between high flow arteries and veins, and Thomasshunts are ideal for hemofiltration, but the necessary blood flow rate between 300 and 500 ml/min can also be achieved by a majority of forearm fistulas. Because of the high bore needles autologous fistulas should be preferred. When used, percutaneous catheters should be short and have a wide inner lumen. With double-lumen catheters a certain amount of recirculation may occur.

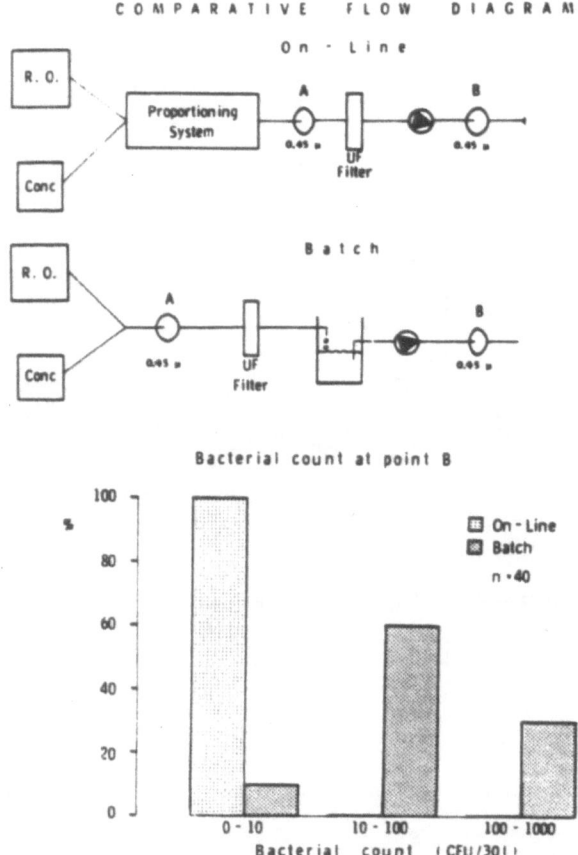

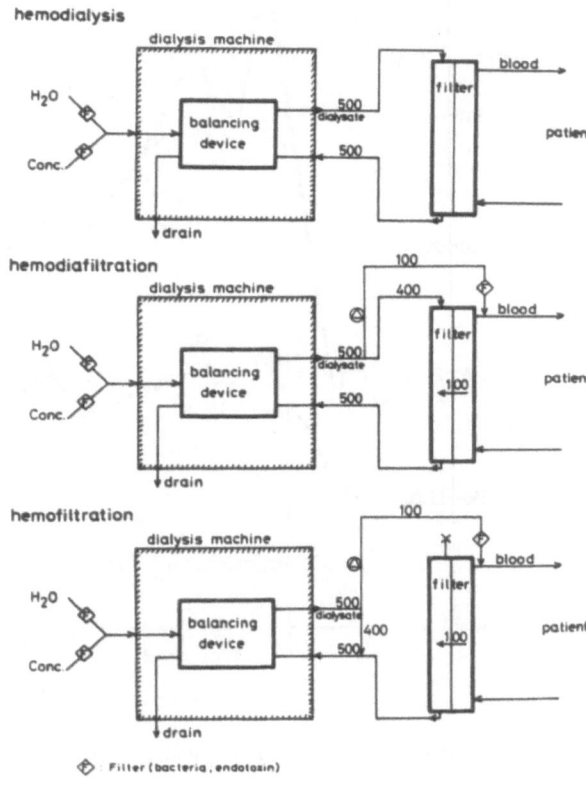

Figure 11. Flow diagram of a hybrid dialysis machine.

Figure 10. Frequency distribution of bacterial counts in colony-forming units (CFU) per 30 l (bottom) of full-stream samples taken at point B using continuous preparation (On-line) and batch-blending preparation (Batch) of substitution fluid.

QUANTITY OF THERAPY

Quantity of treatment should meet hemodialysis standards, i.e. $K \times t/V > 1.0$ with respect to urea removal (K = clearance, t = treatment time, V = distribution volume of urea). For small solutes K is identical with the filtration rate; with regard to higher molecular weight solutes the clearance will be reduced in comparison to the filtration rate by the sieving coefficient which is known for most substances. The term $K \times t$ equals ultrafiltration volume, which should reach urea distribution volume, i.e. approx. 60% of body weight. This target is rarely reached in conventional hemofiltration. Early in hemofiltration, based on the middle molecule hypothesis (100), only 18 l were exchanged per treatment (101). Here protein intake and protein catabolic rate (PCR) deteriorated concomitantly with an increase in pre-treatment BUN levels (PCR: 14 g/kg/day to 8 g/kg/day). Whether this low quantity of therapy leads to a fall in protein intake and protein catabolic rate has been discussed controversially (pro [102, 103], contra [101]). However, increasing the ex-

change volume to 27 l improved protein intake and protein catabolic rate (1.2 g/kg/day) and decreased pre-treatment BUN levels (Figure 12) (102). In clinical routine a protein catabolic rate of 1.0 to 1.2 g/kg/day should be maintained at exchange volume of 40% of body weight. That equals a $K \times t/V = 0.7$. With this empirical regime pre-treatment BUN is reduced during treatment by 50%.

INDICATIONS

The indications for hemofiltration derive from the clinical benefits of this therapy. Patients with cardiomyopathy, autonomic dysfunction, or ischemic heart disease, diabetic patients and the elderly as well as those with excessive weight gain may not tolerate fluid removal during conventional hemodialysis (104) resulting in hypotention, muscle cramps, nausea, and vomiting (105). Here hemofiltration reduces symptomatology impressively (27, 29, 32).

It is still controversial whether hemofiltration is more effective than hemodialysis in controlling hypertension (106, 107). Certainly control of volume-dependent hypertension is a domain of hemofiltration, because fluid removal is more easily achieved. However, whether volume-inde-

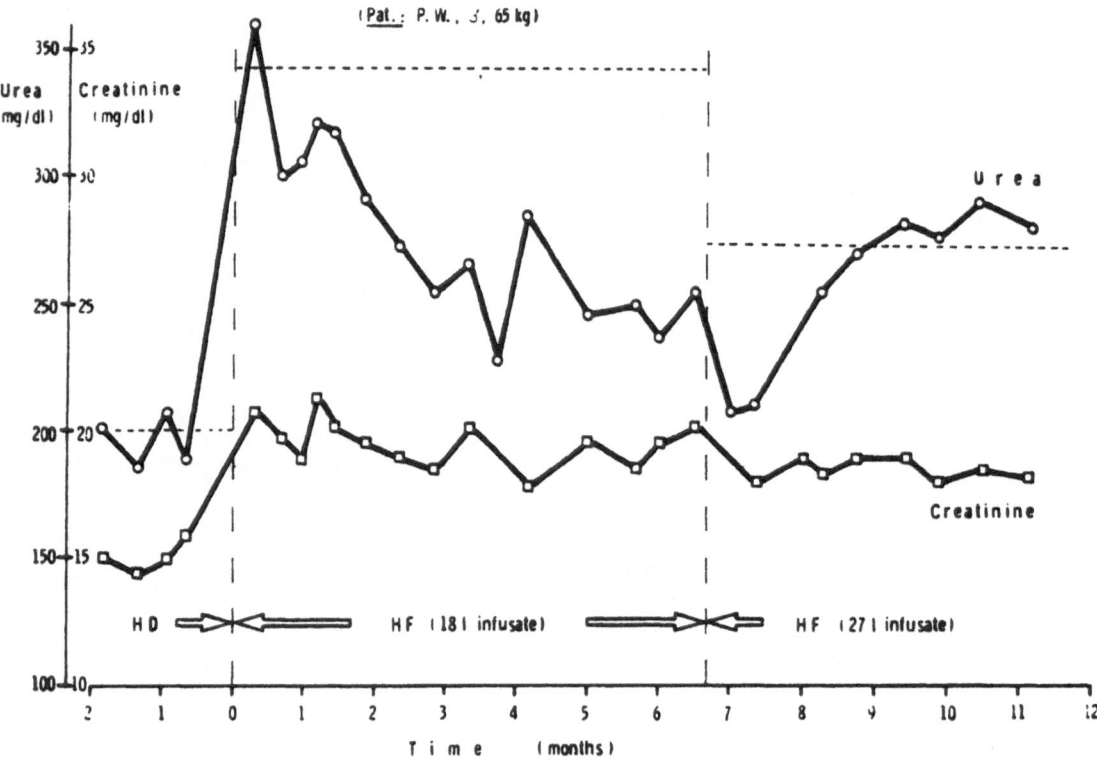

Figure 12. Serum + creatinine levels in a patient transfered from hemodialysis (12 h/week) to hemofiltration (three 18 l- and later three 27 l exchanges).

pendent hypertension is influenced by hemofiltration at all is still a moot point (107).

If beta$_2$ microglobulin has to be removed in order to prevent amyloidosis in long-term ESRD patients, hemofiltration will become the treatment method of choice. If other polypeptides, elevated in end-stage renal failure, become clinically relevant, hemofiltration will also gain.

Removal of iron and aluminum in deferoxamine treated patients is more effective by hemofiltration than by regular hemodialysis (92).

COMPLICATIONS

Technical and medical complications of hemofiltration have to be distinguished (Table 5). Low extracorporeal blood flow is noticed immediately, because a low ultrafiltration rate leads to an intolerably long treatment time.

A low blood flow rate might be caused by low fistula blood flow, but also by the use of small bore fistula needles. The frequency of blood leakage from flat plate or hollow fiber filters has decreased steadily during recent years due to improved manufacturing technique. In most cases blood leaks are detected visually, because the ultrafiltrate is not as diluted as in hemodialysis. Not all blood leaks require a filter replacement, because often they cease spontaneously.

Technical as well as medical complications can result from

the replacement fluid. The risk of erroneous fluid composition is no greater than with hemodialysis. Difficulties can result from inadequate temperature regulation of the infusion fluid, because the temperature of the heating device but not that of the infusion fluid is controlled. At high infusion rates the heating system is overtaxed and cold infusion only leads to subjective discomfort of the patient.

Infusion of fluid from contaminated bags has led to lethal

Table 5. Complications of hemofiltration.

Technical
balancing error
low blood flow
blood leak
replacement fluid
wrong composition
temperature ↑ or ↓
contamination
Medical
septicemia
endotoxin shock
hemolysis
overhydration
hypovolemic shock
inadequate therapy

complications in several instances due to septicemia and endotoxin shock (97).

The insertion of a pyrogen- and bacteria-filter before the venous port and on-line or on-site production of substitution fluid can also solve this problem (95).

Hemolysis may occur if the filters are rinsed improperly, a problem more frequent in the use of flat plate filters than with hollow fibers. It usually happens if filters are replaced. Flat sheet filters must be placed into their clamping device to be rinsed with a blood pump. In manual rinsing not all filter layers are washed by saline. Remaining material like glycerol then causes hemolysis. Dehydration and overhydration due to balancing errors of the hardware are rare with modern hemofiltration hardware. Hypovolemia caused by rapid fluid withdrawal can be compensated easier than in regular hemodialysis (see above). Inadequate treatment can be noticed immediately by checking the ultrafiltration rate and filtered volume. This easy control of treatment quantity is an advantage of hemofiltration.

LONG-TERM OUTCOME

Mainly because of economic reasons long-term hemofiltration treatment is performed in very few centers; hence, reports on long-term survival of patients are based on small numbers (108). Quellhorst (109) has the greatest and longest experience with long-term hemofiltration. Between 1974 and 1978 he randomly admitted his patients either to hemodialysis or hemofiltration treatment. The overall survival rate was equal for both groups amounting to about 90% after 3 years and 80% after 5 years (Figure 13). Survival rates of the French dialysis registry 'Diaphane' (105) and of the European Dialysis and Transplant Association (EDTA) registry for patients aged 40 to 45 years (110) are comparable. Causes of death are listed in Table 6. Myocardial infarction and septicemia were observed in both groups, but congestive heart failure, occurred less frequently in hemofiltration. On the average hemofiltration patients spent 1.3 and hemodialysis patients 1.8 days per month in the hospi-

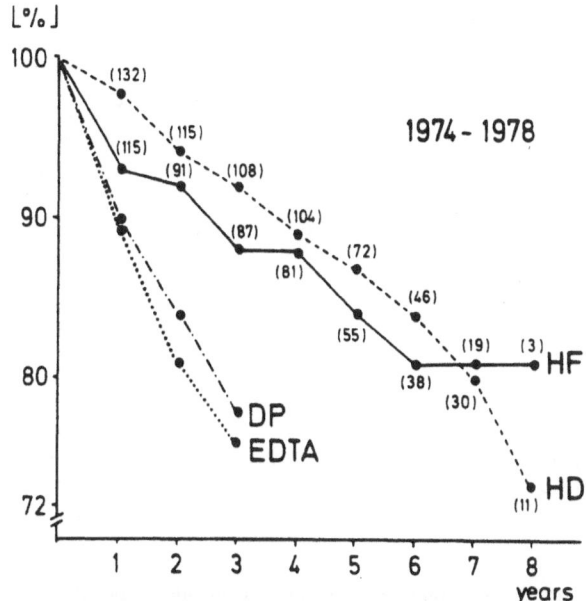

Figure 13. Survival rates of patients starting regular hemofiltration or hemodialysis treatment between 1974 and 1978 ('standard dialysis population'): data of EDTA registry and Diaphene (DP) are shown for comparison.

tal, a significant difference. Technique survival was identical in both groups. Quellhorst (106) also conducted a long-term study in four groups (Figure 14) of patients: 178 patients on hemofiltration (28 diabetics), 168 on intermittent hemodialysis (32 diabetics), 72 treated by CAPD (16 with diabetic nephropathy), and 82 patients on intermittent peritoneal dialysis (IPD) (32 diabetics). The elderly and the diabetic patients showed an improved survival on hemofiltration. Diabetic patients on hemodialysis had the lowest life expectancy. Causes of death were similar in patients on hemofiltration and hemodialysis. Patients on hemofiltration spent fewer days in the hospital. This was also true for the two high risk groups of diabetic and elderly patients.

According to these studies, long-term survival of uncomplicated renal failure patients is identical for hemofiltration and hemodialysis. However, patients with cardiovascular and cerebrovascular complications, the elderly, and diabetic patients seem to profit from hemofiltration.

It is not clear whether patients on long-term hemofiltration suffer less from dialysis associated amyloidosis than patients on hemodialysis. Quellhorst (99) claimed to see less amyloidosis and attributed it to the use of sterile and pyrogen-free solution. Moreover, in hemodialysis patients he found a decrease in beta-2-microglobulin if he used sterile and pyrogen-free dialysate. This points to beta-2-microglobulin generation induced by contaminated fluid.

Table 6. Causes of death in 16 hemofiltration and 18 hemodialysis patients (109).

	Hemofiltration		Hemodialysis	
	Early	Late	Early	Late
Cerebrovascular	2	1	1	2
Myocardial infarction	2	1	2	1
Malignancy	2	–	1	1
Pneumonia	2	1	1	–
Cardiac insufficiency	1	–	1	4
Septicemia	1	–	2	–
Tuberculosis	1	–	1	–
Pancreatitis	1	1	1	–
	12	4	10	8

ECONOMICS

The costs of hemofiltration are significantly higher than

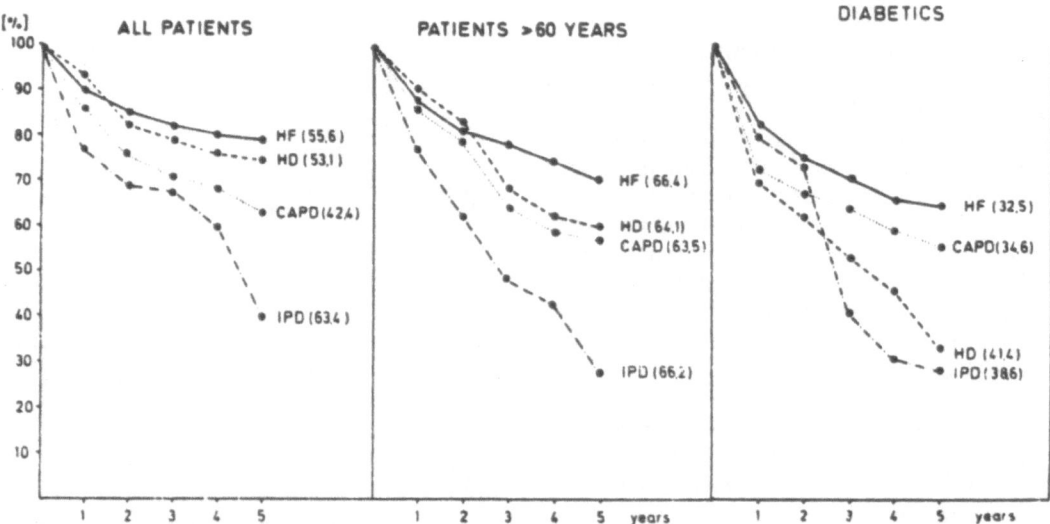

Figure 14. Survival rates for various treatments for end-stage renal failure.

those of hemodialysis even at identical expenditure on hardware. The filters cost nearly twice those of regular dialyzers, but they can be reused. The most expensive part of standard hemofiltration is the substitution fluid. Commercially 4 to 5 l bags are available. The comparative treatment costs for hemofiltration, hemodialysis and CAPD are given in Figure 15 (111). The high costs as well as the medical hazards (97) of hemofiltration substitution fluid in bags has stimulated investigators and industry to improve fluid preparation. On-line preparation of substitution fluid from tap water and concentrate seems to be the best solution (95). Production of hemofilters in large quantities will lower costs too. An important point when discussing economics arises from saving personnel costs based on better intratreatment symptomatology.

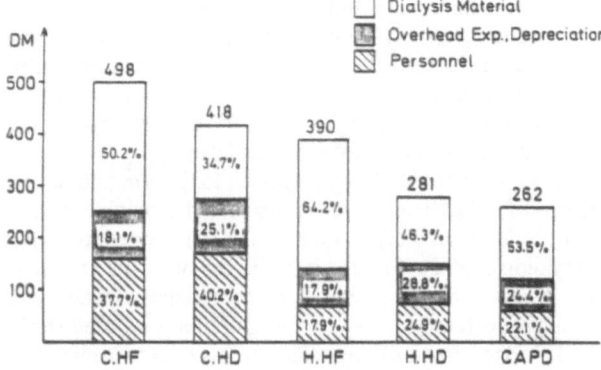

Figure 15. Comparative single treatment costs for center hemofiltration (CHF), center hemodialysis (CHD) home hemofiltration (HHF), home hemodialysis (HHD) and continuous ambulatory peritoneal dialysis (CAPD) including percentages for materials for overhead, depreciation and maintenance and for personnel.

FUTURE DEVELOPMENTS

Industry is developing hybrid machines that perform hemodialysis, hemofiltration and hemodiafiltration (Figure 11). A basic requirement for these machines is the production of a pyrogen-free and sterile fluid which can either be used as dialysate or replacement fluid. Prototypes developed by different manufacturers are in preliminary clinical trials (112).

Filters will be manufactured more economically and membrane technology will aim at high hydraulic permeability and high sieving coefficients for molecules up to 60,000 Daltons mimicking the glomerular basement membrane. These membranes will be charged negatively, in order to impede the passage of albumin and to allow the elimination of neutral and positively charged molecules of even greater molecular size. Increased knowledge of higher molecular weight peptides and of their pathophysiologic role in secondary diseases in renal failure (76) stimulates physicians and industry.

DERIVATIVE TREATMENT MODALITIES

Hemofiltration was stimulated by the experiences of Shaldon (113) and of Bergström (18) in 1986 when they reported that pure ultrafiltration resulted in an improved hemodynamic stability compared with standard hemodialysis.

Pure ultrafiltration is now used in clinical settings such as congestive heart failure and diuretic resistant overhydration (114). In diabetic nephropathy with severe nephrotic syndrome isolated ultrafiltration often succeeds in maintaining patients on conservative treatment for a limited period of time. Iatrogenic overhydration in the immediate postoperative period may also be an indication for isolated ultrafiltra-

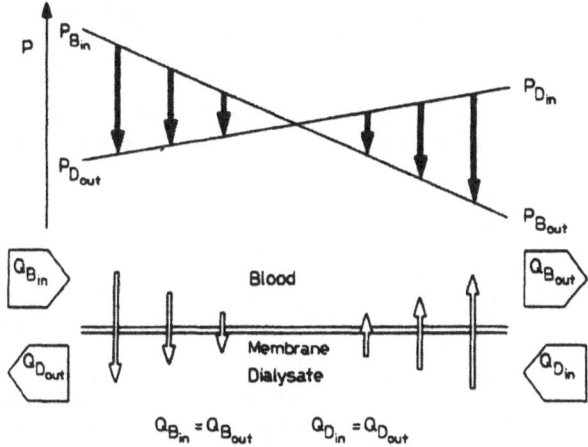

Figure 16. Schematic representation of filtration and backfiltration *in vitro*. Filtration in the first part of the filter equals backfiltration in the second part resulting in a net ultrafiltration rate of zero.

tion. Ultrafiltration is usually performed with a venous to venous extracorporeal circulation using a small roller pump at a blood flow rate of 100 to 150 ml/min. A regular dialyzer, the cheapest filter available, achieves filtration rates between 10 to 30 ml/min.

In open heart surgery hemofiltration is used regularly at the end of the treatment to reconcentrate the patient's blood and to infuse part of the extracorporeal blood without the risk of overhydration.

Hemodiafiltration combines the diffusive process of hemodialysis with the convective solute and water transport of hemofiltration (115). Analysis of hemodynamics during comparative hemodialysis, hemofiltration and hemodiafiltration in the same patients (116) demonstrated a gradual improvement of hemodynamic stability in the sequence hemodialysis – hemodiafiltration – hemofiltration. During hemodiafiltration the filtered volume is replaced by sterile and pyrogen-free fluid as in hemofiltration.

Hemodialysis with high flux hollow fibers guarantees high clearance rates for small and high molecular solutes too. This is due to filtration and back filtration within the dialyzer (117). In a countercurrent flow, pressure differences between blood and dialysate at the blood inlet of the dialyzer result in filtration from blood to dialysate whereas the opposite occurs at the blood outlet (Figure 16). Therefore, dialysis with high flux membranes mimics hemodiafiltration within the dialyzer. Pyrogen reactions during high flux dialysis have been attributed to back filtration of pyrogen or bacteria from contaminated dialysate into blood. Using pyrogen and bacteria-free dialysate, dialyzers with maximal filtration and backfiltration should guarantee a highly efficient treatment.

REFERENCES

1. Henderson L, Besarb A, Michaels A, Bluemle LW: Blood purification by ultrafiltration and fluid replacement (diafiltra-

tion). *Trans Am Soc Artif Intern Organs* 1: 216, 1967
2. Henderson LW, Ford CA, Colton CK, Bluemle LW, Bixler HJ: Uremic blood cleansing by diafiltration using a hollow fiber ultrafilter. *Trans Am Soc Artif Intern Organs* 16: 107, 1970
3. Quellhorst E, Plashues E: Ultrafiltration: Elimination harnpfluchtiger Substanzen mit Hilfe neuartiger Membranen. (Elimination of substances that normally appear in urine with the help of newly developed membranes). in *Aktuelle Probleme der Dialyseverfahren und der Niereninsuffizienz.* (Acute Problems of the Dialysis Procedure and Renal Insufficiency) edited by Ditrich P, Skabal F, Friedberg, Bindernagel, 1971 p 216
4. Quellhorst E, Fernandez F, Scheler F: Treatment of uremia using an ultrafiltration-filtration system. *Proc Eur Dial Transplant Assoc* 9: 584, 1972
5. Reiger J, Quellhorst E, Lowitz HD, Kong RG, Scheler F: Ultrafiltration for middle molecules in uremia. *Proc Eur Dial Transplant Assoc* 11: 158, 1974
6. Quellhorst E, Rieger J, Doht B, Beckmann H, Jacob I, Kraft B, Mietzsch G, Scheler F: Treatment of chronic uremia by an ultrafiltration kidney: first clinical experience. *Proc Eur Dial Transplant Assoc* 13: 314, 1976
7. Markovitz M: An artificial glomerulus. *Ariz Med* 25: 35, 1968
8. Dorson W, Markovitz M: A pulsating artificial kidney. *Chem Eng Prog Symp Ser* 84: 85, 1968
9. Colton CK, Henderson LW, Ford CA, Lysaght MJ: Kinetics of hemofiltration: in vitro transport characteristics of a hollow fiber blood ultrafilter. *J Lab Clin Med* 85: 355, 1975
10. Henderson LW, Colton CK, Ford CA: Kinetics of hemodiafiltration II: clinical characterization of a new blood cleansing modality. *J Lab Clin Med* 85: 372, 1975
11. Dorson WJ, Pizziconi VB: Present status of the hemofiltration molecular separation artificial kidney. *Artif Organs* 3: 6, 1979
12. Symposium on Hemofiltration J Dial 1: 529, 1977
13. v Albertini B: Equipment for hemofiltration. in *Hemofiltration,* edited by Henderson LW, Quellhorst EA, Baldamus CA, Lysaght MJ, Berlin, Heidelberg, New York, Tokyo, Springer-Verlag, 1986, p 83
14. Baldamus CA: Hemodynamics in hemofiltration. in *Hemofiltration,* edited by Henderson LW, Quellhorst EA, Baldamus CA, Lysaght MJ, Berlin, Heidelberg, New York, Tokyo, Springer-Verlag, 1986, p 156
15. Henderson LW, Quellhorst EA, Baldamus CA, Lysaght MJ: *Hemofiltration,* Berlin, Heidelberg, New York, Tokyo, Springer-Verlag, 1986
16. Broyer M, Brunner FP, Brynger H, Fassbinder W, Guillou PJ, Oules R, Rizzoni G, Selwood NH, Wing AJ, Challah S, Dykes SR: EDTA Registry Centre Survey, 1985. *Nephrol Dial Transplant* 2: 475, 1987
17. Henderson LW, Livoti LG, Ford CA, Kelly AB, Lysaght MJ: Clinical experience with intermittent hemofiltration. *Trans Am Soc Artif Intern Organs* 19: 119, 1973
18. Bergström J, Asaba H, Fürst P, Oulés R: Dialysis, ultrafiltration and blood pressure. *Proc Eur Dial Transplant Assoc* 13: 293, 1976
19. Graefe U, Milutinovich J, Follette WC, Babb AL, Scribner BH: Improved tolerance to rapid ultrafiltration with the use of bicarbonate in dialysate. *Proc Eur Dial Transplant Assoc* 14: 153, 1977
20. Brecht HM, Schoeppe W, Scheuermann E, Nassauer A, Baldamus CA, Koch KM: Factors involved in hemodialysis hypotension (Abstract). *7th Congress Int Soc Nephrol,* Montreal 1978

21. Bergström J: Ultrafiltration with simultaneous dialysis for removal of excess fluid. *Proc Eur Dial Transplant Assoc* 15: 260, 1978

22. Wehle B, Asaba H, Castenfors J, Fürst P, Gunnarsson B, Shaldon S, Bergström J: Hemodynamic changes during sequential ultrafiltration and dialysis. *Kidney Int* 15: 411, 1979

23. Pogglitsch H, Holzer H, Waller J, Pristautz H, Leopold H, Katschnigg H: The cause of inadequate hemodynamic reactions during ultradiffusion. *Proc Eur Dial Transplant Assoc* 15: 245, 1978

24. Zucchelli P, Catizone L, Esposti ED, Fusaroli M, Ligabue A, Zuccala A: Influence of ultrafiltration on plasma renin activity and adrenergic system. *Nephron* 21: 317, 1978

25. Zuccala A, Degli Esposti E, Sturani A, Chiarini C, Santoro A, Catizone L, Zuccchelli P: Autonomic function in hemodialyzed patients. *Int J Artif Organs* 1: 76, 1978

26. Canella G, Picotti GB, Mioni G, Cristinelli L, Maiorca R: Blood pressure behaviour during dialysis and ultrafiltration. A pathogenic hypothesis on hemodialysis-induced hypotension. *Int J Artif Organs* 1: 69, 1978

27. Baldamus CA, Schoeppe W, Koch KM: Comparison of hemodialysis and post-dilution hemofiltration on an unselected dialysis population. *Proc Eur Dial Transplant Assoc* 15: 228, 1978

28. Shaldon S, Deschodt G, Beau MC, Claret G, Mion H, Mion C: Vascular stability during high flux hemofiltration. *Proc Eur Dial Transplant Assoc* 16: 695, 1979

29. Quellhorst E: Hämofiltration – Differentialindikation zur Hämodialyse unter Berücksichtigung hämodynamischer und metabolischer Aspekte. (Hemofiltration: differential indication for hemodialysis with reference to the hemodynamic and metabolic aspects.) *Klin Wochenschr* 57: 1061, 1979

30. Quellhorst E, Schuenemann B: Postdilution hemofiltration is rational and preferable. *Proc Clin Dial Transplant Forum* 9: 54, 1979

31. Hampl H, Paeprer H, Unger V, Kessel MW: Hemodynamics during hemodialysis, sequential ultrafiltration and hemofiltration. *J Dial* 3: 51, 1979

32. Hampl H, Paeprer H, Unger V, Fischer C, Resa I, Kessel M: Hemodynamic changes during hemodialysis, sequential ultrafiltration, and hemofiltration. *Kidney Int* 18 (Suppl 10): 583, 1980

33. Baldamus CA, Ernst W, Fassbinder W, Koch KM: Differing hemodynamic stability due to differing sympathetic response: comparison of ultrafiltration, hemodialysis, and hemofiltration. *Proc Eur Dial Transplant Assoc* 17: 205, 1980

34. Baldamus CA, Ernst W, Frei U, Koch KM: Sympathetic and hemodynamic response to volume removal during different forms of renal replacement therapy. *Nephron* 31: 324, 1982

35. Quellhorst E, Schuenemann B, Hildebrand U, Falda Z: Response of the vascular system to different modifications of hemofiltration and hemodialysis. *Proc Eur Dial Transplant Assoc* 17: 197, 1980

36. Shaldon S, Beau MC, Deschodt G, Ramperez P, Mion C: Vascular stability during hemofiltration. *Trans Am Soc Artif Intern Organs* 26: 391, 1980

37. Keshaviah P, Illstrup K, Constantinti E, Berkseth R, Shapiro F: The influence of ultrafiltration and diffusion on cardiovascular parameters. *Trans Am Soc Artif Intern Organs* 26: 328, 1980

38. Henrich WL, Woodard TD, Blachley JD, Gomez-Sanchez C, Pettinger W, Cronin RE: Role of osmolality in blood pressure stability after dialysis and ultrafiltration. *Kidney Int* 18: 480, 1980

39. Wehle B, Asaba H, Castenfors J, Gunnarsson B, Bergström J: Influence of dialysate composition on cardiovascular function in isovolemic hemodialysis. *Proc Eur Dial Transplant Assoc* 18: 153, 1981

40. Aljama P, Martin-Malo A, Sanz R, Pasalodos J, Moreno E, Gomez J, Pérez R, Burdiel LG, Andrés E: Left ventricular function during hemofiltration and hemodialysis: a comparative study. *Proc Eur Dial Transplant Assoc* 19: 281, 1982

41. Cini G, Camici M, Pentimone F, Palla R: Echocardiographic hemodynamic study during ultrafiltration sequential dialysis. *Nephron* 30: 124, 1982

42. Hampl H, Klopp H, Wolfgruber M, Pustelnik A, Schiller R, Hanefeld F, Kessel M: Advantages of bicarbonate hemodialysis. *Artif Organs* 6: 410, 1982

43. Kishimoto T, Sugimura K, Nakatani T, Yamagami S, Ezaki K, Okazaki S, Maekawa M: The effects of diffusion and ultrafiltration on cardiac output and organ blood flows. *Proc Eur Dial Transplant Assoc* 19: 275, 1982

44. Vincent JL, Vanherweghem JL, Degaute JP, Berré J, Dufaye P, Kahn RJ: Acetate-induced myocardial depression during hemodialysis for acute renal failure. *Kidney Int* 22: 653, 1982

45. Schick EC Jr, Idelson BA, Liang C, Redline RC, Bernard DB: Comparison of the hemodynamic response to hemodialysis with acetate or bicarbonate. *Trans Am Soc Artif Intern Organs* 29: 25, 1983

46. Frewin DB, Barholomeusz FDL, Cummings MF, Clarkson AR, Barry LA, Furber B, De Lorenzo C, Jonsson JR, Taylor WB: Changes in plasma catecholamine levels during hemodialysis. *Aust NZ J Med* 14: 31, 1984

47. Leenen FHH, Buda AJ, Smith DL, Farrel S, Levine DZ, Uldall PR: Hemodynamic changes during acetate and bicarbonate hemodialysis. *Artif Organs* 8: 411, 1984

48. Freyschuss U, Asaba H, Danielsson A, Bergström J: Cardiovascular adaptation to dialysis in healthy man. *Contrib Nephrol* 41: 376–379, 1984

49. Zucchelli P, Santoro A, Sturani A, Degli Esposti E, Chiarini C, Zuccala A: Effects of hemodialysis and hemofiltration on the autonomic control of circulation. *Trans Am Soc Artif Intern Organs* 30: 163, 1984

50. Schneider H, Liomin E, Streicher E: Hemodynamic studies of diffusive and convective procedures using a polysulfone membrane. *Contrib Nephrol* 46: 134, 1985

51. Wehle B, Asaba H, Castenfors J, Fürst P, Gunnarsson B, Bergström J: Hämodynamische Veränderungen während Ultrafiltration und Hämodialyse bei Urämikern. (Hemodynamic changes during ultrafiltration and hemodialysis in uremia.) *Z Urol Nephrol* 72: 3, 1979

52. Skillman JJ, Awwad HK, Moore FD: Plasma protein kinetics of the early transcapillary refill after hemorrhage in man. *Surg Gynecol Obstet* 125: 983, 1967

53. Kim KE, Neff M, Cohen B, Somerstein M, Chinitz J, Onesti G, Swartz C: Blood volume changes and hypotension during hemodialysis. *Trans Am Soc Artif Intern Organs* 16: 508, 1970

54. Chaignon M, Chen WT, Tarazi RC, Bravo EL, Nakamoto S: Effect of hemodialysis on blood volume distribution and cardiac output. *Hypertension* 3: 327, 1981

55. Ashkar E, Hamilton WF: Cardiovascular response to graded exercise in the sympathectomized-vagotomized dog. *Am J Physiol* 204: 291, 1963

56. Shaldon S, Deschodt G, Beau MC, Ramperez P, Mion C: The importance of serum osmotic changes in symptomatic hypotension during short hemodialysis. *Proc Clin Dial Transplant Forum* 8: 184, 1978

57. Gotch FA, Sargent JA: Hemofiltration: an unnecessarily

complex method to achieve hypotonic sodium removal and controlled ultrafiltration. *Blood Purif* 1: 9, 1983

58. Baldamus CA: Hemofiltration. in *Nephrology '83* edited by D'Amico G, Colasanti G, Milan, Wichtig, 1983, p 163

59. Brecht HM: Wirkung der Hyponatriämie und der Hypovolämie auf die Sympathikus- und Reninaktivität bei der terminalen Niereninsuffizienz. (Effect of hyponatremia and hypovolemia on sympathetic and renin activity in terminal renal insufficiency). in *Diuretika* (Diuretics) edited by Rosenthal J, Knauf H, Weinheim, Edition Medizin, 1980, p 219

60. Haddy FJ, Scott JB, Emerson TE Jr, Overbeck HW, Daugherty RM: Effects of generalized changes in plasma electrolyte concentration and osmolarity on blood pressure in the anesthetized dog. *Circ Res* 24(Suppl 1): 69, 1959

61. Altura B: Influence of calcium ions on microvascular permeability, contractility, and reactivity. in *Advantages in Microcirculation, vol II,* edited by Altura B, Basel, Karger, 1983, p 62

62. Henrich WI, Hund JM, Nixon JV: Increased ionized calcium and left ventricular contractility during hemodialysis N Engl J Med 310: 19, 1984

63. Keshaviah PR: The role of acetate in the etiology of symptomatic hypotension. *Artif Organs* 6: 378, 1982

64. Canella G, Rodella A, Brunori G, Gaggiotti M, Sandrini M, Maiorca R: Plasma concentrations of atrial natriuretic peptide in relation to body fluid status in chronic uremia. *Nephrol Dial Transplant* 2: 158, 1987

65. Talartschik J, Eisenhauer T, Hansing M, Scheler F: Decrease of atrial natriuretic peptide and cyclic GMP during ultrafiltration in chronic hemodialysis/hemofiltration patients: simple elimination or caused by fluid removal? *Nephrol Dial Transplant* 2: 392, 1987

66. Maggiore Q, Pizzarelli F, Zoccah C, Sisca S, Nicolo F, Parlongo S: Effect of extracorporeal blood cooling on dialytic arterial hypotension. *Proc Eur Dial Transplant Assoc* 18: 597, 1981

67. Maggiore Q, Pizzarelli F, Sisca S, Catalano C, Delfino D: Vascular stability and heat in dialysis patients. *Contrib Nephrol* 41: 398, 1984

68. Maggiore Q, Pizzarelli F, Sisca S, Zoccali C, Parlongo S, Nicolò F, Creazzo G: Blood temperature and vascular stability during hemodialysis and hemofiltration. *Trans Am Soc Artif Intern Organs* 28: 523, 1982

69. Schaefer K, v. Herrath D, Hüfler M: Failure to show a temperature-dependent vascular stability during hemofiltration. *Int J Artif Organs* 6: 75, 1983

70. Vanholder R, Piron M, Ringoir S: Absence of a beneficial hemodynamic effect of bicarbonate versus acetate hemodialysis. *Proc Eur Dial Transplant Assoc* 21: 195, 1984

71. Craddock PR, Fehr J, Brigham KL, Kronenberg RS, Jacob HS: Complement and leukocyte-mediated pulmonary dysfunction in hemodialysis. *N Engl J Med* 296: 769, 1977

72. Arnaout MA, Hakim RM, Todd RF, Dana N, Colton HR: Increased expression of an adhesion-promoting surface glycoprotein in the granulocytopenia of hemodialysis. *N Engl J Med* 312: 457, 1985

73. Hakim RM, Lowrie EG: Hemodialysis-associated neutropenia and hypoxemia: the effect of dialyzer membrane materials. *Nephron* 32: 12, 1982

74. Goodman MG, Chenoweth DE, Wiegle WO: Induction of interleukin-1 secretion and enhancement of humoral immunity by binding of human C5a to macrophage surface C5a receptors. *J Exp Med* 156: 912, 1982

75. Henderson IW, Koch KM, Dinarello CA, Shaldon S: Hemo-

dialysis hypotension: the interleukin hypothesis. *Blood Purif* 1: 3, 1983

76. Shaldon S, Deschodt G, Branger B, Granolleras C, Baldamus CA, Koch KM, Lysaght MJ, Dinarello CA: Hemodialysis hypotension: the interleukin hypothesis restated. *Proc Eur Dial Transplant Assoc Eur Ren Assoc* 22: 229, 1985

77. Lonnemann G, Koch KM, Shaldon S: Induction of interleukin-1 from human monocytes adhering to hemodialysis membranes. *Kidney Int* 31: 238, 1987

78. Luger A, Kovarik J, Stummvoll H-K, Urbanska A, Luger TA: Blood-membrane interaction in hemodialysis leads to increased cytokine production. *Kidney Int* 32: 84, 1987

79. Lonnemann G, Bingel M, Floege J, Koch KM, Shaldon S, Dinarello CA: Detection of endotoxin-like interleukin-1-inducing activity during in vitro dialysis. *Kidney Int* 33: 29, 1988

80. Dinarello CA: Interleukin-1. *Rev Infect Dis* 6: 51, 1984

81. Lazarus JM, Hampers CL, Lowrie EG, Merrill JP: Baroreceptor activity in normotensive and hypertensive uremic patients. *Circulation* 47: 1015, 1973

82. Pickering TG, Gribbin B, Oliver DO: Baroreflex sensitivity in patients on long-term hemodialysis. *Clin Sci* 43: 645, 1972

83. Baldamus CA, Mantz P, Kachel HG, Koch KM, Schoeppe W: Baroreflex in patients undergoing hemodialysis and hemofiltration. *Contrib Nephrol* 41: 409, 1984

84. Gejyo F, Yamada T, Odani S, Nakagawa Y, Kunimoto T, Kataoka H, Suzuki M, Hirasawa Y, Shirahama T, Cohen AS, Schmid K: A new form of amyloid protein associated with hemodialysis was identified as β2-microglobulin. *Biochem Biophys Res Comm* 129: 701, 1985

85. Gorevic PC, Casey TT, Stone WJ, DiRaimondo CR, Prelli FC, Frangione B: Beta-2-microglobulin is an amyloidogenic protein in man. *J Clin Invest* 76: 2425, 1985

86. Bardin T, Zingraff J, Kuntz D, Drüeke T: Dialysis-related amyloidosis. *Nephrol Dial Transplant* 1: 151, 1986

87. Kachel HG, Altmeyer P, Kühn KW, Koch KM, Baldamus CA: Deposition of nonamyloid material in connective tissue in uremia. *Blood Purif* 2: 142, 1984

88. Flöge J, Granolleras C, Bingel M, Deschodt G, Branger B, Oules R, Koch KM: β2-microglobulin kinetics during hemodialysis and hemofiltration. *Nephrol Dial Transplant* 1: 223, 1987

89. Lavaud S, Toupance O, Roujouleh H, Fakir M, Melin JP, Chanard J: Carpal tunnel syndrome in hemodialysis patients: effect of dialysis strategy. *ISAO Press* 308: 125, 1987

90. Lonnemann G, van der Meer JWM, Endres S, Shaldon S, Koch KM, Dinarello CA: Induction and removal of tumor necrosis factor and interleukin-1 during in vitro hemodialysis. *Kidney Int* 33: 229, 1988

91. Colvin RB, Fuller TC, MacKeen L, Kung PC, Ip SH, Cosimi AB: Plasma interleukin-2 receptor levels in renal allograft recipients. *Clin Immunol Immunopathol* 43: 273, 1987

92. Baldamus CA, Schmidt H, Scheuermann E-H, Werner E, Kaltwasser JP, Schoeppe W, Desferrioxamine treatment for aluminium and iron overload in uremic patients by hemodialysis or hemofiltration. *Proc Eur Dial Transplant Assoc* 21: 382, 1984

93. Sargent JA, Gotch FA: Principles and biophysics of dialysis. in *Replacement of Renal Function by Dialysis* 2nd edition, edited by Drukker W, Parsons FM, Maher JF, The Hague, Martinus Nijhoff, 1983, p 53

94. Henderson LW: Biophysics of ultrafiltration and hemofiltration. in *Replacement of Renal Function by Dialysis,* 2nd edition, edited by Drukker W, Parsons FM, Maher JF, The Hague, Martinus Nijhoff, 1983, p 242

95. Eisenbach GM, Shaldon S: Substitution fluid for hemofiltration. in *Hemofiltration,* edited by Henderson LW, Quellhorst EA, Baldamus CA, Lysaght MJ, Berlin, Heidelberg, New York, Tokyo, Springer-Verlag, 1986, p 101

96. Göhl H, Konstantin P: Membranes and filters for hemofiltration. in *Hemofiltration,* edited by Henderson LW, Quellhorst EA, Baldamus CA, Lysaght MJ, Berlin, Heidelberg, New York, Tokyo, Springer-Verlag, 1986, p 42

97. Frei U, Koch KM: Fever and shock during hemofiltration. *Contr Nephrol* 36: 107, 1983

98. Henderson LW, Beans F: Successful production of sterile pyrogen-free electrolyte solution by ultrafiltration. *Kidney Int* 14: 522, 1978

99. Quellhorst EA, Solf A, Meinhold J, Luftner-Nagel S, Schuenemann B: Amyloid osteoarthropathy and hemofiltration. *Blood Purif* 6, in press 1988

100. Babb AL, Strand MJ, Uvelli DA, Milutinovic J, Scribner BH: Quantitative description of dialysis treatment: a dialysis index. *Kidney Int* 7 (Suppl 2): S 23, 1975

101. Quellhorst EA, Schuenemann B, Hildebrand U: Morbidity and mortality in long-term hemofiltration. *asaio J* 6: 185, 1983

102. Baldamus CA: Problems in hemofiltration. *Contr Nephrol* 44: 212, 1985

103. Bosch JP, von Albertini B, Glabman S: Prescription for hemofiltration. *Contr Nephrol* 32: 137, 1982

104. Glabman S, Lauer A: Selection of patients for hemofiltration. in *Hemofiltration,* edited by Henderson LW, Quellhorst EA, Baldamus CA, Lysaght MJ, Berlin, Heidelberg, New York, Tokyo, Springer-Verlag, 1986, p 115

105. Degoulet P, Réach I, Rozenbaum W, Aime F, Devriés C, Berger C, Rojas P, Jacobs C, Legrain M: Programme dialyse-informatique. VI Survie et facteurs de risque. (Dialysis computer program. Survival and risk factors.) *J Urol Nephrol* 85: 909, 1979

106. Quellhorst EA: Blood Pressure Control. in *Hemofiltration,* edited by Henderson LW, Quellhorst EA, Baldamus CA, Lysaght MJ, Berlin, Heidelberg, New York, Tokyo, Springer-Verlag, 1986, p 201

107. Baldamus CA, Koch KM: Hemodialysis/hemofiltration, a comparison of medical, technical, and cost factors. *NIH Annual Progress Report,* 1981

108. Baldamus CA, Quellhorst EA: Outcome of long-term hemofiltration. *Kidney Int* 28: 41, 1985

109. Quellhorst EA: Long-term survival. in *Hemofiltration,* edited by Henderson LW, Quellhorst EA, Baldamus CA, Lysaght MJ, Berlin, Heidelberg, New York, Tokyo, Springer-Verlag, 1986, p 222

110. Broyer M, Brunner FP, Brynger H, Donckerwolcke RA, Jacobs C, Kramer P, Selwood NH, Wing AJ: Combined report on regular dialysis and transplantation in Europe, XI, 1980, *Proc Eur Dial Transplant Assoc* 19: 2, 1982

111. Schuenemann B, Behncke V: Comparative economics of hemofiltration treatment. in *Hemofiltration,* edited by Henderson LW, Quellhorst EA, Baldamus CA, Lysaght MJ, Berlin, Heidelberg, New York, Tokyo, Springer-Verlag, 1986, p 303

112. Shaldon S, Beau MC, Deschodt G, Flavier JL, Nielsson L, Ramperez P, Mion C: Three years of experience with on-line preparation of sterile pyrogen-free infusate for hemofiltration. *Int J Artif Organs* 6: 25, 1983

113. Shaldon S: Sequential ultrafiltration and dialysis. *Proc Eur Dial Transplant Assoc* 13: 300, 1976

114. Bosch J: Continuous arteriovenous hemofiltration. in *Hemofiltration,* edited by Henderson LW, Quellhorst EA, Baldamus CA, Lysaght MJ, Berlin, Heidelberg, New York, Tokyo, Springer-Verlag, 1986, p 233

115. Schmidt M: Hemodiafiltration. in *Hemofiltration,* edited by Henderson LW, Quellhorst EA, Baldamus CA, Lysaght MJ, Berlin, Heidelberg, New York, Tokyo, Springer-Verlag, 1986, p 265

116. Schmidt M, Schoeppe W, Baldamus CA: Hemodynamics during hemodialysis with dialyzer of high hydraulic permeability. *Contr Nephrol* 46: 127, 1985

117. Schmidt M, Baldamus CA, Schoeppe W: Backfiltration in hemodialyzers with highly permeable membranes. *Blood Purif* 2: 108, 1984

CONTINUOUS ARTERIOVENOUS HEMOFILTRATION (CAVH) AND OTHER CONTINUOUS REPLACEMENT THERAPIES: OPERATIONAL CHARACTERISTICS AND CLINICAL USE

JUAN P. BOSCH and CLAUDIO RONCO

INTRODUCTION

Continuous Arteriovenous Hemofiltration (CAVH) is an extracorporeal therapy that can be used for an extended time. In CAVH electrolytes and other small and medium sized solutes are removed from the patient by ultrafiltration. Simultaneously, the blood volume is reconstituted by the administration of a fluid with an electrolyte composition similar to that of normal plasma. A small filter with a membrane highly permeable to water is used and the patient's arterial-to-venous pressure gradient is sufficient to move the blood through the extracorporeal circuit.

CAVH provides uninterrupted renal replacement therapy for patients with acute renal failure. In addition to solute removal, the volume and composition of extracellular fluid can be rapidly modified. The objective of the treatment is to obtain about 12 to 15 l/day of ultrafiltrate (plasma water) which provides the equivalent of a glomerular filtration rate of 8 to 11 ml/min. The ultrafiltrate can be replaced totally, by the administration of substitution fluid, to achieve only solute control replaced partially to control solute concentration and volume or not replaced at all to reduce extracellular volume maximally.

Major advantages of CAVH over hemodialysis

1. CAVH, unlike hemodialysis is a continuous form of therapy and thus achieves a more stable maintenance of the volume and composition of body fluids. The rapid in-tercompartamental fluid shifts observed in hemodialysis are avoided and blood pressure instability is prevented. The marked solute concentration changes observed in intermittent therapy are also avoided.

2. CAVH gives the physician a greater ability to control water and electrolyte balance than hemodialysis. This is especially useful in patients who do not tolerate fluid withdrawal during hemodialysis. CAVH makes possible unlimited use of hyperalimentation in patients with renal failure.

3. CAVH allows the removal or addition of electrolytes independent of changes in total body water. These electrolytes include sodium, potassium, calcium and bicarbonate.

4. The CAVH technique is simple, can be initiated rapidly, and does not require complicated equipment or highly trained personnel.

DEVELOPMENT OF CAVH

The clinical application of ultrafiltration for fluid removal dates from the advent of widespread dialysis therapy. A technique based solely on ultrafiltration for the treatment of renal failure was proposed by Henderson and collaborators (1). In this procedure called hemofiltration, an ultrafiltrate of the plasma was generated by hydrostatic pressure exerted across a semipermeable membrane. A substitution fluid, with a composition similar to that of the extracellular fluid, was used to restore the blood volume. Hemofiltration was proposed as an alternative to hemodialysis. This new methodology stimulated the development of new membranes, filters and most importantly opened the road to the understanding of 'in vivo' ultrafiltration. To enhance fluid withdrawal during dialysis, a modification of the standard hemodialysis circuit was first proposed in 1974 by Silverstein and colleagues (2). In their technique, a filter for ultrafiltration was added to the standard hemodialysis extracorporeal circuit. These authors also suggested the use of a separate system (filter, blood lines and a pump) to ultrafilter patients with fluid overload. In Germany, Kramer and associates (3, 4), using a filter originally designed for hemofiltration eliminated the need for a blood pump by directly connecting a hemofilter to the femoral artery and vein of patients with acute renal failure. This procedure, called Continuous Arteriovenous Hemofiltration was intended to be *a continuous form of therapy for renal failure* as opposed to the intermittence of hemodialysis or hemofiltration. CAVH remained limited to a small group of investigators until 1983 when Lauer et al (5) described the unique operational characteristics of the extracorporeal system and Mault et al (6) emphasized the application of the technique in the treatment of intensive care patients with renal failure. CAVH is presently widely used in the treatment of patients (7), including infants (8), with acute renal failure or fluid overload or both. The use of CAVH to treat other conditions such as congestive heart failure (9), respiratory distress syndrome (10), in association with left or right ventricular assist device (11) or heart-lung bypass (12) is now under investigation.

EQUIPMENT

Filter

A small hollow fiber filter with three ports and a membrane highly permeable to water is most commonly used in CAVH. The inlet and outlet port of the filter are connected to the blood lines. The ultrafiltrate is collected in a graduated bag linked to the ultrafiltrate port by a line. Several filters for CAVH are currently available. They vary in the membrane type, and in the number and length of the fibers. A parallel plate device and a special filter for children are also available (Table 1).

Membrane

Conventional hemodialysis membranes have insufficient hydraulic permeability to provide adequate fluid removal at the pressures available during CAVH (13). Hemodialysis membranes contain interdigitating pores of different sizes extending throughout the whole membrane thickness, resulting in a labyrinth of different diffusion distances. Enlarging the pores would allow protein leakage; a decrease in membrane thickness would reduce the strength below acceptable levels. For hemofiltration and CAVH, procedures that depend on ultrafiltration for solute removal, the membranes used must have a high water permeability and limit the passage of albumin. Such features are fulfilled by asymmetric membranes. These are composite structures that have: 1) a thin skin layer, which is adjacent to the blood and contains pores equal in size and in length (All substances smaller than the membrane pore diameter will pass the membrane unimpeded.) and 2) a substructure which sup-

Table 1. Commercially available devices for CAVH and CAVHD.

Manufacturer	Designation	Membrane material	Area (m^2)	Number of fibers	Length (cm)	Radius (μ)
Amicon Corp. Lexington, MA	Dialfilter 20	Polysulfone	0.25	5000	12.7	100
	Dialfilter 30		0.6	4800	20.0	100
	Dialfilter 10		0.20	6000	9.5	100
	Minifilter		0.005	25	9.0	900
ASAHI Medical Tokyo, Japan	Ultrafilter GS	Polyacrylonitrile	0.5	4300	19.0	100
Fresenius AG Oberusel, FRG	AV-400	Polysulfone	0.7	4500	23.0	110
	AV-600		1.35	9000	23.0	110
Gambro AB Lund, Sweden	FH-55	Polyamide	0.6	6200	14.0	100
Hospal Ltd. Basel, Switzerland	Biospal	Polyacrylonitrile	0.5	*	26.0	*
Renal Systems Minneapolis, MN	Renaflo 0.25	Polysulfone	0.3	3000	14.0	140
	Renaflo 0.50		0.5	3000	22.0	140

* Biospal 1200S has a parallel plate configuration with 15 compartments 6.5 cm wide, 26 cm long, and 250 μ apart.

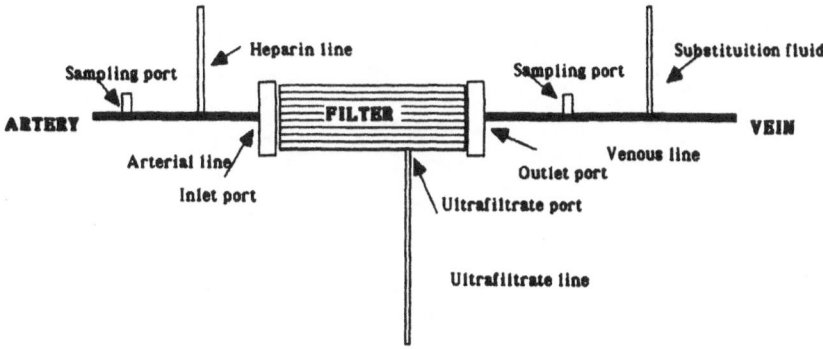

Figure 1. CAVH extracorporeal circuit.

ports the thin layer and provides mechanical integrity, the stroma (14). For processes that use ultrafiltration and diffusion such as continuous arteriovenous hemodialysis, the membranes must have a thinner wall thickness in addition to high water permeability. These are the so called high flux membranes that combine moderately high water flux and high diffusive transport properties.

Extracorporeal circuit

The extracorporeal system is shown in Figure 1. The arterial line should be approximately 50 cm in length, the venous line 75 cm or less with an internal diameter of 0.317 cm. Standard shortened hemodialysis lines can be used. Heparin is administered via the sleeve on the arterial line. The substitution fluid can be given directly to the patient or through the sleeve in the venous line. In both lines, sampling ports are required. The ultrafiltrate line, connecting the ultrafiltrate port and the collection bag, must be 40 to 60 cm long with an internal diameter of 0.474 cm (5).

VASCULAR ACCESS

No special vascular access is required for CAVH; the percutaneous cannulation of an artery and a vein provides adequate circulatory access for CAVH. The femoral artery and vein are particularly suitable for the procedure. In some patients a Scribner shunt may also be used; in this case the arterial and venous branches of the shunt are connected to the arterial and venous lines of the CAVH extracorporeal system. In a patient with an arteriovenous fistula the arterial and venous ends of the fistula can be cannulated percutaneously with standard hemodialysis needles. In the case of an arterial graft, the venous line must be attached to a peripheral vein to achieve an adequate arterio-venous pressure gradient (5).

The blood flow provided by a given vascular access is determined by: the mean arterial pressure of the patient, the type of vascular access (arterial site, shunt, arterio-venous fistula), and the diameter and overall resistance of the device used to achieve the arterial connection (size and length of the needle or catheter) (Figure 2).

Measurement of blood flow

To measure the blood flow through the extracorporeal circuit, blood samples for hematocrit (Hct) are obtained from a sampling sleeve along the arterial (Hct_{inlet}) and venous (Hct_{outlet}) lines. Simultaneously, the ultrafiltration rate (Q_{Uf}), measured from timed volumetric collection in ml/min, is recorded. The blood flow at the inlet (Q_{Bi}) is calculated using the equation:

$$Q_{Bi} = \frac{Q_{Uf} \times Hct_{outlet}}{Hct_{outlet} - Hct_{inlet}} .$$

Plasma flow at the inlet (Q_{Pi}) is calculated from the equation:

$$Q_{Pi} = Q_{Bi} - \text{erythrocyte mass}.$$

Where erythrocyte mass (ml/min) at the inlet =

$$\frac{Q_{Bi} \times Hct_{inlet}}{100} .$$

DETERMINANTS OF THE ULTRAFILTRATION RATE

The ultrafiltration rate in CAVH is determined by the filtration pressure in the filter, that is the net pressure gradient between: 1) those pressures that favor the movement of water across the membrane: the hydraulic and hydrostatic pressure and 2) the pressure that tends to retain the fluid on the blood side of the membrane: the oncotic pressure exerted by the plasma proteins (15).

The blood flow through the extracorporeal circuit is also a critical component in the production of the ultrafiltrate. It determines the hydraulic pressure and also influences the rise in oncotic pressure inside the filter. A given filtration pressure will determine a different increment in oncotic pressure depending on the incoming blood flow. The lower the blood flow the greater the rise in protein concentration for any given ultrafiltration rate. This phenomenon is independent of the plasma protein concentration at the filter inlet.

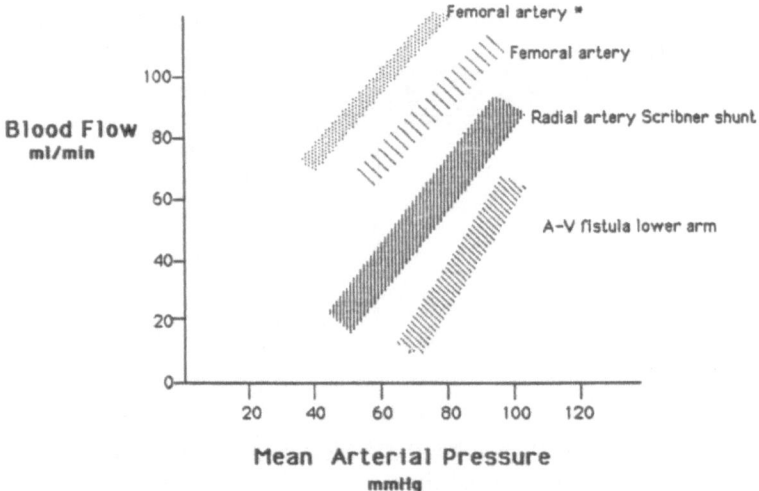

Figure 2. Effect of arterial pressure on blood flow with different vascular accesses. Effect of mean arterial pressure on blood flow rate. In these studies, the length and internal diameter of the blood lines were similar. Cannulation was done via the femoral artery, with a 14 gauge catheter (indicated by *) or a 16 gauge catheter; radial artery Scribner shunt, or arterio-venous (A-V) fistula in the lower arm.

Hydraulic pressure

The hydraulic pressure in the filter is much less than the patient's systemic arterial pressure (Figure 3). Factors responsible for the pressure drop in the extracorporeal circuit are: 1) The type of access and the dimensions of the arterial cannula, 2) The length and internal diameter of the arterial line, and 3) The resistance of the filter.

Hydrostatic pressure

The hydrostatic pressure in the filter is the pressure exerted on the ultrafiltrate side of the membrane. It is generated by the weight of the fluid column inside the ultrafiltrate line. The hydrostatic pressure in the ultrafiltrate compartment (P_f in mm Hg) can be calculated from the height of the column (cm) of the line linking the ultrafiltrate port to the collection bag according to the equation:

Pressure = height × 0.74 mm Hg.

If the filter is above the collection bag, the pressure in the ultrafiltrate is negative. A length of 40 cm is recommended for the ultrafiltrate line (approximately 30 mm Hg). This negative pressure is critically important in the production of the ultrafiltrate because, as pointed out earlier, the hydraulic pressure inside the filter can be very small.

Oncotic pressure

The pressure exerted by the plasma proteins or oncotic pressure at the inlet and outlet of the filter can be calculated from the measured protein concentrations (15).

Filtration pressure or net pressure gradient or transmembrane pressure

The filtration pressure (FP) that determines ultrafiltration is defined by Starling's law:

FP = Hydraulic + Hydrostatic pressure − Mean Oncotic pressure

$$\text{Hydraulic pressure} = \frac{\text{Pre + Post filter pressure}}{2}.$$

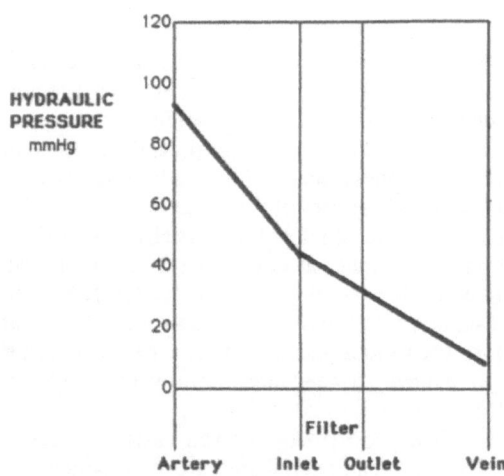

Figure 3. Hydraulic pressure drop in the CAVH extracorporeal circuit. The values represent pressure measurements in a typical case (Amicon Diafilter® 20).

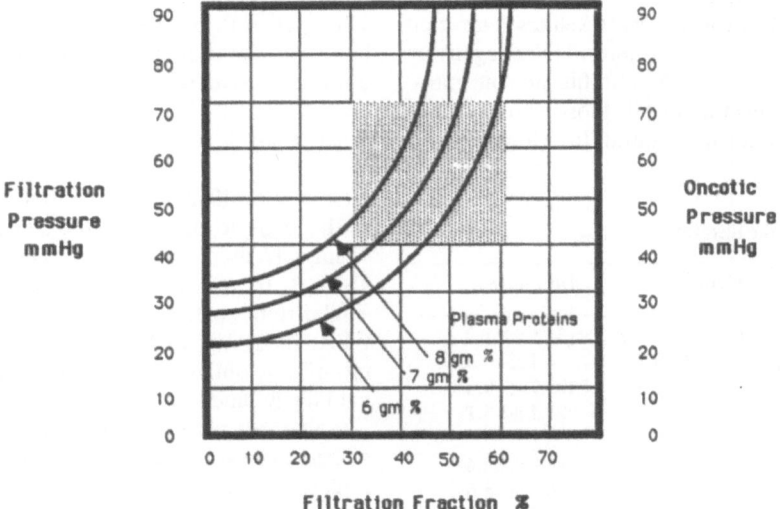

Figure 4. Relationship between filtration pressure and oncotic pressure in the CAVH filter. Shaded area represents range of filtration pressure (hydraulic + hydrostatic pressure). The lines denote the oncotic pressure for different inlet protein concentration.

Hydrostatic pressure (P_f) = Pressure in the ultrafiltrate compartment

Mean Oncotic pressure =

$\dfrac{\text{Post + Pre filter Oncotic pressure}}{2}$.

The oncotic pressure exerted by the plasma proteins inside the filter opposes the hydraulic and hydrostatic pressure. As the blood goes through the filter, plasma water moves across the membrane. The plasma protein concentration increases and the oncotic pressure rises. At some point in the filter, oncotic pressure equals the sum of the hydraulic and hydrostatic pressure, causing ultrafiltration to cease. This equilibrium of pressures is always achieved in CAVH when an Amicon D-20 or similar filter is used. This phenomenon is the result of the low pressure inside and the low blood flow through the filter. When a blood pump is used, greater hydraulic pressure and higher blood flow are obtained. In this case the hydraulic and hydrostatic pressure sum exceeds the oncotic pressure and pressure disequilibrium exists. (Figure 4).

Filtration fraction (FF)

This represents the fraction of the incoming plasma water removed in the ultrafiltrate. It is calculated from the following formulas: (Q_f = ultrafiltrate rate (ml/min), Q_{pi} = plasma flow inlet (ml/min), [P] protein concentration)

$\text{FF (\%)} = \dfrac{Q_f}{Q_{pi}}$

$\text{FF (\%)} = 1 - \dfrac{[P]_{inlet}}{[P]_{outlet}}$

A filtration fraction of 35 to 40% appears to be the maximum that can be achieved during CAVH using the Amicon 20 or similar filters (5). A lower value may be the result of an increase in the inlet protein concentration or more likely, a decrease in filtration pressure. Altering the extracorporeal circuit by using shorter blood lines, larger diameter arterial cannula, and a longer ultrafiltrate line can raise the filtration pressure, thus improving the ultrafiltration rate and increasing the FF. In assessing a low ultrafiltration rate (<5 ml/min) the FF provides useful clinical information. If the FF is greater than 20%, the reduction in ultrafiltration rate is most likely due to a low plasma water flow through the filter secondary to hypotension, blood access problems, high systemic protein concentration, high hematocrit or a partially clotted filter. If the FF is less than 20% the low ultrafiltration rate may be due to a low filtration pressure secondary to hypotension, pressure drop along the circuit or too short an ultrafiltrate line.

COMPOSITION OF THE ULTRAFILTRATE

The fluid removed during CAVH has all the characteristics typical of an ultrafiltrate of plasma water (16). 1) It is protein free. The membranes used in CAVH are impermeable to plasma proteins with a molecular mass of 50,000 daltons or higher. 2) For non-electrolyte solutes, including proteins of lower molecular mass than 50,000 daltons, the ultrafiltrate concentration progressively increases reaching that of the plasma water at a molecular weight of 100 daltons or less. As shown in the rat glomeruli the permeability of molecules with a sieving coefficient less than 1 but greater than 0 is dependent on plasma flow (17). In CAVH the influence of plasma flow on the permeability of solutes with these characteristics has not been determined. 3) The ultrafiltrate concentration of the electrically charged solutes is affected by the negatively charged plasma proteins. Those negatively charged, such as chloride, have an ultrafiltrate concentration greater than in plasma water while those with a positive charge have a concentration in the ultrafiltrate lower than in plasma water. 4) The physicochemical characteristics of the solute, such as protein binding or distribution in the red blood cell water, may result in a lower concentration in the ultrafiltrate than in the plasma water (Table 2).

Drug removal

Golper et al (18–20) have collaborated with several centers in the USA to determine the sieving coefficient of some commonly used medications. Their results are shown in Table 3. In general, the removal of a given drug will be similar to the natural renal excretion of the drug at similar GFR. In CAVH the 'GFR' will be equal to the liters of ultrafiltrate obtained per day divided by 1440 plus the residual kidney function.

Golper has proposed a method to determine the amount of drug to be administered during CAVH or any other renal replacement therapy when the amount of drug removed is not clearly known but there are drug levels to guide management. The volume of distribution (Vd) for that drug must also be known (21).

Table 2. Composition of the ultrafiltrate.

		Plasma	Ultrafiltrate
Sodium	mEq/l	136.2 ± 10.4	135.5 ± 11.2
Potassium	mEq/l	4.1 ± 0.7	4.1 ± 0.3
Chloride	mEq/l	99.3 ± 10.8	103.7 ± 9.6
Carbon dioxide	mEq/l	19.8 ± 4.7	23.1 ± 5.1
Blood urea nitrogen	mg/dl	79.1 ± 36.4	82.9 ± 38.4
Creatinine	mg/dl	6.5 ± 3.9	6.6 ± 4.0
Uric acid	mg/dl	7.4 ± 3.0	7.5 ± 3.3
Phosphorus	mg/dl	3.9 ± 1.1	4.2 ± 1.3
Calcium	mg/dl	8.1 ± 0.6	5.1 ± 0.4
Total bilirubin	mg/dl	12.1 ± 9.5	0.4 ± 0.6
Direct bilirubin	mg/dl	7.4 ± 5.9	0.3 ± 0.3

From reference (16).

Table 3. Sieving coefficient during CAVH.

Drug	Sieving coefficient
Amikacin	0.88 ± 0.03
Amphotericin B	0.35 ± 0.06
Ampicillin	0.69 ± 0.21
Cefoperazone	0.27
Cefotaxime	1.06 ± 0.34
Cefoxitin	0.32
Ceftriaxone	0.82 ± 0.11
Cephapirin	1.48 ± 0.36
Clindamycin	0.49 ± 0.49
Erythromycin	0.37
Gentamicin	0.81 ± 0.02
Imipenen	0.78 ± 0.08
Metronidazole	0.84 ± 0.08
Mezlocillin	0.71 ± 0.10
Nafcillin	0.55 ± 0.12
Oxacillin	0.02
Penicillin	0.68
Streptomycin	0.30
Tobramycin	0.81 ± 0.06
Vancomycin	0.76 ± 0.90
Digoxin	0.96 ± 0.06
N-acetyl procainamide	0.92 ± 0.01
Phenobarbital	0.86 ± 0.01
Phenytoin	0.45 ± 0.06
Procainamide	0.46 ± 0.02
Theophylline	0.86 ± 0.01

From reference (20).

* Mean values $\pm$ SEM. When there is no SEM, only one observation available.

Tobramycin loading

Vd	0.23 l/kg
desired level (peak)	6 mg/l
present level	0 mg/l
difference level	6 mg/l

$$\text{Tobramycin loading} = \text{difference level} \times \text{Vd} \times \text{body weight}$$
$$= 6\,\text{mg/l} \times 0.23\,\text{l/kg} \times 60\,\text{kg}$$
$$= 83\,\text{mg}.$$

Tobramycin maintenance

desired level (peak)	6 mg/l
present level	2 mg/l
difference level	4 mg/l

$$\text{Tobramycin maintenance} = \text{difference level} \times \text{Vd} \times \text{body weight}$$
$$= 4\,\text{mg/l} \times 0.23\,\text{l/kg} \times 60\,\text{kg}$$
$$= 55\,\text{mg}.$$

FLUID AND ELECTROLYTE BALANCE IN CAVH

Fluid balance

CAVH offers almost complete control of the patient's fluid balance. Under most operating conditions 5 to 10 ml/min of ultrafiltrate are produced. By administering a smaller amount of substitution fluid, 2 to 5 ml/min for example, negative fluid balance can be easily established. Most studies have demonstrated that a negative fluid balance induced in this fashion does not cause hypotension. Blood pressure is maintained and cardiac output may even increase over time. The rapidity with which negative fluid balance is attained and the total quantity of fluid removed are important. Hypotension is usually not observed even at net fluid losses of 0.5 ml/min/kg if volume overload preexists. It has been our experience that it is better to achieve the negative fluid balance over an extended period of time. In patients with severe fluid overload we replace only 50% of the ultrafiltrate obtained in the previous hour.

Electrolyte balance

Electrolyte losses during CAVH depend on: 1) the ultrafiltrate electrolyte concentration and 2) the volume of ultrafiltrate obtained. The gain of a given electrolyte depends on: 1) the concentration in the substitution fluid and 2) the rate and volume of fluid administered. For example, the sodium balance during CAVH in a patient that had a weight loss of 2 kg may vary (assuming: plasma and ultrafiltrate [Na] = 140 mEq/l, substitution fluid [Na] = 130 mEq/l) as illustrated in Table 4.

The separation of fluid from the electrolytes losses, permits the administration or removal of a particular electrolyte with ease and allows dissociation of electrolyte losses or gains from changes in total body water. This is useful in the treatment of acidosis (to administer bicarbonate), alkalosis (to remove alkali) or generalized edema (to remove water with or without sodium).

ANTICOAGULATION IN CAVH

Priming of the filter with 2,000 IU of heparin is always required independent of the dose used during the treatment. During the treatment close monitoring of the patient's partial thromboplastin time (PTT) is essential. There are several protocols used to adjust the heparin dose during CAVH. 1) Patients receive a fixed dose of heparin during the treatment (10 IU/kg/h). 2) Adjustment of the heparin dosage according to the blood flow through the filter (heparin dose IU/h = [0.5 or 1.0 IU] × [Q_{bi} ml/min] × 60). The objective of this regimen is to achieve a heparin concentration of 0.5 to 1.0 IU/ml of blood in the filter. At blood flow rates below 70 to 80 ml/min, this schedule may permit the avoidance of systemic anticoagulation (5). 3) In high risk or actively bleeding patients regional heparinization (22) or citrate (23) may be used. In these patients, low resistance filters may diminish the heparin requirement.

A number of alternatives to anticoagulation with heparin

are currently being explored. One of these is the use of prostaglandin I_2 (PGI_2) which is a potent vasodilator (24). Thus, vasodilation and hypotension are complications associated with the use of this agent. Newer analogues of PGI_2, which do not have this side effect are currently being evaluated for anticoagulation. Another promising technique is the development of membranes that may bind heparin. Thus, fiber clotting would be prevented but systemic heparinization would not be necessary (25). The use of low molecular weight heparin with high affinity for antithrombin III (ATIII), yet minimal effect on PTT and the potential removal in the ultrafiltrate could make heparin anticoagulation during CAVH safer (26).

SUBSTITUTION FLUID

In the USA there are no commercially available substitution fluids for hemofiltration or CAVH. We have used Ringer's solution as our standard substitution fluid ([Na] = 130 mEq/l, [K] = 4 mEq/l, [Ca] = 3 mEq/l, [Cl] = 109 mEq/l and [Lactate] = 28 mEq/l). A similar formulation is available with acetate instead of lactate. No clinical problems in lactate or acetate metabolism have been observed by us. It must be pointed out, that the rate of base, acetate or lactate, administered during CAVH is much less than the

Table 5. Clinical indications for CAVH.

---

1. Fluid overload:
A. Hemodialysis patients with pre-existing access
    a) Acute pulmonary edema
    b) Hemodynamic instability
B. Patients with acute renal failure
    a) Hemodynamic instability
    b) Post operative cardiac surgery
    c) Recent myocardial infarct
    d) Sepsis
C. Patients with heart failure (pump failure)
    a) Diuretic resistant
    b) Oliguria despite inotropic support
D. Oliguric states in patients that require large quantities of IV fluids: i.e. hyperalimentation, medications, etc.
E. Chronic fluid overload (?)
    a) Ascites
    b) Nephrotic edema

2. Solute removal
Alternative to hemodialysis or peritoneal dialysis in patients with chronic or acute renal failure and:
A. Hypotension
B. Hemodynamic instability
C. Need for parenteral fluids
D. Associated medical complications

3. Acid-base and electrolyte disturbances
A. Metabolic alkalosis
B. Metabolic acidosis
C. Hyponatremia, etc.

Table 4. Calculations of sodium and fluid balance.

	Case 1	Case 2	Case 3
Volume of ultrafiltrate (ml)	2,000	10,000	15,000
Sodium losses (mEq)	280	1,400	2,100
Substitution fluid given (ml)	0	8,000	13,000
Sodium gain (mEq)	0	1,040	1,690
Weight loss (g)	2,000	2,000	2,000
Sodium balance (mEq)	−280	−360	−410

rate at which acetate intolerance has been described in hemodialysis (± 300 mmol/h). Rather than use a fixed substitution fluid, it is preferable to modify the replacement solution on individual patient's needs.

INDICATIONS

The indications for CAVH are: 1) acute renal failure; 2) fluid overload and 3) electrolyte and acid base disturbances (Table 5). Not all patients with acute renal failure should be treated with CAVH. Hemodialysis or peritoneal dialysis are still the main treatment for patients with acute renal failure. However, in patients with acute renal failure and multiorgan failure (27), vascular instability during hemodialysis, hypercatabolic states, patients that require hyperalimentation, and large amounts of parenteral fluids (28), CAVH offers particular advantages.

The second general indication for CAVH is fluid overload in patients with or without renal failure (29–32). Patients with congestive heart failure refractory to diuretic therapy may benefit from CAVH. Patients with volume overload on maintenance peritoneal dialysis with temporary loss of ultrafiltration capacity and patients on maintenance hemodialysis unable to tolerate fluid withdrawal may also benefit from CAVH. There is an interesting hemodynamic response to fluid withdrawal during CAVH that may partially explain the good clinical tolerance. Table 6 summarizes the hemodynamic response to fluid removal with different therapies. The general response to fluid removal in therapies other than CAVH is a fall in cardiac output. Blood pressure in these treatments will depend on the behavior of the peripheral resistance. In acetate hemodialysis peripheral resistance falls and so does blood pressure. In hemofiltration and bicarbonate hemodialysis peripheral resistance increases and blood pressure remains stable. In CAVH the hemodynamic response is quite different. Cardiac output increases and peripheral resistance decreases. The blood pressure in this case, is maintained by an improvement in myocardial function. The peripheral vasodilation and afterload reduction may in part explain the benefit on the heart function.

The possibility of modifying the extracellular fluid composition with CAVH suggests a third general indication for the treatment, correction of electrolyte and acid base disturbances (33).

Table 6. Hemodynamic response to fluid removal with different therapies.

	Acetate HD	Bicarbonate HD	Hemofiltration	CAVH
Cardiac output	D	D	D	I
Peripheral resistance	DD	I	I	I
Blood pressure	DD	–	–	I

HD = hemodialysis; D = decrease; I = increase; – = no change.

CONTRAINDICATIONS

In patients with systemic bleeding, judgment must be used to weigh the advantages with the risks. In these subjects, the combination of low blood pressure, low blood flow through the circuit and the need for high ultrafiltration rates to control plasma urea nitrogen, makes CAVH a difficult technique to apply.

PROBLEMS ENCOUNTERED IN THE CLINICAL USE OF CAVH

Independent of the vascular access there are two major problems with the clinical use of CAVH. They are 1) frequent clotting of the filter and 2) the inability of the treatment to maintain, in severely catabolic patients, the plasma urea nitrogen concentration below 120 to 150 mg/dl.

Clotting of the filter

Clotting of the filter is in part, a consequence of the performance characteristics of the CAVH extracorporeal system. These features are: a low pressure and a low blood flow.

Low pressure

In CAVH there is a gradual decrease in hydraulic pressure throughout the extracorporeal circuit. The hydraulic pressure falls as the different resistances (the access, tubing and filter) to the blood flow are encountered. The mean hydraulic pressure inside the filter is, therefore, considerably less than the mean arterial pressure of the patient. For example, in a patient with a mean arterial pressure of 90 mm Hg, the hydraulic pressure in the filter may fall to 30 mm Hg or less (Figure 3). The addition of the hydrostatic pressure, generated by the ultrafiltrate column (± 30 mm Hg), results in a filtration pressure that only averages 50 to 60 mm Hg. This pressure is within the range of the oncotic pressure generated by concentrations of plasma proteins observed in clinical medicine.

Low blood flow

The low blood flow is a consequence of the high resistance of the extracorporeal circuit. The blood flow rate in CAVH rarely exceeds 50 to 80 ml/min in patients with a mean arterial pressure of 70 mm Hg or higher.

Inside the filter, as ultrafiltrate is produced, the protein concentration and the oncotic pressure in the blood increase. Since filtration pressure inside the filter is low, a point will be reached in where the rising oncotic pressure will equal the filtration pressure and, due to the absence of a pressure gradient, no further ultrafiltrate will be produced. Filtration pressure equilibrium, always occurs in the present CAVH system. It is not possible to ascertain the point along the length of the filter where this pressure equilibrium takes place. In the Amicon 20, it is probably closer to the arterial

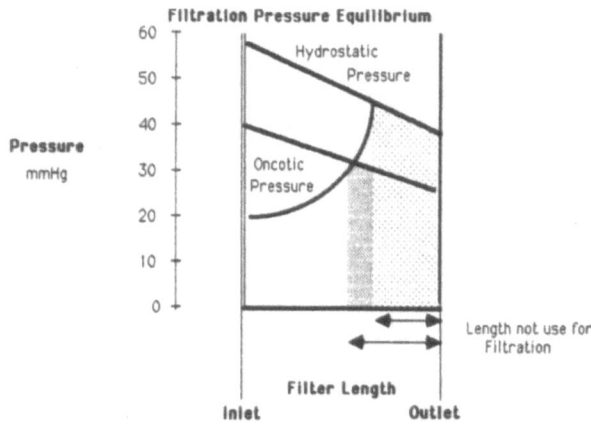

Figure 5. Schematic representation of the filter length. Two different filtration pressures are depicted. The shaded areas represent the filter length not used for filtration. A fall in filtration pressure may result in an increased in the length not used for filtration.

than to the venous port of the filter. With filtration pressure equilibrium a segment of the membrane of the filter is not used for filtration. The blood beyond the filtration pressure equilibrium point is characterized by a higher hematocrit, a higher protein concentration and hence a greater viscosity. The movement of highly viscous blood through an area of the membrane not used for filtration, further increases the resistance of the filter to the blood flow. In patients with a low systemic arterial pressure and thus a low blood flow rate, the higher resistance further decreases hydraulic pressure. As a consequence of the fall in hydraulic pressure filtration pressure falls and the equilibrium point moves closer to the inlet of the filter further increasing the area not used for filtration. A vicious cycle is created and eventually the filter clots (Figure 5).

The resistance of the filter to the blood flow is only partially determined by the intrinsic design of the filter. It is mainly a consequence of the filtration pressure equilibrium. Design modifications may improve the performance of the technique. By shortening the length of the filter, it may be possible to avoid filtration pressure equilibrium. This would decrease the resistance of the filter by avoiding the passage of the blood, with a higher protein concentration, hematocrit and viscosity, through an area of the membrane not used for filtration. By increasing the number of fibers, it may be possible to diminish the resistance of the filter itself and thereby increase the blood flow for a given systemic arterial pressure.

A specially designed filter (Amicon diafilter® 10) has allowed testing of the role of filtration pressure equilibrium in the performance of CAVH (24). This filter was specially designed with a shorter length to have a low resistance to blood flow and to reduce the area of the membrane not used for filtration. The design characteristics are shown in comparison to those of the Amicon diafilter® 20 in Table 7.

In Figures 6 and 7 are shown the performance character-

istics of the two filters. The lower resistance of the AD-10 is apparent in Figure 6. At all levels of systemic blood pressure the blood flow through the AD-10 was higher than observed in the AD-20. At low systemic pressures (60 to 70 mm Hg) the blood flow was 70 ml/min or higher. Figure 7 shows the relationship between the blood flow and the ultrafiltration rate in both filters. On the average the ultrafiltration rate in the AD-10 averaged 8 to 10 ml/min within a wide range of blood flow (50 to 100 ml/min). These ultrafiltration rates are slightly less than those observed with the AD-20 (10 to 12 ml/min). The new design of the AD-10 may represent an improvement in the CAVH technique. The AD-10 does not necessarily replace the other filters used in the treatment but it is a special device to be used in hypotensive patients who cannot be treated with CAVH because of hypotension and/ or low blood flow.

Solute removal during CAVH

In the critically ill patient treated with CAVH it is not infrequent to observe plasma urea nitrogen concentrations exceeding 100 to 120 mg/dl (36 to 43 mmol/l). In some cases, plasma urea nitrogen concentrations may rise to values in excess of 150 to 180 mg/dl (54 to 64 mmol/l) necessitating the additional use of hemodialysis for solute removal. Figure 8 depicts the relationship between the urea generation rate and the liters of ultrafiltrate per day required to maintain a given plasma urea nitrogen concentration. It is apparent that in patients with urea generation rates above 20 g/day, 15 l or less of ultrafiltrate and corresponding quantities of substitution fluid may not be sufficient to maintain plasma urea nitrogen below 120 mg/dl (36 mmol/l) (34).

In patients undergoing CAVH plasma urea nitrogen concentrations depend on: 1) the production of urea nitrogen or urea generation rate. 2) urea nitrogen removal from the body or the ultrafiltration rate and 3) the dilution of the plasma water or the rate of administration of substitution fluid. Several approaches have been used to overcome the inability of CAVH to control plasma urea nitrogen concentration in the critically ill and severely catabolic patient:

Reduction in urea generation rate

The protein catabolic rate of the critically ill patient is often two or three times the normal rate. There are many reasons for this increase in catabolic rate. These patients are usually starving (no oral intake) so that they have an obligatory

Table 7. Diafilter design characteristics.

	AD-20	AD-10
Effective membrane area (m²)	0.25	0.20
Fiber internal diameter (μ)	200	200
Number of fibers	5,000	6,000
Length of fibers (cm)	12.7	9.5
Overall unit length (cm)	17.5	14.0

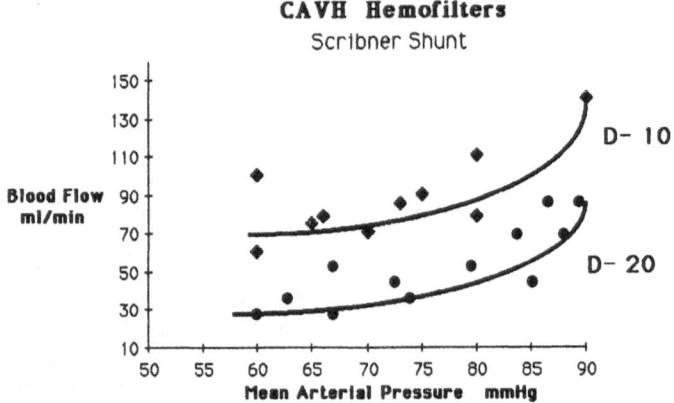

Figure 6. Mean arterial pressure and blood flow in the Amicon 20 and 10. Each observation represents a different patient.

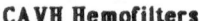

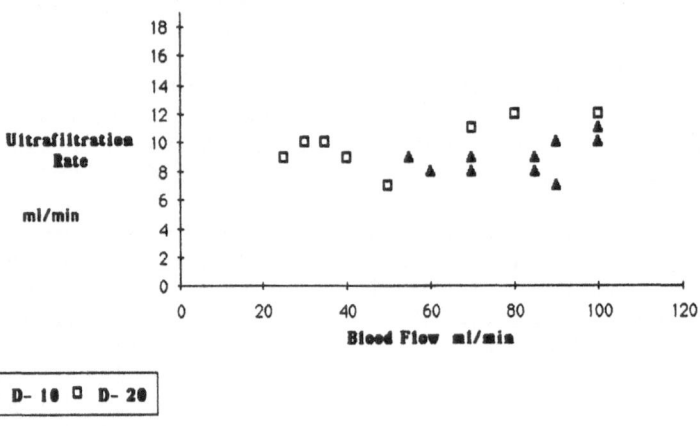

Figure 7. Ultrafiltration rate and blood flow in the Amicon 20 and 10. Systemic pressure in all AD 20 cases was over 70 mm Hg. In all AD 10 cases systemic pressure was less than 70 mm Hg.

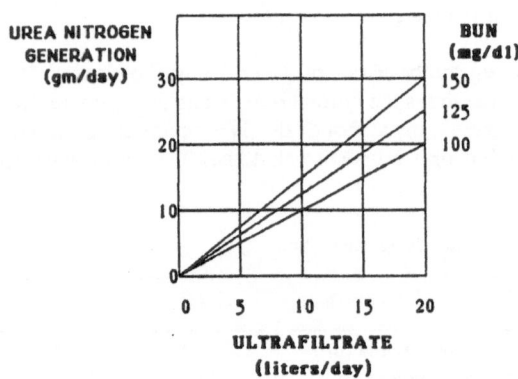

Figure 8. Solute removal rate in CAVH. Relationship between urea generation rate and the liters of ultrafiltrate per day required to maintain a given plasma urea nitrogen concentration.

protein metabolism to supply energy via gluconeogenesis. In addition, circulating hormones (e.g. catecholamines and steroids) and humoral products of the inflammatory state (interleukin 1 and 2, for example) accelerate metabolism. Urea generation can be reduced by treating the underlying process and by supplying energy and proteins by hyperalimentation. Recent preliminary studies suggest that hyperalimentation may have a beneficial impact in the overall mortality of these patients.

Modifications in the CAVH system to increase efficiency

Pre-post dilution mode
Previous studies in hemofiltration (35) demonstrated that it is possible to increase ultrafiltration rate, and thus solute removal, by diluting the blood before it enters the filter. The term pre-post dilution mode in CAVH (36), defines a system in which the substitution fluid is administered to the in-

coming blood as well as to the blood returning to the patient. Predilution is the fraction of the substitution fluid administered at the blood inlet (3 to 10 ml/min). The predilution fluid is usually administered through the heparin line. Postdilution fluid is the majority of the substitution fluid administered in the venous line or into the systemic circulation (8 to 10 ml/min). The lowering, by dilution, of the incoming protein concentration reduces the oncotic pressure inside the filter and therefore, increases the ultrafiltration rate for a constant net filtration pressure. The benefit of this effect is offset by lowering the concentration of urea and other solutes, in the ultrafiltrate. This substitution mode is indicated for patients in whom the blood flow though the extracorporeal circuit is low or the hematocrit is high and clotting of the filter is frequent.

Use of a vacuum pump
Kaplan et al (37) have shown that a vacuum suction attached to the filtrate port may be a useful adjunct to CAVH. The addition of suction increases the net filtration pressure and the ultrafiltration rate. This modification of the technique must be used with caution. Since higher net filtration pressures will produce ultrafiltrate even in the presence of very low blood flows, a filtration fraction in excess of 50% can be obtained. This effect may favor clotting of the filter despite adequate heparin administration.

Combined pre-post dilution mode plus a vacuum pump
In this technique the advantages of both systems are added to increase solute removal (38). Table 8 depicts the results of using pre-post dilution mode and a vacuum pump during CAVH. In the same patient using standard CAVH technique the ultrafiltration rate, and hence the urea clearance, was 12 to 14 ml/min. The urea clearance increased to 18.1 ml/min using pre-post dilution and a vacuum pump. These maneuvers do increase the efficiency of CAVH. The high

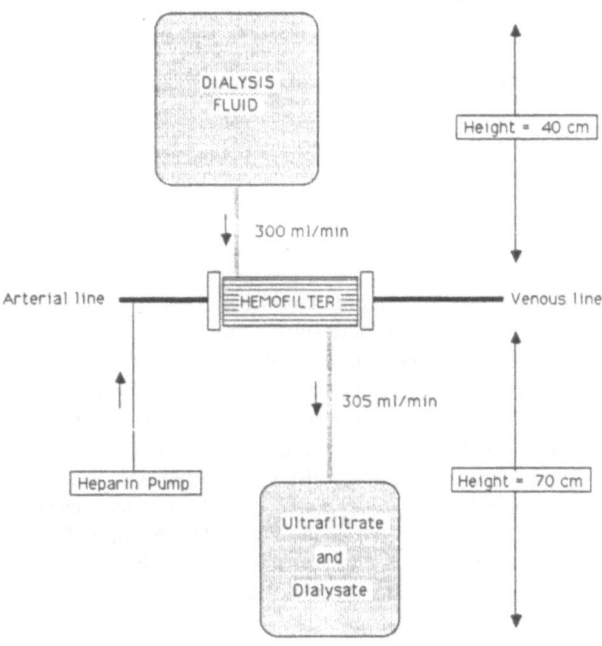

Arterio-Venous Hemodiafiltration

Figure 9. In this system regular CAVH is alternated with periods of arterio-venous hemodiafiltration.

filtration fraction observed, 52%, may limit the application of this technique modification.

Continuous arteriovenous hemodialysis (CAVHD)
Several investigators have sought to improve solute clearance in CAVH by incorporating diffusive transport with convective solute removal. Geronemus et al (39) reported a modification called continuous arteriovenous hemodialysis (CAVHD). In this system a hemodialyzer was connected to the patient using an extracorporeal circuit comparable to CAVH. In addition, dialysate was circulated through the dialyzer using gravity. Solute clearance averaged 10 to 15 ml/min. Cardiovascular stability was excellent. These investigators and others (40, 41) have performed similar studies using a 0.43 m² flat plate PAN membrane dialyzer obtaining urea clearances of 16.9 ml/min.

Siegler et al (41) studied the performance characteristics of CAVHD in a low resistance polyacrylnitrile parallel plate hemodialyzer (Hospal, AN69S; SCU/CAVH). Clearances in CAVHD are calculated using the following formulas:

Blood side clearance

$$K_B = \frac{Q_{Bi}\,C_{Bi} - Q_{Bo}\,C_{Bo}}{C_{Bi}}.$$

Table 8. Pre- postdilution CAVH with vacuum suction.

	Arterial inlet	Pre-dilution ml/min 6.50	Filter	Post filter
Blood flow (ml/min)	50.00		56.50	34.80
Plasma flow (ml/min)	35.00		41.50	19.80
Red cell mass (ml/min)	15.00		15.00	15.00
Hct (%)	30.00		26.50	43.90
[BUN] Plasma (mg/ml)	1.00		.85	.85
[BUN] Blood (mg/ml)	0.96		.84	.84
Ultrafiltrate		21.7	ml/min	
Clearance of urea		18.1	ml/min	
Filtration fraction		52%		

Dialysate clearance

$$K_D = \frac{Q_{Do}\, C_{Do} - Q_{Di}\, C_{Bi}}{C_{Bi}}\ .$$

$Q_{Do} = Q_{Di} + Q_f$ and Q_f = net ultrafiltration rate

Clearance

$$K_D = \frac{QDi\,(CDo - CDi)}{QDi} + \frac{Qf\,CDo}{C_{Bi}}:$$

Continuous arteriovenous hemodiafiltration

Ronco et al (34) (Figure 9) modified the standard AD-20 by adding an extra port to the ultrafiltrate compartment. Dialysate solution circulated through the filter by gravity so that solutes were removed by diffusion and convection simultaneously. The patients were treated with standard CAVH using this device, the extra port occluded. When increased solute clearance was required the added port was opened and, by gravity, the dialysate solution was circulated through the ultrafiltrate compartment of the filter. The addition of diffusion permitted the control of BUN concentration in patients with severe catabolism.

CONCLUSION

CAVH and other continuous therapies are techniques that offer specific clinical advantages. They are easily initiated. They are well tolerated by the patient. They do not require specialized equipment and they are easily adaptable to the patient's needs. The disadvantages are: the need for continuous supervision, the heparin infusion and the risks of the arterial cannulation.

ACKNOWLEDGEMENT

The Authors acknowledge the contributions of the following collaborators and friends that have made these studies possible: Dr. Beat von Albertini, Dr. R. Geronemus, Dr. A. Lauer, and Dr. S. Glabman.

REFERENCES

1. Henderson LW, Besarab A, Michaels A, Bluemle L Jr: Blood purification by ultrafiltration and fluid replacement (Dialfiltration). *Trans Am Soc Artif Intern Organs* 13: 216, 1967
2. Silverstein ME, Ford CA, Lysaght MJ, Henderson LW: The treatment of intractable fluid overload. *N Engl J Med* 291: 747, 1974
3. Kramer P, Wigger W, Rieger J, Matthaei D, Scheler F: Arteriovenous hemofiltration: A new and simple method for treatment of overhydrated patients resistant to diuretics. *Klin Wochenschr* 55: 1121, 1977
4. Kramer P, Kaufhold C, Grone HJ, Wigger W, Rieger J: Management of anuric intensive-care patients with arteriovenous hemofiltration. *Int J Artif Organs* 3: 255, 1980

5. Lauer A, Saccaggi A, Ronco C, Belledonne M, Glabman S, Bosch JP: Continuous arteriovenous hemofiltration in the critically ill patient. *Ann Intern Med* 99: 455, 1983
6. Mault JR, Bartlett RH, Dechert RE, Clark SF, Swartz RD: Starvation: A major contribution to mortality in acute renal failure? *Trans Am Soc Artif Intern Organs* 29: 390, 1983
7. Lieberman KV, Nardi L, Bosch JP: Treatment of acute renal failure in an infant using continuous arteriovenous hemofiltration. *J Pediatr* 106: 646, 1985
8. Paganini EP, Nakamoto S: Continuous slow ultrafiltration in oliguric acute renal failure. *Trans Am Soc Artif Intern Organs* 26: 201, 1980
9. Lauer A, Alvis RC, Avram MM: Hemodynamic consequences of continuous arteriovenous hemofiltration (CAVH) in intractable fluid overload. in *CAVH*, edited by La Greca G, Fabris A, Ronco C, Milan, Wichtig Editore, 1986, p 227
10. Magilligan DJ: Effect of ultrafiltration on lung water. *Proc Third Int Symposium on Acute Continuous Renal Replacement Therapy, Fort Lauderdale, FL* 3: 161, 1987
11. Paganini EP, Suhoza K, Swann S: Continuous renal replacement therapy in patients with acute renal dysfunction undergoing intraaortic balloon pump and/or left ventricular device support. *Trans Am Soc Artif Intern Organs* 32: 414, 1986
12. Coraim F, Wolner E: Management of cardiac surgery patients with continuous arteriovenous hemofiltration. in *Int Conf on CAVH, Aachen*. Karger, Basel 1985
13. Lysaght M, Boggs D, Ritger P, Howard DD, Jensen JJ: Membranes and transport phenomena in CAVH and CAVHD. in *CAVH*, edited by La Greca G, Fabris A, Ronco C, Milan, Wichtig Editore, 1986, p 77
14. Gohl H, Konstantin P, Gulberg CA: Hemofiltration membranes. *Contr Nephrol* 32: 20, 1982
15. Pappenheimer JR: Passage of molecules through capillary walls. *Physiol Rev* 33: 387, 1953
16. Kaplan A, Longnecker R, Folbert VW: Continuous arteriovenous hemofiltration: A report of six month's experience. *Ann Intern Med* 100: 358, 1984
17. Chang RL, Ueki IF, Troy JL, Deen WM, Robertson CR, Brenner BM: Permselectivity of the capillary wall to macromolecules II. Experimental studies in the rat using neutral dextran. *Biophys J* 15: 887, 1975
18. Golper TA, Wedel SK, Kaplan AA, Saad AM, Donta S, Paganini EP: Drug removal during continuous arteriovenous hemofiltration: theory and clinical observation. *Int J Artif Organs* 8: 307, 1985
19. Golper TA: Continuous arteriovenous hemofiltration in acute renal failure. *Am J Kidney Dis* 6: 373, 1985
20. Golper TA: Drug removal during continuous renal replacement therapies in acute renal failure. *Proc Third Int Symposium on Acute Continuous Renal Replacement Therapy, Fort Lauderdale, FL* 3: 135, 1987
21. Bennett WM, Aronoff GR, Morrison G, Golper TA: Drug prescribing in renal failure: Dose guidelines for adults. *Am J Kidney Dis* 3: 155, 1985
22. Maher JF, Lapierre L, Schreiner GE, Geiger M, Westervelt FB: Regional heparinization for hemodialysis. *N Eng J Med* 268: 451, 1963
23. Pinnick RV, Wiegmann TB, Diederich DA: Regional citrate anticoagulation for hemodialysis in patients at high risk for bleeding. *N Eng J Med* 308: 258, 1983
24. Zusman RM, Rubin RH, Cato A: Hemodialysis using prostacyclin instead of heparin as the sole antithrombotic agent. *N Eng J Med* 304: 934, 1981
25. Josefowicz M, Josefowicz J: New approaches to anticoagula-

tion with heparin-like biomaterials. *asaio J* 8: 218, 1985

26. Hirsch J, Ofosu F, Buchanan M: Rationale behind the development of low molecular weight heparin derivatives. *Semin Thromb Hemost* 11: 13, 1985

27. Olbricht C, Mueller C, Schurek HJ, Stolte H: Treatment of acute renal failure in patients with multiple organ failure by continuous spontaneous hemofiltration. *Trans Am Soc Artif Intern Organs* 28: 23, 1982

28. Kramer P, Boehler J, Kehr A, Groene HJ, Schader R, Mattahaei D, Scheler F: Intensive care potential of continuous arteriovenous hemofiltration. *Trans Am Soc Artif Intern Organs* 28: 28, 1982

29. Misler S: Long term ultrafiltration as a treatment of refractory congestive heart failure. *NY State J Med* 10: 518, 1984

30. Morgan SH, Mansell MA, Thompson TD: Fluid removal by hemofiltration in diuretic resistant cardiac failure. *Br Heart J* 54: 218, 1985

31. Lauer A, Alvis R, Beal A, Avram M: Hemodynamic consequences of continuous arteriovenous hemofiltration in intractable fluid overload. (Abstract) *Kidney Int* 29: 218, 1986

32. Kaufman A, Levitt M: The effect of diuretics on systemic and renal hemodynamics in patients with renal insufficiency. *Am J Kidney Dis* 5: A71, 1985

33. Raimondi F, Bianchi T, Emmi V, Braschi A, Iotti G, Bobbio Pallavicini F, Tosi P, Fischetti M, Galli F, Villa S: Use of continuous arteriovenous hemofiltration (CAVH) in lactic acidosis: A case report. in *CAVH,* edited by La Greca G, Fabris A, Ronco C, Milan, Wichtig Editore, 1986, p 135

34. Ronco C, Brendolan S, Bragantini L, Chiaramonti S, Dell'A-

quila R, Fabris A, Feriani M, Milan M, La Greca G: Arteriovenous hemodiafiltration: A combined therapy for acute renal failure in the hypercatabolic patients. in *CAVH,* edited by La Greca G, Fabris A, Ronco C, Milan, Wichtig Editore, 1986, p 171

35. Geronemus R, von Albertini B, Glabman S, Lysaght M, Khan T, Bosch JP: Enhanced molecular clearance in hemofiltration. *Proc Clin Dial Transplant Forum* 8: 147, 1978

36. Kaplan AA: Predilution vs postdilution for continuous arteriovenous hemofiltration. *Trans Am Soc Artif Intern Organs* 31: 28, 1985

37. Kaplan AA, Longnecker R, Folkert VW: Suction-assisted continuous arteriovenous hemofiltration. *Trans Am Soc Artif Intern Organs* 24: 408, 1983

38. Kaplan AA: Enhanced Efficiency During CAVH: Clinical trials with predilution and vacuum suction. in *CAVH,* edited by La Greca G, Fabris A, Ronco C, Milan, Wichtig Editore, 1986, p 49

39. Geronemus R, Schneider N: Continuous arteriovenous hemodialysis: A new modality for treatment of acute renal failure: *Trans Am Soc Artif Intern Organs* 30: 610, 1984

40. Ing TS, Daugirdas JT, Bregman H, Leehey DJ: Continuous arteriovenous hemodialysis. *Int J Artif Organs* 8: 117, 1985

41. Sigler M, Teehan BP: Solute transport in slow continuous arteriovenous hemodialysis: An improved method for treating acute renal failure. *Proc Third Int Symposium on Acute Continuous Renal Replacement Therapy, Fort Lauderdale, FL* 3: 78, 1987

SHORT TREATMENT

JAMES H. SHINABERGER, JOSEPH H. MILLER and PETER W. GARDNER

INTRODUCTION

An examination of the possibility of shortening the time required for dialytic treatment is justified on the basis that patients desire it, and always have. If a time consuming, absolutely necessary treatment can be safely and comfortably applied to meet all currently understood requirements for adequacy in a substantially shorter time than the standard treatment, the potential beneficial effect on the patients' quality of life is beyond debate. As discussed herein, standard therapy is of 4 to 6 h duration. Short treatment strategies should provide equivalent net volume and solute removal in 3 h or less. The intent of this chapter is to create a durable summation of those principles, limitations and constraints which must be understood to create adequate, safe and tolerable shortened treatment strategies. Current strategies and technologies are evolving rapidly and will be presented relatively briefly. Only references to material of basic importance are cited, rather than an encyclopedic review.

DEVELOPMENT OF A RATIONALE FOR SHORT TREATMENT WITHIN THE HISTORICAL EVOLUTION OF DIALYTIC THERAPY

Evolution of early techniques and strategies

Since the classical studies of the Kolff-Brigham Rotating Drum artificial kidney by A.V. Wolf et al (1) and the laboratory and clinical studies by Alwall and colleagues (2), it has been appreciated that high urea clearances could be obtained with high blood flows with large surface area dialyzers. Indeed, in the clinical application of these devices, high blood flows, large surface areas and relatively short treatments of 3 to 6 h were generally employed. Between the early 1950's and the development of true chronic maintenance dialysis in 1960, the Kolff-Travenol twin coil dialyzer utilizing 1.4 to 1.8 m^2 surface area and pumped blood flows of 200 to 300 ml/min was widely employed for both acute, and later, chronic dialyses with 4 to 5 h treatment times (3,

4). With the advent of the Seattle system for chronic maintenance dialysis with $1.0\,m^2$ parallel plate dialyzers, a passive blood flow circuit and sodium acetate buffering, the use of low blood flow rates, small membrane surface areas and, consequently, lower solute clearances was widely introduced (5, 6). Treatment time greatly increased to 20 to 40 h/week. A surface area around $1.0\,m^2$, blood flow rates of 180 to 200 ml/min and dialysis fluid flow rates of 500 ml/min seem to have been 'frozen' into clinical dialysis technology for nearly two decades as a result of this experience.

The introduction of the first dependable commercially produced parallel flow dialyzers and hollow fiber capillary dialyzers led to continuous improvement in dialyzer efficiency, and gradual shortening of dialysis time from 1965 onward (7–9). Investigators were very aware of the possibilities of shortening dialysis time by increasing dialysis efficiency, especially by increasing surface area. Thus, Shaldon et al (10) in 1974, comparing 20 h weekly Kiil dialysis with both 13.5 h weekly of $2\,m^2$ disposable plate dialysis and 15 h of $1\,m^2$ disposable plate dialysis found acceptable solute control in all groups, but noted that 1200 ml/h of ultrafiltration (acetate dialysate) would probably define the limitations of shortened treatment and would limit the utility of large surface area dialysis. Ten years later, this was reconfirmed in a serious prospective study of shortening treatment time (11).

With somewhat better ultrafiltration control, Mirahmadi et al (12) in 1974 made similar studies of $2\,m^2$ dialysis at blood and dialysate flows typical of the time limited to 200 ml/min and 500 ml/min. Urea clearances of 160 ml/min (twice that of Kiil dialyzers) were achieved as was acceptable solute level control on an adequate diet. Undesirable ultrafiltration again required replacement with saline. Treatment time was 12 h per week.

Cambi et al (13), who have provided 4 h thrice weekly dialysis for all their patients since 1974, reported stability of motor nerve conduction velocities, survival and morbidity data equal to or better than that of the European Dialysis and Transplant Association (EDTA) registry over a 9 year period. Dialyzer surface area was generally $1\,m^2$, blood flow rate was 250 to 300 ml/min and predialysis BUN levels were maintained at 21.4 to 28.6 mmol/l (60 to 80 mg/dl). Unfortunately, this therapy cannot be further quantified.

Bosl et al (14) reported in 1975 that a large surface area dialyzer at a blood flow sufficient to produce urea clearances of 240 ml/min caused intolerably severe symptomatology. It now seems almost certain that this represented excessive acetate delivery, not osmotic disequilibrium as the authors had proposed.

Early development of quantified treatment

Manji et al (15) utilized 3 h dialysis with a urea dialysance of 250 ml/min at a blood flow of 400 ml/min to obtain solute removal equal to their standard 6 h treatments. Thus, they were among the first to employ high blood flow and to document equivalent solute removal in shortened treatment. They also used acetate dialysis solution and had to adopt unrealistic means to gain tolerance to ultrafiltration.

In 1975, Babb et al (16) introduced a highly quantitative description of dialysis treatment, the 'dialysis index for middle molecules' (DI_{mm}). Historically, it is relevant if toxins of molecular size of vitamin B_{12} (cyanocobalmin, 1355 daltons) are important in the pathogenesis of uremia. More importantly formulation of the DI included exact measurements of dialyzer clearance, total ultrafiltration, dialysis time, residual renal clearance and patients' body surface area compared to those of standard man to normalize an intuitively perceived 30 l pool of toxic middle molecules requiring weekly clearance. The vitamin B_{12} to urea clearance ratio was so low in all dialyzers available at that time, that it can be confidently calculated that any patient who received a DI_{mm} of 1.0 or more would have achieved adequate small molecule clearance by today's criteria.

During this era, experience with protocols designed to provide selectively high clearance of small molecules in a short time and those designed to retain selectively small molecules, but to remove middle molecules were either unsuccessful or failed to clarify this issue (17,18). Finally, Bergström and Fürst (19), major investigators in identification of middle molecules as uremic toxins declared that no breakthrough in this area had occurred and that endeavors in other fields were justified to determine an optimal dialysis prescription.

A 1977 review 'Short Dialysis, Middle Molecules, and Uremia' noted great difficulty in evaluation of the relevant literature because comparable quantification of the dialysis treatments were not reported (20). The article was a plea for both quantification of therapy and controlled clinical trials.

In contrast to the difficulties and uncertainties experienced by others, Wauters et al (21) reported experience with 259 patients treated between 1976 and 1986 with 3 h thrice weekly dialysis prescribed to maintain midweek predialysis plasma urea concentrations at 28 mmol/l (BUN = 78 mg/dl) and creatinine levels at 1200 μmol/l (13.6 mg/dl). High efficiency capillary dialyzers at blood flows of about 300 ml/min and dialysate flow rates of 500 to 550 ml/min were used. The average age of these patients was 52 years and they apparently were unselected except for a very low incidence of diabetes mellitus compared to the US dialysis population. Patients' weights and dialyzer clearances were not reported. Survival averaged 91% at one year, 76% at 5 years and 60% at 10 years. Morbidity, estimated in 58 patients followed for at least 6 years, was 7 ± 9 hospital days/year (range 2 to 161 days). As reported, this treatment appears to have met the US National Cooperative Dialysis Study (NCDS) criteria for adequate protein intake and midweek blood solute control and represents an important historical bridge spanning the past 10 years of dialysis technology. Although more details of the individual dialysis prescription quantification and residual renal function would be desirable, this report strongly suggests that shortened treatment which adequately controls predialysis solute concentration can achieve longterm success.

Throughout the 1970's the optimal clinical use of dialyzers was restricted by adherence to the original Seattle parameters of blood and dialysate flow and the use of acetate dialysate. Attempts to shorten dialysis were hampered by a lack of generally agreed upon target solute control, inappropriate combinations of blood flow, surface area (permeability) and poorly controlled ultrafiltration (22). Only a few clinical investigators could find an acceptable compromise of these limitations and embark on long-term short dialysis (approximately 3 h) treatment programs. Presumably due to appropriate individualized dialysis prescriptions, guidelines to which have never been published, at least two investigators in Europe appear to have achieved long-term success with such regimens (13, 21).

From the mid 1970's until now, enormous controversy regarding the question of superior cardiovascular stability with bicarbonate buffer has continued. Many of these studies were in stable chronic patients receiving only moderate efficiency dialysis (23). However, with large surface areas and high blood flows it has become clear that most patients demonstrate vascular instability with acetate dialysate (11, 24, 25).

Throughout this time, only those practicing hemofiltration were really aware of the greatest potential for increasing efficiency of treatment, the very high blood flows generally available in patients' angioaccesses (26, 27). Investigators of hemofiltration also commendably observed that cardiovascular stability is best when solute removal is by convection or when ultrafiltration is separated from dialysis (26–30). From these studies it is also apparent that many attempts at moderately high efficiency hemodialysis treatment using acetate buffer were confounded by insufficient vascular stability to permit the required ultrafiltration in the shorter treatment time.

Further development of quantified treatment

In the search for quantified therapy, it is almost embarrassing to realize that in 1974, amid this confusion Gotch, Sargent, Keen and Lee (31) published a paper, 'Individualized, quantified dialysis therapy for uremia' that described the interaction of protein nutrition, urea generation rate, urea distribution volume and dialyzer clearance plus residual renal clearance applied over treatment time to control the target solute, urea, at 28.6 mmol/l (80 mg/dl). Experience with 32 patients who had received urea kinetically modeled (UKM) treatment was reviewed. The mathematical terms used in their modeling and the equations necessary for individual solutions were presented. In 1976, further results with 46 patients receiving UKM treatment of 6 to 2 h were reported (32). Again, all of the terminology in current use and the application of the concepts were described briefly which could have saved 10 to 12 years in the correct application of modeled therapy into predictably adequate short treatment. Presumably, these publications did not receive wide enough attention, the description of the concepts lacked the clarity required by the readers or the mathematical expressions were too formidable for general comprehension.

The design of the subsequent NCDS was based on those principles, and nearly 10 years later, the brilliant, compre-

hensible formulation of fractional clearance of urea volume, $Kt/V \geq 1.0$ at a protein catabolic rate (pcr) of about 1.0 g/kg/day as a definition of an adequate treatment to be applied thrice weekly made it possible to prescribe confidently individualized adequate treatment of very short duration (33, 34). When Manji et al's (15) concept of the equivalences of the total removed solute by the standard and shortened treatment is applied to these treatments, success can be predicted even more confidently. Very strong evidence supporting the fractional clearance of urea volume concept of Gotch and the NCDS was independently supplied by Teschan, Ginn and co-workers at Vanderbilt (35). Between 1978 and 1981, they completed a meticulous 12 month A-B-A prospective study of the effects of shortening dialysis time on six neurobehavioral variables with which they had great experience. The modeling of small molecule (urea) removal was virtually identical to the Gotch concept. The DI_{mm} was included. The results can be directly compared to the work of Gotch and to the NCDS (33, 34). Teschan et al (35) found adequate treatment to be at a total urea clearance of 3 (or more) l/week/l body water, an index exactly equivalent to a Kt/V of 1.0 and a DI_{mm} of 1.0 to 1.1. Treatment was inadequate when urea clearance was at 2.17 l/week/l body water (Kt/V of .67, DI_{mm} of 0.8) (35).

The conclusions from these two idependently designed but comparable studies are so similar and compelling as to mandate universal application of this knowledge, not only in prescribing short treatment, but in reporting dialysis results so that these can be compared on a world-wide basis for on-going analysis of the 'adequacy of dialysis' and for exploration of the areas not covered by the NCDS (34).

This brief historical review of gradually evolving bases for short adequate dialytic treatment suggests that by mid 1983, a fund of knowledge of the technical requirements and goals for treatment was sufficiently established to permit predictably successful entry into this realm.

REQUIREMENTS FOR ADEQUACY OF SHORT TREATMENTS

The essential criterion for the success of shortened dialysis therapy is adequate solute removal so that plasma concentrations remain at apparently non-toxic levels, i.e. sufficiently close to normal that further reduction will not decrease morbidity. Precisely what these levels are, or even which solutes are significant, has not been established. Nevertheless, stringent guidelines for avoiding definitely inadequate therapy do exist.

Modeling considerations for short dialysis

Indices based on the dialysis product (Kt) divided by a measure of patient size are useful. One such index, the Gotch-Sargent Kt/V, uses urea as a marker of low molecular weight solutes and V as body water (34, 36–38). Another index, the DI_{mm}, uses the *in vitro* clearance of vitamin B_{12} of the dialyzer as a surrogate of middle sized molecules and the

Two Compartment Dialysis Model

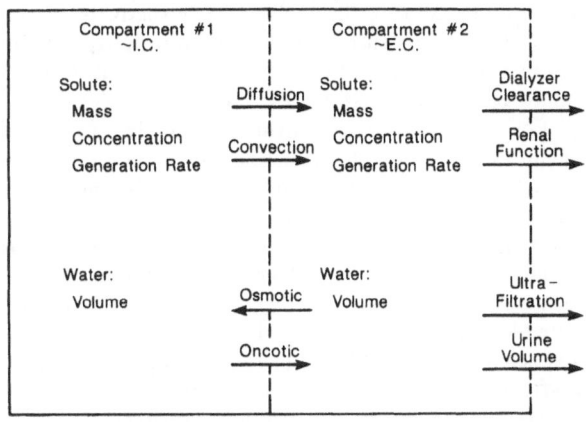

Figure 1. A two compartment dialysis model.

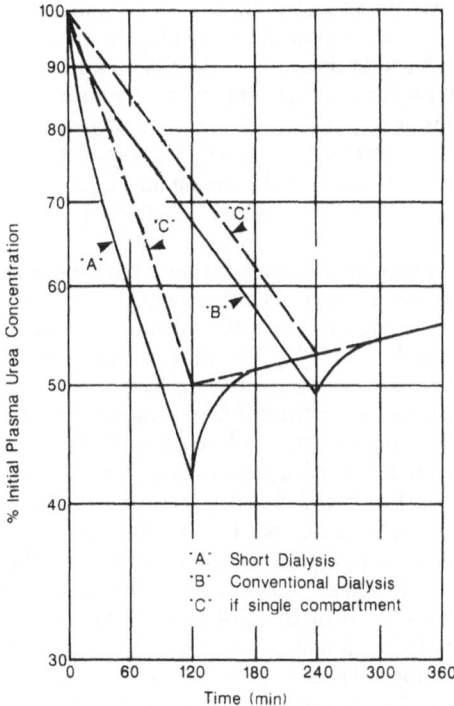

Figure 2. Example of plasma urea concentration during 4 h (line B) and 2 h (line A) dialyses of equivalent urea mass removal. Note the abrupt falls in concentration over the first 30 to 40 min of the dialysis and the rebounds at the end. Lines C depict the changes in concentration with time if the body behaved as a single pool.

body surface area as a measure of body size (16).

These indices consider the body as a single compartment. As will be shown, however, a single compartment model introduces errors when prescribing shortened dialysis treatment. For this purpose, the body's many compartments can best be approximated by a two compartment model, even when using dialyzers of modest performance (39, 40). The compartments can be loosely considered to be the intracellular and extracellular volumes. With ESRD treatment by UKM, neither the inclusion of the erythrocytes as a third compartment nor the division of extracellular into interstitial and plasma water introduce significant differences from the two compartment model (41, 42). Figure 1 exemplifies a two compartment approximation of a complex multicompartmental system used to model solute and water transfer during dialysis. Mass, concentration, volume, osmotic and oncotic forces, solute generation and apparent location of solute generation, as well as dialyzer clearance and ultrafiltration and residual renal function must be considered. Even when so simplified, it can be seen in Figure 2 that the pattern of plasma solute concentrations, lines A and B, differ significantly from those expected for a single compartment, which would be straight lines, C, on this semi-log graph. It can be seen that using dialyzers with sufficiently high clearances to accomplish shorter dialysis, depicted by curve A, intercompartmental solute transfer resistances induce more abrupt falls in plasma solute concentrations with the initiation of dialysis and greater rebounds after dialysis than with conventional dialysis, curve B. These differences are significant. For solute transfer from the intracellular space to the plasma to allow accessibility to the dialyzer for removal, a concentration gradient between these two spaces that is proportional to the rate of removal must be generated by lowering the plasma concentration by dialysis. Consequently, during dialysis, plasma concentrations are less than those of any compartment or of the mean body fluid by increasing amounts as dialysis efficiency rises. Since the rate of mass removal at any instant is the product of clearance and of the concurrent plasma solute concentration, less sol-

ute mass is removed during rapid dialysis than during slow dialysis at the same predialysis concentrations and Kt/V values. Therefore, Kt/V must be *increased* to assure equivalent mass removal.

The blood water clearances needed to achieve equivalent urea removal as dialysis time is abbreviated can be seen in Table 1. These values were generated by mathematical modeling using stepwise integration and verified both by observ-

Table 1. Effect of dialysis duration on urea clearance requirements for modeling adequate short treatment.

Dialysis duration (h)	Blood water urea clearance (ml/min) required for equivalent urea mass removal	Percent increase in minimal target Kt/V required compared to 4 h dialysis
4	169	
3	235	4.3
2	384	13.6

Dialyzer blood water clearances required for the same urea mass removal during dialyses of 3 and 2 h duration compared with one of 4 h. The 4 h clearance results in a Kt/V of 1.0 for a 70 Kg subject with a pcr of 1.0. The third column presents the minimal percent increase in target Kt/V values necessary to achieve the same solute mass removal as with the 4 h dialysis.

ing plasma solute concentrations over extended periods and by solute recovery in the dialysate (43). In Table 1 it can be seen that if a urea clearance of 169 ml/min for 4 h results in a Kt/V of 1.0 for a 70 Kg subject, a clearance of 235, not 225 ml/min is required for the same mass removal in a 3 h dialysis and a clearance of 384 not 338 ml/min is required for 2 h dialyses. In other words, the minimal target Kt/V for 3 h dialyses should be 1.05 and for 2 h dialyses, 1.14 at the same pcr.

Since creatinine and similar solutes have much lower intercompartmental transfer coefficients than urea (approximately 300 vs approximately 900 ml/min), this effect is more marked for them (41, 42). Therefore the target Kt/V values for urea should be increased even further as dialysis time shortens to assure equivalent mass removal of such solutes.

In comparing the pre- and postdialysis urea concentrations as a index of adequacy, as suggested by Jindal et al (44), it must be remembered that the more rapid the dialysis, the greater is the difference between the solute concentration measured in plasma drawn immediately at the end of dialysis and the mean body water concentration. Therefore, if a post/pre ratio of BUN of about 0.45 is indicative of adequacy for a 4 h dialysis, a ratio of about 0.42 would be necessary for a 3 h dialysis and about 0.38 for a 2 h treatment. The longer the delay in sampling the postdialysis blood the greater the equilibration and the more the ratio rises approaching that of a lower efficiency dialysis. For urea, equilibration is essentially complete after 30 min, but delaying that long to obtain the sample is impractical. It is more convenient to withdraw blood from the 'arterial' line within a minute after dialysis is stopped and change the target ratio appropriately.

Modeling treatment to assure adequate middle molecule removal need not be neglected. Since current dialyzers with sufficient urea clearances to meet the requirements of shortened dialysis have B_{12} clearances in the 50 to 100 ml/min range, a DI_{mm} of 1.0 can be relatively easily achieved.

Clearance considerations (K)

When modeling dialyses using Kt/V, errors in estimating any of these factors (K, t, and V) can cause a proportionate error in the product. The effective K_D or dialyzer clearance is particularly susceptible to error in estimation because it depends on blood flow, angioaccess recirculation, blood composition, dialysate flow, dialyzer membrane permeability, flow geometry and ultrafiltration rate.

Angioaccess recirculation

Any recirculation of blood in the angioaccess reduces the benefit of 'clearance' to the patient. Recirculation in the angioaccess reduces clearance according to the formula: Fractional reduction = $R/[R + C_A(1 - R)]/(C_A - C_V)$ (39). A convenient estimate of the effect of recirculation can be obtained from the equation: $K_E = K_M \cdot (1 - 1.05 \cdot R) \cdot (1 - C_V/C_A)$ where K_E = effective clearance, K_M = measured clearance, R = the decimal fraction of recirculation, C_V =

solute concentration leaving the dialyzer and C_A = solute concentration entering the dialyzer. Alternatively, if the systemic blood concentration (C_S) is known, K_E can be found by substituting C_S for C_A as the denominator of the standard clearance equation: $K_E = [C_AQ_i - C_V(Q_i - Q_U)]/C_S$. For large solutes the effect is small, but for small molecules such as urea, the reduction in clearance is approximately $3/4$ the percentage of recirculation. Recirculation percentage can be determined by measuring solute concentrations in the incoming blood, in the blood leaving the dialyzer and systemic blood which can be obtained from a separate blood vessel (preferably contralateral) or by slowing the blood flow to a speed at which no recirculation may be expected and then obtaining a sample from the 'arterial' line after 30 to 60 sec. The equation: $100(C_S - C_A)/(C_S - C_V)$ gives percent recirculation in the angioaccess.

Errors in measurement of whole blood flow

The 'arterial' whole blood flow may differ from that indicated by the meter or setting of the roller blood pump. Sources of error are: (1) miscalibration of the pump in the flow range used for shortened dialysis, (2) variations in the bore (inside diameter) of the pump tubing segment provided by the manufacturer and (3) the effect of the prepump subatmospheric pressure on the ability of the tubing to re-expand fully between rapid compressions by the pump rollers. The latter is especially important at the strongly negative (i.e. −200 mm Hg or lower) pressures often used to obtain high flows. The resulting decrement in blood flow can reach 25% of that indicated. Prepump pressure should be monitored by a gauge with adjustable alarm limits and the blood pump should be calibrated at typical pump speeds with fluid at body temperature at negative prepump pressures duplicating those used clinically. Removing the dialyzer from the circuit after clinical use and connecting the 'arterial' blood line to the joined dialysate lines is a convenient method of obtaining warm fluid at a controllable negative pressure for blood pump calibration in many dialyzing machines.

Effect of blood composition on clearance

The composition of the blood, especially the red blood cell (RBC) mass or hematocrit (Hct), affects dialyzer clearance. Manufacturers usually report *in vitro* aqueous clearances or whole blood clearances at a hematocrit of 25%. Perhaps this was appropriate in the past, but current and future patients should have higher hematocrits due to the availability of erythropoietin. With an increase of hematocrit only from 25% to 35%, actual clearance will be less because of: 1) physical interference with diffusive solute movement by the RBC's, 2) the RBC solute concentration compared to plasma (k) is less than 1.0) and 3) limitations of the rate at which some solutes can move from within the RBC into the plasma water where they can contribute to the concentration gradient which drives transmembrane flux (45). For urea, with its high RBC k of 0.859 and very rapid equilibration between

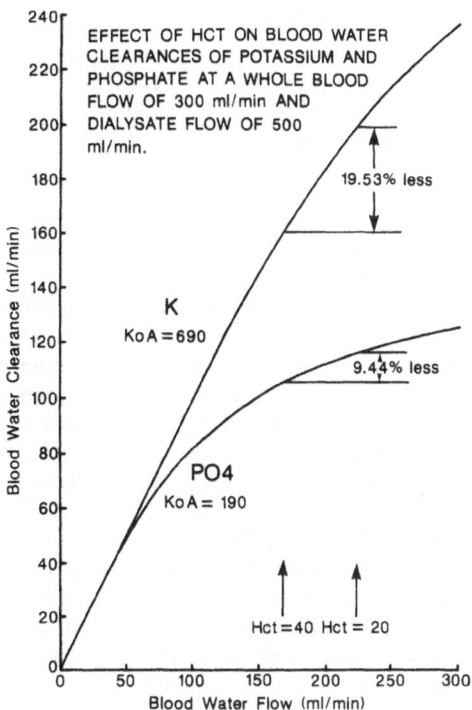

Figure 3. The effect of changes in hematocrit on the blood water clearances of potassium and inorganic phosphate.

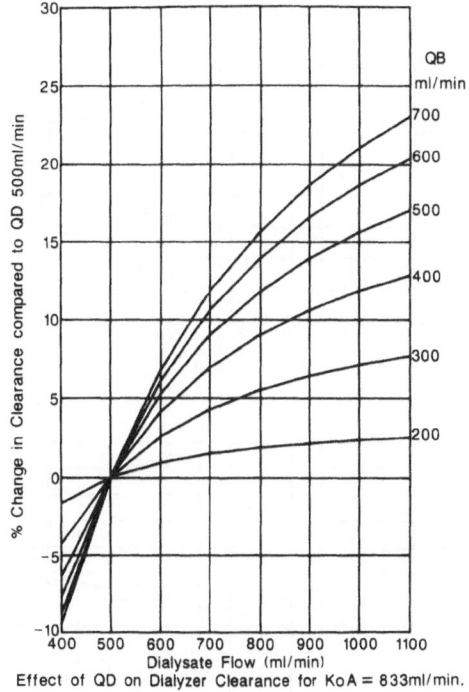

Figure 4. The effect of Q_D (dialysate flow) on urea clearances at different Q_B's (blood flows) in a dialyzer with a KoA of 833 ml/min for urea.

RBC's and plasma, the loss in clearance from these factors is only about 5%. However, with other solutes such as creatinine with a lower red cell solute concentration compared to plasma and a slower rate of RBC to plasma equilibration (k = 0.731, diffusion from RBC. = 4.4%/min), the effect can be 10% to 15% depending on dialyzer performance characteristics (46). Uremic solutes with major potential toxicities, such as potassium and inorganic phosphate, show negligible RBC to plasma diffusion. Should steady state predialysis hematocrit rise from 20% to 40%, at the same dialysis parameters, a decrease of about 19% in potassium dialysance and about 9% in phosphate clearance will result (Figure 3). Thus, steady state predialysis elevations of these blood solute concentrations would occur as hematocrit rises. For example, steady state predialysis serum potassium could rise from 6.0 to 6.95 mEq/l on this basis alone. During rapid dialysis and ultrafiltration, substantial increases in both intradialyzer and whole body hematocrit occur which exacerbate this effect.

When calculating a desired urea clearance based on the Kt/V ratio, it should be remembered that the original concept was based on the clearance of a volume of body water equal to the distribution space of urea three times a week at a pcr equal to about 1.0. Hence, the K of Kt/V should represent blood water urea clearance and not whole blood clearance. Blood water clearance (K_{H2O}) differs from whole blood clearance (K_{WB}) as a function of hematocrit (H), the ratio of the solute concentration in the RBC's compared to that in the plasma (k = 0.859 for urea) and the volume

occupied by the proteins in the plasma (about 7% or 0.0107 times the plasma protein concentration in g/dl) according to the equation, $K_{H2O} = 0.93\ K_{WB}\ (kH + 1 - H)$. For *urea alone*, the equation, $K_{H2O} = 0.9\ K_{WB}$ can be used without introducing errors of clinical importance.

Effect of dialysis fluid flow

The effect of dialysis fluid flow on clearance depends on the magnitude of the dialysis fluid flow, the blood flow and the mass transfer coefficient × area product (KoA) of the dialyzer for that particular solute and blood flow. Figure 4 shows the percentage change in clearance that would occur by changing the dialysis solution flow from 500 ml/min for different blood flows assuming the KoA of the dialyzer is 833 ml/min which is representative for urea transfer by the best of dialyzers currently available. These curves were generated from the equations for the interrelationship of clearance, Q_B, Q_D and KoA developed by Michaels (47) and expanded by Gotch and his committee (48) and assume that the KoA value remains constant with increasing Q_D. However, early work by Miller et al (49) indicated that with some dialyzers, increasing dialysis fluid flow rate reduces the overall mass transfer resistance coefficient. The magnitude of mass transfer augmentation with increased dialysis solution flow with modern hollow fiber dialyzers has not been thoroughly assessed. This effect would vary widely depending on the specific dialyzer, but could result in more than the expected improvement in clearance with increased dialysis solution flow rates.

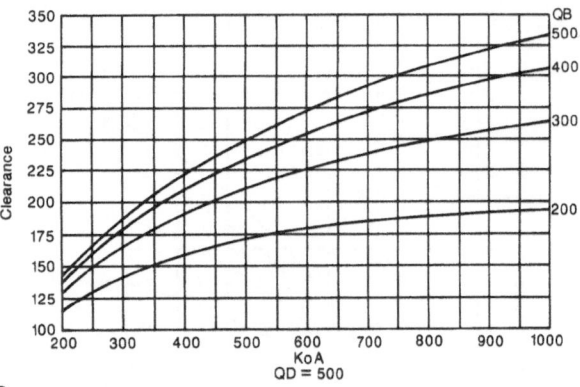

a

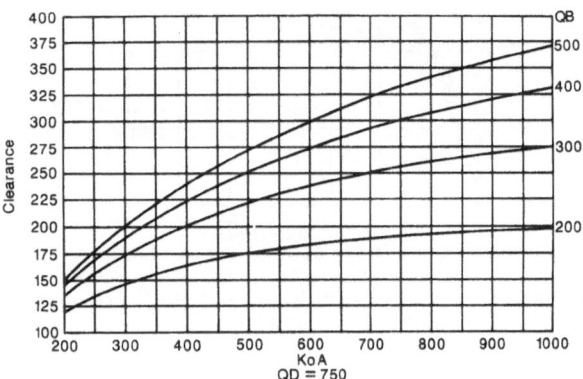

b

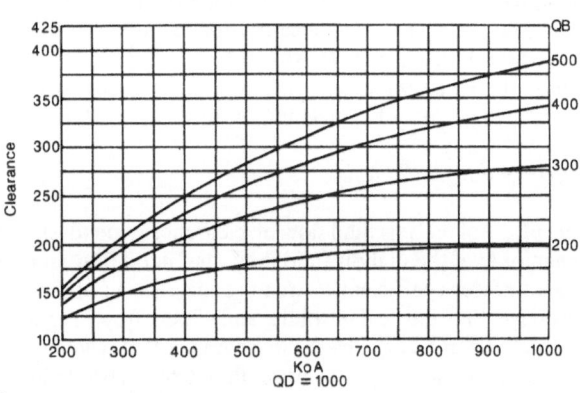

c

Figure 5. The effect of KoA on clearances at various blood flows. All parameters are in ml/min. (a) at a Q_D of 500 ml/min (b) at a Q_D of 750 ml/min (c) at a Q_D of 1000 ml/min.

KoA, Q_B, Q_D relationships

Figures 5 a, b and c show the effective water clearances (K_E) that are expected in counter-current dialyzers on the ordinates, with overall mass transfer coefficient × area product (KoA) on the abscissa at dialysis fluid flows (Q_D) of 500, 750 and 1000 ml/min and at effective blood flow rates as labeled on the right margin (all values are ml/min). These curves were generated using the equations for counter current sys-

tems developed by Michaels (47). These are:

$$KoA = [Q_B/(1 - Z)] \ln[((D/Q_D) - 1)/((D/Q_B) - 1)]$$
if $Q_B = Q_D$, then $KoA = D/[1 - (D/Q_B)]$
$$D = Q_B[1 - \exp((KoA/Q_B)(1 - Z))]/[Z - \exp((KoA/Q_B)(1 - Z))]$$
if $Q_B = Q_D$, then $D = KoA/[(KoA/Q_B) + 1]$
$$Z = Q_B/Q_D.$$

D is equivalent to clearance when $C_{Di} = 0$, which it usually is in counter current dialyses.

The effective flow, Q_E, is the rate of flow of that portion of blood water containing the solute that is accessible for transmembrane transfer. For urea $Q_E = Q_{BH_2}0$. For other solutes that diffuse through the RBC membrane slowly or not at all, Q_E is less than Q_{BH20} and equals plasma volume minus its solid content. The effective water clearance, K_E, is that volume of the effective flow, Q_E, that is cleared of the solute. It should be computed using C_{Bo} ('venous') values of plasma separated from the RBC's before significant equilibration can occur. The clearance calculated by the standard equations will be in terms of whole blood clearance only if the RBC's are separated from plasma after equilibration.

Using these figures, or the equations from which they are derived, the clearance that can be expected from a dialyzer at specified blood and dialysis fluid flow rates can be found by determining the apparent KoA for a known clearance, blood (or effective blood) flow and dialysis fluid flow. Then by using the graph or equation for D, the unknown new clearance can be determined using the computed KoA and the new flows.

For urea, the Q_E generally exceeds 90% of the whole blood flow. Hence, when converting from clearances to KoA and back to a new clearance at a different blood flow, whole blood flow can be used without introducing appreciable errors if ultrafiltration rates are low.

These graphs can be used in planning shortened dialysis because they present the clearances that can be expected when using a particular dialyzer with increased blood or dialysis fluid flows or both. It should be noted that particularly at high blood flow rates the rise in clearance is only a fraction of the increase in blood flow.

Dialyzer variations

A possible source of error in estimating the true dialyzer clearance is variations in clearances between lots and even within lots of dialyzers due to minor variations in membranes and flow geometry.

Ultrafiltration

Ultrafiltration augments the removal of small, highly diffusive solutes in a minor way, but large solute clearance increases, depending on sieving coefficient, nearly equally to the ultrafiltration rate (see hemofiltration and hemodiafiltration).

Residual renal clearance (K_r)

Although having no direct effect on dialyzer clearance per se, residual renal clearance decreases the dialyzer clearance required for prescription of shortened but adequate dialysis (32, 33, 35). Teschan et al (35) provide an expression for thrice weekly dialysis that is equivalent to Kt/V (tot) = K_dt (l/min)/V + 3,36 K_r (ml/min)/V. Gotch (36) presents the equations Kt/V (tot) = K_dt/V + 5.9 K_r for thrice weekly dialysis and Kt/V (tot) = K_dt/V + 10.1 K_r for twice weekly dialysis.

By computing the actual mass of urea removed during a dialysis in which V is 40 l and K_dt/V equals 1.0, compensating for the effect of intercompartmental transfer resistance, water loss and generation rate on the mean body concentration at the end of dialysis, computing the mean plasma concentration during the interdialytic period and the time that K_r acts, it can be shown that the expression is close to: Kt/V (tot) = K_dt/V + 4.0 K_r/V for thrice weekly dialysis. In other words, each 1.0 ml/min of K_r is equivalent to about one tenth of the total urea clearance needed and so reduces the required K_dt. Similarly, if K_r is 2 ml/min, dialysis time could be safely reduced from 240 min to 192 min with a conventional dialyzer and blood flow (i.e. providing a blood water clearance of 166.7 ml/min for a 40 l V).

Treatment duration considerations (t)

When relying on Kt/V for modeling and prescription, time on dialysis (t) critically affects the Kt product and should be as accurate as possible. Initiating treatment with a low blood flow, reducing flow during dialysis or terminating the treatment early will reduce the time of effective dialysis. The shorter the time prescribed for dialysis, the greater is the potential effect of reducing duration by even a few minutes.

Because of the flattening of the K_d vs Q_B curve as Q_B increases, and because of the effect of intercompartmental transfer resistances, the relationship between Q_B and duration of treatment is strongly alinear for equivalent mass removal. Figure 6 depicts this dependency of treatment time (t) on Q_B utilizing a highly permeable circuit with a KoA of 1250 ml/min for ultrashort treatment as described by von Albertini et al (50, 51). With such a high efficiency circuit, a 20% decrease in Q_B from 500 to 400 ml/min increases the required time for equivalent mass removal by only 10%, whereas at low Q_B, i.e. at 250 ml/min, a 20% decrease in blood flow to 200 ml/min would require a 20% increase in treatment time.

Effect of volume of distribution (V)

The same considerations apply concerning 'V' with shortened dialysis as with conventional dialysis. The patient's volume of urea distribution can differ significantly from the average value of 0.58 × body weight. If the patient is very obese, it can be as low as 45%; if lean and heavily muscled, it

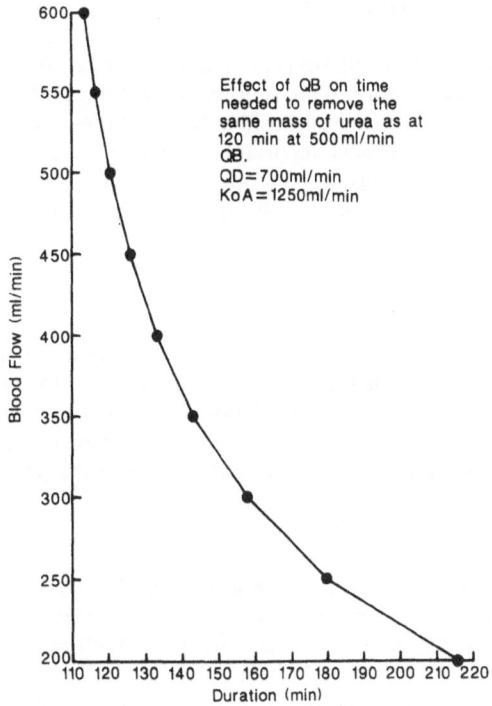

Effect of QB on Dialysis Time

Effect of QB on time needed to remove the same mass of urea as at 120 min at 500 ml/min QB.
QD = 700 ml/min
KoA = 1250 ml/min

Figure 6. The effect of whole blood flow on dialysis time with a highly efficient circuit.

can be as high as 65%. Volume can be determined by methods as described by Gotch (36) or by Farrell (37). An actual determination of V could lead to a safe reduction of dialysis time for some patients. If an unrealistic value for V is estimated or computed, it should be rejected and sources of error sought.

Effect of protein catabolic rate/weight (pcr)

As with conventional dialysis, pcr very strongly influences the Kt/V required to maintain urea levels within acceptable limits. Careful monitoring of pre- and postdialysis BUN levels, corrected for rebound, and exact knowledge of K, t, and V all assist in computing and monitoring pcr accurately (36, 37). As we have emphasized, urea kinetic modeling of short dialysis is subject to many errors and discrepancies. Therefore, attention to accepted BUN concentrations such as the mid-week predialysis concentration (CO_2) and the time-averaged concentration (TAC urea) is especially important (34).

Some of the effects described above are relatively small, and taken singly may not be clinically significant. However, they may be additive and may interact to assist or hinder achieving an adequate short dialysis. They should not be neglected.

CLINICAL CONSIDERATIONS

In addition to the physical considerations which affect adequate solute removal in shortened treatment described above, there are clinical considerations. Of these, hypotension is by far the most important. Others are the possibility of reverse ultrafiltration, problems with the removal of other important solutes and the question of dialysis disequilibrium.

Hypotension

Hypotension, the most probable cause of failure of shortened dialysis, is the result of the patient's inability to tolerate the intravascular volume depletion resulting from the rapid removal of excess fluid gained in the interdialytic interval. Several strategies can be applied to ameliorate this problem.

Automatic UF control

A dialysis fluid preparation machine which provides automatic ultrafiltration control is useful in conventional dialysis and even more so in shortened dialysis. With higher flux dialyzers (KUF>10.0 ml/h/mm Hg TMP), they become essential. With manual transmembrane pressure control, ultrafiltration rates fluctuate. Although the average UF rate may be corrected, periods of high UF result in acute volume depletion which exceeds the poor compensatory cardiovascular response of uremic patients resulting in hypotension (27, 30). A programmed, more linear ultrafiltration rate throughout provides better cardiovascular stability (52).

Dialysate modification

Bicarbonate
We consider it well established that bicarbonate based dialysate is an absolute requirement for short, high efficiency treatment where K_d urea (ml/min) is greater than six times V in liters (36).

Sodium
Another technique for providing better cardiovascular stability is the manipulation of sodium concentration of the dialysis solution. Dialysate sodium concentration at or above 140 mEq/l promotes better vascular refilling (53). The tendency of dialysate sodium concentrations above 145 mEq/l to induce excessive thirst and interdialytic weight gain can be countered by progressively decreasing sodium concentration during the course of the dialysis (54, 55). Many of the newer dialyzers available for high flux dialysis have a sodium modeling feature available. Sequential sodium concentration modeling of dialysate is not as important a factor in maintaining vascular stability as is bicarbonate dialysate at a sodium concentration of 140 mEq/l (53).

Calcium
With very high flux procedures such as hemodiafiltration, it may be necessary to increase the dialysate calcium concentration to offset the additional convective loss of calcium. Plasma ionized calcium concentration is critically important in cardiac performance and systemic vascular resistance during dialysis (56–61). Increasing the dialysate calcium concentration to approximately 4.2 mEq/l increases cardiovascular stability (50, 51).

Purity
Pyrogen free dialysate may play a role in preventing hypotension since pyrogens, even in concentrations too low to evoke chills and other obvious symptomatology, may result in vasodilation when it is critical to increase systemic vascular resistance in response to acute hypovolemia.

Temperature
Lowering dialysate temperature to about 35.5 to 36° C from the usual 37 to 38° C markedly reduces the incidence of hypotension (62, 63). At these temperatures there is no blood to dialysate thermal gradient in uremic patients and clearances are not adversely affected by slightly 'cool' dialysate. Thermo-osmotic diffusion blockade could occur only when dialysate is warmer than blood (64). A much more unfavorable consequence of dialysate warmer than blood is that positive heat exchange occurs favoring peripheral vasodilation when it is least desirable.

Convective transfer

A convective flow of approximately 70 ml/min as was obtained with the earliest clinical application of hemofiltration has enhanced cardiovascular stability compared to conventional hemodialysis (65, 66). The exact mechanism for this is still obscure, but it is clinically supported by the increased stability of the blood pressure observed during hemofiltration and isolated (dry) ultrafiltration procedures at rates of fluid loss that could not be tolerated during hemodialysis (27, 30). Comparing hemofiltration and hemodialysis at equal urea clearance, at equal sodium concentration in dialysate or replacement solution, better intratreatment maintenance and less posttreatment rebound of inulin space occurs with hemofiltration, suggesting better preservation of extracellular volume (52). Catecholamine release and rise in systemic vascular resistance are higher with hemofiltration than with hemodialysis regardless of the buffer base used (27, 67). For these reasons, rapid treatment strategies which employ a convective flow approaching that of hemofiltration are more likely to achieve the vascular stability required to resist the ultrafiltration-induced hypotension of shortened treatment (50, 68). With hemodiafiltration procedures utilizing convective flows over 80 ml/min, fluid losses in excess of 2 l/h can be routinely maintained until the patient reaches his 'dry' weight (69).

Reverse (dialysate to blood) ultrafiltration

The use of dialyzers with higher ultrafiltration coefficients at the high blood and dialysate flows typically required for

PRESSURE RELATIONSHIPS ALONG LENGTH OF DIALYZERS

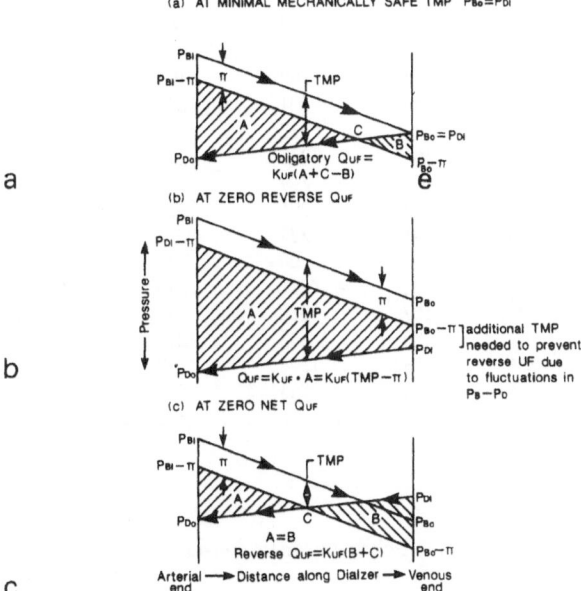

Figure 7. Blood and dialysate compartment pressure relationships along the length of a dialyzer at selected ultrafiltration conditions. For clarity, the changes in the blood compartment pressure and in the oncotic pressure as hemoconcentration and blood viscosity change along the dialyzer are not shown. (In the realm where ultrafiltration rates are in ml/min and blood flows are in hundreds of ml/min, the effects are small). (a) At minimal mechanically safe TMP, i.e. $P_{Bo} = P_{Di}$. The effect of the hydraulic pressure gradient between the blood and dialysate compartments is reduced by the oncotic pressure, π. In area A, blood to dialysate ultrafiltration occurs. In area B, the flux is from dialysate to blood. In region C, periodic reversal of the effective blood compartment pressure, $P_B - \pi$, to dialysate pressure, P_D due to blood pump and dialysate flow balancing valve action result in brief periods of reverse water flux equal to KUF $\times$ C if integrated over time. (b) At zero reverse Q_{UF}, the TMP necessary to prevent all reverse flux depends not only on oncotic pressure, π, at the venous end of the dialyzer, but also on the magnitude of the blood pump and dialysate pressure fluctuations existing at the venous end of the dialyzer. (c) At zero net Q_{UF}, dialysate pressure is such that reverse ultrafiltration, area B, is balanced by blood to dialysate ultrafiltration, area A. The small amount of reverse ultrafiltration that occurs at C is compensated for by a small lowering of P_D. Although there is no net ultrafiltration, reverse flux equals KUF $\times$ (B + C).

shortened treatment forces a difficult clinical dilemma. Either an obligatory net ultrafiltration rate that may exceed the patient's requirement or movement of dialysate into the blood by reverse ultrafiltration must occur. Based on equations developed by Miller et al (70) the mean TMP existing in the dialyzer at which the membrane at the 'venous' end of the dialyzer just becomes back pressured (i.e. $P_{Di} = P_{Bo}$) is a function of the blood and dialysate flows and resistances. This mean TMP is called the minimum mechanically safe TMP since if that pressure is not exceeded, the membranes

of certain dialyzers, of any configuration but especially flat plate dialyzers, are forced together obstructing blood flow. Under this condition, dialysate may enter the blood undetected through a membrane defect (Figure 7). The *obligatory ultrafiltration* is the UFR that occurs at that TMP (Figure 7a). The obligatory ultrafiltration rate of various dialyzers is presented in Table 2.

Although at the minimum mechanically safe TMP, the membrane is not hydraulically back pressured, 1) the plasma oncotic pressure withdraws fluid from the dialysate at all points along the dialyzer length where the local TMP does not exceed it (area B in Figure 7a), and 2) the pulsatile action of the blood pump generates a back and forth surging of fluid across the membrane at those points along the dialyzer length where the local dialysate pressure intermittently exceeds effective blood pressure. This effect cannot be well illustrated in Figure 7, but occurs in the vicinity of the points marked C.

These two phenomena modify the obligatory ultrafiltration based on the minimum mechanically safe TMP and imply that to avoid reverse ultrafiltration the TMP should be maintained above the minimum mechanically safe TMP plus the oncotic pressures at the 'venous' end of the dialyzer (20 to 30 mm Hg), Figure 7b. To these must be added the uncertain amount of additional pressure which depends on blood pump pressure curves and the hydrodynamic buffering of the system just described. When the clinical decision requires reduction of net ultrafiltration to zero, back filtration and forward filtration fluxes are equal (Figure 7c, A = B). These fluxes are equal to: $KUF[(P_{Bi} - P_{Bo}) + (P_{Di} - P_{Do})]/8$ ml/h plus the effects of pulsatile flow. Schmidt et al (71) report that with a highly permeable polysulfone membrane dialyzer, these fluxes are about 20 ml/min, *in vivo*.

During hemofiltration or hemodiafiltration, the TMP required to prevent reverse ultrafiltration is consistently exceeded even when net weight loss is minimal. However, with short hemodialysis, the possibility of dialysate to blood transfer always exists to variable degrees depending on the dialyzer and blood and dialysate pressures, particularly under the conditions depicted in Figures 7a and 7c, in much greater amounts than in conventional hemodialysis because of the high blood flows, dialysate pressures and membrane permeabilities. Reverse UF can also occur under conditions depicted in Figure 7b if the TMP is inadequate to compensate for dynamic pressure fluctuations in the blood and dialysate compartments. These possibilities generate additional requirements for dialysate purity.

Phosphate removal

Adequate removal of phosphate by dialysis alone has never been accomplished with conventional hemodialysis. With newer, more permeable dialyzers with considerably higher phosphate clearances, removal still is not adequate unless dialyses twice as long as needed for urea removal are prescribed. For example, in a study of phosphate removal with shortened high efficiency treatments, only by doubling the

Table 2. In Vivo characteristics of selected high flux dialyzers.

Manufacturer/ distributor	Physical properties			KUF^a	Oblig. QUF^b	Whole blood urea clearances at Q_B (ml/min)			
	Dialyzer	Area m^2	Membrane			200	300	400	450
Hospal	3000-S	1.2	AN69	13	280	152	180	195*	215*
Hospal	Filtral	1.15	AN69	20.5	518	156	201	243	249
Gambro	120-H	1.2	Cu	4.5	63	172	212	236	245*
Gambro	10 N-5	1.1	Cu	5.2	−23	165	225	253*	263*
Asahi	PAN-200	1.4	PAN	42	550	164	199	229	243
CD Medical	DuoFlux	1.4	CA	23	281	162	201	227	232
Toray	B 1–2.0	2.05	PMMA	45	2,500	175*	227	255	265
Fresenius	F-60	1.25	PS	37	1,054	164	200	232	237
Fresenius	F-80	1.9	PS	55	3,000	178	231	270	285
Gambro	180-M	1.8	Cu	5.4	−28	167	210	241	253*
Gambro	180-H	1.8	Cu	7.6	49	180	233	271	287*
Travenol	CA-170	1.7	CA	9.1	264	178	227	259	272*
Travenol	CA-210	2.1	CA	10.3	373	184	244	290	311*

* Extrapolated.
[a] ml/h/mm Hg.
[b] ml/h at Q_B = 300 ml/min.
Q_D = 500 ml/min, Mean Hct = 35 except F-60 (Hct = 40).
AN69, PAN = Polyacrylonitrile, Cu = Cuprophan, CA = Cellulose acetate, PMMA = Polymethylmethacrylate, PS = Polysulfone, Oblig = Obligatory.
The manufacturer or distributor, name, surface area, membrane material, coefficient of ultrafiltration (KUF), obligatory ultrafiltration (i.e. ultrafiltration existing when $P_{Bo} = P_{Di}$) and typical whole blood urea clearances at 200, 300, 400 and 450 ml/min blood flows for dialyzers commonly considered for shortened dialysis at this time.

length (Kt/V≥2) of a high flux hemodiafiltration procedure that achieved otherwise adequate dialysis in only 2 h, could more than one gram of phosphate be removed (72).

Although the phosphate clearances of dialyzers suitable for shortened dialysis are much higher than those of dialyzers commonly used for conventional hemodialysis, the ratios of phosphate clearance to urea clearance do not significantly differ from conventional dialyzers. Furthermore, this ratio decreases with increasing blood and dialysate flow rates (72). Therefore, modeling short dialysis based on Kt urea does not remove more phosphate mass than conventional dialysis with the same type of membrane does, and may actually remove less. The interaction of intercompartmental transfer resistance with dialyzer clearance for phosphate further exacerbates the problem. Short, high efficiency treatments do not solve or even improve the phosphate balance problem

This problem in total mass removed with shortened dialysis will occur with other solutes with low intercompartmental mass transfer coefficients, including RBC to plasma diffusion coefficients, or when clearances are more membrane and less flow limited than with urea.

Dialysis disequilibrium syndrome

Shortened high efficiency treatments should be considered only for patients who are fully stabilized on an adequate dialysis program with acceptable control of BUN level.

These treatments are not proposed for initial dialyses or for critically ill patients in which this application has been insufficiently documented. Severe central nervous system (CNS) symptomatology was originally ascribed to rapid dialysis causing osmotic disequilibrium with fluid shifts (13). In patients stabilized on short dialysis with bicarbonate dialysate, CNS disequilibrium symptomatology has not been reported during hemodialysis treatments of less than 168 min at dialyzer urea clearances of 279 ml/min (73). It has also not been reported in 90 to 120 min high flux hemodiafiltration with urea clearances of up to 514 ml/min (69). With routine use of the latter technique at mean urea clearances of 407 ml/min, and a mean urea concentration fall of 18 mmol/l (51 mg/dl) in an average treatment time of 115 min no evidence of CNS disequilibrium was noted (50). Recently, the inability to demonstrate any pre- to post-treatment brain swelling by computerized axial tomograms and the lack of any adverse effect on power spectrum analyzed electroencephalograms during a 4 h conventional hemodialysis and a 3 h high flux hemodialysis (HFD), each resulting in a fall in BUN of 16 mmol/l (45 mg/dl) was reported. In this study, a smaller decrement in pre – post fall in serum osmolality occurred with hemodiafiltration (HDF) due to a high sodium re-infusion solution (74). No experimental animal studies exist in which the current technologies have been appropriately applied to simulate reasonably this clinical experience.

EQUIPMENT AND SUPPLIES

Because of the higher membrane permeabilities, blood flows, blood circuit pressures, and rates of ultrafiltration required for shortened treatment, and the possibility of back filtration the equipment and supplies may differ from those for conventional dialysis.

Equipment

Water treatment system

Essentially sterile and pyrogen-free water meeting AAMI standards for solutes must be consistently supplied (see Chapter 7).

Bicarbonate concentrate preparation

Should acceptable concentrate not be commercially available, a mixing and distribution system that consistently provides sterile concentrate at the correct solute concentrations and pH is necessary.

Dialysate monitoring and delivery apparatus

The apparatus should be capable of delivering bicarbonate dialysis solution at positive pressures equal to the expected mean blood compartment pressure (i.e. ≥250 mm Hg). At this pressure, dialysate flow, fluid balancing and dialysate mixing functions should not be adversely affected. If reverse ultrafiltration is anticipated or if the dialysis solution is to be infused it must undergo bacterial and pyrogen filtration. Dialysate flow rate in excess of 700 ml/min is recommended (see Figure 4). Continuous pH monitoring of the finished dialysis fluid is recommended. Automatic ultrafiltration control is required. There must be rapid and accurate response to fluctuations in UF requirement or dialysate pressure. The blood pump must be capable of sustained, accurate delivery of high flows for a prolonged period of time without significant reduction in its useful life. There should be a pre-pump pressure monitor with alarm limits, reading to −250 mm Hg and capable of stopping the blood pump upon alarm. If marked hemoconcentration is expected, as in hemofiltration (HF) and HDF, an alarmed, predialyzer blood pressure monitor should be present.

Heparin pump

The heparin infusion line should join the blood line after the blood pump, in the positive pressure region. The heparin pump must be capable of delivering accurately against pressures as high as 1000 mm Hg. If the duration of the treatment is to be 2.5 h or less, consideration should be given to increasing the initial bolus of heparin slightly and not continuously infusing heparin. If this approach is used, the heparin line should be securely clamped to prevent leakage of blood.

Continuous weighing scales

Continuous recordings of body weight are highly desirable for independent verification of the automatic ultrafiltration control.

Dialyzer reuse equipment

Appropriate equipment will be required if reuse is contemplated. This procedure may fall under both national and state regulations.

Supplies

Blood tubing sets

Blood tubing sets including the connections to the dialyzer, heparin reservoir, monitors and access needles must possess the structural integrity to resist disruption or leaks at pressures from −250 to +1000 mm Hg. Other requirements are for prepump, postpump and postdialyzer drip chambers. These should be designed so that the blood may enter the chamber very near the blood-air interface and still retain a volume of air above the interface by which pressures can be monitored and the pulsatile flow be damped. The blood pumping segment should have a wall of such resiliency that blood pump output is not compromised by negative pre-pump pressures more than can be compensated for by simple calibrations. The heparin infusion line should be post-blood pump to prevent aspiration of excess heparin or air.

Angioaccess needles

Fifteen gauge needles generally suffice for blood flows up to 400 ml/min, but 14 gauge needles may be needed at higher blood flows and hematocrits. The needles should be as thin walled and as short as possible since pressure drop through a tube at any particular flow is an inverse function of the fourth power of the bore and a direct function of the first power of the length and of fluid vicosity. Angioaccess needles with both end and side holes ('Back eyes') are helpful in maintaining flow. For the same reason, the small bore tubing that connects the needle itself to the blood line should be as short as possible and of the greatest feasible internal diameter.

Dialyzers

Most dialyzers used for 'conventional' 4 h dialysis have been designed to function at blood flows less than 300 ml/min with urea clearances below 200 ml/min. Because of their relatively small surface areas (about 1.0 m^2) and less permeable membranes (needed for UF control), their clearances do not increase enough with higher blood or dialysate flow rates to allow shortening dialysis time. Dialyzers suitable for short dialysis generally have larger surface areas or greatly increased permeabilities to solutes and water or both. Although they do not function in an outstanding manner at low

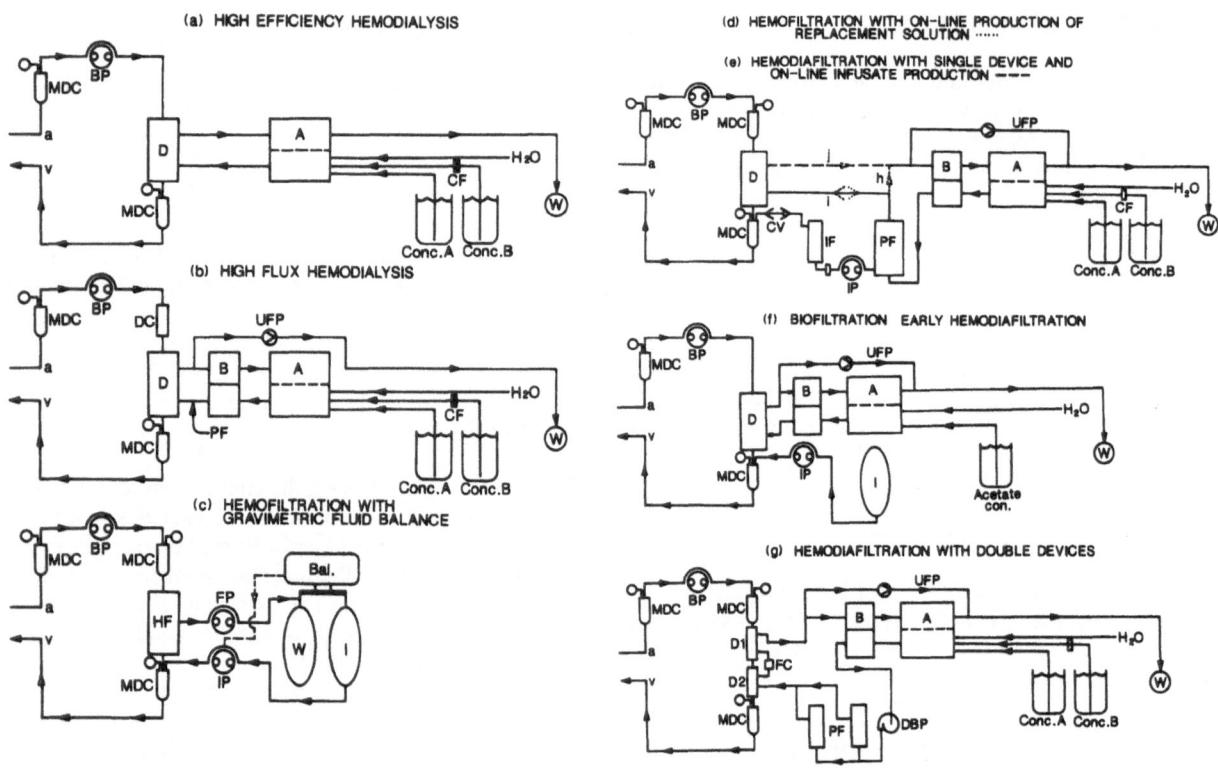

Figure 8. Schematic representations of blood and dialysate circuits for HED, HFD, HF and HDF and variations as labeled. Abbreviations are: a = 'arterial' vascular access, MDC = monitored drip chamber, BP = blood pump, D = dialyzer, v = 'venous' access, A = dialysate preparation and monitoring apparatus, H_2O = purified water inlet, conc A = acidified concentrate, conc B = bicarbonate concentrate, CF = concentrate filter, W = waste. The heparin infusion site (not indicated) is postblood pump if continuous infusion is used rather than single or multiple injections. (a) High Efficiency Hemodialysis with bicarbonate dialysate and manual control of ultrafiltration rate through TMP adjustment. D is a highly efficient hemodialyzer with a KUF below 10 ml/h/mm Hg. (b) High Flux Hemodialysis. Abbreviations are as above plus: B = volume balancing module matching dialysate inflow and outflow by volumetric metering or integration of flow rates so that the dialysate pressure changes to match ultrafiltration to the amount withdrawn from the dialysate circuit by the ultrafiltration pump, UFP. PF = location of a pyrogen filter as in Figure 8g. (c) Hemofiltration with gravimetric fluid replacement metering mechanism. HF = hemofilter, FP = filtrate pump (which generally operates at a constant rate), Bal = mechanism to sum weight of waste, W, and infusate, I, bags and control the infusate pump, IP, so that infusate volume equals filtrate minus desired net weight loss. (d) Hemofiltration using on-line infusion fluid generation. For hemofiltration, line 'h' is present and line 'j' is absent so that dialysate bypasses the hemofilter, 'D', and ultrafiltrate flows through line 'i'. PF = pyrogen filter, IP = infusion pump, IF = infusate filters, CV = check valve (e) Hemodiafiltration with single device and on-line infusate production. Line 'h' is absent and dialysate flow is through lines 'i' then 'j'. Ideally, all dialysate passes through a pyrogen filter as in Figure 8g. (f) Biofiltration and early hemodiafiltration. Fluid balance is achieved by adjusting ultrafiltrate pump to match infusate pump rate plus desired weight loss. Dialysate preparation apparatus, 'A', was, on occasion, a 40 l tank; the flow balance mechanism, 'B', was, on occasion a rigid tank containing a bladder of dialysate. (g) Hemodiafiltration with double devices. Flow controller, FC, generates a large difference between the dialysate pressures in devices D_2 and D_1 so that approximately 100 ml/min of ultrafiltration occurs in device D_1 which is replaced (minus the desired weight loss programmed by the ultrafiltrate pump, UFP) in device D_2 by reverse flux. Dialysate booster pump, DBP, assists the dialysate flow through the pyrogen filters, PF, and the flow controller. Both D_1 and D_2 contribute to diffusive mass transfer.

blood flow rates, they can provide urea clearances of 225 to 300 ml/min with blood flows in excess of 400 ml/min (Table 2). They presently cost two to three times as much as the conventional dialyzers encouraging their reuse.

TECHNIQUES FOR SHORTENED DIALYSIS

Several different technologies have been applied in order to achieve the high clearances and improved vascular stability

required for shortening of treatment time. The ultimate validation of a short treatment strategy requires the demonstration of solute removal equivalent to adequate conventional treatment and careful evaluation of patient outcome over several years. At this time, deficiencies in these areas exist. It is apparent that with any technology shorter times necessitate higher solute fluxes and net ultrafiltration rates. Thus all are, in a sense, equally 'high flux' therapies. In this section 'high flux' will refer to those strategies which cause or permit a much higher transmembrane flux of blood water than that required to achieve ultrafiltration to 'dry weight'. The techniques currently available for short treatments are high efficiency hemodialysis (HED), high flux hemodialysis (HFD), hemofiltration (HF) and hemodiafiltration (HDF). The essentials of these circuits are schematically presented in Figure 8.

High efficiency hemodialysis (HED)

HED is the logical extension of the gradual evolution toward shortened treatment time extensively described in this chapter and of the successful results obtained in group III of the NCDS who received treatment at Kt/V values of approximately 1.0 in approximately 200 min using large surface area dialyzers and conventional acetate delivery systems (33). The essential requirements are conventional cellulosic membrane dialyzers capable of high urea clearances at high blood flows having ultrafiltration rates less than 10 ml/h/mm Hg TMP, bicarbonate based dialysate, blood lines suitable for higher pressures and angioaccess needles suitable for high blood flows (Figure 8a). Keshaviah, Collins and co-workers (75) at the Regional Kidney Disease Program in Minneapolis carefully studied this approach, achieving a mean treatment time of 2.75 h at a mean Kt/V of 1.2. They reported 10 month's experience with 120 patients so treated. It is believed that they currently apply this therapy to over 300 patients and their total experience now greatly exceeds that of the entire NCDS. They have carefully observed intratreatment symptoms and found no evidence whatsoever that high solute flux caused disequilibrium. Although solute mass removal studies were not reported their modeling criteria, blood solute concentration control and ongoing morbidity and psychological assessments established beyond reasonable doubt that by current standards their treatment is adequate. Control of fluid removal presented problems initially, leading to routine use of chair scales, and later, dialysate delivery systems with volumetric control of ultrafiltration. Despite their reported use to date of conventional membranes, they have expressed concern regarding sterility and nonpyrogenicity requirements for bicarbonate dialysate (76). Adequate solute removal by this technique has been confirmed in a small carefully controlled clinical study.(72).

An interesting variation of technology for HED was described by Rotellar et al (77, 78) of Barcelona who divided total Q_B of 500 ml/min and Q_D of 1000 ml/min to perfuse in parallel two 2.5 m^2 dialyzers, each under conventional conditions. Bicarbonate dialysate containing 5 to 10 g/l glucose to prevent 'disequilibrium' and 2.5 mEq/l potassium to prevent 'muscular discomfort' is used. Whole blood urea and phosphate clearances were 436 and 308 ml/min respectively. The therapy is applied to highly selected patients in a 3 × 2 h, a 2 × 3 h, or a single 6 h weekly session depending on residual renal function and dietary compliance. Reported solute control, stable neurophysiologic function and estimated Kt/V indicate that the 3 × 2 h schedule is adequate at one to two years' experience.Values for pcr were not given, but diet was described as 'free' (77, 78).

A brief referral to Table 1 giving dialyzer whole blood urea clearances and Table 2 summarizing clearances required for shortened adequate dialysis reveals an interesting possibility. It can be seen that certain mass produced, conventional Cuprophan dialyzers of high quality are capable of surprisingly high urea clearances at high Q_B. Even when corrected for blood water clearance some of these inexpensive dialyzers can provide adequate shortened treatment for a large percentage of elderly and female dialysis patients with low lean body mass and urea volumes.

On the other hand, to provide a Kt/V of >1.05 for a 'standard', 70 Kg patient with urea V of 40.6 l in 180 min a blood water urea clearance of 235 ml/min is required. Table 2 also indicates that very few dialyzers will provide this clearance, even at unrecirculated blood flows of 400 ml/min. Thus, even the simplest.of the short treatment technologies is not necessarily easy to achieve. There is no known reason for this treatment to provide vascular stability superior to conventional bicarbonate dialysis, and it seems quite probable that this technique is approaching its upper limits of application. A significant 'drop out' rate from HED from inability to keep pace with patients' sodium and water abuse is occurring already and will certainly limit its successful application.

High flux hemodialysis (HFD)

For several years there has been interest in Japan in 'protein leaking dialyzers' in the quest for removal of large molecules associated with uremic toxicity (79). Such solutes are also removed by the very inefficient treatment, CAPD. In 1983, a dialyzer with polysulfone membrane fibers of remarkable permeability to solutes of 10,000 to 60,000 daltons and to water was introduced in Europe. The biocompatibility, permeability and utilization of this new dialyzer in all modalities of convective and diffusive transport was described in 1984 (80). Its mass transfer characteristics in diffusive, convective and combined modes at moderate blood flow rates were described in English in 1985 (81). A subsequent study indicated that the permeability to very large proteins during blood perfusion was essentially lost in the initial few minutes of perfusion through secondary membrane formation, but a useful and enduring sieving coefficient for β_2 microglobulin at 11,400 daltons was confirmed (82). Similar devices utilizing other polymeric membranes are listed in Table 2.

It can also be seen, however, that at equivalent surface area, none of these devices demonstrates a clear superiority over conventional membrane dialyzers in whole blood urea clearance. Their use requires high blood and dialysate flows to accomplish adequate shortened urea kinetic modeled therapy just as do conventional membranes. It is feared that this point has escaped attention and that in their fairly widespread application, very short dialyses have been prescribed without adequate Kt/V studies. Their extreme hydraulic permeabilities absolutely require a volume controlled dialysate delivery device to limit net ultrafiltration to the desired rate (Figure 8b). Depending on flow rates, inlet, outlet and oncotic pressures, gross ultrafiltration and unobserved and unmeasured back filtration of dialysate can occur. Because of the diffusive and convective permeability of these membranes to molecular weight ranges that include many pyrogenic and interleukin-inducing substances, important additional requirements are placed on the sterility and nonpyrogenicity of the bicarbonate dialysate. Complement activation manifested by leukopenia is less with these membranes than with cellulosic ones. Their use is proposed to prevent the accumulation of β_2 microglobulin, amyloid deposition and various types of dialysis-induced osteoarthropathies (83, 84). HFD at higher net ultrafiltration rates has been associated with less nausea and hypotension than conventional dialysis (85). One group has reported a 16% failure rate in the first year due to inability to achieve required net weight loss of 4 to 5 Kg in 2 to 3 h (86).

There are currently unpublished reports of clinically very severe pyrogen reactions associated with the use of these dialyzers and contaminated bicarbonate concentrate (87). These strongly suggest that the entire dialysate should be passed through appropriate pyrogen filters, as is the case with hemofiltration and hemodiafiltration using on-line generated replacement fluid (88). HFD enhances the spectrum of molecular removal from conventional and HED. The use of protein leaking membranes and inevitable reverse ultrafiltration clearly presents new risks and hazards. It will be exciting to observe the long-term effect of this new therapy.

Hemofiltration (HF)

In HF ultrafiltration of plasma water occurs through membranes with permeability spectra similar to the glomerular basement membrane at near maximally obtainable rates. Accompanying this bulk flow of ultrafiltrate, solute is transferred by convection only according to the membrane's sieving coefficient for that solute (89). In HF there is neither dialysate flow nor diffusive solute transfer. For small molecules with high sieving coefficients, clearances closely relate to the filtration rate (Q_F). The rate of mass transfer is the product of the effective plasma water concentration, the sieving coefficient and the filtration rate of plasma water (Chapter 13). An absolutely sterile pyrogen-free replacement or substitution solution similar to dialysate is infused directly into the blood line at a rate, Q_S equal to Q_F minus net ultrafiltration rate. Infusion may be prehemofilter (predilution) posthemofilter (postdilution) or both or between two or more filters in series (mixed hemofiltration). Traditionally, postfilter blood redilution has been almost exclusively used, as this configuration requires the least volume of sterile solution for an arbitrarily defined treatment of 18 to 35 l exchange per session (11, 52) (Figure 8c). We have repeatedly referred to the superior cardiovascular reaction to the acute hypovolemia resulting from intratreatment net ultrafiltration when this is associated with convective rather than diffusive solute transfer. Comparing HF to HD, this is true regardless of the buffer base in the dialysate or replacement solution (27, 52, 67) but the greatest rise in total vascular resistance is seen with HF and bicarbonate replacement solution (67). Hemofiltration has gained recogni-

tion as the treatment probably permitting greatest patient comfort and requiring the least intervention. Most patients who have had both HF and HD would prefer HF even if the treatment time would be one hour longer (90). These positive attributes obviously recommend it for exploration for short treatment.

The use of HF to achieve shortened treatment requires extraordinary effort. For example, Geronemus and coworkers (91) employed three hemofilters in series at a blood flow of 400 ml/min and a replacement fluid flow of 400 ml/min divided into three streams of 125, 125 and 150 ml/min and infused after each hemofilter. Urea clearance rates as high as 282 ml/min were obtained with good cardiovascular stability.

Haas et al (92) treated 12 patients for a year with either a single hemofilter or two hemofilters in series at blood flows of 415 and 485 ml/min respectively and obtained a mean ultrafiltrate volume of 26.8 l per 190 min treatment. Predialysis blood urea nitrogen concentrations were high by current standards (35.4 mmol/l, 99 mg/dl), but not significantly different from those obtained in the same patients with 250 min HD treatments. Better vascular stability at higher net ultrafiltration rates were confirmed. The patients in these two studies had hematocrits under 25%.

Keshaviah et al (11) reported employing two hemofilters, either in parallel or in series, with 10 patients at blood flows of 533 ml/min for 169 ± 6 min. The duration had to be increased for some patients in order to meet prescribed fluid exchange. Because of the high shear rates, visible hemolysis was noted in some patients. Blood circuit leaks occurred, and all connections had to be wrapped with plastic ties to prevent separations. Mean urea clearances (ml/wk/l body water) were $2,730 \pm 150$ compared to 3,600 to 3,810 with HED of the same duration requiring only 405 ml/min blood flow.

Shaldon et al (26) reported results in two patients treated for 18 months with mixed hemofiltration, utilizing two large hemofilters in series with infusion of replacement solution after the first and after the second filter at blood flows of 400 ml/min and filtrate flows of about 400 ml/min. Kt applied to a 56 Kg patient was 26.5 l and to a 100 Kg patient was 34.4 l with clearances of 265 and 260 ml/min for 100 and 140 min. Vascular stability was excellent even though net ultrafiltration rates exceeded 2 l/h. The patients did not have post-treatment fatigue and motor nerve conduction velocities were stable. By current UKM criteria neither patient received adequate treatment. We have been unable to discover adequately described high efficiency hemofiltration studies of under 3 h duration which permitted a Kt/V$\geq$1.0.

These studies illustrate the major reason why HF has been difficult to apply for very short treatments.

Filtration rate is limited by the following physical factors: total blood flow, plasma protein concentration, oncotic pressure, hematocrit, extreme hemoconcentration within the filter fibers, increasing viscosity, high filter inlet pressures and high linear velocities and shear rates that may cause hemolysis. The interactions of these physical forces limit the filtration fraction and therefore the clearance to about 33% of the blood flow at a hematocrit of 25%. In addition, secondary membrane formation reduces both filtration fraction and sieving coefficients, especially of larger molecules (82).

Predilution partially alleviates these physical problems, allowing very high filtration rates but reduces the effective solute concentration depending on the volume of distribution of the solute in the blood and the effect of the predilution on it (93). For example, RBC urea would become immediately available for convection, but most RBC solutes would not.

For adequate urea removal ($V = 40\,l$) in a shortened time, given a hemofilter with an effective KUF of 80 ml/h/mm Hg, a Q_B of 500 ml/min, a Hct of 40%, no net ultrafiltration, Q_E (urea) = 450.8, predilution infusion flow 400 ml/min, Q_F 500 ml/min and postdilution infusion 100 ml/min, a urea clearance of 266 ml/min should permit 'adequate' treatment in 153 min.

Many patients have been maintained by HF in apparent good health for more than 5 years at weekly total urea clearances well below the NCDS recommendations. This raises the question, as CAPD always has, whether the employment of a broader molecular spectrum of clearance than achieved by hemodialysis reduces the requirement for urea removal. Despite the difficulties described above, newer technology such as on-line production of inexpensive bicarbonate based replacement solution should simplify the application of the principle (Figure 8d). This promising modality deserves continued exploration in the realms of dilutions and flows for short treatment.

Hemodiafiltration (HDF)

High small molecular weight solute flux with minimal convection occurs in HED. In HFD accidental back filtration and to and fro convective solute flux is likely to occur during primarily diffusive transport with much more permeable membranes. With these techniques, high rates of solute flux are easily obtained if adequate Q_E is available, but cardiovascular tolerance to net ultrafiltration becomes a problem as 't' is shortened. Hemofiltration, with only convective solute transport results in excellent patient comfort, a different clearance spectrum and cardiovascular stability with rapid net ultrafiltration rates, but high transfer rates of small molecules are extremely difficult to obtain as discussed above.

Hemodiafiltration (HDF), currently using as hemodiafilters, mass transfer devices similar or identical to high flux dialyzers, is an attempt to combine high flux hemodialysis with hemofiltration. The expectation is that the diffusive transport will readily permit short treatments adequate by UKM criteria. When combined with the superior cardiovascular stability associated with the convective transfer of larger solutes in hemofiltration, the favorable aspects of high efficiency diffusion and convection would combine to provide a very high quality treatment which avoids the major limitations of the other modalities. A further expectation

would be that the large blood to dialysate flux would offer some protection against the movement of pyrogenic substances from dialysate to blood and that replacement solution free of all harmful substances could be inexpensively and conveniently supplied by on-line filtration. In the most advanced techniques for HDF, the entire bicarbonate dialysate is subjected to pyrogen filtration, then that portion designated for replacement solution for the gross ultrafiltration is further filter-sterilized by either a separate filter in the infusion line (Figure 8e) or back filtered through the second mass transfer device in a series configuration (Figure 8g).

The degree to which filtrate flux augments the diffusive solute mass transfer under clinical conditions of HDF is extremely complex and is not a simple summation of the two (94, 95). Total clearance depends on the longitudinal and transverse solute concentration gradients in the plasma and the volume of ultrafiltrate at each increment along the length of the membrane, which in turn relies on a pressure gradient which is alinear because of viscosity changes due to local hematocrit and protein concentration. The diffusive component is reduced by hemoconcentration effects and by the reduced concentration gradient resulting from the increase in dialysate solute concentration generated by the convection. The clearance might be estimated using numerical integration as with the expression by Sigdell (95). For a simple estimate, for solutes with sieving coefficients close to one, the diffusive clearance will be augmented by an amount that slightly exceeds the value from Weryński (96) of $Q_F(1 - K'/Q_{Bi})$ where K' is the clearance found at zero Q_F.

The concept and technology for HDF began to evolve as soon as high permeability membranes were incorporated into flat plate or hollow fiber dialyzers-hemofilters reliable enough for clinical testing, and almost immediately after the urea clearance disadvantages of hemofiltration were appreciated (97–100).

In a significant study, Kunitomo et al (97) published in 1976 the results of a combined dialysis – filtration system with volumetric control of dialysate streams and an early high flux polymetylmethacrylate (PMMA) hollow fiber hemodiafilter (KoA urea = 245 ml/min at Q_B = 300 ml/min; Q_F = 40 ml/min at TMP = 400 mm Hg). Predilution of blood augmented urea clearances only 6%, but vitamin B_{12} clearances by 26%. In 1978, using an improved hemodiafilter with postdilution of a sterile solution at up to 55 ml/min, large increases in inulin and vitamin B_{12} clearance over hemodialysis were found (98). Two pool modeling of large solutes was performed and formal UKM was applied to HDF treatments shortened to 3 h and compared to 5 h hemodialyses. This circuit configuration was essentially as depicted in Figure 8f.

Similarly, in 1978 in West Germany, Leber et al (99) and Dieter et al (100) reported on-going clinical studies with postdilution HDF with the goal of improving the clearance spectrum of HD and providing higher urea clearance than was possible using the same flat plate device with AN-69 membrane in pure HF. Leber et al (99) utilized a dialysis fluid flow of 900 ml/min at a Q_F of 55 to 60 ml/min, and demonstrated marked improvement over HF of clearances of urea, creatinine, uric acid, phosphate, inulin, phenols and guanidines. Patient weights were not given. Urea clearance was 140 ml/min; pcr was 0.9 to 1.1 g/Kg/day. Treatment time was 3 h. BUN concentrations averaged 30 mmol/l (84 mg/dl) (99). This or very similar treatment was continued for 6 to 8 years in Giessen during which time, treatment time was further shortened to 2 h (101). It can be calculated that unless the mean patient weight was less than 44 Kg, this treatment could not have achieved Kt/V$\geq$1.0, and was inadequate by current UKM standards. The substitution fluid was usually hyperosmolar, and as experience grew with shorter and shorter treatment times, this group was finally forced to abandon these 'ultrashort' treatmentss due to increasing interdialytic weight gains. Summing up this experience at 8 years, Wizemann (102) expressed discouragement that the hemodiafiltration treatments so described had failed to improve uremic anemia and polyneuropathy. During this experience they did confirm by invasive technique in one chronic stable patient, superior hemodynamic response during a very short treatment of 70 min (101). They additionally confirmed a superior increase in total peripheral resistance as cardiac output fell with both HF and HDF in hemodynamically unstable patients with acute renal failure (102). It is not apparent that the Giessen group ever utilized bicarbonate dialysate or replacement solution in this experience. Nearly equivalent urea and creatinine removal was demonstrated for 2 h HDF and for 4 h conventional HD, but at the expense of increased initial blood solute concentrations in the HDF patients (101).

Ota et al (103) reported 15 months successful experience using 3 h HDF treatments employing about 50 ml/min gross ultrafiltration. The technique was similar to that of Figure 8f. Acetate was used in dialysis fluid, lactate in replacement solution. By their chromatographic technique, a reduction in blood concentration of middle and large molecules exceeding hemodialysis by 20% to 100% was observed. Kt/V cannot be assessed from their published data.

In 1979 Miller et al (104) developed a multipurpose apparatus with volumetrically balanced acetate or bicarbonate dialysate flows up to 1 l/min, high monitored blood flows and on-line production of sterile, pyrogen free replacement fluid. This was suitable for studies of HED, HFD, HF and HDF. It was similar to Figure 8e. This apparatus was employed in 1982 to compare HD, pre- and postdilution HF, and HDF obtainable from the AN-69 membrane in the RP-610 and the 7 + 8 plate dialyzers available at that time. It was found that with blood flows of 300 ml/min at Hct of 36 to 42%, dialysate flows of 0 to 485 ml/min and filtration rates of 85 ml/min with postdilution and 115 ml/min with predilution, adding even small amounts (100 to 200 ml/min) of dialysate flow to HF resulted in marked increases in clearances of urea and creatinine and smaller increases of phosphate and uric acid. When HF was added to HD in the postdilution mode, clearance of urea did not significantly increase, that of creatinine fell and uric acid and phosphate clearances rose significantly. Membrane masking in these flat plate dialyzers probably played a role, emphasizing the need for better hemodiafilter design (105).

A technique extremely similar to the original concept termed 'soft HDF' or biofiltration is currently popular in Italy (Figure 7f). Here a re-infusion solution containing about 145 mEq/l Na$^+$ and 100 mEq/l HCO$_3^-$ is commonly used (106). By our calculation, Kt/V in this report was only 0.85, but this did not substantially differ from the preceding and control period of 4 h hemodialysis.

Using two modern hollow fiber hemodiafilters in parallel, a very high efficiency HDF was described in which 't' ranged from 76 to 121 min and corresponding urea clearances from 527 to 331 ml/min. Excellent tolerance was described. Body weights were not given (107). Use of a volumetric balancing apparatus capable of delivery of 750 ml/min bicarbonate dialysis solution for on-line sterilized high efficiency post-dilution HDF (250 ml/min Q$_S$, 500 ml/min Q$_D$) or two device hemofiltration obtaining 60 l exchange per treatment has been described (108). In this study, with HDF using polysulfone filters, inulin clearance was 125 $\pm$ 15 ml/min and β_2 microglobulin clearance was 100 $\pm$ 36 ml/min. Serum β_2 microglobulin concentration fell from 55 to 25 mg/l.

Preliminary studies of hemodiafiltration employing a Cuprophan dialyzer for diffusive transport and, in parallel, an AN-69 membrane dialyzer for convective transport, both receiving serial dialysate flow have been presented (109). In an attempt to maximize overall diffusive and convective clearances, these two functions were separated in a single hemofilter consisting of a 0.3 m^2 polysulfone segment for convection and a 1.1 m^2 Cuprophan hollow fiber segment for diffusion (110). At blood flows of 500 ml/min and Q$_F$ of 41 ml/min, mass transfer by both methods was impressive.

In 1984 von Albertini et al (50) and Miller et al (51) reported pilot studies of high flux HDF using the apparatus developed earlier by Miller et al (104) in the two hemodiafilter in series configuration shown in Figure 8g. Blood flow rates of 504 $\pm$ 8 ml/min, filtration rates of 116 $\pm$ 20 ml/min and dialysis fluid flows of 1007 $\pm$ 28 ml/min were studied using cellulose acetate hemodiafilters with a surface area of 1.8 m^2 each. Despite the size of the six subjects (86.2 $\pm$ 18.7 Kg) and rates of fluid loss twice those of control 4 h HD (as much as 2 to 3 Kg/h), all treatments, averaging 115 min in duration, were well tolerated and matched 4 h conventional HD in solute removal with urea clearances of 406.7 $\pm$ 14.6 ml/min.

In 1985 studies using two 1.25 m^2 polysulfone (F-60) hemodiafilters were reported at blood flows of 630 ml/min, ultrafiltrate flows of 146 $\pm$ 18 ml/min and dialysate flows of 1006 $\pm$ 11 ml/min. Clearances of 514 $\pm$ 12 ml/min for urea and 431 $\pm$ 7 ml/min for creatinine were obtained with excellent patient tolerance. This illustrated the suitability of high flux hemodiafiltration for shortening the dialysis procedure. These whole blood clearances were validated in one-month cross over studies with conventional hemodialysis in six patients by UKM and measurement of total mass removed in the dialysate (50). Two patients of 79.5 and 75 Kg body weight were reported at more than one year's treatment, and have been continued for 3.5 and 2.5 years meeting all NCDS criteria for adequacy with no morbidity (111).

Another technique that employs reverse flux for the replacement fluid is that of Usuda et al (112) in which fluid is moved back and forth through the dialyzer membrane by rhythmic fluctuation of the dialysate pressure generated by cyclic withdrawal and replacement of dialysate.

Special considerations

HDF presents several special considerations which do not occur with routine hemodialysis or with high efficiency hemodialysis. HDF shares with hemofiltration the concern with the sterility and non-pyrogenicity of large volumes of infusion fluid. If this fluid is prepared on line from dialysate, the concern expands to the quality of the much larger volume of dialysate from which the infusate is made. This need for sterility also applies to the periods between use of the apparatus. Greater efforts must be made to maintain and assure the system's sterility and non-pyrogenicity than with conventional hemodialysis.

The utilization of a portion of the dialysate to produce infusate reduces the diffusive component of the overall urea clearance by amounts as shown in Figure 4. For example if only 500 ml/min of dialysate were available, using 100 of it for infusate would reduce the diffusive component by 7.5% at a Q_B of 500 ml/min and a KoA of 833 ml/min. If 1100 ml/min of dialysate were available, the reduction would be only slightly greater than 1%.

As with hemofiltration, predilution ameliorates the problems of hemoconcentration, but unfortunately, reduces the blood water solute concentration which is the prime driving force for diffusive transfer to such a degree that urea clearances are minimally increased, if at all, over that of hemodialysis alone in spite of the increased effective blood flow and convective flux.

Hemodiafiltration is clearly capable of providing short adequate treatment by UKM. It should provide better vascular stability then HED and HFD.

ADVANTAGES AND DISADVANTAGES OF SHORTENED TREATMENT

The advantages and disadvantages of shortened dialysis can be divided into those for the patient and those for the provider. They are self-explanatory and do not justify extensive elaboration at this stage of development.

Advantages

For the patient

Shorter time is spent in treatment causing less disruption of life style.

Improved techniques such as bicarbonate dialysate, controlled ultrafiltration and more biocompatible membranes allowing a broader spectrum of solute removal are used.

Greater attention given to proper modeling and individualized prescription may result in more patients receiving adequate treatment.

For the provider

Shortened treatment times permit a greater number of treatments per day.

Disadvantages

For the patient

The shorter time available to remove interdialytic weight gain requires better compliance with salt and water restrictions or, at some degree of shortening time, a greater risk of hypotension will ensue.

Higher blood flows result in lower prepump pressures and higher postpump pressures increasing the inherent risks and hazards of the blood circuit.

The 'effective life' of the vascular access may be reduced since high blood flows are always required: progressive stenosis and recirculation are not compatible with shortened treatment time.

There may be added anxiety associated with a new treatment.

For the provider

Supplies, equipment and maintenance will be more expensive.

Dialyzer reuse may be economically necessary.

The need for quality control of water and concentrate is increased.

There will be a greater need for more skilled and dedicated staff.

Increased vigilance with prompt and appropriate responses are required.

Staff-patient contact time is reduced.

Greater compliance with scheduling is required of patients and staff.

The faster work pace and higher performance required may increase staff turnover.

GLOSSARY

BUN	Blood urea nitrogen
C	Solute concentration
CAPD	Continuous ambulatory peritoneal dialysis
CHD	Conventional hemodialysis
CO2	The mid-week pre dialysis level
D	Clearance when C_{Di} is 0
DI_{mm}	Dialysis index for middle molecules
ESRD	End stage renal disease
H	Hematocrit as a decimal fraction
Hct	Hematocrit as a percent
HD	Hemodialysis
HDF	Hemodiafiltration
HED	High efficiency hemodialysis
HF	Hemofiltration
HFD	High flux hemodialysis
K	Clearance
K'	The clearance at zero Q_F

k	The RBC solute concentration compared to plasma
KoA	The mass transfer coefficient – area product
Kt	The dialysis product
KUF	Coefficient of ultrafiltration
m^2	Square meters surface area
NCDS	The USA National Cooperative Dialysis Study
pcr	Protein catabolic rate/weight
PMMA	Polymethylmethacrylate
Q	Flow rate, e.g. Q_B, Q_D, Q_F, Q_s: flow rates of blood, dialysate, filtrate and substitution fluid
R	The decimal fraction of recirculation
RBC	Red blood cell
t	Time on dialysis
TAC	The time-averaged concentration
tot	Total
TMP	Transmembrane pressure
UF	Ultrafiltration
UFR	Ultrafiltration rate
UKM	Urea kinetically modeled
V	Volume as of body water
Z	Q_B/Q_D

Subscripts

A	'Arterial'
B	Blood
BH_2O	Blood water
D	Dialysate
d	Dialyzer (or due to dialyzer)
E	Effective
F	Filtrate
H_2O	Water or blood water
i	In (i.e entering dialyzer)
M	Measured
o	Outgoing (i.e. leaving dialyzer)
r	Residual kidney function
S	Systemic
s	Substitution or replacement fluid
U	Ultrafiltration
V	'Venous'
WB	Whole blood

ACKNOWLEDGMENT

To our former colleague, Beat von Albertini, M.D., our gratitude for the stimulation provided by his conviction that all of the barriers preventing ultra-high efficiency dialytic treatment could be safely and simultaneously broken, for his dedicated participation and for his sharing of knowledge and experience. We sincerely regret the great geographical separation which prevented his active participation in the production of this chapter.

REFERENCES

1. Wolf AV, Remp DG, Kiley JE, Currie GD: Artificial kidney function: kinetics of hemodialysis. *J Clin Invest* 30: 1062, 1951
2. Alwall N, Norviit L, Steins AM: On the artificial kidney, VII, Clinical experiences of dialysis treatment of uremia. *Acta Med Scand* 132: 587, 1948
3. Muehrcke RC: *Acute Renal Failure*, St. Louis, The CV Mosby CO 1969, p 277
4. Maher JF, Schreiner GE, Waters TJ: Successful intermittent hemodialysis-longest reported maintenance of life in true oli-guria (181 days). *Trans Am Soc Artif Intern Organs* 6: 123, 1960
5. Hegstrom RM, Murray JS, Pendras GP, Burnell JM, Scribner BH: Hemodialysis in the treatment of chronic uremia. *Trans Am Soc Artif Intern Organs* 7: 136, 1961
6. Cole JJ, Quinton WE, Williams C, Murray JS, Sherris JC: The pumpless low temperature hemodialysis system. *Trans Am Soc Artif Intern Organs* 8: 209, 1962
7. Alwall N: A new disposable artificial kidney – experimental and clinical experience. *Proc Eur Dial Transplant Assoc* 5: 18, 1968
8. Stewart RD, Lipps BJ, Borella ED, Puring WR, Roth DA, Sargent JA: Short-term hemodialysis with the capillary kidney. *Trans Am Soc Artif Intern Organs* 14: 121, 1968
9. Gotch F, Lipps BJ, Weaver J Jr, Brandes J, Rosin J, Sargent JA, Oja P: Chronic dialysis with the hollow fiber artificial kidney (HFAC). *Trans Am Soc Artif Intern Organs* 15: 87, 1969
10. Shaldon S, Florence P, Fontanuo P, Palito C, Mion C: Comparison of two strategies for short dialysis using $1 M^2$ and $2 M^2$ surface area dialyzers. *Proc Eur Dial Transplant Assoc* 12: 596, 1974
11. Keshaviah P, Berkseth R, Ilstrup K, McMichael C, Collins A: Reduced treatment time: hemodialysis (HD) versus hemofiltration (HF). *Trans Am Soc Artif Intern Organs* 31: 176, 1985
12. Mirahmadi KS, Kay JH, Miller JH, Gorman JJ, Rosen SM: Clinical evaluation of patients dialyzed with double Gambro four hours, three times per week. *Proc Eur Dial Transplant Assoc* 11: 121, 1974
13. Cambi V, Garini G, Sovazzi, Arisi L, David S, Zanelli P, Bono F, Gardini F: Short dialysis. *Proc Eur Dial Transplant Assoc* 20: 111, 1983
14. Bosl R, Shideman JR, Meyer RM, Buselmeier TJ, von Hartitzsch B, Kjellstrand CM: Effects and complications of high efficiency dialysis. *Nephron* 15: 151, 1975
15. Manji T, Maeda K, Kawaguchi S, Kobayashi K, Ohta K, Saito A, Amano I, Shimoi T, Fujisaki Y: Short time dialysis with $2 M^2$ hollow fiber kidney. *Proc Eur Dial Transplant Assoc* 11: 153, 1974
16. Babb AL, Strand MJ, Uvelli DA, Scribner BH: Quantitative description of dialysis treatment: a dialysis index. *Kidney Int* 2(Suppl 2): S23, 1975
17. Ginn HE, Buzel HJ, James L, Hopkins P: Clinical experience with small surface area dialyzers (SSAD). *Proc Clin Dial Transplant Forum* 1: 53, 1971
18. Milutinovich J, Halar EM, Hacker LA, Babb AL, Scribner BH: Further experience with hemodialysis at 100 ml/min dialysate flow. *Proc Clin Dial Transplant Forum* 1: 48, 1971
19. Bergström J, Fürst P: Uremic middle molecules. *Clin Nephrol* 5: 143, 1976
20. Nolph KD: Short dialysis, middle molecules, and uremia. *Ann Intern Med* 86: 99, 1977
21. Wauters JP, Pansiot BC, Gilliard N, Stauffer JC: Short hemodialysis: long-term mortality and morbidity. *Artif Organs* 10: 182, 1986
22. Tolchin N: Acetate metabolism and high efficiency hemodialysis. *Int J Artif Organs* 2: 1, 1979
23. Diamond SM, Henrich WL: Acetate dialysate versus bicarbonate dialysate: a continuing controversy. *Am J Kidney Dis* 9: 3, 1987
24. Tolchin N, Roberts JL, Hayashi J, Lewis EJ: Metabolic consequences of high mass-transfer hemodialysis. *Kidney Int* 11: 366, 1977
25. Graeffe I, Milutinovich J, Follette WC, Vizzo JE, Babb AL:

Less dialysis-induced morbidity and vascular instability with bicarbonate dialysate. *Ann Intern Med* 88: 332, 1978

26. Shaldon S, Beau MC, Deschodt G, Mion C: Mixed hemofiltration (MHF): 18 months experience with ultrashort treatment time. *Trans Am Soc Artif Intern Organs* 27: 610, 1981

27. Baldamus C, Ernst W, Frei U, Koch K: Sympathetic and hemodynamic response to volume removal during different forms of renal replacement therapy. *Nephron* 31: 324, 1982

28. Bergström J, Asaba H, Fürst P, Oules R: Dialysis ultrafiltration and blood pressure. *Proc Eur Dial Transplant Assoc* 13: 293, 1976

29. Asaba H, Bergström J, Fürst P, Lindh K, Mion C, Oules R, Shaldon S: Sequential ultrafiltration and diffusion as alternative to conventional hemodialysis. *Proc Clin Dial Transplant Forum* 6: 129, 1976

30. Rouby J, Rottemberg J, Durande JP, Basset JY, Degoulet P, Glasser P, Legrain M: Hemodynamic changes induced by regular hemodialysis and sequential ultrafiltration hemodialysis: a comparative study. *Kidney Int* 17: 801, 1980

31. Gotch FA, Sargent JA, Keen ML, Lee M: Individualized, quantified dialysis therapy of uremia. *Proc Clin Dial Transplant Forum* 4: 27, 1974

32. Gotch FA, Sargent JA, Keen M, Lam M, Prowitt M, Grady M: Clinical results of intermittent dialysis therapy (IDT) guided by ongoing kinetic analysis of urea metabolism. *Trans Am Soc Artif Intern Organs* 22: 175, 1976

33. Lowrie EG, Laird NM: (editors) The National Cooperative Dialysis Study. *Kidney Int* 23(Suppl 13): S1, 1983

34. Gotch FA, Sargent JH: A mechanistic analysis of the National Cooperative Dialysis Study (NCDS). *Kidney Int* 28: 526, 1985

35. Teschan PE, Ginn HE, Bourne JR, Ward JW, Schaffer JD: A prospective study of reduced dialysis. *asaio J* 6: 108, 1983

36. Gotch FA: Urea kinetic modeling to guide hemodialysis therapy in adults in *Dialysis Therapy*. edited by Nissenson AR, Fine RN, Philadelphia, Hanley & Belfus, Inc, 1986, p 66

37. Farrell PC: Kinetic modeling in hemodialysis in *Clinical Dialysis*. edited by Nissenson AR, Fine RN, Gentile DE, Norwalk, Appleton-Century-Crofts, 1984, p 141

38. Norvit EG, Teschan PE: Principles of prescribing dialysis therapy: implementing recommendations from the National Cooperative Dialysis Study. *Kidney Int* 23(Suppl 13): S113, 1983

39. Ilstrup K, Hanson G, Shapiro W, Keshaviah P: Examining the foundations of urea kinetics. *Trans Am Soc Artif Intern Organs* 3 1: 164, 1985

40. Keshaviah P, Ilstrup K, Shapiro W, Hanson G: Hemodialysis urea kinetics is not single pool. *Abstracts Am Soc Nephrol* 17: 67A, 1984

41. Schindhelm K, Skalsky M, Mahony JF, Farrell PC: Creatinine transfer between interstitial and intracellular fluid: a comparison between normal and uremic subjects. *asaio J* 2: 35, 1979

42. Schindhelm K, Farrell PC: Patient – hemodialyzer interactions. *Trans Am Soc Artif Intern Organs* 24: 357, 1978

43. Miller JH, Gardner PW, Shinaberger JH, von Albertini B: Modeling short treatment: a practical mathematical approach. *Blood Purif* 2: 214, 1984

44. Jindal KK, Manuel A, Goldstein MB: Percent reduction of the blood urea concentration during hemodialysis (PRU), a simple and accurate method to estimate Kt/V urea. *Abstracts Am Soc Artif Intern Organs* 16: 49, 1987

45. Colton CK, Smith DKA, Merrill EW, Reece JM: Diffusion of organic solutes in stagnant plasma and red cell suspensions. *Chem Eng Prog Symp* Ser No 99 66: 85, 1970

46. Babb AL, Popovich RP, Farrell PC, Blagg CR: The effects of erythrocyte mass transfer rates on solute clearance measurements during hemodialysis. *Proc Eur Dial Transplant Assoc* 9: 303, 1972

47. Michaels AS: Operating parameters and performance criteria for hemodialyzers and other membrane – separation devices. *Trans Am Soc Artif Intern Organs* 12: 387, 1966

48. Gotch FA, Autian J, Colton CK, Ginn HE, Lipps BJ, Lowrie E: The evaluation of hemodialyzers. DHEW publication No. (NIH) 72: 103, 1972

49. Miller JH, Shinaberger JH, Gardner PW: Extended mathematical analysis of dialyzer function. *Opuscula Medico-technica Lundensia* X17, 1974

50. von Albertini B, Miller JH, Gardner PW, Shinaberger JH: High-flux hemodiafiltration: under six hours/week treatment. *Trans Am Soc Artif Intern Organs* 30: 227, 1984

51. Miller JH, von Albertini B, Gardner PW, Shinaberger JH: Technical aspects of high-flux hemodiafiltration for adequate short (under 2 hours) treatment. *Trans Am Soc Artif Intern Organs* 30: 377, 1984

52. Quellhorst E, Scheunemann B, Hildebrand U: How to prevent vascular instability: haemofiltration. *Proc Eur Dial Transplant Assoc* 18: 243, 1981

53. Schilling H, Lehman H, Hampl H: Studies on circulatory stability during bicarbonate hemodialysis with constant dialysate sodium versus acetate hemodialysis with sequential dialysate sodium. *Artif Organs* 9: 17, 1985

54. Raja R, Kramer M, Barber K, Chen S: Sequential changes in dialysate sodium (DNa) during hemodialysis. *Trans Am Soc Artif Intern Organs* 29: 649, 1983

55. Muriasco A, France G, LeBlond G, Stroumza P, Durand C, Raynier JP, Crevat A, Elson R: Separation of Na^+ and H_2O transport during hemodialysis and quantification of high-low Na D_1 levels during sequential therapy. *Trans Am Soc Artif Intern Organs* 29: 645, 1983

56. Henrich WL, Hunt JM, Nixon JV: Increased ionized calcium and left ventricular contractibility during hemodialysis. *N Eng J Med* 310: 19, 1985

57. Ginsburg R, Esserman LJ, Brestow MR: Myocardial performance and extracellular ionized calcium in a severely failing human heart. *Ann Intern Med* 98: 603, 1983

58. Chaignon M, Chen WT, Tarazi RC, Nakamoto S, Salcedo E: Acute effects of hemodialysis on echocardiographic-determined cardiac performance: improved contractility resulting from serum increased calcium with reduced potassium despite hypovolemic-reduced cardiac output. *Am Heart J* 103: 374, 1982

59. Schmidt M, Schoeppe W, Baldamus CA: Hemodynamics during dialysis with dialyzers of high hydraulic permeability. *Contr Nephrol* 46: 127, 1985

60. Koon KT, Basile C, Ulan RA, Hetherington MD, Kappagoda T: Effect of hemodialysis and hypertonic hemodiafiltration on cardiac function compared. *Kidney Int* 33: 399, 1987

61. Maynard JC, Cosme C, Kleerkoper M, Levin N: Blood pressure response to changes in serum ionized calcium during hemodialysis. *Ann Intern Med*

62. Mahida BH, Dumler F, Zasuwa G, Flug G, Levin NW: Effect of cooled dialysate on serum catecholamines and blood pressure stability. *Trans Am Soc Artif Intern Organs* 29: 384, 1983

63. Maggiore Q, Pizzarelli F, Zocalli C, Sisca S, Nicolo F, Parlango S: Effect of extracorporeal blood cooling on dialytic arterial hypotension. *Proc Eur Dial Transplant Assoc* 18: 597, 1981

64. Grossman F, Kopp KF: Thermo-osmotic effect and ultrafiltration in the artificial kidney – experience with the 'coil

kidney'. *Proc Eur Dial Transplant Assoc* 3: 299, 1966

65. Quellhorst E, Ruzer J, Doht B, Beckmann H, Jacob I, Kraft B, Mietzsch G, Scheler F: Treatment of chronic uremia by an ultrafiltration kidney – first clinical experience. *Proc Eur Dial Transplant Assoc* 13: 314, 1976

66. Baldamus CA, Schoeppe W, Koch KM: Comparison of hemodialysis (HD) and post dilution hemofiltration (HF) on an unselected dialysis population. *Proc Eur Dial Transplant Assoc* 15: 228, 1978

67. Shaldon S, Beau MC, Deschodt G, Ramperez P, Mion C: Vascular stability during hemofiltration. *Trans Am Soc Artif Intern Organs* 26: 391, 1980

68. Wizemann V, Kramer W, Knopp G, Rawer P, Mueller K, Schuetterle G: Ultrashort hemodiafiltration: efficiency and hemodynamic tolerance. *Clin Nephrol* 19: 24, 1983

69. von Albertini B, Miller JH, Gardner PW, Shinaberger JH: Performance characteristics of the Hemoflow F-60 in high-flux hemodiafiltration. *Contr Nephrol* 46: 169, 1985

70. Miller JH, Shinaberger JH, Gardner PW: Extended ultrafiltration control. *Trans Am Soc Artif Intern Organs* 23: 244, 1977

71. Schmidt M, Baldamus CA, Schoeppe W: Backfiltration in hemodialyzers with highly permeable membranes. *Blood Purif* 2: 108, 1984

72. Shinaberger JH, Miller JH, von Albertini B, Gardner PW, Coburn JW: Phosphate removal by conventional dialysis, high efficiency dialysis and high flux hemodiafiltration. *Kidney Int* 31: 245, 1987

73. Collins A, Ilstrup K, Hanson G, Berkseth R, Keshaviah P: Rapid high efficiency hemodialysis. *Artif Organs* 10: 185, 1986

74. Basile C, Miller JDR, Koles ZJ, Grace M, Ulan RA: The effects of dialysis on brain water and EEG in stable chronic uremia. *Am J Kidney Dis* 9: 462, 1987

75. Keshaviah P, Collins A: Rapid high-efficiency hemodialysis. *Trans Am Soc Artif Intern Organs* 32: 17, 1986

76. Keshaviah P, Luehmann D, Ilstrup K, Collins A: Technical requirements for rapid H-efficiency therapies. *Artif Organs* 10: 189, 1986

77. Rotellar E, Martinez E, Samso JM, Barrios J, Simo R, Mulero JF, Perez D, Bandrés S, Piñol J: Why dialyze more than 6 hours a week? *Trans Am Soc Artif Intern Organs* 31: 538, 1985

78. Rotellar E, Martinez E, Samso JM, Barrios J, Simo R, Mulero JF, Perez MD, Bandrés S, Piñol J: Large-surface Hemodialysis. *Artif Organs* 10: 387, 1986

79. Saito A, Ogawa T, Takugi K, Ohta K, Akasu H, Kawai S, Kubotsu, A: A new approach to glomerular filtration. *Trans Am Soc Artif Intern Organs* 29: 673, 1983

80. Fresenius-Stiftung: *Hochpermeable Membranen für die optimierte Therapie des Nierenversagens.* (Highly permeable membranes for optimal therapy of renal failure.) Beiheft 1, 1985

81. Schneider H, Streicher E: Mass transfer characteristics of a new polysulfone membrane. *Artif Organs* 9: 180, 1985

82. Röckel A, Hertel J, Fiegel P, Abdelhamid S, Panitz N, Walb D: Permeability and secondary membrane formation of a high-flux polysulfone hemofilter. *Kidney Int* 30: 429, 1986

83. Chanard J, Lavaud S, Toupance O, Melin JP, Gillery P: β₂ microglobulin-associated amyloidosis in chronic haemodialysis patients. *Lancet* 1: 1212, 1986

84. Caverle Y, Simon P, Ang K, Cam G, Catheline M: Serum β₂ microglobulin levels in hemodialyzed uremics depend on permeability of dialysis membranes. *Kidney Int* 31: 229, 1987

85. Levin NW, Dumler F, Stella K, Parnell S, Zasuwa BS: High flux dialysis – Henry Ford Hospital approach. *Dial Transplant* 15: 556, 1986

86. Acchiardo S, Burk L, Bannister D: High flux (HF) hemodialysis (HD). One year experience. *Artif Organs* 11: 301, 1987

87. Favero MS: CDC alert to potential microbiological and endotoxin risks. *Nephrol News and Issues* 6: 21, 1987

88. Henderson LW, Beans E: Successful production of sterile pyrogen-free electrolyte solution by ultrafiltration. *Kidney Int* 14: 522, 1978

89. Henderson LW, Besarab A, Michaels AS, Bluemle LW: Blood purification by ultrafiltration and fluid replacement (Diafiltration). *Trans Am Soc Artif Intern Organs* 12: 216, 1967

90. Hüfler M, Asmus G, von Herrath D, Schaefer K: Hemodialysis or hemofiltration – the patients' view. *Blood Purif* 5: 1, 1987

91. Geronemus R, von Albertini B, Glabman S, Bosch JP: High flux hemofiltration: further reduction in treatment time. *Proc Dial Transplant Forum* 9: 125, 1979

92. Haas T, Dongradi G, Villeboeuf F, deViel E, Verrier J, Hillion D: Technical and clinical data on high performance hemofiltration: twelve patients during one year. *Artif Organs* 9: 164, 1985

93. Cheung AK, Alford MF, Wilson MM, Leypoldt JK, Henderson LW: Urea movement across erythrocyte membrane during artificial kidney treatment. *Kidney Int* 23: 866, 1983

94. Villaroel F, Klein E, Holland F: Solute flux in hemodialysis and hemofiltration membranes. *Trans Am Soc Artif Intern Organs* 23: 225, 1977

95. Sigdell JE: Calculation of combined diffusive and convective transfer. *Int J Artif Organs* 5: 361, 1982

96. Weryński A: Evaluation of the impact of ultrafiltration on dialyzer clearance. *Artif Organs* 3: 140, 1979

97. Kunitomo T, Lowrie EG, O'Brien M, Lazarus JM, Gottlieb MN, Kumigawa S, Merrill JP: Performance and clinical use of a convective hemodialysis (HD) -ultrafiltration (HF) system. *Proc Dial Transplant Forum* 6: 120, 1976

98. Kunitomo T, Kirkwood RG, Kumigawa S, Lazarus JM, Gottlieb MN, Lowrie EG: Clinical evaluation of a postdilution dialysis with a combined ultrafiltration (UF) -hemodialysis (HD) system. *Trans Am Soc Artif Intern Organs* 24: 169, 1978

99. Leber HW, Wizemann V, Goubeaud G, Rawer P, Schütterle G: Simultaneous hemofiltration/hemodialysis: an effective alternative to hemofiltration and conventional hemodialysis in the treatment of uremic patients. *Clin Nephrol* 9: 115, 1978

100. Dieter V, Franz HE, Breitag D, Meyer C, Schmidt-Wiederkehr P: Blut detoxification durch simultane Dialyse und Diafiltration. (Blood detoxification by simultaneous dialysis and diafiltration.) *Biomed Techn* 22: 277, 1977

101. Wizemann V, Rawer P, Schütterle G: Ultrashort hemodiafiltration: long term efficiency and hemodynamic tolerance. *Proc Eur Dial Transplant Assoc* 19: 175, 1982

102. Wizemann V: Hemodiafiltration – to be or not to be? The Giessen experience. *Blood Purif* 2: 76, 1984

103. Ota K, Suzuki T, Ozaku Y, Hoshino T, Agishi T, Sugino N: Short – time hemodiafiltration using polymethylmethacrylate hemodiafilter. *Trans Am Soc Artif Intern Organs* 24: 454, 1978

104. Miller JH, Shinaberger JH, Kraut JA, Gardner PW: A volume controlled apparatus for ultrafiltration and hemofiltration with acetate or bicarbonate solutions. *Trans Am Soc Artif Intern Organs* 25: 404, 1979

105. Miller JH: Experience with the RP610 and Filtral 7 + 8 used for simultaneous hemofiltration and hemodialysis. *Proc 1st Am AN69 Membr Sci Exch* 1: 113, 1982

106. Zuchelli P, Santoro A, Raggiotto G, Esposti ED, Sturani A, Capecchi V: Bio-filtration in uremia: preliminary observations. *Blood Purif* 2: 187, 1984

107. Cioni L, Pilone N, Rindi P: Fast safe hemodiafiltration: less than 4 hours/week. *Blood Purif* 2: 206, 1984
108. Wizemann V, Techert F, Schütterle G: High efficiency on line hemofiltration (HF) or hemodiafiltration (HDF) performed with a dialysis machine. *Blood Purif* 2: 206, 1984
109. Rossi R, Farma A, Minoretti C, Colantonio G, Ferradini MA, Martinelli D, Giura C, Quarenghi MI: Short time hemodiafiltration using two joined dialyzers of different membranes: results after 5000 treatments. *Blood Purif* 2: 211, 1984
110. Ghezzi PM, Zucchelli P, Botella J, Koutsikos D, Marazzi F, Canepari G, Nigrelli S, Spongano M, Ziroyannis P, Santaro A: Paired filtration dialysis (PFD), an alternative to classical hemodiafiltration (HDF). *Blood Purif* 2: 203, 1984
111. von Albertini B, Miller JH, Gardner PW, Roberts CE, Shinaberger JH: One year high flux hemodiafiltration: 6 hrs/week. Abstracts *Am Soc Nephrol* 18: 78A, 1985
112. Usuda M, Shinzato T, Sezaki R, Kawanishi A, Maeda K, Kawaguchi S, Shibata M, Toyoda T, Asakura Y, Ohbayashi S: New simultaneous HF and HD with no infusion fluid. *Trans Am Soc Artif Intern Organs* 28: 24, 1982

17

SINGLE NEEDLE HAEMODIALYSIS

R. VANHOLDER, N.A. HOENICH and S. RINGOIR

INTRODUCTION

In 1972 Kopp et al (1) stated 'Access to the blood stream is a problem in chronic hemodialysis. The presently preferred method is via dilated forearm veins which result from a surgically created arteriovenous fistula described by Brescia and co-workers in 1966. Two venipunctures or more in the case of poor puncture are required for dialysis. Since large needles are necessary their insertion requires skill, is painful and is detrimental to the fistula vessels. Usually the insertion of the second needle is considerably more difficult than the first, therefore, if only one venipuncture were necessary it would ease some of the problems'.

This observation, together with parallel evolution of the need to provide access for the treatment of acute renal failure has been fundamental to the development of access techniques that utilise a single needle to withdraw and return blood to the patient's circulation.

Although the principle of single needle dialysis was first published in 1964 (2) it was not applied clinically until some years later (1). It remained unpopular and by 1978 it only accounted for 42.3% of regular treatments in Europe (3). Its limited acceptance for routine use was due to several reasons including poor understanding of the technique and the belief that it was inferior to the more conventional two needle dialysis.

Single needle dialysis or unipuncture may be achieved either by the use of coaxial or dual lumen catheters or needles used with a single pump, or by the use of tidal flow systems with one or two pumps.

CATHETERS FOR SINGLE NEEDLE DIALYSIS

The attainment of adequate and repeated vascular access was a major problem in the early years of haemodialysis. The arteriovenous shunt described by Quinton, Dillard and Scribner (4) was an important step forward since it permitted the survival of chronic renal failure patients. Complications with this method prompted the search for alternative methods of access. The Brescia-Cimino fistula became available in 1966 (5) and was an important landmark in the treatment of renal failure by haemodialysis.

There still remained the difficulty in treating the patient in acute renal failure or those with a damaged vasculature. Femoral vein catheterisation was proposed in the early 1960's by Shaldon (6, 7). The catheters used were withdrawn immediately after each dialysis and a new catheter introduced for the next dialysis (6). Attempts were made to simplify the technique and to allow the catheters to remain in situ between treatments. Continuous femoral vein (6) subclavian vein (8, 9) and deep jugular vein catheters (10) have all been proposed as potential solutions; of these, access via the subclavian vein became the more popular, since it allowed mobilisation of the patient after catheter insertion.

Originally, both femoral and subclavian catheterisations were utilised as a two needle technique. The development of double lumen variants as well as single catheters with single pump devices (11, 12) have superseded this earlier practice.

CATHETER TYPES

The catheter most frequently used is a single lumen catheter (13). Originally, it was made of Teflon and was not radio-opaque but has been largely superseded by polyurethane radioopaque variants which have the added advantage of being less thrombogenic than those made of Teflon (14).

A number of new concepts in catheter design have been recently introduced. Although these are not widely used on a regular basis, they, nevertheless, merit comment.

Double lumen catheters

Double lumen catheters in clinical use may be a single circular catheter with two semi-circular lumens divided by a central septum (dual lumen catheters) (Figure 1), or coaxial in construction consisting of an inner circular and outer circular lumen. The venous or return pathway is the central inner circular position of the catheter while the arterial pathway is the space between the inner and outer catheters (Figure 2).

The idea of using double lumen catheters for haemodialysis has been described by Uldall et al in 1980 (15). Clinical experience with such catheters also has been described (16–19). The advantage of such catheters is that they may be used in a two needle setting allowing their adaptation to sit-uations where expertise with single needle dialysis is unavailable.

Implantable central venous catheters

Although central venous catheterisation is well accepted for short term access, it is unsuitable for long term use. Long term circulatory access by implantable central venous catheters has been described by Francis et al (20) and Reed et al (21, 22). The former used a silicone rubber catheter (2.6 mm internal diameter) with one or two bonded Dacron cuffs which was inserted into the right atrium via an external or internal jugular vein under local or general anaesthesia using full aseptic technique. The latter used a modified Hickman-Broviac catheter, with an identical internal diameter whose overall length was 26 cm, implanted into the superior vena cava through a venotomy in the external or internal jugular vein. Patients with the Francis catheter used it as an access for a mean duration of 11.7 months (5 weeks to 32 months) while for those in Reed's series, the mean catheter survival was 126 days.

Although these catheters are more expensive than those for intermittent use they are valuable in cases where long term treatment by haemodialysis can be expected and vascular access by other routes is difficult; they are also suitable for the treatment of children (23).

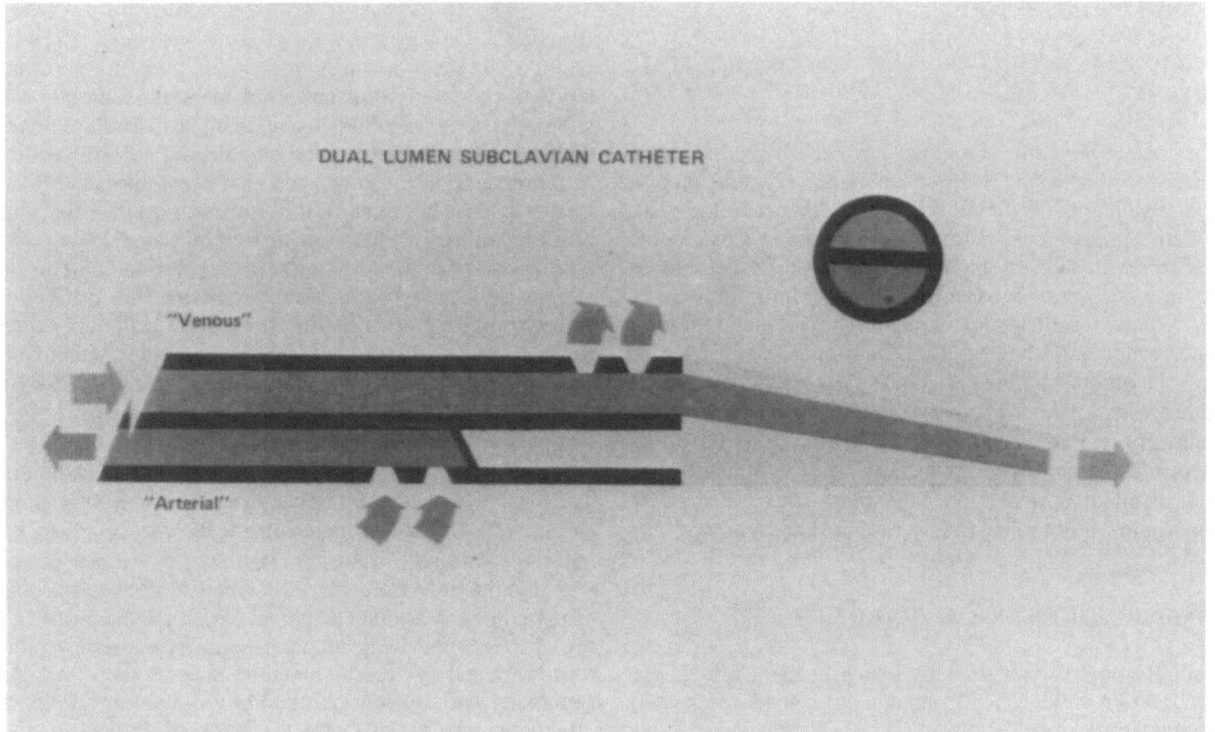

Figure 1. Dual lumen catheter flow pathway.

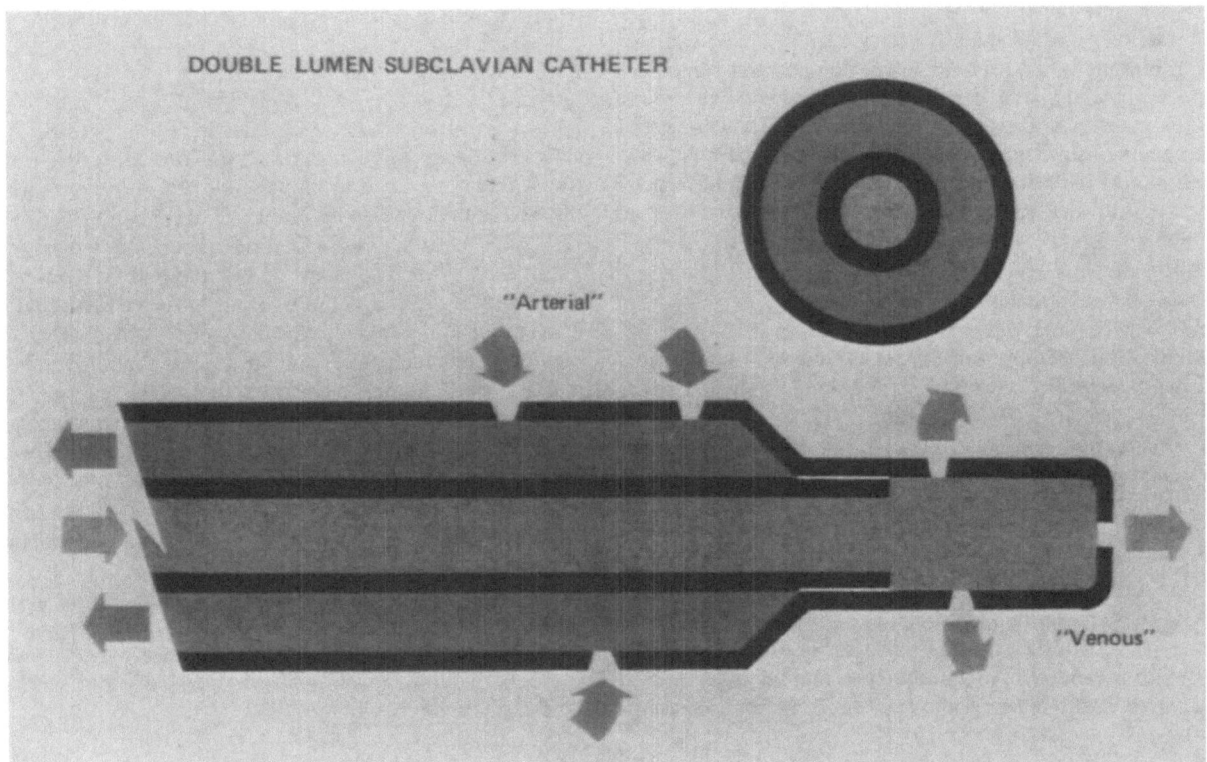

Figure 2. Double lumen catheter flow pathway.

INSERTION TECHNIQUE AND MAINTANANCE OF PATENCY

The correct insertion techniques have been described elsewhere for subclavian (11, 13), deep jugular (24) and femoral (25) as well as those for indwelling long term catheters (20).

Catheter patency is normally maintained by flushing the catheter with saline at the termination of dialysis followed by the injection of heparin (5,000 IU/ml) into the limbs of the catheter by an aseptic technique. The catheter is then left undisturbed until the next use. For permanently implanted Francis catheters before each dialysis the external end of the catheter is suspended in povidone/iodine 10% (aqueous) for 5 min prior to connection to the extracorporeal circuit by aseptic techniques. After each dialysis the catheter is flushed with 10 ml of normal saline and filled with 10,000 IU of heparin in 2 ml of saline before capping and clamping.

COMPLICATIONS OF CATHETER DIALYSIS

Complications of catheter dialysis have been the subject of a number of reviews (26–28). These may be divided into early complications observed at the time of cannulation and late complications developing after days or weeks of use.

Early complications are not unique to dialysis catheters but may be seen following percutaneous puncture or cannulation of the subclavian vein. They include pneumothorax, haemothorax, the inability to cannulate the vessel, puncture of the artery and air or catheter embolism. Perforation of the superior vena cava leading to sudden haemothorax (29) and mediastinal haematoma (30), and perforation of the right atrium leading to haemopericardium (31–33), are two unique complications of long term subclavian catheter usage, many of these complications occurring with stiff Teflon catheters. The inherent stiffness of these catheters causes them to impinge on the wall of the vessel rather than float in the centre of the vessel lumen. During single needle dialysis they are subject to a 'to and fro' motion which is largely responsible for the eventual perforation of the vessel.

Infections are a major concern with subclavian catheters. The incidence of catheter infection varies; some early publications report a much higher incidence (34, 35) than the more recent studies (36, 37). Analysis of the risk factors revealed that infections are more frequent in certain groups of patients such as diabetic patients with chronic renal failure, patients receiving immunosuppressive therapy or in those with staphylococcal infection. Subcutaneous catheter tunnelling was also considered to be a risk factor relating to infections, but a recent study by Dahlberg (38) revealed that this procedure had no influence on catheter bacteremia.

Subclavian vein thrombosis and stenosis may also occur.

Ratcliffe and Oliver (39) described large quantities of thrombus adherent to the catheter and adjacent vessel wall while Davis et al (40) reported suclavian vein stenosis following the use of subclavian catheters, an observation confirmed by others (27, 41).

Nand et al (42) and Kozeny et al (26) both described red cell fragmentation associated with subclavian catheters which they attributed to partial catheter occlusion. Other complications of subclavian catheterisation include occlusion of the subclavian vein (43) and thrombotic arm oedema (44).

NEEDLES FOR SINGLE NEEDLE DIALYSIS

Coaxial counter flow needles of designs comparable with those for catheters have been developed and have seen limited clinical application (45, 46). Their limited use may be attributable to excessive pressure necessary to puncture the skin and fistula and excessive bleeding following the removal of such needles. The more currently used needles for single needle dialysis are single lumen.

DEVICE HAEMODYNAMICS

A haemodynamically efficient catheter or needle may be defined as one which for a minimum diameter and area of puncture provides a clinically acceptable blood flow at a modest pressure gradient.

Access devices in clinical use fall into three major categories, those with a single circular lumen, those of coaxial construction and those consisting of two semi-circular lumens.

Theoretical relationships for the flow pressure characteristics of each of these major types of access device have been developed (47) and are given by:

$$Q = \frac{\prod d^2 \Delta P}{128 \mu L} \quad \text{for circular catheters or needles}$$

$$Q = \frac{\prod [d_o^4 - d_i^4 - (d_o^2 - d_i^2)^2] \; \Delta P}{128 \mu L \quad \quad \text{Log}_e \, d_o/d_i}$$

for coaxial catheters or needles and

$$Q = \frac{\prod^3}{252.24 \mu L \, (\prod + 2)^2} \; \frac{d^4}{} \; \Delta P$$

for catheters or needles consisting of two semi circular lumens

where

$\prod$ = constant
μ = viscosity
L = length
d = diameter
d_o = outer diameter
d_i = inner diameter.

Experimental studies for needles and catheters' haemodynamic characteristics have been performed by a number of investigators (19, 45, 48–50). These have highlighted a wide variability between devices from different manufacturers as well as the ability to attain clinically acceptable flows only at the expense of excessively high pressure by some makes of device.

MECHANICAL SYSTEMS OF SINGLE NEEDLE

Mechanical systems of single needle dialysis break the continuous flow pattern associated with conventional dialysis into an outflow and return phase which results in an intermittent cyclic flow pattern through the extracorporeal circuit. The duration of each phase and the switching from one phase to another is controlled by pressure or time or a combination of the two. Mechanical systems may utilise either one or two pumps.

Single pump mechanical systems

The original single pump mechanical system for single needle dialysis described by Kopp et al (1) was a pressure-time controlled pump. The hydraulic circuit (without electrical control connections) is shown in Figure 3. The blood pump operates continuously in the arterial or aspiration phase and the clamp in the arterial line is open, blood is drawn out from the patient into the extracorporeal circuit, the venous clamp is closed and pressure builds up in the circuit. When the pre-set maximum pressure is reached, the venous clamp is released and the blood in the extracorporeal circuit is returned to the patient, the return phase being controlled by an adjustable timer switch. Upon reaching the pre-selected time, the clamp closes and the cycle is repeated. In a variant of this system the aspiration and return phases are governed by individually adjustable arterial and venous clamp timers.

Figure 4 shows the hydraulic circuit of a pressure-pressure controlled single pump system. In such a system the pump operates intermittently and only a venous clamp is used. In the arterial phase blood is withdrawn from the patient, the venous line clamp is closed and a build up of pressure occurs in the venous drip chamber. When the pre-set maximum pressure is reached the blood pump stops and blood is returned to the patient by the pressure head generated during the arterial cycle. Upon reaching the lower pre-set pressure, the cycle is repeated.

A recently developed variant of single pump systems has been the reciprocating syringe system described by De Virgiliis et al (51) a system which replaces the commonly used blood pump with a specially designed syringe coupled to a reciprocating cam. The unidirectional flow in the system is ensured by the use of mechanical clamps that work in synchronisation with the cam action.

Double pump mechanical systems

The concept of the double pump mechanical system first described by Van Waeleghem and coworkers (52) evolved as a consequence of the desire to overcome the problems ascribed to single pump tidal flow systems during their clin-

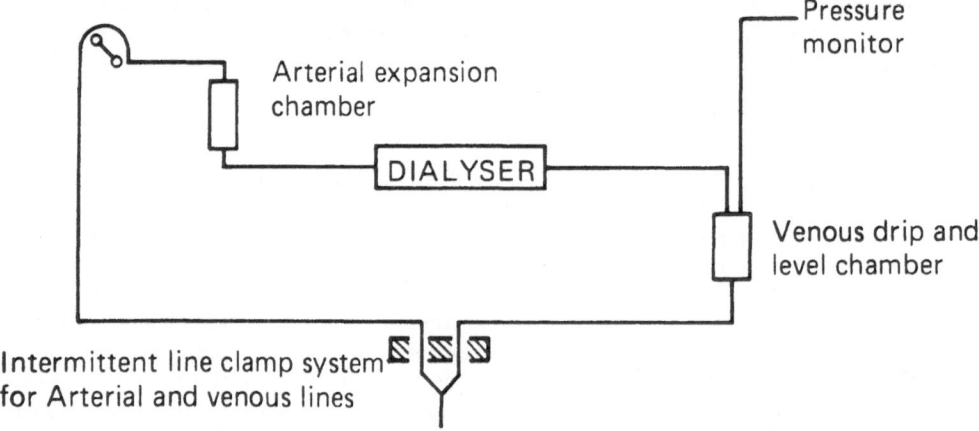

Figure 3. Hydraulic circuit of a pressure-time controlled single pump mechanical system for single needle dialysis.

ical use. In such systems the clamps are replaced by peristaltic pumps and operate on a pressure-pressure cycle. The original system, in production until recently, unlike its more recent variants, used a single electric motor coupled by a clutch mechanism to two pumpheads. This clutch mechanism eliminated the problem of achieving instantaneous flow when starting and stopping the pump heads because the electric motor ran continuously.

Figure 5 shows the hydraulic circuit of such an early system. As with the single pump systems a cyclic mode of operation exists. In the arterial phase, blood is drawn from the patient via the arterial pumphead into the circuit. Since the venous pumphead is occlusive, the pressure in the circuit increases. Upon reaching the pre-set upper pressure limit, the arterial pumphead stops, the venous pumphead is activated and the blood is pumped back to the patient. This causes the pressure to fall in the circuit until the lower pre-set pressure is reached. The cycle is then repeated. The difference between the two pressure limits governs the volume pumped during each cycle. The most recent variant of this system (Figure 6) uses a modified extracorporeal circuit (Figure 7) which allows monitoring of the extracorporeal circuit downstream from the venous pumphead. The insertion of the second drip chamber requires the incorporation of an intermittent line clamp to prevent changes in the drip chamber level during the aspiration phase. This hydraulic circuit forms the basis of the majority of clinically used double pump tidal flow systems of single needle dialysis. Variations of this concept have been produced by Cobe Laboratories (Figure 8) and Travenol (Figure 9), the latter

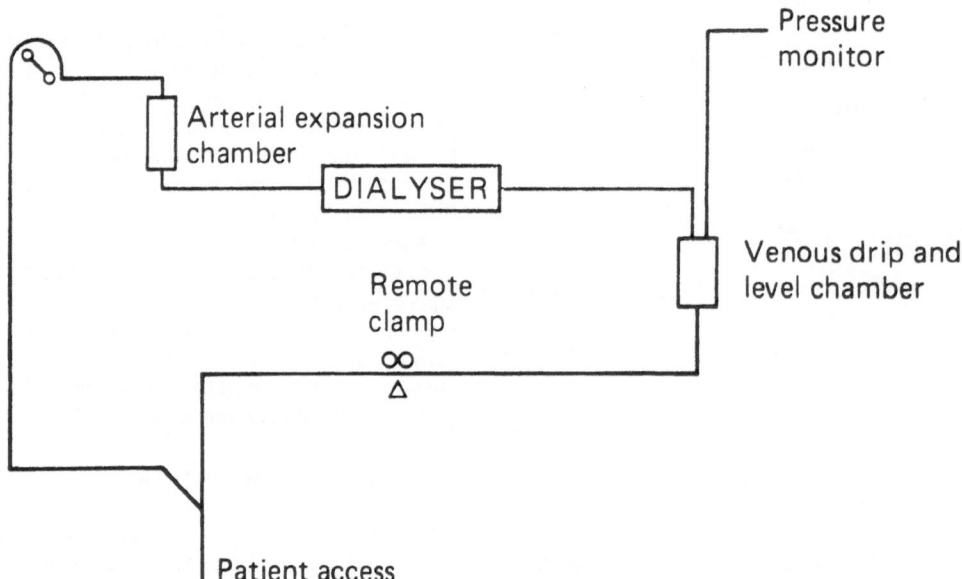

Figure 4. Hydraulic circuit of pressure-pressure controlled single pump mechanical system for single needle dialysis.

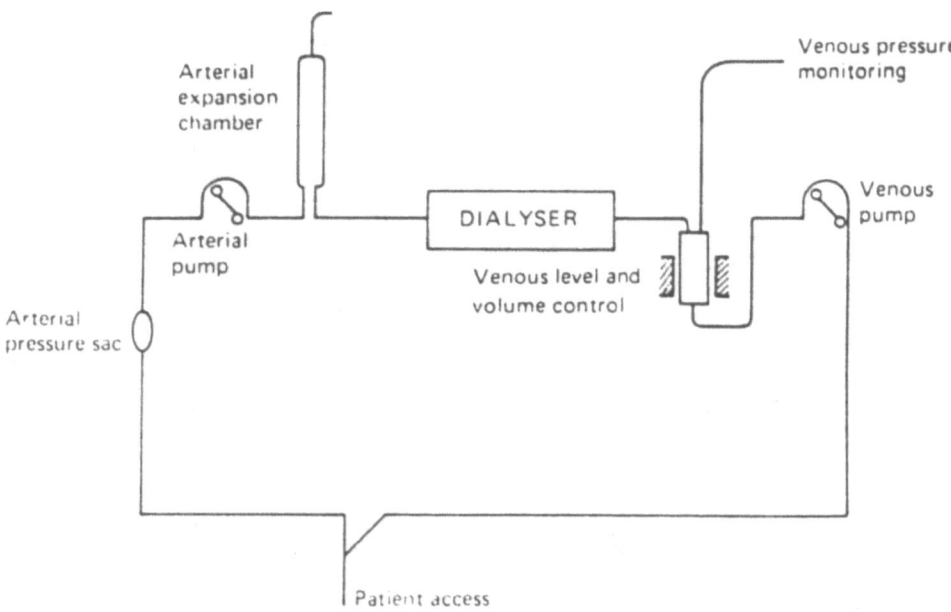

Figure 5. Hydraulic circuit of pressure-pressure controlled double pump mechanical system for single needle dialysis.

involving the use of a microprocessor control system to regulate the blood pump speeds. The use of a compliant accumulator bag after the dialyser eliminates the need to pre-set the upper and lower pressure limits. As the bag is highly compliant and essentially nonelastic when it is full it triggers an electronic pressure sensor switching the arterial pump off and activating the venous pump. The venous pump runs until a pre-set volume (monitored by the microprocessor via the number of venous pumphead revolutions) is returned to the patient. The cycle is then repeated.

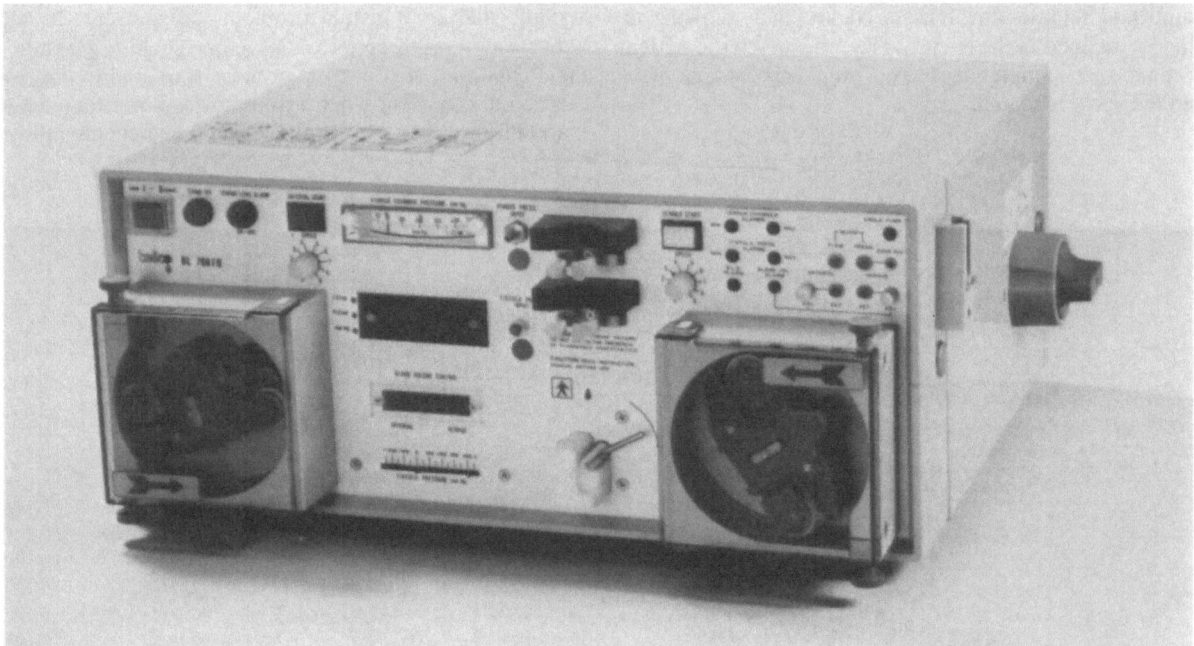

Figure 6. Bellco BL 760 FB double pump mechanical system for single needle dialysis.

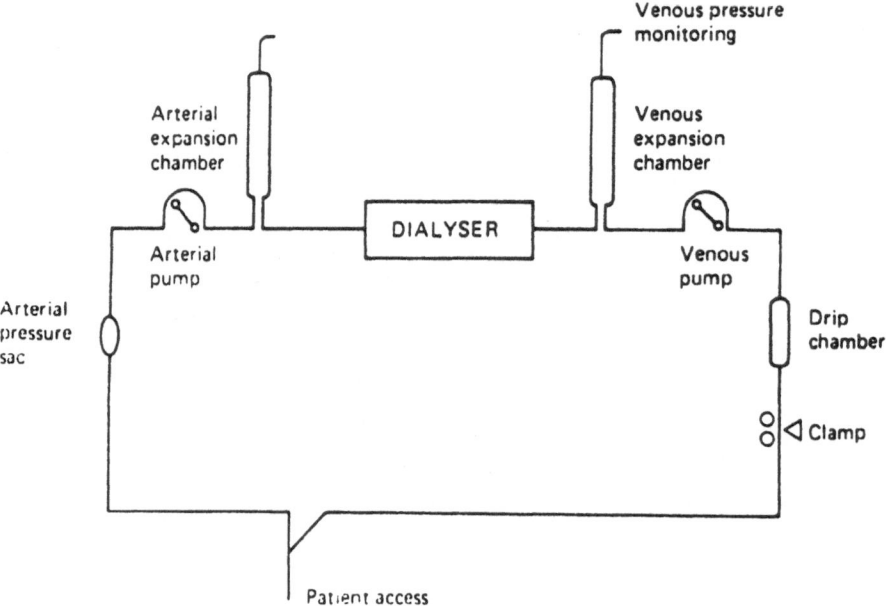

Figure 7. Hydraulic circuit of pressure-pressure controlled double pump mechanical system for single needle dialysis incorporating a secondary venous level and line clamp.

An accumulator bag in conjunction with blood pumps, both in the arterial segment of the extracorporeal circuit has been described by Cunningham et al (53) and is used by the Fresenius A 1008 system. The first pump extracts the blood from the patient and pumps it into the accumulator bag causing the pressure to rise. When it is full the pressure sensor switches the first pump off, activates the second pump and releases the remote clamp, thus allowing the blood contained in the circuit to be returned to the patient. When the accumulator bag is empty the sensor is reactivated and the cycle repeated.

CLINICAL ASPECTS OF SINGLE NEEDLE DIALYSIS

Recirculation

Recirculation or the mixing of purified and nonpurified blood has long been recognised as a feature of single needle dialysis. This type of recirculation may also occur in two needle dialysis if fistula problems are present. In single needle systems three factors have been held responsible for recirculation (54–57). First of these is related to the fistula itself and can occur when fistula flow is lower than dialyser blood flow either as a consequence of inadequate inflow or

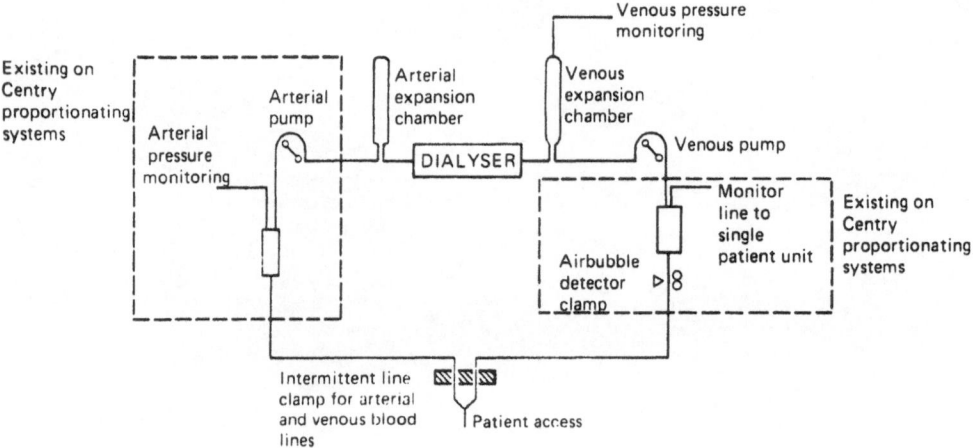

Figure 8. Hydraulic circuit of the Cobe Laboratories pressure-pressure controlled double pump system option for single needle dialysis.

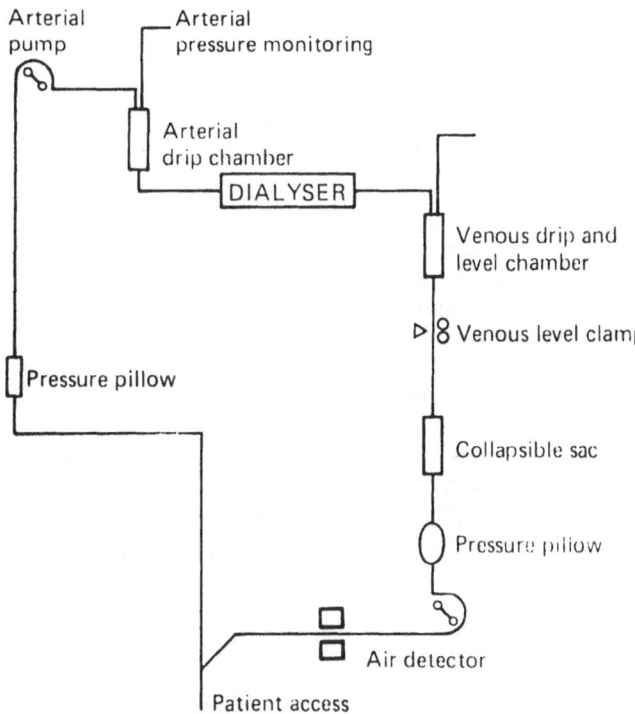

Figure 9. Hydraulic circuit of Travenol SPS system option for single needle dialysis.

outflow. Too often, single needle dialysis is used with a poor fistula, a combination that results in compromised dialytic efficiency. In such circumstances single needle dialysis is an unsuitable option and to avoid compromised dialytic efficiency and flow problems, surgical correction of the arteriovenous fistula is the only suitable solution.

The second cause of recirculation is the use of a common pathway or dead space for the blood entering and leaving the patient. The importance of this dead space varies since it is related to the stroke volume or volume pumped per cycle. As the dead space of the needle or catheter increases, the stroke volume needs to be increased (58).

The third source of recirculation is the extracorporeal circuit compliance resulting from the fluctuating pressures causing the tubing to expand and contract in the aspiration and return phases, this expansion and contraction contributing to the total dead space of their circuit. The use of a long race track to measure blood flow in single needle systems contributes to the compliance and if measurements are made with such a track in situ the result is likely to overestimate true recirculation. In mechanical systems of single needle, a degree of compliance is required for optimal operation and is achieved by the addition of an arterial expansion chamber since in such systems, a further source of recirculation is the frequency of switching from the aspiration to return phases of the cycle.

Estimation of recirculation

Clinical estimation of the total recirculation may be made by

the comparison of solute concentration in peripheral blood (C_p) and the concentrations in the arterial (C_a) and venous (C_v) segments of the extracorporeal circuit by the use of the formula:

$$R = \frac{(C_p - C_a)}{(C_p - C_v)}.$$

Although this relationship is applicable to any solute, it is most commonly performed for urea and creatinine.

Several studies have been described measuring recirculation in single needle dialysis (59–65). These are summarised in Table 1. These indicate that the older single pump tidal flow systems were subject to high (17 to 22%) recirculation rates due to the short cycle times with which they were used. In spite of a low volume and compliance more recent double pump systems show lower recirculation (9 to 17%).

Recirculation with single lumen central venous catheters was markedly higher than with single lumen fistula needles reflecting the differences in dead space between the two (63). The lowest recirculation rates reported (3 to 5%) were attained with double lumen fistula needles (61, 65, 66).

Blood flow in single needle dialysis

Currently used dialysis schedules require the attainment of blood flows in excess of 200 ml/min. In both catheters and mechanical single needle systems the attainment of this ideal poses problems and may not be possible.

Mechanical systems using a single pump are subject to limitations which have resulted in their declining use since the blood flow attainable is at the expense of a high dialyser pressure; this, in turn, leads to a high mandatory ultrafiltration. The amount of blood pumped into the extracorporeal circuit is also a function of the pressure in the system and unless significant compliance is added, the cycle volume is low, leading to high recirculation.

Blood flow depends in part on catheter design. Attainment of clinically acceptable blood flows may be at the expense of excessively high return pressures with resulting poor control of ultrafiltration. Figures 10 and 11 show the blood flow profiles and circuit pressures in single and double pump mechanical systems. In single pump systems clinically acceptable flow is at the expense of a high dialyser pressure. In a double pump mechanical system of single needle the actual flow through the dialyser may be established by considering the relationship between the mean blood flow and that achieved during the arterial and venous cycles. The mean blood flow is a function of the arterial pump speed, the length of time it runs and the number of cycles per minute, such that:

$$Q_B = n \frac{ta}{60} Q_A$$

Similarly, during the venous phase:

$$Q_B = n \frac{tv}{60} Q_V$$

since

$$n = \frac{60}{ta + tv}$$

where Q_B is the mean blood flow, Q_A and Q_V the blood flows obtained during the arterial and venous cycle, ta and tv the duration of the arterial and venous pumping cycle, and n the number of cycles per minute.

Clinically acceptable mean blood flow rates are only possible with patients having sufficient fistula flows since the peak flow rates required during the arterial and venous phases must be twice that of the mean blood flow, because the pumps run only during half of each cycle.

From a practical consideration, the arterial and venous flow rates will only be twice the mean flow rate if the cycle times are equal. As the withdrawal of blood may be more difficult at high flow rates, but the return can generally support high flow rates, adjustment of the arterial and venous cycle times may be necessary.

In mechanical systems of single needle the flow profile varies in different parts of the extracorporeal circuit. The flow fluctuation during operation is maximal at the access site and decreases in amplitude proximal to the dialyser and are largely damped out distal to the dialyser by the dialyser and expansion chamber compliance. This variable flow profile has no clinical significance but is important to bear in mind when measuring blood flow during single needle dialysis for experimental purposes.

For clinical purposes an approximation of the blood flow may be made by timing the blood pump revolutions and applying the formula:

$$\frac{(\text{Number of revolutions}) \times (\text{volume pumped per revolution})}{\text{time taken}}.$$

The volume pumped per revolution may be established experimentally. This calculation is performed automatically and displayed on demand in a number of commercially available systems.

There is an absence of data given in the literature concerning flow rates attained during clinical use of single needle systems. Furthermore, some differences in the ability of some commercially available systems to sustain mean blood flows in excess of 200 ml/min also exist (58). Our own measurements on 76 patients who routinely use a commercially available double pump mechanical system of single needle revealed a mean flow of 284 ± 33 ml/min (Mean ± SD) (64), values which have remained largely unaltered with time (67).

Table 1. Degree of recirculation.

Authors, year	Dialysis system	Vascular access	N	Recirculation
Keshaviah et al (59)	SP	SLN	3	17–19%
Ogden (60)	SP	SLN	20	19–22%
Vanholder et al (61)	DP	SLN	7	16–17%*
Hoenich et al (62)	DP	SLN	5	9–10%
Vanholder et al (63)	DP	SLN	7	12–15%*
Vanholder et al (64)	DP	SLN	76	14%*
Vanholder et al (63)	DP	SC	7	14–25%*
Ogden and Cohen (65)	SP	DLN	42	4.7%
Vanholder et al (61)	DP	DLN	7	3.2%*

N = number of observations; SP: single pump; DP: double pump; SLN: single lumen needle; SC: subclavian catheter; DLN: double lumen needle.

* The values marked by an asterisk were obtained with a 3 m line for bubble flow measurements in place.

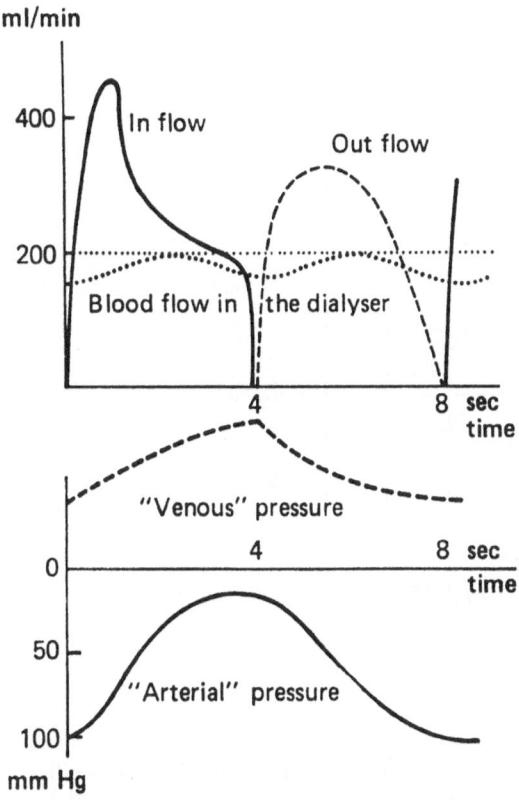

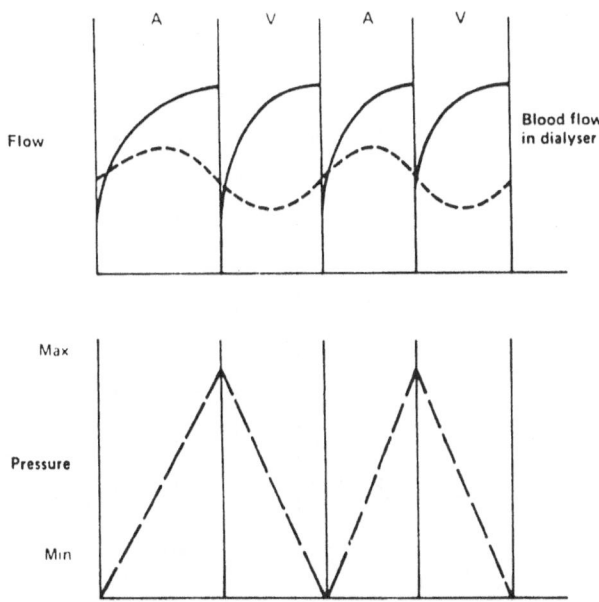

Figure 11. Blood flow profile in extracorporeal circuit when using double pump mechanical system of single needle dialysis (pressure-pressure operation).

Figure 10. Blood flow profile in extracorporeal circuit when using single pump mechanical system of single needle dialysis (time-time operation).

Solute removal during single needle dialysis

Clearance at the dialyser level, as measured by the conventional formula, is unchanged by recirculation. However, with recirculation clearance does not provide a measure of the volumetric rate at which the patient's blood is cleared of the solutes since, due to this recirculation, the systemic blood concentration will be higher than the blood concentration entering the dialyser. Consequently, the clearance must be corrected for this difference. This correction, derived by Gotch (55), is given by:

$$KR: \frac{K(1-R)}{[1-R(1-K/Q_B)]}$$

The percentage decrease clearance may be obtained from rearrangement of the above formula i.e.:

$$[1 - K_R/K] \cdot 100$$

The relationship between K_R and R, shown in Figure 12, shows that solutes with low molecular weights that are cleared during dialysis decrease in clearance, due to this recirculation; the percentual magnitude of the decrease is always less important than the percentual degree of recirculation. Nevertheless, with high efficiency dialysis (high K/Q_B), the impact of recirculation on dialyser clearance is more important than in the case of poorly dialysed large molecular weight solutes.

Since recirculation decreases effective dialyser clearance an adaptation of treatment time might be appropriate.

Recent studies by the US National Cooperative Dialysis Study (72, 73) have suggested than an adequate dialysis

Cell damage

Cell damage by mechanical trauma is well recognised. Such damage during single needle dialysis may arise due to the tidal nature of the flow in such systems and the shear stresses that such flow patterns may generate at the needle or catheter, since at this point in the extracorporeal circuit the flows per unit cross sectional area are the highest. This damage may as well be the consequence of damage from the blood pumps.

A recognised manifestation of cell damage is haemolysis. The factors affecting haemolysis in extracorporeal dialysis circuits have been studied by Veitch et al (68). Hilderson et al (69) studied the indices of haemolysis with the Bellco BL 760 single needle system and observed no difference in measured parameters compared with two needle dialysis. More recently, attention has been focused on platelet aggregation in extracorporeal circuits due to shear stress (70, 71), but little information is available regarding the magnitude of shear stresses in clinically used needles or catheters although Mahurkar (47) has derived estimates of shear values for commonly used catheters.

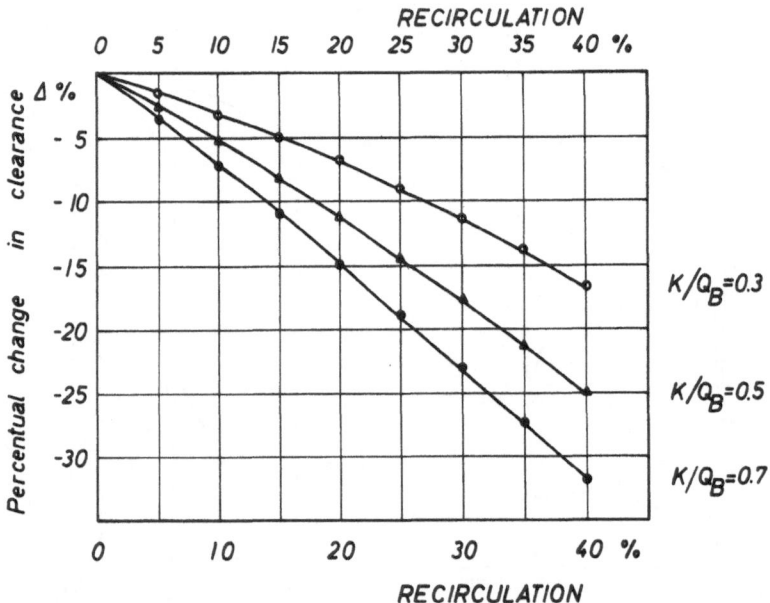

Figure 12. Influence of recirculation on clearance.

prescription during three times weekly dialysis is achieved for urea if:

$$\frac{K \times t}{V} = 1.$$

In the presence of recirculation the above relationship may be written as:

$$\frac{K_R \times t}{V} = 1$$

from which by rearrangement the treatment time as a function of recirculation may be calculated and is shown in Table 2. It is obvious from Table 2 that for a recirculation value of 15% and K/Q_B of 0.5, dialysis duration should be increased by only 8.83% to obtain a comparable dialysis efficiency as with two needle dialysis. For high efficiency dialysers ($K/Q_B = 0.7$), the impact of recirculation is more important.

The clearance of small molecules during haemodialysis is governed principally by the fluid dynamics within the device while those of middle molecules depend on membrane permeability and haemodialyser area. Hilderson et al (69) suggested that the tidal flow generated during single needle dialysis is of benefit as it enhances the clearance of middle molecules, possibly because the periodic flows through the dialyser cause the compliant pathways of the dialyser to flex and contract. Recent studies, which are summarised in Ta-

Table 2. Relationship between recirculation and dialysis time (t).

	Recirculation (%)	Increase t (%)	Increase t (min)		
			A	B	C
$K/Q_B = 0.5$	5	2.63	4.73	6.31*	7.89*
	7.5	4.05	7.31	9.74*	12.18*
	10	5.56	10.01	13.34*	16.68*
	15	8.83	15.89	21.19*	26.49*
$K/Q_B = 0.7$	5	3.69	6.64*	8.86*	11.07
	7.5	5.68	10.22*	13.63*	17.04
	10	7.78	14.00*	18.67*	30.00
	15	12.36	22.25*	29.66*	37.08

t = dialysis time (min); K/Q_B = clearance/flow (filtration fraction). A, B and C: original t-value in the absence of recirculation of 180, 240 and 300 min. respectively.
All calculations are based on a distribution volume of 40 l.
The values, resulting in a K_T/V-value (relation of total clearance over distribution volume) of ± 1 for a blood flow of 300 ml/min are marked by an asterisk.

ble 3, have failed to demonstrate differences in the case of small molecules but showed enhanced inulin clearance confirming Hilderson's original observations.

Fluid removal during single needle dialysis

Clinical dialysis may be performed with proportionating systems not equipped to control ultrafiltration with double pump mechanical systems. In such systems the double pump system may be used to control ultrafiltration since an increase or decrease of the mean hydraulic pressure may be achieved by the alteration of the blood compartment pressure, and this pressure has a constant relationship to the mean hydraulic pressure (Figure 13). A direct consequence of this control is the ability to use high permeability membranes with such systems (74).

When using such a system for controlling ultrafiltration two points must, however, be borne in mind. First, care must be taken to ensure that the blood outlet pressure exceeds the dialysate inlet pressure thus minimising the risk of reverse ultrafiltration particularly in the case of hollow fibre devices. The second relates to the use of ultrafiltration coefficients. The ultrafiltration coefficient of a dialyser represents the slope of the line relating ultrafiltration rate to mean hydraulic pressure such that:

$$UFC = \frac{Q_f}{P_{nett}}$$

by definition P_{nett} is given by:

$$\frac{(P_B in + P_B out)}{2} - \frac{(P_D in + P_D out)}{2}.$$

In clinical practice, all pressures may not be measured and provided the pressure drops in the blood an dialysate pathways are small, P_{nett} approximates the arithmetic sum of the two most commonly measured pressures (P_B out and P_D out). The assumption that the pressure drop in the blood pathway is small is invalid when using double pump mechanical systems of single needle. Hence, a considerable underestimate of the true pressure may exist, when P_{nett} is considered, unless a correction factor is added to the arithmetic sum of the two measured pressures. This correction factor may be derived by consideration of the average hydraulic pressures during a cycle and is given by:

$$\frac{\Delta P_B min \text{ and } \Delta P_B max}{4}$$

where $P_B min$ and $P_B max$ represent the minimum and maximum pressure drops in the blood pathway. Such a correction is valid for noncompliant devices but needs to be modified for use in compliant devices to allow for the changes in the dialysate pathway resistance induced by the changing blood compartment pressure.

Adequacy of treatment

Measurement of urea kinetics has become an accepted and valuable tool in quantifying the adequacy of dialysis treatment (75, 76). Essentially, this technique involves the calculation of the time averaged concentration of urea (TAC_{urea}) together with the protein catabolic rate (PCR), the latter being directly related to dietary protein intake (PI) in equilibriated noncatabolic patients (77). In such patients PCR ranges from 0.8 to 1.4 g/kg/24 h which corresponds to an adequate protein intake (78). The US National Cooperative Dialysis Study showed that a low morbidity in a large multicentre population corresponded to a TAC_{Urea} value (BUN) of 50 mg/100 ml (17.9 mmol/l), whereas a significantly higher morbidity was observed if the TAC_{Urea} was allowed to rise above 70 mg/100 ml (25 mmol/l) either as a result of a decrease in treatment time or dialyser surface area (72).

Despite the availability and use of single needle for routine renal replacement therapy, kinetic modelling has not been used extensively except for a single small study (79). More recently, however, the authors have studied TAC_{Urea} values in a large group of unselected chronic renal failure patients treated continuously with a double pump pressure-pressure controlled single needle system and compared these values with those established by the US National Cooperative Dialysis Study (Figure 14). This shows comparable mid-week predialysis urea concentrations. Furthermore, the values obtained in the course of low efficiency two

Table 3. In vitro solute clearance at a blood flow of 200 ml/min in single and double needle mode. (Dialysate flow 500 ml/min; Temperature 38° C.)

Dialyser	Clearance (ml/min)					
	Urea (60)		Creatinine (113)		^{14}C Inulin (5175)	
	single needle	double needle	single needle	double needle	single needle	double needle
Bellco BL501 Bravo	153 ± 1.5	148 ± 1.0	124 ± 1.7	123 ± 1.7	7.2 ± 2.2	9.6 ± 2.9
Gambro GF 120M	158 ± 1.1	157 ± 1.7	133 ± 0.8	129 ± 1.1	7.5 ± 4.1	3.0 ± 0.8
Toray B1 Filtryzer	172 ± 4.1	167 ± 1.0	146 ± 0.7	138 ± 1.0	20.0 ± 3.0	10.2 ± 1.8

Mean ± standard deviation corrected to zero ultrafiltration.
Number of dialysers studied of each variant = 2.

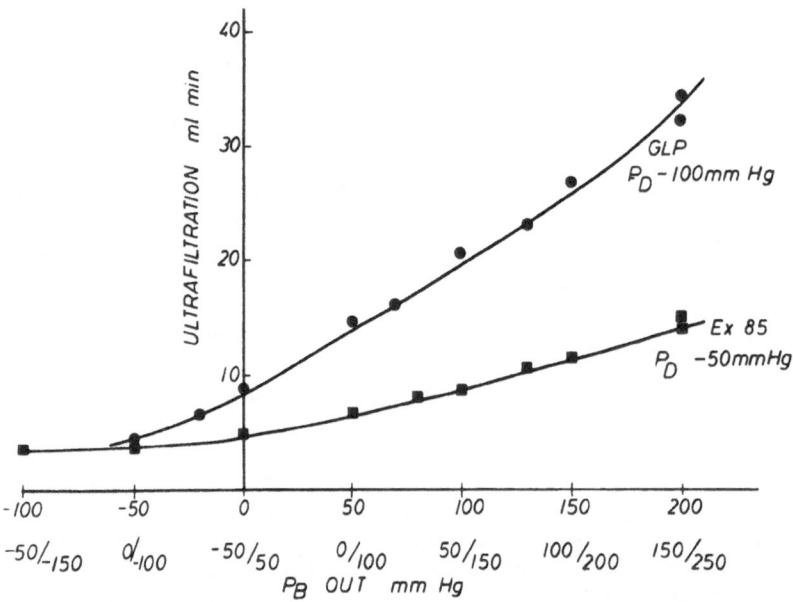

Figure 13. Ultrafiltration control by a pressure-pressure controlled double pump system of single needle dialysis for two dialysers. P_B is pressure in the blood lines, P_D is dialysate pressure.

needle dialysis with a high morbidity, exceeded those observed for single needle dialysis suggesting that provided adequate fistula flow and dialyser blood flow are available, single needle dialysis adequacy is comparable with that attained during adequate dialysis with two needles. Gotch et al (73) suggested that adequate dialysis prescription during three times weekly dialysis is achieved if K_t/V approaches unity. Our own studies with the above patient group have demonstrated close agreement with the above ideal. To our knowledge this is the first study of adequacy of dialysis for a large group of patients using one type of double pump single needle system (Bellco BL 760) (Bellco SpA, Mirandola, Italy). It cannot be taken for granted that other single needle systems yield comparable results, especially if the attainment of clinically acceptable blood flows and low rates of recirculation is not possible.

Patient mortality and morbidity

Patient mortality in those treated with single needle dialysis has only rarely been studied extensively (64, 80, 81). When such data are compared with those in the EDTA-ERA registry (82–84) it appears that the cumulative survival of patients is equal to or better than for those treated by conventional dialysis (Table 4). In our centre, 71 patients have used this modality of treatment continuously for more than 5 years, 13 patients remaining under treatment for more than a decade (85). Two of them were treated for 15 years.

Morbidity data are also scarce. As part of our study on the adequacy of single needle dialysis we compared hospitalisation rate with that reported in the US National Cooperative Dialysis Study. Among our 20 patients 82% remained unhospitalised after 52 weeks, a figure comparable to that obtained in the two groups of the American Study with low morbidity and a TAC_{Urea} between 51.3 and 56 mg/100 ml (18.3 and 20 mmol/l).

In our experience double pump operated single needle dialysis is well tolerated haemodynamically, due to the ability to control ultrafiltration and possibly a reduced incidence of disequilibrium during treatment because of the slower rate of change of small molecular concentration resulting from recirculation (1). This may relate to the observed good mortality and morbidity values.

Fistula survival

The main advantage of single needle dialysis is that the vascular access will be punctured half as frequently than with two needle dialysis, thereby reducing trauma to the fistula and patient discomfort. Cumulative fistula survival during single needle dialysis has received extensive study (86–90).

Reported data are compared with those in two needle dialysis (88, 90–93) in Table 5. These data indicate a better fistula survival for the single needle system.

Single and two needle dialysis have been compared directly with each other in only two studies. Van Waeleghem et al (88) demonstrated that the 5 year vascular access patency was significantly better for single needle dialysis compared with two needle dialysis irrespective of whether Cimino-Brescia fistulas or Xenografts were taken into consideration. Krönung (90), on the other hand, failed to observe any differences between single needle and double needle access. Survival at the end of 4 years in their study of 201 fistulas in four dialysis centres of which 41 were used with single needle, were similar for both techniques, but they did

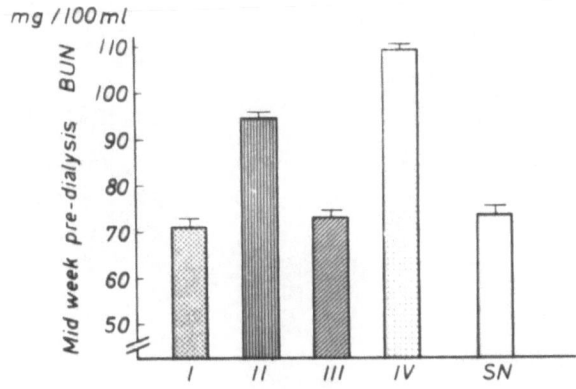

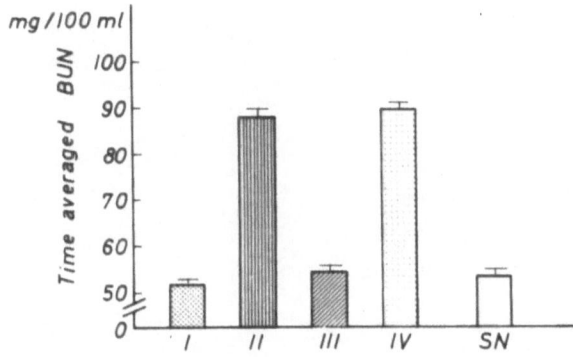

Figure 14. Mid-week pre-dialysis urea (above) and TAC$_{Urea}$-values (below) in patients on single needle dialysis (SN) and in groups I, II, III and IV of the American National Cooperative Dialysis Study (NCDS) (76). The patients on single needle dialysis, and groups I and III of the NCDS-study had a low dialysis-related morbidity, whereas group II and IV had a high morbidity.

note that when each of the centres were separated, significant but discrepant differences were noted.

Although these studies, in general, demonstrate better fistula survival in single needle dialysis, the results are influenced by many parameters independent of puncture, while considerable differences in the quality of puncture technique as well as a variability in the indications for use of single needle techniques make statistical comparisons difficult to interpret.

Table 4. Cumulative patient survival (%).

	1 yr	2 yr	3 yr	5 yr	10 yr
Single needle					
Becaus et al (81)	90	86	77	67	–
Vanholder et al (64)	94	82	76	64	43
Two needle					
EDTA 1980 (82)	87	78	69	54	37
EDTA 1983 (83)	89	80	71	–	–
EDTA 1984 (84)	90	77	69	58	–

Strategy for single needle use

Use of single needle dialysis techniques is helpful in a number of specific situations, e.g. the treatment of acute renal failure since vascular access may be obtained simply, by central venous catheterisation, allowing treatment to be initiated quickly. It is well tolerated by children (94, 95) and suitable for use in small fistulas if the usable length is too small for the insertion of two needles provided that fistula blood flow is sufficiently adequate to yield clinically acceptable flow rates. In routine clinical dialysis, it has often been used as a last resort in patients with poorly functioning fistulae in preference to surgical revision. Use in such situations inevitably leads to compromised dialysis efficiency and is possibly the reason why this technique has failed to gain widespread clinical acceptance until today. Expense and complexity of operation may also contribute to the lack of clinical acceptance of mechanical systems of single needle.

However, one of the benefits of the new generation of double pump mechanical systems is their polyvalence allowing them to be used for all current blood purification strategies and within this context such systems have been used for haemodialysis with devices containing high permeability membranes (74), isolated ultrafiltration in the presence of fluid overload (96), sequential dialysis and ultrafiltration (97), haemofiltration (98, 99), haemodiafiltration (100), plasmapheresis (101–104) and haemoperfusion, all with the same equipment (97). The fact that currently used mechanical systems of single needle dialysis are more complex to operate than conventional two needle dialysis cannot be denied, particularly when such systems are used infrequently. This problem is being resolved by the third generation 'user friendly' systems now becoming available for clinical use such as the Bellco Mimo (Bellco SpA, Mirandola, Italy) (Figure 15). This not only makes use of microprocessor technology to control and monitor operating parameters but

Table 5. Cumulative fistula survival (%) (Hospital dialysis-Brescia-Cimino fistulas).

	1 yr	2 yr	3 yr	5 yr
Single needle				
De Clippele et al (86)	96	89	87	86
Kopp et al (87)	93	89	84	84
Van Waeleghem et al (88)	89	83	–	72
Liu Jing-Duo et al (89)	91	86	86	79
Krönung et al (90)	88	72	65	–
Vanholder et al (64)	94	–	79	74
Two needle				
Haimov et al (91)[a]	68	54	–	–
Rohr et al (92)	61	52	52	–
Raily et al (93)	80	75	72	–
Krönung et al (90)	82	82	72	–
Van Waeleghem et al (88)	84	78	–	62

[a] Cumulative survival calculated from the reported data.

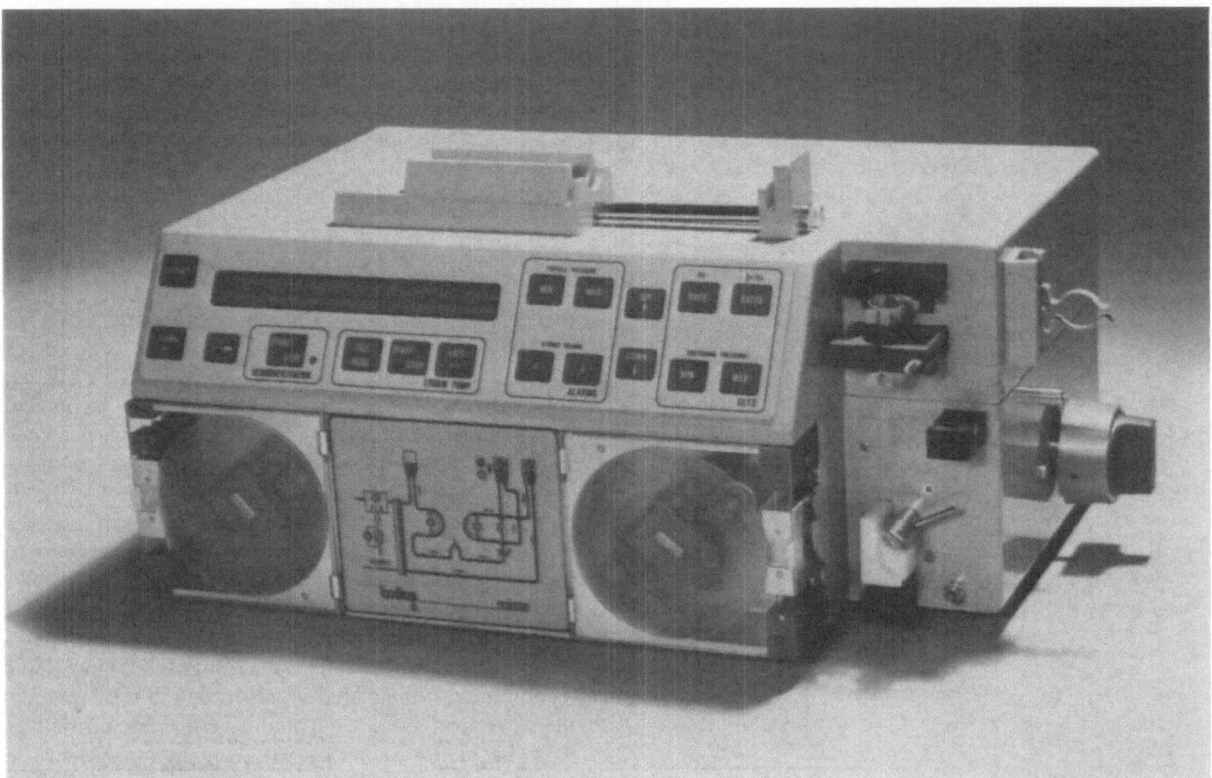

Figure 15. Bellco Mimo new single needle pump system.

also incorporates a liquid crystal display which both displays these parameters and instructs the operator on the nature and remedy of any faults that may develop during clinical use.

CONCLUSION

It is still a widely held belief that the single needle technique is inefficient, and should be reserved for selected patients, e.g. children or persons with an inadequate fistula. The misunderstanding on the efficiency of single needle dialysis can mainly be attributed to the fact that most of the negative experience with single needle dialysis has been obtained with older systems, that are not pressure-pressure monitored. Due to their technical structure, blood flows and clearances are low, whereas recirculation is high, and ultrafiltration control impossible with these older time-time or pressure-time monitored systems.

The pressure-pressure single needle method, that is now currently available, enables adequate dialysis, as delineated by multiple indices of dialysis efficiency, such as dialyzer blood flow, dialyzer clearance, TAC_{Urea}, K_t/V, and patient morbidity that all are highly comparable to the values observed during adequate two needle dialysis.

Furthermore, a number of positive advantages are typical for this single needle system. The perfect ultrafiltration control is reflected in the absence of major changes in cardiac output and arterial oxygen tension. This ultrafiltration control also plays a role in the versatility of this dialysis system, and allows the performance of several other techniques (plasmapheresis, haemofiltration, haemodiafiltration) with the same basic infrastructure; if a two needle system is used on the contrary, it is often necessary to have different machines available for different techniques.

Another positive advantage is that fistula survival is obviously longer with this single needle system. This fact might turn out to be extremely important in an era of treatment where patients can often be expected to remain on dialysis for a decade or more, and where the lack of adequate access may influence patient survival and quality of life in a major way.

Subsequently, we are convinced that the single needle method is at least equivalent to two needle dialysis and that it even should be a method of preference, especially in older and haemodynamically labile persons, and in those where it is expected that dialysis will continue over several years.

REFERENCES

1. Kopp KF, Gutch CF, Kolff WJ: Single needle dialysis. *Trans*

Am Soc Artif Intern Organs 18: 75, 1972

2. Twiss EE: One-cannula haemodialysis. *Lancet* 2: 1106, 1964
3. Brunner FP, Brynger H, Chantler C, Donckerwolcke RA, Hathway RA, Jacobs C, Selwood NH, Wing AJ: Combined report on regular dialysis and transplantation in Europe IX. *Proc Eur Dial Transplant Assoc* 16: 2, 1979
4. Quinton WE, Dillard D, Scribner BH: Cannulation of blood vessels for prolonged hemodialysis. *Trans Am Soc Artif Intern Organs* 6: 104, 1960
5. Brescia MJ, Cimino JE, Appel K, Hurwich BJ: Chronic hemodialysis using venipuncture and a surgically created arteriovenous fistula. *N Engl J Med* 275: 1089, 1966
6. Shaldon S, Chiandussi L, Higgs B: Haemodialysis by percutaneous catheterisation of the femoral artery and vein with regional heparinisation. *Lancet* 2: 857, 1961
7. Shaldon S, Rae AI, Rosen SM, Silva H, Oakley J: Refrigerated femoral venous-venous haemodialysis with coil preservation for rehabilitation of terminal uraemic patients. *Lancet* 1: 1716, 1963
8. Erben J, Kvasnicka J, Bastecky J, Vortel V: Experience with routine use of subclavian vein cannulation in haemodialysis. *Proc Eur Dial Transplant Assoc* 6: 59, 1969
9. Henneman H: Die Vena Subclavia – Akutdialysezugang der ersten Wahl. (The subclavian vein – Access for acute dialysis) *Intensivmed* 15: 236, 1978
10. Bambauer R, Jutzler GA: Erfahrungen mit grosslumigen Verweilkathetern in der V. jugularis interna als Zugang für akute Hämodialysen. (Use of large catheters in the internal jugular vein as an access for acute haemodialysis). *Klin Wocheschr* 60: 285, 1982
11. De Cubber A, De Wolf C, Lameire N, Schurgers M, Ringoir S: Single needle hemodialysis with the double headpump via the subclavian vein. *Dial Transplant* 7: 1261, 1978
12. Schwarzbeck A, Brittinger WD, Von Henning GE, Strauch M: Cannulation of subclavian vein for hemodialysis using Seldinger's technique. *Trans Am Soc Artif Intern Organs* 24: 27, 1978
13. Uldall R: Subclavian cannulation for hemodialysis: the present state of the art. *Artif Organs* 6: 73, 1982
14. Uldall R: Cannula insertion and haemodialysis. *Lancet* 2: 213, 1982
15. Uldall PR, Woods F, Merchant N, Crichton E, Carter H: A double lumen subclavian cannula (DLSC) for temporary hemodialysis access. *Trans Am Soc Artif Intern Organs* 26: 93, 1980
16. Uldall PR, Joy C, Merchant N: Further experience with double lumen subclavian cannula for hemodialysis. *Trans Am Soc Artif Intern Organs* 28: 71, 1982
17. Graber DA, Dinerstein C: The Quinton-Mahurkar dual lumen subclavian catheter-preliminary clinical evaluation. *Dial Transplant* 12: 847, 1983
18. Raja R, Kramer M, Alvis R, Goldstein S, De Los Angeles A: Comparison of double lumen subclavian with single lumen catheter – one year experience. *Trans Am Soc Artif Intern Organs* 30: 508, 1984
19. Hombrouckx R, Leroy F, Larno L, Devos Y, Vanwetter P, De Troch F, Fransaer D: In vitro comparison of five double-lumen catheters on a bipuncture and an unipuncture system in *First Int Symposium on Single-Needle Dialysis*, edited by Ringoir S, Vanholder R, Ivanovich P, Cleveland, ISAO-press, 1984, p 190
20. Francis DMA, Hoenich NA, Taylor RMR, Ward MK, Kerr DNS: An indwelling right atrial catheter for long-term hemodialysis. *Trans Am Soc Artif Intern Organs* 29: 348, 1983

21. Reed WP, Light PF, Sadler JH: Access for hemodialysis by means of long-term central venous catheters. *Kidney Int* 25: 838, 1984
22. Reed WP, Newman KA, De Jongh C, Wade JC, Schimpff SC, Wiernik PH, Mac Laughlin JS: Prolonged venous access for chemotherapy by means of the Hickman catheter. *Cancer* 52: 185, 1983
23. Mahan JD, Mauer SM, Nevins TE: The Hickman-catheter: a new hemodialysis access device for infants and small children. *Kidney Int* 24: 694, 1983
24. Bambauer R, Jutzler GA: Jugular interna-Punktion zur Shaldon-Katheterisierung. Ein neuer Zugang für akute Hämodialysen. (Internal jugular puncture for Shaldon catheter insertion. A new technique for acute hemodialysis). *Nieren- und Hochdruckkrankheiten* 3: 109, 1980
25. Fuchs HJ, Jenett G, Klehr U, Richter G, Wilbrandt R, Frotscher U: Die perkutane Punktion der Vena femoralis zur Hämodialysebehandlung. (Percutaneous puncture of the femoral vein for hemodialysis). *Dtsch Med Wschr* 102: 1280, 1977
26. Kozeny GA, Bansal VK, Vertuno LL, Hurley RM, Hano JE: Complications of subclavian vein dialysis. *Int J Artif Organs* 8: 239, 1985
27. Vanholder R, Lameire N, Verbanck J, Van Rattinghe R, Kunnen H, Ringoir S: Complications of subclavian catheter hemodialysis: a 5 year prospective study in 257 consecutive patients. *Int J Artif Intern Organs* 5: 297, 1982
28. Tapson JS, Uldall R: Avoiding deaths from subclavian cannulation for hemodialysis. *Int J Artif Organs* 6: 227, 1983
29. Tapson JS, Uldall PR: Delayed onset of hemothorax: an unusual complication of subclavian access for hemodialysis. *Nephron* 40: 495, 1985
30. Vaziri ND, Maksy M, Lewis M, Martin D, Edwards K: Massive mediastinal hematoma caused by a double-lumen subclavian catheter. *Artif Organs* 8: 223, 1984
31. Fine A, Churchill D, Gault H, Mathieson G: Fatality due to subclavian dialysis catheter. *Nephron* 29: 99, 1981
32. Merrill RH, Raab SO: Dialysis catheter-induced pericardial tamponade. *Arch Intern Med* 142: 1751, 1982
33. Barton BR, Hermann G, Weill R: Cardiothoracic emergencies associated with subclavian hemodialysis catheters. *JAMA* 250: 2660, 1983
34. Uldall PR, Dyck RF, Woods F, Merchant N, Martin GS, Cardella CJ, Sutton D, Deveber GA: A subclavian cannula for temporary vascular access for hemodialysis or plasmapheresis. *Dial Transplant* 8: 963, 1979
35. Scherertz RJ, Falk RJ, Huffman KA, Thomann CA, Mattern WD: Infections associated with subclavian Uldall catheters. *Arch Intern Med* 143: 52, 1983
36. Kozeny GA, Venezio FR, Bansal VK, Vertuno LL, Hano JE: Incidence of subclavian dialysis catheter-related infections. *Arch Intern Med* 144: 1787, 1984
37. Vanholder R, Hoenich N, Ringoir S: Morbidity and mortality of central vein dialysis catheters. *Nephron*, 47: 274, 1987
38. Dahlberg PJ, Yutuc WR, Newcomer KL: Subclavian hemodialysis catheter infections. *Am J Kidney Dis* 7: 421, 1986
39. Ratcliffe PJ, Oliver DO: Massive thrombosis around subclavian cannulas used for haemodialysis. *Lancet* 1: 1472, 1982
40. Davis D, Petersen J, Feldman R, Cho C, Stevick CA: Subclavian venous stenosis. *JAMA* 252: 3404, 1984
41. Fant GF, Dennis VW, Quarles LD: Late vascular complications of the subclavian dialysis catheter. *Am J Kidney Dis* 7: 225, 1986
42. Nand S, Bansal VK, Kozeny G, Vertuno L, Remlinger KA, Jordan JF: Red cell fragmentation syndrome with the use of

subclavian hemodialysis catheters. *Arch Intern Med* 145: 1421, 1985

43. El-Nachef MW, Rashad F, Ricanati ES: Occlusion of the subclavian vein: a complication of indwelling subclavian venous catheters for hemodialysis. *Clin Nephrol* 24: 42, 1985

44. Glaze RC, Mac Dougall ML, Wiegman TB: Thrombotic arm edema as a complication of subclavian vein catheterization and arteriovenous fistula formation for hemodialysis. *Am J Kidney Dis* 7: 439, 1986

45. Ogden DA, Cohen IM: Hemodialysis with a coaxial counterflow single-needle blood access catheter. *asaio J* 3: 33, 1980

46. Grimsrud L: An improved double lumen needle for single puncture dialysis in *Technical Aspects of Dialysis*, edited by Frost TH, Tunbridge Wells, Pitman Medical Publishing, 1978, p 184

47. Mahurkar SD: The fluid mechanics of hemodialysis catheters. *Trans Am Soc Artif Intern Organs* 31: 124, 1985

48. Tapson JS, Hoenich NA, Ward MK, Wilkinson R: Evaluation of the Shiley dual lumen subclavian hemodialysis catheter. *Trans Am Soc Artif Intern Organs* 31: 140, 1985

49. Tapson JS, Hoenich NA, Wilkinson R, Ward MK: Dual lumen subclavian catheters for haemodialysis. *Int J Artif Organs* 8: 195, 1985

50. Greenwood RN, Lambourn LA, Pavitt L, Cattell WR: Selection of arteriovenous fistula needle sets for hemodialysis. *Dial Transplant* 11: 280, 1982

51. De Virgiliis G, Vanin M, Buoncristiani U: A new single needle dialysis system. *Trans Am Soc Artif Intern Organs* 31: 116, 1985

52. Van Waeleghem JP, Boone L, Ringoir S: New technique on the one needle system during haemodialysis. *Eur Dial Transplant Nurses Assoc* 1: 10, 1973

53. Cunningham J, Sharman VL, Hawkes AP, Goodwin FJ, Marsh FP: New system for single-needle dialysis. *Br Med J* 281: 1109, 1980

54. Meijer JH, Reulen JPH, Schneider H, Koolen MI, Oe PL: Analysis of recirculation in single-needle haemodialysis. *Med Biol Eng Comput* 17: 578, 1979

55. Gotch FA: Models to predict recirculation and its effect on treatment time in single-needle dialysis in *First Int Symposium on Single-Needle Dialysis*, edited by Ringoir S, Vanholder R, Ivanovich P, Cleveland, ISAO Press, 1984, p 47

56. Meijer JH, Aerts MJM, Van Der Meulen J, Schneider H, Oe PL: In vivo analysis of recirculation in single-needle hemodialysis in *First Int Symposium on Single-Needle Dialysis*, edited by Ringoir S, Vanholder R, Ivanovich P, Cleveland, ISAO Press, 1984, p 63

57. Swamy AP, Bernard J, Cestero RVM, Keshaviah P: Determinants of recirculation in a single-lumen needle hemodialysis system. *asaio J* 3: 29, 1980

58. Hoenich NA, Downing N, Pearson S, Woffindin C, Ward MK: Review of mechanical systems for single-needle hemodialysis in *First Int Symposium on Single-Needle Dialysis*, edited by Ringoir S, Vanholder R, Ivanovich P, Cleveland, ISAO Press, 1984, p 22

59. Keshaviah P, Carlson G, Wathen R: In vitro and clinical evaluation of single needle dialysis. *Trans Am Soc Artif Intern Organs* 22: 367, 1976

60. Ogden DA: In vivo measurement of blood recirculation during 'Y' type single needle dialysis. *J Dial* 3: 265, 1979

61. Vanholder R, De Paepe M, Hoenich NA, Ringoir S: Double lumen needle in unipuncture dialysis type double head pump. *Int J Artif Organs* 4: 72, 1981

62. Hoenich NA, Piron M, De Cubber A, Larno L, Ringoir S: A study of the influence of single needle dialysis on the principal parameters of haemodialyzer performance. *Int J Artif Organs* 4: 168, 1981

63. Vanholder R, Hoenich N, Ringoir S: Dialysis performance of single lumen subclavian hemodialysis: a comparative study with single lumen fistula hemodialysis. *Artif Organs* 6: 429, 1982

64. Vanholder R, Hoenich N, Ringoir S: Adequacy studies of fistula single needle dialysis. *Am J Kidney Dis*, 10: 417, 1987

65. Ogden DA, Cohen IM: Blood recirculation during hemodialysis with a coaxial counterflow single needle blood access catheter. *Trans Am Soc Artif Intern Organs* 25: 325, 1979

66. Ogden DA: An in vitro comparison of recirculation in 'Y' flow and coaxial flow single needle dialysis systems. *J Dial* 1: 431, 1977

67. Ringoir S, Piron M, Vanholder R: Conventional single-needle hemodialysis in *First Int Symposium on Single-Needle Dialysis*, edited by Ringoir S, Vanholder R, Ivanovich P, Cleveland, ISAO Press, 1984, p 80

68. Veitch P, Hawkins F, Frost TH, Jolly D, Kerr DNS: Factors affecting haemolysis in extracorporeal dialysis circuits in *Technical Aspects of Renal Dialysis*, edited by Frost TH, Tunbridge Wells, Pitman Medical Publishing, 1978

69. Hilderson J, Van Waeleghem JP, Van Egmond J, Van Haelst JP, Schelstraete K, Ringoir S: Single needle vs double needle dialysis. *Dial Transplant* 3: 10, 1974

70. Leonard EF, Van Vooren C, Hauglustaine D, Haumont S: Shear-induced formation of aggregates during hemodialysis. *Contr Nephrol* 36: 34, 1983

71. Leonard EF: Dialysis membranes. *Proc Eur Dial Transplant Assoc Eur Ren Assoc* 21: 99, 1984

72. Lowrie EG, Laird NM, Parker TF, Sargent JA: Effect of the hemodialysis prescription on patient morbidity. Report from the National Cooperative Dialysis Study. *N Engl J Med* 305: 1176, 1981

73. Gotch FA, Sargent JA: A mechnistic analysis of the national cooperative dialysis studie (NCDS). *Kidney Int* 28: 526, 1985

74. Hilderson J, Ringoir S, Van Waeleghem JP, Van Egmond J, Van Haelst JP, Schelstraete K: Short dialysis with a polyacrylnitril membrane (RP6) without the use of a closed recirculating dialyzate delivery system. *Clin Nephrol* 4: 18, 1975

75. Farrell PC: Kinetic modeling: applications in renal and related diseases. *Kidney Int* 24: 487, 1983

76. Lowrie EG, Sargent JA: Clinical example of pharmacokinetic and metabolic modeling: quantitative and individualized prescription of dialysis therapy. *Kidney Int* 18 (Suppl 10): 511, 1980

77. Cogan MG, Sargent JA, Yarbrough SG, Vincenti F, Ameno WJ: Prevention of prednisone-induced negative nitrogen balance. *Ann Intern Med* 95: 158, 1981

78. Borah MF, Schoenfeld PY, Gotch FA, Sargent JA, Wolfson M, Humphreys MH: Nitrogen balance during intermittent dialysis therapy of uremia. *Kidney Int* 14: 491, 1978

79. Vanholder R, Piron M, De Cubber A, Vermaercke N, Ringoir S: Studies of urea kinetics in single needle hemodialysis. *Life Support Systems* 2: 220, 1984

80. Vanholder R, Hoenich N, Bogaert AM, Ringoir S: Long-term experience with routine single-needle dialysis. *Trans Am Soc Artif Intern Organs* 32: 300, 1986

81. Becaus I, Lornoy W, Martens J, Seghers L, Van Langenhove P, Van Leuven I, De Smet C: Eight years' experience with the single-needle double head-pump in *First Int Symposium on Single-Needle Dialysis*, edited by Ringoir S, Vanholder R, Ivanovich P, Cleveland, ISAO Press, 1984, p 112

82. Brynger H, Brunner FP, Chantler C, Donckerwolcke RA, Jacobs C, Kramer P, Selwood NJ, Wing AJ: Combined report on regular dialysis and transplantation in Europe X. *Proc Eur Dial Transplant Assoc* 17: 2, 1980

83. Wing AJ, Broyer M, Brunner FP, Brynger H, Challah S, Donckerwolcke RA, Gretz N, Jacobs C, Kramer P, Selwood NH: Combined report on regular dialysis and transplantation in Europe XIII. *Proc Eur Dial Transplant Assoc* 20: 5, 1983

84. Kramer P, Broyer M, Brunner FP, Brynger H, Challah S, Oules R, Rizzoni G, Selwood NH, Wing AJ, Balas EA: Combined report on regular dialysis and transplantation in Europe XIV. *Proc Eur Dial Transplant Assoc Eur Ren Assoc* 1: 5, 1984

85. Vanholder R, Hoenich N, Ringoir S: Twelve years experience with continuous single-needle dialysis in *Artificial Organs: The W.J. Kolff Festschrift,* edited by Andrade JD, Brophy J, Kim SW, Normann R, Olsen D, Stephen R, Florida, VCH Publications, 1986, p 225

86. De Clippele M, Vanholder R, De Roose J, Derom F, Ringoir S: Fistula survival in single needle hemodialysis. *Int J Artif Organs* 6: 71, 1983

87. Kopp KF, Sucker A, Schatzle-Schuler G, Pankiewicz T: Fistula survival in single-needle hemodialysis in *First Int Symposium on Single-Needle Dialysis,* edited by Ringoir S, Vanholder R, Ivanovich P, Cleveland, ISAO Press, 1984, p 120

88. Van Waeleghem JP, Elseviers MM, Boone LP, Verpooten GA, Konner K, Cambi V, De Broe ME: A multicenter comparative study of the vascular access in hemodialysis patients treated with single- or double-needle techniques in *First Int Symposium on Single-Needle Dialysis,* edited by Ringoir S, Vanholder R, Ivanovich P, Cleveland, ISAO Press, 1984, p 127

89. Liu Jing Duo, Vanholder R, De Roose J, Derom F, Ringoir S: Fistula survival in chronic single-needle hemodialysis in *First Int Symposium on Single-Needle Dialysis,* edited by Ringoir S, Vanholder R, Ivanovich P, Cleveland, ISAO Press, 1984, p 136

90. Krönung G: Is single-needle dialysis really an advantage for long-term function of vascular access? in *First Int Symposium on Single-Needle Dialysis,* edited by Ringoir S, Vanholder R, Ivanovich P, Cleveland, ISAO Press, 1984, p 142

91. Haimov M, Burrows L, Casey JD, Schupak E: Problems of vascular access for haemodialysis - experience with 214 patients. *Proc Eur Dial Tranplant Assoc* 9: 173, 1973

92. Rohr MS, Browder W, Frentz GD, Mc Donald JC: Arteriovenous fistulas for long-term dialysis. *Arch Surg* 113: 153, 1978

93. Reilly DT, Wood RFM, Bell PRF: Prospective study of dialysis fistulas: problem patients and their treatment. *Br J Surg* 69: 549, 1982

94. Hoenich NA: Single-needle dialysis. *Proc Eur Dial Transplant Assoc Eur Ren Assoc* 22: 341, 1985

95. Eaves JA: Comparison of single access double-pump dialysis and double-needle dialysis in a pediatric unit in *First Int Symposium on Single-Needle Dialysis,* edited by Ringoir S, Vanholder R, Ivanovich P, Cleveland, ISAO Press, 1984, p 77

96. Verbanck J, Schelstraete J, De Paepe M, Hoenich N, Lameire N, Ringoir S: Pure ultrafiltration by repeated puncture of a peripheral arm vein as treatment of refractory edema. *Int J Artif Organs* 3: 342, 1980

97. Vanholder R, Ringoir S: Single-Needle-Hämodialyse. (Single-needle hemodialysis) *Nieren und Hochdruckkrankheiten* 13: 89, 1984

98. De Paepe M, Ringoir S: Evaluation of hemofiltration with different AN 69 membrane devices using a discontinuous flow single needle system. *Int J Artif Organs* 5: 87, 1982

99. Vanholder R, Verbanck J, Schelstraete J, De Smet R, Ringoir S: Unipuncture simultaneous hemofiltration and dialysis in *Hemodiafiltration. Proc 1st Symposium, Giessen 1981,* edited by Schütterle G, Wizemann V, Seyffart G, Oberursel, Verlag Hygieneplan, 1981, p 76

100. Vanholder R, Ringoir S: Single needle hemodiafiltration. *Proc Soc Esp Dial Transplante* 7: 99, 1985

101. Verbanck J, Vanholder R, Schelstraete J, De Clippele M, Wulfrank DA, Deschryver AE, Ringoir SM: Unipuncture membrane plasmapheresis. *Artif Organs* 7: 365, 1983

102. Bambauer R, Jutzler GA, Keller HE, Becker HG: Single needle plasmapheresis in *First Int Symposium on Single-Needle Dialysis,* edited by Ringoir S, Vanholder R, Ivanovich P, Cleveland, ISAO Press, 1984, p 233

103. Vanholder R, De Clippele M, Ringoir S: Membrane plasmapheresis by unipuncture technique in *Plasmapheresis,* edited by Nosé Y, Malchesky Y, Smith JW, Krakauer RS, New York, Raven Press, 1983, p 145

104. Wilms H, Keller F, Offerman G: Membrane plasma exchange by single-needle hemofiltration device. A technical note. *Int J Artif Intern Organs* 7: 236, 1984

MULTIPLE USE OF HEMODIALYZERS

NORMAN DEANE and ROBERT J. WINEMAN

INTRODUCTION

Origin and history

Repeated hemodialysis treatment for chronic renal failure was initiated by Belding Scribner and colleagues (1) in 1960. The earliest dialysis procedures included several features which were soon employed for multiple use of dialyzers. For example, Scribner rinsed the blood and dialysate compartments with water, and sterilized both compartments with formaldehyde, since components of the flat plate dialyzers were not sterile when assembled. The dialyzer remained filled with formalin until the time for dialysis, when it was flushed with saline to remove the formaldehyde. These steps resemble those now employed for multiple use of dialyzers.

Following the initial reports of repeated hemodialysis for chronic renal failure from the Seattle group (1, 2), other nephrologists also initiated chronic treatment programs (3). Disposable coil dialyzers were readily available in many facilities (4), so repetitive hemodialysis was also begun using coil dialyzers despite their large blood compartment volumes (300 to 600 ml). To avoid circulatory instability, blood was needed to prime the coil before each dialysis. After dialysis, the blood left in the coil was discarded. To avoid such waste, Shaldon and colleagues (5), in 1960 refrigerated the coil, with its contained blood, at the end of the dialysis and then used that dialyzer for the next dialysis. This was the first dialyzer reuse. The main problem with this technique was an occasional pyrogenic reaction. The method became outmoded as coil and other types of dialyzers with smaller blood compartments became available.

In 1967, Pollard and co-workers of the Seattle group (6) described a technique for reusing Kiil dialyzers which employed cleaning with sodium hypochlorite, followed by rinsing and sterilization with formaldehyde. Blood handling was avoided since the blood within the dialyzer was returned to the patient at the end of treatment leaving the dialyzer filled with sterile saline. Stimuli for the development of reuse of the Kiil dialyzers were the desires to reduce the time and effort required to assemble the equipment and to conserve materials, thus reducing the cost. Since the sterilization was the same for initial and repeated uses, and the rinsing and cleaning posed no obvious hazards, the safety of the procedure was anticipated and subsequently demonstrated.

Employing variations of the techniques of Shaldon and Scribner, multiple use of dialyzers has continued, and has been applied to coils, parallel plate and hollow fiber dialyzers (7). Factors encouraging multiple use of hemodialyzers have evolved from convenience in 1962, through those of economics, clinical outcome, biocompatibility and performance standards up to the present.

Extent of practice

In the United States, a survey conducted by the National Nephrology Foundation and the Renal Physicians Association in 1984 (8) determined that 55.6% of the patients in responding centers were being treated with multiple usage of dialyzers. Of the surveyed facilities 51.4% practiced multiple use of hemodialyzers in 1984. A general trend was that larger centers more commonly reused dialyzers. Facilities with fewer than 31 patients, however, had a significant minority (38%) involved in reuse during 1984. An independent survey by the Centers for Disease Control (CDC) in December, 1983 reported that a majority of dialysis centers (52%) were reusing hemodialyzers. The reusing centers accounted for 60% of the total hemodialysis patient population (9).

Reuse of hemodialyzers in Europe, based on the published data of the European Dialysis and Transplant Association-European Renal Association (EDTA-ERA) Registry, was just over 10% of the patients in 1982. In the following year the number fell to 9.2%, which was about half of the 1976 level. In the earlier survey (1976) the practice of reuse had been comparable to that in the United States during 1978, where it was estimated that 15.7% of the patients were reusing hemodialyzers. In the 1983 European survey variability among countries was extensive with approximately 76% of the patients in Poland, 36% of those in the United Kingdom, and 35% of those in Switzerland reusing hemodialyzers, while the reuse rates in Germany, the Netherlands and Sweden were approximately 1%. The authors concluded that no single factor can account for the differences in policies among individual countries (10).

STEPS IN HEMODIALYZER REUSE

This section describes briefly each of the component steps of the reuse process. More detailed technical points are covered in the subsequent section, technical aspects of hemodialyzer reuse. The report of the National Workshop on Reuse of Consumables in Hemodialysis (11) described seven individual steps for the reprocessing procedure:
1. Identification of the dialyzer
2. Rinsing
3. Cleaning
4. Functional assessment
5. Sterilization (disinfection)
6. Sterilant removal
7. Monitoring clinical care

The first step primarily concerns documentation and labelling which is discussed in the section on technical aspects. The final step, monitoring clinical care, is normally carried out in dialysis facilities as part of the overall quality control of the dialysis process and is not unique to centers practicing reuse. Clinical care monitoring consists of checking monthly serum chemistries and other data, measuring clearances on a sample basis, and tabulating frequencies of patients' symptoms among other activities. The reuse process itself is concerned primarily with the five steps beginning with rinsing.

Rinsing

The rinsing process begins after the blood has been returned to the patient by displacement with saline. The dialyzer usually is transported to a separate area where the connections are made for rinsing the blood and dialysate compartments. Preferably this should be accomplished within 10 min after the patient has been disconnected. A variety of rinsing techniques have been, and are being used in both automated and manual methods. Water temperature, flow rate, pressure (continuous or pulsatile), use of reverse flushing and, for hollow fiber dialyzers, reverse ultrafiltration are variables in the rinsing procedure.

Cleaning

In the cleaning process a chemical agent is used to remove any blood residues remaining in the dialyzer after the rinse process. The two most common cleaning agents employed in reprocessing hemodialyzers are sodium hypochlorite and hydrogen peroxide. In a series of tests conducted by Deane and Bemis (12), sodium hypochlorite was the only agent that effectively cleaned hollow fiber dialyzers. Caution should be observed in applying sodium hypochlorite because it can weaken certain dialysis membranes and may increase the frequency of blood leaks or ruptures. Use of a specific pre-tested procedure is recommended.

Evaluation

The functional capability of the dialyzer needs to be established in order to know whether the dialyzer should be rejected or sterilized for subsequent use. Hollow fiber dialyzers are most frequently evaluated after reprocessing by measurements of cell volume and ultrafiltration rate and by a pressure test to detect membrane defects. Visual examination of the dialyzer also serves to detect possible mechanical imperfections, as well as the relative number of fibers blocked by blood components. Other methods such as determination of urea or saline clearances are applicable to any type of dialyzer but are more tedious and hence infrequently used.

Sterilization

According to the Renal Physicians Association survey of hemodialyzer reuse practice in the United States – 1984, most facilities that reprocess dialyzers use formaldehyde as a disinfectant (8). In the 1983 CDC Survey (9), 38% of the centers were utilizing 2% formaldehyde and 23% used 4% formaldehyde; the remainder used other disinfectants. The Association for Advancement of Medical Instrumentation (AAMI) recommended practice for reuse (13) and the National Kidney Foundation standards (14) recommend 4% formaldehyde to prevent growth of nontuberculous mycobacteria and other resistant organisms. In normal practice the dialysate and blood compartments of the dialyzer are filled with the chosen chemical disinfectant and the device is stored at room temperature for a minimum of 24 h prior to being prepared for the next use.

Alternative chemical disinfecting agents which are being used or are under investigation are gluteraldehyde-based disinfectants (Cidex® and Sporicidin®), peracetic acid solution (Renalin®) and active chlorine compounds (Warexin® and Amuchina®). Another active chlorine compound (Ren-New-D®) has been withdrawn from the market.

Preparation for subsequent use

Sterilants used for storing the dialyzer must be removed and their concentrations reduced below toxic levels by the flow of sterile saline on the blood side (usually with recirculation) and use of flowing dialysis fluid in the dialysate compartment. For any particular dialyzer and sterilant combination, the detailed kinetics must determine empirically the process required to lower the sterilant level to a negligible concentration. Following use of such a defined procedure, a determination of residual sterilant in each dialyzer should be conducted before its clinical use.

CLINICAL ASPECTS OF HEMODIALYZER REUSE

Indications and contraindications for reuse

The recommended practice for reuse of hemodialyzers developed by AAMI (13) includes a discussion which may be summarized as follows: reprocessing of hemodialyzers should be considered when the quality of and/or access to dialysis is maintained or enhanced because of the cost savings arising from reprocessing of hemodialyzers and/or the patient has the 'first use' syndrome (15), consisting of chest or back pain or respiratory distress and sometimes chills or fever during dialysis with new hemodialyzers. Contraindications are that hemodialyzers should not be reprocessed if any of the following conditions prevail: hepatitis B surface antigen positivity, unexplained abnormal liver function tests indicative of viral hepatitis, AIDS, septicemia, and sensitivity of the patient to materials used in hemodialyzer reprocessing.

Survival

Studies of the survival of patients who reuse versus patients who do not reuse have been conducted by the EDTA Registry (10, 16, 17). The one-year survival of reusers (93.2%) and non-reusers (91.2%) starting renal replacement therapy in 1977, was not significantly different (16). Another study by the EDTA Registry in countries with low reuse versus high reuse practice could not demonstrate an unfavorable effect of reuse on survival (17). Caution should be exercised in interpreting such studies because many confounding factors may influence the results. While age was taken into consideration, other variables may be operating such as the wide differences in acceptance rates for renal replacement therapies among the countries studied. For example, Challah et al (10) pointed out that patients with multisystem diseases are under represented in the dialysis and transplant populations of countries having a low acceptance rate.

In a study of 5-year survival of a cohort of 4,661 USA hemodialysis patients who began treatment in 1977, Held, Pauly and Diamond (18) found that patients whose dialysis unit was a long time reuser of hemodialyzers had a relative risk of death of 0.88, compared to patients whose center never reused (relative risk 1.00), or to those whose center started to reuse after 1980 (relative risk 1.01). Differences between the latter two groups were not significant. The authors state that their results 'clearly suggest that patients whose units were long term reusers had lower mortality than patients whose units did not reuse'. A variety of alternative hypotheses were unable to account for the results. The authors recommend replication and extension of the analyses since the issues are so important and controversial (18).

Certain investigators, while acknowledging that reuse of hemodialyzers is an accepted practice in the United States, and that existing data do not demonstrate any significant mortality effect, believe that additional studies of the impact of reuse on both mortality and morbidity are warranted.

Most experts agree that long term prospective clinical trials of dialyzer reuse would probably not be feasible, because there is a loss to follow up of 15 to 20% of the ESRD population annually. Because mortality and morbidity due to reuse is a low incidence phenomenon, it is probably most appropriately studied through an epidemiological approach. Such studies have been proposed to utilize the consolidated ESRD data system which is now being set up by the National Institute of Arthritis, Diabetes and Digestive and Kidney Diseases (19). This type of a system should enable a low incidence phenomenon to be studied, comparing outcomes between patients who have been treated with reprocessed hemodialyzers and those who undergo single use hemodialyzer treatments.

Morbidity

For dialysis patients morbidity and biocompatibility interrelate closely. A dialyzer, for example, is considered to be biocompatible when patients undergoing therapy with it demonstrate few reactions or symptoms related to its use.

As Ogden has observed (20), new dialyzers are not supplied ready for use because they must first be processed by the facility by flushing the blood compartment. Generally manufacturers' instructions involve flushing the blood compartment with a given volume of sterile saline and possibly at the same time flushing the dialysate compartment with dialysis solution at 500 ml/min. As noted by Ogden (15), failure to pretreat may result in serious and sometimes fatal reactions. Ogden (15, 20) observed that new dialyzers occasionally induced severe reactions in patients and frequent mild to moderate reactions for which he coined the term 'new dialyzer syndrome'. First-use syndromes (21) have subsequently been subdivided into two types: Type A (hypersensitivity related) and Type B (nonspecific) (22, 23). Type A reactions are often severe, but are uncommon with a reported incidence of 3 to 5 per 100,000 dialyzers sold (24), and are associated with ethylene oxide sensitivity. Type B reactions are mild, with an incidence of a few percent of dialyses and with an unknown etiology (22).

In a study by the Food and Drug Administration of the USA with the cooperation of dialyzer manufacturers, Villarroel and Ciarkowski (24) identified 366 reports of first-use syndrome, 85% of which were classified as severe reactions with 11 being fatal. The exact causes of the patient reactions are not known, but most reports implicated dialyzers which contained Cuprophan® hollow fibers.

Nicholls (25) by a mail survey of UK dialysis centers found that severe hypersensitivity reactions occur with an incidence between 1 in 10,000 dialyses to 1 in 50,000 dialyses. Milder reactions occur about 10 times as often, or 1 in 1,000 to 1 in 5,000 dialyses.

Several investigators have compared the frequency of intradialytic symptoms experienced by patients when new or reprocessed hemodialyzers are used in their treatment. Levin and co-workers (26) by a double blind study using new or used hollow fiber dialyzers contained in an opaque box documented the incidence of back pain to be 19.5% for new dialyzers versus 6.5% for reprocessed dialyzers. Similarly the incidence of chest pain was 11% for new versus 2.5% for reprocessed dialyzers. In both cases the more severe reactions were associated with the new rather than the reprocessed dialyzers. Kant, Pollack and associates (27) analyzed hospitalization rates of patients on reuse, compared to those treated by single use of dialyzers. There were no significant differences in the number of days hospitalized for problems unrelated to dialysis but days of hospitalization for dialysis related complications were almost twice as high with single use as with multiple use. These investigators also observed certain symptoms which occurred with greater frequency in patients receiving first use dialyzers as opposed to patients receiving dialysis treatment with reused dialyzers. The symptoms included fever, sweating, chest pains, respiratory distress, hypotension, nausea and vomiting.

Pyrogenic complications have been common in the past with hemodialysis. Chills, fever, muscle cramps, abdominal, chest or back pain constitute the spectrum of pyrogenic reactions which are widely recognized to be associated with hemodialysis. Such episodes have continued with sufficient frequency to be important, clinically. Previously, less effective techniques of source water purification, equipment sterilization and cleaning accounted for many such reactions to dialysis. A clinical pattern of the reactions has been observed which was similar to that caused by intravenous injection of endotoxins isolated from gram negative bacteria (28). Since reactions to treatment were not completely eliminated despite improved methods for water purification and equipment cleansing, attention was focused on the hemodialyzer as a potential source of material causing the morbidity. Studies performed at the CDC, US Public Health Service (29) and later at the Manhattan Kidney Center (30) demonstrated release of LAL[1] reactive material from the blood and dialysate compartments of new dialyzers (15). After a 16-h soak, the leaching rate of endotoxin from the blood compartment of two new dialyzers decreased as dialyzers were flushed on subsequent days. These amounts exceeded 70 ng which is above the threshold level for producing a pyrogenic reaction (29). In the CDC study, endotoxin from new dialyzers was nonpyrogenic, but may affect patients adversely in other ways (29). The source of the LAL reactive material in

new dialyzers has not been determined. One hypothesis is that the LAL reactive material may be incorporated into the membrane during manufacture. Since release of endotoxin when present declines with repeated use of the dialyzer, its presence may be a factor in the 'new dialyzer' syndrome (30, 31). Potentially, a second mechanism may be responsible for release of pyrogenic material: interaction of humoral or formed elements of the blood with the membrane may release pharmacologically active substances. To our knowledge there have been no published confirmatory experimental data concerning the latter hypothesis.

With respect to infectious complications, the incidence of hepatitis B among staff and patients, according to one study done in conjuction with the CDC was no greater in centers that reuse hemodialyzers than in units which do not (32).

Potential morbidity can occur through several different mechanisms when proper procedures are not followed in dialyzer reprocessing. For example, patients may be exposed to acute or chronic toxicity from formaldehyde when inadequate procedures are used to remove residual sterilant formaldehyde from the hemodialyzer prior to the next use. Acute toxicity includes discomfort at the site of venous blood return, characterized by a transient burning sensation (20). Formation of anti-N-like antibodies can occur if residual formaldehyde sterilant levels exceed 10 mg/l (33). (See below.) It is important to minimize the development of anti-N-like antibodies which are associated with hemolysis, increased anemia, and early transplant failure (34). There also is concern that chronic exposure to small amounts of formaldehyde can result in a carcinogenic response. No evidence of such an effect in humans has yet been demonstrated.

Potential morbidity can also arise when proper procedures for hemodialyzer disinfection are not utilized. The most well-known case is the Louisiana incident in which 27 of 140 patients developed bacteremia from Mycobacterium chelonei and M. chelonei-like organisms (35). The organisms are rapidly growing non-tuberculous mycobacteria that are widely distributed in the environment, and are present in many municipal water supplies. They resist chemical disinfection, including 2% formaldehyde. The immediate causes of the infections in the Louisiana incident were attributed to 1) high bacterial counts in the water used for dialysate preparation, and 2) apparent lack of control of the disinfectant concentration (35). Recognition of the widespread distribution of these organisms and their resistance to 2% formaldehyde led the CDC to recommend use of 4% rather than 2% formaldehyde for dialyzer reprocessing (36).

Biocompatibility

After the first pass of a patient's blood through a dialyzer with cellulosic or Cuprophan® membranes, white blood cell counts (Figure 1) and serum complement (Figure 2) decrease (37, 38) more with new dialyzers, than with reprocessed dialyzers (39, 40). Such observations are manifestations of the relative biocompatibility of new and reprocessed hemodialyzers.

---

[1] LAL Limulus amoebocyte lysate, a reagent to detect and quantify bacterial endotoxin.

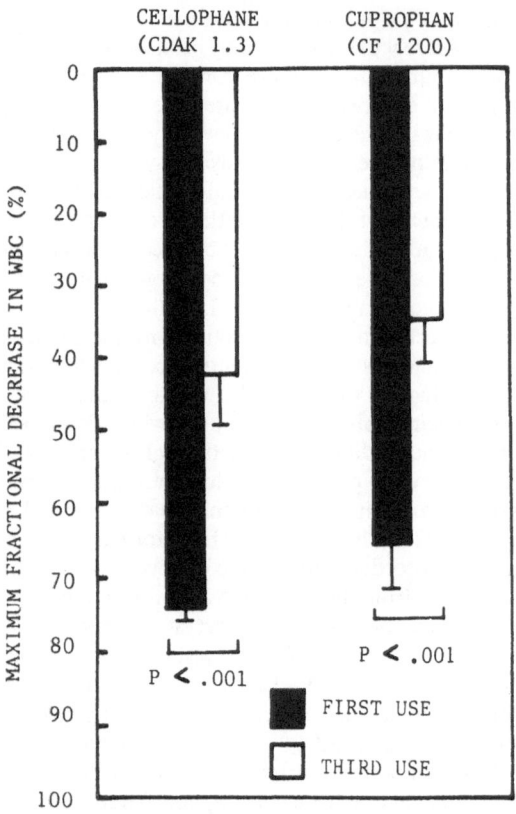

Figure 1. Fractional decrease in white blood cell count with new and reused hollow fiber dialyzers. Reproduced with permission from Lowrie and Hakim (38).

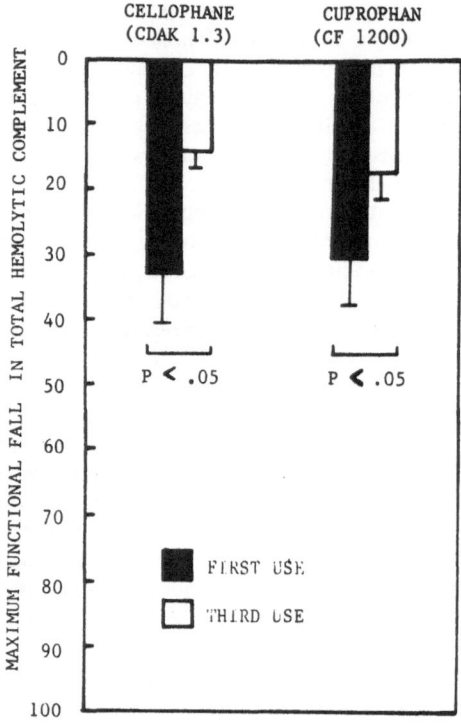

Figure 2. Fractional decrease in serum complement with new and reused hollow fiber dialyzers. Reproduced with permission from Lowrie and Hakim (38).

Recently, several reports on the first use syndrome and on hypersensitivity during hemodialysis have appeared. The relationship between biocompatibility of reprocessed hemodialyzers and the experience with new hemodialyzers provide additional insights into both sets of phenomena.

Charoenpanick and associates (41) reported the incidence of the Type B (see previous section for descriptions of Type A and B responses) first use syndrome and other intradialytic complications in several different periods of their clinical experience. Particularly, pretreating new dialyzers with a manual rinse process during one period, was compared to a pretreatment by machine reprocessing in the second period. The purpose of the preatreatment in all cases was to prevent conventional first use syndrome and in particular to avoid the acute anaphalactic reactions or Type A response. With manual pretreatment of new dialyzers over a total number of dialyses of 1,446, first use syndrome manifested by chest and back pain occurred 10 times. Machine pretreatment was used for 2,843 treatments with new cuprammonium cellulose dialyzers, with the chest and back pain first use syndrome happening once. The manual pretreatment consisted of warm water rinsing of blood and dialysate compartments for 10 min. The automated reprocessing was the conventional Seratronics DRS-4 process which uses a warm water rinse,

reverse ultrafiltration and bleaching followed by another warm water rinse. During their experience with over 32,000 dialyses using cuprammonium cellulose dialyzers, the authors have not noted any severe anaphylactic reaction. They infer that the pretreatment rinse may have eliminated the cause of this severe anaphylactic response. Because of the low frequency of its occurrence, however, additional data will be required.

Dumler, Zasuwa and Levin (42) examined certain other factors involved in intradialytic symptoms related to the hemodialyzer, utilizing a technique in which the subject is blinded with respect to the specific nature of the dialyzer being used. A portion of the study results and experimental design are summarized in Table 1.

These authors compared the intradialytic symptoms experienced by patients with the incidence of chest pain (the most common intradialytic symptom) and a measure of complement activation which occurred. When new dialyzers were machine processed using bleach and formaldehyde, complement activation was greatest. Comparing the means of the three reused dialyzer groups with the two new dialyzer groups, relatively more patients were symptom-free (39%) in the reused dialyzer groups, than in the new hemodialyzer groups (25%). Similarly, chest pain was less frequent in the reprocessed groups (7%) than in the new dialyzer groups (17%). Dumler et al (42) conclude that the type of process used to cleanse reused dialyzers may reduce dialysis-related symptoms, but this effect only partially correlated with reductions in complement activation. The data indicate that other factors (besides complement activation) may be important in the development of the generalized first use syndrome.

Improved biocompatibility was observed by Gagnon, Adkar and Kay (43) in a study of a new active halogen sterilant, REN-NEW-D®. These investigators used the mean decline in percentage of predialysis neutrophil counts as a measure of biocompatibility. While new dialyzers induced a >90% drop in neutrophil counts obtained after 15 min of dialysis, mean neutrophil counts with repeated reuse employing Ren-New-D remained approximately 75 ± 10% of the predialysis values. The dialyzers used were cuprammonium hollow fiber dialyzers.

Vanholder and Ringoir (44) reported five instances of the first use syndrome among 98 patients, when hollow fiber dialyzers replaced flat plate dialyzers, both having cuprammonium membranes. These investigators found that the first use symptoms disappeared when dialyzers were subjected to a reuse-sterilization procedure prior to first use whether formaldehyde, peracetic acid or an active chlorine sterilant, Ren-New-D® was employed. In this study, formaldehyde caused itching in two of the patients, a condition which resolved when the sterilant was changed to peracetic acid.

Thus, based on intradialytic symptoms, complement activation and relative drop in predialysis neutrophil counts, reprocessed hemodialyzers show greater biocompatibility than new hemodialyzers. Additionally, processing prior to first use may avoid the potentially very dangerous Type A anaphylactic response.

Immune response

Three alterations of the immune system may be associated with hemodialysis. In 1972, Howell and Perkins (45) reported anti-N-like antibodies in the sera of patients undergoing chronic hemodialysis. They originated the term 'anti-N-like' antibody and speculated that its formation might be due to the use of formaldehyde for sterilization of the hemodialyzer in the reuse process. The observation was given added importance when Belzer and colleagues (46) detected cold agglutinins in renal transplant recipients and then speculated that their presence may have been responsible for failure

of an attempted transplant. Detailed investigations by Fassbinder and Koch (33) demonstrated that the formation of anti-N-like antibodies in hemodialysis patients is associated with hemodialyzer reuse employing formaldehyde as the sterilant. In the early days of reprocessing Kiil dialyzers, as well as early reuse of hollow fiber dialyzers, the Clinitest® assay was used as recommended by Pollard et al (6) as the accepted test to demonstrate that the bulk of formaldehyde had been removed from the hemodialyzer by rinsing prior to its next use. In 47.3% of 220 Kiil dialyzers prepared for clinical dialysis the residual concentration of formaldehyde was found by Fassbinder and Koch (33) to be 1 mg/dl (10 ppm). Further experimentation demonstrated that the minimum formaldehyde concentration causing the formation of anti-N-like antibodies was 1 mg/dl. This observation was confirmed by Lewis et al (47), who concluded that concentrations below 1 mg/dl do not induce anti-N-like antibody formation.

The presence of anti-N-like antibodies has the following adverse clinical consequences: some difficulties in blood grouping and cross matching of patients with anti-N-like antibodies can occur. Anti-N-like antibodies can decrease the mean red cell half-life. Hence, hematocrits of patients, who are anti-N-like antibody positive, will be lower than those who are negative. Finally, as indicated earlier, anti-N-like antibodies may contribute to early transplant failure (46).

Recently Vanholder and Ringoir (44) compared the development of anti-N-like antibodies in two groups of hemodialysis patients. One group was treated using formaldehyde reprocessed hemodialyzers in which the rinse effluent was kept below 1.0 mg/l of formaldehyde. The second group was treated by hemodialyzers reprocessed with peracetic acid. After 14 months it was found that 4 of the 50 patients in the group exposed to formaldehyde developed anti-N-like antibodies but none of those in the peracetic acid group did. The authors conclude that if patients reuse formaldehyde sterilized hemodialyzers, the blood level of anti-N-like antibodies should be monitored. In view of the complexities of removal of formaldehyde, and its rebound from the potting compound of the tube sheets of hemodialyzers, it would be helpful to have full details of the study, as well as confirmatory studies to determine whether there are significant differences between the exposures of their patients and those

Table 1. Summary of observations on biocompatibility of new and reused hemodialyzers vs reprocessing method (From Dumler, Zasuwa, and Levin [42]).

Dialyzer	Pre treatment	Reagents	% Symptom free	Incidence chest pain	Complement activation
New	None		27		4,700
New	Machine	Bleach/formaldehyde	21		7,300
Mean	New		25	17	
Reused	Machine	Bleach/formaldehyde	33		3,800
Reused	Manual	Formaldehyde	41		800
Reused	Machine	Peracetic acid	44		300
Mean	Reused		39	7	

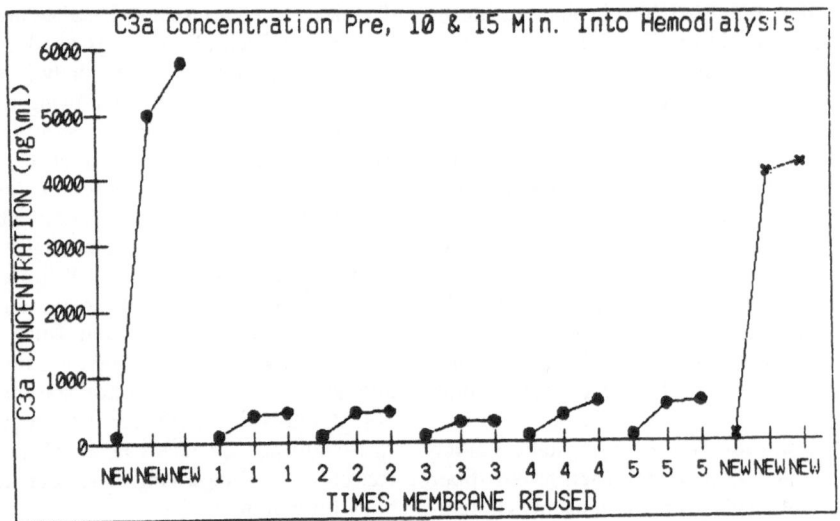

Figure 3. Serum concentrations of C3a are plotted prior to dialysis and at the 10- and 15-min mark for a new membrane, in subsequent reuse on five occasions (closed circles) and reintroduction of a new membrane (xs). The values given are averaged for the 11 subjects studied. Reproduced with permission from Henderson and Chenoweth (48).

of Fassbinder and Koch (33) and of Lewis et al (47).

Complement activation and release of anaphylatoxins, C3a and C5a are other important immune responses to hemodialysis. C5a is a potent mediator of granulocyte responses, including chemotaxis, adherence, aggregation, degranulation and toxic oxygen radical production (48). C5a release is associated with leukocyte accumulation. Thus, the typical leukopenia which occurs within 30 min of initiating Cuprophan® hemodialysis, as observed first by Kaplow and Goffinet (37) is a phenomenon induced by dialyzer membrane activation of the complement system with release of

C5a. The more stable C3a is used rather than C5a as a marker for the extent of complement activation (48). Figure 3 (48) indicates the magnitude of the increase in C3a concentration of a patient exposed to a new Cuprophan® hemodialyzer prepared for clinical use.

Reuse of such a membrane with formaldehyde as a sterilant and appropriate pre-and post-rinses, shows a much lower complement activation. The corresponding white blood cells counts with both new and reprocessed membranes are indicated in Figure 4 (48).

Other membranes such as An-69 polyacrylonitrile mem-

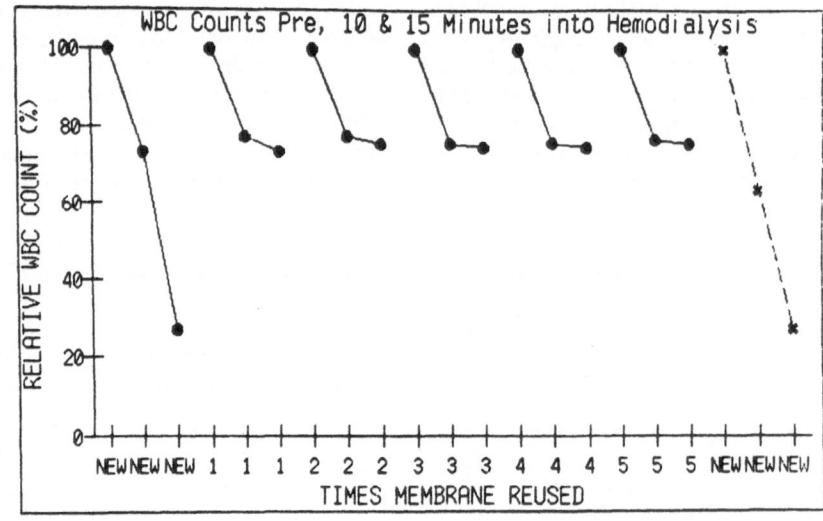

Figure 4. Relative white blood cell counts are plotted predialysis as well as at the 10- and 15-min mark for the 11 subjects studied in figure 3. Reproduced with permission from Henderson and Chenoweth (48).

brane, or polycarbonate membrane activate complement considerably less than Cuprophan®, a cuprammonium cellulose membrane, does. In this instance, measurements of complement activation show that the reused hemodialyzer has higher biocompatibility, as previously discussed, compared to the new device.

As the other side of the coin, Yudis (49) recently reported a hypersensitivity reaction associated with a reused hemodialyzer, which is the first such report. The data suggest residual formaldehyde as the antigen to which this patient was sensitized.

TECHNICAL ASPECTS OF HEMODIALYZER REUSE

General considerations

The dialyzer reprocessing procedures described here and the comments upon them refer to reprocessing procedures specifically for hollow fiber hemodialysis. While reprocessing of both flat plate and coil type dialyzers has been conducted in the past, the lack of availability of a generally accepted, simple test for measuring the functional characteristics of such reprocessed hemodialyzers has inhibited nephrologists from their broader scale use. For hollow fiber dialyzers, the fiber bundle volume (FBV) or the total cell volume can be readily measured; it is directly proportional to the number of functional fibers which relates closely to the clearance of that specific dialyzer. If an individual wishes to reprocess flat plate dialyzers, for example, a measurement of ultrafiltration rate has been utilized by Dorson and coworkers (50) to indicate the function of the specific dialyzer.

Several topics deserve mention although they are not direct steps in the reprocessing of hemodialyzers. Firstly, the anti-coagulation procedures of the center and the care with which each patient's heparin dosage is individually tailored can influence the effectiveness of the dialyzer reprocessing effort of that center.

Another aspect of importance for the reprocessing of hemodialyzers is the specific nature of the dialyzer disconnection procedure used by the center. Rinse back of the patient's residual blood in the hemodialyzer by heparinized saline must be done carefully without allowing air to enter the dialyzer.

It is advantageous that the center develop procedures such that, after completion of dialysis and disconnection of the patient, the used dialyzer is transported to the reprocessing area in a clean and sanitary manner, without undue delay. The interval of time prior to the first dialyzer rinse and the reprocessing procedure correlates inversely with the ease with which a used dialyzer may be restored to its original performance characteristics.

Water quality for reprocessing

Water used for rinsing and cleaning dialyzers and preparation of fluids to do so should be potable water of a quality such that the reprocessed dialyzer meets the specifications required. If the rinsing fluid is tap water or a solution made with tap water, the water should be filtered through a 5 micron filter (13). Previously, it has been recommended that water used for hemodialyzer reprocessing meet the AAMI standards for water used to prepare dialysis solution. This no longer is specified in the AAMI recommended practice (13).

Water used to prepare germicide solution should have a bacterial colony count less than 200/ml as well as a bacterial lipopolysacharide concentration below 1 ng/ml as measured by the LAL assay (13). This has been shown to be necessary specifically for dilution of the formaldehyde germicide solution used in reprocessing to avoid pyrogen reactions from the reprocessed hemodialyzers.

Rinsing procedures

This section refers to more extensive rinsing procedures which are applied to remove blood residues from the blood compartment, and rinse the dialysate compartment, usually through extensive bi-directional rinsing. This process is distinct from the initial prerinse to remove residual blood immediately after the disconnection of the dialyzer and return of blood to the patient. The extensive rinsing procedures often include a so-called 'reverse ultrafiltration' step in which the dialysate compartment is pressurized relative to the blood compartment of the dialyzer. The rationale for this procedure is that blood constituents or residues adhering to the membranes on the interior of the blood compartment fiber surfaces may be lifted from the surfaces and more readily removed. A variety of rinse procedures has been employed including different rinse times, temperatures, pressures and fluid compositions (tap water, saline, reverse osmosis water, and deionized water, with or without heparin). Various flow conditions have also been employed including continuous, or pulsatile uni- or bi-directional flows, and the use of reverse ultrafiltration. An earlier comparison of a simple and complex rinse procedure by Deane and Bemis (51) found that there were no practical differences between performance characteristics of once used dialyzers reprocessed by these two methods. Automated reprocessing devices use a selection of rinse techniques, all of which include at some stage a reverse ultrafiltration component (52).

The rinsing procedure used for manual reprocessing of hemodialyzers at centers operated by the National Nephrology Foundation (51) is the following:

Manual rinse procedure for hollow fiber dialyzers

1. Place the dialyzer in a support rack with the arterial side down.
2. Attach the reverse osmosis (RO) water line to the arterial side of the blood compartment, flush the blood side for 5 min at 3 to 4 l/min., and disconnect the RO line.
3. Attach lines with Hansen connections to the two dialysate ports. Connect the line nearest the arterial side to the RO water outlet and flush the dialy-

sate compartment. Once all air is displaced, clamp the outflow of the dialysate compartment building pressure to a predetermined value[1]. Maintain this pressure for at least 1 h.

4. Fifteen minutes into step 3, release the clamp on the dialysate outflow slowly. Return to step 2, flushing the blood compartment for 2 min.

5. Step 3 is done three (3) more times during the procedure, alternating the direction of flushing. The first and third flushes are with the arterial line connected to the RO water outlet, while the second is with the venous line connected to the RO water outlet. During each 2 min rinse of the blood side, clamp the outflow tubing three times and release.

Cleaning agents

After a rinse procedure, it is optional to apply a chemical cleaning of the hemodialyzer. The cleaning agents most commonly employed are sodium hypochlorite (bleach) and hydrogen peroxide. Certain automated devices use the same chemical as the germicide and as a cleaning agent. For example, the Renal System's Renatron®, utilizes peracetic acid as a cleaning agent; other automated devices employ an active halogen compound, such as a chemical releasing chlorine dioxide as a cleanser and also as a germicide.

In an extensive study of cleaning agents, Deane and Bemis (12) found that the only sodium hypochlorite significantly increased the fiber bundle volume of used hemodialyzers which previously had substantial numbers of clotted fibers. The other cleaning agents evaluated included hydrogen peroxide, seven detergents which included cationic, anionic, non-ionic and zweiter-ionic detergents as well as a calcium chelator, the disodium salt of ethylene diaminetetracetic acid (12).

Sodium hypochlorite has the disadvantage that at higher concentrations and longer exposure times it can attack dialysis membranes, reducing their burst strength, and increasing the ultrafiltration rates and clearances. An important point is that a procedure involving cleaning a dialyzer with sodium hypochlorite needs to be validated not only for its effectiveness, but for its safety, and lack of significant weakening the membrane and/or other structural characteristics of the dialyzer. The effects of sodium hypochlorite have been described by Deane and Bemis (12) and by Dorson et al (50). Sodium hypochlorite may react with regenerated cellulose membranes such as cuprammonium cellulose, and cellulose acetate. Polyacrylonitrile membranes are not effected by sodium hypochlorite, and, in fact, the dialyzer can be stored with sodium hypochlorite for extended time periods (53).

Automated devices for reprocessing hemodialyzers generally employ a cleaning agent. Examples are the following. Sodium hypochlorite is employed by the Seratronics DRS-4, the Lixivitron 2, and the Compudial KP-1, hydrogen perox-

ide is used by the Texas Medical ADR-22 and the Renatron® utilizes peracetic acid, (Renalin®). A cleaning agent is optional in the case of the Mesa Medical's Echo machine (52).

The manual reprocessing procedure of the National Nephrology Foundation does not utilize a cleaning agent.

Biocompatibility of the reprocessed hemodialyzer can be effected by the use of a cleanser, in particular, sodium hypochlorite at higher concentrations or longer exposure times or both. Gagnon and Kaye (54) observed that neutropenia within the first 30 min of hemodialysis reappears (similar to use of a new hemodialyzer of cupro-ammonium cellulose) when more concentrated bleach is used. Other investigators (42) have confirmed this observation.

Methods for testing dialyzer effectiveness

Following the rinsing and cleaning steps in dialyzer reprocessing, either manual or automated, one or more measures of the effectiveness of the reprocessed hemodialyzer is made prior its storage with germicide solution. For hollow fiber dialyzers the assay most commonly utilized either in automated or manually reprocessed devices is a fiber bundle volume test. Other tests which have been employed are measures of the dialyzer's ultrafiltration coefficient, or its inverse, hydraulic resistance (50). Pressure testing has also been recommended for all reprocessed hemodialyzers to minimize or eliminate the possibility of leaking membranes. Reprocessed hemodialyzers, by currently used procedures, have a lower leak rate than new hemodialyzers. For examples, Leuhman et al (55), observed average blood leak rates of 0.16% of reprocessed hemodialyzers compared to 1.38% of new hemodialyzers. Whenever a strong cleaning agent is employed in the reprocessing, it is essential to test each individual dialyzer for leaking. All six of the automated devices previously tested by the National Nephrology Foundation (52) did provide a leak test. A fiber bundle volume test is provided by all six machines, but in one case it is an optional extra. In the case of the Mesa Medical machine, the cell volume must be read visually by the operator. A test of the ultrafiltration rate is also provided by the four more highly automated devices, but not by the simpler single station machines, the Renatron® and the Mesa Echo.

The AAMI Recommemded Practice (13) discusses initial validation of any new reprocessing technique. The validation consists of determining urea and creatinine clearances on representative samples of the reprocessed devices, as well as determining other critical factors on the performance of the dialyzer. Such clearance measures should be done serially on the devices as they are used a number of times. Parallel tests such as fiber bundle volume tests are needed in order to develop the correlation coefficients for clearance with the simpler fiber bundle volume test for subsequent use. Each reprocessing method has to be shown to provide a close correlation between the fiber bundle volume parameter and the urea or sodium chloride clearance. Considerable data have been developed, especially by Gotch (56) demonstrating that if the fiber bundle volume (FBV) is maintained within 80% of the reference volume,

---

[1] The appropriate pressure must be established for each model of hemodialyzer. For example 25 psi is used for the Travenol 1211.

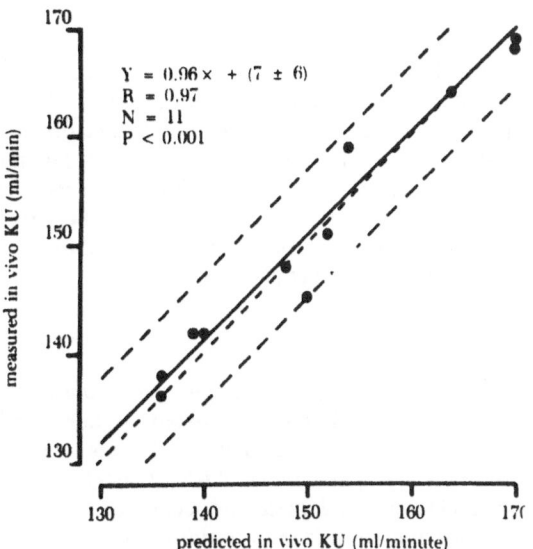

Figure 5. Correlation of measured end dialysis in vivo KU to predicted KU calculated from end dialysis FBV and measured in vitro FBV and KU prior to use. Reprinted with permission of the publisher from Hemodialyzer Reuse: Issues and Solutions (AAMI Technology Assessment Report 10–85), p 38. Copyright 1985 by the Association for the Advancement of Medical Instrumentation, Arlington, Virginia (57).

the hemodialyzer clearance will be 90% or more of the reference value. Gotch (57) found a very tight correlation of the FBV to predicted *in vivo* urea clearances (± 6 ml/min at the 95% confidence level). In the study the individual dialyzer's *in vitro* urea clearance, FBV and effective area were measured prior to its first use. Subsequently, the FBV was measured at the end of each dialysis and each reprocessing period. The predicted *in vivo* clearances were calculated from the standard transport equation of Sargent and Gotch (58). Predicted and measured *in vivo* urea clearances are illustrated in Figure 5.

$$K = \left[1 - e^{\frac{KoA}{QB}\left(1 - \frac{QB}{QD}\right)}\right] \Big/ \left[\frac{QB}{QD} - e^{\frac{KoA}{QB}\left(1 - \frac{QB}{QD}\right)}\right].$$

Ultrafiltration rates should also be measured on a number of reprocessed hemodialyzers as the number of reprocessing procedures increases for validation of the process. According to the AAMI Recommended Practice (13) the *in vitro* ultrafiltration rate should be within 20% of the manufacturer's nominal ultrafilltration rate. Nephrologists are cautioned not to use the *in vitro* ultrafiltration rate as a guide for the *in vivo* performance of the device, since a considerably lower rate is likely to be observed.

Similarly, initial validation of a new reprocessing procedure should include pressure leak tests on the types of dialyzers on which the process is to be employed. Such leak tests should subject dialyzers to a transmembrane pressure

20% above the maximum operating pressure and measure the pressure decay curve, pressure (millimeters) vs time (minutes), comparing it to that of a new, wetted hemodialyzer. Fiber bundle volume tests are readily carried out manually using equipment described by Deane and Bemis (59).

Choice of disinfectant (sterilant) and cycle

Formaldehyde has been the principal disinfectant used to reprocess hemodialyzers since Pollard et al (6) used it to sterilize Kiil dialyzers. Other disinfecting agents used in the past include benzalkonium chloride, other quaternary ammonium detergents, acetic acid, glutaraldehyde, peracetic acid, and active chlorine compounds. By far the greatest experience is with formaldehyde in concentrations from 1.5% to 4%.

The disinfection process which has been used in most dialysis centers is classified as a high level disinfection process (36) designed to inactivate all microorganisms present except bacterial spores. In such a process, both the blood and dialysate compartments are filled with the desired disinfectant solution, and stored for 24 h or more at ambient temperature (20 to 25° C) prior to use for the next dialysis.

In recent years investigators at the CDC, especially Favero, Petersen and Bland, (9, 29, 35, 36, 60, 61) have described the microbiological environment to be considered in dialysis and in dialyzer reprocessing. For some time in the past, concentrations of 2% formaldehyde were considered reasonable, with contact times of 24 or 36 h at 20 to 25° C, because it was assumed that the main microbiologic challenge was due to gram-negative water bacteria. Studies by the CDC demonstrated that when concentrations of gram-negative organisms were reasonably high, there was a risk of pyrogenic reactions in patients undergoing dialysis. This risk persisted even though the organisms had been inactivated, due to the presence of lipopolysacharides or bacterial endotoxins which cause a pyrogenic response. This information led to the recommendation that the total level of microorganisms present in water used to prepare dialysis fluid should not exceed 200/ml and that the contamination in the dialysis fluid itself should not exceed 2000/ml (61, 62). The presence of the endotoxin and/or other LAL active materials led to the recommendation that the maximum concentration of lipopolysacharide in water used for dilution of the germicide should be 1 ng/ml.

In 1982 Petersen of CDC (63) publicized the problems associated with another group of organisms, the non-tuberculous mycobacteria, which also survive and grow rapidly in water, yet resist many chemical disinfectants. Subsequently 27 cases of non-tuberculous mycobacterial infections were identified among 140 patients in two dialysis centers in Louisiana (35). The demonstration that viable non-tuberculous mycobacteria survived 24 h of exposure to 2% formaldehyde led to the recommendation that 4% formaldehyde be used for hemodialyzer disinfection (36). Subsequently, in a CDC study of water samples collected from 115 dialysis centers (representing approximately 1200 centers in the country at the time) 83% tested positive for non-tuberculous mycobacteria (60). In summary, according to Favero (60), 'There is scientific information indicating that 4% formaldehyde for 24 h of exposure at room temperature is at least a high level disinfection, if not a sterilization process. All laboratory data acquired so far show that 24 h of exposure to 4% formaldehyde at room temperature inactivates large numbers of all strains of non-tuberculous mycobacteria tested. Many of the test strains are among the most resistant in our collection.'

The AAMI guidelines (13) limited their recommendation to 4% formaldehyde when formaldehyde is used as a sole germicide, since possible combinations of germicides might also give a satisfactory result. Lower concentrations of formaldehyde and shorter contact times could be employed if adequate disinfection could be shown. Caution should be used in monitoring the disinfection procedure since more sophisticated tests than normally available to a dialysis center are necessary.

The basis of quality control in sterilization should be: adhering rigidly to the established protocol, conducting monthly tests for total bacteria and endotoxin levels in the water used to make up the germicide, testing of the germicide's concentration which is used in the dialyzer, and verifying that each dialyzer was indeed filled with germicide (13).

Despite the history of successful experience with formaldehyde, a number of other potential disinfecting agents have been investigated and are now, or have been on the market in the United States for disinfecting reprocessed hemodialyzers. These include two glutaraldehyde based disinfectants: Cidex-HD® (Surgikos Inc.) and Sporicidin-HD® (Sporicidin Inc.). Renalin® is a peracetic acid based sterilant marketed by Renal Systems Inc. Finally, there are three active chlorine compound sterilants: Warexin® (Mediflex International), Ren-New-D® (Alcide Corporation) and Amuchina® (Amuchina, SpA). Use of these sterilants is discussed briefly by Deane, Maude and Bemis (64)

Concern about the difficulty in removing residual formaldehyde from the reprocessed hemodialyzer when concentrations as high as 4% were used, caused Hakim and associates (65) to investigate incubations of disinfectant filled dialyzers at elevated temperatures and in the presence of

ethanol to increase the bactericidal efficacy of formaldehyde. They found that when dialyzers containing as little as 0.5% formaldehyde were incubated at 40°C for 24 h there were no surviving organisms, after initial innoculation with high concentrations of formaldehyde resistant organisms. These authors also report that exposure to the temperature of 40°C does not change the dialyzer's *in vitro* clearance of small and middle molecules. The comparison between 20° incubation and 40° incubation is demonstrated by Table 2 reproduced from Hakim et al (65).

Sterilant removal

The final part of dialyzer reprocessing is the application of a rinse procedure which has been validated to reduce sterilant residues to safe levels before using the dialyzer for the next procedure on the same patient. AAMI Guidelines recommend that at least a random sample of dialyzers be tested for the presence of germicide prior to rinsing and priming (13). Other procedures might recommend that each individual dialyzer be tested for the presence of adequate sterilant prior to application of the rinsing procedures as a quality control step to insure that adequate disinfection has been applied. When formaldehyde is used as a disinfectant, a positive Clinitest® has been taken to indicate significant levels of formaldehyde present in the hemodialyzer before the rinse procedure (66).

The AAMI recommended practice (13) states the maximum residual level of formaldehyde should be 5 mg/l for the following reasons: anti-N-like antibody formation does not occur below a residual formaldehyde level of 10 mg/l (ppm) (33), the maximum daily dose of formaldehyde due to dialysis is less than the California Occupational Safety and Health Agency daily limit (13), there is no evidence of toxicity due to the long term use of methenamine by mouth for urinary tract infections at doses that release considerably more formaldehyde to the patient than occurs from reused dialyzers (67), and formaldehyde levels below 5 mg/l are difficult to monitor and markedly extended time is required to prepare the dialyzer for dialysis (13).

In one of the more extensive studies of the kinetics of formaldehyde removal from a reprocessed dialyzer, Gotch

Table 2. Number of surviving organisms (CFU/ml) in multiple-use dialyzers.

Organisms (Initial inoculant)	20° C incubation			40° C incubation			
	Formaldehyde concentration			Formaldehyde concentration			
	1%	2%	4%	0.5%	1%	2%	4%
FRO-1 (23 × 10⁶ CFU)	TNTC[a]	900,000	40,000	0	0	0	0
FRO-3 (9 × 10⁵ CFU)	38,700	22,000	1,040	0	0	0	0
FRO-5 (38 × 10⁶ CFU)	TNTC	14,300	1,200	0	0	0	0
FRO-6 (3.2 × 10⁵ CFU)	TNTC	250,000	50,100	0	0	0	0

[a] TNTC, Too numerous to count. FRO, 'formaldehyde resistant organisms'.
Reproduced from Hakim, Freidrich and Lowrie (65) with permission.

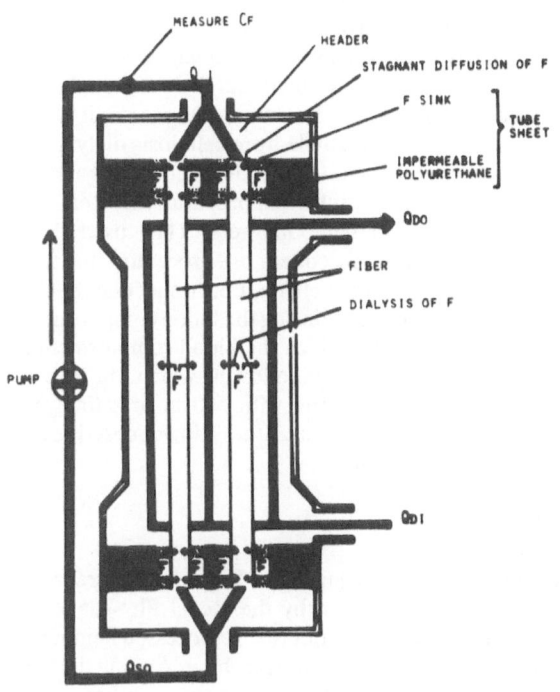

Figure 6. The formaldehyde (F) sink in hollow-fiber dialyzers. Reproduced with permission from Gotch and Keen (67).

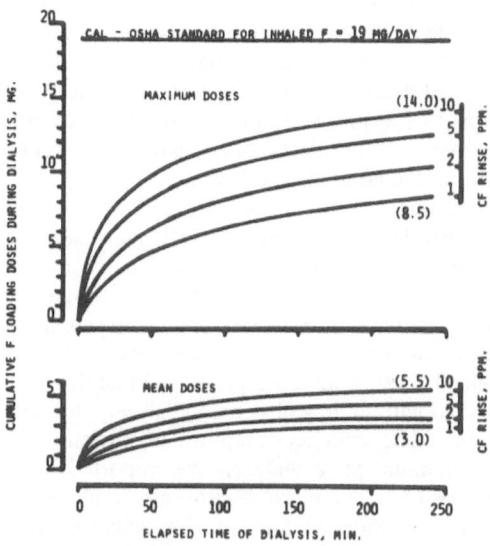

Figure 7. Cumulative mean and maximum formaldehyde loading doses during dialysis as a function of maximal final concentration of formaldehyde in rinse solution, calculated for SCE kidneys. Reproduced with permission from Gotch and Keen (67).

and Keen (67) cited previous work by the Cordis Dow Corporation which demonstrated that the formaldehyde sink in a hollow fiber dialyzer is caused largely by the polyurethane potting compound of the headers. During fabrication, the cellulosic fibers interact with polyurethane to inhibit partially the curing of the latter material resulting in a thin film of polyurethane gel surrounding each fiber, which becomes the formaldehyde sink (See Figure 6).

During storage, formaldehyde diffuses into the gel from which it must be subsequently removed by the rinsing procedure. Because the release of formaldehyde from the tube sheet is relatively slow, Gotch and Keen (67) proposed a rinse procedure whereby the blood compartment saline solution is recirculated while dialysis fluid or water is passed through the dialysate compartment to remove formaldehyde and thus facilitate the rate of stagnant diffusion because of a low concentration of formaldehyde in the blood compartment during the process. To facilitate formaldehyde removal further Gotch and Keen (67) recommend conducting the rinse procedure at 37°C thereby accelerating the diffusion rate. Figure 7 shows the cumulative mean and maximum formaldehyde loading doses during dialysis according to the study of Gotch and Keen (67), as a function of the final concentration of formaldehyde in the rinse solution of Cordis Dow SCE kidneys.

Kaye, Barber, and Gagnon (68) studied the application of a standard rinse procedure to remove 2.7% and 4% formaldehyde from dialyzers. The procedure involved flowing

dialysis fluid at 500 ml/min on the dialysate side, with recirculation of saline in the blood cmpartment presumably at 200 ml/min. The recirculation procedure was continued for 45 min with discard of the wash-out saline prior to connecting the patient. The formaldehyde concentration remaining in the wash-out saline at the conclusion of recirculation in over 96% of all the samples was below 1 mg/l. The few samples with higher concentrations were attributed to improper application of the procedure.

Hakim, Friedrich and Lowrie (65) compared the kinetics of removal of 2% and 4% formaldehyde from new and reprocessed dialyzers. Additionally, they studied the bactericidal effects of these sterilant concentrations against formaldehyde resistant organisms. Importantly, they also examined the effects of increased temperature or addition of ethanol or both as adjuvants for improved bactericidal efficiency of the disinfectant. The standard removal procedure used was recirculation of saline within the blood compartment at 300 ml/min accompanied by single pass dialysis fluid flow at 500 ml/min. In experiments designed to measure the cumulative formaldehyde dose, after a standard rinse of 30 min conducted as described above, and achieving a negative test for formaldehyde by the modified Schiff reagent, dialysate and blood lines were connected together and through a container holding 9.5 l of reverse osmosis (RO) water at room temperature for 24 h. Table 3 shows the total formaldehyde remaining in the dialyzer after the 30-min rinse in milligrams, displayed by whether the dialyzers were new or reused and by the different formaldehyde concentrations and types of dialyzers studied.

The authors conclude that the use of 4% formaldehyde

may be associated with a significant increase in the residual formaldehyde that is potentially infused into the patient. In view of the results which they have demonstrated with incubation of the dialyzer with 2% formaldehyde at 40° C, the solution to the problem appears to be use of the lower formaldehyde concentration and higher temperature, with or without the addition of ethanol.

It is of interest to note the parallel problems associated with removal of trace quantities of ethylene oxide from new dialyzers by rinsing techniques which are somewhat analagous to those used for formaldehyde. Ansorge et al (69) demonstrated that the polyurethane potting compound also acts as a sink for ethylene oxide entrapment which must be removed by a slow diffusion process. While their study was conducted with hollow fiber hemodialyzers, a similar relationship and dependency of removal of ethylene oxide from cuprammonium plate dialyzers was reported by Ing and Daugirdas (70). These investigators also demonstrated that the ethylene oxide retention in new dialyzers after sterilization is considerably enhanced by the polyurethane potting compound. Studies of the removal of ethyle oxide were conducted primarily as part of an effort to determine the causes of the 'first use' syndrome and hypersensitivity reactions during hemodialysis.

Relatively little has been published concerning the details of removal of residues of alternative sterilants (disinfectants). Burkseth et al (71) reported the reprocessing of hemodialyzers using an automated reuse machine, Renatron®, with a proprietary solution of peracetic acid, Renalin®. No details are given of their specific rinse-out procedure, however, a colormetric test insured that the residual Renalin® was less than 2 mg/l. The authors comment that the peracetic acid degrades to acetic acid and water leaving no other residue. Bauer et al (72) reprocessed hemodialyzers using peracetic acid, with a removal process consisting of rinsing the dialysate compartment with warm dialysis solution (38°C) at 500 ml/min for at least 15 min while the blood compartment was rinsed with recirculating saline. The authors state that within 15 min the residual peracetic acid was removed to a level below detection limits with starch iodide paper.

Cidex-HD® is an alkaline solution of glutaraldehyde. According to the manufacturer it washes out from cellulosic

Table 3. Residual amount of formaldehyde (mg) after 30-min rinse.

	New dialyzers		Reused dialyzers	
	Formaldehyde		Formaldehyde	
	2%	4%	2%	4%
Cuprophane	63	151	37	88
Cellulose acetate	98	227	160	280
PMMA	12	47	14	55

Reproduced from Hakim, Freidrich and Lowrie (65) with permission.

dialyzers more easily than formaldehyde does (64). Another glutaraldehyde based disinfectant, Sporicidin-HD® contains both glutaraldehyde and sodium phenate as active ingredients. Gotch (56) determined that the rinse-out kinetics of sodium phenate would be somewhat more difficult than removing 4% formaldehyde from cellulosic dialyzers. Gagnon, Adkar, and Kaye (43) studied one of the new active halogen containing disinfectant preparations, Ren-New-D® for reprocessing of hemodialyzers. They used the same preparation for the subsequent use procedure that they had reported for 4% formaldehyde, i.e. connecting the dialyzer to a delivery system and rinsing the blood compartment with 500 ml of saline, after which the blood compartment saline was recirculated for 45 min following which, the blood compartment was again rinsed with 500 ml of saline prior to connecting the patient. The authors do not describe use of a test for residual sterilant.

Automated reprocessing

According to a 1984 survey of hemodialyzer reuse in the United States conducted by the Renal Physicians Association (8), 39.5% of facilities that reprocessed hemodialyzers used some type of automated machine. Among the facilities using automated devices, the average number of uses of those employing the more complex machines with automated documentation was 9.1 compared to 8.2 in facilities using manual procedures.

During the early 1980's six manufacturers developed automated dialyzer reprocessing devices which were offered to the United States market. Two of these were single station devices: the Mesa 'Echo®' and the Renal Systems 'Renatron®'. The first device was most commonly used with formaldehyde as a sterilant but had been cleared for using other sterilants. The Renatron® was originally developed with formaldehyde as a sterilant, but the emphasis now is for use of peracetic acid in the proprietary formulation, Renalin®. The two single station devices do not automate the recording of a variety of information necessary for reprocessing records (52).

Four more complex multi-station devices feature automated documentation of test results of individual dialyzers; much of the documentation needed for reprocessing is automatically provided. An example of the more complex machine is the Seratronics DRS4 reprocessing device. Most users of the Seratronics device utilize formaldehyde as the disinfectant but the machine has also been cleared for use of Cidex-HD®. All of the devices use a combination of rinse cycles including a reverse ultrafiltration step. Other rinsing cycles, a cleaning step which may employ sodium hypochlorite or hydrogen peroxide, and a test cycle including at least a pressure test and most often a determination of the dialyzer cell volume may also be used. In the most complex devices the ultrafiltration coefficient is also measured (52).

A comparative evaluation of six of the devices was conducted at the Manhattan Kidney Center (73, 74) to determine variability of test measures, the relative retention of original dialyzer properties with number of uses, and patient responses with respect to intradialytic symptoms shown by patients on reuse of the reprocessed hemodialyzers. The intradialytic symptoms recorded in the study included cramps, nausea, pruritus and chest pain. The incidence of intradialytic symptoms recorded for the reprocessed devices was 12.2 per 100 treatments compared with 26 for new hemodialyzers. All devices studied provided reprocessed hemodialyzers that showed biocompatibility equal to or better than that of the new hemodialyzers studied, based upon intradialytic patient response.

Automation will be likely to increase the reliability and reproducibility of the entire reprocessing operation. Manual reprocessing techniques require many repetitive steps which must be conducted in a careful, prescribed manner. Use of a machine has many advantages including facilitated record keeping and a higher reliability of the data. It should be emphasized that the use of an automated device does not eliminate or lessen the need for strict quality control. Continued care is required in a number of areas such as measuring concentrations of reagents, maintaining careful control of raw materials utilized in the process and use of high quality water. With automated reprocessing devices, however, the tasks to be performed are different than those in a manual procedure where a great deal of the quality control depends on motivation of personnel to carry out the highly repetitive process with extreme care.

QUALITY CONTROL AND STANDARDS

The following definitions are given in the AAMI Recommended Practice on Reuse of Hemodialyzers (13):

'Quality assurance: Verification that written policies and procedures have been developed and are being implemented.'

'Quality control: Determination that the materials, process and performance of the final product meet the designated specifications.'

As part of a system for maintaining high quality hemodialyzer reprocessing, and being able to document that such is the case, a detailed system of records is necessary (75). Such records are also needed to meet the requirements of the AAMI Recommended Practice. On December 5, 1986, the Assistant Secretary for Health of the Department of Health and Human Services, USA endorsed the adoption of the AAMI guidelines. On June 17, 1987, the US Health Care Financing Administration published the text of a proposed rule to provide standards for reuse of hemodialyzers and other dialysis supplies (76). In summary, the proposed rule would add standards and conditions for safe and effective hemodialyzer reuse and reprocessing, enforceable as Medicare conditions for coverage. It would incorporate by reference voluntary guidelines and standards adopted by AAMI in July of 1986, the 'Recommended Practice for Reuse of Hemodialyzers'.

The Recommended Practice (13) goes into considerable detail and includes discussions of the following topics: scope, records, personnel qualifications and training, pa-

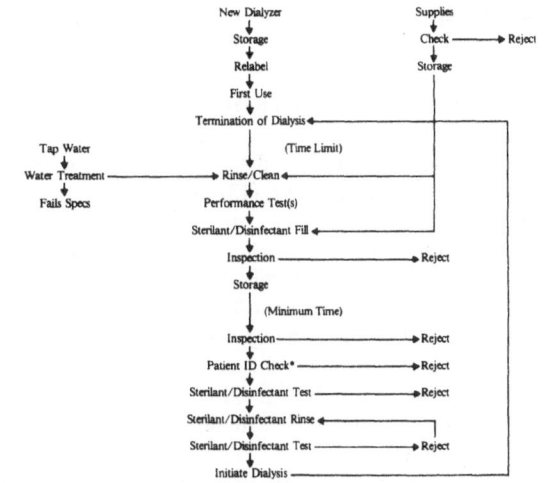

Figure 8. Systems diagram for reprocessing hemodialyzers. Reprinted with permission of the publisher from Recommended Practice for Reuse of Hemodialyzers (AAMI ROH – 1986), p 19. Copyright 1986 by the Association for the Advancement of Medical Instrumentation, Arlington, Virginia (13).

tient considerations, equipment, physical plant and environmental safety considerations, reprocessing supplies, hemodialyzer labeling, reprocessing, preparation for dialysis and testing for potentially toxic residues, monitoring during dialysis, and quality assurance and quality control.

One system of records which has been recommended utilizes seven forms for providing reports and records of the reprocessing process and another set of eight forms which are used for quality assurance (75).

The systems diagram for reprocessing dialyzers in the AAMI Recommended Practice is reproduced in Figure 8. This diagram illustrates some of the detail necessary for quality control of reprocessing (13).

Acquisition of the necessary data and maintenance of records have been helped considerably by the availability and use of automated devices for reprocessing which include the automated documentation features (52).

For an adequate quality control program, activities other than record keeping are required. Periodic control evaluations or audits are necessary and should be scheduled regularly. Such audits should be done by persons not concerned directly with the reprocessing procedure. Reporting of results should be to the physician in charge of the unit and other administrative personnel. The AAMI Recommended Practice (13) specifies the minimum frequency of a number of components of the quality control audit or inspections. For example, the recommendation is made that assurance personnel should audit written procedures for the steps of sterilant (disinfectant) removal and verify their implementation at least quarterly. Quality control personnel should verify the test for the presence of germicide, and the test for residual germicide by the use of positive and negative controls at least quarterly after the process has been established.

ENVIRONMENTAL CONTROLS

Environmental controls are discussed in some detail in the AAMI Standards, Section 6 (13) and in the Deane-Bemis Report (77).

In the proposed guidelines additional rules covering specific points concerning staff exposure to chemical germicides have been added. These rules (76) state that chemical germicides are to be handled in a manner to minimize exposure of staff members involved in reprocessing. Exposure limits for germicides used in dialysis facilities are given in Table 4. Staff exposure to any of these materials must be kept below the stated limits.

According to the AAMI Recommended Practice (13), validation of environmental control equipment must be done when requested by personnel, and should also be done at intervals not exceeding one month. For example, monitoring of formaldehyde vapor should be done at least monthly, and as indicated by personnel discomfort. Precautions for handling of formaldehyde are discussed in considerable detail in Appendix 11 of the Deane-Bemis Report (77).

COMMENTARY ON LONGER RANGE IMPLICATIONS OF HEMODIALYZER REPROCESSING

Currently many dialysis centers in the United States and elsewhere are considering the application of shorter time, high-flux dialysis. High efficiency hemodialysis and related topics have attracted exceptional attention among those in the nephrology community. It has been termed the first major change to benefit patiens in over a decade (78).

Table 4. Exposure limits for active ingredients of chemical germicides used in dialysis facilities according to the US Department of Labor, Occupational Safety and Health Administration (76).

Substance/material	Limits
Formaldehyde	3 ppm
	TWA 5 ppm ceiling
	(1 ppm TWA proposed)
Glutaraldehyde	None developed
Phenol	5 ppm TWA
Glutaraldehyde-phenol	Individual standards should apply
Peracetic acid	None developed
Chlorine dioxide (Chlorine oxide)	100 ppb TWA
Hydrogen peroxide	1 ppm TWA
Chlorine	1 ppm ceiling

Footnotes to Table:

TWA	=	Time weighted average
Ceiling	=	Maximum exposure ceiling
ppm	=	Parts per million (mg/l)
ppb	=	Parts per billion (μg/l)

Patient acceptance of new high-flux dialysis has generally been high because of shortened treatments. Other features of the therapy are improved also: fewer intradialytic and post-dialysis symptoms occur, enhanced biocompatibility has been demonstrated as compared to conventional hemodialysis, improved clearance of high molecular weight substances, especially beta-2 microglobin, which may make the patient less susceptible to dialysis osteoarthropathy (79), and greater tolerance to fluid removal.

In the United States and other countries where economics play a significant role, reprocessing of the hemodialyzers or hemofilters is a key element, which must be in place if a center is to use these improved therapies. Centers which now use shorter treatment state that this practice requires an efficient dialyzer reuse program. The newer dialyzers or hemofilters cost in the range of $ 35.00 to $ 40.00, making single use too expensive to be competitive with conventional hemodialysis.

Thus hemodialyzer reprocessing is, and will continue to be, a significant factor in cost control efforts for delivery of care to the end-stage renal disease population. Availability of reprocessing technology and practice is a key element in determining whether renal replacement therapy may advance to new, more sophisticated levels, on a practical scale in order to benefit significant fractions of patients in the future.

REFERENCES

1. Scribner BH, Buri R, Caner JEZ, Hegstrom R, Burnell JM: The treatment of chronic uremia by means of intermittent dialysis: a preliminary report. *Trans Am Soc Artif Intern Organs* 6: 114, 1960
2. Pendras JP, Cole JJ, Tu WH, Scribner BH: Improved technique of continuous flow hemodialysis. *Trans Am Soc Artif Intern Organs* 7: 27, 1961
3. Brown HW, Maher JF, Lapierre L, Bledsoe FH, Schreiner GE: Clinical problems related to the prolonged artificial maintenance of life by hemodialysis in chronic renal failure. *Trans Am Soc Artif Intern Organs* 8: 281, 1962
4. Merrill JP, Schupak E, Cameron E, Hampers CL: Hemodialysis in the home. *JAMA* 190: 468, 1964
5. Shaldon SH, Silva H, Rosen SM: Technique of refrigerated coil preservation haemodialysis with femoral venous catheterization. *Br Med J* 2: 411, 1964
6. Pollard TL, Barnett BMS, Eschbach JW, Scribner BH: A technique for storage and multiple re-use of the Kiil dialyzer and blood tubing. *Trans Am Soc Artif Intern Organs* 13: 24, 1967
7. Deane N, Bemis JA: *Multiple Use of Hemodialyzers,* New York, Manhattan Kidney Center, National Nephrology Foundation, 1982, Appendices 1, 2
8. Deane N: A survey of dialyzer reuse practice in the United States 1984. in: *Hemodialyzer Reuse; Issues and Solutions,* Arlington, VA, Association for Advancement of Medical Instrumentation, 1985, p 1
9. Bland L, Alter M, Favero M, Carson L, Cusick L: Hemodialyzer reuse: Practices in the United States and implications for infection control. *Trans Am Soc Artif Intern Organs* 31: 556, 1985

10. Challah S, Wing AJ, Brunner FP, Brynger HOA, Oules R, Selwood NH: Use and reuse of dialyzers in Europe. in: *Guide to Reprocessing of Hemodialyzers,* edited by Deane N, Wineman RJ, Bemis JA, Boston, Martinus Nijhoff, 1986, p 99

11. Sadler JH: Reuse workshop report. in: *National Workshop on Reuse of Consumables in Hemodialysis,* Washington, DC, Kidney Disease Coalition, 1982, Appendix A

12. Deane N, Bemis JA: *Multiple Use of Hemodialyzers,* New York, Manhattan Kidney Center, National Nephrology Foundation, 1982, p 64

13. *AAMI Recommended Practices for Reuse of Hemodialyzers.* Arlington, VA, Association for Advancement of Medical Instrumentation, 1986

14. National Kidney Foundation revised standards for reuse of hemodialyzers. *Contemp Dial* 5(2): 29, 37, 1984

15. Ogden DA: New-dialyzer syndrome. *N Engl J Med* 302: 1262, 1980

16. Jacobs C, Brunner FP, Chantler C, Donckerwolcke RA, Gurland HJ, Hathway RA, Selwood NH, Wing AJ: Combined reports on regular dialysis and transplantation in Europe. VII. *Proc Eur Dial Transplant Assoc* 14: 3, 1977

17. Wing AJ, Brunner FP, Brynger H, Chantler C, Donckerwolcke RA, Gurland HJ, Jacobs C, Selwood NH: Mortality and morbidity of re-using dialysers. *Br Med J* 2: 853, 1978

18. Held PJ, Pauly MV, Diamond L: Survival analysis of patients undergoing dialysis. *JAMA* 257: 645, 1987

19. National Institute of Arthritis, Diabetes and Digestive and Kidney Diseases: Briefing paper on NIH response to technology assessment report on dialyzer reuse. In staff report, *Hazards in Reuse of Disposable Dialysis Devices* serial No. 99-K US Govt. Printing Office, 383

20. Ogden DA: Clinical response to new and reprocessed dialyzers. in: *Guide to Reprocessing of Hemodialyzers,* edited by Deane N, Wineman RJ, Bemis JA, Boston, Martinus Nijhoff, 1986, p 87

21. Ing TS, Daugirdas JT, Popli S, Ghandi VC: First-use syndrome with cupro-ammonium cellulose dialyzers. *Int J Artif Organs* 6: 235, 1983

22. Ing TS, Ivanovich PT, Daugirdas JT: First-use syndrome and hypersensitivity during hemodialysis: some pieces of the puzzle are falling into place. *Artif Organs* 11: 79, 1987

23. Daugirdas JT, Ing TS: Classification of first-use reactions. *Int J Artif Organs* 9: 194, 1986

24. Villarroel F, Ciarkowski AA: A survey of hypersensitivity reactions in hemodialysis. *Artif Organs* 9: 231, 1985

25. Nicholls AJ: Hypersensitivity to hemodialysis: The United Kingdom experience. *Artif Organs* 11: 87, 1987

26. Bok DV, Pascual L, Herberger C, Sawyer R, Levin NW: Effect of multiple use of dialyzers on intradialytic symptoms. *Proc Clin Dial Transplant Forum* 10: 92, 1980

27. Kant KS, Pollack VE, Cathey M, Goetz D, Berlin R: Multiple use of dialyzers: safety and efficacy. *Kidney Int* 19: 728, 1981

28. Bennett IL, Cluff LE: Bacterial pyrogens. *Pharmacol Rev* 9: 427, 1957

29. Petersen NJ, Carson LA, Favero MA: Bacterial endotoxin in new and reused hemodialyzers: a potential cause of endotoxemia. *Trans Am Soc Artif Intern Organs* 27: 155, 1981

30. Deane N, Bemis JA: *Multiple Use of Hemodialyzers.* New York, Manhattan Kidney Center, National Nephrology Foundation, 1982, p 99

31. Ogden DA: Clinical response to new and reprocessed dialyzers. in: *Guide to Reprocessing of Hemodialyzers,* edited by Deane N, Wineman RJ, Bemis JA, Boston, Martinus Nijhoff, 1986, p 91

32. Favero MS, Deane N, Leger RT, Sosin AE: Effect of multiple use of hemodialyzers on hepatitis B incidence in patients and staff. *JAMA* 245: 166, 1981

33. Fassbinder W, Koch KM: Immune response to reuse: anti-N-like antibodies. in: *Guide to Reprocessing of Hemodialyzers,* edited by Deane N, Wineman RJ, Bemis JA, Boston, Martinus Nijhoff, 1986, p 135

34. Lewis KJ, Dewar PJ, Ward MK, Kerr DNS: Formation of anti-N-like antibodies in dialysis patients: effect of different methods of dialyser rinsing to remove formaldehyde. *Clin Nephrol* 15: 39, 1981

35. Bolan GA, Reingold AL, Carson LA, Silcox VA, Woodley CL, Hayes PS, Hightower AW, McFarland L, Brown JW III, Petersen NJ, Favero MS, Good RC, Broome CV: Infections with Mycobacterium chelonei in patients receiving dialysis and using processed hemodialyzers. *J Infect Dis* 152: 1013, 1985

36. Favero MS: Distinguishing between high-level disinfection, reprocessing and sterilization. *AAMI Technology Assessment Report No. 6–83.* Arlington, VA, Association for the Advancement of Medical Instrumentation, 1983

37. Kaplow LS, Goffinet JA: Profound neutropenia during the early phase of hemodialysis. *JAMA* 203, 1135, 1968

38. Lowrie EG, Hakim RM: The effect on patient health of using reprocessed artificial kidneys. *Proc Clin Dial Transplant Forum* 10: 86, 1980

39. Savdi E, Bruce L, Vincent PC: Modified neutropenic response to reused dialyzers in patients with chronic renal failure. *Clin Nephrol* 8: 422, 1977

40. Hakim RM, Lowrie EG: Effect of dialyzer reuse on leukopenia, hypoxemia and total hemolytic complement system. *Trans Am Soc Artif Intern Organs* 26: 159, 1980

41. Charoenpanick R, Pollack VE, Kant KS, Robson MD, Cathey M: Effect of first and subsequent use of hemodialyzers on patient well being: The rise and fall of a syndrome associated with new dialyzer use. *Artif Organs* 11: 123, 1987

42. Dumler F, Zasuwa G, Levin NW: Effect of dialyzer reprocessing methods on complement activation and hemodialyzer-related symptoms. *Artif Organs* 11: 128, 1987

43. Gagnon R, Adkar V, Kaye M: Dialyzer reuse following manual reprocessing with a new sterilant, REN-NEW-D. *Artif Organs* 11: 132, 1987

44. Vanholder R, Ringoir S: Influence of reuse and of reuse sterilants on first-use syndrome. *Artif Organs* 11: 137, 1987

45. Howell ED, Perkins HA: Anti-N-like antibodies in the sera of patients undergoing chronic hemodialysis. *Vox Sang* 23: 291, 1972

46. Belzer FO, Kountz SL, Perkins HA: Red cell cold autoagglutinins as a cause of failure of renal allo transplantation. *Transplantation* 11: 422, 1971

47. Lewis KJ, Ward MK, Kerr DNS: Residual formaldehyde in dialyzers: quantity, location and the effect of different methods of rinsing. *Artif Organs* 5: 269, 1981

48. Henderson LW, Chenoweth DE: Immune response to reuse: anaphylactoxins and IgE. in: *Guide to Reprocessing of Hemodialyzers,* edited by Deane N, Wineman RJ, Bemis JA, Boston, Martinus Nijhoff, 1986, p 151

49. Yudis M, Sirota RA, Stein HD: Dialyzer hypersensitivity reactions associated with reuse. *Abstracts Am Soc Artif Inter Organs* 14: 59, 1985

50. Dorson W, Pizziconi V, Hyde G: Technical considerations in multiple use of dialyzers. in: *Proceedings of the National Workshop on the Reuse of Consumables in Hemodialysis,* edited by Sadler J, Washington, DC, Kidney Disease Coalition, 1983, p 11

51. Deane N, Bemis JA: *Multiple Use of Hemodialyzers,* New York, National Nephrology Foundation, 1982, p 31

52. Wineman RJ: Automated reprocessing. in: *Guide to Reprocessing of Hemodialyzers,* edited by Deane N, Wineman RJ, Bemis JA, Boston, Martinus Nijhoff, 1986, p 163

53. Man NK, Lebkiri B, Polo P, De Sainte-Lorette E, Lemaire A, Funck-Brentano JL: Prevention of anti-N-like antibodies development with nonformaldehyde reuse procedure. *Proc Clin Dial Transplant Forum* 10: 18, 1980

54. Gagnon RF, Kaye M: Hemodialysis neutropenia and dialyzer reuse: role of the cleansing agent. *Uremia Invest* 8: 17, 1984

55. Leuhman D, Hirsch D, Carlson G, Constantini E, Keshaviah P: Dialyzer reuse in a large dialysis program. *Trans Am Soc Artif Intern Organs* 28: 76, 1982

56. Gotch FA: Solute and water transport and sterilant removal in reused dialyzers. in: *Guide to Reprocessing of Hemodialyzers,* edited by Deane D, Wineman RJ, Bemis JA, Boston, Martinus Nijhoff, 1986, p 39

57. Gotch FA: Quality control tests for validation of dialyzer performance. in: *Hemodialyzer Reuse: Issues and Solutions, AAMI Technology Assessment Report 10–85,* Arlington, VA, Association for Advancement of Medical Instrumentation, 1985, p 37

58. Sargent J, Gotch F: Principles and biophysics of dialysis. in: *Replacement of Renal Function by Dialysis,* 2nd edition, edited by Drukker W, Parsons FM, Maher JF, The Hague, Martinus Nijhoff, 1983, p 53

59. Deane N, Bemis JA: *Multiple Use of Hemodialyzers.* New York, Manhattan Kidney Center, National Nephrology Foundation, 1982, Appendix 6, p 191

60. Favero MS, Bland LA: Microbiologic principles applied to reprocessing hemodialyzers. in: *Guide to Reprocessing of Hemodialyzers.* edited by Deane N, Wineman RJ, Bemis JA, Boston, Martinus Nijhoff, 1986, p 63

61. Favero MS, Petersen NJ: Microbiological guidelines for hemodialysis systems. *Dial Transplant* 6: 34, 1977

62. Association for the Advancement of Medical Instrumentation: *American National Standards for Hemodialysis Systems,* Arlington, VA, Association for the Advancement of Medical Instrumentation, 1981

63. Petersen NJ: Microbiologic hazards associated with reuse of hemodialyzers. in: *Proceedings of National Workshop on Reuse of Consumables in Hemodialysis,* Baltimore, Kidney Disease Coalition, 1982, p 121

64. Deane N, Maude DL, Bemis JA: Reprocessing techniques. in: *Guide to Reprocessing of Hemodialyzers,* edited by Deane N, Wineman RJ, Bemis JA, Boston, Martinus Nijhoff, 1986, p 28

65. Hakim RM, Friedrich RA, Lowrie EG: Formaldehyde kinetics and bacteriology in dialyzers. *Kidney Int* 28: 936, 1985

66. Deane N, Bemis JA: *Multiple Use of Hemodialyzers,* New York, National Nephrology Foundation, 1982, Appendix 5, p 188

67. Gotch FA, Keen ML: Formaldehyde kinetics in reused dialyzers. *Trans Am Soc Artif Intern Organs* 29: 396, 1983

68. Kaye M, Barber E, Gagnon R: Residual formaldehyde in new and reused dialyzers. *Trans Am Soc Artif Intern Organs* 31: 644, 1985

69. Ansorge W, Pelger M, Dietrich W, Baurmeister U: Ethylene oxide in dialyzer rinsing fluid: Effect of rinsing technique, dialyzer storage time, and potting compound. *Artif Organs* 11: 118, 1987

70. Ing TS, Daugirdas J: Extractable ethylene oxide from cupro-ammonium cellulose plate dialyzers: Importance of potting compound. *Trans Am Soc Artif Intern Organs* 32: 108, 1986

71. Berkseth R, Leuhmann D, McMichael C, Keshaviah P, Kjellstrand C: Peracetic acid for reuse of hemodialyzers: Clinical studies. *Trans Am Soc Artif Intern Organs* 30: 270, 1984

72. Bauer H, Brunner H, Franz HE: Experience with the disinfectant peroxyacetic acid for hemodialyzer reuse. *Trans Am Soc Artif Intern Organs* 29: 662, 1983

73. Deane N, Wineman RJ: Comparative evaluation of automated devices for reprocessing hemodialyzers: Intradialytic patient response. *Trans Am Soc Artif Intern Organs* 30: 498, 1984

74. Wineman RJ: New Technologies in automated reprocessing of hemodialyzers. in: *Hemodialyzer Reuse: Issues and Solutions,* Arlington, VA, Association for Advancement of Medical Instrumentation, 1985, p 50

75. Levin NW, Messana A, Messana MA: Record-keeping procedures for dialyzer reuse. in: *Guide to Reprocessing of Hemodialyzers,* edited by Deane N, Wineman RJ, Bemis JA, Boston, Martinus Nijhoff, 1986, p 75

76. Federal Register Vol 52, No. 116, Wednesday June 17, 1987: Proposed Rules, p 23055

77. Deane N, Bemis JA: *Multiple Use of Hemodialyzers,* New York, National Nephrology Foundation, 1982, Appendix 11, p 219

78. Ogden DA: Quality control and quality assurance are different. Nephrology News and Issues, 24, July, 1987

79. Keshaviah P: Benefits of large solute removal vs pyrogen risk. Nephrology News and Issues, 32, July, 1987

19

DIALYSATE REGENERATION

WILLIAM DRUKKER and ALBERT W.J. VAN DOORN

INTRODUCTION

The ideal of a true, efficient wearable artificial kidney, the *fata morgana* of nephrologists, has kept several groups of investigators busy since dialysis and related forms of uraemia therapy became realities after World War II.

Portable and wearable dialysis systems have been constructed (1–3). They all were a compromise, not meeting the ideal of a truly wearable and effective artificial kidney and did not become popular in contrast with continuous ambulatory peritoneal dialysis (CAPD).

Introduced as a novel portable/wearable peritoneal dialysis technique (4) in 1976, CAPD gained a surprisingly fast acceptance and popularity (see chapters 22–25).

However, certain disadvantages and complications soon became obvious and the main problems of this technique (peritonitis, obesity and hyperlipidaemia [5]) still have to be overcome.

In addition deterioration of the peritoneal membrane, obliteration of the peritoneal cavity and sclerosing peritonitis are (less frequent) complications (see chapter 22) and four exchanges of peritoneal rinsing fluid present a tedious and time consuming routine.

On the other hand conventional single pass haemodialysis performed for 4 h thrice weekly requires slightly less than 400 l of water for preparation of dialysis fluid per week. The usual equipment requires water and drainage connections and is, in practice, immobile.

In certain areas there may be a natural shortage of water; elsewhere plumbing may be inadequate or water may be locally scarce on a periodic basis.

In addition municipal water has to be pretreated (see chapter 7) sometimes with complicated and expensive equipment such as reverse osmosis machines, which are indicated in areas where city water has a high aluminium content, an aluminium precipitation method being used to clear and to remove undesired colour. Aluminium, however, is, on chronic basis, a highly toxic trace element for patients treated by dialysis or haemofiltration.

A first step to a wearable artifical kidney

Not surprisingly, attempts have been going on to construct a truly portable, efficient artificial kidney system, independent of a fixed water supply and drain, with a small amount of dialysis fluid, suitable for regeneration and reuse.

Such a system could be a first step to a truly wearable artificial kidney, a wishful dream of many nephrologists and their patients, which, however, so far has become unrealistic, basically because urea is a chemically unreactive molecule, which is difficult to adsorb.

Nevertheless, activated carbon has been used to treat spent dialysate for reuse (6–10). It was shown that activated carbon effectively adsorbs many urinary nitrogenous waste products, urea remaining the important exception.

Although 100 g of activated carbon is sufficient to adsorb the daily production of creatinine, uric acid and phenols, some 10 to 20 kg would be required to adsorb the daily production of urea (7), unless cooled to 0° C, when activated charcoal binds urea quantitatively but necessitating the additional complication and cost of refrigeration (11).

A new urea sorbent

This problem, however, may be superseded in the future by the work of Smakman and van Doorn (12), who recently developed a new sorbent in which the active principle is ninhydrin and which irreversibly binds urea.

So far this new sorbent has not been used in patients, but it may become an important expedient in the treatment of uraemia.

Finally activated coal has virtually no affinity for mono- and divalent ions and cannot correct abnormalities of sodium, potassium, phosphate, chloride, calcium or magnesium.

This chapter reviews various attempts to develop efficient regeneration of dialysis fluid and describes the only system that has been put into practice and is commercially available.

PREVIOUS ATTEMPTS TO REGENERATE DIALYSATE AND ULTRAFILTRATE

Several attempts have been made to recycle a small volume of dialysate for reuse, making a dialysis system with a small volume of recirculating dialysis fluid possible.

In Japan, Maeda and coworkers (13) in 1971 constructed a portable artificial kidney system, utilising 30 l of dialysate which were regenerated by recirculation through a column containing 500 g of activated charcoal and a second column containing 200 g of alumina. These two substances were selected on the basis of their adsorption rates for creatinine, uric acid and inorganic phosphate. In addition appreciable

amounts of methyl-guanidine and guanidino acetic acid were adsorbed. The adsorbents were tested for the release of potentially toxic trace metals, including aluminium, by atomic absorption spectophotometry and it was concluded that the system was safe. *In vitro* experiments demonstrated satisfactory adsorption of creatinine and uric acid by the activated carbon and of phosphate by the alumina column. It should be mentioned, however, that the investigators did not use the sensitive flameless atomic absorption spectro-photometric technique, as later described by Fuchs and coworkers (14), which is required for accurate aluminium determinations in biological fluids.

The Japanese investigators used their 30 l system for at least 46 months in a number of patients in a comparative study with a single-pass system, which required 210 l of dialysis fluid. Six hundred dialyses were performed and average plasma concentrations were reduced by 59% for creatinine, 67% for uric acid and 58% for phosphate. A rise of blood urea was, however, a matter of concern. Surprisingly in an anuric patient, dialysed 7 h thrice weekly with the new system for 14 months, a fall of the blood urea concentration was observed after an initial rise. The patient was eventually fully rehabilitated.

In 1974 the same investigators (15) reported favourable results in an additional group of patients. At that time, according to the authors, almost all home dialysis patients in Japan were using their system.

Subsequently they changed to a 10 l system, increasing the acetate concentration to 50 mmol/l, which normalised the post-dialysis serum bicarbonate concentration. Equally good results were obtained; pre-dialysis levels of blood urea initially increased but gradually decreased after 6 weeks, stabilising at approximately 420 mg/dl (70 mmol/l). They explained this phenomenon by postulating the incorporation of urea into plasma and tissue proteins.

No further papers on this system have been published in the current literature but the system has been used in Italy.

Italian investigators (16) prepared a sorbent cartridge with a bottom layer of granulated oxidised starch for removal of urea and a layer with aluminium silicate which removed phosphate and substantial amounts of calcium and magnesium. Therefore, a cation exchange resin layer was inserted between the oxystarch and the aluminium silicate layer. This layer served a dual purpose: by exchanging cations, calcium replenishment and potassium removal were obtained. Remaining organic metabolites such as creatinine and uric acid were removed by a terminal layer containing activated carbon. Animal experiments were performed with encouraging results in 1974 but the system had not yet been used in patients. No further reports have been published.

In England dialysate regeneration was reviewed and studied at the Atomic Weapons Research Establishment at Aldermaston by Bultitude and Gower (17). They tried to regenerate the dialysis fluid by circulation through a 4 kg (dry weight) activated charcoal pack. A 30 l batch of a somewhat modified dialysis fluid was used, containing (in mmol/l) sodium 132, potassium 1.3, calcium 1.5, magnesium 0.5, acetate 43 and chloride 94 (without dextrose).

Up to 2.5 l of body water (including solutes) could be removed by ultrafiltration by means of a negative pressure pump situated down stream of the dialyser as is used in a conventional flow-to-waste system. The 30 l volume of dialysis fluid was chosen partly to correct electrolyte imbalance by equilibration with the plasma water across the dialyser and partly to equilibrate urea in a similar manner. A very limited clinical trial was undertaken by Dr. F.M. Parsons at the General Infirmary at Leeds, UK.

Certainly during dialysis, equilibration between plasma water and dialysis fluid occurred, but hypocalcaemia developed and it seemed that with this type of regeneration system, further work on calcium kinetics was required.

The wearable artificial kidney, developed by Stephen and Kolff and coworkers (1) in the mid 1970's, is a somewhat miniaturised haemodialysis system, using a 20 l dialysis fluid batch with (partial) regeneration through a 250 g activated charcoal column, which gives the patient the opportunity of greater mobility by disconnecting himself from the 20 l reservoir for brief periods of time (up to 15 min).

Basically all these designs shared one, crucial problem: the poor removal of urea, which so far had remained unsolved.

Kolff (18, 19) suggested the insertion of an additional dialyser, provided with an asymmetric, positively charged cellulose acetate, anion exchange membrane, attached to a secondary recirculation circuit incorporating a column containing urease and an ion exchange resin. This secondary urea removal system, which originated at the Weizmann Institute of Science in Israel, allowed urea to diffuse through the (secondary) membrane, but electrolytes did not diffuse through the positively charged membrane. Urea was converted by urease into ammonium ions and bicarbonate. The ammonium ions were removed by a cation exchange resin inserted into the secondary circuit. The exchange resin was a zeolite with a high affinity for ammonium ions, which exchanged ammonium for sodium. Neither ammonium nor sodium could diffuse back through the positively charged secondary membrane into the primary dialysis circuit. Insertion of an activated carbon column in the secondary circuit also removed creatinine, uric acid and other organic substances.

Kolff et al (20) later (1979) designed a somewhat simplified system, omitting the secondary circuit with the second dialyser.

This system (Figure 1) incorporated a urease column which hydrolysed urea to ammonium carbonate, and a cation exchange resin (a selective zeolite) which exchanged ammonium ions for sodium. Another cation resin exchanged sodium ions for protons, and, finally, an activated carbon column adsorbed organic wastes such as creatinine, uric acid and others. Sensors monitored pH, calcium and potassium ions and these regulated the bypass flow through the cation resins, to maintain pH between narrow limits.

Another method of removing ammonia generated by urease has been presented by Pişkin and coworkers (21). The dialysis fluid, after passing through a urease column, entered a packed bed gas desorption column, a powerful air

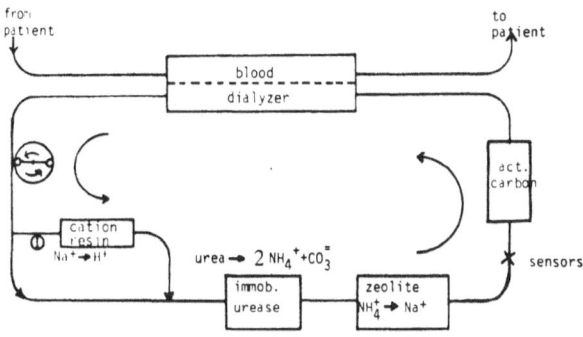

Figure 1. Dialysate regeneration system designed by Kolff and coworkers, incorporating a urease column, an exchange resin (selective zeolite) and an activated carbon column (see text). (From Kolff et al [20] with permission).

stream flowing countercurrently through the degassing column.

Several other ways of removing urea have been suggested. They either derive from animal physiology or from waste-disposal processes (18, 22). One concept, originated by Harmsen and Kolff (23), dates back to 1947. Bacterial cultures were grown inside a cellophane membrane or tube, nutrients coming from the dialysate outside the membrane. It was hoped that microbial enzymes would convert urea into small amino acids, which would dialyse back into the dialysate, finally reaching the patient. Several years later it was demonstrated that decomposition of urea can be achieved by soil bacteria (24) and also by a certain bacterial strain from the rumen of cattle (18).

Malchesky and Nosé (22) studied the removal of nitrogenous waste products in batch reactors, using human urine as substrate, and initially selected bacteria from activated sludge provided by a local sewage treatment plant. They obtained encouraging results, for their cultures removed substantial amounts of urea, creatinine and uric acid from the substrates.

Although the goal of these investigators was to use these 'biological reactors' as renal substitutes (25) their systems could also be used for dialysate regeneration. This was investigated by Ackerman and coworkers (26), who used an immobilised strain of gram positive (presumably non-pyrogenic) bacteria in a bioreactor. The selected bacteria could convert urea to nitrogenous gases with a minimal production of ammonia. They recirculated the dialysate through the bioreactor and used a bacterial filter and a powerful ultraviolet light disinfector to control bacterial contamination (Figure 2). However less desirable bacterial products could also be formed in these systems and reach the patient.

So far these investigators like others have not bridged the gap from laboratory investigations to clinical application. Their *in vitro* results, however, were promising.

The approach of Shaldon and coworkers in 1978–1979 (27, 28) was more realistic. They used a Redy cartridge commonly used in regeneration of spent dialysis fluid, in a closed

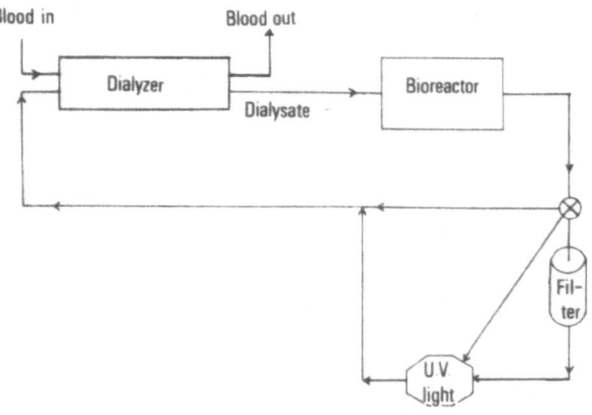

Figure 2. Regeneration of dialysate by bacteria in a 'bioreactor'. In the recirculation circuit are a bacterial filter and a UV disinfector. (From Ackerman et al [26] with permission).

recirculating circuit for regeneration of ultrafiltrate during haemofiltration with an Amicon 0.5 m² filter (see Figure 3). This system was applied to three patients with apparently good results.

When it was shown, however, that the regeneration cartridge released considerable amounts of aluminium in the haemofiltrate the investigations were abandoned.

Another, ingenious approach dates back to the mid 1960's, when Tuwiner (29) reported on the application of electrochemical degradation of organic compounds in urine with the aim of producing potable water for manned space vehicles.

When a direct electric current is passed through a solution containing NaCl, chlorine is produced at the anode and sodium hydroxide and hydrogen at the cathode. The chlorine and sodium hydroxide react to produce sodium hypochlorite, a strong oxidant. It appeared possible to oxidise organic compounds in urine by electrolysis (30, 31). Two French investigators, Bizot and Sausse (32) applied this principle to used dialysate and presented evidence that urea, creatinine and uric acid could be oxidised to nitrogen, water and carbon dioxide.

This work was pursued by Fels (30, 31) in Canada, who showed that the decomposition rate of urea depends strongly on both voltage and current and that for every mole of urea degraded one mole of carbon dioxide, one mole of nitrogen and two moles of hydrogen were produced.

A somewhat similar concept applying electro-oxidation to regenerate haemofiltrate has been pursued by Quellhorst and coworkers (33–37) in the Federal Republic of Germany. An electrochemical cell was developed producing hypochlorite, which, as mentioned above, is a strong oxidant converting urea into CO_2, N_2 and H_2O. Upstream and downstream of the cell a column with activated carbon is inserted, removing creatinine, uric acid and a number of middle molecules.

Excess hypochlorite is removed by a reactor after (upstream of) the electrochemical cell and also by the activated carbon.

The 'purified' (regenerated) haemofiltrate proved to be nontoxic in animal tests. The system appeared to be feasable in animal experiments.

At the time of writing (May 1987) the system was apparently not (yet) applied in human patients.

It is likely that the urea removal problem will be solved with the new ninhydrin sorbent mentioned earlier (12), preempting all other methods briefly described above.

In summary, several groups around the world have tried

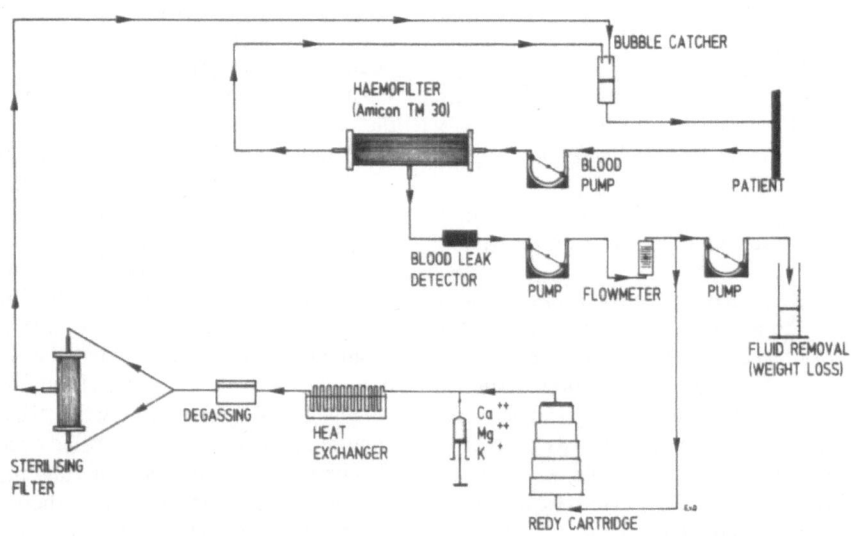

Figure 3. Flow diagram of an on-line regeneration system for haemofiltrate incorporating the old type D11 Redy cartridge, developed by Shaldon and colleagues (1978 [27, 28]). The system was abandoned because of leakage of impermissable quantities of aluminium from the regeneration cartridge. (From Shaldon et al [28], with permission).

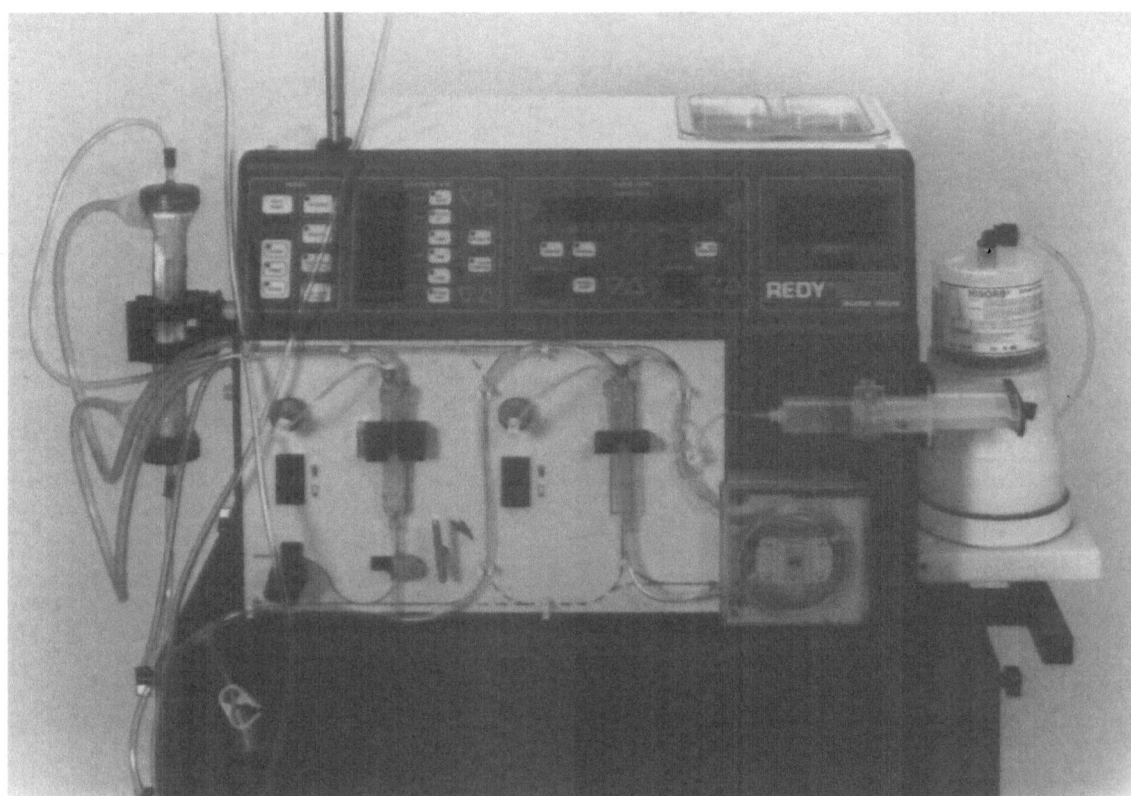

Figure 4. Front view of the Redy 2000 unit.

to develop an efficient system for dialysate regeneration that would eliminate the large quantities of pretreated water, thereby reducing the cost of dialysis, while retaining reliability and safety. So far these efforts have not resulted in systems suitable for clinical application with the single exception of the system described by Maeda (13, 15).

To understand the development of the only practically available dialysate regeneration system we have to recall another approach which originated from manned space flight technology.

In the mid 1960's the aerospace industry in Southern California began to seek diversification by applying aerospace research technology to biomedical engineering, more specifically to dialysis associated engineering. In the absence of a suitable adsorbent, the problem of urea removal could obviously only be solved in an indirect way. An experimental system was designed, using enzymatic hydrolysis of urea by urease, zirconium phosphate (ZP) being selected to bind the produced ammonium.

ZP acts partially as a molecular sieve, but primarily as a cation exchange resin, having a high affinity for ammonium ions exchanging them for H^+ ions and sodium ions, even in the presence of relatively high concentrations of sodium ions. Hydrated zirconium oxide (ZO) was added to bind phosphate by exchange for acetate (in the old type cartridge for chloride).

A sorbent system consisting of urease, ZP, hydrous ZO and activated carbon was subjected to animal testing (3, 38). Initially utilising a total dialysis fluid volume of one litre, anephric dogs were dialysed with this sorbent dialysate regeneration system, resulting in survivals for as long as 37 days without evidence of uraemic or other toxicity. Subsequently two human subjects were dialysed successfully for periods of 9 and 10 months (39, 40).

It was concluded that sorbent regeneration of dialysate provided a realistic approach to a portable dialysis system, independent of a fixed water supply and drain and without the need for pre-treatment of water (41).

PRACTICAL APPLICATION OF DIALYSATE REGENERATION: THE REDY SYSTEM

The system, originally named Redy, which was derived from REcirculating DialYsis system[1] (Figure 4), incorporates a dialysate reservoir containing 6 l of dialysis fluid (Figure 5),

---

1. The name Redy was temporarily changed to Sorb System for unknown (commercial) reasons. The name Redy will be used in this chapter.

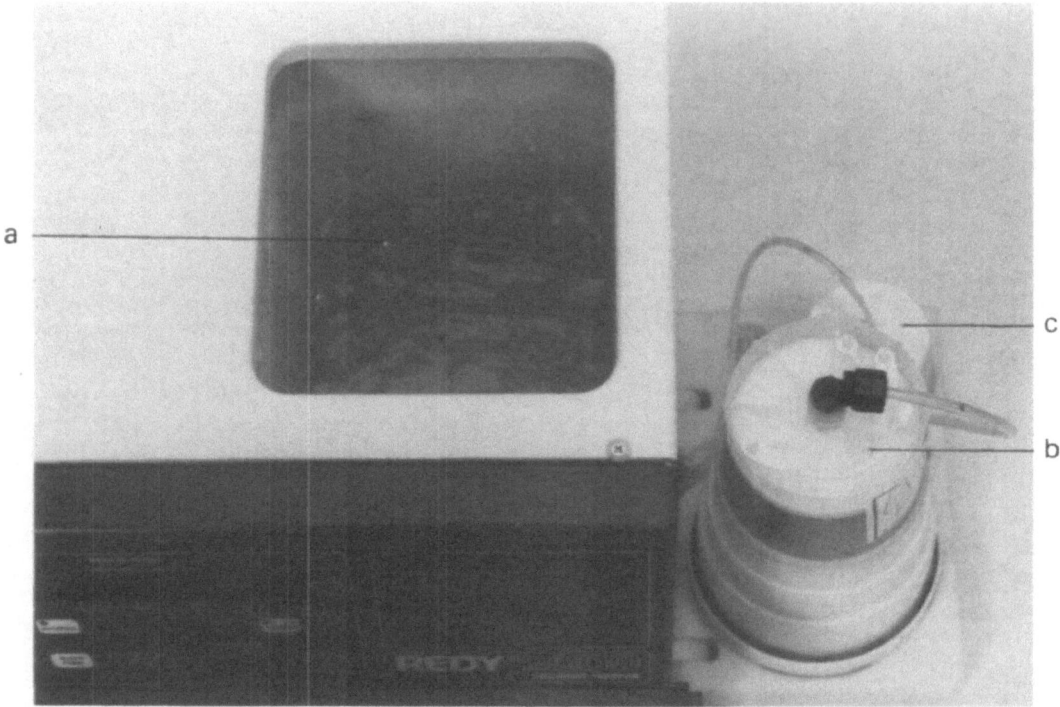

Figure 5. Top view of the Redy 2000: a. dialysate reservoir (61); b. regeneration cartridge; c. infusate container (with [potassium], calcium and magnesium acetate solution).

which is continuously recirculated at a flow rate of 250 ml/min through a disposable five layer cartridge, which regenerates the dialysate.[2]

The apparatus is provided with the usual monitors of temperature and electrical conductivity of the dialysate and a gauge for continuously measuring the volume of ultrafiltrate. Alarm systems include a low pressure alarm for the recirculation circuit, a blood leak detector and an additional safety device, which activates the acoustic alarm in case of failure of the calcium-magnesium acetate infusion pump in delivering the predetermined amount of infusate per minute. A flow diagram of the system is presented in Figure 6.

The kinetics of the regeneration cartridge

The cartridge basically accomplishes three functions:
1. enzymatic decomposition of urea
2. ion exchange
3. adsorption

The first layer

The original cartridge, which had only four layers, was later modified by adding an extra bottom or first layer acting as a

---

2. The amount of dialysis fluid was initially 5.51 but has increased to 61.

scavenger proximal to the urease. This layer consists of activated carbon and hydrated zirconium oxide and prevents inactivation of the urease from trace metal contaminants (especially copper) and oxidising agents such as chlorine, chloramine, sodium hypochlorite and others, which might be present after disinfecting and rinsing the system or in the water used for preparation of dialysis fluid.

The second layer

The second layer contains urease, which catalyses the conversion of urea into ammonia and carbamic acid, which is converted into ammonium ions and bicarbonate ions (42–45) [see equations 1–4]).

$$H_2N\text{-}CO\text{-}NH_2 + 2H_2O \xrightarrow{urease} NH_4^+ + NH_2COO^- + H_2O \quad [1]$$
$$\text{urea} \qquad\qquad\qquad\qquad\qquad \text{carbamic acid}$$

$$NH_4^+ + NH_2COO^- + H_2O \rightleftarrows 2\,NH_4^+ + CO_3^{--}$$
$$2\,NH_4^+ + CO_3^{--} \rightleftarrows NH_4^+ + NH_3 + HCO_3^- \quad [2]$$

Ammonia, in watery solution, will be partially converted into NH_4 staying in equilibrium with ammonium ions and hydroxyl ions:

$$NH_3 + H_2O \rightleftarrows NH_4^+ + OH^-. \quad [3]$$

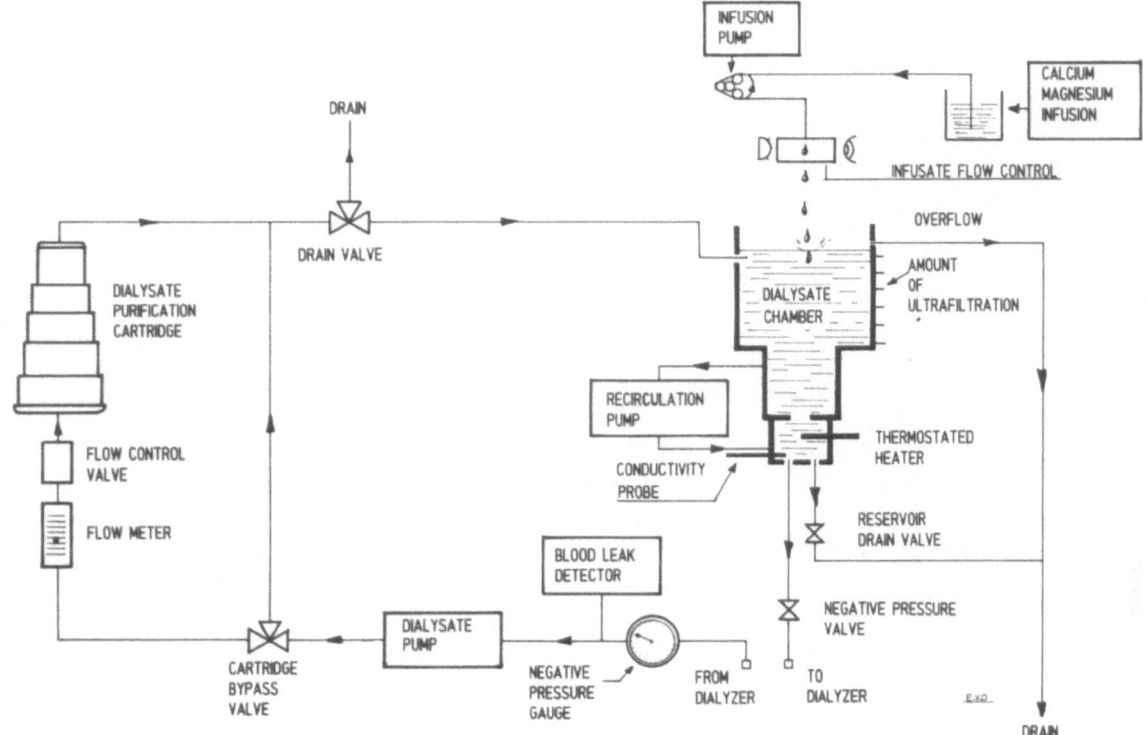

Figure 6. Flow diagram of the Redy system.

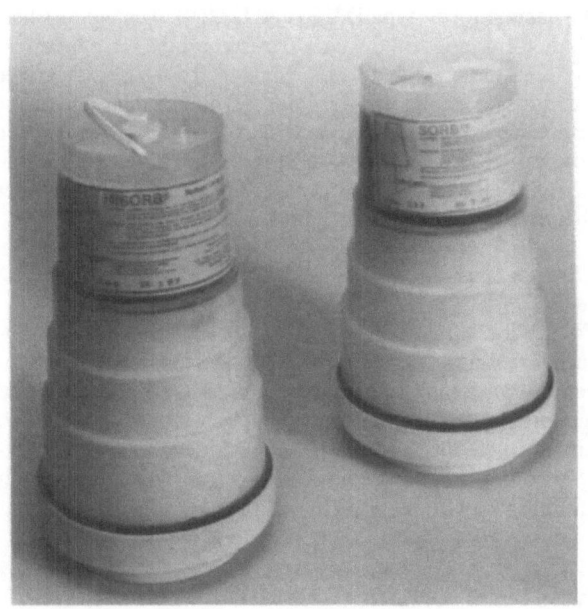

Figure 7. Regeneration cartridges, new model D3160 and D3260, containing reduced amount of aluminium oxide.

The net result of urea splitting may be written as:

$$NH_2\text{-}CO\text{-}NH_2 + 3H_2O \rightarrow 2NH_4^+ + HCO_3^- + OH^-. \quad [4]$$

In addition bicarbonate lost from the patient across the dialyser membrane enters the dialysis fluid. The fluid recirculates through the cartridge which is buffered at a pH of 6 (43–45).

The third layer

The bicarbonate both generated by the conversion of urea and originating from the patient enters the third layer of the cartridge, consisting of buffered zirconium phosphate and reacts with protons delivered by the ZP:

$$ZPH + NaHCO_3 \rightarrow ZPNa + H_2O + \overset{\nearrow}{CO_2}. \quad [5]$$

The stability of the bicarbonate in the dialysis fluid depends on the pH. When pH of this fluid drops below 7 (see Figure 9) bicarbonate decomposes into water and carbon dioxide.

Ammonium ions also enter the ZP layer which acts as a cation exchanger loaded with hydrogen ions and sodium ions, in a ratio of 1:8 (44, 45). The ammonium ions are,

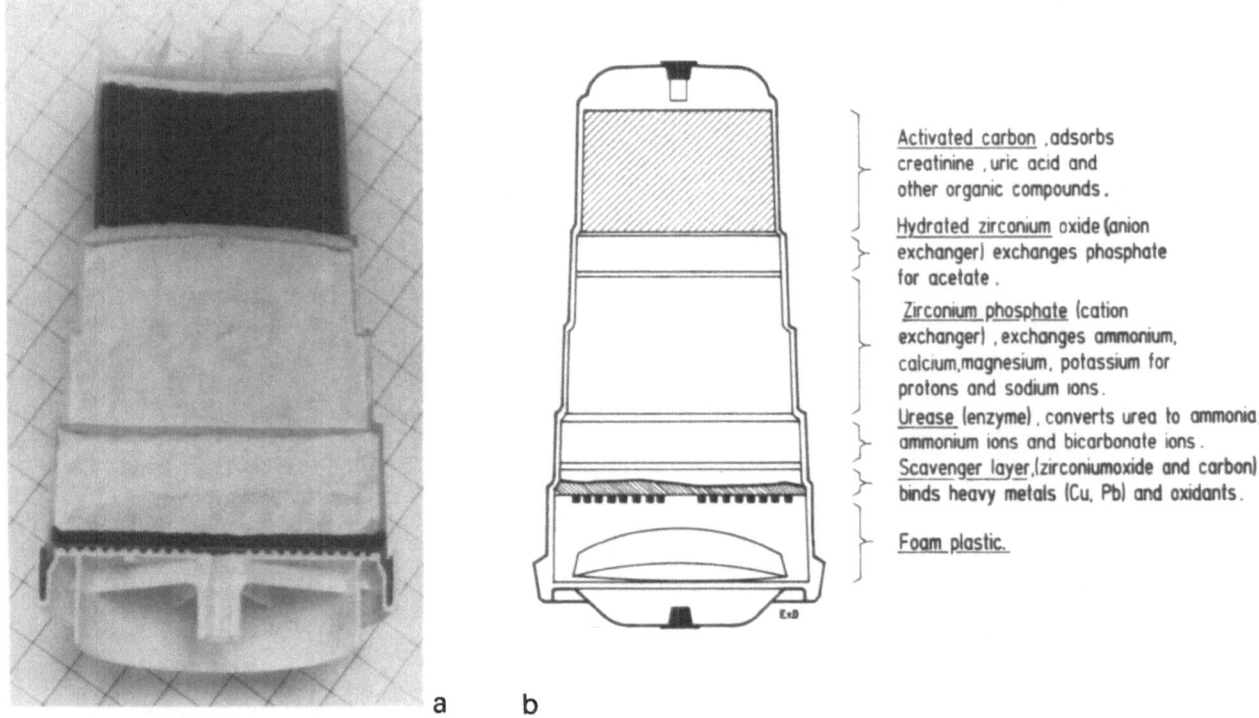

Activated carbon, adsorbs creatinine, uric acid and other organic compounds.

Hydrated zirconium oxide (anion exchanger) exchanges phosphate for acetate.

Zirconium phosphate (cation exchanger), exchanges ammonium, calcium, magnesium, potassium for protons and sodium ions.

Urease (enzyme), converts urea to ammonia, ammonium ions and bicarbonate ions.

Scavenger layer, (zirconium oxide and carbon) binds heavy metals (Cu, Pb) and oxidants.

Foam plastic.

a   b

Figure 8. a. Longitudinal section of new model D3160 cartridge, showing different layers. b. Diagram of a longitudinal section of D3160 cartridge, showing kinetics of different layers.

along with calcium, magnesium and potassium ions, exchanged for hydrogen and sodium ions (3, 38, 39, 44, 45 [Figure 10]). The released hydrogen ions will be buffered partially by the bicarbonate but this does not prevent an initial drop of dialysate pH (see Figure 9), which is caused by the release of hydrogen ions from the third layer and through release of anions from the fourth layer (consisting of hydrated zirconium oxide) in exchange for phosphate.

The release of sodium ions from the ZP layer is responsible for a gradual rise of the dialysate sodium concentration during dialysis.

Because of complete removal of calcium, magnesium and potassium ions from the dialysis fluid by the cartridge, calcium and magnesium ions (and in some cases potassium ions) have to be added continuously to the dialysate. The desired calcium and magnesium concentrations are achieved by continuously infusing a solution of calcium and magnesium acetate (and in some cases also potassium acetate) from a small container by a small Holter-type metering pump (Figure 6) into the main dialysate reservoir.

The fourth layer

The fourth layer of the cartridge consists of hydrous zirconium oxide (ZO), which acts as an anion exchange resin. The early (D11, D44 and D42) cartridges were loaded with chloride. However, the cartridges are now marketed with ZO in

the acetate form (type D3160 and D3260) exchanging phosphate for acetate (in the old cartridges which were taken off the market, phosphate was exchanged for chloride). The cartridge does not remove sulphate from the dialysate to any appreciable degree. Sulphate bypasses the cartridge and accumulates in the dialysate. Plasma sulphate levels in patients treated with the Redy system are, therefore higher than in those treated with single pass dialysis (46, 47).

The fifth layer

Finally the fifth layer, consisting of activated carbon, adsorbs creatinine, uric acid, phenols, indican and other nitrogenous wastes. It also adsorbs amino acids and a limited quantity of dextrose (7.5 to 15 g, [Van Doorn AWJ, 1979, unpublished observations]). The cartridge, however, quickly becomes saturated with dextrose after which the system equilibrates with plasma glucose (45, 48).

PRACTICAL USE OF THE REDY SYSTEM

The practical application of this low volume sorbent regeneration system differs in several aspects from conventional single pass or recirculating dialysis systems. In conventional dialysis the concentration of solutes in the dialysis fluid is the primary chemical variable which the operator must consid-

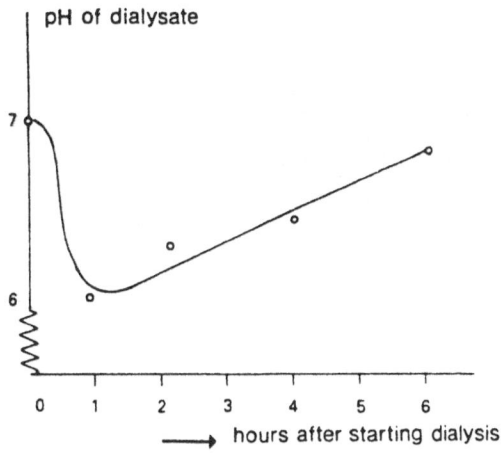

Figure 9. Dialysate pH during the course of dialysis with the Redy apparatus.

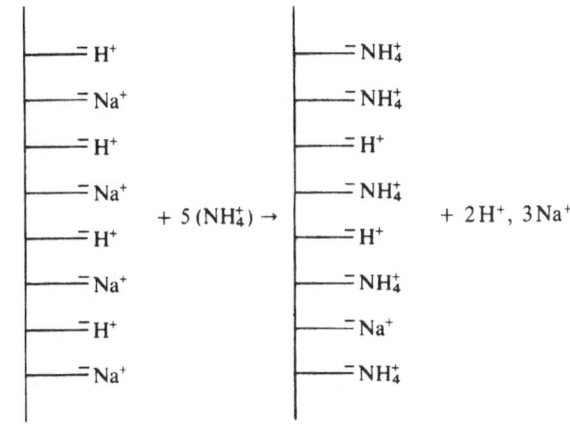

Figure 10. Exchange of NH_4^+ for H^+ and Na^+ in the zirconium phosphate layer. (From Van Doorn and Thomas [44], modified).

er. In Redy dialysis he also must pay attention to the effects of the regeneration cartridge, which extracts waste substances and adds electrolytes continuously. On the other hand the effects of the variable composition of the dialysis fluid are mitigated by the small volume of dialysis fluid as compared with the total body water (see below) and the low dialysate flow rate (45).

Urea removal

The ability to remove urea is basically limited by the capacity of the zirconium phosphate layer of the cartridge to exchange ammonium ions.

Different types of cartridges are available: the D3160 has an average capacity for 20 g urea nitrogen, that is approx. 43 g (approx. 714 mmol) of urea. In muscular patients or (and) after high protein intake or during a hypercatabolic state, when the urea generation rate and the pre-dialysis plasma urea concentration are particularly high, the binding capacity of this cartridge may be exceeded, resulting in free ammonia entering the effluent from the cartridge. When the critical ammonia level of 2 mg/dl (1.11 mmol/l) in the dialysate is exceeded, acute ammonia intoxication may occur, characterised by (rapidly reversible) symptoms of headaches, nausea and vomiting. Ammonia test paper is available, which permits rapid screening of dialysate ammonia levels, whenever an ammonia 'breakthrough' is anticipated or suspected.

A high capacity cartridge (Hisorb D3260) is marketed with an average capacity of 28 g urea nitrogen, that is 60 g (1000 mmol) of urea.

Most patients can be treated by thrice weekly dialysis using three D3160 cartridges per week, provided that the protein intake does not exceed 60 g per day.

Should intercurrent infections occur protein catabolism will increase and either the Hisorb cartridge (D3260) should be used or a conventional dialysis system should be employed temporarily.

Some larger patients routinely require more capacity for urea than provided by the D3160 cartridges and a weekly routine of two D3160 cartridges with one D3260 after the week-end interval may prove satisfactory.

Because there is a linking of the sodium/hydrogen balance to the load of ammonium ions presented to the ZP layer, which in turn depends on the amount of urea removed, the selection of the correct type of cartridge for the individual patient is important.

Low dialysate flow through the circuit

For adequate regeneration of the dialysate by the cartridge the dialysate flow rate through the system, including the dialyser, had to be limited to 250 ml/min (in contrast with the standard flow rate of 500 ml/min through the dialyser in conventional single pass systems). Thus the 6 l volume circulates through the dialyser cartridge ciruit every 24 min. In addition the amount of cations (Ca^{++}, Mg^{++} and K^+) bound by the cartridge (in exchange for sodium ions and protons) would proportionally increase with a higher dialysate flow rate, not only requiring a higher calcium and magnesium infusate flow, but also resulting in a decrease of the ammonium binding capacity and release of an undesirable additional amount of sodium and hydrogen ions.

The effect of low dialysate flow has been studied by Babb and associates (49–51). The clearances of small (readily dialysable) solutes are reduced. Clearances of less dialysable middle molecules are not (or much less) affected. Small molecule clearances (urea, creatinine) using the Redy system are some 10 to 15% less than with standard dialysis systems. This, however, does not influence post-dialysis plasma concentrations of urea and creatinine.

In contrast with conventional single pass dialysis fluid delivery systems both the dialysate pH and the sodium concentration in the rinsing fluid vary during the course of dialysis, as mentioned earlier.

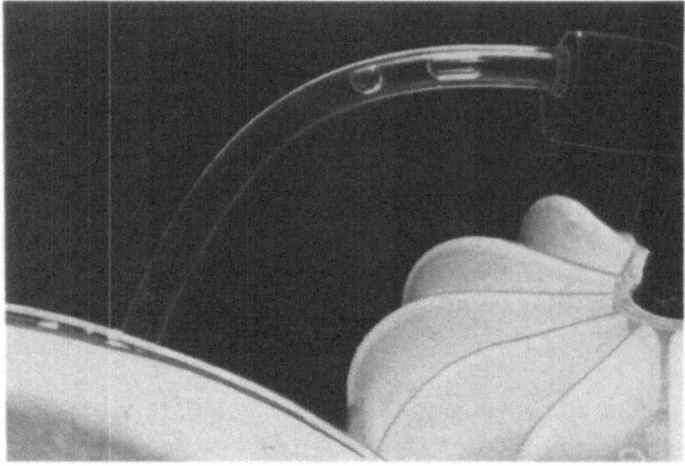

Figure 11. Carbon dioxide produced by the conversion of bicarbonate escaping from the top of the cartridge.

Kinetics of pH and CO$_2$

The ammonium ions produced in the urease layer are exchanged in the ZP layer for hydrogen ions and sodium ions, which are released into the dialysate. In addition, acetate ions are released from the hydrated ZO layer in exchange for phosphate. Obviously both a drop of pH and a progressive increase in sodium concentration in the dialysate occur during dialysis (Figures 9 and 10). The drop in pH, however, is partially buffered by bicarbonate and has no significant effect on the acidity of the blood perfusing the dialyser. Any hydrogen ions passing through the membrane into the patient's blood will be immediately buffered. But as the dialysate pH drops below 7 during recirculation through the cartridge, a further conversion of the bicarbonate will occur, producing CO$_2$ and H$_2$O. Gaseous carbon dioxide escapes from the top of the cartridge (Figure 11). The dialysate leaves the cartridge supersaturated with carbon dioxide (the excess escaping in the air). A very high pCO$_2$ is generated in the dialysate (200 mm Hg at 120 min [52, 53]). Consequently total CO$_2$ of the blood perfusing the dialyser rises. Simultaneously, there is a loss of bicarbonate (see below).

The blood leaving the dialyser in a Redy system is, therefore, hypercapnic and because of combined 'respiratory' and 'metabolic' acidosis has a very low pH (45, 53–55).

In conventional dialysis systems using acetate in place of bicarbonate, the blood leaving the dialyser also has a low bicarbonate concentration, but a normal pH, because of a simultaneous loss of carbon dioxide to the dialysate (which goes to drain).

The blood leaving the dialyser in a Redy system rapidly mixes with the patient's blood-pool and any excess of CO$_2$ is immediately lost in the expired air. Therefore, this interesting phenomenon seems to have little if any clinical significance (45, 55).

However, when the blood circuit during dialysis is switched into the 'dialyser bypass' mode, while continuing the dialysate circulation through the cartridge and the dialyser,[3] the stagnant blood in the dialyser will be saturated with CO$_2$, resulting in extreme hyercapnia.

When the blood circuit is restored and the hypercapnic blood reaches the respiratory centre, rather unpleasant side effects occur, such as hyperventilation with facial flushing, feelings of oppression and acute headaches.

Excess CO$_2$ in the dialysis fluid of the Redy system requires degassing of the bath fluid (52, 55): the CO$_2$ (and also nitrogen from dissolved air) will escape from the blood when negative pressure on the dialysate is applied. This causes foaming of the blood leaving the dialyser and could adversely interfere with mass transfer and also increase fibrin deposition in hollow fibre dialysers. These effects can be minimised by degassing of the dialysis fluid (55; see also chapter 8).

Degassing of the dialysis fluid

Partial degassing may be achieved by replacing the standard pump in the recirculation circuit by a small high power (Micro Giant) pump and inserting an adjustable constriction in the circuit (Figure 12), thus creating a negative pressure area (55, 56). To prevent temperature instability a simple stirrer has to be added in the reservoir (Figure 12). This modification has not been incorporated by the manufacturers. Alternatively, it seems possible to insert a device with a degassing membrane for removal of CO$_2$ and nitrogen (28).

Sodium kinetics

Ammonium ions produced by the enzymatic conversion of

---

3. This is sometimes done while correcting positions of fistula needles.

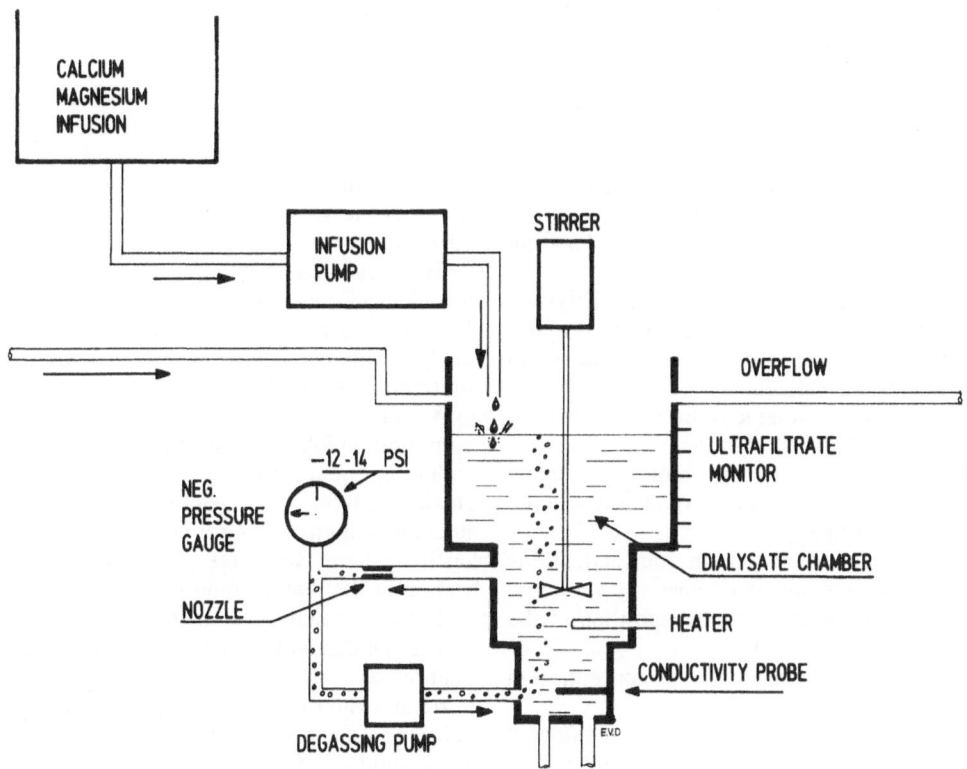

Figure 12. Partial flow diagram of the Redy system (see also Figure 6) with degassing of the dialysate by negative pressure (12–15 PSI = approx. 0.82–0.95 atmosphere).

urea are exchanged in the ZP layer for hydrogen ions and sodium ions, increasing dialysate sodium during dialysis. The increase depends on the amount of urea removed from the patient. Removal of 18.7 g of urea nitrogen or 40 g of urea (668 mmol) releases from the cartridge some 200 mmol sodium, so that the sodium concentration in the 6 l dialysis fluid increases about 8.25 mmol/l/h.

In addition about 50 mmol of Na are liberated from the cartridge during the first passage of the dialysis fluid (57). When hard water is used for preparation of the priming dialysis fluid the release of Na (because of exchange of Ca and Mg) will be greater.

The initial circulation of the dialysis fluid through the dialyser which is primed with normal saline (155 mmol/l of sodium) increases dialysate Na by 3 to 5 mmol/l.

Further the calcium, magnesium and potassium ions from the infusate will be exchanged for sodium ions (and hydrogen ions). The dialysate Na increases from this source some 10 to 12.5 mmol/l/h.

Obviously, a substantial increase of dialysate Na occurs before and during a Redy dialysis, which can be observed with the conductivity meter.

This increase of sodium in the dialysate relates to the amount of urea removed from the patient and presented to the cartridge, as mentioned above.

The gradual increase of the dialysate Na during dialysis

requires a low initial sodium concentration in the dialysis fluid and a starting concentration of 100 to 110 mmol/l is usually recommended.

Thus a negative sodium concentration gradient exists between dialysate and plasma during the first hours of dialysis, sodium being transferred from plasma to dialysate. Subsequent to a brief period of equilibrium with zero transfer, Na transfer occurs in the opposite direction (from dialysate to the patient), counteracted of course by convective Na loss from the patient during ultrafiltration. It should be kept in mind that an unsuitably large urea load (in excess of that for which the cartridge was designed) additionally increases sodium ion release by the cartridge with a further rise of dialysate sodium. The selection of a suitable cartridge and the initial sodium concentration in the dialysis fluid are, therefore, of importance.

Recently, the relationship between urea removal and sodium release has been expressed in a somewhat complicated equation (Schilb and coworkers [58]), allowing a calculation of the sodium increase, using predialysis plasma urea concentration and dialysis time as parameters.

Several clinical investigators have now confirmed that in practice there is no difference in hypertension control between the Redy system and conventional dialysis systems (55, 57, 59). During Redy dialysis diffusion of sodium clearly varies with the concentration gradient and is, therefore, a dynamic variable; but the effects are mitigated by the small volume of dialysis fluid and the low dialysate flow.

The ratio between the 6 l of dialysis fluid in the Redy system and the 34 to 45 l of total body water of an adult patient is approximately 1:6 to 7 and contrasts with a ratio of about 2.7 to 3.4:1 in a conventional 4 h single pass dialysis. The 250 ml dialysis fluid flow in the Redy also means less impact on the body sodium concentration (content) than in a single pass dialysis (with a dialysis fluid flow rate of 500 ml/min).

As discussed earlier, the dialysate Na in the Redy system may increase some 30 to 33 mmol/l during dialysis and a hypernatric bath late in dialysis may add about 50 to 100 mmol of sodium to the patient.

This, however, is amply counteracted by a convective Na loss of about 135 mmol/l with ultrafiltrate.

Clearly net sodium balance is much more importantly influenced by convective than by diffusive factors and the 'metabolism' of the cartridge.

Summarising, dialysate sodium concentration in the Redy system is a variable (rising) parameter. Obviously, the initial sodium concentration depends on the composition of the dialysis fluid placed in the reservoir.

The degree and tempo of the rise in sodium concentration depend on the following factors:
1. The equilibration time between commencing the flow of the dialysis fluid through the cartridge and the start of dialysis.
2. The amount of urea extracted from the patient (in turn depending on predialysis plasma urea concentration, the clearance rate of the dialyser and the 'urea' capacity of the cartridge).
3. Duration of dialysis, which will determine the amount of sodium released by the cartridge in exchange for ammonium ions (derived from urea) and calcium, magnesium and potassium ions supplied by the infusate and removed from the dialysate by the cartridge.
4. The accuracies of both the flow meter and infusion pump. When both are not entirely satisfactory this causes variations of the rate of cation exchange in the cartridge, which in turn affects sodium release.

Clearly anion release (acetate) will vary between different patients, depending on the amount of anions (predominantly phosphate) exchanged.

Fortunately, in practice the majority of the above conditions is remarkably constant in the individual stable chronic dialysis patient; the major factors affecting the final dialysate composition are the initial concentrations in the dialysis fluid, timing of the commencement of dialysis, the duration of dialysis and the amount of urea, removed from the patient.

Thus each dialysis unit should ascertain these variables and adjust the initial dialysis fluid composition accordingly. As a guide it would be reasonable to use an initial dialysis fluid of the following composition:

Sodium: 100–110 mmol/l
Potassium: 0–1 mmol/l
Calcium: 1.5–1.75 mmol/l
Magnesium: 0.5–0.85 mmol/l
Chloride: 65–75 mmol/l
Acetate: 35–45 mmol/l
Dextrose monohydrate: 0–10.1 mmol/l (0–200 mg/dl).

Moreover, the correct cartridge 'size' either with normal or with 'high' urea capacity should be selected.

As explained earlier because of the 1:6 to 7 relationship of the dialysate volume to the patient's total body water and also because of the low dialysate flow (45) the impact of the dialysis fluid on the patient's body fluid composition is much less than in conventional 500 ml/min single pass dialysis. Nevertheless pre- and post-dialysis plasma and dialysate analyses should be undertaken in patients not yet stabilised on treatment with the Redy system.

An adult patient can commence dialysis after a 30 min equilibration following insertion of the cartridge,[4] when the sodium in the dialysis fluid is usually 115 to 120 mmol/l. A small or paediatric patient should not commence dialysis until the sodium concentration reaches 125 mmol/l. The conductivity meter can be used to estimate the sodium concentration in the dialysis fluid (115 to 120 mmol Na/l = 11 to 11.5 mMhos readings on the meter).

The conductivity meter should, however, be properly calibrated.

If hard water is used for preparation of dialysis fluid, the calcium in the initial fluid placed in the reservoir should be either omitted or much reduced.

Calcium, magnesium and potassium kinetics

Calcium and magnesium ions are completely removed by the cartridge from the dialysis fluid. Therefore, they must be added continuously. The manufacturer supplies Ca and Mg as acetate salts in the appropriate amounts as dry powder with each cartridge (Sorb 10 pack). This is dissolved in warm water to the graduated 300 ml mark in a suitable container. This solution is infused into the dialysate at a rate of 19.6 mmol Ca plus 6.5 mmol Mg (and 52.2 mmol of acetate) per hour with the calibrated infusion pump.

Attention should be paid to maintaining the correct dialysate flow rate of 250 ml/min for which the infusate pump has been calibrated, in order to maintain the correct Ca and Mg concentrations of 1.5 mmol/l (6 mg/dl) and 0.5 mmol/l (1.2 mg/dl) respectively. Obviously, it is possible to alter the calcium and magnesium concentrations in the dialysate by varying the infusate concentrations. Potassium is also completely removed from the dialysis fluid and, if potassium-free dialysate is undesirable for a particular patient, potassium acetate should also be added via the infusate system. For this purpose commercially prepared packages are available containing the correct amount of potassium acetate to increase dialysate potassium concentration in increments of 1 mmol/l.

---

4. To reduce the dialysis fluid aluminium content to safe levels (see further) a minimal equilibration time of 30 min is indicated (see p 432).

Acetate kinetics and correction of metabolic acidosis

In conventional dialysis correction of acidosis occurs by metabolic conversion of acetate into bicarbonate (60). Several clinical investigators noted incomplete correction of metabolic acidosis in patients treated with the Redy system with the old type cartridges containing chloride loaded ZO (52, 54, 55, 61). This was particularly obvious in so called 'short dialysis' when large ($2 m^2$) surface area dialysers were used (54). Various explanations have been presented (55).

In the Redy system with the present D3160 or D3260 cartridges containing acetate loaded hydrous ZO about 100 mmol of acetate is exchanged for phosphate. In the 6 l dialysis fluid with an initial sodium concentration of 105 to 110 mmol/l and 25 to 30 mmol acetate/l some 150 to 180 mmol acetate become available to the patient during a 4 h Redy dialysis.

Finally the infusion of the acetate salts of Ca and Mg adds an additional 209 mmol of acetate in a 4 h dialysis. This totals 360 to 390 mmol of acetate available to the patient during a 4 h dialysis with the Redy machine.

During an entire 4 h Redy dialysis the patient is exposed to some 460 to 490 mmol of acetate.

In contrast in a single 4 h haemodialysis with a standard single pass system 120 l dialysis fluid containing 35 mmol/l acetate traverse the dialyser, exposing the patient to 4200 mmol acetate, nine times more than in a Redy dialysis.

On the other hand the enzymatic conversion of urea generates bicarbonate and during a 4 h dialysis of an average adult patient the cartridge delivers some 150 mmol bicarbonate to the dialysis fluid.

In addition during dialysis with a bicarbonate free dialysis fluid, such as in a single pass system (with acetate) and in the early stage of Redy dialysis the patient loses bicarbonate which goes to the drain.

In the recirculating Redy system no bicarbonate is lost to drain: most of the bicarbonate, initially dialysed out of the patient and produced by the cartridge remains in the dialysate and remains available to the patient.

It has to be expected that with the present 'acetate loaded' D3160 and D3260 cartridges a satisfactory correction of the metabolic acidosis in the uraemic patient is obtained.

On the other hand it is now generally accepted that an excess acetate load during conventional dialysis may cause dialysis associated problems and side effects, such as vascular instability with hypotension and post-dialysis hangover (see chapter 8).

The pre-dialysis plasma bicarbonate values achieved with the acetate loaded cartridges seem to be comparable to those achieved with standard single pass dialysis techniques (62).

The Redy system in patients with normal or low plasma urea concentration

As discussed earlier an unexpectedly low urea load or a cartridge with an unsuitable high urea binding capacity may cause persistence or aggravation of metabolic acidosis. Unless sufficient urea enters the cartridge, it adsorbs dialysate sodium and severe hyponatraemia and acidosis may develop, the concentration of chloride in the dialysate remaining unaltered. Obviously the Redy system should not be used with the standard cartridges (containing urease) in patients with normal or only marginally raised plasma urea (e.g. in cases of drug overdose).

For (haemoperfusion) treatment of patients who have taken an overdose of a dialysable poison that is adsorbed by charcoal, a special sorbent cartridge (type D13) is available, containing activated carbon only. (This system is, however, not as efficient as a standard haemoperfusion system, without a dialyser).

Long-term treatment with the Redy system

The Redy system was commercially introduced in 1972. Until recently, only a few reports have been published on the results of long-term treatment, in particular compared with treatment with conventional dialysis systems (55, 57, 63–65).

In the earlier years with the 'chloride loaded' cartridges an incomplete correction of metabolic acidosis was noted. Since the introduction of 'acetate loaded' cartridges (i.e. with the acetate form of hydrous zirconium) predialysis serum bicarbonate values have been comparable to those achieved with standard single pass dialysis techniques (66).

In a retrospective study Odell and coworkers (66) compared 24 patients dialysed with the Redy system for longer than 4 years with a group of age matched controls treated by conventional single-pass haemodialysis. Both groups had identical electrolyte, urea and creatinine profiles.

Mean systolic blood pressure readings were slightly higher in the Redy patients, diastolic readings, however, were somewhat lower.

Hospitalisation data indicated no major difference.

Of the measured parameters only serum alkaline phosphatase values were significantly higher in the Redy patients, a finding which was also reported by Whalen et al (67), who found elevated serum alkaline phosphatase values in 12 of 19 patients after being treated with the Redy system for 12 months or longer with peak values after 2 years. All patients responded to therapy with vitamin D derivatives and the authors concluded that their findings indicated early renal osteodystrophy, which might have eventually caused symptoms and radiographic abnormalities had the patients been left untreated with a vitamin D metabolite for a longer time.

It has been suggested (46) that as the sorbent cartridge does not remove sulphate (47) elevated plasma concentrations of sulphate (twice as high as in single pass dialysis patients) could have played a role in bone metabolism.

Prevention of ammonia 'break through'

In chronic long-term patients sometimes an unusual high blood urea level may be anticipated, for example when the patient reports a dietary indiscretion with an unusual high protein intake or during an intercurrent febrile complication and temporarily increased protein catabolism. An episode of ammonia 'break through' may then be prevented by a rapid predialysis blood urea test and selection of a high capacity sorbent cartridge.

Alternatively if an unusual high blood urea is suspected, repeated ammonia testing of the cartridge effluent in the third and fourth hour of dialysis is indicated.

If the test becomes positive the dialysis should be terminated and repeated the following day.

Insertion of a fresh cartridge has to be discouraged because of the initial release of aluminium.

Choice of the Redy system

Reasons for choice of the Redy system have mostly arisen from the disadvantages of using a conventional single pass system, requiring formal installation for regular dialysis at home (68). The use of a portable system solved the delay and problems of adapting or extending the house or even rehousing the family (69).

Some factors influencing the choice of the system have now altered: continuous ambulatory peritoneal dialysis (CAPD) has become an important alternative therapy (see also chapters 22, 24 and 25).

Cost of treatment with the Redy system exceeds that with conventional systems, because of the cost of cartridges (61, 69) but this is balanced by savings made on home adaptations and by reducing time on hospital haemodialysis. (The extra cost of Redy home dialysis for 2 years has proved equivalent to the price of one of the more expensive home conversions or the cost difference between 6 months hospital dialysis as opposed to 6 months conventional home dialysis [69]).

The greatest advantage is the mobility of the equipment as dialysis can be performed without being in the immediate vicinity of either a water tap or (and) a drain.

The system makes travelling for holiday and business purposes possible. It has been used for dialysis in hotels, in a caravan, on camping sites and even in a sailing boat (65), and while sunbathing on the beach. If necessary the Redy can be operated from a small electric power generator driven by a petrol engine.

Airlines have agreed to accept the monitor without freight charge and in many countries the required rather bulky disposables can be obtained through the manufacturers' local representatives.

These advantages of the Redy system have been largely fading away after the introduction and rapid evolution of the simple 'machine free' ambulatory method for replacement of renal function, i.e. CAPD (see chapters 22, 24, 25) in 1976–1978 (4, 70).

Undesired side effects or unexpected complications with the Redy system

The suitability of the Redy system, in particular for long-

term haemodialysis treatment has often been questioned (66), but irrespective of brief and rapidly reversible episodes of acute ammonia intoxication undesirable acute or chronic side effects have only rarely been reported.

Unexplained weakness

Gault and coworkers (71) described a syndrome of progressive fatigue, incapacitating weakness, vomiting and loss of weight in two patients after 15 and 32 months on Redy dialysis, respectively.

After institution of conventional single pass (acetate) dialysis improvement was rapid and dramatic; the pathogenesis of this unusual syndrome remains unexplained.

Unexpected metabolic acidosis in Redy bicarbonate dialysis

Brozis and Brown (72) observed severe metabolic acidosis in a patient with end stage renal disease and an intercurrent upper respiratory tract infection during Redy dialysis in the bicarbonate mode. It was shown that dialysate bicarbonate during dialysis had dropped from the initial 60 mmol/l to 15 mmol/l.

The authors measured bicarbonate values in blood and dialysis fluid in an additional five chronic patients during 15 bicarbonate dialyses with the Redy system, using the 'acetate' loaded 31 type sorbent cartridge and the Ca/Mg/K infusate with the chloride anion instead of acetate. The bicarbonate concentration in the dialysate was noted to be quite low and variable (mean $16.5 +/- 8.3$ mmol/l, instead of the original 60 mmol/l). The low dialysate bicarbonate values failed to correct and often even worsened the metabolic acidosis of the patients.

Obviously the release of protons from the ZP layer of the regeneration cartridge and the consequent pH decrease of the dialysis fluid caused a considerable loss of bicarbonate during the first 30 (or 60) minutes of recirculation and a further bicarbonate loss occurred during the actual clinical dialysis.

Because the Redy system was used with the infusate in the chloride mode the patients were deprived of a certain amount of acetate, which could have contributed to the correction of their metabolic acidosis. A calcium/magnesium/potassium acetate infusate would have supplied some 480 mmol acetate during a 5 h Redy dialysis (73), not enough to correct acidosis fully, but better than nothing.

In addition it should be appreciated that with the Redy system the loss of bicarbonate from the dialysis fluid will be more or less proportional to the amount of urea removed from the patient. The more urea enters the cartridge, the more protons will be released (74).

Unexpected respiratory acidosis

As described above the blood leaving the dialyser of the Redy system has a high pCO_2 (and a low pH) because CO_2 is generated from bicarbonate in the cartridge (see Figure 11) and also in the dialysate reservoir.

This hypercapnic blood rapidly mixes with the patient's circulating blood when leaving the dialyser, pH being buffered and CO_2 being lost with the expired air.

However, in patients with pulmonary diseases such as chronic emphysema and (asthmatic) bronchitis and in those who are mechanically ventilated, a limited excretion of the CO_2 generated in the Redy circuit may in extreme situations be responsible for a respiratory acidosis, for instance because of a mismatch between the high pCO_2 produced in the dialyser and the fixed mechanical ventilation as in the case of Hamm and coworkers (75). This phenomenon will be rare in patients treated with the Redy in the acetate mode, but there may be an increased risk with bicarbonate dialysis, which obviously enhances production and release of greater volumes of CO_2. Obviously efficient degassing would help to solve this, but the manufacturers have so far not provided the machine with a simple and efficient degassing device (see page 426 and 427, Figure 12).

What NOT to do

It needs no explaining that the unusual properties of the Redy system with its continuously changing composition and pH of the dialysis fluid, willy-nilly at the beginning and at the end of a dialysis session beyond physiological limits, and its excessive production of CO_2 makes a profound study of the system mandatory.

The risk of undesired even dangerous side effects such as metabolic acidosis or insufficient correction of metabolic acidosis (72), the occurrence of respiratory acidosis (75) and other electrolyte or acid-base abnormalities or both requires in acute, non adapted uraemic patients careful planning of each dialysis and also in chronic, well adapted patients should acute intercurrent complications occur.

The use of the Redy system for bicarbonate dialysis with an initial concentration of 135 mmol sodium bicarbonate (72, 76) should certainly be disouraged; 60 mmol added immediately before the beginning of dialysis is enough (77).

Bicarbonate dialysis requires a 3160 or 3260 type 'aluminium poor' cartridge, but is not recommended (see further). The use of a dialysis machine (Redy or not) in hospitals without dialysis facilities (61) and with a staff without adequate dialysis training and experience should be likewise strongly dissuaded.

THE REDY SYSTEM IN ACUTE RENAL FAILURE AND IN PATIENTS WITH GROSS ELECTROLYTE ABNORMALITIES

Sodium gradient

In a 4 h conventional single pass dialysis some 120 l of dialysis fluid perfuses the dialyser at 500 ml/min. In a patient with a plasma sodium concentration within normal limits an initial dialysis fluid sodium of 100 mmol/l (as used in the Redy system) would be dangerous even deleterious to the patient in a single pass system. On the other hand an initial dialysis fluid Na 120 mmol/l matched with the patient, for example in a case of acute renal failure, increasing during dialysis with the Redy system to 155 mmol/l or more at the end of dialysis, would also be dangerous indeed.

Correction of sodium abnormalities (both hypo- and hypernatraemia) should be gradual to avoid transcellular fluid shifts and neurologic complications or worsening of neurologic symptoms (78–82). Specific correction of asymptomatic hyponatraemia is often unnecessary and occasionally hazardous (82). It has therefore always been a good thumb rule to equilibrate dialysis fluid sodium concentration in cases of acute renal failure or in new, not yet adapted patients with chronic renal failure to the patient's plasma sodium level and to avoid Na gradients and transcellular fluid shifts during dialysis. With the Redy system this is obviously impossible: the diffusion of Na will vary with the changing sodium concentration in the dialysis fluid and the continuously varying Na gradient.

Nevertheless mismatched sodium concentrations with the Redy system are much less dangerous than in a conventional single pass system, because of the small dialysis fluid volume (and the low dialysate flow rate).

A built in safeguard

A 4 h conventional single pass dialysis exposes the patient to some 120 l dialysis fluid that pass the dialyser with a flow rate of 500 ml/min.

Exchange of electrolytes occurs along a concentration gradient between the dialysis fluid and the extracellular fluid of the patient, which osmotically equilibrates with total body water.

The ratio between the 120 l volume of dialysis fluid and the patient's total body water depends on body weight and sex and may be anywhere between 2 and 4:1. Obviously the dialysis fluid 'dominates' the patient.

In Redy dialysis the volume relationship is reversed and varies from 1:4.7 in a small woman to 1:9 in a large man. Volumetrically the patient 'dominates' the dialysis system. This is more or less a 'built in safeguard' of the regeneration system.

For example: a 7 mmol increase of dialysate sodium in the Redy causes only a 1 mmol increase in the 42 l body fluid of a standard 70 kg male dialysis patient.

The choice of the dialysis system

The choice to dialyse a patient in acute renal failure (often critically ill and with multiple organ system failure) with either a conventional single pass machine or a Redy system depends on personal experience and preference. It is clear that the doctor in charge should be perfectly acquainted with the system he is going to use and should also be perfectly familiar with the clinical condition of the patient and his pathophysiology.

A careful planning and detailed lay-out of the renal function replacement therapy, e.g. dialysis or haemofiltration, the type of machine, the composition of the dialysis fluid, the heparinisation, the monitoring systems required and the duration of dialysis are essential.

The responsible physician(s) should personally attend the entire procedure.

Presently in many dialysis centres patients in acute renal failure are preferably treated with haemofiltration in particular with continuous arterial-venous haemofiltration (CAVH, see chapter 15).

TOXICOLOGY OF THE REDY SYSTEM

Zirconium

Toxicology studies have been performed by Møller et al (83). Their primary concern was a potential toxicity of zirconium, which as they indicated is an essential human trace metal. Using emission spectrochemical analysis they found in a series of Redy dialysate samples, values far below normal serum values. Other trace elements analysed (copper, silicon, aluminium) gave similar results. Only boron levels appeared to be three times normal, which the investigators explained either by high plasma boron levels in uraemic patients or by release from the cartridge. Boron seems to be toxic to man, but the Danish investigators concluded that the Redy system carried no obvious toxicological risk.

Møller and coworkers, using formaldehyde as a sterilising agent found however 'alarmingly high' formaldehyde concentrations, even after an extra (third) rinse of the system, when the Clinitest check (which is notoriously insensitive) was negative. This, however, is obviously not a specific Redy problem: many dialysis systems presently in use are disinfected with formaldehyde (see also chapters 12 and 18 for formaldehyde toxicity), and may present a similar problem.

Aluminium

It should be emphasised that Møller and his colleagues (83) did study the early release of aluminium from the cartridge (see following pages) but their flame emission analysis had a sensitivity limit of $100 \mu g/l$ ($3.7 \mu mol/l$), obviously far too insensitive for measuring Al in dialysate and biological fluids, which require a minimal sensitivity of $5 \mu g/l$ ($0.18 \mu mol/l$). It is now appreciated that flameless spectrophotometric analysis[5] using a high temperature graphite furnace, is required to measure low concentrations of aluminium (14).

Chronic aluminium intoxication

Aluminium transfer from the dialysis fluid into the patient by reverse dialysis is the main causative factor of chronic aluminium intoxication in dialysis patients, resulting in dialysis encephalopathy (84–86) and fracturing osteomalacia (so called Newcastle bone disease), which responds poorly or

---

5. Inductively Coupled Plasma (ICP) emission spectrometry seems to be a promising new analytical technique (84).

---

not at all to vitamin D derivates (87, 88), see also chapters 3 and 50.

Oral aluminium containing phosphate binders, routinely administered to dialysis patients, contribute to the aluminium load of the patients and the safety of these compounds is at least questionable (89–91).

It was initially not generally known that the Redy cartridges contained in addition to the active reactants considerable amounts of aluminium oxide (Al_2O_3), which until the mid seventies was considered an inert non reactive, non toxic and harmless filling and binding substance for the active compounds in the cartridge (27, 28, 92).

In addition activated carbon, which forms the top layer of the cartridge (see Figures 7 and 8) is commonly contaminated with substantial amounts of aluminium oxide (AWJ Van Doorn, unpublished data).

Obviously leakage of Al from the cartridge into the recirculating dialysate seemed a potential hazard of the system for chronic dialysis patients.

Kinetics and dialysability of aluminium

Conflicting and confusing opinions concerning solubility and dialysability of aluminium ions have been reported (93–97), but confusion was clarified by a Seattle group of investigators (98).

It was demonstrated that both solubility and dialysability of aluminium ions are strongly pH dependent; aluminium solubility and (reverse) clearances appeared negligible at pH values ranging from 6.5 to 7.6, but increased dramatically at pH below 6.5 and above 7.6.

Initial dialysis fluid pH clearly depends on the pH of the water used for preparation, however, pH decreases during dialysis for reasons explained earlier, rising again towards the end of the dialysis (see Figure 9). Apparently the risk of substantial leakage of Al from the cartridge and reverse dialysis into the patients seems to be small as long as dialysate pH fluctuates between 6.5 and 7.6 (98).

Release and removal of aluminium ions by the Redy cartridge

The cartridge with its large amounts of Al potentially not only releases Al but the cation exchange (ZP) layer also removes aluminium ions, exchanging them for protons and sodium ions. Consequently Al released from the urease layer will be bound in the zirconium phosphate layer but Al leaked from the top layer will enter the dialysis fluid. It will be removed by the ZP layer during recirculation.

A toxic 'bomb'

The original aluminium oxide loaded cartridges, however, resembled a potential toxic 'bomb' for chronic dialysis patients in particular when dialysate pH deviated from the limits of 6.5 to 7.6.

This was soon confirmed by Shaldon (27, 28), who reported in 1978 and 1979 that aluminium was leaking from the cartridge in large quantities after rinsing with a weak

(1/6 molar = 0.2%) bicarbonate solution. (In these investigations the old [presently outdated] chloride and aluminium oxide loaded D11 cartridge was used).

Subsequently Branger and associates (99) confirming Shaldon's observations, demonstrated not only a 'significant' release of Al from the cartridge after bicarbonate rinsing, but also a substantial transfer of Al across the dialyser membrane in simulated (*in vitro*) dialyses.

Shortly afterwards several cases of dialysis dementia and dialysis osteomalacia were reported from the USA and France (92, 99).

Case reports of chronic aluminium intoxication in Redy patients

In 1981 Pierides and Frohnert (92) reported on six patients from the Mayo Clinic, Rochester, MN with endstage renal failure who were dialysed with the Redy system for periods of 18 to 34 months and who developed symptoms of dialysis encephalopathy and osteomalacia with pathological fractures.

This was the first report on aluminium intoxication in patients dialysed with the Redy system. No details were given by Pierides and Frohnert on the administration of oral aluminium containing phosphate binders and on previous dialysis treatment with other systems.

Several years later (1984) Pierides and Myli (100) reported on two additional cases who developed fatal dialysis dementia. Ultimately, six out of eight of their patients had died.

Several patients underwent bone biopsies, which were analysed for Al which appeared very high (135 to 160 mg/kg, normal in the authors' unit <10 mg/kg).

Mion and associates (101) observed three cases of fracturing osteomalacia with very high bone Al values after being treated with regular haemofiltration for 15 to 20 months, the haemofiltrate being regenerated by passage via a bicarbonate rinsed Redy cartridge and reinfused into the patient.

'Safe' dialysis fluid aluminium levels

Safe levels of Al in dialysis fluid cannot be given: according to Graf and coworkers (102) the 'ideal' dialysis fluid should contain less than $5.4 \mu g/l$ ($0.2 \mu mol/l$), which, however, is often difficult to obtain, in particular with the Redy system.

The maximum permissable Al concentration in dialysis fluid was in Europe more or less arbitrarily set for $50 \mu g/l$ (50 ppb or $1.9 \mu mol/l$), which was later no longer considered being 'safe'.

In April 1982 the British Department of Health and Social Security recommended an upper level of $30 \mu g/l$ for the Redy system (102) but in the same year the upper limit for Europe was set at 10 to $15 \mu g/l$ (0.37 to $0.56 \mu mol/l$) (96).

The maximum permissable limit in the USA has been set to $10 \mu g/l$ ($0.37 \mu mol/l$).

Dialysis fluid aluminium concentrations with the Redy system

Several groups of investigators studied aluminium levels in the dialysate of the Redy system (95, 98–100, 102–108), both with regular acetate loaded dialysis fluid and with bicarbonate dialysate and with the (old) D31 cartridge and the more recent D3160 and D3260 cartridges.

As mentioned above the originally designed Redy cartridges, either with chloride loaded zirconium oxide (D11, D41, D42) or with acetate loaded ZO (D31, D32, D3150 and D3250), were stabilised with large amounts of alumina (aluminium oxide), both as filling substance and as binding compound for urease.

Later in the early 1980's, when it was learned that substantial amounts of Al leaked from the cartridges in particular when rinsed with bicarbonate solution or when bicarbonate dialysis fluid was used or both and that several long term Redy patients developed fatal aluminium toxicity of the brain and aluminium osteomalacia, the manufacturers developed the D3160 and D3260 cartridges. The aluminium oxide content of these cartridges has been substantially reduced by removing all except that specifically indispensable for binding urease.

The geometry of this improved cartridge is somewhat different from the previous models.

Glass beads are used in the zirconium oxide layer and a polystyrene spacer is used below the urease layer instead of the aluminium oxide in previous models (103).

This filling compound was omitted from all layers above the urease and in addition a different type of activated carbon, less contaminated with aluminium, was used in the top layer. It was expected that Al released from the urease layer was bound in the ZP layer and that any Al that leaked from the top (carbon) layer, was bound in the 'scavenger' layer and the zirconium phosphate during recirculation.

The D3160 and 3260 cartridges became available in 1982.

Dialysate aluminium concentration with the old, aluminium loaded cartridges

Pierides and Frohnert (92) performed perfusion studies with the old D31 cartridges and with acetate containing dialysis fluid and observed a variable but 'highly significant' release of Al from all cartridges. The majority of the tested cartridges released most of the aluminium during the first hour of perfusion. Some cartridges continued to leak and Al values below $50 \mu g/l$ ($1.9 \mu mol/l$) were only obtained after recirculating the dialysate for 90 to 120 min and some continued to leak substantial quantities, even throughout the full 4 h of the test.

In addition it went out that aluminium released from some cartridges readily diffused across the Cuprophane membrane into the blood compartment in appreciable quantities.

Similar results were obtained by Van Doorn (93), who studied also aluminium release from the D31 cartridge with acetate dialysis fluid, both *in vitro* and *in vivo*.

Branger and associates (99) used both bicarbonate and

acetate loaded dialysis fluid for their *in vitro* recirculation studies with the D41 and D31 cartridges. The leakage with bicarbonate dialysate was enormous, rising to $1153 \pm 90\,\mu g/l$ within 20 min and slowly falling to $174 \pm 40\,\mu g/l$ at 60 min of recirculation (still 6 times too high).

The highest value with acetate was $38 \pm 5\,\mu g/l$ ($1.41 \pm 0.19\,\mu mol/l$) at 20 min, being $7 \pm 7\,\mu g/l$ ($0.26 \pm 0.26\,\mu mol/l$) at 60 min.

There was also considerable transfer of Al across the cellulose acetate membrane during *in vitro* dialysis.

The obvious comment of the authors was 'it seems preferable to avoid bicarbonate dialysis with the Redy system in maintenance haemodialysis. Total elimination of Al_2O_3 from the Redy sorbent cartridge should resolve this important problem' (99).

Aluminium kinetics with the 'aluminium poor' D3160 (and D3260) cartridges

Several groups studied aluminium kinetics with the D3160 and 3260 cartridges both *in vitro* and *in vivo* (103–107).

Divergent, even conflicting results have been reported, probably because of different experimental designs and perhaps less accurate Al analytical technology.

Odell et al (104) analysed Al release from the D3160 *in vitro* with an acetate 'dialysate' test solution and pH values ranging from 6.26 to 6.46: the cartridge initially released some Al (25 to 29 μg [1 $\mu mol/l$]), which rapidly decreased in 30 min to 'safe' values (5.8 to 6.8 μg [0.22 to 0.25 $\mu mol/l$]).[6]

In vivo three different dialysis fluid formulations were tested with 27.5 mmol acetate, 60 mmol bicarbonate and 135 mmol bicarbonate, all containing 20 μg (0.74 μmol) Al/l in the original bath. The D3160 reduced this concentration to less than 10 μg (0.37 μmol)/l within 30 min with each dialysate.

Culpepper and coworkers (105) compared the old fully Al loaded D3250 and the D3160 both *in vitro* and *in vivo* using acetate dialysis fluid and found similar results: the D3160 initially released a peak of aluminium and within 15 to 20 min the concentration decreased to 0.5 $\mu g/l$.

In vivo somewhat higher values were noted, Al in the dialysis reservoir rising slowly to 27 μg (1 μmol)/l.

The old 3250 cartridge yielded inadmissable high aluminium figures with net uptake by the patient in the fourth and fifth hours of dialysis.

Shapiro and associates (106) obtained in the haemofiltration setting very low figures with the D3160 cartridge both *in vitro* (Al averages in the cartridge effluent 4 to 6 μg [0.15 to 0.22 $\mu mol/l$]) and *in vivo* (dog) Al averages of 3.5 to 8.0 μg [0.13 to 0.30 $\mu mol/l$]).

Mion's group from Montpellier, France (107) studied aluminium release from the modified, so called 'aluminium poor' D3160 cartridge with bicarbonate dialysis fluid both *in vitro* and *in vivo*. They found a minimal aluminium release,

---

6. 'Safe' levels of aluminium: in England (DHSS): $\leqslant 30\,\mu g = 1.11\,\mu mol/l$. In the USA (AAMI/ASAIO) $\leqslant 10\,\mu g = 0.37\,\mu mol/l$.

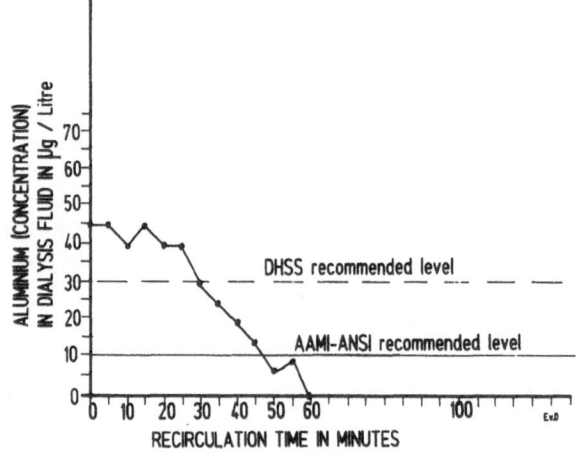

Figure 13. Aluminium analyses of the reservoir dialysate with the D3160 cartridge. The additive to the test 'dialysate' was 50 μg ($= 1.85\,\mu mol$)/l aluminium. Data derived from Drury et al (103 [1986]. With permission.

despite a priming bath solution with relatively high pH values (7.70 ± 0.06).

Aluminium concentrations in the dialysate outflow from the cartridge remained in or below the 10 μg (0.37 $\mu mol/l$) range, with a few exceptions (of 12 to 19 [0.44 to 0.70 μmol]/l), concentrations remaining 5 to 10 times lower than those reported by Branger et al (99) in 1980 with the (old) D41 cartridge.

Nevertheless the authors concluded that the persistent release of Al even in low concentrations by the D3160 cartridge should be considered a risk factor in patients on long-term treatment with Redy cartridges.

They strongly recommended also replacing aluminium oxide in the urease layer by aluminium-free material.

Drury et al (103) assessed the ability of the D3160 and 3260 cartridges to remove Al from the dialysis fluid prepared with aluminium free (reverse osmosis) water and provided with Al in different concentrations (0, 50, 200 and 1000 μg/l). Possible release by the cartridge itself was also examined.

These studies were carried out with and without the manufacturers pretreatment protocol.

The results of these carefully designed investigations contradicted those of Culpepper: without pretreatment substantial amounts of aluminium leaked initially from the cartridges, ranging between 550 and 1800 μg (20 and 67 μmol)/l. When the recommended pretreatment procedure was carried out some cartridges still produced inadmissible levels of aluminium (40 to 150 μg [1.48 to 5.6 μmol]/l) at the start of dialysis. An additional 45 to 60 min of recirculation were required to reach the 'safe' British level of less than 30 $\mu g/l$ and another 20 min to reach the American upper limit of 10 $\mu g/l$ (see Figures 13 and 14). Is should be mentioned that a preparation period of 60 min causes a loss of 1.5 g urea capacity of the cartridges.

Finally VanDeVijver and associates (108) compared 15

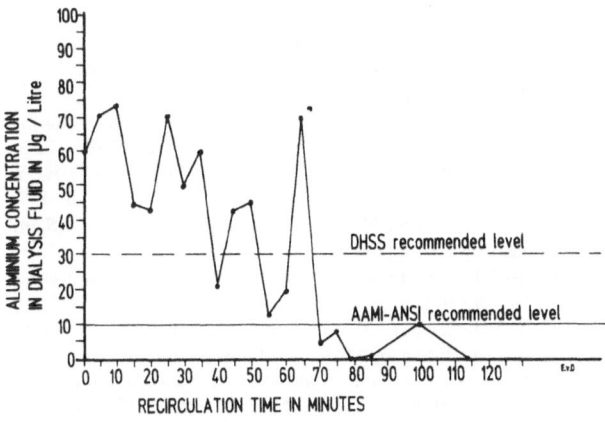

Figure 14. Aluminium analyses of the reservoir fluid with the D3260 Redy cartridge. The test 'dialysate' was 'spiked' with $50\,\mu g$ ($1.85\,\mu mol$)/l aluminium. Data derived from Drury et al (103 [1986]). With permission.

long-term Redy patients with 15 single pass dialysis patients. Because both groups were treated in different centres and the Redy group was dialysed with special precautions they were not comparable. In both groups pathologic fractures occurred and bone Al was increased in several patients in both groups ($>20\,\mu g/g$). Their results remained inconclusive.

SUMMARY

1. The 'heart' of the Redy (Sorb-) system is the cartridge which regenerates spent dialysate by enzymatic decomposition of urea, cation exchange in the zirconium phosphate layer and anion exchange in the zirconium oxide layer. Creatinine, uric acid, phenols and other waste metabolites are adsorbed in an activated carbon layer.

2. Sodium concentration and pH in the regenerated dialysate change continuously during dialysis, because sodium ions and protons are released by the cartridge in exchange for ammonium ions produced from urea.

3. Potassium ions and divalent cations (calcium, magnesium) are also exchanged for sodium and H^+ ions and must be continuously added to the dialysate from a potassium/calcium/magnesium acetate solution by a small metering pump.

4. Regenerated dialysate has a high pCO_2 because CO_2 is produced from bicarbonate originating both from urea degradation and from plasma bicarbonate reacting with protons released by the zirconium phosphate layer in exchange for ammonium ions also produced from the decomposition of urea.

5. Since its introduction in 1972 ample evidence has shown that blood chemistry and clinical parameters in long-term Redy patients are comparable with those from chronic dialysis patients treated with conventional single pass dialysis.

6. Redy dialysis requires careful study of the specific properties and the chemistry of the system to avoid compli-

cations and side effects which are inherent in its unusual characteristics (104).

7. Originally aluminium oxide was used as a filling and binding substance in the cartridge and cases of often fatal chronic aluminium intoxication (dialysis encephalopathy and vitamin D resistant osteomalacia) have been observed.

8. From the new model cartridges (D3160 and 3260, marketed in 1982) aluminium oxide has been largely removed except from the urease layer, where it apparently is required as a 'carrier' and binder of urease.

9. According to several investigators the D3160 and 3260 leak considerably less aluminium. Aluminium levels with acetate 'loaded' dialysate remain below the maximum permissible level in England ($30\,\mu g$ [$1.1\,\mu mol$]/l) and usually even below $10\,\mu g/l$ ($0.37\,\mu mol/l$) as required in the USA.

10. With bicarbonate loaded dialysate solubility of aluminium increases and release from the cartridge may be substantial higher, exceeding permissible levels. Bicarbonate dialysis with the Redy system is discouraged.

11. Because of conflicting opinions and divergent data from the current literature on aluminium release from the D3160 and 3260 cartridges (both with acetate and bicarbonate dialysate) more carefully designed investigations with accurate aluminium analyses and long-term follow-up of chronic 'Redy' patients are required (107) with regular aluminium analyses of the dialysis fluid and, if possible, of bone biopsies.

12. Wherever regular dialysis with the Redy system is considered, the final comment of Branger and associates (99) is stil valid: 'It seems preferable to avoid bicarbonate dialysis with the Redy system in maintenance haemodialysis. Total elimination of Al_2O_3 from the Redy sorbent cartridge should resolve potentially dangerous aluminium problems.'

13. Redy dialysis is more expensive than conventional single pass haemodialysis and CAPD because of the cost of the cartridge. On the other hand in the home dialysis setting, special plumbing and special drainage facilities are not required.

14. For travelling (65, 110) Redy dialysis has been superseded by CAPD.

SPECIAL RECOMMENDATIONS (108):

1. Either in the hospital or in the home setting an analysis of the drinking water to be used for preparation of dialysis for the Redy apparatus is required. If aluminium content or hardness is substantial, pretreatment (with reverse osmosis) is required.

2. To obtain a safe aluminium level in the dialysate special precautions are indicated:
a. discard the first cartridge efluent (during 5 min)
b. a recirculation period of 60 min is recommended before patient contact
c. this causes a loss of 1.5 g or urea capacity of the cartridge.

3. Once again:
a. Exclusively acetate dialysis should be used and never

bicarbonate dialysis, until aluminium oxide is totally removed from the cartridge.

b. The Redy cartridge should *not* be used for regeneration of haemofiltrate.

ACKNOWLEDGMENTS

The authors are indebted to Mr. David Suk of Organon Teknika Corporation, Turnhout, Belgium, who made the photographs available of the newest model of the Redy 2000 system (Figures 4, 5, 7 and 8a).

Figures 3, 6, 8b, 12, 13 and 14 were prepared (and partially revised) by Mr. Emile Van Doorn, Arnhem, The Netherlands.

REFERENCES

1. Stephen RL, Jacobson SC, Atkin-Thor E, Kolff WJ: Portable/wearable artificial kidney (WAK) – initial evaluation. *Proc Eur Dial Transplant Assoc* 12: 511, 1975

2. Briefel GR, Hutchisson JT, Galonsky RS, Hessert RL, Friedman EA: Compact travel hemodialysis system. *Proc Clin Dial Transplant Forum* 5: 61, 1975

3. Gordon A, Greenbaum MA, Marantz LB, McArthur MJ, Maxwell MH: A sorbent-based low volume dialysate system. *Trans Am Soc Artif Intern Organs* 15: 347, 1969

4. Popovich RP, Moncrief JW, Decherd JB, Bomar JB, Pyle WK: The definition of a novel portable/wearable equilibrium peritoneal dialysis technique. *Abstracts Am Soc Artif Intern Organs* 5: 64. 1976

5. Nolph KD: The status of continuous ambulatory peritoneal dialysis. *Int J Artif Organs* 3: 235, 1980

6. Blaney TL, Lindan O, Sparks RE: Adsorption: a step forwards to a wearable artificial kidney. *Trans Am Soc Artif Intern Organs* 12: 7, 1966

7. Jutzler GA, Keller HE, Klein J, Carius J, Floss K, Dijckmans J, Fürsattel L, Leppla W: Physico-chemical investigations in regeneration of the dialysis fluid. *Proc Eur Dial Transplant Assoc* 3: 265, 1966

8. Twiss EE, Paulsen MMP: Dialysis-system incorporating the use of activated carbon. *Proc Eur Dial Transplant Assoc* 3: 262, 1966

9. Van Leer E: *Hemodialyse met koolstof adsorptie.* (Haemodialysis with carbon adsorption). MD Thesis 1970 University of Rotterdam, the Netherlands. Rotterdam, Bronder-Offset N.V., 1970 (in Dutch)

10. Kolobow T, Dedrick RL: Dialysate capacity augmentation with activated carbon slurry. *Proc Eur Dial Transplant Assoc* 3: 375, 1966

11. Burton BT: Overview of blood purification in uremia. *Int J Artif Organs* 3: 204, 1980

12. Smakman R, van Doorn AWJ: Urea removal by means of direct binding. *Clin Nephrol* 26 (Suppl 1): S58, 1986

13. Maeda K, Kawaguchi S, Manji T, Kobayashi K, Ohta K, Saito A, Shimoji T, Yui T, Hori M: Portable artifical kidney system with adsorbents. *Proc Eur Dial Transplant Assoc* 10: 298, 1973

14. Fuchs C, Brasche M, Paschev K, Nordbeck H, Quellhorst E: Aluminium-Bestimmung in Serum mit flammenloser Atomabsorption. (Determination of aluminium in serum with flameless atomic absorption). *Clin Chim Acta* 52: 71, 1974 (in German)

15. Maeda K, Kawaguchi S, Shimizu K, Manji T, Kobayashi K, Ohta K, Saito A, Amano I, Yoshiyama N, Nakagawa S, Koshikawa S: Ten-litre dialysate supply system with adsorbents. *Proc Eur Dial Transplant Assoc* 11: 180, 1974

16. Petrella E, Orlandini GC, Bigi L: Regeneration of dialysis fluid. *Proc Eur Dial Transplant Assoc* 11: 173, 1974

17. Bultitude FW, Gower RP: Sorption based haemodialysis system. In *Renal Dialysis,* edited by Whelpton D, London, UK, Sector Publishing Ltd., 1974, p 74 (distributed in the US and Canada by JB Lippincott Company)

18. Kolff WJ: Longitudinal perspectives on sorbents in uremia. *Kidney Int* 10 (Suppl 7): S211, 1976

19. Kolff WJ, Walker JM, Gregonis D, Klein E: A membrane system to remove urea from the dialyzing fluid of the artificial kidney. *Proc 11th Annu Contractors' Conf Artif Kidney Program* NIAMDD, edited by Mackey BB, DHEW publ no (NIH) 79–1442, 1978, p 162

20. Kolff WJ, Gregonis D, Wisniewski S, Klein E, Wendt R: A membrane system to remove urea from dialysate. *Proc 12th Annu Contractors' Conf Artif Kidney Program NIAMDD,* edited by Mackey BB, DHEW publ no (NIH) 81–1979, 1981, p 215

21. Pişkin E, Evren V, Azdural AR, Chang TMS: Design of a packed bed gas desorption column for the removal of urea as ammonia. *Artif Organs* 5 (Abstracts): 56, 1981

22. Malchesky PS, Nosé Y: Biological reactors for renal support. *Trans Am Soc Artif Intern Organs* 23: 726, 1977

23. Harmsen GW, Kolff WJ: Cultivation of micro organisms with the aid of cellophane membranes. *Science* 105: 582, 1947

24. Setälä K, Heinonen H, Schreck-Pulona I: Uraemic waste recovery II: *in vitro* studies. *Proc Eur Dial Transplant Assoc* 9: 514, 1972

25. Malchesky PS, Nosé Y: Biological reactors as renal substitutes. *Artif Organs* 3: 8, 1979

26. Ackerman RA, Crosby SC, Morefield EF, Stevenson RS: Dialysate delivery and regenerative system. *Trans Am Soc Artif Intern Organs* 25: 398, 1979

27. Shaldon S, Beau MC, Claret G, Deschodt G, Mion H, Oulès R, Ramperez P, Mion C: Sorbent regeneration of ultrafiltrate as a long-term treatment of end-stage renal failure. *Artif Organs* 2: 343, 1978

28. Shaldon S: Early clinical trial of hemofiltrate recycling via sorbents. *Proc 12th Annu Contractors' Conf Artif Kidney program NIAMDD,* edited by Mackey BB,, DHEW publ no (NIH) 81–1979, 1981, p 265

29. Tuwiner SB: Research, design and development of an improved water reclamation system for manned space vehicles. *RAI Research Corp Report 364 for NASA Contract NASA-4373* (cited in reference 31)

30. Fels M: Electrochemnical degradation of waste metabolites in dialysate solution, in *Technical Aspects of Renal Dialysis,* edited by Frost TH, Tunbridge Wells, UK, Pitman Medical Publishing Company 1978, p 226

31. Fels M: Recycling of dialysate from the artificial kidney by electrochemical degradation of waste metabolites: small-scale laboratory investigation. *Med Biol Eng Comput* 16: 25, 1978

32. Bizot J, Sausse A, German patent no 2261220. French patent application no 7144868 (cited in reference 30)

33. Quellhorst E, Rieger J, Doht B, Beckmann H, Jacob I, Kraft B, Mietsch G, Scheler F: Treatment of chronic uraemia by an ultrafiltration kidney. First clinical experience. *Proc Eur Dial Transplant Assoc* 13: 314, 1976

34. Quellhorst E, Schuenemann B: Regeneration of hemofiltrate by using charcoal-coated membranes and electro-oxidation. *Int J Artif Organs* 4: 265, 1981

35. Köster K, Wendt H, Gallus J, Krisam G, Lehmann HD: Regeneration of hemofiltrate by anodic oxidation of urea. *Int J Artif Organs* 4: 264, 1981

36. Schuenemann B, Nebendahl K, Schunk O, Quellhorst E, Mundt K, Richter G: Regeneration of hemofiltrate using an absorption and electro-chemical oxidation system. *Contrib Nephrol* 32: 192, 1982

37. Schuenemann B, Quellhorst E, Kaiser H, Richter G, Mundt K, Weidlich E, Loeffler G, Zacharial M, Schunk O: Regeneration of filtrate and dialysis fluid by electro-oxidation and absorption. *Trans Am Soc Artif Intern Organs* 28: 49, 1982

38. Gordon A, Popovitzer M, Greenbaum MA, Marantz LB, McArthur MJ, DePalma JR, Maxwell MH: Zirconium phosphate – a potentially useful adsorbent in the treatment of chronic uraemia. *Proc Eur Dial Transplant Assoc* 5: 86, 1969

39. Gordon A, Gral T, DePalma JR, Greenbaum MA, Marantz LB, McArthur MJ, Maxwell MH: A sorbent-based low volume dialysate system: preliminary studies in human subjects. *Proc Eur Dial Transplant Assoc* 7: 63, 1970

40. Gordon A, Better OS, Greenbaum MA, Marantz LB, Gral T, Maxwell MH: Clinical maintenance hemodialysis with a sorbent-based, low volume dialysate regeneration system. *Trans Am Soc Artif Intern Organs* 17: 253, 1971

41. Greenbaum MA, Gordon A: A regenerative dialysis supply system. *Dial Transplant* 1(1): 18, 1972

42. Reithel FJ: Ureases, in *The Enzymes*, edited by Boyer PD, volume IV: Hydrolysis, 3rd edition, New York, London, Academic Press, 1971, p 1

43. Better OS, Gordon A, Greenbaum MA, Marantz LB, Maxwell MH: Acid-base balance in patients on sorbent hemodialysis. Role of bicarbonate generation in dialysate. *Am Soc Nephrol (Abstracts)* 4: 8, 1970

44. Van Doorn AWJ, Thomas HCL: The working of the cartridge, with special regard to bicarbonate and acetate aspects. *Nieren- u Hochdruckkrankheiten 5 (Suppl 1)*: 9, 1976

45. Henderson LW: Redy or not. *asaio J* 2: 49, 1979

46. Van Doorn AWJ, Drukker W, Thomas HCL, Verdickt L: Regeneration dialysis; handling of sulfate by the cartridge. *Eur Dial Transplant Assoc (Abstracts)* 5: 177, 1976

47. Freeman RM, Richards CJ: Studies on sulfate in end-stage renal disease. *Kidney Int* 15: 167, 1979

48. Lewin AJ, Gordon A, Greenbaum MA, Maxwell MH: Sorbent based regenerative delivery system for use in peritoneal dialysis. *Proc Eur Clin Dial Transplant Forum* 3: 126, 1973

49. Babb AL, Popovich RP, Christopher TG, Scribner BH: The genesis of the square meter-hour hypothesis. *Trans Am Soc Artif Intern Organs* 17: 81, 1971

50. Christopher TG, Cambi V, Harker LA, Hurst PE, Popovich RP, Babb AL, Scribner BH: A study of hemodialysis with lowered dialysate flow. *Trans Am Soc Artif Intern Organs* 17: 92, 1971

51. Eberhard K, Thomae U, Von Frowein G, Kuhlmann H: Anwendung der Adsorptionsmethode zur Regeneration von Spüllösungen in der Hämodialysebehandlung (Redy System). (Application of the adsorption method to regeneration of rinsing fluids used in haemodialysis (Redy System). *Med Klin* 70: 323, 1975 (in German)

52. Farrell PC, Hone PW, Ward RA, Abernethy PE, Mahony JF: Development of a sorbent-based wearable artifical kidney. *Second Australasian Conference on Heat and Mass Transfer*. The University of Sidney, 1977 (February) p 207

53. Rohmer D, Nassri M, Sherlock J, Letteri J, Ledwith J: A comparison of the respiratory dynamics during hemodialysis using acetate and bicarbonate dialysate in a sorbent regenerative system. *Trans Am Soc Artif Intern Organs* 27: 176, 1981

54. Farrell PC, Mahony JF, Jones BV, Mathew TH, Dawborn JK, Disney AP: Clinical evaluation of a dialysate regeneration system for maintenance haemodialysis. *Aust NZ J Med* 6: 292, 1976

55. Drukker W: Introduction to the Redy System. Two long-term patients. *Nieren- u Hochdruckkrankheiten 5 (Suppl 1)*: 5, 1976

56. Drukker W, Van der Werff B, Meinsma K: De-aeration of dialysis fluid. *Dial Transplant* 3(3): 33, 1974

57. Roberts M, Pecker EA, Lewin AJ, Gordon A, Maxwell MH: Clinical experience with adsorptive recirculation dialysis. *Dial Transplant* 6(5): 16, 1977

58. Schilb Th, Shapiro W, Porush J: Sodium kinetics of the Redy sorbent cartridge (RSC) when used to recycle ultrafiltrate (UF). *Artif Organs (Abstracts)* 5: 61, 1981

59. Bisson P: Redy System for home haemodialysis. *Nieren- u Hochdruckkrankheiten 5 (Suppl 1)*: 9, 1976

60. Mudge GH, Manning JA, Gilman A: Sodium acetate as a source of fixed base. *Proc Soc Exp Biol Med* 71: 136, 1949

61. Roberts M, Daugirdas JT: Redy sorbent hemodialysis. In *Handbook of Nephrology* edited by Daugirdas JT, Ing TS, Boston, Little, Brown and Co, 1987 p 146

62. Hampl H, Kessel M, Horn G: Short duration dialysis employing the Redy System with special consideration of buffer capacity. *Nieren- u Hochdruckkrankheiten 5 (Suppl 1)*: 34, 1976

63. Lewin AJ, Greenbaum MA, Gordon A, Maxwell MH: Current status of the clinical application of the Redy® dialysate delivery system. *Proc Clin Dial Transplant Forum* 2: 52, 1972

64. Mansell MA, Wing AJ: Long term experience of home dialysis with sorbent regeneration of dialysate. *Proc Eur Dial Transplant Assoc* 13: 275, 1977

65. Drukker W, Parsons FM, Gordon A: Practical application of dialysate regeneration: the Redy system. in *Replacement of Renal Fuction by Dialysis*, edited by Drukker W, Parsons FM, Maher JF, (1st edition), The Hague, Boston, London, Martinus Nijhoff Publishers, 1978, p 255

66. Odell RA, George CRP, Farrell PC: Redy sorbsystem dialysis: a long term study. *Contemp Dial* 4: 1983

67. Whalen JE, Freeman RM, Richards CJ: Elevated serum alkaline phosphatse in patients receiving sorbent cartridge hemodialysis. *asaio J* 4: 9, 1981

68. Wing AJ: Discussion in *Proc Eur Dial Transplant Assoc* 11: 550, 1975

69. Wing AJ, Mansell MA: Home dialysis with the Redy system – socio-economic and biochemical observations. *Nieren- u Hochdruckkrankheiten 5 (Suppl 1)*: 21, 1976

70. Popovich RP, Moncrief JW, Nolph KD, Ghods AJ, Twardowski ZJ, Pyle WK: Continuous ambulatory peritoneal dialysis. *Ann Intern Med* 88: 449, 1978

71. Gault MH, Ryan B, Chalker J, Ronayne D, Fine A, Churchill DN: Symptoms on sorbent dialysis reversed by conventional dialysis. *Nephron* 32: 162, 1982

72. Brozis M, Brown RS: An unexpected cause for metabolic acidosis in chronic renal failure: sorbent system hemodialysis. *Am J Kidney Dis* 6: 425, 1985

73. Shapiro WB: Letter to the editor. *Am J Kidney Dis* 8: 277, 1986

74. Blumenkrantz M: Letter to the editor. *Am J Kidney Dis* 8: 278, 1986

75. Hamm LL, Lawrence G, DuBose Jr ThD: Sorbent regenerative hemodialysis as a potential cause of acute hypercapnia. *Kidney Int* 21: 416, 1982

76. Richards CJ, Newhouse CE, Freeman RM: Bicarbonate hemodialysis using a sorbent regenerative system. *Clin Nephrol*

11: 289, 1979

77. Raja RM, Henriquez M, Knamex N, Rosenbaum JL: Improved dialysis tolerance using Redy sorbent dialysis system with bicarbonate dialysate in critically ill patient. *Dial Transplant* 8: 241, 1979

78. Jamieson MJ: Hyponatremia. *Br Med J* 290: 1723, 1985

79. Arieff AI: Hyponatremia convulsions, respiratory arrest and permanent brain damage after elective surgery in healthy women. *N Engl J Med* 314: 1529, 1986

80. Sterns RH, Riggs JE, Schoghet Jr S: Osmotic demyelination syndrome following correction of hyponatremia. *N Engl J Med* 314: 1535, 1986

81. Narins RG: Therapy of hyponatremia: does haste make waste? *N Engl J Med* 314: 1573, 1986

82. Levinsky NG: Sodium and water. in *Harrison's Principles of Internal Medicine,* edited by Braunwald E, Isselbacher KJ, Petersdorf RG, Wilson JD, Martin JB, Fauci AS, 11th edition, New York, McGraw-Hill Book Co, 1987, p 198

83. Møller BB, Bahnsen M, Solgaard P, Sørensen E: Toxicological problems with the Redy System. *Scand J Urol Nephrol (Suppl)* 30: 23, 1976

84. Alfrey AC, LeGendre GR, Kaehny WD: The dialysis encephalopathy syndrome. Possible aluminum intoxication. *N Engl J Med* 294: 184, 1976

85. Flendrig JA, Kruis H, Das AH: Aluminium intoxication: the cause of dialysis dementia? *Proc Eur Dial Transplant Assoc* 13: 355, 1976

86. Flendrig JA, Kruis H, Das AH: Aluminium and dialysis dementia. *Lancet* 1: 1235, 1976

87. Platts MM, Goode GC, Hislop JS: Composition of domestic water supply and the incidence of fractures and encephalopathy. *Br Med J* 2: 657, 1977

88. Ott SM, Maloney NA, Coburn JW, Alfrey AC, Sherrard DJ: The prevalence of aluminum deposition in renal osteodystrophy and its relation to the response to calcitriol therapy. *N Engl J Med* 307: 709, 1982

89. Berlyne GM, Ben-Ari J, Pest D, Weinberger J, Stern M, Gilmore GR, Levine R: Hyperaluminaemia from aluminium resins in renal failure. *Lancet* 2: 494, 1970

90. Berlyne GM: Aluminium toxicity in renal failure. *Int J Artif Organs* 3: 60, 1980

91. Ulmer DD: Toxicity from aluminum antacids (Editorial). *N Engl J Med* 294: 184, 1976

92. Pierides AM, Frohnert PP: Aluminum related dialysis osteomalacia and dementia, after prolonged use of the Redy cartridge. *Trans Am Soc Artif Intern Organs* 27: 629, 1981

93. Van Doorn AWJ, unpublished data cited in (110)

94. Whittier FC, Hurwitz A, Scott JA: Aluminum toxicity in uremia, a preliminary report. *Abstracts Am Soc Artif Intern Organs* 2: 72, 1973

95. Knepshield JH, Schreiner GE, Lowenthal DT, Gelfland MC: Dialysis of poisons and drugs – annual review. *Trans Am Soc Artif Intern Organs* 19: 609, 1973

96. Kaehny WD, Alfrey AC, Holman RE, Shorr WJ: Aluminum transfer during hemodialysis. *Kidney Int* 12: 361, 1977

97. Savory J, Berlin A: *Memorandum on the summary and conclusions of the International Workshop on the role of biological monitoring in the prevention of aluminium toxicity in man (aluminium analysis in biological fluids),* Luxembourg, 1982. Commission of the European Communities Directorate-General of Employment, Social Affairs and Education, Luxembourg, 1982

98. Gacek EM, Babb AL, Uvelli DA, Fry DL, Scribner BH: Dialysis dementia: the role of dialysate pH in altering the dialyzability of aluminum. *Trans Am Soc Artif Intern Organs* 25: 409, 1979

99. Branger B, Ramperez P, Marigliano N, Mion H, Shaldon S, Mion C: Aluminium transfer in bicarbonate dialysis using a sorbent regenerative system: an in vitro study. *Proc Eur Dial Transplant Assoc* 17: 213, 1980

100. Pierides AM, Myli MP: Therapy of aluminum overload (I). *Contrib Nephrol* 38: 65, 1984

101. Mion C, Branger B, Issautier R, Ellis HA, Rodier M, Shaldon S: Dialysis fracturing osteomalacia without hyperparathyroidism in patients treated with HCO_3^- rinsed Redy cartridge. *Trans Am Soc Artif Intern Organs* 27: 634, 1981

102. Graf H, Stummvoll HK, Meisinger V: Dialysate aluminium concentration and aluminium transfer during haemodialysis. *Lancet* 1: 46, 1982

103. Drury JP, Harston GA, Ineson PR, Smith S, Stoves JL, Bray CS, Black MM: Aluminium release from the Sorbsystem D-3160 and D-3260 cartridges. *Life Support Systems* (J Eur Soc for Artif Organs) 4: 211, 1986

104. Odell RA, Yang J, George ChR, Farrell PC: Aluminum kinetics during sorbent (Redy) dialysis. *Contemp Dial* 3 (no 7): 57, 1982

105. Culpepper CP, Cummings R, Westervelt FB, Savory J, Wills MR: Aluminum kinetics of the Redy system: a study of the impact of deferoxamine therapy. *Trans Am Soc Artif Intern Organs* 29: 76, 1983

106. Shapiro WB, Schilb ThP, Waltrous CL, Levy SR, Porush JG: Aluminum leakage from Redy sorbent cartridge. *Kidney Int* 23: 536, 1983

107. Mourad G, Roura R, Misse P, Mauras Y, Allain P, Mion C: Bicarbonate dialysis using a modified sorbent regenerative system with low aluminium release. *Abstracts Eur Dial Transplant Assoc Eur Renal Assoc* 20: 89, 1983

108. VanDeVijver FL, Visser WJ, Silva SJ, D'Haese PC, Thomas H, De Broe M: Risk of aluminium intoxication in long-term closed-circuit Redy dialysis. *Nephrol Dial Transplant* In press

109. Kelleher SP, Nolan ChR: Complications of sorbent regenerative hemodialysis. *Dial Transplant* 16: 323, 1987

110. Wing AJ, Parsons FM, Drukker W: Dialysate regeneration. in *Replacement of Renal Function by Dialysis,* edited by Drukker W, Parsons FM, Maher JF, (2nd edition), Dordrecht, Boston, London, Martinus Nijhoff Publishers, 1983 p 337

HEMOPERFUSION

JAMES F. WINCHESTER

INTRODUCTION

Treatment of chronic uremia has focused on reducing the generation of nitrogenous end products of protein breakdown, or on their removal by dialysis techniques. Treatment of many thousands of patients with chronic uremia has demonstrated that diet and dialysis can sustain life, although they do not correct all the metabolic consequences of renal failure and many features of uremia continue unabated. Attention has been directed over the last two decades to the properties of sorbents in an attempt to increase the efficiency of the dialysis technique. Oral sorbents such as oxystarch and charcoal, have been of considerable interest, but as yet remain of unproven value as the sole treatment for severe uremia. However, sorbent regeneration of dialysate (see Chapter 19), is now accepted in the clinical management of uremia. This chapter will deal with direct contact of blood with sorbents within cartridges (columns), primarily reviewing the potential use of hemoperfusion in uremia, but also discussing the application of hemoperfusion in drug intoxication, hepatic encephalopathy, and other potential uses (Figure 1).

PRINCIPLES OF HEMOPERFUSION

The term, hemoperfusion, implies the direct contact of blood from the patient or animal with a sorbent system. Clinically available devices consist of plastic housings incorporating particulate sorbent materials within them, through which system blood percolates in a laminar flow. The sorbent system must be sufficiently biocompatible to allow direct blood contact without allowing appreciable destruction of blood elements. To overcome the problem of incompatibility of early hemoperfusion systems (1, 2), Chang (3) introduced a microencapsulation process by which the sorbent particles were coated with a polymer membrane, such as collodion (cellulose nitrate). Many other encapsulation polymers have been introduced subsequently for clinical use as outlined below. The basic requirements for clinical hemoperfusion are the following: the hemoperfusion device with inlet and outlet blood lines; vascular

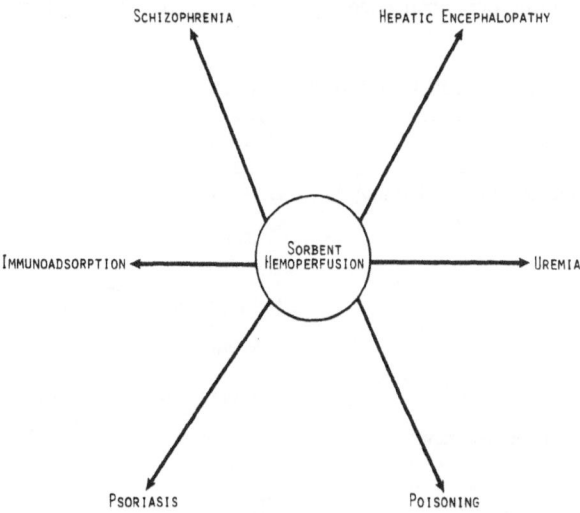

Figure 1. Uses of sorbent hemoperfusion.

access to the patient, a blood pump sufficient to maintain blood flow of 200 to 300 ml/min; gauges to detect pressure drops across the column indicating clotting with the device; intermittent or continuous use of heparin sufficient to maintain whole blood clotting time greater than 30 min (or prostacyclin [epoprostenol or PGI_2]); and facilities for monitoring safety (platelet and white blood cell counts, plasma calcium and glucose concentrations) and efficiency (plasma solute or drug levels).

SORBENTS

Typical sorbents used in hemoperfusion devices are the activated carbons (charcoals), ion-exchange resins or non-ionic macroporous resins. Activated charcoals are available in many forms, but initially consisted of uncoated granular carbons in the loose-bed form, or fixed-bed form (whereby the particles are fixed to a polyethylene backing and wound in a spiral as in the Hemodetoxifier [Becton-Dickinson, USA, now unavailable]).

All devices now available use coated activated charcoal, either as granular charcoal coated with albumin cellulose nitrate (collodion) polymer (Chang's previous research model) or with acrylic hydrogel polymer (Hemocol [Smith and Nephew, UK]), or heparinised copolymer (Clark, USA). Other devices containing charcoals are prepared from extruded charcoal coated with cellulose acetate (Ab Gambro, Sweden), or with methacrylic hydrogel (Technologie Biomediche, Italy, Organon Teknika, Netherlands). Other columns contain spherical charcoals derived from pyrolized macroporous resins (uncoated with polymer: XE-336 [previously available from Extracorporeal Medical Specialties Inc, USA]) or spherical charcoals derived from petroleum and coated with albumin-collodion solutions (Hemosorba [Asahi Medical Inc, Japan]). In addition columns containing petroleum based charcoal coated with cellulose nitrate are now available in North America (DiaKart [Biomicroencapsulation Technology, Canada] and Hemo-

kart or Alukart [Erika, USA]). Two other cartridges contain cellulose/collodion coated petroleum based spherical charcoal (Teijin Co, Ltd, Japan) or pitch-based polyhema coated spherical charcoal (Kuraray Co, Japan). Ion-exchange resins have been used in various studies but are not yet available for clinical use; they include the amberlite series, Zerolit 225 and the Zeolite series. The non-ionic resins consist of macroporous crosslinked polystyrene amberlite series such as XAD-2, and XAD-4 which had been clinically available for several years (XR-004 cartridge, [Extracorporeal Medical Specialties Inc, USA], which is no longer available in the USA, but is available in Europe [Braun, Germany]). The latter contains 650 g (wet weight) of washed, heat sterilized, pyrogen free XAD-4.

The devices used in clinical studies commonly contain 70 to 300 g of activated charcoal coated with polymer membranes ranging in thickness from 0.05 to 0.5 μm. The details of each sorbent device are given below in the section on clinical studies of hemoperfusion in uremia, and in Table 1. Activated carbons are prepared from biological substances (e.g. coconut shells, peach pits, sawdust, coal, peat or molasses), or from non-biological substances (petroleum or pitch). Although the physical properties of activated carbons are more influenced by the activation process, the choice of starting material produces such characteristics as fine pore distribution, for example, with coconut shell carbons. Activation is induced by controlled oxidation in air, carbon dioxide or steam. Maximal adsorptive capacity is achieved by inducing a high surface porosity and large surface area (approximately 1,000 m²/g). The pores are classified by the size of the radius which principally determines the efficiency of adsorption, into micropores (less than 20 Å), transitional pores (20 to 500 Å) and macropores (radius equal to or greater than 500 Å). The removal of solutes or toxic compounds from the perfusion solution depends on complex physical forces where the solute is trapped at the liquid-sorbent interface and adsorption fits with the Freundlich or Langmuir isotherms (4). Some carbons also possess the ability for chemisorption (with the

Table 1. Available hemoperfusion devices.

Manufacturer	Device	Sorbent type	Amount of sorbent	Polymer coating
Bioencapsulation Technology	DiaKart	Petroleum based charcoal	70 g	collodion
Clark	Biocompatible system	Charcoal	50, 100, 250 cc	heparinized polymer
Erika	Hemokart or Alukart	Petroleum based charcoal	60 or 155 g	collodion
Gambro	Adsorba	Norit	100 or 300 g	cellulose acetate
Organon-Teknika	Hemopur 260	Norit extruded charcoal	250	cellulose acetate
Smith and Nephew*	Hemocol or Haemocol	Sutcliffe Speakman charcoal	100 or 300 g	acrylic hydrogel
Extracorporeal*	XR-004	XAD-4 resin	350 g	none

* = No longer available in U.S.A.

formation of chemical bonds) or chemical conversion of some compounds. In general, non-polar solutes are better adsorbed from aqueous solution than are polar solutes. With activated carbon, solutes must diffuse, externally through the liquid phase (from plasma and from within red blood cells) to the carbon particles and are then subject to several rate limiting steps. If the carbon is coated with polymer, diffusion must occur through the membrane, through the macropores, then into the micropores where the adsorption process is finalized. For uncoated carbon, the rate limiting step is pore diffusion, while with coated carbon the rate limiting step is diffusion through the polymer coating. For medical use in hemoperfusion devices, activated carbons must possess the following qualities: freedom from microparticulate fines, easy washability, resistance to attrition within devices, high adsorptive capacity, smooth surface morphology, low microparticle generation, minimal elution of toxic ions, high blood compatibility, and easy sterilization, low toxicity and low pyrogenicity. All these qualities determine the manufacturers' choice of charcoal for hemoperfusion cartridges and such properties have been reviewed by Denti and Walker (5). Ion exchange resins possess the ability to exchange one ion for another, the same quantity of charge being removed and replaced by another, to maintain electrical neutrality. Some of the materials used for ion exchange also function as adsorbents, but presently no system has been developed for continuous hemoperfusion because of the prohibitive side effects of removal of biologically important ions such as calcium and magnesium, although the removal of such compounds can be minimized by pretreating the ion exchange resin with appropriate electrolyte solutions. Chemical adsorbents (chemisorbents) depend on the formation of chemical bonds between the solute and the adsorbent, and although not yet clinically accepted, it has been demonstrated in man that oral polyaldehydes (oxy-starch and oxy-cellulose) are able to remove urea and ammonia from the gastrointestinal tract under physiologic circumstances. The macroporous resins are non-ionic, gel type resins which are formed in beads by an agglomerate of microspheres that are cross-linked to a high degree, thereby producing less swelling of the beads in physiologic solutions. The macroporous resins have a high ability to adsorb organic solutes on the surfaces of the microspheres, which possess surface areas of 300 to 500 m²/g. Uncharged macroporous resins (e.g. XAD-4 and XAD-7) are similar to activated charcoal, however, they adsorb solutes with less energetic forces and consequently, the adsorption is more reversible than that with organic sorbents such as activated carbon. The elution of organic solutes (such as barbiturates, methaqualone and glutethimide) from XAD-4 is more readily obtained with the use of methanol or ethanol than can ever be achieved using similar elution techniques with activated carbon.

Solute spectrum adsorbed and effects of coating of sorbent

The solute spectrum adsorbed, particularly with activated charcoal and with special regard to uremic solutes, is shown in Table 2. Removal by activated carbon of solutes ranging in molecular mass from 60 to 21,500 daltons has been demonstrated *in vitro* and *in vivo*. As mentioned above, diffusion of solutes into the microporous structure of coated carbon depends on the polymer membrane thickness and for substances of low molecular mass (creatinine [113 daltons], uric acid [168 daltons], hippuran [363 daltons], vitamin B$_{12}$ [1,355 daltons]) a thin cellulose coating reduces the adsorption only slightly. At higher molecular weights (above 3,500 daltons), however, substantial reduction of adsorption occurs with polymer coating (6). Nevertheless, it is this capacity to adsorb molecules of the 'middle molecular weight' size (300 to 1,500 daltons) that has stimulated interest in activated charcoal hemoperfusion in uremia. Adsorption of molecules larger than most middle molecular mass solutes (>1,500 daltons) is limited by the pore structure of the specific semipermeable membrane coating. It must be borne in mind, however, that adsorption of biologically important small solutes also occurs. This is most noticeable clinically with adsorption of glucose, calcium, amino acids, and middle molecules, all of which exhibit finite saturation rates for adsorption. Even 25-hydroxycholecalciferol and other hormones (7, 8) have been removed by charcoal hemoperfusion *in vivo,* and important trace metals such as arsenic, cobalt, chromium, and selenium are also removed *in vitro* with perfusion of protein solutions through activated charcoal devices (9). No experience with long term effects of such removal is available, but these observations indicate the wide spectrum adsorbent capacity of activated carbon.

Table 2. Putative uremic toxins removed by sorbents (Molecular weight range 60 to 21,500 daltons).

Adrenocorticotrophin	Middle molecule peaks*
(Aldosterone)*	Myoinositol
Amino acids*	Non-protein nitrogen
Calcium*	Norepinephrine
25,OH cholecalciferol*	Organic acids*
Creatinine*	Oxalate*
Cyclic AMP	Parathyroid hormone*
Epinephrine	Phenols*
Folic acid**	(Phosphate)*
Fibronectin	Polyamino acids
Gastrin*	(Renin)*
Glucagon	Ribonuclease
Glucose*	Serotonin
(Growth hormone)*	Thyroxine*
Guanidines	Trace metals: As, Co, Cr, Se
Indoles*	Triglycerides*
Insulin*	Triiodothyronine*
L-dopamine	(Urea)*
Lysozyme	Uric acid*
(Magnesium)*	Vitamin B$_{12}$

* Studied during hemoperfusion in uremic patients.
** Unpublished.
( ) Incompletely removed.

SIDE EFFECTS OF HEMOPERFUSION

Particle embolization was a feature of the early poorly washed hemoperfusion devices. This problem has been essentially improved by selecting charcoal resistant to attrition by using polymer coating techniques, and by washing procedures applied on a commercial scale, each of which reduces particulate matter to acceptable infusion fluid limits (required by Federal or other agencies). Similarly, profound platelet depletion seen with early uncoated charcoal hemoperfusion devices (1, 2, 10) has been overcome with the introduction of microencapsulation techniques, and in uremia, current hemoperfusion devices produce platelet losses of 30% or less (11). Chang's techniques, as used by his own team (12) or by others (13, 14 and Tables 3 and 4), is particularly notable for being the most hemocompatible, and the recent selection and use of a hydrophilic methacrylate membrane coating for extruded charcoal hemoperfusion has been associated with minimal change in platelets (15) during treatment. Transient leukopenia, similar to that observed during hemodialysis, occurs during hemoperfusion in man, and may be a result of complement activation by surface contact, with margination of leukocytes similar to that observed during hemodialysis (16). Adsorption or activation of coagulation factors has also been observed during clinical hemoperfusion. The most significant change is a minor reduction in the fibrinogen concentration (1, 2), and fibronectin (17) even with polymer coated activated charcoal devices (7), but no appreciable changes in coagulation factors II-XII have been observed as a response to charcoal hemoperfusion in uremic patients (7). The side effects outlined above, although minor in nature, have stimulated the search for more biocompatible activated carbon adsorbents in the form of carbon containing membranes, and fibers (18–21).

The hemostatic changes may be particularly severe in patients with hepatic failure (see below) and may be associated with the production of platelet aggregates (22), although this has not been observed in uremic patients treated with charcoal hemoperfusion (7). There is the possibility that these platelets aggregates produce vasoactive amines responsible for hypotension observed during hemoperfusion in hepatic coma (22). This has led to the selection of agents to reduce platelet aggregability. Prior administration of sulfinpyrazone or aspirin can reduce platelet adhesion to activated charcoal in an ex-vivo hemoperfusion test system (23) and prostacyclin can serve as an adjunctive agent to heparin, or as the sole agent for anti-coagulation both in animals (24) and in man undergoing hemoperfusion for hepatic coma (25, 26). In hemoperfusion for hepatic failure, hypotension, and platelet aggregation or depletion, were prevented with prostacyclin (25, 26). Additionally, other coagulation disturbances may be prevented with prostacyclin (27).

Other side effects of hemoperfusion such as removal of calcium or glucose, exhibit finite saturation characteristics and are usually easily overcome. Reduction of body temperature occurring during hemoperfusion may result from rein-fusion of a large unheated, extracorporeal blood volume, but this problem is also easily managed by appropriate measures such as heating blankets. In children it is possible to use large (adult) extracorporeal blood volume containing devices, provided that the devices are primed with anti-coagulated whole blood (28). Pyrogenic reactions observed with the initial charcoal hemoperfusion devices introduced by Yatzidis in 1964 (1) are not seen with modern hemoperfusion devices which have been subjected to commercial washing techniques, as outlined above. The use of ion exchange resins and non-ionic resins which are not specifically prepared for medical use, can be associated with pyrogenic events, however, in this regard XAD-4 resin is pyrogen free. Recent observations that hormones and trace metals can be adsorbed by activated charcoal devices (7–15) should raise the possibility that deficiency states may be induced in the long term, with activated charcoal hemoperfusion. Another postulated complication of repetitive therapy relates to the effect of charcoal residuals, particularly hydrocarbons on those charcoals prepared from petroleum or pitch. In addition, metallic or other contaminants within the carbon may theoretically produce cumulative toxicity, although these contaminants can be substantially reduced with special washing techniques (29). Another concern is that the charcoal hemoperfusion device may possess a large residual blood volume which in long-term treatment of uremia may give rise to anemia of blood loss, as has been shown in hemodialysis (30). Where measured, however, by Chang et al (31) and Stefoni et al (32), clinically acceptable mean residual blood volumes of 7 ml and 3.1 ml, respectively, were observed.

HEMOPERFUSION IN UREMIA

Historical background

The first publication on blood contact with sorbents was in 1948 by Muirhead and Reid (33), who used a mixture of cation and anion exchange resins (amberlite IR-100 H and deacidite) contained in a hemoperfusion device. They demonstrated in animals and *in vitro*, that this system was able to adsorb 3.5 g urea; however, these initial experiments were associated with severe side effects and further use of this resin was not pursued. In 1958, Schreiner (34) reported lactated anion exchange resin column hemoperfusion in a patient with pentobarbital poisoning. The column was used for two 15 min periods during which substantial drug removal was demonstrated. These early resin studies, however, were complicated by pyrogenic reactions, electrolyte disturbances and hemolysis (33, 35), and although electrolyte abnormalities could be reduced by pre-treating the resins with electrolyte solutions (36, 37), the other side effects were considered too dangerous for continued use. In 1964, Yatzidis (1) reported that a column containing 200 g of uncoated activated charcoal, derived from coconut shells could adsorb, *in vitro* from plasma, approximately 2 g of barbital, phenobarbital and pentobarbital, and 2.6 g of salicylic acid

Table 3. Short term clinical studies of sorbent hemoperfusion in uremia.

Sorbent system and method	Solute removed (clearance ml/min or % ↓ in plasma level)	Adverse effects, % ↓ in concentration, and comments	First author (ref.)
Uncoated Merck 200 g HP alone	U (100), Cr (220), UA (227), P (175), G (191), I (190), O (167)	platelets 50%, fibrinogen 40%, proteins, pyrexia hypotension	Yatzidis (1, 217)
Uncoated Union Carbide charcoal 200 g HP alone	Cr (160), Ca, Gl, UA	platelets 50%, blood loss hemolysis	Dunea (2)
Fisher albumin collodion coated charcoal (ACAC) 300 g charcoal HP alone	Cr (160), UA (180)	platelets 92%, of control pyrexia	Chang (39)
ACAC 300 g with HD or with ultrafiltration	HP/HD Cr (163), UA (153), MMS (99)	–	Chang (31, 40)
Norit cellulose acetate coated charcoal 150 g HP alone	Cr, UA, P, G	platelets 40%	Yatzidis (218)
Uncoated fixed bed charcoal 100 g HP alone or with HD	Cr (100 HP/HD), UA, Ca, triglycerides	platelets 53% or 26%	Dunea (219)
Petroleum based ACAC 300 g HP with HD	Cr (65%), UA (68%)	platelets variable	Ota (14)
Sutcliffe Speakman acrylic hydrogel coated charcoal or XAD-4 resin HP alone	Cr (67% charcoal), Cr (95% XAD-4), U, G, P, MMS, amines	MMS removal, XAD-4, charcoal	Leber (220)
Norit cellulose acetate coated charcoal 300 g HP alone	Cr (180), UA (180), MMS (50%), AAS	leukopenia, hypotension	Oules (42)
Sutcliffe Speakman acrylic hydrogel coated charcoal 300 g HP alone or with HD	Cr (180), UA (115), MMS, AAS, hormones	platelets 30%, fibrinogen 30%, dialysis, encephalopathy, unchanged	Winchester (7)
Norit cellulose acetate coated charcoal 300 g HP alone or with HD	Cr (180), UA (180), P (110)	–	Martin (221)
Norit cellulose acetate coated charcoal 300 g HP alone or with HD	MMS (59%), U (6%), Cr (32%), US (42%), Myoinositol (27%), Ca (8%)	platelets 20%	Trznadel (46)
Norit cellulose acetate coated charcoal 300 g HP alone or with HD	–	cardiac function improved 24 h after HP	Trznadel (50)
Sutcliffe Speakman acrylic hydrogel coated charcoal 300 g HP alone	–	platelets fell 33%	Mydlik (222)
Uncoated pyrolized resin XE-336 200 g HP alone	Cr (220), UA (220), Ca	platelets fell 40%, leukocytes 80%, bioincompatible	Rosenbaum (44)
Norit cellulose acetate coated charcoal 300 g HP alone	–	MMS molecule removal equal to PAN dialysis	Asaba (49)
Norit cellulose acetate coated charcoal 300 g HP alone	–	MMS fell 52–86%	Asaba (51)

Abbreviations: HP = hemoperfusion, HD = hemodialysis, U = urea, Cr = creatinine, UA = uric acid, P = phosphate, G = guanidines, I = indoles, O = organic acids, Ca = calcium, Gl = glucose, MMS = middle molecular weight substances, AAS = amino acids.

Table 4. Long term clinical studies of HP in uremia.

First author (ref.)	Duration	(HP h/wk)	Number of subjects	Sorbent system and methods	Solute removed (clearance ml/min or % ↓ in plasma level)	Adverse effects and comments
Chang (31)	3 mo 1 HD/HP/week 2 HD/week	2	1	ACAC 300 g with HD or ultrafiltration	HP/HD Cr (163), UA (153), MMS (99)	Nerve conduction velocity improved
Odaka (49)	3–19 mo 3 HD/HP/week	9	3	petroleum based ACAC 130 with HD	Cr (50%), UA (62%)	disequilibrium headache, pyrexia platelets rose
Siemsen (57)	5–6 mo 1 or 3 HP/HD/week 2 HD/week	3–7.5	6	Uncoated fixed bed charcoal 100 g alone and with HD	Cr (100 HP/HD), Cr (25%), UA (22%), Ca (10%)	hypotension, platelets 26%–50%, depending on priming
Otsubo (53)	2–3 mo 3 HD/HP/week	9	9	Hydron coated petroleum based charcoal 170 g HP with HD	–	improved neuropathy and electromyogram
Agishi (54)	1–2 mo 3 HD/HP/week	15	6	ACAC coated coconut or petroleum based charcoal 300 g HP with HD	–	Nerve conduction velocity improved
Stefoni (32)	1–12 mo 1 or 2 HP/HD/week	3–5	18	hydroxymethacrylate coated Norit charcoal initially 300 g then 150 g with HD	HP Cr (77), UA (55), Vitamin B$_{12}$ (31), HP/HD Cr (174), UA (119)	Platelets unchanged hypotension, cramps, headache, pyrexia, improved neuropathy, and wellbeing
Stefoni (61)	12 mo 2 HP/HD/week or 2 HP/HD/week plus 1 HD/week	8	18 34 6	hydroxymethacrylate coated Norit charcoal 150 g with HD	11–15% drop out for fluid overload	No changes in hematology, biochemistry, nerve conduction, reduction in treatment time
Stefoni (60)	6 mo 2 or 3 HD/HP/week	15	6–8	hydroxymethacrylate coated Norit charcoal 150 g with HD	–	No difference in lymphocyte number and function compared to HD
Bonomini (59)	1–36 mo (mean 7.5 mo) 2 HP/HD/week	8–10	27	hydroxymethacrylate coated Norit charcoal 150 g with HD	Water retention (9/27) solute clearances as in (32)	Stable MNCV other side effects as in (32)
Bonomini (60)	variable 1 HP/HD/week 2 HD/week	4–5	64	as in (61)	Cost increase 30%	30% reduction in treatment time
Henderson (56)	10 mo 3 HP/HD/week (controls 3 HD)	15	9	Sutcliffe Speakman acrylic hydrogel coated charcoal 100 g HP with HD	–	Improved well being
Chang (55)	6 mo crossover with 12 h HD/week 3 HP/HD/week	8	4	ACAC Diakart petroleum based 70 g with HD	–	No change in biochemistry, hematology, etc.
Espinosa (63)	1–6 mo 2 HP/HD/week	10	3	ACAC Diakart petroleum based 70 g with HD	–	No change in biochemistry compared to HD

Table 4. (Continued).

First author (ref.)	Duration	(HP h/wk)	Number of subjects	Sorbent system and methods	Solute removed (clearance ml/min or % ↓ in plasma level)	Adverse effects and comments
Barre (62)	4–6 mo 2 or 3 HD/HP/week	8	5	ACAC Diakart petroleum based 70 g with HD	–	No increased heparin requirement, cost effective, improved pericarditis, neuropathy, hypercoagulability
Splendiani (223)	16 mo 2 HP/HD/week	8	14	polymethacrylate coated charcoal	HP/HD Cr (228), U (236)	Reduced dialysis frequency, improved neuropathy, insomnia, pruritus

Abbreviations: ACAC = albumin collodion (= cellulose nitrate) coated charcoal, HP = hemoperfusion, HD = hemodialysis, Cr = creatinine, UA = uric acid, Ca = calcium, MMS = middle molecular weight substances.

and glutethimide. Extension of the *in vitro* work to uremic patients (1), demonstrated that the putative uremic toxins creatinine, uric acid, guanidine, indoles, phenolic compounds and organic acids could be removed more efficiently than with the dialysis equipment then available. In 1965, Yatzidis et al (38) used activated uncoated carbon hemoperfusion to treat two patients with barbiturate poisoning, both of whom recovered consciousness after three and five hemoperfusions lasting 1 h each. Transient side effects seen with this device were facial flushing, dyspnea, and a burning sensation. It was also demonstrated that in animals and man, hemoperfusion was accompanied by platelet depletion and reduction of plasma fibrinogen concentrations (1). Hagstam et al (10) confirmed that in animals, drug removal was possible, but extensive carbon particle embolization to the lungs (on histology), and platelet depletion occurred with the use of uncoated activated charcoal hemoperfusion devices. Dunea and Kolff (2), also confirmed a 50% reduction of platelet count as well as significant hemolysis in their experiments with hemoperfusion using uncoated charcoal. They confirmed Yatzidis' observations on the removal of uremic solutes. It was not until 1966, when Chang (3) demonstrated that microencapsulation of charcoal within polymers prevented embolization of charcoal particles and reduced platelet depletion, that the process was reinvestigated for use for uremia and poisoning. Chang et al (39), confirmed that in uremic man charcoal hemoperfusion could remove putative uremic toxins as reported earlier by Yatzidis (1), but also could remove polyamino acids (40) and medium molecular weight substances (40, 41). In addition, Chang and co-workers (40, 41) demonstrated both *in vitro* and *in vivo* that plasma creatinine and urate clearances with hemoperfusion alone in man were greater than with conventional hemodialysis. These reports noted, however, that urea could not be adsorbed in the quantities thought necessary for the treatment of uremia. Stimulated by Yatzidis' work in Greece and Chang's work in Canada, many others throughout the world have become involved in the development and use of charcoal hemoperfusion devices in ex-

perimental uremia and also in the treatment of uremic man. These studies are outlined in detail in Tables 3 and 4.

Short-term clinical studies

Table 3 shows that in short-term studies (repetitive studies over a period of time less than 3 months) there is a wide variability, in terms of solute clearance and response to hemoperfusion, depending on the clinical device used. It is apparent, however, that creatinine and uric acid are cleared efficiently by charcoal hemoperfusion alone in contrast with urea which is much better removed by standard hemodialysis. The addition of charcoal hemoperfusion to hemodialysis increases the total clearance rates of creatinine, urate and middle molecules. While there is some question as to the total quantity of middle molecules removed by hemoperfusion (42), middle molecular weight substance clearances approach 144 ml/min at a blood flow rate of 300 ml/min as reported by Chang (43).

Oules et al (42) examining specific subpeaks of middle molecular weight substances reported that extraction of peaks 7a-d was initially 60 to 70% of blood flow rates, but decreased to 10 to 30% during the course of a 2 to 3 h hemoperfusion. Rosenbaum et al (44) obtained with XE-336 hemoperfusion a middle molecular weight substance removal of 273 ml/min at blood flow rates of 300 ml/min in uremic animals. Analysis of the total solute removed during hemoperfusion (7), has shown that total solute removal with a 2 h hemoperfusion alone or combined with hemodialysis for standard markers of uremia such as creatinine and urate is substantially less than achieved during a 5 h standard hemodialysis. Subsequent analysis (45), has shown that small molecular weight substances (urea, urate, guanidines, and phenols) with the exception of creatinine are not removed by hemoperfusion alone with any substantially greater efficiency than by hemodialysis. Creatinine and urate clearances *in vitro* are close to blood flow rates, but these values are reduced *in vivo* due to the competitive adsorption of other thio-compounds. Significant quantities of organic acids, indoles, and myoinositol (46) are also removed by hemoperfusion *in vivo* and *in vitro*.

The structure of amino acids determines their adsorption to activated carbon. Amino acids with aromatic groups are more efficiently adsorbed than branched chain amino acids (47). In studies of uremia, amino acids not only are removed by charcoal hemoperfusion (7, 32) but are also released from charcoal or other body pools after initial adsorption (42). Appreciable alterations in plasma insulin, plasma growth hormone, plasma total thyroxine and total triiodothyronine concentrations during hemoperfusion in uremic patients (7, 15), with some differences from that occurring during hemodialysis, have been observed. Other hormones and metabolites removed during *in vitro* or *in vivo* hemoperfusion are listed in Table 2. Most short term studies have not reported any clinical improvement with the use of charcoal hemoperfusion in uremia, although the initial observation of Yatzidis and coworkers (1), suggested that improvement in pericarditis, gastrointestinal symptoms and lethargy occurred. Martin and associates (48) and Odaka et al (49), also reported that pericarditis appeared to resolve faster when patients are treated with short term charcoal hemoperfusion, than when treated with hemodialysis. Trznadel et al (50) reported improvement in cardiac function, measured by systolic time intervals, at 24 h after a 4 h hemoperfusion, the delay in effect being postulated as being due to slow tissue reduction in middle molecules. This may be so, since middle molecule removal with charcoal hemoperfusion is equivalent to polyacrylonitrile hemodialysis (51), and the rebound in plasma concentrations is delayed, indicating release of middle molecules from more than one body pool (52).

Long-term clinical studies

It has become appreciated that charcoal hemoperfusion alone is insufficient for the control of symptoms or removal of water in uremic subjects (Table 4). For sufficient removal of water, charcoal hemoperfusion is generally combined with hemodialysis or ultrafiltration devices. Several long-term studies have shown an improvement in mean nerve conduction velocity (32, 43, 53, 54). In addition, others have (53) demonstrated improvement in the electromyogram, in pruritus, and pericarditis. Stefoni and colleagues (32) and Chang et al (55) have demonstrated that with combined hemoperfusion-hemodialysis, a substantial reduction in dialysis time could be achieved without the development of any significant symptomatology. In another 9 month study of thrice weekly hemoperfusion added to hemodialysis in nine uremic patients there was no change however in nerve conduction velocity (56). The adverse reactions associated with intermittent prolonged hemoperfusion have been hypotension (32, 57), flushing, fever, chills, nausea and headaches (32, 58–61). An inability to maintain fluid balance in a modest percentage of patients, with reduced ultrafiltration during reduced dialysis time and falling residual renal function (59–61), or a rise in biochemical parameters of uremia (62) consequent on reduced residual renal function. Poor fluid balance was not a features of the studies of Chang et al

(55), nor those of Henderson and Kennedy (56).

Bio-incompatibility was not of any clinical significance, except that clinically unimportant falls in platelet and leucocyte count occurred indicating that the foreign surface interaction between blood cells and the charcoal particles is present but minimal.

Clinical improvements in 'well being' were mentioned in several studies (32, 56, 59–61), only one of which was a controlled study (56). Improvement in mean nerve conduction velocity (32) stabilised on continuation of the studies in the same patients (59), while Barre et al (62) noted improvement in pericarditis, peripheral neuropathy and hypercoagulability, as well as a reduction in dialysis time. Others (63) have used combined hemoperfusion/hemodialysis, to reduce successfully dialysis frequency in patients with vascular access problems. A fall in blood urea was observed by Stefoni et al (32), and attributed to reduction in catabolism (59), but this was not a feature of other studies (55, 56). Interestingly, a reduction in plasma aluminum was observed, and speculated to be due to adsorption on proteins adsorbed on charcoal (56). In addition a transient fall in lymphocyte transformation to poke week mitogen was observed (56), but other studies of lymphocyte count and function revealed no significant differences from hemodialysis subjects (64).

Specifically, Stefoni et al (32) and Bonomini et al (59) have commented on a 30% added annual cost for dialysis, with combined hemoperfusion/hemodialysis, while Barre et al (62) have found the addition of hemoperfusion to hemodialysis be cost effective. Capodicasa et al (65), have commented on the improvement in outcome from continuous ambulatory peritoneal dialysis (CAPD) by adding one hemoperfusion treatment to the weekly CAPD regimen.

Comparison of devices

Based on the experience to date, no particular device has substantial advantage over another in term of solute removal, although Chang's coating technique does appear to produce the most biocompatible surface attainable with these devices (12–14, 54, 62, 63). Stefoni et al, and other Italian studies (15, 32, 59–61, 65, 66) have shown that, with prolonged hemoperfusion, a high degree of compatibility, similar to that observed by Chang, can also be achieved using methacrylate hydrophilic membrane coated charcoal.

Solute clearance values for devices used in the major studies of combined hemoperfusion/hemodialysis are as follows; urea 143 to 160 ml/min, creatinine 168 to 174 ml/min, urate 119 to 194 ml/min, and 'middle molecules' 51 to 165 ml/min; hemoperfusion alone accounted for solute clearances as follows; urea 11 ml/min (32), creatinine 77 (32) to 86 (56) ml/min, and urate 55 ml/min (32, 56), with all blood flow rates being approximately 200 ml/min.

Potential clinical benefits and present role in treatment of end-stage renal disease

The potential clinical benefits of charcoal hemoperfusion

relate to the wide spectrum adsorptive qualities of charcoal and the improvements in uremic symptomatology reported by Yatzidis initially, and now by others. These suggest that hemoperfusion may have a role in the treatment of uremia. The absence of urea, water, electrolyte and hydrogen ion removal, however, renders it necessary to combine hemosorbent removal of solutes with dialysis or ultrafiltration and many investigators are examining urea removing devices combining different physical-chemical processes. It is likely that in the future sorbents will be used in a hybrid device which will combine all the properties achieved by hemodialysis but in greater efficiency and capacity (67–69). Such devices should be capable of removing water, urea, uric acid, creatinine, and other products of nitrogenous breakdown. At present the hemoperfusion devices available are biocompatible for repetitive use, although it is still unclear whether long term repetitive use of hemoperfusion might induce deficiency states.

It has recently been shown that in short term studies addition of charcoal HP to HD, improves upon the removal of iron-deferoxamine complex, or iron-aluminum complex in patients with metal overload syndromes (70–72) (see below).

A major reason for HP not being widely used relates to cost. Hemoperfusion devices range in cost from $80 to $500 for a single device, which is unacceptable for continual use in the long term, even taking into account some cost saving with reduction in dialysis time. Should the cost of hemoperfusion devices be reduced to values approaching those of conventional hemodialyzers, then hemoperfusion might be used widely. At present it seems justifiable to use these high cost devices in the treatment of specific problems of dialysis, i.e. treatment of iron and aluminum overload syndromes, and specific complications such as peripheral neuropathy and pericarditis.

HEMOPERFUSION AND DRUG INTOXICATION

A fairly large number of patients present as medical emergencies to hospitals as a result of acute self-poisoning, with 40% requiring admission for treatment. Probably 10% require intensive care management, while about 5% require methods to eliminate poisons (73). About 85% of cases referred to American poison control centers can be managed by telephone consultation and follow-up (74). In the United Kingdom, over the 10 year period 1975–1984, 38,024 died as a result of poisoning (75), while in the United States in 1985, 900,513 poisoning cases were referred to 56 poison control centers covering a population base of 113.6 million (76). Extrapolation to the entire United States estimates that the number of poisoning cases in 1985 was 1.9 million. There were 328 deaths from poisoning, reported to these poison control centers (76). Interestingly, hemodialysis was used in 217 cases and hemoperfusion in 56 (76).

Treatment of poisoned patients should follow well tested management guidelines (77). Intensive supportive management without the use of central stimulants (78), reduced the mortality from acute sedative drug overdosage from 25% in 1945 to less than 1% in 1966 (79). Moreover, depending on the severity, sedative self-poisoning causing Grade III or Grade IV coma (80) carries a mortality ranging from 8.3% to 34% (81). In very severely poisoned patients recourse has often been made, under the guidelines proposed by Maher and Schreiner (82), to the use of dialytic techniques for removing drugs. Because of its simplicity and efficiency, attention has been directed to the use of sorbent hemoperfusion in the treatment of severely drug intoxicated patients. This subject has been reviewed in depth (81, 83–85). While hemodialysis is a most effective method for removing highly diffusible substances, it has become clear that hemoperfusion is more efficient with regard to certain other poisons. Lipid soluble drugs and protein bound drugs which are inefficiently removed by hemodialysis can be removed more efficiently by hemoperfusion. Drugs such as salicylates and barbiturates can also be removed more effectively by hemoperfusion, *in vitro* and *in vivo*, than by hemodialysis under the same conditions of blood flow rate and plasma drug concentrations.

Clinical and laboratory studies

Table 5 lists the drugs removed by various hemoperfusion devices *in vitro* and *in vivo*. Most studies have dealt principally with activated charcoal hemoperfusion, less commonly with non-ionic macroporous resin hemoperfusion, and rarely with ion exchange resin hemoperfusion. Table 6 gives, for similar conditions of blood flow rate and drug concentrations, the extraction ratio for certain drugs (inlet concentration – outlet concentration divided by inlet concentration) and indicates that for lipid soluble drugs that the most effective removal is with the macroporous, non-ionic resin XAD-4. In terms of spectrum of activity, however, although XAD-4 can remove lipid soluble drugs particularly well, activated charcoal is more non-specific and can be used in a wide variety of clinical poisonings.

Following the initial use of pharmacokinetic modeling (86), which demonstrated that drug elimination could be substantially enhanced with hemoperfusion, several reports (87–90) and reviews (91–93) have confirmed that, for certain drugs in both animal and clinical studies, elimination rates can be substantially increased during the hemoperfusion periods. Pharmacokinetic studies have become an important aspect of determining efficiency and utility of hemoperfusion in poisoning.

Adverse reactions observed during hemoperfusion in poisoning are similar to those seen in treatment of uremia. Side effects are less troublesome since repetitive hemoperfusion is rarely required, except in glutethimide, ethchlorvynol, or other poisoning by drugs which possess slow intercompartmental transfer rates and large volumes of distribution (81). Thrombocytopenia developing during hemoperfusion in poisoning cases usually recovers within 24 to 28 h and very rarely is associated with hemostatic problems (81).

Several authors oppose the use of hemoperfusion in poisoning on kinetic grounds for certain drugs (94, 95), or arguing that conservative management alone is almost invariably associated with a favorable clinical outcome (95, 96). It must, however, be pointed out that the geographic and other variations in poisoning severity and type are such (97) that consideration should be given to hemoperfusion or dialysis in severe cases with specific toxic agents. Small retrospective (98) and prospective (99) studies of hemoperfusion in poisoning have suggested benefit from hemoperfusion, but is has not been possible to conduct a large scale controlled clinical trial of hemoperfusion in poisoning, and reliance on clinical judgement and to the guidelines given below is recommended, when considering hemoperfusion (or hemodialysis) in poisoning.

In general, patients that are poisoned with agents that cause metabolic abnormalities such as acidosis, should be treated by hemodialysis, or combined hemodialysis/hemoperfusion (100), since correction of the acidosis is more rapidly attained with dialysis (101, 102). Hemodialysis is recommended as the treatment of choice for severely poisoned patients with ethanol poisoning (sorbent devices saturate rapidly with ethanol), methanol (because of formaldehyde and formic acid formation and profound acidosis), ethylene glycol (acidosis and oxalate formation) and salicylate (acidosis [103–106]) and the risk of bleeding from the effect on platelets.

There are several controversial areas where the indications for hemoperfusion remain, as yet, unproven. Acetaminophen (paracetamol) poisoning is best treated by administering sulfhydryl compounds, such as oral (107), or intravenous (108; still under investigation in USA) n-acetylcysteine within 14 h of ingestion. The only controlled clinical trial of hemoperfusion in acetaminophen poisoning started within the first 14 h of ingestion did not demonstrate clinical benefit (109). Similarly in patients treated later than 14 h after ingestion hemoperfusion may be associated with a lesser rise in hepatic enzyme (SGOT, SGPT) concentrations, than occurs with conservative management alone (110, 111). The value of hemoperfusion in acetaminophen poisoning remains, nevertheless, unproven. Clinical benefit of hemoperfusion for amitriptyline poisoning has been reported using either activated charcoal (112) or resin hemoperfusion (113–115). Others have not supported this contention (116). Tricyclic drugs have large volumes of distribution and intoxication occurs at low plasma concentrations. Although a 60% (activated charcoal) to 90% (XAD-4 resin) extraction of nortriptyline occurs during hemoperfusion, in severe cases no substantial alteration in arterial plasma drug concentrations occurs (116, 117). Several studies attest to the beneficial effects of hemoperfusion in digitalis poisoning in animals (87, 118–120) and in man (121–123), showing increased drug elimination rates and reduction in plasma digitalis concentrations; but other clinical studies of hemoperfusion in digoxin poisoning have reported somewhat disappointing results (124–126). Certainly, in renal failure subjects, who

Table 5. Drugs and chemicals removed with hemoperfusion.

Barbiturates	Antimicrobials/anticancer	Cardiovascular
amobarbital	(adriamycin)	digoxin
butabarbital	ampicillin	diltiazem
hexabarbital	carmustine	(disopyramide)
pentobarbital	chloramphenicol	metoprolol
phenobarbital	chloroquine	n-acetylprocainamide
quinalbital	clindamycin	procainamide
secobarbital	dapsone	quinidine
thiopental	doxorubicin	(aluminum)*
vinalbital	gentamicin	(iron)*
	isoniazid	
Nonbarbiturate	(methotrexate)	*Miscellaneous*
hypnotics, sedatives,	thiabendazole	aminophylline
tranquilizers		cimetidine
carbromal	*Antidepressants*	(fluoroacetamide)
chloral hydrate	(amitryptiline)	(phencyclidine)
chlorpromazine	(imipramine)	phenols
(diazepam)	(tricyclics)	(podophyllin)
diphenhydramine		theophylline
ethchlorvynol	*Plants, animals,*	
glutethimide	*herbicides,*	*Solvents, gases*
meprobamate	*insecticides*	carbon tetrachloride
methaqualone	amanitin	ethylene oxide
methsuximide	chlordane	trichloroethanol
methyprylon	demeton sulfoxide	
promazine	dimethoate	
promethazine	diquat	
	methylparathion	
Analgesics,	nitrostigmine	
antirheumatic	organophosphates	
acetaminophen	phalloidin	
acetylsalicylic acid	polychlorinated	
colchicine	biphenyls	
d-propoxyphyene	paraquat	
methylsalicylate	parathion	
phenylbutazone		
salicylic acid		

( ) Not well removed; ( )* Removed with chelating agent.

Table 6. Plasma drug extraction ratios with different devices.*

	Standard hemodialysis	Coated OR uncoated charcoal hemoperfusion	XAD-2 or XAD-4 resin hemoperfusion
Acetaminophen	0.4	0.5	0.7
Amobarbital	0.26	0.3	0.9
Acetylsalicylic acid	0.5	0.5	–
Carbromal	0.31	0.55	1.0
Digoxin	0.2	0.3–0.6	0.4
Ethchlorvynol	0.32	0.7	1.0
Glutethimide	0.16	0.65	0.8
Paraquat	0.5	0.6	0.9**
Phenobarbital	0.27	0.5	0.85
Theophylline	0.5	0.7	0.75
Tricyclics	0.35	0.35	0.8

* Calculated for blood flow rate 200 ml/min.
** Ion exchange resin.

are at particular risk of developing digoxin intoxication, the benefits of hemoperfusion (123) might outweigh the benefits and cost of administration of Fab fragments of digitalis antibodies (127, 128). Despite initial removal of paraquat by hemoperfusion (129), disappointing results were obtained with hemoperfusion in man (130–132). In very severe poisoning, death may supervene despite all therapy including hemoperfusion (132), but in certain situations repetitive (almost continuous) activated charcoal hemoperfusion treatment, can prevent pulmonary fibrosis, and induce a favorable clinical outcome (130, 133). In theophylline poisoning, seizures and other complications of high plasma concentration of theophylline, can be abolished with the rapid reduction of plasma theophylline concentrations with charcoal (89, 134–136), and resin (137, 138) hemoperfusion.

Indications for hemoperfusion in intoxication

Patients should only be considered for sorbent hemoperfusion if, in addition to fulfilling clinical criteria (Table 7), they also have been poisoned with adsorbable drugs such as those outlined in Table 5, and in Chapter 51. Drug concentrations may help as a guide to determining severity of toxicity (Table 7), but for some drugs the toxic concentration may be unknown (diquat, amanita phalloides), and often hemoperfusion may need to be considered at lower individual plasma drug concentrations, since in mixed poisonings drug effects may be additive. As mentioned above, it is probably more correct to use hemodialysis for severe drug intoxication with ethanol, methanol, ethylene glycol and salicylates in view of the rapid correction of both the drug intoxication and the associated metabolic abnormalities.

Since renal function is the primary determinant of the excretion of water soluble drugs, renal insufficiency or failure is associated with a high prevalence of drug side effects. Dialysis or hemoperfusion may be useful, where an excessive dosage is administered of drugs such as antibiotics aminoglycosides, chloramphenicol, digitalis glycosides, and possibly in the distribution phase after anticancer drug administration. Digoxin intoxication is commonly encoun-

tered and may require a judgement whether to use hemoperfusion or immunopharmacology in dialysis patients. In addition drug dosage adjustments are required for drugs that are removed with hemodialysis (e.g. antibiotics, [see also Chapter 51]).

Poison removal in conjunction with chelates

Aluminum overload syndromes associated with refractory bone disease (osteomalacia) or dialysis dementia, has seen the widespread use of deferoxamine in conjunction with continuous ambulatory peritoneal dialysis (139) hemodialysis (140) or hemoperfusion (70, 71) for removal of the deferoxamine-aluminum complex. Clinical improvement in the osteomalacic component of renal osteodystrophy (140, 141), and in encephalopathy (142) have been reported.

Iron overload in chronic dialysis patients, particularly those that possess the hemochromatosis alleles (HLA A_3, B_7, B_{14}) is also fairly common. Dialysis (70, 144), hemofiltration (145) or hemoperfusion (70–72) also in conjunction with deferoxamine may also be useful in these iron overload syndromes, since in hemoglobinopathy subjects long term iron deposition responsible for cardiomyopathy, diabetes, and other complications may improve with chelation treatment (146, 147).

Heavy metals and their salts are not removed efficiently by dialysis or hemoperfusion alone (148–150), while in hemodialysis metal removal may be enhanced with certain chelating agents, such as n-acetylcysteine (151), or cysteine (152). On the other hand, mercury (148), and thallium (149, 150) removal with hemoperfusion appears modest at best. Development of chelating microspheres (153) or chelate-metal groups for adsorption (152, 154) may prove useful clinically in the future for heavy metal removal.

HEMOPERFUSION IN HEPATIC ENCEPHALOPATHY

The pathogenesis of hepatic encephalopathy in fulminant hepatic failure, like that of uremia, is poorly understood and

Table 7. Clinical and drug concentration* criteria for hemoperfusion in poisoning.

Clinical	Drug	Serum conc ($\mu g/ml$)	($\mu mol/l$)	Method of choice
1. Progressive deterioration despite intensive care.	Phenobarbital	100	430	HP > HD
	Other barbiturates	50	200	HP
	Glutethimide	40	180	HP
2. Severe intoxication with mid-brain dysfunction.	Methaqualone	40	160	HP
	Salicylates	800	5,000	HD
	Theophylline	400	2,200	HP > HD
3. Development of complications of coma.	Paraquat	0.1	0.5	HP > HD
	Trichloroethanol	50	335	HP > HD
	Meprobamate	100	460	HP
4. Impairment of normal drug excretory function.				
5. Intoxication with agents producing metabolic and/or delayed effects.				
6. Intoxication with an extractable drug which can be removed at a greater rate than endogenous elimination.				

* Suggested concentrations only: Clinical condition may warrant intervention at lower concentrations, e.g. in mixed intoxications.

consequently therapy directed at removing specific toxins has been limited. Current hypotheses on pathogenesis, center arround excessive production of mercaptans (155), ammonia (156), false neurotransmitters (156), altered circulating plasma branched chain to aromatic amino acid ratio (156), and excessive production of gamma-aminobutyric acid which contributes to neural inhibition (157).

In 1972, Chang (158) reported improvement in consciousness in a 50 year old woman treated with charcoal hemoperfusion. This report stimulated the application of charcoal hemoperfusion in the management of fulminant hepatic encephalopathy in the most severe grade of coma (stage IV). Initial studies of small groups of patients, reported high success (49, 58, 159–162). In the earliest largest series of

patients, (163) the results were highly encouraging. Subsequent studies by the same group were dissappointing and felt to be due to a change in the bioengineering design (164, 165) and attention was for some time directed to the use of hemodialysis with polyacrylonitrile membrane dialyzers (164–167). Chang et al 9168) demonstrated that the optimum time for hemoperfusion to be initiated for increased survival in an experimental animal model, was stage III coma. Following this, human studies confirmed that the timing of hemoperfusion was critical in determining outcome (26), particularly since the deepest coma (stage IV) was associated with a high incidence of irreversible cerebral edema (78% in stage IV versus 49% in stage III) despite deepening of coma from grade III to grade IV after hemoperfusion was initiated.

Table 8. Effect of hemoperfusion in fulminant hepatic encephalopathy.

Study (year) (ref)	# of patients	Recovery of consciousness	Survival	Biochemical changes, and comments	Device/anticoagulant
Chang (1972) (158)	1	100%	100%	–	ACAC, heparin
Gazzard et al (1974) (163)	31	48%	39%	amino acids removed	Hemocol 300, heparin
Chang et al (1976) (159)	6	66%	16%	–	ACAC, heparin
Blume et al (1976) (160)	2	100%	100%	–	Hemocol 300, heparin
Yamazaki et al (1977) (224)	13	69%	38.5%	–	
Bartels et al (1977, 1981) (162, 225)	19	–	28%	hormones removed	Hemocol 300, heparin
Silk & Williams (1978) (165)	71	–	23.9%	–	Hemocol 300, heparin
Amano et al (1978) (174)	15	40%	20%	amino acids fell in blood and csf	Petroleum based collodion coated (200 g), heparin
Gelfand et al (1978) (173)	10	90%	40%	amino acid B/A** ratio rose, csf cAMP rose	Hemocol 300, heparin
Odaka et al (1978) (49)	10*	70%	30%	amino acids removed	petroleum based, ACAC coated (130 g), heparin
Agishi et al (1980) (54)	18	70%	22%	–	4 types used, heparin
Gimson et al (1980) (25)	12	nr	nr	–	Hemocol 100, heparin, prostacyclin
Gimson et al (1982) (26)	31 Grade III	68%	65%	cerebral edema 49%	Hemocol 100, heparin,
	45 Grade IV	22%	20%	cerebral edema 78%	prostacyclin
Takahashi (1983) (169)	123		Early 41% Late 21%		Not given, heparin
Cordopatri et al (1982) (181)	2	100%	100%	BTG, platelets preserved	Adsorba 300C, prostacyclin
Williams (1983) (226)	as in (26)			MMS removed which inhibit Na/K ATPase	Hemocol 100, heparin, prostacyclin
Bihari et al (1983) (185)	13 Grade IV		42%		XAD-7 albumin coated resin 260 g
	6 Grade III				
Kennedy et al (1985) (182)	12 Grade IV		33%	platelets fell 50%	Hemocol 100, heparin

** Includes 5 patients in Stage III coma, BTG = beta-thromboglobulin.
** B/A ratio = branched chain-aromatic acid ratio (see text).

Studies reporting the use of charcoal hemoperfusion in fulminant hepatic encephalopathy are shown in Table 8. In comparison to conservative therapy alone, which is associated with a 17.6% (169) to 18.7% (170) survival, in some series a substantially greater survival was achieved, with 65% survival of those in stage III coma being reported (26). Berk (171) however, pointed out that survival with charcoal hemoperfusion may not differ significantly from that achieved with conservative management. The focus on survival, however, fails to emphasize that in most series a large number of patients recover consciousness at some point during the hemoperfusion treatment schedule, perhaps indicating alteration (or removal) of factors responsible for induction of coma. The main goal of therapy is to induce reversal of coma for sufficiently long to allow spontaneous hepatocellular regeneration, since experimentally it has been shown that substances which are cytotoxic to hepatocytes *in vitro* are absorbed onto charcoal (172). Attention should now be directed at instituting hemoperfusion at a much earlier stage of hepatic encephalopathy (prior to stage IV, when irreversible changes, most likely cerebral edema with brain-stem herniation, may have already occurred).

The substances which may be relevant to the development of hepatic encephalopathy and that are removed by sorbent hemoperfusion are shown in Table 9. Gazzard et al (163), demonstrated that the aromatic amino acids, particularly methionine, were reduced with charcoal hemoperfusion, while Gelfand et al (173) demonstrated in plasma and also in cerebrospinal fluid that the ratio of branched chain to aromatic amino acids increased after hemoperfusion. (The ratio of branched chain to aromatic amino acids holds an inverse correlation with the degree of hepatic coma). Amino acid removal has also been demonstrated by Amano et al (174), and Odaka et al (58), while it has been demonstrated that after hemoperfusion in man, serum inhibitors of brain Na+ K+ ATPase are reduced with charcoal and resin hemoperfusion (175). Serum inhibitors of the enzyme are thought to play a role in the production of hepatic coma (176, 177).

Coagulation abnormalities, including increased platelet aggregation (22, 27, 178, 179), release of platelet factors and increased heparin consumption (180) are associated with fulminant hepatic failure itself. Hemoperfusion may induce

Table 9. Substances relevant to hepatic failure removed with sorbent hemoperfusion.

Amino acids*	Fatty acids – oleic, hexanoic, octanoic
Aromatic > branched chain	N-valeric
(Ammonia)*	(Glucose)*
Bile acids*	Mercaptan
Bilirubin*	Middle molecules
(Calcium)*	Norepinephrine
Coagulation factors*	Octopamine
(Cyclic AMP)*	Phenols*
Dopamine	Protein bound molecules
Epinephrine	Inhibitor of Na/K ATPase*

* Studied *in vivo*; ( ) Ineffectively removed.

coagulation disturbances in hepatic encephalopathy, leading some investigators to use routine infusions of platelets and fresh frozen plasma following hemoperfusion (173), and others to use prostacyclin (26, 181) to prevent the primary as well as the secondary coagulation disturbances from hemoperfusion for hepatic encephalopathy. However, others have disputed the need for prostacyclin (182).

Controlled clinical trials of hemoperfusion are, at present, logistically impossible, while optimal timing and frequency of hemoperfusion have not been determined. It has been suggested by Berk (171), on the basis of kinetic modeling, that hepatic toxins move in a slowly equilibrating pool and for optimal results detoxification procedures should be performed every 12 h. Charcoal hemoperfusion does not supply nutritive or reparative properties associated with normal hepatic function, nor does it adsorb all the protein bound substances thought to produce hepatic coma. For this reason, some investigators have suggested the use of resin hemoperfusion (183, 184), and introduced this in man on a pilot basis (185), and others have designed plasma perfusion apparatus to adsorb protein bound materials and to avoid contact with blood to circumvent the hemostatic abnormalities (186), induced with hemoperfusion. It is not yet possible to design a specific sorbent for removing the hepatic failure 'toxin'. Like uremia, hepatic encephalopathy is more likely of multifactorial origin and, at present, the design of a specific sorbent cannot be undertaken.

On the basis of the results shown in Table 8, it is reasonable to suggest that hemoperfusion be performed for fulminant hepatic encephalopathy, especially in drug induced liver disease (187) where the outcome is better than for hepatic failure associated with viral infections. Consideration of hemoperfusion might also be part of a vigorous liver transplant program.

Indications for hemoperfusion

At present, it is impossible to give definitive criteria for the adoption of charcoal hemoperfusion in fulminant hepatic encephalopathy, since survival from this disorder depends on many factors such as the etiology of the liver disease, age and sex. Clear results will only emerge from a large, well-conducted controlled clinical trial. However, until alternative approaches are better defined, hemoperfusion should be used in carefully selected patients, at an early stage of coma (stage III) and perhaps more frequently than has been the position so far, since hemoperfusion probably represents the most effective available treatment for acute fulminant hepatic failure at the present time.

OTHER USES OF SORBENT HEMOPERFUSION

Schizophrenia

In 1977 Wagemaker and Cade (188) reported dramatic improvement of five of six schizophrenic patients treated with regular (once weekly) hemodialysis; later they observed similar beneficial results in an additional series of patients (in 16 out of 23). They attributed the therapeutic effect to removal of leucine-endorphin by dialysis (189), although this was not confirmed by others (190). Several clinical investigators were stimulated to apply other treatment techniques such as hemoperfusion and hemofiltration in the treatment of this serious psychiatric disorder (191–194). Controlled clinical trials of dialysis in schizophrenia have shown little clinical improvement in psychiatric symptoms (195).

Psoriasis

In a similar fashion favorable results have been found in patients with severe psoriasis treated with peritoneal dialysis (196) and hemodialysis (197). Others, however, have observed psoriasis developing during regular dialysis (198) and have noted negative results with hemodialysis treatment (199). Patients with psoriasis have also been treated with hemoperfusion and hemofiltration (200, 201). As with schizophrenia controlled clinical trials using hemodialysis have demonstrated little value (199).

Anti-cancer drug removal

Since the use of anti-cancer drugs may be limited by the presence of hepatic or renal dysfunction, the full benefits of such drugs as adriamycin or methotrexate may be curtailed in patients with diseases of these systems. Several authors have attempted to remove anti-cancer drugs from patients with inadvertent excessive dosage of these drugs. On the other hand, exposure of patients to a high therapeutic drug load with subsequent rapid removal might obviate the known tissue toxicity of high dose anti-cancer drug therapy (90, 202).

Although initial reports of uncoated charcoal hemoperfusion in removal of methotrexate were encouraging, subsequent reports of XAD-4 resin or uncoated charcoal hemoperfusion and hemodialysis or peritoneal dialysis have been somewhat disappointing (202, 203). Methotrexate removal is more efficiently achieved with the use of uncoated charcoal hemoperfusion, than with XAD-4 resin hemoperfusion or with hemodialysis or peritoneal dialysis. But, although substantial methotrexate clearance is initially achieved, the charcoal columns rapidly saturate and become inactive. Therefore, there is no substantial change in drug elimination kinetics (202). It is unlikely, consequently, that tissue concentrations of methotrexate can be substantially reduced, although intensive charcoal hemoperfusion has been successful in reducing plasma methotrexate concentrations in man (204).

Similarly, substantial removal of the anthracycline antibiotic and anti-cancer drug adriamycin can be achieved with charcoal hemoperfusion and substantial increases in drug elimination rates can be achieved (90). However, reduction of tissue levels of this drug with hemoperfusion probably would require prolonged hemoperfusion.

Regional hemoperfusion for removal of anticancer drugs after intracarotid chemotherapy for brain tumors, has been associated with reduction of systemic exposure and of consequent side effects in man (205).

Immunoadsorption

Specific adsorption of immune proteins on antigen or antibody coated carrier particles, in hemoperfusion columns, has also been developed. This technique was introduced by Terman and co-workers (206), who have shown that it is possible to remove antibodies to such proteins or polypeptides as bovine serum albumin, deoxyribonucleic acid and antiglomerular basement membrane antibody from blood percolated through immunoadsorbent systems. DNA-collodion coated charcoal in an extracorporeal column removed significant quantities of single stranded anti-DNA antibodies and immune complexes from the circulating blood of a patient with systemic lupus erythematosus, with reduction of subendothelial glomerular deposits on comparison of pre- and post-treatment renal biopsy specimens (207). The technique may also benefit hyperacute renal xenograft rejection in animals (208). In a dog model with spontaneous breast cancer, passage of blood over a column containing Staphylococcal A protein was associated with regression and complete disappearance of the breast cancer lesions (209). Studies of this technique in human cancer are underway (210–211) and the results are awaited with considerable interest. The technique has also been extended to the removal of poisons by immunoadsorption, with successful reversal of digoxin poisoning in dogs (212) and in man (213) after hemoperfusion of blood through digoxin antibody-coated polyacrolein microsphere beads.

Miscellaneous

Hemoperfusion has also been used in the removal of bilirubin (214), and plasma lipids (215) as well as in a variety of other conditions including sepsis (216). The role of hemoperfusion in these conditions is not yet defined.

FUTURE DEVELOPMENTS

It is likely that the future development of treatment of uremia will involve the hybridization of sorbent technology in conjunction with dialysis/hemofiltration techniques. The wide spectrum, of uremic toxins is a major barrier to development in this field. Current interest in this complex area centers around the removal of middle molecules and recent attention has also been directed toward the removal of urea, which has been the classical 'marker' of uremia. Urea sorbents which combine the necessary properties of effectiveness and biocompatibility along with control of pH and electrolyte abnormalities are a feasible prospect for the treatment of uremia. At present, however, no sorbents have been developed which have all of these desirable properties.

Hemoperfusion has a definitive role in the management of acute drug intoxication, less so in the management of uremia, and hepatic encephalopathy. It is likely that the specific extracorporeal immunoadsorbent columns will be developed, which not only offer the prospect of treatment of severe refractory immune mediated diseases but theoretically may allow examination of the role specific antibodies in the mediation of such diseases, and in the area of drug neutralization.

REFERENCES

1. Yatzidis H: A convenient haemoperfusion micro-apparatus over charcoal for the treatment of endogenous and exogenous intoxications. Its use as an artificial kidney. *Proc Eur Dial Transplant Assoc* 1: 83, 1964

2. Dunea G, Kolff WJ: Clinical experience with the Yatzidis charcoal artificial kidney. *Trans Am Soc Artif Intern Organs* 11: 178, 1965

3. Chang TMS: Semipermeable aqueous microcapsules (artifical cells): with emphasis on experiments in an extracorporeal shunt system. *Trans Am Soc Artif Intern Organs* 12: 13, 1966

4. Asher WJ: Introduction to sorbents. in *Sorbents and Their Clinical Applications*, edited by Giordano C, New York, Academic Press Inc, 1980, p 3

5. Denti E, Walker JM: Activated carbon: properties, selection and evaluation. in *Sorbents and Their Clinical Applications*, edited by Giordano C, New York, Academic Press Inc, 1980, p 101

6. Denti E, Luboz MP, Tessore V: Adsorption characteristics of cellulose acetate coated charcoals. *J Biomed Mater Res* 9: 143, 1975

7. Winchester JF, Ratcliffe JG, Carlyle E, Kennedy AC: Solute, amino acid, and hormone changes with coated charcoal hemoperfusion in uremia. *Kidney Int* 14: 74, 1978

8. Kokot F, Pietrek J, Seredynski M: Influence of haemoperfusion on plasma levels of hormones and B-methyldigoxin. *Proc Eur Dial Transplant Assoc* 15: 604, 1978

9. Cornelis R, Ringoir S, Mees L, Hoste J: Behavior of trace metals during hemoperfusion. *Miner Electrolyte Metab* 4: 123, 1980

10. Hagstam KE, Larsson LE, Thysell H: Experimental studies on charcoal haemoperfusion in phenobarbital intoxication and uraemia, including histopathologic findings. *Acta Med Scand* 180: 593, 1966

11. Winchester JF: Hemoperfusion in uremia. in: *Sorbents and Thier Clinical Applications*, edited by Giordano C, New York, Academic Press Inc, 1980, p 387

12. Chang TMS: Microcapsule artificial kidney in replacement of renal function. With emphasis on adsorbent hemoperfusion. in: *Replacement of Renal Function by Dialysis*, First Edition, edited by Drukker W, Parsons FM, Maher JF, The Hague, Boston, London, Martinus Nijhoff, 1978, p 217

13. Odaka M, Tabata Y, Kobayashi H, Nomura Y, Soma M, Hirasawa H, Sato H, Suenaga E, Nabeta K: Three hour maintenance haemodialysis combining direct haemoperfusion and haemodialysis. *Proc Eur Dial Transplant Assoc* 13: 257, 1976

14. Ota K, Ohta T, Kobayashi M, Yoshida S, Kaneko I, Agishi T, Sugihara M: Petroleum based activated charcoal for direct haemoperfusion. *Proc Eur Dial Transplant Assoc* 13: 250, 1976

15. Stefoni S, Feliciangeli G, Coli L, Bonomini V: Evaluation of a new coated charcoal for hemoperfusion in uremia. *Int J Artif*

Organs 2: 320, 1979

16. Craddock PR, Fehr J, Brigham KL, Kronenberg R, Jacobs HS: Complement and leukocyte-mediated pulmonary dysfunction in hemodialysis. *N Engl J Med* 296: 769, 1977

17. Pott G, Voss B, Lohmann J, Zundorf P: Loss of fibronectin in plasma of patients with shock and septicaemia, and after haemoperfusion in patients with severe poisoning. *J Clin Chem Clin Biochem* 20: 333, 1982

18. Gurland HJ, Fernandez JC, Samtleben W, Castro LA: Sorbent membranes used in a conventional dialyzer format: In vitro and clinical evaluation. *Artif Organs* 2: 372, 1978

19. Davis TA, Cowsar DR, Harrison SD, Tanquary AC: Artificial carbon fibers for hemoperfusion. *Trans Am Soc Artif Intern Organs* 20: 353, 1974

20. Malchesky PS, Varnes WG, Nokoff R, Nose Y: The charcoal capillary haemoperfusion system. *Proc Eur Dial Transplant Assoc* 13: 242, 1976

21. van Berlo AMW, Poelmans AP, van der Pols, Aarts PJM, Verkooyen AHM: Comparing in vitro adsorption studies with the filmadsorber and other haemoperfusion devices. in: *Biomaterials in Artificial Organs*, edited by Paul JP, Gaylor JDS, Courtney JM, Gilchrist T, London, Basingstoke, The Macmillan Press Ltd, 1984, p 155

22. Weston MJ, Langley PG, Rubin MH, Hanid MA, Mellon P, Williams R: Platelet function in fulminant hepatic failure and effect of charcoal haemoperfusion. *Gut* 18: 897, 1977

23. Winchester JF, Forbes CD, Courtney JM, Reavey M, Prentice CRM: Effect of sulphinpyrazone and aspirin on platelet adhesion to activated charcoal and dialysis membranes in vitro. *Thromb Res* 11: 443, 1977

24. Bunting S, Moncada S, Vane JR, Woods HF, Weston MJ: Prostacyclin improves haemocompatibility during charcoal haemoperfusion. in: *Prostacyclin*, edited by Vane JR, Bergstrom S, New York, Raven Press, 1979, p 361

25. Gimson AES, Langley PG, Hughes RD, Canalese J, Mellon PG, Williams R, Woods HF, Weston MJ: Prostaclyclin to prevent platelet activation during charcoal haemoperfusion in fulminant hepatic failure. *Lancet* 1: 173, 1980

26. Gimson AES, Braude S, Mellon PJ, Canalese J, Williams R: Earlier charcoal haemoperfusion in fulminant hepatic failure. *Lancet* 2: 681, 1982

27. Woods HF, Weston MJ, Bunting S, Moncada S, Vane J: Prostacyclin eliminates the thrombocytopenia associated with charcoal hemoperfusion and minimizes heparin and fibrinogen consumption. *Artif Organs* 4: 176, 1980

28. Mauer S, Chavers BM, Kjellstrand CM: Treatment of an infant with severe chloramphenicol intoxication, using charcoal-column hemoperfusion. *J Pediatr* 96: 136, 1980

29. Winchester JF: *Evaluation of Sorbent Haemoperfusion in Poisoning and Uraemia*. MD Thesis, University of Glasgow, Scotland, 1980

30. Lindsay RM, Prentice CRM, Davidson JF, Burton JA, McNicol GP: Haemostatic changes during dialysis associated with thrombus formation on dialysis membranes. *Br Med J* 4: 454, 1972

31. Chang TMS, Chirito E, Barre B, Cole C, Hewish M: Clinical performance-characteristics of a new combined system for simultaneous hemoperfusion-hemodialysis-ultrafiltration in series. *Trans Am Soc Artif Intern Organs* 21: 502, 1975

32. Stefoni S, Coli L, Feliciangeli G, Baldrati L, Bonomini V: Regular hemoperfusion in regular dialysis treatment. A long-term study. *Int J Artif Organs* 3: 348, 1980

33. Muirhead EE, Reid AF: Resin artificial kidney. *J Lab Clin Med* 33: 841, 1948

34. Schreiner GE: The role of hemodialysis (artificial kidney) in acute poisoning. *Arch Intern Med* 102: 896, 1958

35. Rosenbaum JL, Onesti G, Heider C: The removal of cation from dogs with an ion-exchange column. *JAMA* 180: 762, 1962

36. Kissack AS, Gliedman L, Karlson KE: Studies with ion exchange resins. *Trans Am Soc Artif Intern Organs* 8: 219, 1962

37. Nealon TF Jr, Ching N: An extracorporeal device to lower blood ammonia levels in hepatic coma. *Trans Am Soc Artif Intern Organs* 8: 226, 1962

38. Yatzidis H, Voudiclari S, Oreopoulos D, Tsaparas N, Triantaphyllidis D, Gavras C, Stavroulaki A: Treatment of severe barbiturate poisoning. *Lancet* 2: 216, 1965

39. Chang TMS, Gonda A, Dirks JH, Malave N: Clinical evaluation of chronic intermittent and short term hemoperfusion in patients with chronic renal failure using semipermeable microcapsules (artificial cells) formed from membrane coated activated charcoal. *Trans Am Soc Artif Intern Organs* 17: 246, 1971

40. Chang TMS, Migchelsen M: Characterization of possible 'toxic' metabolites in uremia and hepatic coma based on the clearance spectrum for larger molecules by the ACAC microcapsule artificial kidney. *Trans Am Soc Artif Intern Organs* 19: 314, 1973

41. Chang TMS, Migchelsen M, Coffey JF, Stark R: Serum middle molecule levels in uremia during long term intermittent hemoperfusion with ACAD (coated charcoal) microcapsule artificial kidney. *Trans Am Soc Artif Intern Organs* 20: 364, 1974

42. Oules R, Asaba H, Neuhauser M, Yahiel V, Gunnarsson B, Bergström J, Fürst P: Removal of uremic small and middle molecules and free amino acids by carbon hemoperfusion. *Trans Am Soc Artif Intern Organs* 23: 583, 1977

43. Chang TMS: Assessment of clinical trials of charcoal hemoperfusion in uremic patients. *Clin Nephrol* 11: 111, 1979

44. Rosenbaum JL, Kramer MS, Raja R, Henriques M: Hemoperfusion in uremia: Effect of time, solute competition and biocompatibility on column adsorption. in: *Hemoperfusion, Kidney and Liver Support and Detoxification,* edited by Sideman S, Chang TMS, Washington DC, Hemisphere Publishing Corp, 1980, p 245

45. Gelfand MC, Winchester JF: Hemoperfusion results in uremia. *Clin Nephrol* 1: 107, 1979

46. Trznadel K, Walasek L, Kidawa Z, Lutz W: Comparative studies on the effect of hemoperfusion and hemodialysis on the elimination of some uremic toxins. *Clin Nephrol* 10: 229, 1978

47. Weber WJ, Morris JC: Kinetics of adsorption on carbon from solutions. *Proc Am Soc Civil Eng* 89: 31, 1963

48. Martin AM, Gibbins JK, Kimmitt J, Rennie F: Hemodialysis and hemoperfusion in the treatment of uremic pericarditis. A study of 13 cases. *Dial Transplant* 8: 135, 1979

49. Odaka M, Kirasawa H, Kobayashi H, Ohkawa M, Soeda K, Tabata Y, Soma M, Sato H: Clinical and fundamental studies of cellulose coated bead-shaped charcoal haemoperfusion in chronic renal failure. in: *Hemoperfusion, Kidney and Liver Support and Detoxification,* edited by Sideman S, Chang TMS, Washington DC, Hemisphere Publishing Corp, 1980, p 45

50. Trznadel K, Luciak M, Wyszogrodzka M: Effect of haemoperfusion on the left ventricular systolic function in patients with chronic uraemia. *Acta Med Pol* 22: 75, 1981

51. Asaba H: Uremic middle molecules. Accumulation, renal excretion and elimination by extracorporeal treatment. *Scand J Urol Nephrol* Supplement 67: 1, 1982

52. Asaba H, Bergström J, Fürst P, Gunnarsson B, Neuhauser M, Oules R, Yahile V: Removal of endogenous middle molecules by hemoperfusion. *Artif Organs* 3: 132, 1979

53. Otsubo O, Kuzuhara K, Simada Y, Yamauchi Y, Takahashi I, Yamada Y, Otsubo K, Inou T: Treatment of uraemic peripheral neuritis by direct haemoperfusion with activated charcoal. *Proc Eur Dial Transplant Assoc* 16: 731, 1979

54. Agishi T, Yamashita N, Ota K: Clinical results of direct charcoal hemoperfusion for endogenous and exogenous intoxication. in: *Hemoperfusion, Kidney and Liver Support and Detoxification,* edited by Sideman S, Chang TMS, Washington DC, Hemisphere Publishing Corp, 1980, p 255

55. Chang TMS, Barre P, Kuruvilla S: Long-term reduced time hemoperfusion-hemodialysis compared to standard dialysis. A preliminary crossover analysis. *Trans Am Soc Artif Intern Organs* 31: 572, 1985

56. Henderson IS, Kennedy AC: Long-term evaluation of charcoal haemoperfusion combined with dialysis for uraemic patients. in: *Biomaterials in Artificial Organs,* edited by Paul JP, Gaylor JDS, Courtney JM, Gilchrist T, London, Basingstoke, The Macmillan Press Ltd, 1984, p 72

57. Siemsen AW, Dunea G, Mamdani BH, Guruprakash G: Charcoal hemoperfusion for chronic renal failure. *Nephron* 22: 386, 1978

58. Odaka M, Tabata Y, Kabayashi H, Nomura Y, Soma A, Hirasawa A, Sato H: Clinical experience of bead-shaped charcoal hemoperfusion in chronic renal failure and fulminant hepatic failure. in: *Artificial Kidney, Artificial Liver and Artificial Cells,* edited by Chang TMS, New York, Plenum Press, 1978, p 79

59. Bonomini V, Stefoni S, Feliciangeli G, Coli L, Scolari MP, Orsi C, Nanni Costa A, Prandini R, Galanti S: Shortened treatment time by combined hemodialysis and hemoperfusion. *Contr Nephrol* 44: 57, 1985

60. Bonomini V, Stefoni S, Feliciangeli G, Coli L, Scolari MP, Prandini R, Casciani CU, Taccone Gallucci, Albertazzi A, Mioli V, Mastrangelo F: Present status of hemoperfusion/hemodialysis in Italy. *Appl Biochem Biotechnol* 10: 157, 1984

61. Stefoni S, Coli L, Feliciangeli G, Scolari MP, Bonomini V: Hemoperfusion in reduced-time programmes for chronic uremia. Long term results. *Int J Artif Organs* 9: 297, 1986

62. Barre PE, Gonda A, Chang TMS: Routine clinical applications of hemodialysis-hemoperfusion in chronic renal failure: case reports. *Int J Artif Organs* 9: 305, 1986

63. Espinosa-Melendez E, Bourgouin PA, Chang TMS: Combined hemoperfusion-hemodialysis in the treatment of uremic patients with vascular access problems: case reports. *Int J Artif Organs* 9: 309, 1986

64. Stefoni S, Nanni Costa A, Liviano D'Arcangelo G, Biavati M, Ianelli S, Bonomini V: Biocompatibility of charcoal hemoperfusion. Effects of long-term treatment on lymphocyte characteristics and function. *Int J Artif Organs* 9: 301, 1986

65. Capodicasa G, De Santo NG, Galione A, Bellavia C, Annaloro R, Vaccaro F, Picone F, Vinti V, Davi G, Rapisarda LM, Giordano C: CAPD plus hemoperfusion once a week for end stage renal disease. *Int J Artif Organs* 5: 125, 1981

66. Capodicasa G, Davi G, Picone F, Mattina A, Gianetto V, Vinti V, Vaccaro F, Strano A, De Santo NG, Giordano C: Platelet thromboxane formation and BTG levels after intensive charcoal hemoperfusion in uremia or regular hemodialysis treatment. *Int J Artif Organs* 6: 241, 1983

67. Winchester JF, Ash SR: Hemoperfusion for uremia: Past present and future. *Kidney Int* 28 (Suppl 17): S127, 1985

68. Hone PWE, Farrell PC: Urea adsorption capacity of sulfonat-

ed polystyrenes. *asaio J* 3: 1, 1980

69. Ash SR, Barile RG, Wilcox PG, Wright DL, Thornhill JA, Dhein CR, Kessler DP, Wang N-HL: The sorbent suspension reciprocating dialyzer: a device with minimal sorbent saturation. *asaio J* 4: 28, 1981

70. Chang TMS, Barre P: Effect of desferrioxamine on removal of aluminium and iron by coated charcoal haemoperfusion and haemodialysis. *Lancet* 2: 1051, 1983

71. Hakim RM, Schulman JM, Lazarus JM: Hemoperfusion in the treatment of aluminum (Al) and iron (Fe) induced bone disease. *Abstracts Am Soc Nephrol*, 18: 65A, 1985

72. Winchester JF: Management of iron overload. *Semin Nephrol* 4 (suppl 1): 22, 1986

73. Vale JA, Meredith T, Buckley B: ABC of poisoning. Eliminating poisons. *Br Med J* 289: 366, 1984

74. Litovitz T, Veltri J: 1984 Annual report of the American Association of Poison Control Centers. *Am J Emerg Med* 3: 423, 1985

75. Henry JA, Cassidy SL: Membrane stabilising ability: A major cause of fatal poisoning. *Lancet* 1: 1414, 1986

76. Litovitz TL, Normann SA, Veltri JC: 1985 Annual report of the American Association of Poison Control Centers National Data Collection System. *Am J Emerg Med* 4: 427, 1986

77. Haddad LM: A general approach to poisoning. in: *Office Procedures: Office Management of Poisoning*, edited by Winchester JF, Philadelphia, Hanley and Belfus Inc, 1986, p 325

78. Clemmesen C, Nilsson E: Therapeutic trends in the treatment of barbiturate poisoning: The Scandinavian method. *Clin Pharmacol Ther* 2: 220, 1961

79. Lawson AA, Mitchell I: Patients with acute poisoning seen in a general medical unit (1960–1971). *Br Med J* 4 153, 1972

80. Reed CE, Driggs MF, Foote CC: Acute barbiturate intoxication: A study of 300 cases based on a physiologic system of classification of the severity of the intoxication. *Ann Intern Med* 37: 290, 1952

81. Winchester JF, Gelfand MC, Tilstone WJ: Hemoperfusion in drug intoxication – Clinical and laboratory aspects. *Drug Metab Rev* 8: 69, 1978

82. Maher JF, Schreiner GE: The dialysis of poisons and drugs. *Trans Am Soc Artif Intern Organs* 13: 369, 1967

83. Winchester JF, Gelfand MC, Knepshield JH, Schreiner GE: Dialysis and hemoperfusion of poisons and drugs – Update. *Trans Am Soc Artif Intern Organs* 23: 762, 1977

84. Cohan SL, Winchester JF, Gelfand MC: Treatment of intoxications by charcoal hemadsorption. *Drug Metab Rev* 13: 681, 1982

85. Rosenbaum JL, Kramer MS, Raja RM, Krug MJ, Boliday CG: Current status of hemoperfusion in toxicology. *Clin Toxicol* 17: 493, 1980

86. Winchester JF, Tilstone WJ, Edwards RO, Gilchrist T, Kennedy AC: Hemoperfusion for enhanced drug elimination – A kinetic analysis in paracetamol poisoning. *Trans Am Soc Artif Intern Organs* 20: 358, 1974

87. Gibson TP, Atkinson AJ: Effect of changes in intercompartmental rate constants on drug removal during hemoperfusion. *J Pharm Sci* 67: 1178, 1978

88. Zmuda MJ: Resin hemoperfusion in dogs intoxicated with ethychlorvynol (Placidyl), *Kidney Int* 17: 303, 1980

89. Ehlers SM, Zaske DE, Sawchuck RJ: Massive theophylline overdose. Rapid elimination by charcoal hemoperfusion. *JAMA* 240: 474, 1978

90. Winchester JF, Rahman A, Tilstone WJ, Kessler A, Mortensen L, Schreiner GE, Schein PS: Sorbent removal of adriamycin in vitro and in vivo. *Cancer Treat Rep* 63: 1787, 1979

91. Pond S, Rosenberg J, Benowitz NL, Takki S: Pharmacokinetics of haemoperfusion in drug overdose. *Clin Pharmacokinet* 4: 329, 1979

92. Verpooten GA, De Broe ME: Combined hemoperfusion – hemodialysis in severe poisoning: Kinetics of drug extraction. *Resuscitation* 11: 275, 1984

93. Cutler RE, Forland SC, St John Hammond PG, Evans RJ: Extracorporeal removal of drugs and poisons by hemodialysis and hemoperfusion. *Annu Rev Pharmacol Toxicol* 27: 169, 1987

94. Farrell PC: Commentary: Acute drug intoxication and extracorporeal intervention. *asaio J* 3: 39, 1980

95. De Broe ME, Bismuth C, De Groot G, Heath A, Okonek S, Ritz DR, Verpooten GA, Volans GN, Widdop B: Haemoperfusion: a useful therapy for a severly poisoned patient? *Hum Toxicol* 5: 11, 1986

96. Lorch JA, Garella S: Hemoperfusion to treat intoxications. *Ann Intern Med* 91: 301, 1979

97. Maher JF: In discussion in hemoperfusion for poisoning – Is it really necessary? in: *Controversies in Nephrology*, Volume 2, edited by Schreiner GE, Winchester JF, Washington DC, Georgetown Nephrology Press, 1980, p 228

98. Hampel G, Crome P, Widdop B, Goulding R: Experience with fixed-bed charcoal haemoperfusion in the treatment of severe drug intoxication. *Arch Toxicol* 45: 133, 1980

99. Uldall PR: Controlled trial of resin hemoperfusion for the treatment of drug overdose at Toronto Western Hospital (TWH). *Trans Am Soc Artif Intern Organs* 28: 676, 1982

100. De Broe ME, Verpooten BA, Van Haesebrouck B: Recent experience with prolonged hemoperfusion-hemodialysis treatment. *Artif Organs* 3: 188, 1979

101. Winchester JF: Methanol, isopropyl alcohol, higher alcohols, ethylene glycol, cellosolves, acetone and oxalate, in: *Clinical Management of Poisoning and Drug Overdose*, edited by Haddad LM, Winchester JF, Philadelphia, WB Saunders Co, 1983, p 393

102. Winchester JF: Active methods for detoxification: Oral sorbents, forced diuresis, hemoperfusion, and hemodialysis, in: *Clinical Management of Poisoning and Drug Overdose*, edited by Haddad LM, Winchester JF, Philadelphia, WB Saunders Co, 1983, p 154

103. Proudfoot AT: Salicylates and salicylamides, in: *Clinical Management of Poisoning and Drug Overdose*, edited by Haddad LM, Winchester JF, Philadelphia, WB Saunders, 1983, p 575

104. Winters RW, White JS, Hughes MC, Ordway NC: Disturbances of acid-base equilibrium in salicylate intoxication. *Pediatrics* 23: 260, 1959

105. Gabow PA, Anderson RJ, Potts DE, Schrier RW: Acid-base disturbances in the salicylate-intoxicated adult. *Arch Intern Med* 138: 1481, 1978

106. Anderson RJ, Potts DE, Gabow PA, Rumack BH, Schrier RW: Unrecognized adult salicylate intoxication. *Ann Intern Med* 85: 745, 1976

107. Rumack BH, Peterson RG: Acetaminophen overdose: Incidence, diagnosis, and management in 416 patients. *Pediatrics* 62: 898, 1978

108. Prescott LF, Illingworth RR, Critchley JA, Stewart MJ, Adam RD, Proudfoot AT: Intravenous N-acetylcysteine. *Br Med J* 2: 1097, 1979

109. Gazzard BG, Willson RA, Weston MJ, Thompson R, Williams R: Charcoal haemoperfusion for paracetamol overdose. *Br J Clin Pharmacol* 1: 217, 1974

110. Winchester JF, Gelfand MC, Helliwell M, Vale JA, Goulding R, Schreiner GE: Extracorporeal treatment of salicylate or

acetaminiphen poisoning – Is there a role? *Arch Intern Med* 141: 370, 1981

111. Helliwell M, Vale JA, Goulding R: Hemoperfusion in 'late' paracetamol poisoning. *Hum Toxicol* 1: 25, 1981

112. Diaz-Buxo JA, Farmer CD, Chandler TY: Hemoperfusion in the treatment of amitriptyline poisoning. *Trans Am Soc Artif Intern Organs* 24: 699, 1978

113. Trafford JAP, Jones RH, Evans R, Sharp P, Sharpstone P, Cook J: Haemoperfusion with R-004 amberlite resin for treating acute poisoning. *Br Med J* 2: 1453, 1977

114. Trafford A, Sharpstone P, O'Neal H: Haemoperfusion in tricyclic antidepressant poisoning. *Lancet* 1: 155, 1980

115. Heath A, Wickstrom I, Ahlmen J: Haemoperfusion in tricyclic antidepressant poisoning. *Lancet* 1: 155, 1980

116. Crome P, Braithwaite RA, Widdop B, Medd RK: Haemoperfusion in clinical and experimental tricyclic antidepressant poisoning. in: *Hemoperfusion, Kidney and Liver Support and Detoxification*, edited by Sideman S, Chang TMS, Washington DC, Hemisphere Publishing Corp, 1980, p 301

117. Pedersen RS: Haemoperfusion in tricyclic antidepressant poisoning. *Lancet* 1: 154, 1980

118. Carvallo A, Ramirez B, Honig H, Knepshield J, Schreiner GE, Gelfand MC: Treatment of digitalis intoxication by charcoal hemoperfusion. *Trans Am Soc Artif Intern Organs* 22: 718, 1976

119. Gibson TP, Lucas SV, Nelson HA, Atkinson AJ, Okita GT, Ivanovich P: Hemoperfusion removal of digoxin from dogs. *J Lab Clin Med* 91: 673, 1978

120. Shah G, Nelson HA, Atkinson AJ, Okita GT, Ivanovich P, Gibson TP: Effect of hemoperfusion on the pharmacokinetics of digitoxin in dogs. *J Lab Clin Med* 93: 370, 1979

121. Marbury T, Mahoney J, Juncos L, Conti R, Cade R: Advanced digoxin toxicity in renal failure – Treatment with charcoal hemoperfusion. *South Med J* 72: 279, 1979

122. Tobin M, Cerra F, Steinvach J, Mookerjee B: Hemoperfusion in digitalis intoxication: A comparative study of coated versus uncoated charcoal. *Trans Am Soc Artif Intern Organs* 23: 730, 1977

123. Hoy WE, Gibson TP, Rivero AJ, Jain JK, Talley TT, Bayer RM, Montondo DF, Freeman RB: XAD-4 resin hemoperfusion for digitoxic patients with renal failure. *Kidney Int* 23: 79, 1983

124. Warren SE, Fanestil DF: Digoxin overdose: Limitations of hemoperfusion – hemodialysis treatment. *JAMA* 242: 2100, 1979

125. Freed CR, Gerber JG, Cal J, Rumak BH, Nies AS: Hemoperfusion in drug overdose. *JAMA* 241: 1575, 1979

126. Slattery JR, Koup JR: Hemoperfusion in the management of digoxin toxicity. Is it warranted? *Clin Pharmacokinet* 4: 395, 1979

127. Wenger TL, Butler VP Jr, Haber E, Smith TW: Treatment of 63 severely digitalis-toxic patients with digoxin specific antibody fragments. *J Am Coll Cardiol* 5 ([5] Suppl A): 118A, 1985

128. Colburn WA: Specific antibodies and Fab fragments to alter the pharmacokinetics and reverse the pharmacologic/toxicologic effects of drugs. *Drug Metab Rev* 11: 233, 1980

129. Maini R, Winchester JF: Removal of paraquat from blood by haemoperfusion over sorbent materials. *Br Med J* 3: 281, 1975

130. Gelfand MC, Winchester JF, Knepshield JH, Hanson KM, Cohan SL, Strauch BS, Geoly KL, Kennedy AC, Schreiner GE: Treatment of severe drug overdose with charcoal hemoperfusion. *Trans Am Soc Artif Intern Organs* 23: 599, 1977

131. Van de Vyver FL, Giuliano RA, Paulus GJ, Verpooten GA,

Franke JP, De Zeeuw RA, Van Gaal LF, De Broe ME: Hemoperfusion-hemodialysis ineffective for paraquat removal in life-threatening poisoning? *J Toxicol Clin Toxicol* 23: 117, 1985

132. Mascie-Taylor BH, Thompson J, Davison AM: Haemoperfusion ineffective for paraquat removal in life-threatening poisoning. *Lancet* 1: 1376, 1983

133. Okonek S, Baldamus CA, Hofman A, Schuster CJ, Bechstein PB, Zoller B: Two survivors of severe paraquat intoxication by 'continuous hemoperfusion.' *Klin Wochenschr* 57: 957, 1979

134. Sahney S, Abarzua J, Sessums L: Hemoperfusion in theophylline neurotoxicity. *Pediatrics* 71: 615, 1983

135. Park GD, Spector R, Roberts RJ, Goldberg MJ, Weissman D, Stillerman A, Flanigan MJ: Use of hemoperfusion for treatment of theophylline intoxication. *Am J Med* 74: 961, 1983

136. Connell JM, McGeachie JF, Knepil J, Thomson A, Junor B: Self-poisoning with sustained-release aminophylline: secondary rise in serum theophylline concentration after charcoal haemoperfusion. *Br Med J* 284: 943, 1982

137. Woo OF, Pond S, Benowitz NL, Olson KR: Benefit of hemoperfusion in acute theophylline intoxication. *J Toxicol Clin Toxicol* 22: 411, 1984

138. Ahlmen J, Heath A, Herlitz H, Kvist L, Mellstrand T: Treatment of oral theophylline poisoning. *Acta Med Scand* 216: 423, 1984

139. Schwartz RD: Deferoxamine and aluminum removal. *Am J Kidney Dis* 6: 358, 1985

140. Brown DJ, Dawborn JK, Ham KN, Xipell JM: Treatment of dialysis osteomalacia with desferrioxamine. *Lancet* 2: 343, 1982

141. Andress DL, Maloney NA, Endres DB, Sherrard DJ: Aluminum-associated bone disease in chronic renal failure: high prevalence in a long-term dialysis population. *J Bone Miner Res* 1: 391, 1986

142. Arieff AI: Aluminum and the pathogenesis of dialysis encephalopathy. *Am J Kidney Dis* 6: 317, 1985

143. Bregman H, Gelfand MC, Winchester JF, Manz HJ, Knepshield JH, Schreiner GE: Iron overload-associated myopathy in patients on maintenance haemodialysis. A histocompatibility linked disorder. *Lancet* 2: 882, 1980

144. Falk RJ, Mattern WD, Lamanna RW, Gitelman HJ, Parker NC, Cross RE, Rastall JR: Iron removal during continuous ambulatory peritoneal dialysis using deferoxamine. *Kidney Int* 24: 110, 1983

145. McCarthy JT, Libertin Cr, Mitchell JC III, Fairbanks VF: Hemosiderosis in a dialysis patient. Treatment with hemofiltration and deferoxamine chelation therapy. *Mayo Clin Proc* 57: 439, 1982

146. Marcus RE, Davies SC, Bantock HM, Underwood SR, Walton S, Huehns ER: Desferrioxamine to improve cardiac function in iron overloaded patients with thalassemia major. *Lancet* 1: 392, 1984

147. Wolfe L, Olivieri N, Sallan D, Colan S, Rose V, Propper R, Freedman M, Nathan DG: Prevention of cardiac disease by subcutaneous deferoxamine in patients with thalassemia major. *N Engl J Med* 312: 1600, 1985

148. Worth DP, Davison AM, Lewins AM, Ledgerwood MJ, Taylor A: Haemodialysis and charcoal haemoperfusion in acute inorganic mercury poisoning. *Postgrad Med J* 60: 636, 1984

149. De Backer W, Zachee P, Verpooten GA, Majelyne W, Vanheule A, De Broe ME: Thallium intoxication treated with combined hemoperfusion-hemodialysis. *J Toxicol Clin Tox-*

icol 19: 259, 1982

150. De Groot G, van Heijst AN, van Kesteren RG, Maes RA: An evaluation of the efficacy of charcoal haemoperfusion in the treatment of three cases of acute thallium poisoning. *Arch Toxicol* 57: 61, 1985

151. Lund ME, Banner W, Clarkson TW, Berlin M: Treatment of acute methylmercury ingestion by hemodialysis with n-acetyl-cysteine (Mucomyst) infusion and 2,3-dimercaptopropane sulfonate. *J Toxicol Clin Toxicol* 22: 31, 1984

152. Al-Abassi AH, Kostyniak PJ, Clarkson TW: An extracorporeal complexing hemodialysis system for the treatment of methylmercury poisoning. III Clinical applications. *J Pharmacol Exp Ther* 207: 249, 1978

153. Margel S: A novel approach for heavy metal poisoning treatment, a model. Mercury poisoning by means of chelating microspheres; hemoperfusion and oral administration. *J Med Chem* 24: 1263, 1981

154. Banner W, Koch M, Capin DM, Hopf SB, Chang S, Tong TG: Experimental chelation therapy in chromium, lead and boron intoxication with n-acetylcysteine and other compounds. *Toxicol Appl Pharmacol* 83: 142, 1986

155. Zieve L, Doizeki WM, Zieve FJ: Synergism between mercaptans and ammonia or fatty acids in the production of coma; a possible role for mercaptans in the pathogenesis of hepatic coma. *J Lab Clin Med* 83: 16, 1974

156. James TH, Ziparo V, Jeppsson B, Fischer JE: Hyperammonaemia, plasma aminoacid imbalance, and blood-brain aminoacid transport: A unified theory of portal-systemic encephalopathy. *Lancet* 2: 772, 1979

157. Schafer DF, Jones EA: Hepatic encephalopathy and the gamma-aminobutyric-acid neurotransmitter system. *Lancet* 1: 18, 1982

158. Chang TMS: Haemoperfusion over microencapsulated adsorbent in a patient with hepatic coma. *Lancet* 2: 1371, 1972

159. Chang TMS: Hemoperfusion alone and in series with ultrafiltration or dialysis for uremia, poisoning and liver failure. *Kidney Int* 10 (Suppl 7): S305, 1976

160. Blume U, Helmstaedt D, Sybrecht G, Baldamus C, Sussmann P, Heyer U, Schmidt E, Schmidt FW: Hamoperfusions-therapie des acuten Leberversagens. (Hemoperfusion treatment for acute hepatic failure) *Dtsch Med Wochenschr* 101: 559, 1976

161. Colon AR, Gelfand MC, Winchester JF: Hemocarboperfusion (HCP) in hepatic decompensation and cerebral edema. in: *Reye's Syndrome II*, edited by Crocker JFS, New York, San Francisco, London, Grune and Stratton, 1978, p 139

162. Bartels O, Neidhardt B, Neidhardt M, Schellberger H, Issel W, Waldherr AM, Demling L: Untersuchungen und Entahrungen mit der Kohlehaemoperfusion bei Leber-koma. in: *Entgiftung mit Hamoperfusion*, (Investigation and experience with carbon hemoperfusion for liver coma. in: Detoxification by Hemoperfusion) edited by Demling L, Bartels O, Freiburg, Bundernagel-Verlag, 1977, p 119

163. Gazzard BG, Portmann BA, Weston MJ, Langley PG, Murray-Lyon IM, Dunlop EH, Flax H, Mellon PJ, Record CO, Ward MB, Williams R: Charcoal haemoperfusion in the treatment of fulminant hepatic failure. *Lancet* 1: 1301, 1974

164. Silk DBA, Williams R: Sorbents in hepatic failure. in: *Sorbents and Their Clinical Applications*, edited by Giordano C, New York, Academic Press Inc, 1980, p 415

165. Silk DBA, Williams R: Experiences in the treatment of fulminant hepatic failure by conservative therapy, charcoal haemoperfusion and polyacrylonitrile haemodialysis. *Int J Artif Organs* 1: 29, 1978

166. Opolon P, Rapin JR, Huguet C, Granger A, Delorme ML, Boschat M, Sausee A: Hepatic failure coma treated by polyacrylonitrile membrane hemodialysis. *Trans Am Soc Artif Intern Organs* 22: 701, 1976

167. Silk DBA, Trewby PN, Chase RA, Mellon PJ, Hanid MA, Davies M, Langley PG, Wheeler PG, Williams R: Treatment of fulminant hepatic failure by polyacrylonitrile membrane haemodialysis. *Lancet* 2: 1, 1977

168. Chang TMS, Lister C, Chirito E, O'Keefe P, Resurreccion E: Effects of hemoperfusion rate and time of initiation of ACAC charcoal hemoperfusion on the survival of fulminant hepatic failure rats. *Trans Am Soc Artif Intern Organs* 24: 243, 1978

169. Takahashi Y: Acute hepatic failure – in special relation to treatment. *Jpn Med J* 22: 140, 1983

170. Tygstrup N, Ranek L: Fulminant hepatic failure. *Clin Gastroenterol* 10: 191, 1986

171. Berk PD: A computer simulation study relating to the treatment of fulminant hepatic failure by hemoperfusion. *Proc Soc Exp Biol Med* 155: 535, 1977

172. Hughes RD, Cochrane AMD, Thomson AD, Murray-Lyon, Williams R: Cytotoxicity of plasma from patients with acute hepatic failure to isolated rabbit hepatocytes. *Br J Exp Pathol* 57: 348, 1976

173. Gelfand MC, Winchester JF, Knepshield JH, Cohan SL, Schreiner GE: Reversal of hepatic coma by coated charcoal hemoperfusion: Clinical and biochemical observations. *asaio J* 1: 73, 1978

174. Amano I, Kano H, Takahira H, Yamamoto Y, Itoh K, Iwatsuki S, Maeda K, Ohta K: Hepatic assist system using bead type charcoal, in: *Artificial Kidney, Artificial Liver and Artificial Cells*, edited by Chang TMS, New York, Plenum Press, 1978, p 89

175. Seda HWM, Hughes RD, Give CD, Williams R: Removal of inhibitors of brain Na+ K+ ATPase by haemoperfusion in fulminant hepatic failure. *Artif Organs* 8: 174, 1984

176. Foster D, Ahmed K, Zieve L: Action of methanethiol on membrane Na+ K+ ATPase: Implications for hepatic coma. *Ann NY Acad Sci* 242, 573, 1974

177. Seda HWM, Hughes RD, Give CD, Williams R: Inhibition of rat brain Na+ K+ ATPase activity by serum from patients with fulminant hepatic failure. *Hepatology* 4: 74, 1984

178. Langley PG, Hughes RD, Ton HY, Silk DBA, Williams R: The effect of prostaglandin E₁ and adenosine on adverse platelet reactions during charcoal haemoperfusion. *Thromb Res* 13: 351, 1978

179. Rubin MH, Weston MJ, Bullock G, Roberts J, Langley PG, White YS, Williams R: Abnormal platelet function and ultrastructure in fulminant hepatic failure. *Q J Med* 46: 339, 1977

180. Sette H, Hughes RD, Langley PG, Gimson AE, Williams R: Heparin response and clearance in acute and chronic liver disease. *thromb Haemostas* 54: 591, 1985

181. Cordopatri F, Boncinelli S, Marsili M, Lorenzi P, Fabbri LP, Paci P, Salvadori M, Morfini M, Cinoti S, Casparini P: Effects of charcoal haemoperfusion with prostacyclin on the coagulation-fibrinolysis system and platelets of patients with fulminant hepatic failure – preliminary observation. *Int J Artif Organs* 5: 243, 1982

182. Kennedy HJ, Greaves M, Triger DR: Clinical experience with the use of charcoal haemoperfusion: Is prostacyclin required? *Life Support syst* 3: 115, 1985

183. Ton HY, Hughes RD, Silk DBA, Williams R: Adsorption of human serum albumin to Amberlite XAD-7 resin. *J Biomed Mater Res* 13: 403, 1979

184. Hughes RD, Ton HY, Langley PG, Davis M, Hanid MA,

Mellon PS, Silk DBA, Williams R: Albumin-coated Amberlite XAD-7 resin for hemoperfusion in acute liver failure. Part II. In vivo evaluation. *Artif Organs* 3: 23, 1979

185. Bihari D, Hughes RD, Gimson AES, Langley PG, Ede RJ, Eder G, Williams R: Effects of serial resin haemoperfusion in fulminant hepatic failure. *Int J Artif Organs* 6: 299, 1983

186. Maini R, Gaylor JDS, Courtney JM, Wozniak A: Removal of protein-bound bilirubin from plasma using small particle size anion exchange resin and microfiltration. in: *Biomaterials in Artificial Organs,* edited by Paul JP, Gaylor JDS, Courtney JM, Gilchrist T, London, Basingstoke, The Macmillan Press Ltd, 1984, p 186

187. Hughes R, Williams R: Clinical experience with charcoal and resin hemoperfusion. *Semin Liver Dis* 6: 164, 1986

188. Wagemaker H, Cade R: The use of hemodialysis in chronic schizophrenia. *Am J Psychiatr* 134: 684, 1977

189. Cade R, Wagemaker H: The use of hemodialysis in chronic schizophrenia. *Abstracts Am Soc Artif Intern Organs* 7: 1, 1978

190. Kolff WJ: Dialysis of schizophrenics. Weird and novel applications of dialysis, hemofiltration, hemoperfusion, and peritoneal dialysis: Witchcraft? *Artif Organs* 2: 277, 1978

191. Gurland HJ: Chronic schizophrenia. in: *The S. Neaman Workshop on Hemoperfusion: Devices and Clinical Applications,* edited by Sideman S, Chang TMS, Haifa, Publication No. 01/108/80, Technion-Israel Institute of Technology, 1980, p 123

192. Chang TMS: Hemoperfusion in chronic schizophrenia. *Int J Artif Organs* 1: 253, 1978

193. Kinney MJ: Hemoperfusion for chronic schizophrenia: Preliminary psychiatric results (Cited in Gurland [191])

194. Nedipil N, Dieterle D, Gurland HJ: Blood purification treatment of schizophrenia. *Int J Artif Organs* 3: 76, 1980

195. Schulz SC, VanKammen DP, Balow JE, Flye NW, Bunney WE: Dialysis in schizophrenia: A double blind evaluation. *Science* 211: 1066, 1981

196. Twardowski AJ, Nolph KD, Rubin J, Anderson PC: Peritoneal dialysis for psoriasis. *Ann Intern Med* 88: 349, 1978

197. McEvoy J, Kelly AMT: Psoriatic clearance during hemodialysis. *Ulster Med J* 76: 1976

198. Breathnach SM, Boon NA, Black MM, Jones NF, Wing AJ: Psoriasis developing during dialysis. *Br Med J* 1: 236, 1979

199. Nissensson AB, Rapaport M, Gordon A, Narins RG: Controlled study demonstrates that psoriasis is not improved by hemodialysis. *Kidney Int* 14: 682, 1978

200. Maeda K, Asada H, Yamamoto Y, Ohta K: Psoriasis treatment with direct hemoperfusion. in: *Hemoperfusion, Kidney and Liver Support and Detoxification,* edited by Sideman S, Chang TMS, Washington DC, Hemisphere Publishing Corp, 1980, p 349

201. Tagami H, Ofuji S: Leukotactic properties of soluble substances in psoriasis scale. *Br J Dermatol* 95: 1, 1978

202. Winchester JF, Rahman A, Bregman H, Mortensen LM, Gelfand MC, Schein PS, Schreiner GE: Role of hemoperfusion in anticancer drug removal. in: *Hemoperfusion, Kidney and Liver Support and Detoxification,* edited by Sideman S, Chang TMS, Washington DC, Hemisphere Publishing Corp, 1980, p 369

203. Hande KR, Balow JE, Draje JC, Rosenberg SA, Chabner BA: Methotrexate and hemodialysis. *Ann Intern Med* 87: 496, 1977

204. Molina R, Fabian C, Cowley B Jr: Use of charcoal hemoperfusion to reduce serum methotrexate levels in a patient with acute renal insufficiency. *Am J Med* 82: 350, 1987

205. Oldfield EH, Dedrick RL, Yeager RL, Clark WC, DeVroom

HL, Chatterji DC, Doppman JL: Reduced systemic drug exposure by continuous intra-arterial chemotherapy with hemoperfusion of regional venous drainage. *J Neurosurg* 163: 726, 1985

206. Terman DS: Extracorporeal immunoadsorbents for extraction of circulating immune reactants. in: *Sorbents and Their Clinical Applications,* edited by Giordano C, New York, Academic Press Inc, 1980, p 470

207. Terman DS, Buffaloe G, Mattioli C, Cook G, Tillquist R, Sullivan M, Ayus JC: Extracorporeal immunoabsorption: Initial experience in human systemic lupus erythematosus. *Lancet* 2: 824, 1979

208. Terman DS, Garcia-Rinaldi R, McCalman R, Crumb CC, Mattioli C, Cook G, Poser R: Modification of hyperacute renal xenograft rejection after extracorporeal immunoadsorption of heterospecific antibody. *Int J Artif Organs* 2: 35, 1979

209. Terman DS, Yamamoto T, Mattioli M, Cook G, Tillquis R, Henry J, Poser Daskal Y: Extensive necrosis of spontaneous canine mammary adenocarcinoma after extracorporeal perfusion over Staphylococcus aureus Cowans I. *J Immunol* 124: 795, 1980

210. Terman DS, Betram HJ: Antitumor effects of immobilized protein A and Staphylococcal products: Linkage between toxicity and efficacy and tumoricidal reagents. *Eur J Cancer Clin Oncol* 21: 1115, 1985

211. Langone JJ, Das C, Bennett D, Terman DS: Generation of human C_{3a}, C_{4a}, and C_{5a} anaphylotoxin by protein A of Staphylococcus aureus and immobilized protein A reagents in serotherapy of cancer. *J Immunol* 133: 1057, 1984

212. Marcus L, Margel S, Savin H, Ofarim M, Ravid M: Therapy of digoxin intoxication in dogs by specific hemoperfusion through agarose polyacrolein microsphere beads-antidigoxin antibodies. *Am Heart J* 110: 30, 1985

213. Savin H, Marcus L, Margel S, Ofarim M, Ravid M: Treatment of adverse digitalis effects by hemoperfusion through columns with antidigoxin antibodies bound to agarose polyacrolein microsphere beads. *Am Heart J* 113: 1078, 1987

214. Sideman S, Mor L, Rousseau I, Brandes JM: Ben-Arie D: Removal of bilirubin from the blood of jaundiced infants. in: *Artificial Organs,* edited by Kenedi RM, Courtney JM, Gaylor JDS, Gilchrist T, London, Basingstoke, Macmillan, 1971, p 413

215. Odaka M, Kobayashi H, Tabata Y, Soeda K, Hayashi H, Ito S, Murotani N, Saito Y, Nishide Y, Shinomiya M, Yoshida S: Long term results of LDL selective plasma adsorption therapy on familial hypercholesterolemia. *Biomater Artif Cells Artif Organs* 15: 113, 1987

216. Chang TMS, Nicolaev VG: Hemoperfusion, sorbents and immobilized bioreactants. *Biomater Artif Cells Artif Organs* 15 (special issue), 1987

217. Yatzidis H, Oreopoulos D: Early clinical trials with sorbents. *Kidney Int* 10 (Suppl 7): S215, 1976

218. Yatzidis H, Yullis G, Digenis P: Hemocarboperfusion-haemodialysis treatment in terminal renal failure. *Kidney Int* 10 (Suppl 7): S312, 1976

219. Dunea G, Rizvii ZH, Mamdani BH, Anicama HJ, Mahurkar SK: Charcoal hemoperfusion and combination dialysis-hemoperfusion in chronic renal failure. *Abstracts Am Soc Artif Intern Organs* 5: 22, 1975

220. Leber HE, Neuhauser M, Goubeaud G: Chronic uraemia: haemodialysis or haemoperfusion? in: *Artificial Organs,* edited by Kenedi RM, Courtney JM, Gaylor JDS, Gilchrist T, London, Basingstoke, Macmillan Press Ltd, 1977, p 220

221. Martin AM, Gibbins JK, Oduro M, Herbert R: Clinical expe-

rience with cellulose coated carbon hemoperfusion. in: *Artificial Liver, Artificial Kidney, and Artificial Cells*, edited by Chang TMS, Plenum Press, New York, 1978, p 143

222. Mydlik M, Bucek J, Derzsiova K, Jarcuska J, Takac M: Influence of charcoal haemoperfusion on platelet count in acute poisoning and during regular dialysis treatment. *Int Urol Nephrol* 13: 387, 1981

223. Splendiani G, Albano V, Trancredi M, Daniele M, Pignatelli F: Our experience with combined hemodialysis-hemoperfusion treatment in chronic uremia. *Biomater Artif Cells Artif Organs* 15: 175, 1987

224. Yamazaki Z, Fujimori Y, Sanjo K, Kojima Y, Sugiura M, Wada T, Inoue N, Sakai T, Oda T, Kominami N, Fujisake U, Kataoka K: New artificial liver support system (Plasma perfusion detoxification) for hepatic coma. *Artif Organs* 1: 148, 1977

225. Bartels O, Neidhardt M, Schellberger H: Hormone losses by charcoal haemoperfusion. in: *Artificial Liver Support*, edited by Brunner G, Schmidt FW, Berlin, Springer-Verlag, 1981, p 121

226. Williams R: Fulminant hepatic failure. *Postgrad Med J* 59 (Suppl 4): 33, 1983

PLASMA EXCHANGE: PRINCIPLES AND PRACTICE

WALTER SAMTLEBEN and HANS J. GURLAND

INTRODUCTION

Circulating pathogens are instrumental in the pathogenesis of several disorders or the presence of these substances is responsible for subsequent organ dysfunctions. Examples include:

1) uremic toxins (molecular weight range 60 up to 5,000 or more daltons) in renal failure;
2) circulating toxins in drug intoxications as well as exogenous and endogenous poisonings;
3) autoantibodies of the IgG or IgM class (molecular weight 150,000 and 970,000 daltons respectively) with subsequent binding to antigens in autoimmune disorders (e.g. Goodpasture's syndrome, myasthenia gravis, immune thrombocytopenia);
4) circulating immune complexes (molecular weight about 500,000 daltons up to 3,000 kilodaltons) which cause tissue lesions by deposition;
5) excessive low density lipoprotein concentrations (molecular weight about 2,400 kilodaltons) in type II hyperlipidemia and
6) paraproteins (intact immunoglobulins as well as free light or heavy chains) with subsequent disturbances, e.g.

renal paraprotein deposition, hyperviscosity, and polyneuropathy.

Depending on the molecular size of the offending substances and their distribution within the body, a battery of more or less specific extracorporeal procedures is available for their removal from the patient's circulation (Figure 1). The choice of procedure is determined by the molecular size of the substance and its intracorporeal location.

Blood letting, performed for several hundred years, can be considered a very crude precursor of more recent blood purification systems. Today a variety of techniques based on centrifugation, membrane separation, adsorption, other physico-chemical fractionation procedures or interactions with enzymes is available experimentally or in routine therapeutic applications.

A blood purification system ideally should remove only the pathogen (high selectivity). It should have a high removal capacity and its clinical application should be free of side effects. These three assumptions have been realized for only a few systems applicable in some distinct clinical entities with well characterized pathogens (e.g. LDL removal systems). This chapter summarizes the application of macromolecular separation processes regarding both the technical

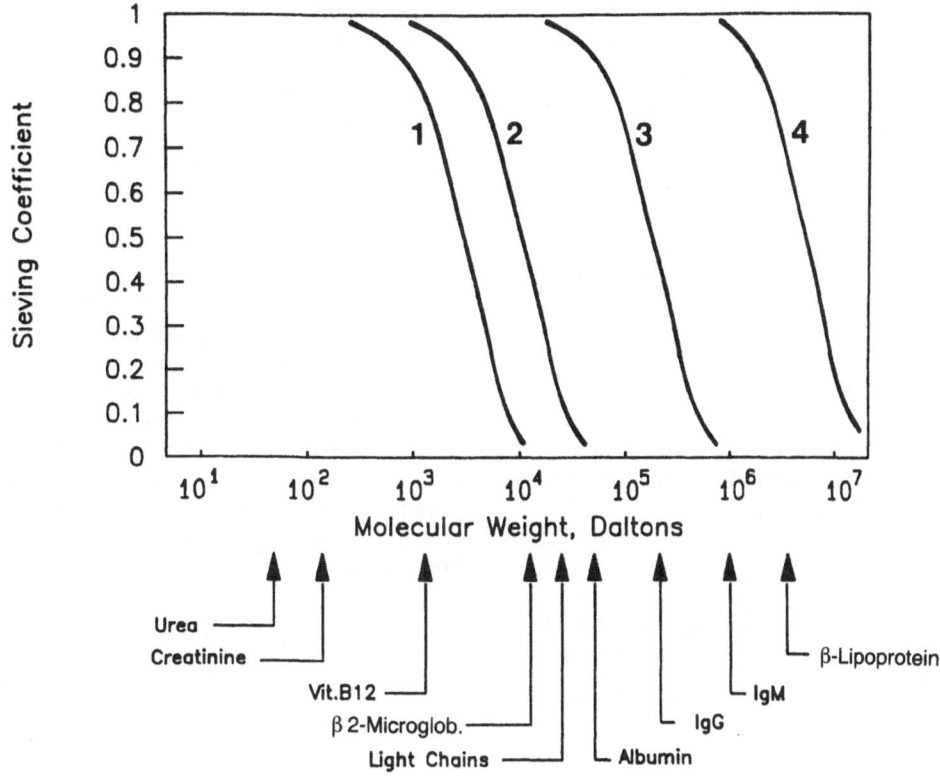

Figure 1. Permeability properties (sieving coefficients) of filters used for various extracorporeal procedures with reference to molecular weight of several plasma constituents. Curves represent: 1 – standard dialysis membrane; 2 – hemofiltration membrane; 3 – cascade filtration membrane; 4 – plasma separation membrane.

possibilities of unselective and selective protein separation and their clinical application.

METHODS FOR UNSELECTIVE PLASMA EXCHANGE

Separation techniques

The simplest way to harvest an adequate volume of plasma from whole blood is to collect a bag of anticoagulated blood, centrifuge it and collect the plasma supernatant (1). This plasma containing the target pathogen(s) is discarded while the cells are resuspended in a (proteinaceous) solution and returned to the patient. When repeated several times this batch process provides effective removal of those plasma constituents primarily confined within the vasculature, e.g. IgM paraproteins (2).

In the late 1960s closed centrifugal apheresis equipment was developed, originally with the aim of collecting blood cells for bone marrow transplant recipients (3). Without significant technical adaptation these centrifuges could also be used for continuous separation of plasma from blood. Originally such equipment was quite bulky. Newly developed centrifuges for therapeutic plasmapheresis have become more compact and require smaller extracorporeal

priming volumes and a few are capable of performing apheresis with a single venous access. Centrifugal plasmapheresis is the domain of hematologists and blood banks; therefore, technical details will not be discussed here.

Clinical on-line plasma separation employing membranes became available in 1978 (4). These highly permeable membranes were developed originally to recover a cell free filtrate of ascitic fluid for reinfusion in patients with advanced liver disease. These early filters were not ideal in respect to their protein permeability (5). Within a few years, membrane filters made from a variety of polymers became available for clinical on line plasma separation (6). All of these filters exhibit nearly ideal permeability properties without significant retention of high molecular weight proteins. Furthermore, the design of membrane filters has been improved so that devices with smaller surface areas permit plasma exchanges at low blood flow rates obviating the need for central venous access (7). In parallel, membrane filters and hardware for plasma donation have been designed and are already in use. (This topic, however, will not be covered in this chapter).

Membrane materials and device configuration

Polymers used for hollow fiber and flat sheet plasma separation membranes are summarized in Table 1. The diameter of all hollow fiber membranes is between 270 and 370 μm with a wall thickness of about 50 μm. The nominal pore size is 0.5 μm which prevents a transfer of normal sized platelets through the membrane. The effective fiber length chosen by the different manufacturers is between 13.5 and 26 cm. Two flat sheet devices for plasma separation (in 1987) are also commercially available. They employ polyvinyl chloride and polyvinylidene fluoride respectively as membrane materials. Several other polymers have been used in vitro for characterization of the transmembrane transport of solutes (8).

Factors governing mass transport in membrane plasma separation

The transport of plasma through plasma separation membranes depends primarily on:
1) membrane filter design (flat sheet or hollow fiber, pore size, filter length, fiber diameter in hollow fiber filters or channel heights in flat sheet devices, membrane surface area);
2) blood composition (hematocrit, blood and plasma viscosity, platelet count, plasma protein composition), and
3) operating conditions (blood flow, transmembrane pressure, filtrate flux, shear rate, filtration fraction).

Membrane filter design

When the blood passes through a highly permeable hollow fiber filter, red cells and platelets together with the plasma move towards the wall and accumulate to form a secondary membrane which limits the filtration efficiency. Blood flow tangetial to the membrane surface removes these blood cells from the wall by particle diffusion (8). This dynamic process is called cellular concentration polarization and may, in extreme situations, completely block further plasma filtration through the membrane if the cells cannot be moved from the wall.

Table 1. Description of membrane plasma separation filters (selection of currently available filters).

Membrane material	Trade name, (manufacturer)	Surface area (m^2)	Fiber diameter (μm)
Cellulose-diacetate	Plasmaflo AP-06-H (ASAHI)	0.50	330
Polyethylene	MPS 0.250 (Mitsubishi)	0.50	270
	OP-T-1 (ASAHI)	0.40	340
Polymethylmethacrylate	Plasmax PS-05 (Toray)	0.50	370
	Plasmax PS-02 (Toray)	0.20	370
Polymer alloy (cellulose diacetate based)	TP 50 (Teijin)	0.30	320
Polypropylene	CPS-10 (Travenol)	0.20	330
	Curesis (Organon)	0.12	330
	Fiber Plasmafilter (Gambro)	0.40	330
	Fiber Plasmafilter PF 1000 (Gambro)	0.14	330
	Hemaplex BT 900 (Dideco)	0.20	320
	Plasmaflux P1 (Fresenius)	0.25	330
	Plasmaflux P2 (Fresenius)	0.50	330
Polysulfone	Sulflux (Kanegafuchi)	0.5	340
Polyvinyl alcohole	Plasmacure (Kuraray)	0.50	300
Polyvinyl chloride	TPE (COBE)	0.13	(flat sheet)
Polyvinylidene fluoride	Therapore (3M)	0.056	(flat sheet)

Cellular concentration polarization is enhanced by the following operating conditions (see below): a high filtration fraction, a high transmembrane pressure, and a low shear rate.

With regard to plasma filtration efficiency, flat sheet devices are superior to hollow fiber filters. At hematocrits usually found in the plasma exchange population (20 to 40%), hollow fiber filters can be operated at a filtration fraction not exceeding 0.3 (8). This means that a plasma flux of 30 volume % of the blood input is filtered through the membrane. This increases the filter outlet hematocrit, the value achieved depending on the filter inlet hematocrit. To prevent fiber plugging, outlet hematocrit should be kept below 70% by decreasing the filtration fraction (8).

Flat sheet devices offer the advantage of allowing a far higher filtration fraction. This is especially true when an automated fluid cycler (e.g. Cobe TPE) is used. This equipment automatically adjusts the channel height and the filtration rate to give an optimal shear rate and transmembrane pressure for a given blood flow. The maximum filtration fraction which can be achieved in flat sheet devices is 0.6 (8) allowing high yield plasma separations even at low blood flow rates when peripheral veins serve as vascular access.

Surface areas of commercial membrane plasma separators for therapeutic purposes are in the range of 0.12 to 0.6 m² in hollow fiber devices and 0.06 to 0.13 m² for flat sheets (6).

Under appropriate operating conditions all recently available membrane plasma separation modules exhibit nearly ideal protein permeability properties without significant protein retention (6). Protein permeability can be best described by the sieving coefficient which is calculated according to the following equation:

$$SC = \frac{2\,C_f}{C_{in} + C_{out}} \qquad [1]$$

where SC = dimensionless sieving coefficient, C_{in} = protein inlet concentration, C_{out} = protein outlet concentration and C_f = protein concentration in the filtrate.

For characterization of a plasma separation module it is necessary to have sieving coefficients for a spectrum of proteins which cover a wide molecular weight range. This should at least include the following globularly shaped proteins (molecular weight): albumin (66,000), IgG (150,000), IgM (970,000), and β-lipoprotein (2,400,000). A sieving coefficient of 1.0 would represent the same protein concentration in the filtrate as in the blood fed into the filter. At a sieving coefficient of 0 the protein under investigation cannot be detected in the plasma filtrate. Sieving coefficients of at least 0.95 for all proteins mentioned above are standard for membrane plasma separators currently available on the market (6). Furthermore, the optimal sieving coefficient should be stable during the run to allow an exchange of at least one patient's plasma volume (about 31). Appropriate anticoagulation and optimal operating conditions (see below) are the assumptions for stable flux and protein permeability during clinical plasmapheresis.

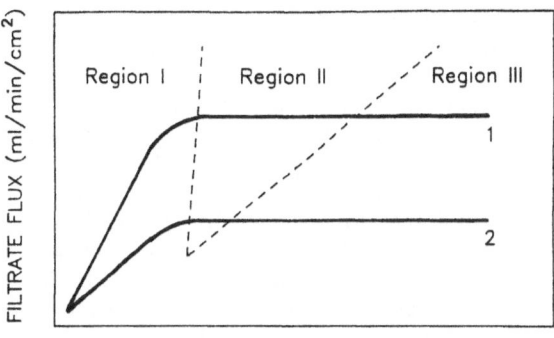

Figure 2. Schematic showing filtration behavior in membrane plasmapheresis. For details see text. Curve 1 represents high shear rates, curve 2 shows low shear rates.

Blood composition

The plasma filtration flux is independent of hematocrit in the range of 0 to 60% (8). The platelet count affects the filtration rate by causing a decrease at nonphysiologically high concentrations. Furthermore, high molecular weight plasma constituents when present in extremely high plasma concentrations can also limit filtration efficiency. This is true for IgM (paraproteinemia) and for β-lipoprotein. Those cryoglobulins (mostly of type I = monoclonal) which already dissolve a few degrees centigrades below the physiologic temperature, might precipitate immediately after blood withdrawal resulting in membrane plugging of the plasma separation filter. This phenomenon can be prevented by warming the entire extracorporeal circuit including the filtering device to 37 to 38°C.

Operating conditions

Early on it was noted that membrane plasmapheresis can be performed safely only at a 'narrow window of operating conditions' (8), which is determined primarily by the transmembrane pressure (TMP), the shear rate and the filtrate flux per unit filtering area (Figure 2). For a hollow fiber device the wall shear rate, γ, is directly proportional to the blood flow rate and inversely correlated to the number of fibers and to the third power of the fiber radius. It is calculated according to the following equation (9):

$$\gamma = \frac{4 \times Q_B}{n \times \pi \times R^3} \qquad [2]$$

where Q_B = inlet blood flow (ml/sec), n = number of fibers and R = internal fiber radius (cm).

Consequently, for a given device geometry the shear rate is determined only by the blood flow rate.

The mean TMP represents the pressure difference between the blood and the filtrate compartment:

$$TMP = \tfrac{1}{2}(P_{in} + P_{out}) - P_{filtr} \qquad [3]$$

where P_{in} = pressure at the filter blood inlet, P_{out} = pressure at the filter blood outlet and P_{filtr} = pressure at the filtrate side.

At very low TMPs, there is a nearly linear increase of the filtrate flux (per unit surface area) with increasing TMP (Figure 2, Region I). At intermediate TMPs, the plasma filtration reaches a plateau (Region II) with a filtrate flux independent of the TMP. If the TMP is further increased, this does not influence the filtrate flux positively but induces hemolysis resulting in free hemoglobin in the plasma filtrate (Region III). Region III represents unstable operating conditions with flux decay, worsening of the protein permeability of the filter and hemolysis as already mentioned (6, 7).

Sterilization of membrane plasma separators

In general, sterilization procedures used for hemodialyzers are also used for membrane plasma separators. Most are sterilized with ethylene oxide gas. However, at least one anaphylactoid reaction during a clinical plasma exchange treatment has been attributed to residual ethylene oxide as is well known from hollow fiber dialysis (10). Gamma radiation (e.g. KNS-05® from Kanegafuchi) and steam autoclavation (e.g. Plasmacure ®, Kuraray Co, Ltd, Japan) are also employed.

Reuse

Because membrane plasma separators were expensive when first introduced commercially, reuse of these filters in the same patient has been investigated by several groups (11, 12). When performed properly the filter can be reused a few times without significant loss in flux or protein permeability (12). However, as a result of considerations of additional manual labor and the obligation of the responsible physician for device safety, coupled with decreasing filter costs, reuse never became an issue in clinical plasmapheresis.

Hardware

Equipment for membrane plasmapheresis is available from several companies. Safety standards for this extracorporeal treatment are similar to those for hemodialysis. There are, however, some differences in safety requirements inherent in the membrane plasma separation process. Figure 3 illustrates a fully equipped membrane plasmapheresis flow diagram. An ideal system should include (labels in brackets relate to Figure 3):

1) negative pressure monitor in the blood drawing line (P1);
2) blood pump (BP) which can be operated at low blood flow rates (minimum 40, maximum 200 ml/min);
3) continuous infusion of the anticoagulant (heparin or citrate) with the option of different anticoagulant to blood application ratios (AC);
4) filter inlet and outlet pressure monitors (P2, P4);
5) air bubble detector and clamp (C1) in the venous return line;

6) pressure gauge in the plasma filtrate line (P3);
7) controlled plasma filtration via a pump in the plasma line (PP);
8) hemoglobin detector in the plasma filtrate line (HbD);
9) substitution pump (SP) adjustable to different substitution ratios in relation to the separated plasma, and
10) low volume warmers (H) in the replacement and venous return lines.

The optional equipment should display the transmembrane pressure. Adequate alarms should be included for all essential parameters (inadequate blood withdrawal, TMP, and air).

Technical aspects of membrane plasma exchange

Vascular access

For most membrane plasma separation devices a stable blood flow of 50 to 80 ml/min is sufficient. Consequently, in those patients with adequate peripheral veins these can be used for access. Newly developed filters and hardware (e.g. Therapore System®) can also be operated at blood aspiration rates as low as 20 ml/min. Large surface area hollow fiber plasma separators (0.5 to 0.6 m²) can be operated at blood flow rates up to 300 ml/min or more, resulting in a plasma flow of up to 100 ml/min. As some side effects of plasma exchange procedures probably relate to the rate of the infused proteinaceous substitution fluid, reinfusion rates not exceeding 30 to 50 ml/min are preferred.

In patients with potentially irreversible renal disease with the risk of complete loss of kidney function (e.g. all forms of rapidly progressive glomerulonephritis) a large bore central venous catheter for plasma exchange is preferred. This alternative access preserves peripheral veins for fistula placement should renal replacement therapy be required later.

Anticoagulation

For anticoagulation in a routine membrane plasma exchange a bolus of heparin (2,000 to 5,000 IU) is combined with continuous heparin (300 to 1,200 IU/h) or citrate infusion (ACD-A 1 ml per 15 to 30 ml of blood). In patients at a high risk for bleeding (e.g. pulmonary hemorrhage in Goodpasture's syndrome), the actual dose of the anticoagulant should be reduced to avoid bleeding complications. In those cases the anticoagulant regimen should be monitored during treatment by an appropriate test (aPTT when heparin is used).

Replacement solutions

Albumin, the bulk protein and the main determinant of oncotic pressure should be kept constant to avoid potentially life threatening intracorporeal fluid shifts. The separated plasma has to be replaced isovolumetrically and isooncotically. Most centers prefer an albumin solution as replacement (4 to 5% human albumin solution). Commercial albumin preparations have low potassium, calcium and magnesi-

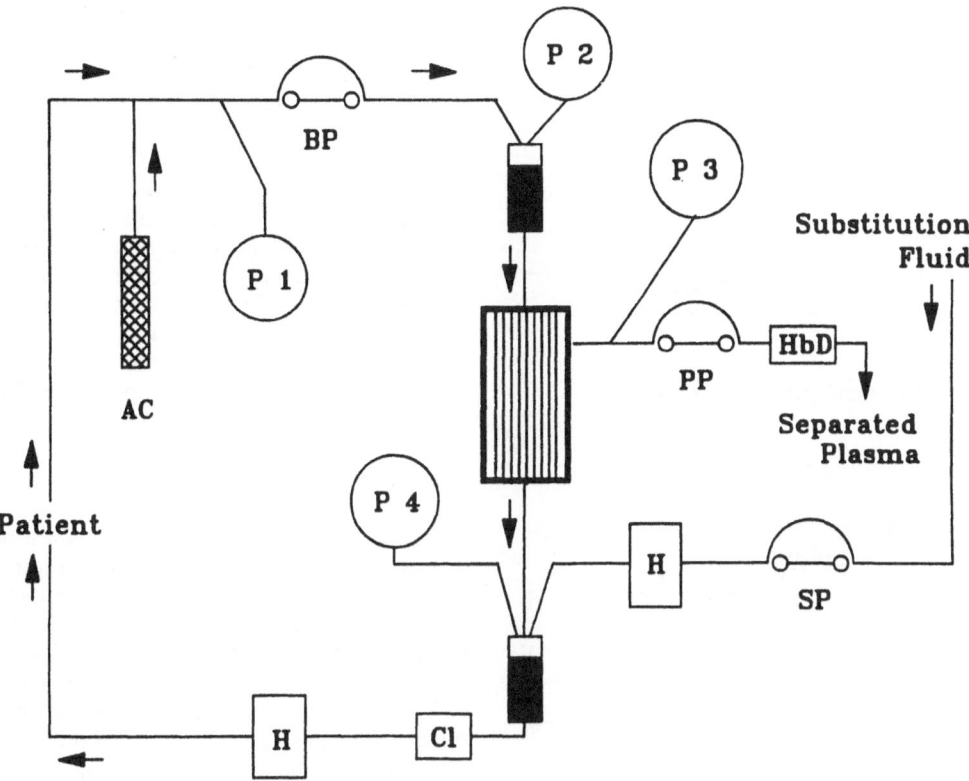

Figure 3. Schematic illustration of a membrane plasma separation circuit.

um concentrations. Calcium should be adjusted to a physiologic concentration to avoid hypocalcemic symptoms especially when citrate is used for anticoagulation. In large volume plasma exchanges with rapid reinfusion via a catheter placed in the superior caval vein, cardiac arrhythmias have been attributed to substitution fluid low in potassium (13).

Colloid isooncotic replacement fluids (dextran, gelatin, hydroxyethyl starch) have been used in plasma exchange with the intention of cost reduction. This can be done without a high risk as long as it is used for replacing the first 20% of the volume to be exchanged (e.g. first 500 ml in a 3 l plasma exchange). It should be taken into account that (semi-)synthetic colloidal substitutes are rapidly cleaved with a serum half-life of hours compared to 10 to 18 days for albumin.

In patients where a decrease of coagulation factors or other blood proteins (e.g. immunoglobulins, complement) is thought to influence the disease course negatively, fresh (frozen) plasma (FFP) is recommended for replacement of the separated plasma. However, FFP still has an intrinsic risk of transmitting (viral) infections. Furthermore, the incidence of immediate side reactions is highest with this type of volume replacement. Finally, as citrate is the anticoagulant in FFP, calcium must be replaced when FFP is infused.

Exchange volume and protein kinetics

Assuming a single pool model, the reduction of plasma proteins not returned with the replacement fluid can be predicted by the following equation (14):

$$C = C_0 \exp(-V/P) \qquad [4]$$

where C = protein concentration after the volume, V, has been exchanged; C_0 = initial protein concentration (g/l); P = total patient's plasma volume (l) and V = plasma volume actually exchanged (l).

The concentration of a given protein at the end of a plasma exchange session depends on the plasma volume exchanged. As exchange volumes increase the overall removal efficiency decreases. Also as a result of redistribution and resynthesis the predicted protein concentration decrease is usually not completely reached (15). The described removal kinetics have been proven for immunglobulins, coagulation factors, complement proteins and lipoproteins. Conflicting data have been published for circulating immune complexes mostly with a far more pronounced decrease than expected from equation 4. This phenomenon has been explained by 1) an enhanced endogenous catabolism (16, 17), 2) the formation of new immune complexes in the changed protein milieu which behave differently both

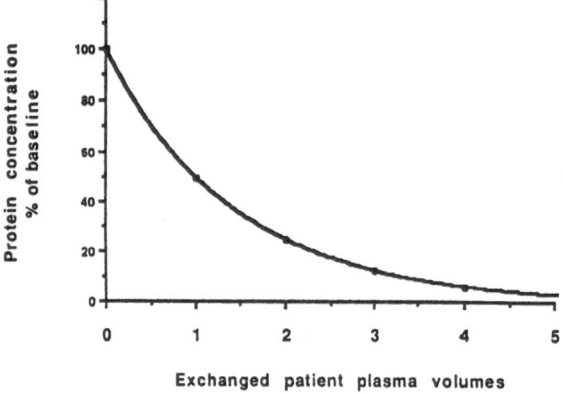

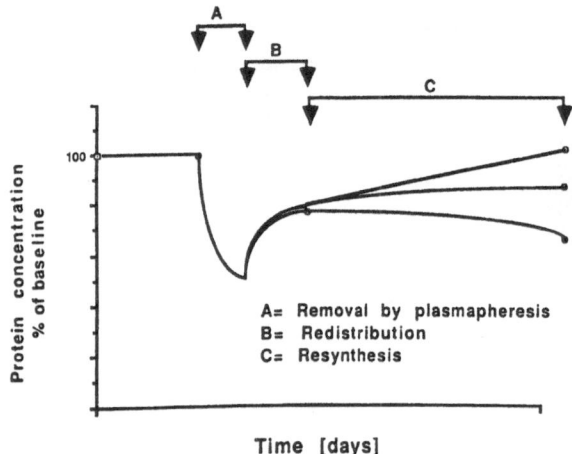

Figure 4. Protein kinetics in plasmapheresis. Upper: Protein concentration as dependent variable of the exchanged plasma volumes. Lower: Protein kinetics with respect to its removal, redistribution and resynthesis.

biologically in the patient and biochemically in the assays used compared to the original ones, and 3) methodological problems with the detection of circulating immune complexes due to multiple interactions (18).

The plasma concentration of most proteins increases fol-

lowing a plasma exchange session. The first phase of this increment is governed primarily by a reequilibration of the plasma protein with that of the extravascular compartment (redistribution). This phase lasts about 6 to 12 h. Its amplitude depends on the distribution space of the particular protein within the body. Only 25% of the total body IgM content is located extravascularly compared to about half of the total body IgG. Consequently, the post exchange increase of IgM is lower than that of IgG. The further time course of the plasma protein concentrations mostly depends on the resynthesis (Figure 4). In the case of (pathogenic) immunoglobulins (autoantibodies, paraproteins) synthesis can be reduced by cytotoxic drugs to deplete selectively B lymphocytes stimulated by the plasma exchange induced immunoglobulin depletion (19).

Side effects

Side effects observed in plasma exchange are independent of the method used (membrane based or centrifugal plasmapheresis) and can be attributed to the risks of the substitution fluid, the anticoagulant used and the extracorporeal procedure itself, including technical failures. Common side effects of plasma exchange together with their estimated incidence and the proposed medical management are summarized in Table 2 (13, 20–27). Severe side reactions are rare. Death has been reported to occur once in about 3,000 treatments or once per 500 patients (28, 29).

Traces of macroaggregates of altered serum proteins and activators of the kinin system probably present in some commercial albumin solutions, as well as the nonphysiologic electrolyte milieu (which can be corrected before use) have been incriminated for the majority of side effects. The incidence of reactions when FFP is used is even greater than for albumin replacement. Therefore, FFP administration should be limited to those cases where it is definitely indicated.

The fact that albumin is administered at a far faster rate (10 to 40 ml/min) in plasma exchange instead of the recommended maximum 8 to 10 ml/min may explain the high incidence of side reactions seen in this treatment compared to the infusion of albumin in the common hospitalized population where albumin related side effects are rare (about 0.01%) (30).

If plasma exchange is performed within 3 days prior to anaesthesia, the depletion of cholinesterase can cause pro-

Table 2. Incidence and management of immediate side reactions observed in therapeutic plasma exchange (13, 20–27).

Side reaction	Incidence	Management
Allergic and quasiallergic reactions	0–12%	steroids, antihistamines, (calcium)
Hypotension, vaso-vagal reactions	0–12%	atropine
Febrile reactions	1–18%	steroids, antipyretics
Hypocalcemic symptoms	0–9%	calcium
Arrhythmias	about 3%	depending on the type of arrhythmia, correction of electrolyte imbalances
Citrate intoxication	(rare)	calcium, decrease of citrate infusion rate

longed postoperative apnea requiring assisted ventilation (31).

Few publications deal with the removal of therapeutic drugs during plasma exchange (32, 33). In general, the fractional removal of substances with a large volume of distribution is low regardless of the drug ratio bound to plasma proteins. When exchanging one patient's plasma volume usually less than 1 to 3% of the total body store of a particular drug is removed. Consequently, an additional dose to compensate for the removed fraction is usually unnecessary. Whenever possible drug monitoring should be performed especially in drugs with a narrow therapeutic range as for example phenytoin. Such samples should be drawn before rather than after plasma exchange. Furthermore, drugs should be administered after and not before plasmapheresis. Based on this information plasma exchange is an inadequate method to remove sufficient amounts of protein bound drugs or toxins when performed with the intention of treating severe intoxications.

Alternative plasma exchange procedures

The application of (hollow fiber) membrane plasma separation modules is not necessarily limited to centers equipped with sophisticated hardware. These filters can be used in pumpless circuits either in a spontaneous arteriovenous pathway or in a one access set-up with gravity as the driving force for blood and plasma separation (34–36). Furthermore, membrane plasma separation can also be combined with routine hemodialysis (37) as has also been described for centrifuges (38, 39).

PLASMA FRACTIONATION

Several procedures have been developed recently with the aim of removing selectively disease specific circulating macromolecular pathogens. Altogether these procedures are termed plasma fractionation or closed loop plasmapheresis. A few have already become routine in some institutions. The incentives for a procedure which removes only the pathogen and returns the 'normal' proteins back to the patient are to minimize 1) side reactions (immediate reactions during the procedure and long term effects, e.g. infection) mostly related to the exogenous protein replacement, and 2) costs and sourcing of commercial plasma proteins.

In diseases in which the circulating macromolecular pathogen is known and chemically or immunologically defined or both a selective removal should offer at least two advantages: 1) The patient's normal proteins are recovered and reinfused. 2) The incidence of side reactions should be lower than in unselective plasma exchange. All plasma fractionation procedures employ routine laboratory protein separation techniques adapted to the requirements of an on line extracorporeal circuit. Currently, four strategies are used (40, 41).

Cascade filtration

With the help of a membrane filter the separated plasma is divided into a high and a low molecular weight fraction. The low molecular weight fraction containing most of the albumin is returned to the patient. The pathogen accumulates in the high molecular weight fraction retained by the filter. With filters currently available, cascade filtration can be applied under the assumption that the target pathogen has a molecular weight which is ten times higher than that of albumin. Hyperviscosity due to macroglobulinemia (IgM 970,000 dalton) and familial hypercholesterolemia (β-lipoproteins 2,400,000 dalton) are clinical conditions in which cascade filtration offers a more selective treatment than unselective plasma exchange. Since many high molecular weight proteins are removed in addition to the pathogen, cascade filtration does not result in specific pathogen removal. It does, however, recover sufficient albumin to obviate exogenous replacement.

Since membrane sieving alone has been the basis for fractionation the desired separation of albumin from IgG necessary for treatment of most autoimmune diseases has not been possible. The differences of the molecular shape are too neglible to allow a discrimination between these two proteins with membranes only. Filtering devices employing charged membranes probably might have better fractionation characteristics than currently available membranes.

Adsorption techniques

With on-line adsorption the plasma is processed through an adsorption column which contains a ligand capable of binding the target pathogen. This process is analogous to affinity chromatography. Three main types of ligands have been utilized for on-line plasma processing:

1) In the case of removal of antibodies of known specificity, the corresponding (multivalent) antigens when fixed to a solid matrix can trap the antibodies from the perfusate. This has been described for DNA antibodies with a DNA-containing column in SLE (42).
2) In some instances, the pathogenic protein's chemical affinity for another substance is employed for extraction. Low density lipoproteins (LDL) which are known to have an affinity for heparin or dextran sulfate can be removed from plasma by column perfusion using these ligands (43, 44). Other ligands under investigation are protein A (for binding of IgG 1, 2, 4 and probably IgG-containing immune complexes), phenylalanine (for immune complexes) and tryptophan (for anti-acetylcholine receptor antibodies in myasthenia gravis).
3) Immunoadsorption uses specific antibodies fixed to a solid matrix support. This technique offers a high degree of selectivity and specificity when compared with chemical affinity systems. Currently, columns with antibodies directed against LDL are already beyond the experimental stage and are undergoing clinical evaluation (45).

Plasma electrophoresis

In plasma electrophoresis, the fractionation process is based on differences in molecular charge and protein mobility. This technique should offer a higher degree of versatility than the fractionation processes mentioned above. At present, plasma electrophoresis is still in an experimental preclinical stage (46).

Combination of physicochemical separation techniques

An excellent example of physicochemical separation and plasmapheresis is the selective LDL removal from plasma by heparin precipitation without cations followed by membrane separation. This technique employs the property of the LDL-heparin complex to form a precipitate at low pH, which then can be removed by filtration from the plasma. Following readjustment of pH and electrolyte levels by dialysis and ultrafiltration, the LDL-free plasma is then recombined with the main bloodstream. This technique is presently under clinical investigation (47).

APPLICATION OF PLASMA EXCHANGE IN RENAL DISEASES

In the mid-1970s spectacular results following plasma exchange treatment were reported in diseases known to have poor prognoses (e.g. Goodpasture's syndrome, rapidly progressive glomerulonephritis, myasthenic crisis, thrombotic thrombocytopenic purpura) (48–51). These dramatic results stimulated widespread application of this new therapeutic approach for more than 200 different disease entities resulting in the publication of over 2,400 articles by 1984. These dealt primarily with the clinical results of plasma exchange (52). Several editorials and overview articles tried to summarize the overall clinical application of macromolecular separation (53–60). However, the recommendations provided were in part still controversial. According to the 'American Society for Apheresis', the role of plasma exchange in the therapeutic regimen of disorders can be classified as (60):

1) acceptable therapy under appropriate circumstances (e.g. in Goodpasture's syndrome),
2) sufficient data warrant a preliminary position (e.g. in hemolytic uremic syndrome),
3) requires further investigation (e.g. in idiopathic thrombocytopenic purpura), and
4) plasma exchange has been adequately tested and found to be of no benefit beyond conventional therapy (e.g. in schizophrenia).

The rationale for the application of plasma exchange in renal diseases is the elimination of those circulating pathogenic proteins involved in the renal inflammatory process. These immune factors are circulating autoantibodies (anti-glomerular basement membrane (GBM) antibodies, anti-DNA antibodies, and C3 nephritic factor), circulating immune complexes and free antigens and antibodies capable of forming immune complexes in situ in the kidney. They also include paraproteins, unknown circulating factors responsible for microvascular lesions in hemolytic uremic syndrome and thrombotic thrombocytopenic purpura, anti-graft antibodies in vascular kidney transplant rejection, and mediators of inflammatory processes (e.g. fibrinogen and complement components).

Anti-glomerular basement membrane antibody mediated nephritis

This disorder is mediated by autoantibodies directed against a 26 kilodalton (kD) monomeric peptide (and a 48 kD dimeric aggregate) present in one of the two noncollagenous parts of type IV collagen which is the main constituent of glomerular basement membrane (61, 62). Type IV collagen and hence the Goodpasture antigen is present not only in the kidney but also in other vascular regions (e.g. lungs). Because of the shaded intramolecular location of the Goodpasture antigen in the extrarenal vessels, additional factors (such as cigarette smoke, viral infections) are necessary to enable the autoantibodies to obtain access to the normally cryptic antigen (63). Anti-GBM nephritis makes up but 5% of all glomerulonephritides. Usually, its clinical course is associated with a rapid decline of kidney function (rapidly progressive glomerulonephritis). In early publications (64), poor prognosis of renal function was reported. None of the 39 untreated and only one of the 29 patients treated with drugs retained adequate renal function (65). However, improved diagnostic tools (indirect immunofluorescence available at most hospitals, anti-GBM antibody radioimmunoassay, direct immunofluorescence of kidney biopsy specimens) have made it possible to identify early stages of this disease with a limited expression and more benign course. About 70% of cases with anti-GBM mediated nephritis present with pulmonary hemorrhage (Goodpasture's syndrome) (63, 66).

Based on publications from the Hammersmith Hospital, London, UK (67), the therapeutic regimen in patients with progressive renal failure due to anti-GBM nephritis should include daily plasma exchanges together with cytotoxic drugs (cyclophosphamide 3 mg/kg and azathioprine 1 mg/kg) as well as prednisone (starting dose 60 mg/day). This combined therapy resulted in improvement of renal function in 15 of 17 patients presenting with a serum creatinine below 600 μmol/l. Patients with an advanced disease (serum creatinine exceeding 600 μmol/l or oligo-anuric at presentation) exhibited a far poorer response with improvement in but one of 27 patients. Furthermore, most of the deaths occurred in this latter group. A similar response to treatment has been reported by others (68). Mortality, therefore, should be considered when discussing initiation of treatment in patients with advanced disease and minimal likelihood of recovering renal function. Pulmonary hemorrhage can be readily controlled by plasmapheresis in about 90% of cases (67). As the lung infiltrates resolve there is parallel improvement in pulmonary gas exchange. An inadequate response of pulmonary hemorrhage to plasmapheresis should make one suspect a superimposed infection or fluid overload both of which radiographically can enhance the appearance of the pulmonary lesions. Specific antibiotic treatment of the infection, volume reduction by diuretics or by ultrafiltration and, if necessary, positive pressure ventilation are the appropriate therapeutic measures in such cases.

Circulating anti-GBM antibodies (measured by a sensitive radioimmunoassay rather than by indirect immunofluorescence) finally disappear in the shortest period in those patients most aggressively treated (daily plasma exchanges for 14 days and immunosuppression as described above). In most individuals, antibody synthesis is switched off within 6 weeks. After the circulating antibody disappears, it does not usually reappear (69).

During the later course of the disease, infections of the upper respiratory tract and the vascular access site (AV shunt) may be associated with pulmonary and renal deterioration, however, without recurrence of the autoantibody (70). In these cases, the organs primarily involved in the disease process seem to be highly sensitive to all types of inflammatory lesions which mimic the original disorder. Pulmonary hemorrhage without renal relapse also has been observed in acutely overhydrated patients in whom the antibody production had been controlled. As both types of relapses are not caused by autoimmunity, antibiotics and/or volume reduction or removal are the treatments of choice.

Non anti-glomerular basement membrane crescentic nephritis

This entity represents those cases of rapidly progressive glomerulonephritis which are not mediated by anti-GBM antibodies. Without treatment rapid decline of kidney function within weeks is the usual course of disease. There is evidence that immune complexes are involved in disease pathogenesis, either via deposition of circulating preformed complexes or by in situ formation of these complexes in glomeruli (71). Nephritis of this type is often associated with systemic diseases such as polyarteritis, Wegener's granulomatosis, and other types of vasculitis. Also it may be seen following such infections as streptococcal sore throat, visceral abscesses, or infected ventriculo-atrial shunts. In other cases, an initiating event cannot be identified ('idiopathic'). Non anti-GBM nephritis, therefore, comprises several forms of nephritides of quite different etiology and pathogenesis. As the natural course and response to therapy in the subsets of non anti-GBM nephritis are variable, reported treatment results should be analyzed with respect to the underlying disease.

In groups of patients with idiopathic and secondary forms of non anti-GBM mediated rapidly progressive glomerulonephritis serving as historical controls, immunosuppressive medication resulted in improved renal function in up to 50% of the patients (72). In reported trials comparing pulse methylprednisolone or plasma exchange in combination with immunosuppressive therapy, improved renal function was seen in 60 and 64% respectively (72). One controlled study analyzed the survival time without dialysis in 27 patients treated with either pulse methylprednisolone or plasma exchange and found both therapies to be equal (73). Similar results were described for 24 patients randomly treated either by immunosuppressive therapy or additional plasma exchange (72). In another prospective study which included 14 patients (pulse methylprednisolone, immunosuppressive drugs and anticoagulants versus additional plasma exchange), renal function statistically improved after 2 months in the latter group. However, no difference in recovery was seen in long term follow-up (74). The largest group of patients with non anti-GBM nephritis treated in a single center (Hammersmith Hospital, London) indicates that patients who present with oligo-anuria or a serum creatinine exceeding 600 μmol/l have a good chance to regain adequate renal function without requiring renal replacement therapy (67). According to the Hammersmith data, patients with advanced renal damage (oligo-anuria or creatinine >600 μmol/l at presentation) in non anti-GBM disease may regain adequate renal function when plasma exchange is performed early in the course of the disease. Patients suffering from less advanced disease (creatinine <600 μmol/l) appear not to require an aggressive therapeutic regimen which includes plasma exchange but should be treated with standard immunosuppressive therapy. Judging by the above reported results the prognosis in patients with rapidly progressive glomerulonephritis is better if it is not associated with autoantibodies against glomerular basement membrane.

Other types of glomerulonephritis

IgA nephropathy

The renal and extrarenal deposition of IgA 1 polymers in both primary and secondary IgA nephropathy appears to be the pathogenetic event (75, 76) which initiates a chronic glomerular lesion that may lead to a less than favorable prognosis. About one quarter of such patients develop end-stage renal disease within 6 years. Both immunosuppressive and phenytoin therapy have shown disappointing results of renal outcome. Plasma exchange has been performed with some success in those patients in whom primary IgA nephropathy (Berger's disease) or Henoch Schönlein nephritis are associated with rapidly progressive deterioration of renal function (77, 78).

Membranoproliferative glomerulonephritis type II

C3 nephritic factor, an IgG autoantibody directed against the C3-B-complex stabilizing the C3 convertase activity of the alternative complement pathway, plays the central pathogenic role in membranoproliferative glomerulonephritis type II. Usually this disease progresses slowly to end-stage renal failure. Its course is uninfluenced by the use of cytotoxic drugs. Several anecdotal reports have been published showing moderate response to treatment with plasma exchange performed in patients with this form of glomerulonephritis (79).

Lupus nephritis

In situ immune complex formation (71) and the deposition of circulating immune complexes are involved in the renal lesions of lupus nephritis. Among the different types of glomerulonephritis, diffuse proliferative lupus nephritis has the poorest prognosis both in respect to renal function and to overall patient survival (22% 5-year survival) (80). The application of plasma exchange in systemic lupus erythematosus was first reported in 1976 (81). Since then hundreds of patients have undergone plasma exchange even though, in most cases, they were treated outside of randomized protocols. Logically there appear to be two reasons to justify the use of plasma exchange in patients with lupus erythematosus. Such therapy can be expected to remove circulating autoantibodies directed against DNA, peripheral blood cells and coagulation factors (82) or to remove circulating immune complexes present in lupus sera. Also deficient complement proteins, e.g. C3 and C4 are usually decreased in active disease and may be replaced by the use of fresh frozen plasma as substitution fluid. These considerations form the basis for applying plasma exchange in systemic lupus (82). Reported indications for plasma exchange in SLE are: progressive renal and extrarenal organ involvement, including leuko- and thrombocytopenia, and the requirement of high dose steroid to control disease activity.

Progressive renal failure responded to standard immunosuppression combined with plasma exchange in a mean of 69% in uncontrolled studies (82). In a prospective controlled trial, 86 patients were randomly treated either by plasma exchange or by standard therapy (regimen not explained) (83). The mean serum creatinine in both groups pretreatment was 2.0 ± 0.2 mg/dl. At 9, 32, 56 and 104 weeks the mean serum creatinine concentration decreased continuously to 1.0 mg/dl in the group receiving standard therapy but increased to 3.5 mg/dl in the plasma exchange group at 2 years. The authors concluded that plasmapheresis had no beneficial effect upon the clinical, renal and serologic course of patients suffering from severe SLE nephritis (83).

Other controlled studies (84, 85) failed to confirm significant differences in the outcome of plasma exchange groups when compared to control groups. Despite those results, plasma exchange is useful in the management of progressive disease and in life threatening complications (82).

Wegener's granulomatosis

Wegener's granulomatosis is a systemic necrotizing granulomatous vasculitis of unknown etiology which primarily involves the kidney (rapidly progressive glomerulonephritis) and the upper and lower respiratory tract. It may also involve skin, joints, heart, and other organs. Polyclonal B cell activation, elevated immunoglobulins and detectable circulating immune complexes support evidence that a humoral immune mechanism is operative in this disease (86). Recently, autoantibodies directed against an intracytoplasmatic antigen of neutrophils and monocytes were identified in sera

of patients with active disease (87) but not in other systemic vasculitides (88).

Cyclophosphamide (2 mg/kg/day) combined with oral steroids is the treatment of choice and can induce remission in about 90% of patients (86). Azathioprine is far less effective than cyclophosphamide. Plasmapheresis together with immunosuppressive therapy (either cyclophosphamide or azathioprine) used in progressive and otherwise resistant disease resulted in a 74% improvement of renal function (23 cases, uncontrolled observations) (78).

Renal involvement in polyarteritis

Polyarteritis in both macroscopic and microscopic varieties causes a rapid decline of renal function in some patients. The overall response to plasma exchange in polyarteritis in uncontrolled studies showed improvement of renal function in 69% of the patients analyzed (78). A controlled two-arm study (with 30 patients enrolled, not all with renal involvement) compared corticosteroid therapy and long-term intermittent plasma exchange (12 treatments in 6 months) with a second group whose therapy was identical except for the addition of cyclophosphamide. No significant difference could be confirmed between the two treatment groups (89). Patients presenting with severe and progressive renal involvement in polyarteritis may benefit from a course of plasma exchange combined with immunsuppression.

Hemolytic uremic syndrome; thrombotic thrombocytopenic purpura

Hemolytic uremic syndrome (HUS) and thrombotic thrombocytopenic purpura (TTP) represent expressions of an endotheliotropic hemolytic angiopathy with severe renal involvement (90). HUS is more common in children than in adults. Clinically they present with progressive renal failure associated with hemolytic anemia and thrombocytopenia. In addition to the above mentioned findings, fluctuating neurological symptoms and fever are characteristic for TTP. The typical histological lesions result from microthrombi consisting primarily of platelets. These can be found in the capillaries of virtually every tissue including skin and kidneys (90, 91). Both diseases develop as a result of extensive endothelial injury with not only renal (HUS, TTP) but also generalized (TTP) organ involvement. Etiology remains unknown in most cases. Triggering mechanisms include: preceding bacterial or viral infections, post partum and drug exposure (cyclosporine A, antineoplastic drugs, and contraceptives) (90, 91). Several mechanisms have been proposed to be operative in the pathogenesis of HUS and TTP (90–92): 1) lack of prostacyclin or a releasing factor from the vascular endothelium to prevent generalized intravascular coagulation, 2) lack of a plasma factor necessary to degrade factor VIII: von Willebrand factor multimers (which potently trigger platelet agglutination under certain circumstances), 3) lack of a plasma factor (probably an IgG) which inactivates a 'platelet aggregating factor' and 4) endothelial injury mediated by free radicals due to their reduced degradation (e.g. vitamin E deficiency).

In the late 1940's, the mortality rate of HUS in children was nearly 50%. It has decreased to 4 to 13% during recent years, primarily related to better supportive care (90). Generally, a favorable prognosis can be anticipated in children with either HUS or TTP. Plasma infusion therapy in children has influenced neither acute mortality nor long term prognosis (93).

The prognosis of TTP has also improved in adults. Previously, patient survival rate was but 28% at 3 months (94). Recently, using different therapeutic regimens, remissions can be induced in 80 to 90% of the afflicted patients (94). Most published treatment regimens for HUS and TTP include infusion of fresh frozen plasma (FFP) or plasma exchange with FFP replacement. Each is combined with antiplatelet agents and/or corticosteroids. The replacement of a missing as yet unidentified serum factor is the rationale for FFP infusions.

Plasma exchange has the advantage of avoiding the risk of volume overload which limits plasma infusion in adults to a maximum of 0.5 to 1.0 l per day.

TTP is rare; however, it remains a life threatening disease. Before data from controlled clinical studies become available, a polypragmatic therapeutic regimen including plasma exchange with FFP replacement, platelet aggregation inhibitors and corticosteroids is recommended for TTP as soon as the diagnosis is confirmed.

Renal involvement in paraproteinemia

About one half of the patients with multiple myeloma develop renal failure. These patients usually have a poor prognosis. Factors pathogenetically involved in myeloma renal failure include tubular and glomerular damage by light chains, amyloid deposition, hypercalcemia, hyperuricemia, hyperviscosity (rarely), interstitial infiltration by plasma cells, and acute renal failure following intravenous contrast media. The major fraction of the free light chains (22,000 daltons) which are filtered by the glomeruli is reabsorbed and catabolized by tubular cells. Precipitation of light chains in the distal tubules and a direct toxic effect on tubular cells are the pathogenetic mechanisms in paraproteinemic acute renal failure. Hypercalcemia, present in about 50% of these cases, (95, 96) can also precipitate acute renal failure.

Paraproteinemic acute renal failure is one of the established indications for therapeutic plasma exchange. Of 142 patients suffering from this condition, 40% retained adequate renal function following plasma exchange (97). To reduce light chain synthesis, concomitant cytotoxic therapy should be administered.

Removal efficiency for Bence Jones proteins with plasma exchange (4 to 5 l exchanged) is 10 times greater than with peritoneal dialysis (98). Elimination of monomeric light chains should also be possible with hemofiltration which would offer the advantage of protein-free substitution of plasma filtrate. However, no conclusive data are available concerning light chain removal efficiency to support this therapy in favor of standard plasma exchange.

If renal failure in paraproteinemia fails to respond to an adequate course of plasma exchange, factors other than light chain toxicity may be involved in kidney damage (e.g. amyloidosis, hypercalcemia, hyperuricemia).

Plasmapheresis in renal transplantation

Removal of preformed lymphocytotoxic antibodies prior to transplantation

The presence of lymphocytotoxic antibodies against multiple HLA antigens may limit kidney transplantation in some dialysis patients. Plasma exchange has been performed in some highly sensitized individuals with the aim of removing these antibodies. To suppress further antibody synthesis, plasma exchange was combined with an immunosuppressive regimen. Nine of 18 patients showed a significant decrease in cytotoxic anti-HLA antibodies (99, 100) and were transplanted, six of them successfully. However, there are too few published case reports to allow a general statement to be made about the role of plasma exchange in highly sensitized dialysis patients at this time.

Plasma exchange in transplant rejections

Plasma exchange has been used for treatment of acute and chronic rejection during the post transplant course. The type of rejection (cellular or humoral/vascular) was confirmed by biopsy in but a few studies. According to a literature overview (101), 127 of 214 acute (59%) and five of 26 chronic (19%) rejections responded to plasma exchange. The response rate of 0 to 93% at different centers may be explained by differences in entry criteria and treatment protocols.

Controlled studies of acute rejections exhibited an overall successful outcome (61%) in the plasma exchange group compared to 51% in the controls (101). One prospective controlled trial used plasma exchange randomly in all acute transplant rejection episodes (85 patients). During the entire 4 year study period, the graft survival rate was better in the plasma exchange group than in the patients treated with conventional antirejection therapy (102). Paying special attention to anti-HLA antibodies an Italian group treated steroid resistant rejections in 44 patients in a randomized protocol, either by plasmapheresis or by pharmacological therapy alone. The rate of graft failures was lower in the plasma exchange group (7/23) than in the controls (17/21) (103).

In conclusion, some patients benefit from plasma exchange performed in acute kidney transplant rejection of either vascular or cellular variety. However, the data as a whole are derived from quite different entry and treatment protocols and do not yet allow a specification of subgroups for whom plasmapheresis can be recommended as standard therapy.

Recurrent glomerular disease in the transplanted kidney

A recurrence of primary renal disease in the transplanted

organ was the reason for plasma exchange in five patients suffering from lupus nephritis, mesangial proliferative glomerulonephritis, and anti-GBM nephritis. In three cases, renal function or proteinuria improved. Thus, therapeutic plasma exchange can be attempted for those rare cases of recurrent primary renal disease in a transplant recipient (78).

CONCLUSION

During the past decade plasma exchange performed either by centrifuge or membrane-based equipment has become routine therapy in many hospitals. Its application is still accompanied by a certain risk posed by administration of substitution fluids. Plasma fractionation procedures offer more selective plasma manipulation especially in diseases with well characterized macromolecular circulating pathogens. The ability to remove specific pathogens exceeds by far our knowledge of disease processes. This may, however, contribute to better understanding of disease pathogenesis.

Data are available from but a few conclusive controlled studies for some distinct situations in several disorders. Consequently, the physician's therapeutic decision must be influenced not only by published data but also by his experience with the disease process and extracorporeal immunomodulating therapy.

REFERENCES

1. Adams WS, Blahd WH, Bassett SH: A method of human plasmapheresis. *Proc Soc Exp Biol Med* 80: 377, 1952
2. Conway N, Walker JM: Treatment of macroglobulinaemia. *Br Med J* 2: 1296, 1962
3. Millward BL, Hoeltge GA: The historical development of automated hemapheresis. *J Clin Apheresis* 1: 25, 1982
4. Gloeckner WM, Sieberth HG: Plasma filtration, a new method of plasma exchange. *Proc Eur Soc Artif Organs* 4: 214, 1978
5. Gurland HJ, Samtleben W, Blumenstein M, Randerson DH, Schmidt B: Clinical applications of macromolecular separations. *Trans Am Soc Artif Intern Organs* 27: 356, 1981
6. Gurland HJ, Lysaght MJ, Samtleben W, Schmidt B: Comparative evaluation of filters used in membrane plasmapheresis. *Nephron* 36: 173, 1984
7. Lysaght MJ, Samtleben W, Schmidt B, Gurland HJ: Contemporary technical issues in membrane plasmapheresis: Controversies and reconciliation. in: *Plasma Separation and Plasma Fractionation,* edited by Lysaght MJ, Gurland HJ, Basel, Karger, 1983, p 315
8. Lysaght MJ, Schmidt B, Samtleben W, Gurland HJ: Transport considerations in flat sheet microporous membrane plasmapheresis. *Plasma Ther Transfus Technol* 4: 373, 1983
9. Colton CK, Henderson LW, Ford CA, Lysaght MJ: Kinetics of hemodiafiltration. I. In vitro transport characteristics of a hollow-fiber blood ultrafilter. *J Lab Clin Med* 85: 355, 1975
10. Nicholls AJ, Platts MM: Anaphylactoid reactions due to haemodialysis, haemofiltration, or membrane plasma separation. *Br Med J* 285: 1607, 1982
11. Klinkmann H, Schmitt E, Falkenhagen D, Schmidt R, Osten B, Ahrenholz P, Tessenow D: Reuse of membrane plasma

12. Randerson DH, Blumenstein M, Samtleben W, Schmidt B, Gurland HJ: Reuse of membrane plasma separators. in: *Plasmapheresis,* edited by Nose Y, Malchesky PS, Smith JW, Krakauer RS, New York, Raven Press, 1983, p 161
13. Sutton DMC, Cardella CJ, Uldall PR, DeVeber GA: Complications of intensive plasma exchange. *Plasma Ther* 2: 19, 1981
14. Roberts CG, Schindhelm K, Smeby LC, Farrell PC: Kinetic analysis of plasma separation: Use of an animal model. in: *Plasma Separation and Plasma Fractionation,* edited by Lysaght MJ, Gurland HJ, Basel, Karger, 1983, p 25
15. Samtleben W, Randerson DH, Blumenstein M, Habersetzer R, Schmidt B, Gurland HJ: Membrane plasma exchange: Principles and application techniques. *J Clin Apheresis* 2: 163, 1984
16. Frank MM, Hamburger MI, Lawley TJ, Kimberly RP, Plotz PH: Defective reticuloendothelial system Fc-receptor function in systemic lupus erythematosus. *N Engl J Med* 300: 518, 1979
17. Lockwood CM, Worlledge S, Nicholas A, Cotton C, Peters DK: Reversal of impaired splenic function in patients with nephritis or vasculitis (or both) by plasma exchange. *N Engl J Med* 300: 524, 1979
18. Samtleben W, Schmidt B, Bosch T, Gurland HJ: Are immune complex assays an appropriate tool for quantitation of plasma exchange? *Plasma Ther Transfus Technol* 6: 523, 1985
19. Schroeder JO, Euler HH, Loeffler H: Synchronization of plasmapheresis and pulse cyclophosphamide in severe systemic lupus erythematosus. *Ann Intern Med* 107: 344, 1987
20. Aufeuvre JP, Morin-Hertel F, Cohen-Solal M, Lefloch A, Baudelot J: Hazards of plasma exchange. A nation-wide study of 3431 exchanges in 592 patients. in: *Plasma Exchange,* edited by Sieberth HG, Stuttgart, New York, Schattauer, 1980, p 149
21. Das PC, Smit Sibinga CT: Complications of therapeutic plasma exchange. *Lancet* 2: 455, 1983
22. Borberg H: Problems of plasma exchange therapy. in: *Therapeutic Plasma Exchange,* edited by Gurland HJ, Heinze V, Lee HA, Berlin, Heidelberg, New York, Springer, 1981, p 191
23. Bussel A, Sitthy X, Reviron J: Aspects technologiques et complications des exchanges plasmatiques. (Technical aspects and complications of plasma exchange.) *Rev Fr Transfus Immunohematol* 25: 547, 1982
24. Fabre M, Andreu G, Mannoni P: Some biological modifications and clinical hazards observed during plasma exchange. in: *Plasma Exchange,* edited by Sieberth HG, Stuttgart, New York, Schattauer, 1980, p 143
25. Gajdos P, Pourrat J, Elkharrat D, Terre C: National register for plasma exchange – The French Society for Hemapheresis. Results for 1985. *Plasma Ther Transfus Technol* 8: 137, 1987
26. Samtleben W, Hillebrand G, Krumme D, Gurland HJ: Membrane plasma separation: Clinical experience with more than 120 plasma exchanges. in: *Plasma Exchange,* edited by Sieberth HG, Stuttgart, New York, Schattauer, 1980, p 175
27. Tindall RSA, Walker JE, Ehle AL, Near L, Rolins J, Becker D: Plasmapheresis in multiple sclerosis: Prospective trial of pheresis and immunosuppression versus immunosuppression alone. *Neurology* 32: 739, 1982
28. Editorial: Hazards of apheresis. *Lancet* 2: 1025, 1982
29. Huestis DW: Mortality in therapeutic haemapheresis. *Lancet* 1: 1043, 1983
30. Ring J, Messmer K: Incidence and severity of anaphylactoid reactions to colloid volume substitutes. *Lancet* 1: 466, 1977

filters. in: *Plasmapheresis,* edited by Nose Y, Malchesky PS, Smith JW, Krakauer RS, New York, Raven Press, 1983, p 107

31. Evans RT, MacDonald R, Robinson EAE: Suxamethonium apnoea associated with plasmapheresis. *Anaesthesia* 35: 198, 1980

32. Jones JV, Parker WA, Sketris IS: The effect of plasmapheresis on therapeutic drugs. *Dial Transplant* 14: 225, 1985

33. Sketris IS, Parker WA, Jones JV: Plasmapheresis: Its effect on toxic agents and drugs. *Plasma Ther Transfus Technol* 5: 305, 1984

34. Schmidt B, Lysaght MJ, Samtleben W, Gurland HJ: Plasmapheresis without pumps for therapeutic and donor purposes. in: *Plasma Separation and Plasma Fractionation,* edited by Lysaght MJ, Gurland HJ, Basel, Karger, 1983, p 188

35. Samtleben W, Lysaght MJ, Schmidt B, Gurland HJ: A very simple technique for spontaneous membrane plasma exchange without arterial access. *Blood Purif* 1: 90, 1983

36. Landini S, Coli U, Lucatello S, Fracasso A, Morachiello P, Righetto F, Scanferla F, Bazzato G: Spontaneous plasma exchange by gravity. *Int J Artif Organs* 7: 137, 1984

37. Samtleben W, Lysaght MJ, Banthien F, Hillebrand G, Gurland HJ: Simultaneous combined hemodialysis and membrane plasmapheresis. in: *Plasma Separation and Plasma Fractionation,* edited by Lysaght MJ, Gurland HJ, Basel, Karger, 1983, p 213

38. Scheiner E, Reich L, Isaacs M, Vanamee P, Fombaum CD, van Strien S, Gulati SC: Simultaneous hemodialysis and plasmapheresis: Ten years experience. *Kidney Int* (abstract) 23: 160, 1983

39. Gross MLP, Baillod RA, Sweny P, Pearson RM: (Letter) *Plasma Ther* 2: 255, 1981

40. Lysaght MJ, Samtleben W, Schmidt B, Gurland HJ: Closed-loop plasmapheresis. in: *Therapeutic Hemapheresis,* edited by MacPherson JL, Kasprisin DO, Boca Raton, CRC Press, 1985, Volume I, p 149

41. Samtleben W, Schindhelm K: Therapeutic plasmapheresis (Editorial). *Biomed Pharmacother* 40: 281, 1986

42. Terman DS, Stewart I, Robinetti J, Carr R, Harbeck R: Specific removal of DNA antibodies in vivo with an extracorporeal immunoadsorbent. *Clin Exp Immunol* 24: 231, 1976

43. Lupien PJ, Moorjani S, Awad J: A new approach to the management of familial hypercholesterolemia: removal of plasma cholesterol based on the principle of affinity chromatography. *Lancet* 1: 1261, 1976

44. Yokoyama S, Hayashi R, Kikkawa T, Tani N, Takada S, Hatanaba K, Yamamoto A: Specific sorbent of apolipoprotein B-containing lipoproteins of plasmapheresis. Characterization and experimental use in hypercholesterolemic rabbits. *Arteriosclerosis* 4: 276, 1984

45. Stoffel W, Borberg H, Greve V: Application of specific extracorporeal removal of low density lipoprotein in familial hypercholesterolaemia. *Lancet* 2: 1005, 1981

46. Pourrat JP, Sanchez V, Conte JJ, Man NK: On-line plasma reprocessing by convective electrophoresis. in: *Plasma Separating and Plasma Fractionation,* edited by Lysaght MJ, Gurland HJ, Basel, Karger, 1983, p 303

47. Fuchs C, Windisch M, Wieland H, Armstrong VW, Rieger J, Koestering H, Scheler F, Seidel D: Selective continuous extracorporeal elimination of low-density lipoproteins from plasma by heparin precipitation without cations. in: *Plasma Separation and Plasma Fractionation,* edited by Lysaght MJ, Gurland HJ, Basel, Karger, 1983, p 272

48. Lockwood CM, Rees AJ, Pearson TA, Evans DJ, Peters DK, Wilson CB: Immunosuppression and plasma-exchange in the treatment of Goodpasture's syndrome. *Lancet* 1: 711, 1976

49. Lockwood CM, Rees AJ, Pinching AJ, Pussell B, Sweny P,

Uff J, Peters DK: Plasma-exchange and immunosuppression in the treatment of fulminating immune-complex crescentic nephritis. *Lancet* 1: 63, 1977

50. Pinching AJ, Peters DK, Newsom Davis J: Remission of myasthenia gravis following plasma-exchange. *Lancet* 2: 1373, 1976

51. Bukowski RM, King JW, Hewlett JS: Plasmapheresis in the treatment of thrombotic thrombocytopenic purpura. *Blood* 50: 413, 1977

52. Kambic H, Hyslop L, Nose Y: *Topics in Plasmapheresis. A Bibliography of Therapeutic Applications and New Techniques.* Cleveland, ISAO Press, 1985

53. Conference report: Plasma exchange. *Ann Rheum Dis* 39: 95, 1980

54. Wysenbeck AJ, Smith JW, Krakauer RS: Plasmapheresis II: Review of clinical experience. *Plasma Ther* 2: 61, 1981

55. Wenz B, Barland P: Therapeutic intensive plasmapheresis. *Sem Hematol* 18: 147, 1981

56. International Forum: What are the established clinical indications for therapeutic plasma exchange and how important is the choice of replacement for efficacy of therapeutic plasma exchange in these situations? *Vox Sang* 43: 270, 1982

57. Kennedy MS, Domen RE: Therapeutic apheresis. Applications and future directions. *Vox Sang* 45: 261, 1983

58. Shumak KH, Rock GA: Therapeutic plasma exchange. *N Engl J Med* 310: 762, 1984

59. Council on Scientific Affairs: Current status of therapeutic plasmapheresis and related techniques. Report of the AMA panel on therapeutic plasmapheresis. *JAMA* 253: 819, 1985

60. Klein HG, Balow JE, Dau PC, Hamburger MI, Leitmann SF, Pineda AA, Tindall RSA: Clinical applications of therapeutic apheresis. Report of the Clinical Applications Committee. American Society for Apheresis. *J Clin Apheresis* 3 (special issue): 1986

61. Fish AJ, Lockwood MC, Wong M, Price RG: Detection of Goodpasture antigen in fractions prepared from collagenase digest of human glomerular basement membrane. *Clin Exp Immunol* 55: 58, 1984

62. Wieslander J, Byrgen P, Heinegard D: Isolation of the specific glomerular basement membrane antigen involved in Goodpasture syndrome. *Proc Natl Acad Sci USA* 81: 1544, 1984

63. Salant DJ: Immunopathogenesis of crescentic glomerulonephritis and lung purpura (Nephrology Forum). *Kidney Int* 32: 408, 1987

64. Wilson CB, Dixon FJ: Anti-glomerular basement membrane antibody-induced glomerulonephritis. *Kidney Int* 3: 74, 1973

65. Wilson CB, Dixon FJ: The renal response to immunological injury. in: *The Kidney,* edited by Brenner BM, Rector FC, Philadelphia, London, Toronto, Saunders, 1981, p 1237

66. Rees AJ, Lockwood CM, Peters DK: Nephritis due to antibodies to GBM. in: *Progress in Glomerulonephritis,* edited by Kincaid-Smith P, D'Apice AJF, Atkins RJ, New York, John Wiley, 1980, p 348

67. Lockwood CM, Pusey CD, Peters DK: Indications for plasma exchange: renal diseases. in: *Plasma Separation and Plasma Fractionation,* edited by Lysaght MJ, Gurland HJ, Basel, Karger, 1983, p 145

68. Swainson CP, Winney RJ, Urbaniak SJ, Robinson JS: Plasma exchange in severe glomerulonephritis – who benefits? *Proc Eur Dial Transplant Assoc* 19: 732, 1982

69. Peters DK, Pusey CD, Lockwood CM: Immunomodulation by plasma exchange: Therapeutic objectives. in: *Plasma Separation and Plasma Fractionation,* edited by Lysaght MJ, Gurland HJ, Basel, Karger, 1983, p 1

70. Rees AJ, Lockwood CM, Peters DK: Enhanced allergic tissue injury in Goodpasture's syndrome by interccurrent infection. *Br Med J* 2: 723, 1977

71. Couser WG, Salant DJ: In situ immune complex formation and glomerular injury. *Kidney Int* 17: 1, 1980

72. Sieberth H-G, Maurin N: The therapy of rapidly progressive glomerulonephritis. *Klin Wochenschr* 61: 1001, 1983

73. Stevens ME, McConnel M, Bone JM: Aggressive treatment with pulse methylprednisolone or plasma exchange is justified in rapidly progressive glomerulonephritis. *Proc Eur Dial Transplant Assoc* 19: 724, 1982

74. Rifle G, Chalopin JM, Zech P, Deteix P, Ducret F, Vialtel P, Cordonnier D: Treatment of idiopathic acute crescentic glomerulonephritis by immunodepression and plasma-exchanges. A prospective randomized study. *Proc Eur Dial Transplant Assoc* 18: 493, 1980

75. Kauffmann RH, van Es LA, Daha MR: The specific detection of IgA immune complexes. *J Immunol Meth* 40: 117, 1981

76. Valentijn RM, Kauffmann RH, De La Riviere GB, Daha MR, van Es LA: Presence of circulating macromolecular IgA in patients with hematuria due to primary IgA nephropathy. *Am J Med* 74: 375, 1983

77. Hene RJ, Kater L: Plasmapheresis in nephritis associated with Henoch-Schoenlein purpura and in primary IgA nephropathy. *Plasma Ther Transfus Technol* 4: 165, 1983

78. Samtleben W, Gurland HJ: Plasma exchange in nephrological diseases. in: *Therapeutic Hemapheresis,* edited by Valbonesi M, Pineda AA, Biggs JC, Milan, Wichtig Editore, 1986, p 29

79. Chalopin JM, Rifle G, Tanter Y, Besancent JF, Cabanne JF, Justrabo E: Treatment of IgA nephropathy by plasma exchanges alone. *Artif Organs* 5 (Suppl): 138, 1981

80. Schwarzt RS: Immunologic and genetic aspects of systemic lupus erythematosus. *Kidney Int* 19: 474, 1981

81. Jones JV, Cumming RH, Bucknall RC, Asplin CM, Fraser ID, Bothamley J, Davis P, Hamblin TJ: Plasmapheresis in the management of acute systemic lupus erythematosus? *Lancet* 1: 709, 1976

82. Samtleben W, Lysaght MJ, Gurland HJ: Plasma exchange in lupus nephritis: Rationale and clinical experiences. *Dial Transplant* 14: 213, 1985

83. Herbert L, Nielsen E, Pohl M, Lachin J, Hunsicker L, Lewis E: Clinical course of severe lupus nephritis during the controlled clinical trial of plasmapheresis therapy (PPT). *Kidney Int* (abstract) 31: 201, 1987

84. Wei N, Klippel JH, Huston DP, Hall RP, Lawley TJ, Balow JE, Steinberg AD, Decker JL: Randomized trial of plasma exchange in mild systemic lupus erythematosus. *Lancet* 1: 17, 1983

85. Clark WF, Balfe JW, Cattran DC, Williams W, Koval JJ, Arnott M, Chodirker WB, Lindsay RM, Linton AL: Long-term plasma exchange in patients with systemic lupus erythematosus and diffuse proliferative glomerulonephritis. *Plasma Ther Transfus Technol* 5: 353, 1984

86. Fauci AS, Haynes BF, Katz P, Wolff SM: Wegener's granulomatosis: Prospective clinical and therapeutic experience with 85 patients for 21 years. *Ann Intern Med* 98: 76, 1983

87. van der Woude FJ, Rasmussen N, Lobatto S, Wiik A, Permin H, van Es LA, van der Giessen M, van der Hem GK, The TH: Autoantibodies against neutrophils and monocytes: tool for diagnosis and marker of disease activity in Wegener's granulomatosis. *Lancet* 1: 425, 1985

88. Gross WL, Luedermann G, Kiefer G, Lehmann: Anticy-toplasmatic antibodies in Wegener's granulomatosis. *Lancet* 1: 806, 1986

89. Guillevin L, Bussel A, Andreu G: Treatment of polyarteritis nodosa with plasma exchange, corticosteroids and a randomized trial of cyclophosphamide. One year results in 30 cases. *Eur J Clin Invest* (abstract) 13: A43, 1983

90. Remuzzi G: HUS and TTP: Variable expressions of a single entity. *Kidney Int* 32: 292, 1987

91. Neild G: The haemolytic uremic syndrome: A review. *Q J Med* 241: 367, 1987

92. Aster RH: Plasma therapy for thrombotic thrombocytopenic purpura. Sometimes it works, but why (Editorial retrospective). *N Engl J Med* 312: 985, 1985

93. Rizzoni G, Pavanelle L, Claris-Appiani A, Edefonti A, Facchin P, Franchini F, Gussmano R, Imbasciati E, Perfumo F, Remuzzi G: Treatment of children with hemolytic uremic syndrome (HUS) with plasma: A multicenter controlled trial (abstract). *Helv Paediatr Acta* 41: 114, 1986

94. Stoffner D, Banthien FCA, Habersetzer R, Samtleben W, Clemm C, Unterburger P, Zaehringer J, Gurland HJ: Plasma exchange and concommitant therapy in TTP. *Int J Artif Organs* 7: 223, 1984

95. Pourrat JP, Dueymes JM, Conte JJ, Pourrat O, Alcalay D, Touchard G, Patte D: Plasma exchange in myeloma renal failure. in: *Plasmapheresis,* edited by Nose Y, Malchesky PS, Smith JW, Krakauer RS, New York, Raven Press, 1983, p 349

96. Blumenstein M, Samtleben W, Gurland HJ: Die Behandlung des paraproteinämischen Nierenversagens mit Plasmapherese (Plasma therapy for treatment of renal failure in patients with plasma cell diseases.) *Nieren- und Hochdruckkrankh* 16: 140, 1987

97. Blumberg A, Buergi W, Marti HR: Plasmapheresebehandlung bei multiplem Myelom mit Niereninsuffizienz. (Plasmapheresis therapy for multiple myeloma with renal insufficiency.) *Schweiz Med Wochenschr* 113: 398, 1983

98. Russell JA, Fitz-Harris BM, Corringham R, Darcy DA, Powles RL: Plasma exchange versus peritoneal dialysis for removing Bence Jones protein. *Br Med J* 2: 1397, 1978

99. Hillebrand G, Castro LA, Samtleben W, Albert E, Scholz S, Illner WD, Land W, Gurland HJ: Removal of preformed cytotoxic antibodies in highly sensitized patients using plasma exchange and immunosuppressive therapy, azathioprine, or cyclosporine prior to renal transplantation. *Transplant Proc* 18: 1033, 1986

100. Minakuchi J, Takahashi K, Toma H, Teroaka S, Hayasaka Y, Ota K: Removal of preformed antibodies by plasmapheresis prior to kidney transplantation. *Transplant Proc* 18: 1083, 1986

101. Gurland HJ, Blumenstein M, Lysaght MJ, Samtleben W, Stoffner D: Plasmapheresis in renal transplantation. *Kidney Int* 23 (Suppl 14): S82, 1983

102. Cardella CJ, Sutton DMC, Uldall PR, Cook GT, deVeber GA: Factors influencing the effect of intensive plasma exchange on acute transplant rejection. *Transplant Proc* 17: 2777, 1985

103. Bonomini V, Vangelista A, Frasca GM, Di Felice A, Liviano D'Arcangelo G: Effects of plasmapheresis in renal transplant rejection. A controlled study. in: *Therapeutic Plasma Exchange and Selective Plasma Separation,* edited by Bambauer R, Malchesky PS, Falkenhagen D, Stuttgart, New York, 1987, p 69

PERITONEAL DIALYSIS: A HISTORICAL REVIEW

WILLIAM DRUKKER

INTRODUCTION: THE INVENTION OF PERITONEAL LAVAGE (1744–1745)

For several centuries the peritoneum has enchanted physiologists, pathologists, surgeons, gynaecologists and internists. More recently nephrologists joined the teams of clinical investigators.

The concept of peritoneal lavage goes back almost 150 years (1) when it served a purpose totally different from removal of toxins.

Actually the idea came from a clergyman, the Reverend Stephen Hales, a man with great interest in biology (Figure 1). It so happened that the reverend gentleman in the year 1744 during his pastorate at Teddington in the London District of Richmond, attended a Thursday meeting of the Royal Society of Medicine in London and learned about a new – rather drastic – method of treating recurrent ascites, presented by Christopher Warrick, a surgeon from Truro in Cornwall, England (2).

Mr. Warrick was called to the assistance of a lady named Jane Roman, near 50 years old, who was confined to bed by recurrent ascites. He performed paracentesis and drew 36 pints[1] of fluid from her abdominal cavity, being aware that this would not be an absolute cure for the ascites of the lady. Therefore he took some part of the extracted 'lymph' to his own home and started a number of experimental investigations with the withdrawn fluid, looking for a method whereby the 'ruptured lymphatics must close their mouths' so as to prevent recurrence of the ascites. As expected the relief of the lady was only of short duration: 10 days after the first paracentesis 'an inundation alarmed her again' and within 14 days the patient again desired Mr. Warrick's assistance for relief. By this time he had drawn some conclusions from his experimental work and resolved to try their efficiency. With another paracentesis he removed more than 20 pints of clear briny lymph as before, which quantity did not exceed 2/3 of the whole. Ten he replaced the 'ascitic lymph' by a blood-warm mixture of equal parts of fresh Bristol water and cohore claret (a Bordeaux wine). After injection of 10–12 pints of the claret-water mixture the patient collapsed and apparently went into an alarming condition. She recovered however and Mr Warrick, who had interrupted the injection, and expected that this partial instillation of the therapeutical fluid would not be effective enough, asked the lady if she thought herself capable of undergoing the procedure a second time. She was apparently a courageous patient and she answered him 'in the affirmative'. He then prepared a stronger mixture for the second injection, the claret being in a double proportion of the water and drew off the whole contents of the abdomen and repeated the injection as before. The patient complained of 'heavy pungent pain, darting through all the viscera' and Warrick became alarmed because her breathing became difficult, her pulse faltered, the syncope returned and the patient became speechless. He withdrew the cannula, ended the procedure and much to his relief the patient recovered.

---

[1] 1 pint (British) = 0.568 l.

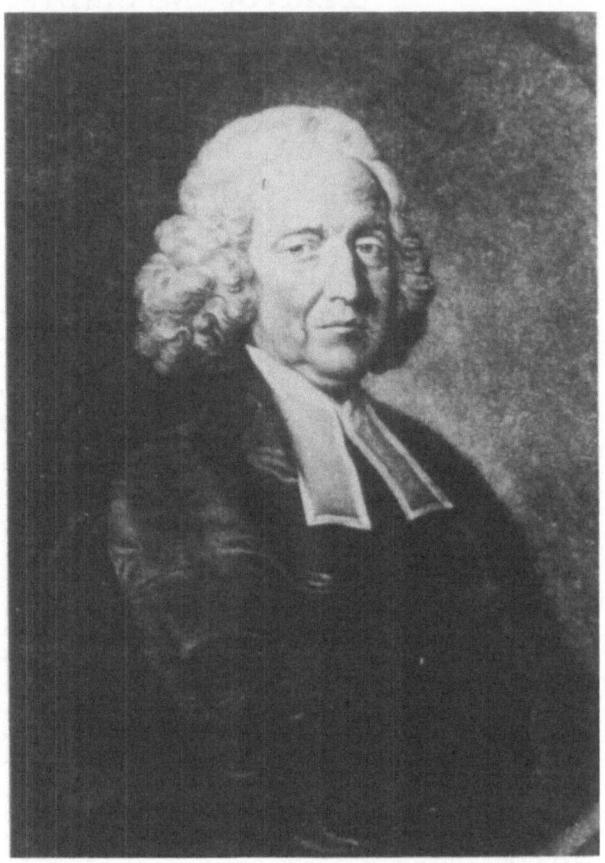

Figure 1. The Rev. Stephen Hales: 'A Method of conveying Liquors into the Abdomen during the Operation of Tapping; ... communicated in a Letter to Cromwell Mortimer, M.D. Secr. R.S. (Feb 22, 1744)'. (From the Library of the Royal Society of Medicine, London, England).

During a 1 month follow-up the ascites did not recur. 'Apparently the mouths of the lymphatics had been closed'.

The Reverend Stephen Hales (3) obviously felt pity for the poor lady and wrote a letter to the secretary of the Royal Society, Dr. Cromwell Mortimer, which was published in the Philosophical Transactions, suggesting a more gentle modification of Mr. Warrick's method for 'an absolute cure for an ascites'.

'By having two trochars fixed at the same time, one on each side of the belly; one of them having a communication with a vessel full of the medicinal liquor by means of a small leathern pipe: this liquor might flow into the abdomen, as fast as the dropsical lympha passed off through the other trochar; by which the dropsical lympha might be conveyed off to what degree it shall be thought proper; and that without any danger of a syncope from inanition; because the abdomen would, through the whole operation, continue distended with liquor, in such a degree as should be found proper; by raising or lowering the vessel with the medicinal liquor in it'.

IV. *A Method of conveying* Liquors *into the* Abdomen *during the Operation of* Tapping; *proposed by the Reverend* Stephen Hales, *D. D. and F. R. S. on Occasion of the preceding Paper; communicated in a Letter to* Cromwell Mortimer, *M. D. Secr. R. S.*

S I R,   Feb. 22. 1743-4.

Read Feb. 23. 1743-4.

IT occurred to me, on your reading, *Thursday* last, before the Society, the Case of the Woman at *Truro* in *Cornwall*, who was cured of a Dropsy, by injecting into the *Abdomen Bristol* Water and *Cohore* Wine, after having drawn off a good Quantity of the dropsical *Lympha*; that, in case of further Trial, that, or any other Liquor, shall be found effectual to the Purpose, it might be more commodiously injected in the following Manner; *viz.*

By having Two *Trochars* fixed at the same time, one on each Side of the Belly; one of them having a Communication with a Vessel full of the medicinal Liquor by means of a small leathern Pipe: This Liquor might flow into the *Abdomen*, as fast as the dropsical *Lympha* passed off through the other *Trochar*; whereby the dropsical *Lympha* might be conveyed off, to what Degree it shall be thought proper; and that without any Danger of a *Syncope* from Inanition; because the *Abdomen* would, through the whole Operation, continue distended with Liquor, in such a Degree as shall be found proper, by raising or lowering the Vessel with the medicinal Liquor in it.

It is probable, that, if the Surface of the medicinal Liquor be about a Foot higher than the *Abdomen*, it may be sufficient for the Purpose.

It were easy to find the Force with which the *Abdomen* is distended by the dropsical *Lympha*, by seeing to what Height it arose in a Glass Tube fixed to the *Trochar*; which Tube being taken away, it might, I suppose, be sufficient to have the medicinal Liquor flow in from a lesser perpendicular Height, than that to which the dropsical *Lympha* arose in the Glass Tube. I am,

S I R,

Your humble Servant,

Stephen Hales.

Figure 2. The Rev. Stephen Hales' letter to the Secretary of the Royal Society (3).

This first description of peritoneal lavage was essentially identical with continuous peritoneal lavage, later to be used for the treatment of uraemia.

In retrospect Mr. Warrick's method 'for an absolute cure' of recurrent ascites obviously served the purpose of obliterating the abdominal cavity, something that should definitely be avoided in peritoneal dialysis ... At Mr. Warrick's last

visit to the patient he 'left her in pursuit of that health which she soon acquired and continued to enjoy ...'

EARLY STUDIES OF THE PERITONEUM (1877–1922/23)

Nothing is known of the fate of subsequent patients with recurrent ascites; the next publication on experimental peritoneal lavage was published more than 130 years later and came from Wegner (4), a German investigator, who published in 1877 the results of a series of animal experiments, perfusing the abdominal cavity of rabbits with cold saline solution, observing a decrease of the animals' body temperature.

The peritoneum as a semi-permeable membrane

The results of other animal experiments of Wegner were more important: he observed an increase in volume of concentrated sugar solutions or glycerol during a dwell period in the abdominal cavity.

This phenomenon was studied again by a group of English physiologists, headed by Starling in 1894 and 1895. Starling and his co-workers (5, 6) confirmed Wegner's observations and also demonstrated a decrease in volume of a hypotonic solution, whereas the volume of isotonic solutions or serum remained unaltered for several hours.

Similar observations were reported by Orlow (7) from Germany: solutions with a low sodium chloride concentration (0.3% [51 mmol/l]) when injected in the peritoneal cavity, decreased in volume with an increase of the salt concentration. Hypertonic salt solutions (1.5% [256 mmol/l] or more) caused transfer of fluid from the blood and an increase of plasma chloride. Solutions with sodium chloride concentrations between 0.4 and 0.9% (68 and 154 mmol/l) decreased slowly in volume, the chloride concentrations equilibrating with the chloride concentration of the blood serum.

The experimental work of Clark (8) showed that after introduction of a sodium chloride solution first absorption occurs and later slower diffusible substances enter the peritoneal fluid from the blood with an increase of the osmotic pressure of the peritoneal fluid, slowing the absorption. When dextrose was introduced (8, 9), making the fluid hypertonic and preventing absorption of fluid, water and crystalloids entered the peritoneal fluid. Because of the slow diffusion of dextrose this effect was rather long lasting. Dextrose appeared therefore an excellent substance to remove fluid from the blood into the peritoneal cavity.

Finally Clark (8) showed that the rate of absorption through the peritoneum was increased by elevating the temperature of the solution and decreased by introducing a cold solution. A similar effect was noted by application of heat to the abdominal wall, which apparently increased the permeability of the peritoneum. Cooling the abdominal wall had the opposite effect (10).

Other investigators (11) noted an increase in absorption from the peritoneal cavity by increasing intestinal mobility (e.g. by means of physostigmin). When intestinal peristalsis

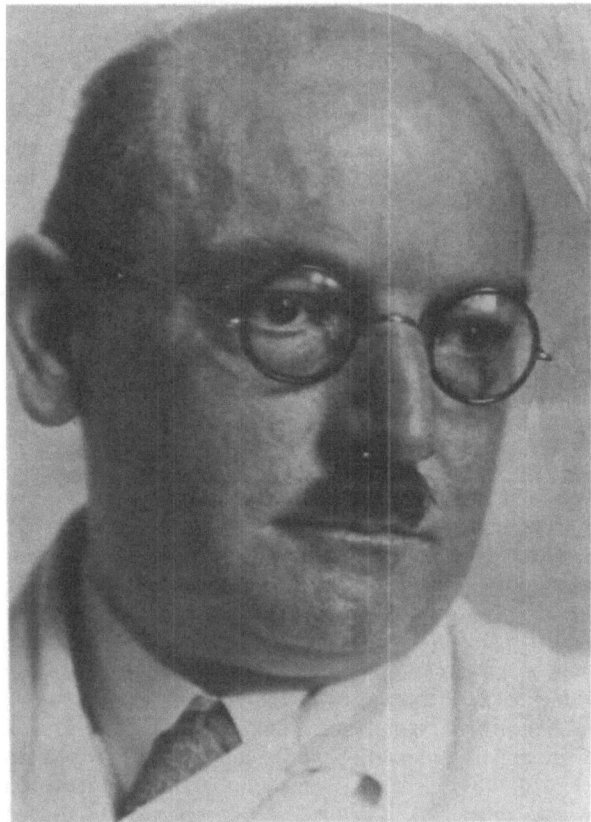

Figure 3. G. Ganter, M.D. (1885–1940), professor of medicine at Würzburg, Germany, who introduced the concept of intermittent peritoneal dialysis (1923 [24]).

was inhibited with opiates absorption was delayed.

Putman (12) demonstrated that his experimental animals tolerated the intraperitoneal introduction of sodium chloride solutions of less than 1% (170 mmol/l) reasonably well, being initially uncomfortable but rapidly recovering. However solutions of more than 1% sodium chloride were tolerated poorly: the animals frequently died within a few hours.

Permeability of the peritoneum

Many of these early investigations and other experimental data from ancient literature (9, 10, 12–14) presented convincing evidence that the peritoneal membrane is permeable in two directions, acting *in vivo* in a similar way as a pig's bladder membrane *in vitro* or a membrane of nonbiological material like parchment (15). Starling and Tubby (5) and several other investigators (10, 16) also demonstrated a bidirectional permeability of the peritoneum for larger solutes in the range of the so called middle molecules (see chapters 2, 3 and 13). Methylene blue (molecular weight 374), indigo carmine (M.W. 466) or eosin (M.W. 624), when introduced in the peritoneal fluid, pass rapidly into the blood and ap-

pear subsequently in the urine.

When these substances are injected intravenously, they pass rapidly through the peritoneum in the opposite direction to appear promptly in the peritoneal fluid. The permeability of the peritoneum for molecules in the middle molecular weight range was rediscovered in 1965 and plays presently an important role in the clinical application of the peritoneum as a dialysis membrane in uraemia.

As early as 1923 Putman (12) described the living peritoneum as a membrane with holes punched in it, permitting the passage of larger molecules than ordinary, non-living dialysis membranes do.

In addition, a living membrane like the peritoneum is subject to inflammation which changes the permeability drastically (17–19), permitting the passage of protein molecules.

Comprehensive surveys of the earlier literature and historical studies on the physiology and permeability of the peritoneum have been published previously. The reader who is interested in these early investigations is referred to these reviews (20–22).

Further progress and practical application of the acquired knowledge was relatively slow, mainly because most work was undertaken by scientists. The clinical investigators had not appreciated a medical application so far.

Furthermore World War I delayed and interrupted progress in medical work. In 1918 two American paediatricians, Blackfan and Maxcy (23), were the first to utilise the peritoneal cavity for the administration of fluids to dehydrated children. The first attempt to use the peritoneal membrane the other way, namely to remove uraemic substances from the body of a human patient, dates back to 1923.

EXPERIMENTAL PERITONEAL DIALYSIS (1923)

Ganter (24), a German clinical investigator, is traditionally credited with the first attempts of peritoneal dialysis in a human being. Originally (in 1918) he removed a pleural effusion from a uraemic man, replacing the fluid with 0,75 l of a sodium chloride solution. He observed some improvement of the patient's condition during the next two days.

Subsequently he performed a series of experimental peritoneal dialysis in rabbits and guinea pigs, made uraemic by ligation of the ureters. Injecting 40 to 60 ml of saline into the peritoneal cavity of a guinea pig, Ganter removed the remaining fluid after approximately 3 h and then instilled fresh salt solution. The procedure was repeated every 3 h, up to 4 times, thereby sometimes 'rinsing' the peritoneal cavity several times without a dwell time.

Actually Ganter performed in his animals what later became intermittent peritoneal dialysis.

He observed an almost complete equilibration of the non-protein nitrogen content of the peritoneal fluid with the blood in 3 h and noted that some 2/5 to 4/5 of the injected quantity was absorbed: often only 10 ml could be recovered.

Ganter noted a definite improvement of the animal's condition after each session of peritoneal lavage.

INTERMITTENT PERITONEAL DIALYSIS: THE FIRST ATTEMPT

Finally Ganter instilled 1,5 l of physiological saline in the peritoneal cavity of a patient who became rather acutely uraemic from a bilateral obstruction of the ureters caused by a uterine carcinoma. He observed a slight, transient improvement in the patient's condition (1923).

In another patient who was deeply comatose from diabetic keto-acidosis, 3 l of saline was injected into the peritoneal cavity: a striking but transient improvement was noted, the patient waking up, temporarily communicating with this relatives.

After these observations Ganter published his investigations in the Münchener Medizinische Wochenschrift in December 1923, but ended his work for unknown reasons.

In the years after World War I several German investigators were active in the field of replacement of renal function either with still experimental extracorporeal haemodialysis (so called 'external dialysis' [22, 25–27]) or with peritoneal dialysis (so called 'internal dialysis' [22]), probably because of the numerous cases of trench nephritis observed during the war, some of them leading to fatal uraemia and, on the other hand, because of the numerous victims of acute renal failure complicating battle field injuries, also usually dying from uraemia.

Necheles' criticism (1924)

One of these investigators, Heinrich Necheles (25, 26) from Hamburg, Germany, who was in touch with John Jacob Abel in Baltimore, the inventor of the vividiffusion apparatus (see chapter 3), read Ganter's paper and repeated his animal experiments with negative results. Apparently, not very happy with Ganter's work he wrote to John Abel in June 1924 (without mentioning Ganter's name):

> 'zZ Berlin 16/6, 1924 ... Ich habe jetzt seine Methode nachgeprüft, die unter Kritik meiner Arbeiten vor einigen Monaten in der Münchener Medizin. Wochenschift erschienen ist; hier wurde als physiologischerer Weg vorgeschlagen, das Peritoneum der Bauchhöhle als Dialysiermembran zu benutzen und zu durchspülen; in einigen klinischen Fällen will er vorübergehend Erfolg gesehen haben, in Tierexperimenten nicht. Ich habe diese Frage an einem grösseren Material nephrectomierter Katzen und Hunde nachgeprüft, ohne irgend einen Erfolg gesehen zu haben. In der Tat stellt sich das Peritoneum eine ausgedehnte Fläche vor, es findet auch Dialyse statt, der Reststickstoff der Durchspülungsflüssigkeit ist erhöht, der klinische Erfolg ist aber eher als negativ zu bezeichnen, wahrscheinlich weil der Eingriff ein zu schweres ist.'*

Necheles abandoned his peritoneal experiments and returned to his own experimental work with a dialyser with semipermeable conical tubes prepared from visceral animal peritoneum (gold-beaters' skin), which apparently was a good dialysis membrane (25, 26, see also chapter 3).

CONTINUOUS PERITONEAL DIALYSIS (1927)

Three years later, in 1927, two other German investigators reported their attempts to save the lives of three uraemic patients with acute renal failure, caused by mercury bichloride, with peritoneal dialysis (Heusser and Werder [28], 1927). They modified Ganter's technique, inserting two catheters and perfusing the peritoneal cavity continuously, using one catheter (located between the diaphragm and the liver) for the inflow and the other one (placed in the pelvic area) for the outflow. They observed that not only nitrogenous substances were extracted but also mercury and noted some protein loss in the dialysis fluid. Their attempts were unsuccessful.

OTHER UNSUCCESSFUL EARLY ATTEMPTS (1930–1940)

In the late twenties and early thirties peritoneal dialysis remained a new and relatively unknown method of treatment: experience with the new procedure was minimal. Nothing was known about the efficiency of peritoneal dialysis, about optimal flow rate of the dialysis solution or peritoneal clearances. In the 1930's peritoneal dialysis remained an ill investigated, experimental, more or less 'hit and miss' treatment of uraemia.

Seven years passed before another report was published by Balazs and Rosenak (1934), [29]). They also dialysed three cases of acute renal failure with anuria, caused by mercury bichloride, using a similar technique. Their attempts were also futile: obviously those groups of clinical investigators used too little dialysis fluid and their rinsings were too short.

Somewhat more successful were Wear and co-workers (30) in 1938. They treated five patients, dialysed longer (2 to 5 h) and noted a fall in serum creatinine and non protein nitrogen. One patient improved enough to tolerate surgical removal of bladder stones. This patient recovered.

In the same year Rhoads (31) treated two uraemic patients with chronic renal failure with peritoneal dialysis, using for the first time the intermittent method, as used by Ganter in his animal experiments 14 years earlier. He instilled 1,5 l of dialysate through a single catheter, removing the fluid after a 'dwell' time of approximately 15 min through the same tube, repeating the procedure several

---

* Translation: 'Temporarily in Berlin, June 16, 1924 ... I have now tried a method which was published a few months ago in the Münchener Medizin. Wochenschrift simultaneously criticising my own work. The author suggests using the peritoneum as a dialysis membrane and to perfuse the peritoneal cavity because this would be more physiological. The author states that he, in a few clinical

cases transient favourable results has observed, but not in his animal experiments. I repeated these experiments on a rather large number of bilaterally nephrectomised cats and dogs without any result. The peritoneum has indeed a large surface area and dialysis does occur for the non-protein nitrogen in the perfusion fluid is increased, but the clinical results are negative. Probably because the intervention is too drastic.'

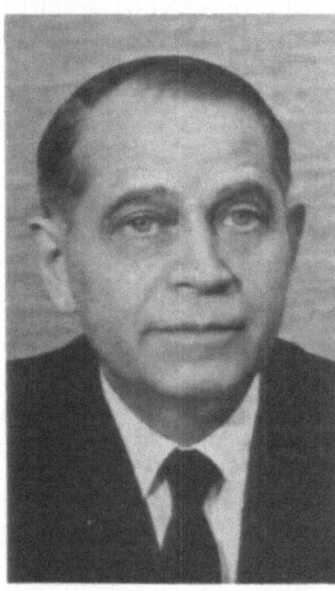

Figure 4. Stephen Rosenak (born 1900). Early pioneer of peritoneal lavage and designer of a flexible drainage tube (29, 45, 49)'.

times. The outflow fluid contained substantial amounts of urea.

During World War II thousands of cases of acute renal shutdown caused by severe trauma both in the military and in the civilian population in Europe, the Far East and in other scenes of war, harshly alerted surgeons, internists and nephrologists (at that time a new budding specialism) to the problem.

In this context it is worth quoting the remark made by Dr. Edward D. Churchill from Boston MA at a meeting of the American Surgical Association held in April, 1946, in Hot Springs VA after Dr. Fine (32) presented his classical paper on the treatment of acute renal failure by peritoneal dialysis:
... 'despite all the optimistic reports on the successful management of shock in this war, renal shutdown was the stonewall against which we butted our heads many times. ... The surgeons caring for these patients with anuria tried many forms of treatment: high spinal anesthesia; alkalies to the point of severe alkalosis; and many other measures. Still the patients died in uraemia. Dr. Fine's methods represent one more procedure, that may be applicable to men suffering from renal shutdown following severe trauma. I hope it will prove successful ...'.

THE TURNING OF THE TIDE: THE INVESTIGATIONS OF FRANK, SELIGMAN AND FINE (1946–1948)

After an interval of 8 years (1938–1946) the method finally started catching up. The pioneering investigations of Frank, Seligman and Fine (32–35) from Boston, MA were published in 1946 and 1948 and the experiences from the Mayo Clinic were made public by Odel and associates (22) in 1948.

The Boston investigators were convinced that the peritoneum was an efficient dialysis membrane, which, so far had been utilised for the treatment of uraemia without success. They decided to determine systematically whether peritoneal dialysis could be made practical for clinical use. They made numerous studies on nephrectomised dogs before turning to peritoneal dialysis for the treatment of uraemic patients.

Emphasising the importance of a meticulous technique and observing a painstaking sterility, not only in human patients but also in experiments on the dog, they adopted the continuous flow-technique as Heusser and Werder in 1927 and Balazs and Rosenak in 1934 had done.

Their irrigation fluid, originally Ringer solution with dextrose was later changed to Tyrode solution prepared in 5 gallon (appr. 19l) Pyrex carboys. In the dog experiments they determined the optimal flow rates of the dialysis fluid and achieved urea clearances ranging 5 to 11 ml/minute (depending on the position of the dog) with flow rates of 25 to 50 ml/minute. The survival of bilateral nephrectomised dogs was prolonged from 3 to 10 days and the animals did not die from uraemia, but from bacterial infection along the catheter tracts.

SUCCESSFUL TREATMENT OF ACUTE RENAL FAILURE WITH PERITONEAL DIALYSIS (1946)

In March 1946, Frank, Seligman and Fine reported a successful application of peritoneal irrigation in a patient with severe uraemia from sulphathiazol induced anuria. The patient survived after 4 days of continuous peritoneal lavage. The investigations of the Boston team were the first in the field of peritoneal lavage, to be based on sound scientific evidence; they attracted considerable interest and should be considered as a landmark in the history of treatment of uraemia. From then on the tide turned.

In 1948, Odel and co-workers (22) collected a total of 53 uraemic patients previously reported in the literature and treated by peritoneal dialysis. In this group they noted 27 cases with reversible, and 13 with irreversible lesions. Thirteen others had undetermined kidney disease. Seventeen survived, the majority being cases with acute renal failure, caused by incompatible blood transfusions, sulphonamide intoxications or toxaemia of pregnancy.

Muehrcke (36) found in the literature until 1948 a total of 101 uraemic patients treated by peritoneal dialysis: 63 were diagnosed as having acute renal failure, 32 had irreversible, chronic lesions and 6 were cases of poisoning. Of those with acute renal failure 32 survived. In the Netherlands, an early series of 21 patients was reported by Kop (37), who worked with Kolff in Kampen between July 1945 and November 1947. Five had acute renal failure; three of them survived.

Nevertheless in the early 1950's peritoneal dialysis was still an experimental procedure, considered by many to be used as a last resort in cases with terminal uraemia. Side effects and complications were observed during and after treatment. They could be dangerous, sometimes leading to death from pulmonary oedema or peritonitis.

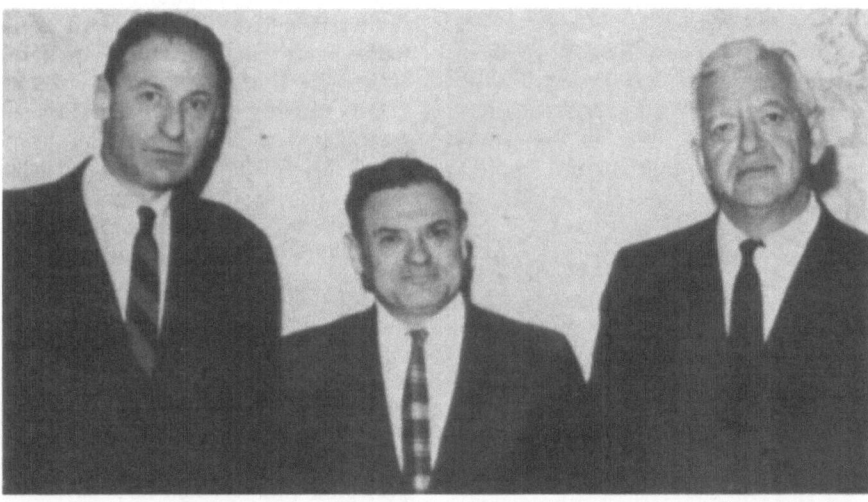

Figure 5. Left to right: Howard Frank, Arnold Seligman, Jacob Fine, the Boston investigators, whose clinical work in the field of peritoneal lavage was based on scientific evidence (32–35).

THE COMPOSITION OF THE PERITONEAL DIALYSIS FLUID

Complications and undesirable side effects were often observed and in retrospect they could be readily explained by the unsuitable compositions of different dialysis fluids used by various investigators until the mid 1960's.

Odel and associates (22) reviewed the literature until 1948, and calculated the electrolyte composition of dialysis solutions reported by a number of clinical investigators, as far as data were available. When studying Table 1 (which is partly derived from Odel and associates [22]), it is not surprising that hyperchloraemic metabolic acidosis was a frequently observed side effect of peritoneal dialysis with Locke-Ringer and modified Tyrode solutions and 'normal' or 'twice normal' saline. Obviously these fluids contained excessive chloride concentrations and were deficient in bicarbonate (or acetate and lactate, which also serve as a source for fixed base) or even did not contain bicarbonate at all.

Sodium concentration

Peripheral oedema, pulmonary oedema and hypertension frequently accompanied peritoneal dialysis in the earlier days of its use (until the early fifties): high dialysis fluid sodium concentrations up to 156 mmol/l, were used rather commonly. Reid and co-workers (38) who performed the first peritoneal dialysis in England (in March 1946) used a rinsing fluid consisting of 'twice normal saline'. The patient, a lady of 36 suffering from acute renal failure caused by a mismatched blood transfusion, tolerated bilateral renal decapsulation and 2 days of peritoneal dialysis with a solution containing 306 mmol Na and Cl per liter. She survived and made a full recovery.

In the late fifties and early sixties it became apparent that lower dialysis fluid sodium and chloride values were indicated and that appropriate amounts of bicarbonate (or acetate or lactate) were indicated to avoid (or to correct) electrolyte abnormalities in the patients (39, 40), see Table 1.

Dextrose concentration (See footnote to table 1)

For adequate dehydration of the patients the osmolality of the rinsing fluid was often increased by adding dextrose in different concentrations (up to about 6 g/100 ml). It appeared however that the sodium concentration of the excess fluid removed from the extracellular fluid compartment was much lower than the normal concentration in the extracellular fluid (80 to 115 mmol [mean 110 mol/l] versus 140 mmol/l, Moriarty and Parsons [41], 1966. See also Chapter 23).

The sodium concentration in the ultrafiltrate is dependent on the dwell time of the dialysate in the peritoneal cavity (Parsons FM & Moriarty MV personal communication). In rats (Figure 4) using hypertonic, dehydrating glucose concentrations in dialysis solution the sodium concentration in the dialysis fluid falls reaching the lowest value in about 45 min. After a 2.5 h dwell time sodium has equilibrated across the peritoneum (Figure 6) but by this time some of the ultrafiltered water has started to be reabsorbed. In order to remove not only water but also an adequate amount of sodium during 'hypertonic' peritoneal dialysis with the conventional hourly exchange time the sodium content of the dialysate should be below the normal extracellular concentration of 140 mmol/l, e.g. 110 to 125 mmol/l, depending on the dextrose content of the dialysis fluid (41).

These observations have been confirmed more recently by Nolph and associates (42–44). Obviously the disadvantage of dextrose to achieve water removal by osmotic ultra-

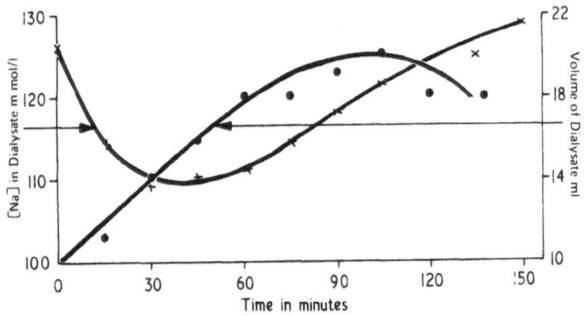

Figure 6. The change in volume (●—●) and sodium concentration (×—×) in hypertonic peritoneal dialysis fluid with time in the rat. Initially 10 ml of dialysis fluid was injected. (Parsons and Moriarty, unpublished observation).

filtration is the absorption of this solute from the peritoneal cavity. In addition hypertonic dextrose solution may be damaging to the peritoneal membrane (see further p. 500–501).

Other solutes have been used for increasing dialysis fluid osmolality without the risk of causing hyperglycaemia: dextran, fructose, sorbitol, xylitol and gelatin (42, 45). All had disadvantages, either being toxic or too expensive or both. Glucose (dextrose monohydrate), usually in concentrations of 1,5–4,25% is still preferred.

Even presently the optimal composition of peritoneal dialysis solution is a matter of debate. In 1959 Doolan and co-workers (39) used a dialysis solution with a low sodium concentration of 128 mmol/l, a chloride concentration equal to the blood (100 mmol/l) and a bicarbonate concentration of 28 mmol/l. By administering calcium parenterally and omitting calcium from the dialysis fluid they avoided the precipitation of calcium carbonate. The potassium content was adapted to the clinical setting and the plasma potassium

Table 1. Composition of solutions for peritoneal dialysis used by some previous investigators* (Partly derived from Odel and associates [22] with permission).

	Na mmol/l	K mmol/l	Cl mmol/l	Ca mmol/l	bicarb mmol/l	acet/lact. mmol/l	glucose** g/100 ml	osmolal m osm/l		Ref
Ganter 1923	136	0	136	0	0	0	0	272	–	24
Balasz, Rosenak 1934	136	0	136	0	0	0	0	272	–	29
	0	0	0	0	0	0	4.2	233		
Wear, Sisk, Trinkle 1938	130	4	110	2	28	0	0	274	Hartmann sol	30
	156	3	165	4	2	0	0.09	326	Locke/Ringer sol	
Fine, Frank, Seligman 1946	151	3	145	1	12	0	1.5	321	Mod. Tyrode	32
Reid, Penfold, Jones 1946	306	0	306	0	0	0	0	612	Twice normal saline	38
Kop 1946–1947	135	5.4	109	2.5	23	0	1–3	–		37
Odel, Ferris, Power 1948	151	3	145	1	12	0	1.5	321	Mod. Tyrode	22
	139	3	109	1	36	0	1–2	344–400	'P' solution	
	140	3	109	1	24	13	1–2		Mod. 'P' sol	
Maxwell, Rockney, Kleeman, Twiss 1959	140	0–4	101–105	2	0	45	1.5	372–380	–	40
Doolan and coworkers 1959	128	as indicated	100	parent- erally	28	0	3.25	400	–	39
Moriarty, Parsons 1966	141	0	101	1.8	0	45	1.36–6.36	372–667	–	41
Presently	130–135	0	99–101	1.75–2.0	0	35–45	1.5–4.25	334–350	–	42

* Magnesium values in these fluids fluctuate between 0 and 1.5 mmol/l

Na, K, Cl, bicarbonate, acetate, lactate: mmol/l = mEq/l

Ca, Mg: mmol/l × 2 = mEq/l, Ca mmol/l × 4 = mg/dl, mg mmol/l × 2.4 = mg/dl.

** Glucose = dextrose monohydrate; 1.5 g/dl of dextrose monohydrate = $\frac{180 \times 1.5}{198}$ = 1.36 g/dl anhydrous dextrose.

Presently for most commercially made peritoneal dialysis fluids the term dextrose (which is anhydrous) is used.

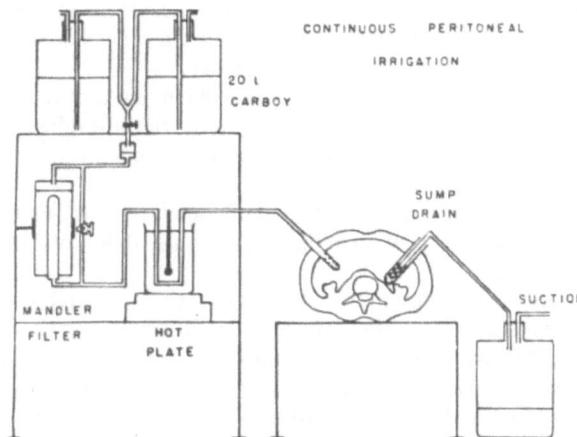

Figure 7. Flow diagram of Dr. Fine's closed circuit for continuous peritoneal irrigation. Dialysis fluid supply came from two 20 l Pyrex carboys (1946 [32]). (With permission of the publishers of the *Ann Surg.*)

values of the patient. Maxwell and co-workers, also in 1959 (40), utilised a fluid with 140 mmol/l sodium and 101–105 mmol/l chloride, depending on the amount of potassium chloride to be added and 2 mmol/l calcium.

Lactate and acetate vs. bicarbonate

Others (32) sterilised bicarbonate solution separately which then was added aseptically to the rinsing fluid, after cooling. Acetate poses problems when sterilised together with glucose, because caramelisation takes place. Presently other dialysis solutions are prepared, however, either with lactate or acetate at a pH adjusted to below 5.5, which prevents caramelisation but may also be damaging to the peritoneum. In this context it should be mentioned that lactate, if the racemic mixture is used, will only partly be metabolised into bicarbonate: the laevo-isomer will be converted only (21). Strict sterility of course is obligatory and when large amounts of fluid (40 l/day) are required, problems may occur when peritoneal rinsing fluid is prepared in bottles of 1 or 2 l, which have to be replaced every 1 or 2 h. Obviously the disconnections endanger the sterility of the circuit. Fine and co-workers (32) prepared the dialysis fluid in 20 l Pyrex carboys. This made the creation of a closed administration system possible. Two elevated carboys were joined by a Y-tube and the fluid flowed by gravity through syphon tubes into the peritoneal cavity (Figure 7). This system however – presumably because of the many technical problems – never gained popularity.

Maxwell and associates (40) circumvented these problems by introducing commercially prepared solutions in 1 l infusion bottles, which came together with sterile Y-type administration tubing (1959, [Figure 8]). Obviously the continuity of this system had to be broken hourly; for every exchange two fresh bottles had to be connected. This endangered sterility every hour.

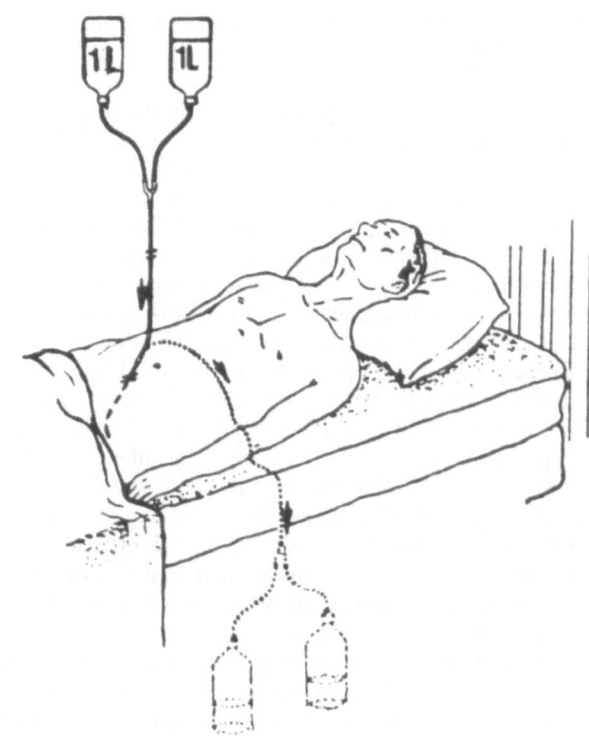

Figure 8. 'Hanging bottle' peritoneal dialysis (Maxwell et al 1959 [40]). (With permission of the authors and the publishers of the *JAMA*).

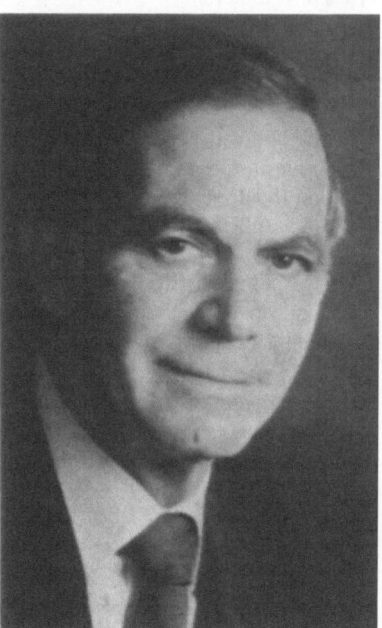

Figure 9. Morton Maxwell (born 1924). He standardised the technique with commercially prepared dialysis fluid and administration sets and introduced hanging bottle peritoneal dialysis (40).

CONTINUOUS vs INTERMITTENT PERITONEAL DIALYSIS

Another controversy concerned the technique of peritoneal dialysis. Many early investigators (3, 4, 30, 32, 34, 45) were advocates of the continuous flow method. This method involved the (surgical) insertion of two catheters: one in the right upper quadrant (between liver and diaphragm) and the other in either lower quadrant of the abdomen, often being located in the cul de sac. Continuous lavage was then instituted: the dialysis fluid was instilled through one catheter, leaving the peritoneal cavity through the other (Figure 7). Channelling of the dialysis fluid between the inflow and outflow catheters was predictable and common. Leakage occurred frequently and obviously the risk of peritonitis was appreciably greater than with the 'one catheter, intermittent' technique. With this method, advocated by Rhoads (31), Reid, Penfold and Jones (38), Grollman and associates (46, 47) and others, only one catheter is inserted in the peritoneal cavity, the rinsing fluid being instilled and drained after a certain dwell time through the same catheter, usually by the syphon effect.

In the 1950's the continuous method was gradually abandoned and in 1959 the matter was settled in favour of the intermittent method by the introduction of a nylon non-irritating flexible catheter by Maxwell and co-workers (40), which was relatively easily introduced through the linea alba with a trocar.

PERITONEAL ACCESS

Different types of catheters

Actually the access to the peritoneal cavity has been a problem for years (48) and a multitude of access devices has been used: Foley catheters (38), mushroom tip catheters, whistle tip catheters (34), polyethylene tubes (45), stainless steel sump drains (similar to the metal-perforated suction tubes, used in operating theatres (32) and even glass drains. Also simple soft rubber tubes with or without side holes were utilised.

Leakage was a common problem opening the way for infection and often mattress sutures were applied to eliminate this problem. Rosenak and Oppenheimer (49) de-signed a double lumen catheter with a flexible distal extension, made of coiled stainless wire. It had a collar which was sewn in the subcutis to prevent leakage.

Obstruction was common because of kinking of the catheter or from blood clots or plugging of the outflow tube with tiny bits of omental fat, sucked into the lumen through the side perforations (40). Another common cause of catheter failure was the wrapping of the omentum around the catheter blocking outflow, sometimes causing also inflow obstruction.

Doolan (39) described in 1959 a new PVC catheter, constructed by his associate Murphy. This catheter, which had multiple small side holes, was transversely ridged with spiral grooves. The ridging helped to prevent blockage by the omentum and kinking. Introduction, however, was somewhat laborious and had to be performed either with a #22 gall bladder trocar or by laparotomy. It did not become widely used (Figure 10).

The stylet catheter (1965)

A major advance was made by Weston and Roberts (50), who improved the Maxwell catheter (1965). Roberts, a research biochemist, happened to visit Dr. Weston at the Cedars-Sinai Medical Center in Los Angeles in 1964 and saw him struggling to pierce the abdominal wall of a sick patient with a 17F trocar to insert a Maxwell catheter. Roberts made a simple modification by inserting a pointed stylet within the Maxwell catheter (Figures 11a, b and c), thus eliminating the need for a trocar and sutures. The stylet catheter (Trocath) soon became commercially available. It simplified temporary peritoneal access considerably. The use of the stylet catheter is now standard practice for acute dialysis and for temporary access in case of catheter failure in chronic patients treated with periodic peritoneal dialysis.

STANDARDISING THE TECHNIQUE (1959)

In the late fifties and early sixties intermittent peritoneal dialysis became gradually a safe and standardised procedure, in particular by the work of Doolan and his coworkers (39) and Maxwell and associates (40). Both groups contributed much to the improvement and perfection of peritoneal dialysis technique.

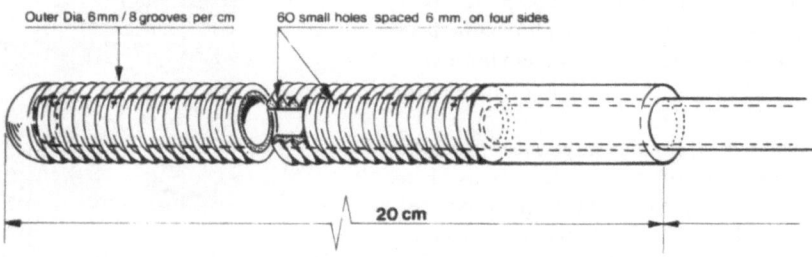

Figure 10. Murphy-Doolan implantable peritoneal lavage tube, made from transversely ridged polyvinylchloride, with 60 small hand-punched holes (1959 [39]). (With permission of the authors and the publishers of the *Am J Med*).

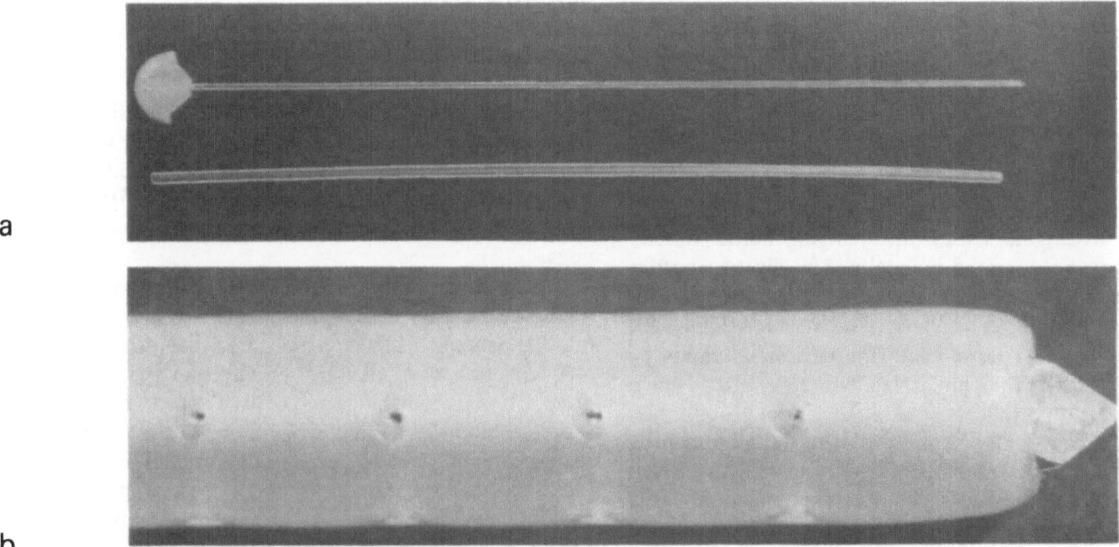

a

b

Figure 11 (a and b). Stylet catheter ('Trocath') (Weston and Roberts, 1965 [50]).

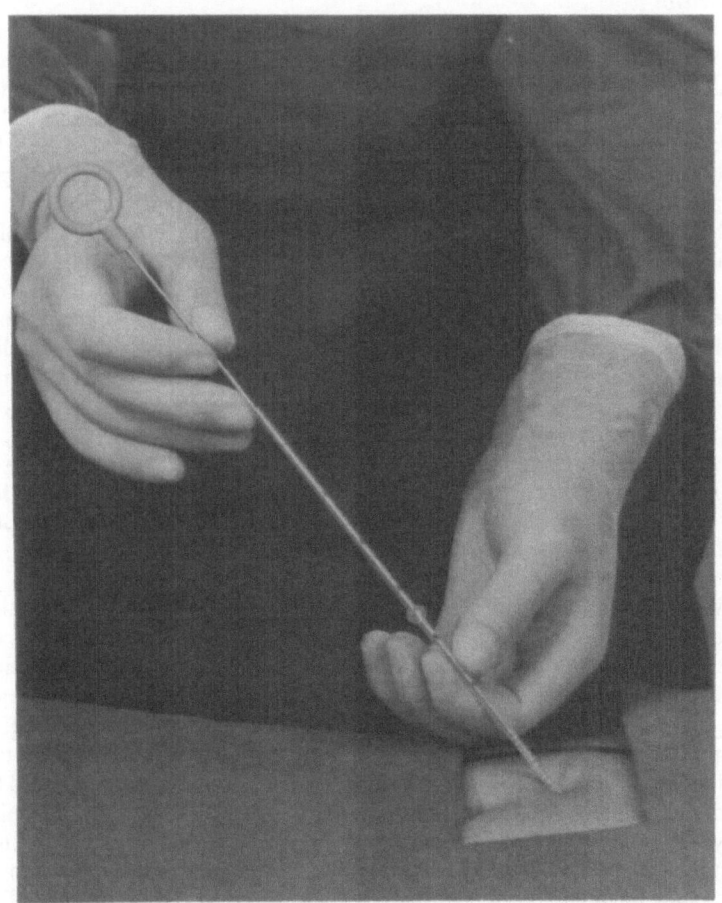

c

Figure 11c. Insertion of a stylet catheter.

Development of 'hanging bottle' peritoneal dialysis (1959)

Commercial preparation of dialysis fluid and tubing

The Maxwell and Doolan groups both used commercially prepared rinsing fluids which considerably simplified the procedure and also contributed appreciably to the popularisation of peritoneal dialysis in the hospital setting. Both groups of investigators used the 'hanging bottle system' which had to be operated manually. Usually two bottles each containing 1 l of dialysis fluid were used with a Y type of administration tubing connected to the catheter (Figure 8). The rinsing solution flowed into the peritoneal cavity by gravity as rapidly as possible (usually taking 5 to 10 min). After a dwell time (30 min to 1 h), the inflow tubing was clamped and the fluid was drained from the abdomen by syphon effect into the original bottles which were lowered to the floor besides the patient's bed. The system could easily be operated by nurses but obviously carried the risk of bacterial contamination and peritonitis because the inflow circuit had to be broken every hour.

Closed administration systems

Years before (in 1946) Fine and co-workers (32) created a closed dialysate administration system by introducing 5 gallons (appr. 19 l) Pyrex carboys for sterilising the rinsing solution. Two of these large bottles made a peritoneal dialysis possible lasting 20 h. The Seattle group used these carboys later (1962) with an automatic peritoneal cycling machine (51). However the need for special requirements (a large autoclave, special caps, special Pyrex bottles) made this system expensive. Later 12 gallon (45 l) carboys were used permitting a single carboy for each dialysis (51). Cost, transport problems and explosion risks of the large carboys restricted the use of these large bottles to local use in Seattle.

SEMI-AUTOMATIC PERITONEAL DIALYSIS MACHINES ('CYCLERS') (1964–1966)

Bosch et al (52) constructed a semi-automatic supply system, consisting of 15 or more, commercially available 3 l bottles with sterile dialysis solution, interconnected by sterile polyethylene tubes and wide bore needles. A somewhat similar commercially produced apparatus made in West-Germany was modified by the author (1967). Instead of multiple 3 l bottles, six interconnected 10 l plastic containers, also commercially produced, were utilised (Figure 12).

These semi-automatic peritoneal dialysis systems, called cyclers, were bacteriologically much safer than the hanging bottle systems. The 'cycler' (53) was the precursor of the modern automatic peritoneal dialysis machines which were introduced in the mid sixties for home peritoneal dialysis (54) (see page 492). Obviously, peritoneal dialysis technique and practical application of the procedure made considerable progress in the 1950's and 1960's.

FURTHER PROGRESS

Clearance studies

The kinetics and biophysics of peritoneal dialysis have been studied by several groups of investigators; their work significantly improved the effectiveness of the procedure.

In 1945–46 Frank, Seligman, and Fine (32–35) studied the effect of irrigation flow rate on peritoneal urea clearance in dogs.

Grollman and co-workers (46, 47) determined, also in dogs, the rapidity with which substances like urea passed into the peritoneal cavity. They noted that after intraperitoneal injection of 1 l of fluid, equilibrium was complete in about 2 h. An identical period of time appeared to be necessary in the human subject when 2 or 3 l were introduced in the peritoneal cavity. They also determined in dog experiments the disappearance rate of dextrose from the peritoneal fluid and the amount of fluid that was removed from the extracellular space with different concentrations of dextrose.

Significance of dialysate flow rates

Boen (20, 21) investigated the relationship between dialysate flow rates and peritoneal clearances of urea and several other substances. Optimal clearances were obtained with a flow rate of 3.5 l/h. For practical purposes he advised 2.5 l/h, the gain with higher flow rates being only minimal. Tenckhoff and associates (55) repeating Boen's original investigations obtained different results: the peritoneal clearance of urea could be increased 2 to 3 fold by increasing the dialysate flow rate from 2 to 12 l/h, which was well tolerated by the patient. Several other groups of investigators (42, 56–58) studied peritoneal clearances and mass transfer kinetics and factors influencing peritoneal dialysis efficiency.

So far these investigators limited their studies with a few exceptions to so called small molecules up to the size of uric acid (molecular weight 168).

THE PERMEABILITY OF THE PERITONEUM TO LARGER SOLUTES (SO CALLED MIDDLE MOLECULES)

Scribner (59) noticed in 1965, that patients on chronic periodic peritoneal dialysis, which controls plasma chemistries of small molecules less efficiently than haemodialysis does often feel better than when treated by haemodialysis. Notwithstanding a certain amount of 'underdialysis' of small molecules, peripheral neuropathy either did not develop, or did not progress. He presented the hypothesis that the peritoneum, that is more permeable for proteins, is also more permeable for substances of higher molecular weight than the artificial membranes commonly used for haemodialysis. He suggested that peritoneal dialysis removed larger molecules (molecular weight 300–2000), the so called 'middle molecules', more efficiently than haemodialysis. Scribner's hypothesis was confirmed by the work of Babb et al. (60)

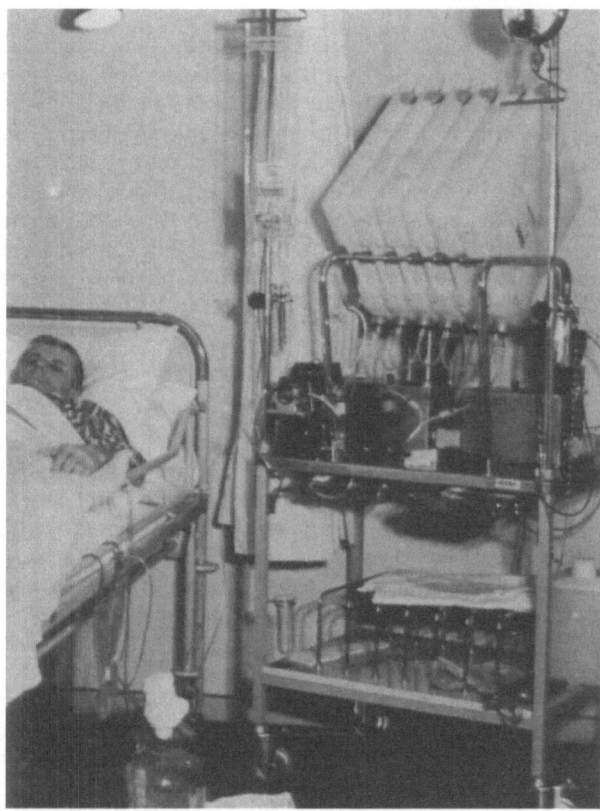

Figure 12. Cycler with six interconnected 10 l plastic containers.

who in 1973 reported on the mass transfer characteristics of the human peritoneum during peritoneal dialysis with special respect to solutes with different molecular weights. They demonstrated that clearances of small molecules were only 1/4 to 1/6 of those with haemodialysers. Higher molecular weight solutes (e.g. vitamin B_{12} [1355], inulin [5200]) were removed at relatively higher rates than urea and other small molecules compared with haemodialysis using conventional membranes. The longer peritoneal dialysis times served primarily to reduce small molecule concentrations to acceptable levels. According to some reports (61–63) solutes up to a molecular mass of 30,000 daltons may diffuse through the peritoneum. Interestingly, so far no cases of dialysis amyloidosis have been reported in patients treated with peritoneal dialysis. It has been demonstrated that this syndrome is caused by retention of a specific protein, β_2-microglobulin, which does not permeate the Cuprophan membrane commonly used in haemodialysis and has a molecular mass of 11,800 daltons.

On the other hand dialysis amyloidosis occurs only in patients treated at least 5 to 10 years and most chronic patients treated by intermittent peritoneal dialysis are trans-ferred to transplantation or haemodialysis after a shorter period of time and CAPD treatment was only introduced in 1978.

THE FIRST CHRONIC CASE SUCCESSFULLY TREATED WITH INTERMITTENT PERITONEAL DIALYSIS (1959–1960)

The successful application of intermittent peritoneal dialysis in cases with acute renal failure (38–40) lead to a trial of repeated peritoneal dialysis in a patient with terminal, chronic, irreversible renal failure shortly before Scribner and collaborators in Seattle WA (64) initiated intermittent haemodialysis treatment in their first two chronic patients (March, 1960, see chapter 3). The patient, Willie Mae Stewart, a 33 year old black female, was first seen by the end of December, 1959 by Dr. R.F. Ruben at the Mount Zion Hospital in San Francisco CA as an outpatient who came back for a post partum check-up. She was not doing too well and was found to be uraemic. Dr. Ruben, who was an assistant resident of Dr. Paul Doolan at the US Naval Hospital at Oakland CA, admitted the patient to the Clinical Investigation Center at the Naval Hospital. The decision was made to perform an initial peritoneal dialysis to improve her condition and a Murphy-Doolan peritoneal catheter was inserted. After the first dialysis further examination revealed bilateral shrunken end-stage kidneys and, obviously, the patient was a case of end-stage chronic renal failure. But after the first dialysis she thrived so well that it was decided to leave the tube in, to clamp it and await events. She deteriorated in a week or so and a second dialysis was done. And after the second dialysis Ruben and Doolan wondered why not a third, not a fourth and after the fourth why not a fifth . . .? They decided to start what became later 'periodic' peritoneal dialysis and dialysed her as an outpatient every time the blood creatinine level reached 20 mg/dl (1770 μmol/l). The dialysis were termed when creatinine was about 13 mg/dl (1150 μmol/l). The patient went home after each dialysis and remained symptom free somewhat restricting her physical activities to housework, shopping and helping with the care of her children and enjoying television.

After 3 months and 12 peritoneal dialyses the catheter failed and a new catheter was inserted through a small laporatomy. Periodic peritoneal dialysis was continued, but by the end of April, 1960 pericarditis developed with fever and a psychotic syndrome. The patient refused further treatment and died on the 4th of June, 1960, after 6 months of periodic peritoneal dialysis. The post mortem revealed pericarditis, peritonitis, bilateral bronchopneumonia and chronic glomerular nephritis with contracted kidneys.

This was actually the first chronic patient successfully treated with periodic peritoneal dialysis. The case report has never been published in the literature; it was presented for publication but a reviewer rejected it, probably because it was a single case and survival was relatively short.

REPEATED ACCESS TO THE ABDOMINAL CAVITY IN CHRONIC CASES

Indwelling plastic conduits (1962–1963)

Merrill and collaborators (65) attempted repeated peritoneal irrigation in four patients with end-stage irreversible renal failure and also in one with acute renal failure, utilising a plastic conduit for repeated insertion of the catheter. They had little success: a number of technical problems necessitated revision or removal of the conduits in periods from 2 weeks to 4 months. In one patient the use of the device however permitted peritoneal irrigation to be carried out temporarily at home.

The successful introduction of intermittent haemodialysis for terminal irreversible chronic renal failure in April 1960 by Scribner and co-workers (64) led the Seattle team to attempt periodic peritoneal dialysis in a patient who clotted all his cannulae and eventually ran out of cannulation sites. By the end of January 1965, periodic peritoneal dialysis was started. Originally, an indwelling plastic conduit was implanted, to facilitate repeated insertion of a plastic or Silastic catheter.

The condition of the patient, a 28 year old male with end-stage chronic glomerulonephritis, remained good during 4 months. Thereafter infections started around the plastic conduit and recurrent peritonitis and adhesions became more and more of a problem. The patient died 9 months after the first peritoneal dialysis.

In the early 1960's many centres attempted periodic peritoneal dialysis for end-stage chronic renal failure using various implanted devices for repeated access to the peritoneal cavity. The reports, however, were discouraging (66), the main problem being peritonitis from infection along the channel of the indwelling devices and from manually changing bottles. Repeated episodes of peritonitis were often followed by the development of adhesions with partial or more extensive obliteration of the peritoneal cavity, decreasing the dialysis efficiency. Most patients died within a few months to a year.

The approach of the Seattle group was different; instead of the hanging bottle method they reintroduced 20 l Pyrex carboys (originally used by Fine and co-workers [32–35]), which soon were replaced by larger bottles with a volume of 45 l [21, 66]). In addition Boen and co-workers used the automatic cycling machine, constructed by Mr. James Sisley (21, 53) of the Medical Instrument Facility of the University of Washington, Seattle. Later an improved cycling machine was designed and constructed by Boen and Curtis et al (53, 66), which was easily transportable. This improved system facilitated uninterrupted cycling without breaking the continuity of the closed sterile fluid administration circuit. In addition, the problem of nursing time was largely solved; but sterilisation and handling of the large carboys remained a drawback.

Repeated puncture technique (1964)

Because of the bad results obtained with implanted 'buttons' or other conduits, the Seattle group changed to a so called repeated puncture technique, introducing a catheter in the peritoneal cavity for each dialysis and removing it at the end of each treatment (53, 66, 67). Satisfactory results were obtained with this technique in a 28 year old woman with end-stage chronic pyelonephritis and a residual creatinine clearance of 0.7 ml/min. She was rehabilitated with once weekly ambulatory peritoneal dialysis, originally lasting 14 h, later 22 h (53).

INTERMITTENT PERITONEAL DIALYSIS IN THE HOME (1964)

Using similar equipment and repeated puncture access Tenckhoff, Shilipetar and Boen (67) trained a 32 year old housewife for intermittent peritoneal dialysis in the home. She started home treatment in May 1964 with once weekly, later twice weekly dialysis. Forty l carboys were shipped in special creates from the hospital to the patient's home, and obviously, a doctor's visit, once or twice weekly was necessary to insert the peritoneal catheter. Initially, this was performed by using a trocar described by McDonald (68); later the stylet catheter ('Trocath' [50]) was utilised. The treatment was reasonably successful but frequent bleeding episodes from the abdominal wall occurred. The treatment caused apparently considerable stress: the husband reacted with two depressive episodes for the first time in his life.

Because of the many technical problems, the workload of preparing large amounts of sterile rinsing fluid, the transport problems of the heavy carboys filled with dialysis fluid and the peritoneal access problem in the home setting, requiring regular doctor's visits, periodic peritoneal dialysis remained for the time being an experimental procedure, not only in the home but also in the hospital (67). Yet, Boen, Mion and other members of Scribner's team (53, 54) had convincingly demonstrated that periodic peritoneal dialysis as replacement of renal function for end-stage chronic kidney disease was feasible and could basically be further developed into an acceptable alternative for regular haemodialysis treatment, but sterilisation and handling of the large carboys hampered large scale application.

CONSERVATIVE TREATMENT OF ACUTE RENAL FAILURE vs PERITONEAL DIALYSIS (1948–1949)

After many years of quite irrational conservative treatment of uraemia (in particular of uraemia caused by acute renal failure) the Bull-Joekes-Lowe regimen developed in the UK and the Borst treatment based on the same principle developed in the Netherlands (69, 70) seemed to provide in the late 40's a rational and rather easy conservative means of treating acute renal failure.

In many centres these regimens became standard practice with occasional use of the artificial kidney, which was developed some years before by Kolff and Berk (see chapter 3) and of peritoneal dialysis.

Notwithstanding the successes reported by Fine and co-workers (32–35) and by Grollman et al (46, 47) and the work reported from Scribner's group in Seattle (51, 53, 55, 66, 67), peritoneal dialysis was only slowly and hesitatingly accepted as treatment for acute renal failure in centres which had no artificial kidney available.

The use of peritoneal dialysis in cases of acute renal failure became, however, more wide spread as it became clear, with increasing experience, that the conservative regimen in cases with prolonged oliguria or (and) severe catabolism failed. In addition the application of peritoneal dialysis was facilitated by the introduction of commercially prepared dialysis solutions and the stylet catheter.

HAEMODIALYSIS vs PERITONEAL DIALYSIS IN ACUTE RENAL FAILURE

On the other hand it became apparent that even peritoneal dialysis failed in highly catabolic cases of acute renal failure, requiring early and frequent (daily) haemodialysis (71). But in numerous cases of acute renal failure peritoneal dialysis became the treatment of choice, in others haemodialysis was preferred. The choice often depended on personal preference and experience, on available equipment and of course on contra-indications to either method.

In recent years peritoneal dialysis (either intermittent or continuous [CAPD]) has been combined with haemodialysis or continuous arteriovenous haemofiltration in acute renal failure cases with severe catabolism and in patients on chronic dialysis with acute complications causing also severe catabolism.

PERITONEAL DIALYSIS BECOMES A GOOD 'LEADEN BULLET' FOR TREATING ACUTE URAEMIA; IT REMAINS A 'CINDERELLA' TREATMENT FOR CHRONIC URAEMIA

With growing experience indications and contra-indications both for peritoneal and haemodialysis became gradually clear. Peritoneal dialysis appeared to be particularly useful in patients with recent wounds and where there was a haemorrhagic risk because systemic heparinisation is not required and also in cases where slower chemical change than that brought about by the artificial kidney was required (e.g. in advanced uraemia with very high levels of blood urea, in which haemodialysis may cause severe disequilibrium).

Peritoneal dialysis was also utilised as a 'holding procedure' for patients waiting for a place in a chronic haemodialysis programme or while waiting for vascular access to mature and as a holding procedure whilst waiting for a kidney transplant (73).

The Editor of the Lancet (72) stated in 1959:

'Peritoneal dialysis is obviously no "silver bullet" for renal failure, but in suitable cases it is a good leaden bullet, which

should perhaps be more commonly fired'.

But the rapid technical improvement of haemodialysis and the increasing success of renal transplantation made these treatments in the past 20 years the 'Glamour Stars' of the medical world (74). Peritoneal dialysis lagged technically behind and remained the 'Cinderella' treatment for chronic renal failure. Longterm treatment was frequently associated with recurrent episodes of peritonitis, with protein loss, malnutrition, progressive wasting and poor rehabilitation.

In the late sixties and early seventies, however, two technical developments changed the 'Cinderella' aspect of intermittent peritoneal dialysis, dramatically.

So far peritoneal access was one of the bottle-necks of long-term peritoneal dialysis. The stylet catheter, mentioned before, was an important technical step forwards, but was impractical for long-term periodic peritoneal dialysis in chronic cases.

INTRODUCTION OF THE TENCKHOFF CATHETER (1968)

Numerous indwelling devices, both access conduits (51, 65, 75–77) and catheters (78–81), had been designed. Some were made of ordinary rubber, glass or stainless steel such as the sump drain of Fine and associates (1948 [35]), others were flexible and made from coiled wire such as the catheter of Rosenak (1948 [49]), which was a two channel device with an in- and outflow tracts.

None appeared to be completely satisfactory: either dislocations or obstruction (by kinking or by the omentum) caused problems and sooner or later infection occurred leading to loss of the device and usually to peritonitis. It was shown that silicone rubber (Silastic) was a more suitable material for implantable access devices and the curled catheter designed by Palmer and Quinton (1964 [80]) was one of the first made from this material. It had a triflanged button which had to be sutured to the peritoneum and also to the deep abdominal fascia.

This catheter and also the simpler, straight Silastic catheter of Gutch (1966 [79]) were more successful.

But the Tenckhoff catheter (82), introduced in 1968 did even better and is still faring well. This catheter or its subsequent modifications are now accepted as the only practical access devices. The original Tenckhoff catheter, made from Silastic (Figure 13), is basically a modification of the curled Palmer catheter (80). It has an open end and numerous side holes in its terminal part of 15 cm (6 inch). Two Dacron felt cuffs should protect against infection along the subcutaneous tract: one just outside the peritoneum, the other in the subcutaneous tissue. The curled section of the Palmer catheter was replaced by a straight intra-abdominal part. The Tenckhoff catheter is inserted either surgically through a mini-laparotomy or with local anaesthesia and the aid of a special trocar at the bedside.

Subsequently a modification of the Tenckhoff catheter with a single Dacron felt cuff became available which can be inserted with a pointed stylet like the Weston-Roberts catheter (83 [see Figure 14]).

The Tenckhoff catheter appeared to be a major advance

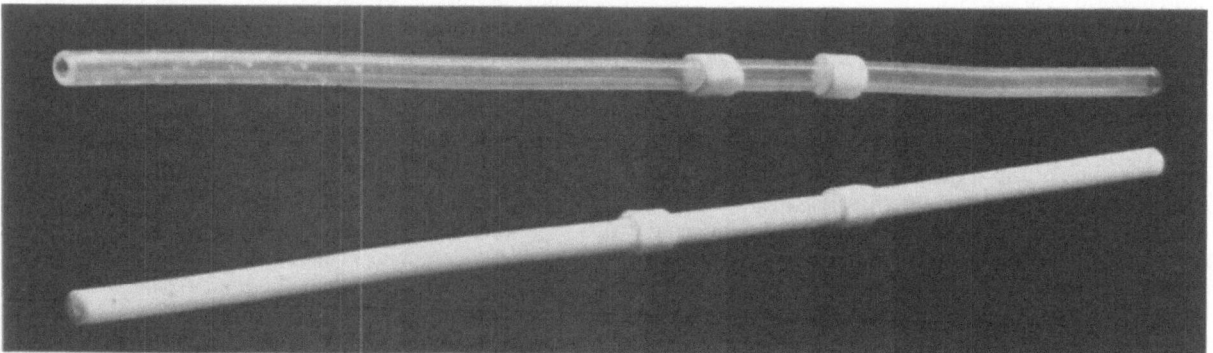

Figure 13. Tenckhoff catheter, clear and radio-opaque model (1968 [82]).

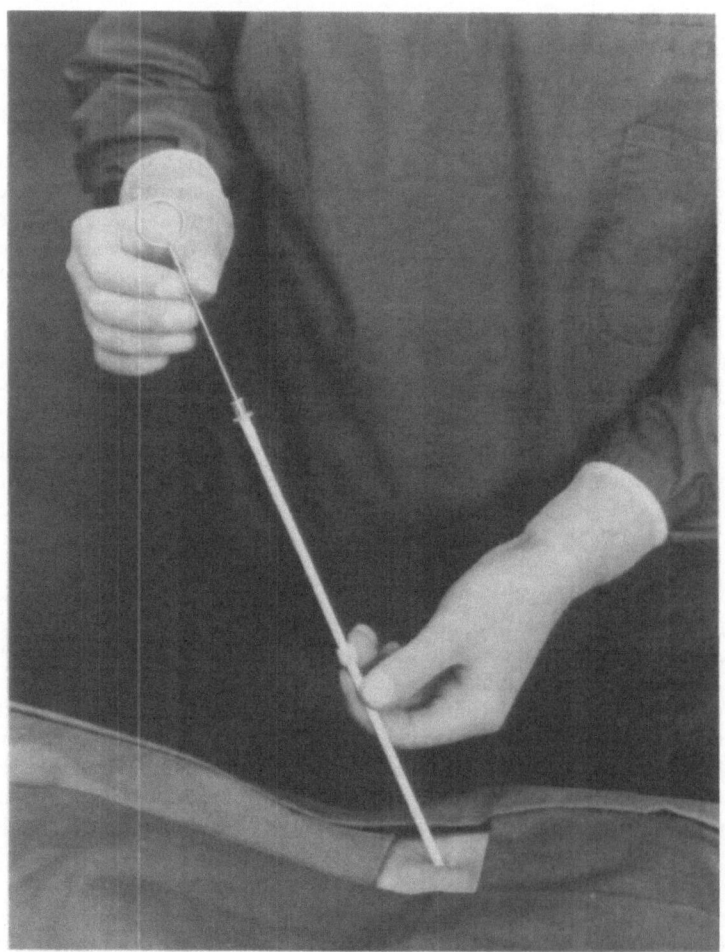

Figure 14. Introduction of a modified, single cuff Tenckhoff catheter with a pointed stylet inserted (83).

for intermittent peritoneal dialysis; it allows longterm access to the abdominal cavity. Still dislocation and obstruction may occur.* Several investigators therefore modified the design (84–87). Goldberg and Hill (86) designed a catheter somewhat similar to the Tenckhoff device, but with a blunt formed tip, facilitating the introduction with an internal obturator and provided the catheter with an inflatable balloon, some distance from the distal end. After insertion the balloon was inflated with sterile saline to prevent occlusion of the drainage holes by the peritoneal contents (omentum) and to keep the catheter down in the pelvis.

For the same reason the catheter developed by Oreopoulos and Zellerman (88, 89) (the Toronto Western Hospital catheter) has two Silastic discs near the distal end (and two Dacron cuffs more proximally localised).

A design somewhat similar to the Goldberg-Hill catheter has recently been described by an Italian group (Valli et al [90]); the intraabdominal end is provided with a perforated balloon which is kept distended by a Silastic ring and cords.

Other designs still prefer the curled configuration of the original Palmer-Quinton catheter (for example the Quinton CurlCath) or are provided with two Silastic discs with multiple columns in between. The proximal disc should stay anchored against the anterior abdominal wall (91) (see Figure 16).

Some of these indwelling catheters can be introduced with a trocar; others can be inserted at the bed side by simple puncture by means of an internal obturator. Some, however, have the disadvantage of requiring surgical implantation (e.g. the Toronto Western Hospital catheter).

The 'life span' of different indwelling catheters has been evaluated: divergent results were reported (88, 89, 92).

Not only the choice but also the survival of the different peritoneal catheters usually depends on personal experience, preference, catheter care and technique of insertion. The 'classic' Tenckhoff catheter is still widely used and has a good longevity.

Still dislocation and obstruction may occur, which sometimes can be corrected, sometimes require removal of the catheter and re-insertion of a new one (for instance in cases with persistent peritonitis).

Visual implantation of a peritoneal catheter or exact replacement of a dislodged catheter is presently possible by means of a (small bore) peritoneoscope.

AUTOMATIC CYCLING MACHINES

Cyclers (1962)

Another major advance which made periodic peritoneal

---

* Evaluation of the cause of obstruction is facilitated by using a radio-opaque model (Quinton Instrument Co, Seattle, WA, USA). This obviates filling with contrast fluid, which may be harmful for the peritoneum, but obviously has the disadvantage that filling defects caused e.g. by fibrin clots (which can be removed by urokinase) cannot be demonstrated. Clear models with a longitudinal radio-opaque mark are presently available and are being preferred.

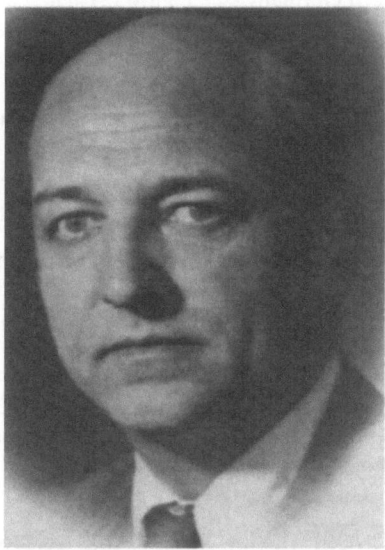

Figure 15. Henry Tenckhoff. Who designed with Schechter a successful chronic peritoneal catheter (82).

dialysis much more dependable was the introduction of automatic cycling machines by Boen and co-workers in 1962 (51–53). These cyclers were later (1972) combined with automatic machines which produce sterile rinsing fluid from concentrate and pre-treated water.

Several models of automatic 'cyclers' have been described in previous years (1962–1968 [51–54, 93–96]). These peritoneal cyclers are relatively simple apparatus with timers which are set for inflow time, dwell period and outflow, freeing nurses from manual operation. Premixed sterile dialysis fluid is supplied either from 19 to 45 l Pyrex carboys (51, 53) or small (1 to 2 l) interconnected bottles (52, 94) or from interconnected plastic containers with 10 l sterile dialysis fluid each. These containers and the cycling machine are commercially available from Messrs. Braun A.G., Melsun-

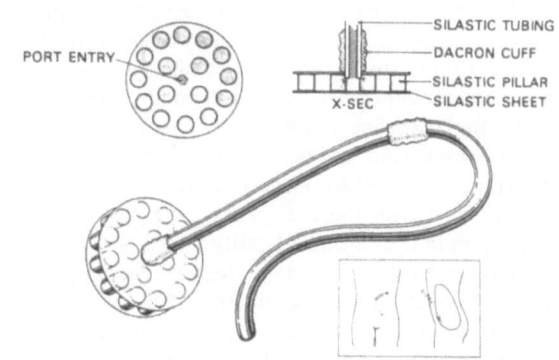

Figure 16. Column disc peritoneal catheter. (Ash, Johnson, Hartman et al [91]). The proximal disc should stay anchored against the anterior abdominal wall in the peritoneal cavity.

gen, Western Germany (see Figure 12). The Lasker system (93) is also commercially produced (American Medical Products, Fairfield, NJ, USA). Other cyclers are marketed by Gambro Inc., Lund, Sweden, an English firm named RA Scientific in London and others. In the McDonald machine (95), non-sterile rinsing fluid is pumped through a Millipore filter to obtain sterility. A similar system, also incorporating a Millipore filter was constructed by Vercellone et al in 1968 (96).

These cyclers are simple to operate and relatively cheap. But because large quantities of sterile rinsing fluid have to be stored and transported, the operating cost is relatively high. The most serious objection however is that sterility of the system cannot be guaranteed, because containers or bottles have to be changed or (and) interconnected manually. In addition systems depending for sterility on bacterial filters do not seem very reliable and safe.

CLOSED LOOP, REVERSE OSMOSIS AUTOMATIC PERITONEAL DIALYSIS MACHINES (1972)

A prototype of a proportioning peritoneal dialysis system was constructed and described by Tenckhoff and coworkers in 1969 (97). Sterile dialysate was prepared from a concentrate and locally produced distilled water with an occlusive roller pump. Because of the necessity of a water still and a rather large stainless steel water sterilisation tank it was a bulky system, requiring a considerable amount of floor space.

An automatic peritoneal dialysis system using reverse osmosis (RO) for tapwater purification and sterilisation was designed years later also by Tenckhoff and co-workers (1972 [98]). The purified sterile water was mixed with sterile concentrate at a ratio of 20 to 1, also by an occlusive roller pump. A commercial model of this system (with different proportioning pumps) was manufactured by Physio-Control Corporation of Seattle, WA and was marketed in 1973. A machine of somewhat different design was designed by Curtis and Scollard (unpublished)* and was marketed by Drake-Willock Corporation from Portland, OR (Figures 17 and 18). Both systems deionise, sterilise and polish the water by reverse osmosis. They have both a proportioning ratio of about 1 to 19, the Drake-Willock machine using roller pumps and the other machine piston pumps. Both use more or less similar cycling and monitor systems. The machines are bacteriologically and technically safe but both have the disadvantage of cold sterilisation with formaldehyde solution, which carries the risk of accidental infusion of the disinfectant in the peritoneal cavity.

The reverse osmosis machines are expensive but running cost is relatively low being limited to the cost of sterile concentrate and concentrated dextrose solutions, sterile administration tubing sets and electrical power for driving the

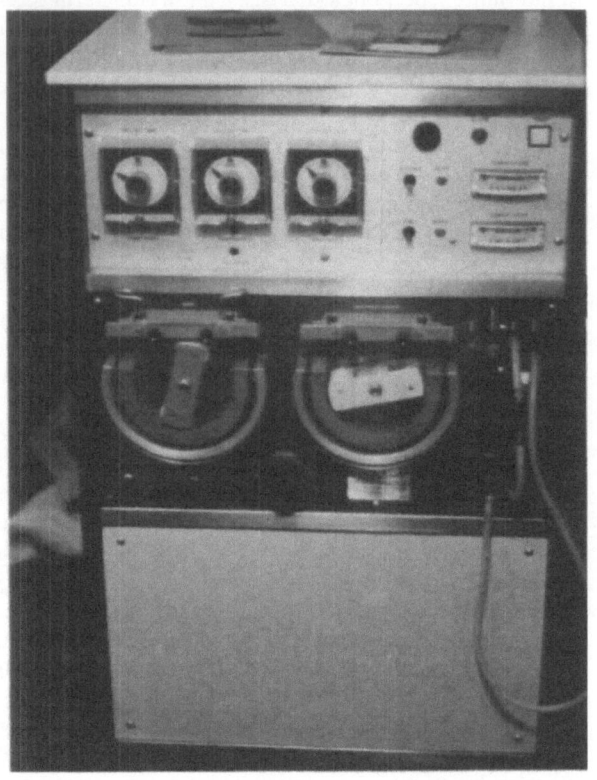

Figure 17. Reverse osmosis automatic peritoneal machine, 1972, (98).

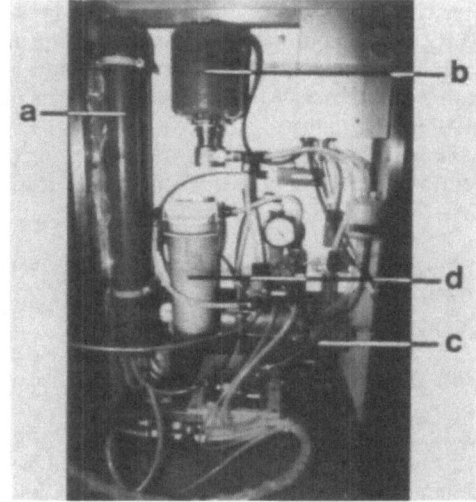

Figure 18. Reverse osmosis unit of automatic peritoneal dialysis machine. a. R.O. filter, b. high pressure pump, c. heat exchanger, d. water filter.

---

* Cited from McBride P, Pioneers in peritoneal dialysis (Peritoneal Dial Bull 3: 47, 1983)

Table 2. Comparison of typical haemodialysis and peritoneal dialysis clearance values.

	Exchange area	C_{urea} ml/min	C_{creat} ml/min	C_{inulin} ml/min	Q_B ml/min	Q_D ml/min
Haemodialysis	1–2 m^2	150	110	5	200–250	350–500
Peritoneal dialysis	1.5–2 m^2 (?)	20–26	15	5	?	30–70

From: Barbour (101 and Nolph et al 102).
Urea: 60 daltons. Creatinine: 113 daltons. Inulin: 5200 daltons.

reverse osmosis compressor, proportioning pumps and the heater.

These machines have the important advantage that the fluid factory and the peritoneal circuit form a closed system and that this continuity is not broken during the dialysis procedure, in contrast with the simpler (and cheaper) cyclers. The risk of bacteriological contamination of the sterile circuit or the rinsing fluid is practically eliminated. The incidence of peritonitis with these machines is therefore minimal. On the other hand they are much more complicated, requiring training for adequate operation and maintenance. These machines became increasingly popular for periodic maintenance peritoneal dialysis, in particular in the United States, Canada and in European countries, until the introduction of CAPD in 1978.

Presently our knowledge of the (patho-)physiology of the peritoneum and of the peritoneal transport, the introduction of the new indwelling catheters and the new automatic R.O. proportioning-cycling machines have doubtless made intermittent peritoneal dialysis a safe and efficient method for long-term replacement of renal function. Rehabilitation and quality of life and presumably survival rates are comparable with those obtained with extracorporeal haemodialysis (99), in particular when peritoneal dialysis is performed overnightly in the home.

Nevertheless CAPD, being a 'machine free' system and a home therapy which is easy to learn within a short training time (1 to 2 weeks compared with 8 to 12 weeks for home haemodialysis) gained in the late 1970's and the 1980's rapidly in popularity. It also is popular because it requires no partner. In addition CAPD is apparently cheaper than hospital haemodialysis and perhaps also cheaper than home haemodialysis. It soon superseded both intermittent peritoneal dialysis with RO proportioning machines and home haemodialysis (100 [see Tables 14 and 15, and Figure 30, p. 507 and 508]).

ENHANCEMENT OF PERITONEAL DIALYSIS EFFICIENCY

With peritoneal dialysis, clearances of small molecules (urea, creatinine, uric acid) are appreciably lower than with the artificial membranes of haemodialysers, even when the clearances of so called middle molecules are more or less similar (101, 102 [see table 2]).

Understandably, much work has been done to enhance the efficiency of peritoneal dialysis, in particular to increase the removal of small solutes.

Hydrodynamic and physical methods

Different approaches have been summarised by Gutman (103 [see table 3]).

The influence of dialysis fluid flow and exchange volumes have been studied by several early investigators in the 1940's and 50's (20, 21, 34, 40, 55). Fine and coworkers (1946 [32]), while using the continuous flow method found maximum clearances of urea with dialysis fluid flow rates of 40 to 60 ml/min (2.4 to 3.6 l/h); using the intermittent technique Boen (1959–1961 [20, 21, 104]) found optimal clearances with exchange volumes of 3 to 4 l/h (50 to 67 ml/min), admitting that these figures could be wrong. Later Tenckhoff and co-workers, including Boen (55), using automated equipment demonstrated that the urea clearance could be doubled (to 40 ml/min) with a dialysis fluid flow rate of 200 ml/min, or an exchange volume of 12 l/h. Obviously these high flow rates led to better mixing diminishing stagnant dialysate layers.

Nevertheless, the small solute clearances obtained with these very high flow rates fall far short of the clearances obtained with extracorporeal haemodialysis (101, 102 [Table 2]). In addition these high exchange volumes are expensive and often uncomfortable for the patients.

Robson and co-workers (105) recently confirmed a substantial increase in small solute clearances with exchange volumes up to 6 l/h (see table 4). Since patients could not tolerate a flow rate of 6 l/h or 100 ml/min, a volume of 4 l/h was considered a satisfactory compromise and this is presently accepted as the standard exchange volume with automatic RO equipment, yielding urea clearance values of 24 to 28 ml/min (see table 5).

Table 3. Enhancement of the effectiveness of peritoneal dialysis.

1. Increase of dialysate flow
2. Optimalisation of dialysate temperature
3. Increase of solute transfer by diffusion by optimalisation of 'dwell' time and 'dwell' volume
4. Increase of solute transfer by convection (increase of ultrafiltration)
5. Vasodilatation
   Increase of peritoneal blood flow?
   Opening of peritoneal capillaries?
6. Increase of membrane permeability

From: Gutman (103) 1979 with permission (slightly modified).

Table 4. Small solute clearances with different peritoneal dialysate flow rates.

Mean clearances, ml/min (2 l exchange volume)

Flow rate l/h	Creat.	Urea	Uric acid
2	13	22	10
3	14	22	10
4	19	26	14
6	23	30	17

From: Robson et al (105) with permission.

The effect of temperature has been studied by Gross and McDonald (56) in 1967. Lowering dialysate temperature decreases peritoneal clearance values (and may be uncomfortable to the patient). Obviously, the upper limit is close to 38° C at the abdominal inflow point.

Optimalisation of dwell time. Several investigators have demonstrated that complete equilibration of small molecules between peritoneal fluid and the blood occurs in 2 to 3 h (20, 21, 105, 106). Dwell times with 4 l hourly exchanges are necessarily much shorter (15 to 20 min), optimal extraction of waste metabolites therefore does not occur; maximum extractions being only accomplished with dwell times of 4 h and longer, as occur in chronic ambulatory peritoneal dialysis. Data of Robson (105) and Gutman (103) suggest that some enhancement is obtained by using two exchanges of 2 l/h, with a residual fluid volume of 1 l remaining in the peritoneal cavity between two exchanges, which is well tolerated by the patient.

Increase of solute transfer by convection was studied by Henderson and Nolph (107, 108). They demonstrated that hypertonicity of the peritoneal fluid not only increases ultrafiltration but also enhances clearances of small and middle molecules (e.g. inulin). This has to be explained by the solvent drag effect of (osmotically induced) ultrafiltration (see also chapter 13). This phenomenon has been used for augmentation of peritoneal dialysis efficiency in animal experiments by Zelman and associates (109). In practice increased ultrafiltration by more liberal use of hypertonic rinsing fluid for more efficient solute clearing could be com-

Table 5. Mean peritoneal clearances ± SEM in ml/min at a flow rate of 4 l/h and an exchange volume of 2 l.

Creatinine	18.6 ± 3.2
Urea	26.2 ± 2.4
Uric acid	13.2 ± 2.8
Phosphate	14.0 ± 2.7
Potassium	20.4 ± 2.2

From: Robson et al (105) with permission.

pensated by increasing fluid intake and a more liberal salt intake by the patient.

Increase of solute clearances by increasing peritoneal blood flow and membrane permeability has been achieved with various drugs.

Pharmacological methods

Although some early investigations date back to some 10 years ago or more (106, 110, 111), the classic investigations on this subject from Nolph, Maher and collaborators (112–118) and others (119–120) are from recent years. The aim of these investigations was to study the effect of small amounts of vasoactive drugs in the dialysis solution. This provides relatively high concentrations of the pharmacological agent adjacent to and within the peritoneal membrane with minimal systemic effects. Slow resorption and passage through the liver via the portal venous circulation also results in minimal concentrations in the systemic circulation (112). Several drugs were studied; two (diazoxide and nitroprusside) increased creatinine clearances by 20 to 25%, which could reduce dialysis time by 6 to 8 h; with nitroprusside a doubling of inulin clearance was observed. It is unlikely that the enhancing effects can be explained by simple vasodilatation and an increase of peritoneal blood flow rate. A direct effect on the permeability of the peritoneal membrane is more likely.

Other drugs (ethacrynic acid, furosemide and others) have been studied both in rabbits and patients. Some are effective in the dialysis solution. Others work only on the blood side (glucagon). These investigations are also helpful in clarifying some issues about mesenteric blood flow and mechanisms of transport and to identify which drugs are deleterious, e.g. norepinephrine, which causes vasoconstriction. For similar reasons peritoneal dialysis clearances are very low in shock, i.e. when there is generalised vasoconstriction (see table 6). So far drug enhancement of peritoneal dialysis efficiency has not (yet) found clinical application.

Table 6. Vasodilators that augment peritoneal clearances.

Effective intraperitoneally only
　Intravenously nonselective vasodilation:
　　Isoprenaline, nitroprusside, tolazoline
　Intravenously immediately degraded:
　　Prostaglandins PGE_2, PGA_1

Preferential splanchnic vasodilation
　Effective intravenously or intraperitoneally:
　　Dopamine (high dose), dipyridamole (transient)
　Effective intravenously only:
　　Glucagon (poorly absorbed intraperitoneally)

From: Maher and Hirszel (121).

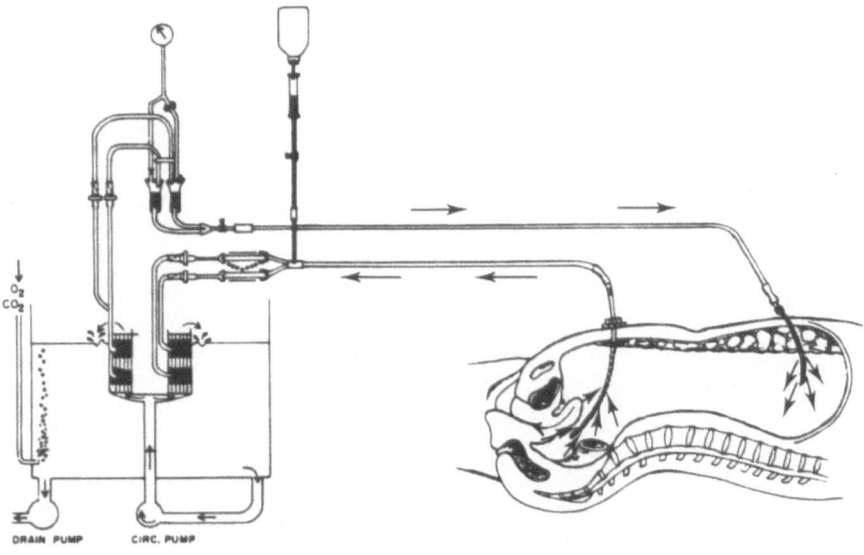

Figure 19. Peritoneal-extracorporeal recirculation dialysis (Shinaberger, 1965 [122]), using Twin Coil artificial kidney. (With permission of the authors and the publishers of the *Trans Am Soc Artif Intern Organs*).

OTHER HISTORICAL PERITONEAL DIALYSIS MODIFICATIONS

Recirculation peritoneal dialysis (1965)

Recently interest in recirculation dialysis originally described in 1965, another approach to enhance peritoneal dialysis efficiency, has been revived by Kolff's group (87). For reasons discussed previously continuous flow peritoneal dialysis was gradually replaced by intermittent dialysis in the 1950's. But in 1965 Shinaberger, Shear and Barry (122) reported urea- and creatinine clearances which were two to three times greater with recirculation peritoneal dialysis than with standard intermittent lavage. With this method (peritoneal-extracorporeal recirculation dialysis) 3 to 4 l of sterile peritoneal dialysis fluid were recirculated through a twin coil dialyser; this apparently appreciably increased the efficiency of peritoneal dialysis (Figure 19). A similar system was described by Lange, Freser and Mangalat from Western Germany in 1968 (123). Stephen and co-workers (87) using a newly developed ⌐-shaped, two way implantable peritoneal catheter, modified the Shinaberger design. The sterile (primary) dialysate was recirculated through the blood path of a hollow fibre dialyser. The 'secondary' (non-sterile) dialysate was recirculated from a 20 l reservoir through a charcoal module for (partial) regeneration (Figure 20 and 21). This non-sterile bath fluid had to be changed at least once during dialysis. The peritoneal flow rates had to be limited to 200 ml/min or less, higher flow rates resulting in abdominal pain. Clearance values were somewhat higher than with conventional intermittent peritoneal dialysis, but the results were slightly disappointing. Apparently streaming or recirculation of the dialysis fluid sometimes occurred in the peritoneal cavity. In addition, problems of infection, often with peritonitis occurred with the two way subcutaneous catheter.

These, per se, ingenious methods did not gain application in other centres.

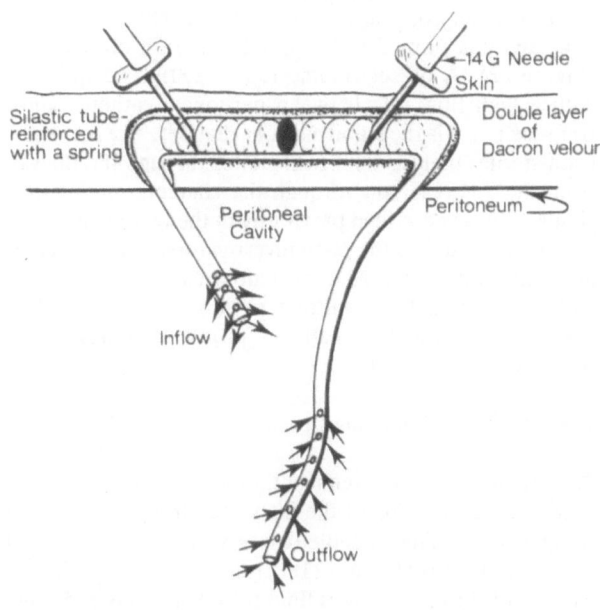

Figure 20. Two way subcutaneous catheter used for recirculation peritoneal dialysis (Stephen et al 1976 [87]).

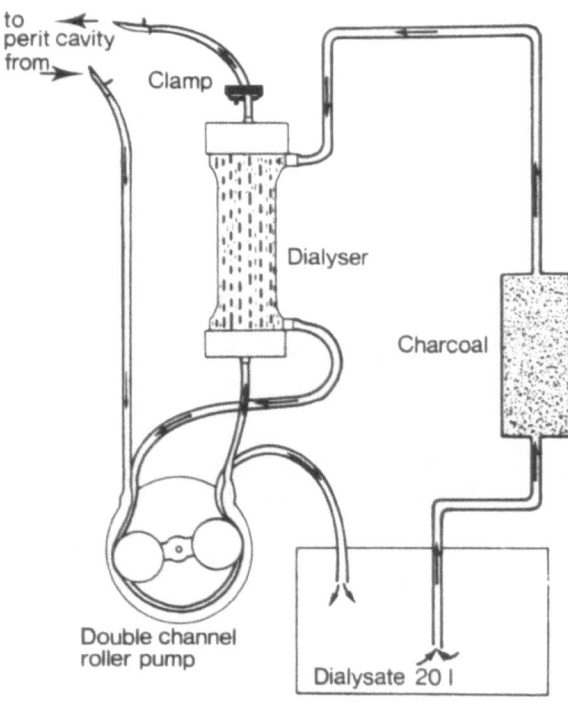

Figure 21. Peritoneal-extracorporeal recirculation dialysis with partial regeneration of dialysis fluid (Stephen et al 1976 [87]).

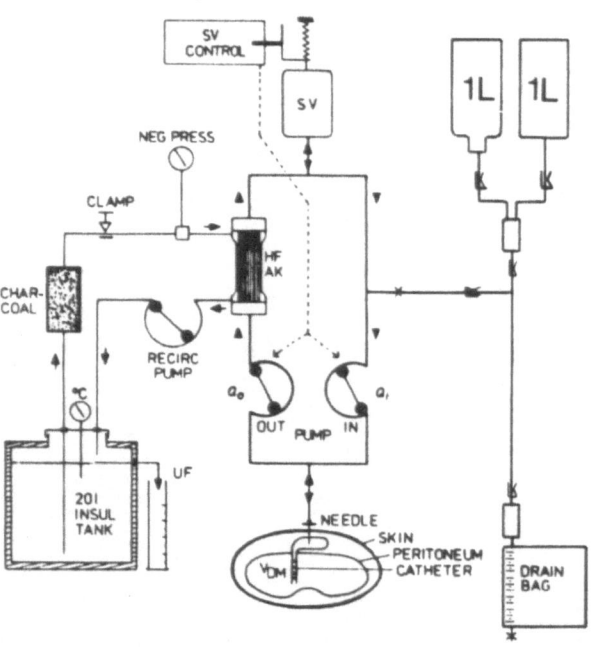

Figure 22. Reciprocating peritoneal dialysis (1978) [124]).
SV   : Transpak bag containing preset stroke volume
VDM   : intraperitoneal volume (appr. 2 l)
CLAMP   : screw clamp for regulating negative pressure of secondary dialysis fluid.
(Figures 20, 21 and 22 are reproduced with permission of the authors and the publishers of the *Trans Am Soc Artif Intern Organs* and *Dial Transplant*).

Reciprocating peritoneal dialysis (1978)

Another approach to augmentation of peritoneal clearances was called reciprocating peritoneal dialysis (124): the peritoneal cavity is primed with appr. 1 l of fresh dialysis fluid (Figure 22). A preset volume (appr. 200 ml) reciprocates with a high flow rate between peritoneal catheter and a transpak bag, via the blood path of a dialyser. The secondary (non-sterile) dialysis fluid recirculates through the dialyser from the 20 l reservoir through the charcoal module in a similar way as described previously in the recirculating system, constructed by the same investigators. The urea clearance increased some 29% over urea clearances obtained with conventional intermittent peritoneal dialysis. However, in this procedure catheter problems (plugging, infection) were frequent.

Fresh fluid, semicontinuous peritoneal dialysis (1978)

A simpler system of 'semicontinuous' peritoneal dialysis (without regeneration of the dialysate through a dialyser), using a simple single needle device was constructed by Di Paolo (125) in 1978 (Figure 23). After priming the peritoneal cavity with 1 to 1.5 l dialysis fluid 100 ml dialysate is drained every minute and an equal amount of fresh rinsing fluid is introduced. In 8 h approximately 50 l are exchanged and several litres of ultrafiltrate are simultaneously drained. Total dialysis time could be shortened by 50%: with three 8 h

'semi-continuous' peritoneal dialysis sessions per week, serum levels of urea, creatinine and uric acid were similar to the levels obtained with twice weekly 24 hours of 'conventional' intermittent peritoneal dialysis.

Commercial closed loop RO delivery machines can be converted to 'fresh fluid' semicontinuous systems, delivering a stroke volume of 200 ml fresh dialysis solution (126 [Figure 24]). Because the peritoneal cavity is initially 'primed' with 2 l rinsing fluid, a certain amount of dialysate remains in the abdomen during the dialysis procedure. Dialysate flow rates of 160 ml/min are obtained (9.6 l/hour) and urea clearance is boosted to about 40 ml/min.

Obviously it is presently possible to enhance peritoneal dialysis efficiency by 25 to 50% both by pharmacological or hydrodynamical methods, which makes shortening of total dialysis hours per week possible. But one of the problems resulting from increasing efficiency of peritoneal dialysis by drugs or high flow rates (and also from high dextrose concentrations to correct overhydration) is the inevitable increase of loss of plasma proteins which can cause a state of protein malnutrition (Dr. F.M. Parsons, Leeds UK, personal communication).

The different procedures to enhance peritoneal clearances are still in an experimental stage and are not yet accepted for practical application. The pro's and con's

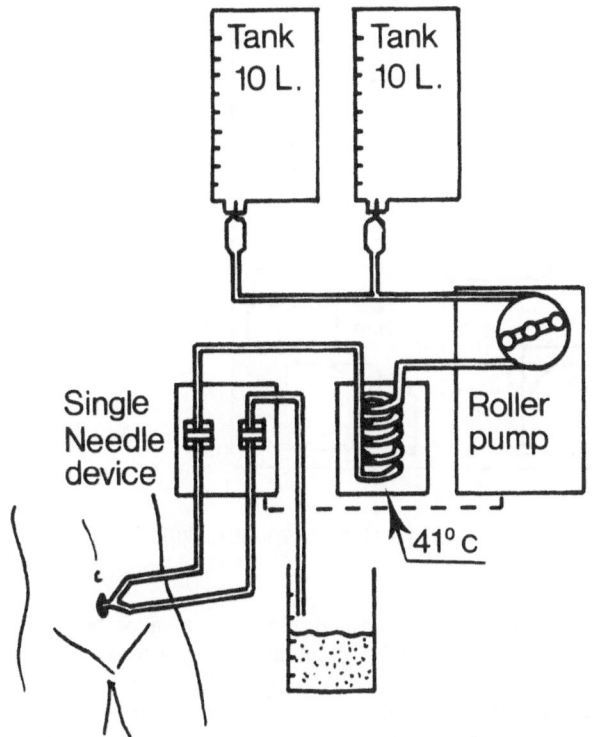

Figure 23. Fresh fluid, semicontinous peritoneal dialysis (1978 [125]).

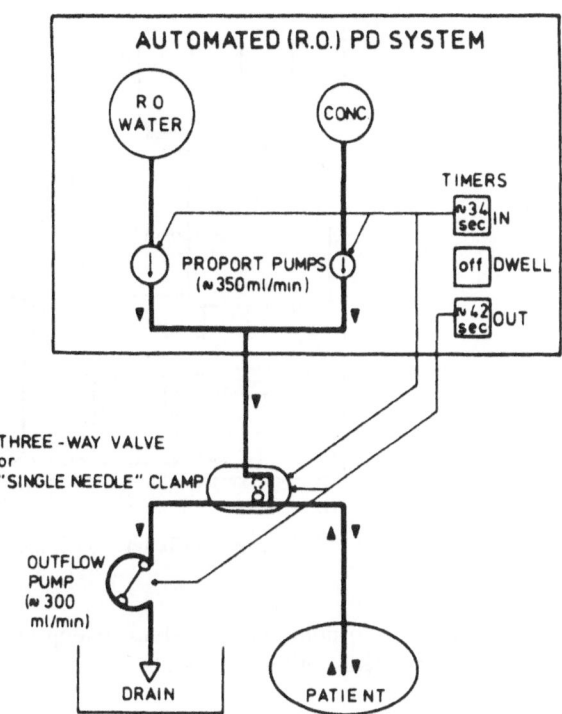

Figure 24. Fresh fluid, semicontinous peritoneal dialysis with a reverse osmosis dialysis fluid delivery machine (126).

should be carefully balanced: shortening of dialysis time versus the frequency of technical break-downs, catheter problems, the risk of infection, the increased loss of plasma proteins and the possibility of discomfort for the patient. In addition these technologies are taking away the simplicity, which has always been one of the advantages and features of peritoneal dialysis compared with extracorporeal haemodialysis.

Further development and practical application have been overshadowed by the introduction of CAPD.

Regeneration peritoneal dialysis (1974–1978)

Regeneration of peritoneal dialysate (Figure 25) has been attempted by Gordon and Maxwell and co-workers (127, 128) and by Lai and collaborators (129). Both systems employed urease, charcoal and ion exchange resins and have been tested in series of animal experiments. The former system has been utilised in a number of clinical trials (128, 130); 41 of fresh dialysis fluid was used and the outflowing perfusate was regenerated by recirculation through a gamma-ray sterilised sorbent cartridge as used in the Redy system (see chapter 19) and after passage through a bacterial filter re-introduced in the peritoneal cavity (see Figure 25). Several problems were encountered, such as adequate sterilisation of the dialysate pathway including the cartridge ensuring a sterile rinsing fluid, the preparation of pyrogen free urease and the production of regenerated rinsing fluid

with an adequate, non-irritating pH. According to Lewin (130) these problems were successfully solved.

Since fluid quantities with this system were not a problem, it seemed possible to produce dialysis fluid flow rates of 6 l/h or more, which should provide augmented small molecule clearances compared with conventional intermittent peritoneal dialysis. The system had the advantage of portability, like the original Redy system for haemodialysis. Transportability e.g. for travelling purposes, was more of a problem. For each dialysis 4 l of sterile fresh dialysate and a fresh sterile sorbent cartridge (weighing several kg) was required. For one week of travelling (three dialyses) an extra weight of about 20 kg plus the machine had to be carried on. For additional protection against bacterial contamination it seemed wise to insert a photochemical reactor, producing ultraviolet light in the inflow line before the indwelling peritoneal catheter as described by Eisinger in 1980 (131).

Further development and clinical trials have been halted because of the unexpected sudden death of the principal investigator and probably because of the introduction of CAPD.

MODERN MACHINE-FREE PERITONEAL DIALYSIS: CAPD (CONTINUOUS AMBULATORY PERITONEAL DIALYSIS) (1976–1978)

Manual hanging bottle peritoneal dialysis of the 1960's and 1970's has moved away from a simple 'machine free' system

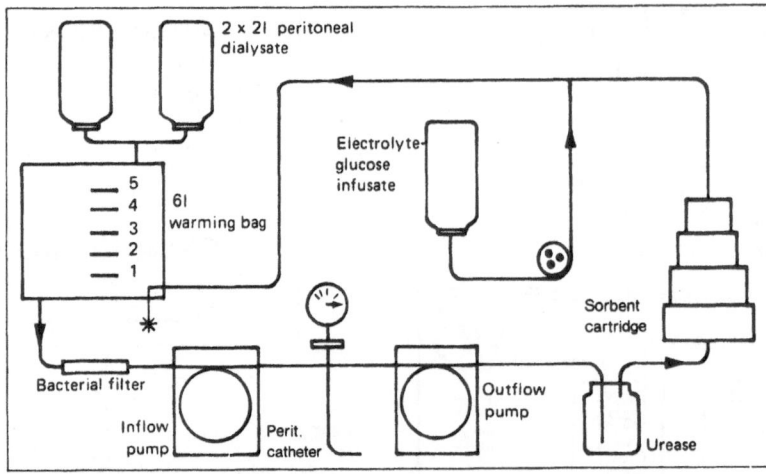

Figure 25. Flow diagram of the Sorbsystem (Redy) regenerating peritoneal dialysis system (1974 [127], 1978 [128, 130]).

via automatic cyclers to more complicated closed loop automatic peritoneal systems with RO machines.

Introduction of CAPD (1976–1978)

It has been suggested that back to nature activists, conservationists, pollution fighters and similar groups also have influenced the nephrologic mind particularly in the field of replacement of renal function (Diaz Buxo [132]). The way back to a simple, machine free, power free, natural membrane mediated replacement of renal function originated in Austin, Texas and was pointed out by Popovich and colleagues (133). Their paper was originally not accepted for presentation at the San Fancisco ASAIO meetings in 1976, but the method, by the originators called 'continuous ambulatory peritoneal dialysis (CAPD)' was briefly described in an abstract (133) and later in 1978 published in full (134–137). Their method aroused considerable interest in many centres in North America, Europe and Australia. Basically this treatment modality resembles intermittent 'hanging bottle' peritoneal dialysis. Dwell periods however are extended to 4 to 6 h by day and 8 h overnight (allowing the

patient uninterrupted sleep). In place of glass bottles 3 l capacity plastic bags containing 2 l of peritoneal dialysis solution became available commercially. With completion of the inflow the empty bag and administration set are folded in a small container or a cloth waist pocket. When the dwell time has elapsed the used dialysate is drained into the empty plastic bag by gravity, which is then discarded and replaced by a bag with fresh dialysis fluid, the Tenckhoff catheter or one of its modifications being used for peritoneal access (138).

Treatment is carried out 7 days a week and most patients exchange four or five bags a day at intervals of 4 h, extending the interval to 8 h during the night.

CAPD does not require major capital investment for a machine or special plumbing and other (often expensive) provisions in the house as for haemodialysis. It is performed as self-treatment and training time is short: 1 to 2 weeks (100, 139–145).

Efficiency of CAPD

Removal of small molecules (urea) with CAPD is approxi-

Table 7. Clearances (l/week) for different solutes by various dialysis techniques.

	Haemodialysis 15 h/week	IPD 40 h/week	CAPD continuous	CCPD			Normal kidney
				Nocturnal	Diurnal	Total	
Urea (60 daltons)	135	60	76–84	54	12.7	66.7	604
Creatinine (113 daltons)	90	28	58	46.2	12.5	58.7	1200
B_{12} (1350 daltons)	30	15–16	50	34.8	10.1	44.9	1200
Inulin (5200 daltons)	5	12	30	–	–	–	1200

From: Moncrief et al (137) and Diaz-Buxo et al (147). With permission (slightly modified).
IPD   : Intermittent peritoneal dialysis.
CAPD : Continuous ambulant peritoneal dialysis.
CCPD : Continuous cyclic peritoneal dialysis (see text).

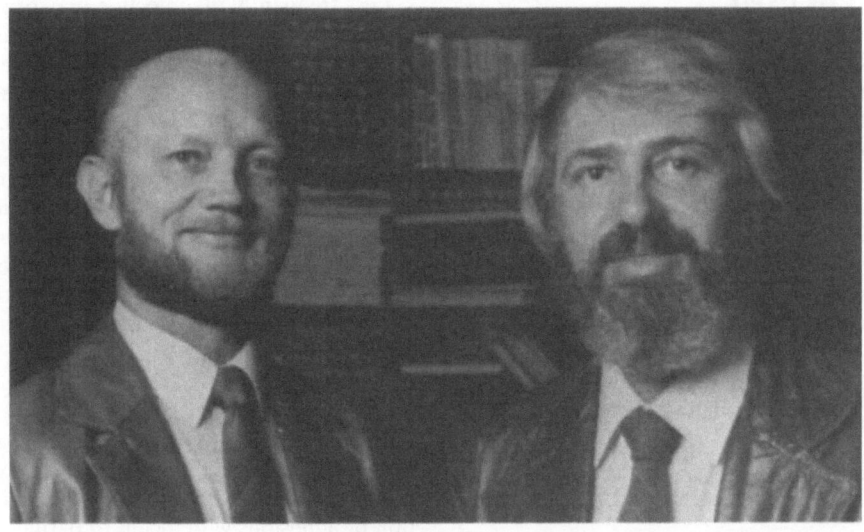

Figure 26. Jack W Moncrief (left) and Robert P Popovich (right) from Austin, TX, who introduced Continuous Ambulatory Peritoneal Dialysis (CAPD) (1976–'78 [133, 134]).

mately 1/3 less efficient than with haemodialysis (15 h/week), but more efficient than with intermittent peritoneal dialysis (40 h/week [see table 7]).

Removal of middle molecules with CAPD however (as illustrated by B_{12} and inulin) is more efficient as compared with intermittent peritoneal dialysis and haemodialysis.

Continuous cyclic peritoneal dialysis (CCPD) (1981)

Two groups of investigators (146–148) introduced a modified CAPD technique, called continuous cyclic peritoneal dialysis (CCPD) or automated long cycle peritoneal dialysis.

Both methods (which are identical) reintroduce a machine: a cycler is programmed to deliver three or four exchanges of 2 l over 9 to 10 h during the night. At disconnection in the morning 2 l dialysis fluid remain in the peritoneal cavity for 12 to 14 h

The results (see table 7) are comparable to CAPD and better than with intermittent peritoneal dialysis. Only one connection at night and one disconnection in the morning are required, which according to the originators should 'significantly reduce the incidence of peritonitis' (147, 148).

Although at the time of writing the place of CAPD and CCPD for short- and medium-term treatment of end-stage renal disease is secure (149), the long-term success rate is less certain.

Cost of CAPD

According to several clinical investigators, cost of CAPD is considerably less than of regular haemodialysis, either at the hospital or at the home (140–143). According to Robson and Oreopoulos (140) the expenses of CAPD are (in Canada) only one third of the yearly cost of intermittent peritoneal dialysis with an automatic cycler.

It has therefore been suggested that CAPD could potentially be a mode of treatment to alleviate the staggering and still escalating cost of treatment for end-stage renal failure (135, 149, 150). In addition, it does not require major capital investment for a machine. The short training period and the treatment outside hospital are also cost saving elements. As has been mentioned before no special plumbing and other costly provisions at the patient's home are required. But cost calculations in other centres have been different: in the USA maintenance cost of CAPD was approximately equivalent to the cost of home haemodialysis (151). However, in Canada, in Australia and the UK CAPD seems to be the cheapest form of all types of dialysis treatment (152). But when one includes the cost of hospitalisations for catheter problems and treatment of peritonitis the true cost of CAPD will be substantially higher.

Moreover CAPD is applicable to a wider range of patients than haemodialysis, including the elderly and the diabetic. This element may out-weigh the cheaper maintenance cost of CAPD, because a much greater number of patients can (and will be) treated (149), increasing the necessary ESRD budget. When the CCPD technique is preferred, giving the patient a better utilisation of time and a higher degree of freedom and mobility with a potential of lower incidence of peritonitis (153) the cost saving element of low capital investment will be partially lost because either a cycler or a (expensive) RO proportioning machine is a necessary piece of equipment.

COMPLICATIONS OF CAPD

But all that glitters is not gold: the success and advantages of CAPD have been overshadowed by certain drawbacks, characteristic for this type of dialysis therapy.

The three major complications are peritonitis, exit/tunnel infection and catheter replacement (154–157 [see Table 8]).

Initial enthousiasm after the introduction of CAPD in 1976–1978 (156, 157) soon tempered because of an unacceptable high incidence of peritonitis; the originators initially reported an incidence of one peritonitis episode every 10 weeks (157). This contrasted sharply with one episode every 54 months, reported by Slingeneyer and Mion (158, 159) in patients receiving intermittent peritoneal dialysis with a closed loop system and an automatic RO delivery machine.

Table 8. Complications of CAPD.

Peritonitis
Exit/tunnel infection
Catheter replacement
Loss of ultrafiltration
Loss of peritoneal surface
Sclerosing peritonitis

Peritonitis

Infection of the peritoneum has been called the Achilles heel of CAPD and at the time of writing (May, 1987) peritonitis is still the main complication (160–162).

The most common routes of infection are the lumina of the transfer-set and the catheter. They may become infected when the bag or the transfer set or both are changed (156, 158–160). If four exchanges daily are used the system is broken at least 28 times per week. (In intermittent peritoneal dialysis, which is usually carried out three times per week, the closed loop system is opened only six times per week).

Even meticulous aseptic technique cannot always prevent contamination: skin scales carrying bacteria (usually Staph. epidermidis, sometimes Staph. aureus or other micro-organisms [162]) are constantly shed by the patient (and others in the surroundings). These scales float around in the air and are attracted into the lumina of the tubing system and the catheter both by electrostatic forces and a minute negative pressure generated by opening of the circuit. On reconnection the minute airpocket with the contaminated skin scales is trapped and flushed into the abdominal cavity (156, 163, 164).

Other routes of infection of the peritoneum (see Table 9) are around the catheter along the subcutaneous catheter tract originating from the skin exit. Tunnel infections seem to be less frequent with double cuff catheters of any kind (165) but partial exteriorising and prolapse of the subcutaneous cuff open the port for catheter exit and tunnel infection. This cuff should be buried sufficiently deeply in the subcutaneous tissue to prevent this complication.

Less frequently the infection may originate in the bowel through a perforation or by transmural migration of the bacteria, as may occur in bowel inflammation for instance in diverticulitis. Patients with recurrent diverticulitis seem less suitable candidates for CAPD or CCPD.

Ascending infection via the female genital tract or via a vaginal fistula may occur but is less common.

Uncommon are also haematogenous infections of the peritoneum as may occur in septicaemia or in tuberculosis. The skin, however, is the main source of infection: some 45% of the infections is caused by a common skin bacteria such as Staph. epidermidis and by Staph. aureus (14%) (162).

Sequelae of peritonitis

Although most peritonitis episodes can be managed successfully without disruption of dialysis, they may damage the peritoneal membrane (see further) and may lead to formation of adhesions with loculi, to partial or complete loss of the peritoneal cavity and of course to loss of active exchange surface of the membrane.

A fatal outcome through the infection *per se* has occurred. Recurrent peritonitis may contribute to the development of sclerosing peritonis (see below), a condition which usually proves fatal.

Peritonitis may impair the ultrafiltrating capability of the peritoneal membrane (166).

Peritonitis is certainly the most feared complication of CAPD both by the patient, the nurses and the doctors and it is also the most frequent complication. According to the National CAPD Registry in the US, covering the 3 year period 1981 through 1983 (167) with data from some 7,400 patients, in nearly one half of the patients treated with CAPD during that period peritonitis occurred with a mean frequency of 1.7 times per patient year and exit-site/tunnel infections 0.7 times per patient year.

Prevention of peritonitis

The cornerstone of peritonitis prophylaxis is a meticulous, aseptic bag exchange technique. Patients should be trained by experienced nurses, specialised in CAPD. Training facilities need sufficient staff and space which should be prefer-

Table 9. Various routes of bacterial invasion of the peritoneal cavity.

Through the lumina of the transfer system and the peritoneal catheter (exogenous contamination during disconnection and connection)
Across the abdominal wall, through the catheter exit-site and along the subcutaneous catheter tunnel
Across the bowel wall, through perforation (faecal peritonitis) or by transmural migration (diverticulosis, -itis)
Haematogenous (from nasopharynx? from teeth?)
Ascending via the female genital tract

From Oreopoulos DG et al (154) and Mion CM (155) with permission.

ably separated from the hospital dialysis unit.

But even scrupulous aseptic technique cannot always prevent intraluminal infection by airborne skin squames carrying bacteria, when the circuit is opened.

In addition one should be aware, that with three or four rather time consuming exchange procedures per day, 7 days per week, week in, week out, psychologically from time to time some negligence may occur, even in patients who have been rigorously trained, are dedicated to their treatment and are anxious about their own well-being.

'Connectology'

Various transfer systems and a multitude of special 'safe' connectors have been designed to prevent bacterial contamination or to eliminate contamination with antiseptic solutions like povidone-iodine, sodium hypochlorite or chlorhexidene (163, 164, 168–171).

Ingenious devices were invented by industrial firms, depending on physical methods of decontamination such as bag connection by heat welding (172) or UV irradiation of the connectors and the surrounding air (Travenol Laboratories [154, 156]). Infection of the peritoneum may also be prevented by a bacteriological filter (e.g. $0,22\,\mu$ Micropore filter) inserted in the inflow line (173–177).

The fear of contamination and peritonitis culminated in the late 1970's and early 1980's in a kind of anxiety neurosis ('If the problem of peritonitis can be overcome, CAPD may offer a new dimension in dialysis technology '[Moncrief et al, (137)]. It is obvious that 'connectology' turned CAPD into a gadgeteer's paradise . . . (178).

Incidence of peritonitis

With growing experience of doctors and nurses, with scrupulous aseptic technology of bag exchanges and replacements of administration sets and in particular with rigorous training of patients the infection rate of the peritoneum has gradually come down (see Table 10).

Very low figures were reported by Italian groups (179, 180) with the Y connector system and hypochlorite disinfection and by Parsons and associates (164) in Leeds, UK

with Luer-Lok connectors and a Betadine spray.

However, it seems reasonable to consider the recent data reported from the UK by the Working Party chaired by Bint (162) and published in 1987 as an acceptable average: one episode per patient year. In some patients recurrent peritonitis presents a serious problem which may lead to structural and functional changes of the peritoneum which were briefly mentioned above. Although in many centres, in particular in those which have specialised in the peritonitis problem a substantial reduction of the incidence has been obtained, peritonitis remains the most common complication in CAPD.

STRUCTURAL AND FUNCTIONAL CHANGES OF THE PERITONEAL MEMBRANE FROM IPD OR CAPD

The peritoneal membrane is a delicate structure made up of a single layer of flat mesothelial cells, separated from the capillaries by a thin layer of fibrous tissue and clearly separated from the underlying fat tissue. The peritoneal membrane is certainly not designed for repetitive or even permanent contact with unphysiological and potentially noxious fluids containing acetate or lactate, often high dextrose concentrations and having low pH values.

Verger and associates (181, 182) took biopsies of the peritoneal membrane in patients treated by CAPD and noted hypervascularisation and considerable increase of the thickness of the fibrous layer. In addition they noted patchy destruction of the mesothelial cell layer in particular when peritonitis had occurred. In some patients the mesothelium was totally destroyed and only a thin layer of fibrous tissue had been left.

Loss of ultrafiltration capability

These structural changes explain the decrease or loss of ultrafiltration capability in a number of CAPD patients who had experienced peritonitis, in particular in those who had resistant or recurrent episodes. The phenomenon is explained by increasingly fast resorbtion of dextrose with decrease or loss of the osmotic gradient (183, 184). This manifests itself by an increase of the number of hyperosmolar

Table 10. Peritonitis.

Year	First author	Episodes/patient mo	Particulars	Ref.
1978	Popovich	1/2.5	USA	134
1980–'83	Nolph	1/7.1	USA	167
1985	Bint	1/12	UK	162
1982	Slingeneyer	1/18	$0.22\,\mu$ filter	174
1984	Slingeneyer	1/24	$0.22\,\mu$ filter	175
1984	Buoncristiani	1/47.8	Y connector Na hypochlorite	179
1984	Cantaluppi	1/53.3	Y connector Na hypochlorite	180
1986	Parsons	1/86	Luer-Lok connector Betadine spray	164

bags (2.5 and 4.0% dextrose) over the month (166), which is necessary to obtain sufficient ultrafiltration.

A similar loss of ultrafiltration capability occurs in some patients, who never had peritonitis (166). The phenomenon usually occurs between 6 and 24 months of CAPD treatment and has also been observed in patients treated with IPD. These 'changes' may lay the foundation of thickening and sclerosis of the peritoneum which is known to occur in patients treated by IPD or CAPD (166, 185–187).

The increasing number of exchanges with hyperosmolar bags may enhance further structural and functional deterioration of the peritoneal membrane, finally necessitating transfer of the patient to haemodialysis, because of total loss of ultrafiltration capability.

Interestingly, if this vicious circle is broken and it still appears possible to place the patient on hypoosmolar bags the ultrafiltration capability of some patients returns (166).

Loss of effective surface of the peritoneal membrane

Recurrent peritonitis may result in formation of adhesions and loculi leading to reduction of the peritoneal space resulting in abdominal pain during exchanges and necessitating termination of peritoneal dialysis therapy.

Loss of effective surface area may result in decreasing clearance figures and ineffective dialysis also leading to transfer to haemodialysis (188).

Table 11. Sclerosing peritonitis (SP). Case reports 1978–1986.

Author, Country	Year	SP patients	Total patients	%	IPD or CAPD	Duration PD (mo)	Acetate (A) or (L) lactate	Peritonitis	β blocking drug	Survival	Ref
Gandhi, USA	1978–1980	5	30	17	4 IPD 1 CAPD	3–48	A	++	no (?)	4 alive 1 dead	185–187
Denis, France	1980	1	?	?	CAPD	8	A	+	no (?)	dead	191
Thomson, Australia	1981	2	54	3.7	CAPD	8–16	L	–	no (?)	1 alive 1 dead	192
Heale, Australia	1981	12*	50	24	IPD or CAPD 4 both	7–75	?	++	no (?)	1 alive 11 dead	193
Grefberg, Sweden	1983	1**	?	?	CAPD	22	L	+	+ metoprolol atenolol	dead	194
Hauglustaine, Belgium	1983	1	?	?	CAPD	37	L	++	+ labetalol	dead	195
McWinnie, Scotland	1984–1986	9	80	11.3	CAPD	14–40	L	++	+ propranolol oxprenolol atenolol	2 alive 7 dead	189 196 197
Rottembourg, France	1984–1986	12	163	7.4	CAPD	7–42	A	++	+ acebutolol propranolol	5 alive 7 dead	190 198
Slingeneyer, France	1984	6	431	1.4	CAPD	1.2–46	A 5 L 1	+	+ acebutolol propranolol	2 alive 4 dead	199 200
Manos, UK	1986	2	97	2	CAPD (+ IPD)	7–14	L	+	no (?)	1 alive 1 dead	188
Total	1978–1986	51	–	–	–	–	–	–	–	16 alive 35 dead = ±70%	–

Updated from (203), with permission of the publishers of Dialysis and Transplantation.
* 4 membrane failure 7 catheter malfunct. (no transfer to haemodialysis).
** SP manifest 22 mo after transplant.

SCLEROSING PERITONITIS

The structural changes of the membrane described by Verger and associates are probably the basic pathology for the loss of ultrafiltration capability, leading finally to the macroscopic milky thickening of the peritoneal membrane observed at autopsy or laparatomy in a number of long-term CAPD cases.

However, in 1978 and 1980 Gandhi and colleagues from Chicago, IL (185, 186) reported on observations in five patients treated by IPD with automatic (RO) machines who all suffered from repeated peritonitis episodes and who all underwent laparatomies for catheter failure or persistent abdominal pains or peritonitis.

The findings in all cases were similar: numerous adhesions and a thick shaggy peritoneal membrane covering the entire small bowel or parts of it. Biopsies showed marked thickening of the peritoneum due to proliferation of fibro-connective tissue with infiltration mostly of mononuclear inflammatory cells.

One patient died, the other four were returned to haemodialysis. Later the same investigators described two more patients and demonstrated a marked reduction of peritoneal clearances after the onset of peritoneal sclerosis (187).

Soon other cases were reported in the literature (188–202) and in 1984 45 cases could be reviewed (203).

Two years later 6 additional cases were reported and a total of 51 cases of this dramatic complication is summarised in Table 11.

Clinical manifestations and pathology

Sclerosing peritonitis usually develops insidiously in ESRD patients treated by CAPD or IPD (186, 199) with nonspecific abdominal symptoms and abdominal pains, vomiting, anorexia, weight loss and low grade fever. Protein malnutrition usually develops and an abdominal mass becomes palpable, consisting of intestinal loops grown together by tight fibrous tissue and covered by a milkish white fibrous shield. This cocoon is considered characteristic and diagnostic for the syndrome (198). As the disease progresses colicky abdominal cramps occur with signs of total or partial bowel obstruction urging surgery.

At laparatomy both visceral and parietal peritoneum are thickened by deposition of a dense layer of fibrous tissue covering the small bowel or parts of it. The colon may also be involved. The small bowel is in typical cases totally or partially encapsulated by a dense fibrous cocoon which often causes intestinal obstruction (196 [see Figure 27]). At operation (often to be performed as an emergency procedure) the bowel loops should be freed and released from the constricting cocoon.

In early cases a line of cleavage may be found but in longer standing cases freeing the bowel is difficult or impossible and multiple intestinal perforations may occur. Many patients therefore die soon after the operation.

The histology of biopsies is not specific, presenting proliferation of bland connective tissue with infiltration by mononuclear cells and increased vascularity.

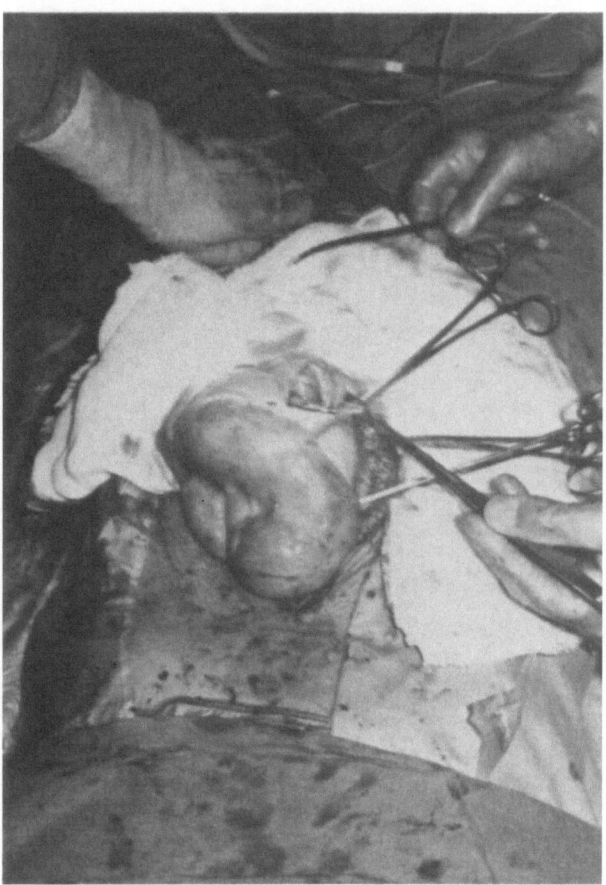

Figure 27. Sclerosing peritonitis (picture taken during laparatomy). Small bowel loops distended and cocooned in a bag of thickenend peritoneum. Part of membrane opened, freeing bowel loops. (Courtesy Dr. Alain Slingeneyer, Montpellier, France [199, 200]).

The mesenteric cell layer is disrupted or entirely absent (Figures 28 and 29).

Prognosis and diagnosis of sclerosing peritonitis

The prognosis is poor: of the 51 cases reviewed in 1987 35 have died (about 70%).

The diagnosis is usually based on the history, the clinical signs and symptoms, the presence of a palpable mass in the abdomen and the occurrence of partial or total bowel obstruction.

Finally the findings at laparatomy with biopsies of the thickened, milky peritoneum confirm the diagnosis.

A plain film of the abdomen showing dilatation of the duodenum and jejunal loops may support the diagnosis.

An early diagnosis is extremely important: early surgery may be successful and early transfer to haemodialysis may arrest the condition but does not always prevent progression.

An early sign which may raise suspicion of the condition is

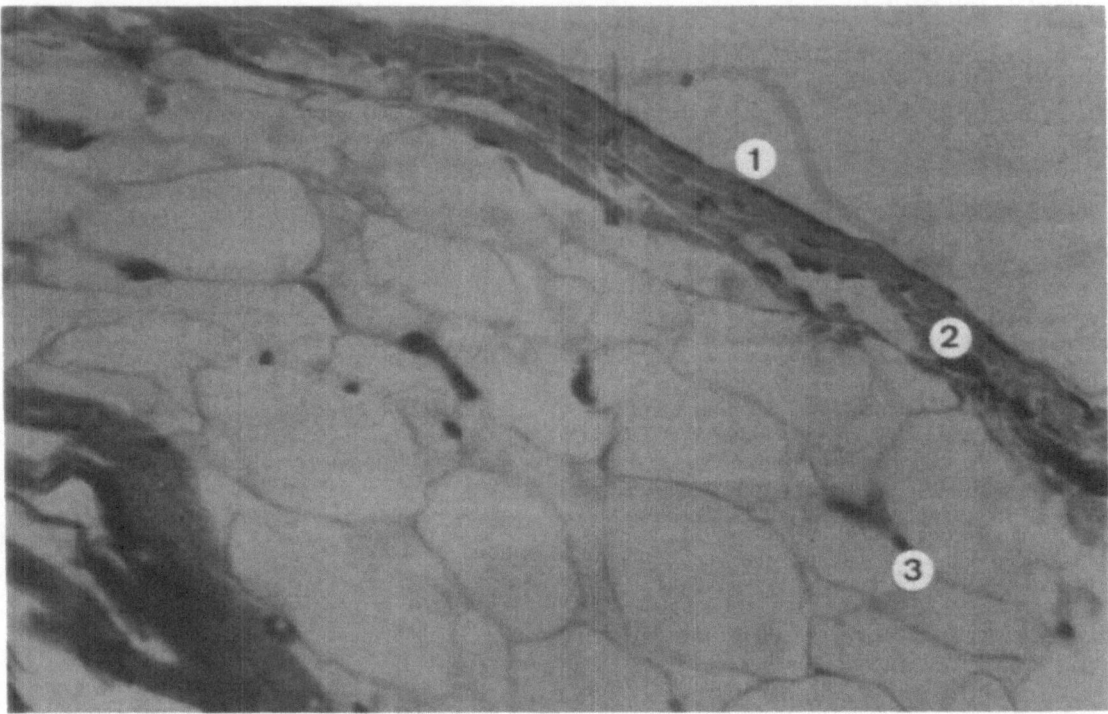

Figure 28. Normal peritoneal membrane. 1. Monolayer of mesothelial cells 2. Submesothelial fibrous tissue 3. Adipocytes (Hematoxylin-eosin, × 100). (Courtesy Dr. Alain Slingeneyer, Montpellier, France [200]).

loss of ultrafiltration capability of the peritoneum and sometimes also loss of active surface area occurs with decrease of urea and creatinine clearances (166, 199, 200). A transverse sonogram of the abdomen can be of diagnostic help by showing the enveloping membrane (199).

There is no correlation between the duration of peritoneal dialysis therapy and the occurrence of sclerosing peritonitis; cases have been reported after 40 to 75 months of treatment but also after less than 12 months (190, [Table 11]), but usually the patients have been treated for at least 2 years.

The disease may become manifest months, sometimes years after cessation of peritoneal dialysis after transfer to haemodialysis or transplantation.

In 1984 the Registration Committee of the EDTA-ERA

asked dialysis units in Europe and adjacent countries to report the number of patients (either living or expired) with sclerosing peritonitis diagnosed up until the end of 1984 (204). Some 70 cases appeared to have the characteristic cocoon and 55 could be studied in some detail.

By the end of 1984 the mortality (66%) was almost equal to that reported in Table 11.

The age and sex distribution was comparable to the general dialysis population with a preponderance of the middle aged and elderly age groups of 50 to 70 years.

It went out that the prevalence of sclerosing peritonitis was 1.5 to 1.6 per 1,000 patients at risk, somewhat higher in Belgium and France (3.1 and 2.1 per 1,000) and lower in Spain (0.3 per 1,000).

Aetiology

A number of possible causative factors have been mentioned by clinical investigators (See Table 12). These include peritonitis, chemical sterilants used for bag and tubing connections (hypochlorite solution, chlorhexidene or formaldehyde used for disinfecting automatic peritoneal dialysis machines). Small amounts may enter the peritoneal cavity damaging the peritoneal membrane.

Buffers (acetate, lactate) and hypertonic dextrose solutions may also be damaging to the membrane (191, 198, 200).

Table 12. Sclerosing peritonitis: Possible causative factors.

1. Peritonitis
2. Chemical sterilants
   (hypochlorite, chlorhexidene, formaldehyde)
3. Buffers (acetate, lactate)
4. Hypertonic dextrose
5. Beta blocking agents
6. Low pH of dialysis fluid
7. Drugs added to dialysis fluid
8. Inflow filters (IL 1)

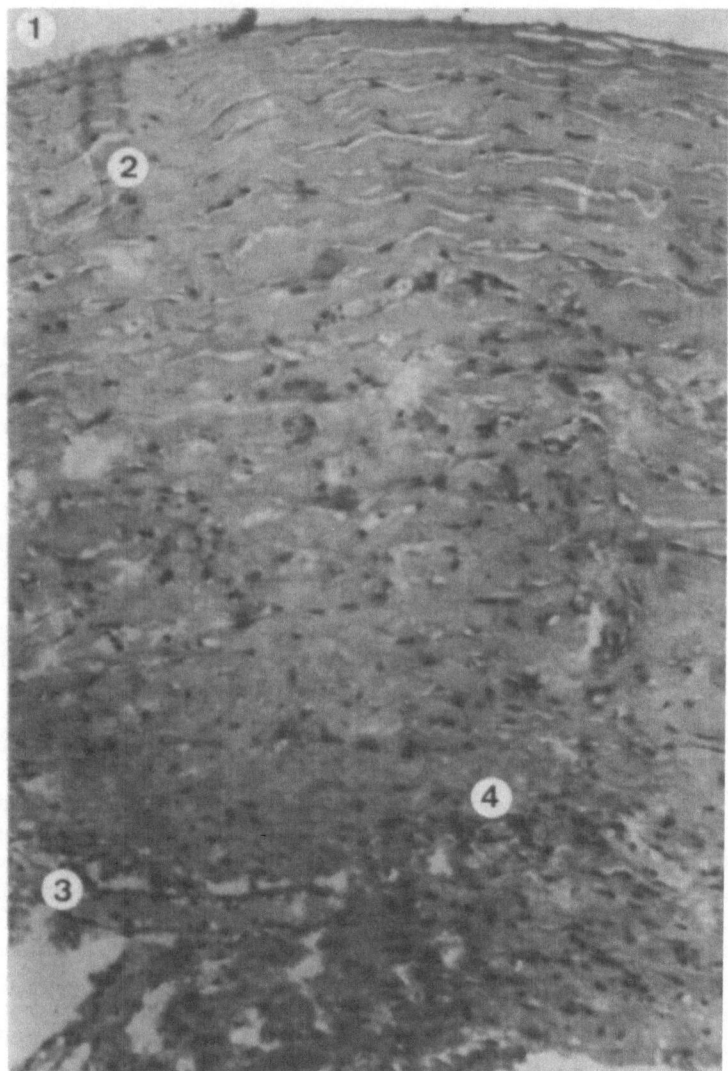

Figure 29. Biopsy of peritoneal membrane from a patient on intermittent peritoneal dialysis with sclerosing peritonitis. Mesothelial cell layer is missing. 1. Fibrin deposit 2. Hyaline fibrous tissue 3. Widened capillary 4. Cellular inflammatory infiltrate. The peritoneal membrane is grossly thickened (Hematoxylin-eosin, × 100). (Courtesy Dr. Alain Slingeneyer, Montpellier, France [200]).

Beta blocking agents have been suspected because the wide spectrum of effects of these agents on the gastrointestinal system (205, 206) and the similarity between sclerosing peritonitis and the peritoneal sclerosis caused by practolol (207, 208).

Peritoneal sclerosis has also been observed in patients treated with other β-blocking agents (propranolol, oxprenolol, atenolol, metoprolol [209–214]).

In this context it is important that the half-life of some β-blockers is considerably increased in patients with terminal renal failure (215 [see Table 13] which may enhance undesired side effects.

As has been demonstrated by Danish investigators (216) β

adrenergic stimulation increases intracellular cyclic AMP. Blocking of this effect may lead to cell proliferation and leads to thickening of fibrosis tissue. These observations may be a key to the solution of the mystery of some undesired side-effects of β-blocking agents.

The pH of the dialysis fluid is usually maintained at unphysiological low values (pH 5 to 6) to avoid caramelisation of dextrose during autoclaving. This may be damaging to the peritoneal membrane. The addition of metabisulfite serves the same purpose but may be noxious to the membrane as well.

Drugs added to the dialysis fluid – often in unphysiological concentrations – may have an adverse effect on the delicate and vulnerable peritoneal membrane.

Finally an interesting hypothesis has been brought forward by Shaldon and colleagues (217), explaining a paradoxical double role of bacterial filters in the inflow line (158, 159, 174). A 0.22 μ filter prevents bacterial contamination of the peritoneal cavity, decreasing efficiently the frequency of peritonitis, but it permits bacteria to multiply on the upstream side of the filter. They produce pyrogens which pass the filter.

The pyrogen stimulates monocytes (peritoneal macrophages) after a suitable period of incubation, for instance during the overnight dwell. The monocytes produce interleukin 1, which stimulates fibroblast formation, inducing fibrous tissue proliferation in the peritoneum.

Preliminary experiments have supported this hypothesis (217, 218).

Nevertheless it remains unexplained that the majority of patients with sclerosing peritonitis were not treated with an inline bacterial filter and so far only 10% of the patients treated with a filter developed sclerosing peritonitis (217, 218).

The EDTA-ERA Registration committee published in the 1985 report a statistical analysis of the possible causative factors of sclerosing peritonitis using the 55 identified patients on the Registry file and a control group of CAPD patients without this complication. For only one exposure a statistically significant difference was found, namely the use of chlorhexidene (204).

It seemed advisable to halt the use of this disinfectant for tubing connections.

Nevertheless it seems justified to conclude that the aetiology of sclerosing peritonitis is not yet satisfactorily elucidated and that the definite cause of this complication remains mysterious.

Probably the aetiology is multifactorial with (recurrent) peritonitis, chlorhexidene and inline bacterial filters high on the list of suspects.

SOME SUMMARISING REFLECTIONS AND SOME ADDITIONAL DATA

The first primitive attempt of a peritoneal dialysis in a human being was performed by a German doctor early in 1923 (24), one and a half year before the first human extracorporeal haemodialysis was carried out, also in Germany, in October 1924 (27).

Peritoneal dialysis evolved slowly and did not gain very much practical application until the work of Doolan (39) and Maxwell (40) in the USA in 1959. In particular the introduction of commercially prepared dialysis solution and tubing and the disposable stylet catheter by Weston and Roberts in 1965 (50) were major steps forward and in the 1960's, peritoneal dialysis gained ground for treatment of acute renal failure.

It was however overshadowed by haemodialysis which made rapid technical and practical progress in the late 1950's and early 1960's in particular when Scribner and co-workers (64) reported their successful haemodialysis treatment of chronic irreversible uraemia in the early 1960's.

Many considered chronic intermittent peritoneal dialysis as a less efficient, time consuming, cheap, second class treatment of chronic uraemia. It was more or less the 'Cinderella treatment' of chronic patients used temporarily for patients on the waiting list for haemodialysis treatment or transplantation (219). Only a few mastered the painstaking technique of chronic peritoneal dialysis and were able to provide patients with irreversible end-stage kidney disease a good quality of life. Many other patients who were treated by chronic peritoneal dialysis in the 1960's faced a treatment which only delayed death.

In 1965 Scribner (59) stirred the dialysis world again: he had noted that patients on chronic peritoneal dialysis which controlled traditional blood chemistries less well than haemodialysis often felt better. In addition peripheral neuropathy did not occur or did not progress despite a certain amount of 'underdialysis'. Scribner then presented the hypothesis that the peritoneal membrane was more permeable than Cuprophan and that peritoneal dialysis removed substances of higher molecular weight more efficiently than haemodialysis. This hypothesis led to the middle molecule hypothesis (220) which greatly influenced dialysis strategy and technology and led to a growing interest in chronic intermittent peritoneal dialysis.

The break-through came also from Seattle when Tenckhoff and co-workers (82) in the late '60's introduced the indwelling Silastic catheter, which solved the problem of repeated peritoneal access and when the closed loop reverse osmosis dialysis fluid factories with automatic cyclers became available in 1972 (98). With these innovations chronic intermittent peritoneal dialysis came of age (221). Chronic intermittent peritoneal dialysis with a 'closed loop, reverse osmosis automatic system' has been widely accepted as an adequate mode of replacement of renal function, offering satisfactory rehabilitation. Morbidity and mortality compared well with regular haemodialysis and the economics seemed to be competitive. But intermittent peritoneal dialysis was in the late 1970's rapidly superseded by CAPD.

Advantages of CAPD

Introduced in 1976–1978 by Popovich et al (133, 134) and improved by Oreopoulos and associates (1978 [138]), who

Table 13. Half-lives of β blocking agents in terminal renal failure (h).

Drug	Normal	Anephric
Propranolol	3.5	3.5
Sotalol	6	50
Practolol	9	60
Acebutolol	4	4
Atenolol	6	75
Metoprolol	4	4

From Maher JF (215), with permission.

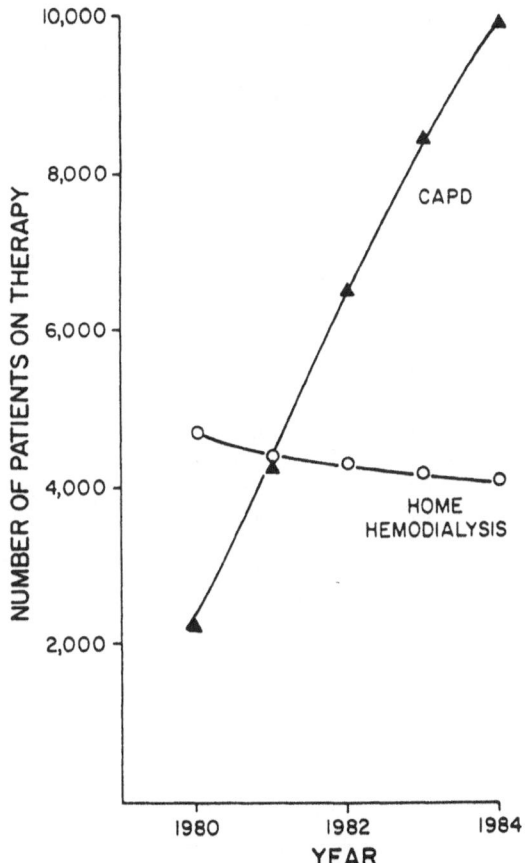

Figure 30. Decline of the number of home haemodialysis patients in the US after introduction of CAPD. The number of CAPD patients increased rapidly (100) (1980–1984 data from health Care Financing Administration, Dept. of Health and Human Service, Washington DC).

replaced the original glass bottles by plastic bags, it appeared to be a simple, easy to learn self-treatment in the home. The training time is short (1 to 2 weeks) and a partner is – in contrast with home haemodialysis – usually not required.

It gives to the patient freedom to go where he prefers and offers freedom to travel.

CAPD is better tolerated by older patients than haemodialysis and is also more suitable for diabetic uraemic patients.

CAPD is according to many paedriatic nephrologists the preferred therapy for juvenile patients. Finally, CAPD presently is often the primary choice of new ESRD patients themselves.

Acceptance of CAPD

CAPD gained popularity surprisingly fast and with its tremendous growth a simultanous decline of home haemodialysis occurred, which has been evident both in the USA (100 [Figure 30]) and in Europe (Tables 14, 15 see also Table 4, chapter 3).

In the USA in 1979 fewer than 1,000 patients were treated by CAPD; by the end of 1985 this number had multiplied 12 fold to 12,189 (including CCPD) (100, 222), that made 14,4% of the total dialysis population in the USA.

The number of home haemodialysis patients decreased in the same period from 4,720 (1980) to 3,983 (1985).

In Europe the number of CAPD/CCPD patients multiplied 9 to 10 fold between 1978 and 1985 from 779 to 7,529, the percentage increasing from 1.9% in 1979 to 9.2% of the total dialysis population.

The number of IPD patients remained stable, in the same period numbering somewhat less than 1,000.

The percentage of IPD decreased gradually to 1.2% of the total dialysis population.

Likewise CAPD rapidly superseded home haemodialysis in Europe, the percentage of patients declining from 21 to 24% in the mid-seventies to 9.1% in 1986 (Table 14, see also Table 4, chapter 3).

In scarcely populated countries like Australia and Canada CAPD/CCPD, being a home dialysis treatment, also gained popularity rapidly reaching 30% of the total dialysis patient population by 1984. In 1985 37% of the total dialysis population in the UK was treated by CAPD (204).

More detailed statistics became available from the NIH-CAPD Registry in the USA (167, [1981–1983]) and from the EDTA-ERA Registry Reports in Europe (204, 223–226).

In the USA the number of patients treated by CAPD/CCPD increased from 2,440 in 1980 (4.7%) to 8,688 in 1983 (12.1% of the dialysis population [157]). In Europe (and adjacent countries) CAPD patients increased from 779 (1.9%) in 1979 to 7,529 (9.2%) in 1985 (Table 15, see also Table 4, chapter 3).

It had been prophecied that the CAPD/CCPD population world-wide would be 22,000 by the end of 1984 (157).

This remarkably rapid growth of CAPD has been explained by the enthousiastic approach of the pioneers of the

Table 14. Europe (1972–1985). Home haemodialysis and CAPD/CCPD. (Percentages of total dialysis patients).

	Home HD	CAPD/CCPD
1972	17.7%	–
1973	22.4%	–
1974	22.9%	–
1975	21.6%	–
1976	24.4%	–
1977	23.5%	–
1978	18.4%	–
1979	19.9%	1.9%
1980	16.2%	3.8%
1981	15.1%	5.7%
1982	12.5%	6.2%
1983	12.2%	7.9%
1984	9.8%	8.1%
1985	9.0%	9.2%
1986	7.3%	9.1%

Data derived from the annual statistical reports of the EDTA-ERA.

Table 15. Europe 1971–1985. Chronic peritoneal dialysis patients (1971–1985) (see also Table 4, chapter 3).

	Total chronic dialysis patients	Total chronic PD patients	% of total dialysis patients	Total IPD patients	% of total dialysis patients	Total CAPD/ CCPD patients	% of total dialysis patients
Mar. 1971	5,133	102	2.0	102	2.0	–	–
Dec. 31 1971	7,499	159	2.1	159	2.1	–	–
Dec. 31 1972	10,496	175	1.7	175	1.7	–	–
Dec. 31 1973	14,171	196	1.4	196	1.4	–	–
Dec. 31 1974	17,927	268	1.5	268	1.5	–	–
Dec. 31 1975	22,757	336	1.6	336	1.6	–	–
Dec. 31 1976*	27,779	436	1.6	436	1.6	–	–
Dec. 31 1977	31,842	545	1.7	545	1.7	–	–
Dec. 31 1978**	35.840	839	2.3	839	2.3	–	–
Dec. 31 1979	42,228	1,583	3.9	804	1.9	779	1.9
Dec. 31 1980	51.157	2,749	5.4	910	1.8	1,839	3.6
Dec. 31 1981***	52,758	3,953	7.5	951	1.8	3,002	5.7
Dec. 31 1982	58,305	4,431	7.6	824	1.4	3,607	6.2
Dec. 31 1983	70,845	6,547	9.2	984	1.4	5,563	7.9
Dec. 31 1984	78,999	7,418	10.3	968	1.2	6,450	8.2
Dec. 31 1985	82,283	8,514	10.4	985	1.2	7,529	9.2
Dec. 31 1986	92,568	9,360	10.1	869	1.1	8,491	9.1

* Introduction of automatic RO equipment.
** Introduction of CAPD.
*** Introduction of CCPD.
Data derived from the annual statistical reports of the EDTA-ERA.

Table 16. Patient survival (Europe).

Age at 1st dialysis yr	Year of 1st dialysis 1980–84				Year of 1st dialysis 1981–84		
	% survivial				% survival		
	Hospital haemodialysis				CAPD		
	1 yr	2 yr	3 yr	4 yr	1 yr	2 yr	3 yr
0–14	94	90	89	85	96	89	–
15–44	93	86	82	77	94	88	83
45–64	89	78	70	63	87	74	63
≥65	80	64	53	43	78	58	44

Source: EDTA-ERA Registry Report 1985 (204).

method and the efficient efforts of the 'new medical industrial complex' (227, 228) to launch the new technique with technical support and unprecedented financial support for publishing. In addition CAPD is relatively cheap and this has been an important aspect in an episode of global economical recession.

Patient survival with CAPD therapy

The survival figures are presented in Table 16. The differences with hospital haemodialysis are only marginal.

The hospitalisation data in the large CAPD population group by Nolph et al (167) averaged 10.2 hospital days for CAPD related complications and 22.3 days per year for all causes, not much different from the data of Charytan and coworkers (151), who noted an average of 17.2 hospital

Table 17. CAPD.

Plus	Minus
Machine free technique	Frequent peritonitis
Capital investment negligible	Exit/tunnel infections
Relatively cheap	Catheter replacements
Brief training period	Damage to the peritoneal
Essentially home dialysis	membrane
Quality of life better than	a. loss of ultrafiltration
with home haemodialysis?	b. loss of active membrane surface
	c. sclerosing peritonitis
	Limited technique survival (transfer to haemodialysis or transplantation)

Table 18. CAPD complications (162, 167).

	3 mo	*12 mo*	*24 mo*
Peritonitis	25%	66%	–
Exit/tunnel infection	16%	40%	–
Catheter replacement	8%	20%	–
Left therapy (USA)	–	33%	55% (1981–'83)
Left therapy (Europe)	–	43%	60% (1981)
Sclerosing peritonitis	–	1 per 1000 patients at risk	–

days/year for their CAPD patients (diabetics excluded) and 18.7 days for their hospital haemodialysis patients.

The pluses and minuses of CAPD and the frequency of complications are summarised in Tables 17 and 18.

SOME QUESTIONS REGARDING CAPD, WHICH REMAINED UNANSWERED IN THE PREVIOUS EDITION OF THIS BOOK (229), CAN PRESENTLY (MAY 1987) BE ANSWERED, SOME, HOWEVER, CANNOT; AND A SUMMARY CONCERNING CAPD

In the previous edition of this book a number of questions remained unanswered.

CAPD (and CCP/D) has certainly come of age (144) but the peritonitis problem is not yet satisfactorily solved.

The risk of irreversable damage to the membrane by recurrent peritonitis and (or) hypertonic dextrose solutions with loss of ultrafiltration capability has remained and the development of sclerosing peritonitis is a 'sword of Damocles' above the heads of the patients (230).

The cause of sclerosing peritonitis is still mysterious and the risk of this usually deadly complication is not yet eliminated.

The drop out rate from CAPD is still too high and long-term CAPD will probably not be tolerated by the peritoneal membrane.

So far CAPD has not become the 'silver bullet' for treatment of end-stage chronic renal disease – and it will certainly not be a viable long-term treatment comparable with haemodialysis that still should be considered the 'gold standard' (231).

But CAPD (and CCPD) is certainly another milestone in the history of dialysis, which will not fade away from the firmament of medicine.

It is presently the treatment of choice for children and young patients who are expecting a transplant in the foreseeable future, for diabetics and for older and brittle patients.

CAPD is also an acceptable therapy for older patients if it is their own preference and if no alternative facilities are available, but for a limited period of time. Back-up facilities for transfer to haemodialysis should always be available.

Optimal technique and optimal training with periodic supervision after the patient has gone home and avoidance

of any 'risk factors' are prerequisites for an acceptable rehabilitation and an acceptable quality of life of the CAPD patients and also for those on regular IPD therapy (229).

ACKNOWLEDGEMENTS

The author gratefully acknowledges the courtesy of Mr D.W.C. Stewart, librarian, The Royal Society of Medicine, London UK, for the picture of the Rev. Stephen Hales (*Figure 1*) and the facsimile of the Reverend's letter to the secretary of the Royal Society of Medicine (*Figure 2*).

Mr. David Hamilton, PhD, FRCS, consultant surgeon Dept. of Surgery, Western Infirmary, Glasgow, Scotland, kindly provided the author with a photocopy of the original letter from Heinrich Necheles to John Jacob Abel, dated June 16, 1924, which the author gratefully acknowledges. The original letter is in the archives of the Johns Hopkins Hospital, Baltimore MD, USA.

Dr. Ganter's picture (*Figure 3*) and his biographical data were kindly supplied by the editors of the Münchener Medizinische Wochenschrift (Mr. H. Lichtenstern).

Figure 4 is reproduced from a paper by Patrick McBride in the *Peritoneal Dial Bull* 1: 75, 1981, with permission.

Figure 5 is reproduced from a paper by Patrick McBride in the *Peritoneal Dial Bull* 3: 146, 1982, with permission.

Figure 6 was kindly supplied by Dr. F.M. Parsons, Leeds UK.

Figure 9 is reproduced from Patrick McBride's paper in *Peritoneal Dial Bull* 4: 58, 1984, with permission.

Figures 11c and 14 are reproduced from photographs made available by B. Braun Melsungen AG, W. Germany and kindly supplied by Messrs. Soho BV, Purmerend, The Netherlands.

The author gratefully acknowledges the courtesy of Dr. Paul D. Doolan, St. Mary's Hospital, Waterbury CT and Dr. Richard F. Ruben, San Francisco CA, USA who sent him a photocopy of the case history report and further particulars of the first chronic patient maintained with periodic peritoneal dialysis.

Figure 13 is reproduced from a photograph made available by Messrs. Quinton Instrument Co., Seattle WA, USA, which is gratefully acknowledged.

Figure 15 is reproduced from Patrick McBride's paper 'Pioneers in Peritoneal Dialysis' in *Peritoneal Dial Bull* 3: 47, 1983

Figure 16 is reproduced from the *asaio Journal* 3: 109, 1980, with permission.

Figure 26 is taken from the article by RA Palmer: 'As it was in the beginning: a history of peritoneal dialysis'. (*Peritoneal Dial Bull* 2: 16, 1982), with permission (Photograph kindly supplied by Dr. D.G. Oreopoulos, Toronto, Can.)

Figures 27, 28 and 29 were kindly supplied by Dr. Alain Slingeneyer from Montpellier, France.

Figure 30 is reproduced from the editorial by Dr. B.G. Delano in the ASAIO Transactions 32 (1): 1, 1987 (100), with permission.

REFERENCES

1. Earle DP: An eighteenth century suggestion for peritoneal dialysis? *Int J Artif Organs* 3: 67, 1980
2. Warrick Ch: An improvement on the practice of tapping; by which that operation instead of a relief for symptoms, becomes an absolute cure for an ascites. *Philos Trans R Soc Lond* (Biol) 43: 5, 1744–1745
3. Hales S: A method of conveying liquors into the abdomen during the operation of tapping. *Philos Trans R Soc Lond* (Biol) 43: 8, 1744–1745

4. Wegner G: Chirurgische Bermerkungen über die Peritoneal-höhle mit besonderer Berücksichtigung der Ovariotomie (Surgical considerations regarding the peritoneal cavity with special attention to ovariotomy). *Langenbecks Arch Chir* 20: 51, 1877 (in German)

5. Starling EH, Tubby EH: On absorption from and secretion into the serous cavities. *J Physiol* (*Lond*) 16: 140, 1894

6. Leathes JB, Starling EH: On the absorption of salt solutions from the pleural cavities. *J Physiol* (*Lond*) 18: 106, 1895

7. Orlow WN: Einige Versuche über die Resorption in der Bauchhöhle (Some experiments on the resorption in the peritoneal cavity). *Pflügers Arch* 59: 170, 1895 (in German)

8. Clark AJ: Absorption from the peritoneal cavity. *J Pharmacol Exp Ther* 16: 415, 1921

9. Cunningham RS: Studies on absorption from serous cavities. *Am J Physiol* 53: 488, 1920

10. Klapp R: Über Bauchfellresorption (On resorption by the peritoneum). *Mitt Grenzgeb Med Chir* 10: 254, 1902 (in German)

11. Clairmont P, von Haberer H: Experimentelle Untersuchungen zur Physiologie und Pathologie des Peritoneums (Experimental investigations on the physiology and pathology of the peritoneum). *Langebecks Arch Chir* 76: 1, 1905 (in German)

12. Putnam T: The living peritoneum as a dialyzing membrane. *Am J Physiol* 63: 548, 1922–1923

13. Hertzler AE: *The Peritoneum Structure and Function in Relation to Principles of Abdominal Surgery*. St Louis, MO, CV Mosby Company, 1919, vol I, p 379

14. Schechter AJ, Cary MK, Carpentieri AL, Darrow DC: Changes in composition of fluids injected into the peritoneal cavity. *Am J Dis Child* 46: 1015, 1933

15. Graham T: Liquid diffusion applied to analysis. *Philos Trans R Soc Lond* (Biol) 151: 183, 1861

16. Prima C: Über die Resorptionsfähigkeit des Bauchfells bei gesteigerten Darmperistaltik (On the resorption activity of the peritoneum during increased intestinal peristalsis). *Mitt Grenzgeb Med Chir* 36: 678, 1923 (in German)

17. Fleisher MS, Loeb L: Studies in edema II. The influence of adrenalin on absorption from the peritoneal cavity, with remarks on the influence of calcium chloride on absorption. *J Exp Med* 12: 288, 1910

18. Fleischer MS, Loeb L: Studies in edema VII. The influence of nephrectomy and other surgical operations and of the lesions produced by uranium-nitrate upon resorption from the peritoneal cavity. *J Exp Med* 12: 487, 1910

19. Fleischer MS, Loeb L: Studies in edema VIII. The influence of caffeine on absorption from the peritoneal cavity and the influence of diuresis on edema. *J Exp Med* 12: 510, 1910

20. Boen ST: *Peritoneal dialysis. A clinical Study of Factors Governing its Effectiveness*. MD Thesis 1959 Univ of Amsterdam, Assen, van Gorcum and Comp NV – Dr. HJ Prakke and HMG Prakke

21. Boen ST: *Peritoneal Dialysis in Clinical Medicine*. American Lecture series, Springfield, IL, Charles C Thomas, 1964

22. Odel HM, Ferris DO, Power MH: Clinical considerations of the problem of extrarenal excretion: peritoneal lavage. *Med Clin North Am* 32: 989, 1948

23. Blackfan KD, Maxcy KF: The intraperitoneal injection of saline solution. *Am J Dis Child* 2: 1257, 1918

24. Ganter G: Über die Beseitigung giftiger Stoffe aus dem Blute durch Dialyse (On the elimination of toxic substances from the blood by dialysis). *Munch Med Wochenschr* 70: 1478, 1923 (in German)

25. Necheles H: Über dialysieren des strömenden Blutes am Le-benden (On dialysis of the circulating blood in vivo). *Klin Wochenschr* 2: 1257, 1923 (in German)

26. Necheles H: Erwiderung zu vorstehender Bermerkung (Commentary on the above remark) *Klin Wochenschr* 2: 1888, 1923 (in German)

27. Haas G: Dialysieren des strömenden Blutes am Lebenden (Dialysing the circulating blood). *Klin Wochenschr* 4: 13, 1925 (in German)

28. Heusser H, Werder H: Untersuchungen über die Peritoneal-dialyse (Investigations on peritoneal dialysis). *Brun's Beitr Klin Chir* 141: 38, 1927 (in German)

29. Balazs J, Rosenak S: Zur behandlung der Sublimatanurie durch peritoneale Dialyse (On the treatment of anuria caused by mercury bichloride with peritoneal dialysis), *Wien Klin Wochenschr* 47: 851, 1934 (in German)

30. Wear JB, Sisk IR, Trinkle AJ: Peritoneal lavage in the treatment of uremia. *J Urol* 39: 53, 1938

31. Rhoads JE: Peritoneal lavage in the treatment of renal insufficiency. *Am J Med Sci* 196: 642, 1938

32. Fine J, Frank HA, Seligman AM: The treatment of acute renal failure by peritoneal irrigation. *Ann Surg* 124: 857, 1946

33. Frank HA, Seligman AM, Fine J: Treatment of uremia after acute renal failure by peritoneal irrigation. *JAMA* 130: 703, 1946

34. Seligman AM, Frank HA, Fine J: Treatment of experimental uremia by peritoneal irrigation. *J Clin Invest* 25: 211, 1946

35. Fine J, Frank HA, Seligman AM: Further experiences with peritoneal irrigation for acute renal failure. *Ann Surg* 128: 561, 1948

36. Muehrcke RC: *Acute Renal Failure*, St Louis, MO, The CV Mosby Company, 1969, p 274

37. Kop PSM: *Peritoneaal Dialyse* (Peritoneal Dialysis). MD Thesis Groningen, Kampen (The Netherlands), JH Kok NV, 1948 (in Dutch, with summaries in English, French and German)

38. Reid R, Penfold JB, Jones RN: Anuria treated by renal decapsulation and peritoneal dialysis. *Lancet* 2: 749, 1946

39. Doolan PD, Murphy WP, Wiggins RA, Carter NW, Cooper WC, Watten RH, Alpen EL: An evaluation of intermittent peritoneal lavage. *Am J Med* 26: 831, 1959

40. Maxwell MH, Rockney RE, Kleeman CR, Twiss MR: Peritoneal dialysis. *JAMA* 170: 917, 1959

41. Moriarty MV, Parsons FM: Intermittent peritoneal dialysis. *Proc Eur Dial Transplant Assoc* 3: 359, 1966

42. Nolph KD, Hano JE, Teschan PE: Peritoneal sodium transport during hypertonic peritoneal dialysis: physiologic mechanism and clinical implications. *Ann Intern Med* 75: 253, 1971

43. Ahearn DJ, Nolph KD: Controlled sodium removal with peritoneal dialysis. *Trans Am Soc Artif Intern Organs* 18: 423, 1972

44. Nolph KD: Peritoneal dialysis: In *Replacement of Renal Function by Dialysis*, edited by Drukker W, Parsons FM, Maher JF, 1st edition, The Hague, Boston, London, Martinus Nijhoff, Medical Division, 1978, p 285

45. Rosenak S, Siwon P: Experimentelle Untersuchungen über die peritoneal Ausscheidung harnpflichtiger Substanzen aus dem Blut (Experimental investigations on peritoneal excretion of uraemic products from the blood). *Mitt Grenzgeb Med Chir* 39: 391, 1925 (in German)

46. Grollman A, Turner LB, McLean JA: Intermittent peritoneal lavage in nephrectomized dogs and its application to the human being. *Arch Int Med* 87: 379, 1951

47. Grollman A: *Acute Renal Failure*. Springfield, IL, Charles C. Thomas, 1954

48. Blumenkrantz MJ, Roberts M: Progress in peritoneal dialysis: a historical prospective. *Contrib Nephrol* 17: 101, 1979

49. Rosenak SS, Oppenheimer GD: An improved drain for peritoneal lavage, *Surgery* 23: 832, 1948

50. Weston RE, Roberts M: Clinical use of stylet catheter for peritoneal dialysis. *Arch Int Med* 15: 659, 1965

51. Boen ST, Mulinari AS, Dillard DH, Scribner BH: Periodic peritoneal dialysis in the management of chronic uremia. *Trans Am Soc Artif Intern Organs* 8: 256, 1962

52. Bosch E, De Vries LA, Boen ST: A simplified automatic peritoneal dialysis system. *Proc Eur Dial Transplant Assoc* 3: 362, 1966

53. Boen ST, Mion CM, Curtis FK, Shilipetar G: Periodic peritoneal dialysis using repeated puncture technique and an automatic cycling machine. *Trans Am Soc Artif Intern Organs* 10: 409, 1964

54. Tenckhoff H, Boen ST: Long term peritoneal dialysis in the home, the first one and one half years. *Proc Eur Dial Transplant Assoc* 2: 104, 1965

55. Tenckhoff H, Ward G, Boen ST: The influence of dialysate volume and flow rate on peritoneal clearance. *Proc Eur Dial Transplant Assoc* 2: 113, 1965

56. Gross M, McDonald HP Jr: Effects of dialysate temperature and flow rate on peritoneal clearance. *JAMA* 202: 215, 1967

57. Nolph KD, Stoltz ML, Maher JF: Altered peritoneal permeability in patients with systemic vasculitis. *Ann Intern Med* 75: 753, 1971

58. Henderson LW: Peritoneal dialysis. In *Clinical Aspects of Uremia and Dialysis* (chapter 19), edited by Massry SG, Sellers AL, Springfield, IL, Charles C Thomas, 1976, p 561

59. Scribner BH: Discussion. *Trans Am Soc Artif Intern Organs* 15: 87, 1965

60. Babb AL, Johansen PJ, Strand MJ, Tenckhoff H, Scribner BH: Bi-directional permeability of the human peritoneum to middle molecules. *Proc Eur Dial Transplant Assoc* 10: 247, 1973

61. Nolph KD: Peritoneal anatomy and transport physiology. in *Replacement of Renal Function by Dialysis*, edited by Drukker W, Parsons FM, Maher JF, 2nd edition, Dordrecht (the Netherlands), Boston, MA, Lancaster, UK, Martinus Nijhoff, Publishers, 1983, p 491

62. Hirszel P, Maher JF, Chakrabarti E, Bennett RR: Maximal peritoneal pore size determined by dextran transport. in *Frontiers in Peritoneal Dialysis* edited by Maher JF and Winchester JF, New York, Field, Rich and Assoc, 1986, p 37

63. Boesken WH, Schuppe HC, Seidler A, Schollmeyer P: Peritoneal membrane permeability for high and low molecular proteins (H/LMWP) in CAPD. in *Frontiers in Peritoneal Dialysis* edited by Maher JF and Winchester JF, New York, Field, Rich and Assoc, 1986, p 47

64. Scribner BH, Buri R, Caner JEZ, Hegstrom R, Burnell JM: The treatment of chronic uremia by means of intermittent dialysis. *Trans Am Soc Artif Intern Organs* 6: 114, 1960

65. Merrill JP, Sabbaga E, Welzant W, Crane C: The use of an indwelling plastic conduit for chronic peritoneal irrigation. *Trans Am Soc Artif Intern Organs* 8: 252, 1962

66. Boen ST, Curtis FK, Tenckhoff H, Scribner BH: Chronic hemodialysis and peritoneal dialysis. *Proc Eur Dial Transplant Assoc* 1: 221, 1964

67. Tenckhoff H, Shilipetar G, Boen ST: One year's experience with home peritoneal dialysis. *Trans Am Soc Artif Intern Organs* 11: 11, 1965

68. McDonald HP Jr: A peritoneal dialysis trocar. *J Urol* 89: 946, 1963

69. Bull GM, Joekes AM, Lowe KG: Conservative treatment of anuric uraemia. *Lancet* 2: 229, 1949

70. Borst JCG: Protein katabolism in uraemia. *Lancet* 1: 824, 1948

71. Teschan PE, Baxter MD, O'Brien TF, Freyhof JN, Hall WH: Prophylactic hemodialysis in the treatment of acute renal failure. *Ann Intern Med* 53: 992, 1960

72. Leading article (anonymous): Intermittent peritoneal lavage. *Lancet* 2: 551, 1959

73. Mowbray JF: Peritoneal dialysis for pre- and postoperative management in a cadaveric transplantation program. *Trans Am Soc Artif Intern Organs* 13: 46, 1967

74. Matthews DE: Beyond survival. *Dial Transplant* 9: 657, 1980

75. Barry KG, Shambaugh GE, Goler D: A new flexible cannula and seal to provide prolonged access for peritoneal drainage and other procedures. *J Urol* 90: 125, 1963

76. Malette WG, MacPaul JJ, Bledsoe F, MacIntosh DA, Koegel E: A clinical successful subcutaneous peritoneal access button for repeated peritoneal dialysis. *Trans Am Soc Artif Intern Organs* 10: 396, 1964

77. Jacob GB, Deane N: Repeated peritoneal dialysis by the catheter replacement method: description of technique and a replaceable prosthesis for chronic access to the peritoneal cavity. *Proc Eur Dial Transplant Assoc* 4: 136, 1967

78. Gutch CF: Peritoneal dialysis. *Trans Am Soc Artif Intern Organs* 10: 406, 1964

79. Gutch CF, Stevens SC: Silastic catheter for peritoneal dialysis. *Trans Am Soc Artif Intern Organs* 12: 106, 1966

80. Palmer RA, Quinton WE, Gray JE: Prolonged peritoneal dialysis for chronic renal failure. *Lancet* 1: 700, 1964

81. McDonald HP Jr, Gerber N, Mischra D, Wolm L, Peng B, Waterhouse K: Subcutaneous Dacron and Teflon cloth adjuncts for Silastic arteriovenous shunts and peritoneal dialysis catheters. *Trans Am Soc Artif Intern Organs* 15: 176, 1968

82. Tenckhoff H, Schechter H: A bacteriologically safe peritoneal access device. *Trans Am Soc Artif Intern Organs* 14: 181, 1968

83. Gahl GM, Kessel M: The indwelling stylet catheter for peritoneal dialysis. *Clin Nephrol* 6: 414, 1976

84. Lewkonia RM: Simple indwelling cannula for repeated peritoneal dialysis. *Lancet* 2: 134, 1970

85. Heal MR, England AG, Goldstein HJ: Four years experience with indwelling silastic cannulae for long-term peritoneal dialysis. *Br Med J* 4: 596, 1973

86. Goldberg EM, Hill W: A new peritoneal access prosthesis. *Proc Clin Dial Transplant Forum* 3: 122, 1973

87. Stephen RL, Atkin-Thor E, Kolff WJ: Recirculation peritoneal dialysis with subcutaneous catheter. *Trans Am Soc Artif Intern Organs* 22: 575, 1976

88. Oreopoulos DG, Izatt S, Zellerman G, Karanicolas S, Matheus RE: A prospective study of the effectiveness of three permanent peritoneal catheters. *Proc Clin Dial Transplant Forum* 4: 96, 1976

89. Khanna R, Izatt S, Burke D, Matheus R, Vas S, Oreopoulos DG: Experience with the Toronto Western Hospital permanent peritoneal catheter. *Peritoneal Dial Bull* 4: 95, 1984

90. Valli A, Crescimanno U, Midiri O, Arw K, Riegla P, Huber W, Cabassa N: 18 months experience with a new (Valli) catheter for peritoneal dialysis. *Peritoneal Dial Bull* 3: 22, 1983

91. Ash SR, Johnson H, Hartman J, Granger J, Koshuta J, Sell L, Dhein Ch, Blevins W, Thornhill JA: The column disc peritoneal catheter: a peritoneal access device with improved drainage. *asaio J* 3: 109, 1980

92. Flanigan MJ, Ngheim DD, Schulak JA, Ullrich GE, Freeman

RM: The use and complications of three peritoneal catheters designs. A retrospective analysis. *ASAIO Transactions* 32(1): 33, 1987

93. Lasker N, McCauley EP, Passarotte CT: Chronic peritoneal dialysis. *Trans Am Soc Artif Int Organs* 12: 94, 1966

94. Jarrel B, Lasker N, Roberts M: A simple system of automated peritoneal dialysis. *Dial Transplant* 3(2): 36, 1974

95. McDonald H Jr: An automatic peritoneal dialysis machine: preliminary report. *Trans Am Soc Artif Intern Organs* 11: 83, 1965

96. Vercellone A, Piccoli G, Cavalli PL, Ragni R, Alloatte S: A new automatic peritoneal dialysis system. *Proc Eur Dial Transplant Assoc* 5: 344, 1968

97. Tenckhoff H, Shilipetar G, van Paasschen WH, Swanson E: A home peritoneal dialysate delivery system. *Trans Am Soc Intern Artif Organs* 15: 103, 1969

98. Tenckhoff H, Meston B, Shilipetar G: A simplified automatic peritoneal dialysis system. *Trans Am Soc Artif Intern Organs* 18: 436, 1972

99. Blagg CR: Peritoneal dialysis and the Medicare ESRD program. *Dial Transplant* 8: 1081, 1979

100. Delano BG: The failure of home hemodialysis (editorial). *ASAIO Transactions* 32(1): 1, 1987

101. Barbour GL: The kinetics of peritoneal dialysis. *Dial Transplant* 8: 1055, 1979

102. Nolph KD, Popovich RP, Ghods AJ, Twardowski Z: Determinants of low clearances of small solutes during peritoneal dialysis. *Kidney Int* 13: 117, 1978

103. Gutman RA: Toward enhancement of peritoneal clearance. *Dial Transplant* 8: 1072, 1979

104. Boen ST: Kinetics of peritoneal dialysis. *Medicine* 40: 243, 1961

105. Robson M, Oreopoulos DG, Izatt S, Ogilvie R, Rapoport A, DeVeber GA: Influence of exchange volume and dialysate flow rate on solute clearance in peritoneal dialysis. *Kidney Int* 14: 486, 1978

106. Giordano C: Studies on peritoneal dialysis. *Dial Transplant* 7: 828, 1978

107. Henderson L: Peritoneal ultrafiltration dialysis. Enhanced urea transfer using hypertonic peritoneal dialysis fluid. *J Clin Invest* 45: 950, 1964

108. Henderson L, Nolph KD: Altered permeability of the peritoneal membrane after using hypertonic peritoneal dialysis fluid. *J Clin Invest* 48: 992, 1969

109. Zelman A, Gisser D, Whittam PJ, Parsons RH, Schuyler R: Augmentation of peritoneal dialysis efficiency with programmed hyper/hypo-osmotic dialysates. *Trans Am Soc Artif Intern Organs* 23: 203, 1977

110. Hazel HG, Valtin H, Gosselin RE: Effects of drugs on peritoneal dialysis in the dog. *J Pharmacol Exp Ther* 145: 122, 1964

111. Henderson LW, Kintzel JE: Influence of antidiuretic hormone on peritoneal membrane area and permeability. *J Clin Invest* 50: 2437, 1971

112. Nolph KD, Ghods AJ, van Stone JC, Brown P: Effect of intraperitoneal vasodilators on peritoneal clearances. *Proc 9th Annu Contractors Conf Artif Kidney-Chronic Uremia Program of NIAMDD* edited by Mackey BB, DHEW publ no (NIH) 77, 1167: 118, 1976

113. Nolph KD, Ghods AJ, van Stone J, Brown PA: The effects of intraperitoneal vasodilators on peritoneal clearances. *Trans Am Soc Artif Intern Organs* 22: 586, 1976

114. Maher JF, Hirszel P, Abraham JE, Galen MA, Chamberlin M, Hohnadel DC: The effect of dipyrimadole on peritoneal transport. *Trans Am Soc Artif Intern Organs* 23: 219, 1977

115. Maher JF, Hohnadel DC, Shea CD, Sanzo F, Cassetta M: Effect of intraperitoneal diuretics on solute transport during hypertonic dialysis. *Clin Nephrol* 7: 96, 1977

116. Hirszel P, Maher JF, LeGrow W: Increased peritoneal mass transport with glucagon acting at the vascular surface. *Trans Am Soc Artif Intern Organs* 24: 136, 1978

117. Maher JF, Hirszel P, Lasrich M: Modulation of peritoneal transport rates by prostaglandins. *Adv Prostaglandin Thromboxane Res* 7: 695, 1980

118. Maher JF: Peritoneal transport rates: mechanisms, limitations, and methods for augmentation. *Kidney Int* 18, (Suppl 10): S 117, 1980

119. Raja RM, Kramer SM, Rosenbaum JL: Enhanced clearance with intraperitoneal nitroprusside in high flow recirculation peritoneal dialysis. *Trans Am Soc Artif Intern Organs* 24: 133, 1978

120. Hirszel P, Lasrich M, Maher JF: Augmentation of peritoneal mass transport by dopamine. Comparison with norephinephrine and evaluation of pharmacologic mechanism. *J Lab Clin Med* 94: 747, 1979

121. Maher JF, Hirszel P: Augmentation of peritoneal clearances by drugs. in *Continuous Ambulatory Peritoneal Dialysis*, edited by Legrain M, Amsterdam, Oxford, Princeton, Excerpta Medica, Amsterdam, 1980, p 42

122. Shinaberger J, Shear L, Barry KG: Increasing efficiency of peritoneal dialysis: experience with peritoneal-extracorporeal recirculation dialysis. *Trans Am Soc Artif Intern Organs* 11: 76, 1965

123. Lange K, Freser G, Mangalat J: Automatic continuous high flow rate peritoneal dialysis. *Arch Klin Med* 214: 201, 1968

124. Stephen RL: Reciprocating peritoneal dialysis with a subcutaneous peritoneal catheter. *Dial Transplant* 7: 834, 1978

125. Di Paolo N: Semicontinuous peritoneal dialysis. *Dial Transplant* 7: 839, 1978

126. Kablitz C, Stephen RL, Duffy DP, Jacobsen SC, Zelman A, Kolff WJ: Technological augmentation of peritoneal urea clearance, Past, present, future. *Dial Transplant* 9: 741, 1980

127. Gordon A, Greenbaum M, Maxwell MH: Sorbent regeneration of peritoneal dialysate. *Trans Am Soc Artif Intern Organs* 20A: 130, 1974

128. Blumenkrantz MJ, Lewin AJ, Gordon A, Roberts M, Pecker EA, Coburn JW, Maxwell MH: Development of a sorbent peritoneal dialysate regeneration system – a progress report. *Proc Eur Dial Transplant Assoc* 15: 213, 1978

129. Lai F, Scott R, Tankersley R, Wayt H, Green L, Rhodes R, Zelman A: Third generation artificial kidney. *Trans Am Soc Artif Intern Organs* 21: 346, 1975

130. Lewin AJ: Sorbent based regenerative peritoneal dialysis system. *Dial Transplant* 7: 831, 1978

131. Eisinger AJ: A simple method of lessening the incidence of peritonitis in peritoneal dialysis using a photochemical reactor. *Clin Nephrol* 14: 42, 1980

132. Diaz Buxo JA: Introduction: Peritoneal dialysis 1979. *Dial Transplant* 8: 1054, 1979

133. Popovich RP, Moncrief JW, Decherd JB, Bomar JB, Pyle WK: The definition of a novel portable/wearable equilibrium peritoneal dialysis technique. *Abstracts Trans Am Soc Artif Intern Organs* 5: 64, 1976

134. Popovich RP, Moncrief JW, Nolph KD, Ghods AJ, Twardowski ZJ, Pyle WK: Continuous ambulatory peritoneal dialysis. *Ann Intern Med* 88: 449, 1978

135. Leading article (anonymous): Chronic ambulatory peritoneal dialysis. *Br Med J* 2: 229, 1979

136. Thomson NM, Walker RG, Whiteside C, Scott DF, Atkins

RC: Continuous ambulatory dialysis (CAPD) in the treatment of end stage renal failure. *Proc Eur Dial Transplant Assoc* 16: 171, 1979

137. Moncrief JW, Nolph KD, Rubin J, Popovich RP: Additional experience with continuous ambulatory peritoneal dialysis (CAPD). *Trans Am Soc Artif Intern Organs* 24: 476, 1978

138. Oreopoulos DG, Robson M, Izatt S, Clayton S, DeVeber GA: A simple and safe technique for continuous ambulatory peritoneal dialysis (CAPD). *Trans Am Soc Artif Intern Organs* 24: 482, 1978

139. Moncrief JW: Continuous ambulatory peritoneal dialysis. *Dial Transplant* 7: 809, 1978

140. Robson MD, Oreopoulous DG: Continuous ambulatory peritoneal dialysis. A revolution in the treatment of chronic renal failure. *Dial Transplant* 7: 999, 1978

141. Khanna R, Oreopoulos DG, Dombros N, Vas S, Williams P, Meema HE, Husdan H, Ogilvie R, Zellerman G, Roncari DAK, Clayton S, Izatt S: Continuous ambulatory peritoneal dialysis (CAPD) after three years: still a promising treatment. *Peritoneal Dialysis Bull* (Publ Toronto Western Hosp, Can) 1: 24, 1981

142. Gokal R, McHugh M, Fryer R, Ward MK, Kerr DNS: Continuous ambulatory peritoneal dialysis: one year's experience in a UK dialysis unit. *Br Med J* 281: 474, 1980

143. Chan MK, Chuah P, Raftery MJ, Baillod RA, Sweny P, Varghese Z, Moorhead JF: Three years' experience of continuous peritoneal dialysis. *Lancet* 1: 1409, 1981

144. Oreopoulos DG: The coming of age of continuous ambulatory peritoneal dialysis (CAPD). *Dial Transplant* 8: 460, 1979

145. Moncrief JW: Continuous ambulatory peritoneal dialysis. *Dial Transplant* 8: 1077, 1979

146. Diaz-Buxo JA, Walker PJ, Farmer CD, Chandler JT, Holt KL: Continuous cyclic peritoneal dialysis (CCPD). *Kidney Int* (Abstract) 19: 145, 1981

147. Diaz-Buxo JA, Farmer CD, Walker PJ, Chandler JT, Holt KL: Continuous cyclic peritoneal dialysis: a preliminary report. *Artif Organs* 5: 157, 1981

148. Adams FF, Brunt JR, Pucker CT, Williams AV: Automated long cycle peritoneal dialysis (ALCPD). *Kidney Int* (Abstract) 19: 144, 1981

149. Anonymous: CAPD for chronic renal failure. *Lancet* 2: 1172, 1980

150. Anonymous: Renal failure – who cares? *Lancet* 1: 1011, 1982

151. Charytan C, Spinowitz BS, Galler M: A comparative study of CAPD and center haemodialysis. *Arch Intern Med* 146: 1138, 1986

152. Bulgin RH: Comparative costs of various dialysis treatments. *Peritoneal Dial Bull* 1: 88, 1981

153. Diaz-Buxo JA, Walker PJ, Farmer CD, Chandler JT, Holt KL, Cox P: Continuous cyclic peritoneal dialysis. *Trans Am Soc Artif Intern Organs* 27: 51, 1981

154. Oreopoulos DG, Vas SI, Khanna R: Prevention of peritonitis during continuous ambulatory peritoneal dialysis. *Peritoneal Dial Bull* 3 (Suppl 3): S 18, 1983

155. Mion ChM. Practical use of peritoneal dialysis. in *Replacement of Renal Function by Dialysis*, edited by Drukker W, Parsons FM, Maher JF, 2nd edition Boston, The Hague, Dordrecht, Lancaster UK: Martinus Nijhoff, 1983, p 457

156. Drukker W: CAPD and the peritonitis problem. Can it be overcome? *Dial Transplant Int* 13: 570A, 1984

157. Twardowski ZJ, Nolph KD: USA CAPD Registry with special emphasis on diabetes mellitus. in *Continuous Ambulatory Peritoneal Dialysis (Proc of the fourth Benelux Symposium, November 1984, edited by Weimar W, Fieren MWJA, Dider-*

ich PPNM, op de Hoek CT, 1984 p 41 (obtainable from last editor, Diatel Rijnmond, 1a Meeuwensingel, 2903 TA Capelle a/d IJssel, the Netherlands

158. Slingeneyer A, Liendo-Liendo C, Mion C: Continuous ambulatory peritoneal dialysis with a bacteriological filter on the dialysate infusion line. in *Continuous Ambulatory Peritoneal Dialysis. Proc Int Symp Paris*, edited by M Legrain, Amsterdam, Oxford, Princeton: Excerpta Medica, 1979, p 59

159. Mion C, Slingeneyer A, Liendo-Liendo C, Perez C, Despaux E: Reduction in incidence of peritonitis (P) associated with continuous ambulatory peritoneal dialysis (CAPD). *Proc Clin Dial Transplant Forum* 9: 9, 1979

160. Gokal R, Ramos JM, Francis DMA, Ferner DE, Goodship TH, Proud G, Bint AJ, Ward MK, Kerr DNS: Peritonitis in continuous ambulatory peritoneal dialysis. *Lancet* 2: 1388, 1982

161. Anonymous: Ambulatory peritonitis. *Lancet* 1: 1104, 1982 (editorial)

162. Bint AJ, Finch RG, Gokal R, Goldsmith HJ, Junor B, Oliver D: Diagnosis and management of peritonitis in continuous ambulatory peritoneal dialysis (Report of a working party of the British Society for Antimicrobial Chemotherapy). *Lancet* 1: 845, 1987

163. Parsons FM, Ahmed-Jushuf IH, Brownjohn AM, Coltman SJ, Gibson J, Young GA, Young JB: Preventing CAPD peritonitis. *Lancet* 2: 907, 1983

164. Parsons FM, Brownjohn AM, Turney JH, Young GA, Young JB, Ahmed-Jushuf IH, Gibson J, Coltman S: Profound reduction in peritonitis in CAPD using Travenol system IIR connectors and betadine. in *Frontiers in Peritoneal Dialysis*, edited by Maher JF, Winchester JF, New York, Field, Rich and Assoc, 1986, p 183

165. Smith C: CAPD: one cuff vs two cuff catheters in reference to incidence of infection. in *Frontiers in Peritoneal Dialysis*, edited by Maher JF, Winchester JF, New York, NY, Field, Rich and Assoc, 1986, p 181

166. Ota K, Mineshima M, Watanabe N, Naganuma S: Functional deterioration of the peritoneum. Does it occur in the absence of peritonitis? *Nephrol Dial Transplant* 1987, 2: 30

167. Nolph KD, Cutler SJ, Steinberg SM, Novak JW: Continuous ambulatory peritoneal dialysis in the United States. A three year study. *Kidney Int* 28: 198, 1985

168. Buoncristiani U, Cozzari M, Carobi C, Quintaliani G, Barbarossa D, Di Paolo N: Semicontinuous semi-ambulatory peritoneal dialysis. *Proc Eur Dial Transplant Assoc* 17: 328, 1979

169. Buoncristiani U, Cozzari M, Quintaliani G, Carobi C: Abatement of exogenous peritonitis risk using the Perugia CAPD system. *Dial Transplant* 12: 14, 1983

170. Maiorca R, Cancarini GC, Broccoli R, Brasa S, Cantaluppi A, Scalamogna A, Graziani G, Ponticelli C: Prospective controlled trial of a Y connector and disinfectant to prevent peritonitis in continuous ambulatory peritoneal dialysis. *Lancet* 2: 642, 1983

171. Maiorca R, Cantaluppi A, Cancarini GC, Scalamogna A, Strada A, Graziani G, Brasa S, Ponticelli C: 'Y' connector system for prevention of peritonitis in CAPD: a controlled study. *Proc Eur Dial Transplant Assoc* 20: 223, 1983

172. Hamilton RW, Disher BA, Dillingham GA, Nicholas AF: The sterile weld: a new method for connection in continuous ambulatory peritoneal dialysis. *Peritoneal Dial Bull* 3 (Suppl 4): S8, 1983

173. Gokal R, Ramos JM, Francis DMA, Ferner RE, Goodship THJ, Proud G, Bint AJ, Ward MK, Kerr DNS: Peritonitis in continuous ambulatory peritoneal dialysis. *Lancet* 2: 1388, 1982

174. Slingeneyer A, Mion C: Peritonitis prevention in continuous ambulatory peritoneal dialysis: long-term efficacy of a bacteriological filter. *Proc Eur Dial Transplant Assoc* 19: 388, 1982

175. Slingeneyer A, Mion C: Peritonitis (PE) prevention in CAPD: long-term efficacy of a bacteriological filter. *Abstracts Eur Dial Transplant Assoc* p 134, 1982

176. Sarles HE, Lindley JD, Fish JC, Biggers JA, Cottom DL, Cotton JE, Mader JT, Dunaway JF, Remmers AR Jr: Peritoneal dialysis utilizing a Millipore filter. *Kidney Int* 9: 54, 1976

177. Ash SR, Horswell Jr R, Heeter EM, Bloch R: Effect of the Peridex filter on peritonitis rates in a CAPD population. *Peritoneal Dial Bull* 3: 89, 1983

178. Shaldon S: Discussion remark at a round table discussion. In *Continuous Ambulatory Peritoneal Dialysis. Proc Int Symp Paris*, edited by Legrain M. Amsterdam, Oxford , Princeton, Excerpta Medica 1979, p 91

179. Buoncristiani U, Carobi C, Cozzari M, Di Paolo N: Clinical application of a miniaturized variant of the Perugia CAPD connection system. *Peritoneal Dial Bull* 4 (Suppl): 59, 1984

180. Cantaluppi A, Scalamogna A, Guerra L, Castelnovo C, Graziani G, Ponticelli C: Peritonitis prevention in CAPD: efficacy of a Y-connector and disinfectant. *Peritoneal Dial Bull* 4 (Suppl): S10, 1984

181. Verger C, Brunschvicq O, Le Charpentier Y, Lavergne A: Structural and ultrastructural peritoneal membrane changes and permeability alterations during continuous ambulatory peritoneal dialysis. *Proc Eur Dial Transplant Assoc* 18: 199, 1981

182. Verger C, Luger A, Moore H, Nolph KD: Acute changes in peritoneal morphology and transport properties with infectious peritonitis and mechanical injury. *Kidney Int* 23: 823, 1983

183. Verger C: Relationship between peritoneal membrane structure and its permeability: clinical complications. in *Advances in Peritoneal Dialysis*, edited by Gahl GM, Kessel M, Nolph KD, Amsterdam, Oxford, UK, Princeton, NJ, Excerpta Medica, 1981, p 87

184. Smeby LC, Wideroe T-E, Svartas TM, Jorstad S: Changes in water removal due to peritonitis during continuous peritoneal dialysis. in *Advances in Peritoneal Dialysis*, edited by Gahl GM, Kessel M, Nolph KD, Amsterdam, Oxford, UK, Princeton, NJ, Excerpta Medica, 1981, p 287

185. Gandhi VC, Ing TS, Jablokow VR, Daugirdas JT, Iwatsuki S, Geis WP, Hano JE: Thickened peritoneal membrane in maintenance peritoneal dialysis patients. *Kidney Int* 14: 675, 1978 (Abstract)

186. Gandhi VC, Humayun MH, Ing TS, Daugirdas JT, Jablokow VR, Swatsuki S, Geis WP, Hano JE: Sclerotic thickening of the peritoneal membrane in maintenance peritoneal dialysis patients. *Arch Intern Med* 140: 1201, 1980

187. Gandhi VC, Ing TS, Daugirdas JT, Hagen C, Blumenkrantz MJ, Jablokow VR: Failure of peritoneal dialysis due to peritoneal sclerosis. *Int J Artif Organs* 6: 97, 1983 (Letter to the Editor)

188. Manos J, Postlethwaite RJ, Mallick NP, Gokal R: Sclerosing encapsulating peritonitis and other complications of CAPD peritonitis. in *Frontiers in Peritoneal Dialysis*, edited by Maher JF, Winchester JF, New York, Field, Rich and Assoc, 1986, p 634

189. McWinnie DL, Bradley JA, Bramwell SP, Hamilton DNH, Macpherson SG, Cram LP, More SAR, Forwell MA, Smith WGJ, Briggs JD, Junor BJR: Sclerosing peritonitis a further complication of CAPD. in *Frontiers in Peritoneal Dialysis*, edited by Maher JF, Winchester JF, New York, Field, Rich and Assoc, 1986, p 838

190. Rottembourg J, Issad B, Langlois P, deGroc F, Legrain M: Sclerosing encapsulating peritonitis during CAPD. Evaluation of potential risk factors. in *Frontiers in Peritoneal Dialysis*, edited by Maher JF, Winchester JF, New York, Field, Rich and Assoc, 1986, p 643

191. Denis J, Paineau J, Potel G, Fontenaille Ch, Guenel J: Continuous ambulatory peritoneal dialysis. *Ann Intern Med* 93: 508, 1980

192. Thomson NM, Atkins RC, Hooke D, Maydom B, Scott DF: Efficacy and clinical experience of continuous ambulatory peritoneal dialysis. Long term clinical experience in Australia. in *Peritoneal Dialysis*, edited by Atkins RC, Thomson NM, Farrell PC, Edinburgh, London, Melbourne, New York, Churchill Livingstone, 1981, p 93

193. Heale WF, Letch KA, Dawborn JK, Evans SM: Longterm complications of peritonitis. in *Peritoneal Dialysis*, edited by Atkins RC, Thomson NM, Farrell PC, Edinburgh, London, Melbourne, New York, Churchill Livingstone, 1981, p 284

194. Grefberg N, Nilsson P, Andréen Th: Sclerosing obstructive peritonitis, beta blockers and continuous ambulatory peritoneal dialysis. *Lancet* 2: 733, 1983

195. Hauglustaine D, Monballyu J, van Meerbeek J, Godeeris P, Lauwerijns J, Michielsen P: Sclerosing obstructive peritonitis, beta blockers and continuous ambulatory peritoneal dialysis. *Lancet* 2: 734, 1983

196. Bradley JA, McWinnie DL, Hamilton DNH, Starnes F, Macpherson SG, Seywright M, Briggs JD, Junor BJR: Sclerosing obstructive peritonitis after continuous ambulatory peritoneal dialysis. *Lancet* 2: 113, 1983

197. Bradley JA, Hamilton DNH, McWinnie DL, Briggs JD, Junor BJR: Sclerosing peritonitis after CAPD. *Lancet* 2: 572, 1983

198. Rottembourg J, Gahl GM, Poignet JL, Mertani E, Strippoli P, Langlois P, Tranbaloc P, Legrain M: Severe abdominal complications in patients undergoing continuous ambulatory peritoneal dialysis. *Proc Eur Dial Transplant Assoc-Eur Ren Assoc* 20: 236, 1983

199. Slingeneyer A, Mion C, Mourad G, Canaud B, Béraud JJ: Progressive sclerosing peritonitis: a late and severe complication of maintenance peritoneal dialysis. *Trans Am Soc Artif Intern Organs* 29: 633, 1983

200. Slingeneyer A: Une complication grave de la dialyse péritonéale: la péritonite progressive encapsulante à propos de six cas (A severe complication of peritoneal dialysis: progressive encapsulating peritonits. Observations in six cases). *A report presented to the Medical Faculty of the University of Montpellier, France* 1983 (in French)

201. Oreopoulos DG, Khanna R, Wu G: Sclerosing obstructive peritonitis after CAPD. *Lancet* 2: 409, 1983

202. Dunea G: ASAIO 1984. *Int J Artif Organs* 7: 169, 1984

203. Drukker W: Sclerosing peritonitis. *Dial Transplant Int* 13: 768A, 1984

204. Oulès R, Fassbinder W, Broyer M, Brunner FP, Brynger H, Challah S, Guillon PJ, Rizzoni G, Selwood NH, Wing AJ: Combined report on regular dialysis and transplantation in Europe XVI, 1985. (Available from Ms Sheila R Dykes, Administrator of the EDTA-ERA Registration Committee, St. Thomas' Hospital, Lambeth Palace Road, London SE1 7EH, UK).

205. Jacob H, Brandt LJ, Farkas P, Frishman W: Beta-adrenergic blockade and the gastrointestinal system. *Am J Med* 74: 1042, 1983

206. Smith B, Butler M: The effects of long-term propranolol on the salivary glands and intestinal serosa of the mouse. *J Pathol* 124: 185, 1974

207. Brown P, Baddeley H, Read AE, Davies JD, McGarry J: Sclerosing peritonitis: an unusual reaction to a beta adrenergic blocking drug (practolol). *Lancet* 2: 1477, 1974

208. Marshall AJ, Baddeley H, Barritt DW, Davies JD, Lee REJ, Low-Beer TS, Read AE: Practolol peritonitis. *Q J Med* 181: 135, 1977

209. Doherty CC, McGeown MG, Donaldson RA: Retroperitoneal fibrosis after treatment with atenolol. *Br Med J* 2: 1786, 1978

210. Harty HF: Sclerosing peritonitis and propranolol. *Arch Intern Med* 138: 1424, 1978

211. Ahmed S: Sclerosing peritonitis and propranolol. *Chest* 79: 361, 1981

212. Thompson J, Julian DG: Retroperitoneal fibrosis associated with metoprolol. *Br Med J* 284: 83, 1982

213. Marigold JH, Pounder RE, Pemberton J, Thompson RPH: Propranolol, oxprenolol and sclerosing peritonitis. *Br Med J* 284: 870, 1982

214. Clark CV, Terris R: Sclerosing peritonitis associated with metoprolol. *Lancet* 1: 937, 1983

215. Maher JF: Pharmacological aspects of renal failure and dialysis. in *Replacement of Renal Function by Dialysis*, 2nd edn, edited by Drukker W, Parsons FM, Maher JF, Boston, The Hague, Dordrecht, Lancaster, Martinus Nijhoff Publishers, 1983, p 773

216. Madsen SN, Søndergaard J: Cyclic nucleotides, practolol and the peritoneum. *Lancet* 1: 1055, 1977

217. Shaldon S, Koch KM, Quellhorst E, Dinarello CA: Hazards of CAPD: Interleukin-1 production. in *Frontiers in Peritoneal Dialysis*, edited by Maher JF, Winchester JF, New York, Field, Rich and Assoc, 1986, p 630

218. Shaldon, Koch KM, Quellhorst E, Dinarello CA: Pathogenesis of sclerosing peritonitis in CAPD. *Trans Am Soc Artif Intern Organs* 30: 193, 1984

219. Mowbray JF: Human cadaveric transplantation: report of twenty cases. *Br Med J* 2: 1387, 1967

220. Babb AL, Farrell PC, Uvelli DA, Scribner BH: Hemodialyzer evaluation by examination of solute molecular spectra. *Trans Am Soc Artif Intern Organs* 18: 98, 1972

221. Diaz Buxo JA, Haas VF: The influence of automated peritoneal dialysis on an established dialysis system. *Dial Transplant* 8: 531, 1979

222. Anonymous: Statistics Health Care Financing Administration, Dept. of Health and Human Services, Washington DC. *Dial Transplant* 15: 544, 1986

223. Brynger H, Brunner FP, Chantler C, Donckerwolcke RA, Jacobs C, Kramer P, Selwood NH, Wing AJ: Combined report on regular dialysis and transplantation X, 1979. *Proc Eur Dial Transplant Assoc* 17: 4, 1980

224. Jacobs C, Broyer M, Brunner FP, Brynger H, Donckerwolcke RA, Kramer P, Selwood NH, Wing AJ, Blake PH: Combined report on regular dialysis and transplantation in Europe, XI, 1980. *Proc Eur Dial Transplant Assoc* 18: 38, 1981

225. Broyer M, Brunner FP, Brynger H, Donckerwolcke RA, Jacobs C, Kramer P, Selwood NH, Wing AJ: Combined report on regular dialysis and transplantation in Europe, XII, 1981. *Proc Eur Dial Transplant Assoc* 19: 4, 1982

226. Brynger H, Challah S, Donckerwolcke RA, Gretz N, Jacobs C, Kramer P, Selwood NH: Combined report on regular dialysis and transplantation in Europe, XIII, 1982. *Proc Eur Dial Transplant Assoc-Eur Renal Assoc* 20: 5, 1983

227. Relman AS: The new medical industrial complex. *N Engl J Med* 303: 963, 1980

228. Shaldon S, Koch KM, Quellhorst E, Lonnemann G, Dinarello ChA: CAPD is a second class treatment. *Contr Nephrol* 44: 163, 1985

229. Drukker W: Peritoneal dialysis: a historical review. in *Replacement of Renal Function by Dialysis*, 2nd edition, edited by Drukker W, Parsons FM, Maher JF, Dordrecht, Boston, Lancaster, Martinus Nijhoff Publishers, 1983, p 434

230. Schmidt RW, Blumenkrantz M: Peritoneal sclerosis. A 'sword of Damocles' for peritoneal dialysis? *Arch Intern Med* 141: 1265, 1981

231. Parsons FM, Ogg C (editors): *Renal Failure – Who cares?* (*Symposium Proceedings*). Lancaster, UK, MTP, Medical and Technical Publ Co Ltd 1982

PERITONEAL ANATOMY AND TRANSPORT PHYSIOLOGY

KARL D. NOLPH

ANATOMY AND HISTOLOGY OF THE PERITONEAL DIALYSIS SYSTEM

The peritoneum and the peritoneal cavity

The peritoneum (Figure 1) is a living membrane that covers visceral organs, forms the visceral mesentery that connects loops of bowel, and reflects over the inner surface of the abdominal wall (1, 2). The peritoneum is continuous and forms a closed sack, which, because the space within contains only small amounts of fluid (probably less than 100 ml), usually is nearly collapsed. In an adult of normal size, the space can be enlarged by instillation of fluid; two or more liters of fluid can be accommodated without causing discomfort. The surface of the membrane is a shiny layer of mesothelial cells, beneath which lie supporting interstitium containing extracellular fluid, connective tissue fibers, blood vessels, and lymphatics. The visceral peritoneum is that part of the membrane that courses over the surface of visceral organs. As visceral peritoneum reflects from loops of bowel to form the visceral mesentery (connecting adjacent loops of

bowel), the interstitium becomes interspersed between adjacent mesothelial layers. The parietal peritoneum is that portion of the membrane that covers the inner surface of the abdominal wall. The total surface area of the peritoneal mesothelium (parietal and visceral) is believed to approximate the surface area of skin, which, in most adults, is 1 to $2\,m^2$ (3).

The parietal peritoneum

The parietal peritoneum represents only a small portion of the total mesothelial surface area and receives its blood supply from the vasculature of the abdominal wall. The exact ratio of parietal to visceral peritoneal surface area is unknown, but the many folds of visceral mesentery obviously represent a larger fraction of the total peritoneal surface area; therefore, parietal peritoneal participation in solute transport during peritoneal dialysis usually is considered to be less than that of visceral peritoneum. Portions of the parietal peritoneum, however, may be more vascular than some of the early avascular sections of mesentery, and the

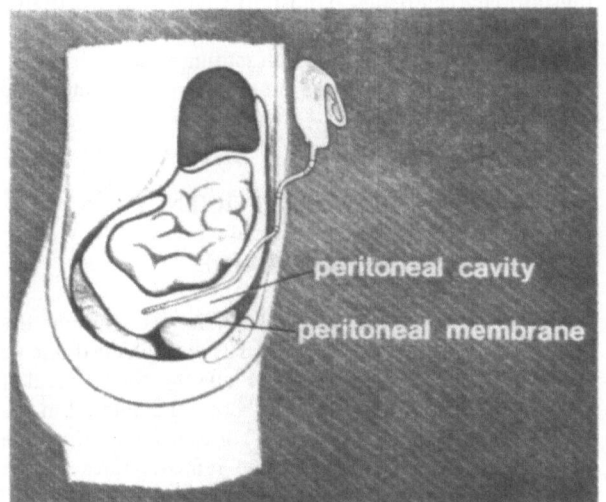

Figure 1. A diagrammatic sketch of the peritoneal cavity and the membrane lining the cavity. A peritoneal catheter is in place.

true fractional contributions of parietal and visceral peritoneum to solute transport during peritoneal dialysis have not yet been determined.

During peritoneal dialysis, solutes moving from capillaries in the parietal peritoneum must traverse capillary endothelial walls, parietal peritoneal interstitium, and the parietal peritoneal mesothelial layer (4, 5). Relative contributions of parietal lymphatics versus capillaries to net transport during peritoneal dialysis are unknown, but it is assumed that blood vessels are a more important source because of the relatively slow flow through lymphatics (4, 5). A very specialized system of lymphatics on the under surface of the diaphragm absorbs fluid and solutes from the peritoneal

cavity; these subdiaphragmatic lymphatics will be discussed in detail in a later section.

The visceral peritoneum

The visceral mesentery contains many relatively large blood vessels on their way to visceral organs. Arteriolar and capillary beds capable of participating in exchange of solutes during peritoneal dialysis are located primarily where mesentery and large blood vessels reflect over loops of bowel and then divide into smaller (less than 10 microns in diameter) arterioles and capillaries on the bowel surface (6). Lymphatics also are plentiful in the visceral mesentery, but their participation in peritoneal dialysis is unknown.

As in the parietal peritoneum, solutes moving from the visceral peritoneal microcirculation into dialysis solution must cross capillary endothelium, interstitium, and mesothelium.

Membrane resistances to solute movement

Pathways for solute movement from peritoneal capillaries into the peritoneal cavity can be subdivided into at least six resistance sites (5): R_1: stagnant fluid films within peritoneal capillaries, R_2: capillary endothelium, R_3: capillary basement membranes, R_4: interstitium, R_5: mesothelium, R_6: stagnant fluid films within the peritoneal cavity. These sites and their hypothesized dimensions are diagrammatically shown in Figure 2.

Anatomy and permeability characteristics of the peritoneum

The exact route taken by solutes traversing the peritoneal cellular layers has not been established. Some reports suggest that solutes up to a molecular mass of 30,000 daltons diffuse across biological membranes, primarily through in-

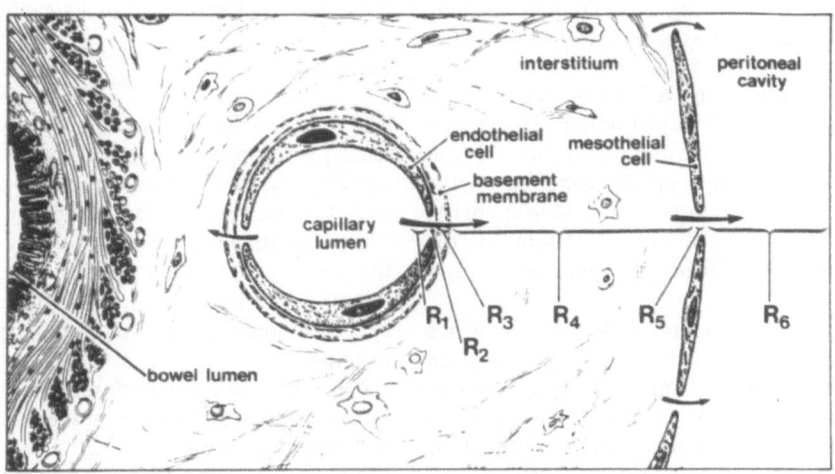

Figure 2. Resistances (R_1–R_6) to solute movement during peritoneal dialysis (see text). (From Nolph et al. [5] with permission of the publisher).

tercellular channels, as indicated in Figure 2 (7, 8). The results of a study of isolated rat mesentery, however, indicate that transcellular movement of some solutes may occur, at least across mesothelium (9). Capillary endothelial cells in the human peritoneum are usually not fenestrated as are glomerular capillaries (10). An analysis of vascular profiles in biopsies of the human peritoneum suggests a 1.7% incidence of fenestrated capillaries (11).

The basement membrane seems to offer little resistance to solute diffusion when molecular mass is less than 30,000 daltons (7, 8). Patients on chronic peritoneal dialysis may develop a multi-layered basal lamina in postcapillary venules and mesothelium of the parietal peritoneum (12). It is not known whether these reduplications of the peritoneal basement membranes affect transport.

Mesothelium appears to be more permeable than endothelium, possibly because of the larger intercellular gaps, between mesothelial cells (13). The permeability of the peritoneal mesothelium apparently is not uniform; it has been suggested that the visceral portion is more permeable than the parietal portion (14).

Recent studies in rabbits have noted very tight intercellular mesothelial cell junctions and numerous intravital plasmic vesicles (15, 16). Following intravenous injection of iron dextran, an electron dense tracer, it was found mainly in vesicles in the peritoneum of the rabbit. Additional work is needed to determine the relative roles of intercellular gaps and vesicles in passive solute transport across the peritoneum. This may vary from species to species in different areas of the peritoneum and for solutes of different molecular weight. It is not clear how peritoneal morphology and solute transport in animals relate to humans, nor how tissue processing may artifactually misrepresent the number of vesicles and/or the dimensions of the intercellular gaps in vivo. Finally, in vivo inflammation such as with peritonitis may widen intercellular gaps misrepresenting the situation under noninfected conditions (17).

In peritonitis, peritoneal clearances, glucose absorption, and protein losses increase (17, 18). In addition to widening of intercellular gaps there is a loss of mesothelial microvilli; there may also be interstital edema, vasodilation and interstital cellular infiltration. Thus, it is impossible to determine whether transport changes result primarily from mesothelial, interstital or vascular alterations. In the rat, heat injury, which morphologically appears confined to the mesothelium, also enhances transport (17). Morphological changes resemble those of peritonitis. This supports the contention that mesothelial integrity may influence peritoneal transport.

It is not known whether mesothelial microvilli influence transport. In mice, these are usually 1.5 to 3.0 μm long and 400 to 900 Å wide (19). Microvilli markedly increase gross surface area. Surface charges may trap water between microvilli and prevent friction of adjacent surfaces (20). At the base of microvilli the open ends of surface vesicles can be seen (21).

Much needs to be learned about the importance of various components of the peritoneal ultrastructure to membrane transport characteristics. Transport changes are associated with diseases or injuries that cause morphological alterations of the microcirculation, interstitum and/or mesothelium. Detailed reviews of this subject have been published (22).

ASSESSMENT OF DIALYSIS EFFICIENCY

Net solute removal rate (mass transfer)

For solutes not present in instilled dialysis solution, the amount removed can be determined by multiplying drainage volume by solute concentration in dialysate. Net removal of solutes can be calculated by subtracting the amount in the instilled dialysis fluid (volume X concentration) from the total amount removed. Net solute removal rates can be expressed as the amount removed between the time dialysis solution is instilled and the time drainage is completed. Such a cycle usually is referred to as one exchange, and the removal rate per exchange or per minute can be expressed in milligrams, milliequivalents, or millimoles. The net removal rate often is referred to as the mass transfer rate.

The net rate of solute diffusion into dialysis solution, however, depends on the concentration gradient from blood to dialysis fluid. The instilled dialysis solution approximates normal diffusible plasma concentrations of electrolytes. Hence, net electrolyte removal (in the absence of ultrafiltration) is small when plasma values are normal. The dialysis fluid concentration of other solutes such as urea and creatinine is zero, and the initial concentration gradient for diffusion depends on the plasma concentration, assuming that peripheral blood reflects concentrations in peritoneal capillary inflow. (The latter may not be so for solutes such as lipids or glucose in the process of being absorbed from gastrointestinal tract or dialysate (23, 24). Because net removal rates of nonelectrolytes depend primarily on blood concentrations, the quantities removed per unit time are not good indices of peritoneal dialysis efficiency.

Clearances

The efficiency index most commonly used (at least by clinicians) is the plasma clearance rate. This is calculated by dividing the amount of solute removed per unit time, the mass transfer rate, by the concentration of solute in plasma. This calculation expresses the volume of plasma cleared of that solute per unit time (usually expressed in milliliters per minute). The clearance term is independent of the solute concentration in plasma water and expresses the efficiency of removal.

Clearance, so calculated, represents the mean clearance rate per exchange. The instantaneous clearance is highest at the beginning of an exchange when the dialysis solution solute concentration is near zero and the diffusion gradient is maximum. The instantaneous clearance approaches zero exponentially as the dialysis solution concentration approaches equilibrium with blood.

The mean clearance rate, though independent of blood solute concentration, is influenced by effective peritoneal membrane area, blood flow rate to the peritoneum, flow rate of dialysis fluid, the physical characteristics of the dialysis solution, the size and number of distribution spaces of the solute, fluid films adjacent to endothelium and mesothelium, and the permeability characteristics of the peritoneal membrane.

Dialysance, instantaneous clearance, and mass transfer coefficient

Estimates of the theoretical instantaneous clearance at the beginning of an exchange have been developed. Such a derivation (often called a dialysance, or a mass transfer coefficient) is thought to be primarily or solely a function of peritoneal diffusive permeability (cm/min) and the effective surface area (cm^2) (25–27). Henderson and Nolph (26) proposed that ratios of dialysance or mass transfer coefficients for different solutes are the same as ratios of respective permeability coefficients when effective membrane pore area is the same for both solutes. For example:

$$\frac{\text{dialysance inulin}}{\text{dialysance urea}} =$$

$$= \frac{\text{Membrane area} \times \text{inulin permeability coefficient}}{\text{Membrane area} \times \text{urea permeability coefficient}}.$$

The use of such terms often incorporates assumptions as to the movement of solutes within body spaces, contributions of convective transport, absence of blood flow limitations on solute movement, and simplifications relative to inflow time and drainage time. These primarily research terms are used to determine more precisely the effective area and permeability characteristics of the peritoneal membrane. Clinically, the mean clearance rate is a direct calculation of what is actually accomplished, is more readily understood, and is more commonly used. The discussion of factors affecting peritoneal dialysis efficiency will deal primarily with their relation to peritoneal clearances.

FACTORS AFFECTING DIALYSIS EFFICIENCY

Flow-rate and other physical characteristics of dialysis solution

Dialysate flow rate

In adults when peritoneal dialysis solution is instilled and drained by gravity rather than by automated equipment, it is customary to use 2.0 l exchanges with an inflow duration of 10 min, a dwell of 30 min, and a drainage period of 20 to 30 min. Thus, dialysate flow rate is a potential limitation on peritoneal dialysis clearance of small highly diffusible solutes. With 1.5% dextrose* dialysis solution (which is usually

slightly hypertonic to azotemic plasma), a typical drainage volume is 2,100 to 2,200 ml per exchange. With a 70 min exchange, this represents an average dialysate turnover rate near 30 ml/min. If a solute equilibrated totally between plasma and dialysate during such an exchange (and even urea does not), the maximum clearance possible would be 30 ml/min. Urea clearance usually is 18 to 20 ml/min with this type of exchange.

Clearances of small solutes can be increased by more rapid exchanges. As dwell time is shortened, however, the portion of exchange time occupied by inflow and drainage increases. During inflow and drainage, there is less volume in the peritoneal cavity, which reduces clearances during those times and so reduces the final average clearance per exchange. Thus, although clearances can be increased by increasing dialysate flow, with the usual manual method a point of diminishing gains is eventually reached. Boen (28, 29), using a 10 min inflow, 5 min dwell time, and 15 min drain cycle, has shown that urea clearance decreases at flow rates above 3.5 l/h. Studies by Penzotti and Mattocks (30) support this finding. Tenckhoff, Ward, and Boen (31), using automated cycling equipment, later showed that urea clearance may increase to over 40 ml/min with dialysate flow rates of 12 l/h. By using automatic peritoneal dialysis equipment to reduce inflow and drainage time, short exchanges may be more efficient. The nursing time required for more rapid exchanges (when performed manually) also is a major limiting factor.

It is possible to achieve higher dialysis solution flow rates without increasing inflow and drainage times by continuous flow through two catheters or a double-lumen catheter (32–37). Clearances of urea may approach 40 ml/min using an 10 l/h dialysate flow (34). Dialysis solution may be utilized single pass (33) or be recycled after passage through an extracorporeal dialysis system (34, 36). A danger limiting this approach is channeling, whereby dialysis solution streams from lumen to lumen. Abdominal pain is common at flow rates above 12 l/h, presumably due to mechanical irritation (34).

Another way to increase the dialysate flow rate is to increase the volume per exchange. Dialysis solutions are marketed primarily in 2 l containers, making this an easy choice for manual methods. Many adults, however, find intraperitoneal volumes exceeding 2 l uncomfortable, and some patients cannot even tolerate 2 l exchanges. Some normal size adults tolerate up to 4 l of intraperitoneal volume without discomfort and such patients have been maintained on continuous ambulatory peritoneal dialysis with 3 l exchanges (38). Clearance increase with 3 l volumes as compared to 2 l volumes at fixed cycle times mainly as a function of the increased dialysis solution flow rate rather than increased fluid membrane contact (39).

Reciprocating peritoneal dialysis (Chapter 22) involves rapid in-and-out cycling of dialysate (100–200 ml, in one min and out the next), with an intraperitoneal residual dialysate reservoir of usually 2 l (40, 41). This can accommodate net flow rates of 6 l/h or more with better patient tolerance and without the manipulations of patient position often required

---

* 1.5% dextrose dialysis solution equals 15 g/l of dextrose monohydrate or 13.6 g/l of anhydrous dextrose (d-glucose) which equals 76 mmol/l.

for complete drainage. Urea clearances of 30 to 40 ml/min may be achieved. Dialysate regeneration (with sorbents or by dialysis of used dialysate) is often attempted at high dialysate flow rates (42).

Dialysis solution distribution

Manipulations of dialysate flow rate minimally affect the clearances of larger solutes that are limited by membrane area and permeability; however, the mechanics of moving dialysis solution in and out of the peritoneal cavity may improve the clearances of larger solutes when optimal distribution of dialysis solution is assured (so as to minimize large pools and distribute the solution in thin layers with maximum membrane contact). Total membrane resistance also includes blood and dialysate films adjacent to the membrane. Currently there are no techniques that assure optimal intraperitoneal distribution of dialysate, and good catheter placement and patient positioning often are achieved only after trial and error.

Temperature

Dialysis solution temperature influences solute movement into the peritoneal cavity, and higher temperatures presumably enhance solute diffusion and cause vasodilation (43–45). Theoretically, very cold solutions should reduce clearances. However, no significant differences in peritoneal clearances at room temperature as compared to body temperature have been found (45). Perhaps this reflects rapid heat exchange between dialysis solutions and body fluids so that temperature differences are not sustained. Thus, the instilled solution temperature may be of little clinical importance relative to its impact on peritoneal transport. This should be particularly true for long dwell exchanges where any temperature differences would exist for only a small portion of the exchange time. With rapid cycling techniques, it has been customary to heat peritoneal dialysis solutions to body temperature before instillation. Patients on continuous ambulatory peritoneal dialysis often choose not to warm the solution, particularly in warmer environments. If commercially prepared solutions are warmed prior to instillations, dry heat is recommended. Warming baths soon develop high bacterial counts and enhance the risk of contamination while handling the wet containers (46).

pH

A high dialysate pH may increase net clearances of anions of weak acids such as urate and barbiturate. As these acids diffuse into more alkaline dialysate, fractions are converted to the charged, less diffusible anionic salts. This helps keep the diffusible acid concentration low on the dialysate side and tends to 'trap' the solute in less diffusible form (47–49).

The addition of protein to dialysis solution

For solutes bound to protein, the addition of protein to dialysis solution may enhance clearances (49). The diffusible free solute binds to protein in dialysate maintaining a very low dialysate water concentration of the free diffusible form and a high efflux gradient.

Osmolality

Peritoneal dialysis solutions made hypertonic with dextrose increase clearances (26). This is partly due to the solvent drag effects of osmotically induced ultrafiltration during such exchanges. But clearances often remain elevated when less hypertonic exchanges are resumed, which may be due to vasodilatory effects of the hyperosmolar solutions. Absorption of dextrose during hypertonic exchanges may cause extracellular fluid space expansion which in turn could enhance peritoneal perfusion and transport. In rabbits with intact kidneys undergoing peritoneal dialysis, hypertonic exchanges result in polyuria minimizing volume expansion; clearances were similar to those with less hypertonic exchanges (50). Volume expansion with rapid intravenous administration of dextrose solutions did increase clearances. However, since ultrafiltration into the peritoneal cavity may offset glucose mobilization of intracellular fluid and its effects on plasma volume, the relative contributions of convection, vasodilatation, other membrane changes, and volume expansion in explaining increased clearances during hypertonic exchanges in humans are unknown.

Subdiaphragmatic lymphatics

Many of the factors discussed may also affect the flow of intraperitoneal fluid into the subdiaphragmatic lymphatics. The importance of this will be discussed in a separate section.

Microcirculatory factors

Peritoneal capillary blood as the major source of solutes and fluid removed

Pertitoneal capillary blood may be the major source of solutes, cells, and water removed during peritoneal dialysis. Most evidence for this is indirect and can be summarized as follows (also, see Table 1).

1. Hypertonic peritoneal dialysis solution (4.25% dextrose monohydrate) can generate net ultrafiltration in excess of 500 ml/h (51). Many liters per day of ultrafiltration can be tolerated with the rapid resolution of edema. If hypertonic exchanges are used intermittently, so avoiding severe hyperglycemia or hypotension, net ultrafiltration per hypertonic exchange remains consistent (52). It seems unlikely that mesothelial cells, interstitium, or lymphatics could yield so much ultrafiltrate over short periods of time; it is more reasonable to assume that ultrafiltrate comes from the capillaries.

2. Dramatic falls in blood pressure sometimes occur after one or two hypertonic exchanges, which suggests that ultrafiltration without adequate mobilization of extravascular

fluid can jeopardize blood volume.

3. Hypotension can decrease peritoneal clearances (53). Although such clearance reductions often are modest, even in severe shock (for reasons discussed below), the findings suggest that solute clearances are affected by peritoneal capillary blood flow (4).

4. Intraperitoneal or systemic use of vasoconstrictors reduces peritoneal clearances (54–57) and decreases both the number of peritoneal capillaries perfused and peritoneal capillary blood flow (6, 58, 59), which supports the conjecture that the status of the microcirculation influences peritoneal clearances.

5. Peritoneal clearances increase with intraperitoneal administration of vasodilators (54, 60–68). These agents increase peritoneal capillary blood flow, as well as the number of capillaries perfused (58, 61). Vasodilation and/or direct effects of these agents may increase capillary permeability (69). The point, however, is that vasoactive agents affect peritoneal clearances in the expected direction if clearances relate directly to blood flow, number of capillaries, and vascular permeability.

6. Histamine topically applied to the rat peritoneum widens the intercellular gaps in small venules (70), as assessed by serial section studies of the peritoneum with electron microscopy, computerized reconstruction of venular intercellular gaps, and direct observations of fluorescein-tagged albumin movement across the walls of small vessels in the rat mesentery, using a laser beam microscope. Miller and co-workers (71) have observed a similar extravasation of albumin with nitroprusside. In clinical studies, nitroprusside added to peritoneal dialysis solution also markedly increased protein losses (58–62). Studies with dextrans and albumin in rats suggest that substances injected intravenously have a net transport from blood capillaries to the peritoneal cavity (72). In contrast, absorption from the peritoneal

Table 1. Indirect evidence that peritoneal capillary blood is a major source of solutes, cells, and water removal during peritoneal dialysis.

1. Sustained ultrafiltration with repeated hypertonic exchanges
2. Hypotension with repeated hypertonic exchanges
3. Decreased clearances with hypotension
4. Decreased clearances with vasoconstrictors
5. Increased clearances with vasodilators
6. Drugs known to increase protein leaking from venules increase protein losses during peritoneal dialysis
7. Decreased clearances with vasculitis
8. Decreased clearances with diabetic vascular disease
9. Dialysate potassium concentrations approach Gibbs-Donnan equilibrium with plasma, not with intracellular fluid
10. Convective removal of potassium per liter of ultrafiltrate does not exceed extracellular concentrations
11. Limited pools of fluid and solutes in peritoneal mesothelium and interstitium are quickly exhausted unless rapidly replaced
12. Lymphatic flow presumably quite low; drainage not chylous
13. Dialysate leukocyte counts and fibrin increase rapidly with inflammation

cavity to plasma is via peritoneal lymphatics for substances of molecular weight greater than 39,000 daltons. Below a molecular weight of 19,400 substances are absorbed from the peritoneal cavity primarily via lymphatics with some blood capillary uptake.

7. Patients with severe systemic vasculitis, presumably involving the peritoneal microcirculation, can have significantly reduced peritoneal clearances (73, 74). To date, there are reports of reduced clearances in patients with systemic lupus erythematosus, diffuse scleroderma (progressive systemic sclerosis), and malignant hypertension.

8. Some patients with widespread diabetic vascular disease have significantly reduced clearances (73). This is not a universal finding in all diabetics, but may be related to capillary basement membrane thickening and to vascular disease as it exists in the peritoneum. Early diabetic changes in the microcirculation may be associated with increased permeability similar to early glomerular findings (75).

9. The concentration of potassium in the intracellular fluid of mesothelial cells is near 140 mEq/l (76–78); dialysis solution in the peritoneal cavity, however, approaches Gibbs-Donnan equilibrium with the potassium concentration in plasma water (79, 80). Because the composition of dialysis solution is similar to that of extracellular fluid, it is not surprising that the mesothelial cells can maintain their normal internal milieu even though bathed with dialysis solution. The fact that intracellular electrolytes do not participate in peritoneal dialysis exchange to any great extent, however, does not exclude the possibility that some creatinine and urea are removed from the intracellular fluid.

10. Solutes can be removed by convection in the absence of a diffusion gradient when hypertonic solutions induce ultrafiltration (81–83). The net removal of potassium by convection per liter of ultrafiltrate does not exceed potassium concentration in extracellular fluid (79, 84–85), and therefore even hypertonic exchanges do not appear to mobilize much, if any, intracellular potassium.

11. Diffusible solutes probably are removed from peritoneal interstitium and perhaps to some extent from mesothelial intracellular fluid (4, 5, 83, 86). Ultrafiltrate would of course involve water movement through the interstitium and perhaps to some extent through or from mesothelial cells (82). Mesothelial cells can tolerate only a modest degree of dehydration, however, and interstitial pools of water and solute would be exhausted quickly without rapid replacement from peritoneal capillaries. Hence, most of the water and solutes removed during peritoneal dialysis must represent water and solute movement from peritoneal capillaries into the peritoneal cavity via pathways through the interstitium and mesothelial layer.

12. Solutes and water could move into the peritoneal interstitium from peritoneal lymphatics (87). The portions of removal of solutes or water that come from peritoneal lymphatics are unknown, but have been assumed to be minimal because flow rates in mesenteric lymphatics are presumably low and drainage usually is not chylous. We have followed one patient on continuous ambulatory peritoneal dialysis whose drainage contained lymph for nearly 3

years after an episode of streptococcal peritonitis. Drainage was milky, particularly after meals, and contained high triglyceride concentrations. There was no evidence of inflammation (dialysate white counts were low and there were no symptoms). This finding, however, is extremely unusual.

13. The finding that dialysate leukocyte counts in the presence of infection can increase over several hours from less than 100 to many thousands of white cells per cubic millimeter is additional evidence that peritoneal capillary blood can rapidly and significantly contribute to what is removed in peritoneal dialysis solution (88, 89). In the presence of inflammation, an outpouring of fibrinogen with formation of fibrin in dialysate apparently often occurs quickly.

Thus, indirect evidence supports the hypothesis that peritoneal dialysis represents fluid and solute exchange between peritoneal capillary blood and dialysis solution in the peritoneal cavity. The capillary, the endothelium, the peritoneal interstitium, and the mesothelium represent the resistance sites that fluid and solutes must cross for exchange to take place.

Peritoneal capillary blood flow

The absolute peritoneal capillary blood flow that participates in peritoneal dialysis exchange is not known. Total splanchnic blood flow in adult humans may exceed 1,200 ml/min (90). Most of this blood, however, perfuses visceral organs, not the peritoneum. In fact, our observations of the rat peritoneum suggest that the mesentery itself is not particularly vascular and that most of the small vessels capable of participating in exchange are located at sites where peritoneum reflects over loops of bowel (91, 92).

Maximum urea clearances in adult humans usually do not exceed 30 ml/min, even with the most rapid cycling (31, 34, 93). A possible explanation may be that maximum urea clearances are approaching effective peritoneal capillary blood flow and that is blood flow does not exceed 30 to 40 ml/min. Abundant indirect evidence, however, suggests that such is not the case. Rather, indirect evidence suggests that maximum peritoneal urea clearances are not primarily blood flow-limited. This evidence (summarized in Table 2) is as follows:

1. Animal studies have shown that urea clearances remain above 70% of control values even with severe shock and 38% reduction in splanchnic blood flow (53). This observation suggests that although the magnitude of change in peritoneal capillary flow from control to shock conditions is not known, effective peritoneal capillary flow is well above urea clearance in the control state and falls into a modest flow-limiting range only in the presence of severe hypotension.

2. Urea clearances increase only modestly (usually less than 20%) with intraperitoneal vasodilators (58–63). Vasodilators influence the number of capillaries perfused, induce venodilation, and alter vascular permeability directly (6, 91, 92). Because these latter effects could account for the modest increases in small solute clearances observed with vasodilator use, any increases in effective capillary flow so induced have little or no effect on urea clearances indicating that there is no major blood flow limitation on urea clearances.

3. In fact, vasodilators primarily increase clearances of larger solutes (59, 60). Such increments may exceed 100% for solutes above 5,200 daltons. These observations support the contention that vasodilator effects may relate more to venodilation and alterations in permeability than to blood flow, per se (70, 92, 94), but do not negate the very likely possibility that vasodilators increase effective peritoneal capillary flow. However, if this was the major effect of the drugs, and if urea clearances were flow-limited, proportionally greater increases should occur in urea clearances than in clearances of larger solutes.

4. Peritoneal clearances of CO_2 gas in humans and hydrogen gas in rabbits are two-to-three times the maximum urea clearances (4, 95). Gas clearances also should be limited by effective peritoneal capillary flow and should not exceed urea clearances to any great extent if capillary flow was the main determinant of urea clearance; on the other hand, gases should diffuse across all membrane resistances more rapidly. Gases also might use transcellular routes, whereas the path taken by nongaseous solutes is primarily through intercellular gaps and extracellular pathways (35, 36, 96). The fact that gas clearances can be two-to-three times urea clearances suggests that urea clearances are limited by total membrane resistances, including fluid films, rather than by peritoneal capillary flow.

5. If urea clearances are only one-third to one-half of the effective capillary blood flow, then kinetic modeling analyses and in vitro simulations of peritoneal dialysis suggest that under such conditions effective capillary flow would exert only modest limitations on peritoneal urea clearances and that the relationship between urea clearance and effective capillary flow would be in the 'plateau' portion of the clearance-to-blood flow relationship (4). Figure 3 shows a hypothetical relationship of urea clearance to blood flow at high dialysis solution flow rates for peritoneal dialysis, compared with typical findings with a hollow-fiber artificial kidney. With the hollow-fiber kidney, dialysate flow would be near 500 ml/min; with peritoneal dialysis, flow rates would exceed 4 l/h. If effective peritoneal capillary flow rate is near 70 ml/min (as CO_2 gas diffusion studies suggest), urea clear-

Table 2. Indirect evidence that maximum* peritoneal urea clearances are not primarily blood-flow-limited.

1.	Urea clearances remain 70% of control even in shock
2.	Urea clearances increase < 20% with vasodilators
3.	Vasodilators increase clearances of larger solutes more than urea clearances
4.	Clearances of CO_2 and H_2 gases are nearly three times maximum urea clearances
5.	Urea clearances, if only 1/3 of effective capillary blood flow (as gas clearances suggest), would be minimally flow-limited according to kinetic modelling analyses and *in vitro* simulations

* Very high dialysate flow, > 4 l/h, yields urea clearances in man < 40 ml/min.

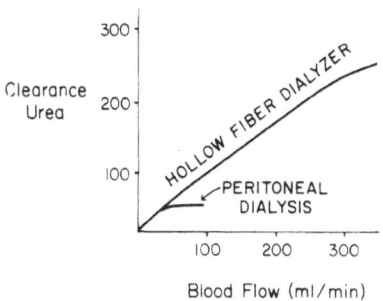

Figure 3. Urea clearances are related to blood flow in a hollow-fiber dialyzer and during peritoneal dialysis (at high dialysis solution flow rates). Peritoneal blood flow values are theoretical, based on gas diffusion studies.

ances would show a nearly 'plateau' relationship with effective blood flow. This plateau presumably represents effects of membrane and fluid film resistances. On the other hand, the hollow-fiber dialyzer fluid film and membrane resistance to urea transport are so low that the system is primarily blood-flow limited. Urea clearance remains at a very high fraction of blood flow up to very high blood flows.

Capillary permeability

In contrast to the situation for small solutes, where interstitial and fluid films appear to be major determinants of maximum clearances, the permeability of the microcirculation appears to be a major influence on clearances of larger solutes (59, 63, 94). The evidence for this is summarized below and in Table 3).

1. As previously mentioned, protein losses increase when agents known to increase venular permeability are topically applied to the mesentery (70). Intraperitoneal nitroprusside, for example, markedly increases protein losses.

2. Vasoactive drugs causes proportionally larger increases in inulin clearances than in urea clearances (59–63). Evidence suggests that vasoactive drugs alter vascular permeability (70, 71), which would explain the proportionally greater effects on larger solutes, where vascular permeability has a major effect on clearances.

3. Protein losses increase with peritoneal inflammation from any cause (17–18), which stimulates an outpouring of white blood cells into the peritoneal dialysate (89). Inflam-

mation in other tissues of the body usually is associated with vasodilation; therefore, it would be reasonable to assume that this also would occur in the peritoneum. Thus, the protein losses with inflammation may merely reflect endogenous mechanisms that induce vasodilation. Vasodilation, per se, may result in perfusion of more permeable capillaries (69). Local release of histamine may increase vascular permeability. In rats activation of the alternative pathway of complement by intraperitoneal or intraarterial injections of endotoxin or zymosine – activated rat serum produced a dramatic increase in dialysate protein concentrations (101). There is also recent evidence that prostaglandins which are known to alter vascular permeability may help to mediate loss of proteins during peritonitis in continuous ambulatory peritoneal dialysis patients (102).

4. After injection of fluorescein-tagged albumin into the rat, the albumin remains within the microcirculation over many minutes of observation without obvious leaking into the interstitium (10). There is an almost explosive outpouring of albumin from the microcirculation into the interstitium within seconds after agents that alter vascular permeability are topically applied peritoneally.

Interstitial factors and fluid films

Indirect evidence suggests that fluid films and interstitial resistance are important in limiting urea clearances during peritoneal dialysis (Table 4).

1. As previously mentioned, maximum urea clearances usually do not exceed 30 ml/min, even with rapid cycling or use of intraperitoneal vasodilators (31, 34, 93). The rapid cycling should minimize limitations due to dialysis solution flow rate. Vasodilators, which presumably increase the number of capillaries perfused and alter capillary permeability, should minimize endothelial resistance. Studies in isolated mesentery suggest that mesothelium should offer little resistance to solute and water transport (9, 10, 13, 14, 103, 104). However, in vivo mesentery may offer more resistance than suggested by these in vitro studies of isolated membranes (17). Thus, under the conditions of rapid cycling and use of intraperitoneal vasodilators (and assuming that effective peritoneal capillary flow is not limiting), major resistance sites that explain the limits on urea clearances should be the interstitium and the stagnant fluid films in the peritoneal cavity.

Table 3. Evidence that vascular permeability is a major resistance for large solutes.

1. Increased protein losses with agents known to increase venular permeability
2. Proportionately larger increases in inulin clearances (compared with urea clearances) with vasoactive drugs
3. Increased protein losses with peritoneal inflammation
4. Laser studies with fluorescein-tagged albumin in the rat microcirculation

Table 4. Indirect evidence that fluid films and/or interstitial resistance limit urea clearances during peritoneal dialysis.

1. Maximum urea clearances near 30 ml/min even with rapid cycling or with vasodilators
2. Dialysate relatively stagnant
3. Probably very wide dialysate channels
4. Interstital solute path; potentially long distance
5. *In vitro* simulations of peritoneal dialysis demonstrate high fluid film resistances
6. Little evidence to support blood flow limitation
7. Vascular resistance appears low for small solutes.

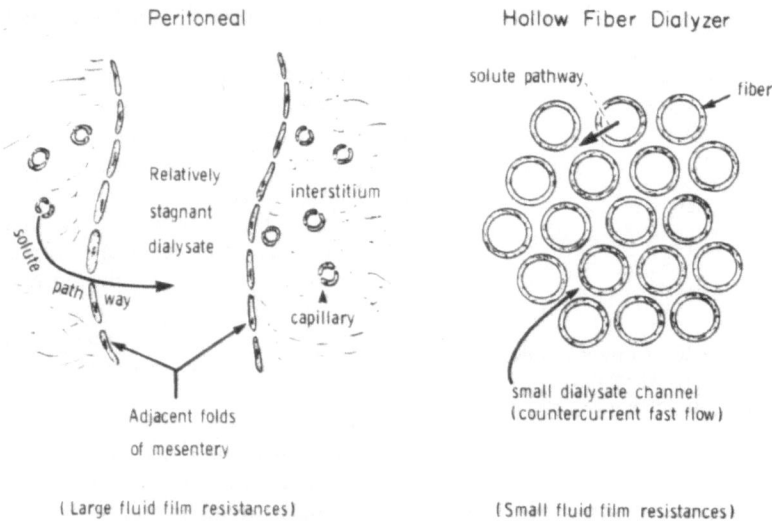

Figure 4. Dialysate channel configurations in peritoneal and hollow-fiber dialysis.

2. Dialysate in the peritoneal cavity within the many folds of the mesentery always remains relatively stagnant, even with rapid cycling (31, 34, 93). External massage of the abdomen increases clearances in rats (105).

3. Dialysate channels probably are relatively wide (93). Figure 4 is a comparison between dialysate channel dimensions during peritoneal dialysis and those in a man-made hollow-fiber dialyzer. Note that in the hollow-fiber dialyzers much of the cross-section represents blood path. In small dialysate channels there is rapid couter-current flow and minimal fluid film resistance (106, 107). In contrast, in the peritoneal system the interstitium and stagnant pools of fluid between folds of mesentery represent substantial fluid film resistances.

4. The interstitital solute path probably represents a relatively long distance (5), and, as shown in Figure 2, may be 100 microns or more. Figure 5 shows that the situation may be even more complex. Wayland (70) suggests that the interstitium may represent a network of aqueous channels through mucopolysaccharide and collagenous gels. Hypertonic peritoneal dialysis solutions may dehydrate the interstitium and, although the total distance may be shortened, the aqueous network of channels could become more tortuous and the resistance to solute movement could actually increase (92, 108).

5. In vitro simulations of peritoneal dialysis (using hollow-fiber dialyzers with the outer shell removed placed in stagnant pools of fluid) demonstrate rapid deterioration in urea

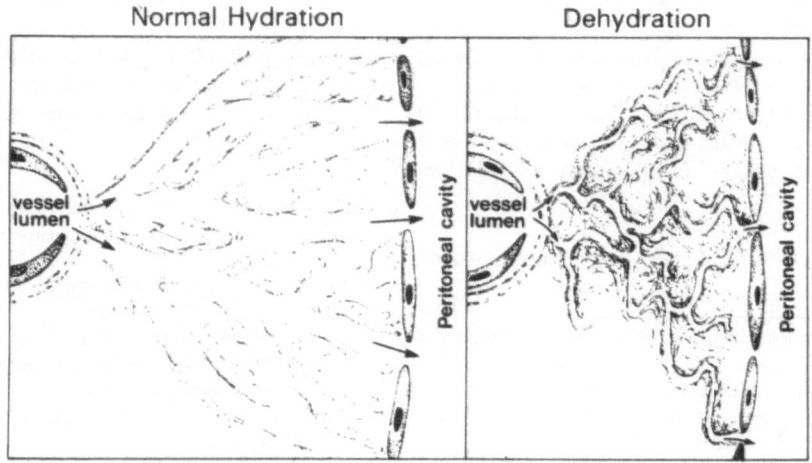

Figure 5. Hypothetical changes in interstitial aqueous channel dimensions during peritoneal dialysis and interstitial dehydration.

clearances attributable to high fluid film resistances (4, 109). Even with the most rapid cycling in and out of the simulated peritoneal cavity, clearances cannot be restored. Vigorous shaking of the cavity and improved mixing diminish the effects of fluid film resistances to some extent, but never approach the performance that can be achieved with rapid counter-current flow of dialysis fluid in the usual manner (109).

6. As mentioned previously, because there is little evidence in support of a blood flow limitation, the importance of fluid film is implied.

7. Wayland (70) suggests that endothelium offers very little resistance to small solute movement from peritoneal capillary blood into peritoneal dialysis solution. When rats are injected with fluorescein-tagged small solutes, extensive migration of the solute into the interstitium is observed. This contrasts with observations after injection of fluorescein-tagged albumin, where movement of albumin across vascular walls is not obvious over many minutes unless agents that increase vascular permeability are administered in solutions bathing the peritoneum (70).

Mesothelial factors

Mesothelial permeability

Results of functional and morphological studies in isolated mesentery suggest that gaps between adjacent mesothelial cells may form very loose junctions, particularly over the diaphragmatic surface (13). Intercellular gaps 500 Å wide have been observed. Transport studies in isolated mesentery also suggest the presence of pores of similar dimensions (103, 104). Some mesothelial intercellular junctions may be tighter, however, and may influence peritoneal transport (15–17). Diuretics (110) and inhibitors of cellular metabolic pathways (9) may influence diffusion rates through isolated mesentery and during peritoneal dialysis. Alterations in mesothelial metabolic functions may alter dimensions of intercellular gaps or cell surface charges; both factors could influence the permeability characteristics of the mesothelium to passive solute movement. Cell surface charges in particular might influence the movement of charged solutes. Whether the active transport of electrolytes across mesothelial cell walls influence net electrolyte removal or uptake during peritoneal dialysis remains unknown.

Total pore area across mesothelium

Studies by Karnovsky (7, 96) indicate that intercellular gaps between mesothelial cells may be pathways for solute movement; if so, the total pore area would be well below the total gross surface area of the mesothelial layer, and the magnitude of the transmesothelial total pore area could be influenced by the extent of solution/mesothelial contact within the abdominal cavity.

Ultrafiltration factors

Ultrafiltration can increase solute clearances (26, 81). Solutes may accompany the bulk flow of water from peritoneal capillary blood into the peritoneal cavity by convection. Most solutes do not accompany the bulk flow of water in concentrations comparable to those in extracellular water (26, 61, 79, 83, 111). Thus, the concentration gradient for net diffusion of a solute from blood to dialysis solution may be enhanced by ultrafiltration. With longer dwell times, the sieving effects of disproportionate water removal would be obliterated by greater net diffusion into the peritoneal dialysis solution. At equilibrium greater amounts of solute are removed with hypertonic exchanges because of increased drainage volumes (112).

Convective net removal of sodium and potassium per liter of ultrafiltrate usually is well below respective extracellular fluid concentrations (79, 83, 111). The convective component of sodium and potassium removal can be calculated by subtracting net removal accountable to diffusion from the net total removal. Another way to estimate convective transport is to instill solutions with sodium and potassium concentration in Gibbs-Donnan equilibrium with serum water. Although a sieving effect creates a concentration gradient for some diffusion, net electrolyte removal per liter of ultrafiltrate remains far below that in extracellular fluids with 1 to 2 hr cycles (112). Severe hypernatremia can result from overly zealous peritoneal ultrafiltration and removal of water without amounts of sodium equal to extracellular concentrations (113, 114).

Hypothesis to explain solute sieving during ultrafiltration

How is it possible that a membrane as permeable as the peritoneum (which, in terms of protein losses, is more permeable than the membrane of hollow-fiber dialyzers (115, 116)) can hinder convective movement of electrolytes with ultrafiltration? The answer to this question is not known. Possible mechanisms for the net electrolyte sieving effect with peritoneal ultrafiltration are summarized in Table 5 and Figure 6.

1. There is substantial evidence that the width of intercellular gaps progressively increases from proximal to distal portions of the capillaries, with the most permeable

Table 5. Possible mechanisms for the net electrolyte sieving effect with peritoneal ultrafiltration.

1.	Ultrafiltration through narrow intercellular gaps in proximal capillaries
2.	Endothelial cell surface charges in intercellular gaps
3.	Transendothelial cell water movement
4.	Interstitial gel surface charges along aqueous channels
5.	Mesothelial cell surface charges in intercellular gaps
6.	Transmesothelial cell water movement
7.	Dextrose interaction with cations in intercellular gaps or interstitial channels

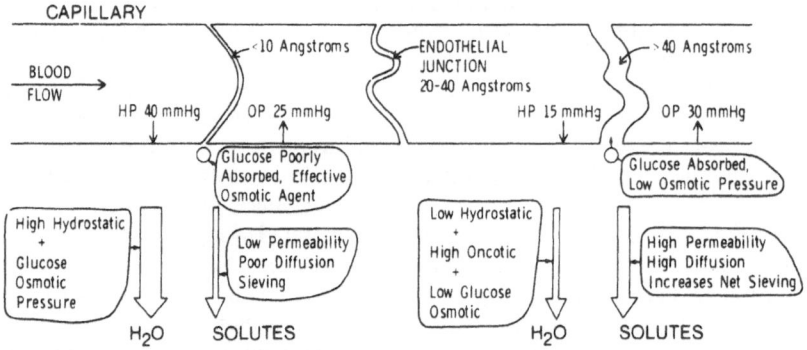

HYPOTHESIS: PROXIMAL CAPILLARY ULTRAFILTRATION AT LOW PERMEABILITY
AND DISTAL DIFFUSION AT HIGH PERMEABILITY DURING PERITONEAL DIALYSIS

Figure 6. Hypothetical diagrammatic summary of factors influencing ultrafiltration during peritoneal dialysis (see text). (From Nolph et al. [120], with permission of the publisher). HP = Hydrostatic pressure; OP = Osmotic pressure.

portions being in the small venules (70). Peritoneal capillaries may differ from man-made fibers in having a progressive increase in pore width along the capillary, whereas man-made fibers are more homogenous. At the proximal end of the capillaries, hydrostatic pressure should be higher (69). Dextrose should be more osmotically effective across this tighter portion of the capillary than in the distal portion, where it may be readily absorbed and exert little osmotic pressure. Thus, combined hydrostatic and osmotic pressures could induce maximum ultrafiltration rates across portions of the capillary that are least permeable.

2. If most of the water flows through the intercellular gap where junctions are rather narrow, then endothelial cell surfaces in close proximity and their respective charges could impede electrolyte movement through the gap.

3. Perhaps when transmembrane hydrostatic and osmotic pressures are high enough, some transendothelial cell water movement does occur (82). Such net movement of water across the cell may occur without proportional movement of electrolytes through the very complex internal cell milieu.

4. Surface charges on the capillary basement membrane or on the surfaces of interstitial gels may impede the movement of charged solutes, which would be akin to the charge interference by polar molecules in the glomerulus (117). That passage of albumin is restrained more by charge than by pore dimensions has been suggested (117).

5. Mesothelial cell surface charges in intercellular gaps could influence electrolyte movements. If mesothelial permeability is much greater than endothelial permeability, however, this could be less important than the same phenomenon in the endothelium.

6. The movement of ultrafiltrate from the interstitium into the peritoneal cavity could occur by hydrostatic pressure, with the build-up of fluid in the interstitium and with some osmotic pressure induced by glucose gradients across the mesothelium. If the mesothelium is indeed more permeable than the endothelium, then the major glucose gradient could be across the vessel wall, with only a modest dextrose gra-

dient maintained across the mesothelium. Nevertheless, if water does move through mesothelial cells, this could interfere with the convective transport of electrolytes.

7. We have reported studies showing that even neutral molecules may not accompany ultrafiltration induced by glucose osmotic pressure in the same proportions as when ultrafiltration is induced by hydraulic pressure across the same membrane (118). This is not an effect of osmotic pressure, per se, but perhaps is due to the use of a solute (e.g. dextrose) that can enter the membrane and move upstream against the flow of ultrafiltrate (119). We have hypothesized that molecular interaction within the membrane may alter net sieving effects (119).

Figure 6 summarizes these ultrafiltration characteristics during peritoneal dialysis. We have previously presented a hypothesis to explain the net sieving effects (120). The primary assumption is that most ultrafiltration is across the proximal capillary where the effective pore width is small compared to that in the distal capillary. It is also known that neutral solutes may be subjected to sieving with peritoneal ultrafiltration (111). Here the explanations for sieving are based on 'pore width' or intramembranous solute interaction rather than charge effects.

Lymphatic factors

The anatomy of peritoneal lymphatics has recently been reviewed (121). The lymphatics which probably have the greatest impact on peritoneal transport kinetics are those immediately below the mesothelial layer on the caudal surface of the diaphragm. Mesenteric lymphatics drain fluid and nutrients from the intestine; diffusive and convective movement of solutes and water from mesenteric lymphatics into the peritoneal cavity may occur during peritoneal dialysis. The extent of such lymphatic contributions is unknown but assumed to be small. In contrast, diaphragmatic contractions may actively pump fluid from the peritoneal cavity into and through the diaphragmatic lymphatics and mainly via the right lymphatic duct into the venous circulation.

On the under surface of the diaphragm there are intercellular gaps or stomata located between lateral borders of the mesothelial cells that overlie lymphatic lacunae (122). Erythrocytes or particles introduced in the peritoneal cavity pass through mesothelium at the point of separation of these cells (122, 123). Submesothelial connective tissue is interrupted at the site of the stoma and contains masses of microfibrils. The cytoplasm of mesothelial cells and lymphatic endothelial cells beneath the stomata have abundant fine filaments (124, 126, 127). When the diaphragm is relaxed with succinylcholine, numerous patent stomata are observed (128); when the diaphragm is contracted with carbachol, the stomata are less apparent and often appear nonpatent (128). Flaps of mesothelial and underlying lymphatic endothelial cells may influence the patency of the stomata based on the status of the actin components in the cytoplasm of these cellular extensions. Lymphatic endothelium forms a continuous layer in the roof of each lacuna. It appears that overlapping lymphatic endothelial cell junctions may separate to allow passage of cells or particles into the lymphatic vessels (123, 129). Overlapping cell junctions may act as flap valves preventing the passage of lucunae contents back into the peritoneal cavity (129).

When the diaphragm relaxes in expiration, the lacuni are thought to dilate; during contraction in inspiration the lacuna are compressed and the lymph they contain is expelled into the connecting lymph vessels (122). Mesothelial and lymphatic endothelial cells in the walls of the lacunae seem to separate and come together with each respiratory cycle (130, 131). The diaphragm and the lymphatics therein act as pumps with the mesothelial and endothelial flaps as 'inlet valves'. The flow of fluid from the peritoneal cavity into and through this system would thus represent a convective transport system with little or no molecular size discrimination. Recent studies have examined the complexity of the diffusion of small solutes through the tissues of the peritoneum (132) and the absorption of macromolecules from the peritoneal cavity (133, 134). The absorption of macromolecules is probably by convective transport through subdiaphragmatic lymphatics with little or no molecular size discrimination. Isoosmotic solutions may be absorbed primarily by convective movement into this same system (135).

The absorption of fluid from the peritoneal cavity through subdiagphragmatic lymphatics can be measured by monitoring the absorption of albumin (136–139). By instilling dialysis solutions containing albumin (at concentrations so high that effects of albumin entering the peritoneal cavity from plasma on dialysate albumin concentrations are negligible), and knowing 1) average concentrations of albumin during an interval, 2) intraperitoneal volumes and 3) the net amount of removal of albumin from the peritoneal cavity, one can calculate lymphatic absorption.

Figure 7 shows mean cumulative lymphatic absorption in six rats undergoing 6 h exchanges with 16 ml of 15% dextrose dialysis solutions. Mean values for net cumulative ultrafiltration are also shown. At any point, the sum of the two volumes would estimate the actual cumulative total transca-

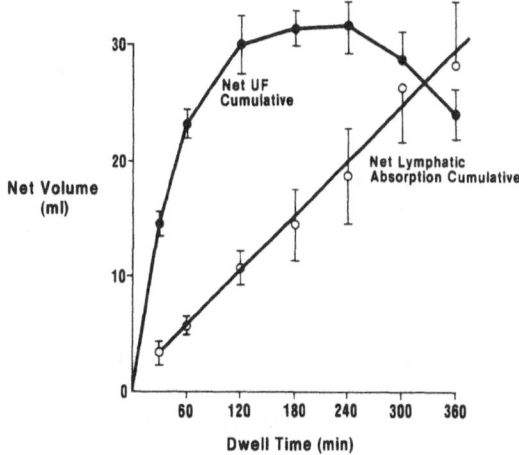

Figure 7. Mean (± SEM) cumulative net lymphatic absorption (open circles) and mean (± SEM) cumulative net ultrafiltration (closed circles) in 6 rats during 6 hours exchanges with 16 ml instillations of a 15% dextrose dialysis solution. (From reference 139.)

pillary ultrafiltration. In these studies, rats were anesthetized and lymphatic absorption rate appeared almost constant. Figure 8 summarizes mean transcapillary total ultrafiltration rate over the 6 h period based on these same studies. Mean lymphatic reabsorption rate is shown as fixed. The difference between transcapillary ultrafiltration and mean lymphatic reabsorption rate is the net ultrafiltration rate. The peak intraperitoneal volume is actually reached before the point of osmotic equilibrium when transcapillary UF rate no longer exceeds the mean lymphatic reabsorption rate. In these studies, it was noted that osmotic equilibrium occurs while glucose concentration is still substantially higher in dialysate than in serum. This is presumably due to the low electrolyte content of the ultrafiltrate and the subsequent relatively low osmolality of the ultrafiltrate producing a transient hypoosmolar dialysate. Low grade transcapillary ultrafiltration persisted when the dialysate was hypoosmolar because the glucose gradient still existed between dialysate and serum and the reflection coefficient for glucose is presumably higher than those of electrolytes. Later, as osmotic equilibrium and glucose equilibrium are approached transcapillary ultrafiltration rate approaches zero and the net reabsorption of isosmotic fluid from the peritoneal cavity approaches that of lymphatic reabsorption rate.

Studies of lymphatic absorption during peritoneal dialysis in humans have recently been performed (140, 141). The methodology of these studies again depends on the monitoring the kinetics of albumin absorption from the peritoneal cavity and the assumption that this is primarily by subdiaphragmatic lymphatics. Figure 9 shows the mean intraperitoneal volumes (using corrected intraperitoneal albumin content as a marker), mean dialysate and serum osmolalities, and mean dialysate and serum glucose concentrations in ten patients undergoing 4 h exchanges with 2 l of 2.5% dextrose dialysis solution. Note in humans, as mentioned for rats, that peak intraperitoneal volume occurs before osmotic

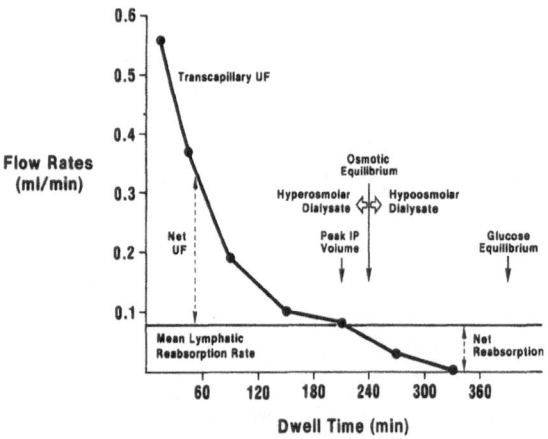

Figure 8. Mean transcapillary ultrafiltration rate (solid circles) and mean lymphatic absorption rate (solid horizontal line) during exchanges in figure 7. The periods of net ultrafiltration and net reabsorption as well as other events during the exchanges are indicated. (From reference 139.)

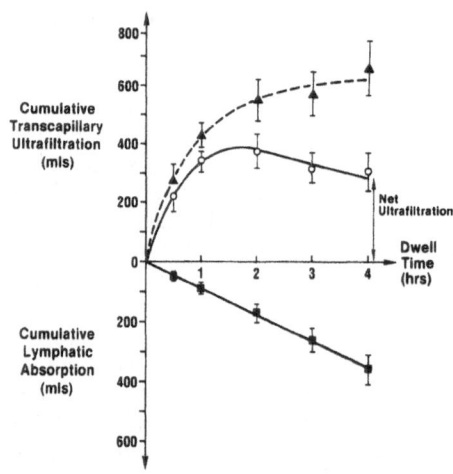

Figure 10. Mean (± SEM) cumulative transcapillary ultrafiltration (triangles), cumulative lymphatic absorption (squares), and net ultrafiltration (circles) from the same studies as in Figure 9. (From reference 140.)

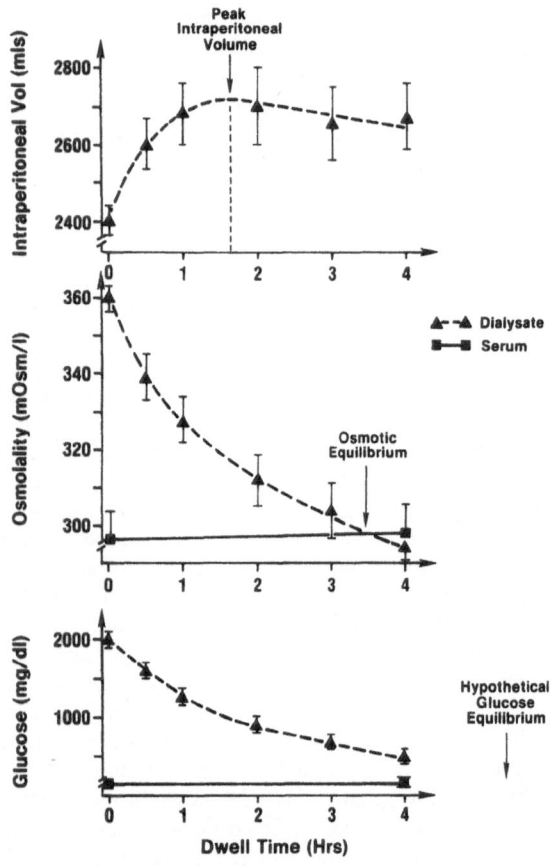

Figure 9. Mean (± SEM) intraperitoneal volumes, dialysate and serum osmolalities, and dialysate and serum glucose concentrations during 4 hr exchanges with 2.5% dextrose dialysis solutions in ten patients. (From reference 140.)

equilibrium and that osmotic equilibrium occurs before glucose equilibrium. Note also the late slightly hypoosmolar phase of the dialysate (140). Figure 10 summarizes cumulative transcapillary ultrafiltration, the cumulative lymphatic absorption and the net ultrafiltration over the 4 h in these same studies. Overall, the cumulative lymphatic absorption during the 4 h exchanges represented 58% of the total transcapillary ultrafiltration that should have been present in the peritoneal cavity prior to drainage in the absence of lymphatic reabsorption. These studies were performed in the supine position which may have optimized fluid subdiaphragmatic contact and may have exaggerated lymphatic reabsorption compared to what occurs in upright active patients. Further studies are necessary to determine this.

Nevertheless, it would appear that the convective movement of fluid in the peritoneal cavity into the subdiaphragmatic lymphatics along with dissolved solutes, particles and cells has an important impact on the net efficiency of peritoneal dialysis. Future studies are necessary to see if intraperitoneal drugs could be used clinically to reduce lymphatic outflow and yield more net ultrafiltration, higher drainage volumes (and accordingly higher clearances) at any given dextrose concentration in the dialysis solution. The potential for capturing adequate ultrafiltration at lower dialysis solution glucose concentrations is very attractive.

Other factors

Solute distribution volumes

Larger body fluid spaces (e.g., when body size is large) are associated with less rapid decreases in blood solute concentrations during dialysis (for solutes that can diffuse readily from extravascular pools into blood (142). When concentrations decrease rapidly, clearances calculated by using a pre-exchange blood sample rather than a midpoint sample will

Peritoneal   Hollow Fiber Dialyzer

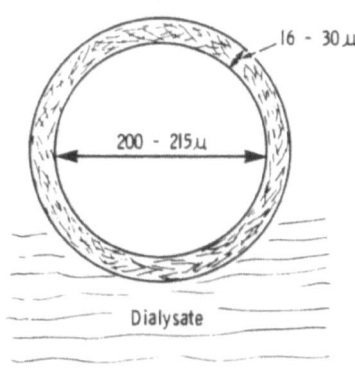

Figure 11. Scaled comparison of peritoneal and hollow-fiber capillaries.

be spuriously low. Blood concentration changes following an hourly exchange usually are small and within the limits of the laboratory methods. On the other hand, large patients also have greater peritoneal surface area (143). They may have more fluid membrane contact per exchange volume and may have higher clearances.

Protein binding of solutes

Total clearances of solutes bound to plasma proteins such as calcium are lower than their molecular size would suggest (28). Total clearance may change if fractions of bound and free solute are altered.

Intracellular trapping

Some solutes are not readily mobilized from the intracellular space. This may represent slow diffusion across cell membranes or binding to intracellular constituents. Plasma clearances usually are not affected, but plasma concentrations may rapidly decrease during dialysis and increase immediately postdialysis for such solutes. With diffusion disequilibrium, plasma clearances overestimate the true clearance from the total space of distribution. Also, if blood samples are allowed to set for any time prior to separation of erythrocytes, concentrations in serum or plasma may increase as in vitro re-equilibration occurs. Calculated clearances will be lower than actual plasma clearances *in vivo* if separation is delayed.

Lipid solubility

Lipid-soluble substances may be removed in peritoneal dialysis drainage at concentrations higher than in serum (144). Possible explanations include facilitated transport through lipid layers of the cell wall or direct removal of lipid substances from cell surfaces of the peritoneum and cells of the mesentery.

COMPARISONS WITH HOLLOW-FIBER DIALYZERS

Capillary dimensions, configurations, and permeability

Figure 11 shows cross-sections of a peritoneal capillary and a synthetic fiber in a hollow-fiber dialyzer. The dimensions are drawn to scale, as indicated. Even though the synthetic fiber wall is much thicker, a high fraction of the wall luminal surface may represent 'pore' area. The fiber wall is a mesh of synthetic material with many spaces between interstices. In contrast, the peritoneal capillary may have not only a very small relative total luminal surface, but only a small fraction (less than 0.2%, according to Pappenheimer (145) of that surface may represent 'pore' area. This is true, of course, only if intercellular gaps are indeed the major pathways for solute and water movement from the capillary.

Figure 12 shows lateral views of the fiber walls. This demonstrates even more clearly the great distance that may exist between intercellular slits in capillary endothelium and in contrast, the high fraction of synthetic fiber walls representing space available for solute exchange between the molecules, composing the wall.

Figure 13 shows lateral views of the course of capillaries in the peritoneal membrane and synthetic fibers in a hollow-fiber dialyzer. Notice that the capillary network in the peritoneal system is complex, with many interconnections. The total number of capillaries participating in exchange is unknown. In contrast, each fiber in the hollow-fiber dialyzers is a separate entity. There are no interconnections and the numbers are well known, depending on the type of hollow-fiber dialyzer. In the peritoneal system, only a portion of capillaries may be perfused at any one time, as others may essentially be closed down by precapillary sphincter tone (5). In contrast, most fibers in the hollow-fiber dialyzer are perfused simultaneously unless fiber plugging occurs (146).

Dialysate flow characteristics

Figure 14 compares typical dialysate flow rates in milliliters

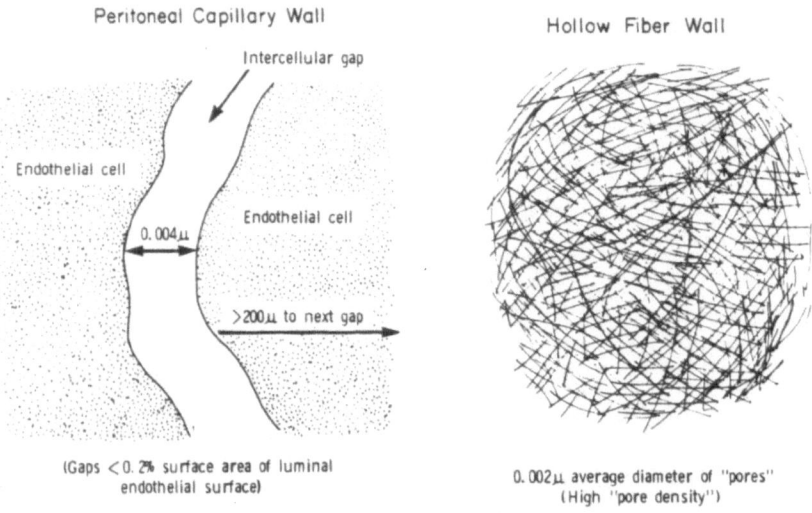

Figure 12. Luminal view of transcapillary pathways for solute movement.

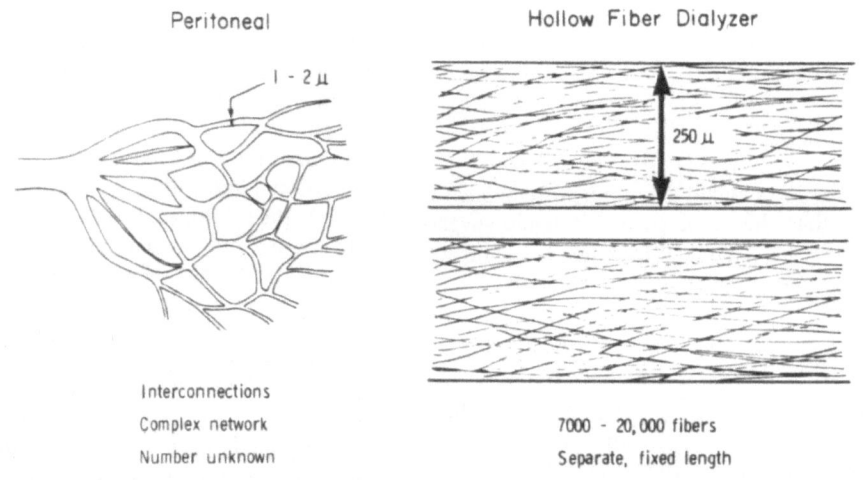

Figure 13. Lateral view of capillaries in peritoneal and hollow-fiber dialysis.

per minute and in liters per week for dialysis with a hollow-fiber dialyzer (12 h per week), intermittent peritoneal dialysis (40 h per week), and continuous ambulatory peritoneal dialysis (four 2 l exchanges per day). This figure does not include ultrafiltration rates that have little impact on the values for hollow-fiber dialysis and intermittent peritoneal dialysis but add substantially to total flow for continuous ambulatory peritoneal dialysis.

With hollow-fiber dialysis, urea clearances are primarily blood-flow-limited; with intermittent peritoneal dialysis, urea clearances probably are limited primarily by fluid resistances, for the reasons discussed above; with continuous ambulatory peritoneal dialysis, the urea clearances are limited by dialysis solution flow rate and are nearly identical to dialysis solution flow rate.

Figure 15 shows that typical urea clearances during treatment sessions are nearly one-third of the dialysis solution rate for both hollow-fiber dialysis and intermittent peritoneal dialysis. During continuous ambulatory peritoneal dialysis, the ratio of urea clearance to flow rate of dialysis solution approaches 1.0 (52, 146–151).

Comparisons of resistances for large and small solutes during hollow-fiber dialysis and peritoneal dialysis

Figure 16 is a summary of the important resistance sites during peritoneal dialysis and during hollow-fiber dialysis. The height of each bar is a hypothetical value, since the actual numbers are for the most part unknown.

The upper portions of the figure reflect the importance of

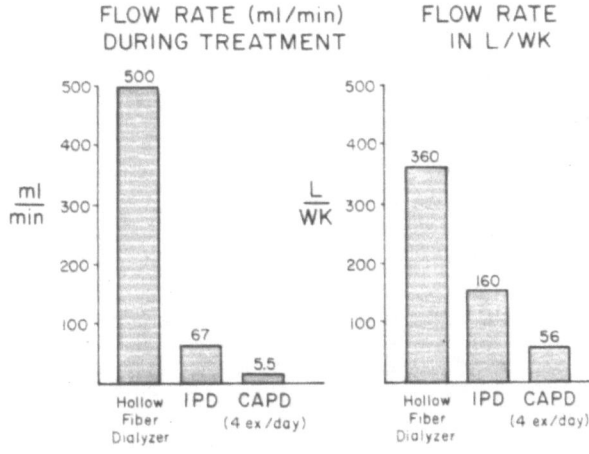

Figure 14. Dialysate flow rates for hollow-fiber dialyzers, intermittent peritoneal dialysis (IPD) and continuous ambulatory peritoneal dialysis (CAPD) are compared in ml/min and l/wk.

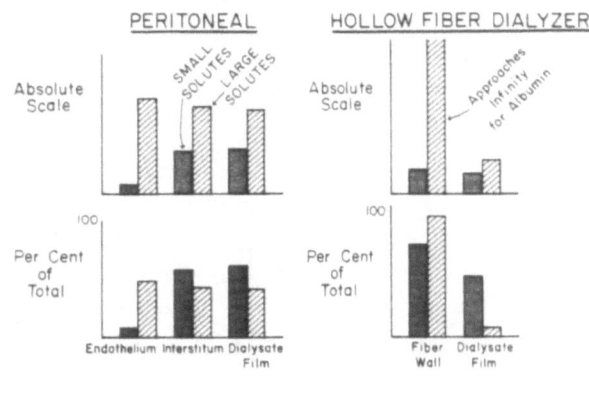

Figure 16. Hypothetical absolute and relative magnitudes of various resistances in peritoneal dialysis and hollow-fiber dialysis for small (< 100 daltons) and large (> 5,000 daltons) solutes (see text). Blood film resistances are not compared but are especially important in extracorporeal dialyzers.

various resistance sites on an absolute scale. In peritoneal dialysis, the vascular wall probably offers substantial resistance only to solutes larger than 1,000 daltons (70). For smaller solutes, this is a short distance to traverse with a relatively large mean pore size (perhaps greater than 40 Å in width at the venular end of the capillary) (7, 8, 96). The interstitial resistance is substantial for both small and large solutes. Again, this would be an even greater resistance for large solutes, since they must diffuse across this distance and greater hindrance by the dimensions of the aqueous channels (if such truly exists) would be expected. The fluid films in the peritoneal cavity offer substantial resistance to both small and large solutes. The resistance to the latter would be greater because of the distances involved and their poorer diffusibility. Mesothelial resistance is not shown, since in-

tercellular gaps may be 500 Å or more in diameter and there is little evidence to suggest that mesothelium is a major resistance site (9, 103, 104). Intracapillary stagnant fluid films and capillary basement membranes are not shown, since they also are not known to be major resistance sites.

Below these hypothetical absolute resistance values for peritoneal dialysis are figures showing relative resistances. In the case of urea clearance, the interstitium and the fluid films are proportionately greater resistances. Because the vascular wall is a major resistance site for large solutes, interstitial and dialysis solution fluid films are proportionally shown as less important.

In the hollow-fiber dialyzer, there are only two major resistance sites: the fiber wall and fluid films. The mean pore size of the fiber wall may be 20 Å or less (152). Synthetic fiber resistance to very large solutes such as albumin approach infinity, since fibers are impermeable to solutes of such a size. The thickness of the fiber wall makes the fiber an important resistance site for urea, primarily, perhaps, because of the distance involved. Dialysis solution fluid film resistances are much smaller than in peritoneal dialysis for reasons discussed. Thus, on a relative scale, the fiber wall would offer a high proportion of the total resistance to movement of both small and large solutes.

Blood flow comparisons

Figure 3 relates the clearance of urea to blood flow during hollow-fiber dialysis and to hypothetical effective peritoneal capillary blood flows during peritoneal dialysis. Hollow-fiber dialyzers are so efficient that urea clearance is limited markedly by blood flow. Gas diffusion studies previously mentioned suggest that effective peritoneal capillary blood flow during peritoneal dialysis in adults of a normal size is near 60 to 70 ml/min and do not explain maximum urea clearances during rapid cycling peritoneal dialysis of only near 30 ml/min (4, 95).

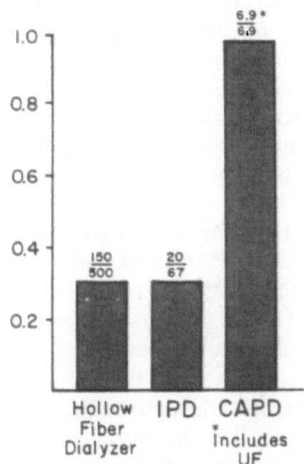

Figure 15. The ratios of urea clearance/dialysate flow for different techniques are compared, as in Figure 14.

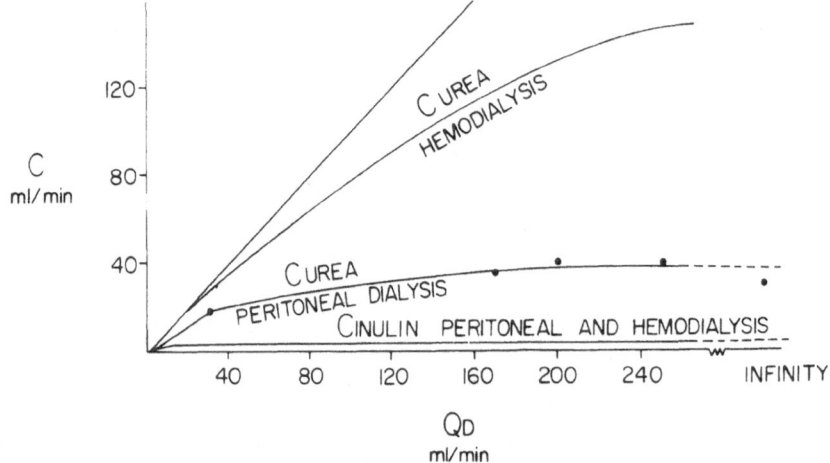

Figure 17. Typical clearances of urea and inulin during peritoneal and hemodialysis related to dialysate flow rate (Q_D). (From Nolph et al. [4] with permission of the publisher).

Table 6. Substances reportedly affecting peritoneal clearances.

Albumin
Aminoproprionate
Anthranilic acid
Bradykinin
Calcium
Cetyl trimethyl NH_4CL
Cholecystokinin
Dialysate alkalinization
Diazoxide
Dioctyl sodium sulfosuccinate
Dipyridamole
Dopamine
Ethacrynic acid, furosemide
Glucagon
Histamine
Hypertonic glucose
Insulin
Isoproterenol
Lipid in dialysate
Methylprednisolone
Nitroprusside
N-Myristyl alanine
Norepinephrine
PGA_1, PGE_1, PGE_2
PGF_{2a}
Phenazine-methosulfate
Phentolamine
Protamine
Paromycin
Secretin
Serotonin
Specific chelate
Streptokinase
THAM
Tolazoline
Vasopressin

MANIPULATING PERITONEAL TRANSPORT

Cycling time

Figure 17 shows the effects of dialysate flow rates on peritoneal clearances of urea. At rates above 4 l/h peritoneal clearances are only moderately dialysate flow rate-limited and approach maximum clearances. Many techniques for increasing dialysis solution flow rate have been described (22, 97). Although studies suggest that clearances relate to flow rate in a fairly fixed manner regardless of the cycle or residual volumes used, further investigation is needed.

Vasoactive substances

Table 6 summarizes the substances that reportedly alter the status of the peritoneal microcirculation by intraperitoneal or systemic administration (22, 65–66, 153). Vasodilatory drugs presumably increase clearances by increasing the number of capillaries perfused, opening more permeable capillaries, and minimizing blood flow limitations, if present. Vasoconstrictors tend to decrease the number of capillaries perfused and close down more permeable capillaries, and may introduce some blood flow limitations on small solute clearances.

All commercial peritoneal dialysis solutions appear to cause a transient constriction of the microvasculature of the parietal peritoneum (lasting 1 to 3 min), but subsequently cause a marked (150 to 200%), sustained vasodilation of parietal, as well as visceral, peritoneal vessels (59). The vasoconstrictive component of the solutions has not been identified, but does not appear to be the pH (59). Studies in rats strongly suggest that the vasodilatory components of solutions are the hyperosmolality and nonbicarbonate buffer anions (91). Very high molecular weight vasodilators may not be effective if administered intraperitoneally. Glucagon, for example, increases clearances only when given intravenously unless dosage is very high by the intraperitoneal route (154). It has been suggested that glucagon is too large to cross the mesothelium and interstitium effectively and achieve high concentrations at vascular receptor sites (154). (Very large doses overcome the slow absorption from the peritoneum and are effective). Whether other agents exert their vasodilatory effects by reaching receptor sites from the luminal side of the vessel or from the extraluminal side when administered intraperitoneally is unclear.

Manipulating the interstitium

Preliminary studies suggest that hypo-osmolar solution may reduce interstitial resistance and increase protein losses (108). Figure 5 demonstrates the hypothesis to explain such an observation. The number and dimensions of aqueous channels through the interstitium may be increased by better hydration, since hyperosmolar solutions could cause interstitial dehydration leading to an increased resistance to passive solute movement through the interstitium.

Other drug effects

Diuretics seem to have a slight influence on the net removal of electrolytes during peritoneal dialysis (110). The mechanisms to explain this are not known, but possibly relate to alterations in mesothelial cell surface charges.

Surface-acting agents

Surface-acting agents such as dioctyl sodium sulfosuccinate reportedly increase clearances when administered intraperitoneally (155). Whether these agents alter the status of the microcirculation or influence the other components of resistance in the peritoneal membrane is not known. And whether the dimensions of aqueous channels through the interstitium or fluid films adjacent to the mesothelium could be changed by altering surface tensions also is not known.

REFERENCES

1. Cunningham RS: The physiology of the serous membranes. *Physiol Rev* 6: 242, 1926
2. Putnam TJ: The living peritoneum as a dialyzing membrane. *Am J Physiol* 63: 547, 1922–1923
3. Henderson LW: Peritoneal dialysis. In: *Clinical Aspects of Uremia and Dialysis,* edited by Massry SG, Sellers AL. Springfield IL, Charles C Thomas. 1976, p 555
4. Nolph KD, Popovich RP, Ghods AJ, Twardowski Z: Determinants of low clearances of small solutes during peritoneal dialysis. *Kidney Int* 13: 117, 1978
5. Nolph KD, Miller F, Rubin J, Popovich RP: New directions in peritoneal dialysis concepts and applications. *Kidney Int* 18 (Suppl 10): S111, 1980
6. Nolph KD, Ghods AJ, Brown P, Van Stone J, Miller FN, Wiegman DL, Harris PD: Factors affecting peritoneal dialysis efficiency. *Dial Transplant* 6: 52, 1977
7. Karnovsky MJ: The ultrastructural basis of capillary permeability studied with peroxides as a tracer. *J Cell Biol* 3: 213, 1967
8. Cotran RS: The fine structure of the microvasculature in relation to normal and altered permeability. In: *Physical Bases of Circulatory Transport:* Regulation and Exchange, edited by Reeve EB, Guyton AC. Philadelphia, PA, WB Saunders Co, 1967
9. Rasio EA: Metabolic control of permeability in isolated mesentery. *Am J Physiol* 276: 962, 1974
10. Miller F: The peritoneal microcirculation. In: *Peritoneal Dialysis,* edited by Nolph KD, The Hague, Boston, London, Martinus Nijhoff, 1981
11. Gotloib L, Shostak A, Bar-Sella P, Eiali V: Fenestrated capillaries in human parietal and rabbit diaphragmatic peritoneum, *Nephron* 41: 200, 1985
12. Gotloib L, Bar-Sella P, Shostak A: Reduplicated basal lamina of small venules and mesothelium of human parietal peritoneum: ultrastructural changes of reduplicated peritoneal basement membrane. *Peritoneal Dial Bull* 5: 212, 1985
13. Tsilibary EC, Wissig SL: Absorption from the peritoneal cavity: SEM study of the mesothelium covering the peritoneal surface of the muscular portion of the diaphragm. *Am J Anat* 149: 127, 1977
14. Cascarano J, Rubin AD, Chick WL, Sweifach BW: Metabolically induced permeability changes across mesothelium and endothelium. *Am J Physiol* 206: 373, 1964
15. Gotloib L, Digenis GE, Rabinovich S, Medline A, Oreopoulos DG: Ultrastructure of normal rabbit mesentery. *Nephron* 34: 248, 1983
16. Digenis GE, Rabinovich S, Medline A, Rodella H, WvG, Oreopoulos DG: Electron microscopic study of the peritoneal kinetics of iron dextran during peritoneal dialysis in the rabbit. *Nephron* 37: 108, 1984
17. Verger C, Luger A, Moore H, Nolph K: Acute changes in peritoneal morphology and transport properties with infectious peritonitis and mechanical injury. *Kidney Int* 23: 823, 1983
18. Rubin J, McFarland S, Hellems EW, Bower JP: Peritoneal dialysis during peritonitis. *Kidney Int* 19: 460, 1981
19. Baradi AF, Rao SN: A scanning electron microscope study of mouse peritoneal mesothelium. *Tissue Cell* 8: 159, 1976
20. Andrews PM, Porter KR: The ultrastructure morphology and possible functional significance of mesothelial microvilli. *Anat Res* 177: 409, 1973
21. Baradi AF, Rayns DJ: Mesothelial intercellular junctions and pathways. *Cell Tissue Res* 173: 133, 1976
22. Nolph KD: Peritoneal dialysis. In: *The Kidney* edited by Brenner BM, Rector FC Jr, 3rd ed Philadelphia, PA, WB Saunders Co, 1986, p 1847
23. Nolph KD, Rosenfeld PS, Powell JT, Danforth E Jr: Peritoneal glucose transport in hyperglycemia during peritoneal dialysis. *Am J Med Sci* 259: 272, 1970
24. Maher JF: Principles of dialysis and dialysis of drugs. *Am J Med* 62: 475, 1977
25. Bomar JB, Decker JS, Dechard JF, Hlavinka DJ, Moncrief JW, Popovich RP: The elucidation of maximum efficiency minimum cost peritoneal dialysis protocols. *Trans Am Soc Artif Intern Organs* 20: 120, 1974
26. Henderson LW, Nolph KD: Altered permeability of the peritoneal membrane after using hypertonic peritoneal dialysis fluid. *J Clin Invest* 48: 992, 1969
27. Babb AL, Johansen PF, Strand MJ, Tenckhoff H, Scribner BH: Bidirectional permeability of the human peritoneum to middle molecules. *Proc Eur Dial Transplant Assoc* 10: 247, 1973

28. Boen ST: *Peritoneal Dialysis in Clinical Medicine,* Springfield, JL, Charles C Thomas, 1964

29. Boen ST: Kinetics of peritoneal dialysis, comparison with artificial kidney. *Medicine* 40: 243, 1961

30. Penzotti SC, Mattocks AM: Effects of dwell time, volume of dialysis fluid, and added accelerators on peritoneal dialysis of urea. *J Pharm Sci* 60: 1520, 1971

31. Tenckhoff H, Ward G, Boen ST: The influence of dialysate volume and flow rate on peritoneal clearance. *Proc Eur Dial Transplant Assoc* 2: 113, 1965

32. Lange K, Treser G: Automatic continuous high flow peritoneal dialysis, *Trans Am Soc Artif Intern Organs* 13: 164, 1967

33. Lange K, Treser H, Managalap J: Automatic continuous high flow rate peritoneal dialysis. *Arch Klin Med* 214: 201, 1968

34. Stephen RL, Atkin-Thor E, Kolff WJ: Recirculating peritoneal dialysis with subcutaneous catheter. *Trans Am Soc Artif Intern Organs* 22: 575, 1976

35. Lewin AK, Greenbaum MA, Gordon A, Maxwell MH: Sorbent based regenerating delivery system for use in peritoneal dialysis. *Trans Am Soc Artif Intern Organs* 20: 130, 1974

36. Shinaberger JH, Shear L, Barry KG: Increasing efficiency of peritoneal dialysis-experience with peritoneal extracorporeal recirculation dialysis. *Trans Am Soc Artif Intern Organs* 11: 76, 1965

37. Kablitz C, Stephen RL, Duffy DP: Technological augmentation of peritoneal urea clearance: past, present and future. *Dial Transplant* 9: 741, 1980

38. Twardowski ZJ, Prowant BF, Nolph KD, Martinez AJ, Lamton LM: High volume, low frequency continuous ambulatory peritoneal dialysis. *Kidney Int* 23: 64, 1983

39. Twardowski ZJ, Nolph KD, Prowant B, Moore HL: Efficiency of high volume, low frequency CAPD. *Trans Am Soc Artif Intern Organs* 29: 53, 1983

40. Finkelstein FO, Kliger AS: Enhanced efficiency of peritoneal dialysis using rapid, small-volume exchanges. *asaio J* 2: 103, 1979

41. Warden GD, Maxwell JG, Stephen RL: The use of reciprocating peritoneal dialysis with a subcutaneous peritoneal catheter in end-stage renal failure in diabetes mellitus. *J Surg Res* 24: 495, 1978

42. Blumenkrantz MJ, Gordon A, Roberts M: Applications of the Redy sorbent system to hemodialysis and peritoneal dialysis. *Artif Organs* 3: 230, 1979

43. Gross M, McDonald HP Jr: Effects of dialysate temperature and flow rate on peritoneal clearance. *JAMA* 202: 215, 1967

44. De Santo NG, Capodicasa G, Capasso G, Giordano C: Development of means to augment peritoneal urea clearances: The synergistic effects of combining high dialysate temperature and high dialysate flow rates with dextrose and nitroprusside. *Artif Organs* 5: 409, 1981

45. Indraprasit S, Namwongprom A, Sooksriwongse CO, Buri PS: Effect of dialysate temperature on peritoneal clearances. *Nephron* 34: 45, 1983

46. Mader JT, Reinarz JA: Peritonitis during peritoneal dialysis – the role of the preheating water bath. *J Chronic Dis* 31: 635, 1978

47. Knochel JP, Mason AD: Effect of alkalinization on peritoneal diffusion of uric acid. *Am J Physiol* 210: 1160, 1966

48. Deger GE, Wagoner RD: Peritoneal dialysis in acute uric acid nephropathy. *Mayo Clin Proc* 47: 189, 1972

49. Campion DS, North JP: Effect of protein binding of barbiturates on their rate of removal during peritoneal dialysis. *J Lab Clin Med* 66: 549, 1965

50. Maher JF, Bennett RR, Hirszel P, Chakrabarti E: The mechanism of dextrose-enhanced peritoneal mass transport rates. *Kidney Int* 28: 16, 1985

51. Rubin J, Nolph KD, Popovich RP, Moncrief J, Prowant B: Drainage volumes during CAPD. *Asaio J* 2: 2, 1979

52. Popovich RP, Moncrief JW, Nolph KD, Ghods AJ, Twardowski ZJ, Pyle WK: Continuous ambulatory peritoneal dialysis. *Ann Intern Med* 88: 449, 1978

53. Erbe RW, Greene JA Jr, Weller JM: Peritoneal dialysis during hemorrhagic shock. *J Appl Physiol* 22: 131, 1967

54. Hare HG, Valtin H, Gosselin RE: Effects of drugs on peritoneal dialysis in the dog. *J Pharmacol Exp Ther* 145: 122, 1964

55. Henderson LW, Kintzel JE: Influence of antidiuretic hormone on peritoneal membrane area and permeability. *J Clin Invest* 50: 2437, 1971

56. Chan MK, Varghese Z, Baillod RA, Moorhead JF: Peritoneal dialysis effect of intraperitoneal dopamine. *Dial Transplant* 9: 382, 1980

57. Gutman RA, Nixon WP, McRae RL, Spencer HW: Effect of intraperitoneal and intravenous vasoactive amines on peritoneal dialysis: study in anephric dogs. *Trans Am Soc Artif Intern Organs* 22: 570, 1976

58. Miller FN, Nolph KD, Harris PD, Rubin J, Wiegman DL, Joshua IG: Effects of peritoneal dialysis solutions on human clearances and rat arterioles. *Trans Am Soc Artif Intern Organs* 24: 131, 1978

59. Miller FN, Nolph KD, Harris PD, Rubin J, Wiegman DL, Joshua IG, Twardowski ZJ, Ghods AJ: Microvascular and clinical effects of altered peritoneal dialysis solutions. *Kidney Int* 15: 630, 1979

60. Nolph KD, Ghods AJ, Van Stone J, Brown PA: The effects of intraperitoneal vasodilators on peritoneal clearances. *Trans Am Soc Artif Intern Organs* 22: 586, 1976

61. Nolph KD, Ghods AJ, Brown PA, Miller FN, Harris P, Pyle K, Popovich R: Effects of nitroprusside on peritoneal mass transfer coefficients and microvascular physiology. *Trans Am Soc Artif Intern Organs* 23: 210, 1977

62. Nolph KD, Ghods AJ, Brown PA, Twardowski ZJ: Effects of intraperitoneal nitroprusside on peritoneal clearances with variations in dose, frequency of administration, and dwell times. *Nephron* 24: 114, 1979

63. Nolph KD: Effects of intraperitoneal vasodilators on peritoneal clearances. *Dial Transplant* 7: 812, 1978

64. Hirszel P, Lasrich M, Maher JF: Augmentation of peritoneal mass transport by dopamine. *J Lab Clin Med* 94: 747, 1979

65. Gutman RA: Toward enhancement of peritoneal clearances. *Dial Transplant* 8: 1072, 1979

66. Maher JF: Acceleration of peritoneal mass transport by drugs and hormones. *Artif Organs* 3: 224, 1979

67. Felt J, Richard E, McCaffrey C, Levy M: Peritoneal clearance of creatinine and inulin during dialysis in dogs: Effect of splanchnic vasodilators. *Kidney Int* 16: 459, 1979

68. Maher JF, Hirszel P, Lasrich M: Modulation of peritoneal transport rates by prostaglandins. *Adv Prostaglandin Thromboxane Res* 7: 695, 1980

69. Renkin EM: Exchange of substances through capillary walls: Circulatory and respiratory mass transport. In: *Ciba Foundation Symposium,* edited by Wolstenholme GEW, Boston, Little Brown, 1969, p 50

70. Wayland H: Transmural and interstitial molecular transport. Action of histamine. In: *Continuous Ambulatory Peritoneal Dialysis,* edited by Legrain M, Amsterdam, Excerpta Medica, 1980, p 20

71. Miller FN, Joshua IG, Harris PD, Wiegman DL, Jauchem JR: Peritoneal dialysis solutions and the microcirculation. *Contrib Nephrol* 17: 51, 1979

72. Flessner MF, Dedrick RL, Schultz JS: Exchange of macromolecules between peritoneal cavity and plasma. *Am J Physiol* 248: H15, 1985

73. Nolph KD, Stoltz M, Maher JF: Altered peritoneal permeability in patients with systemic vasculitis. *Ann Intern Med* 75: 513, 1971

74. Brown ST, Ahearn DJ, Nolph KD: Reduced peritoneal clearances in scleroderma increased by intraperitoneal isoproterenol. *Ann Intern Med* 78: 891, 1973

75. Zimmerman AL, Sablay LB, Aynedjian HS, Bank N: Increased peritoneal permeability in rats with alloxan-induced diabetes mellitus. *J Lab Clin Med* 103: 720, 1984

76. Manery JF: Water and electrolyte metabolism. *Physiol Rev* 34: 334, 1954

77. Tarail R, Hacker ES, Taylor R: The ultrafilterability of potassium and sodium in human serum. *J Clin Invest* 31: 23, 1952

78. Folk BP, Zierler KL, Lilienthal JL: Distribution of potassium and sodium between serum and certain extracellular fluids in man. *Am J Physiol* 153: 381, 1948

79. Brown ST, Ahearn DJ, Nolph KD: Potassium removal with peritoneal dialysis. *Kidney Int* 4: 67, 1973

80. Kelton JG, Vlan R, Stiller C, Holmes E: Comparison of chemical composition of peritoneal fluid and serum. *Ann Intern Med* 89: 67, 1978

81. Henderson LW: Peritoneal ultrafiltration dialysis: Enhanced urea transfer using hypertonic peritoneal dialysis fluid. *J Clin Invest* 45: 950, 1966

82. Ahearn DJ, Nolph KD: Controlled sodium removal with peritoneal dialysis. *Trans Am Soc Artif Intern Organs* 18: 423, 1972

83. Nolph KD, Hano JE, Teschan PE: Peritoneal sodium transport during hypertonic peritoneal dialysis: Physiologic mechanisms and clinical implications. *Ann Intern Med* 70: 931, 1969

84. Nolph KD, Sorkin MI, Moore H: Autoregulation of sodium and potassium removal during continuous ambulatory peritoneal dialysis. *Trans Am Soc Artif Intern Organs* 26: 334, 1980

85. Maher JF, Chakrabarti E: Ultrafiltration by hyperosmotic peritoneal dialysis fluid excludes intracellular solutes. *Am J Nephrol* 4: 169, 1984

86. Nolph KD: CAPD – A logical approach to peritoneal dialysis limitations (A comparison of the peritoneal dialysis system and hollow fiber kidneys). *Int J Nephrol Urol Androl* 1: 5, 1980

87. Wayland H, Silberberg A: Blood to lymph transport. *Microvasc Res* 15: 367, 1978

88. Nolph KD, Prowant B: Complications during continuous ambulatory peritoneal dialysis. In: *Continuous Ambulatory Peritoneal Dialysis,* edited by Legrain M, Amsterdam, Excerpta Medica, 1980, p 258

89. Rubin J, Rogers WA, Taylor HM, Everett ED, Prowant BP, Fruto LV, Nolph KD: Peritonitis during continuous ambulatory peritoneal dialysis. *Ann Intern Med* 92: 7, 1980

90. Wade OL, Combes B, Childs AW, Wheeler HO, Dournand D, Bradley SE: The effect of exercise on the splanchnic blood flow and splanchnic blood volume in normal man. *Clin Sci* 15: 457, 1956

91. Miller FN, Nolph KD, Johsua IG: The osmolality component of peritoneal dialysis solutions. In: *Continuous Ambulatory Peritoneal Dialysis,* edited by Legrain M, Amsterdam, Excerpta Medica, 1980, p 12

92. Nolph KD: Introductory remarks: Anatomy, physiology and kinetics of peritoneal transport during peritoneal diaglysis. In: *Continuous Ambulatory Peritoneal Dialysis,* edited by Legrain M, Amsterdam, Excerpta Medica, 1980, p 7

93. Goldschmidt ZH, Pote HH, Katz MA, Shear L: Effect of dialysate volume on peritoneal dialysis kinetics. *Kidney Int* 5: 240, 1975

94. Miller FN, Wiegman DL, Joshua IG, Nolph KD, Rubin J: Effects of vasodilators and peritoneal dialysis solution on the microcirculation of the rat cecum. *Proc Soc Exp Biol Med* 161: 605, 1979

95. Aune S: Transperitoneal exchange. II. Peritoneal blood flow estimated by hydrogen gas clearance. *Scand J Gastroenterol* 5: 99, 1970

96. Karnovsky JF: The ultrastructural basis of transcapillary exchanges. In: *Biological Interfaces: Flows and Exchanges,* Boston, Little Brown, 1968, p 64

97. Nolph KD: Peritoneal dialysis. In: *Replacement of Renal Function by Dialysis,* edited by Drukker W, Parsons FM, Maher JF, The Hague, Boston, London, Martinus Nijhoff, First edition, 1978, p 277

98. Blumenkrantz MJ, Roberts CE, Card B: Nutritional management of the adult patient undergoing peritoneal dialysis. *J Am Diet Assoc* 73: 351, 1978

99. Giordano C, De Santo NG: Dietary management of patients on peritoneal dialysis. *Contrib Nephrol* 17: 77, 1979

100. Kobayashi K, Manji T, Hiramatsu S: Nitrogen metabolism in patients on peritoneal dialysis. *Contrib Nephrol* 17: 93, 1979

101. Miller FN, Hammerschmidt DE, Anderson GI, Moore JN: Protein loss induced by complement activation during peritoneal dialysis. *Kidney Int* 25: 480, 1984

102. Steinhauer HB, Schollmeyer P: Prostaglandin-mediated loss of proteins during peritonitis in continuous ambulatory peritoneal dialysis. *Kidney Int* 29: 584, 1986

103. Nagel W, Kuschinsky W: Study of the permeability of isolated dog mesentery. *Eur J Clin Invest* 1: 149, 1970

104. Gosselin RE, Berndt WO: Diffusional transport of solutes through mesentery and peritoneum. *J Theor Biol* 3: 487, 1962

105. Rubin J, Kirchner K, Bower J: Evaluation of stagnant fluid films during simulated peritoneal dialysis: In vitro and in vivo studies. *Clin Exper Dial Apheresis* 5: 285, 1981

106. Maher JF, Nolph KD: Factors affecting optimal performance of coil dialyzers. *Proc 6th Int Congr Nephrol,* edited by Giovannetti S, Bonomini V, D'Amico G, Basel, S Karger 6: 657, 1976

107. Maher JF, Nolph KD: Resistance to diffusion in dialyzers. *Clin Nephrol* 1: 333, 1974

108. Rubin J, Nolph KD, Arfania D, Miller FM, Wiegman DL, Joshua IG, Harris PD: Studies on non-vasoactive peritoneal dialysis solutions. *J Lab Clin Med* 93: 910, 1979

109. McGary TJ, Nolph KD, Rubin J: In vitro simulations of peritoneal dialysis: A technique for demonstrating limitations on solute clearances due to stagnant fluid films and poor mixing. *J Lab Clin Med* 96: 148, 1980

110. Maher JF, Hohndel DG, Shea C, Di Sanzo F, Cassetta M: Effects of intraperitoneal diuretics on solute transport during hypertonic dialysis. *Clin Nephrol* 7: 96, 1977

111. Rubin J, Klein F, Bower JD: Investigation of the net sieving coefficient of the peritoneal membrane during peritoneal dialysis. *asaio J* 5: 9, 1982

112. Nolph KD, Twardowski ZJ, Popovich RP, Rubin J: Equilibration of peritoneal dialysis solutions during long dwell exchanges. *J Lab Clin Med* 246: 256, 1979

113. Boyer J, Gill GN, Epstein FH: Hyperglycemia and hyperosmolality complicating peritoneal dialysis. *Ann Intern Med* 67: 568, 1967

114. Smith RJ, Block MR, Arieff AI, Blumenkrantz MJ, Coburn JW: Hypernatremic, hyperosmolar coma complicating chronic peritoneal dialysis. *Proc Clin Dial Transplant Forum* 4: 96, 1974

115. Nolph KD, New DL: Effects of ultrafiltration on solute clearances in hollow fiber artificial kidneys. *J Lab Clin Med* 88: 593, 1976

116. Nolph KD, Stoltz ML, Maher JF: Electrolyte transport during ultrafiltration of protein solutions. *Nephron* 9: 473, 1971

117. Glassock RJ: The nephrotic syndrome. *Hosp Pract* 14: 105, 1979

118. Nolph KD, Hopkins CA, New D, Antwiler GD, Popovich RP: Differences in solute sieving with osmotic vs. hydrostatic ultrafiltration. *Trans Am Soc Artif Intern Organs* 22: 618, 1976

119. Twardowski ZJ, Nolph KD, Popovich RP, Hopkins CA: Comparison of polymer, glucose, and hydrostatic pressure induced ultrafiltration in a hollow fiber dialyzer: Effects on convective solute transport. *J Lab Clin Med* 92: 619, 1978

120. Nolph KD, Miller FN, Pyle K, Popovich RP, Sorkin MI: A hypothesis to explain the characteristics of peritoneal ultrafiltration. *Kidney Int* 20: 543, 1981

121. Khanna R, Mactier R, Twardowski Z, Nolph K: Peritoneal cavity lymphatics. *Peritoneal Dial Bull* 6: 113, 1986

122. Yoffey JM, Courtice FC: The peritoneal and pleural cavities. In: *Lymphatics, Lymph and the Lymphomyeloid Complex*, edited by Yoffey JM, Courtice FC, London, Academic Press, 1970, p 295

123. French JE, Florey HW, Morris B: The absorption of particles by the lymphatics of the diaphragm. *Q J Exp Physiol* 45: 88, 1960

124. Tsilibary EC, Wissig SL: Structural plasticity in the pathway for lymphatic drainage from the peritoneal cavity. *Microvasc Res* 17: S144, 1979

125. Bettendorf U: Lymph flow mechanism of the subperitoneal diaphragmatic lymphatics. *Lymphology* 11: 111, 1978

126. Leak LV: Permeability of peritoneal mesothelium: A TEM and SEM study. *J Cell Biol* 70: 423, 1976

127. Tsilibary EC, Wissig SL: Cytochalasin D modifies the cell surface and actin distribution of cells in vivo. *J Cell Biol* 83: 328, 1979

128. Tsilibary EC, Wissig SL: Lymphatic absorption from the peritoneal cavity: Regulation of patency of mesothelial stomata. *Microvasc Res* 25: 22, 1983

129. Casley-Smith JR: Endothelial permeability. The passage of particles into and out of diaphragmatic lymphatics. *Q J Exp Physiol* 49: 365, 1964

130. Allen L: On the penetrability of the lymphatics of the diaphragm. *Anat Rec* 124: 639, 1956

131. Allen L, Vogt E: A mechanism of lymphatic absorption from serous cavities. *Am J Physiol* 119: 776, 1937

132. Flessner MF, Dedrick RL, Schultz JS: A distributed model of peritoneal-plasma transport: theoretical considerations. *Am J Physiol* 246: R597, 1984

133. Flessner MF, Dedrick RL, Schultz JS: Exchange of macromolecules between peritoneal cavity and plasma. *Am J Physiol* 248: H15, 1985

134. Flessner MF, Fenstermacher JD, Blasberg RG, Dedrick RL: Peritoneal absorption of macromolecules studies by quantitative autoradiography. *Am J Physiol* 248: H26, 1985

135. Shear L, Castellot JJ, Barry KG: Peritoneal fluid absorption. I. Effect of dehydration on kinetics. *J Lab Clin Med* 66: 232, 1965

136. Courtice FC, Steinbeck AW: The lymphatic drainage of plasma from the peritoneal cavity of the cat. *Austr J Exp Biol Med Sci* 27: 161, 1950

137. Lill SR, Parsons RH, Buhac I: Permeability of the diaphragm and fluid resorption from the peritoneal cavity in the rat. *Gastroenterology* 76: 997, 1979

138. Anne S: Transperitoneal exchange IV. The effect of transperitoneal fluid transport on the transfer of solutes. *Scand J Gastroenterol* 5: 241, 1970

139. Nolph KD, Mactier RA, Khanna R, Twardowski Z, Moore H, McGary T: The kinetics of ultrafiltration during peritoneal dialysis: The role of lymphatics. *Kidney Int* 32: 219, 1987

140. Mactier RA, Khanna R, Twardowski Z, Nolph KD: Contribution of lymphatic absorption to loss of ultrafiltration and solute clearances in continuous ambulatory peritoneal dialysis. *J Clin Invest* 80: 1311, 1987

141. Rippe BG, Stelin, and Ahlem J: Lymph flow from the peritoneal cavity in CAPD patients. In: *Frontiers in Peritoneal Dialysis*, edited by Maher JF, Winchester JF, New York, Field, Rich and Assoc, 1986, p 24

142. Nolph KD, Whitcomb ME, Schrier RW: Mechanisms for inefficient peritoneal dialysis in acute renal failure associated with heat stress and exercise. *Ann Intern Med* 71: 317, 1969

143. Rubin J, Nolph K, Arfania D, Brown P, Moore H, Rust P: Influence of patient characteristics on peritoneal clearances. *Nephron* 27: 118, 1981

144. Maher JF, Hirszel P, Hohnadel DC, Abraham J, Lasrich M: Fatty acid removal during peritoneal dialysis: mechanisms, rates and significance. *Asaio J* 1: 8, 1978

145. Pappenheimer JR: Passage of molecules through capillary walls. *Physiol Rev* 33: 387, 1953

146. Nolph KD, Ahearn DJ, Esterly JA, Maher JF: Irreversible morphological and functional changes in hollow fiber kidneys with a single dialysis. *Trans Am Soc Artif Intern Organs* 20: 604, 1974

147. Nolph KD: Peritoneal clearances. *J Lab Clin Med* 94: 519, 1979

148. Nolph KD, Popovich RP, Moncrief JW: Theoretical and practical implications of continuous ambulatory peritoneal dialysis. *Nephron* 21: 117, 1978

149. Popovich RP, Moncrief JW: Kinetic modeling of peritonal transport. *Contrib Nephrol* 17: 59, 1979

150. Popovich RP, Pyle WK, Moncrief JW: Peritoneal dialysis. *Am Inst Chem Eng Symp Series* 75: 31, 1979

151. Popovich RP, Pyle WK, Hiatt MP, McCollough WS, Moncrief JW: Metabolite transport kinetics in peritoneal dialysis. In: *Continuous Ambulatory Peritoneal Dialysis*, edited by Legrain M, Amsterdam, Excerpta Medica, 1980, p 28

152. Green DM, Antwiler GD, Moncrief JW, Decherd JF, Popovich RP: Measurement of the transmittance coefficient spectrum of cuprophan. *Trans Am Soc Artif Intern Organs* 22: 627, 1976

153. Maher JF, Hirszel P: Pharmacologic manipulation of peritoneal transport. In: *Peritoneal Dialysis*, edited by Nolph KD. The Hague, Boston, London, Martinus Nijhoff, 1985, p 267

154. Hirszel P, Maher JF, LeGrow W: Increased peritoneal mass transport with glucagon acting at the vascular surface. *Trans Am Soc Artif Intern Organs* 24: 136, 1979

155. Mattocks AM, Penzotti SC: Acceleration of peritoneal dialysis with minimum amounts of dioctyl sodium sulfosuccinate. *J Pharm Sci* 61: 475, 1972

PRACTICAL USE OF PERITONEAL DIALYSIS

CHARLES MION

INTRODUCTION

The modern era of clinical peritoneal dialysis started in 1959 with the introduction of a simplified method based on the intermittent irrigation of the peritoneal cavity using a single disposable catheter and commercially prepared dialysis solutions (1). Peritoneal dialysis then became an established method for the treatment of acute renal failure, but many clinicians were reluctant to use it in spite of its technical simplicity, because of a high incidence of peritonitis, a lower efficacy in comparison with hemodialysis and the high cost of commercially prepared dialysis solutions. In the 1960s and the early 1970s, these shortcomings were partly overcome due to many conceptual technical advances including: a better understanding of solute peritoneal transfer kinetics, which gave a scientific basis for improving peritoneal clearances (2–4); the development of automated closed circuit dialysate delivery systems which simplified nursing procedures and strikingly reduced the incidence of peritoneal infection (5, 6); the introduction of a bacteriologically safe peritoneal access device which eliminated the difficulty and hazard of the repeated puncture technique (7) and finally simplified logistics and reduced costs which were obtained when the reverse osmosis machines became available for the continuous production of sterile, apyrogenic dialysis fluid at the bedside (8). Despite these improvements and long term clinical studies demonstrating its feasibility and efficiency in patients with chronic uremia (9, 10), periodic (intermittent) peritoneal dialysis (IPD) was long regarded as having little place in the treatment of end-stage renal disease (ESRD), except in a few dedicated dialysis centers (11, 12). In 1976, the concept of a 'portable/wearable equilibrium' peritoneal dialysis technique was introduced (13). This new approach, resulting in steady low blood levels of uremic metabolites was later developed as continuous ambulatory peritoneal dialysis (CAPD), the technique being simplified with the introduction of dialysis solutions in plastic bags (14, 15). In contrast with periodic peritoneal dialysis, CAPD gained very rapidly an almost universal acceptance and is at present widely prescribed as a major treatment modality of ESRD. Several thousands of ESRD patients are now receiving CAPD in Europe (16) and in the United States (17). The extensive use of CAPD in the treatment of chronic uremia has stimulated many studies on the structure (18–20) and the physiology of the peritoneum (21, 22), on local host defense mechanisms (23) and mass transfer kinetics across the peritoneal membrane (24–26), and also the effects of drugs in influencing the efficacy of peritoneal dialysis (27). Progress in tubing connections have lowered to acceptable levels the incidence of peritonitis in CAPD (28). Simultaneously, new indications for peritoneal dialysis, such as refractory congestive cardiac failure (29) or the local administration of chemotherapeutic agents (30) enlarged the field of its clinical applications.

In this chapter, the practical aspects common to all peritoneal dialysis regimens will be discussed, except for the specific items related to CAPD that are reviewed in chapter 25. Our aim is to provide updated information on the clinical use of peritoneal dialysis and also to present a balanced view on the advantages and inherent limitations of this dialysis modality.

TECHNICAL ASPECTS OF PERITONEAL DIALYSIS

The three main components indispensable to perform peritoneal dialysis include a peritoneal access, various formulations of sterile pyrogen free dialysis solutions and an adequate tubing set for peritoneal irrigation. Although these components remain basically the same as those used in the early 1960s (1), the technique of peritoneal dialysis has evolved over the past three decades from a rather crude and agressive method (1, 9) to a variety of more sophisticated systems (7, 8, 10, 15, 28) developed to improve the safety of this dialysis modality, to decrease the incidence of peritoneal infection and to ameliorate patients comfort and tolerance.

Aseptic procedures and use of antiseptics

When starting a peritoneal dialysis program, the nephrologist should keep in mind that bacterial contamination of the peritoneum is a constant risk as long as an indwelling catheter is present in the peritoneal cavity (31). Although peritonitis complicating peritoneal dialysis most often follows a benign course, it should be seen as a potentially lethal complication (32) and every effort should be made to prevent it. Asepsis remains the corner-stone of a successful peritoneal dialysis program; it is the safest and most cost effective approach for infection prophylaxis (31). In most dialysis units, peritoneal dialysis (PD) procedures are performed and/or taught to patients by competent and experienced nurses (33, 34); nevertheless, it remains the physician's responsibility to review frequently aseptic procedures with the nursing staff and to maintain a high degree of awareness in this key area. Furthermore, the allocation of adequate space and personnel is a prerequisite to permit the everyday practice of asepsis in a clean environment and out of unnecessary stress (33–35). Although rigid 'non-touch' aseptic techniques are of greater importance than any chemical degerming agents (36), the use of antiseptic solutions is mandatory to disinfect hands and connectors when assembling intermittent peritoneal dialysis equipment and during all connect-disconnect procedures required for peritoneal irrigation. The use of povidone iodine solutions has long been advocated as the safest antiseptic (31) and this recommendation appears to hold true in most circumstances (37). The superiority of iodophors over 70% ethanol solutions, however, has been questioned (38, 39). Doubts about the safety of iodophors aqueous solutions arose from the following facts: an epidemic of Pseudomonas aeruginosa peritonitis was found to have originated in contaminated poloxamer-iodine solutions (40); commercial 10% povidone iodine aqueous solutions contaminated with Pseudomonas cepacia during the manufacturing process brought about epidemics of pseudobacteremia in several hospitals (41, 42); commercial iodophors prepared according to USP recommendations demonstrate a lower bactericidal activity than more diluted solutions (36, 43); many factors such as evaporation, alkalinity, presence of blood, glucose, glycols or other organic matter can reduce the concentration of free iodine released by iodophors, thereby reducing their efficacy (36). Whenever antiseptics are used, several important points should be kept in mind: a minimum contact time, which varies with the type of disinfectant, is necessary to kill organisms; repeated accidental introduction of antiseptics in the dialysate circuit may induce severe long term peritoneal complications: this process was suspected in cases of sclerosing peritonitis occurring in CAPD patients using routinely chlorhexidine solutions in 70% alcohol (44). In the absence of an ideal antiseptic, the use of 70% ethanol (containing 1% glycerol as emollient when used as a skin disinfectant) appears commendable because of a lower toxicity and a more reproducible efficacy than other disinfectants (38, 39).

Access to the peritoneal cavity

Today, peritoneal dialysis is always done with a single catheter. This technique, which permits the tidal irrigation of the peritoneum and prevents fluid channelling, prevailed over the two-catheter approach proposed during the pioneering era (45) because of its simplicity and safety.

The key to successful chronic peritoneal dialysis is a permanent and safe access to the peritoneal cavity. Mastering all the aspects of peritoneal catheter implantation and utilisation should be the major concern of the nephrologist contemplating the use of PD in his patients. Adherence to current recommendations on peritoneal catheter management will promote success (46).

Disposable versus permanent catheters

Two main types of peritoneal catheters are available: the disposable stylet catheter (Trocath, McGaw Laboratories, Irvine, CA, USA) and the permanent Silastic catheter. Extensive clinical experience indicates that permanent indwelling Silastic catheters have many advantages over disposable catheters and should be preferred even in acute renal failure. These advantages include avoidance of repeated puncture if several dialysis sessions are required, ease of instituting dialysis, excellent irrigation characteristics independent of patient's position, no pain during and between dialysis, few restrictions in physical and recreational activities leading to excellent patient's acceptance and suitability to self dialysis (31). However, there are still some specific indications for the use of disposable catheters, e.g. in the setting of severe extracellular volume overload and severe hyperkalemia when dialysis should be quickly instituted, because of one way obstruction of the Silastic catheter with abdominal distension (drainage of the peritoneal cavity can be accomplished through a stylet catheter), in situations where only one dialysis session is contemplated or during antibiotic treatment of a skin infection of the abdominal wall before implanting a permanent Silastic catheter. It should be mentioned, however, that many nephrologists, when faced with such conditions, would institute hemodialysis with the use of a temporary vascular access (i.e. subclavian [47] or internal jugular vein catheter [48]) rather than resorting to peritoneal dialysis.

Recommendations for placement of peritoneal catheters and preparation of the patient

Before inserting a peritoneal catheter, the bladder should be emptied. If the patient cannot void, urethral catheterization should be done. Constipated patients should have an enema prior to the procedure. Abdominal hair should be removed preferably with an electric shaver, from xyphoid to symphysis pubis and a large area of skin disinfected. The physician should examine carefully the patient's abdomen to detect abnormalities which may cause difficulties (e.g. previous surgery, skin infection or organomegaly). The operator should wear mask, cap, sterile gown and gloves; the sterile field is shielded to isolate the patient; all assistants and bystanders should wear masks and caps. If the patient is conscious, the physician should give him a detailed description of the procedure to relieve anxiety and obtain his cooperation. As the procedure progresses, each step of the operation has to be explained to the patient. This will allow catheter implantation under mild sedation (diazepam 10% intramuscularly, atropine 0.25 mg intramuscularly) and local anaesthesia (1 to 2% lidocaine) in most patients.

Disposable stylet catheter (Trocath): description, technique of implantation and withdrawal

Description
The disposable stylet catheter (Trocath) consists of two parts: a rigid plastic catheter of approximately 3 mm overall diameter and 25 to 30 cm in length, with multiple small holes on its distal 8 cm; a metal stylet protruding from the end of the catheter, providing a sharp cutting tip to penetrate the abdominal wall.

Technique of insertion
To reduce the hazards of catheter implantation, filling the abdomen with prewarmed dialysis solutions is recommended prior to catheter insertion. Enough fluid is infused to distend the abdomen moderately without causing discomfort or respiratory embarrassment to the patient. Priming may be done through a large bore (14 to 15 gauge) short bevel spinal needle (8 to 10 cm long) or during the procedure itself, after introducing the perforated segment of the catheter within the peritoneal cavity. Priming the abdomen with fluid increases the safety of introducing the stylet catheter; it creates a fluid cushion which maintains the parietal peritoneum against the abdominal wall, it reduces the risk of bowel perforation and facilitates catheter positioning as the intestinal loops float freely in a fluid medium.

The usual insertion site is on the midline 3 to 6 cm below the umbilicus. The catheter may also be located in either iliac fossa. After local anaesthesia, a 2 mm skin incision is made with a # 11 blade; the catheter should fit snugly in the wound to prevent leakage and to reduce the risk of infection. Nicking the fascia of the linea alba with the blade reduces the force needed to carry the catheter through. The stylet catheter is inserted perpendicular to the abdominal wall, while the patient tightens his abdominal musculature; a sudden decrease in resistance occurs when the stylet catheter passes the parietal peritoneum and enters the peritoneal cavity. The stylet is then withdrawn about 2 cm to sheathe its cutting tip. If the abdomen has not been primed with fluid prior to the procedure, the catheter should be advanced until all perforations are within the peritoneal cavity; the stylet should then be withdrawn and 2,000 ml of dialysis fluid infused into the abdominal cavity. At this point, the catheter, with reinserted stylet but with shielded cutting tip is advanced at 45 degrees into the true pelvis; the stylet is then removed. The dialysis fluid should well up into the catheter lumen confirming that the catheter is in the peritoneal space; the administration set is attached to the catheter and the dialysate is allowed to drain out. Careful positioning of the catheter is essential to achieve a technically statisfactory dialysis. Final placement is made by assessing drainage and by positioning the tip of the catheter according to the patient's comfort. The catheter is fixed to the abdominal wall with nonallergic surgical tape. The entry site is protected with several sterile 10 cm gauze squares cut to fit around the catheter, that are then taped to the skin.

Stylet catheter withdrawal

When dialysis is completed, the peritoneal cavity is emptied and the catheter is removed under strict aseptic conditions. Occasionally, catheter withdrawal may be uncomfortable and painful to the patient due to the penetration of omental fringes into the holes in the distal segment of the catheter. When this occurs, the catheter should be gently mobilised and freed by a slow axial rotation after infusing 2 ml of 1% procaine into the lumen of the catheter. After withdrawing the catheter, the stab wound is closed with surgical tape strips and dressed for 48 h.

Complications related to insertion of stylet catheters

Numerous complications (Table 1) have been described with the use of the stylet catheter (49, 50). Most of them are due to inexperience, and can be avoided by following accurately the correct implantation procedure.

Bleeding is frequently observed after catheter implantation and clears spontaneously after a few dialysate exchanges. The addition of heparin (500 UI/l) to the dialysis solution is recommended to prevent early catheter clotting. Major bleeding is diagnosed when effluent dialysate is grossly bloody (hematocrit >5%). In most circumstances, the site of bleeding is in the abdominal wall, the blood seeping into the peritoneal cavity at the peritoneal entry site. At-

tempts to stop bleeding include the following: pressure dressing, placement of a deep purse string around the catheter, injection of epinephrine in the tissues surrounding the catheter, and discontinuation of heparin in the dialysis fluid (with the associated risk of catheter plugging by blood clots). It is often difficult to assess the efficiency of such measures since bleeding has a tendency to stop spontaneously. A transfusion is rarely needed and the necessity for laparotomy is exceptional.

Bowel perforation is a rare complication. This accident is best prevented by priming the abdomen with fluid prior to catheter insertion; during placement, the catheter should never be forced into the peritoneal cavity whenever intra-abdominal resistance occurs. Previous abdominal surgery (with peritoneal adhesions), distension of the bowel with gas, or a scaphoid abdomen are the usual predisposing factors. The risk of perforation is also high when the patient is unconscious or cachectic. In these circumstances, surgical placement should be preferred to blind implantation. A perforation of the gut has to be suspected in case of failure of dialysate to drain, cloudy, malodorous or frankly faeculent returning fluid or watery diarrhoea (51); the stool has then a strongly positive Clinistix test for glucose. Early signs of peritoneal irritation are common. Two therapeutic approaches have been equally successful: firstly conservative management with local and systemic antibiotics and continued peritoneal dialysis through another abdominal entry site (51, 52), secondly laparotomy and surgical repair of the perforation, followed by continuous antibiotic lavage to prevent formation of peritoneal adhesions and loss of peritoneal surface area (31).

Perforation of the bladder has also been reported (51); after continuous drainage of the bladder with a Foley catheter and inserting a new peritoneal catheter, the dialyses were continued uneventfully.

Leakage of dialysis fluid around the catheter is a consequence of too large an incision of the skin and/or the peritoneum. This apparently benign complication should be prevented as leaking interferes with accurate fluid balance, causes abdominal wall and scrotal edema and carries the risk of infection. Catheter re-insertion through a new small incision and avoidance of abdominal overdistension with dialysis fluid are effective measures.

Inadequate drainage of peritoneal fluid is often encountered when a hurried operator does not take the necessary time to position the catheter properly and to check the adequacy of the drainage at the time of implantation. Other possible causes of inadequate drainage are: disruption of the siphon effect due to air gaining access into the peritoneal cavity, blockage of side-holes by omentum, intraperitoneal pooling of fluid by adhesions, and fibrin or blood clots plugging the catheter lumen (49, 50). Manipulating (or) flushing the catheter may restore a proper drainage; in case of failure, catheter replacement is mandatory. When plugging of the catheter by blood clots is suspected, catheter disobstruction may be achieved by instilling a fibrinolytic agent (streptokinase 250,000 U) in the catheter lumen and waiting 1.0 h before resuming dialysis.

Table 1. Complications related to insertion and use of stylet catheters.

A) *During percutaneous insertion procedures*
   Preperitoneal catheter placement
   Perforation of a hollow viscus:
      small bowel, colon, urinary bladder
   Injury to a splanchnic vessel
   Subcutaneous bleeding

B) *During peritoneal dialysis*
   Leakage of peritoneal dialysis fluid
   Pelvic pain (perineal, rectal, vaginal)
   Persistent intraperitoneal bleeding
   One or two-way catheter obstruction (clot, omental wrapping)
   Accidental pulling out of the catheter
   Failure to drain by loss of siphon effect
   Hematoma of the pouch of Douglas
   Loss of catheter in the peritoneal cavity

C) *Discontinuation of peritoneal dialysis*
   Peritoneal fluid seeping at the catheter insertion site
   Skin infection at the site of catheter implantation

Pain in a localised area (e.g. rectum, vagina), may result from mechanical trauma by the catheter tip. Relief will be obtained by withdrawing slowly the semirigid catheter a few centimeters.

Skin infection at the site of the stylet catheter (49) implantation is seldom reported, but is rather common. It should be prevented by careful cleansing of the skin stab wound after catheter removal; if successive catheter placements are necessary, repeated puncture at the same site should be avoided.

Other complications related to catheter placement include loss of catheter into the peritoneal cavity (49, 50), preperitoneal catheter placement with creation of a preperitoneal space due to not perforating the linea alba and peritoneum with the stylet (50), and accidental pulling out of the catheter during dialysis by an agitated patient (49).

Permanent (indwelling) Silastic peritoneal catheters

As shown in Figure 1, several types of permanent peritoneal catheters are currently available. The original straight Tenckhoff catheter introduced in 1968 (7), remains, two decades later, the golden standard for peritoneal access (53). This prosthesis is made of silicone rubber tubing, a material well tolerated by the peritoneal serosa (54). Other types of peritoneal catheters were developed in an attempt to prevent the most common complications of the Tenckhoff catheters, but they are basically modified versions of the original prototype.

The standard Tenckhoff peritoneal catheter
Made of straight Silastic tubing (35 to 45 cm long, 3 mm inner diameter), the Tenckhoff catheter is fitted with one or two Dacron felt cuffs. The double cuff model seems to satisfy the needs of most patients and is used most widely. The usual intercuff distance is 5 cm for non obese patients, it should be increased to 7 cm for use in obese subjects to permit correct positioning of the catheter in the presence of excessive abdominal wall adipose tissue. The two Dacron cuffs delineate three segments: the intraperitoneal portion (20 cm overall length), perforated with side holes on its distal 15 cm to improve dialysate flow; the subcutaneous portion, 5 to 7 cm long; the external segment, 20 to 30 cm long. The inner (distal) cuff is placed deeply at the entry point of the catheter in the peritoneal cavity; the outer (proximal) cuff should be located in the subcutaneous tissue 2 cm inside the skin exit; the segment between the two cuffs lies in a tunnel of subcutaneous tissue.

Other permanent catheters
Alternative models of peritoneal access devices were developed in an attempt to avoid three major complications of the standard Tenckhoff catheter, namely exit site and/or tunnel infections, external cuff extrusion, and migration of the catheter tip out of the true pelvis. Four peritoneal catheters were specifically designed to avoid the migration of intraperitoneal portion of the catheter and consequent omental wrapping: the Coil-Cath catheters (55), the Oreopoulos-

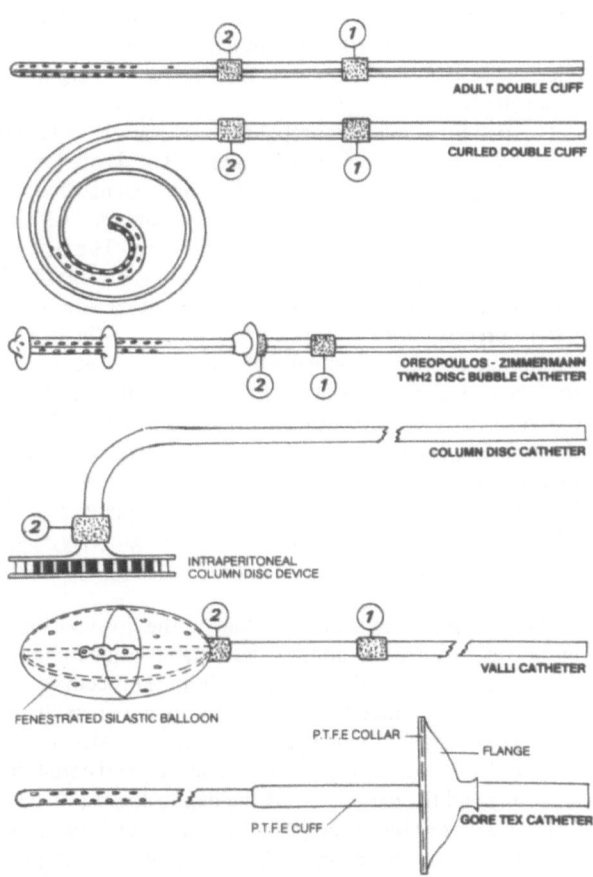

Figure 1. Main types of peritoneal catheters; 'adult double cuff' refers to the standard double cuff Tenckhoff catheter.

Zellerman (TWH) catheter (56), the Valli catheter (57) and the Column Disc catheter (58). The main distinguishing features of these various catheters lie with modifications of the intra-abdominal portion including 1) a curled shape for the Coil-Cath catheter, 2) the presence of two flat silicone rubber disks glued 5 cm apart perpendicular to the tubing for the TWH catheter, 3) a perforated balloon surrounding the perforated part of the intra-abdominal segment for the Valli catheter and 4) the replacement of the intra-abdominal portion by a distribution head made of two silicone rubber discs separated by Silastic columns for the Column Disk catheter. Two other prostheses were developed with the aim of reducing the incidence of exit site infection and external cuff extrusion: the Gore-Tex catheter (59) has a polytetrafluoroethylene (PTFE) disc lying immediately beneath the skin and is surrounded by a long PTFE sheath extending down to the peritoneum; the Swan Neck Missouri catheter (60) is characterised by its permanently bent subcutaneous segment.

Catheter implantation techniques
The long-term survival of the peritoneal catheter depends

essentially upon the competence and experience of the catheter insertion team. Implantation procedures should be done exclusively by an experienced operator (surgeon or nephrologist).

The patient should be prepared as previously described for stylet catheter insertion (vide supra). The day before the operation, the exit site should be identified and marked with a skin marker; it should be above or below the belt line, taking into account the patient's preference. The exit site should not be placed on a scar and should be above fat folds, the extent of which is determined in a sitting position (46).

The prescription of prophylactic antibiotics before implantation appears commendable in view of the general surgical experience indicating that perioperative antibiotics diminish the incidence of wound infection, particularly in the presence of a foreign body. It is recommended that 1 g of first generation cephalosporin be given intravenously one hour before the operation and two subsequent doses of 500 mg each given 8 and 12 h later. Alternatively, 1 g of vancomycin can be administered intravenously the day before the operation (46).

Catheter insertion should be done in the hospital setting under strict sterile conditions. The catheter can be implanted as a surgical (open) or a bedside (blind) procedure. The choice of the implantation modality ('open' versus 'blind') depends mostly upon logistics (e.g. easy access to an operating theatre, availability of an experienced and committed surgeon) and the experience of the nephrologist (46, 53).

Bedside insertion of the peritoneal catheter is often preferred when a nephrologist is in charge of catheter placement (61). Bedside insertion is contraindicated in extremely obese patients or in those who have had previous abdominal surgery, since peritoneal adhesions increase the risk of accidental viscus perforation. In addition, it should be preferably avoided in cachectic patients, in those treated with corticosteroids or in children. To facilitate assessment of catheter function during and immediately after completion of insertion, the abdomen may be filled with 1.5% dextrose solution containing heparin (1,000 U/l) (see section on placement of stylet catheter).

Under local anaesthesia, a 4 to 6 cm midline skin incision is made below the umbilicus. The linea alba is exposed by blunt dissection with a hemostat. A special trocar with a bivalved tip is used (31). Trocar insertion is made easier by a stab incision of the fascia and is performed perpendicular to the abdominal wall asking the patient to tighten his musculature. The permanent catheter, stiffened by an obturator, is then introduced in the peritoneal space using the trocar which is directed caudally; for this maneuver the obturator should not protrude at the tip of the catheter to prevent injury to intra-abdominal structures. The catheter should be gently advanced toward the pelvis without strain. If progression of the catheter is impeded by elastic resistance, omental entanglement of the catheter tip must be suspected. The catheter should then be withdrawn and reinserted at a different angle. When the catheter tip reaches the deeper pelvis, the patient notes a sense of pressure at the rectum. At this point, the obturator is withdrawn and the catheter is

checked for easy irrigation. In case of persisting pain, indicating that the intra-abdominal catheter portion is too long or too far in, the catheter is pulled back on a few centimeters or removed and reinserted after trimming away up to 5 cm of its distal end. Careful attention should be given to obtain a satisfactory catheter position allowing painless easy irrigation lest continuing pain necessitates early catheter replacement or leads to the patient's refusal of peritoneal dialysis. The trocar is then removed. The deeper cuff is tightly anchored to the peritoneum and to the linea alba in a 45 degree position maintaining the intra-abdominal catheter segment in a caudal direction. A lateral subcutaneous tunnel with an arcuate course should be created; a 5 mm stab incision is made at its external end to give way to the external catheter segment. The exit site should be caudally oriented and properly dimensioned to fit nicely around the Silastic tube. If the exit site is too large infection may develop or if it is too small sloughing may occur. The subcutaneous Dacron felt cuff should be placed about 2 cm inside the skin exit to prevent skin erosion. The catheter is then placed into the subcutaneous tunnel and its external segment pulled through the skin exit with the aid of a metal guide. The optimal post-operative position of the Tenckhoff catheter is depicted on Figure 2. The catheter should be irrigated with heparinised saline and closed with a rubber cap. The midline incision is closed and dressed. Dialysis should be started as soon as possible adding heparin (500 U/l) to the dialysis fluid.

Other methods are available for the percutaneous insertion of straight or curled Tenckhoff catheters at the bedside. One approach utilises a wire-guide for the lateral implantation of the catheter in the right or left lower quadrant (McBurney or contralateral point) (62). Another procedure consists in the midline insertion of the catheter using an angiotcath and a disposable dilator and introducer sheath inserted into the peritoneal space over a wire-guide (63). Finally, another appraoch advocates the placement of the Tenckhoff catheter under direct peritoneoscopic control after insufflation of air into the peritoneal cavity (64).

Whenever possible, 'open' surgical implantation of the peritoneal catheter should be preferred to 'blind' bedside procedures (53). Reasons for this preference are: priming the abdomen with fluid prior to the operation is not necessary; a better catheter positioning is obtained under direct vision; entanglement of the catheter tip with the omentum is easily prevented by pulling the omentum towards the upper abdomen with a finger or a smooth hemostat during catheter insertion; adhesions when present can be freed to prevent subsequent loculation of dialysis fluid; finally, surgical implantation may obtain longer catheter survival than bedside implantation of the Tenckhoff catheter (56).

The catheter can be implanted either in the midline or in a lateral paramedian position. The lateral approach, however, is considered as the procedure of choice because it reduces dialysate leakage and hernia (46, 56, 65).

Surgical insertion can be done under either local or general anaesthesia. General anaesthesia should be preferred in the pusillanimous patient, the obese patient, or those with previous abdominal surgery as well as in children. With the

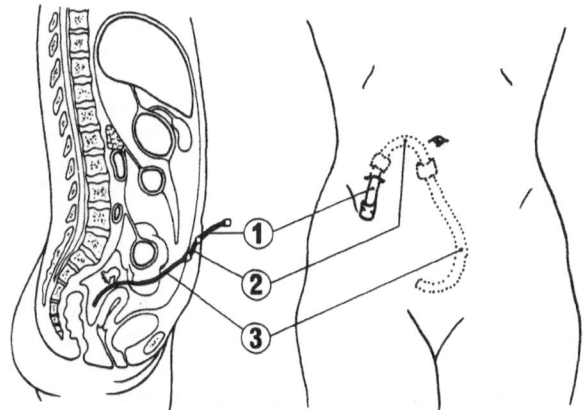

Figure 2. Double-cuffed Tenckhoff catheter placed as recommended by Tenckhoff (31): 1) external segment (note the downwards orientation of the exit site on the right side of the figure); 2) subcutaneous segment with its two Dacron felt cuffs; 3) intraperitoneal segment. As shown on the postero-anterior section, the tip of the intraperitoneal segment should lie deep into the pouch of Douglas.

simultaneous administration of a sedative, local anaesthesia is adequate for the 'open' surgical implantation of the double cuff straight Tenckhoff catheter.

The main aspects of surgical implantation of the peritoneal catheters are presented in this section. Two approaches are possible: midline and lateral. They differ by the position given to the preperitoneal (distal) Dacron cuff: between the peritoneum and linea alba with the midline insertion, and lying in the rectus abdominis muscle in the lateral approach. The midline approach is technically simpler and may be mastered more easily by a trained nephrologist (53) whereas the lateral approach will rather require the competence of an experienced surgeon (66–69).

For *midline surgical implantation,* under local anaesthesia, a 4 to 6 cm midline skin incision is made below the umbilicus. The incision is deepened down to the linea alba which is incised. The peritoneum is identified, incised and marked with haemostats. The catheter, stiffened by an obturator and previously moistened with heparinised saline is gently introduced in the peritoneal cavity. For this manoeuvre, the obturator should not protrude at the tip of the catheter to prevent injury to intra-abdominal structures. The catheter is slowly inserted without strain in the depth of the pelvis. If progression of the catheter is hindered by elastic resistence, omental entanglement or abutement against a bowel loop of the catheter must be suspected. The catheter should be withdrawn: the absence of adhesions should be checked with the index finger or under direct visual control. The catheter should be reinserted at a different angle and the intra-abdominal segment placed in the depth of the true pelvis. When the catheter reaches the deeper pelvis, the patient notes a sense of pressure at the rectum. At this point, the obturator is withdrawn and the catheter is checked for ease of irrigation. In case of persisting pain indicating that the intra-abdominal portion of the catheter is too long or too far in, the catheter is pulled back

on a few centimetres or removed and reinserted after triming away up to 5 cm of its distal end. Careful attention should be given to obtain a satisfactory catheter position allowing painless, easy irrigation. When a satisfactory position of the intra-abdominal portion is obtained, the peritoneum should be tightly closed around the catheter to prevent dialysate leak. The deeper cuff is anchored to the peritoneum in a 45 degree angle maintaining the intra-abdominal catheter segment in a caudal direction. The subcutaneous tunnel is fashioned as for the 'bedside' blind insertion. The catheter subcutaneous segment is carefully positioned into the tunnel. After checking that dialysis solution inflow and outflow are freely obtained, the skin is closed as described for the 'bedside' technique. Dialysis may be started soon after implantation, but it may also be delayed using one of the break-in techniques described below (46).

Some groups advocate *lateral surgical implantation* as the procedure of choice, because it reduces the incidence of dialysate leakage and hernia (46, 56, 65, 68). A 4 to 6 cm horizontal (68) or vertical (69) paramedian incision is made into the skin overlying the rectus sheath below the level of the umbilicus. Care should be taken to prevent injury to the inferior epigastric vessels. The rectus abdominis muscle is then exposed to an horizontal incision of the anterior rectus sheath. The fibers of the rectus abdominis are separated carefully in the direction of the fibers to expose the peritoneum. The peritoneal catheter with its guide is inserted through a small swab incision. The guide is removed and the peritoneal opening is tightly closed with a pass of the sutures through the internal Dacron cuff which is then buried within the rectus muscle. The catheter is pulled through a stab incision made in the superior flap of the anterior rectus sheath 5 cm above the incision of the posterior rectus sheath. A subcutaneous tunnel is created, up to the lateral exit site chosen earlier by the patient. Great care should be taken to give the tunnel the arcuate shape and to orient the exit site caudally to allow free drainage of the external segment of the tunnel and reduce the risk of infection (31). The exit site should be placed superior to the fascial insertion site so as to minimise the potential for catheter displacement secondary to the Silastic tubing resilience. The catheter is then placed into the subcutaneous tunnel and its external segment pulled through the skin. The final stages of lateral catheter insertion are similar to those of the midline approach. Whichever method of catheter insertion is used, great care must be taken to achieve complete hemostasis and a watertight wound (66–69).

Post operative care and break in procedures

Catheter care is as follows. The exit site of the catheter should be kept clean and dry at all times. It should be protected by a 8 × 8 cm sterile gauze dressing which also prevents direct contact of the catheter with the skin. Before and after each dialysis, the exit site is cleaned with sterile applicators dipped into povidone-iodine (Betadine) or hydrogen peroxide. When the wound and exit site are healed, a daily shower is recommended after removing the dressing; after the shower, the exit site is carefully dried and cleaned with Betadine. For the long term, the patient may chose either to cover the skin exit site with an occlusive dressing, or to leave it exposed between the showers, as the incidence of skin exit infection and of peritonitis is similar whether or not a dressing is used (70).

During the immediate post operative period, several approaches of catheter break-in have been proposed. Some authors, following Tenckhoff's recommendation (31) institute small volume rapid exchange intermittent peritoneal dialysis for 2 to 3 days. An outpatient irrigation technique has been developed in which the content of a single bag of 0.5 l heparinised dialysis solution is sequentially infused, drained from and reinfused into the peritoneal cavity three times a day by the patient himself. This in and out close circuit rinsing procedure does not require aseptic precautions and the dialysis bag is changed every day by nursing personnel until CAPD training can be initiated (71). Another post operative approach consists in flushing the peritoneal cavity with 0.5 l of dialysis solutions until the effluent return is clear of blood. Once this is achieved, 100 to 200 ml of heparinised dialysis solution should be left in the peritoneal cavity and the catheter capped (46). The first dialysis should preferably be delayed for 2 to 3 days to allow for good healing. If dialysis must be initiated immediately after implantation, IPD with a reduced exchange volume (500 ml) should be utilised. To prevent early dialysate leakage, CAPD should not start for about 2 weeks after catheter insertion. Meanwhile, the patient should be maintained on IPD with gradually increasing exchange volumes or on hemodialysis, unless adequate residual renal function permits dispensing with dialysis (46).

Complications of peritoneal catheters

Numerous complications listed in Table 2, have been described following the implantation of indwelling peritoneal catheters and during their long term use. Most of them may be prevented by adhering to sterile procedures and by giving careful attention to important details during catheter insertion and postoperative care. Adequate patient training plays the major role in this prevention. The patient should be thoroughly informed on safe catheter utilization procedures and the need to maintain excellent personal hygiene. He should also be taught about the early detection of catheter related problems. The patient should be instructed to report problems without delay to a member of the peritoneal dialysis team, as prompt medical intervention may often avoid catheter loss (72).

Early post operative complications
Pain may occur in the perineal area, urinary bladder or in the rectum, following the introduction of the catheter into the true pelvis. Encountered in 3 to 8% of the patients (73), this painful sensation is usually mild and tends to resolve spontaneously during the fortnight following catheter placement. On rare occasions, however, persistent or more intense pain due to the permanent pressure of the catheter tip on the parietal peritoneum may require a laparotomy to shorten a straight Tenckhoff catheter or to position the intraperitoneal segment of the prosthesis in a different location.

Leakage of dialysis fluid occurs when the peritoneum is not tightly closed at the point of entry of the catheter. The incidence of this complication varies from 3 to 30% according to the series (53, 56, 73, 74). Significant risk factors for leakage include age over 60 years, obesity, diabetes mellitus, chronic use of steroids, previous catheter implantation and multiparity in women (73). An anti-leakage technique, consisting in the placement of a double purse string suture around the peritoneal catheter and the distal Dacron cuff, reduced the dialysate leakage rate to below 1.0% in one series (75). Leakage presents itself as discharge of dialysis fluid at the catheter exit site or as an infiltration of subcutaneous tissue of the anterior abdominal wall, resulting in scrotal swelling. When a leak occurs, CAPD should be discontinued. The patient should be maintained on IPD with small exchange volumes, or transferred to hemodialysis for 1 or 2 weeks, giving enough time for the leak to seal off. Leakage may be effectively prevented by a careful surgical technique, the lateral placement of the catheter and by waiting several days after catheter insertion before initiating peritoneal dialysis (46, 56, 65).

Table 2. Complications of peritoneal catheters.

A) *Operative and early post-operative complications*
   Pain in the perineal area (rectum, vagina, urinary bladder)
   Leakage of dialysis fluid
      external dialysate leak
      subcutaneous infiltration
      scrotal edema
   Reflex ileus
   Bleeding
      exit site oozing, tunnel hematoma
      intraperitoneal bleeding
      severe hemorrhage from mesenteric vessel injury
   Perforation of hollow viscus
      small bowel or colon
      urinary bladder
   Exit site infection

B) *Complications occurring during long term use*
   Skin exit-site infection
   Tunnel infection
   Catheter cuff erosion and prolapse
   Catheter malfunction (one way obstruction)
   Functional failure to drain (constipation)
   Two-way obstruction
      intraluminal clot
      catheter kinking
   Pericatheter hernia or pseudohernia
   Perforation of posterior peritoneum
   Severing of Silastic tubing

C) *Complications occurring after interruption of peritoneal dialysis*
   Ileal or colonic perforation
   Intraabdominal hematoma with superinfection

Reflex ileus following catheter implantation is common but rarely persists beyond 24 to 36 h. In an occasional patient, a persistent paralytic ileus with major abdominal distension will occur, even when implantation has been uneventful. Oral mannitol in a 10% solution and hypertonic enemas help to restore intestinal motility. Oral feeding should be delayed until bowel function returns, to prevent vomiting that could result in an undue stress to the healing tissues (70).

Bleeding is observed occasionally during the first few exchanges following catheter implantation. This rare complication is easily eliminated by careful hemostasis during surgical placement. In patients with major abdominal operations prior to catheter insertion, the need to divide existing peritoneal adhesions increases significantly the risk of bleeding (76).

Perforation of a hollow viscus or injury to other intraperitoneal structures (such as the mesenteric vessels) are exceptional with a surgical technique. They occur mainly when the peritoneal catheter is placed with a 'blind' method. They are best prevented by avoiding forceful insertion against intraabdominal resistence and by making sure that the catheter guide is sheathed within the Silastic tube for introducing the catheter into the peritoneal cavity.

Infection of the exit site in the postoperative period complicates 3 to 5% of catheter placements (65, 73). Strict adhesion to aseptic precautions in the care of operative wound and exit site is a major step in the prevention of this complication. During catheter placement, the cuffs should be soaked in saline solution. Air is expelled from the Dacron felt of the cuffs, a procedure that enhances fibroblast ingrowth and tissue fixation (72). Prophylactic antibiotics are also considered a useful adjunct to the prevention of early exit site infection (46). An occlusive dressing should be applied in the operating room and changed daily by competent personnel until healing is complete (72). The catheter, anchored to the abdominal wall with adhesive tape should be immobilised at all times.

Late complications

Skin exit infection and catheter malfunction are the two most common complications occurring during long term utilization of the indwelling peritoneal catheter. Both alike alter significantly catheter survival.

Skin exit infection is observed in 15 to 30% of the patients (73–76). Its early recognition is essential to prevent contiguous contamination of the subcutaneous Dacron cuff and subsequent tunnel infection. Most infections are caused either by external contamination or by microtrauma due to repeated tension and tugging of the catheter external segment. Numerous factors may trigger exit site infection including: 1) a poorly drained tunnel; 2) poor exit site selection and placement; 3) poor tunnel and exit site construction; 4) improper subcutaneous (proximal) cuff placement; 5) improper post operative wound or exit site cleansing or 6) improper maintenance of the exit site (72). Dialysate leakage around the catheter, skin reactivity against the catheter with the production of foreign body granuloma (77), allergic

dermatitis (53, 78), or patient's susceptibility to infection due to depressed immunity may also contribute in the genesis of this complication. Divergent opinions exist about the effect of single versus double cuff catheters on exit site infection rates. Some studies reported a similar incidence of infections with both types of catheters (79, 80), while other groups observed a reduced rate with the double cuff catheter (81, 82). Staphylococcus aureus is the most common infecting agent, followed by Staphylococcus epidermidis, Pseudomonas aeruginosa, Enterobacteriacae and Corynebacterium species (53, 83–85). Continued moisture or slight bleeding at the exit site may be the first indication of an infection at this site. Pain and redness are manifestations of a progressing infection, while the presence of granulation tissue implies an advanced infection (72). Once infection is suspected, a culture should be taken and antistaphylococcal antibiotherapy should be started without delay, later adapted according to microbiologic data and maintained for at least two weeks. Infection of the exit site is frequently associated with peritonitis and tunnel infections (53, 84–86). Considered as an indication for catheter removal, this complication is an important cause of catheter loss (86). Infection should be cured before implanting a new catheter. Meanwhile, the patient is maintained on haemodialysis. With double cuff catheters, skin exit site infection may be cured by externalization and shaving of the infected cuff (53, 65), but this approach was found unsuccessful in one series (83).

Tunnel infection is often associated to exit site infection, but it can occur even in the presence of a normal exit site. The skin over the tunnel is erythematous, indurated and tender. Tunnel infection may extend deeply into the abdominal wall and may cause persisting peritonitis by intraperitoneal bacterial seeding. It may also evolve in cellulitis by the contiguous invasion of surrounding tissues. In addition to aggressive antibiotic treatment and surgical drainage of the subcutaneous tunnel, catheter removal is always necessary.

Catheter cuff erosion and prolapse are due to pressure necrosis or to infection of the skin at the catheter exit site or both. To prevent this complication, the subcutaneous catheter tunnel should be of an appropriate length and the subcutaneous Dacron cuff should lie into the subcutaneous tissue at about 2 cm from the exit site. The use of a Swan Neck peritoneal catheter is also advocated to prevent cuff extrusion; the arcuate shape of this permanently bent prosthesis decreases the pressure exerted by the Silastic tubing on the skin around the exit site (81). Cuff extrusion requires elective catheter removal and replacement with one cuff catheter, while two cuff catheters may be left in situ after shaving the external cuff (65).

Catheter malfunction is a frequent complication occurring in about 15 to 20% of implanted peritoneal catheters (73) and representing up to 43% of catheter failures (79). Two way obstruction is usually due to intraluminal occlusion by blood or fibrin clots, particularly following catheter placement or during peritonitis episodes. The clots can be dislodged by forceful irrigation with a syringe or dissolved by instillation of streptokinase (87). Kinking of the catheter can also be a cause of inflow obstruction requiring surgical exploration (46). One way obstruction presents itself as a reduction in drainage flow rates or complete failure to drain. Causes of outflow obstruction include 1) displacement of the intraperitoneal segment in the upper abdomen (31, 81, 88), 2) omental wrapping of the catheter (31), 3) incarceration of fatty peritoneal fringes within catheter side holes (31), 4) catheter encasement by adhesions, or 5) fungal invasion of the catheter (89). The careful construction of an arcuate subcutaneous tunnel that is convex upwards is essential to prevent the translocation of the intraperitoneal portion of the catheter (31). The caudal direction of the internal segment of the tunnel tends to keep the catheter in the true pelvis and prevents omental wrapping (81). Partial omentectomy is another measure proposed to prevent the capture of the intraperitoneal segment by the omentum (65). Early observations suggesting that curled (55) or TWH catheters (90) could prevent catheter tip dislodgement were not confirmed in larger series (81, 88, 91, 92). Outflow obstruction due to catheter tip translocation may respond to catheter manipulation and relocation in the true pelvis following intraluminal insertion of a bent stiff trocar (88, 93). Spontaneous relocation of a migrated catheter tip may also occur. Other causes of outflow obstruction require surgical revision and relocation of the peritoneal catheter or its removal and replacement. Before contemplating surgery, a catheterography may help to identify the cause of obstruction and decide on the appropriate treatment (94).

Failure to drain may be also of functional, reversible origin. This common complication of chronic peritoneal dialysis responds readily to bowel stimulation by oral administration of mannitol or by enema. This treatment should always be tried before seeking a mechanical cause of catheter failure (31).

Pericatheter hernia or pseudohernia is a complication most commonly observed with the single cuff catheters. Pseudohernia consists in a dilatation of the fibrous tract surrounding the catheter subcutaneous segment by intra-abdominal dialysate, rather than an eventration of the peritoneum through a weakness of the anterior abdominal wall (79). Pericatheter hernia may be related to poor surgical technique or to suboptimal tissue healing. The lateral paramedian technique for catheter insertion (46, 65, 68) and the use of double cuff catheters (79) markedly decreased the frequency of pseudohernia.

Other complications include the perforation of the posterior peritoneum by the catheter tip (95), the accidental severing of the external segment of the Silastic tubing, the rupture of the Silastic tubing in its subcutaneous segment due to accidental brisk tugging of the dialysate tubing or the late occurrence of localised abdominal pain exacerbated during dialysis fluid infusion (53). The latter is suggestive of adhesion formation around the catheter tip and should be treated by catheter revision and relocation (53).

Complications occurring after discontinuation of peritoneal dialysis

Erosion of the ileum (96) or of the sigmoid (97, 98) and superinfection of an intra-abdominal hematoma (99) were observed in patients with indwelling peritoneal catheters left in situ after CAPD discontinuation. These complications, although exceptional, raise the issue of timely catheter removal when CAPD is interrupted (46, 99).

Management of peritoneal catheters after transplantation

Renal transplantation can successfully be performed in patients receiving CAPD (100–102). In cadaveric transplantation, the peritoneal catheter should be left in place at the time of transplantation provided the skin exit site is not infected. This practice will allow easy resumption of CAPD in case of early posttransplant failure; it makes also possible to dialyze the patient during post operative acute renal failure if the peritoneum has not been transected at operation. If exit site infection is present, the catheter should be removed at the end of the operation. With living related transplants, the catheter should be treated in the same way as in cadaveric transplant for one haplotype 'matches', as the results are similar in both cases; on the other hand, two haplotypes 'matches' should have their catheter removed as the chance of achieving a successful graft is greater than 90% (46). Post transplant catheter care includes once weekly change of dressing until the catheter is removed. Cultures of peritoneal fluid are taken once a week while in the hospital but not thereafter, unless clinically indicated. If the graft functions satisfactorily, the peritoneal catheter should be removed in 2 to 3 months (46).

Catheter revision, removal and replacement

Catheter revision is indicated in the presence of catheter malfunction or persistent localized abdominal pain suspected to originate from the catheter tip. Under local anaesthesia, the original incision is reopened: the abdominal wall is dissected down through the fascia to the point of entry of the catheter into the peritoneal cavity; below this point, the peritoneum is incised over about 3 to 4 cm; the intraperitoneal segment is pulled out from the peritoneal space with a finger or a smooth forceps and freed from surrounding adhesions or incarcerated tissues. The intraperitoneal segment is then shortened if necessary and properly positioned into the true pelvis (53). The operation is completed by water tight closure of the peritoneum and of the abdominal incision.

Catheter removal is indicated in the following circumstances; 1) peritonitis recurring with the same organism 10 to 15 days after cessation of adequate antibiotherapy, 2) peritonitis not responding to treatment for 5 to 7 days, 3) fecal peritonitis, 4) persisting dialysate leakage, 5) one way obstruction not cured by manipulations or catheter revision, 6) complete catheter obstruction, 7) interruption of PD following improvement in renal function, transfer to hemodialysis or renal transplantation (103, 104). Catheter removal is commonly considered as absolutely indicated in recurrent peritonitis; several groups, however, achieved the cure of this complication by local infusion of streptokinase (105,

106) or urokinase (107, 108) without removing the permanent catheter. Fungal or tuberculous peritonitis are also considered as indications for catheter removal (103), but they may be regarded as relative indications because the definitive cure of peritoneal infection due to yeasts or to Mycobacterium tuberculosis may be obtained with a catheter left in situ (104). Removal and replacement of Tenckhoff catheter at a single operation is recommended, even in cases of resistent peritonitis in CAPD provided the exit site is not infected (109); this approach reduces the demand which temporary haemodialysis of CAPD patients makes on centre dialysis facilities and may prevent the formation of adhesions when the catheter is removed for persistent peritonitis (31, 109). Single cuff catheters are easily removed by a single skin incision around the catheter exit site. Two skin incisions are required for removal of double cuff catheters (one incision for each cuff); to reduce the risk of peritoneal infection, it is prefereable to dissect down first to the deep cuff, remove the catheter from the peritoneal cavity, and then close this first incision before approaching the potentially contaminated subcutaneous cuff (31).

Catheter replacement is a procedure similar to first implantation. However, careful attention should be paid to the possible persistence of infectious foci on or in the abdominal wall. In case of doubt, the new catheter should be implanted at least 5 cm away from the suspected area (31).

Catheter survival

A peritoneal access with excellent hydraulic characteristics and functioning over long periods without complication is essential to the success of CAPD and the patient's quality of life. The actuarial survival of indwelling peritoneal catheters is in range of 40 to 90% at one year, and 30 to 80% at 2 years (53, 61, 73, 75, 79, 91, 92, 110), and of 20 to 75% at 3 years (53, 61, 91, 110). The wide scatter of reported actuarial survivals suggests that long term results depend mostly on local factors such as the competence and experience of the catheter insertion team and the careful management of the catheter. As shown in Figure 3, the type of implanted catheter appears to play some role in catheter outcome (73, 91, 92, 111): the longest survivals were reported mainly by groups using double cuff straight Tenckoff catheters (53, 61, 91, 110).

Automatic machines, dialysis solutions and disposables for intermittent (periodic) peritoneal dialysis (IPD) and continuous cyclic peritoneal dialysis (CCPD)

The various technical aspects of CAPD, including ready to use peritoneal dialysis solutions, tubing sets for dialysate infusion and drainage, and connectors are described in chapter 25. This section, therefore, will only deal with the equipment and disposables necessary to perform IPD and CCPD.

Dialysis solutions for IPD and CCPD

The formulation of peritoneal dialysis solutions used for

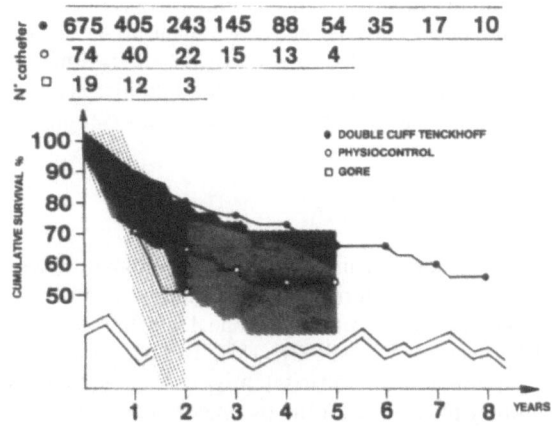

Figure 3. Compared actuarial survival of three types of peritoneal catheters. 'Physiocontrol' refers to the disk-column catheter, and 'Gore' to the Gore-Tex catheter shown in Figure 1. The grey areas indicate the 95% confidence limit for each curve (Courtesy Dr A Slingeneyer).

CAPD are also appropriate for IPD and CCPD. The problems related to their composition, contaminants, shelf life and possible additives will not be discussed in this section. The reader will find detailed information on this subject in chapter 25.

Ready to use dialysis solutions are available in 2 or 4.5 l plastic bags and in 10 l plastic containers. Two-liter bags are usually preferred for CCPD, while 4.5 l bags or 10 l plastic containers are more convenient for IPD. Plastic bags, made of transparent polyvinyl chloride, are protected by an external envelope, made of a thicker more resistent plastic material. A vacuum is created during sterilisation between the bag and its external envelope. The persistence of this vacuum and the absence of fluid in the interstice are reliable indicators of an intact package and preserves sterility of the solution. Checking carefully the clearness of the solution before use is recommended as contamination of the fluid during storage can occur (112). Rigid 10 l plastic containers are not transparent and the clarity of their contents is difficult to check even with transillumination. Although rare, fungal contamination of dialysis solutions may occur through pin holes and/or small cracks formed during transportation and storage. An in line microbiologic filter on the dialysate delivery circuit is recommended when this type of container is utilised (113).

Concentrated solutions are prepared for use with automatic reverse osmosis (RO) machines. Two formulations of concentrates are necessary: 1) an electrolyte solution with a concentration of 20 to 1 giving a final sodium concentration of 140 mmol/l; 2) a 50% dextrose concentrate which permits the preparation of final dialysis solutions with dextrose concentrations ranging from 27.5 to 275 mmol/l (5 to 50 g/l). The addition of dextrose concentrate to diluted electrolyte concentrate permits lowering the final sodium concentration in the range of 128 to 135 mmol/l (31). The separated preparation of the dextrose and electrolyte concentrates prevents the occurrence of heavy caramelization observed when electrolytes and dextrose are mixed together in a single concentrate (114). Concentrated solutions are conditioned in 2.5 l plastic bags protected by an external envelope.

Automatic cyclers

Since the introduction in 1962 of the first automatic machine for the delivery of sterile premixed dialysis solution via a closed circuit (5), the rate of peritoneal infection complicating IPD decreased drastically (115). Today, automatic cyclers are commonly found in intensive care units where IPD is routinely prescribed for the treatment of acute renal failure or various complications of CAPD; they are also utilized to perform other modalities of maintenance peritoneal dialysis in the home (i.e. IPD or CCPD). Automatic cyclers offer the advantage of technical simplicity, moderate capital cost and inexpensive maintenance. Their main drawback is the need for commercial solutions that are expensive, bulky and may become contaminated during storage. Automatic cyclers reduce the workload of the nursing staff and improve the efficiency of IPD because they allow the irrigation of the peritoneum at fixed intervals.

Cyclers are designed to carry on repeatedly a series of dialysis cycles, programmed at the beginning of each session. The main functions of the cycler are 1) to deliver a prescribed volume of dialysate to the peritoneal cavity, 2) to monitor the duration of the dwell time during which the dialysis fluid remains in the abdomen, and 3) to provide a period of drainage. In addition, cyclers incorporate a heater warming the dialysis fluid up to 38°C before infusion, and many of them are equiped with ultrafiltration monitors. The design of available cyclers is derived from the original concepts presented in the early sixties (5, 6). In most types of cyclers, gravity is utilized for infusion and drainage of dialysate, ensuring the safety of peritoneal irrigation procedures. The hydraulic circuits of two models of cyclers are schematised in Figures 4 and 5. Before dialysis, the sterile tubing set used as dialysate circuit should be installed on the cycler and connected to dialysate containers. The monitors should be set to determine the volume of exchanges, length of intra-abdominal dwell and the duration of drainage. After eliminating air from the dialysate delivery circuit and connecting it to the patient, the cycler is activated to initiate dialysis. The dialysate flows from the container to a heating cabinet that will also set the volume of inflow. When a temperature of about 38°C is reached, dialysate is delivered to the peritoneal cavity. Once the prescribed dwell time is completed, the cycler automatically shifts to a drain cycle. The peritoneal fluid, draining out by gravity, is collected in a weight bag to monitor adequate drainage. The spent dialysate is finally transferred in a large disposable drain bag.

Another type of cycler depicted in Figure 5, designed for using large dialysate containers, uses a roller pump to fill up a heating bag placed 30 to 40 cm over the patient's abdomen. The heated dialysate is delivered by gravity to the peritoneal

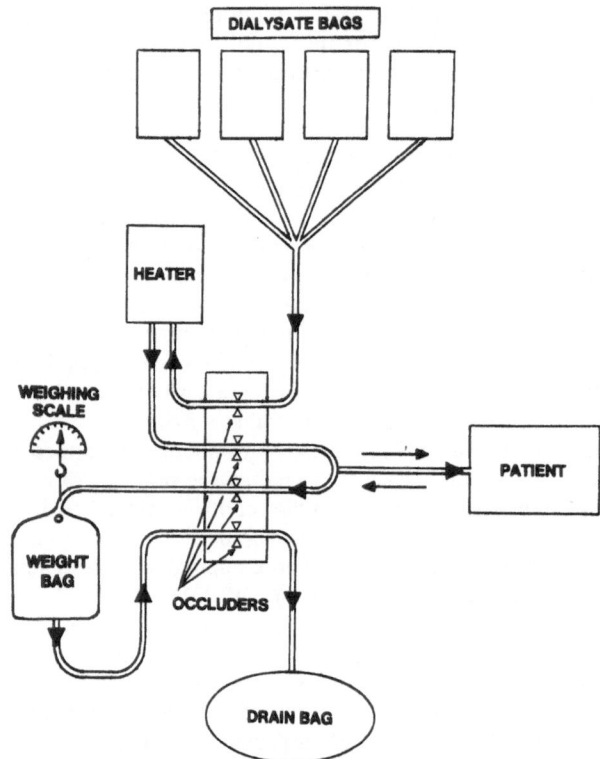

Figure 4. Schematic representation of the hydraulic circuit of a standard cycler system utilising gravity infusion and drainage.

cavity. The roller pump delivers a prescribed volume of dialysate to the heating bag while transferring simultaneously the used dialysate from the weight bag to the final drain container.

Cyclers can also be equipped with a microcomputer programmed to assess the cumulative balance of infused and drained volumes. This permits close monitoring of net ultrafiltration. The complexity and cost of this added monitor is not always justified, particularly in ESRD patients with a well functioning peritoneal catheter receiving maintenance IPD (31).

Reverse osmosis machines

In 1972, a major advance in peritoneal dialysis consisted in the development of automatic, so called reverse osmosis (RO) peritoneal dialysis systems capable of producing unlimited quantities of sterile pyrogen free dialysate from tap water and sterile concentrate (8). With this equipment, sterile, apyrogenic water is obtained by reverse osmosis; dialysis solution is prepared by mixing one volume of dextrose/electrolyte concentrate and 19 volumes of reverse osmosis treated, sterile water; to this mixture, a variable amount of dextrose concentrate is added to adapt the dextrose concentration of the final dialysis fluid to the patient needs. The safety of these systems depends on the perfect quality of the reverse osmosis modules, including intactness

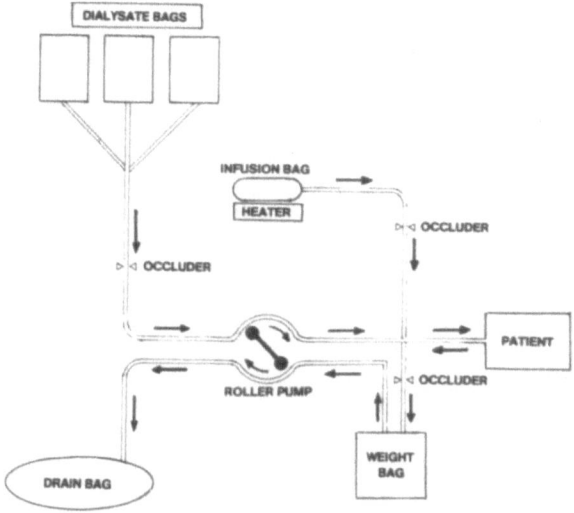

Figure 5. Schematic representation of the hydraulic circuit of a modified cycler system utilizing a roller pump for active transfer of solution from dialysate bags to the infusion bag and insuring infusion and drainage by gravity.

of the spiral acetate cellulose or nylon hollow fiber membranes and the tightness of the assembled permeators (116). It has been shown that bacteria from supply water may cross most currently available reverse osmosis modules and may colonise the downstream portion of the system (117). Accordingly, the safe use of reverse osmosis modules for the production of water includes the following requirements: 1) pretreatment of tap water should comply with the recommendations of the manufacturers of the reverse osmosis module, keeping in mind that pretreatment devices such as carbon filters, softeners, prefilters and storage tanks may promote bacterial growth (117, 118); 2) the use of bacterial filters and ultrafilters to ensure downstream apyrogenicity and sterility during dialysis fluid production (119); 3) the routine disinfection of the reverse osmosis modules and dialysate circuit with 3 to 4% formaldehyde after each dialysis (119, 120); and 4) the timely change of reverse osmosis modules when their ion rejection capability decreases (120). Although the safety of the RO machines has been proven in most published series (121–123) the recommended preventive measures should be strictly applied lest a high incidence of peritoneal infection be observed (124).

The only peritoneal dialysis system currently available for the bedside production of dialysis solutions (Perisart, Sartorius GmbH, Göttingen, FRG) is depicted on Figure 6 and its hydraulic circuit is schematically represented in Figure 7. This equipment, which does not incorporate a RO module, should be fed with RO treated water. Gravimetry is used for the batch preparation of diluted dialysis solutions from an electrolyte concentrate (concentration ratio 20 to 1), a 50% glucose concentrate and RO treated water, filtered on a 0.2 μm microbiologic filter at the water inlet. A weighing scale, monitored by a microcomputer, measures the appro-

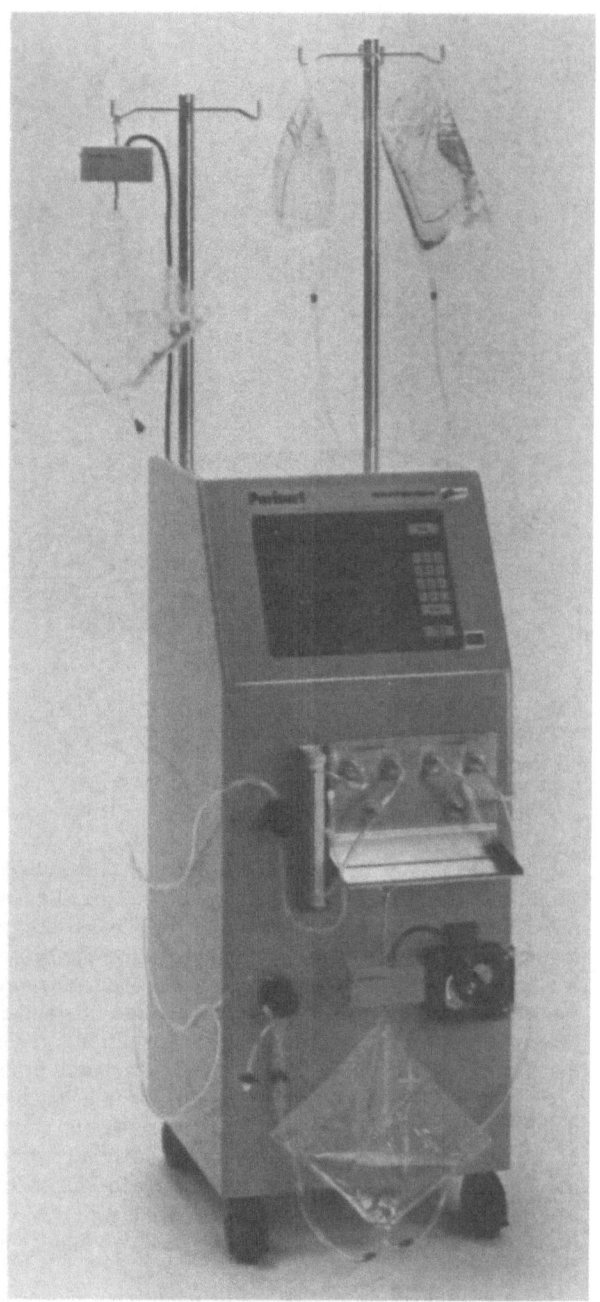

Figure 6. Peritoneal dialysis system for the bedside preparation and distribution of sterile apyrogenic dialysis solution. The bags and tubing sets are disposable (Perisart®, Sartorius GmbH, Göttingen, FRG).

priate amounts of electrolyte and glucose concentrate and water admitted into the mixing vessel. Mixing and heating of the 5 l batch is obtained by recirculating the solution in a closed loop equiped with an in line conductivity meter and a heater. When the conductivity stabilizes at the prescribed

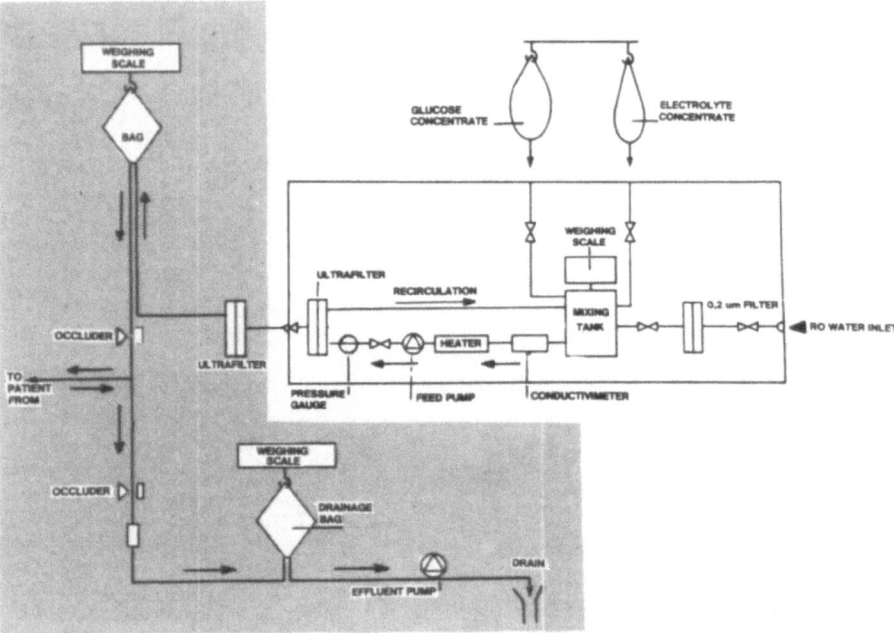

Figure 7. Diagrammatic representation of the hydraulic circuit of peritoneal dialysis solution supply system Perisart®, Sartorius. This equipment must be fed with reverse osmosis treated water. The homogeneity of each batch of dialysis solution is obtained by recirculating the mixture of water and concentrates in the circulation loop. The disposable infusion and drainage set (including a disposable ultrafilter) is represented in the grey insert.

value, the solution is infused into the dialysate delivery circuit through a permanent $0.2\ \mu$m microbiologic filter and a disposable depyrogenating ultrafilter (cellulose triacetate membrane with a cut off point of 20,000 daltons: Sartocon®, Sartorius). The disposable dialysate delivery circuit represented in Figure 7 is similar to the sets used in standard cyclers except for the presence of the in line ultrafilter. The machine monitors the duration of inflow, dwell and drainage times as well as net ultrafiltration. Once a batch of dialysis fluid is used up, the machine prepares automatically another batch and the dialysis session can go uninterrupted as long as needed. At the end of the session, the disposable set used for dialysate infusion and drainage is removed and the system is disinfected with peracetic acid or sodium hypochlorite.

Since the advent of CAPD, most nephrologists lost interest in treating ESRD patients with IPD. As a consequence, the potential market for automatic RO peritoneal dialysis machines vanished, and companies previously involved in their manufacture gave up. New modalities of periodic peritoneal dialysis, such as nightly peritoneal dialysis and tidal peritoneal dialysis are under clinical evaluation. In the present economic constraints, the clinical application of these new peritoneal dialysis regimens will require the use of an automatic machine producing cheap sterile apyrogenic peritoneal dialysis solutions. This renewed interest in IPD should encourage manufacturers to develop new peritoneal dialysis systems for on site production of dialysis fluid.

Disposable sets for delivery and drainage of peritoneal dialysis fluids

Peritoneal dialysis solutions are infused into the peritoneal cavity during dialysis using disposable sterile apyrogenic sets made of polyvinyl chloride, packaged in plastic bags, strengthened against accidental pin holes and tears by an external envelope. These sets, specifically designed to suit each type of equipment, are sterilized with ethylene oxide. Aseptically installed on the cycler or automatic RO machine before initiating dialysis, they should be discarded after each use. These disposables are expensive and contribute to the high cost of IPD or CCPD. Most of these sets are manufactured according to the closed circuit concept (5), including a large drainage bag where spent dialysate is collected. Although the use of a closed circuit increases the bacteriologic safety of peritoneal dialysis, in vitro studies demonstrate a low risk of retrograde bacterial contamination when peritoneal effluent is directly drained into an infected sink (125); these studies suggest that the suppression of the draining bag could significantly lower the cost of disposables used in CCPD and IPD without compromising the safety of these procedures.

Peritoneal dialysis regimens

The basic technique of peritoneal dialysis rests on the intermittent irrigation of the peritoneal cavity with dialysis solutions through a single peritoneal catheter (1). Peritoneal irrigation is accomplished according to a cycle that includes three sequential periods: 1) inflow of dialysis fluid into the abdomen by gravity or under the action of a roller pump (infusion time); 2) dwelling of fluid into the peritoneal cavity for a variable duration (diffusion time); 3) draining of the peritoneal fluid to empty the peritoneal cavity (drainage time). As soon as a cycle is completed, it may be repeated as many times as needed. In clinical practice, this basic procedure is applied in many different ways, resulting in a variety of peritoneal dialysis regimens that can be classified under two main categories: periodic or intermittent, and continuous peritoneal dialysis.

Intermittent (periodic) peritoneal dialysis (IPD)

This mode of peritoneal dialysis alternates dialyses of various duration (8 to 12 h or longer) with interdialytic phases lasting 14 h to several days according to patient's needs (i.e. residual renal function, protein catabolic rate). Originally, the term periodic peritoneal dialysis was used to describe this regimen (5). It was later replaced by the current terminology of intermittent peritoneal dialysis, which previously referred to the process of peritoneal irrigation itself.

Standard IPD regimens

An inflow volume of 2 l is commonly used in adults. The exchange volume can be adjusted, however, from 1 to 3 l according to patient's size, abdominal capacity and cardiopulmonary tolerance (126, 127). Peritoneal clearances increase slightly with increments in dialysate flow rates (128). At a value of 35 ml/min, however, peritoneal urea clearances tend clearly to level off in spite of dialysate flow rates of 40 ml/min or more. In these circumstances, the low mass tranfer area coefficient (MTAC) of the peritoneal membrane becomes the limiting factor of IPD, because dialysate flow rates reach a value equal or superior to the MTAC (129). A standard protocol uses exchange cycles with 5 to 10 min infusion time (200 to 400 ml/min), 5 to 15 min dwell time, 10 to 20 min drainage time. This corresponds to dialysate flow rate of 30 to 66 ml/min (1.8 to 4.0 l/h) maintaining urea and creatinine clearances around 20 to 25 ml/min and 12 to 20 ml/min respectively (130). To maintain higher peritoneal clearances for a given dialysate flow rate, the drainage time should be set without aiming at a complete drainage of the residual intraperitoneal fluid (131), an unnecessary step that results in lower peritoneal clearances and longer dialysis duration (132).

With manual techniques, it is difficult to maintain an hourly dialysate exchange rate at more than 2 l. The use of automated techniques not only makes IPD easier and safer, but it also improves the effectiveness of this dialysis mode by ensuring the repetition of exchange cycles at regular intervals. In a cost effectiveness analysis of various IPD protocols, increasing dwell time from 0 to 15 min resulted in a considerable saving of dialysate with little reduction of net urea transfer (4), a fact of major economic importance when premixed commercial solutions are used (133).

Nightly peritoneal dialysis and tidal peritoneal dialysis

To compensate for the intrinsic limitations of transperitoneal transport encountered in IPD, two major approaches are utilized. The first approach consists in increasing the total weekly dialysis time. This increment in weekly treatment duration can be obtained either with longer dialysis sessions at fixed intervals or with more frequent shorter dialyses. This resulted in a great variety of dialysis schedules: 10 to 12 hours two to three times a week (10), 10 hrs four times a week (21, 134), 9 hours three times a week (135), 5 to 7 overnight dialyses (136) and short daily dialyses (137). The weekly amount of dialysate used with these schedules ranged from 70 to 240 l at a dialysate flow rate of 2 to 4 l/h.

Among these various protocols, it was suggested that *nightly peritoneal dialysis* may evolve as the method of choice because it has the potential to maximize the advantages of both IPD and CAPD while minimizing their disadvantages (138). Nightly IPD performed over 8 h using 26 l of dialysis solutions and 21 exchanges, obtained mean urea and creatinine clearances of 8.4 and 5.3 l per day'respectively (139, 140). In patients with low or average peritoneal permeability, however, 10 to 12 h are required to match CAPD clearances (139).

The second approach consists in various attempts to maximize the effeciency of IPD by increasing the time of contact between the dialysate and the peritoneal membrane. Initially described as reciprocating peritoneal dialysis (141), this protocol is now reported as *tidal peritoneal dialysis* (140). With this method, a constant volume of dialysis fluid remains in the peritoneal cavity on top of which a tidal volume of dialysis solution is cycled. Tidal peritoneal dialysis obtains the best values of urea and creatinine clearances (i.e. 8.5 and 6.3 l/day respectively) when both the residual and tidal volumes are of 1.5 l (140).

Continuous peritoneal dialysis

Continuous peritoneal dialysis overcomes the problem of low efficiency inherent in peritoneal dialysis by making continuous operation an integral part of the procedure (129). According to the position of the patient during dialysis, continuous peritoneal dialysis can be ambulatory or supine. It is almost exclusively performed as CAPD in ESRD patients (14–17), but it has been also utilised in supine patients for the treatment of acute renal failure (142–146).

The various schedules utilized in CAPD are discussed in Chapter 25. In acute renal failure, the protocols for continuous peritoneal dialysis, also described as equilibration (142) or low flow (144) peritoneal dialysis, consist in 6 to 8 daily exchanges of 2 l of dialysate left in situ for 3 to 4 h each. In terms of peritoneal transport kinetics, continuous peritoneal dialysis is a flow rate limited system, with a maximum urea clearance of no more than 10 to 12 ml/min. To avoid multiple daily manipulations of the dialysate infusion lines, special tubing sets designed as manifolds with 6 to 8 'spikes' are utilised to connect in the morning the dialysate bags necessary for 24 h treatment time. With this system, the nurse easily performs the sequential dialysate exchanges by activating manual clamps according to the prescribed dialysis schedules (146).

Continuous cyclic peritoneal dialysis

To alleviate the day time work load resulting from the daily exchanges of continuous ambulatory peritoneal dialysis and to prevent peritonitis or patient's burn out, an alternative approach preserving the concept of continuous peritoneal dialysis was developed. Defined as continuous cyclic peritoneal dialysis, this regimen includes several short dialysate exchanges (usually 4 to 6) realized during the night, and a single long daytime exchange. An automatic cycler is necessary to effect the nocturnal exchanges that characterize CCPD (147). Before the patient goes to bed, the equipment is set up in about 20 min and the peritoneal catheter is connected to the cycler dialysate circuit with great aseptic care. Three or four 2 l exchanges take place automatically during the night, each lasting 2 to 3 h. In the morning, 2 l of dialysis solution are infused prior to disconnection, and allowed to dwell intraperitoneally for the rest of the day (approximately 13 to 15 h) with the catheter capped. All connect-disconnect procedures take place at night and in the early morning in the convenience of patient's home, facilitating adherence to strict sterile procedures.

As significant dialysate absorption is expected during the daytime long dwell exchange, dialysis solutions containing 2.5 to 4.25 g/dl dextrose are recommended. Some clinicians have proposed to eliminate the long diurnal cycle of CCPD to prevent complications related to increased intra-abdominal pressure or to avoid excessive fluid absorption from the peritoneal cavity in patients with increased peritoneal permeability. The suppression of the diurnal cycle results in a significant reduction in urea and creatinine clearances (148).

Table 3. Undesirable effects of peritoneal dialysis.

I	Disturbances in the physiology of the peritoneum
	Suppressed upwards circulation of normal peritoneal fluid
	Removal of surface acting material
II	Continuous mesothelial injury and regeneration
III	Interference with local host defense mechanisms
	Open peritoneal cavity
	Dilution of immunoglobulins and C3
	Functional alterations of peritoneal phagocytes
IV	Increase in intraabdominal pressure
V	Effect on hemodynamics and pulmonary function
VI	Metabolic consequences
	Protein losses
	Amino acid losses
	Glucose loading
	Hyperlipemic and atherogenic changes
	Loss of carnitine
	Loss of free fatty acids
	Loss of vitamins
VII	Gastrointestinal side effects
VIII	Air under the diaphragm
IX	Duration of peritoneal dialysis procedures

UNDESIRABLE EFFECTS OF PERITONEAL DIALYSIS

Technically, peritoneal dialysis presents itself as the simplest among the various dialysis therapies presently available. Using the peritoneal cavity as an artificial kidney, however, does not go without inherent undesirable effects. Although not life-threatening on the short term, some of these side effects (e.g. protein losses, glucose load) are potentially harmful to the patient on the long term. In spite of the extensive use of CAPD over the last decade, their clinical significance has not yet been fully elucidated.

The main undesirable effects of peritoneal dialysis are listed in Table 3. This list illustrates the numerous consequences of peritoneal dialysis which interfere locally with the physiology, the ultrastructure and the immunology of the peritoneum. Beyond its local actions, the irrigation of the peritoneal cavity with unphysiologic dialysis solutions (e.g. hyperosmolar and acidic) containing high dextrose concentrations, is also associated with metabolic disturbances while inducing subtle changes in cardiovascular and respiratory functions.

Interferences with the normal physiology of the peritoneum

In a healthy subject, the peritoneum is a potential space containing about 50 ml of peritoneal fluid which provides lubrication of the abdominal viscera as they slide over one another (149). The normal peritoneal fluid, which contains phagocytic cells (mainly macrophages), immunoglobulins and complement (150, 151), flows continuously upwards from the pelvis to the subdiaphragmatic area, where it drains off into the lacunae of diaphragmatic lymphatics through small intercellular openings called the mesothelial stomata (152). This upward circulation of peritoneal fluid is induced by diaphragmatic contractions during respiration (152). This permanent flux sweeps the mesothelial surface and permits the rapid elimination from the peritoneal cavity of particulate matter up to 20 μm in size (including bacteria) through the diaphragmatic lymphatics and the thoracic duct to the systemic circulation (153). When the peritoneal cavity is filled with dialysate, the infused volume, 10 to 60 times larger than normal peritoneal fluid, presumably disrupts the physiologic intraperitoneal circulation. This disturbance may explain why bacteremia, a common finding in secondary bacterial peritonitis (149) is a rare observation among patients with CAPD peritonitis (103).

Removal of surface-active material is another adverse effect of peritoneal dialysis (154). This material is composed of phospholipids, with a predominance of phosphatidylcholine. This substance, isolated from dialysate effluent was studied *in vitro;* it demonstrated a moderate degree of repellency and surface activity. In addition to surface-tension reduction, this surface-active material may have lubrication properties (154) and confers water repellency to the mesothelial surface by its attachment to the anionic sites of the peritoneum (155). As shown in *in vitro* studies, the peritoneum is capable of synthesizing phosphatidylcholine in amounts equivalent to lung tissue (22). Among CAPD patients, phospholipid levels in the dialysis effluent were lower in those receiving CAPD for 8 to 48 months than in patients starting treatment. Spent dialysate phospholipid levels were even lower in patients with low ultrafiltration rates or during an episode of peritonitis (156). Addition of phosphatidylcholine to fresh dialysis fluid raised ultrafiltration in patients with previously reduced ultrafiltration rates (156). Furthermore, administration of oral phosphatidylcholine (300 mg/day for one year) appeared as an efficient prophylaxis of reduced peritoneal ultrafiltration in ten patients (157). These findings suggest that permanent lavage of the mesothelium with dialysis solutions could deplete surface-active material, which could alter permeability of the peritoneum eventually resulting in clinically significant loss of ultrafiltration (158).

Continuous injury and regeneration of the mesothelium

Ultrastructural studies of the peritoneum demonstrate that, even in the absence of infection, mesothelial cells and submesothelial tissues are affected by exposure to dialysis solutions. Patchy open intercellular clefts, presumably due to cell shrinkage (18, 19, 159), increased density of the cell cytoplasm and a striking development of the rough endoplasmic reticulum are observed after only a few days exposure to dialysate. Micropinocytotic vesicles are larger but less numerous than in normal peritoneum. Minimal edema of the submesothelial tissue may be evident, and active fibroblasts begin to appear under the mesothelium (18). A progressive reduction and subsequent disappearance of microvilli is another striking modification of the peritoneum in CAPD patients (159). Peritoneal dialysis induces a process of continuous mesothelial injury and regeneration, the whole sequence of which can be observed on histological sections coming from the same peritoneal biopsy (160). The ultrastructural changes of the mesothelium and submesothelial tissues become more pronounced following long term exposure to dialysis solutions and episodes of peritonitis (18, 159). These changes are indicative of reactive fibroplasia (18). Whether the structural changes of the peritoneum associated with long term exposure to the dialysate can induce progressive functional deterioration in some patients, even in the absence of peritonitis, is still an unanswered question (161–164).

Interference with local host defense mechanisms

Peritoneal dialysis alters local host defense mechanisms of the peritoneum in a complex way. This interference is more pronounced in CAPD, where the peritoneal cavity is almost constantly filled with dialysis fluid, transforming it in an immunocompromised site. Over the last decade, the multifaceted factors contributing to the increased risk of opportunistic infection in peritoneal dialysis have been identified. These factors have been thoroughly discussed in several reviews (23, 104, 165–170). These undesirable effects are summarised in this section.

An indwelling peritoneal catheter creates a permanent breach through the skin and the peritoneal serosa, becoming the main port of entry for microorganisms. The lumen of the Silastic tubing is also a site for biofilm formation (171–173) and colonisation of bacteria (174) and fungi (174, 175). It has been hypothesized that the catheter material could activate peritoneal macrophages (176) or the complement system (177), or induce by direct contact a granulocyte phagocytic defect (178). These possibilities, however, have not been explored.

The multiple exchanges of dialysis solutions represent the main factor which alters the physiologic environment of the peritoneal cavity. Peritoneal irrigation disturbs local host defense mechanisms, not only by diluting the existing opsonins, but also by depleting the peritoneum of phagocytic cells and by adversely affecting the function of peritoneal macrophages and polymorphonuclear neutrophils.

By diluting the normal peritoneal fluid, the large volume of dialysate infused at each exchange lowers 50 to 100 fold the concentration of opsonins (i.e. immunoglobulins G, C3 and fibronectin) (168, 179–186). The function of opsonins is to react with foreign particles and render these more susceptible to ingestion by phagocytosis. The low concentration of these substances in the peritoneal fluid creates a state of opsonic deficiency (168, 169). A positive correlation has been observed in CAPD patients between the opsonizing capacity of drained dialysate and IgG and C3 concentrations (180–184). Complement-mediated opsonization, however, was found defective in commercial peritoneal dialysis solutions, whereas antibody-mediated opsonization was little affected. Inactivation of complement by CAPD solutions was mainly due to the low pH of these solutions (185). Several studies have demonstrated that patients can be divided prospectively into high risk and low risk groups for Staphylococcus epidermidis infection, based on the concentration of IgG, C3 and opsonic activity, as measured by phagocytosis, of the dialysis fluid (169, 179, 183). The incidence of S epidermidis peritonitis was decreased in patients with higher IgG and C3 concentration and opsonic activity in their dialysis effluents (169, 179, 182, 184). In one study, bacterial growth of S epidermidis was superior in peritoneal effluent than in normal serum or fresh dialysis solution, and was negatively correlated with the concentration of transferrin (184). Transferrin, which is not an opsonin, may provide an important antimicrobial defence mechanism by rendering iron unavailable to microorganisms in vivo (184, 187). Fibronectin levels in noninfected peritoneal fluid were 20 fold lower than those found in normal plasma (181, 182, 186). The concentration of this opsonin increased in the peritoneal fluid in case of peritonitis and returned to normal a few days after the clearing of peritoneal infection (186). The influence of peritoneal fluid fibronectin concentration on subsequent peritonitis is not known.

Peritoneal irrigation with unphysiologic dialysis solutions not only dilutes various components of humoral immunity, but it also interferes with local cellular immunity and polymorphonuclear leucocyte defense (166, 188). By diluting the number of peritoneal phagocytic cells, the technique of peritoneal dialysis decreases the ability to eliminate bacteria as the cell per volume ratio is reduced (166). The changing of peritoneal fluid at regular intervals depletes the peritoneal cavity of large numbers of phagocytic cells. In the absence of infection, 80 to 90% of the cells lost in dialysis effluent are peritoneal macrophages and monocytes (151, 189–191). During peritonitis, a predominance of polymorphonuclear neutrophils characterizes the cellular pattern of drained dialysate (189, 190). The viability of the cells removed with spent dialysate is usually preserved (165, 166). The cytotoxicity of fresh commercial dialysis solutions, however, has been repeatedly demonstrated towards peripheral blood leukocytes (166, 167) and peritoneal macrophages in man (191–193) as well as in chronically uremic mice (194). Worthy of note is that 60% of human peritoneal macrophages are still viable after 60 min exposure to fresh dialysis fluid whereas most polymorphonuclear leukocytes have died during a similar time exposure. Surviving macrophages, however, demonstrate a marked decrease in phagocytosis (192). The low pH of these solutions appears to be the main cytotoxic factor (166, 194). Dialysate hyperosmolality was found to adversely affect peripheral blood leukocytes (165, 166), but it did not appear to have a major cytotoxic effect towards peritoneal macrophages in man (192) or in the mouse (194). The degree of suppression of peritoneal macrophage function depends largely of dwell time duration. Macrophages showed markedly depressed phagocytosis after dwell time of 30 to 180 min (192), but demonstrated a normal phagocyte function after an overnight dwell (192, 193). This improvement in phagocytic function with longer dwell times results from the modification of peritoneal dialysis fluid composition (i.e. higher pH, lower osmolality) occurring during diffusion (166). It may also reflect the invasion of the peritoneal cavity with a new population of monocytes and polymorphonuclear leucocytes derived from the blood (177, 191). Depressed macrophage function may result also in decreased intracellular killing (193). Intracellular bacteria, including S epidermidis, can survive and grow within human peritoneal macrophages and monocytes even in the presence of antibiotics (195). Similar observations were made for Candida albicans (196). There is some evidence that such intraleukocytic sequestration may be of clinical importance in CAPD patients (197). Another aspect of disturbed cellular immunity concerns the possible activation of macrophages by peritoneal dialysis procedures. Fresh dialysate appears to have a stimulating effect towards peritoneal macrophages. If in one study resting nonstimulated monocytes were observed in spent dialysate (191), several groups brought direct evidence of macrophage activation. One group observed a strong predominance of exudate macrophages in the peritoneal effluent of noninfected CAPD patients, a cellular pattern reflecting a permanent state of peritonitis (198). Another group isolated variable amounts of interleukin-1 (IL-1) on the overnight dialysate effluent of noninfected CAPD patients, whether or not an in-line bacteriological filter was utilized (199, 200). The presence of IL-1 in the peritoneal fluids may have some bearing on the development of sclerosing peritonitis (104, 176, 197). Other workers suggested that abnormal macrophage production of IL-1 and prostaglanding E_2 (PGE_2) could result in a higher incidence of peritoneal infection. A low IL-1 production and the release of large amounts of PGE_2 by peritoneal macrophages were observed in CAPD patients with a high incidence of peritonitis, by comparison with a group of patients with a low incidence of peritoneal infection. It was concluded that an imbalance in the production of humoral factors by peritoneal macrophages (i.e. decreased IL-1, increased PGE_2) induced a suppressor activity facilitating bacterial invasion of the peritoneal fluid in patients with a high incidence of peritonitis (201).

In summary, the technique of peritoneal dialysis adversely affects peritoneal host defense mechanisms through several mechanisms. The factors involved in this detrimental process include the following: 1) *The physicochemical composition of fresh peritoneal dialysis solutions,* altering the viability of polymorphonuclear leukocytes, the phagocytic capacity of macrophages and inducing defective complement mediated immunity; 2) *the washout effect of repeated peritoneal fluid drainage,* removing numerous phagocytic cells (particularly during peritonitis) and significant amounts of IgG; 3) *the dilutional effect of the large volume* of fluid infused for each exchange, inducing a local state of opsonic deficiency and impairing the bactericidal efficiency of peritoneal phagocytes; 4) *the activation of peritoneal macrophages* entailing the production of humoral factors (i.e. IL-1, PGE_2) susceptible to modify the local resistance to infection or to stimulate reactive fibroplasia. The full blown effects of these factors are obtained during CAPD as a consequence of the continuous irrigation of the peritoneal cavity. The practical consequences of these observations was a modification of the treatment approach for CAPD associated peritonitis (202). Instead of the time honored rapid peritoneal lavage (31), the new approach recommended to continue CAPD with low dialysate volumes and long dwell times to facilitate the rapid equilibration of peritoneal fluid pH and osmolality with splanchnic blood, and to prevent the dissipation of opsonins and phagocytic cells indispensable to contain the bacterial invasion of the peritoneum. Likewise, transient interruption of CAPD by emptying the abdomen during the night was shown to improve the prognosis of CAPD associated peritonitis (203). Finally, the periodic nature of IPD, where the normal physiology of the peritoneum is restored during the interdialytic period, explains, at least in part, the lower peritonitis incidence observed with this treatment modality (115).

Increased intra-abdominal pressure

The intra-abdominal pressure of the empty abdominal cavity ranges between 0.5 and 1.5 cm of water (204) and increases linearly with the volume of dialysis fluid present in the peritoneal cavity (204–206). Each liter of intraperitoneal fluid increases the intra-abdominal pressure by 2 to 3 cm of water and the abdominal girth by 1.81 cm. Coughing and straining generate the highest intra-abdominal pressures in every position. The pressures, generally higher with greater dialysate volumes, vary with physical activity; bicycle training produces lower pressure than jogging or jumping. Intra-abdominal pressures are higher with most maneuvers in obese patients and in elderly (206). Raised intra-abdominal pressure is a major risk factor in CAPD and CCPD; it may create dialysate leaks, hernia, cardiopulmonary compromise and hemorrhoids. It may also accentuate gastroesophageal reflux and urinary incontinence. To reduce the risk of these complications, useful recommendations to the patient include 1) a reduction in voluntary coughing, particularly after catheter insertion; 2) careful prevention of constipation to prevent excessive straining; 3) emptying of the abdomen for strenuous exercises (i.e. tennis, weight lifting) (206).

Effects on the cardiovascular system

Instillation of 2 to 3 l of dialysis solution in the peritoneal cavity induces a 98% increase in the inferior vena cava pressure (207). Two hemodynamic studies conducted in CAPD patients gave slightly divergent results (204, 208). In one study, graded increases in exchange volume from 15 to 26 ml/kg/body weight in supine patients produced a decreased cardiac output of 25% when intra-abdominal pressure reached 15 cm of water. At the same time, heart rate, mean arterial blood pressure and total peripheral resistance showed significant increases, whereas a 35% reduction in stroke volume was observed (204). In another study, comparing hemodynamic changes induced by 2 l of intraperitoneal dialysate in the standing versus supine position, significant falls in blood pressure, stroke volume and cardiac output, accompanied by an increase in heart rate, were observed only in the upright position, with no change in peripheral resistance (208). Differences in methodology may account for the discrepancy observed in these two studies. Both groups, however, concluded that the observed hemodynamic changes have little clinical consequence in the uncomplicated patients (204) and that the ability of the patient to cope with postural stress was preserved (208). The cardiovascular effects of CAPD were studied in patients with left ventricular hypertrophy; a progressive decrease in left ventricular function occurred with incremental infusion of intraperitoneal dialysate, both in the supine and standing position but this abnormality had no clinical consequence (209).

Effects on pulmonary function

Most studies of pulmonary function during peritoneal dialysis, comparing data obtained with an empty or full abdomen, report a reduction in functional residual capacity (FRC) following dialysis fluid infusion, both in the supine and sitting positions (210–212). A reduction in vital capacity, however, is a less common finding (213, 214). In fact, when interpreting the results of pulmonary function tests in patients receiving peritoneal dialysis, several parameters should be taken into account, including the volume of infusate and the resulting intraperitoneal pressure (214) as well as the patient's position (i.e. supine, sitting or upright)

and the compliance of the abdominal wall (205). During IPD, performed with 2 l dialysis solution infusion in a recumbent patient, a significant drop in FRC was observed and resulted in air ways closure as the FRC values were lower than the closure capacity (210). Similar findings were obtained in CAPD patients, in whom airway closure induced a significant decrease in PaO_2 (212). This hypoxemia was abolished a few months later, suggesting the development of compensatory mechanisms in long term CAPD (212). This observation may account for the absence of abnormalities in pulmonary function observed by one group in CAPD patients studied in the sitting position (215). In normal operating conditions, the procedure of PD does not induce respiratory distress. Severe discomfort or dyspnea, however, can occur when the dialysate volume is increased above 2 l, particularly when the patient is lying flat in his bed both with IPD (212) or CAPD (205). In practice, exchange volumes and respiratory tolerance should be carefully monitored in patients with borderline respiratory function. On the other hand, improvement in pulmonary function during the second half of an IPD session was noted in one study and attributed to extracellular volume and pulmonary water removal during dialysis (210).

Metabolic interactions with ventilation were observed in CAPD patients. They were ascribed to a high input of glucose and lactate due to transperitoneal transfer, resulting in a marked elevation of minute ventilation and O_2 consumption ($V O_2$) (216). Such an increase in $V O_2$ was compatible with the stoichiometry of the oxidation of glucose and lactate (217). These findings, however, were not confirmed by others who reported normal ventilation and low O_2 consumption, together with normal 2,3 diphosphoglycerate and P_{50} (218).

Metabolic disturbances

Protein losses are inherent in peritoneal dialysis due to the high permeability of the peritoneal membrane (2, 129, 219). In IPD, the protein loss per dialysis depends on the nature and type of peritoneal catheter, the length of dwell time, the osmolality and the temperature of dialysis solutions as well as the duration of dialysis (220). During periods of peritoneal infection, protein losses may increase 3–10 fold (220, 221). This increased protein loss during peritoneal infection reflects an increased permeability of the peritoneal membrane mediated by the vasoactive prostaglandins PGI_2 and PGE_2 (222). Protein concentration is usually highest in the first drainage; this washout phenomenon may be explained by the remaining 'ascites' in the peritoneal cavity during interdialytic intervals (210). Published figures on total protein loss during IPD diverge widely. This is explained by wide variations between individual patients; it also depends on the techniques of peritoneal dialysis utilised (e.g. disposable rigid stylet catheter versus indwelling Silastic catheters) (220). When IPD was performed with a permanent Silastic catheter and 40 l of dialysate per session, the average total protein losses reported were ranging from 4 to 22.3 g per dialysis (223–225). In CAPD, total protein loss ranged from 5 to 12 g/24 h and albumin accounted for about 65% and IgG for 15% of protein loss. IgA, IgM and C3 were also found in small quantities in the peritoneal effluent. The losses of IgG and IgM correlated with the serum concentration of these immunoglobulins (226). During a single dialysate exchange, the amount of protein loss increased from 1.3 g after a 4 h dwell to 1.6 and 1.8 g after 6 and 8 h dwells respectively. Protein losses increased considerably during peritonitis and remained elevated for several weeks, after curing the peritoneal infection (226). When protein concentrations were measured during successive dialysate exchanges, dialysate protein content was higher during the first exchange and then, decreased progressively to stabilize after the third exchange. Steady state protein levels in the peritoneal fluid were not altered by the osmolality of dialysis solutions (227). In spite of the considerable amount of total protein lost in the dialysate, most CAPD patients maintain stable serum total protein and albumin levels that are only slightly reduced (228–230). The total albumin mass and the plasma albumin mass as well as the distribution of albumin are normal in CAPD patients because decreased catabolism and increased synthesis of albumin maintain albumin homeostasis (228). Besides the immunoglobulins, several other proteins are found in spent dialysate, including fibrinogen and antithrombin III (231, 232), beta-2 microglobulin (230, 233–235), haptoglobin and ceruloplasmin (230).

Amino acid losses during IPD averaged 4.96 g/27 l (236, 237); the concentrations of most amino acid in dialysate were proportional to their plasma concentrations (237). In CAPD, the daily loss of amino acids amounted to 2 g when patients drained a total dialysate volume of 10 l, an average weekly loss of 12 g (229, 238–240). CAPD did not correct the plasma amino acid abnormalities of uremia (229). During dialysis, the dialysate to plasma concentration ratio approached unity for most amino acids (with two notable exceptions of aspartic acid and tryptophan), suggesting a trend toward equilibrium due to a passive diffusion gradient (229).

Glucose loading is a major side effect of peritoneal dialysis. Glucose diffuses continuously from dialysate to blood due to a favorable concentration gradient. In IPD, the total amount of glucose absorbed during a dialysis depends on dialysate glucose concentration and flow rate, and also on dialysis duration (241). In CAPD, daily absorption varies roughly between 100 and 200 g per 24 h. This amount represents 70 to 75% of glucose supplied with the dialysis fluid (229). During a 6 h cycle, 45 to 50 g of glucose are absorbed from the 4.25 g% dialysis solution while 25 to 40 and 15 to 22 are absorbed, respectively, from 2.5 and 1.5% dialysis solutions (242). Large differences in the rate of glucose absorption exist between patients (161, 243, 244). In the same patient, glucose absorption may increase with time on CAPD leading to poor ultrafiltration (161, 163, 243). The energy intake from dialysate glucose absorption represents on average approximately 8 kcal/kg/day and accounts for about 20% of total energy intake (229). During CAPD, a single dialysis cycle with hypertonic fluid (glucose monohydrate 4.25 g/dl) induces a rise in blood glucose and plasma

insulin levels to peak values within 45 to 90 min, whereas serum glucagon levels decrease only slightly (229). Studies on oral glucose tolerance after 6 and 12 months on CAPD show that blood glucose, serum insulin and serum glucagon responses to an oral glucose load remain abnormal, but are not further impaired during CAPD in most patients (229). However, insulin response to oral glucose has been reported to deteriorate with time in some patients (245), while some others may become insulin-dependent de novo during CAPD due to the permanent hyperglycemic stress (246).

Hyperlipidemic effects are also observed during IPD and CAPD (229, 247, 248). In CAPD during the first year of treatment, both serum triglycerides and serum cholesterol levels usually increase and show a later tendency to stabilize and even to decrease (248). Circulating triglycerides levels appear to be affected by energy intake and many centers recommend to their patients a restricted use of hypertonic dialysis fluid as well as a decreased dietary energy intake (247, 249). Both decreased removal and increased production of triglycerides contribute to the hyperlipidemia of patients receiving IPD or CAPD, and insulin resistance is presumably the cause of the defective triglyceride removal (247). The fractional removal rate of exogenous triglyceride from the blood (K_2) evaluated during intravenous fat tolerance tests appears to be an important parameter to identify the patients at risk of developing hypertriglyceridemia as increasing K_2 values were observed in patients with stable or decreasing triglyceride levels (229, 247).

Hypercholesterolemia results from increased levels of both VLDL cholesterol and LDL cholesterol. Glucose absorption from dialysis fluid, increased dietary protein intake and protein losses in the dialysate may all contribute to this abnormality (229). Changes in serum lipid concentration during CAPD are transitory except in a small group of patients with steadily increasing concentrations. In most patients, the uremic dyslipoproteinemia is essentially unchanged after one year of CAPD compared to pretreatment status (229, 248).

Potentially *atherogenic changes* are induced by CAPD, especially during the initial months of treatment. Atherogenic indices, such as the ratio between VLDL and HDL cholesterol as well as the ratio between VLDL plus LDL cholesterol and HDL cholesterol, have been shown to increase significantly in CAPD patients (229). The long term effects of the deterioration of uremic dyslipoproteinemia during CAPD are difficult to assess due to high drop-out rates (250). However, the incidence of cardiovascular deaths appears to be similar among CAPD and hemodialysis patients in spite of a better control of hypertension with CAPD (102, 251, 252). The possibility that CAPD is atherogenic cannot presently be ruled out, and it is, therefore, warranted to develop and evaluate therapeutic approaches to lower serum lipid levels in CAPD patients, such as dietary modifications, the restricted use of hypertonic dialysis fluids, exercise, the replacement of dextrose with new osmotic agents and the use of lipid lowering agents including L-carnitine (229).

Significant increases in serum concentrations of both

HDL$_2$ cholesterol and total HDL cholesterol, associated with a marked reduction in triglycerides, have been obtained in CAPD patients by the daily use of omega-3 polyinsaturated fatty acid (253). If these results are confirmed, fish oil containing eicosapentaenoic and docosahexaenoic acids will represent a major prophylactic approach to protect CAPD patients against further progression of atherosclerosis (254).

Vitamin loss in the dialysate has been evaluated in patients undergoing CAPD. Significant losses of hydrosoluble vitamins result in lower serum levels of vitamin B$_1$, B$_6$, folic acid and vitamin C in some patients, while vitamin B$_2$ and B$_{12}$ remain normal in short term studies (255). Daily supplementation with 30 mg vitamin B$_1$, 10 mg vitamin B$_6$, 0.5 folic acid, 100 mg vitamin C is advised (255). Decreasing serum vitamin B$_{12}$ levels may also occur over longer periods of treatment and supplementation with this vitamin appears warranted (256, 257). Fat soluble vitamin D derivatives are also removed by peritoneal dialysis. The permeability of the peritoneal membrane leads to significant loss of 25-hydroxycholecalciferol (25-OH-D$_3$) binding capacity, with loss of 25-OH-D in the dialysate (258). In CAPD patients, the serum concentrations of 1,25 dihydroxy-cholecalciférol (1,25-(OH)$_2$-D$_3$) are undetectable and those of 24,25(OH)$_2$-D$_3$ are considerably lower than in HD patients. The losses of both metabolites in the peritoneal fluid amount to 6 to 8% of the plasma pool per day (259). Increased replacement doses of vitamin D metabolites are clearly needed in CAPD patients.

Loss of carnitine occurs during both IPD and CAPD (260, 261). In spite of this loss, serum total carnitine concentrations remain normal during CAPD, whereas IPD patients demonstrate increased serum levels due to elevated concentrations of esterified carnitine. These abnormalities suggest limited carnitine utilization in the patients receiving maintenance peritoneal dialysis (261). Although normal plasma and muscle carnitine levels were reported during IPD and CAPD (260), one study suggests that carnitine depletion may occur during long term CAPD (262).

Free fatty acid loss during IPD was more important than expected on the basis of a transport mechanism involving simple diffusion. Free fatty acid concentration in dialysate exceeded those of plasma water, suggesting a tissue-lipase mediated release of fatty acid into peritoneal dialysate from adjacent adipose tissue (263). In two studies, plasma free fatty acid levels were measured during an IPD session: one group observed no variations (263) while a significant rise in serum fatty acid concentrations were consistently observed by the other (264).

Digestive symptoms

Nausea and vomiting are observed in about 35% of the patients receiving maintenance IPD in the home; these symptoms occur mainly during the first few dialysate exchanges (265). A decreased appetite is not exceptional in patients undergoing CAPD, particularly during the early stages of the treatment (229, 265). This side effect results in a selective reduction in dietary carbohydrate intake and in low protein consumption (266). Poor appetite may be due to continuous glucose absorption or to abdominal distension by peritoneal fluid. Obviously, inadequate dialysis as a cause of anorexia should be first ruled out before considering the loss of appetite as a side effect of CAPD.

Air under the diaphragm

Free air under the diaphragm is a common finding in patients undergoing IPD. As subdiaphragmatic air usually indicates bowel perforation in the context of peritonitis, this finding should be interpreted with caution in peritoneal dialysis patients. Small amounts of air are introduced at initiation of dialysis. When gravity is used to infuse heat sterilised solutions which do not contain dissolved gas, sufficient air to cause discomfort may enter the peritoneal cavity only if administration tubing sets repeatedly run dry and air is pushed into the abdomen by dialysate. When IPD is performed using a reverse osmosis machine, inadequately deaerated water may cause abdominal air accumulation. This phenomenon occurs primarily during the winter months, since cold water contains considerably more dissolved gas. An in-line bubble trap will retain efficiently most of the air (31).

In CAPD, the technique of bag exchange does not predispose to air instillation. Consequently, air is seen under the diaphragm with a very low incidence (267). Subdiaphragmatic air is mainly observed after specific procedures such as catheter reinsertion or extension tube changes, and also during transient use of IPD performed with an automatic equipment (reverse osmosis or cycler) (267). Small amounts of intraperitoneal air are innocuous. Large volumes of instilled air may cause peritoneal pleocytosis with eosinophilia and/or monocytosis (268) and shoulder pain (31, 268). The time required for the resorption of air from the peritoneal cavity varies with the amount of instilled air from 4 days for 100 ml to 7 weeks for 500 ml (268).

Duration of peritoneal dialysis procedures

One of the most prominent side effects of peritoneal dialysis, and also one of the most neglected, is the time required to obtain adequacy of treatment with this dialysis modality. By comparison with the urea clearance of modern hemodialysers, the instantaneous peritoneal clearance of urea is 10 to 15 times lower with IPD and 30 to 40 times lower with CAPD (129). The only way to compensate for the low efficiency of IPD is to lengthen the duration or to increase the frequency of dialysis or both. This unavoidable side effect has long been seen as a major obstacle to a wider use of IPD in the treatment of end-stage renal disease.

With CAPD, the benefit of living without a machine was partly spoiled by the inconvenience of daily multiple bag exchanges. With four exchanges per day, the never ending manual labour of CAPD (269) is tantamount to about 2 to 2.5 h/day. Accumulated time of 14 h/week devoted to CAPD procedures is clearly longer than present days' schedules of rapid high efficiency hemodialysis (270). Weariness induced by repetition and time committment required for CAPD is not an exceptional cause of drop-out (17).

COMPLICATIONS OF PERITONEAL DIALYSIS

Since its use became a routine, peritoneal dialysis has been plagued by a great variety of mechanical, inflammatory and metabolic complications, some of them potentially lethal. These complications have been thoroughly reviewed (48, 49, 271, 272). Table 4 presents the complications that may acutely occur during peritoneal dialysis, and Table 5 lists those observed in the course of maintenance peritoneal dialysis. Although arbitrary, this classification offers some practicality to the clinician faced with an unexpected problem in a patient undergoing peritoneal dialysis, whatever the indication or the utilized procedure. The complications related to the insertion or the use of the peritoneal catheter are discussed in the section dealing with peritoneal access (vide supra). Peritonitis, loss of ultrafiltration and sclerosing peritonitis, are not dealt with in this section as they are discussed at length in chapter 25.

Acute complications (other than peritonitis)

The term acute complications includes all unusual events that may happen during peritoneal dialysis, exposing the patient to an unexpected hazard. These complications supervene most often during IPD, but they may also occur at the initiation of CAPD (e.g. massive hydrothorax) or during the course of long term, previously uneventful CAPD (e.g. pancreatitis).

Table 4. Acute complications of peritoneal dialysis other than peritonitis.

I	Abdominal pain
II	Inadequately rewarmed dialysis fluid
III	Water and electrolyte imbalances
	Hypernatremia
	Hypo- or hypervolemia
	Hypo- or hyperkalemia
IV	Acid-base disorders
	Metabolic alkalosis
	Metabolic acidosis
V	Disequilibrium syndrome
VI	Acute metabolic changes
	Hyper- or hypoglycemia
	D-lactate toxicity (?)
VII	Pulmonary complications
	Basal atelectasis pneumonia
	Massive hydrothorax
VIII	Cardiovascular complications
	Arrhythmias
IX	Acute pneumoperitoneum
X	Pancreatitis (?)

Pain

Although much less common with the permanent Silastic catheter than with the disposable catheter (7, 31), pain occurring during dialysis is always distressing to the patient. Localization and timing of pain should be carefully studied.

Pain occurring during inflow can be caused by low temperature of the dialysis solution or by a low pH of the solution requiring adequate sodium hydroxide buffering (31, 273, 274). Pain can be caused by a pulsatile fluid inflow due to infusion by a peristaltic pump. This pain may be alleviated by infusion by gravity or by using special flow dampeners (275). Pain during infusion is also more frequent with acetate than lactate containing dialysis solutions (276). Pain can also be caused by a high inflow rate, particularly in case of peritoneal catheter encasement. Pain may be also a symptom of low grade peritonitis and peritoneal adhesion formation (31). Painful abdominal distension at the end of infusion should be relieved by immediate drainage and reduction of exchange volumes.

Outflow pain is much less common. It may be due to entrapment of omentum in the catheter lumen during drainage; incomplete emptying of the abdominal cavity, longer dwell-times and analgesics will help the patient. *Permanent pain* occurring after several hours of dialysis is suggestive of mechanical or chemical peritoneal irritation and improves quickly with oral indomethacin (50 to 100 mg). Constant pain persisting after dialysis completion is almost always indicative of peritonitis (except during the period following catheter implantation). Catheter related pain has been discussed previously.

Inadequately rewarmed dialysis fluid

Infusion of *inadequately rewarmed* dialysis solution has been a cause of severe complications. Infusion of cold dialysis fluid can induce acrocyanosis or cardiac arrhythmias (271). This resulted in a cardiac arrest in two children (31). Overheated dialysate is a cause of severe intra-abdominal pain that may be quickly relieved by immediate drainage of the dialysate; however, it has been followed in one occasion by a persistent paralytic ileus and metabolic acidosis (272). Fail safe temperature monitoring is mandatory for automatic and semi-automatic peritoneal dialysis equipment.

Water and electrolyte imbalances

Peritoneal dialysis disturbs the metabolism of water and electrolytes and of carbohydrates. Electrolyte imbalance due to renal failure is usually satisfactorily corrected by peritoneal dialysis; however, difficulties with dialysate outflow, excessive administration of dialysis solutions with high osmolality or unusual permeability characteristics of the peritoneal membrane observed in certain patients (161, 243) may all induce metabolic complications.

Hypernatremia
Hypernatremia is a special hazard of IPD, resulting from

short diffusing times and prolonged use of hyperosmolar dialysis solutions. Plasma Na concentrations over 150 mmol/l have been reported in 3 to 10% of dialyses (49, 277). This complication is induced by osmotic ultrafiltration with the production of a hyponatric ultrafiltrate (278). It can be prevented by giving to the patient adequate amounts of free water orally or 5% dextrose solution intravenously depending on his clinical status. Hypernatremia can also result from the accidental instillation of hypernatric dialysis fluid due to a malfunctioning reverse osmosis machine (268).

Hypovolemia

Hypovolemia resulting in acute hypotension and even shock because of excessive ultrafiltration has been observed. To prevent this, it is wise to test the ultrafiltration capacity of each patient by measuring the ultrafiltration obtained in a certain period of time with different dialysis solutions. It is also preferable to avoid more than two or three consecutive highly hypertonic exchanges to prevent this complication.

Hypervolemia

Hypervolemia can be caused by the accumulation of dialysate in the peritoneal cavity due to poor drainage or to a peritoneal fluid leak into the subcutaneous tissues caused by a rupture of the peritoneal membrane, in particular after recent abdominal surgery. The subsequent extracellular fluid overload can lead to hypervolemia with pulmonary edema or hypertension or both (48, 49). In this situation, extracorporeal ultrafiltration is mandatory.

Hypokalemia

Hypokalemia has been observed in 10 to 19% of peritoneal dialysis (49, 277); it is usually moderate and without clinical significance, but may cause severe arrhythmias in a digitalised patient. Severe hypokalemia can occur with prolonged peritoneal lavage in the anorectic patient (e.g. with peritonitis) and may be aggravated by dextrose loading and correction of acidosis. To prevent this risk, 2 to 4 mmol/l KCl should be added to dialysis solutions.

Hyperkalaemia

Hyperkalaemia results from the inappropriate use of potassium containing dialysate (48) or from ineffective dialysis in a highly catabolic patient. A sudden rise of serum K has been noted shortly after termination of peritoneal dialysis and has been attributed to the breakdown of glycogen (49); it never reached levels requiring the resumption of dialysis.

Acid-base disorders

Metabolic alkalosis

Metabolic alkalosis with serum bicarbonate level over 30 mmol/l has been observed both in IPD (279) and in CAPD (280). This disorder was due to the use of dialysis solutions containing 42 to 45 mmol/l lactate in patients undergoing IPD (279). Contraction alkalosis was suggested as the mechanism explaining elevated plasma bicarbonate levels in two diabetic patients receiving CAPD (280). In one patient undergoing CCPD, two episodes of severe respiratory alkalemia were observed due to the lack of physiologic renal response (281).

Metabolic acidosis

Metabolic acidosis may also occur when peritoneal dialysis is performed with lactate containing dialysis solutions in patients with liver failure. This can be corrected by intravenous bicarbonate or continuation of dialysis with a solution containing acetate (48, 282) or bicarbonate (283).

Disequilibrium syndrome

Neurologic complications including confusion, headache, neuromuscular irritability, transient cerebral abnormalities or seizures during IPD have been noted in 6 to 18% of dialyses (49, 277). They have been attributed to the *dialysis disequilibrium syndrome*, but metabolic disturbances (hyperosmolality, hypoglycemia, alkalosis) may cause similar manifestations and should be excluded. Convulsions have also been observed 6 to 12 h after termination of dialysis (49, 277); in one series this was associated with impaired lactate metabolism (284). Cerebral dysfunction associated with hyperventilation and respiratory alkalosis due to increased level of D-lactate may also be misdiagnosed as dialysis disequilibrium syndrome (285). Studies on lactate metabolism in IPD and CAPD demonstrate, however, that lactate is rapidly utilised in dialysed uremics (286). They also suggest that the risk of D-lactate toxicity is low during peritoneal dialysis because D-lactate appears to be as important a source of bicarbonate as its L isomer (287, 288).

Acute blood glucose level variations

Disorders of blood glucose regulation may occur both in IPD (49, 277) and in CAPD (229, 289). With IPD, blood sugar levels over 11 mmol/l (200 mg/dl) have been observed in 10 to 15% of dialyses (49, 277). *Severe hyperglycemia* may occur even in the non diabetic patient with the prolonged use of 215 mmol/l (4.25%) concentration of dextrose monohydrate in dialysis solutions because of rapid loading with dextrose, absence of glycosuria and uremic carbohydrate intolerance (241). This rare complication (occurring in 1 to 3% of dialyses) can result in hyperosmolar (nonketotic) coma with convulsions and death. However, serum glucose levels over 60 mmol/l with serum sodium of 125 mmol/l were reported to occur without associated neurologic impairment (289). It was suggested that the absence of osmotic diuresis and the reduced peritoneal osmotic ultrafiltration resulting from hyperglycemia prevented the development of hypernatremia and hyperosmolar coma. Close monitoring of blood sugar levels is mandatory when serial exchanges with high dextrose concentrations are needed and insulin should be given intraperitoneally (290) or subcutaneously to maintain blood sugar levels below 16.5 mmol/l (300 mg/dl).

Severe hypoglycemia may occur after cessation of dialysis in patients receiving insulin during IPD. Convulsions with irreversible brain damage can complicate such hypoglycemic episodes (48). Prevention is best accomplished by omitting intraperitoneal insulin for the last four exchanges or by leaving a final volume of 500 ml of 215 mmol/l (4.25 g/dl) dextrose monohydrate dialysate in the peritoneal cavity at the end of dialysis (272); with subcutaneous insulin, the last injection should be administered at least 6 h before terminating dialysis. Spontaneous hypoglycemia was also observed in a CAPD patient during an episode of peritonitis. Acute liver failure accounted for this accident which occurred in spite of the presence of glucose containing dialysate in the abdomen (291). Fatal hypoglycemia was also observed during CAPD in a young diabetic not receiving insulin (292).

Pulmonary complications

Pneumonitis following basal atelectasis may occur during prolonged peritoneal dialysis, particularly in the overhydrated patients with acute renal failure receiving IPD in the supine position (213). Prophylactic measures include dialyzing the patient with reduced exchange volumes in a sitting position, adequate ultrafiltration and physical respiratory therapy (213).

Acute massive hydrothorax

This complication has been reported with an increasing frequency in patients undergoing IPD (293–297) or CAPD (298–306), with an estimated incidence of 5% among the patients and an apparent female preponderance (305). Commonly revealed by an increasing shortness of breath occurring within hours to a few days after the onset of CAPD, the massive hydrothorax is easily recognised upon clinical examination and chest roentgenogram. It is usually right-sided with only a few exceptions. The passage of dialysis solution in the pleural cavity may be confirmed by the high dextrose concentration or the presence of D-lactate in the pleural fluid (305). The passage of methylene blue (298–300) or of technetium-99m-labelled macro aggregated albumin (298, 299) from the peritoneal cavity to the pleural space, have also been advocated to confirm the peritoneal origin of the pleural fluid.

The pathogenesis of this complication is still unclear, but the acute onset of hydrothorax following the initiation of peritoneal dialysis and its rapid resolution after discontinuation, suggest that the dialysis fluid reaches the pleural space through a pre-existing diaphragmatic defect co-existing with anatomical pleuro-peritoneal communication. The defects, usually too small to be detected on gross examination, could be seen in one case at thoracotomy (304) and in another case at careful dissection done at autopsy (302). When massive hydrothorax occurs, CAPD should be discontinued without delay after complete drainage of the peritoneal cavity. The pleural effusion should be tapped to give functional relief and the patient should be transferred to hemodialysis. If continuation of peritoneal dialysis is deemed necessary, some patients will do well on IPD. Pleurodesis obtained by pleural poudrage, a painful procedure

(300), or intrapleural tetracycline (305), or surgical closure of the diaphragmatic cleft (304) may be indicated if the patient refuses transfer to hemodialysis. Before resorting to these treatment approaches, it should be kept in mind that massive hydrothorax may resolve spontaneously after transient cessation of CAPD (306).

In posttraumatic acute renal failure, acute hydrothorax has been ascribed to the seeping of fluid through a rent in the diaphragm (271).

Cardiovascular complications

A high incidence of tachyarrhythmias and cardiac arrest has been reported in patients treated with acute peritoneal dialysis (277). Possible mechanisms leading to these dangerous arrhythmias include hypovolemia the rapid correction of hyperkalemia, hypocalcemia, hyponatremia or acidosis and digoxin intoxication (272). The inappropriate ventilation and hypoxemia which occur during peritoneal dialysis (210–212) may also contribute to triggering cardiac arrhythmias (307).

Bradyarrhythmias during IPD using a stylet catheter were attributed to a vasovagal reflex induced by abdominal distension or the manipulation of the peritoneal catheter (308).

In patients undergoing CAPD, a prospective study using 24 h Holter monitoring did not reveal any difference in arrhythmia type or frequency whether the monitoring was done concurrently with the performance of CAPD or with an empty abdomen while interrupting CAPD for 24 h (309). Left ventricular hypertrophy, frequently observed among dialysed uremic patients (310), may account for atrial and/or ventricular premature beats commonly observed in CAPD patients.

Acute abdominal events

Wound dehiscence with evisceration is a real hazard when acute peritoneal dialysis is performed following recent abdominal surgery (48, 271). In long term IPD and CAPD, it may be facilitated by protein malnutrition. This severe complication should be prevented by sealing tightly the abdominal incision at the termination of the surgical procedure, by providing total parenteral nutrition pre- and post-operatively and by using small volume exchanges (272, 311); it is often safer to treat the patient with hemodialysis until the abdominal wound heals.

Acute pneumoperitoneum may be observed after accidental air infusion at the end of dialysis when an automatic cycler with a roller pump is used for dialysate infusion or when a reverse osmosis machine is fed with poorly deaerated water. Acute pneumoperitoneum may cause persistent epigastric and shoulder pain in the upright position; air removal should be attempted by infusing 1 or 2 l dialysis fluid in the peritoneal cavity and asking the patient to resume Trendelenburg or chest-knee position (31).

Hemoperitoneum is characterized by red discoloration of peritoneal effluent. Peritoneal bleeding of minor importance was observed with an incidence of 31%, while bleeding requiring transfusion occurred in 1% of the cases in acute peritoneal dialysis (49). In CAPD, hemoperitoneum is not exceptional. Predominant among female patients, it usually follows a benign course with spontaneous resolution (312). Sometimes of unknown etiology, hemoperitoneum may result from various causes, including menstruation, enema, trauma (313), thrombocytopenia, peritonitis, ovarian tumor, ruptured polycystic kidney (312), radiation induced peritoneal injury (314), ruptured hepatic artery aneurism (315), erosion of a small artery by the peritoneal catheter (316), acute cholecystitis, colonoscopy (317) and rupture of the spleen (318). Recurring bloody dialysate, usually observed in female patients during menses (319) was associated to upper respiratory tract infection in a CAPD patient with mesangial IgE glomerulonephritis (320) and followed extracorporeal shock wave lithotripsy in another (321). A case of fatal massive hemoperitoneum occurring 9 months after CAPD cessation was attributed to the formation of chronic inflammatory tissue around bowel adhesions (322).

Acute pancreatitis
The incidence of pancreatitis is thought to be greatly increased in chronic uremia (323) and a high prevalence of pancreatic pathology has been demonstrated in patients sustained on long term hemodialysis (324). Several reports suggest that acute pancreatitis may be a specific complication of IPD or CAPD (325–330). In one case, pancreatitis abated when CAPD was witheld and recurred on its resumption, necessitating termination of this therapy (327). The disease usually occurs in nonalcoholic patients without gallstones or biliary tree abnormality. The clinical picture is commonly suggestive of peritonitis (326). The diagnosis of pancreatitis should be considered when abdominal pain and a cloudy dialysate persist in spite of appropriate antibiotic therapy. A brownish-black colored peritoneal effluent, due to the presence of methemalbumin was found of diagnostic value in one case (329), while a nonketotic hyperosmolar diabetic pre-coma associated to peritonitis led to the recognition of acute hemorragic pancreatitis in a boy undergoing CAPD (330). Serum amylase levels and amylase activity of dialysate show marked elevations which differentiate pancreatitis from infectious peritonitis (331). Computerized tomography, a more sensitive method than ultrasound to detect pancreatitis, should be performed to confirm this diagnosis in patients with persistent unexplained abdominal symptoms (326).

The acute abdomen in maintenance peritoneal dialysis
Besides peritonitis, which is discussed in chapter 25, intercurrent acute visceral diseases are commonly observed in patients undergoing IPD or CAPD (32, 311, 332). Acute abdominal pain, nausea and vomiting, sometimes associated with fever, are usually the initial symptoms. The differential diagnosis is made difficult because the clinical picture is obscured by the irrigation of the peritoneal cavity (311). The association of a cloudy peritoneal effluent may further confuse the diagnosis. An acute abdomen should be suspected in the presence of peritonitis resistant to adequate antibiotic

treatment. Appendicitis (332), diverticulitis (333), cholecystitis (334) and bowel perforation (32, 311) are the most common etiologies, requiring early diagnosis and timely surgery (311). Acute bowel occlusion is not a rare cause of the acute abdomen; it may result from bowel incarceration in a parietal defect (335) or in the catheter tract (336, 337), or from an internal hernia (338) (see also section on hernia). Acute abdominal symptoms may also result from ischemic colitis due to hypotensive episodes (339, 340) and from transient choleperitoneum (341).

Miscellaneous acute complications

Other acute complications include various rare clinical entities. Two cases of *chyloperitoneum* were reported one in a 8 year old girl who received acute IPD for extensive burns complicated with acute renal failure (342) and the other in a 13 year old girl during the course of CAPD (343).

Fournier's syndrome, characterised by fulminant necrotising subcutaneous infection of the male genitalia, was observed in two CAPD patients as a consequence of massive scrotal edema (344). *Subcutaneous necrosis of the skin of the anterior abdominal wall* resulted from a leak of heparin containing dialysate into the area in a patient undergoing CAPD (345).

A case of *acute aluminum intoxication* was also observed in a CAPD patient (346) resulting in non specific symptoms such as lethargy, mental changes, vomiting and headache. Discontinuation of all aluminum containing medicine was associated with a rapid fall in serum Al concentration and a considerable improvement in the general health and intellectual state of the patient. This favorable outcome obtained without CAPD cessation pointed out the major role of oral Al containing phosphate binders in the acute toxicity of aluminum (346). *Acute aluminum intoxication* resulting in digestive symptoms, cramp-like abdominal pain and general malaise was also observed as a consequence of accidentally contaminated peritoneal dialysis fluid (347).

Chronic complications of maintenance peritoneal dialysis

Long term peritoneal dialysis, whatever the utilized technique, may result in five main groups of chronic complications (excluding loss of ultrafiltration and sclerosing peritonitis) which are presented in Table 5: 1) deterioration of the peritoneal membrane, 2) parietal complications, 3) cardiovascular complications, 4) metabolic complications, 5) miscellaneous.

Deterioration of the peritoneal membrane

The peritoneum is a living membrane. During long term peritoneal dialysis, not only is this serosa submitted to the undesirable effects of this procedure but also the mesothelium and the submesothelial tissues suffer from repeated attacks of peritonitis. As a consequence, the peritoneal membrane may deteriorate with time resulting in a partial or total loss of dialysis efficacy. Unfortunately, short of sensitive and easily reproducible tests of peritoneal function, epidemiologic data studying the prevalence of this complication in large numbers of patients are lacking.

Peritoneal adhesions, peritoneal fibrosis and loss of peritoneal membrane surface area

When numerous peritoneal adhesions develop loculation of peritoneal fluid or complete obliteration of the peritoneal cavity will result in inadequate dialysis, requiring cessation of PD. The reported prevalence of this complication is difficult to assess, although histological studies of the peritoneum have documented a frequent development of scar tissue following peritonitis (348, 349). Inadequate dialysis that may reflect peritoneal membrane failure was more commonly reported among IPD patients (350–353) than in those undergoing CAPD (17). In a large Canadian series, membrane failure was recognised as the cause of CAPD discontinuation in 2.5% of the patients (354). In another series, a progressive decline of peritoneal urea clearances was observed in a subgroup of patients with a high peritonitis incidence (355). However, it should be noted that a drop in mass transfer area coefficient (MTAC) to less than half the average value would be required before membrane properties could exert a significant effect on clearances (129). Sequential measurement of peritoneal clearances are therefore insensitive methods to detect slight changes of the transport ability of reflecting structural alterations of the peritoneal membrane. In two series, repeated measurement of MTAC, a more sensitive method for evaluating peritoneal function, were performed in CAPD patients (162, 356); progressive deterioration of this parameter was observed in 20 (355) and 26% (162) of the patients, respectively. On the other hand, long term preservation of peritoneal function in patients undergoing CAPD for 5 or more years was reported in small groups of patients (258, 357). Another degenerative

Table 5. Chronic complications of peritoneal dialysis other than loss of ultrafiltration and sclerosing peritonitis.

I	Deterioration of the peritoneal membrane
	Adhesion formation
	Peritoneal calcifications
	Loss of membrane surface area and inadequate dialysis
II	Parietal complications
	Dialysate leaks
	Abdominal hernias
	Back pain
III	Cardiovascular complications
	Chronic hypotension
	Exacerbation of peripheral vascular disease
IV	Metabolic complications
	Protein malnutrition
	Disorders of glucose and lipid metabolism
	Permanent diabetes mellitus
	Obesity
	Hypertriglyceridemia
V	Psychological complications
	Patient's or helper's burnout
	Chronic depression

change of the peritoneal structure in CAPD patients relates to small peritoneal vessels. Replication of the basal lamina of mesenteric capillaries has been observed after a certain period of CAPD in non-diabetic patients (349).

Peritoneal calcifications

Peritoneal calcifications were described in patients receiving long term IPD and/or CAPD (358, 359). On plain X-rays of the abdomen, they had an eggshell-like appearance and prevailed in the pelvic area, lining the pouch of Douglas. Major clinical findings included hemoperitoneum, repeated subocclusive episodes, and infectious peritonitis, but about 25% of the patients were asymptomatic. The precise cause of peritoneal calcifications remains unknown; acetate containing peritoneal dialysis solutions, frequent episodes of peritonitis and hyperparathyroidism were suggested as possible etiological factors (358, 359). The deposition of calcium and phosphorus in the peritoneal serosa presumably represents an example of dystrophic calcifications. In this type of calcifications, serum Ca and P levels are within the normal range and the site of calcifications are areas that are already abnormal before the pathological mineralization occurs. Necrotic tissues or scarred tissues, especially if of long standing, may both undergo progressive calcification. The mineral is usually in the form of hydroxyapatite Ca_{10} $(PO_4)_6$ $(OH)_2$ (360).

Parietal complications

Due to the increased intra-abdominal pressure induced by the volume of intraperitoneal fluid (204, 206), the various structures of the anterior abdominal wall, the lumbo-sacral spine and the diaphragm are submitted to unusual mechanical strains that can produce three major parietal problems: 1) dialysate leaks, 2) abdominal hernias, 3) back pain.

Dialysate leaks

Besides the external dialysate leaks that occur following catheter implantation (vide supra section on complications of peritoneal catheters), late dialysate leaks may occur at any time in the course of peritoneal dialysis. Rare with IPD, their incidence in CAPD ranges from 2 to 10% of the patients (73). External leaks through the skin exit site are easily recognised. Internal leaks may be difficult to diagnose when the peritoneal fluid diffuses evenly throughout the layers of the abdominal wall. The most common site of leak is around the catheter entrance to the peritoneum, but leaks may also occur through previous surgical incisions or areas of brittle peritoneal tissue difficult to localize. Rapid weight gain unexplained by dietary indiscretion and the sudden reduction in the drainage volume are early evidence of internal dialysate leaks. Localized edema of the abdominal wall and/or subcutaneous accumulation of dialysis fluid in the external genitalia, the buttocks and the thighs are pathognomonic of dialysate leakage (361). Unusual presentations include massive and painless swelling of the penis and the scrotum that may reveal a latent open processus vaginalis (362) and pseudonecrotizing fasciitis due to simultaneous air and dialysate leakage (363). Computerized tomography performed after intraperitoneal infusion of dialysis solution added with contrast material (361, 364, 365) or peritoneal scintigraphy (366) may help to localize the site of leakage. After a 2 week period of temporary discontinuation, CAPD can usually be resumed but relapsing episodes of leakage have also been reported (366). Cure may also be obtained by surgical correction of the parietal defect (367). If the leak reappears after surgery, the patient should definitely be transferred to hemodialysis.

Abdominal hernias
The incidence of newly formed abdominal hernias among CAPD patients ranges from 10 (368) to 25% (369). Hernias may form at usual sites (i.e. inguinal, umbilical, epigastric), but approximately half of them develop through a healed incision or at the site of the catheter insertion. In one series, two thirds of patients with incisional hernias had a temporary dialysate leak following catheter placement (368). A predominance of women, often multiparous, is observed among patients who develop hernias. Significant risk factors in the development of hernias include age greater than 40 years, three or more laparotomies, three or more pregnancies and a hernia repaired prior to commencing CAPD (369).

The most common initial presentation is localized painless swelling, but acute bowel obstruction is not exceptional (368–372). Acute abdominal pain and peritonitis may reveal incarcerated small bowel loops or omentum (369). Isolated genital edema is another unusual presentation of inguinal or umbilical hernias (373, 374). Subclinical inguinal hernias are best demonstrated by peritoneal scintigraphy (366, 375). Insertion of the peritoneal catheter through the midline appears to facilitate the formation of incisional hernias. The use of a paramedian incision through the rectus muscle (65, 73), as well as the placement of double cuff peritoneal catheters (79) may reduce the incidence of this complication. The surgical repair of abdominal hernias does not necessitate discontinuation of maintenance peritoneal dialysis. After the operation, intermittent peritoneal dialysis with small dialysate volumes can be used as temporary treatment for 10 to 15 days until CAPD is resumed (365). Pre-existing abdominal hernias do not contraindicate CAPD, but they should preferably be repaired before CAPD is begun (376).

Back pain
In CAPD, the permanent presence of 2 to 3 l of dialysate in the peritoneal cavity alters body posture and causes low back strain. CAPD patients are therefore prone to the development of recurrence of a low back pain syndrome, which can lead to the discontinuation of CAPD (377). In fact, among the few patients who develop back pain while on CAPD, most have a history of back disorders and present degenerative spinal disease or metabolic bone disease, and/or extraspinal diseases affecting the normal spinal mechanics (e.g. obesity, weak abdominal muscles, arthritis of the hip) (378). Prevention of back pain is the best therapeutic approach. Back education, performed during the training

period of CAPD, will teach simple and graded exercises (e.g. pelvic tilt in lying or standing) adapted to the exercise tolerance of the individual patient (377).

Cardiovascular complications

Chronic hypotension
Chronic hypotension usually associated with symptomatic orthostatic hypotension develops in a small number of patients undergoing CAPD (246, 379, 380). This fall in arterial pressure results from a failure to adjust the 'dry weight' of the patient. Underestimation of the 'dry weight' is not uncommon during CAPD because a rapid increase in body mass is observed after initiation of the treatment and because hypoproteinemia, frequent in these patients, may cause peripheral edema which can be misinterpreted as intravascular fluid overload despite chronic hypovolemia. A state of extracellular volume depletion is also facilitated during the first weeks of CAPD by a low Na intake due to anorexia (252, 379). Furthermore, the reactivity of the sympathetic nervous system to standing may be inadequate in these patients (381). Chronic hypotension can be efficiently corrected by salt loading which produces an increase in extracellular volume and in sympathetic tone (381).

Symptomatic exacerbation of peripheral vascular disease
This complication, that may lead to gangrene of the lower limbs, was reported in CAPD patients with pre-existing peripheral atherosclerosis. Presumably related to chronic hypovolemia, it should be feared in the patients with previous intermittent claudication and may force a change from CAPD to intermittent peritoneal dialysis or hemodialysis (391) if ischemic symptoms worsen after initiating CAPD.

Metabolic complications

Protein malnutrition
Severe malnutrition was a major cause of transfer to hemodialysis among patients undergoing IPD (350–353). On the other hand, clinically overt protein energy malnutrition or severe hypoproteinemia are rarely reported among CAPD patients. Accumulating evidence indicates that protein malnutrition may be more common in CAPD than initially believed (229). Dietary surveys reveal that daily dietary protein intakes are often lower than recommended ranging from 0.7 to 1.0 g/kg (266, 383) and show a tendency to decrease with time on CAPD (229).

Muscle biopsy studies show that muscle content in non-collagen alkaline soluble protein (ASP) is significantly reduced as well as the ratio of ASP/DNA (229, 384, 385). Skeletal muscle intracellular concentration of free amino acids are abnormal and indicate a marked depletion of taurine and tyrosine (229) that may contribute to muscle fatigue, a frequent complaint in CAPD patients (380). Persistent protein depletion was also suggested by the association of cell overhydration, a low muscle nitrogen content and a reduced exchangeable protein pool (385). Similarly, a prospective study of total body nitrogen, which is an index of total body protein mass, identified a gradual deterioration of the nutritional status of patients undergoing CAPD for more than 2 years, particularly in men and those of large body size (383). Frequent assessment of nutritional status is mandatory, particularly during the first year of treatment, to obtain optimal nutrition of the CAPD patients (386).

Disorders of glucose and lipid metabolism
Severe disorders of glucose and lipid metabolism are seldom observed among CAPD patients (229). However, some may develop permanent hyperglycemia and become insulin-dependent de novo during CAPD as a consequence of the continuous glucose load (248).

Similarly, very high serum triglyceride concentrations may develop particularly in thos who show no improvement in the fractional removal rate of exogenous triglycerides during the intravenous fat tolerance test repeated after one year on CAPD (229). Obesity is also reported to occur in individual patients in whom the weight gain has been found to correlate with the use of hypertonic dialysis fluid (387, 388).

Miscellaneous chronic complications

Ascites
Ascites accumulation was described in patients receiving IPD (31, 389). This complication is more likely to happen with the use of highly hypertonic dialysis solutions, or in patients with low residual urine volume. Longer interdialytic intervals or sudden discontinuation of IPD (as for transplantation or transfer to hemodialysis), expose the patient to' the risk of ascites formation to the point of respiratory embarrassment. In one IPD series, repeated paracentesis was required to relieve respiratory discomfort. Biopsy of the peritoneum showed lesions typical of chronic inflammation (389). In most cases, however, ascites formation ceased spontaneously after several weeks to months (31). In a few cases, a laparotomy with complete removal of ascitic fluid appeared to obtain a dramatic improvement (389).

Ascites with elevated concentrations of protein and fibrin was a constant finding in cases of sclerosing encapsulating peritonitis (205, 390).

Ascites was also observed after transplantation in patients treated with CAPD, in adults (391) as well as in children (392, 393) with an incidence of 25 to 30% of the patients. The possibility that post transplant ascites represents a sign of acute rejection has been suggested (394).

Chronic aluminum intoxication
Aluminum concentration is commonly below 10 μg/l in peritoneal dialysis solutions (395–399), although a range from 2 to 50 μg/l was observed in two studies (396, 399). Effective removal of Al was observed during CAPD suggesting that the risk of chronic aluminum intoxication was very low in CAPD (395, 398). However, two cases of dialysis encephalopathy (400, 401) and one case of fracturing osteomalacia (402) were reported: the source of Al in these cases was suspected to be via gastrointestinal absorption. A study on risk factors for hyperaluminemia in CAPD concluded that

the Al intake from aluminum containing phosphate binders is a major factor in the evolution of hyperaluminemia and, potentially, aluminum toxicity in CAPD patients (403).

Other miscellaneous complications
Transmission of hepatitis B virus is a recognised hazard of hemodialysis procedures and precautionary measures to prevent antigen transmission are well established in dialysis units (404). Because peritoneal dialysis obviates the need for extracorporeal circulation, this treatment modality offers the theoretical benefit of reducing antigen exposure. In fact, HBsAg has been detected in the peritoneal effluent of infected patients (405). Two epidemics have demonstrated that contaminated peritoneal dialysis fluid may serve as a source of viral spread (406, 407). To reduce the risk of hepatitis B transmission in dialysis units, the transfer of HBsAg positive patients to CAPD is recommended (408).

Kidney stone formation occurred with an incidence 5.4% in CAPD patients (409). A consistent elevation of urine oxalate concentration and a relative increase in urine Ca were responsible for the rise in urine calcium oxalate activity product and stone formation. Treatment with 1,25-$(OH)_2$ cholecalciferol was the cause of increased urinary Ca concentration in these patients. Plasma oxalate levels in CAPD patients were found to be as elevated as those in hemodialysis patients before dialysis and may be a contributing factor to kidney stone formation (410).

Pseudoporphyria cutanea tarda (PCT), a bullous dermatosis, described in patients receiving maintenance hemodialysis (411), was observed in a CAPD patient (412). This disease developed in temporal association with non-A non-B hepatitis suggesting that the histopathological lesions of pseudo-PCT can be triggered by hepatocellular damage.

Finally, a case of *nonbacterial thrombotic endocarditis*, involving a partially calcified tricuspid aortic valve, has been observed in a CAPD patient (413). The disease progressed slowly over a period of one year. Repeated echocardiograms identified a tricuspid aortic valve with marked vegetations, the presence of which was confirmed at post-mortem examination. Non bacterial thrombotic endocarditis is usually associated with wasting diseases; it was suggested that the severe protein malnutrition observed in this patient was the causative factor.

INDICATIONS FOR PERITONEAL DIALYSIS

Due to its clinical simplicity and to its almost universal availability, peritoneal dialysis has been used not only in the treatment of acute and chronic renal failure, but also in various clinical states, most often but not always associated with renal dysfunction (414). The great diversity of peritoneal dialysis uses goes far beyond the conventional problems of solute removal from blood. In an attempt to present a full spectrum of its therapeutic applications in adults, the numerous uses of peritoneal dialysis are presented in Tables 6 and 7 under the two major headings of acute and chronic peritoneal dialysis.

Acute peritoneal dialysis

Peritoneal dialysis was initially proposed as an alternative to hemodialysis in the treatment of acute renal failure (ARF) (1, 2, 45). Although endogenous toxin removal remained over the years the major indication for PD, the field of its application was progressively enlarged to a variety of acute clinical situations shown in Table 6 including the treatment of acute poisoning and drug overdose, the correction of fluid electrolyte and acid-base disorders, the correction of acute metabolic disorders, the treatment of acute pancreatitis, and finally the administration of drugs and nutriments via the peritoneal route.

Peritoneal dialysis in acute renal failure

Intermittent PD is well established as an effective treatment of ARF (415). By comparison with hemodialysis, IPD admittedly offers some advantages such as technical simplicity, safety due to the absence of the extracorporeal circuit, no bleeding risk, excellent cardiovascular tolerance and low risk of disequilibrium syndrome. IPD has also recognized limitations with a lower effectiveness, the risk of peritoneal infection, the occurrence of obligatory protein loss, the need

Table 6. Indications for acute peritoneal dialysis.

A) *Toxin removal*
  1 Endogenous toxins
      Acute renal failure
      Fulminant hepatic failure
  2 Exogenous toxins
      Acute poisoning
      Drug overdose

B) *Fluid-electrolyte and acid-base disorders*
  1 Extracellular volume excess or depletion
  2 Hypo- or hyperkalemia
  3 Metabolic acidosis or metabolic alkalosis

C) *Acute metabolic disorders*
  1 Hypercalcemia
  2 Hypoglycemia
  3 Hyperuricemia
  4 Profound hypothermia

D) *Acute pancreatitis*

E) *Administration of drugs or nutrients*
  1 Local and systemic action: antibiotics
  2 Local action
      Standard heparin
      Chemotherapy (ovarian cancer)
  3 Systemic action
      Insulin (artificial pancreas)
      Deferoxamine
      Potassium, calcium
      Low molecular weight heparin
      Angiotensin I
  4 Nutritional support
      Artificial gut

---

for an intact peritoneal cavity ensuring an adequate membrane surface area and the required tightness for intermittent dialysate flow. Following the large scale use of CAPD in ESRD patients, continuous equilibration peritoneal dialysis (CEPD) has been proposed as a substitute to IPD in the management or ARF (143–146). Performed easily and safely without an automatic cycler, CEPD requires a smaller daily amount of sterile apyrogenic dialysis solutions and is therefore less costly than IPD.

Peritoneal dialysis versus hemodialysis in acute renal failure

During the past decade, indications for peritoneal dialysis became less common in ARF. Many reasons may explain this trend, including the practical problems of logistics, the availability of adequate nursing staff and the physicians prior training and personal biases. In fact, the less frequent use of peritoneal dialysis presumably results from multiple technological advances in extracorporeal dialysis. The introduction of various techniques such as bicarbonate hemodialysis with controlled ultrafiltration (416, 417), continuous arteriovenous (418, 419) or venovenous (420) hemofiltration and continuous hemodialysis (421) resulted in a better cardiovascular stability during treatment. Temporary blood accesses were easily obtained with the cutaneous implantation of cannulae in central veins including subclavian (47) or internal jugular veins (48). The bleeding risk of extracorporeal dialysis was effectively reduced by new anticoagulation techniques including low dose heparinization (422). HD without heparin (423), low molecular weight heparin (424) or regional citrate anticoagulation (425). Furthermore, extracorporeal dialysis offers the potential for higher ultrafiltration rates facilitating excellent control of extracellular volume when total parenteral nutrition is required. These developments in extracorporeal hemodialysis techniques opened a new field of investigation that attracted the interest of nephrologists, while PD fell in a relative disfavor. However, PD should not be neglected; the effectiveness of this method in the management of ARF has been confirmed over the years. No data are presently available to prove the superiority of more intensive dialysis on the eventual outcome of patients with acute uremia (426). As this syndrome is observed in patients of all ages (427) and is associated with a variety of risk factors (428), PD and HD should be seen as complementary to each other. By having both dialysis methods available in the intensive care unit, the nephrologist may provide his patients with the most suitable treatment at any given time.

General indications

Clearly, peritoneal dialysis may be utilized in all varieties of ARF. In case of obstruction of the urinary tract, it is the technique of choice to correct hyperkalemia or pulmonary edema in a patient requiring general anesthesia for urologic or surgical procedures. In cases of prerenal ARF associated with high blood urea levels, PD can be used to permit a faster control of uremia and to correct persisting fluid and electrolyte imbalances. However, PD finds it main indications in acute tubular necrosis. In adults, PD should be preferred in cases of ARF without hypercatabolism, in patients with bleeding complications, or in those with predominant extracellular volume excess, hypervolemia, and cardiopulmonary overload, particularly in case of associated cardiac failure. When there is a doubt as to the nature of the renal disease, PD is an excellent approach since it corrects the main acid-base and fluid electrolyte disorders, prevents or improves the bleeding tendency or uremia, and buys time to assess the patient's status before deciding whether to resort to hemodialysis or to continue with PD. Patients with severe cardiac disease or with a disease of the central nervous system are supposed to fare better with PD. However, a high incidence of arrhythmia and cardiac arrest was observed among ARF patients with pre existing heart disease who received PD (277). This observation suggested that PD may not be as safe in this group of patients, as previously contended.

Special indications

Hypercatabolic acute renal failure, defined by a high urea apparition rate with a daily rise in blood urea levels greater than 15 mmol/l, is observed in about 35% of the cases of acute tubular necrosis, particularly those complicating accidental trauma, post-operative surgery, severe burns, and leptospirosis (428). In such cases, early institution of dialysis, maintenance of adequate nitrogen and caloric intake during the period of illness, and continuation of periodic PD with elevated dialysate flow rates maintained blood urea levels below 30 mmol/l (429). Hypercatabolic ARF was also managed successfully by continuous equilibration peritoneal dialysis using 3 to 4 h dialysate dwell times (430). Successful treatment of ARF was also obtained with CAPD in cases of severe rhabdomyolysis (431). If peritoneal dialysis does not satisfactorily control uremia, hemodialysis should be instituted as soon as possible to meet the patient's dialysis needs.

ARF frequently complicates *surgery with cardiopulmonary bypass.* When this complication is severe enough to require dialysis, it is said to be highly lethal (432). Early institution of dialysis, as little as 24 h after oliguria, has been recommended to improve the outcome. Although hemodialysis can also be conducted without major complications, in such cases the less vigorous IPD or CEPD will give better results in patients with extremely unstable cardiovascular status (143, 433).

Acute renal failure after major abdominal surgery is another special indication for PD. Several reports confirm that peritoneal dialysis is technically possible after major abdominal surgery (including abdominal aortic grafts) and that it can obtain satisfactory results (434, 435). However, the occurrence of specific complications might be expected, particularly when the posterior peritoneum has been opened or when abdominal drains or colostomy are in place. Dissection of dialysis fluid in the subcutaneous tissue of the retroperitoneal space can lead to scrotal edema and later to pulmonary edema when the fluid is mobilized into the vascular space. Dialysate leakage around drains and enterostomies are almost unavoidable and result in grossly inaccurate

fluid balance. Wound dehiscence from abdominal distention can occur if too large a volume of dialysate is infused with each exchange or if dialysis fluid accumulates due to incomplete drainage during several cycles. In our experience, this complication carries a significant mortality. These potential problems are often seen as strong arguments to recommend hemodialysis in such patients (436).

An approach to the management of patients with *secondary bacterial peritonitis complicated by acute tubular necrosis* is to use PD to treat both peritoneal infection and ARF (149). At the end of abdominal surgery and after careful peritoneal toilet, a Silastic catheter is implanted and peritoneal irrigation is immediately initiated. Heparin and appropriate antibiotics should be added to dialysis solutions. This approach, however, is a source of potential dangers that should not be underestimated. The respiratory failure that often accompanies peritonitis may be aggravated, requiring mechanical respiratory assistance via an endotracheal tube during the lavage (149). Peritoneal irrigation, per se, and the considerable protein loss observed in case of peritoneal inflammation may interfere with wound healing of enterostomies and anastomoses. Finally, a positive fluid balance may result from the decreased capacity of the peritoneum to ultrafilter during peritonitis (437). In this context, extracorporeal dialysis together with adequate total parenteral nutrition seems preferable.

ARF has been reported with an increasing frequency following *large doses of iodinated contrast material.* In these cases, early institution of peritoneal dialysis is recommended to prevent uremia and pulmonary edema, which may result from intravascular infusion of osmotically active contrast media. Actually, it is an effective method to remove the offending agent. In one study, the peritoneal clearance of iodide was 12 ml/min with 2.0 l/60 min exchanges, and 56% of iodide was removed during 64 h of intermittent peritoneal dialysis (438).

ARF may cause death in *falciparum malaria.* Hemodialysis, though effective, is not commonly available in endemic malarial areas. PD is eminently suitable for hospitals in the tropics (439) and has been successful in the treatment of ARF following malarial hemoglobinuria (440). Studies of peritoneal function in these patients have shown that urea and creatinine clearances were low during the early acute stage of illness and returned to normal by the time the second dialysis was performed 48 h later. This phenomenon might be explained by the known occurrence of disseminated intravascular coagulation and red blood cells sludging in malaria or by a reduction in splanchnic blood flow during the acute illness (440). Such a problem was not encountered in another series, where falciparum malaria complicated by ARF was successfully managed by continuous peritoneal dialysis with a favorable outcome (441).

Peritoneal dialysis in fulminant hepatic failure and hepatic coma

Fulminant hepatic failure (FHF) is the acute failure of liver function occurring in a patient with no antecedent liver disease and in whom hepatic encephalopathy supervenes within 8 weeks after the onset of clinical symptoms (442). ARF frequently complicates this syndrome. The rate of survival from FHF in patients with stage IV hepatic encephalopathy (hepatic coma), which was approximately 10 to 20% in the early 1970s (443) was estimated to be 20 to 35% with modern supportive care (442). This high mortality rate justified the evaluation of various artificial liver support techniques, including charcoal hemoperfusion (444), hemodialysis with high permeability membrane (445) and post dilution hemofiltration (446). No single technique, however, has been widely applied or generally accepted. In the early 1960s, case reports suggested that IPD may have a beneficial role in the management of FHF (1, 447, 448). More recently, full recovery of FHF with hepatic coma was obtained by IPD in three of five patients (449). Potentially, IPD in FHF has both advantages and shortcomings. Automated IPD is easy to perform continuously during several days without increasing the bleeding risk of FHF due to prolonged prothrombin time and thrombocytopenia. Furthermore, adverse metabolic and hemodynamic factors that may worsen hepatic coma, including hyponatremia, hypoglycemia, hypokalemia or hypotension, can easily be prevented (449) or corrected (450) by peritoneal dialysis. Conversely, IPD may induce protein depletion, necessitating albumin infusion to maintain baseline serum albumin levels (450). Another shortcoming of IPD is the risk of peritonitis, which should be reduced by the use of an automatic cycler (115). The limited number of patients studied with IPD or with alternative artificial liver support does not permit a conclusion as to the relative value of these methods (442).

Peritoneal dialysis in acute poisoning and drug overdose

Numerous reports concerning the removal of drugs and poisons with peritoneal dialysis have been published (414, 451).Due to its relatively low efficiency, however, peritoneal dialysis does not permit the rapid removal of poisonous substances from the body. In fact, the clearances of small molecular weight toxins are consistently lower with peritoneal dialysis than with hemodialysis or hemoperfusion. The addition of various substances such as albumin (452), lipids (453) or furosemide (454) to the peritoneal fluid has been shown to enhance peritoneal clearances but not to the level achieved with hemodialysis. Therefore, most authors agree that peritoneal dialysis has a minor role if any to play in today's treatment of poisoning (455).

Occasionally, the use of IPD may be justified to treat accidental drug overdose in a patient receiving CAPD. This approach was successful in a case of tobramycin overdose, where the peritoneal aminoglycoside clearance reached 14.2 ml/min with a dialysate flow rate of approximately 4 l/h. The patient recovered without ototoxic sequellae (456). Resorting to IPD in such a setting was required because clearances by CAPD are 8 ml or less and do not affect appreciably the elimination of most drugs (457).

Peritoneal dialysis for the correction of acute fluid, electrolyte and acid-base disorders

Peritoneal dialysis effectively corrects a variety of fluid/electrolyte disorders (279). *Repletion of the extracellular volume* can be induced with 0.5 g/l dextrose dialysis solutions in cases of prerenal azotemia due to sodium depletion (279, 458, 459). Conversely, *removal of large amounts of extracellular fluid* can readily be obtained in cases of severe Na overload with hypervolemia and pulmonary edema, using hypertonic dialysis solutions (40 g/l dextrose) and dwell times of 15 to 30 min (279). *Hyperkalemia* is also effectively corrected by PD albeit more slowly than with HD. Besides K removal, which is limited to about 10 to 15 mmol/h, PD may lower serum K levels by the correction of metabolic acidosis and diffusion of glucose from dialysate to blood, which favor the shift of potassium into the cells (460). In cases of *hypokalemia*, peritoneal dialysis solutions have been shown to be a safe and effective route for acute potassium repletion provided the dialysis solution K does not exceed 20 mmol/l (461).

The correction of *metabolic acidosis* in ARF with peritoneal dialysis is due to the diffusion of a buffer anion, commonly lactate or acetate, more exceptionnally bicarbonate, from dialysate to blood. PD has been proposed as an adjunctive therapy for lactic acidosis for which dialysis solutions containing acetate (281) or bicarbonate (282) are recommended.

Peritoneal dialysis in the treatment of acute metabolic disorders

A role for peritoneal dialysis has been suggested in the management of a variety of acute metabolic disorders. In *hypercalcemia* due to vitamin D intoxication, calcium-free peritoneal dialysis solutions can significantly decrease serum Ca (462–464).

Hyperuricemia complicating leukemia has been successfully treated with peritoneal dialysis (465–467). Experiments in dogs suggested that the diffusion of uric acid across the peritoneal membrane was enhanced when the pH of peritoneal dialysate was increased by the addition of bicarbonate (468).

Severe protracted hypoglycemia due to acetohexamide in a patient with chronic renal failure was effectively corrected by peritoneal dialysis, which acted both by removing acetohexamide and its metabolites, and by providing glucose (469).

Peritoneal dialysis is also considered a safe treatment approach for core rewarming of patients with *profound hypothermia* (470–473).

Acute pancreatitis

Since the early 1960s peritoneal dialysis has been repeatedly advocated for the management of acute pancreatitis (473, 474), in an attempt to remove pancreatic enzymes from the peripancreatic tissues by peritoneal lavage and to curtail necrotic processes. Peritoneal clearances of lipase and amylase range from 5 to 13.5 ml/min with short dwell times (475); these values are five times those predicted from the molecular weight of these enzymes. This suggests direct spilling of lipase and amylase into the dialysate from necrotic pancreas and surrounding inflamed tissues.

In the absence of randomised prospective studies, the possible benefits of PD in the management of acute pancreatitis are difficult to evaluate. Numerous experimental and clinical studies, however, suggest that the use of PD in this context improves the prognosis and is associated with a lower morbidity and mortality (476, 477).

Administration of drugs and nutriments

The peritoneal cavity has been used as a route for the administration of numerous drugs. The expected effect of the administered drug may be predominantly local, systemic or both as shown in Table 6. However, due to the large pore size of the peritoneal membrane, most drugs given intraperitoneally diffuse into the blood. Care should be therefore be taken to use appropriate drug concentrations in the dialysate, lest toxic serum levels be reached (457). The drugs most commonly added to peritoneal dialysis solutions include various antibiotics for treating peritonitis complicating CAPD or IPD (103, 104), heparin to prevent the formation of fibrin clots in the dialysate (31, 478, 479) and insulin to obtain a better control of blood glucose levels in diabetics undergoing maintenance PD (480–482). In patients undergoing CAPD, medications indicated for intercurrent diseases have been occasionally administered via the peritoneal route, including deferoxamine for aluminum (483, 484) or iron (485) chelation, angiotensin I in a case of crippling orthostatic hypotension (486), and low molecular weight heparin in a case of deep vein thrombosis (487). Intraperitoneal chemotherapy has also been extensively used in the treatment of ovarian carcinomas (30, 488, 489).

Finally, both clinical (490) and experimental (491) studies have demonstrated that the peritoneal cavity may be used as a simplified gut for the administration of nutrients (i.e. dextrose and amino acids) in adults and children with acute renal failure.

Special indications in infants and children

It is often observed that peritoneal dialysis is a safer procedure in infants (492) and children (493) in whom it is more comfortable and easier to implement than hemodialysis. It has been commonly used in acute renal failure (494–498) including the hemolytic-uremic syndrome (499, 500), ARF following cardiopulmonary bypass (501) and after extensive resection of the small intestine (502), as well as in acute poisoning (503, 504). Peritoneal dialysis has also been used successfully in various diseases of infancy and childhood such as cystic fibrosis with congestive renal failure (505), Reyes' syndrome (506, 507), severe hydrops foetalis (508), the respiratory distress syndrome (509) and hyaline membrane disease of newborn premature infants (510). Encou-

raging results have also been obtained in the management of maple syrup urine disease (511), propionic acidemia (512), hyperbilirubinemia using albumin in dialysate (513), and neonatal lactic acidosis (514).

Chronic peritoneal dialysis

As shown in Table 7, peritoneal dialysis finds a wide field of application in chronic diseases, predominantly in chronic renal failure, today's major indication for this dialysis modality, more exceptionally in chronic conditions such as refractory congestive heart failure or multiple myeloma.

Peritoneal dialysis in chronic renal failure

Over the past decade, peritoneal dialysis has been increasingly used in the treatment of end stage renal disease following the advent of CAPD (14–17). In some geographical areas, the number of ESRD patients receiving CAPD has increased up to 45 to 65% of the total number of new patients admitted in an ESRD treatment program (17, 515, 516).

General indications

Peritoneal dialysis may be used in the context of chronic renal failure both as a temporary treatment and as long term maintenance therapy.

Table 7. Indications for chronic peritoneal dialysis.

A)   *End stage renal disease: maintenance peritoneal dialysis*
  1   Intermittent peritoneal dialysis
         Temporary treatment of ESRD
         Maintenance IPD
  2   CAPD
         Temporary: waiting for a transplant
         Long term:
             Independent patient – Home dialysis
             Special indications:
                 Diabetics
                 Children, elderly, spinal cord injury
             Special problems in hemodialysed patients:
                 severe cardiovascular instability
                 repeated blood connection failures
                 refractory hypertension, severe anemia
                 recurrent hepatic coma in hemodialysed
                 ESRD patients
  3   CCPD
         Dependent patients requiring a helper
             Children, elderly
         Independent patients requiring freedom from
         daytime exchanges: adolescents, workers

B)   *Refractory congestive cardiac failure*

C)   *Special indications*
  1   Multiple myeloma
  2   Amyloidosis
  3   Psoriasis

The temporary use of PD may be indicated in cases of sudden deterioration in renal function occurring in patients with chronic renal insufficiency from various etiologies (e.g. drug nephrotoxicity, urinary tract infection), in particular in patients with polycystic kidneys or chronic pyelonephritis, where prolonged remissions may be observed after a single PD (517). Temporary PD is also indicated in conjunction with a hemodialysis program in the following circumstances: 1) in preparation for blood access surgery in the bleeding uremic patient, 2) during maturation of a recently created arteriovenous fistula, 3) in patients with repeated thrombosis of the blood connection until a new access is created, 4) during an episode of dialysis-associated pericarditis, 5) as a holding procedure until a place becomes available in a hemodialysis unit, 6) in conjunction with an active transplantation program both to maintain the patient before transplantation and to manage post transplant acute renal failure (100–102).

Maintenance peritoneal dialysis is recognized as one of the major treatment modality of ESRD patients. However, in Europe, the use of CAPD varies from 2% in the Federal Republic of Germany to 47% in the United Kingdom, two countries with similar populations (516). Such a discrepancy in prescription habits among nephrologists of different countries reflects the fact that there is no absolute indication for PD. The rates and extent of application of CAPD will therefore be influenced by many factors, including 1) availability of hemodialysis units, 2) improvement in technology and equipment, 3) reimbursement mechanisms, 4) biases and committments of the nephrologists and the nursing team towards CAPD, 5) patients' referral patterns and 6) patients' preference, which may be influenced by a host of factors such as preconceived ideas, age, medical complications, psychosocial factors including home setting, family status and independency desires, convenience including time committment to therapy and distance between home and the dialysis unit, and finally patients' desire for professional rehabilitation (518).

In fact, the main impetus for the development of CAPD in ESRD treatment program came in some countries from an inadequate number of hemodialysis centers to face the demand (519) and in others from the wish to promote home dialysis and independence among ESRD patients as well as from economical constraints resulting from reimbursement practices. Some groups of patients, however, are conventionally considered as being especially benefitted by peritoneal dialysis, including 1) older patients, aged usually over 65 years, 2) patients with preexisting cardiovascular disease, so called high cardiovascular risk patients (e.g. patients with angina pectoris, previous myocardial infarction, cardiomyopathies, arrhythmias or previous cerebrovascular accident), 3) insulin and noninsulin dependent diabetic patients, 4) children, 5) patients with frequent blood access failure and those with severe bleeding risks and 6) Jehovah's witnesses.

Periodic peritoneal dialysis versus CAPD/CCPD
In the late 1970s a reappraisal of periodic (intermittent) peritoneal dialysis clearly demonstrated the limitations and potential dangers of this mode of dialysis (350–353). At the same time, the introduction of CAPD resulted in an almost complete lack of interest in IPD with few exceptions (520–522). Besides these two major factors, the constraints of IPD (i.e. long dialysis hours) and the high cost of the method due to the consumption of large volumes of commercially available peritoneal dialysis solutions with cyclers or to the high maintainance expenses with RO machines (523), contributed to the withdrawal of IPD from the armamentarium of ESRD therapy.

The extensive clinical experience acquired during the early 1980s with CAPD demonstrated beyond doubt its effectiveness and superiority over IPD. However, the latter still should keep a role in an ESRD treatment program. As a complement of CAPD and/or HD, conventional IPD (i.e. three dialyses per week, 10 to 12 h per dialysis) provides the nephrologist with a therapeutic technique that helps to solve a variety of clinical situations including 1) temporary IPD following the implantation of the peritoneal catheter before initiation of CAPD (46), 2) during a peritonitis episode secondary to diverticulitis in a CAPD patient (333), 3) home IPD in patients requiring a helper, in patients with high peritoneal transport rates of creatinine, glucose and sodium at the equilibration test (243, 244), who are not able to continue on standard CAPD schedule due to poor ultrafiltration and in CAPD patients with a progressive loss of ultrafiltration (158), 4) in-center ambulatory IPD (522) and 5) maintenance PD in a patient with a large inguino-scrotal hernia not accessible to surgery (31) or in a diabetic with lower limb peripheral vascular disease (382).

The clinician who prescribes IPD, however, should keep in mind its low efficiency. IPD may be safely used as long as the patient's residual renal function is over 3 ml/min. Careful monitoring of residual renal function is, therefore, of paramount importance in a patient dialysed three times weekly with IPD (524). This parameter should be controlled monthly and the dialysis duration should be increased by 9 h/week for each 1 ml/min decrement in glomerular filtration rate (525). Worth noting is the fact that the progressive loss in renal function observed in dialysed ESRD patients occurs faster with IPD than CAPD (526). The need to increase the weekly dialysis duration to compensate for the reduced GFR stimulated the interest in new IPD schedules, such as nightly IPD (139) or tidal IPD (140), which offer interesting alternatives to standard CAPD/CCPD or to maintenance HD.

Peritoneal dialysis in end stage diabetic nephropathy
Since the early days of maintenance peritoneal dialysis, IPD has been used in diabetic patients (527–531). It was then felt that IPD might be superior to HD for insulin dependent diabetic patients, as the prognosis with hemodialysis was deemed very poor (532). Indeed, very good results have been obtained with IPD, particularly in type I diabetes with actuarial survival rates of 60% at 5 years (531, 533). During the same period, however, remarkable improvement in the outcome of hemodialysed diabetic patients was also observed, with a 4 year cumulative actuarial survival of 60% in

patients less than 60 years of age (534). Since the early 1980s CAPD/CCPD replaced IPD in most centers as the treatment of choice for uremic diabetic patients (535). In the absence of prospective randomised studies, it is impossible to confirm the purported superiority of peritoneal dialysis over hemodialysis (530, 535). Nonetheless, CAPD offers several potential advantages to the diabetic patient (533). By suppressing the need for vascular access, CAPD obviates the difficulties and complications that may arise as a consequence of vascular surgery in the patients with peripheral atherosclerosis (536, 537). The control of blood pressure is made easier and only a few patients require antihypertensive therapy. The intraperitoneal administration of insulin added to dialysate (480–482) results in a better blood glucose normalisation. Both diabetic retinopathy and neuropathy may improve in some patients, but stabilization is more common, and only few patients show a progression of these complications (533). Inspite of frequent visual impairment, 70% of diabetics perform CAPD without assistance (535) and even some blind patients can master CAPD procedures to become independent (538). Most series indicate that the incidence of peritonitis is no higher in diabetic than in non-diabetic patients (533, 535). Peripheral vascular disease may, however, be aggravated by CAPD, resulting in lower limb gangrene (382).

First and second year actuarial cumulative survival reached 90 and 80% respectively in two series (533, 535); in another series, a cumulative survival of 70 and 44% at 1 and 5 years, respectively, was observed (53). These data confirm the effectiveness of CAPD as a long term treatment of end-stage diabetic nephropathy.

Peritoneal dialysis in children and adolescents
Peritoneal dialysis is particularly adapted to the treatment of ESRD in infants, children (540) and adolescents (541). Two major advantages by comparison with HD are the absence of an extracorporeal circuit, which obviates the need for repeated venipuncture often feared by children, and the simplicity of the PD techniques, making home dialysis an acceptable choice for most families (10, 540). Furthermore, an increased efficiency of peritoneal dialysis is favoured in children by smaller body weights (129). The main technical and clinical aspects of peritoneal dialysis in children are briefly reviewed here.

In large children or adolescents, PD techniques do not differ from adults. In smaller children and infants, however, peritoneal catheters and dialysate infusion volumes should be adapted to the body weight. Adult Tenckhoff catheters can be used in children weighing over 30 kg, while pediatric catheters (intraperitoneal segment [IPS] 12 to 14 cm length, 1.8 mm inner diameter [ID]) are recommended in children weighing 30 kg or less and neonatal catheters (IPS 10 to 12 cm length, 0.5 mm ID) in those weighing less than 5 kg (542). One cuff catheters, said to be associated with a lower incidence of tunnel infection, are preferred by some authors (542, 543), but equally good results have been reported with double cuff catheters (544). To reduce the rate of dialysate leaks, special care should be taken to create a water tight seal at the entry point of the catheter into the peritoneal cavity, using a permanent peritoneal purse-string suture anchored to the base of the catheter cuff (543). Both partial omentectomy (543) or the implantation of a TWH2 catheter (542, 545, 546) have obtained low rates of one way catheter obstruction, a frequent cause of catheter failure in the absence of these preventive measures. Dialysate leaks, exit site and tunnel infections as well as hernias are more frequently observed among children than in adults (542, 547).

The prescribed dialysate volume averages 35 to 50 ml/kg/ exchange (543, 548). Studies of mass transfer properties of the peritoneum have shown that they were similar in adults and in children, and that they could be related to body weight (129). Empiric observations suggest that adequate dialysis should usually be obtained with a CAPD regimen providing a total urea clearance (dialysate + residual GFR) of a least 210 ml/kg/day when dietary protein intake is 2.0 g/ kg/day (543).

In the 1970s several reports emphasised the clinical effectiveness of IPD in the treatment of children with end-stage uremia. IPD was found particularly suitable when performed overnight in the home under parents' supervision (10, 549, 550). As for the population of adult ESRD patients, however, in the early 1980s, CAPD/CCPD quickly superseded IPD in the care of children and adolescents (551–555). Many pediatric nephrologists consider this treatment modality as first choice in their patients awaiting renal transplantation (556, 557). The medical advantages resulting from the continuous nature of CAPD are even more conspicuous in children than in adults. However, the endless routine of CAPD often results in a syndrome of parents' fatigue with small children or in patients' burnout in the case of adolescents (540). CCPD offers a practical solution to the psychological impediment of CAPD and an increasing number of children and adolescents are shifting from CAPD to CCPD in many pediatric centers (552–555). CAPD or CCPD results in improved control of hypertension. With CCPD, however, the long dwell daytime exchange (12 to 14 h) may be associated with peritoneal fluid resorption and extracellular volume excess, requiring an increased use of hypertonic solutions during automated night time exchanges to maintain sodium balance and normotension (147). In some patients, suppression of the diurnal dwell is required because of excessive resorption of peritoneal dialysis fluid (148). Hemoglobin levels are maintained resulting in reduced transfusion requirement. As a consequence, exercise tolerance is improved fostering rehabilitation. Decreased dietary restrictions facilitate improved nutritional status. Moreover, CAPD (or CCPD) avoids wide fluctuations in biochemical abnormalities due to uremia and the biological stability eliminates the fatigue generally seen during and after hemodialysis sessions. More importantly, normal or accelerated growth occurs in roughly 50% of children undergoing CAPD (552, 558, 559). However, control of serum parathormone levels and adequate protein energy nutrition (over 2.0 g protein/kg/day and energy intakes in excess of 100% recommended dietary allowances) are essential determinants of growth rates. Renal osteodystrophy often progresses in children treated with CAPD (551). The prescription of 1-25-dihydroxycholecalciferol is recommended to control bone disease, and the dosage of this hormone should be increased until serum parathormone and alkaline phosphatase levels approach normal or the serum Ca exceeds 2.9 mmol/l (11.5 mg/dl). Oral phosphate binding agents are required to maintain the serum P between 1.2 to 1.8 mmol/l (4.0 and 6.0 mg/dl), particularly in those children who have high protein intakes (560). The dangers of high doses of aluminum containing phosphate binding agents, however, should be emphasized as younger and smaller children are at increased risk for accumulation of aluminum (561). A combined peritonitis incidence in children of 1.70 episodes per patient treatment year, calculated from various reports, does not differ from that in adult CAPD patients (543). Finally, the most impressive feature of CAPD is a remarkable improvement in the quality of life of patients and their families. Not only does CAPD (or CCPD) free the patient from the constraint of in-center hemodialysis and from repeated painful venipunctures, but it promotes independence and self-reliance. It also gives the family an opportunity to take an active part in the treatment of their children, an essential step to avoid the creeping conflict which so often opposes the families to the nursing team during in-center HD (540).

Peritoneal dialysis in elderly patients
Peritoneal dialysis has been used with an increasing frequency in patients over 60 years of age. This trend is due to three major factors: 1) the excellent cardiovascular stability obtained with PD, 2) the simplicity of the technique facilitating the promotion of home dialysis in this group of patients and 3) the scarcity of beds for hospital hemodialysis in many countries (519–521, 562).

With intermittent peritoneal dialysis, the results obtained in elderly patients were comparable to those of hemodialysis in the first year of treatment, but declined, thereafter in three retrospective studies (265, 562, 563). An excess mortality due to peritonitis was observed among PD patients but these data are difficult to interpret because atherosclerotic cardiovascular diseases were more frequently observed in patients receiving IPD (562, 563).

Although some groups refer older patients to center HD on the basis of untrainability (564), CAPD is considered a reasonable alternative treatment for elderly patients (519, 565–567). Except for an inordinately long time to learn the technique successfully in some patients (519), a more frequent change in dialysis modality (567) and the expected increase in death in this age group, the elderly compared favorably in morbidity to younger patients receiving this modality of therapy. Particular attention should be paid, however, to some intercurrent disorders more commonly encountered among elderly patients, including 1) a tendency to constipation, that may result in bowel impaction and trigger an attack of diverticulitis (333), 2) depressive episodes that may be induced by the endless repetition of dialysate bag exchanges or by social neglect or both and 3) the cunning installation of protein malnutrition, observed in

about 10% of elderly (568), which is facilitated by the anorexia often associated with CAPD procedures and with depression.

Peritoneal dialysis in refractory congestive heart failure

Acute intermittent peritoneal dialysis has been recommended for many years to remove fluid from patients with intractable edema due to heart failure (569–572). When diuretics and vasodilating agents are no longer effective, osmotic ultrafiltration with peritoneal dialysis can accomplish significant weight reduction, fluid removal reaching 10 to 15 l during a single dialysis (572). Invariably acute IPD ameliorates the symptoms of heart failure. Hemodynamic studies showed a decrease in venous pressure and blood volume; cardiac output rose in a majority of patients in one study (571), but no change in cardiac index was observed in another study (570). The improvement obtained with IPD is temporary and the long term results disappointing. Edema returns between dialyses which become necessary at shorter intervals. Other drawbacks of IPD in these patients include hypotension due to rapid intravascular volume depletion, hyperglycemia due to large glucose load and aggravation of pulmonary edema due to interdialytic weight gain.

CAPD offers some advantages over IPD (29, 573–575). By allowing gradual removal of sodium and water, it prevents thirst and hypotension, that accompany rapid ultrafiltration. As the intravascular compartment stabilizes with CAPD, initial clinical improvement is maintained on a longer follow-up period. The highly effective ultrafiltration allows the patients to eat a more liberal diet. CAPD also provides adequate dialysis in case of renal failure due to inadequate renal perfusion (575).

Miscellaneous indications of chronic peritoneal dialysis

Chronic peritoneal dialysis has been advocated in various disease states, such as multiple myeloma or scleroderma and also in diseases not associated with renal failure such as severe psoriasis.

Multiple myeloma, paraproteinemia and amyloidosis
Significant amounts of immunoglobulins are lost in the dialysate (225, 226). It has been suggested that this side effect of peritoneal dialysis could be utilised in the prevention or treatment of renal failure secondary to multiple myeloma and other protein disorders (576). Actually, peritoneal dialysis has been used in cases of acute renal failure complicating multiple myeloma (577–581). In one series, recovery of renal function was more frequent in patients receiving peritoneal dialysis than in those treated with hemodialysis (577). Successful reversal of ARF was also obtained in two other series (578, 579), while others found peritoneal dialysis of no benefit in their patients (580, 581). In this context, plasma exchange appears as the method of choice (582) as it removes immunoglobulins and light chains 100 times more effectively than peritoneal dialysis (576, 580, 582).

Experience with long term CAPD in the management of

multiple myeloma remains limited, with survival of 18 (583) and 54 months (584) respectively in two case reports.

CAPD has also been recommended in the treatment of end stage renal amyloidosis (585).

Peritoneal dialysis in rare causes of end stage renal disease
Successful use of IPD (586) or CAPD (587, 588) has been reported in *scleroderma,* in spite of previous studies suggesting reduced peritoneal clearances of urea and creatinine with this disease (589). Except for the triggering of Raynaud's phenomenon by unheated dialysate (588), blood pressure was easily controlled and adequate dialysis readily obtained. CAPD, by eliminating the blood access problems commonly encountered with hemodialysis (590) in this disease appears as a first choice treatment for scleroderma with end stage renal failure.

Temporary IPD (591) and long term CAPD (592, 593) have also been used successfully in renal failure associated with *spinal cord injury.* Peritoneal dialysis appeared as a satisfactory alternative to hemodialysis in these patients.

Finally, *recurrent hepatic coma* complicating the course of maintenance hemodialysis in a case of post hepatitic liver cirrhosis improved dramatically when the patient was transferred to CAPD (594).

Peritoneal dialysis in psoriasis
Prompt and dramatic remissions of long standing psoriasis have been noted in patients undergoing peritoneal dialysis (595, 596). In a double blind prospective study, sham dialysis procedure had no effect on psoriasis, whereas the partial or complete clearing of severe disabling plaque type psoriasis was obtained by true peritoneal dialysis in four out of five patients (597). In spite of these encouraging results, the small number of patients does not allow drawing firm conclusions from these studies as to the role of peritoneal dialysis in the management of severe psoriasis.

CONTRAINDICATIONS

The remarkable technical simplicity of peritoneal dialysis favored its use in almost all types of clinical situations. As a consequence, it has become almost proverbial to state that there is no contraindication to this mode of dialysis (376). Today, such an attitude is warranted only in places where the lack of alternative dialytic techniques may occasionnally justify desperate attempts to institute peritoneal dialysis under the most difficult circumstances. On the other hand, a more critical approach, taking into account the limitations inherent to peritoneal dialysis, seems more appropriate in places where extracorporeal hemodialysis methods are available.

Contraindications may be analysed under the dual perspective of 1) factors reducing the effectiveness of the method, and 2) associated diseases susceptible to be decompensated by or to increase the intrinsic hazards of dialysis procedures. For sake of clarity, the contraindications are presented in the following section under four headings: 1) absolute contraindications to all peritoneal dialysis regimens, 2) relative contraindications due to associated abdominal abnormalities, 3) relative contraindications to CAPD and 4) contraindications to self dialysis.

Absolute contraindications

Abdominal conditions associated with reduced peritoneal clearances of urea and creatinine, the presence of peritoneal defects and severe chronic respiratory failure are the three major absolute contraindications to peritoneal dialysis.

Peritoneal clearances may be drastically affected, particularly with IPD (129) in case of large mesenteric resection (e.g. following mesenteric infarction), multiple adhesions with peritoneal fluid loculation and abdominal distension due to bowel loop dilatation (e.g. intestinal ileus). These anatomical or functional abnormalities result in reduced peritoneal membrane surface area and/or poor dialysate flow characteristics. As a consequence, reduced peritoneal clearances of urea and creatinine lead to inadequate dialysis and transfer to HD is mandatory.

Acquired peritoneal defects that may follow abdominal or retroperitoneal (e.g. abdominal aorta) surgery or congenital defect (e.g. peritoneo-pleural communication) may result in external, intraparietal or intrapleural fluid accumulation (269, 270). This complication renders difficult the maintainance of an adequate extracellular volume or entails inacceptable risks of respiratory compromise. It should therefore be considered as an absolute contraindication for peritoneal dialysis.

Finally, patients with severe chronic obstructive bronchopneumopathy are at risk of decompensating acutely a borderline respiratory function during the intraperitoneal infusion of dialysis fluid (204, 205). It appears preferable to consider severe chronic respiratory insufficiency as absolute contraindication to peritoneal dialysis.

Relative contraindications due to associated abdominal abnormalities

In *severe obesity,* catheter implantation is made difficult due to the thickness of the subcutaneous tissues and dialysate leakage is more common (73). Similarly, multiple scars of the abdominal wall due to previous surgery renders catheter placement more hazardous. In both cases, this difficulty may be overcome by surgical implantation done under general anesthesia (31, 76).

In patients with *polycystic kidneys,* the presence of large renal masses reducing the volume of the peritoneal cavity may cause discomfort during dialysate infusion. Actually, polycystic kidney disease is not an obstacle to peritoneal dialysis and is the cause of renal failure in about 10% of patients receiving CAPD (17).

Finally, peritoneal dialysis should preferably be avoided in the presence of *enterostomies* or *urostomies* because of the increased risk of peritoneal infection.

Relative contraindications to CAPD

Patients with *severe peripheral vascular disease* are at increased risk to develop gangrene of their distal extremities during CAPD (382). Careful monitoring of ultrafiltration and prevention of hypotensive episodes will avoid this serious complication.

Diverticulosis of the colon should be suspected in a high percentage of patients aged over 50 (598). As fecal peritonitis may result from attacks of diverticulitis, it has been suggested that CAPD was contraindicated in patients with diverticulosis. In fact, with careful prevention of constipation, there is no evidence, to date, that CAPD increases the incidence of diverticulitis (333).

Chronic lower back pain may be aggravated by permanent abdominal distension during CAPD. This can effectively be prevented be appropriate exercises strengthening the abdominal wall muscles (377, 378).

Elevated intra-abdominal pressure due to dialysate infusion in the peritoneal cavity aggravates *pre-existing abdominal wall hernias* and favors the formation of hernias in CAPD patients (367–375). Surgical repair of hernias can readily be performed while the patient receives temporary IPD or HD (311).

Finally, cessation of CAPD is considered as essential in the management of recurrent bacterial peritonitis as well as fungal or tuberculous peritoneal infection (104, 105).

Contraindications of self dialysis

The success of home peritoneal dialysis depends on the patient's strict adhesion to sterile procedures and prescribed regimen. A highly motivated patient is a prerequisite for self dialysis (70). The lack of motivation or the inability to learn or memorize the necessary procedures by psychotic, mentally retarded or demented patients is, therefore, an absolute contraindication to independent dialysis in the home.

Physical handicaps are also to be considered as contraindicating self dialysis. In elderly patients, crippling arthritis of the fingers, hand tremor or poor vision, will often compromise patients' independence. In the diabetic patients, blindness is a major obstacle to self treatment although properly trained blind patients have been able to master CAPD techniques (538).

CONCLUSIONS

During the past 5 years, the field of peritoneal dialysis has expanded impressively in both the clinical and the research areas. The clinical utilization of peritoneal dialysis has spread worldwide in almost every nephrology center. Continuous ambulatory peritoneal dialysis has become an established treatment modality for end-stage renal disease (17, 599). Technologic progress has permitted a striking decrease in the incidence of peritonitis, the major complication of CAPD (28). While clinical experience is accumulating and basic knowledge in the physiology and immunology of the peritoneum is rapidly growing, several major problems remain unsolved requiring further progress. The central question, which has not yet been answered, relates to the long term durability of the peritoneal membrane (600). Studies on the morphology of the peritoneum during CAPD have constantly revealed the presence of mesothelial and submesothelial lesions (19, 29, 159, 160, 348, 349). The clinical significance of these anomalies has been questioned and cannot be presently elucidated due to the scarcity of available data. Ultrafiltration failure, characterized by an increasing need for hypertonic exchanges with time on CAPD, is observed in about 5% of patients undergoing CAPD (17, 272). This well identified chronic complication of CAPD presumably reflects the progressive alteration of peritoneal structures as a consequence of permanent bathing with highly unphysiologic dialysis solutions. Besides the long term viability of the peritoneum, many side effects of peritoneal dialysis should be improved. Main areas for progress include the preparation of more physiologic dialysis solutions, with a better compatibility to the peritoneal serosa and less nutritional consequences, and the development of simpler, safer connectors facilitating quick dialysate bag exchanges with a low risk of contamination. Furthermore, the development of reliable and easy to maintain machines for the bedside preparation of sterile apyrogenic solutions should be encouraged to permit the utilization of intermittent dialysis schedules (including nightly and tidal peritoneal dialysis) at an acceptable cost.

After almost three decades of extensive use of peritoneal dialysis in acute and chronic renal failure, the nephrologist should remain aware of the intrinsic limitations and hazards of this dialysis modality. He should also be convinced that the best approach to manage severe complications of peritoneal dialysis may often be the early transfer of the patient to hemodialysis (601). To be utilized adequately and prescribed safely, peritoneal dialysis should be considered as a medium term treatment for chronic renal failure (601). Clearly, CAPD and its alternatives cannot be the only dialytic method available in a nephrologic center, particularly in the management of end-stage renal disease. CAPD and IPD should be integrated with extracorporeal hemodialysis methods and transplantation in a program insuring the patients with an easy transfer from one method to the other according to the changing needs of a lifetime.

REFERENCES

1. Maxwell MH, Rockney RE, Kleeman CR, Twiss MR: Peritoneal dialysis. 1. Technique and application. *JAMA* 170: 917, 1959
2. Boen ST: Kinetics of peritoneal dialysis. A comparison with the artificial kidney. *Medicine* 40: 243, 1961
3. Henderson LW: Peritoneal ultrafiltration dialysis: enhanced urea transfer using hypertonic dialysis fluid. *J Clin Invest* 49: 950, 1966
4. Bomar JB, Decherd JF, Hlavinka DJ, Moncrief JW, Popovich RP: The elucidation of maximum efficiency – minimum cost peritoneal dialysis protocols. *Trans Am Soc Artif Intern Organs* 20: 120, 1974

5. Boen ST, Mulinari AS, Dillard DH, Scribner BH: Periodic peritoneal dialysis in the management of chronic uremia. *Trans Am Soc Artif Intern Organs* 8: 256, 1962

6. Jarrell B, Lasker N, Roberts M: A simple system of automated peritoneal dialysis. *Dial Transplant* 3(2): 36, 1974

7. Tenckhoff H, Schechter H: A bacteriologically safe peritoneal access device for repeated peritoneal dialysis. *Trans Am Soc Artif Intern Organs* 14: 181, 1968

8. Tenckhoff H, Meston B, Shilipetar RG: A simplified automatic peritoneal dialysis system. *Trans Am Soc Artif Intern Organs* 18: 436, 1972

9. Boen ST, Mion CM, Curtis FK, Shilipetar G: Periodic peritoneal dialysis using the repeated puncture technique and an automatic cycling machine. *Trans Am Soc Artif Intern Organs* 10: 409, 1964

10. Tenckhoff H, Blagg CR, Curtis KF, Hickman RO: Chronic peritoneal dialysis. *Proc Eur Dial Transplant Assoc* 10: 363, 1973

11. Gurland HJ, Brunner FP, Chantler C, Jacobs C, Schärer K, Selwood NA, Spies G, Wing AJ: Combined report on regular dialysis and transplantation in Europe, VI, 1975. *Proc Eur Dial Transplant Assoc* 13: 3, 1976

12. Scribner BH, Giordano C, Oreopoulos DG, Mion C, Buoncristiani U, Davids SG, Gahl GM, Jones KM: Long term peritoneal dialysis. *Proc Eur Dial Transplant Assoc* 12: 131, 1975

13. Popovich RP, Moncrief JW, Decherd JB, Bomar JB, Pyle WK: The definition of a novel portable/wearable equilibrium peritoneal dialysis technique. *Abstracts Am Soc Artif Intern Organs* 5: 64, 1976

14. Popovich RP, Moncrief JW, Nolph KD, Ghods AJ, Twardowski ZJ, Pyle WK: Continuous ambulatory peritoneal dialysis. *Ann Intern Med* 88: 449, 1978

15. Oreopoulos DG, Robson M, Izatt S, Clayton S, De Veber GA: A simple and safe technique for continuous ambulatory peritoneal dialysis. *Trans Am Soc Artif Intern Organs* 24: 484, 1978

16. Broyer M, Brunner FP, Brynger H, Fassbinder N, Guillou PJ, Oulès R, Rizzoni G, Selwood NH, Wing AJ, Challah S, Dykes SR: Demography of dialysis and transplantation in Europe, 1984. *Nephrol Dial Transpl* 1: 1, 1986

17. Nolph KD, Cutler SJ, Steinberg SM, Novak JW: Continuous ambulatory peritoneal dialysis in the United States: a three-year study. *Kidney Int* 28: 198, 1985

18. Verger C, Brunschvicg O, Le Carpentier Y, Lavergne A, Vantelon J: Structural and ultrastructural peritoneal membrane changes and permeability alterations during continuous ambulatory peritoneal dialysis. *Proc Eur Dial Transplant Assoc* 18: 199, 1981

19. Dobbie JW, Zaki MA: The ultrastructure of the parietal peritoneum in normal and uremic man and in patients on CAPD. in: *Frontiers in Peritoneal Dialysis*, edited by Maher JF, Winchester JF, New York, Field, Rich and Assoc, 1986, p 3

20. Gotloib L: Morphological and functional aspects of the peritoneal membrane. in: *Peritoneal Dialysis*, edited by La Greca G, Chiaramonte S, Fabris A, Feriani M, Ronco C, Milan, Wichtig, 1988, p 7

21. Mactier RA, Khanna R, Twardowski ZJ, Nolph KD: Role of peritoneal cavity lymphatic absorption in peritoneal dialysis. *Kidney Int* 32: 165, 1987

22. Pavlina T, Lloyd J, Johnson R, Dobbie JW: Phosphatidylcholine synthesis by rat peritoneum. *Kidney Int* 33: 248, 1988

23. Keane WF, Peterson PK: Host defense mechanisms of the peritoneal cavity and continuous ambulatory peritoneal dialysis. *Peretoneal Dial Bull* 4: 122, 1984

24. Flessner MF, Dedrick RL, Schultz JS: A distributed model of peritoneal-plasma transport: theoretical considerations. *Am J Physiol* 246: R597, 1984

25. Maher JF, Chakrabarti E: Ultrafiltration by hyperosmotic peritoneal dialysis fluid excludes intracellular solutes. *Am J Nephrol* 4: 169, 1984

26. Hirszel P, Maher JF, Chakrabarti E, Bennett RR: Maximal peritoneal pore size determined by dextran transport. in: *Frontiers in Peritoneal Dialysis*, edited by Maher JF, Winchester JF, New York, Field, Rich and Assoc, 1986, p. 37

27. Maher JF, Hirszel P: Pharmacologic manipulations of peritoneal transport. in: *Peritoneal Dialysis*, edited by Nolph KD, 2nd edition, Boston, Dordrecht, Lancaster, Martinus Nijhoff, 1985, p 267

28. Maiorca R, Cantaluppi A, Cancarini GC, Scalamogna A, Broccoli R, Graziani G, Brasa S, Ponticelli C: Prospective controlled trial of a Y-connector and disinfectant to prevent peritonitis in continuous ambulatory peritoneal dialysis. *Lancet* 2: 642, 1983

29. Kim D, Khanna R, Wu G, Fountas P, Druck M, Oreopoulos DG: Successful use of CAPD in refractory heart failure. in: *Frontiers in Peritoneal Dialysis*, edited by Maher JF, Winchester JF, New York, Field, Rich and Assoc Inc, 1986, p 382

30. Dedrick RL, Myers CE, Bungay PM, De Vita VT: Pharmacokinetic rationale for peritoneal drug administration in the treatment of ovarian cancer. *Cancer Treat Rep* 62: 1, 1978

31. Tenckhoff H: Home peritoneal dialysis. in: *Clinical Aspects of Uremia and Dialysis*, edited by Massry SG, Sellers AL, Springfield IL, Charles C Thomas, 1976, p 583

32. Slingeneyer A, Mion C, Béraud JJ, Oulès R, Branger B, Balmes M: Peritonitis, a frequently lethal complication of intermittent and continuous ambulatory peritoneal dialysis. *Proc Eur Dial Transplant Assoc* 18: 212, 1981

33. Clayton S: The organisation and implementation of a peritoneal dialysis program. *Pertioneal Dial Bull* 1: 134, 1981

34. Uttley L, Gokal R: Organisation of a CAPD programme: the nurses' role. in: *Continuous Ambulatory Peritoneal Dialysis*, edited by Gokal R, Edinburgh, Churchill Livingstone, 1986, p 145

35. Oreopoulos DG: Requirements for the organisation of a continuous ambulatory peritoneal dialysis program. *Nephron* 24: 261, 1979

36. Furman K, Doehring RO, Galasko GTF, Kleiman MS, Rudnick J: Suitability of povidone-iodine formulations for CAPD. in: *Frontiers in Peritoneal Dialysis*, edited by Maher JF, Winchester JF, New York, Field, Rich and Assoc Inc, 1986, p 619

37. Golper TA, Sewell DL, West L, Trinklein M: Povidone-iodine sterilisation of contaminated CAPD – exchange spikes. *Peritoneal Dial Bull* 5: 24, 1985

38. Gruer LD, Babb JR, Davies JG, Ayliffe GAJ, Adu D, Michael J: Disinfection of hands and tubing of CAPD patients. *J Hosp Infect* 5: 305, 1984

39. Werner HP: Disinfectants in dialysis: dangers, drawbacks and disinformation. *Nephron* 49: 1, 1988

40. Parrott PL, Terry PM, Whitworth EN, Franley LW, Coble RS, Wachsmuth IK, McGowan JE: Pseudomonas aeruginosa peritonitis associated with contaminated poloxamer-iodine solutions. *Lancet* 2: 683, 1982

41. Berkelman RL, Lewin S, Allen JR, Anderson RL, Budnick LD, Shapiro S, Friedman SM, Nicholas P, Holzman RS, Haley RW: Pseudo bacteremia attributed to contamination of povidone-iodine with Pseudomonas cepacia. *Ann Intern Med* 95: 32, 1981

42. Craven DE, Moody D, Connoly MG, Kollisch NR, Strott-meier KD, McCabe WR: Pseudobacteremia caused by povi-done-iodine solution contaminated with Pseudomonas cepa-cia. *N Engl J Med* 305: 621, 1981

43. Berkelman RL, Holland BW, Anderson RL: Increased bac-tericidal activity of dilute preparations of povidone-iodine solutions. *J Clin Microbiol* 15: 635, 1982

44. Junor BJR, Briggs JP, Forwell MA, Dobbie JW, Henderson IS: Sclerosing peritonitis. The contribution of chlorhexidine in alcohol. *Peritoneal Dial Bull* 5: 101, 1985

45. Frank HA: Experimental and clinical origins of peritoneal dialysis for renal failure. in: *Frontiers in Peritoneal Dialysis*, edited by Maher JF, Winchester JF, New York, Field, Rich and Assoc Inc, 1986, p 143

46. Oreopoulos DG, Helfrich GB, Khanna R, Lum GM, Mat-thews R, Paulsen K, Twardowski ZJ, Vas SI: Peritoneal cath-eters and exit-site practices. Peritoneal Dial Bull 7: 130, 1987

47. Uldall R: Subclavian cannulation for hemodialysis: the pre-sent state of the art. *Artif Organs* 6: 73, 1982

48. Canaud B, Béraud JJ, Joyeux H, Mion C: Internal jugular vein cannulation using 2 silastic catheters: a new, simple and safe long term vascular access for extracorporeal treatment. *Nephron* 43: 133, 1986

49. Ribot S, Jacobs MG, Frankel HJ, Bernstein A: Complications of peritoneal dialysis. *Am J Med Sci* 35: 505, 1966

50. Vaamonde CA, Michael GP, Metzger RR, Carroll KE: Com-plications of acute peritoneal dialysis. *J Chron Dis* 20: 637, 1975

51. Simkin EP, Wright FC: Perforating injuries of the bowel complicating peritoneal catheter insertion. *Lancet* 1: 64, 1968

52. Rubin J, Oreopoulos DG, Lio TT, Mathews R, de Veber GA: Management of peritonitis and bowel perforation during peri-toneal dialysis. *Nephron* 16: 220, 1976

53. Slingeneyer A, Mion C, Charpiat A, Balmès M: Is an alterna-tive to the Tenckhoff catheter necessary? in: *Advances in Peritoneal Dialysis*, edited by Gahl G, Kessel M, Nolph KD, Amsterdam, Excerpta Medica, 1981, p 179

54. Mion CM, Boen ST, Scribner P: An analysis of the factors responsible for the formation of adhesions during chronic peritoneal dialysis. *Am J Med Sci* 250: 675, 1965

55. Rottembourg J, Jacq D, Vonlanthen M, Issad B, El Shahat Y: Straight or curled Tenckhoff peritoneal catheters for contin-uous ambulatory peritoneal dialysis. *Peritoneal Dial Bull* 2: 123, 1982

56. Khanna R, Izatt S, Burke D, Mathews R, Vas SI, Oreopoulos DG: Experience with the Toronto Western Hospital perma-nent peritoneal catheter. *Peritoneal Dial Bull* 4: 95, 1984

57. Valli A, Crescimanno U, Mioiri O, Arw K, Riegler P, Huber W, Cabassa N: 18 months experience with a new (Valli) catheter for peritoneal dialysis. *Peritoneal Dial Bull* 3: 22, 1983

58. Ash SR, Johnson H, Hartmann J, Granger J, Koszuta J, Sell L, Dhein S, Blevins W, Thornhill JA: The Column Disc peritoneal catheter: a peritoneal access device with improved drainage. *asaio J* 3: 110, 1980

59. Erlich LF, Powell SL: Care of the patient with a Gore-Tex peritoneal dialysis catheter. *Dial Transplant* 12: 572, 1983

60. Twardowski ZJ, Khanna R, Nolph KD, Nichols WK, Ryan LP: Preliminary experience with the Swan Neck peritoneal dialysis catheters. *Trans Am Soc Artif Intern Organs* 32: 64, 1986

61. Henao J, Mejia G, Arbelaez M, Sus A, Arango JL, Aramburo O, Sanchez J: A new approach for catheter placement and care in CAPD. *Peritoneal Dial Bull* 5: 223, 1985

62. Nakanishi T, Yanase M, Fujii M, Tanaka Y, Orita Y, Abe H: New acute peritoneal dialysis technique: wire guide insertion and long term indwelling of peritoneal catheter. *Nephron* 37: 1281, 1984

63. Allon M, Soucie JM, Macon EJ: Complications with perito-neal dialysis catheters: experience with 154 percutaneously placed catheters. *Nephron* 48: 8, 1988

64. Ash SR, Handt AE, Block R: Peritoneoscopic placement of the Tenckhoff catheter: further clinical experience. *Peritoneal Dial Bull* 3: 8, 1983

65. Helfrich GB, Pechan BW, Alijani MR, Barnard WF, Rakow-ski TA, Winchester JF: Reduction of catheter complications with lateral placement. *Peritoneal Dial Bull* 3 (Suppl): S2, 1983

66. Scott DF, Marshall VC: Insertion and complications of Tenckhoff catheters: surgical aspects. in: *Peritoneal Dialysis*, edited by Atkins RC, Thomson NP, Farrell PC, Edinburgh, Churchill Livingstone, 1981, p 61

67. Olcott C, Feldman CA, Coplon NY, Oppenheimer ML, Me-higan JT: Continuous ambulatory peritoneal dialysis: tech-nique of catheter insertion and management of associated surgical complications. *Am J Surg* 146: 98, 1983

68. Lovinggood JP: Peritoneal catheter implantation for CAPD. *Peritoneal Dial Bull* 4 (Suppl): S106, 1984

69. Veitch P: Surgical aspects of CAPD. in: *Continuous Ambula-tory Peritoneal Dialysis*, edited by Gokal R, Edinburgh, Chur-chill Livingstone, 1986, p 110

70. Oreopoulos DG, Vas SI, Khanna R: Prevention of peritonitis during continuous ambulatory peritoneal dialysis. *Peritoneal Dial Bull* 3 (Suppl): S18, 1983

71. Moncrief JW, Popovich RP: Continuous ambulatory perito-neal dialysis. in: *Peritoneal Dialysis*, edited by Nolph KD, 2nd edition, Boston, Dordrecht, Lancaster, Martinus Nijhoff, 1985, p 209

72. Copley JB: Prevention of peritoneal dialysis catheter related infections. *Am J Kidney Dis* 10: 401, 1987

73. Ponce PE, Pierratos A, Izatt S, Mathews R, Khanna R, Zellerman G, Oreopoulos DG: Comparison of the survival and complications of three permanent peritoneal dialysis cath-eters. *Peritoneal Dial Bull* 2: 82, 1982

74. Swarz RD: Chronic peritoneal dialysis: mechanical and in-fectious complications. *Nephron* 40: 29, 1985

75. Odor A, Alessio-Robles LP, Leuchter J, Mendoza A, Bordes J, Wadjymar A, Gonzalez RF, Chaves Peon F: Experience with 150 consecutive permanent peritoneal catheters in pa-tients on CAPD. *Peritoneal Dial Bull* 5: 226, 1985

76. Levey AS, Simon GM. McCauley J, Smith TJ, Cho SI, Har-rington JT: Outcome of peritoneal catheter placement in the high risk patient. *Peritoneal Dial Bull* 4 (Suppl): S112, 1984

77. Amair P, De Camejo O, Dominguez O, Boissiere M: Skin reaction against the catheter: an explanation for exit site in-fection in CAPD. in: *Frontiers in Peritoneal Dialysis*, edited by Maher JF, Winchester JF, New York, Field, Rich and Assoc Inc, 1986, p 207

78. Kurihara S, Tani Y, Tateischi K, Yuri T, Kitada H, Sugishita N, Fukuda Y, Ishikaua I, Shinoda A, Hayakawa Y: Allergic eosinophilic dermatitis due to silicone rubber: a new but trou-blesome complication of the Tenckhoff catheter. *Peritoneal Dial Bull* 5: 65, 1985

79. Diaz-Buxo JA, Geissinger WT: Single cuff versus double cuff Tenckhoff catheter. *Peritoneal Dial Bull* 4 (Suppl): S100, 1984

80. Kim D, Burke D, Izatt S, Mathews R, Wu G, Khanna R, Vas SI, Oreopoulos DG: Single- or double-cuff peritoneal cathe-ters? A prospective comparison. *Trans Am Soc Artif Intern Organs* 30: 232, 1984

81. Twardowszki ZJ, Nolph KD, Khanna R, Prowant BF, Ryan LP, Nichols WK: The need for a 'Swan neck' permanently bent, arcuate peritoneal dialysis catheter. *Peritoneal Dial Bull* 5: 219, 1985

82. Smith C: CAPD: one-cuff versus two-cuff catheters in reference to the incidence of infection. in: *Frontiers in Peritoneal Dialysis,* edited by Maher JF, Winchester JF, New York, Field, Rich and Assoc Inc, 1986, p 181

83. Piraino B, Bernardini J, Peitzman A, Sorkin M: Failure of peritoneal cuff shaving to eradicate infection. *Peritoneal Dial Bull* 7: 179, 1987

84. Krothapalli R, Duffy WB, Lacke C, Payne W, Patel H, Perez V, Senekhian HO: Pseudomonas peritonitis and continuous ambulatory peritoneal dialysis. *Arch Intern Med* 142: 1862, 1982

85. Leung ACT, Orange G, Henderson IS, Kennedy AC: Diphteroid peritonitis associated with continuous ambulatory peritoneal dialysis. *Clin Nephrol* 22: 200, 1984

86. Piraino B, Bernardini J, Sorkin M: The influence of peritoneal catheter exit site infections on peritonitis, tunnel infections and catheter loss in patients on continuous ambulatory peritoneal dialysis. *Am J Kidney Dis* 8: 436, 1986

87. Wiegman TB, Stuewe B, Duncan KA, Chonko A, Diederich DA, Grantham JJ, Savin VJ, MacDougall ML: Effective use of streptokinase for peritoneal catheter failure. *Am J Kidney Dis* 6: 119, 1985

88. Schleifer CR, Ziemek H, Teehan BP, Benz RL, Sigler MH, Gilgore GS: Migration of peritoneal catheters: personal experience and a survey of 72 other units. *Peritoneal Dial Bull* 7: 189, 1987

89. DeVault GA, Brown IIIrd ST, King JW, Fowler M, Oberle A: Tenckhoff catheter obstruction resulting from invasion by Curvularia lunata in the absence of peritonitis. *Am J Kidney Dis* 6: 124, 1985

90. Oreopoulos DG, Izatt S, Zellerman G, Karanicolas S, Mathews RE: A prospective study of the effectiveness of three permanent catheters. *Proc Clin Dial Transplant Forum* 6: 96, 1976

91. Flanigan MJ, Ngheim DD, Schulak JA, Ulurich GE, Freeman RM: The use and complications of three peritoneal dialysis catheter designs. A retrospective analysis. *Trans Am Soc Artif Intern Organs* 33: 33, 1987

92. Bierman MH, Kasperbauer J, Kusek A, HJammeke MD, Fitzgibbons Jr RJ, Egan JD: Peritoneal catheter survival and complications in end stage renal disease. *Peritoneal Dial Bull* 5: 229, 1985

93. Davis R, Young J, Diamond D, Bourke E: Management of chronic peritoneal catheter malfunction. *Am J Nephrol* 2: 85, 1982

94. Hemmeloff Hendersen KE, Damgard-Morch P: Catheterography in the diagnosis of catheter failure in peritoneal dialysis. *Clin Nephrol* 16: 142, 1981

95. Rodriguez-Perez JC, Palop L, Plaza C, Arrieta J: Perforation and/or laceration of posterior peritoneum in continuous ambulatory peritoneal dialysis. *Peritoneal Dial Bull* 5: 141, 1985

96. Parvin SD, Beaman M: Ileal erosion by the Tenckhoff catheter. *Peritoneal Dial Bull* 5: 82, 1985

97. Watson LC, Thomson J: Erosion of the colon by a long dwelling peritoneal dialysis catheter. *JAMA* 234: 2156, 1980

98. Della Volpe M, Iberti M, Ortensi A, Veronesi GV: Erosion of the sigmoid by a permanent peritoneal catheter. *Peritoneal Dial Bull* 4: 108, 1984

99. Braden GL, Germain MJ, Guardione VA, Fitzgibbons JP: Infected intraabdominal hematoma associated with an in-

dwelling Tenckhoff catheter. *Peritoneal Dial Bull* 4: 248, 1984

100. Donnelly PK, Lennard TN, Proud G, Taylor RMR, Henderson R, Fletcher K, Elliot W, Ward MR, Wilkinson R: Continuous ambulatory peritoneal dialysis and renal transplantation: a five year experience. *Br Med J* 291: 1001, 1985

101. Evangelista IB, Bennett-Jones D, Cameron JS, Ogg C, Williams DG, Taube DH, Neild G, Rudge C: Renal transplantation in patients treated with hemodialysis and short term or long term continuous ambulatory peritoneal dialysis. *Br Med J* 291: 1004, 1985

102. Gokal R, Baillod R, Bogle S, Hunt L, Jakubowski C, Marsh F, Ogg C, Oliver D, Ward M, Wilkinson R: Multi-centre study on outcome of treatment in patients on continuous ambulatory peritoneal dialysis and hemodialysis. *Nephrol Dial Transplant* 2: 172, 1987

103. Vas SI: Microbiologic aspects of chronic ambulatory peritoneal dialysis. *Kidney Int* 23: 83, 1982

104. Mion C, Slingeneyer A, Canaud B: Peritonitis. in: *Continuous Ambulatory Peritoneal Dialysis,* edited by Gokal R, Edinburgh, Churchill Livingstone, 1986, p 163

105. Block RA, Taylor B, Frederich G: Intraperitoneal infusion of streptokinase in the treatment of recurrent peritonitis. *Peritoneal Dial Bull* 3: 162, 1983

106. Norris KC, Shinaberger JH, Reyes GD, Kraut JA: The use of intracatheter instillation of streptokinase in the treatment of recurrent bacterial peritonitis in continuous ambulatory peritoneal dialysis. *Am J Kidney Dis* 10: 62, 1987

107. Benevent D, Peyronnet P, Brignon P, Leroux-Robert C: Urokinase infusion for obstructed catheters and peritonitis. *Peritoneal Dial Bull* 5: 77, 1985

108. Pickering SJ, Bowley JA, Fleming SJ, Oppenheim BA, Ralston AJ, Sissons P, Ackrill P, Burnie J: Urokinase for recurrent CAPD peritonitis. *Lancet* 1: 1258, 1987

109. Paterson AD, Bishop MC, Morgan AG, Burden RS: Removal and replacement of Tenckhoff catheter at a single operation: successful treatment of resistant peritonitis in continuous ambulatory peritoneal dialysis. *Lancet* 2: 1245. 1986

110. Vogt K, Binswanger U, Buchmann P, Baumgartner O, Keusch G, Largiader F: Catheter related complications during continuous ambulatory peritoneal dialysis: a retrospective study on sixty-two double cuff Tenckhoff catheters. *Am J Kidney Dis* 10: 47, 1987

111. Boss HP, Ganger KH, Gurck Z: Goretex versus Oreopoulos peritoneal catheters: a clinical evaluation and comparison (letter). *Peritoneal Dial Bull* 7: 209, 1987

112. Stewart WK, Anderson DC, Wilson MI: Hazard of peritoneal dialysis: contaminated fluid. *Br Med J* 1: 606, 1967

113. Slingeneyer A, Mion C, Despaux E, Perez C, Duport J, Dansette AM: Use of a bacteriologic filter in the prevention of peritonitis associated with peritoneal dialysis: long term clinical results in intermittent and continuous ambulatory peritoneal dialysis. in: *Peritoneal Dialysis,* edited by Atkins RC, Thomson NM, Farrell PC, Edinburgh, Churchill Livingstone, 1981, p 301

114. Tenckhoff H: Solutions and equipment. *Dial Transplant* 6: 24, 1977

115. Boen ST: Overview and history of peritoneal dialysis. *Dial Transplant* 6: 12, 1977

116. Kabei N, Kolff WJ, Foux A: Evaluation of hollow-fiber reverse osmosis filtration permeators for use in peritoneal dialysis. *Dial Transplant* 6: 59, 1977

117. Petersen NJ, Carson LA, Favero MS: Microbiological quality of water in an automatic peritoneal dialysis system. *Dial Transplant* 6: 38, 1977

118. Mayr HU, Stec F, Canaud B, Mion C, Shaldon S: Microbiological aspects of the batch preparation of replacement fluid for hemofiltration. *Blood Purif* 2: 158, 1984

119. Mion C, Canaud B: 'On-site' preparation of sterile apyrogenic electrolyte solutions for hemofiltration and hemodiafiltration. in: *Short Dialysis*, edited by Cambi V, Boston, Dordrecht, Lancaster, Martinus Nijhoff, 1987, p 261

120. Gutman RA, Shelburne JD: An outbreak of cryptogenic peritonitis: implications for reverse osmosis production of biologically safe water. *Dial Transplant* 6: 35, 1977

121. Gutman RA: Automated peritoneal dialysis for home use. *Q J Med* 47: 261, 1978

122. Karanicolas S, Oreopoulos DG, Pylypchuck G, Fenton SSA, Cattran DC, Rapoport A, de Veber GA: Home peritoneal dialysis: three years' experience in Toronto. *Can Med Assoc J* 116: 226, 1977

123. Diaz-Buxo JA, Chandler JT, Farmer CD, Smith DU: Chronic peritoneal dialysis at home: a comparison with hemodialysis. *Trans Am Soc Artif Intern Organs* 23: 191, 1977

124. Furman KI, Koornhof HJ, Frizelle K, Block CK, Van Wyck H, Allcock R: Unsafe automatic peritoneal dialysis in Johannesburg. *Kidney Int* 16: 86, 1979

125. Sommer A: Open drain in cycling peritoneal dialysis. *Peritoneal Dial Bull* 6: 41, 1986

126. Pirpasopoulos M, Lindsay RM, Rahman M, Kennedy AC: A cost-effectiveness study of dwell times in peritoneal dialysis. *Lancet* 2: 1135, 1972

127. Goldschmidt ZH, Pote HH, Katz MA, Shear L: Effect of dialysate volume on peritoneal dialysis kinetics. *Kidney Int* 5: 240, 1974

128. Tenckhoff H, Ward G, Boen ST: The influence of dialysate volume and flow rate on peritoneal clearance. *Proc Eur Dial Transplant Assoc* 2: 113, 1965

129. Popovich RP, Moncrief JW: Transport kinetics. in: *Peritoneal Dialysis*, edited by Nolph KD, 2nd edition, Boston, Dordrecht, Lancaster, Martinus Nijhoff, 1985, p 115

130. Robson M, Oreopoulos DG, Izatt S, Ogilvie R, Rapoport A, de Veber GA: Influence of exchange volume and dialysate flow rate on solute clearance in peritoneal dialysis. *Kidney Int* 14: 486, 1978

131. Bennett RR, Hirszel P, Chakrabarti E, Maher JF: Residual intraperitoneal fluid: volume and effect on peritoneal clearances (abstract). *Peritoneal Dial Bull* 4 (Suppl): S4, 1984

132. Indraprasit S, Taramas W, Panparde O: Complete dialysate drainage: an unnecessary step in intermittent peritoneal dialysis. *Peritoneal Dial Bull* 5: 233, 1985

133. Mani MK, Raibagi MH, Dincankar AD: The economics of peritoneal dialysis. A cost-efficiency study. *Nephron* 17: 130, 1976

134. Blumenkrantz MJ, Shapiro DJ, Miller JH, Barshay M, Kopple JD, Shinaberger JO, Friedler RM, Coburn JW: Chronic peritoneal dialysis for the management of chronic renal failure. *Proc Clin Dial Transplant Forum* 3: 117, 1973

135. Von Hartitzsch B, Hill AVL, Medlock TR: Nine hour peritoneal dialysis, three times weekly. An alternative to conventional hemodialysis. *Proc Eur Dial Transplant Assoc* 13: 306, 1976

136. Sherrard DJ, Curtis FK, Lindner A, Scollard D, Merritt A: Peritoneal dialysis, a feasible alternative. *Proc Clin Dial Transplant Forum* 3: 114, 1973

137. Giordano C, De Santo NG, Cirillo O: Short daily peritoneal dialysis. *Nephron* 21: 131, 1978

138. Scribner BH: Foreword to second edition. in: *Peritoneal Dialysis*, edited by Nolph KD, 2nd edition, Boston, Dordrecht, Lancaster, Martinus Nijhoff, 1985

139. Twardowski Z, Nolph KD, Khanna R, Gluck Z, Prowant BF, Ryan LP: Daily clearances with continuous ambulatory peritoneal dialysis and nightly peritoneal dialysis. *Trans Am Soc Artif Intern Organs* 32: 575, 1986

140. Twardowski Z, Nolph K, Khanna R, Prowant B, Frock J, Dobbie J, Serkes K, Kenley R, Witsoe D, Garber J: Eight hour tidal peritoneal dialysis matches 24 hour CAPD and surpasses 8 hour nightly intermittent peritoneal dialysis clearances (abstract). *Peritoneal Dial Bull* 7 (Suppl 2): S79, 1987

141. Stephen RC: Reciprocating peritoneal dialysis with a subcutaneous peritoneal catheter. *Dial Transplant* 7: 834, 1978

142. Posen GA, Luisiello J: Continuous equilibration peritoneal dialysis in the treatment of acute renal failure. *Peritoneal Dial Bull* 1: 6, 1980

143. Fraedrich G, Scholz R, Mulch B, Leber HW, Hehrlein FW: Continuous peritoneal dialysis. An alternative to hemodialysis in acute renal failure after cardiovascular operations. *Thorac Cardiovasc Surg* 28: 246, 1980

144. Gastaldi L, Baratelli L, Castani D, Cinquepalmi M: Low flow continuous peritoneal dialysis in acute renal failure (letter). *Nephron* 29: 101, 1981

145. Pomeranz A, Reichenberg Y, Schurr D, Drukker A: Acute renal failure in a burnt patient: the advantage of continuous peritoneal dialysis. *Burns Incl Therm Inj* 11: 367, 1985

146. Sorrels-Akar 'P'AJ, Bobbitt M, Aguirre F, Moncrief JW, Popovich RP: Peritoneal dialysis for in-hospital patients. in: *Frontiers in Peritoneal Dialysis*, edited by Maher JF, Winchester JF, New York, Field, Rich and Assoc Inc, 1986, p 347

147. Diaz-Buxo JA: Continuous cyclic peritoneal dialysis. in: *Peritoneal Dialysis*, edited by Nolph KD, 2nd edition, Boston, Dordrecht, Lancaster, Martinus Nijhoff, 1985, p 247

148. Diaz-Buxo JA, Farmer CD, Chandler JT, Walker PJ, Burgess WP: CCPD: 'wet' is better than 'dry' (abstract). *Peritoneal Dial Bull* 7 (Suppl 2): S22, 1987

149. Hau T, Ahrenholz DH, Simmons RL: Secondary bacterial peritonitis: the biologic basis of treatment. *Curr Prob Surg* 16: 1, 1979

150. Haney AF, Muscato JJ, Weinberg JB: Peritoneal fluid cell populations in infertility patients. *Fertil Steril* 35: 696, 1981

151. Simberkoff MS, Moldover NH, Weiss G: Bactericidal and opsonic activity of cirrhotic ascites and non ascitic peritoneal fluid. *J Lab Clin Med* 91: 831, 1978

152. Allen L: The peritoneal stomata. *Anat Rec* 67: 89, 1936

153. Allen L, Weatherford T: Role of fenestrated basement membrane in lymphatic absorption from peritoneal cavity. *Am J Physiol* 197: 551, 1959

154. Grahame GR, Torchia MG, Dankewich KA, Fergusson IA: Surface-active material in peritoneal effluent of CAPD patients. *Peritoneal Dial Bull* 5: 109, 1985

155. Breborowicz A, Sombolos K, Rodela H, Ogilvie R, Bargman J, Oreopoulos DG: Mechanism of phosphatidylcholine action during peritoneal dialysis. *Peritoneal Dial Bull* 7; 6, 1987

156. Di Paolo N, Buoncristiani U, Capotondo L, Gaggiotti E, De Mia M, Rossi P, Sansoni E, Bernini M: Phosphatidylcholine and peritoneal transport during peritoneal dialysis. *Nephron* 44: 365, 1986

157. Di Paolo N, Sacchi G, Capotondo L: Physiological role of phosphatidylcholine in peritoneal function. in: *Peritoneal Dialysis*, edited by La Greca G, Chiaramonte S, Fabris A, Feriani M, Ronco C, Milan, Wichtig, 1988, p 49

158. Slingeneyer A, Canaud B, Mion C: Permanent loss of ultrafiltration capacity of the peritoneum in long-term peritoneal dialysis: an epidemiological study. *Nephron* 33: 133, 1983

159. Di Paolo N, Sacchi G, Buoncristiani U, Rossi P, Gaggiotti E,

Alessandrini C, Ibba L, Pucci RA: The morphology of the peritoneum in CAPD patients. in: *Frontiers in Peritoneal Dialysis,* edited by Maher JF, Winchester JF, New York, Field, Rich and Assoc Inc, 1986, p 11

160. Gotloib L, Shostack A, Bar-Sela P, Cohen R: Continuous mesothelial injury and regeneration during long term peritoneal dialysis. *Peritoneal Dial Bull* 7: 148, 1987

161. Randerson DH, Farrell PC: Mass transfer properties of the human peritoneum. *asaio J* 3: 140, 1980

162. Selgas R, Rodriguez-Carmona A, Martinez ME, Perez-Fontan M, Salinas M, Escuin F, Rinon C, Martinez-Ara J, Sanchez-Sicilia L: Peritoneal mass transfer in patients on long-term CAPD. *Peritoneal Dial Bull* 4: 153, 1984

163. Wideroe TE, Smeby LC, Mjaland F, Dahl K, Berg KJ, Aas TN: Long term changes in transperitoneal water transport during continuous ambulatory peritoneal dialysis. *Nephron* 33: 238, 1984

164. Ota K, Mineshima M, Watanabe N, Naganuma S: Functional deterioration of the peritoneum: does it occur in the absence of peritonitis? *Nephrol Dial Transplant* 2: 30, 1987

165. Duwe A, Vas SI, Weatherhead JW: Effects of the composition of peritoneal dialysis fluid on chemiluminescence, phagocytes and bactericidal activity in vitro. *Infect Immun* 33: 130, 1981

166. Vas SI, Duwe A, Weatherhead J: Natural defence mechanisms of the peritoneum: the effect of peritoneal dialysis fluid on polymorphonuclear cells. in: *Peritoneal Dialysis,* edited by Atkins RC, Thomson NM, Farrell PC, Edinburgh, Churchill Livingstone, 1981

167. Vas SI: Peritonitis. in: *Peritoneal Dialysis,* edited by Nolph KD, 2nd edition, Boston, Dordrecht, Lancaster, Martinus Nijhoff, 1985, p 411

168. Verbrugh HA, Keane WF, Hoidal JF, Freibert MR, Elliott GR, Peterson PK: Peritoneal macrophages and opsonins: antibacterial defences in patients undergoing chronic peritoneal dialysis. *J Infect Dis* 147: 1018, 1983

169. Keane WF, Comty CM, Verbrugh HA, Peterson PK: Opsonic deficiency of peritoneal dialysis effluent in continuous ambulatory peritoneal dialysis. *Kidney Int* 25: 539, 1984

170. Lewis SL, Van Epps DE: Neutrophil and monocyte alterations in chronic dialysis patients. *Am J Kidney Dis* 9: 381, 1987

171. Holmes CJ, Evans R: Biofilm and foreign body infection. The significance to CAPD-associated peritonitis. *Peritoneal Dial Bull* 6: 168, 1986

172. Dasgupta MK, Bettcher KB, Ulan RA, Burns V, Lam K, Dossetor JB, Costerton JW: Relationship of adherent bacterial biofilms to peritonitis in chronic ambulatory peritoneal dialysis. *Peritoneal Dial Bull* 7: 168, 1987

173. Verger C, Chesneau AM, Thibault M, Bataille N: Biofilm on Tenckhoff catheters: a negligible source of contamination. *Peritoneal Dial Bull* 7: 174, 1987

174. Schünemann B, Schwartz P, Quellhorst E: Results of electromicroscopic studies of peritoneal dialysis catheters: conclusions for peritonitis therapy. *Contr Nephrol* 57: 122, 1987

175. Lukowski KJ, Peters G, Finke K, Locci R, Pulverer G: Morphological observation in an indwelling peritoneal catheter infected with Candida albicans. *Peritoneal Dial Bull* 2: 44, 1982

176. Shaldon S: Peritoneal macrophage: the first line of defence. in: *Peritoneal Dialysis,* edited by La Greca G, Fabris A, Chiaramonte S, Feriani M, Ronco C, Milano, Wichtig Editore, 1986, p 201

177. Lewis SL, Van Epps DE, Chenoweth DE: C5a receptor modulation on neutrophils and monocytes from chronic hemodialysis and peritoneal dialysis patients. *Clin Nephrol* 26: 37, 1986

178. Zimmerli W, Lew PD, Waldvogel FA: Pathogenesis of foreign body infection. Evidence for a local granulocyte defect. *J Clin Invest* 73: 1191, 1983

179. Lamperi S, Carozzi S: Defective opsonic activity of peritoneal effluent during continuous ambulatory peritoneal dialysis: importance and prevention. *Peritoneal Dial Bull* 6: 87, 1986

180. Steen S, Brenchley P, Manos J, Pumphrey R, Gokal R: Opsonizing capacity of peritoneal fluid and relationship to peritonitis in CAPD. in: *Frontiers in Peritoneal Dialysis,* edited by Maher JF, Winchester JF, New York, Field, Rich and Assoc Inc, 1986, p 565

181. Giacchino F, Rotunno M, Pozzato M, Formica M, Belardi P, Bonello F, Piccoli G: Opsonization capacity of plasma and peritoneal dialysate in CAPD patients. in: *Frontiers in Peritoneal Dialysis,* edited by Maher JF, Winchester JF, New York, Field, Rich and Assoc Inc, 1986, p 569

182. Yewdall VMA, Bennett-Jones DN, Cameron JS, Ogg CS, Williams DG: Opsonically-active proteins in CAPD. in: *Frontiers in Peritoneal Dialysis,* edited by Maher JF, Winchester JF, New York, Field, Rich and Assoc Inc, 1986, p 573

183. Coles GA, Alobaidi HMM, Topley N, Davies M: Opsonic activity of dialysis effluent predicts those at risk of Staphylococcus epidermidis infection. *Nephrol Dial Transplant* 2: 359, 1987

184. McGregor SJ, Brock JH, Briggs JD, Junor BJR: Relationship of IgG, C3 and transferrin with opsonising and bacteriostatic activity of peritoneal fluid from CAPD patients and the incidence of peritonitis. *Nephrol Dial Transplant* 2: 551, 1987

185. Verbrugh HA, Verkooyen RP, Verhoef J, Oe PL, Van der Meulen J: Defective complement-mediated opsonization and lysis of bacteria in commercial peritoneal dialysis solutions. in: *Frontiers in Peritoneal Dialysis,* edited by Maher JF, Winchester JF, New York, Field, Rich and Assoc Inc, 1986, p 559

186. Khan RH, Klein M, Vas SI: Fibronectin in the normal peritoneal fluids of patients on chronic ambulatory peritoneal dialysis and during peritonitis. *Peritoneal Dial Bull* 7: 69, 1987

187. Brock JH: Iron and the outcome of infection. *Br Med J* 293: 518, 1986

188. Peterson PK: Host defence abnormalities predisposing the patient to infection. *Am J Med* 76: (5A): 2, 1984

189. Hurley RM, Muogabo D, Wilson GW, Ali MAM: Cellular composition of peritoneal effluent: response to bacterial peritonitis. *Can Med Assoc J* 117: 1061, 1977

190. Flanigan MJ, Freeman RM, Lim VS: Cellular response to peritonitis among peritoneal dialysis patients. *Am J Kidney Dis* 6: 420, 1985

191. Goldstein CS, Bomalaski JS, Zurier RB, Neilson EG, Douglas SD: Analysis of peritoneal macrophages in continuous ambulatory peritoneal dialysis patients. *Kidney Int* 26: 733, 1984

192. Alobaidi HM, Coles GA, Davies M, Lloyd D: Host defence in continuous ambulatory peritoneal dialysis: the effect of dialysate on phagocyte function. *Nephrol Dial Transplant* 1: 16, 1986

193. McGregor SJ, Brock JH, Briggs JD, Junor BJT: Bactericidal activity of peritoneal macrophages for continuous ambulatory dialysis patients. *Nephrol Dial Transplant* 2: 104, 1987

194. Gallimore B, Gagnon RF, Stevenson MM: Cytotoxicity of commercial peritoneal dialysis solutions toward peritoneal cells of chronically uremic mice. *Nephron* 43: 283, 1986

195. Verbrugh HA, Van Bronswijk H, Van der Meulen J, Oe PL, Verhoef J: Phagocytic defence against CAPD peritonitis. The

bacterium, the phagocyte and the doctor. *Contr Nephrol* 57: 85, 1987

196. Peterson PK, Lee D, Suh HJ, Devalon M, Nelson RD, Keane WF: Intracellular survival of Candida albicans in peritoneal macrophages from chronic peritoneal dialysis patients. *Am J Kidney Dis* 7: 146, 1986

197. Buggy BP, Schaberg DR, Swartz RD: Intraleucocytic sequestration as a cause of persistant Staphylococcus aureus peritonitis in continuous ambulatory peritoneal dialysis. *Am J Med* 76: 1035, 1984

198. Beelen RHJ, Van der Meulen J, Verbruck HA, Oe PL, Verhoef J: CAPD, a permanent state of peritonitis: a study on peroxidase activity. in: *Frontiers in Peritoneal Dialysis,* edited by Maher JF, Winchester JF, New York, Field, Rich and Assoc Inc, 1986, p 524

199. Shaldon S, Koch KM, Quellhorst E, Dinarello CA: Pathogenesis of sclerosing peritonitis in CAPD. *Trans Am Soc Artif Intern Organs* 30: 193, 1984

200. Dinarello CA, Wyler DJ: Isolation of interleukin I from CAPD lavage fluid: lymphocytes and fibroblast activating properties of interleukin I (abstract). *Blood Purif* 2: 48, 1984

201. Lamperi S, Carozzi S: Suppressor resident peritoneal macrophages and peritonitis incidence in continuous ambulatory peritoneal dialysis. *Nephron* 44: 219, 1986

202. Williams P, Khanna R, Vas S, Layne S, Pantalony D, Oreopoulos DG: The treatment of peritonitis in patients on CAPD: to lavage or not? *Peritoneal Dial Bull* 1: 14, 1980

203. Guiberteau R, Le Chapois D, Nony A, Talin d'Eyzac A: Treatment of peritoneal infection by the natural defences of the peritoneal cavity. *Contr Nephrol* 57: 92, 1987

204. Gotloib L, Mines M, Garmizo L, Varka I: Hemodynamic effects of increasing intra-abdominal pressure in peritoneal dialysis. *Peritoneal Dial Bull* 1: 41, 1981

205. Twardowski ZJ, Prowant BF, Nolph KD, Martinez AJ, Lampton LM: High volume, low frequency continuous ambulatory peritoneal dialysis. *Kidney Int* 23: 64, 1983

206. Twardowski ZJ, Khanna R, Nolph KD, Scalamogna A, Metzler MH, Schneider TW, Prowant BF, Ryan LP: Intra-abdominal pressures during natural activities in patients treated with continuous ambulatory peritoneal dialysis. *Nephron* 44: 129, 1986

207. Schurig R, Gahl G, Schartl M, Becker H, Kessel M: Central and peripheral hemodynamics in long term peritoneal dialysis patients. *Proc Eur Dial Transplant Assoc* 16: 165, 1979

208. Kong CH, Raval U, Thompson FD: Effect of 2 liters of intraperitoneal dialysate on the cardiovascular system. *Clin Nephrol* 26: 134, 1986

209. Franklin JO, Alpert MA, Twardowski ZHJ, Khanna R: Effect of intraperitoneal infusion volume and posture on left ventricular systolic function in patients on continuous ambulatory peritoneal dialysis. *Trans Am Soc Artif Intern Organs* 32: 554, 1986

210. Prefaut C, Monteil A, Ramonatko M, Slingeneyer A, Chardon G, Mirouze J: Closing volume and pulmonary gas exchange during peritoneal dialysis. *Bull Eur Physiopath Resp* 14: 755, 1978

211. Ahluwalia M, Ishjikawa S, Gellman M, Shah T, Sekar T, Mac Donnell KF: Pulmonary functions during peritoneal dialysis. *Clin Nephrol* 18: 251, 1982

212. Taveira da Silva AM, Davies WB, Winchester JF, Coleman DE, Weir CN: Peritonitis, dialysate infusion and lung function in continuous ambulatory peritoneal dialysis. *Clin Nephrol* 24: 79, 1985

213. Berlyne GM, Lee HA, Ralston AJ, Woolcock JA: Pulmonary

complications of peritoneal dialysis. *Lancet* 2: 75, 1966

214. Gotloib L, Garmizo L, Varak I, Mines M: Reduction of vital capacity due to increased intra-abdominal pressure during peritoneal dialysis. *Peritoneal Dial Bull* 1: 63, 1981

215. Epstein SN, Inouye T, Robson M, Oreopoulos DG: Effect of peritoneal dialysis fluid on ventilatory function. *Peritoneal Dial Bull* 2: 120, 1982

216. Fabris A, Biasioli S, Chiaramonte C, Feriani M, Pisani E, Ronco C, Cantarella G, La Greca G: Buffer metabolism in continuous ambulatory peritoneal dialysis: relationship with respiratory dynamics. *Trans Am Soc Artif Intern Organs* 28: 270, 1982

217. Eiser AR: Pulmonary gas exchange during hemodialysis and peritoneal dialysis: interaction between respiration and metabolism. *Am J Kidney Dis* 6: 131, 1985

218. Blumberg A, Keller R, Marti HR: Oxygen affinity of erythrocytes and pulmonary gas exchange in patients on continuous ambulatory peritoneal dialysis. *Nephron* 38: 248, 1984

219. Krediet RT, Boeschoten EW, Zuyderhoudt FMJ, Arisz L: Peritoneal transport characteristics of water, low molecular weight solutes and proteins during long term continuous ambulatory peritoneal dialysis. *Peritoneal Dial Bull* 6: 61, 1986

220. Strauch M, Walzer P, v Henning GE, Roettger G, Christ H: Factors influencing protein loss during peritoneal dialysis. *Trans Am Soc Artif Intern Organs* 13: 172, 1967

221. Rubin J, McFarland S, Hellems EW, Bower JD: Peritoneal dialysis during peritonitis. *Kidney Int* 19: 460, 1981

222. Steinhauer HB, Schollmeyer P: Prostaglandin-mediated loss of proteins during peritonitis in continuous ambulatory peritoneal dialysis. *Kidney Int* 29: 584, 1986

223. Lindner A, Tenckhoff H: Nitrogen balance in patients on maintenance peritoneal dialysis. *Trans Am Soc Artif Intern Organs* 16: 255, 1970

224. Scarpioni L, Poisetti P, Ballocchi S, Bergonzi G, Mistraletti C: Protein loss and compensation in uremic patients during peritoneal dialysis. *Int J Artif Organs* 1: 76, 1979

225. Blumenkrantz MJ, Gahl GM, Kopple JD, Kamdar AV, Jones MR, Kessel M, Coburn JW: Protein losses during peritoneal dialysis. *Kidney Int* 19: 53, 1981

226. Dulaney JT, Hatch FE Jr: Peritoneal dialysis and loss of proteins: a review. *Kidney Int* 26: 253, 1986

227. Miller FN, Nolph KD, Joshua JG, Wiegman DL, Harris PD, Andersen DB: Hyperosmolality, acetate and lactate: dilatory factors during peritoneal dialysis. *Kidney Int* 20: 397, 1981

228. Kaysen GA, Schoenfeld PY: Albumin homeostasis in patients undergoing continuous ambulatory peritoneal dialysis. *Kidney Int* 25: 107, 1984

229. Lindholm B, Bergstrom J: Nutritional aspects of CAPD, in: *Continuous Ambulatory Peritoneal Dialysis,* edited by Gokal R, Edinburgh, Churchill Livingstone, 1986, p 228

230. Young GA, Brownjohn AM, Parsons FM: Protein losses in patients receiving continuous ambulatory peritoneal dialysis. *Nephron* 45: 196, 1987

231. Gries E, Paar D, Graben N, Bock KD: Intraperitoneal fibrin formation and its inhibition in CAPD. *Clin Nephrol* 26: 209, 1986

232. De Stefano V, Triolo L, De Martini D, Ferrelli R, Mori R, Leone G: Antithrombin III loss in patients with the nephrotic syndrome or receiving continuous ambulatory peritoneal dialysis. Evidence of inactive antithrombin III in urine of patient with nephrotic syndrome. *J Lab Clin Med* 109: 550, 1987

233. Lillo-Ferez M, Dupommereille C, Prieur P, Allain B, Petrover M: Beta 2 microglobulin clearance by chronic intermittent peritoneal dialysis. *Peritoneal Dial Bull* 6: 215, 1986

234. Blumberg A, Bürgi W: Behavior of beta 2 microglobulin in patients with chronic renal failure undergoing hemodialysis, hemodiafiltration and continuous ambulatory peritoneal dialysis. *Clin Nephrol* 27: 45, 1987

235. Gagnon RF, Somerville P, Kaye M: Beta 2 microglobulin serum levels in patients on long term dialysis. *Peritoneal Dial Bull* 7: 29, 1987

236. Berlyne GM, Lee HA, Giordano C, de Pascale C, Esposito R: Amino acid loss in peritoneal dialysis. *Lancet* 1: 1339, 1967

237. Young GA, Parsons FM: The effect of peritoneal dialysis upon the amino acids and other nitrogenous compounds in the blood and dialysates from patients with renal failure. *Clin Sci* 37: 1, 1969

238. De Santo NG, Capodicasa G, Dileo V, Di Stefano A, Cirillo D, Esposito R, Fiore R, Cucciniello E, Damiano M, Buonadonna L, Di Iorio R, Capasso G, Giordano C: Kinetics of amino acids equilibration in the dialysate during CAPD. *Int J Artif Organs* 4: 23, 1981

239. Dombros N, Oren A, Marliss EB, Anderson GA, Stein AN, Khanna R, Petit J, Brandes L, Rodella H, Leibel BS, Oreopoulos DG: Plasma amino acid profiles and amino acid loss in patients undergoing CAPD. *Peritoneal Dial Bull* 2: 27, 1982

240. Kopple JD, Blumenkrantz MJ, Jones MR, Horan JK, Coburn JW: Plasma amino acid levels and amino acid losses during continuous ambulatory peritoneal dialysis. *Am J Clin Nutr* 36: 295, 1982

241. Nolph KD, Rosenfield PS, Powell JT, Danforth E Jr: Peritoneal glucose transport and hyperglycemia during peritoneal dialysis. *Am J Med Sci* 259: 272, 1970

242. Grodstein GP, Blumenkrantz MJ, Kopple JD, Moran JK, Coburn JW: Glucose absorption during continuous ambulatory peritoneal dialysis. *Kidney Int* 19: 564, 1981

243. Verger C, Larpent L, Dumontet M: Prognostic value of peritoneal equilibration curves in CAPD patients. in: *Frontiers in Peritoneal Dialysis*, edited by Maher JF, Winchester JF, New York, Field, Rich Assoc, 1986, p 88

244. Twardowski ZJ, Nolph KD, Khanna R, Prowant BF, Ryan LP, Moore HL, Nielsen MP: Peritoneal equilibration test. *Peritoneal Dial Bull* 7: 113, 1987

245. Armstrong VW, Creutzfeldt N, Ebert R, Fuchs C, Hilgers R, Scherer F: Effect of dialysate glucose load on plasma glucose and glucoregulatory hormones in CAPD patients. *Nephron* 39: 141, 1985

246. Kurtz SB, Wong G, Anderson CF, Vogel J, McCarthy JT, Mitchell JC, Kumar R, Johnson WJ: Continuous ambulatory peritoneal dialysis: three years' experience at the Mayo Clinic. *Mayo Clinic Proc* 58: 633, 1983

247. Chan MK, Varghese Z, Persaud JW, Baillod RA, Moorhead JF: Hyperlipidemia in patients on maintenance hemo- and peritoneal dialysis: the relative pathogenetic roles of triglyceride production and triglyceride removal. *Clin Nephrol* 17: 183, 1984

248. Khanna R, Breckenridge C, Roncari D, Digenis G, Oreopoulos DG: Lipid abnormalities in patients undergoing continuous ambulatory peritoneal dialysis. *Peritoneal Dial Bull* 3 (Suppl): S13, 1983

249. Turgan C, Flehally J, Bennett S, Davies TJ, Walls J: Accelerated hypertriglyceridemia in patients on continuous ambulatory peritoneal dialysis. A preventable abnormality. *Int J Artif Organs* 4: 158, 1981

250. Ramos JM, Heaton A, McGurk JG, Ward MK, Kerr DNS: Sequential changes in serum lipids and their subfractions in patients receiving continuous ambulatory peritoneal dialysis. *Nephron* 35: 20, 1983

251. Wu G & the University of Toronto Collaborative Dialysis Group: Cardiovascular deaths among CAPD patients. *Peritoneal Dial Bull* 3 (Suppl): S23, 1983

252. Mion C, Slingeneyer A, Canaud B: Pathophysiology and management of hypertension in continuous ambulatory peritoneal dialysis. *Contr Nephrol* 54: 202, 1986

253. Van Acker BAC, Bilo HJG, Popp-Snijders C, Van Bronswijk H, Oe PL, Donker AJM: The effect of fish oil on lipid profile and viscosity or erythrocyte suspensions in CAPD patients. *Nephrol Dial Transpl* 2: 557, 1987

254. Bang HO, Dyerberg J: Fish consumption and mortality from coronary heart disease. *N Engl J Med* 313: 822, 1985

255. Blumberg A, Hanck A, Sander G: Vitamin nutrition in patients on continuous ambulatory peritoneal dialysis. *Clin Nephrol* 20: 244, 1983

256. Gilmour J, Wu G, Khanna R, Schilling H, Mitwalli A, Oreopoulos DG: Long term continuous ambulatory peritoneal dialysis. *Peritoneal Dial Bull* 5: 112, 1985

257. Digenis GE, Dombros N, Charytan C, Oreopoulos DG: Supplements for the CAPD patient (vitamins, folic acid, zinc, iron and anabolic steroids). *Peritoneal Dial Bull* 7: 219, 1987

258. Aloni Y, Shany S, Chaimovitz C: Losses of 25-hydroxyvitamin D in peritoneal fluid: possible mechanism for bone disease in uremic patients treated with chronic ambulatory peritoneal dialysis. *Miner Electrolyte Metab* 9: 82, 1983

259. Shany S, Rapoport J, Goligorsky M, Yankowitz N, Zuici I, Chaimovitz C: Losses of 1,25- and 24,25-dihydroxycholecalciferol in the peritoneal fluid of patients treated with continuous ambulatory peritoneal dialysis. *Nephron* 36: 111, 1984

260. Moorthy AV, Rosenblum M, Rajaram R, Shug AL: A comparison of plasma and muscle carnitine levels in patients on peritoneal or hemodialysis for chronic renal failure. *Am J Nephrol* 3: 205, 1983

261. Wanner C, Förstner-Wanner S, Schaeffer G, Schollmeyer P, Hörl WH: Serum free carnitine, carnitine esters and lipids in patients on peritoneal dialysis and hemodialysis. *Am J Nephrol* 6: 206, 1986

262. Buoncristiani U, Carobi C, Di Paolo N, Cozzari M, Brugnaro R: Progression of carnitine depletion in patients on long-term CAPD. *Peritoneal Dial Bull* 4 (Suppl): S10, 1984

263. Maher JF, Hirszel P, Hohnadel DC, Abraham J, Lasrich M: Fatty acid removal during peritoneal dialysis: mechanisms, rate and significance. *asaio J* 1: 8, 1978

264. Bartel LL, Hussey JL, Shrago E: Effect of dialysis on serum carnitine, free fatty acids, and triglyceride levels in man and the rat. *Metabolism* 31: 944, 1982

265. Mion C, Slingeneyer A, Huchard G, Deschodt G, Polito C, Issautier R, Florence P: Traitement de suppléance chez l'insuffisant rénal chronique à haut risque: hémodialyse ou dialyse péritonéale? (Maintenance dialysis in high risk patients: hemo- or peritoneal dialysis?). in: *Actualités Néphrologiques de l'Hôpital Necker*, edited by Hamburger J, Crosnier J, Funck-Brentano JL, Paris, Flammarion Médicine Sciences, 1979, p 71 (in French)

266. Von Bayer H, Gahl GM, Riedinger H, Borowzak R, Averdunk R, Schurig R, Kessel M: Adaptation of CAPD patients to the continuous peritoneal energy uptake. *Kidney Int* 23: 29, 1983

267. Lampeinnen E, Khanna R, Schaeffer R, Twardowski ZJ, Nolph KD: Is air under the diaphragm a significant finding in CAPD patients? *Trans Am Soc Artif Intern Organs* 32: 581, 1986

268. Daugirdas JT, Leehey DJ, Popli S, Hoffman W, Zayas I, Gandhi VC, Ing TS: Induction of peritoneal fluid eosinophilia

and/or monocytosis by intraperitoneal air injection. *Am J Nephrol* 7: 116, 1987

269. Shaldon S: A cynical critique of continuous ambulatory peritoneal dialysis. in: *Continuous Ambulatory Peritoneal Dialysis*, edited by Legrain M, Amsterdam, Oxford, Princeton, Excerpta Medica, 1980, p 137
270. Keshaviah P, Collins A: Rapid high-efficiency bicarbonate hemodialysis. *Trans Am Soc Artif Intern Organs* 32: 17, 1986
271. Maher JF, Schreiner GE: Hazards and complications of dialysis. *N Engl J Med* 273: 370, 1965
272. Khanna R, Oreopoulos DG: Complications of peritoneal dialysis other than peritonitis in peritoneal dialysis. in: *Peritoneal Dialysis*, edited by Nolph KD, 2nd edition, Boston, Dordrecht, Lancaster, Martinus Nijhoff, 1985, p 441
273. Pauli HG, Büttikofer E, Vorburger CH: Clinical experience with peritoneal dialysis. *Helv Med Acta* 1: 51, 1966
274. Romagnoni M, Beccari M, Faiolo S, Granello E, Scalia P, Paleardi P: Abdominal pain with infusion of the peritoneal dialysis solutions relieved by alkalinisation (letter). *Peritoneal Dial Bull* 4: 188, 1984
275. Ivanovich P, Jones KM, Borsanyi A: Relief of pain associated with automated peritoneal dialysis. *Proc Eur Dial Transplant Assoc* 12: 156, 1976
276. Pedersen FB, Ryttov N, Deleuran D, Dragsholt C, Koldeberg P: Acetate versus lactate in peritoneal dialysis solutions. *Nephron* 39: 55, 1985
277. Swartz RD, Valk TW, Brain AJP, Hsu CH: Complications of hemodialysis and peritoneal dialysis in acute renal failure. *Asaio J* 3: 98, 1980
278. Raja RM, Cantor RE, Beoryko C, Busherhi H, Kramer MS, Rosenbaum JL: Sodium transport during ultrafiltration peritoneal dialysis. *Trans Am Soc Artif Intern Organs* 18: 429, 1972
279. Gault MH, Fergusson EL, Sidhu JS, Corbin RP: Fluid and electrolyte complications of peritoneal dialysis. *Ann Intern Med* 75: 253, 1971
280. Tzamaloukas AH: Contraction alkalosis during treatment of hyperglycemia in CAPD patients. *Peritoneal Dial Bull* 3: 196, 1983
281. Kenamonde TG, Graves JW, Lempert KD, Moss AH, Whittier FC: Severe recurrent alkalemia in a patient undergoing continuous cyclic peritoneal dialysis. *Am J Med* 81: 548, 1986
282. Naparstek Y, Rubinger D, Friedlander MM, Popovtzer MM: Lactic acidosis and peritoneal dialysis. *Isr J Med Sci* 18: 513, 1982
283. Foulks CJ, Wright LF: Successful repletion of bicarbonate stores in ongoing lactic acidosis: a role for bicarbonate-buffered peritoneal dialysis. *South Med J* 74: 1162, 1981
284. Lee HA, Hill LF, Hewitt V, Ralston AJ, Berlyne GM: Lactic-acidaemia in peritoneal dialysis. *Proc Eur Dial Transplant Assoc* 4: 150, 1967
285. Veech RL, Fowler RC: Cerebral dysfunction and respiratory alkalosis during peritoneal dialysis with D-lactate containing dialysis fluids (letter). *Am J Med* 82: 572, 1987
286. La Greca G, Biasioli S, Chiaramonte S, Davi M, Fabris A, Feriani M, Pisani E, Ronco C, Zen F: Acid-base balance on peritoneal dialysis. *Clin Nephrol* 16: 1, 1981
287. Teehan BP, Schleifer CR, Reichard GA, Lupit MC, Sigler MH, Haff AC: Acid-base studies in continuous ambulatory peritoneal dialysis. in: *CAPD Update – Continuous Ambulatory Peritoneal Dialysis*, edited by Moncrief JW, Popovich RP, New York, Masson Publishing USA, Inc, 1981, p 95
288. Richardson RMA, Roscoe JM: Bicarbonate, L-lactate and D-lactate balance in intermittent peritoneal dialysis. *Peritoneal Dial Bull* 6: 178, 1986

289. Al-Kudsi RR, Daugirdas JT, Ing TS, Kheirbek AO, Popli S, Hano JE, Gandhi VC: Extreme hyperglycemia in dialysis patients. *Clin Nephrol* 17: 228, 1982
290. Flynn CT, Hibbard J, Dohrmann B: Advantages of continuous ambulatory peritoneal dialysis to the diabetic with renal failure. *Proc Eur Dial Transplant Assoc* 16: 184, 1979
291. Smithard D, Khanna R, Ryan D, From G, Oreopoulos DG: Spontaneous hypoglycemia during continuous ambulatory peritoneal dialysis. *Peritoneal Dial Bull* 3: 191, 1983
292. Tchetagni J, Ngu JL: Fatal hypoglycemia during CAPD in a young diabetic not receiving insulin. *Peritoneal Dial Bull* 7: 109, 1987
293. Edwards S, Unger H: Acute hydrothorax – a new complication of peritoneal dialysis. *JAMA* 199: 189, 1967
294. Finn R, Jewett E: Acute hydrothorax complicating peritoneal dialysis. *Br Med J* 277: 94, 1970
295. Holm J, Lieden B, Lindquist B: Unilateral pleural effusion, a rare complication of peritoneal dialysis. *Scand J Urol Nephrol* 5: 84, 1971
296. Rudnick M, Coyle J, Beck L, McCurdy D: Acute massive hydrothorax complicating peritoneal dialysis, report of two cases and review of the literature. *Clin Nephrol* 12: 38, 1979
297. Milutinovic J, Wu W, Lindholm D, Lapp N: Acute massive unilateral hydrothorax: a rare complication of chronic peritoneal dialysis. *South Med J* 73: 827, 1980
298. O'Connor J, Rutland M: Demonstration of a pleuro-peritoneal communication with radionuclide imaging in a CAPD patient (letter). *Peritoneal Dial Bull* 1: 153, 1981
299. Spadaro JJ, Thakur V, Nolph KD: Technetium-99m-labelled macroaggregated albumin in demonstration of trans-diaphragmatic leakage of dialysate in peritoneal dialysis. *Am J Nephrol* 2: 36, 1982
300. Scheldewaert R, Bogaerts Y, Pauwels R, Van der Straeten M, Ringoir S, Lameire N: Management of a massive hydrothorax in a CAPD patient: a case report and a review of the literature. *Peritoneal Dial Bull* 2: 69, 1982
301. Nässberger L: Left-sided pleural effusion secondary to continuous ambulatory peritoneal dialysis. *Acta Med Scand* 211: 219, 1982
302. Grefberg N, Danielson BG, Benson L, Pitkänen P: Right-sided hydrothorax complicating peritoneal dialysis. Report of 2 cases. *Nephron* 34: 130, 1983
303. Singh S, Vaidya P, Dale A, Morgan B: Massive hydrothorax complicating continuous ambulatory peritoneal dialysis. *Nephron* 34: 168, 1983
304. Pattison CW, Rodger RSC, Adu D, Michael J, Matthews HR: Surgical treatment of hydrothorax complicating continuous ambulatory peritoneal dialysis. *Clin Nephrol* 21: 191, 1984
305. Benz RL, Schleifer CR: Hydrothorax in continuous ambulatory peritoneal dialysis: successful treatment with intrapleural tetracycline and a review of the literature. *Am J Kidney Dis* 5: 136, 1985
306. Vezina D, Winchester JF, Rakowski TA: Spontaneous resolution of massive hydrothorax in a CAPD patient. *Peritoneal Dial Bull* 7: 212, 1987
307. Ayres SM, Grace WJ: Inappropriate ventilation and hypoxemia as causes of cardiac arrhythmias: the control of arrhythmias without antiarrhythmic drugs. *Am J Med* 46: 496, 1969
308. Kutsky EA: Bradycardic rhythms during peritoneal dialysis. *Arch Intern Med* 128: 445, 1971
309. Peer G, Korzets A, Hochauzer E, Eschchar Y, Blum M, Aviram A: Cardiac arrhythmia during chronic ambulatory peritoneal dialysis. *Nephron* 45: 192, 1987
310. Morrison G, Michelson EL, Brown S, Morganroth J: Mecha-

nisms and prevention of cardiac arrhythmias in chronic hemodialysis patients. *Kidney Int* 17: 811, 1980

311. Moffat FL, Deitel M, Thompson DA: Abdominal surgery in patients undergoing long-term peritoneal dialysis. *Surgery* 92: 598, 1982

312. Niemiera RM, Winchester JF, Rakowski TA, Rahmat J, Argy WP, Gelfand ML, Barnard WF, Schreiner GE: Hemoperitoneum: a frequent complication of CAPD (abstract). *Peritoneal Dial Bull* 4 (Suppl 2): S44, 1984

313. Oreopoulos DG, Khanna R, Williams P, Vas SI: Continuous ambulatory peritoneal dialysis – 1981. *Nephron* 30: 293, 1982

314. Hassell LH, Moore J Jr, Conklin JJ: Hemoperitoneum during continuous ambulatory peritoneal dialysis: a possible complication of radiation induced peritoneal injury. *Clin Nephrol* 21: 241, 1984

315. Flapan AD, Brown CB, Hamilton DV: Rupture of hepatic artery aneurysm: an unusual cause of death during acute peritoneal dialysis. *Peritoneal Dial Bull* 4: 268, 1984

316. Shoat J, Shapira Z, Yussim A, Boner G: An unusual cause of massive intraperitoneal bleeding in CAPD. *Peritoneal Dial Bull* 4: 257, 1984

317. Nace GS, George Al Jr, Stone W: Hemoperitoneum: a red flag in CAPD. *Peritoneal Dial Bull* 5: 42, 1985

318. de los Santos A, von Eye O, d'Avilla D, Mottin CC: Rupture of the spleen: a complication of continuous ambulatory peritoneal dialysis. *Peritoneal Dial Bull* 6: 203, 1986

319. Coronel F, Maranjo P, Torrente J, Pratz D: The risk of retrograde menstruation in CAPD patients. *Peritoneal Dial Bull* 4: 190, 1984

320. Rambausek M, Ritz E, Waldherr R: Recurrent blood dialysate during upper respiratory tract infection in mesangial IgA glomerulonephritis. *Nephron* 46: 213, 1987

321. Husserl F, Tapia N: Peritoneal bleeding in a CAPD patient after extracorporeal lithotripsy. *Peritoneal Dial Bull* 7: 262, 1987

322. Modi KB, Henderson IS: Fatal massive hemoperitoneum after cessation of CAPD (letter). *Clin Nephrol* 27: 47, 1987

323. Avram MM: High prevalence of pancreatic disease in chronic renal failure. *Nephron* 18: 68, 1977

324. Vaziri ND, Dure-Smith B, Miller R, Mirahmadi M: Pancreatic pathology in chronic dialysis patients – an autopsy study of 28 cases. *Nephron* 46: 347, 1987

325. Pitrone F, Pellegrino E, Mileto G, Consolo F: May pancreatitis represent a CAPD complication? Report of two cases with a rapid evolution to death. *Int J Artif Organs* 8: 235, 1985

326. Caruando RJ, Wolfman NT, Karstaedt N, Wilson DJ: Pancreatitis: an important cause of abdominal symptoms in patients on peritoneal dialysis. *Am J Kidney Dis* 7: 135, 1986

327. Flynn CT, Chandran PKG, Shadur CA: Recurrent pancreatitis in a patient on CAPD. *Peritoneal Dial Bull* 6: 106, 1986

328. Singh S, Wadhwa N: Peritonitis, pancreatitis, and infected pseudocyst in a continuous ambulatory peritoneal dialysis patient. *Am J Kidney Dis* 9: 84, 1987

329. Connacher AA, Steward WK: Pancreatitis causes brownish-black peritoneal dialysate due to the presence of methamalbumin. *Nephrol Dial Transplant* 2: 45, 1987

330. Emder PJ, Howard NJ, Rosenberg AR: Non-ketotic hyperosmolar diabetic pre-coma due to pancreatitis in a boy on continuous ambulatory peritoneal dialysis. *Nephron* 44: 355, 1987

331. Caruana RJ, Burkart J, Segraves D, Smallwood S, Haymore J, Disher B: Serum and peritoneal fluid amylase levels in CAPD. Normal values and clinical usefulness. *Am J Nephrol* 7: 169, 1987

332. Vogt K, Hess B, Baumgartner D, Maass D, Keusch G, Bing-

swanger U: Appendicitis perforata in CAPD patients: report of two cases. *Peritoneal Dial Bull* 5: 237, 1985

333. Wu G, Khanna R, Vas S, Oreopoulos DG: Is extensive diverticulosis of the colon a contraindication to CAPD? *Peritoneal Dial Bull* 3: 180, 1983

334. Nelson W, Khanna R, Mathews R, Yeung H, Wu G, Vas S, Oreopoulos DG: Gallbladder stones, cholecystitis and cholecystectomy in patients on continuous ambulatory peritoneal dialysis. *Peritoneal Dial Bull* 4: 245, 1984

335. Power DA, Edward N, Catto GRD, Muirhead N, MacLeod A, Engeset J: Richter's hernia: an unrecognised complication of chronic ambulatory peritoneal dialysis. *Br Med J* 283: 528, 1981

336. Madden MA, Beirne GJ, Zimmerman W, Sollinger H: Acute bowel obstruction: an unusual complication of chronic peritoneal dialysis. *Am J Kidney Dis* 1: 219, 1982

337. Shenouda AN, Puckett W, Burns R, Miller FJ: Acute intestinal obstruction complicating CAPD. *Peritoneal Dial Bull* 2: 49, 1982

338. Ramos JM, Burke DA, Veitch PS: Hernia of Morgagni in patients on continuous ambulatory peritoneal dialysis. *Lancet* 1: 161, 1982

339. Koren G, Aladjem M, Militiano J, Seegal B, Jonash A, Boichis H: Ischemic colitis in chronic intermittent peritoneal dialysis. *Nephron* 36: 272, 1984

340. Wehling M, Jenni R, Steurer J, Buhler H, Siegenthaler W, Kuhlman U: Ischemic colitis in a patient undergoing continuous ambulatory peritoneal dialysis. *Peritoneal Dial Bull* 2: 123, 1982

341. Steiner RW: Acute abdominal events other than primary peritonitis in CAPD patients (letter). *Peritoneal Dial Bull* 7: 107, 1987

342. Pomeranz A, Reichenberg Y, Schurr D, Drukker A: Chyloperitoneum: a rare complication of peritoneal dialysis. *Peritoneal Dial Bull* 4: 35, 1984

343. Roodhooft AM, Van Acker KJ, De Broe ME: Chylous peritonitis: an infrequent complication of peritoneal dialysis. *Peritoneal Dial Bull* 7: 195, 1987

344. Walshe JJ, Reddy PV: Continuous ambulatory peritoneal dialysis complicated by Fournier's syndrome. *Peritoneal Dial Bull* 7: 193, 1987

345. Somerville PJ, O'Brien E, Kaye M: Possible heparin-induced subcutaneous necrosis in a CAPD patient. *Peritoneal Dial Bull* 7: 187, 1987

346. Dibble JB, Coltman SJ, Gibson J, Brownjohn AM: Acute aluminum toxicity in a CAPD patient: the role of oral aluminum hydroxide. *Peritoneal Dial Bull* 7: 207, 1987

347. Cumming AD, Simpson G, Bell D, Cowie J, Winney RJ: Acute aluminium intoxication in patients on continuous ambulatory peritoneal dialysis (letter). *Lancet* 1: 103, 1982

348. Di Paolo N, Sacchi G, De Mia M, Gaggiotti E, Capotondo L, Rossi P, Bernini M, Puggi AM, Ibba L, Sabatelli P, Alessandrini C: Morphology of the peritoneal membrane during peritoneal dialysis. *Nephron* 44: 204, 1986

349. Di Paolo N: The morphology of peritoneal membrane during peritoneal dialysis. in: *Peritoneal Dialysis*, edited by La Greca G, Chiaramonte S, Fabris A, Feriani M, Ronco C, Milan, Wichtig, 1988, p 3

350. Tenckhoff H: Advantages and shortcomings of peritoneal dialysis in the management of chronic renal failure. in: *Seminaires d'Uro-Néphrologie Pitié-Salpétrière, Troisième Série 1977*, edited by Küss R, Legrain M, Paris, Masson, 1977, p 107

351. Ahmad S, Gallagher N, Shen F: Intermittent peritoneal dialysis – status reassessed. *Trans Am Soc Artif Intern Organs* 25: 86, 1979

352. Ganthous WN, Salkin MS, Adelson BH, Ghantous S, McGinnis K, Valenziano A, Cronin M: Limitations of peritoneal dialysis in the treatment of ESRD patients. *Trans Am Soc Artif Intern Organs* 25: 100, 1979

353. Heale WF, Letch KA, Dawborn JK, Evans SM: Long term complications of peritonitis. in: *Peritoneal Dialysis,* edited by Atkins RC, Thomson NP, Farrell PC, Edinburg, Churchill Livingstone, 1981, p 284

354. Williams CC & The University of Toronto Collaborative Dialysis Group: CAPD in Toronto, an overview. *Peritoneal Dial Bull* 3 (Suppl): S6, 1983

355. Rubin J, Kirchner K, Barnes T, Neal N, Ray R, Bower JD: Evaluation of continuous ambulatory peritoneal dialysis. *Am J Kidney Dis* 3: 199, 1983

356. Spencer PC, Farrell PC: Peritoneal membrane stability and the kinetics of peritoneal mass transfer. in: *Peritoneal Dialysis,* edited by Nolph KD, 2nd edition, Boston, The Hague, Dordrecht, Lancaster, Martinus Nijhoff, 1985, p 581

357. Oreopoulos DG: Duration of peritoneal dialysis – ten years or more. *Peritoneal Dial Bull* 4: 61, 1984

358. Marichal JF, Faller B, Brignon P, Wagner D, Straub P: Progressive calcifying peritonitis: a new complication of CAPD. Report of two cases. *Nephron* 45: 229, 1987

359. Slingeneyer A, Canaud B, Mion C, Elie M: Peritoneal calcifications in maintenance peritoneal dialysis: a search for etiological factors. in: *Proc IVth Congr Int Soc Peritoneal Dial,* Venice, July 1987, (in press).

360. Glynn LE: The pathology of scar tissue formation. in: *Tissue Repair and Regeneration, Handbook of Inflammation,* volume 3, edited by Glynn LE, Houck JC, Weissmann G, Amsterdam, New York, Oxford, Elsevier/North Holland, Biomedical Press, 1981, p 285

361. Singal K, Segel DP, Bruns FJ, Fraley DS, Adler S, Julian TB: Genital edema in patients on continuous ambulatory peritoneal dialysis. *Am J Nephrol* 6: 471, 1986

362. Schurgers MCL, Bopelaert JRO, Daneels RFS, Robbens EJ, Vandelanotte MMJ: Open processus vaginalis. *Peritoneal Dial Bull* 3: 30, 1983

363. Graves J, Cella C, Peacock JE Jr, Plonk G: Pseudonecrotizing fasciitis due to dialysate and air leak in a peritoneal dialysis patient. *Am J Nephrol* 7: 241, 1987

364. Twardowski ZJ, Tully RJ, Nichols WK, Sunderrajan S: Computerized tomography in the diagnosis of subcutaneous leak sites during continuous ambulatory peritoneal dialysis. *Peritoneal Dial Bull* 4: 163, 1984

365. Schultz SG, Harmon TM, Nachtnebel KL: Computerized tomographic scanning with intraperitoneal contrast enhancement in a CAPD patient with localized edema. *Peritoneal Dial Bull* 4: 253, 1984

366. Kopecky RT, Frymoyer PA, Witanowski LS, Thomas FD: Complications of continuous ambulatory peritoneal dialysis: diagnostic value of peritoneal scintigraphy. *Am J Kidney Dis* 10: 123, 1987

367. Schleifer CR, Morfesis FA, Cupit M, Chen C, Smink RD: Management of hernias and Tenckhoff catheter complications in CAPD. *Peritoneal Dial Bull* 4: 146, 1984

368. Digenis GE, Khanna R, Mathews R, Oreopoulos DG: Abdominal hernias in patients undergoing continuous ambulatory peritoneal dialysis. *Peritoneal Dial Bull* 2: 115, 1982

369. O'Connor JP, Rigby RJ, Hardie IR, Wall DR, Strong RW, Woodruff PWH, Petrie JJB: Abdominal hernias complicating continuous ambulatory peritoneal dialysis. *Am J Nephrol* 6: 271, 1986

370. Chan MK, Baillod RA, Tanner A, Raftery M, Sweny P,

Fernando ON, Moorhead JF: Abdominal hernias in patients receiving continuous ambulatory peritoneal dialysis. *Br Med J* 283: 826, 1981

371. Rubin J, Raju S, Teal N, Hellems E, Bower JD: Abdominal hernia in patients undergoing continuous ambulatory peritoneal dialysis. *Arch Intern Med* 142: 1453, 1982

372. Jorkasky, Goldfarb S: Abdominal wall hernia complicating chronic ambulatory peritoneal dialysis. *Am J Nephrol* 2: 323, 1982

373. Cooper JC, Nicholls AJ, Simms JM, Platts MM, Brown CB, Johnson AG: Genital edema in patients treated by continuous ambulatory peritoneal dialysis: an unusual presentation of inguinal hernia. *Br Med J* 286: 1923, 1983

374. Orfei R, Seybold K, Blumberg A: Genital edema in patients undergoing continuous ambulatory peritoneal dialysis. *Peritoneal Dial Bull* 4: 251, 1981

375. Johnson BF, Segasby CA, Holroyd AM, Brown CB, Cohen GL, Raftery AT: A method for demonstrating subclinical inguinal herniae in patients undergoing peritoneal dialysis: the isotope 'peritoneoscrotogram'. *Nephrol Dial Transplant* 2: 254, 1987

376. Nolph KD: What are the contra-indications for CAPD if any? *Peritoneal Dial Bull* 2: 182, 1982

377. Goodman CE, Husserl FE: Etiology, prevention and treatment of back pain in patients undergoing continuous ambulatory peritoneal dialysis. *Peritoneal Dial Bull* 1: 119, 1981.

378. Hamodraka-Mailis A: Pathogenesis and treatment of back pain in peritoneal dialysis patients. *Peritoneal Dial Bull* 3 (Suppl): S41, 1983

379. Canaud B, Mimran A, Liendo-Liendo C, Slingeneyer A, Mion C: Blood pressure control in patients treated by continuous ambulatory peritoneal dialysis. in: *Continuous Ambulatory Peritoneal Dialysis,* edited by Legrain M, Amsterdam, Excerpta Medica, 1980, p 212

380. Khanna R, Oreopoulos DG, Dombros N, Vas S, Williams P, Meema HE, Husdan H, Ogilvie R, Zellerman G, Roncari DAK, Clayton S, Izatt S: Continuous ambulatory peritoneal dialysis after three years: still a promising treatment. *Perit Dial Bull* 1: 24, 1981

381. Leenen FHH, Shah P, Boer WK, Khanna R, Oreopoulos DG: Hypotension on CAPD: an approach to treatment. *Peritoneal Dial Bull* 3 (Suppl): S33, 1983

382. Brown PM, Johnston KW, Fenton SS, Cattran DC: Symptomatic exacerbation of peripheral vascular disease with chronic ambulatory peritoneal dialysis. *Clin Nephrol* 16: 258, 1981

383. Shilling H, Wu G, Pettit J, Harrisson J, McNeil K, Siccion Z, Oreopoulos DG: Nutritional status of patients on long term CAPD. *Peritoneal Dial Bull* 5: 12, 1985

384. Guarnieri G, Toigo G, Situlin R, Faccini L, Coli U, Landini S, Bazzato G, Dardi F, Campanacci L: Muscle biopsy studies in chronically uremic patients: evidence for malnutrition. *Kidney Int* 24 (Suppl 16): S 187, 1983

385. Panzetta G, Guerra U, D'Angelo A, Sandrini S, Terzi A, Oldrizzi L, Maiorca R: Body composition and nutritional status in patients on continuous ambulatory peritoneal dialysis. *Clin Nephrol* 23: 18, 1985

386. Marckmann P: Nutritional status of patients on hemodialysis and peritoneal dialysis. *Clin Nephrol* 29: 75, 1988

387. Young GA, Hobson SM, Young SM, Young JP, Hildreth B, Gibson J, Coltman SJ, Brownjohn AM, Parsons FM: Adverse effects of hypertonic dialysis fluid during CAPD (letter). *Lancet* 2: 1421, 1983

388. Bouma SF, Dwyer JT: Glucose absorption and weight chang-

584   *Charles Mion*

es in 18 months of continuous ambulatory peritoneal dialysis. *J Am Diet Assoc* 84: 194, 1984

389. Rodriguez HJ, Walls J, Slatopolsky E, Klahr S: Recurrent ascitis following peritoneal dialysis. *Arch Intern Med* 134: 283, 1974

390. Slingeneyer A, Mion C, Mourad G, Canaud B, Faller B, Béraud JJ: Progressive sclerosing peritonitis: a late and severe complication of maintenance peritoneal dialysis. *Trans Am Soc Artif Intern Organs* 29: 633, 1983

391. Dutton S: Ascites in the CAPD patient post-transplant. *Peritoneal Dial Bull* 4 (Suppl): S146, 1984

392. Stefanidis CJ, Balfe JW, Arbus GS, Hardy BE, Churchill BM, Rance CP: Renal transplantation in children treated with continuous ambulatory peritoneal dialysis. *Peritoneal Dial Bull* 5: 5, 1985

393. Watson AR, Vigneux A, Balfe JW: Renal transplantation in children on CAPD and post transplant ascites. *Peritoneal Dial Bull* 4: 189, 1984

394. Gomez Campdera FJ, Lopez Gomez JM, Luque de Pabos A: Is post-transplant ascites a sign of rejection? *Peritoneal Dial Bull* 4: 107, 1984

395. Sorkin MI, Nolph KD, Anderson HO, Morris JS, Kennedy J, Prowant B, Moore H: Aluminum mass transfer during continuous ambulatory peritoneal dialysis. *Peritoneal Dial Bull* 1: 91, 1981

396. Thomson NM, Stevens BJ, Humphery TJ, Atkins RC: Comparison of trace elements in peritoneal dialysis, hemodialysis, and uremia. *Kidney Int* 23: 9, 1983

397. Gokal R, Ramos JM, Ellis HA, Parkinson I, Sweetman V, Dewar J, Ward MK, Kerr DNS: Histological renal osteodystrophy, 25-hydroxycholecalciferol and aluminum levels in patients on CAPD. *Kidney Int* 23: 15, 1983

398. Rottembourg J, Gallego JL, Jaudon MC, Clavel JP, Legrain M: Serum concentration and peritoneal transfer of aluminum during treatment by continuous ambulatory peritoneal dialysis. *Kidney Int* 25: 919, 1984

399. Mion C: Aluminium in continuous ambulatory peritoneal dialysis and post dilutional hemofiltration. *Clin Nephrol* 24 (Suppl 1): 588, 1985

400. Williams P, Khanna R, Crapper MacLaghlan DR: Enhancement of aluminum removal in a patient on CAPD with dementia. *Peritoneal Dial Bull* 1: 73, 1981

401. Bertholf RL, Roman JM, Brown S, Savory J, Wills MR: Aluminum hydroxide-induced osteomalacia, encephalopathy and hyperaluminemia in CAPD. Treatment with desferrioxamine. *Peritoneal Dial Bull* 4: 30, 1984

402. Kingswood C, Banks RA, Bunker T, Harrison P, Mackenzie C: Fracture osteomalacia, CAPD, and aluminium. *Lancet* 1: 70, 1983

403. Mactier RA, Nolph KD, Khanna R, Twardowski Z: Risk factors for hyperaluminemia in continuous ambulatory peritoneal dialysis. *Peritoneal Dial Bull* 6: 188, 1986

404. Marmion BP, Tonkin CP: Control of hepatitis in dialysis units. *Br Med Bull* 28: 169, 1972

405. Oreopoulos DG: Hepatitis and treatment of chronic renal failure by peritoneal dialysis (letter). *Lancet* 2: 1255, 1972

406. Spector D: Hepatitis B mini epidemic in a peritoneal dialysis unit. *Arch Intern Med* 137: 1030, 1977

407. Goodman W, Gallagher N, Sherrard DJ: Peritoneal dialysis fluid as a source of hepatitis antigen. *Nephron* 29: 107, 1981

408. Vas SI, Oreopoulos DG: Handle with care: hepatitis B antigen carriers in peritoneal dialysis units. *Nephron* 29: 105, 1981

409. Oren A, Husdan H, Cheng PT, Khanna R, Pierratos A, Digenis G, Oreopoulos DG: Calcium oxalate kidney stones in patients on continuous ambulatory peritoneal dialysis. *Kidney Int* 25: 534, 1984

410. Yamauchi A, Fujii M, Shirai D, Mikami H, Okada A, Imai E, Ando A, Orita Y, Kamada T: Plasma concentration and peritoneal clearance of oxalate in patients on continuous ambulatory peritoneal dialysis. *Clin Nephrol* 25: 181, 1986

411. Gilchrest B, Rowe JW, Mihm MC Jr: Bullous dermatosis of hemodialysis. *Ann Intern Med* 83: 480, 1985

412. Zeier M, Doss M, Ziegler T, Ritz E, Rambausek M: Pseudoporphyria cutanea tarda and non-A non-B hepatitis in a CAPD patient. *Peritoneal Dial Bull* 7: 231, 1987

413. Modi KB, Henderson IS: Nonbacterial thrombotic endocarditis in a CAPD patient. *Nephron* 46: 392, 1987

414. Nolph KD: Peritoneal dialysis. in: *The Kidney,* edited by Brenner BM, Rector FC, third edition, Philadelphia, WB Saunders Co, 1986 p 1847

415. Mion CM, Béraud JJ: Treatment of acute renal failure by peritoneal dialysis. in: *Acute Renal Failure, Pathophysiology, Prevention and Treatment,* edited by Andreucci V, Boston, The Hague, Dordrecht, Lancaster, Martinus Nijhoff, 1984, p 463

416. Scribner BH: Substitution of bicarbonate for acetate in the dialysate for care of a critically ill patient. *Dial Transplant* 6: 26, 1977

417. Leunissen KML, Hoorntje SJ, Fiers HA, Dekkers WT, Mulder AW: Acetate versus bicarbonate hemodialysis in critically ill patients. *Nephron* 42: 146, 1986

418. Golper TA: Continuous arteriovenous hemofiltration in acute renal failure. *Am J Kidney Dis* 6: 373, 1985

419. Bosch JP: Continuous arteriovenous hemofiltration. in: *CAVH, Proceedings of the International Symposium on Continuous Arteriovenous Hemofiltration,* edited by La Greca G, Fabris A, Ronco C, Milano, Wichtig, 1986, p 9

420. Canaud B, Béraud JJ, Mion C: Pump assisted continuous veno-venous hemofiltration (PA-CVVH): a more flexible mode of acute uremia treatment in severely ill patients. in: *CAVH, Proceedings of the International Symposium on Continuous Arteriovenous Hemofiltration,* edited by La Greca G, Fabris A, Ronco C, Milano, Wichtig, 1986, p 185

421. Geronemus R, Schneider W: Continuous arteriovenous hemodialysis: a new modality for the treatment of acute renal failure. *Trans Am Soc Artif Intern Organs* 30: 423, 1984

422. Vogel GE, Kopp KF: Minimal dose heparinization for hemodialysis patients with high bleeding risk. *Kidney Int* 8: 436, 1975

423. Casati S, Ponticelli C: Hemodialysis in patients with a risk of bleeding. *N Engl J Med* 305: 521, 1981

424. Schrader J, Stibbe W, Armstrong VW, Kant M, Muche R, Köstering H, Seidel D, Scheler F: Comparison of low molecular weight heparin to standard heparin in hemodialysis/hemofiltration. *Kidney Int* 33: 890, 1988

425. Pinnich RV, Weighmann TB, Diederich DO: Regional citrate anticoagulation for hemodialysis in the patient at high risk of bleeding. *N Engl J Med* 304: 934, 1981

426. Gillum DM, Dixon BS, Yanover MJ, Kelleher SP, Shapiro MD, Benedetti RG, Dillingham MA, Paller MS, Goldberg JP, Tomford RC, Gordon JA, Conger JD: The role of intensive dialysis in acute renal failure. *Clin Nephrol* 25: 249, 1986

427. Lameire N, Matthys E, Vanholder R, De Keyser K, Pauwels W, Nachtergaele H, Lambrecht L, Ringoir S: Causes and prognosis of acute renal failure in elderly patients. *Nephrol Dial Transplant* 2: 316, 1987

428. Bullock ML, Umen AJ, Finkelstein M, Keane WF: The as-

sessment of risk factors in 462 patients with acute renal failure. *Am J Kidney Dis* 5: 97, 1985

429. Cameron JS, Ogg C, Trounce JR: Peritoneal dialysis in hypercatabolic acute renal failure. *Lancet* 1: 1188, 1967

430. Katirtzoglou A, Kontesis P, Myopoulou-Symvoulidis D, Digenis GE, Symvoulidis A, Komminos Z: Continuous equilibration peritoneal dialysis in hypercatabolic renal failure. *Peritoneal Dial Bull* 3: 178, 1983

431. Trevino-Becerra A, Munoz P, Avilez C, Maimone MAS, Lopez MLE: Equilibrium peritoneal dialysis in acute renal failure secondary to rhabdomyolysis. *Peritoneal Dial Bull* 7: 244, 1987

432. Abel RM, Buckley MJ, Austen WG, Barnett GO, Beck CH, Fischer JE: Etiology, incidence and prognosis of renal failure following cardiac operations. *J Thorac Cardiovas Surg* 71: 323, 1976

433. Gailiunas P Jr, Chawla R, Lazarus JM, Cohn L, Sanders J, Merrill JP: Acute renal failure following cardiac operations. *J Thorac Cardiovasc Surg* 79: 241, 1980

434. Kanter A, Nadler N, Vertel RM, Pollak VE: Peritoneal dialysis: indications and technique in the surgical patient. *Surg Clin North Am* 48: 47, 1968

435. Tzamaloukas AH, Garella S, Chazan JA: Peritoneal dialysis for acute renal failure after major abdominal surgery. *Arch Surg* 106: 639, 1973

436. Berne TW, Barbour BH: Acute renal failure in general surgical patients. *Arch Surg* 102: 594, 1971

437. Raja RH, Kramer MS, Rosenbaum J, Bolisay C, Krug M: Contrasting changes in solute transport and ultrafiltration with peritonitis in CAPD patients. *Trans Am Soc Artif Intern Organs* 27: 68, 1981

438. Brooks MH, Barry KG: Removal of iodinated material by peritoneal dialysis. *Nephron* 12: 10, 1973

439. Akinkugbe OO: Nephrology in the tropical setting. *Nephron* 22: 249, 1978

440. Donadio JV, Wheldon A, Kazyak L: Quinine therapy and peritoneal dialysis in acute renal failure complicating malarial haemoglobinuria. *Lancet* 1: 375, 1968

441. Indraprasit S, Charoenpan P, Suvachittanont O, Mavichak V, Kiatboonsri S, Tanomsup S: Continuous peritoneal dialysis in acute renal failure for severe falciparum malaria. *Clin Nephrol* 29: 137, 1988

442. Pappas SC: Fulminant hepatic failure and the need for artificial liver support. *Mayo Clin Proc* 63: 198, 1988

443. Trey C, Lipworth L, Davidson CS: Parameters influencing survival in the first 318 patients reported to the fulminant hepatic failure surveillance study (abstract). *Gastroenterology* 58: 306, 1970

444. Gazzard BG, Weston MJ, Murray-Lyon AM, Flax H, Record CO, Portmann B, Langley PG, Dunlop EH, Mellon PJ, Ward MB, Williams R: Charcoal hemoperfusion in the treatment of fulminant hepatic failure. *Lancet* 1: 1301, 1974

445. Denis J, Opolon P, Nusinovici V, Granger A, Darnis F: Treatment of encephalopathy during fulminant hepatic failure by haemodialysis with high permeability membrane. *Gut* 19: 787, 1978

446. Rakela J, Kurtz SB, McCarthy JT, Krom RA, Baldus WP, McGill DB, Perrault J, Milliner DS: Post dilution hemofiltration in the management of acute hepatic failure: a pilot study. *Mayo Clin Proc* 63: 113, 1988

447. Nienhuis LI, Mulmed EL, Kelley JW: Hepatic coma. *Am J Surg* 106: 980, 1963

448. Krebs R, Flynn M: Treatment of hepatic coma with exchange transfusion and peritoneal dialysis. *JAMA* 199: 430, 1967

449. Mactier RA, Dobbie JW, Khanna R: Peritoneal dialysis in fulminant hepatic failure. *Peritoneal Dial Bull* 6: 199, 1986

450. Ring-Larsen H, Clausen E, Ramek L: Peritoneal dialysis in hyponatremia due to liver failure. *Scand J Gastroenterol* 8: 33, 1972

451. Winchester JF, Gelfand MC, Knepshield JH, Schreiner GE: Dialysis and hemoperfusion of poison and drugs – update. *Trans Am Soc Artif Intern Organs* 23: 762, 1977

452. Berman LB, Vogelsang P: Removal rates for barbiturates using two types of peritoneal dialysis. *N Engl J Med* 270: 77, 1964

453. Shinaberger JH, Shear L, Clayton LE, Barry KG, Knowlton M, Goldbaum LR: Dialysis for intoxications with lipid soluble drugs: enhancement of glutethimide extraction with lipid dialysate. *Trans Am Soc Artif Intern Organs* 10: 345, 1964

454. Exaire E, Trevino-Becerra A, Monteon F: An overview of treatment with peritoneal dialysis in drug poisoning. *Contr Nephrol* 17: 39, 1979

455. Blye E, Lorch J, Cortell S: Extracorporeal therapy in the treatment of intoxication. *Am J Kidney Dis* 3: 321, 1984

456. Cujec B, Wu G, Vas S, Lawson V, Khanna R: Accidental tobramycin overdose in a CAPD patient treated by intermittent peritoneal dialysis. *Peritoneal Dial Bull* 4: 266, 1984

457. Maher JF: Influence of continuous ambulatory peritoneal dialysis on elimination of drugs. *Peritoneal Dial Bull* 7: 159, 1987

458. Shear L, Swartz C, Shinaberger JA, Barry KG: Kinetics of peritoneal fluid absorption in adult man. *N Engl J Med* 272: 123, 1965

459. Shear L, Harvey JD, Barry KG: Peritoneum sodium transport: enhancement by pharmacologic and physical agents. *J Lab Clin Med* 67: 181, 1966

460. Brown ST, Ahearn DJ, Nolph KD: Potassium removal with peritoneal dialysis. *Kidney Int* 4: 67, 1973

461. Spital A, Sterns RH: Potassium supplementation via the dialysate in continuous ambulatory peritoneal dialysis. *Am J Kidney Dis* 6: 173, 1985

462. Nolph KD, Stoltz M, Maher JF: Calcium free peritoneal dialysis. Treatment of vitamin D intoxication. *Arch Intern Med* 128: 809, 1971

463. Counts SJO, Baylink DJ, Shen F, Sherrard DJ, Hickman RO: Vitamin D intoxication in an anephric child. *Ann Intern Med* 82: 196, 1975

464. Stoltz ML, Nolph KD, Maher JF: Factors affecting calcium removal with calcium free peritoneal dialysis. *J Lab Clin Med* 78: 389, 1971

465. Barry KG, Hunter RH, Davis TE, Crosby WH: Acute uric acid nephropathy. *Arch Intern Med* 111: 452, 1963

466. Weintraub LR, Penner JA, Meyers MC: Acute uric acid nephropathy in leukemia. *Arch Intern Med* 113: 111, 1964

467. Maher JF, Rath CE, Schreiner GE: Hyperuricemia complicating leukemia. Treatment with allopurinol and dialysis. *Arch Intern Med* 123: 198, 1969

468. Knochel JP, Mason AD: Effect of alkalinization on peritoneal diffusion of uric acid. *Am J Physiol* 210: 1160, 1966

469. Lampe WT: Hypoglycemia due to acetohexamide. *Arch Intern Med* 120: 239, 1967

470. Reuler JB, Parker RA: Peritoneal dialysis in the management of hypothermia. *JAMA* 240: 2289, 1978

471. Zawada ET: Treatment of profound hypothermia with peritoneal dialysis. *Dial Transplant* 9: 255, 1980

472. O'Connor J: The treatment of profound hypothermia with peritoneal dialysis. *Peritoneal Dial Bull* 2: 171, 1982

473. Wall AJ: Peritoneal dialysis in the treatment of severe acute pancreatitis. *Med J Austr* 52: 481, 1965

474. Gliedman ML: Bolooki H, Rosen RG: Acute pancreatitis. *Cur Prob Surg* 7: 1, 1970

475. Glenn LD, Nolph KD: Treatment of acute pancreatitis with peritoneal dialysis. *Peritoneal Dial Bull* 2: 63, 1982

476. Ranson JHC: Acute pancreatitis. *Cur Prob Surg* 16: 1, 1979

477. De Jode LRJ: The management of acute pancreatitis. *Br J Clin Pract* 34: 37, 1980

478. Furman KL, Gomperts ED, Hockley J: Activity of intraperitoneal heparin during peritoneal dialysis. *Clin Nephrol* 9: 15, 1978

479. Canavese C, Salomone M, Mangiarotti G, Pacitti A, Trucco S, Scaglia C, Assone F, Lunghi F, Vercellone A: Heparin transfer across the rabbit peritoneal membrane. *Clin Nephrol* 26: 116, 1986

480. Crossley K, Kjellstrand CM: Intraperitoneal insulin for control of blood sugar in diabetic patients during peritoneal dialysis. *Br Med J* 1: 269, 1971

481. Shapiro DJ, Blumenkrantz MJ, Levin SR, Coburn JW: Absorption and action of insulin added to peritoneal dialysate in dogs. *Nephron* 23: 174, 1979

482. Flynn CT, Nanson J: Intraperitoneal insulin with CAPD: an artificial pancreas. *Trans Am Soc Artif Intern Organs* 25: 114, 1979

483. O'Brien AAJ, McParland C, Keogh JAB: The use of intravenous and intraperitoneal desferrioxamine in aluminium osteomalacia. *Nephrol Dial Transplant* 2: 117, 1987

484. Taber T, Hegeman T, York S, Miller R: Removal of aluminum with intraperitoneal deferoxamine. *Peritoneal Dial Bull* 6: 213, 1986

485. Stanbaugh GH, Holmes AW, Gillit D, Reichel GW, Stranz M: Iron chelation therapy in CAPD: a new and effective treatment of iron overload disease in ESRD patients. *Peritoneal Dial Bull* 3: 99, 1983

486. Bonner C, Lukowski K: Angiotensin I in peritoneal dialysis fluid improved hypotension: a case report. *Clin Nephrol* 27: 99, 1987

487. Schrader J, Tönnis HJ, Scheler F: Long-term intraperitoneal application of low molecular weight heparin in a continuous ambulatory peritoneal dialysis patient with deep vein thrombosis. *Nephron* 42: 83, 1986

488. Howell SB, Pfeifle CL, Wung WE, Olshen RA, Lucas WE, Yon JL, Green M: Intraperitoneal cisplatin with systemic thiosulfate protection. *Ann Intern Med* 97: 845, 1982

489. Knapp RC, St John E, Bast RC Jr: A review of intraperitoneal therapy of human ovarian carcinoma. *Peritoneal Dial Bull* 3: 59, 1983

490. Giordano C, De Santo NG, Capodicasa G, Di Iorio B, De Simone V, Capasso G, Arico C, Castellino P, Nuzzi F, Trasente I, Alinei P: CAPD in acute renal failure. The usability of the peritoneal cavity as a simplified gut for total parenteral nutrition. in: *Acute Renal Failure,* edited by Eliahou HE, London, John Libbey, 1982, p 186

491. De Alvaro F, Jimeno A, Perez-Diaz V, Largo E, Ibanes E, Mertin del Rio R, Latorre A, Anllo F, Ortiz O: Parenteral nutrition via the peritoneum with dextrose and amino acids. *Nephron* 46: 49, 1987

492. Donaldson MDC, Spurgeon P, Haycock GB, Chantler C: Peritoneal dialysis in infants. *Br Med J* 286: 759, 1983

493. Lattouf OM, Ricketts RR: Peritoneal dialysis in infants and children. *Ann Surg* 52: 66, 1986

494. Joly JB, Bouhanna A, Boigne N. Huault C, Kachaner J, Saint-Martin J, Thieffry ST: Results of 62 peritoneal dialyses in neo-nates infants and children. Applications to emergency pediatrics (Résultats de 62 dialyses péritonéales chez le nou-

veau-né, le nourrisson et l'enfant). *Arch Franc Ped* 27: 237, 1970 (in French)

495. Chan JC: Peritoneal dialysis for renal failure in childhood. Clinical aspects and electrolyte changes as observed in 20 cases. *Clin Pediatr* 17: 349, 1978

496. Ellis D, Gartner JC, Galvis AG: Acute renal failure in infants and children: diagnosis, complications and treatment. *Crit Care Med* 9: 607, 1981

497. Schurig R, Paust H, Gahl GM, Becker H, Park W: Continuous peritoneal dialysis as treatment of acute renal failure in early childhood. in: *Advances in Peritoneal Dialysis,* edited by Gahl GM, Kessel M, Nolph KD, Amsterdam, Oxford, Princeton, Excerpta Medica, 1981, p 256

498. Offner G, Brodehl J, Galaske R, Rutt T: Acute renal failure in children: prognostic features after treatment with acute dialysis. *Eur J Pediatr* 144: 482, 1986

499. Coulthard MG: An evaluation of treatment with heparin in the hemotylic-uremic syndrome successfully treated with peritoneal dialysis. *Arch Dis Child* 54: 962, 1979

500. Gianantonio CA: Hemolytic uremic syndrome. in: *Acute Renal Failure, Pathophysiology, Prevention and Treatment,* edited by Andreucci V, Boston, The Hague, Dordrecht, Lancaster, Martinus Nijhoff, p 327

501. Baxter P, Rigby ML, Jones OD, Lincoln C, Shinebourne EA: Acute renal failure following cardiopulmonary bypass in children: results of treatment. *Int J Cardiol* 7: 235, 1985

502. Alon U, Bar-Maor JA, Bar-Joseph G: Effective peritoneal dialysis in an infant with extensive resection of the small intestine. *Am J Nephrol* 8: 65, 1988

503. Baliah T, Mac Leish H, Drummond KN: Acute boric poisoning. Report of an infant successfully treated with peritoneal dialysis. *Can Med Assoc J* 101: 166, 1969

504. Grubbauer HM, Schwartz R: Peritoneal dialysis in alcohol intoxication in a child. *Arch Toxicol* 43: 317, 1980

505. Stamm SJ, Doctor J, Rose R, Isbister J, Hickman RO: Peritoneal dialysis in the treatment of cystic fibrosis with congestive heart failure. *Clin Pediatr* 5: 755, 1966

506. Pross DC, Bradford WD, Krueger RP: Reye's syndrome treated by peritoneal dialysis. *Pediatrics* 45: 845, 1970

507. Samaha FJ, Blan E, Berardinelli JL: Reye's syndrome. Clinical diagnosis and treatment with peritoneal dialysis. *Pediatrics* 53: 336, 1974

508. Nathan E: Severe hydrops foetalis treated with peritoneal dialysis and positive-pressure ventilation. *Lancet* 1: 1393, 1968

509. Collip PJ: Peritoneal dialysis for the respiratory distress syndrome. *JAMA* 203: 169, 1968

510. Boda D, Muranyi L, Veress I, Pataki L, Streitmann K, Hencz P: Peritoneal dialysis in the treatment of hyaline membrane disease of newborn premature infants. *Acta Pediatr Scand* 60: 90, 1971

511. Sallan SE, Cottom D: Peritoneal dialysis in maple syrup urine disease. *Lancet* 2: 1423, 1969

512. Russell G, Thom H, Tarlow MJ, Gomperz D: Reduction of plasma propionate by peritoneal dialysis. *Pediatrics* 53: 281, 1974

513. Hobolth N, Devantier M: Removal of indirect reacting bilirubin by albumin binding during intermittent peritoneal dialysis in the newborn. *Acta Pediatr Scand* 58: 171, 1969

514. Nash MA, Russo JC: Neonatal lactic acidosis and renal failure: The role of peritoneal dialysis. *J Pediatr* 91: 101, 1977

515. Posen G, Lam E, Rappaport A: CAPD in Canada in 1982. *Peritoneal Dial Bull* 4: 72, 1984

516. Wing AJ, Moore R, Brunner FP, Jacobs C, Kramer P, Selwood NH: The demography of CAPD in Europe. *Peritoneal*

Dial Bull 4 (Suppl): S80, 1984

517. Maher JF, Ahearn DJ, Bryan CW, Nolph KD: Prognosis of chronic renal failure. III. Survival after one peritoneal dialysis. *Nephron* 15: 8, 1975

518. Shapiro FL: Hemodialysis and alternative treatments. A look into the near future. *Nephron* 24: 2, 1979

519. Nicholls AJ, Waldek S, Platts MM, Moorhead PJ, Brown CB: Impact of continuous ambulatory peritoneal dialysis on treatment of renal failure in patients aged over 60. *Br Med J* 288: 18, 1984

520. Mion CM: Integration of peritoneal dialysis in a regional end stage renal disease programme: a French experience in Languedoc-Roussillon. in: *Peritoneal Dialysis*, edited by Atkins RC, Thomson NM, Farrell PC, Edinburgh, Churchill Livingstone, 1981, p 395

521. Mion C, Slingeneyer A, Canaud B, Elie M: A review of seven years' home peritoneal dialysis. *Proc Eur Dial Transplant Assoc* 18: 91, 1981

522. Rashid HU, Azhar MA, Rahman A: Management of end stage renal disease with intermittent peritoneal dialysis. *Peritoneal Dial Bull* 6: 214, 1986

523. Blagg CR: Seattle experience with peritoneal dialysis. *Dial Transplant* 7: 790, 1978

524. Milutinovic J, Cutler RE, Hoover P, Meijsen B, Scribner BH: Measurement of residual glomerular filtration rate in the patient receiving repetitive dialysis. *Kidney Int* 8: 185, 1975

525. Ahmad S, Shen FH, Blagg CR: Intermittent peritoneal dialysis as renal replacement therapy. in: *Peritoneal Dialysis*, edited by Nolph KD, 2nd edition, Boston, Dordrecht, Lancaster, Martinus Nijhoff, 1985, p 179

526. Rottembourg J, Issad B, Gallero JL, Degoulet P, Aimé F, Gueffaf B, Legrain M: Evaluation of residual renal function in patients undergoing maintenance hemodialysis or continuous ambulatory peritoneal dialysis. *Proc Eur Dial Transplant Assoc* 19: 397, 1982

527. Blumenkrantz MJ, Shapiro DJ, Mimura N, Oreopoulos DG, Friedler RM, Levin S, Tenckhoff H, Coburn JW: Maintenance peritoneal dialysis as an alternative in the patient with diabetes mellitus and end-stage uremia. *Kidney Int* 6 (Suppl 1): S108, 1974

528. Finkelstein FO, Kliger AS, Bastl C, Yap P, Goffinet J: Chronic peritoneal dialysis in diabetic patients with end-stage renal failure. *Proc Clin Dial Transplant Forum* 5: 142, 1975

529. Quellhorst E, Schuenemann B, Mietzsch G, Jacob I: Haemo- and peritoneal dialysis treatment of patients with diabetic nephropathy – a comparative study. *Proc Eur Dial Transplant Assoc* 15: 205, 1978

530. Hood SA, Frohnert PP, Mitchell JC, Kurtz SB: Home peritoneal dialysis: dialysis therapy of choice in chronic renal failure of juvenile onset diabetes mellitus. *Dial Transplant* 9: 843, 1980

531. Mion C, Slingeneyer A, Oulès R, Branger B, Chong G, Mourad G: Home intermittent peritoneal dialysis in the treatment of end-stage diabetic nephropathy. 1982 update. in: *Prevention and Treatment of Diabetic Nephropathy*, edited by Keen H, Legrain M, Boston, MTP Press Ltd. 1983, p 263

532. Ghavanian M, Gutch CF, Kopp KF, Kolff WJ: The sad truth about diabetic nephropathy. *JAMA* 222: 1386, 1972

533. Mion C, Slingeneyer A, Canaud B, Mourad G: Optimized dialytic therapy for insulin-dependent diabetics. in: *Diabetic Renal-Retinal Syndrome, Therapy*, volume 3, edited by Friedman EA, L'Esperance FA, Orlando, Grune and Stratton, 1986, p 383

534. Whitley KY, Shapiro FL: Hemodialysis for end-stage diabetic nephropathy. in: *Diabetic Renal-Retinal Syndrome, Therapy*, volume 3, edited by Friedman EA, L'Esperance FA, Orlando, Grune and Stratton, 1986, p 349

535. Khanna R, Wu G, Prowant B, Jastrzebska J, Nolph KD, Oreopoulos DG: Continuous ambulatory peritoneal dialysis in diabetics with end-stage renal disease: a combined experience of two North American centers. in: *Diabetic Renal-Retinal Syndrome, Therapy*, volume 3, edited by Friedman EA, L'Esperance FA, Orlando, Grüne and Stratton, 1986, p 363

536. Butt KMH, Ortega-Gaytan M, Shirani K, Hong JH, Adamsons RJ, Manis T, Friedman EA: Angioaccess in uremic diabetics. in: *Diabetic Renal-Retinal Syndrome, Therapy*, volume 3, edited by Friedman EA, L'Esperance FA, Orlando, Grüne and Stratton, 1986, p 209

537. Buselmeier TJ, Najarian JS, Simmons RL, Rattazzi LC, Von Hartitzsch B, Callender CO, Goetz FC, Kjellstrand CM: A-V fistulas and the diabetic: ischemia and gangrene may result in amputation. *Trans Am Soc Artif Intern Organs* 19: 49, 1973

538. Flynn CT: The role of CAPD in the treatment of diabetic patients with renal failure. in: *Nephrology '83*, edited by D'Amico G, Colasanti G, Milan, Wichtig, 1983, p 91

539. Zimmerman SW, Johnson CA, O'Brien M: Survival of diabetic patients on continuous ambulatory peritoneal dialysis for over five years. *Peritoneal Dial Bull* 7: 26, 1987

540. Fine RN: Choosing a dialysis therapy for children with end stage renal disease. *Am J Kidney Dis* 4: 249, 1983

541. Fine RN: The adolescent with end-stage renal disease. *Am J Kidney Dis* 6: 81, 1985

542. Watson AR, Vigneux A, Hardy BE, Balfe JW: Six-year experience with CAPD catheters in children. *Peritoneal Dial Bull* 5: 119, 1985

543. Alexander SR: Pediatric CAPD update – 1983. *Peritoneal Dial Bull* (Suppl 4): S15, 1983

544. Hymes LC, Clowers B, Mitchell C, Warshaw BL: Peritoneal catheter survival in children. *Peritoneal Dial Bull* 6: 185, 1986

545. Hogg RJ, Coln D, Chang J, Arant BS Jr, Houser M: The Toronto Western Hospital catheter in a pediatric dialysis program. *Am J Kidney Dis* 3: 219, 1983

546. Stone MM, Fonkalsrud EW, Salusky IB, Takiff H, Hall T, Fine RN: Surgical management of peritoneal dialysis catheters in children: five-year experience with 1,800 patient-month follow-up. *J Pediatr Surg* 21: 1177, 1986

547. von Lilien T, Salusky IB, Yap HK, Fonkalsrud EW, Fine RN: Hernias: a frequent complication in children treated with continuous peritoneal dialysis. *Am J Kidney Dis* 10: 356, 1987

548. Salusky IB, Davidson D, Wilson M, Hall T, Jordan SC, Ettenger RB, Fine RN: CAPD/CCPD in children: update 1984. *Peritoneal Dial Bull* 4 (Suppl): S152, 1984

549. Hickman RO: Nine years experience with chronic peritoneal dialysis in childhood. *Dial Transplant* 7: 803, 1978

550. Brouhard BH, Berger M, Cunningham RJ, Petrusick T, Allen W, Lynch RE, Travis LB: Home peritoneal dialysis in children. *Trans Am Soc Artif Intern Organs* 25: 90, 1979

551. Balfe JW, Vigneux A, Willumsen J, Hardy BE: The use of CAPD in the treatment of children with end-stage renal disease. *Peritoneal Dial Bull* 1: 35, 1981

552. Hogg RJ, Roy III S, Travis L, Wenzl J, Reisch JS, Fox W, Green K: Continuous ambulatory and continuous cycling peritoneal dialysis in children. A report of the Southwest Pediatric Nephrology Study Group. *Kidney Int* 27: 558, 1985

553. Zaontz MR, Cohn RA, Moel DI, Majkowski N, Firlit CF: Continuous ambulatory peritoneal dialysis: the pediatric experience. *J Urol* 138: 353, 1987

554. Brem AS, Toscano AM: Continuous-cycling peritoneal dialysis for children: an alternative to hemodialysis treatment. *Pediatrics* 74: 254, 1984

555. Alliapoulos JC, Salusky IB, Hall T, Nelson P. Fine RN: Comparison of continuous cycling peritoneal dialysis with continuous ambulatory peritoneal dialysis in children. *J Pediatr* 105: 721, 1984

556. Hymes LC, Warshaw BL: Renal transplantation in children undergoing peritoneal dialysis. *Peritoneal Dial Bull* 6: 74, 1986

557. Leichter HE, Salusky IB, Ettenger RB, Jordan SC, Hall TL, Marik J, Fine RN: Experience with renal transplantation in children undergoing peritoneal dialysis. *Am J Kidney Dis* 8: 181, 1986

558. Kohaut EC: Growth in children with end-stage renal disease treated with continuous ambulatory peritoneal dialysis for at least one year. *Peritoneal Dial Bull* 2: 159, 1982

559. Fennell RS, Orak JK, Hudson T, Garin EH, Iravani A, Van Deusen WJ, Howard R, Pfaff WW, Walker RD, Richard GA: Growth in children with various therapies for end-stage renal disease. *Am J Dis Child* 138: 28, 1984

560. Paunier L, Salusky IB, Slatopolskly E, Kangarloo H, Kopple JD, Horst RL, Coburn JW, Fine RN: Renal osteodystrophy in children undergoing continuous ambulatory peritoneal dialysis. *Pediatr Res* 18: 742, 1984

561. Milliner DW, Malekzadeh M, Lieberman E, Coburn JW: Plasma aluminum levels in pediatric dialysis patients: comparison of hemodialysis and continuous ambulatory peritoneal dialysis. *Mayo Clin Proc* 62: 269, 1987

562. Mion M, Oulès F, Canaud B, Branger B, Granolleras C, Alsabadani B, Florence P, Chouzenoux R, Maurice F, Issautier R, Slingeneyer A, Flavier JL, Polito C, Saunier F, Marty L, Fontanier P, Emond C, Ramtoollah H, de Cornelissen F, Huchard G, Fitte H, Boudet R: Maintenance dialysis in the elderly. A review of fifteen years experience in Languedoc-Roussillon. *Proc Eur Dial Transplant Assoc* 21: 490, 1984

563. Marai A, Rathaus M, Gibor Y, Bernheim J: Chronic dialysis in the elderly: intermittent peritoneal dialysis or hemodialysis? *Peritoneal Dial Bull* 3: 183, 1983

564. Mackow RC, Argy WP: Chronic ambulatory peritoneal dialysis in the elderly. in: *Geriatric Nephrology,* edited by Michelis MF, Davis BB, Preuss HG, New York, Field, Rich and Assoc, 1986, p 135

565. Kaye M, Pajel PA, Somerville PJ: Four years' experience with continuous ambulatory peritoneal dialysis in the elderly. *Peritoneal Dial Bull* 3: 17, 1983

566. Steinberg SM, Cutler SJ, Nolph KD: A comprehensive report on the experience of patients on continuous ambulatory peritoneal dialysis for the treatment of end-stage renal disease. *Am J Kidney Dis* 4: 233, 1984

567. Nissenson AR, Gentile DC, Soderblom R, Brax C: CAPD in the elderly – Regional experience. in: *Frontiers in Peritoneal Dialysis,* edited by Maher JF, Winchester JF, New York, Field, Rich and Assoc, 1986, p 312

568. Dombros NV, Oreopoulos DG: Nutritional aspects of patients on CAPD. in: *Peritoneal Dialysis,* edited by La Greca G, Chiaramonte S, Fabris A, Feriani M, Ronco C, Milan, Wichtig, 1988, p 117

569. Schneison SJ: Continuous peritoneal irrigation in the treatment of intractable edema of cardiac origin. *Am J Med Sci* 218: 76, 1949

570. Mailloux LU, Swartz CD, Onesti G, Heider C, Ramirez O, Brest AN: Peritoneal dialysis for refractory congestive heart failure. *JAMA* 199: 873, 1967

571. Cairns KB, Porter GA, Kloster FE, Bristow JD, Griswold HE: Clinical and hemodynamic results of peritoneal dialysis for severe cardiac failure. *Am Heart J* 76: 227, 1968

572. Shapira J, Lang R, Jutrin I, Robson M, Ravid M: Peritoneal dialysis in refractory congestive heart failure. Part I: intermittent peritoneal dialysis. *Peritoneal Dial Bull* 3: 130, 1983

573. Robson M, Biro A, Knobel B, Schai G, Ravid M: Peritoneal dialysis in refractory congestive heart failure. Part II: continuous ambulatory peritoneal dialysis. *Peritoneal Dial Bull* 3: 133, 1983

574. Page D, Hierlihy PJ, Couture RA, Levine DZ: CAPD in the treatment of severe congestive heart failure (letter). *Peritoneal Dial Bull* 4: 56, 1984

575. Rubin J, Ball R: Continuous ambulatory peritoneal dialysis as treatment of severe congestive heart failure in the face of chronic renal failure. *Arch Intern Med* 146: 1533, 1986

576. Rosansky SJ, Richards FW: Use of peritoneal dialysis in the treatment of patients with renal failure and paraproteinemia. *Am J Nephrol* 5: 361, 1985

577. Cosio FG, Pence TV, Shapiro FLM, Kjellstrand CM: Severe renal failure in multiple myeloma. *Clin Nephrol* 15: 206, 1981

578. Yium J, Martinez-Maldonado M, Eknoyan G, Suki WN: Peritoneal dialysis in the treatment of renal failure in multiple myeloma. *South Med J* 64: 1403, 1971

579. Bear RA, Colme EH, Lang A, Johnson M: Treatment of acute renal failure due to myeloma kidney. *Can Med Assoc J* 123: 750, 1980

580. Russell JA, Fitzharris BM, Corringham R, Darcy DA, Powles RL: Plasma exchange versus peritoneal dialysis for removing Bence Jones proteins. *Br Med J* 2: 1397, 1978

581. Cohen DJ, Sherman WH, Osserman EF, Appel GB: Acute renal failure in patients with multiple myeloma. *Am J Med* 76: 247, 1984

582. Zucchelli P, Pasquali S, Cagnoli L, Ferrari G: Controlled plasma exchange trial in acute renal failure due to multiple myeloma. *Kidney Int* 33: 1175, 1988

583. Boyce NW, Holdsworth SR, Thomson NM, Atkins RC: 'Long-term' survival in light-chain myeloma with dialysis therapy alone. *Aust NZ J Med* 15: 676, 1984

584. Agostini L, Leon I, Rojas M: Treatment with CAPD for 54 months of a patient with end stage renal disease due to multiple myeloma (letter). *Peritoneal Dial Bull* 6: 46, 1986

585. Browning MJ, Banks RA, Harrison P, Mackenzie JC: Continuous ambulatory peritoneal dialysis in systemic amyloidosis end-stage renal disease. *J R Soc Med* 77: 189, 1984

586. Robson M, Oreopoulos DG: Dialysis in scleroderma. *Ann Intern Med* 83: 843, 1978

587. Winfield J, Khanna R, Reynolds NJ, Gordon DA, Finkelstein S, Oreopoulos DG: Management of end-stage scleroderma renal disease with continuous ambulatory peritoneal dialysis. Report of two cases. *Peritoneal Dial Bull* 2: 174, 1982

588. Copley JB, Smith BJ: Continuous ambulatory peritoneal dialysis and scleroderma. *Nephron* 40: 353, 1985

589. Brown ST, Ahearn DJ, Nolph KD: Reduced peritoneal clearances in scleroderma increased by intraperitoneal isoproterenol. *Ann Intern Med* 78: 891, 1973

590. Dichoso CC: The kidney in progressive sclerosis (scleroderma). in: *The Kidney in Systemic Disease,* edited by Suki WN, Eknoyan G, New York, Wiley, 1976, p 57

591. Vaziri ND, Lopez G, Nikakhtar B, Gordon S, Penera N: Peritoneal dialysis in renal failure associated with spinal cord injury. *J Am Paraplegia Soc* 7: 63, 1984

592. Smith B, Sica DA, Stacy W: Peritoneal dialysis in spinal cord injury. *Nephron* 44: 245, 1986

593. Chandran KG, Lane T: Peritoneal dialysis in spinal cord

injury. *Nephron* 47: 155, 1987

594. Segaert MF, Carlier B, Verbanck J: Recurrent hepatic coma in a chronic hemodialysis patient: successful treatment by CAPD. *Peritoneal Dial Bull* 4: 32, 1984

595. Twardowski ZJ: Abatement of psoriasis and repeated dialysis. *Ann Intern Med* 86: 509, 1977

596. Twardowski ZJ, Nolph KD, Rubin J, Anderson PC: Peritoneal dialysis for psoriasis: an uncontrolled study. *Ann Intern Med* 88: 399, 1978

597. Whittier FC, Evans DH, Anderson PC, Nolph KD: Peritoneal dialysis for psoriasis. Controlled study. *Ann Intern Med* 99: 165, 1983

598. Almy TP, Howell DA: Diverticular disease of the colon. *N Engl J Med* 302: 324, 1980

599. Oreopoulos DG: Continuous ambulatory peritoneal dialysis: present and future. *Semin Nephrol* 1: 11, 1988

600. Diaz-Buxo JA: The durability of the peritoneal membrane. *Peritoneal Dial Bull* 4 (Suppl): S85, 1984

601. Mion C, Slingeneyer A, Elie M, Canaud B, Mourad G, Flavier JL, Oulès R, Branger B, Florence P: Transfers from maintenance peritoneal dialysis to hemodialysis: causes and outcome. in: *Peritoneal Dialysis*, edited by La Greca G, Chiaramonte S, Fabris A, Feriani M, Ronco C, Milan, Wichtig, 1988, p 223

25

CONTINUOUS AMBULATORY PERITONEAL DIALYSIS

RAM GOKAL

INTRODUCTION

Although successful long term treatment with peritoneal dialysis was first reported by Boen et al (1), it was not until the introduction of continuous ambulatory peritoneal dialysis (CAPD) by Popovich, Moncrief and colleagues in 1976 (2), that the use of peritoneal dialysis for the management of patients in end-stage renal failure increased explosively. After about 10 years experience with this technique the role of CAPD in renal replacement programmes has now become more clearly defined whilst patient and technique survival have steadily improved (3). The exciting mush-

rooming of scientific knowledge on various aspects of peritoneal dialysis has led to a better understanding of the technique; the current state of the art portrayed in this chapter, has been a combination of painstaking efforts on the part of several innovative pioneers in the field (4).

CAPD has proved to be an effective mode of dialysis and has gained increasing acceptance as a first choice dialysis treatment for many patients. This review outlines the more recent advances in the technique of CAPD and in the understanding of its impact on pathophysiological processes and attempts to correlate these with the clinical results and use of CAPD in chronic renal failure.

THE CONCEPT OF CAPD – PHYSIOLOGICAL CONSIDERATIONS

When an aqueous solution is instilled into the peritoneal cavity, the solute composition equilibrates with that of plasma water by passive diffusion along electrochemical concentration gradients. In addition the flux of fluid across the peritoneum in response to an osmotic agent moves solutes in the absence of a concentration gradient, leading to the concept that solute transport occurs partly by convection or 'solvent drag' (5). Removal of excess fluid is a critical component of dialysis treatment that is achieved in CAPD by adding to the solution various concentrations of an osmotic agent (usually dextrose). Ultrafiltration continues until the dialysate becomes virtually isotonic, after which the rate that fluid is absorbed into the circulation exceeds that of the ultrafiltration induced by transcapillary hydrostatic pressure gradient alone. Net solute and water removal during CAPD have been shown to be reduced by dialysate absorption (6) (see Chapter 23). Through these two processes, diffusion and osmotic ultrafiltration, appropriate quantities of solute metabolites and fluid need to be removed to maintain the patient's body fluid volumes and composition within appropriate limits.

Several mathematical models have been used to describe peritoneal transport phenomena. Whatever the model, peritoneal clearance is a complex function of blood and dialysate flow rates and the mass transfer area coefficient. The Homogenous (or membrane) Theory (7, 8) utilises a two compartment model with a simple exponential decay of concentration gradient between body fluids and dialysate. Moncrief et al (9) expanded the model to include the effects of metabolite generation, protein binding and non-equilibrium distribution. To account for the convective element of solute transport the relationship between solute and membrane 'pore size' (Staverman's reflection co-efficient) was incorporated into the mathematical model. Using this model, Popovich and Moncrief theorised that a patient will maintain a steady blood urea level of about 30 mmol/l if 10 l of peritoneal dialysis fluid was allowed to equilibrate with body fluids and exchanged daily. Hence was born the CAPD technique of 4 daily exchanges of 2 l volumes to produce with ultrafiltration a total dialysate volume of 10 l over a 24 h period with 4 to 8 h dwell periods to fit into the patients daily routine. Daily dialysis without interruption was advocated.

TECHNIQUE AND SYSTEMS

CAPD entails a 'closed system' whereby fluid is initially instilled by gravity into the peritoneal cavity and drained out after a dwell period of several hours (Figure 1). The initial use of glass bottles was associated with unacceptable peritonitis rates (10), but with the introduction of plastic bags by Oreopoulos et al (11) there was a dramatic improvement. The basic CAPD system which, to this day remains unchanged, consists of the plastic bag containing 0.5 to 3 l peritoneal dialysis fluid, a transfer set and a permanent

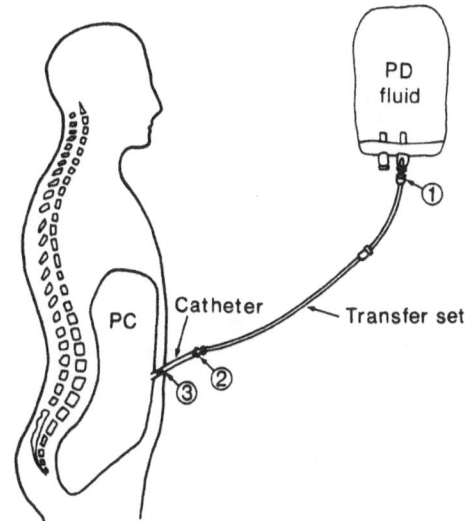

Figure 1. Diagramatic representation of the standard CAPD system: 1: The connection between plastic bag and transfer set. This is connected/disconnected 3 to 4 times dialy. 2: Attachment of transfer set to Tenckhoff catheter via a titanium adapter. 3: Exit site – point of entry of catheter into peritoneal cavity.

indwelling Silastic Tenckhoff catheter. The connection between the bag and transfer set (Figure 1, site 1) is broken 3 to 4 times a day and the procedure must be performed using a strict, sterile non-touch technique (about 1,500 exchanges/year). To prevent touch contamination various connection devices have been developed; none have eliminated peritonitis (12). The commonest devices (at site 1) have been the spike and luer lock formats. More recent innovations such as the ultraviolet Germicidal exchange system (Travenol®) the Sterile connection device (Dupont®) safelock connector (Fresenius®) or incorporation of a micropore filter in the transfer set (13) have not substantially improved peritonitis rates except in high risk groups (14, 15).

A major departure from the above technique was the development of the 'Y' connection system by Italian workers (16, 17). This entails drainage of the effluent after the connection is made with a new bag, thereby enabling any touch contamination to be 'flushed' out before new fluid is instilled into the peritoneal cavity (Figure 2). The Y piece is then filled with a sodium hypochlorite disinfectant solution. This system has dramatically reduced the peritonitis rate, but its use outside of Italy is sadly lacking. The Travenol 'O' and 'Y' and the Fresenius '5F' systems are based on the 'Y' system concept and have lowered peritonitis rates compared to standard luer lock set ups. These systems, however, do not have a disinfectant step as they are essentially disconnect systems leaving the patient free from the empty bag and transfer set.

Solutions

Several large pharmaceutical (dialysis) companies supply

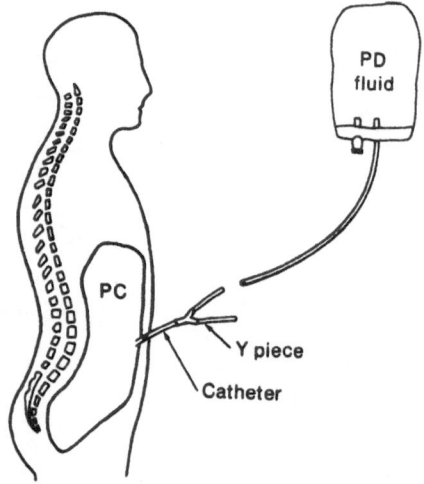

PD
fluid

PC

Y piece

Catheter

Figure 2. Diagramatic representation of the Italian 'Y' set system. The tubing from the new plastic bag is connected to one arm of the 'Y' which is normally kept filled with disinfectant. A bolus of fresh solution usually flushes this out followed by drainage of effluent through the other arm of the 'Y'. The final steps involve draining the fresh fluid into the peritoneal cavity and filling the 'Y' with a disinfectant.

peritoneal dialysis solutions, sterilised in varying volumes with different concentrations of dextrose as an osmotic agent. Table 1 gives the usual electrolyte and anhydrous dextrose concentrations (approximately 10% less than the hydrated dextrose concentrations). All the available solutions are similar in their constituent concentrations mainly differing in the lactate, sodium and potassium concentrations. The effects of these are discussed in the sections on electrolyte and mineral balance. Acetate usage as a buffer has now been discontinued because of its association with loss of ultrafiltration and sclerosing peritonitis (18, 19).

Lactate in dialysis solutions is a mixture of the D and L forms both of which appear to be readily metabolised. The use of lactate does not lower the pH of the solution but autoclaving requires a low pH to reduce dextrose caramelization. The ideal buffer for peritoneal dialysis would be sodium bicarbonate, but solutions containing mixtures of bicarbonate, calcium and glucose are difficult to prepare, sterilise and store because of the formation of insoluble calcium salts (20). This has been made possible by Italian workers (21), who produced the Vicenza bag for bicarbonate peritoneal dialysis. This consists of a double chamber bag, to accommodate the bicarbonate and acid solutions. These chambers are connected via a valve, which is opened when the bag is ready for use. The solution pH at use is 7.17 (21).

Current peritoneal dialysis solutions have considerable limitations in terms of the goals that need to be achieved. There are factors other than the bare essentials of adequate ultrafiltration and uraemic solute clearance, that are necessary. These are outlined in Table 2.

Osmotic agents

At the end of the 19th century it was demonstrated in animals that hypertonic solutions placed into the peritoneal cavity initially increased in volume whereas isotonic fluids were absorbed (22). In the 1940s it was realised that the most suitable dialysis solutions should have a chemical composition similar to that of interstital fluid and be slightly hypertonic which was achieved by adding dextrose (23). The use of dextrose as an osmotic driving force, became established and remains so to this day.

Dextrose

There are several disadvantages to dextrose (d-glucose). The rapid absorption of glucose and dilution by ultrafiltration leads to progressive diminution of the osmotic gradient,

Table 1. Chemical composition of fluids for CAPD.

Na (mmol/l)	130–135
K (mmol/l)	0– 2
Cl (mmol/l)	96–102
Mg (mmol/l)	0.5–0.75
Ca (mmol/l)	1.5–2.0 (usually 1.75)
Lactate (mmol/l)	35–40 (usually 35)
Dextrose (g/dl)*	1.36/2.27/3.86
Osmolality (mOsm/kg)**	346/396/485
pH	5.0–5.5
Volumes (ml)	500–3000

* Anhydrous dextrose concentration.

** Each osmolal value corresponds to equivalent dextrose concentration.

Table 2. Characteristics of an 'ideal' peritoneal dialysis solution.

Physiological considerations
1. Sustained, predictable solute clearance and ultrafiltration.
2. Supply deficient solutes (e.g. Ca++, amino acids) and remove uraemic toxins at rates equal to or exceeding those achieved with haemodialysis.
3. Supply part of nutrition without promoting metabolic complications.
4. Minimal or no absorption of osmotic agent.
5. Adequate correction of acidosis.
6. Physiological pH.

Bacteriological considerations
1. Pyrogen-free, sterile.
2. Inhibit bacterial and fungal growth.
3. Does not impair host defence mechanisms.

Toxiological considerations
1. Free of particulate matter and plasticisers.
2. Free of toxic trace metals (e.g. Al, Cu, Cr).
3. Nontoxic osmotic agent.
4. No toxic breakdown product from chemicals or osmotic agent on storage.
5. Inert with regard to peritoneal membrane.

so that effective ultrafiltration lasts only 2 to 3 h. This effect is of little consequence during short dwell (3 to 60 min) intermittent peritoneal dialysis. However, in CAPD, the long dwell periods allow net fluid absorption, especially during the long overnight exchanges, necessitating the use of a higher concentration of dextrose. Furthermore, a daily absorption of 150 to 300 g of glucose from the dialysate aggravates the metabolic complications of hyperinsulinaemia, hyperlipidaemia and obesity (24). Moreover, hypertonic solutions may be detrimental to the peritoneum (25). In spite of several advantages of dextrose the search for an alternative osmotic agent capable of sustained ultrafiltration with minimal absorption has continued. The search has followed two pathways. One has been the use of low molecular weight agents (Table 3) in an attempt to minimise the metabolic side effects of glucose without altering the ultrafiltration profile. Only two such agents have had reasonable success:

Glycerol

Long term use of glycerol has been evaluated in 13 diabetic patients for a mean period of 18 months (29). Although hyperinsulinaemia does not occur the ultrafiltration rate is less than that obtained with glucose.

Amino acids

Use of amino acids has been limited with the longest experience of 4 weeks in six patients (30). Major disadvantages (Table 3) seem to have been overcome by Bergström (unpublished observations) by combining their use with dextrose. The major advantage is an increase in total body nitrogen.

High molecular weight solutes

A variety of large solutes have been studied to try and minimise the metabolic side effects of absorbed small solutes and to achieve sustained ultrafiltration. None have been found to be suitable osmotic agents for peritoneal dialysis. These agents need to be dissolved in higher percentage mass concentrations to obtain the same osmolality as achieved by low molecular weight agents (31), thus making them hyperviscous, non-physiological, allergenic and toxic to the peritoneum.

In biological systems, where transport requirements similar to those of CAPD exist across many permeable membranes, the osmotic effectiveness of albumin (68,000 daltons) is well recognised. The capillary wall is freely permeable to plasma crystalloids but restricts passage of albumin, which exerts a weak but effective 'colloid' osmotic pressure even though its molar concentration (0.66 mmol/l) represents a fraction of total plasma solutes (295 mmol/l). It also is negatively charged at physiological pH and, therefore, influences the distribution of diffusible ions by the Donnan effect resulting in colloidal osmotic pressure much greater than that predicted by its molar concentration. Human albumin would thus be an ideal osmotic agent (31), but the high cost limits its clinical use.

Glucose polymer

Is it necessary to have a very high molar concentration for an osmolality gradient to induce ultrafiltration? Recently Mistry et al (34) using glucose polymers suggested that this is not necessary. A 16,000 dalton preparation containing dextrins on chain length in excess of 12 glucose units induced sustained ultrafiltration in spite of the solution being isosmotic to plasma. The phenomenon resembles the 'colloid' osmosis concept based on the permeable nature of the membrane, the large size of the polymer with an appropriately high reflection coefficient. A problem with glucose polymers is the 7.9 fold increase of maltose levels already present in uraemic serum (35). Long term studies are needed to evaluate this product fully.

Table 3. Osmotic agents studied in CAPD patients.

Agent (Daltons)	Side effects	Ref.
Low molecular weight agents		
Fructose (182)	Hypertriglyceridaemia	(26)
Sorbitol (182)	Hyperosmolality and retention	(27)
Xylitol (152)	Lactic acidosis	(28)
Glycerol (92)	Short UF, retention of glycerol	(29)
Amino Acids (100–200)	Expensive, optimal formula and use unknown. Increased N_2 load, sterilisation	
High molecular weight agents		
Dextrans (60,000–250,000)	Intraperitoneal bleeding, retention	(32)
Polyanions (40,000–90,000)	Cardiovascular instability	(33)
Gelatin (20,000–35,000)	Prolonged half-life, immunogenecity	(31)
Glucose polymer (250–250,000)	Retention of maltose	(34)

CLINICAL RESULTS

Some of the relative advantages and disadvantages of CAPD as compared to haemodialysis are listed in Table 4 and discussed below. Because CAPD is a continuous therapy, it provides stable blood concentrations of electrolytes and nitrogenous waste products. The actual blood levels achieved depend on the residual kidney function, the daily dialysate volume and the rate of production of the waste products which reflects in part dietary intake. In addition the signs and symptoms associated with high efficiency intermittent procedures such as haemodialysis are infrequent in CAPD patients.

Electrolyte and fluid balance

Sodium and water balance

Relatively large amounts of sodium and water can be removed with the use of hypertonic dextrose dialysis fluid. Rapid ultrafiltration causes movement of relatively sodium free water from blood to the peritoneum. However, the resulting hypernatraemia is short lived as the prolonged dwell time allows near equilibrium of sodium (36). If 2 l of ultrafiltrate are produced daily a considerable negative sodium balance would arise; in practice a removal of 140 to 175 mmol sodium/day occurs (37).

Ultrafiltration is brought about by crystalloid or colloid osmotic agents. With anhydrous dextrose this occurs over the first 2 to 4 h with standard 1.36 g/dl (76 mmol/l) solutions, after which a gradual fall in intraperitoneal volume occurs because of a diminished osmotic gradient and lymphatic reabsorption.

Potassium

Most dialysis solutions contain no potassium and CAPD patients can lose up to 30 mmol/day via the dialysate. This is considerably lower than the usual daily intake of 70 to 80 mmol. In spite of this most patients have a normal serum level, which can be explained by an increased excretion of potassium in the stools (38); there appears to be enhanced large interstinal potassium excretion, which is particularly important at higher potassium intakes and is sensitive to changes in plasma concentrations (39). Insulin also promotes cellular uptake of potassium.

Acid base control

With a dialysis fluid lactate level of 35 mmol/l most patients are in a negative peritoneal bicarbonate balance and CAPD patients display a chronic mild metabolic acidosis. Teehan et al (40) showed that lactate uptake from the peritoneal dialysis fluid was efficient (70%) but was often exceeded by the bicarbonate loss and hydrogen ion generation. This negative buffer balance could be corrected by an increase in dialysis fluid lactate to 40 mmol/l, which raises the serum bicarbonate level from 24 to 27 mmol/l (41). Alternatively the use of bicarbonate containing solutions corrects the acidosis completely (21) and also minimises the lactate related derangements of the Krebs cycle (increased malate) (42).

Anaemia

The increase in well being of patients after starting CAPD is probably in part due to the rise in haematocrit which occurs within a few months of initiating treatment (43), although the response can vary considerably among patients. There is some evidence that the improvement in anaemia may not be wholly sustained after 2 years and that levels beyond this time may not differ from predialysis values or from those in patients on haemodialysis (44).

The mechanism of anemia of chronic renal failure includes deficiency of erythropoietin, accumulation of inhibitors of erythropoiesis and shortened red cell survival. The increase in haematocrit with CAPD is associated with a fall in plasma volume and an increase in red cell mass (43, 45). To date there have not been any serial studies of ferrokinetics in CAPD patients other than one report of a reduced red cell lifespan (46). Most show a normal (44) mixed (47) or increased (48) red cell survival after the onset of CAPD with a correlation of this parameter and red cell mass (46). In-

Table 4. Relative advantages and disadvantages of CAPD as compared to haemodialysis and intermittent peritoneal dialysis.

Advantages	*Disadvantages*
1. Well being	1. Peritonitis
2. Easier dietary management	2. Mechanical problems with catheter and connectors
3. Freedom to travel	3. Hernias
4. Steady state biochemistry; better middle molecular removal	4. Patient dislikes and 'fatigue'
5. Improved anaemia	5. Obesity and hyperlipidaemia
6. More appropriate for children elderly and diabetics; better growth in children	6. Loss of UF and clearance
7. Lower costs	7. Malnutrition
8. ? Improved bone disease	8. ? Lower long term technique success
9. Rapidity and ease of establishing home dialysis	
10. Freedom from complex machinery	
11. No vascular access	

creased red cell survival almost certainly contributes to the rise in red cell mass.

Measurements of iron utilisation and erythrocyte turn-over suggest that red cell production is also an important determinant of red cell mass in CAPD (44), with increased proliferation of bone marrow erythroid progenitor cells after starting CAPD (49). This improved erythropoiesis could relate to an increase in erythropoietin production or to removal of inhibitors of erythropoiesis by dialysis. Predialysis erythropoietin levels are normal but inappropriately low for the degree of anaemia (47, 50) without a consistent increase with duration of CAPD (45, 47, 49). Increase in erythropoietin production is, therefore, unlikely to be a cause of the rise in red cell mass.

Inhibitors of erythropoiesis have been studied by observing the effect of uraemic serum on erythroid progenator cells *in vitro*. In CAPD patients haematocrit correlated inversely with the level of inhibitors in serum (50) and directly with peritoneal clearance of 'middle molecules' (51). Whilst the removal of these inhibitors may be important, other factors must contribute to the improvement of anemia. These may be enhanced iron utilisation in CAPD and decreased blood loss noted especially in those haemodialysis patients switching to CAPD (52).

Although a few CAPD patients achieve a normal haematocrit most continue somewhat anaemic. However, the availability of human recombinant erythropoietin and its successful use in haemodialysis patients (53) is likely to change the outlook for CAPD patients. As yet, there are no reports relating to its use in patients treated by CAPD and studies of intravenous, intraperitoneal and subcutaneous administration are awaited (54).

Whereas there is an early and significant increase in haematocrit over the initial 12 months of CAPD with an increase in red cell mass, persisting improvement thereafter is multifactoral. The use of recombinant erythropoietin almost certainly will change this and bring about increased well being from normalisation of the anaemia. The consequences however, on peritoneal clearances, hypertension and blood flow will need careful study.

Renal osteodystrophy and aluminium bone disease

Renal osteodystrophy is virtually a universal complication of renal failure. It encompasses the histological lesions of osteitis fibrosa (OF) osteomalacia (OM), mixed lesions and aplasia. The pathogenetic mechanisms for OF (related to secondary hyperparathyroidism) and OM (the majority due to aluminium) are complex and reviewed in Chapters 44 and 50.

The use of CAPD in the management of end-stage renal failure affects the complex interrelationship between calcium-phosphate, parathyroid hormone (PTH), vitamin D and aluminium metabolism. Initial short term experience (less than 5 years) based on bone histomorphology, is encouraging and has enabled the development of a rational approach for the prevention and treatment of renal osteodystrophy during CAPD therapy.

Calcium, phosphorus and magnesium metabolism

There is a wide disparity in the literature concerning mineral mass transfer during peritoneal dialysis with a calcium concentration in dialysis solution of 1.75 mmol/l. Calcium balance was positive (84 to 300 mg/day) in two studies where ionised calcium levels were not measured (38, 55). Delmez et al (56) showed that the transfer of calcium depended not only on the serum ionised Ca levels but also on the ultrafiltration volume. Thus, an exchange with a 1.36% dextrose dialysis solution resulted in a 9.8 mg calcium uptake whilst use of a 3.86% solution led to a net loss of 21 mg, findings that were confirmed by others (57). Also it is not surprising that peritoneal dialysis fluid calcium concentration affects mass transfer. A negative balance resulted if the dialysis solution concentration was 1.5 mmol/l (6 mg/dl) (58) but balance was highly positive using a level of 2.0 mmol/l (8 mg/dl) (59).

Overall, calcium mass transfer is a function of the dialysis solution Ca concentration, the ionised serum Ca level and the rate of ultrafiltration. Nevertheless, serum total and ionised calcium levels rapidly become normal using a daily CAPD regime of four 2l exchanges (1.75 mmol/l calcium, 1.36% glucose) (60). The desired ionised calcium level, however, appears to be at the upper limit of normal to suppress PTH overactivity (61) and can be achieved by altering the dialysis solution calcium level and by oral calcium and vitamin D supplements.

The hyperphosphataemia of renal failure is rapidly improved by CAPD though the serum phosphate fails to normalize once on CAPD because an intake of 1.2 to 1.4 g/kg of protein which is recommended to maintain positive nitrogen balance is high in phosphate. This obligatory ingestion of 800 to 1200 mg/day (26 to 38 mmol/day) would require removal of 100 to 200 mg of phosphate by binding agents assuming a 50% gut absorption and a 250 to 350 mg/day removal in the peritoneal dialysate (56). The need to control serum phosphate levels (between 1 to 1.5 mmol/l) is crucial and can be achieved by a combination of dietary phosphate restriction (limited in view of the protein intake) calcium carbonate orally, and finally aluminium containing binders; the latter should only be used when serum phosphate levels exceed 2 mmol/l.

The appropriate concentration of magnesium in CAPD dialysis solutions has not been established. A level of 0.75 mmol/l causes hypermagnesaemia (55, 56) though no pathological consequences have been identified. Solutions with a lower concentration (0.5 mmol/l [1.0 mEq/l]) have normalised serum magnesium levels (41).

Vitamin D metabolism

Levels of 1,25-dihydroxy-vitamin D_3 (1,25 [OH]$_2D_3$) are reported to be low in CAPD patients as in others with renal failure (57, 62). However, 25-hydroxy-vitamin D_3 (25[OH]D_3) levels, which are usually normal at the start of CAPD, may decline with time to reach subnormal values (63–65) or remain stable (56, 59, 62). This discrepancy may be related to the amount of sunlight exposure in the study populations (Cassidy et al [66] have shown a seasonal variation in the level of $25[OH]D_3$), the availability of adequate amounts of parent vitamin D_2 (58) and the duration of therapy (66).

Although $25[OH]D_3$ and its binding protein are lost in the dialysate (63, 64), there is no universal agreement on a routine vitamin D supplement to replace these losses. The potential problems of hypercalcaemia and hyperphosphataemia with routine supplementation mean that therapy should be based on clinical indications such as hypocalcaemia and hyperparathryoid bone disease. The appropriate replacement form of vitamin D is $1,25\text{-}(OH)_2D_3$ or 1 hydroxyvitamin D_3. Whilst vitamin D supplementation can lead to a rise in $25(OH)D_3$ and $24,25\text{-}(OH)_2D_3$ (67), the clinical significance of these changes in CAPD is not apparent as levels of $1,25\text{-}(OH)_2D_3$ remain subnormal. Of much greater interest is the work relating to the use of intraperitoneal $1,25\text{-}(OH)_2D_3$ (59). This route raised ionised serum Ca levels, with marked suppression of PTH, greater than that from an increased dialysate Ca of 2 mmol/l (8 mg/dl). Whether this route is superior to oral calcium or oral vitamin D therapy awaits further study.

Finally, a recent report relates the *in vitro* synthesis of $1,25\text{-}(OH)_2D_3$ by peritoneal macrophages of CAPD patients (68). Although it has been postulated that this may be a source of this active vitamin D stimulated by CAPD its clinical relevance has not been proven.

Parathryoid hormone

CAPD removes substantial quantities of PTH, which circulates as inactive carboxy-terminal fragments; a peritoneal clearance of this fragment of 1.5 ml/min has been reported (56). Despite this removal, interpreting the effects of CAPD on PTH levels is extremely difficult. Calcium and phosphate control and use of vitamin D analogues vary from centre to centre as do PTH radioimmunoassay techniques which recognise different portions of the molecule.

Studies from Newcastle upon Tyne in England show a steady decline in PTH levels with time of CAPD treatment (63, 66) and this trend has been confirmed by others (69–71). Other reports show either no change (56), an increase in PTH levels (62, 72) or a variable response (57) to CAPD treatment.

The simplest way to suppress PTH secretion is by increasing the serum ionised Ca levels by raising Ca intake or vitamin D supplements or both given orally or intraperitoneally (59). Because of the shift in the set point for calcium induced suppression of PTH (61) higher than normal serum Ca levels need to be achieved to lower PTH. In paediatric patients this has been shown to be so; by using high doses of calciferol to raise serum Ca to 2.75 mmol/l (11 mg/dl), PTH and alkaline phosphatase levels declined with concomitant improvement in radiological evidence of bone disease (73).

Similar results were achieved with intraperitoneal administration of $1,25\text{-}(OH)_2D_3$ which led to a decrease in PTH, related to an increased serum ionised Ca level (59).

Aluminium

The main sources of aluminium in CAPD patients are oral ingestion (aluminium containing phosphate binders [ACPB]) and transfer from peritoneal dialysis fluid. A significant elevation of serum Al has been found in CAPD patients with concentrations steadying at 30 to 40 ug/l (1.1 to 1.5 umol/l) after about 24 months on CAPD (66, 74). A rise in red blood cell Al levels has also been reported in patients not exposed to ACPB (75). It is doubtful whether peritoneal dialysis fluid Al contributes significantly to this rise because most manufacturers can produce fluids with Al levels below 10 ug/l; whether this is still above the level at which aluminium transfers across the peritoneum is unknown.

Twice as much aluminium is removed by CAPD as by haemodialysis on a weekly basis (76). Although, only a few cases of aluminium related osteomalcia have been described in CAPD patients, this may well increase with prolonged use of ACPB. The removal of aluminium is thus important and is substantially enhanced by the use of deferoxamine given either intravenously or intraperitoneally (77). Although the serum Al level that causes significant toxicity has not been defined a concentration above 60 ug/l may be cause for concern. The deferoxamine test has not proved a reliable indicator of the tissue stores of aluminium nor of the development of osteomalacia (78).

Avoidance of ACPB by using other binders is vital in minimising the problem of aluminium intoxication.

Metastic calcification

In CAPD patients metastatic calcification in small and large vessels as well as soft tissues has been reported (66). No correlation was found with vitamin D supplements nor the calcium-phosphate product, but the modest hypermagnesaemia found in CAPD patients may play a protective role in retarding the development of arterial calcification (79).

Renal bone disease

Does the introduction of CAPD influence the expression of renal osteodystrophy and if so does it differ from that seen in haemodialysis patients? A few studies would seem to support the view that careful medical management can prevent symptomatic bone disease (63, 66, 80, 81). However, the picture is confusing (Table 5) as there are very few studies large enough and carried out for a sufficient length of time to draw any firm conclusion.

The Newcastle group have consistently maintained that after initiating CAPD a vast majority of their patients with secondary hyperparathyroidism showed histological improvement on repeat biopsy (63, 66, 82); all patients with non-aluminium related osteomalacia improved. The experiences from the Toronto group (58, 72) would make one believe that renal bone disease deteriorates with CAPD as assessed radiologically. Similar results are reported by Kurtz et al (57, 83), Bucciante et al (84), and Loschiavo et al (71). Others reported no change in the histological parameters of osteitis fibrosa (85, 86) or a variable response (87).

Why this apparent conflict in reports? I attribute it to the heterogeneity of the patients and their management. The differing management practices in the use of calcium carbonate, ACPB, vitamin D analogues and the concentration of calcium and magnesium in the dialysis fluid all play a role. The true picture may not emerge for some time and will necessitate comprehensive documentation over many years of plasma biochemistry measurements (total and ionised calcium, phosphate), PTH and vitamin D values, radiological studies and bone histology. However, it does seem that when serum PTH levels decline with time, osteitis fibrosa concomitantly improves. Suppression of PTH has not been universally reported but is unlikely unless high serum ionised Ca levels are achieved with 'normal' phosphate levels.

Recommendations for managing renal osteodystrophy

The avoidance of aluminium intoxication and the concurrent calcium phosphate and PTH control are the goals of any therapeutic regime. Restricting dietary phosphate intake may be difficult in the face of the high dietary protein requirements. Whilst the use of calcium carbonate as a phosphate binding agent may be limited by development of hypercalcaemia in a few; this could be overcome by using dialysis fluid with a Ca level of 1.25 to 1.5 mmol/l. Within these confines recommendations include (76):
1. Dietary phosphate reduced as much as possible within the 1.2 g/kg/day protein diet.
2. Serum phosphate should be controlled by diet and oral calcium carbonate, to maintain a level <1.5 mmol/l. For levels >2.0 mmol/l it may be necessary to control the phosphate first by aluminium containing phosphate binders.
3. Serum ionised calcium levels need to be maintained at the upper limit of normal by judicious use of calcium carbonate; low calcium peritoneal dialysis fluids may be needed and should be available.
4. Routine administration of vitamin D or its analogues is not necessary and should be prescribed when clinically indicated for osteitis fibrosa, osteomalacia (not aluminium related) or hypocalcaemia.
5. Monitoring of PTH and aluminium levels is mandatory and if the patient develops evidence of aluminium intoxication, deferoxamine may be administered.

Nutritional aspects of CAPD

Chronic renal failure is associated with a variety of metabolic and endocrine disturbances that contribute to protein energy malnutrition and protein wasting (89). These abnormalities are altered substantially with dialysis and sometimes for the worse. CAPD is no exception. In the first few years of CAPD several favourable effects on nutrition were reported. Patients appeared to thrive, their body weights and haemoglobin increased, control of serum biochemistry, acid base equilibrium and fluid balance was equal to or better than on haemodialysis; all suggesting an anabolic state (90). However, potentially harmful metabolic factors have also been identified. These include inferior removal of small sized nitrogenous waste products, protein losses in the dialysate, constant absorption of glucose from the dialysate and inadequate protein intake. These observations raise questions about the long term consequences of CAPD and adverse effects which may limit its more widespread use.

Table 5. Renal bone disease on CAPD.

Authors	Ref.	Type of study		Comments
Calderaro	(58)	R		RO worse, Dialysate Ca 1.5 mmol/l
Tielemans	(65)	R		RO worse
Teitelbaum	(69)		H	OM improves; OF improves (depends on PTH)
Gokal	(63)	R + H		OM and OF improve
Llach	(85)	R		No change
Digenis	(72)	R + H		RO worse, minority improve (depends on PTH)
Zuccelli	(80)	R + H		RO improves > in haemodialysis
Kurtz	(83)	R		RO worse similar to haemodialysis
Cassidy	(66)	R + H		OF, OM improve
Loschiavo	(71)		H	OM no improvement; OF slight improvement
Rahman	(82)	R + H		OM, OF improve
Delmez	(87)		H	Variable change
Shusterman	(86)		H	OM improves, OF no change
Buccianti	(84)	R + H		OF worse
Giangrande	(81)		H	OF improves
Nilsson	(88)	R + H		OF, OM improve but variable

OF   Osteitis fibrosa.
OM   Osteomalacia.
RO   Renal osteodystrophy.
R   Radiological.
H   Histological.

Carbohydrate metabolism and glucose absorption

Uraemia is associated with glucose intolerance and abnormalities reflecting impaired glucose metabolism, the predominant one being peripheral resistance to the action of insulin attributed to the postreceptor defect in insulin action (92). These alterations are of particular importance for CAPD patients in view of the glucose absorption from the dialysate.

Glucose absorption is reported to average between 100 and 200 g daily with marked variation between individuals (52 to 316 g) (24); intraindividual absorption is fairly constant. During a 6 h dwell 45 to 60 g are absorbed from a 3.86% dextrose dialysis solution and 15 to 22 g from a 1.36% solution. This accounts for about 20% of total energy intake which in reported studies averaged 37 kCal/kg (24, 90). Glucose absorption is enchanced during peritonitis (93).

The adverse effects of glucose absorption relate to hyperglycaemia, accentuated hyperinsulinaemia (94), reduced appetite (90), excessive weight gain in some patients (95) and aggravation of lipid and lipoprotein abnormalities. The hyperinsulinaemia is reflected by increased plasma C peptide levels indicating increased production of proinsulin. The continuous hyperglycaemic stress and hyperinsulinaemia may result in β cell exhaustion with diabetes mellitus (96), increased body weight and obesity. The latter appears to be related to increase in body fat (95, 96), substantiated by increase in mean fat cell size during the initial year of CAPD (90).

Metabolic effects of a single CAPD cycle: Heaton et al (94) reported that the elevated glucagon levels in uraemia decreased only slightly whilst basal lactate and alanine levels were elevated but did not change during the CAPD cycle. This may indicate that the endogenous production of lactate is increased in CAPD, perhaps due to increased glycolysis, coupled with reduced lactate utilisation by gluconeogenesis. The concentration of ketone bodies and non-esterified fatty acids were lowered throughout dialysis, indicating suppression of both lipolysis and ketogenesis.

Lipid metabolism

Patients with chronic renal failure demonstrate several signs of deranged lipid metabolism all culminating in elevated serum triglyceride but normal cholesterol levels (97). There is concommitant decreased HDL cholesterol, altered apoprotein content of lipoproteins (98) and abnormal accumulation of cholesterol in VLDL remnants, all thought to be atherogenic factors (99). The aetiological factors are varied but an important cause is thought to relate to the excessive supply of carbohydrate which in CAPD is secondary to absorption of glucose by the peritoneal route. One study has correlated mean daily peritoneal glucose absorption and total VLDL and triglycerides (90).

A hyperlipidaemic effect of CAPD has indeed been confirmed by several studies, with the hypertriglyceridaemia and lipoprotein abnormalities being accentuated within the first months of treatment (90, 100, 101). Thereafter, the results appear to differ because of large variations among patients varying energy intakes and individual fluctuations with time. The overall results can be roughly summarised to indicate that 60 to 80% of patients show hypertriglyceridaemia at some stage but especially during the early months of CAPD, that serum cholesterol levels are normal and that the changes are more marked in patients already hyperlipidaemic at the start of CAPD.

The magnitude of the changes seem to relate to the individual's reaction to the treatment. Thus, the fractional removal rate of exogenous triglycerides from the blood (K2) during intravenous fat tolerance tests varies considerably among patients with increasing K2 values in those showing a fall in triglycerides and vice versa (90).

About 20 to 30% of patients develop hypercholesterolaemia de novo during the first year of CAPD (102), including increases in VLDL cholesterol. However, increased LDL cholesterol levels have also been observed (103).

Overall the uraemic dyslipoproteinaemia remains essentially unchanged after one year of CAPD compared to the pretreatment status except in a small group of patients in whom triglyceride levels increase significantly. Lameire et al (104) have reported on long term lipoprotein abnormalities in groups of 10 patients on CAPD for greater than 6 years. They report on a tendency to hypertriglyceridaemia after the first year which persists, whilst total HDL, HDL_2 and HDL_3 cholesterols remain in the low normal range. Apolipoprotein A_1 levels increase after one year and remain normal, thereafter.

Protein and amino acid metabolism

Multiple studies have demonstrated that protein energy malnutrition and protein wasting are common complications of uraemia. CAPD influences many facets of protein metabolism.

Protein losses and serum levels
During CAPD protein losses are a major drawback of CAPD, with the average loss of 5 to 15 g/day (doubled during peritonitis) (105) with large differences among patients. Protein losses are stable during long term treatment. The major fractions found in the effluent are albumin (48 to 65%) and IgG (15%) but most proteins are lost. Protein losses depend on the molecular weight and size, peritoneal permability and plasma concentrations (106). Despite the losses, most patients maintain stable total protein and albumin levels, although in the low normal range. Serum transferrin and C_3 may even increase to normal values during the initial anabolic months of CAPD. In addition, Kaysen and Schoenfield (107) reported that plasma albumin mass, total albumin mass and the distribution of albumin are normal in CAPD and homeostasis is maintained through decreased catabolism and increased synthesis. Although plasma protein levels are commonly used as indicators of nutritional status, many factors other than dialysate loss affect these (nutritonal intake, peritonitis).

Amino acid abnormalities

Patients on CAPD exhibit plasma amino acid abnormalities that resemble those in other uraemic patients; there is a decreased sum of essential amino acids, decreased ratio between valine/glycine and tyrosine/phenylalaline and this in part reflects losses in the dialysate of 1.2 to 3.4 g/day (29% essential; 53% of total nitrogenous losses) (38). Since the size of most amino acids (about 140 daltons) is only slightly higher than that of creatinine (113 daltons) the peritoneal clearances for amino acids are 20% lower than for creatinine. However, large variations exist between different amino acids and for some, the dialysate/plasma ratios may exceed one, suggesting that active transport may play a role (108).

Muscle free amino acids are abnormal with reduced levels of tyrosine and taurine and increased levels of lysine, asparagine, aspartic acid, glutamic and citrulline (91). Taurine may be an essential amino acid in uraemia and its low levels may reflect low levels of the enzyme cysteine sulphinic acid decarboxylase possibly due to pyridoxine deficiency.

Protein and energy requirements

During the first 6 to 12 months of CAPD there appears to be nitrogen equilibrium or even positive nitrogen balance, which correlates positively with protein and total energy intakes. Whereas Lindholm and Bergström (90) found this to be linear others have shown this relationship to be curvilinear (38); nitrogen balance rose as protein intake increased up to 1.1 g/kg day, but no additonal increase in nitrogen balance was observed with further increases in dietary protein.

During long term CAPD, few patients develop overt protein malnutrition (except in severe peritonitis). But there is a gradual decrease in nutritional intake with time with decrease in nitrogen balance after 3 to 5 years of CAPD (90, 91). Protein and calorie intake decline significantly after 1 year (protein 1.2 g/kg/day to less than 1; calories 35 kCal/kg/day to below 30). This reduced intake reflects decreased appetite, abdominal distension, delayed gastric emptying and glucose absorption. Some CAPD patients show subtle indices of malnutrition and a significant proportion have a low nitrogen index (91).

Table 6. Dietary nutritional requirements in CAPD.

Energy	– 30 to 50 Kcals/kg/day (including that from glucose absorption) 30 to 35 for obese patients
Protein	– 1.2 g/kg/day
Lipids	– P:S ratio 1.5:1
Potassium	– 60 to 80 mmol/day
Magnesium	– 200 to 300 mg/day
Calcium	– 1 4 g/day (includes oral calcium supplements)
Phosphate	– 0.7 to 1.2g/day
Vitamins	– Oral supplements: C (100 to 200 mg/day)
	B_1 (10 to 40 mg/day)
	B_6 (5 to 15 mg/day)
	Folic acid (0.5 to 1.0 mg/day)

Using dialysis fluid with zero K, 0.75 mmol/l Mg, 1.75 mmol/l Ca.

Adequacy of dialysis and nutritional therapy

Adequacy of dialysis is still difficult to define and no one measure has proven acceptable. Blood urea, creatinine, albumin and haemoglobin concentrations are all influenced by nutritonal factors. Whereas there are some signs that CAPD provides adequate dialysis (improved platelet function, immunological competence and anaemia) other uraemic symptoms are not adequately controlled, increasing tiredness, insomnia, muscle weakness and anorexia, which in turn leads to inadequate nutrient intake. Single measurements of plasma urea and creatinine concentrations are far from ideal in determining adequacy of dialysis or protein intake. To overcome this, use is made of the linear and predictable relationship between urea nitrogen appearance and total nitrogen output; dietary protein can thus be estimated assuming neutral nitrogen balance (109) (urea nitrogen appearance g/24 h = urea nitrogen in dialysate and urine; 1.0 g N_2 = 6.25 g protein).

The recommended dietary and nutritional requirements in CAPD patients are shown in Table 6. Individualised dietary prescriptions are necessary and ad libitum diets should be discouraged.

Vitamins and carnitine

Several studies have looked at vitamin status in CAPD patients (110, 111). These results show that depletion of vitamin C, B_1, B_6 and folic acid may occur and that patients should receive supplements of these vitamins (Table 6). Vitamin D has been discussed earlier.

Carnitine is a quaternary amine essential for the transport of fatty acids across inner mitochondrial membranes to their oxidation sites in the mitochondria. Recent studies have reported a deficiency of carnitine in CAPD patients related to dialysate losses, deficient stores of the precursors, lysine and methionine and inadequate protein intake (112, 113). This deficiency may enhance the uraemic hypertriglyceridaemia and carnitine repletion in haemodialysis patients has been shown to ameliorate this abnormality and increase the haemoglobin level (114).

$β_2$ Microglobulin and amyloidosis

It has become evident that patients maintained on long term dialysis may develop serious joint and soft tissue problems related to a new type of amyloidosis; its clinical manifestations include carpal tunnel syndrome, destructive arthropathy and pathological fractures (115). This haemodialysis associated amyloid contains, as a major component, a new form of amyloid fibril protein that is homologous to $β_2$ microglobulin ($β_2$M) (116). The reason why amyloid fibrils are preferentially located in these tissues is not yet elucidated but the retention of $β_2$M with massively elevated serum levels is undoubtedly an important pathogenetic factor.

Levels of $β_2$M in CAPD patients are elevated to about the same extent as in hemodialysis patients (115–117). Levels of up to 30 to 40 mg/l (normal about 1.2 mg/l) have been reported. Peritoneal clearance of this protein on CAPD amounts to about 30 to 40 mg/day. This is rather low compared to about 150 mg/day filtered and metabolised by the normal kidney. With the use of glucose polymers as osmotic agents in peritoneal dialysis fluid the removal of β_2M can be enhanced twofold related to the higher ultrafiltration rate (118) but even this is not likely to prevent amyloid problems in long term CAPD patients, whose β_2M pool is large and whose levels are related to the residual renal function.

This type of amyloid complicating CAPD has been mentioned in a report on β_2M in CAPD (119) but the paucity of this complication may indicate there are few long term CAPD patients. However, a patient who has been on long term dialysis (8 years of haemodialysis followed by 2 years of CAPD) developed the amyloid related carpal tunnel syndrome in my unit. Therefore the problem, though not of the same magnitude as in long term haemodialysis population is nevertheless potentially worrisome for long term CAPD patients.

Hypertension and cardiovascular effects

The level of blood pressure is an important influence on the quality and duration of life on dialysis. Most attention has been paid to the role of sodium balance and the activity of the renin angiotensin-aldosterone system in determining blood pressure in chronic renal failure although other factors may be important (120).

During CAPD, most of the sodium movement occurs by convective transfer and with a net ultrafiltration of 1.5 to 2.0 l, sodium loss of up to 200 to 250 mmol/day can be achieved. Salt and water overload need not be a problem. In a more detailed study of 44 patients, mean exchangeable sodium was no different from normal controls or patients on haemodialysis (121) and in a smaller study total body water was found to be normal on CAPD, with reduction in the extra-cellular component (122).

As a consequence of the avoidance of sodium overload, the control of blood pressure is generally good and comparable to that achieved by haemodialysis (123, 124). In one study (121) whilst there was a significant fall in the blood pressure at 6 months, none occured thereafter. In the same report, plasma renin activity and plasma aldosterone were elevated above normal controls and related to fluid status, a finding confirmed by Zabetakis et al (125). This latter group also demonstrated elevated catecholamine and vasopressin levels which were partly causative in the elevation of renin and aldosterone. The vasopressin elevation correlated with an increased plasma osmolality whilst that of catecholamines was felt to result from a variety of factors including glucose loading. Another pathogenetic mechanism was suggested by the finding of reduced vascular sensitivity to infused angiotensin II, implying that CAPD removes putative vasopressor substances (126).

The most important factor influencing blood pressure in CAPD would appear to be the salt and fluid status. In fact postural hypotension in non-diabetic CAPD patients has been reported and related to sodium depletion (or use of low

sodium dialysate) with improvement after oral salt loading (127).

Effect of intraperitoneal fluid on cardiovascular and respiratory systems

The presence of 2.0 l of intraperitoneal fluid did not adversely affect cardiovascular haemodynamics in the supine or upright positions or the ability to cope with postural stress even though the pattern of response to tilt was abnormal (128). Similar results were reported specifically on left ventricular function in CAPD patients (129). Symptoms of peripheral vascular disease show some worsening on CAPD (130) related perhaps to decreased venous return and increased peripheral vasconstriction from elevated levels of pressor hormones (125). In addition CAPD does not seem to provoke or aggravate cardiac arrhythmias even in elderly or cardiac patients (131).

Intra-abdominal pressures have been measured by several workers; some show a correlation with exchange volume (132) while others do not (133). This relates to respiratory function, in particular the vital capacity which limits the intra-peritoneal volume. Twardowski et al (134) studied this relationship in supine, sitting and upright positions; forced vital capacity in the supine position seemed the most sensitive indicator of tolerance of large volumes of fluid. There is no doubt that pulmonary function deteriorates in those CAPD patients with inherent respiratory disorders and in these patients intraperitoneal volumes may well need to be decreased so as to minimise further embarrassment of the vital capacity (135). CAPD patients with previously normal lungs do not show major derangement of pulmonary function or significant hypoxia on serial studies; the nature of the mechanism compensating for the fluid suggests that patients with chest disease should be able to tolerate CAPD (136, 137).

Neuropathy

The aetiology of uraemic polyneuropathy is unknown but it is commonly assumed that the accumulation of uraemic toxins, particularly middle molecules, directly or indirectly damages the peripheral neurons. Because of the superior middle molecular clearance on CAPD, one would expect a low incidence of neuropathy in these patients.

There are now several reports on the occurence of neuropathy on CAPD (138–140). Most report that nerve conduction velocites do not deteriorate during long term CAPD e.g. over 3 to 5 years (138, 139). Others have found the opposite result (140). The discrepancy was thought to relate to a greater number of women in the study populations reporting a favourable outcome. Lindholm and Bergström (90) report on a controlled study comparing male haemodialysis and CAPD patients. Using the vibratory perception thresholds and nerve conduction velocities over a 30 month period there was a slight but significant deterioration in the latter in both groups; the former parameter increased markedly in CAPD patients only. Clinical signs of neuropathy worsened in haemodialysis patients but not with CAPD. They conclude that peripheral neuropathy deteriorates during both modalities but in different ways, indicating that several pathogenetic mechanisms operate. The neuropathy remains mild except in those with secondary hyperparathryoidism. Elevated PTH and protein malnutrition may be important causes of uraemic neuropathy.

Marsh et al (141) reported on central nervous system function with haemodialysis and CAPD treatments using a battery of evoked and event related brain potential measures. CAPD patients were more similar to normal than those undergoing haemodialysis in indices of attention and the efficiency of cognitive processing.

PERITONITIS

Since the introduction of CAPD, peritonitis has remained its most significant complication. The original CAPD technique utilising bottled peritoneal dialysis fluid gave unacceptably high rates but then there was a dramatic reduction with the introduction of fluid in plastic bags (11). Further development of adequate delivery systems and connectors especially designed to prevent touch contamination have further reduced the incidence of peritonitis (12). However, in spite of the experience gained by CAPD units there has been little improvement in the prevention of peritonitis, which occurs at a rate 3 to 5 times that observed in patients treated intermittently (142). Recent reports using the Italian Y system bring considerable hope that effective prevention of peritonitis will become a reality in the not too distant future (16, 17).

Several factors distinguish CAPD peritonitis from classical surgical peritonitis. The constant presence of peritoneal fluid in the peritoneal cavity modifies the host response and alters the pathogenesis of the infection. For example minor episodes of contamination in CAPD lead to peritonitis whilst in surgical cases gross contamination is needed for overt peritonitis to develop. Toxic manifestation with CAPD peritonitis are unusual and symptoms can be mild. A positive blood cultures is a rarity and the repeated drainage of peritoneal fluid offers an unique opportunity for the early detection of peritoneal inflammation – the turbidity of the effluent still remains the earliest sign for both patient and doctors of a probable infection.

Definitions and clinical diagnosis

As yet there is no clear cut definition of peritonitis in CAPD. The initial one proposed by Vas (143) entailed any two of three features: signs or symptoms, cloudy dialysate with >100 cells/mm^3, and microorganisms in the effluent. Others have, however, stressed the diagnostic value of a turbid dialysate and its microscopic examination (144).

Based on replies of the members of the Editorial Board of the Peritoneal Dialysis Bulletin (145) several definitions were formulated. These, modified by the authors own experience and review of the literature, are shown in Table 7.

One cannot stress enough the need for standardisation and uniformity of definition when comparative and scientific work is undertaken.

For practical purposes, the cloudiness of the dialysate is the earliest sign of peritoneal inflammation, which can be identified by the patient (even in the absence of abdominal signs) who is taught to report to the dialysis unit promptly.

Signs and symptoms

From a review of the literature (146) it would seem that a cloudy dialysate is present in 97 to 100% of all episodes; other symptoms at presentation are abdominal pain (80 to 95%) and nausea, vomiting or diarrohea (7 to 30%). In contrast with peritonitis, the most frequent of clinical signs is tenderness (75%) whilst a fever was present in only 20 to 35% of cases. Drainage problems occur frequently.

The cloudiness of the effluent, if related to cells, is usually visible to the patient at a cell count of >100 mm^3. On the other hand, the observation of a cloudy dialysate is not synonymous with peritoneal infection and other causes need to be excluded (Table 7) and this can only be done by performing an absolute cell count of the cloudy effluent. Normal uninfected CAPD effluents have cell counts which are rarely above 50 mm^3 (143); however, when cultured intensively these clear effluents have been shown to grow microorganism in about 7% of effluents (147). During infections, the counts range from a few hundred to over $10,000$ mm^3 with the increase in cellularity being similar whatever the bacterial organism.

The differential cell count during an episode reveals a striking change from the normal distribution and cell type seen in uninfected effluents. In bacterial peritonitis $>50\%$ of cells are neutrophils with a striking increasing in pleomorphism. The cell count differentiation is also important in identifying unusual patterns of cellularity, chiefly eosinophilia (148) or lymphocytosis. The syndrome of peritoneal eosinophilia presents with a cloudy effluent in an asymptomatic patient with persistently negative cultures. It occurs during

Table 7. Definitions related to peritonitis.

Peritonitis: greater than 100 cells/mm with $>50\%$ neutrophils, with or without the signs of peritonitis or a positive culture.

Relapse: Return of signs and symptoms of peritonitis with the same (or culture negative) organism within 15 days of stopping antibiotic therapy.

Cure: Complete resolution of signs and symptoms of peritonitis without having to resort to catheter removal.

Persistent: Peritonitis that does not improve within 5 days of appropriate antibiotic therapy and requires catheter removal for cure.

Cloudy Effluent caused by: Infectious Peritonitis
　　　　　　　　　　　　　　Blood tinged dialysate
　　　　　　　　　　　　　　Fibrin filaments
　　　　　　　　　　　　　　Intra-abdominal pathologies
　　　　　　　　　　　　　　Diarrhoea

the initial stages of CAPD and resolves spontaneously within 8 weeks. The aetiology appears to be an allergy to the constituents of the CAPD system.

Cause of peritonitis

The main pathways for infection of the peritoneal cavity are exogenous contamination (through the lumen of the catheter, across the abdominal wall) or endogenous contamination. The most common portal of entry is the lumen of the peritoneal catheter, which gets contaminated while performing a bag exchange. Contaminations during an exchange procedure (done 3 to 4 times a day) of the connection between the dialysis bag and the transfer set (Figure 1) is the most important cause of peritonitis. In the standard procedure the effluent fluid is first drained out, the transfer set connected to a new bag and fluid (plus any contamination) is drained into the peritoneal cavity; in the Y set the potential contamination is flushed out before fresh fluid is drained into the peritoneal cavity. This must undoubtedly be the major difference in the marked improvement in peritonitis with the Y system.

Whilst touch contamination is the commonest cause, infection with infected skin scales attracted to plastic surfaces by electrostatic charges may also be important (149) as is penetration of microorganisms from defects (cracks, malfunctioning clamps) in the delivery system (150).

Infection of the catheter exit site usually starts in the short sinus between the exit and the subcutaneous Dacron cuff. This coupled with tunnel infection has been estimated to give rise to 2.0 to 8.6% of peritonitis episodes (146). Endogenous contamination from the bowel is not an infrequent source of peritonitis especially in the elderly with diverticulosis coli (151). The passage of bacteria across the wall of the bowel (152) may be enhanced in acute vesical diseases such as appendicitis and diverticulitis whilst catheter erosion from pressure necrosis may also be possible (153). Finally endogenous contamination via the blood stream has been identified for some *Streptococcus viridans* infections (154) as has vaginal leak of peritoneal fluid (155) or retrograde infection via the fallopian tubes.

Microbiological aspects of CAPD peritonitis

Causative organisms

The microorganisms isolated from infected peritoneal fluid are listed in Table 8. Gram positive organisms are found in 50 to 70% of isolates. *Staphylococcus epidermidis* causes 40 to 50% of all episodes of confirmed peritonitis. This organism is found on swabs of skin and nasopharynx of most dialysis patients (143). The importance of the skin as a source of infective organisms is indicated by the fact that many of the others (e.g. *Staph aureus*, streptococci and dipheroids) are likewise skin commensals. Whilst *Staph epidermidis* infection is usually mild and cure is readily obtained with appropriate antibiotic therapy, *Staph aureus* is associated with a much more severe picture with tendency to

abscess formation and a significant risk of death (156).

Two major groups of gram negative bacteria are responsible for 15 to 20% of peritonitis: the enterobacteriacae and *Pseudomonas* species. The latter are responsible for 4 to 5% of peritonitis episodes but usually associated with severe disease, difficulty in eradication and loss of peritoneal cavity (157). Fungal peritonitis is uncommon (2 to 5%) and is generally caused by yeasts especially *Candida* species. There is a wide range of other less common and miscellaneous organisms causing peritonitis and these are detailed in several extensive reports (146, 158).

Microbiological methods

The two major steps for the identification of the causative organism are the microscopic examination of the gram stain and the innoculation of culture media with the peritoneal fluid. When peritonitis is suspected microbiological studies should be completed in the shortest possible time to identify the responsible organisms and to help in the treatment. The importance of adequate bacteriological methods is now well recognised and has led to reports of elimination of 'sterile peritonitis' (143). Figure 3 represents the standard diagnostic methods in the format of a flow chart.

A cell count indicates whether the turbidity is due to increased white cells. The gram stain though only positive in 30% of cases (159) may be of immediate value in identifying broadly the sort of organism which would aid in the choice of antibiotics. The culture technique is crucial to identifying an organism. Since the concentration of bacteria may be less than one colony forming unit per cubic millimeter (158), sensitivity can be increased by centrifugation filtration and enrichment culture of the effluent (143, 157, 159). The filtration of the dialysate is most easily done with an Addicheck system (143). In addition 10 ml of effluent is injected into aerobic and anaerobic blood culture bottles. This method yeilds the highest percentage of positive cultures (159) and this positivity is not enhanced any further by using cell lysis procedures such as 'Triton X' to release intracellular organism (160).

Table 8. Organisms causing peritonitis in CAPD.

Organism	%
Staphylococcus epidermidis	45
Staphylococcus aureus	14
Streptococci	9
Strep faecalis	4
Diphtheroids	1.5
E Coli	8.0
Enterobacter spp	1.5
Klebsiella spp	2.5
Acinetobacter spp	2.0
Pseudomonas aeroginosa	4.5
Fungi	2.0
Miscellaneous	6.0

Completed from various series.

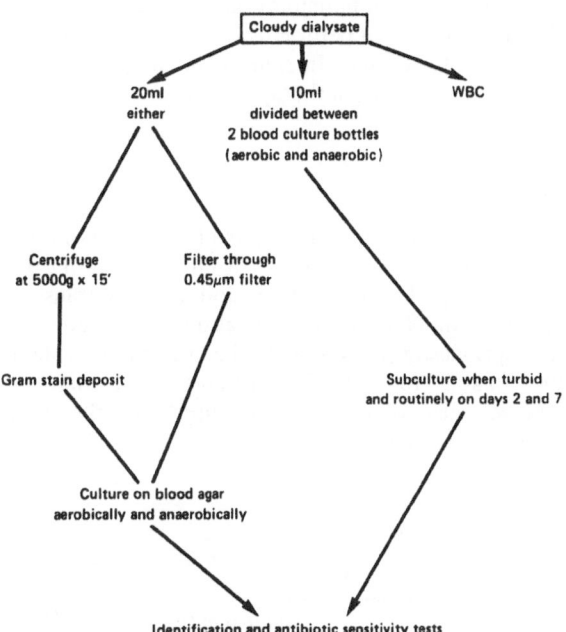

CAPD PERITONITIS
Flow chart of diagnostic procedures

Figure 3. Flow chart of diagnostic procedures for microbiological work up of a potentially infected effluent.

'Culture negative' or 'sterile' peritonitis

There is a varying incidence of culture negative peritonitis among published series ranging from 0 to 50% (146). Whilst some investigators believe that this entity does not exist but is solely the result of inadequate culture methods (143, 144) there are indeed genuine causes for sterile peritonitis as listed in Table 9. Nevertheless, in the authors opinion, culture negative peritonitis should not exceed 10% of episodes; where it does microbiological methods should be reviewed (158, 161). In the presence of a peritonitis episode that does not yield organisms with standard cultures (Figure 3), more sophisticated methods with prolonged incubation must be used.

Management of peritonitis

When peritonitis occurs in a patient on CAPD, treatment should be started immediately after completion of the appropriate microbiological workup. Many protocols for antibiotic treatment have been proposed. They differ in dose duration and route of administration. The management of CAPD peritonitis, therefore, remains empirical. However, there is an increasing consensus towards a standardised approach combining continuation of CAPD (perhaps after an initial short lavage period), intraperitoneal antibiotics and management of patient at home if possible (143, 157, 158, 161, 162). In this respect the recent reports of two working parties give excellent recommendation in manage-

ment with appropriate antibiotic doseage and the reader is referred to these for detailed knowledge (158, 161).

Peritoneal lavage

The evidence of the detrimental effects of fresh dialysis solution on local host defence mechanisms (163) has convinced most nephrologists to abandon for peritonitis treatment high flux peritoneal lavage which would also necessitate hospitalisation. CAPD is continued, after a few rapid exchanges in severe cases, although the dwell time may have to be shortened in cases of ultrafiltration difficulties (related to rapid influx of glucose into the blood stream) or drainage problems (which may be avoided by adding heparin 500 IU/l to reduce fibrin clots).

Antibiotic regime

Various combinations and modes of antibiotic administration for peritonitis have been tried (164). Most would now use the intraperitoneal route with a single broad spectrum or combination of antibiotics to give the widest possible cover against the major organisms encountered in CAPD peritonitis (Table 8).

The choice of antibiotics differs from centre to centre. The initial first line regimen should cure about 80% of episodes without catheter removal and a further 10% should respond to a change in antibiotics. The most commonly used antibiotics are vancomycin and cephalosporins (for gram positive organism) and cephalosporins and aminoglycosides (for gram negative). Their dose and routes vary; the principle of minimizing toxicity but at the same time providing a high degree of efficacy is essential. Table 10 gives some details of the commonly used antibiotics with loading and maintenance doses and approximate safe blood levels.

Table 9. Causes of 'sterile' or 'culture negative' peritonitis.

1. *True 'sterile' peritonitis*
   'Chemical' irritants
   Peritoneal irritation from dialysis fluid
     High osmolality, low pH
     Acetate buffer
     Particulate matter
     5-Hydroxymethylfurfurol
     Preservative (metabisulphate)
     Plasticisers
   Peritoneal irritation from contaminants
     Endotoxins
     Antiseptics: Chlorhexidine

2. *Undiagnosed infectious peritonitis*
   Microbiological deficiencies
     Inadequate culture media
     Short incubation time
     Small volume of unconcentrated dialysate
   Inadvertant use of antibiotics by patient prior to culture

Practical antibiotic regime

For the empirical treatment of peritonitis the two working parties have produced differing recommendations (158, 161). The UK study advocates a combination of vancomycin and an aminoglycoside, a regime that would cover most of the pathogens. As an alternative, cefuroxime or ceftazidime may be used (158). The American study (161) advocates vancomycin or a first generation cephalosporin (cefazolin) as the first line approach for a regime utilising a single agent: for a two antimicrobial regime, they advocate the combination of a first generation cephalosporin and an aminoglycoside. The potential additive oto- and vestibular toxicity of vancomycin and an aminoglycoside has not been substantiated in reports using an intermittent dosing regime (165).

The chosen regime is modified according to the pathogen and its sensitivities and the subsequent clinical response. For unresponsive *Staph* peritonitis episodes managed by vancomycin, the addition of oral rifampicin has been of benefit (161). For *Pseudomonas* infections a combination of azlocil-lin or ticarcillin with an aminoglycoside is recommended (158). Catheter removal should be prompt, within 48 h, where there has been no clinical improvement. Although the incidence of fungal peritonitis is low the morbidity and mortality are high (166). In spite of reports of successful intraperitoneal antifungal therapy, catheter removal is advocated (158).

Catheter removal

Indications for catheter removal include, catheter or tunnel infection; fungal, tuberculous, persistent and relapsing peritonitis, bowel perforation, cuff erosions and post transplant peritonitis. Catheter removal may also be indicated for repeated episodes of peritonitis. Catheter reinsertion should be undertaken 7 to 21 days later although there are reports of relatively successful immediate reinsertion at the time of catheter removal (167).

Table 10. Commonly used antibiotics in CAPD peritonitis.

Antibiotic	Loading dose mg	Maintenance mg/l	Approximate maximum safe blood level mg/l
Penicillins			
Ampicillin	1000	125	300
Ticarcillin	2000	250	300
Azlocillin	2000	250	300
Cephalsporins			
Cefuroxime	750	125	100
Cephalothin	1000	250	100
Cefotaxime	1000	250	100
Ceftazidime	1000	125	100
Cefazolin	1000	125	100
Cefoxitin	1000	100	100
Cephradine	500	125	100
Aminoglycosides			
Gentamicin	1.7 mg/kg	4–8	steady state
Tobramycin	1.7 mg/kg	4–8	4
Netilmicin	2.5 mg/kg	4–8	
Amikacin	7.5 mg/kg	25	10
Others			
Vancomycin	500	25	60–80
Aztreonam	1000	250	–
Rifampicin	600 PO	600 PO	–
Ciprofloxacin	750 PO	NK	NK
Sulphamethoxasole	1600 PO	100–200	
Trimethoprim	320 PO	20–40	
Antifungal			
Amphotericin B	–	5	NK
Miconazole	100	50	NK
Flucytosine	200	50	80
Ketoconazole	400 PO	400 PO	NK

PO Per oral.
NK Not known.
Adapted from (158, 161).

Incidence, outcome and prevention of peritonitis

Incidence

The incidence of peritonitis varies among centres and depends on the type of system utilised. The standard set up (Figure 1) is notorious for its high peritonitis rates which generally have not been lower than one episode every 20 months, in spite of innovation in connection techniques (UV devices, sterile cutting device, etc [12]). The cummulative probability of experiencing the first episode of peritonitis was 87% at 3 years in the NIH-USA CAPD Registry; the overall peritonitis rate was 1.4 episodes/patient year (168). In the United Kingdom the prospective seven centre study revealed similar peritonitis rate with only 10% remaining peritonitis free at 3 years (169). This contrasts sharply with data from the Italian studies on the Y set (Figure 2) when peritonitis rates between one episode every 33 to 50 patient months have been reported (17, 170). Interestingly, these individual Italian centre reports are not borne out by the Italian multicentre study whose overall peritonitis rate in the Y set patients was one episode/21 patient months (171), raising some doubt about the results.

Outcome

The complications of peritonitis though rare, can be serious. In the acute stage in severe episodes, pulmonary oedema, basal atelectasis and pneumonia, and protein malnutrition can occur. *Clostridium difficile* – related colitis has been reported as a sequel to treatment of peritonitis (157). In the later stages peritoneal fibrosis may develop and lead to progressive peritoneal failure and loss of ultrafiltration especially after *Staph aureus* and *Pseudomonas* infections. Hospitalisation for peritonitis amounts to 5 days/patient year of therapy (169) whilst change to other modes of therapy because of peritonitis is extremely high at around 30% of all cause of treatment change (168, 169, 171). Mortality from peritonitis is reported at 2 to 12% (146).

Prevention of peritonitis

The various factors that are directly or indirectly implicated in the pathogenesis of CAPD peritonitis are listed in Table 11. Prevention of peritonitis can therefore be approached in several ways.

Table 11. Factors implicated in pathogenesis of CAPD peritonitis.

CAPD System	Renal unit	Patient
Connectors	Training programme	Compliance
Catheters	Enthusiasm	Motivation
Lines	Adequate staff	Depression
Fluid	Training area	Age
	Back up haemodialysis	Social support
	Bacteriology	Host defence
		Mechanism

The organisation of a CAPD programme is crucial to prevent peritonitis. This demands adequate staff (1 nurse/10 to 15 CAPD patients), space for training, a clear concise patient training programme and back up facilities (172). Medical staff enthusiasm is essential; to set up a programme and hope it will 'run on autopilot' will have deleterious effects. Patient selection is important (see later) and improvements in the equipment, though improving the rates have not totally eliminated peritonitis. Recent advances in the pathogenesis throw an encouraging light. These include the work on catheter colonisation by the *Staphylococci*, protected by the extracellular slime substance they release (173); the host defence mechanism and way to enhance these by intraperitoneal IgG (174) and the probability of developing a vaccine against coagulase negative *Staphylococci* (175).

LOSS OF ULTRAFILTRATION

Peritoneal ultrafiltration (UF) is primarily an osmotically driven phenomenon currently achieved by addition of appropriate concentrations of dextrose to the fluid. When it is not possible to achieve sufficient UF to attain 'dry weight', control blood pressure and remove oedema, then clinically there is loss of UF, which may necessitate transfer to hemodialysis or intermittent peritoneal dialysis. In absolute terms loss of UF can be defined as significant dimunition of effluent volume from a 4 h hypertonic (3.86%) cycle in successive measurements over time. Loss of UF in some cases may only be apparent in that UF capacity of the membrane actually remains intact, but fluid overload results from increased oral fluid, loss of residual renal function and other causes of loss of drainage volumes (e.g. catheter malfunction).

Aetiology and pathogenesis

The structural changes which increase peritoneal permeability to glucose are unknown. Introduction of dialysis fluid into the peritoneal cavity induces structural changes which include, the development of mesothelial intracellular oedema, disruption of organelles, interstitial oedema and submesothelial deposition of collagen fibres (176, 177). In patients with loss of UF the appearances are of increased mesothelial cell separation, loss of microvilli and submesothelial oedema. Verger et al (178) correlated these changes with increased glucose transport indicating that the mesothelium may play an important role in preserving UF.

Shaldon (179) recently put forward a hypothesis to explain the development of both loss of UF and sclerosing peritonitis. He suggests that the peritoneal macrophages are in a state 'over stimulation' from exogenous factors such as peritoneal dialysis fluid, glucose metabolites, peritonitis, acetate and disinfectants. These macrophages release interleukin-1, which at the peritoneal level stimulates fibroblasts to produce more collagen and initiate fibrosis; it also induces endothelial cells to release prostacyclin which leads to a loss of ultrafiltration from a rapid loss of glucose gradient. Shaldon has further suggested that the so called sleep factor – maramyl dipeptide which enters from the colon, can also influence macrocytes and macrophages to release interleukin-1, especially in the presence of endotoxins; in a sterile pyrogen and endotoxin free environment there would be no problem.

Another factor that is important in the loss of UF is related to the lymphatic reabsorption of fluid (see Chapter 23). Various agents have been implicated in the initiation of loss of UF: acetate (180), glucose metabolites (aldelyde, 5-hydroxymethylfurfural, formic acid) (181), chlorhexidine (182) and the constant use of hypertonic solutions (25).

There are permeability changes in patients who suffer from loss of ultrafiltration and Verger (184) has delineated two patterns. Type I corresponds to a hyperpermeable membrane (assessed by the dialysate/plasma ratio of glucose and urea) which histologically shows loss of mesothelial microvilli and increased cell separation. Type II occurs when the permeability is low and is associated with multiple adhesions or sclerosing encapsulating peritonitis. Of particular importance is the observation that Type I is reversable on cessation of peritoneal dialysis, but if continued Type II changes, which are irreversible, may supervine (185). Verger (184) advocates 6 monthly permeability 'curves' in the management of CAPD patients.

Reversal of loss of ultrafiltration

Is there any cure for loss of UF? Other than discontinuing CAPD, using less hypertonic solutions and leaving the peritoneum empty overnight to allow mesothelial regeneration, there are no obvious answers and even these are empirical. However, initial reports along two lines appear promising. Lamperi and Carozzi (186) have used calcium channel antagonists to improve ultrafiltration. In some CAPD patients peritoneal macrophages and lymphocytes become hyperactiviated by a calcium dependent mechanism and secrete high amounts of lymphomonokines (1L-1 and interferon) which have a stimulating effect on fibroblast proliferation. Calcium channel antagonists block endocellular calcium leading to a reversal of these abnormalities.

The other approach has been to add phosphatidyl choline to the dialysis fluid (187). Phosphatidylcholine is a surface active material (surfactant) entrapped normally between the microvilli of the mesothelium; with dialysis this is washed away into the dialysate. In studies in rabbits, Breborowicz et al (188) also showed the effectiveness of this compound; they related its action to a decrease in the thickness of the unstirred fluid layers at the surface of the mesothelium. However, intact mesothelial cells with enough anionic sites on their surface may be necessary to bind this drug. Thus phosphotidylcholine may have little or no effect in patients with totally injured or desquamated mesothelium.

SCLEROSING PERITONITIS

Whilst episodes of peritonitis can result in scar tissue, fibrous adhesion and areas of peritoneal sclerosis, the extent to which this occurs is difficult to assess. Multiple adhesions can obliterate the peritoneal cavity (146). By contrast sclerosing peritonitis is a clinico-pathologic entity characterised by diffuse peritoneal sclerosis occurring in the context of continuing inflammation. The commonest form is the sclerosing encapsulating peritonitis (SEP), a lethal condition of which over 85 cases have been described (189).

The disease is characterised by the development of a new membrane that encases wholly or partially the small bowel such that the appearances resemble a cocoon. Histologically this neomembrane (0.2 to 4.0 mm thick) comprises laminated fibrous tissue with superimposed sclerotic layers; the mesothelium has disappeared and the deeper layers contain mononuclear cells and new vessels.

Repeated attacks of peritonitis, use of acetate and disinfectants (chlorhexidine) are important causative factors. Based on histological examinations of peritoneal biopsies, Dobbie et al (190) point to the irreversibility of damage observed after repeated episodes of peritonitis from the outpouring of fibrinous exudate secondary to changes mediated by mast cells. They have put forward the theory that excessive fibrosis associated with healing is strongly linked to massive or prolonged fibrin deposition and failure to remesothelialise. Whatever the aetiological factors or pathogenetic mechanisms (179, 190), the end result is devastating with high mortality from intestinal obstruction, anorexia and wasting (146). Upon diagnosis, which can require explorative laporotomy, CAPD must be stopped. Attempts at removing the neomembrane in the advanced stages of the disease are of no value.

PATIENT SELECTION AND QUALITY OF LIFE

Patients can be maintained in excellent condition by CAPD in the short term. Certain patients do better with this treatment than with haemodialysis and factors that need to be taken into account in selecting patients for CAPD are shown in Table 12. Patients with cardiovascular disease, diabetes mellitus, small children and the elderly, do relatively well on

Table 12. Factors influencing choice of CAPD in new patients.

Medical factors	Psychological factors
Age	Patient preference
Ischaemic heart disease	Motivation
Diabetes mellitus	Compliance
Ease of transplantation	Family support
Extensive abdominal surgery	Distance from centre
Blindness	Occupation
Severe pulmonary disease	Concern with body image
Lumbar disc problems	Travel
Extensive diverticulitis?	

CAPD. Renal transplantation has an important bearing on the choice of type of dialysis for a patient in end-stage renal failure. For those suitable, CAPD before transplantation would seem to be the most appropriate approach. Haemodialysis (in particular at home) could then be for those in whom transplantation is impossible or is going to be delayed beyond 3 years or so. In the United Kingdom where this policy pertains patients unable to perform home haemodialysis require in centre (hospital) dialysis, for which facilities are limited. This approach presupposes that availability of kidneys and transplantation results are both good, that successful transplantation is regarded as the renal replacement treatment of choice and that grafts are allocated on the basis of HLA matching (191).

What about the quality of life achieved in CAPD? Several studies have addressed this question. A multicentre report in the United States (192) involving 859 patients on renal replacement therapy (only 80 were CAPD) showed that 79% of transplant recipients were able to function at nearly normal levels, as opposed to 47.5% for CAPD and 59% for home haemodialysis patients. In-centre haemodialysis patients appeared to do least well. On three subjective measures (life satisfaction, well being and psychological effect) the transplant patient had a higher quality of life than those receiving treatment in hospital; they perceived their lives to be only slightly inferior to those of the general population. A UK study involving patients from two renal units (193) reached similar conclusions. In addition the report classified patients above and below 60 years of age, with or without risk factors (diabetes mellitus, cerebro-cardio-vascular disease, severe disability, mental illness, social isolation, unemployment, IQ, and health care compliance). The patients that did least well were males below 60 years with risk factors. On a few psychological assessment scales CAPD patients percieved life better than haemodialysis patients did. An important finding was that patients over 60, even in the presence of risk factors perceived life to be good. In a smaller comparative study of matched in-centre haemodialysis and home CAPD patients, who were medically comparable, CAPD was associated with marginally to moderately superior psychological and social adaptation (194). Centre haemodialysis patients reported a high level of personal stress from certain physical symptoms and regimen requirements and high levels of illness related stress in family members.

Employment status suffers significantly once patients start treatment. Fragola et al (195) found that only 27% of the patients were able to continue their employment, which they held prior to the start of CAPD, while the UK study (193) showed that only half those previously employed or fit to work were able to do so after treatment. In the large multicentre USA study (192) only 25% of those employed were working after starting CAPD, compared with 60% for home haemodialysis and 75% for transplant recipients. These differences to some extent reflect patient selection with a bias towards placing high risk patients onto CAPD or hospital haemodialysis. Although these patients can adapt to very adverse life circumstances and perceive good quality

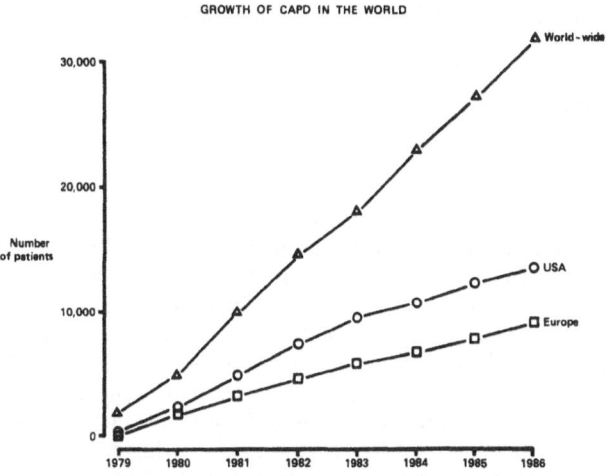

Figure 4. Growth of CAPD in the world – actual numbers on treatment up to end of 1986. (Data provided by Travenol).

of life, objective evidence of successful rehabilitation does not exist except in transplant recipients and some dialysis patients.

THE USE AND OUTCOME OF CAPD

The numbers of patients on CAPD over the last decade has shown a dramatic but steady increase throughout the world (Figure 4). At the end of 1986, there were over 32,000 patients alive on this treatment, representing about 11% of the total dialysis population. This percentage varies from country to country depending on local factors; in the UK for instance the figure of 41% is related partly to the lack of in centre haemodialysis facilities whilst in West Germany, the heavy emphasis on centre haemodialysis means only 3% are on CAPD.

Despite this growth of CAPD in the last 10 years (3) the long term outlook of patients on this modality is still uncertain (196). The earliest reports from the European Dialysis and Transplant Registry on patient survival and technique 'drop out' were such that only a quarter of the patients starting CAPD were still on it at 2 years (197). These results undoubtedly reflected a learning phase in a rapidly expanding modality. It is interesting that the early haemodialysis experience, in the late 1960s, showed very similar outcome patterns; a two year drop out of about 60% was reported (198). The problems of CAPD have therefore been compared with current haemodialysis results, telescoping its learning experience to within 5 to 10 years what haemodialysis took more than 20 years to achieve.

Recent individual centre and national registry reports are more encouraging with medium term survival (up to 5 years) being comparable to that on haemodialysis (183). Most units now have a few patients who are into their seventh, eight and even ninth year of treatment by CAPD but only a few. The longest survivor has now been on CAPD for 10 years (with an additional 3 years of intermittent peritoneal dialysis (199).)

Treatment outcomes

USA-NIH-Study

The largest data base on CAPD in the world is that of the National Institute of Health in the USA. The CAPD Registry had follow-up data on over 16,000 patients at the end of 1986 (168). The most recent data from the Registry gives probabilities of various events at yearly intervals up to 3 years (Table 13). A cumulative probability of death at 3 years of 42% is not too dissimilar from that of haemodialysis, whilst that of transfer to haemodialysis or to intermittent peritoneal dialysis of 44% may well reflect a higher percentage than haemodialysis populations shift. Peritonitis (in 29%) was the commonest cause of transfer. Other causes (medical 25%, patient abuse 14%) were important as were factors such as distance of home from centre, social circumstances and previous dialysis therapy. The cumulative probability of death increased twofold if the patients were greater than 60 years or were diabetic. Diabetic patients formed 31% of all patients taken on for CAPD in the Registry.

Best demonstrated practice

In the United States, Travenol sponsored this programme (200) with the purpose of improving CAPD retention by following carefully patient retention and causes of failure and trying to improve clinical practice by sharing the lessons from successful programmes to others that were less successful. The study incorporated 150 centres with over 7,500 patients (30% Diabetics, 38% cerebro-cardio-vascular disease at start).

The actuarial technique survival at 6 years was about 50%, the main reasons for transfer from CAPD were peritonitis (27%) other medical reasons (24%) psychological (14%) catheter related (14%) non-compliance (11%) and inadequate dialysis (<10%). The disparity between the best (80% at 3 years) and worst centres (10% at 2 years) in technique survival was striking. When the experience from the derived best demonstrated practices was then applied from the centres of excellence to these that had high drop

Table 13. NIH National CAPD Registry 1986 – cumulative probabilities (%).

Year	1	2	3
Peritonitis	60	78	87
Exit/tunnel infection	31	46	54
Catheter loss	19	33	43
Drop out	30	62	75
Transplant	10	18	23
Transfer	18	32	44
Deaths	16	30	42

Drop out – all causes of change including transplantation and death.

out rates, there was a dramatic improvement in the failure rate (29%/year reduced to 14.5%/year).

Europe – EDTA data

A report from the European Dialysis and Transplant Association (EDTA) on the contribution of CAPD to overall survival on renal replacement therapy in Europe was presented at the International Congress of Nephrology 1987 (209). Whilst CAPD had made a growing contribution, especially for the elderly and diabetics, this was not uniformly so; Nordic countries and the UK have used CAPD for a larger proportion of patients. Because of bias introduced by differing approaches to patient selection, it was difficult to make survival comparison with modalities. However, over the 2 years of follow up for patients starting therapy in 1983, CAPD use did not affect patient survival on renal replacement therapy (Table 14).

United Kingdom

The data from the UK relate predominantly to the recently reported seven centre prospective study on the outcome of new patients starting either CAPD or haemodialysis in 1983 to 1985 and followed up for up to 4 years (169). Actuarial patient survival at 4 years was 74% (haemodialysis) 62% (CAPD) whilst that for change of therapy revealed figures of 92% on haemodialysis compared to 62% on CAPD. Using Cox's multivariate analysis age >60 years, cardio-cerebro-vascular disease, diabetes mellitus and amyloid at start of CAPD were adverse risk factors for survival in

Table 14. Comparison of the contribution of CAPD in different groups of countries: proportions of patients on CAPD at start of first treatment in 1983 and at the first and second anniversaries with overall cummulative survival. Patients are aged 15 to 55 with 'standard' primary renal diseases.

Groups of countries	Patients N	Percentage of patients on CAPD			Overall survival %	
		Start	1 yr	2 yr	1 yr	2 yr
Latin	2570	6	7	6	97.6	94.6
Nordic	271	18	18	15	95.9	91.0
Britain	776	19	23	19	94.7	90.9
Austria, W. Germany	1472	2	2	2	95.6	90.1

CAPD but none of these were associated with a change of therapy to haemodialysis. In half of those who changed to haemodialysis peritonitis was the cause. Overall hospitalisation was similar for CAPD (14.8/days/patient year of therapy) and haemodialysis (12.8 days) patients. With the 10%/year drop out and frequent temporary use of haemodialysis (for periods of <2 months) a significant haemodialysis back up was necessary as was the equivalent of 8 inpatient beds for hospitalisation in a large CAPD programme of 100 patients.

Italy

The Italian CAPD Study group involving 33 centres recently reported its data on outcome over 5 years (171). The study comprised 1,364 patients. Technique survival was 56.6% at 5 years with 30% of drop out secondary to peritonitis. The annual drop out rate has shown steady improvement with a level of 7.5% in 1985.

Prevention of drop out

Overall results from the above as well as those not discussed here, now show similar outcomes with patient survival of 50 to 60% at 5 years, not too dissimilar from haemodialysis populations. Technique failure rate on CAPD may well be higher than on haemodialysis but undoubtedly reflects widely varying conditions in its deployment in individual countries. Nevertheless, technique survival of 50% at 5 years is readily achievable. Improvement in the retention rate, must, therefore, concentrate on the major reasons for drop out, peritonitis which is related to the organisation of a programme, patient factors and catheter problems.

In terms of peritonitis the exciting developments in the understanding of host defence, catheter colonisation and the possibility of a vaccine raise hopes that the retention rate will improve with time. The organisation of the CAPD programme will still remain the cornerstone of success (172); improvements in catheter design, placement and reduction in exit infection (see Chapter 24) are urgently needed. Should these come about there is no reason to doubt that CAPD will be a viable long term therapy.

COST AND COST EFFECTIVENESS

Whilst longevity and quality of life differ among the various treatment modalities, an overriding factor that governs avialability of treatment is cost. Renal replacement therapy is expensive and consumes a large proportion of any countries health budget relative to the number of patients treated. Several attempts have been made to cost the treatment accurately (201). However, the estimates vary because some items defy accurate costing (191). In 1979 in the USA Manis and Friedman (202) reported on annual costs as centre haemodialysis $27,000, home haemodialysis $17,000 first year and $9,000 subsequently. Nolph (203) in 1983 costed CAPD at $8,300 annually. In 1984 the UK Department of Health and Social Security (DHSS) costed home haemodialysis to be £9,000 annually, CAPD £8,700 and hospital haemodialysis £12,500 (204). The resources necessary to achieve an intake of 40 new patients/million of population (five of these considered high risk, 80% considered to be standard risk assumed transplantable and 70% suitable for independant home dialysis) were considered by a working party of the Renal Association in England (205). In a steady state situation the national model predicted an outlay of £3.1 million/million of population rising to £4.2 million for an intake of 60 new patients/million (1983 prices). This model took into account life expectancy, effect of transplantation, staff overheads and hospitalisation as obtained from EDTA statistics.

For a country such as the United Kingdom the estimated annual expenditures would be £252 million (steady state: 60 new patients/million) whilst for the USA this would amount to about £1.8 billion. Is this expenditure cost effective? To a nephrologist the question is not whether CAPD is more cost effective than haemodialysis but whether adequate resources are available to treat an individual. Yet funding bodies, such as governments who claim to have only a finite sum for health, may well wish to have a yardstick by which to measure the cost effectiveness of a treatment to help it in resource allocation. Economists have recently attempted this by creating measures of the quality and quantity of life to evaluate health improvements (206). Using various grades of physical mobility and freedom from pain as quality of life and combining this with life expectancy, a single unit of measure – the quality adjusted life year (QALY) i.e. gaining one year of life devoid of disability or pain) was obtained. This concept has been used to value alternative procedures on the basis of cost/QALY. Within renal replacement therapy, CAPD (£47,000 cost/QALY) was deemed more cost effective than haemodialysis (£54,000) but much less so than cadaveric renal transplantation (207). Williams (206) has ranked the various therapies in order of priority given the resources in working out a scale of extra service cost per extra QALY gained; hip replacement compared most favourably, followed by coronary artery bypass graft surgery, before transplantation and dialysis make an impact. If these data are accepted as indicating the relative order of magnitude of the cost effectiveness of treatment treatments they point to several 'best buys' if resources have to be restricted.

However, the data upon which the analysis are based (Rosser Scale [208]) are at best crude and need considerable refining. They, nevertheless, point to areas of high expenditure and ways in which future allocations may proceed.

CONCLUSION

Survival of patients on haemodialysis beyond 10 years is common place and raises no excitement. However, no patient has gone beyond this on CAPD. Is CAPD going to be a viable long term therapy? The answer lies in the long term viability of the peritoneal membrane. The future of CAPD therefore rests in research and further development in various areas.

1. Peritoneal membrane, long term clearance and ultrafiltration capacity.
2. Osmotic agents to replace glucose.
3. Peritonitis (connections, catheters, host defence).
4. Nutritional and metabolic (malnutrition and bone).
5. Patient acceptability.

Although, its long term future may be in some doubt, there is no question about the immediate and medium term viability of CAPD. Indeed in some countries, many patients have been treated by CAPD who would have previously been denied any therapy. It seems futile to compare it with other treatments; rather CAPD needs to be fully integrated into a renal replacement programme as an equal partner to haemodialysis and renal transplantation. Various integration patterns have been reported (191, 201).

CAPD has not been a panacea for end-stage renal failure patients. But CAPD does provide the nephrologist with an additional means to manage renal failure. The treatment choice needs to be tailored to meet the patients medical and social needs. CAPD has enabled many patients to live who would otherwise have died. For these the therapy has been particularly invaluable. CAPD is here to stay and one can be cautiously optimistic about its future.

ACKNOWLEDGEMENT

I am grateful to Miss K. Hulme and Mrs T. Drucker for typing the manuscript.

REFERENCES

1. Boen ST, Mulinari AS, Dillard DH, Scribner BH: Periodic peritoneal dialysis in the management of chronic uremia. *Trans Am Soc Artif Intern Organs* 8: 256, 1962
2. Popovich RP, Moncrief JW, Decherd JF, Bomar JB, Pyle WK: Definition of a novel portable wearable equilibrium dialysis technique. *Abstracts Am Soc Artif Intern Organs* 5: 64, 1976
3. Gokal R: Continuous ambulatory peritoneal dialysis (CAPD) – Ten years on. *Q J Med* 63: 465, 1987
4. Gokal R: Historical development and clinical use of continuous ambulatory peritoneal dialysis. in: *Continuous Ambulatory Peritoneal Dialysis*, edited by Gokal R, Edinburgh, Churchill Livingstone, 1986, p 1
5. Henderson LW: Peritoneal ultrafiltration dialysis: enhanced urea transfer using hypertonic peritoneal fluid. *J Clin Invest* 45: 950, 1966
6. Mactier RA, Khanna R, Twardowski ZJ, Nolph KD: Role of peritoneal cavity lymphatic absorption in peritoneal dialysis. *Kidney Int* 32: 164, 1987
7. Kallen RJ: A method for approximating the efficacy of peritoneal dialysis for uremia. *Am J Dis Child* 111: 156, 1966
8. Miller JH, Gipstein R, Maroules R, Swartz M, Rubini ME: Automated peritoneal dialysis: Analysis of several methods of peritoneal dialysis. *Trans Am Soc Artif Intern Organs* 12: 98, 1966
9. Moncrief JW, Popovich RP, Okutan M, Decherd JF: A model of the peritoneal dialysis system. *Proc 25th Annu Cong Eng Med Biol* 14: 142, 1976
10. Popovich RP, Moncrief JW, Nolph KD, Ghods AJ, Twardowski Z, Pyle WK: Continuous ambulatory peritoneal dialysis. *Ann Intern Med* 88: 449, 1978
11. Oreopoulos DG, Robinson M, Izatt S, Clayton S, de Veber GA: A simple and safe technique for continuous ambulatory peritoneal dialysis (CAPD). *Trans Am Soc Artif Intern Organs* 24: 484, 1978
12. Winchester JF: CAPD systems and solutions. in: *Continuous Ambulatory Peritoneal Dialysis*, edited by Gokal R, Edinburgh, Churchill Livingstone, 1986, p 94
13. Slingeneyer A, Mion C: Peritonitis prevention in continuous ambulatory peritoneal dialysis: Long term efficacy of a bacteriologic filter. *Proc Eur Dial Transplant Assoc* 19: 388, 1983
14. Popovich RP, Moncrief JW, Sorrels-Akar AJ, Mullins-Blackson C, Pyle K: The ultraviolet germicidal system: the elimination of distal contamination in CAPD. in: *Frontiers in Peritoneal Dialysis*, edited by Maher JF, Winchester JF, New York, Field, Rich and Assoc, 1986, p 169
15. Ogden DA: Multi-center field evaluation of the sterile connection device (SCD) in CAPD in the prevention of peritonitis. *Peritoneal Dial Bull* 4: 846, 1984
16. Buoncristiani U, Bianchi P, Cozzari M, Carobi C, Quitaliani G, Barbarassa D: A new, safe, simple connection system for CAPD. *Int J Nephrol Urol Androl* 1: 50, 1980
17. Maiorca R, Cantaluppi A, Cancarini GC, Scalamogna A, Broccoli R, Graziani G, Brasa S, Ponticelli C: Prospective controlled trial of a Y-connector and disinfectant in CAPD. *Lancet* 2: 642, 1983
18. Faller B, Marichal JF: Loss of ultrafiltration in continuous ambulatory peritoneal dialysis: A role for acetate. *Peritoneal Dial Bull* 4: 10, 1984
19. International Study Group: A survey of ultrafiltration in continuous ambulatory peritoneal dialysis: A second report on an international cooperative study. *Peritoneal Dial Bull* 4: 137, 1984
20. Ing TS, Quon MJ, Daugirdas JT: Preparation of bicarbonate containing peritoneal dialysate using an automated dialysate delivery system. *Int J Artif Organs* 4: 148, 1981
21. Feriani M, Biasioli S, Chiaramonte S, Fabris A, Ronco C, Brendolan A, Bragantini L, Dell'aquila R, Zambello A, LaGreca G: Substitution of sodium bicarbonate for sodium acetate/lactate in CAPD fluid. in: *Advances in Continuous Ambulatory Peritoneal Dialysis*, 1986, edited by Khanna R, Nolph K, Prowant B, Twardowski ZJ, Oreopoulos DG, Toronto, Peritoneal Dialysis Bull Inc, 1986, p 16
22. Wegner G: Chirurgische Bemerkungen über die Peritonealhöhle, mit besonderer Berücksichtigung der Ovariotomie. (Surgical considerations regarding the peritoneal cavity with special attention to ovariotomg.) *Arch Klin Chir* 20: 51, 1977.
23. Odel HM, Ferris DO, Paver MH: Peritoneal lavage as an effective means of external excretion. *Am J Med* 9: 63, 1950
24. Grodstein GP, Blumenkrantz MJ, Kopple JD, Moran JK, Coburn JW: Glucose absorption during continuous ambulatory peritoneal dialysis. *Kidney Int* 19: 564, 1981
25. Ota K, Mineshima M, Watanabe N, Naganuma S: Functional deterioration of the peritoneum: does it occur in the absence of peritonitis? *Nephrol Dial Transpl* 2: 30, 1987
26. Raja RM, Kramer MS, Manchanda R, Lazaro N, Rosenbaum JL: Peritoneal dialysis with fructose dialysate – prevention of hyperglycemia and hypermolality. *Ann Intern Med* 79: 511, 1973
27. Yutuc W, Ward G, Shilipetar G, Tenckhoff H: Substitution of sorbitol for dextrose in peritoneal irrigation fluid: a preliminary report. *Trans Am Soc Artif Intern Organs* 13: 168, 1967

28. Bazzato G, Coli U, Landini S, Fracasso A, Morachiello P, Righetto F, Scanferla F: Xylitol and low doses of insulin: new perspectives for diabetic uremic patients on CAPD. *Peritoneal Dial Bull* 2: 161, 1982

29. Matthys E, Dolkart R, Lameire N: Extended use of a glycerol-containing dialysate in diabetic CAPD patients. *Peritoneal Dial Bull* 7: 10, 1987

30. Khanna R, Wu G, Rodella H, Oreopoulos DG: Use of amino acid containing solution in CAPD patients. *Peritoneal Dial Bull* 4: S121, 1984

31. Twardowski ZJ, Khanna R, Nolph KD: Osmotic agents and ultrafiltration in peritoneal dialysis. *Nephron* 42: 93, 1986

32. Gjessing J: The use of dextran as a dialysing fluid in peritoneal dialysis. *Acta Med Scand* 185: 237, 1969

33. Twardowski ZJ, Moore HL, McGary TJ, Poskuta M, Hirszel P, Stathakis C: Polymers as osmotic agents for peritoneal dialysis. *Peritoneal Dial Bull* 4: S125, 1984

34. Mistry CD, Mallick NP, Gokal R: Ultrafiltration with an isosmotic solution during long peritoneal dialysis exchanges. *Lancet* 2: 178, 1987

35. Mistry CD, Fox JE, Mallick NP, Gokal R: Circulating maltose and isomaltose in chronic renal failure. *Kidney Int* 32: S210, 1987

36. Gokal R, Prescott R, Fryer R, Petty R, Ward MK, Kerr DNS: Plasma and dialysate correlations for small solutes after overnight dwell in CAPD patients. *Dial Transplant* 11: 406, 1982

37. Nolph KD, Sorkin MI, Moore H: Autoregulation of sodium and potassium removal during continuous ambulatory peritoneal dialysis. *Trans Am Soc Artif Intern Organs* 26: 334, 1980

38. Blumenkrantz M, Kopple J, Moran J, Coburn JW: Metabolic balance studies and dietary protein requirements in patients undergoing continuous ambulatory peritoneal dialysis. *Kidney Int* 21: 849, 1982

39. Sandle GI, Gaiger E, Tapster S, Goodship THJ: Evidence for large intestinal control of potassium homeostasis in uraemic patients undergoing CAPD. *Clin Sci* 73: 247, 1987

40. Teehan BP, Schleifer CR, Reichard GA, Cupit MC, Sigler MH, Haff AC: Acid base sudies in continuous ambulatory peritoneal dialysis. in: *CAPD Update*, edited by Moncrief JW, Popovich RP, New York, Masson Publ, 1981, p 95

41. Nolph KD, Prowant B, Serkes KD, Morgan L, Baker B, Charytan C, Gham C, Hamburger R, Husserl F, Kleit S, McGuiness J, Moore H, Warren T: Multicenter evaluation of a new peritoneal dialysis solution with a high lactate and a low magnesium concentration. *Peritoneal Dial Bull* 3: 63, 1983

42. Feriani M, Biasioli S, Fabris A, Brendolan A, Bragantini L, Chiaramonte S, Ronco C, La Greca G: The Krebs cycle derangements in CAPD patients. *Peritoneal Dial Bull* 7: S30, 1987

43. De Paepe MB, Schelstraete KHG, Ringoir SM, Lameire NH: Influence of continuous ambulatory peritoneal dialysis on the anemia of end stage renal disease. *Kidney Int* 23: 744, 1983

44. Salahudeen AK, Keavy PM, Hawkins T, Wilkinson R: Is anaemia during CAPD really better than during haemodialysis? *Lancet* 2: 1046, 1983

45. Saltissi D, Coles GA, Napier JAF, Bentley P: The hematological response to continuous ambulatory peritoneal dialysis. *Clin Nephrol* 22: 21, 1984

46. Hefti JE, Blumberg A, Masti HR: Red cell survival and red cell enzymes in patients on continuous ambulatory peritoneal dialysis (CAPD). *Clin Nephrol* 19: 232, 1983

47. Coles GA, Cavill I: Erythropoiesis in the anaemia of chronic renal failure: the response to CAPD. *Nephrol Dial Transplant* 1: 170, 1986

48. Summerfield GP, Gyde OHB, Forbes AMW, Goldsmith HJ, Bellingham AJ: Haemoglobin concentration and serum erythropoietin in renal dialysis and transplant patients. *Scand J Haematol* 30: 389, 1983

49. Lamperi S, Carrozzi S, Icardia A: In vitro and in vivo studies of erythropoies during continuous ambulatory peritoneal dialysis. *Peritoneal Dial Bull* 3: 94, 1983

50. McGonigle RJS, Husserl F, Wallin JD, Fisher JW: Hemodialysis and continuous ambulatory peritoneal dialysis effects on erythropoiesis in renal failure. *Kidney Int* 25: 430, 1984

51. Lamperi S, Carozzi S, Icardi A: Improvement of erythropoiesis in uremic patients on CAPD. *Int J Artif Organs* 6: 191, 1983

52. Movilli E, Natale C, Cancarini G, Maiorca R: Improvement of iron utilisation and anemia in uremic patients switched from hemodialysis to continuous ambulatory peritoneal dialysis. *Peritoneal Dial Bull* 6: 147, 1986

53. Eschbach JW, Egrie JC, Downing MR, Browne JK, Adamson JW: Correction of anemia of end stage renal disease with recombinant human erythropoietin. *N Engl J Med* 316: 73, 1987

54. Boelaert J, Schurgers N, Matthys E, Daneels R: Recombinant Human erythropoietin pharmacokinetics in CAPD patients comparison of intravenous, subcutaneous and intraperitoneal routes. *Nephrol Dial Transplant* 3: 493, 1988

55. Parker A, Nolph KD: Magnesium and calcium transfer during continuous ambulatory peritoneal dialysis. *Trans Am Soc Artif Intern Organs* 26: 194, 1980

56. Delmez JA, Slatopolsky E, Martin KT, Gearing BK, Harter HR: Minerals, vitamin D and parathyroid hormone in continuous ambulatory peritoneal dialysis. *Kidney Int* 21: 862, 1982

57. Kurtz SB, McCarthy JT, Kumar R: Hypercalcaemia in continuous ambulatory peritoneal dialysis (C.A.P.D.) patients: Observations on parameters of calcium metabolism. in: *Advances in Peritoneal Dialysis*, edited by Gahl G, Kessel M, Nolph KD, Amsterdam, Excerpta Medica, 1981, p 467

58. Calderaro V, Oreopoulos DG, Meema HE, Husdan H, Khanna R, Quinton C, Murray T, Carmichael D: The evolution of renal osteodystrophy in patients undergoing continuous ambulatory peritoneal dialysis (CAPD). *Proc Eur Dial Transplant Assoc* 17: 533, 1980

59. Delmez JA, Dougan CS, Gearing BK, Rothstein M, Windus DW, Rapp N, Slatopolsky E: The effects of intraperitoneal calciferol on calcium and parathyroid hormone. *Kidney Int* 31: 795, 1987

60. Gokal K: Renal osteodystrophy in continuous ambulatory peritoneal dialysis. *Peritoneal Dial Bull* 2: 111, 1982

61. Slatopolsky E, Martin KJ, Mirrisseg JJ, Hruska KA: Parathyroid hormone: alterations in chronic renal failure. in: *Nephrology* Vol II, edited by Robinson RR, New York, Springer-Verlag, 1985, p 1292

62. Nolph KD, Ryan L, Prowant B, Twardowski Z: A cross sectional assessment of serum vitamin D and triglyceride concentrations in a CAPD population. *Peritoneal Dial Bull* 4: 232, 1984

63. Gokal R, Ramos JM, Ellis HA, Parkinson I, Sweetman V, Dewar J, Ward MK, Kerr DNS: Histological renal osteodystrophy, 25 hydroxycholecalciferol and aluminum levels in patients on continuous ambulatory peritoneal dialysis. *Kidney Int* 23: 15, 1983

64. Aloni Y, Shany S, Chaimovitz C: Losses of 25 hydroxyvitamin D in peritoneal fluid: Possible mechanism for bone disease in uremic patients treated with CAPD. *Miner Electrolyte Metab* 9: 82, 1983

65. Tielemans C, Aubrey C, Dratwa M: The effects of continuous

ambulatory peritoneal dialysis (CAPD) on renal osteodystrophy. in: *Advances in Peritoneal Dialysis*, edited by Gahl G, Kessel M, Nolph KD, Amsterdam, Excerpta Medica, 1981, p 455

66. Cassidy MJD, Owen JS, Ellis HA, Dewar J, Robinson CJ, Wilkinson R, Ward MK, Kerr DNS: Renal osteodystrophy and metastatic calcification in long term CAPD. *Q J Med* 54: 29, 1985

67. Shany S, Rapoport J, Zuili I, Yankovitz N, Chaimovitz C: Enhancement of 24,25-dihydroxyvitamin D levels in patients treated with continuous ambulatory peritoneal dialysis. *Nephron* 42: 141, 1986

68. Chaimovitz C, Rapoport J, Zuili R, Yankovitz N, Shany S: In vitro synthesis of 1, 25(OH)$_2$ D$_3$ by peritoneal macrophages of CAPD patients. *Nephrol Dial Transplant* 1: 113, 1986

69. Teitelbaum SL, Fallon MD, Gearing BK, Dougan CS, Delmez JA: The effects of continuous ambulatory peritoneal dialyses (CAPD) on bone histomorphology. *Kidney Int* 21: 180, 1982

70. deFremont JF, Morinière P, Decourcelle PH, Roussel A, Makdassi R, Kaczmareck P, Fievet P, Bataille P, Fournier A: Control of hyperparathyroidism by continuous ambulatory peritoneal dialysis (CAPD). *Kidney Int* 21: 122, 1982

71. Loschiavo C, Fabris A, Adami J, Tomelleri L, Tessitore N, Valio E, Lupo A, Oldrizzi L, Ruqui C, Gammaro L, Mascio G: Effects of continuous ambulatory peritoneal dialysis on renal osteodystrophy. *Peritoneal Dial Bull* 5: 53, 1985

72. Digenis G, Khanna R, Pierretos A, Meema HE, Rabinovich S, Pettit J, Oreopoulos DG: Renal osteodystrophy in patients maintained on CAPD for more than three years. *Peritoneal Dial Bull* 3: 81, 1983

73. Salusky IB, Fine RN, Kangarloo H, Gold R, Paunier L, Goodman WG, Brill JE, Gilli G, Slatopolsky E, Coburn JW: 'High dose' calcitriol for control of renal osteodystrophy in children on CAPD. *Kidney Int* 32: 89, 1987

74. Rottembourg J, Gallego JL, Jaudon M, Clavel J, Legrain M: Serum concentration and peritoneal transfer of aluminum during treatment by continuous ambulatory peritoneal dialysis. *Kidney Int* 25: 919, 1984

75. Umeda M, Umimoto K, Kamizuru M, Izumi N, Nishio S, Kishimoto T, Maekawa M: Aluminium accummulation in red blood cells of CAPD and chronic nephritis patients. *Nephrol Dial Transplant* 2: 408, 1987

76. Delmez J: Renal osteodystrophy and aluminium bone disease in CAPD patients. in: *Advances in Continuous Ambulatory Peritoneal Dialysis 1987*, edited by Khanna R, Nolph K, Prowant B, Twardowski Z, Oreopoulos DG, Toronto, University of Toronto Press, 1987, p 38

77. Hercz G, Salusky IB, Norris KC, Fine RN, Coburn JW: Aluminum removal by peritoneal dialysis: intravenous vs intraperitoneal deferoxamine. *Kidney Int* 30: 944, 1986

78. Milliner DS, Nebeker HG, Ott SM, Sherrard DJ, Andress OL, Alfrey AC, Coburn JW: Desferrioxamine infusion tests for diagnosis of aluminum osteomalacia. *Kidney Int* 25: 149, 1984

79. Meema HG, Oreopoulos DG, Rapoport A: Serum magnesium level and arterial calcification in end-stage renal disease. *Kidney Int* 32: 388, 1987

80. Zuccelli P, Fusaroli M, Casanova S, Fabbri L, Catizone L: Renal osteodystrophy on CAPD patients. in: *Peritoneal Dialysis*, edited by LaGreca G, Biasioli S, Ronco C, Milan, Wichtig Editore, 1982, p 409

81. Giangrande A, Castiglioni A, Ballanti P, Constantini S, Pisoni I, Bonucci E, Giordano R: Renal osteodystrophy during long term CAPD. in: *Proc IV Congr Int Soc Peritoneal Dial 1987 Venice*, edited by Giordano G, Bazzato G, DeSanto N, Milan, Wichtig Editore (in press)

82. Rahman H, Heaton A, Goodship T, Rodger R, Tapson J, Sellars L, Ellis H, Wilkinson R, Ward MK: Renal osteodystrophy in patients on continuous ambulatory peritoneal dialysis; a five year study. *Peritoneal Dial Bull* 7: 20, 1987

83. Kurtz SB: Clinical parameters of renal bone disease: a comparison of CAPD and HD. *Dial Transplant* 14: 30, 1985

84. Buccianti G, Bianchi ML, Valenti G: Progress of renal osteodystrophy during continuous ambulatory peritoneal dialysis. *Clin Nephrol* 22: 279, 1984

85. Llach F: Metabolic bone disease in CAPD patients. *Peritoneal Dial Bull* 3: S24, 1983

86. Shusterman N, Fallon M, Kaplan F, Audet P, Morrison A, Wowserstein A: Favorable response of renal osteodystrophy in CAPD patients. *Abstracts Am Soc Nephrol* 18: 88A, 1985

87. Delmez JA, Fallon MD, Bergfeld MA, Gearing BK, Donegan CS, Teitelbaum SL: Continuous ambulatory peritoneal dialysis and bone. *Kidney Int* 30: 379, 1986

88. Nilsson P, Danielsson BG, Grefberg N, Wide L: Secondary hyperparathyroidism in diabetic and non-diabetic patients on long term CAPD. *Scand J Urol Nephrol* 19: 59, 1985

89. Kopple JD: Abnormal amino acid and protein metabolism in uremia. *Kidney Int* 14: 340, 1978

90. Lindholm B, Bergström J: Nutritional aspects of CAPD. in: *Continuous Ambulatory Peritoneal Dialysis*, edited by Gokal R, Edinburgh, Churchill Livingstone, 1986, p 228

91. Sombolis K, Berkelhammer C, Baker J, Wu G, McNamee P, Oreopoulos D: Nutritional assessment and skeletal muscle function in patients on continuous ambulatory peritoneal dialysis. *Peritoneal Dial Bull* 6: 53, 1986

92. Defronzo RA, Alverstrad A, Smith D, Hendler R, Hindler E, Wahren J: Insulin resistance in uremia. *J Clin Invest* 67: 563, 1981

93. Rubin J, Ray R, Barnes T, Bower J: Peritoneal abnormalities during infectious episodes of continuous ambulatory peritoneal dialysis. *Nephron* 29: 124, 1981

94. Heaton A, Johnston DG, Burren JM, Orskor H, Ward MK, Alberti KGM, Kerr DNS: Carbohydrate and lipid metabolism during CAPD: the effect of a single dialysis cycle. *Clin Sci* 65: 539, 1983

95. Bouma SF, Dwyer JT: Glucose absorption and weight change in 18 months of CAPD. *J Am Diet Assoc* 84: 194, 1984

96. Kurtz SB, Wong VH, Anderson CF, Vogel JP, McCarthy JT, Mitchell JC: CAPD – three years experience at the Mayo Clinic. *Mayo Clin Proc* 58: 633, 1983

97. Bagdade JD, Albers JJ: Plasma high-density lipoprotein concentrations in chronic hemodialysis and renal transplant patients. *N Engl J Med* 296: 1436, 1977

98. Wertel PJ, Fidgi NH, Tan MH: Increased lipoprotein-remnant formation in chronic renal failure. *N Engl J Med* 307: 329, 1982

99. Kannel WB, Castilli WP, Gordon T: Cholesterol in the prediction of atherosclerotic disease. New prospectives based on Framingham Study. *Ann Intern Med* 90: 85, 1979

100. Lindholm B, Karlander SG, Norbeck HE, Bergström J: Glucose and lipid metabolism in peritoneal dialysis. in: *Peritoneal Dialysis*, edited by La Greca G, Biasioli S, Ronco C, Milan, Wichtig Editore, 1982, 219

101. Gokal R, Ramos JM, McGurk JG, Ward MK, Kerr DNS: Hyperlipidaemia in patients on continuous ambulatory peritoneal dialysis. in: *Advances in Peritoneal Dialysis*, edited by Gahl G, Kessel M, Nolph K, Amsterdam, Excerpta Medica, 1982, p 430

102. Ramos JM, Heaton A, McGurk JG, Ward MK, Kerr DNS: Sequential changes in serum lipids and their subfractions in patients receiving CAPD. *Nephron* 35: 20, 1983

103. Brekenridge WC, Roncari DAK, Khanna R, Oreopoulos DG: The influence of CAPD on plasma lipoproteins. *Atherosclerosis* 45: 249, 1982

104. Lameire N, Matthys E, Matthys E, Beheydt R: Effects of long term CAPD on carbohydrate and lipid metabolism. *Clin Nephrol* (in press)

105. Rubin J, Nolph KD, Arfania D, Prowant B, Fruto L, Brown P, Moore H: Protein losses in continuous ambulatory peritoneal dialysis. *Nephron* 28: 218, 1981

106. Dulaney JT, Hatch FE: Peritoneal dialysis and loss of proteins: a review. *Kidney Int* 26: 253, 1984

107. Kayson GA, Schoenfield PY: Albumin homeostasis in patients undergoing continuous ambulatory peritoneal dialysis. *Kidney Int* 25: 107, 1984

108. De Santo NG, Capodicasa G, Di Leo VA, Di Serafino A, Grillo D, Esponto R, Fiore R, Cucciniello E, Damiano M, Buonadonna L, Di Iono R, Capasso G, Giordano C: Kinetics of amino acid equilibration in the dialysate during CAPD. *Int J Artif Organs* 4: 23, 1981

109. Blumenkrantz MJ, Kopple JD, Moran K, Grodstein G, Coburn J: Nitrogen and urea metabolism during continuous ambulatory peritoneal dialysis. *Kidney Int* 20: 78, 1981

110. Blumberg A, Hanck A, Sander G: Vitamin nutrition in patients on continuous ambulatory peritoneal dialysis (CAPD). *Clin Nephrol* 20: 244, 1983

111. Henderson IS, Leung ACT, Shenkin A: Vitamin status in continuous ambulatory peritoneal dialysis. *Peritoneal Dial Bull* 4: 143, 1984

112. Moorthy V, Rosenblum M, Rajaram R, Shing AL: A comparison of plasma and muscle carnitine levels in patients on peritoneal or haemodialysis for chronic renal failure. *Am J Nephrol* 3: 205, 1983

113. Lescke M, Rumpf W, Eisenhauer T, Fuchs C, Becker K, Koethe U, Scheler F: Quantitative assessment of carnitine loss during hemodialysis and hemofiltration. *Kidney Int* 24: S143, 1983

114. Trovoto GM, Ginardi V, Marco V, Dellaire A, Corsi M: Long term carnitine treatment of chronic anaemia of patients with end stage renal failure. *Curr Therap Res* 31: 1042, 1982

115. Noel LH, Zingraff J, Barden T, Atienza C, Kuntz D, Drüeke T: Tissue distribution of dialysis amyloidosis. *Clin Nephrol* 27: 175, 1987

116. Blumberg A, Burgi W: Behavior of B2 microglobulin in patients with chronic renal failure undergoing hemodialysis hemofiltration and continuous ambulatory peritoneal dialysis. *Clin Nephrol* 27: 245, 1987

117. Ballardie FW, Kerr DNS, Tennet G, Pepys MB: HD versus CAPD: Equal predisposition to amyloidosis? *Lancet* 1: 795, 1986

118. Mistry CD, O'Donoghue DJ, Gokal R, Pepys MB, Tennant G, Ballardie FW: Transperitoneal removal of β_2 microglobulin using glucose and glucose polymer solutions. *Nephrol Dial Transplant* 2: 455, 1987

119. Gagnon RF, Sommerville P, Kaye M: β_2 microglobulin serum levels in patients on long term dialysis. *Peritoneal Dial Bull* 7: 29, 1987

120. McGrath BP, Ledingham JGG: Renin blood volume and response to saralasin in patients in HD: evidence against volume and renin dependent hypertension. *Clin Sci Mol Med* 54: 305, 1978

121. Youmbissi J, Sellars L, Shore AC, Poon T, Wilkinson R: Blood pressures on CAPD: relationship to sodium status, renin and aldosterone compared with hemodialysis. in: *Frontiers in Peritoneal Dialysis*, edited by Maher JF, Winchester JF, New York, Field, Rich & Assoc, 1986, p 450

122. Panzetta G, Guerra U, D'Angelo A, Sondrini S, Terzi A, Oldrizzi L, Maiorca R: Body fluid spaces in in patients on CAPD. *Int J Artif Organs* 7: 89, 1984

123. Ramos J, Gokal R, Siamopoulos K, Ward MK, Wilkinson R, Kerr DNS: CAPD: three years experience. *Q J Med* 206: 165, 1983

124. Young MA, Nolph KD, Dulton S, Prowant B: Antihypertensive drug requirements in continuous ambulatory peritoneal dialysis. *Peritoneal Dial Bull* 4: 85, 1984

125. Zabetakis PM, Kumar DN, Gleim GW, Gardenswartz MH, Agrawal M, Robinson AG, Michells TNF: Increased levels of plasma renin, aldosterone, catecholamines and vasopressin in chronic ambulatory peritoneal dialysis (CAPD) patients. *Clin Nephrol* 28: 147, 1987

126. Olasson PH, Favre H, Vallotton MB: Response of blood pressure and the renin-angiotensin-aldosterone system to CAPD in hypertensive end stage renal failure. *Clin Sci* 63: S207, 1982

127. Leenan FH, Shah P, Boer WH, Khanna R, Oreopoulos DG: Hypotension on CAPD: an approach to treatment. *Peritoneal Dial Bull* 3: S33, 1983

128. Kong CH, Raval H, Thompson FD: Effect of 2 liters of intraperitoneal dialysate on the cardiovascular system. *Clin Nephrol* 26: 134, 1984

129. Franklin JO, Alpert MA, Twardowski ZJ, Khanna R: Effect of intraperitoneal infusion volume and posture on left ventricular function in patients on continuous ambulatory peritoneal dialysis. *Trans Am Soc Artif Intern Organs* 32: 554, 1986

130. Brown PM, Johnston KW, Fenton SSA, Cattran DC: Symptomatic exacerbation of peripheral vascular disease with chronic ambulatory peritoneal dialysis. *Clin Nephrol* 16: 258, 1981

131. Peer G, Korzets A, Hochhauzer E, Eschchar Y, Blum M, Aviram A: Cardiac arrhythmia during chronic ambulatory peritoneal dialysis. *Nephron* 45: 192, 1987

132. Gotloib L, Mines M, Garnnizo L, Varka I: Haemodynamic effects of increasing intraabdominal pressure in peritoneal dialysis. *Peritoneal Dial Bull* 1: 41, 1981

133. Twardowski Z, Nolph KD: Optimal exchange volume for continuous ambulatory peritoneal dialysis (CAPD). *Peritoneal Dial Bull* 2: 154, 1982

134. Twardowski ZJ, Prowant BF, Nolph KD, Martine AJ, Lampton LM: High volume low frelquency continuous ambulatory peritoneal dialysis. *Kidney Int* 23: 64, 1983

135. Beasley CRW, Ripley JM, Smith DA, Neale TJ: Pulmonary function in chronic renal failure patients managed by CAPD. *NZ Med J* 99: 313, 1986

136. Singh S, Dale A, Morgan B, Sahebjami H: Serial studies of pulmonary function in CAPD – prospective study. *Chest* 86: 874, 1984

137. Bush A, Miller J, Peacock AJ, Sopwith T, Gabriel R, Denison D: Some observations on the role of the abdomen in breathing in patients on peritoneal dialysis. *Clin Sci* 68: 401, 1985

138. Kim D, Blair G, Wu G, Ayiomamitis A, Oreopoulos DG: Electrophysiological studies of nerve function in patients on CAPD over long periods. *Peritoneal Dial Bull* 5: 45, 1985

139. Sunderrajan S, Nolph KD: Longitudinal study of nerve conduction velocities during continuous ambulatory peritoneal dialysis. *Peritoneal Dial Bull* 5: 48, 1985

140. Lindholm B, Tegner R: Deterioration of peripheral nerve

function during continuous ambulatory peritoneal dialysis. *Peritoneal Dial Bull* 6: 20, 1986

141. Marsh JT, Brown WS, Wolcott D, Landsverk J, Nissenson AR: Electrophysiological indices of CNS function in hemodialysis and CAPD. *Kidney Int* 30: 957, 1986

142. Editorial: Ambulatory peritonitis. *Lancet* 1: 1104, 1982

143. Vas SI: Microbiological aspects of chronic ambulatory peritoneal dialysis. *Kidney Int* 23: 83, 1983

144. Prowant B, Nolph KD: Five years experience with peritonitis in a CAPD program. *Peritoneal Dial Bull* 2: 169, 1982

145. Pierratos A: Peritoneal dialysis glossary. *Peritoneal Dial Bull* 4: 2, 1984

146. Mion C, Slingeneyer A, Canard B: Peritonitis. in: *Continuous Ambulatory Peritoneal Dialysis,* edited by Gokal R, Edinburgh, Churchill Livingstone, 1986, p 163

147. Sombolos K, Vas S, Rifkin A, Ayiomamitis A, McNamee P, Oreopoulos D: Propioni-bacteria isolates and asymptomatic infections of the peritoneal effluent in CAPD patients. *Nephrol Dial Transplant* 1: 175, 1986

148. Gokal R, Ramos J, Ward MK, Kerr DNS: 'Eosinophilic peritonitis' in continuous ambulatory peritoneal dialysis (CAPD). *Clin Nephrol* 15: 328, 1981

149. Parsons F, Ahmed IH, Brownjohn A, Coltman S, Gibson J, Young G, Young J: CAPD peritonitis. *Lancet* 1: 348, 1983

150. Gokal R, Manos J, Walker C, Mallick NP: Peritonitis related to defective CAPD equipment. *Lancet* 2: 382, 1982

151. Wu G, Khanna R, Vas S, Oreopoulos DG: Is extensive diverticulosis of the colon a contraindication to CAPD? *Peritoneal Dial Bull* 3: 180, 1983

152. Schweinburg FB, Seligman A, Fine J: Transmural migration of intestinal bacteria. A study based on the use of radioactive Escherichia coli. *N Engl J Med* 242: 747, 1950

153. Della Volpe M, Iberti M, Ortensia A, Veronesi GV: Erosion of the sigmoid by a permanent peritoneal catheter. *Peritoneal Dial Bull* 4: 108, 1984

154. Kiddy K, Brown P, Michael J, Adu D: Peritonitis due to Streptococcus viridans in CAPD. *Br Med J* 290: 969, 1985

155. Coward R, Gokal R, Wise M, Mallick NP, Warrell D: Peritonitis associated with vaginal leakage of dialysis fluid in CAPD. *Br Med J* 284: 1529, 1982

156. Kim D, Tapson J, Wu G, Khanna R, Vas SI, Oreopoulos DG: Staphylococcus aureus peritonitis in patients on CAPD. *Trans Am Soc Artif Intern Organs* 30: 494, 1984

157. Gokal R, Ramos J, Frances DMA, Ferner RE, Goodship T, Proud G, Bint A, Ward MK: Peritonitis in CAPD. *Lancet* 2: 1388, 1982

158. Working Party of the BSAC: Diagnosis and management of peritonitis in CAPD. *Lancet* 1: 845, 1987

159. Knight KR, Polak A, Crump J, Maskell R: Laboratory diagnosis and oral treatment of CAPD peritonitis. *Lancet* 2: 1301, 1982

160. Gould I, Casewell M: Laboratory diagnosis of peritonitis during CAPD. *J Hosp Infect* 7: 155, 1986

161. Keane WF, Everett ED, Fine RN, Golper TA, Vas SI, Peterson PK: CAPD related peritonitis management and antibiotic therapy recommendations. *Peritoneal Dial Bull* 7: 55, 1987

162. Rubin J, Ray R, Barnes T, Teal N, Hellenus E, Humphries J, Bower JD: Peritonitis in CAPD patients. *Am J Kidney Dis* 2: 602, 1983

163. Duwe AK, Vas SI, Weatherhead JW: Effects of the component of peritoneal dialysis fluid on chemiluminescence, phagocytosis and bacterial activity in vitro. *Infect Immun* 33: 134, 1981

164. Gokal R, Marsh FP: Survey of continuous ambulatory peritoneal dialysis in the United Kingdom, 1982. *Peritoneal Dial Bull* 4: 240, 1984

165. Mistry CD, Salgia P, Manos J, Marsden A, Tooth A, Ramsden RT, Gokal R: Netilmicin and vancomycin in the treatment of peritonitis in patients on CAPD. in: *Advances in Continuous Ambulatory Peritoneal Dialysis, 1986,* edited by Khanna R, Nolph KD, Prowant B, Twardowski Z, Oreopoulos D, Peritoneal Dial Bull Inc, Toronto, 1986, p 129

166. Fabris A, Biasioli S, Borin D: Fungal peritonitis in peritoneal dialysis: our experience and review of treatments. *Peritoneal Dial Bull* 4: 75, 1984

167. Paterson AD, Morgan GA, Bishop MC, Burden RP: Removal and replacement of Tenckhoff catheter at a single operation: Successful treatment of resistant peritonitis in CAPD. *Lancet* 2: 1245, 1987

168. *Report of the National CAPD Registry of the National Institutes of Health.* Characteristics of participants and selected outcome measures for the period 1.1.81 to 31.8.86. 1987 p 4–8

169. Gokal R, Jakubowski C, King J, Bogle S, Hunt L, Baillod R, Marsh FP, Ogg C, Oliver D, Ward M, Wilkinson R: Outcome in patients in HD and CAPD: 4 years analysis of a prospective study. *Lancet* 2: 1105, 1987

170. Maiorca R, Cancarine G, Colombrita D, Manili L, Camerini C: Further experience with Y-system in CAPD. in: *Advances in Continuous Ambulatory Peritoneal Dialysis 1986,* edited by Khanna R, Nolph KD, Prowant B, Twardowski Z, Oreopoulos D, Peritoneal Dial Bull Inc, Toronto, 1986, p 172

171. Tarchini R, Segoloni P, Gentile M, Lupo A, Cancarini G, Salomoni M, D'Amico G, Mioli V, Vercillone A, Zucchelli P: The role of experience and Y transfer set in preventing dropouts: a report from the Italian CAPD study group. in: *Advances in Continuous Ambulatory Peritoneal Dialysis 1987,* edited by Khanna R, Nolph KD, Prowant B, Twardowski Z, Oreopoulos D, Peritoneal Dial Bull Inc, Toronto, 1987, p 192

172. Uttley L, Gokal R: Organisation of a CAPD programme – the nurses role. in: *Continuous Ambulatory Peritoneal Dialysis,* edited by Gokal R, Edinburgh, Churchill Livingstone, 1986, p 145

173. Dasgupta M, Ulan RA, Beltcher KB, Burns V, Lam K, Dosseter JB, Casterton JW: Effect of exit site infection, and peritonitis on the distribution of biofilm encased adherent bacterial microcolonies on Tenckhoff catheter in patients on CAPD. in: *Advances in Continuous Ambulatory Peritoneal Dialysis 1986,* edited by Khanna R, Nolph KD, Prowant B, Twardowski Z, Oreopoulos D, Toronto, Peritoneal Dial Bull Inc, 1986, p 102

174. Lamperi S, Carozzi S, Nasine M: Pharmacokinetics of intraperitoneal Immunoglobulins (Ig) in CAPD patients. in: *Advances in Continuous Ambulatory Peritoneal Dialysis 1987,* edited by Khanna R, Nolph KD, Prowant B, Twardowski Z, Oreopoulos D, Toronto, Peritoneal Dial Bull Inc, 1987, p 18

175. Ballardie FW, Barsham S, Clutterbuck EJ, Brenchley PE, Bayston R: IgG antibodies to coagulase negative staphylococci in CAPD patients. Detection and role as potential opsonins. in: *Advances in Continuous Ambulatory Peritoneal Dialysis 1987,* edited by Khanna R, Nolph KD, Prowant B, Twardowski Z, Oreopoulos D, Toronto, Peritoneal Dial Bull Inc, 1987, p 130

176. Verger C, Brunschweig O, Le Charpentier Y: Peritoneal structural alterations in CAPD. in: *Advances in Peritoneal Dialysis,* edited by Gahl G, Nolph K, Kessel M, Amsterdam, Excerpta Medica, 1981, p 10

177. Dobbie J, Zaki M, Wilson L: Ultrastructural studies on the

peritoneum with special reference to CAPD. *Scott Med J* 26: 213, 1981

178. Verger C, Luger A, Moore J, Nolph KD: Acute changes in peritoneal morphology and transport properties with infectious peritonitis and mechanical injury. *Kidney Int* 23: 823, 1983

179. Shaldon S: Peritoneal macrophages – the first line of defence. in: *Peritoneal Dialysis*, edited by La Greca G, Chiaramonte S, Fabris A, Feriani M, Ronco C, Milan, Wichtig Editore, 1986, p 201

180. Faller B, Marichal JF: Loss of ultrafiltration in CAPD: a role for acetate. *Peritoneal Dial Bull* 4: 10, 1984

181. Henderson IS, Couper IA, Lumsden A: The effect of shelf-life of peritoneal dialysis fluid in ultrafiltration in CAPD. in: *Peritoneal Dialysis*, edited by La Greca G, Chiaramonte S, Fabris A, Feriani M, Ronco C, Milan, Wichtig Editore, 1986, p 85

182. Junor BR, Briggs JD, Forewill MA, Dobbie JW, Henderson I: Sclerosing peritonitis – the contribution of chlorhexidine in alcohol. *Peritoneal Dial Bull* 5: 101, 1985

183. Burton P, Walls J: Selection adjusted comparison of life expectancy of patients on CAPD, haemodialysis and renal transplant. *Lancet* 1: 1115, 1987

184. Verger C: Clinical significance of ultrafiltration alterations on CAPD. in: *Peritoneal Dialysis*, edited by La Greca G, Chiaramonte S, Fabris A, Feriani M, Ronco C, Milan, Wichtig Editore, 1986, p 91

185. Verger C, Celicont B: Peritoneal permeability and encapsulating peritonitis. *Lancet* 1: 486, 1985

186. Lamperi S, Carozzi S: Lympho-monokine disorders and ultrafiltration loss in CAPD patients. in: *Advances in Continuous Ambulatory Peritoneal Dialysis 1987*, edited by Khanna R, Nolph KD, Prowant B, Twardowski Z, Oreopoulos D, Toronto, Peritoneal Dial Bull Inc, 1987, p 7

187. DiPaolo N, Buoncristiani U, Gaggiotti E: Improvement of impaired ultrafiltration after addition of phosphatidylcholine in patients on CAPD. *Peritoneal Dial Bull* 6: 44, 1986

188. Breborowicz A, Sambolos K, Rodela H, Ogilvie R, Bargman J, Oreopoulos D: Mechanisms of phosphatidylcholine action during peritoneal dialysis. *Peritoneal Dial Bull* 7: 6, 1987

189. Slingeneyer A, Elie M, Mion C: Sclerosing encapsulating peritonitis: results of an international survey. *Nephrol Dial Transplant* 1: 112, 1986

190. Dobbie J, Henderson I, Wilson L: New evidence on the pathogenesis of sclerosing encapsulating peritonitis obtained from serial biopsies. in: *Advances in Continuous Ambulatory Peritoneal Dialysis 1987*, edited by Khanna R, Nolph KD, Prowant B, Twardowski Z, Oreopoulos D, Toronto, Peritoneal Dial Bull Inc, 1987, p 138

191. Kerr DNS: Dialysis strategy: cost and effectiveness. *Proc Eur Dial Transplant Assoc* 118: 664, 1981

192. Evans RW, Manninen DL, Garrison LP, Hart LG, Blagg C, Gutman R, Hull AR, Lorne E: The quality of life of patients with end-stage renal disease. *N Engl J Med* 312, 553, 1985

193. Gokal R, Stout JP, Hillier V, Kincey J, Auer J, Oliver D,

Simon G: The quality of life of high risk and elderly dialysis patients (with particular reference to medical risk factors). in: *Advances in Continuous Ambulatory Peritoneal Dialysis 1987*, edited by Khanna R, Nolph KD, Prowant B, Twardowski Z, Oreopoulos D, Toronto, Peritoneal Dial Bull Inc, 1987, p 56

194. Nissenson AR, Maida CA, Katz AH, Wolcott DI, Landsverk J, Strauss G, Coleman W: Psychosocial adaptation of CAPD and center hemodialysis patients. in: *Advances in Continuous Ambulatory Peritoneal Dialysis 1986*, edited by Khanna R, Nolph KD, Prowant B, Twardowski Z, Oreopoulos D, Toronto, Peritoneal Dial Bull Inc, 1986, p 47

195. Fragola J, Grube J, Van Block L, Bourke E: Multicentre study of physical activity and employment status on CAPD patients in the USA. *Proc Eur Dial Transplant Assoc* 20: 243, 1983

196. Coles GA: Is peritoneal dialysis a good long term treatment? *Br Med J* 290: 1164, 1985

197. Broyer M, Brunner F, Brynger H, Donckerwolcke R, Jacobs C, Kramer P, Selwood NH, Wing A: Combined report on regular dialysis and transplantation in Europe 1981. *Proc Eur Dial Transplant Assoc* 19: 4, 1982

198. Drukker W, Schonten W, Alberts C: Report on regular dialysis treatment in Europe. *Proc Eur Dial Transplant Assoc* 5: 3, 1968

199. Oreopoulos DG: Duration of peritoneal dialysis ten years and more. *Peritoneal Dial Bull* 4: 61, 1984

200. Holden AL, Gaumer G: Best demonstrated practices program promoting CAPD patient retention in the United States. in: *Advances in Continuous Ambulatory Peritoneal Dialysis 1987*, edited by Khanna R, Nolph KD, Prowant B, Twardowski Z, Oreopoulos D, Toronto, Peritoneal Dial Bull Inc, 1987, p 186

201. Gokal R: World wide experience, cost effectiveness and future of CAPD – its role in renal replacement therapy. in: *Continuous Ambulatory Peritoneal Dialysis*, edited by Gokal R, Edinburgh, Churchill Livingstone, 1986, p 349.

202. Manis T, Friedman E: Dialytic therapy for irreversible uremia. *N Engl J Med* 301: 1260, 1979

203. Nolph KD: Dialysis and transplantation in the USA and impact of CAPD. in: *Renal Failure Who Cares?* edited by Parsons F, Ogg C, Lancaster, MTP Press, 1983, p 75

204. Mancini PV: *The Cost of Treating ESRF*. Draft paper for DHSS. London, Elephant and Castle, June 1984

205. Wood IT, Mallick NP, Wing AJ: Prediction of resources needed to achieve the national target for the treatment of renal failure. *Br Med J* 294: 1467, 1987

206. Williams A: Economics of coronary artery bypass grafting. *Br Med J* 291: 326, 1985

207. Churchill DN, Lemon BL, Torrance GW: Quality of life in end-stage renal disease. *Peritoneal Dial Bull* 4: 20, 1984

208. Rosse R, Kind P: Evaluation of status of illness: is there a social mechanism? *Int J Epidemiol* 7: 347, 1978

209. Geerlings W, Selwood NH, Brunner FP: The contribution of CAPD to overall survival on renal replacement therapy in Europe. *Proc Int Congr Nephrol* London, July, 1987 (in press)

REPLACEMENT OF RENAL FUNCTION BY DIALYSIS

REPLACEMENT OF RENAL FUNCTION BY DIALYSIS

A textbook of dialysis

Third edition

Updated and enlarged

Edited by

JOHN F. MAHER

KLUWER ACADEMIC PUBLISHERS

DORDRECHT / BOSTON / LANCASTER

Library of Congress Cataloging-in-Publication Data

Replacement of renal function by dialysis: a textbook of dialysis /
  edited by John F. Maher. – 3rd ed., updated and enl.
     p.   cm.
  Includes bibliographies and index.
  ISBN 978-94-010-6979-3
  1. Hemodialysis. 2. Chronic renal failure – Treatment. 3. Maher, John F. (John Francis), 1929–
  [DNLM: 1. Hemodialysis.   WJ 378 R425]
  RC901.7.H45R46 1988
  617′.461059 – dc19
  DNLM/DLC
  for Library of Congress
  ISBN 978-94-010-6979-3   88-13539
                                                                       CIP

First edition 1978
Second, revised and enlarged edition 1983
Third edition, updated and enlarged 1989

Cover illustration: the characteristic chromatogram showing peak 7C from the studies
of Dr. J. Bergström and Dr. J. Fürst.

Published by Kluwer Academic Publishers
P.O. Box 17, 3300 AA Dordrecht, Holland.

Kluwer Academic Publishers incorporates the publishing programmes of
D. Reidel, Martinus Nijhoff, Dr W. Junk and MTP Press.

Sold and distributed in the U.S.A. and Canada
by Kluwer Academic Publishers,
101 Philip Drive, Norwell, MA 02061, U.S.A.

In all other countries, sold and distributed
by Kluwer Academic Publishers Group,
P.O. Box 322, 3300 AH Dordrecht, Holland.

To Marge

It is difficult to say what is impossible,
for the dream of yesterday is the hope of
to-day and the reality of to-morrow.

ROBERT H. GODDARD

FOREWORD TO THE THIRD EDITION

BELDING H. SCRIBNER

The foreword to this edition is more difficult for me to write than that for the first edition because we are just entering a new era in the use of hemodialysis to treat end-stage kidney disease. This new era results from a substantial increase in our knowledge of the pathophysiology of renal failure and its therapy (see below). Consequently, I feel I must become bolder in my speculations.

Last spring (1987), the second patient to enter the Seattle hemodialysis program which began in 1960, died suddenly of a myocardial infarction on a golf course in Palm Springs, California. He was in his 28th year of renal replacement therapy, having received a transplant from his mother in 1968. Patient #5 of the original Seattle group remains on dialysis and is beginning his 27th year. Dr. Robin Eady, an academic dermatologist in London, began dialysis in Seattle in February of 1963. After 25 years on dialysis, he recently had his first renal transplant at Oxford. He had waited four and one-half years for a negative cross match. Since he reacted to 100% of the test panel, this successful transplant exemplifies the great advances being made in transplant immunology.

These three patients are among the several hundred worldwide who have survived more than 20 years on renal replacement therapy. Based on the unexpectedly long survival of these original patients and considering the fact that by today's standards their dialysis therapy during the first 5 years was terrible, one can entertain the following important prediction: A patient with end-stage renal failure who is in the 20 to 50 year age range and is otherwise well who starts renal replacement therapy in the 1980's *should have a nearly normal life expectancy*. There are, however, two caveats that must be fulfilled: 1) circulatory access must be maintained and 2) hypertension must be controlled beginning with the onset of chronic renal failure.

The subject of control of hypertension raises immediately my concern over the long-term effects of so called 'high flux' dialysis. That term, from the patients' perspective, translates into less time on dialysis which accounts for the current enormous popularity worldwide and its enthusiastic promotion by the manufacturers of the numerous devices needed to provide the required technology. On the plus side, I must admit that I am amazed that urea can be removed at these high transfer rates without causing CNS complications. After all, the neurosurgeons used to use urea to shrink the brain. Nevertheless, very high urea clearances and dialysis times as short as 120 min seem to be well tolerated with less post-dialysis morbidity. The latter benefit could be due to the fact that the membranes used for high flux dialysis cause less immunologic insult as discussed below.

The down side of high flux dialysis lies in two areas. The first is a concern over the increase in morbidity and mortality that seems inevitable as a result of placing the required 'high tech' equipment in inexperienced hands. Any time you push a system toward its technological and physiological limits, the chance of malfunction increases dramatically. I fear that such malfunction may increase as the use of high clearance dialysis becomes widespread. Of even greater concern is the adverse effect that shortening dialysis time has on extracellular fluid removal and hence adequate control of blood pressure. In the February 1983 issue of *Nephron*, Bernard Charra and his colleagues presented a classic paper that is yet to be fully appreciated. They showed that by using long, slow 'low flux' dialysis, blood pressure control was excellent, toxic anti-hypertensive drugs could be eliminated, and the risk of accelerated atherosclerosis was reduced to near zero. High flux dialysis represents the opposite end of the spectrum. One simply cannot remove enough fluid to achieve good control of blood pressure in so short a time, especially in patients who have poor compliance with a low salt diet. The net result is either poor control of blood pressure or high doses of anti-hypertensive medication or both, which in my view, in the long-term represents a dangerous trend.

The above prediction of a nearly normal life expectancy for patients on renal replacement therapy, even if it is overly optimistic, has important implications for the future.

Unfortunately, the economic implications head the list. Longer survival means that the total number of patients on renal replacement therapy (dialysis plus renal homografts) will continue to increase for several more decades. At the same time, the percent of the gross national product devoted to health care continues to increase, at least in the United States, despite serious efforts to reverse the trend. A conflict between these two trends appears inevitable and will not be easy to resolve. One possibility is a return to 'do it yourself' home hemodialysis but with easy to use, fully automated equipment. Home peritoneal dialysis with on-line preparation of the dialysis fluid at the bedside, may become another good alternative.

The implications of long survival for a patient's chances of obtaining a kidney transplant are more difficult to predict. On the one hand, longer survival translates into more demand for grafts. On the other hand, as Dr. Eady's case demonstrates, improvement in transplant matching and immunotherapy undoubtedly will increase the number of successful grafts as well as their longevity, decreasing the need for second transplants. Therefore, the situation probably will remain indefinitely as it is today, namely, a chronic shortage of renal homografts. Hence, various forms of dialysis will continue to carry the major burden.

A NEW ERA FOR DIALYSIS THERAPY

About 20 years after the discovery of insulin, the various degenerative complications of diabetes became manifest. It, therefore, is an interesting historical parallel that beginning in 1980 as we passed the 20-year mark for the use of dialysis to treat end-stage renal disease, several problems began to emerge that were new and unexpected. Two have been particularly worrisome. The first, chronic aluminum intoxication, is covered in depth in this edition, and shows promise of being prevented in the future. The second, dialysis amyloid syndrome, first was described by Laurent and colleagues in 1981. This complication also is dealt with in detail herein. However, we are just beginning to understand the possible relationship between this disease and the hemodialysis process itself. Indeed, a whole new area of investigation, the immunologic impact of the hemodialysis process, is just now being investigated and much of the early work is covered in this edition.

I am not an immunologist, so I will try to summarize the current situation as I understand it in clinical terms because I believe the implications for the future are very great indeed.

Each time a patient undergoes hemodialysis, the immunologic systems are stimulated by at least three factors: 1) blood-membrane interaction, 2) acetate infusion and 3) pyrogens in dialysis fluid. There may be additional factors as yet unidentified. The consequences of this stimulation include the familiar sequestration of leukocytes in the lung, increased production of β_2 microglobulin and a newly discovered severe catabolic reaction in skeletal muscle. This catabolic reaction was described by Jonas Bergström in a landmark presentation at the International Congress of Nephrology in London last summer (1987). Bergström and his colleagues demonstrated that sham dialysis in normal individuals caused destruction of skeletal muscle. The effect occurred at the end of the 2 h sham dialysis and persisted for at least 2 additional hours; it could account for the postdialysis fatigue syndrome. This catabolic effect was prevented when dialysis membranes that do not stimulate the immune system were substituted for cellulose membranes.

Closely related to Bergström's observation are the unpublished data from Seattle of Robertson and Ahmad. They have demonstrated a remarkable muscle weakness in even the healthiest dialysis patients. Using the maximum exercise test, they showed that muscle weakness was the limiting factor to exercise, unlike normal individuals for whom cardiac output is limiting. Furthermore, they found that curing the anemia with erythropoietin did not fully correct exercise ability, providing further confirmation of the marked degree muscle weakness of the hemodialysis patient.

Since the factors in a dialysis that are known to stimulate the immune response are all amenable to correction, they will be altered in the future provided costs per dialysis can be kept down. Thus, using compatible membranes that do not stimulate the immune system will help reduce β_2 microglobulin production and also, unlike cellulose membranes, will remove some β_2 microglobulin with each dialysis. These new membranes also will reduce the catabolic effect of each dialysis on skeletal muscle. Switching to bicarbonate dialysate and making it pyrogen-free also may further reduce the immune response to a dialysis.

The question of whether or not reducing the immune response to dialysis will help in the long run to prevent the amyloid problem, improve muscle strength and perhaps benefit the patient in other as yet unidentified ways will undoubtedly be answered in the pages of the 4th edition of this book. However, other developments of this new dialysis era already are underway and are sure to improve the quality of life of the dialysis patient by correcting hormonal deficiencies of chronic renal failure. The first of these, the introduction of $1,25-(OH)_2$ vitamin D_3, which has so greatly improved management of renal osteodystrophy is covered in detail in this edition. The second more recent development, the introduction of the renal hormone, erythropoietin, will have a major impact on patients' well being, as described in the chapter by Eschbach. As this volume goes to press, the magnitude of that impact is not yet fully appreciated because so little time has elapsed since human recombinant erythropoietin became available. Suffice it to say that the combined impact of all these developments of this new dialysis era could be so beneficial to the quality of life of dialysis patients that the decision to go for a transplant, especially a second transplant, could become very difficult indeed.

FOREWORD TO THE FIRST EDITION

BELDING H. SCRIBNER

The year was 1942 and William Kolff was hard at work perfecting the device that would not only revolutionize the treatment of renal failure, but more importantly point the way to the development of the entire field of extracorporeal devices in general and cardiac bypass devices in particular.

The enormity of the impact that Kolff's contribution was to have on medicine was revealed retrospectively to me when I recalled that in that same year, 1942, I was a second year medical student at Stanford University, taking among other things, P.J. Hanzlik's required course in pharmacology. I have two memories of that course. One was the requirement that we students learn to recognize 64 old time drugs by appearance, smell and taste. For better or worse, almost all of the 64 have disappeared from the scene. The other memory is the more pertinent one. I can still visualize the scene in the small classroom in the attic of the old red brick Stanford Lane building at Webster and Sacramento Streets. Professor Hanzlik had a pigeon for a 'patient' and had planned a dramatic demonstration. I can still hear him command one of my fellow students to 'Seize the patient!', which the student did in fear and uncertainty as the poor bird struggled against its fate. Hanzlik then proceeded with great flair and ceremony to inject some drug intended for intravenous use into the poor pigeon, where upon the bird promptly expired and Hanzlik drove home the point that intravenous therapy of any kind was dangerous and should be avoided at all costs. This 'conservative' attitude was quite consistent with that prevailing throughout the practice of medicine in that era. If intravenous therapy was dangerous, then a device for extracorporeal circulation must be an invention of the devil! Indeed, for the decade after the first clinical dialysis in Europe and Canada, acceptance was painfully slow and often resisted by all the usual techniques of those in power. During the early 60's, we encountered exactly the same kind of resistance to the concept of chronic dialysis. But as has happened over and over again in all of science, the heresy of one decade becomes the practice of the next – a phenomenon that the young heretics among the third generation readers of this volume should not forget.

And so, today Drukker, Parsons and Maher have successfully undertaken the very difficult task of bringing together in one volume all the diverse elements of dialysis therapy. The size of the volume reflects not only the magnitude of the interdisciplinary effort that brought about the technical and clinical advances, but also the many clinical and other ramifications of dialysis therapy.

In 1977, this therapy will cost the United States taxpayer nearly one billion dollars as the number of dialysis patients in the United States soars above 30,000, while the projection of the ultimate number increases from 40,000 to 60,000 and the cost projection to two billion per year by 1985. Concurrently, in the United States, the percentage of patients on home dialysis has dropped from a high of 41% in 1973 to just under 15%. This trend away from home dialysis cost the United States taxpayer an additional 150 million dollars in 1976. In an effort to control costs, the United Kingdom has increased the percentage of patients on home care to nearly 70%. In addition, the United Kingdom and perhaps other Western countries are beginning to exert subtle but effective cost control on dialyses by limiting the numbers of dialysis patients (1). In contrast, in the United States in 1977, there is no cost control on dialysis. What this contrast means to me is that dialysis is having an impact on Western medicine far beyond its significant impact on the patients, family, physicians and staff who are directly involved.

The nature and enormity of this impact began to become apparent to me in 1962 when magazine writer Shana Alexander came to Seattle to do a story on the artificial kidney. I shall always remember how incredulous I was that she did not want to see or hear about the patients whose lives had been saved – no interest there. She wanted to find out all about the 'life and death committee'. As a result, her article on the Seattle Life and Death Committee appeared in *Life Magazine* that fall (2) and set off discussion and controversy that have persisted to the present (3); indeed, the current British versus American approach to chronic dialysis is but a dramatic extension to international medicine of the basic 'who shall live' issue that was raised by the Seattle Life and Death Committee. I believe that what has happened is that dialysis has greatly accelerated the process of bringing to the forefront a basic issue in Western medicine that up to now has been kept hidden. That issue is *priorities*. Can the United States really afford to spend two billion dollars per year on dialysis? If not, who will decide to curtail expenses, and how will the decision be implemented? Significant curtailment already is being implemented in the United Kingdom by limiting the dialysis population (1). The question is how are they able to 'get away with it', and if the real truth were known, could they get away with it?

To put this issue in a different context, I believe the rapid development of dialysis marks the beginning of the end for unrestrained expansion of expensive medical technology – just as surely as the energy crisis tells us that unlimited expansion of a petroleum based Western civilization is about to come to an end. I believe that the energy crisis poses the greatest threat to democracy that has ever been posed in peacetime because the basic inability of the democratic process to cope with decisions about priorities in times of crises. Does dialysis and other very expensive technology pose a similar threat to medical free enterprise as still practiced mainly in the United States? Unless we put our house in order, I believe it does.

Let us take a brief look at another example of costly medical technology that already has overtaken dialysis in terms of total cost. Coronary by-pass surgery is currently costing Americans nearly two billion dollars per year. Preston, in a just published critique of the operation (4), points out that not only is its efficacy unproven, but he makes a strong case for the point that the economic incentives of the free enterprise system rather than medical efficacy explain why in 1975 the operation was performed on 28 patients/100,000 population in the United States in contrast to 2.1 patients/100,000 population in Western Europe.

Dialysis doctors can take comfort in the fact that at least the question of efficacy is not an issue with our expensive technology. But important and unresolved issues nag at our conscience with respect to the cost-benefit ratio of dialysis. These issues are far too complex to be resolved during the life-time of the first generation of readers of this volume and pose the ultimate challenge to the younger generations. The

clinical and technological aspects of dialysis must not remain static at the state of the art level described in this volume while the demand for costly services increases. Rather, we must build on the knowledge reviewed in this book to improve the cost-benefit ratio of our services. Meanwhile, we function as our technological advances create new social problems. And so my advice to all three generations is to try and understand and cope with a new responsibility that dialysis, because of its high cost, has introduced into the basic doctor-patient relationship. How can each of us fulfill our basic responsibility to our patients while at the same time doing everything possible to reduce the overall cost to society of this very expensive treatment?

REFERENCES

1. Distribution of nephrological services for adults in Great Britain. Report of the Executive Committee of the Renal Association. *Br Med J* 2: 903, October 16, 1976
2. Alexander S: They decide who lives, who dies. *Life Magazine*, p. 102, November 9, 1962
3. Fox RC, Swazey JP: *The courage to fail – A social view of organ transplants and dialysis*. Chapters 8, 9 and 10. University of Chicago Press, 1974
4. Preston TA: *Coronary by-pass surgery: A critical review*. Raven Press, New York, 1977

PREFACE

In this rapidly evolving field it is appropriate to update frequently our state of the art knowledge of uremia therapy. Hence, this third edition of *Replacement of Renal Function by Dialysis* appears before many of its predecessors have been destroyed by normal wear and tear over 11 and 6 years of use, respectively.

The first two editions of this book were designed to be integrated comprehensive reviews of the pertinent aspects of dialysis and related fields with sufficient clarity for the novice to learn, yet adequate depth for the expert to rely on them as encyclopedic desk references on renal replacement therapy. Based on the favorable readers' comments and reviewers' opinions these editions achieved their goal. The success of those editions is a tribute to the expertise of the authors and to the skill and dedication of my coeditors Dr. William Drukker and Dr. Frank M. Parsons, with whom it was an honor, an education and a pleasure to associate (Figure 1). When Dr. Drukker and Dr. Parsons announced their retirements, I was somewhat reluctant to undertake the task of editing this text again, especially without their capable association. Nevertheless, I felt that it was important to proceed with another edition as new information

developed. When I did not identify European colleagues who had the expertise who could expend the time and with whom I could work so smoothly, I began alone.

Although I was tempted to ask all the same authors as had written so well previously to contribute again, I realized that the new edition must be revitalized. Accordingly a fraction of the authors changed, some new topics have been added and others have been deleted. The multinational character of authorship has been maintained. Existing chapters have been rewritten thoroughly, and new authors have provided as requested a full discussion and bibliography in keeping with the previous editions.

As previously, the first half of the book emphasizes the techniques and procedures for blood purification, while clinical considerations of various types follow in the latter pages. This edition begins with a description of uremia toxicity and includes the classical chapters on the history of dialysis, now updated. New chapters dealing with technical aspects of renal replacement therapy are those on continuous arteriovenous hemofiltration, short treatment, single-needle hemodialysis and continuous ambulatory peritoneal dialysis. Other new chapters relate to the complement sys-

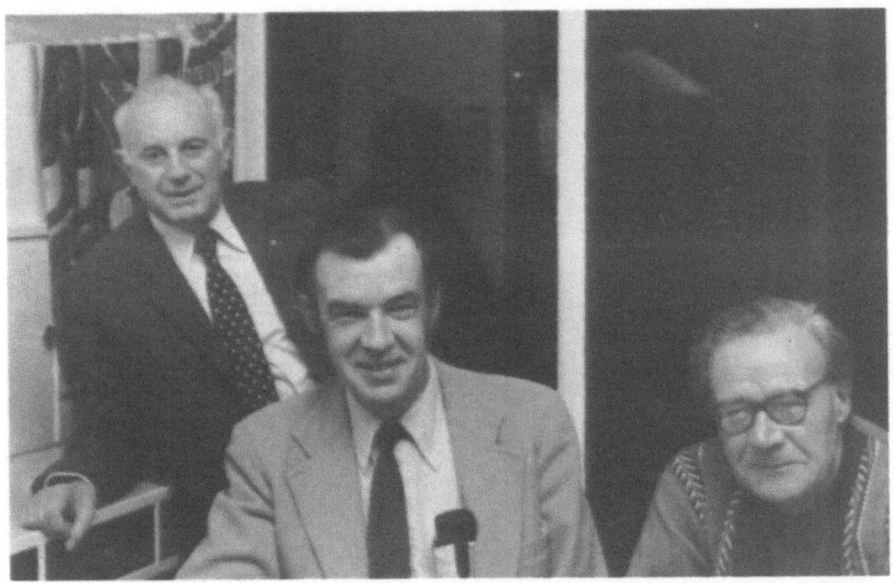

Figure 1. Dr. Drukker (standing), Dr. Parsons (sitting right), and Dr. Maher (center) during an editorial meeting in Amsterdam in 1981.

tem, acid-base homeostasis and pulmonary, gastrointestinal and oral aspects of renal failure and dialysis. The changing dialysis patient population can be appreciated by the chapters devoted to long-term survivors of dialysis treatment, diabetes mellitus, and acquired immunodeficiency syndrome. Importantly, a chapter has been added about the prevention of end-stage renal failure. Nephrologists should all strive to prevent uremia, the treatment of which provides their income.

The editor acknowledges with gratitude the excellent contributions of over 100 distinguished colleagues without whom the book would not be a reality. Included among the authors are a group of peers who have enlightened me considerably about these topics over the past few decades, as well as some younger colleagues who provide fresh insights.

The characteristic chromatogram showing peak 7C from the studies of Dr. Jonas Bergström and Dr. Peter Fürst has been kept as the symbolic cover illustration. It represents the success of our therapy and advances in our knowledge of uremia as well as the limitations of our insights and the need for further research.

The production and publication by Kluwer Academic Publishers (Martinus Nijhoff) has also been integral to the success of the book and is appreciated. Mr. B.F. Commandeur has been primarily responsible for this effort which has assisted the editor appreciably.

My colleagues, particularly Dr. P. Hirszel and Dr. E. Marks, graciously abided the distractions that editing created.

I am especially grateful to Mrs. Barbara Fitzgerald who provided outstanding secretarial assistance throughout the preparation of this edition.

Finally, adding an editing task to an already full agenda takes personal time from those who are most giving and understanding, from family. Thus, the patience, tolerance, encouragement and devotion of my wife, Marge, is most appreciated, for without it this publication would not have occurred.

JOHN F. MAHER

TABLE OF CONTENTS

CONTRIBUTING AUTHORS

Michael Adler, M.D.
Associate Professor
Department of Gastroenterology
Université Libre de Bruxelles
Chef de Clinique
Department of Gastroenterology
C.U.B. Hôpital Erasme
Brussels, Belgium
Chapter 39

Allen C. Alfrey, M.D.
Professor of Medicine
University of Colorado
Chief of Renal Section
Veterans Administration Medical Center
Denver, CO USA
Chapter 49

Anthony J.F. d'Apice, M.D., FRACP, FRCPA
Assistant Director
Department of Nephrology
Royal Melbourne Hospital
Victoria, Australia
Chapter 27

Conrad A. Baldamus, M.D.
Professor, Internal Medicine and Nephrology
Medizinische Universitätsklinik I
University Hospital
Cologne, FRG
Chapter 14

Claudio Bazzi, M.D.
Assistant, Division of Nephrology
San Carlo Hospital
Milan, Italy
Chapter 30

Christopher R. Blagg, M.D., FRCP
Professor of Medicine
University of Washington, Seattle
Director Northwest Kidney Center
Seattle, WA USA
Chapter 33

Juan Bosch, M.D.
Professor of Medicine
Director of Renal Diseases
George Washington University Medical Center
Washington, DC USA
Chapter 15

Michel J.C. Broyer, M.D.
Professor of Pediatrics
Necker's School of Medicine
Université Paris V
Director, Pediatric Nephrology
Hôpital des Enfants Malades-Necker
Paris, France
Chapter 32

Felix P. Brunner, M.D.
Professor of Medicine
University of Basel
Department of Internal Medicine
Kantonsspital
Basel, Switzerland
Chapter 31

Hans O.A. Brynger, M.D., Ph. D.
Associate Professor of Surgery
University of Göteborg
Director Transplant Unit
Sahlgren's Hospital
Göteborg, Sweden
Chapter 31

Vardaman M. Buckalew, Jr., M.D.
Professor of Medicine and Physiology
Chief of Nephrology
Department of Medicine
Bowman Gray School of Medicine
of Wake Forest University
Winston-Salem, NC USA
Chapter 55

John M. Burkart, M.D.
Assistant Professor of Medicine
Bowman Gray School of Medicine
of Wake Forest University
Medical Director, Piedmont Dialysis Center
Winston-Salem, NC USA
Chapter 55

Cyril Chantler, M.A., M.D., FRCP
Professor Paediatric Nephrology
Evelina Children's Department
United Medical and Dental Schools of
Guy's and St. Thomas's Hospitals
Guy's Hospital
London, England
Chapter 32

Stefano Chiaramonte, M.D.
Associate of Clinical Nephrology
Department of Nephrology
St. Bortolo Hospital
Vicenza, Italy
Chapter 37

Jack W. Coburn, M.D.
Professor of Medicine
University of California, Los Angeles
Nephrology Section
Veterans Administration Wadsworth Medical Center
Los Angeles, CA USA
Chapter 44

Jean Crosnier, M.D.
Professeur
Université René Descartes
Faculte de Médecine Necker Enfants-Malades
Clinique Néphrologique
Hôpital Necker
Paris, Cedex, France
Chapter 42

Nancy Boucot Cummings, M.D.
Associate Director for Research
and Assessment, NIDDK
National Institutes of Health
Bethesda, MD USA
Chapter 57

Giuseppe D'Amico, M.D.
Professor of Medicine
University of Milan
Head, Division of Nephrology
San Carlo Hospital
Milan, Italy
Chapter 30

Norman Deane, M.D.
Chairman, Section on Nephrology
Doctors Hospital
Director Manhattan Kidney Center
New York, NY USA
Chapter 18

Wilfried A. De Backer, M.D.
Pulmonary Medicine Division
University Hospital Antwerp
Antwerp, Belgium
Chapter 38

Marc E. De Broe, M.D., Ph. D.
Professor of Medicine
University of Antwerp
Director Nephrology Division
University Hospital Antwerp
Antwerp, Belgium
Chapter 38

Françoise Degos M.D.
Service d'Hépatologie
Hôpital Beaujon
Clichy, France
Chapter 42

Barbara G. Delano, M.D.
Associate Professor of Clinical Medicine
Director-Home Dialysis Program
State University of New York
Health Science Center at Brooklyn
Brooklyn, NY USA
Chapter 29

Raymond A. Donckerwolcke, M.D.
Pediatric Nephrologist
Department of Pediatrics
University of Utrecht
Director, Dialysis and Transplant Program
Wilhelmina Children's Hospital
Utrecht, The Netherlands
Chapter 32

William Drukker, M.D.
Formerly Reader in Dialysis
Department of Medicine Queen Wilhelmina
University Hospital, Amsterdam
Emeritus Director Department of Nephrology and Dialysis
St. Lucas Hospital, Amsterdam
Present Address: De Lairessestraat 75
1071 NV Amsterdam, The Netherlands
Chapters 3, 19, 22

Sheila R. Dykes
Administrator
EDTA Registry
St. Thomas Hospital
London, England
Chapter 31

Joseph W. Eschbach, M.D.
Clinical Professor of Medicine
Division of Nephrology
Department of Medicine
University of Washington
Seattle, WA USA
Chapter 40

Aldo Fabris, M.D.
Associate of Clinical Nephrology
Department of Nephrology
St. Bortolo Hospital
Vicenza, Italy
Chapter 37

Winfried Fassbinder, M.D.
Professor of Nephrology
University Hospital
Frankfurt am Main
Head, Department of Nephrology
Städtische Klinikum
Fulda, FRG
Chapter 31

Mariano Feriani, M.D.
Associate of Clinical Nephrology
Department of Nephrology
St. Bortolo Hospital
Vicenza, Italy
Chapter 37

Eli A. Friedman, M.D.
Professor of Medicine
Chief, Renal Diseases Division
State University of New York
Health Science Center at Brooklyn
Brooklyn, NY USA
Chapter 54

Peter W. Gardner, B.S.
Chief Research Technician
Dialysis Unit, Nephrology Section
Medical Service, Wadsworth Division
West Los Angeles Veterans Administration Medical Center
Los Angeles, CA USA
Chapter 16

Ram Gokal, M.D., FRCP
Consultant Nephrologist
Honorary Lecturer
University of Manchester
Manchester Royal Infirmary
Manchester, England
Chapter 25

Frank A. Gotch, M.D.
Associate Clinical Professor of Medicine
University of California, San Francisco
Medical Director
Dialysis Treatment and Research Center
Davies Medical Center
San Francisco, CA USA
Chapter 4

Hans J. Gurland, M.D.
Professor, Director Nephrology Division
Medical Department I. Klinikum Grosshadern
University of Munich
München, FRG
Chapter 21

Robert W. Hamilton, M.D.
Associate Professor of Medicine
Bowman Gray School of Medicine
of Wake Forest University
Medical Director, Dialysis Unit
North Carolina Baptist Hospital
Winston-Salem, NC USA
Chapter 55

Lee W. Henderson, M.D.
Professor of Medicine
University of California, San Diego
Veterans Administration Medical Center
San Diego, CA USA
Chapter 13

Robert J. Heyka, M.D.
Medical Director – CCF West Side Dialysis Center
Department of Hypertension/Nephrology
The Cleveland Clinic Foundation
Cleveland, OH USA
Chapter 34

Nicholas A. Hoenich, Ph.D.
Lecturer in Clinical Science
Department of Medicine
Medical School
Newcastle upon Tyne, England
Chapters 5, 17

Peter Ivanovich, M.D.
Professor of Medicine
Section of Nephrology
Northwestern University Medical School
Director of Hemodialysis
Department of Medicine, Section of Nephrology
Veterans Administration Lakeside Medical Center
Chicago, IL USA
Chapter 6

Stefan Jacobson, M.D., Ph.D.
Assistant Professor, Institute of Medicine
Karolinska Institute
Associate Physician
Division of Nephrology, Department of Medicine
Karolinska Hospital
Stockholm, Sweden
Chapter 26

Frans G.I. Jennekens, M.D.
Senior Neurologist
Head of the Laboratory for Neuromuscular Diseases
Department of Neurology
University Hospital Utrecht
Utrecht, The Netherlands
Chapter 46

Aagje Jennekens-Schinkel, M.D.
Neuropsychologist, Department of Neuropsychology
University Hospital Leiden
Leiden, The Netherlands
Chapter 46

Paul Jungers, M.D.
Départment de Néphrologie
Hôpital Necker
Paris, France
Chapter 42

William F. Keane, M.D.
Professor of Medicine
University of Minnesota School of Medicine
Division of Nephrology
Hennepin County Medical Center
Minneapolis, MN USA
Chapter 41

Prakash R. Keshaviah, Ph.D.
Senior Research Associate
University of Minnesota, Department of Medicine
Director of Dialysis Regional Kidney Disease Program
Hennepin County Medical Center
Minneapolis, MN USA
Chapters 7, 12

Carl M. Kjellstrand, M.D., FACP
Professor of Medicine and Surgery
University of Minnesota
Chief, Division of Nephrology
Department of Medicine
Karolinska Hospital
Stockholm, Sweden
Chapter 26

Franciszek Kokot, M.D.
Professor of Medicine
Department of Nephrology
Silesian School of Medicine
Katowice, Poland
Chapter 45

Giuseppe La Greca, M.D.
Professor of Medicine
Director of Department of Nephrology
St. Bortolo Hospital
Vicenza, Italy
Chapter 37

Robert MacGregor Lindsay, M.D., FRCP(E), FRCP(C), FACP
Professor, Department of Medicine
The University of Western Ontario
Director of the Renal Unit
Department of Medicine
Victoria Hospital Corporation
London, Ontario, Canada
Chapter 11

Lars-Eric Lins, M.D., Ph.D.
Associate Professor, Institute of Medicine
Karolinska Institute
Senior Physician
Division of Nephrology, Department of Medicine
Karolinska Hospital
Stockholm, Sweden
Chapter 26

Robert R. Lins, M.D.
Director Nephrology Division
General Hospital Stuivenberg
Antwerp, Belgium
Chapter 38

Francisco Llach, M.D.
Professor of Medicine
University of Oklahoma Health Sciences Center
Veterans Administration Hospital
Nephrology Section
Oklahoma City, OK USA
Chapter 44

A. Peter Lundin, M.D.
Associate Professor of Medicine
State University of New York
Health Science Center at Brooklyn
Brooklyn, NY USA
Chapter 56

Michael M. Maddy, M.D.
Fellow in Nephrology
Department of Medicine
Hennepin County Medical Center
Minneapolis, MN USA
Chapter 41

John F. Maher, M.D., FACP
Professor of Medicine
Director, Nephrology Division
F. Edward Hébert School of Medicine
Uniformed Services University of the Health Sciences
Bethesda, MD USA
Chapters 1, 35, 51

Timothy H. Mathew, M.D., B.S., FRACP
Director Renal Unit
Queen Elizabeth Hospital
Adelaide, S.A., Australia
Chapter 28

Joseph H. Miller, M.D.
Associate Research Renologist
Department of Medicine
University of California at Los Angeles
Chief, Dialysis Instrumentation
Dialysis Unit, Nephrology Section
Medical Service, Wadsworth Division
West Los Angeles Veterans Administration Medical Center
Los Angeles, CA USA
Chapter 16

Charles M. Mion, M.D.
Professor of Medicine, Head Division of Nephrology
University Hospital Montpellier
Service de Néphrologie, Hôpital Saint-Charles
Montpellier, France
Chapter 24

William E. Mitch, M.D.
Professor of Medicine
Director, Renal Division
Department of Medicine
Emory University School of Medicine
Atlanta, GA USA
Chapter 53

S. Fazal Mohammad, Ph.D
Associate Professor of Pathology
University of Utah
Director, Hematology Laboratories
Institute for Biomedical Engineering
Division of Artificial Organs
Salt Lake City, UT USA
Chapter 10

John F. Moorhead, FRCP
Director
Department of Nephrology and Transplantation
The Royal Free Hospital
London, England
Chapter 36

Salim K. Mujais, M.D.
Assistant Professor of Medicine
Section of Nephrology
Northwestern University Medical School
Staff Physician
Department of Medicine, Section of Nephrology
Veterans Administration Lakeside Medical Center
Chicago, IL USA
Chapter 6

Karl D. Nolph, M.D.
Professor of Medicine
Director, Division of Nephrology
University of Missouri Health Sciences Center
Harry S. Truman Memorial Veterans Administration Hospital
Columbia, MO USA
Chapter 23

Emil Paganini, M.D., FACP
Head, Section of Dialysis and Extracorporeal Therapy
Department of Hypertension/Nephrology
The Cleveland Clinic Foundation
Cleveland, OH USA
Chapter 34

Bettine C.P. Polak, M.D.
Lecturer in Opthalmology
Erasmus University
Eye Hospital
Rotterdam, The Netherlands
Chapter 47

Manfred Pollok, M.D.
Senior Resident
Department of Nephrology
Medizinische Klinik I.
University Hospital
Cologne, FRG
Chapter 14

David S. Precious, M.D.
Chairman, Department of Oral Diagnosis and Oral Surgery
Dalhousie University
Halifax, Nova Scotia, Canada
Chapter 48

T.K. Sreepada Rao, M.D., FACP
Associate Professor of Medicine
Director of Hemodialysis
State University of New York
Brooklyn, NY USA
Chapter 43

Severin G. Ringoir, M.D.
Professor of Medicine
University of Ghent
Director, Division of Nephrology
University Hospital
Ghent, Belgium
Chapters 2, 17

Gianfranco Rizzoni M.D.
Head, Division of Nephrology and Dialysis
Department of Pediatric Research and Teaching
Ospedale Bambino Jesu
Rome, Italy
Chapter 32

Claudio Ronco, M.D.
Associate of Clinical Nephrology
Department of Nephrology
St. Bortolo Hospital
Vicenza, Italy
Chapters 15, 37

Walter Samtleben, M.D.
Privat Dozent, Nephrology Division
Medical Department I. Klinikum Grosshadern
University of Munich
München, FRG
Chapter 21

John A. Sargent, Ph.D.
Quantitative Medical Systems, Inc.
Emeryville, CA USA
Chapter 4

Ad C. Schoots, Ph.D.
Senior Researcher Analytical Biochemistry
Laboratory for Instrumental Analysis
Faculty of Chemical Engineering
Eindhoven University of Technology
Eindhoven, The Netherlands
Chapter 2

Belding H. Scribner, M.D.
Professor of Medicine
Division of Nephrology
University of Washington
Seattle, WA USA
Forewords to the First and Third Edition

Neville H. Selwood, M.D.
Deputy Director
UK Transplant Service
Southmead Hospital
Bristol, England
Chapter 31

Stanley Shaldon, M.A., M.D. (Cantab), MRCP
Professor of Nephrology
Université de Nimes
Centre Hospitalier Regional, Service de Néphrologie
Nimes, France
Chapter 12

James H. Shinaberger, M.D.
Adjunct Professor of Medicine
University of California, Los Angeles
Chief, Dialysis Program
Dialysis Unit, Nephrology Section
Medical Service, Wadsworth Division
West Los Angeles Veterans Administration Medical Center
Los Angeles, CA USA
Chapter 16

Anne M. Smith, B.Sc., M.B.Ch.B.; MRCP(UK), FRCP(C)
Clinical Assistant Professor of Medicine
The University of Western Ontario
Laboratory Hematology, and Oncology
Victoria Hospital Corporation
London Regional Cancer Centre
London, Ontario, Canada
Chapter 11

Theodore I. Steinman, M.D.
Associate Clinical Professor of Medicine
Harvard Medical School
Director Dialysis Unit
Beth Israel Hospital
Boston, MA USA
Chapter 53

William Kinnear Stewart, M.D., Ph.D., FRCP(Lond), FRCP(Edin)
Reader in Medicine
University of Dundee
Hon. Consultant Physician
General Medicine (special interest Nephrology)
Royal Infirmary
Dundee, Scotland
Chapter 8

Paul Sweny, M.D., FRCP
Senior Lecturer
Department of Nephrology and Transplantation
Royal Free Hospital Medical School
London, England
Chapter 36

Nicholas E. Tawa Jr., M.D.
Clinical Fellow in Surgery
Harvard Medical School
Resident in Surgery
Brigham and Women's Hospital
Boston, MA USA
Chapter 7

Nicholas L. Tilney, M.D.
Professor of Surgery
Director, Surgical Research Laboratories
Harvard Medical School
Director, Transplant Service
Brigham and Women's Hospital
Boston, MA USA
Chapter 9

Charles R.V. Tomson, M.B., B.S., MRCP
Medical Research Council Training Fellow
Department of Medicine
University of Newcastle upon Tyne
Royal Victoria Infirmary
Newcastle upon Tyne, England
Chapter 50

Charles Toussaint, M.D.
Professor
Department of Clinical Medicine, Nephrology
Université Libre de Bruxelles
Head, Nephrology Department
C.U.B. Hôpital Erasme
Brussels, Belgium
Chapter 39

John E. Utting, M.A. M.B., B. Chir., FFARCS
Professor of Anaesthesia
The University of Liverpool
The University Department of Anaesthesia
Royal Liverpool Hospital
Liverpool, England
Chapter 52

Albert W.J. van Doorn, Ph.D.
Scientific Consultant
Arnhem, The Netherlands
Chapter 19

Raymond Vanholder, M.D., Ph.D.
Instructor, Renal Division
University of Ghent
Associate, Renal Division
University Hospital
Ghent, Belgium
Chapters 2, 17

Zachariah Varghese, Ph.D.
Associate Director
Renal Research Unit
Royal Free Hospital
London, England
Chapter 36

Rowan G. Walker, M.D., B.S., FRACP
Director, Dialysis and Transplantation
Royal Childrens Hospital
Victoria, Australia
Chapter 27

Michael K. Ward, M.B., B.S., FRCP
Consultant Physician/Senior Lecturer in Medicine
University of Newcastle upon Tyne
Royal Victoria Infirmary
Newcastle upon Tyne, England
Chapter 50

David C. Wheeler, M.B., Ch.B., MRCP
MRC Training Fellow
Renal Research Unit
Department of Nephrology and Transplantation
The Royal Free Hospital
London, England
Chapter 36

Andrzej Wiȩcek, M.D.
Department of Nephrology
Silesian School of Medicine
Katowice, Poland
Chapter 45

James F. Winchester, M.D.
Professor of Medicine
Director of Dialysis
Division of Nephrology
Georgetown University Medical Center
Washington, DC USA
Chapter 20

Robert Wineman, Ph.D.
Director of Special Projects
National Nephrology Foundation
New York, NY USA
Chapter 18

Antony J. Wing, M.A., D.M., FRCP
Consulting Physcian
St. Thomas' Hospital
London, England
Chapter 31

Celia Woffindin, B.Sc.
Scientific Officer
Renal Unit
Royal Victoria Infirmary
Newcastle upon Tyne, England
Chapter 5

26

ACUTE RENAL FAILURE

CARL M. KJELLSTRAND, STEFAN JACOBSON and LARS-ERIC LINS

INTRODUCTION

The introduction of the artificial kidney into clinical practice in 1943 by Kolff in the Netherlands, and in 1947 by Alwall in Sweden and Murray in Canada was an astounding technical breakthrough in modern medicine (1–3). Subsequently, the most frequent abnormality for which dialysis had been used acutely, has been acute tubular necrosis. It accounts for approximately two-thirds of all patients dialyzed for acute renal failure.

Since 1950 many groups have presented their clinical experiences with large series of patients (4–10). (The historical development of dialysis is described in Chapters 3 and 22.)

Despite many technical improvements in the care of these patients, the basic treatment with dialysis has remained the same. Unfortunately, the mortality rate in patients with acute tubular necrosis, except for some early gains (11), has not improved. It remains between 30 and 80% depending mainly on the severity of the underlying precipitating event. On the other hand, the one year mortality rate of patients dialyzed for chronic renal failure has decreased from 50% to 15% over the last 20 years. The lower mortality rate in patients treated by dialysis for chronic renal failure reflects technical improvements of the dialysis procedure. The lack of improvement of mortality in patients with acute renal failure can probably be explained by a much sicker patient population now, than those treated in the early days of hemodialysis. Many milder cases of acute tubular necrosis are now treated with improved fluid management, cardiovascular monitoring and potent diuretics. Thus, the patients who now come to dialysis have more serious disease.

This chapter touches on the major causes and treatments for acute renal failure. Most of the discussion however, will center on acute tubular necrosis, on dialysis treatment and important aspects of conservative management of patients with this disease.

INCIDENCE OF ACUTE RENAL FAILURE, NEED FOR DIALYSIS

The European Dialysis and Transplant Association, in a 1982 survey, from 32 countries, found a mean of 28.9 (range 0.4 to 177.1) patients per million population per year who required dialysis for acute renal failure (17). As only centers, performing chronic dialysis were questioned, the true incidence is probably higher. Several studies of acute renal failure, have concluded that 30 to 60 patients per million population need dialysis yearly (12–16).

The clinical course of these patients is swift, typically requiring only four dialysis (10) before death or recovery occurs, almost always within one month. Thus, in industrialised countries approximately 200 dialyses per million population per year are needed for acute renal failure.

For every patient with acute renal failure who requires dialysis, 10 to 12 patients with milder forms of renal insufficiency are managable by conservative treatment (17).

CAUSES OF ACUTE RENAL FAILURE, GENERAL WORKUP OF PATIENTS

The most common disease, leading to acute renal failure, is acute tubular necrosis, responsible for about 80% of such cases. Of these $^{1}/_{4}$ acutely exacerbate underlying chronic renal disease. Approximately 12% of these patients have primary parenchymal disease (glomerulonephritis, vasculitis, other immunological diseases, hemolytic – uremic syndrome, interstitial nephritis). Five percent of the patients (Figure 1) have postrenal obstruction (4–15).

Over the 4 decades acute dialysis has been available, there has been little change in the relative frequency of the diseases causing acute renal failure. However, with time there has been a marked change in the causes of acute tubular necrosis (Figure 2). Before the mid-1970's, surgery and trauma were the most common cause of acute tubular necrosis (18). Now it is usually secondary to such medical disorders as volume contraction and decreased cardiac output) and from

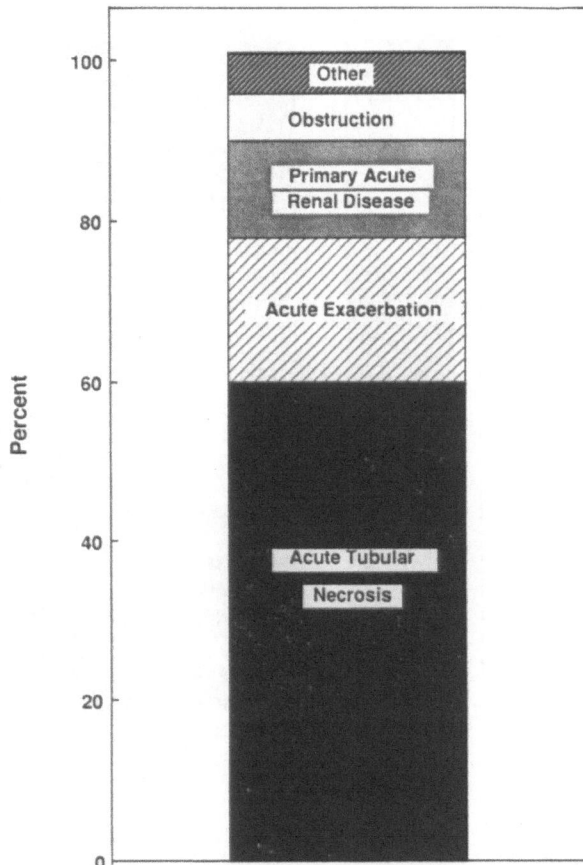

Figure 1. The most common cause of acute renal failure is acute tubular necrosis followed by acute exacerbation of chronic underlying renal failure. Data from over 1,000 patients dialyzed at University of Lund and Minnesota. The causes of acute renal failure are the same in the mid-1950's and late 1970's.

iatrogenic toxins: antibiotics, nonsteroidal anti-inflammatory drugs, contrast media and antihypertensives (17, 18).

Symptomatic and supportive treatments are usually all that can be offered to patients with acute renal failure. Despite suggestions that early treatment of tubular necrosis may change its natural course, the main-stay of treatment is supportive while awaiting spontaneous recovery of renal function. The same is true for most patients with an acute exacerbation of chronic renal failure. When urinary obstruction occurs, urinary flow must be reestablished, e.g. through surgery, in order to achieve return of renal function. Similarly, when the kidney is underperfused, this abnormality must be corrected.

Renal cortical necrosis exemplifies lesions that begin acutely, require considerable supportive management, do not respond to any treatment and result in severe persistent impairment of renal function.

Patients who suffer from such parenchymal renal diseases as glomerulonephritis, Goodpasture's syndrome, hemolyt-

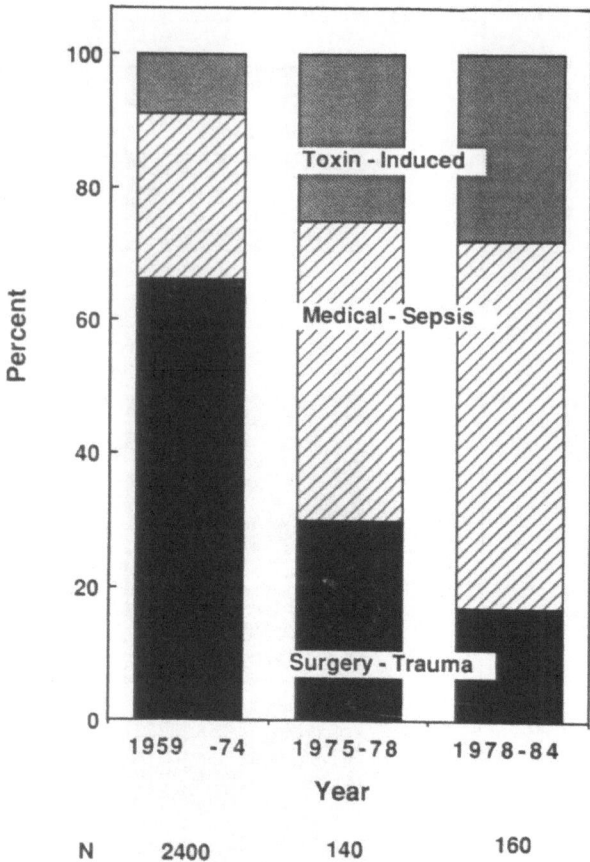

Figure 2. The most common cause of acute tubular necrosis has changed from surgery and trauma to medical including sepsis and toxin-induced renal failure. In the early days, patients with surgery and trauma made up two-thirds of all patients with acute tubular necrosis. Now two-thirds are due to medical disease. Own data and from references (4–19).

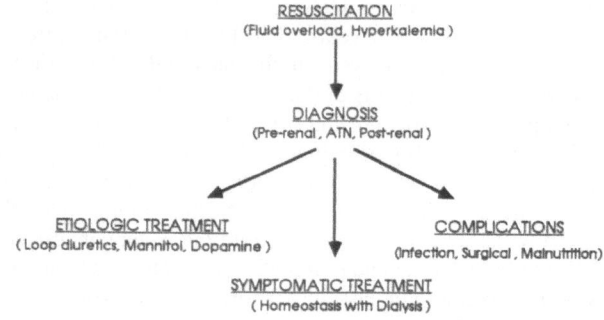

Figure 3. Schedule of approach to management of patients with acute renal failure.

The rest of this chapter will be devoted to acute tubular necrosis. However, the symptomatic and supportive treatments apply to all patients with acute renal failure.

Figure 3 outlines the basic approach when a patient develops acute renal failure. Immediate dangers in such patients include fluid overload with pulmonary edema and hyperkalemia with cardiac arrest. After guarding against these, the diagnosis is ascertained, differentiating pre-and post-renal failure from acute tubular necrosis. Treatment with fluid or cardiotonics or both in the patients with pre-renal failure, removal of obstruction in those with post-renal failure, and possibly a trial of renal vasodilator-diuretics in the patient with tubular necrosis is then undertaken. Should these efforts fail, homeostasis is maintained with dialysis, and a constant watch for specific complications is instituted.

PATHOGENESIS, PATHOPHYSIOLOGY, AND DIFFERENTIAL DIAGNOSIS OF ACUTE RENAL FAILURE

Experimental studies

The etiology, pathogenesis and pathophysiology of acute tubular necrosis are of interest in experimental research. Ideally, an animal model should meet several criteria. The initiating factors should be identical to those operating in acute tubular necrosis in humans, a situation where multiple factors are usually involved. Secondly, it should be possible to determine the transition point from subclinical renal illness to clinical acute renal failure, the point of no return. Five models presently used frequently are: renal artery constriction, intrarenal norepinephrine, intramuscular glycerol, mercuric chloride and uranyl nitrate. None of these models mimics accurately most situations causing tubular necrosis in humans and the interpretation of the results is still a matter of debate. The pathogenesis of acute renal failure could involve perpetuated renal ischemia, decreased filtration through a changed glomerular membrane or tubular dysfunction with a backleak of normally filtered tubular fluid, alone or in various combinations. Acute renal failure can occur with morphologically preserved but functionally dam-

ic-uremic syndrome, acute interstitial nephritis or vasculitis, pose a particularly difficult and unresolved dilemma. All etiologic treatments of these disorders, such as immunosuppression, corticosteroids, anticoagulation, and plasmapheresis, carry considerable risk in both morbidity and mortality. There is as yet no satisfactory answer of what treatment is best for most of these patients. In the rare patient who suffers from systemic disease with life threatening involvement of other organs systems, the solution is easy. Almost any form of treatment that may benefit the patient, should be tried.

When the manifestations of the disease are only renal, however, the benefits and dangers of combinations of immunosuppression, prednisone, anticoagulation and plasma and cyta-pheresis must be weighed against the low mortality rate in patients with chronic renal failure treated by dialysis. Astounding successes have been achieved in individual cases but mortality has also resulted from such treatment.

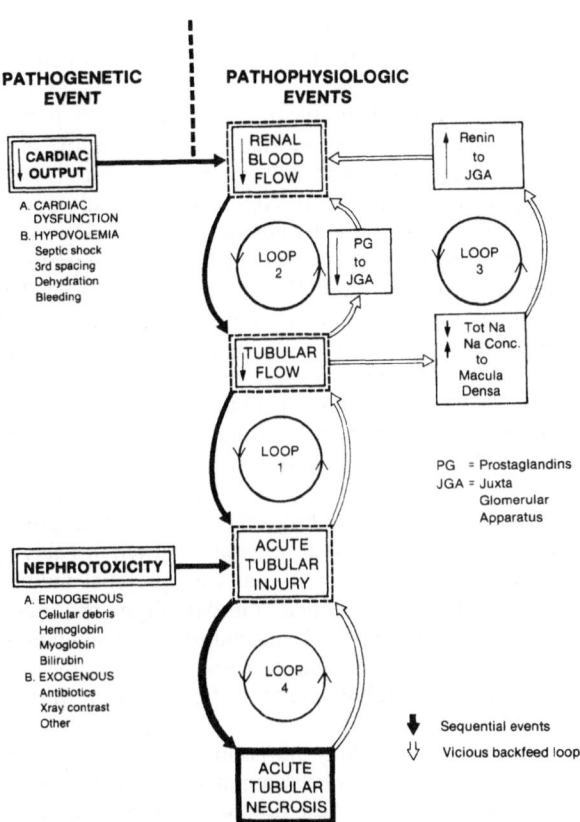

PG = Prostaglandins
JGA = Juxta
        Glomerular
        Apparatus

Figure 4. A summary of the pathogenic and pathyphysiologic events that follow ischemic or nephrotoxic insult to the kidneys in the clinical situation. Four vicious feedback loops perpetuate or aggravate decreased tubular flow and tubular cell injury. Through loop 2 and loop 3, the renal ischemia may be perpetuated. Nephrotoxicity can feed back through loop 1 to decrease tubular flow and then decrease renal blood flow. Loop 4 consists of intracellular perpetuating mechanisms such as oxygen-free radicals, influx of calcium ions with mitochondrial damage and further calcium influx.

aged tubules, or involve frank necrosis of the tubular epithelium. When tubular cell necrosis occurs, the tubular cell may be shed off its basement membrane and potentially cause obstruction with increased intraluminal hydrostatic pressure. Almost any of these events can be found at one point or another in the various models described above. It has become clear that none of them very faithfully mimic the human situation, that seems to evolve through many stages (19–25). However, at least two animal models combine ischemia and nephrotoxicity; both show a synergistic detrimental effect on renal function (26, 27).

Clinical studies

Figure 4 summarizes factors precipitating and perpetuating acute tubular necrosis. There may be two principal initiating events, ischemia and nephrotoxicity. Clinically, there is almost always a mixture of these factors. Thus, nephrotoxic proteins such as myoglobin and hemoglobin may cause both

direct tubular damage and ischemia or obstruction. Conversely, factors that cause ischemia may lead to release of nephrotoxic substances such as myoglobin or nephrotoxic drugs may be given to the patient.

A number of factors cause renal ischemia without necessarily decreasing systemic blood pressure. These include dehydration secondary to burns, edema into nontraumatized tissue, diarrhea, vomiting and sequestration of extracellular fluid due to ileus or retroperitoneally in such conditions as acute pancreatitis or after surgery. Similarly, any decrement in cardiac output following myocardial dysfunction or reduction of the circulating blood volume or the ratio of blood volume to capacitance of the vascular system such as may occur in gram negative bacterial sepsis, endotoxemia or anaphylactic reactions, can also cause tubular necrosis. Surgery and general anesthesia uniformly decrease renal blood flow.

Almost no critically ill patients escape treatment with drugs that are potentially nephrotoxic. Aminoglycoside and cephalosporin antibiotics are used especially frequently in this circumstance. Increasingly, diagnostic procedures also cause problems such as nephropathy following contrast radiography (28). Self inflicted intoxication with such substances as ethylene glycol and carbon tetrachloride is less frequent. Certain endogenously produced substances such as uric acid, calcium, myoglobin and hemoglobin, are also potentially nephrotoxic.

Patients developing tubular necrosis are usually exposed to several pathogenic factors. For example, after cardiovascular surgery, where both the operation and the anesthesia contribute to decreased renal blood flow, cardiac output may be decreased and nephrotoxic drugs may be administered. After cross clamping the aorta for repair of an abdominal aneurysm, nephrotoxic antibiotics are frequently used, sequestration of fluid may decrease cardiac output, internal hemorrhage may occur and ischemic muscle may release myoglobin.

In a clinical analysis of 145 patients who developed acute tubular necrosis, there was more than one insult in 74% of them (29).

Differential diagnosis

In most instances, tubular necrosis is easily distinguished from prerenal failure and obstruction. The differential diagnosis is made by history, review of the patient's charts, clinical investigation and frequently confirmed by a series of radiological and laboratory tests.

The history and the patient's records often reveal clues to identify the correct diagnosis. For example, patients with prerenal failure may have had water and electrolyte losses from diarrhea and have received insufficient fluid in relation to losses. If body weight has been recorded, it shows a decrease. A previous history of stones or cancer in or near the genitourinary tract should raise the suspicion of urinary obstruction. Joint pain, rashes, or other organ involvement should suggest such diagnoses as lupus erythematous, vasculitis, anaphylactoid purpura or acute interstitial nephritis

Cathastrophic surgical events, sepsis, shock and oliguria, in spite of marked weight gain due to inappropriate fluid management, often precede tubular necrosis.

It used to be believed that urinary volume was a good indicator of kidney function and that acute tubular necrosis was usually signalled by oliguria. It has been increasingly recognized, however, that polyuria is common in acute tubular necrosis, particularly when caused by antibiotics. Even more confusing is the finding that patients with severe dehydration and prerenal failure may continue to make large amounts of urine (30). Patients with partial urinary tract obstruction also may have normal or increased urinary output. However, absolute anuria, particularly when interspersed with episodes of polyuria, suggests obstruction.

On physical examination, the patient with marked prerenal failure shows sunken eyes, central venous and pulmonary wedge pressures are low, skin turgor is decreased and orthostatic hypotension is present. These classical findings of extracellular fluid volume depletion may be absent, however, in some patients who have prerenal azotemia due to a decreased cardiac output (with markedly increased total body water because of edema). This is most commonly encountered in patients with heart failure secondary to myocardial infarction or after heart surgery for valve replacement or coronary artery bypass. A septic patient also may suffer a sudden decrease in effective blood volume secondary to decreased tone of capacitance vessels without a decrease in total body fluid volume.

There is no typical physical finding in patients with tubular necrosis. Many such patients, however, have signs of fluid overload (edema, fluid lung or frank pulmonary edema) secondary to inappropriate fluid management. Patients with urinary obstruction may have a large urinary bladder or a pelvic mass or both.

Radiological procedures are often helpful, particularly in diagnosing obstruction. Thus, ultrasonography, intravenous pyelography, computerized axial tomography or radioisotope renography with or without furosemide administration demonstrate a dilated renal pelvis, particularly when delayed imaging is also used.

Ultrasonography of the obstructed kidney gives particularly accurate diagnostic information. It has a low incidence of false positive and false negative findings. Some cases, however, require cystoscopy and retrograde or antegrade pyelography for a definite diagnosis (31–33).

Radiologic tests are less useful in differentiating prerenal failure and tubular necrosis. The kidneys tend to be small in prerenal failure and enlarged in acute tubular necrosis, but this is an unreliable sign. Radiologic examination of the chest is very important, however, for the diagnosis of fluid overload in the lungs. Some patients have a low cardiac output but marked increase in total body water so that, paradoxically, they suffer both fluid excess and prerenal failure.

The numerous diagnostic tests used to differentiate prerenal failure from acute tubular necrosis are listed in Table 1. The physiologic hypothesis is that with prerenal failure, glomerular filtrate is modified considerably by the intact tubules under maximum ADH and aldosterone stimulation. To the contrary, with tubular necrosis or urinary tract obstruction, the renal tubule modifies the glomerular filtrate very little.

The literature regarding the accuracy of these tests is confusing and has recently been summarized (34, 35). When first described, many of these tests were considered highly accurate, but later were found to be of very limited or no use, a frequent fate of medical tests (36). There is also no unanimity regarding the values that differentiate acute tubular necrosis from prerenal failure. For example, the urine sodium concentration or the urine to plasma creatinine concentration ratio reported to be suggestive of acute tubular necrosis varies almost ten-fold.

The fractional excretion of sodium (FE_{Na}) was earlier thought to be an almost infalliable test to differentiate acute

Table 1. Differential diagnosis between pre-renal failure and acute tubular necrosis.

Test	Pre-renal failure	Acute tubular necrosis
Urinary specific gravity	>1.030	<1.020
Urinary osmolality	>400 mOsm/kg/H_2O	<350 mOsm/kg/H_2O
Urine/plasma osmolal ratio	>1.4	<1.1
Urine/plasma creatinine ratio	>30	<20
Urine/plasma urea ratio	>7	<5
Serum urea N/creatinine ratio	>10	<10
Urinary sodium concentration	<30 mmol/l	>30 mmol/l
Excreted/filtered sodium	<1%	>2%
Renal failure index	<1	>1
Free water clearance	Negative	Rising to 0
2 h creatinine clearance	Stable	Falling
Urinary sediment	Hyaline or finely granular casts	Tubular cell casts Coarse granular casts
Proteinuria	0+ to 1+	1+ to 2+

These tests for distinguishing between pre-renal failure and acute tubular necrosis are nonspecific and should be used only as a part of the global clinical evaluation of the patients.

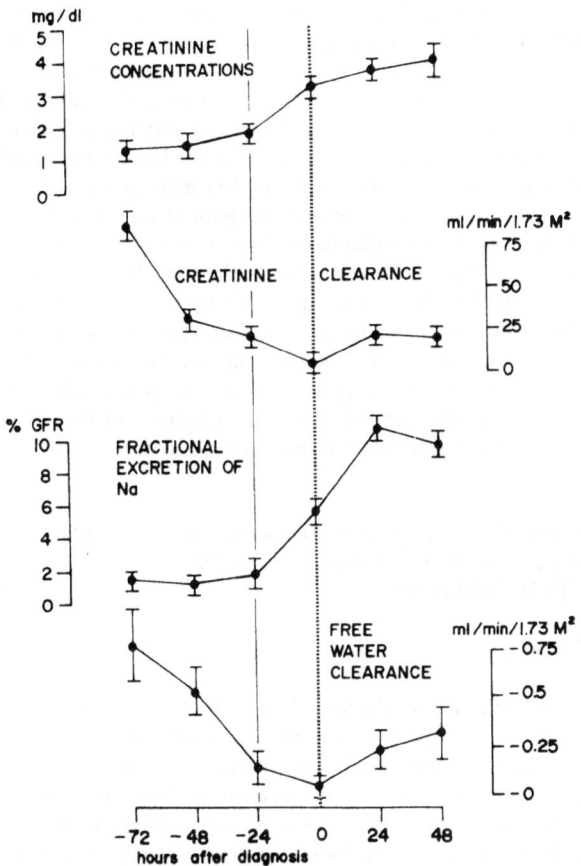

Figure 5. Serial changes in tests of renal function in 13 patients followed prospectively and who developed acute renal failure. The dotted vertical line indicates the time when three of the four criteria for renal failure were met (free water clearance higher than 0 ml/min, creatinine clearance less than 30 ml/min, FE_{Na} more than 3%, and persistently rising serum creatinine). The solid vertical line indicates the time, 24 hours earlier, when the diagnosis of acute renal failure was established by changes in creatinine clearance and free water clearance. These two latter parameters change earlier than FE_{Na} or serum creatinine concentration. One must do repeated tests for the earliest possible diagnosis. Figure reproduced from reference (37) with permission.

tubular necrosis and prerenal failure. Recent experience, however, suggests that this test is of limited value in differentiating the patient who will need dialysis from the one who will recover renal function, when given fluids. Serial free water and creatinine clearances may be the best tests differentiating prerenal failure from acute tubular necrosis. Figure 5 (37). Prerenal failure very commonly precedes acute tubular necrosis. Prerenal failure and acute tubular necrosis may succeed each other or even co-exist in a patient (35). Often therefore, a specific diagnosis of either tubular necrosis or prerenal failure can not be made definitively; many patients have findings that fluctuate between the two entities.

The urinary sediment should be a good test to differ-

entiate between tubular necrosis and prerenal failure but has not been rigorously evaluated in recent years. Early urine from patients with obstruction tends to have a chemical composition similar to urine from patients with prerenal failure. After 2 or 3 days it resembles urine from patients with tubular necrosis (34).

The studies summarized in Table 1 are all easy to perform and should be available in any hospital dealing with patients with acute renal failure. They should be done on these patients, with the understanding that the results should be interpreted as only one part of the total clinical picture. No test is infallible; most are only clues to the correct diagnosis; they are most reliable when employed serially.

AVOIDING DIALYSIS – ETIOLOGIC TREATMENT

Only the treatment of acute tubular necrosis will be reviewed in detail.

The etiologic treatment of dehydration is a vigorous rehydration, and of obstruction, operative or percutaneous nephrostomy drainage. The dangerous and poorly controlled treatments of acute renal failure due to primary parenchymal renal disease include treatment with corticosteroids, various cytostatics, anticoagulation, antiplatelet drugs, plasma infusion, plasmapheresis and cytapheresis will not be further examined.

The aim of the treatment of acute tubular necrosis is to stop the progress of the renal failure and inhibit the feedback loops, restore renal blood flow, increase tubular flow of urine and repair ongoing intracellular injury.

Figure 4 summarizes a possible scheme for the etiology, pathogenesis and pathophysiology of acute tubular necrosis. In the clinical situation, as noted above, there are almost always several factors operative. The first step in treatment is to review the patients medications. If possible, those that are potentially nephrotoxic should be discontinued.

The key element in the ischemic pathway leading to tubular necrosis, is decreased renal blood flow and a final common pathway for acute renal failure, independent of nephrotoxicity or ischemia, is a decrease in tubular fluid flow.

Changes in the rate of delivery of salt and water to the distal tubules, sensed at the macula densa, also can stimulate renin release, causing renal ischemia. A decrease in renal medullary vasodilator prostaglandin activity can also contribute to the decrease in renal blood flow. These factors may perpetuate renal ischemia. Drugs that increase renal blood flow or tubular fluid flow or both, could thus theoretically influence the development of tubular necrosis. Finally, drugs that stabilize the intracellular milieu could be beneficial.

Loop diuretics increase both renal blood flow and tubular fluid flow rates. Mannitol, ethacrynic acid and furosemide have each been used clinically a) prophylactically b) as a treatment for aborting incipient acute tubular necrosis or shortening its clinical course and c) to change oliguria to non-oliguria. Several clinical trials of these drugs have been undertaken; few of these have been controlled or randomized. Controlled trials have shown that furosemide in a daily dose up to 4,000 mg, which has been investigated most recently, is either ineffective, can change oliguric acute tubular necrosis to non-oliguria, thus easing management or will appreciably shorten both the anuric period and the time it takes for the plasma creatinine concentration, to return to normal. These drugs are potentially effective only when used early during the development of acute renal failure. In many patients they induce diuresis. Reports of treatment of acute tubular necrosis with diuretics and mannitol suggest that many patients respond by changing from oliguria to a diuresis but that mortality rates do not decrease (38, 39).

Clinical and experimental data suggest that low-dose intravenous dopamine, infused at a rate of $1 \mu g/kg/min$, may also change oliguria to diuresis (40, 41). Experimental studies suggest that a combination of dopamine and furosemide may be more effective (42). Recent experiments also indicate that atrial natriuretic factor, a potent diuretic and vasodilator of the renal bed, is of benefit in renal ischemic injury (43). Finally, damage can theoretically be repaired by the use of xanthine oxidase inhibitors, calcium channel blockers, free oxygen radical scavengers, and the infusions of intracellular substances, particularly magnesium, nucleotides, and amino acids (44–51). Both the experimental and clinical studies of this approach are controversial. Many drugs can not be used in patients because of the risk of toxicity. One exception is the use of intravenous amino acids. Some have found that they decrease the creatinine elevation and lower the mortality rate in patients with tubular necrosis. Others have found them useless (52–55). Amino acids in experimental acute renal failure have been reported both to improve and worsen renal function and lower and increase mortality.

The clinical management of acute tubular necrosis is also obviously controversial. Some nephrologists believe there is no true etiologic treatment and, after fluid volumes have been restored, and cardiac output maximized, will do nothing further. Others use dopamine, mannitol, and furosemide alone or in combination. We suggest that a patient with a serum creatinine below 5 mg/dl (442 μmol/l) should be treated with dopamine infused at a rate of $1 \mu g/kg/minute$ and with rapidly increasing doses of furosemide, approximately 2 to 5 to 10 mg/kg infused at hourly intervals over a 15 to 20 min period to decrease the ototoxicity of a high peak level. If diuresis occurs it can often be maintained by continued infusion of mannitol and furosemide. For a 60 kg adult, infusion of 500 ml of 20% mannitol to which has been added the furosemide dose to which the patient responded, at a rate of 20 ml/h often maintains diuresis and sometimes also decreases creatinine levels. Even without a fall in creatinine, diuresis makes the conservative management of such a patient much easier. Actual and calculated plasma osomolality must frequently be checked to avoid mannitol intoxication (56). Rare side effects of furosemide are pancreatitis and deafness. Some cases of acute renal failure resolve, if an increased abdominal pressure is reduced to normal (57, 58).

MORTALITY, CAUSE OF DEATH, PROGNOSTIC FACTORS AND AVOIDING DIALYSIS – NONTREATMENT

Mortality

Table 2 summarizes the disorders leading to tubular necrosis during the 35 years between 1945 and 1980 while hemodialysis treatment has been clinically available. Surgery and trauma have always been the most common causative incidents preceding severe acute tubular necrosis requiring dialysis. Medical causes account for between one-fourth to one-third of the cases. Although not expressed in the Table, there has been a marked decline in tubular necrosis complicating obstetrical and gynecological disease during the 35 years that dialysis has been available.

These figures apply only to highly technologically developed countries. In other parts of the world, acute renal failure is mostly secondary to acute infections, snakebites and abortions. In a review of 577 cases of acute renal failure in India, 63% were secondary to medical diseases, mostly due to gastrointestinal infections, 23% complicated obstet-

Table 2. Outcome and mean age of patients with acute tubular necrosis in the early, middle and late years of acute dialysis.

Initiating disorder	University of Minnesota 1968–1979			Glasgow Royal Infirmary 1959–1970			University of Lund 1945–1961		
	n	Mortality (%)	Mean age	n	Mortality (%)	Mean age	n	Mortality (%)	Mean age
Medical diseases intoxications	140	63	41	56	36	48	225	35	50
Gastrointestinal surgery	95	78	55	97	58	51	87	56	50
Cardiovascular surgery	135	73	52	6	–	–	12	83	50
Obstetrical, gynecologic, other surgery, trauma	62	68	45	92	–	–	236	46	50
Total	432	69	48	251	44	–	560	44	50

Results of dialysis treatment of acute renal failure from the early years (1945–61), the middle years (1959–70), and the recent years of acute dialysis (1968–79). Surgical disease has always been the most common cause of acute tubular necrosis. The mortality rate has not improved, nor has the mean age of the patients increased.

rical/gynecological disorders and only 14% followed surgery. In figures from Asia, Africa and India the findings were similar and markedly different from those published from North America and Europe, where surgical complications were causative in 50% of the cases that need dialysis. (4–15, 59–61).

There has been no tendency for improvement in the mortality rate with time (Table 2), nor has there been an increase in the patient's mean age in the later series (4–10).

It is difficult to compare patients who are treated by dialysis now to those dialyzed almost 40 years ago. It seems clear that patients with acute tubular necrosis now have much more serious underlying disorders in each etiological category. Milder disorders, such as gastroenteritis, no longer give rise to tubular necrosis, because of improved resuscitation and electrolyte and fluid management. Presently, cancer, catastrophic septicemia and major surgery are increasingly more common antecedents of tubular necrosis.

The comparative survival rate of groups of patients that are well defined as to age and basic disease, such as a young man with acute renal failure sustained during war, is not encouraging. Teschan et al (6, 11) reported a 32% overall survival in soldiers dialyzed for tubular necrosis during the Korean war 1950 to 1953. The survival rate for such soldiers in Viet Nam in the 1960's was 23 to 37% (62–64). Barsoum and coworkers (65) reported a 37% survival rate in young soldiers dialyzed for acute renal failure resulting from the 6-day war in the Middle East in 1973. These figures do not show any substantial improvement in survival. It is believed, however, that improved resuscitation and transportation enabled much more severely traumatized soldiers to reach dialysis units during the Viet Nam and Middle East Wars, than during the Korean conflict. Thus, shifts in patient population towards more severely traumatized cases may conceal actual improvements in the management of acute tubular necrosis (66).

Cause of death

The causes of death in patients dialyzed for acute renal failure are depicted in Figure 6. Infections are the most common cause of death in almost all reports. Infection is often complicated by progressive multisystem failure. Cardiac disease is the next most common cause of death. Death occurs secondary to acute myocardial infarction, or irreversible cardiac failure in the old patient with degenerative vascular disease. Gastrointestinal disease (hemorrhage or perforation) and pulmonary insufficiency come next but intestinal hemorrhage has decreased with early more frequent dialysis. Some patients die from irreversible central nervous disease, secondary to bleeding, brain edema or unexplained coma. A few patients die from hyperkalemia, digitalis intoxication, and technical dialysis mishaps. Although these latter tend to be under-reported (67) they should occur in less than 1 of 50,000 dialyses (68, 69). Thus, most patients die of infections, multiorgan system failure or irreversible, underlying diseases. The exact role of each is poorly understood. Infection often seems complicated by multiorgan system failure.

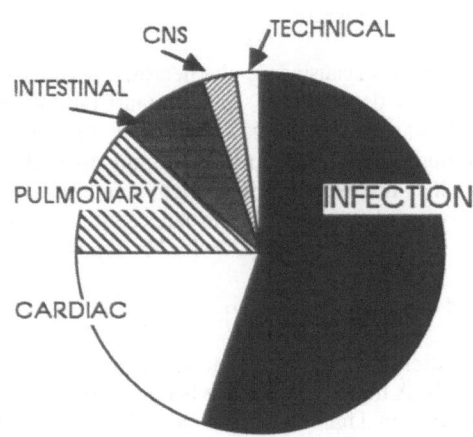

Figure 6. Summary of causes of death in approximately 2,000 reported patients dialysed for acute renal failure (4–18, 62–66).

Prognostic factors

Patients with acute renal failure are often extremely ill and need high technology medicine in an intensive care setting. This treatment is often extremely uncomfortable to patients, frightening to relatives, expensive and the beds in the intensive care units are limited. Exact prognosis, so one could avoid treating unnecessarily those patients, who are invariably going to die of their acute illness, would thus be of great benefit to all. Attempts to establish prognostic factors are summarized in this section. Controversy surrounds almost every factor studied.

Demographic factors

Sex has not been found to influence the outcome in patients dialyzed for acute renal failure.

The influence of age is controversial. Some have found a direct relationship between age and mortality (4, 66). In one series the mortality in patients below age 29 was 39% and rose to almost 80% in patients over the age of 80. Some groups reported a U-shaped relationship between survival and age: the lowest survival was encountered in the youngest and the very oldest patients (10, 70). Most have found age to be of no importance for survival in patients dialyzed for acute renal failure (17, 71).

The time period of dialysis is of no importance (4, 7, 17, 71–73). There has been no improvement in survival in war-induced acute renal failure.

Comorbid condition

Most have found a history of pre-existing disease to be of no importance (71, 74, 75).

Basic underlying disease

The basic disease, causing tubular necrosis, is a most important factor in determining survival. Gastrointestinal and cardiovascular surgery have particularly high mortality rates, around 80%. The mortality in patients with underlying medical disease is now also high. Acute renal failure, secondary to obstruction and urological surgery, usually carries a low mortality rate (4, 7–10, 70, 72).

Type and degree of renal failure

Survival after toxic and ischemic acute tubular necrosis is similar (17). A higher survival has been reported by some in non-oliguric renal failure. A 26% mortality rate occurred in nonoliguric patients compared to 50% in those with oliguria. The figures were 58% and 82% in another study (66, 74, 76). Others have found no difference in mortality between oliguric or nonoliguric patients when stratifying for age and underlying disease (71, 75).

In one study, there was a direct, linear correlation between the degree of creatininemia and mortality in nondialyzed patients with acute renal failure. It was the most important factor associated with death, of six factors studied (17).

Infections

Infections are the most common cause of death in acute renal failure. The number of infections and the mortality rate are related directly. Survival was 80% in the noninfected patient and less than 30% in patients with four or more infections (70). In 50 patients with acute renal failure, after aortic aneurysm surgery, there was decreased survival in patients who had a temperature over 100°F or a white blood cell count over 10,000 mm³, if persisting 2 weeks after the onset of renal failure. No patient with positive blood cultures during antibiotic treatment survived (71). Many others have similar findings of a dismal outcome in septic patients (77–80), but in others it was of no importance (75, 81).

Complicating disorders, 'organ system failure'

'Organ system failure' is a poor prognostic sign in patients dialyzed for acute renal failure. It is often secondary to severe infection (80–83). In one study, over 90% of the patients survived if no other organ system than the kidneys failed, but less than 30% of those with more than seven organs failing, survived (70, 73). In particular, pulmonary complications and central nervous system dysfunction (66, 71, 74, 75, 78–80) occur more often in patients who die than in those who survive. The influence on survival of cardiac problems or gastrointestinal problems is less certain. It is difficult to know whether 'organ system failure' is due to primary incurable disease, or occurs secondary to infections (80).

Type and quantity of dialysis

Since the introduction of early start and the use of daily or alternate day dialysis, there is no difference in predialysis chemistries between survivors and patients who die (17, 84). There was no difference in survival, at any time, between comparable patients, who had immediate renal function and those who needed dialysis for acute renal failure following transplantation (85).

In the most thorough, recent comparison of daily, to every-other-day dialysis, survival was equivalent, 41% in daily, 53% in the every-other-day group. BUN was 60 mg/dl (21.4 mmol/l), creatinine 5.3 mg/dl (469 μmol/l), bicarbonate 23 mmol/l, PO$_4$ 4.3 mg/dl (1.4 mmol/l) and pH 7.42 in the daily vs. 101 mg/dl (36.1 mmol/l), 9.1 mg/dl (80.5 μmol/l), 18 mmol/l, 6.7 mg/dl (2.2 mmol/l) and 7.35 respectively (86). Thus, dialysis, per se, is almost never a cause of death and present alternative day treatment schedules seem to achieve maximal survival.

In several comparisons of peritoneal to hemodialysis for acute renal failure, there is no difference in survival (84, 87–89).

Multifactorial prognostic formulae

Using multifactorial statistical analysis, several teams have tried to create formulas predicting death and survival. In one study of 17 factors influencing survival in 300 patients with postoperative acute renal failure, a linear discriminant function was derived. It included 7 factors (age, transfusions, cardiac surgery, cardiac failure, sex, vascular surgery and interval to dialysis). The only variable that could be influenced was the serum creatinine level before the first dialysis. It was 6.6 ± 1.7 mg/dl (584 μmol/l) in survivors and 8.6 ± 7.8 mg/dl (761 μmol/l) in patients who died (81).

The combination of sepsis, respiratory failure and oliguria in 151 patients, was associated with almost no survival (79). In another study of 58 dialysed patients, central nervous sytem (CNS) dysfunction, the use of inotropic drugs and old age were bad prognosticators (75). In a third study of 148 patients, seen by a nephrologist, 10 factors (acute cardiac illness, cancer, oliguria, pancreatitis, trauma, pre-existing renal- and heart disease, CNS and respiratory failure and surgery) could be used for an accurate discriminatory score predicting death.

Summary of prognostic factors

No group has derived a perfect predictive index in patients who develop acute renal failure. However, the combination of sepsis, CNS and respiratory failure in patients with acute renal failure, particularly if the patient is elderly and postoperative, should make one strongly consider using only conservative management.

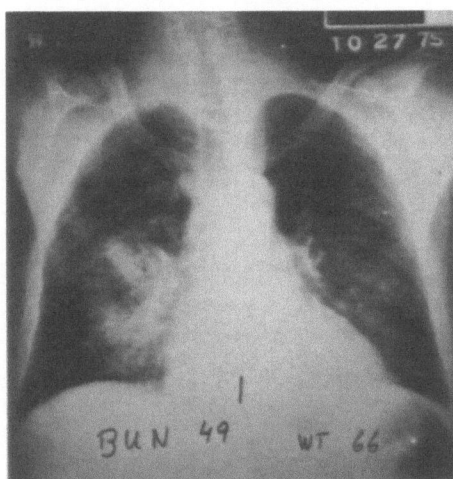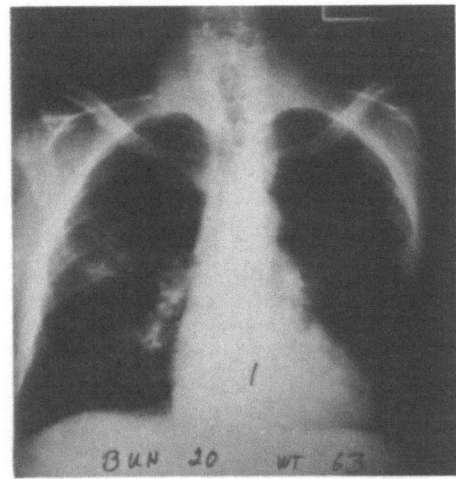

Figure 7. Classical appearance of fluid overload in a uremic patient. Note the occurrence of the central (butterfly or bat wing pattern) pulmonary edema. The infiltration rapidly clears with fluid removal by ultrafiltration in this patient. The first chest x-ray taken in the morning before dialysis, the second one on the evening on the same day after dialysis with a 3 kg fluid removal (From Kjellstrand et al [92] with permission of the publishers).

TREATMENT EARLY: RESCUSITATION

Patients with acute renal failure are frequently very ill, often suffer iatrogenic disease and half of them will die. Time is running fast and there is little margin for error. The differential diagnosis may be impossible without an extended time to evaluate the situation and the psychological pressure on the nephrologist is heavy. It is, therefore, necessary to approach and solve the problems in a logical order as described in Figure 3.

First immediate dangers to life must be removed. Then the differential diagnosis resolved and etiological treatment tried, as outlined above. If this fails, one must decrease the chance of complications, particularly infectious and metabolic, by conservative and dialysis treatment.

Immediately after the onset of acute renal failure, two main threats to the patient's life arise. One is fluid overload, almost always iatrogenic, as excessive fluids are often used to treat real or imagined dehydration. The second problem is hyperkalemia, due both to the release of potassium from traumatized, damaged tissue and hematomata as well as from shifts from the intracellular to the extracellular space, because of the acidosis that is almost uniformly present in such patients.

Fluid overload

Assessment of a patient's fluid state requires daily measurements of body weight, an accurate review of intake and output and continuous monitoring of fluid balance. Even when all these data are available, it is difficult to deal with such patients because of the impossibility of quantifying third spaced (sequestered) fluid volume acurately.

The most dangerous complication of fluid overload is fluid lung (pulmonary edema, uremic 'pneumonitis').

Patients with acute renal failure, frequently have a decreased plasma oncotic pressure, an increased hydrostatic pressure in pulmonary capillaries, because of fluid overload and subtle capillary injury in their lungs, particularly in the perihilar region. All these factors make such patients susceptible to pulmonary edema (4, 90, 91). Figure 7 shows the typical perihilar x-ray localization of fluid. The edema is rarely atypical but may then be difficult to differentiate from infections or pulmonary emboli (4, 92, 93) and may cause hemoptysis. The x-rays of one such patient with lobar pulmonary edema, indistinguishable from pneumonia, are shown in Figure 8.

During the acute restoration phase invasive monitoring of blood pressure, central venous pressure (CVP), cardiac output and pulmonary arterial and wedge pressures are often necessary to maximize volumes without causing pulmonary edema (94, 95).

A mild degree of fluid overload can sometimes be treated simply by not replacing ongoing output. In more urgent situations, oral sorbitol (70% solution, 2 ml/kg) or rectal sorbitol (20% solution, 10 ml/kg) can be used, provided that the gastrointestinal tract is functional (4, 96). Up to 5 kg per day of fluid can be removed this way. Furosemide may contribute to clearing of the pulmonary edema even in oliguric patients by increasing venous capacitance (96). Severe fluid overload is a classical indication for emergency dialysis with ultrafiltration.

Hyperkalemia

The second lethal threat to a patient with acute renal failure is hyperkalemia. It is frequently associated with acidosis and necrosis of large organs or muscle (97). It is disproportional-

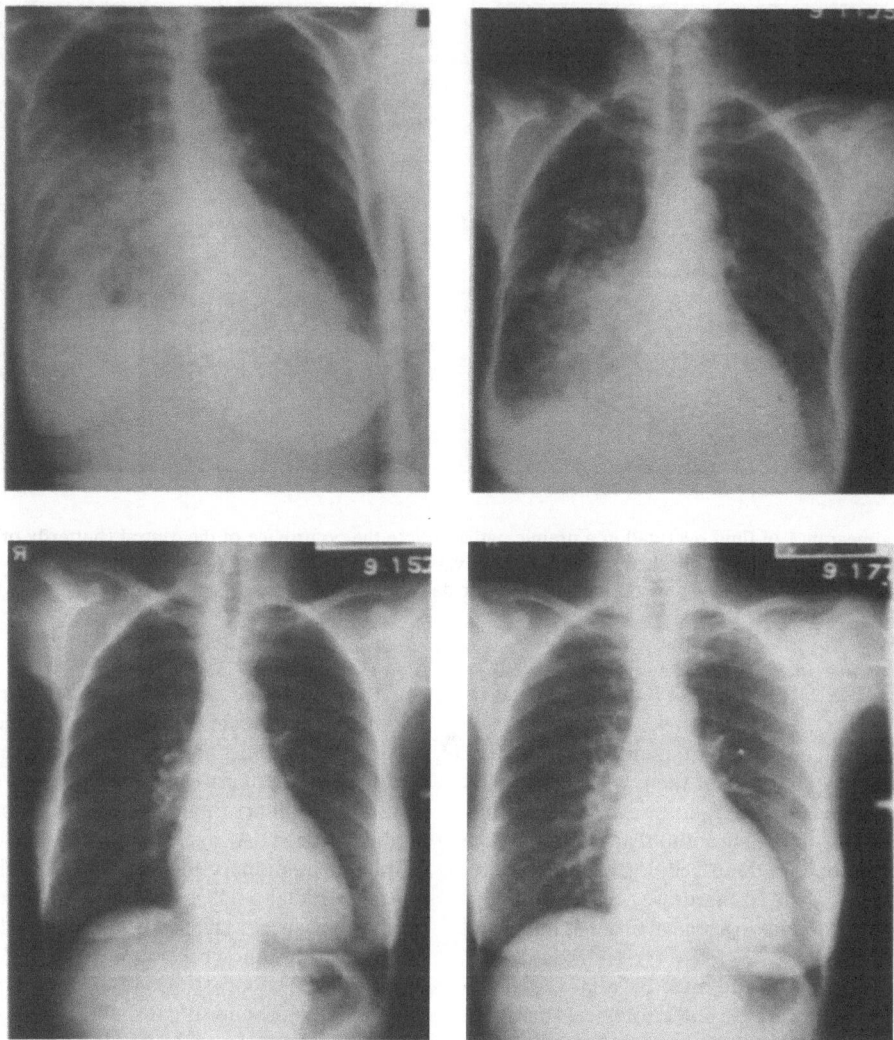

Figure 8. Lobar pulmonary edema in a patient with renal failure. Top left picture was taken immediately before dialysis, the second top right picture 5 hours later a 5 kg fluid removal with dialysis. The lower left picture was taken the next morning with a further 1 kg weight loss induced by diarrhea. The bottom right picture was taken 3 days after dialysis with no further fluid removal.

ly high in acute renal failure caused by nonsteroidal anti-inflammatory drugs (98). Hyperkalemia causes cardiac conduction defects, leading to ectopic rhythms ending in ventricular fibrillation or asystole. Figure 9 illustrates the electrocardiographic changes encountered in hyperkalemia and the approximate plasma potassium levels at which they occur. Rarely, electrocardiographic changes in extreme hyperkalemia are indistinguishable from those of myocardial infarction (99). The treatment of hyperkalemia consists of antagonizing the effects on the myocardium, shifting potassium to the intracellular space and removing it (90, 92).

Both calcium and sodium ions directly antagonize the cardiotoxic effect of potassium. Calcium should be infused under electrocardiographic monitoring. In less urgent sit-

uations, infusion of a mixture of glucose, insulin, calcium and sodium lactate (bicarbonate cannot be mixed with calcium) is started. This promotes flux of the potassium ion from the extracellular to the intracellular space. Lactate is converted (in patients not suffering from lactic acidosis) to bicarbonate in the body. β-adrenergic stimuli also facilitate movement of K^+ to the intracellular space. An infusion of 0.5 mg albuterol sulfate will decrease the K^+ approximately 1 mmol/l in 20 min (100). Removal of potassium is achieved through the oral or rectal administration of exchange resins or by dialysis. Table 3 summarizes the treatment for hyperkalemia and Figure 10 exemplifies the use of all treatment modalities.

K⁺ in Serum mEq./L

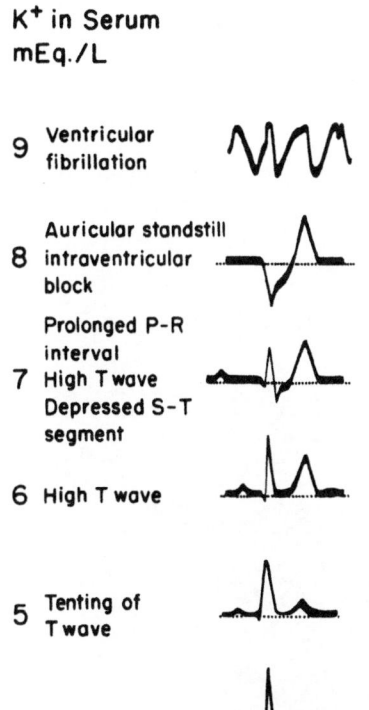

9   Ventricular fibrillation

8   Auricular standstill intraventricular block

7   Prolonged P-R interval High T wave Depressed S-T segment

6   High T wave

5   Tenting of T wave

4   Normal

Figure 9. Electrocardiographic change seen at various plasma potassium levels. Note that the plasma levels are only approximate and electrocardiographic changes only roughly correlate to the plasma potassium levels (From Kjellstrand et al [92] with permission of the publishers).

TREATMENT LATE: CONSERVATIVE

Once the restoration phase in a patient with acute tubular necrosis is over, treatment directed against commonly occurring complications and problems, is instituted. Included are prophylaxis against infections, a watch for surgical complications and bleeding.

Avoiding infections

The number of infections that occur in a patient with acute renal failure correlates directly with mortality. While, 85% of the patients without infections survived in one series, 75% of those with four infections died (70). The urinary tract is infected in 80% of patients with acute renal failure, the lungs in 60%, clinical septicemia is present in 30%, and positive blood cultures in 15% (4). Almost all patients who develop positive blood cultures, while on broad-spectrum antibiotics die (4, 71, 84).

The diagnosis of infections is difficult, because urea is a strong antipyretic. The temperature increases less in infection in patients with uremia. While a patient with normal blood urea level, will develop fever exceeding 103° F during culture-verified septicemia, a patient with a creatinine clearance of less than 30 ml/min, will rarely raise their temperature over 102° F (101).

The white blood cell response to culture-verified septicemia, is also decreased. Only 5/17 patients on chronic dialysis raised their segmented neutrophils count to over 5,000 cells/mm³. Nonsegmented neutrophils/mm³ may be more accurate, as 13/17 patients had a count of more than 400 nonsegmented neutrophils/mm³ during septicemia (102, 103).

Most patients with tubular necrosis are oliguric or develop oliguria when started on dialysis. An indwelling urinary catheter is not necessary and very dangerous in oliguric patients. As soon as the patient is obviously oliguric, the catheter should be removed and the bladder palpated and percussed daily. Straight catheterization can be performed if retention of urine is suspected. If a catheter is deemed necessary, a condom catheter should be tried. A closed system should always be utilized. Almost all bladders with indwelling catheters are infected after 4 days. Pyelonephritis and sepsis may result (104, 105).

As soon as the restoration phase is over, all intravascular catheters, not absolutely necessary for hemodynamic monitoring, should be removed. There is almost never a reason to measure intra-arterial blood pressure in any patient. Nor should there be any need for continued measurements of

Table 3. Treatment of hyperkalemia.

Urgency	Treatment	Dose	Mechanism	Time for effect
Hyperacute	Calcium intravenously	10 ml 10% calcium gluconate/1–5 min until EKG improves May need 100 ml	Antagonism	Immediate
Acute	A. Insulin-glucose-lactate-calcium	500 ml 30% dextrose 30 units insulin 100 mmol Na lactate 30 ml 10% calcium gluconate; 100 ml in 1st h	Shifts K⁺ to intracellular space	30 min
	B. Bicarbonate intravenously			Minutes
	C. Albuterol sulfate	0.5 mg iv in 10 min		
Less urgent	A. Exchange resin	50 g Kayexalate orally in 100 ml 20% sorbitol solution or 60 g Kayexalate as an enema in 500 ml 10% sorbitol solution	Removes K⁺ from body	1 to 2 h
	B. Dialysis			Immediate

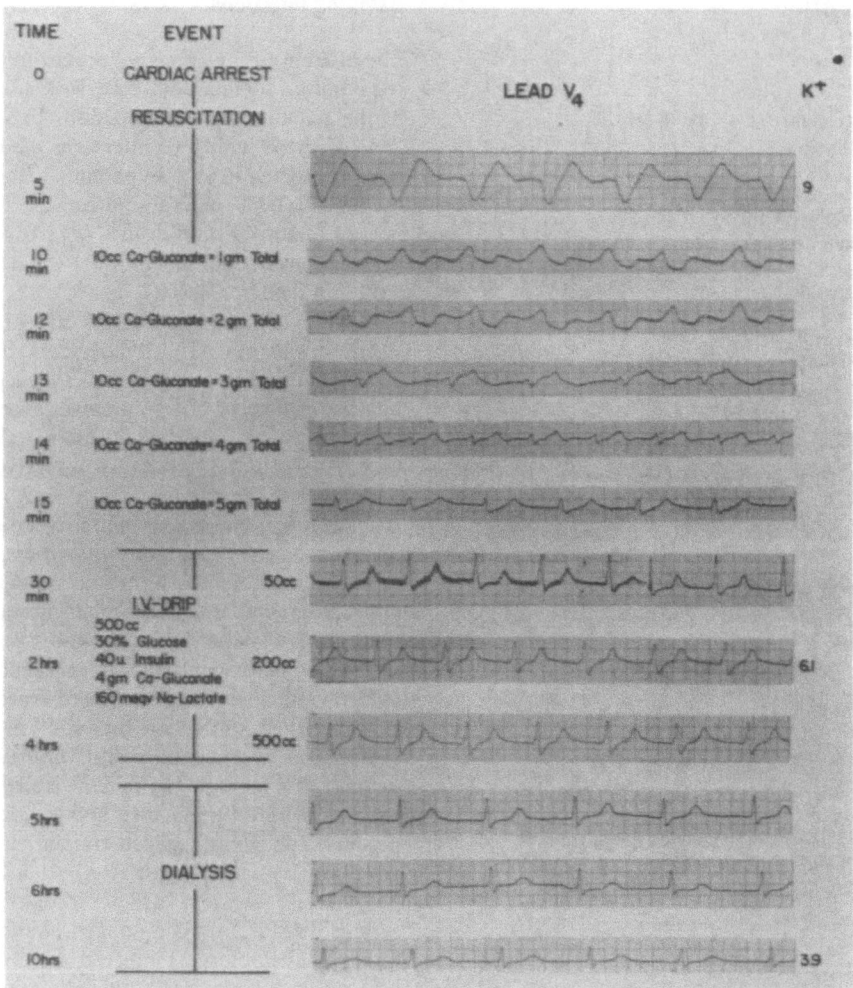

Figure 10. Electrocardiographic changes in a patient with hyperkalemia treated with rapid infusion of calcium gluconate, antagonizing potassium toxicity, followed by shifting of potassium to intracellular space through insulin, glucose, calcium and lactate infusion, and finally by dialysis (From [92] with permission).

central venous or wedge pressures. Clinical examination and chest x-ray suffice. Intravascular catheters become infected with increased frequency beyond the 4th day. Of patients with flow-directed pulmonary artery catheters, 53% showed endocardial lesions, 19% of the catheter tips had positive cultures and 7% of the patients developed infective endocarditis after 1 to 2 weeks (106). A central catheter may be necessary for hyperalimentation, but it may be safer to hyperaliment through an arteriovenous shunt. We have successfully hyperalimented many patients through their shunts and believe infections are infrequent and easier to diagnose with this approach.

As the lungs are very prone to infection, patients should be extubated as soon as possible and mobilized. Physical therapy, breathing and coughing exercises are instituted, although their value is controversial.

Indwelling catheters and treatment with broad spectrum antibiotics are often complicated by fungal infections, particularly Candida. Prophylaxis is indicated with nystatin or clotrimazole, swish and swallow, every 4 h or administered through a nasogastric tube. Specimens for culture should be obtained frequently. Isolation of the patient is probably of little help.

Re-operation and surgical complications

Almost all patients who develop tubular necrosis after abdominal operations, have neglected complications of surgery. Thus, Marshall (107) describing post-operative acute renal failure, re-explored 18 of 118 such patients; 17 had a gross surgical complication. All nine patients, who developed acute tubular necrosis after a large bowel surgery, had developed a fecal leak. Postoperative shock was common in these patients. Kornhall (108), reviewing 298 surgical patients with tubular necrosis, found that 98 (33%) had neglected surgical complications; 81 of these 98 (83%) died. An aggressive surgical approach to these patients is necessary. Marshall comments: '. . . these patients are invariably too ill not to be operated on, rather than the reverse . . .' In spite of reoperation, most patients died in both series. Such patients can not survive without re-operation, but they also tolerate the operations poorly. Perhaps newer methods of percutaneous drainage of abscesses can improve this dismal survival rate.

Gallium or indium scans, sonograms, computerized tomographic and (CAT)scans of the operative areas of the body, should be done early, when acute renal failure develops and then repeated frequently. Changes in masses may then be detected early and further investigated by percutaneous aspirations or exploration. In one investigation, of such an approach survival of patients in an intensive care unit (ICU), increased from 19% to 31% (109).

Nutrition, hyperalimentation

Many patients with acute tubular necrosis are critically ill and under maximal stress. They may utilize 5,000 calories and 200 g of protein per day (110).

Malnourished patients suffer from increased post-operative complications including deficient wound healing, immunological defects and increased rates of infections. It is therefore important to supply adequate calories and protein to such patients (111–113).

For feeding, the gastrointestinal route is much safer than intravenous hyperalimentation and should be used whenever possible. New techniques include small diameter soft nasogastric tubes, operative and percutaneous gastrostomy and ileostomy. An elemental oral diet is no more effective than regular homogenized high calorie, high quality protein, normal food. To the contrary, use of the elemental diet, because of the higher osmotic load, is complicated by diarrhea more often (114–116).

Intravenous hyperalimentation causes a number of clinical problems. Plasma electrolyte concentrations may change rapidly and need to be measured frequently. Hypoglycemia and hyperglycemia can occur, contributing to water shifts and intracellular edema or dehydration. Finally, even with new concentrated solutions, hyperalimentation invariably causes periodic fluid overload and full hyperalimentation in the oliguric patient almost always necessitates daily hemodialysis or continuous ultrafiltration to remove the 'carrier water'. Present regimens of hyperalimentation include 0.5 to 1.5 g/kg/day of an amino acid solution. The patient should also receive between 40 and 100 calories/kg/day (117). Ten percent of the calories are supplied by the amino acid solution, 50% by dextrose and the remaining 40% by intravenous fat. The 20% fat solution contains more calories/volume and less osmoles/calorie than any other intravenous solution.

It should be understood, that the exact needs, dangers and benefits of intravenous hyperalimentation for the patient with acute tubular necrosis are not yet fully evaluated. Feinstein et al (110) could not find any definite advantage of dextrose plus essential amino acids over dextrose plus essential and non-essential amino acids over dextrose also, a finding also noted by Leonard, Luke and Siegel (55, 106).

Abel et al (52, 117), however, found more rapid recovery of renal function and increased survival in patients with acute renal failure, when given essential amino acid containing hyperalimentation solutions. Baek et al (53), found no difference in renal recovery, but better survival in hyperalimental patients, than in those not receiving hyperalimentation. Others have found neither an increase in renal recovery rate nor a decrease in mortality rate, with intravenous hyperalimentation (54, 55). Traumatic, thrombotic and septic complications occur, but can be minimized with experience and caution (116). Nevertheless, intravenous hyperalimentation decreases hypercatabolism and does help some individual patients survive. An example is shown in Figure 11.

It seems best to avoid hyperalimentation for the first 3 or 4 days of acute renal failure, because it can complicate the restoration treatment. Even the most enthusiastic advocates of hyperalimentation, conclude that recovery is enhanced even when initiated first on the 4th day after the onset of acute renal failure (52). After resuscitation and stabilization, parenteral hyperalimentation should be started if oral feeding is impossible. Full hyperalimentation should be reached in 3 to 4 days. Smaller amounts can be given through peripheral veins (114).

Sargent and Gotch (118), suggest that urea appearance (generation) rate should be measured, and used to titrate individual hyperalimentation requirements. Their data in patients treated by chronic dialysis, show that protein catabolic rate = $6.4 \times$ BUN generation + 11, and are similar to those of patients with acute renal failure ($6.75 \times$ BUN generation + 5.1) reported by others (110). The factors (11 or 5.1) derive from obligatory extrarenal nitrogen losses in the feces and elsewhere in grams per day and represent the breakdown of 11 or 5.1 g of protein. The urea generation rate can be calculated by multiplying total body water of a patient, derived from clinical examination and tables, by the change in blood urea nitrogen concentration, measured at two different times, e.g. over a 24 h interval. When plotting protein catabolic rate against caloric intake in acutely ill patients, it becomes clear that some patients respond with a large decrease in protein catabolism as the calories are increased, whereas other show less response. In clinical use, this approach can be simplified to calculating the rise in blood urea nitrogen concentration during 24 h while giving increasing amounts of calories. Whether the protein sparing achieved in an individual patient, is worth the increased technical and metabolic problems, caused by giving more calories, can then be determined.

Recent development and improvement in alimentation may change the uncertain clinical approach to these patients (120).

Anabolic steroids are often given to patients with renal failure and can decrease protein catabolic rate (119).

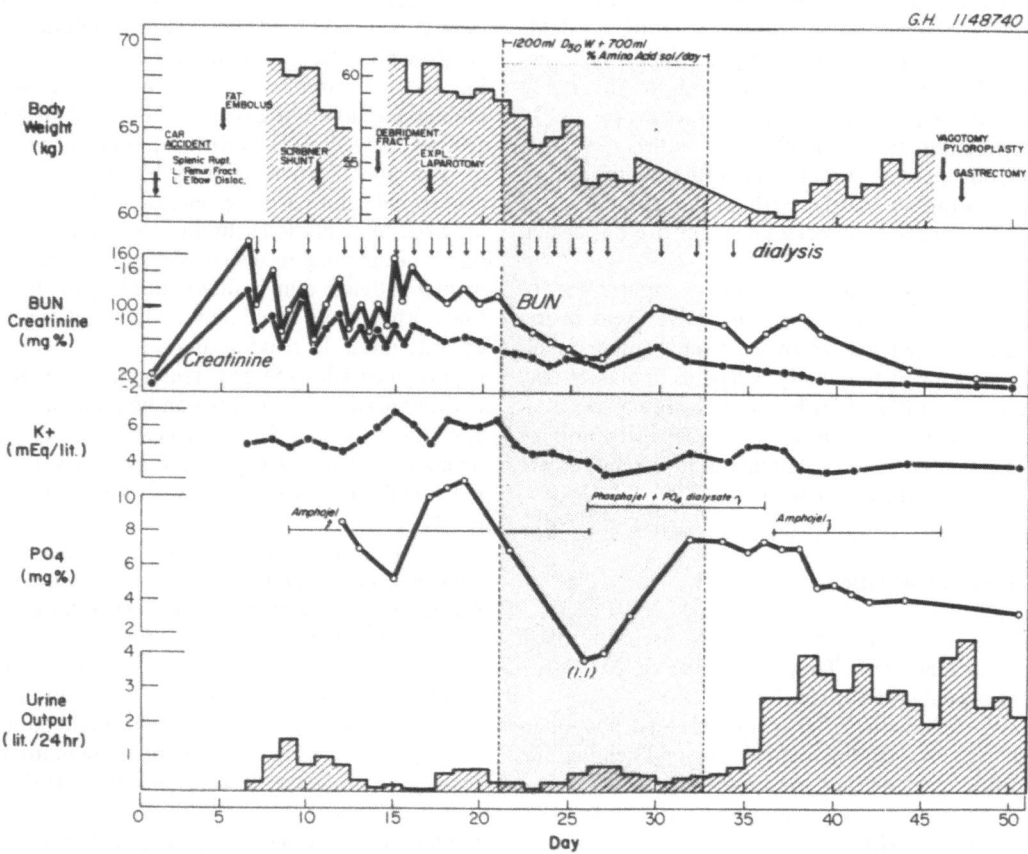

Figure 11. The influences of hyperalimentation and of catabolism in a patient requiring dialysis for acute renal failure following trauma. Before hyperalimentation, BUN ranged from 36 to 54 mmol/l despite daily dialysis. Plasma potassium varied between 5 and 7 mmol/l and phosphorus remained between 3.3 and 5.5 mmol/l. During hyperalimentation these values decreased and supplements of both potassium and phosphorus were required. (From [94], with permission). (BUN mmol/l – mg/dl: multiply by 2.8 creatinine umol/l – mg/dl: multiply by 0.0113 PO$_4$ mmol/l – mg/dl: multiply by 3.1).

Bleeding

Guanidinosuccinic acid and phenolic acid increase in uremic plasma and impair platelet production, adhesiveness, and factor III. Because they are small molecules they are removed by dialysis.

The level of guanidinosuccinic acid level is related to that of urea (121). It seems unlikely that guanidinosuccinic acid should cause bleeding at a BUN less than 60 mg/dl (21.4 mmol/l), but is a problem if the BUN exceeds 100 mg/dl (35.7 mmol/l) (121). Platelet counts fall a mean of 30%, but sometimes more during dialysis and this may cause significant bleeding (122, 123).

Some defects in the clotting cascade are not improved by dialysis. Sometimes prolonged bleeding can be normalized by cryoprecipitate, approximately 10 units (124). Deamino-arginine vasopressin 0.3 µg/kg can rapidly improve bleeding time in some uremic patients (125). Progesterone in high doses (10 to 30 mg daily), for several days, may also help (126). Bleeding is more common if the hematocrit is less than 30% (127, 128). Other postoperative complications are also increased when the hematocrit is below this level (127, 128). Prostacyclin is increased in blood vessel walls in patients on dialysis (129). It is unknown if this contributes to bleeding. The best clinical tests for bleeding include: platelet count, Ivy bleeding time, thrombin time and prothrombin time. If they are abnormal and surgery is planned, vitamin K deficiency and thrombocytopenia should be corrected, the hematocrit should be over 30%, and the patient's BUN decreased to less than 60 mg/dl (21.4 mmol/l). If bleeding parameters still are abnormal, cryoprecipitate, deamino-arginine-vasopressin and progesterone may normalize them.

Other metabolic problems

Although gastrointestinal bleeding is now less common, patients with acute renal failure are stressed and serum gastrin is elevated. Aluminum hydroxide suspension 15 to 60 ml should be used and gastric acidity should be titrated to pH above 3.5. Besides decreasing gastric acidity, it decreases serum levels of phosphorus and hydrogen ion. The formation of bezoar is a side effect of aluminum hydroxide and small and large bowel ischemia, perforation and death have been described. Sorbitol in a final concentration of 20% can prevent this complication. Phosphorus adsorption by aluminum hydroxide rarely leads to severe hypophosphatemia, but it may occur if the patient is also hyperalimented. Aluminum phosphate antacid can then be used to decrease gastric acidity without causing hypophosphatemia. Histamine receptor inhibitors are probably as effective as aluminum hydroxide antacids in stress ulceration (130). The dose of histamine receptor antagonists must be reduced in uremia. Magnesium-containing antacids should not be used, as serum magnesium may rise to toxic levels.

The onset of acute uremia causes several endocrine-metabolic problems (see Chapter 45). Peripheral insulin sensitivity is decreased in uremia and many such patients have hyperinsulinemia. Furthermore, glucose metabolism becomes impaired, with septicemia hyperglycemia often occurs. Glucose levels, therefore must be carefully monitored to prevent marked fluid shifts (117).

Shortly after the onset of acute renal failure, plasma calcium levels start to decrease. This is not due to increased excretion, but reflects a shift of calcium out of the extracellular space (see also Chapter 44). Calcitonin increases to extremely high levels (131), and secondary to the decline in plasma calcium concentration, parathyroid hormone levels rise (132). Calcium and magnesium levels in the brain increase which may contribute to the stupor and confusion often observed in such patients (133). Plasma phorphorus levels usually rise and may also contribute to the secondary hyperparathyroidism, the decline in plasma calcium concentration and the increase in calcitonin levels. The hypocalcemia and hyperphosphatemia can be particularly marked in patients with rhabdomyolysis and acute renal failure. When uremia subsides, some patients with acute renal failure (especially those with rhabdomyolysis) develop marked hypercalcemia (134–137). Many other hormonal abnormalities occur, but are insufficiently studied. Plasma gastrin levels increase and may contribute to the stress ulcers that patients develop.

Anemia develops quickly, possibly secondary to a decreased erythropoietin level or decreased peripheral sensitivity to it. As mentioned above, these patients should be transfused to a hematocrit of approximately 30% (127). Plasma uric acid levels rise; particularly high levels are seen in patients with neoplasms or rhabdomyolysis. Excess uric acid may perpetuate acute renal failure by precipitating in renal tubules (138, 139). In such patients, the ratio of uric acid to creatinine in uric exceeds 1.0 (140). Many of these metabolic problems, e.g. plasma calcium, phosphorus and uric acid levels, improve with dialysis. They rarely need special treatment (141, 142).

Use of drugs

The elimination of most drugs is modified in patients with acute renal failure and by dialysis treatment, necessitating adjustment of dosages. Many drugs are normally excreted in urine, many are removed by dialysis and protein binding of drugs, and hepatic metabolism may change in patients with uremia and sepsis. Chapter 51 of this book, excellent monographs and frequently updated reviews should be consulted (143).

TREATMENT – DIALYSIS

Overview of methods

Dialysis effectively removes small solutes and efficiently corrects electrolyte abnormalities and excess body water. But all dialysis procedures are time consuming and take the patient away from other therapeutic and diagnostic procedures, and have specific complications, although they rarely are life-threatening.

One can choose between three methods of blood purification in acute uremia: hemodialysis, hemofiltration, and peritoneal dialysis. They can be combined or used in succession. Each method can be used intermittent or continuously. Clinically established are: intermittent hemodialysis, continuous peritoneal dialysis and slow continuous hemofiltration. There is only anecdotal experience in acute uremia, with slow continuous hemodialysis, intermittent hemofiltration or hemodiafiltration in acute renal failure. Intermittent peritoneal dialysis has largely been replaced by continuous peritoneal dialysis.

Comparison of dialysis methods

There are no randomized clinical studies comparing intermittent hemodialysis, peritoneal dialysis and slow contunous hemofiltration. The relative indications in patients with acute renal failure are therefore speculative.

Nonrandomized interinstitutional comparisons of hemodialysis to intermittent peritoneal dialysis in acute renal failure have shown similar mortality (66, 87, 88, 89). No comparison to other methods of slow continuous hemofiltration has been done. The mortality report for this procedure has been comparable to that of hemodialysis (144–146). In one randomized comparison of slow continuous hemofiltration to hemodialysis, there were more side effects per treatment time during hemodialysis but more side effects per treatment efficiency (measured as total BUN clearance) with slow continuous hemofiltration (147).

The main advantage of hemodialysis is that it is between 10 and 20 times more efficient than peritoneal dialysis and slow continuous hemofiltration. Treatment time is short and thus more time can be spent on other therapeutic or diagnostic procedures. The main disadvantages are the cardiovascular side effects, particularly hypotension that occur in between 10 and 50% of treatments. Anticoagulation is required during treatment, but this is less than that necessary for hemofiltration.

The main advantages of peritoneal dialysis are the absence of need for anticoagulation and minimal effect on the cardiovascular system. The cleaning of the abdominal cavity may be an advantage in a patient with a soiled peritoneal cavity. The main disadvantages are the low efficiency, the requirement for an intact peritoneum and the risk of peritonitis.

The main advantage of slow continuous hemofiltration, is the remarkable absence of cardiovascular effects, at least early during the treatment. The main disadvantages are the need for continuous anticoagulation in most patients, its relatively low efficiency, and possibly cardiovascular complications occurring later in treatment.

The relative merits of each procedure, depend on the special complications of the patient and the timing of the procedure. Most cardiovascular instability occurs early in treatment. Therefore, peritoneal dialysis or slow continuous hemofiltration, may then be best. Later, patients will usually be more stable and it is important to mobilize them. Intermittent hemodialysis is then best. Patients with unstable cardiovascular systems, are best treated with peritoneal dialysis and slow continuous hemofiltration; for those who are stable, hemodialysis is best. Peritoneal dialysis is least risky in patients prone to bleeding, slow continuous hemofiltration the worst, and intermittent hemodialysis in between. The hypercatabolic patient may be treatable only with hemodialysis because of the low clearances of the other methods. The continuous methods make fluid and electrolyte balance more even in oliguric patients that need large amounts of intravenous fluids i.e. during hyperalimentation. The absence of brain edema and anticoagulation during continuous peritoneal dialysis makes this method preferable in patients with brain damage.

In most instances, the differences between the various methods are trivial and best settled by the technical expertise of the treating center. In some patients it may be best to oscillate between methods. A traumatized patient with severe hyperkalemia may need emergency hemodialysis to regulate homeostasis preoperatively, then best be treated with continuous peritoneal dialysis to cleanse the peritoneal cavity, avoid anticoagulation and maintain him over a time of instability and later return to hemodialysis to allow mobilization.

Start and frequency of dialysis

Urgent indications for dialysis in acute renal failure are plasma potassium concentrations above 7 mmol/l, plasma bicarbonate levels of 15 mmol/l or less, blood urea nitrogen concentrations over 150 mg/dl (54 mmol/l) and plasma creatinine values above 10 mg/dl (885 μmol/l). *Dialysis should be started long before such concentrations occur.*

Electrolyte and fluid disturbances, often due to inappropriate conservative treatment, should not progress until their severity precipitates the need for emergency dialysis. In the well-managed patient with acute tubular necrosis, the decision to start dialysis will then be based on the degree of azotemia that should not be harmful to the patient.

The general trend has been towards early and more frequent dialysis. This strategy should protect the patient with acute renal failure, who is often struggling with extremely severe underlying basic problems, from taking on the additional burden of severe uremia and electrolyte and fluid disturbances. Clinical observations and calculation of BUN levels, based on protein catabolic rate and dialyzer urea clearance, can be used for guidelines for when dialysis should be started, and how often and long it should be used.

Teschan et al (11) introduced the concept of 'prophylactic hemodialysis' during the Korean War. When dialysis was used only on clinical indications, such as coma or severe electrolyte and fluid disturbances, the mortality was over 70%. When dialysis was performed prophylactically to keep the predialysis BUN below 120 mg/dl (42.9 mmol/l), the mortality was 30%. In another study mortality decreased from 77% to 51%, when predialyses BUN was 152 mg/dl (54.3 mmol/l) instead of 231 mg/dl (82.5 mmol/l) (63, 148). In a third study, the mortality decreased from 42% to 29%, when more frequent and earlier dialysis was used and the predialysis BUN was decreased from 163 to 93 mg/dl (58.2 to 33.2 mmol/l) (87). The early observations make it clear, that predialysis BUN should not exceed 100 to 120 mg/dl (35.7 to 42.9 mmol/l). Gillum and coworkers (86), have recently carefully investigated whether even more intensive dialysis could further lower mortality. They randomized 34 patients to intensive daily dialysis, keeping the serum creatinine at 5.3 mg/dl (469 μmol/l) and the BUN at 60 mg/dl (21.4 mmol/l) or 'ordinary dialysis' where the mean predialysis serum creatinine was 9.1 mg/dl (805 μmol/l) and the BUN 101 mg/dl (36.1 mmol/l). There was no difference in mortality or complication rates. Others have made similar observations (71, 84). In one study, 236 patients who needed dialysis for postoperative acute renal failure, immediately following renal transplantation, were compared to matched controls with good renal function. There was no difference in mortality, indicating that dialysis, which was used every other day, had maximally lowered mortality (85). Both continuous peritoneal dialysis and hemofiltration have a urea clearance of approximately 15 ml/min. This is also the *mean,* time average, clearance achieved with hemodialysis, used 4 h every other day, with a blood flow that gives a urea clearance of 180 ml/min (180 ml/min × 4/48).

The following formula, allows calculation of frequency and duration needed for dialysis (149):

1. Protein catabolic rate (PCR) ÷ 6 = Nitrogen production = BUN removal at steady state.

2. BUN removal = Mean blood concentration of BUN × Clearance of dialyzer × time. Dialysis supplied = Total body water × (predialysis BUN − postdialysis BUN).

At a PCR of 70 g protein/day, the two continuous methods, assuming a clearance of 15 ml/min, result in a mean BUN concentration of 55 mg/dl (19.6 mmol/l). If the PCR exceeds 120 g/day, a constant clearance of 15 ml/min is insufficient to keep BUN below 100 mg/dl. At such a PCR, it is necessary to dialyze 7 h every other day with intermittent hemodialysis with a clearance of 180 ml/min to keep the predialysis BUN concentration below 100 mg/dl, post dialysis BUN level is then 45 mg/dl (16.1 mmol/l). Two hours of daily hemodialysis at the same clearance would also keep predialysis BUN below 100 mg/dl (35.7 mmol/l).

These clinical observations and the analyses of the relation of PCR and dialysis clearance, indicate that hemodialysis should be started when the patient's BUN is 100 mg/dl. It is then performed every- or every other day, for between 2 and 5 h depending on the PCR, estimated by predialysis BUN levels that should not exceed 100 mg/dl. Continuous peritoneal dialysis or hemofiltration are started when the blood urea nitrogen level is approximately 60 mg/dl (21.4 mmol/l). Continuous peritoneal dialysis is not sufficient if the urea nitrogen level continues to rise. The clearance of slow continuous hemofiltration can be increased by applying suction on the dialysate side, but then very large fluid shifts and difficult problems with fluid balance occur. Slow continuous hemodiafiltration can overcome these problems, but there is no large clinical study of this procedure in patients with acute renal failure.

HEMODIALYSIS

Vascular access

Vascular access for acute hemodialysis is usually obtained by percutanous cannulation of the femoral or subclavian veins or operative insertion of the Scribner shunt. Arteriovenous subcutaneous fistula or vessel bridging artificial blood vessel has no place because of the time required for maturation. The Scribner shunt can be changed to a fistula later if the patient does not regain renal function (150). Single need technique can be used with any blood access, with only little loss of dialysis efficiency (see also chapter 17).

The femoral vein has the advantage of being technically easier and anatomically safer than the subclavian vein. It has the disadvantage of being a 'dirtier' area, close to the perineum. Femoral catheters can not be left in place, because of risk of infection. Complications of femoral vein catheterization consist of femoral vein thrombosis with pulmonary emboli, when the catheter is left in situ more than 24 h, infections and inadvertent arterial punctures with hematoma and rarely arteriovenous fistula formation. Accidental perforation of the femoral vein by a Seldinger wire and then by the catheter, a rare occurrence, can cause a massive retroperitoneal hematoma and shock on initiation of hemodialysis. Yet, skilled operators have used repeated puncture of the femoral vein for several years. It is contraindicated to leave the catheter in situ more than 24 to 36 h (151).

Subclavian vein catheterization is being used with increasing frequency. It is the most convenient, but also the most dangerous, blood access. There have been several deaths, secondary to perforation of the heart or blood vessels, with hemothorax, both during and several days after insertion of the catheter (152, 153). Other complications are subclavian thrombosis (154) and sepsis (155, 156).

The safest method of blood access for acute dialysis, is the Scribner shunt. There are no lethal complications during insertion. Infection, during the short time required for acute dialysis, is rare. It can also be used for hyperalimentation and blood gas sampling, simplifying patient care.

An arteriovenous shunt can usually be achieved in small children, weighing more than 3 to 4 kg, utilizing special pediatric shunt material to connect the radial artery and cephalic vein in the forearm. Children smaller than 3 kg can either undergo dialysis with an arteriovenous shunt in the groin or in the upper arm, or preferably can be dialyzed with vein-to-vein access with catheters placed with the tip centrally. In children smaller than 3 kg, a blood flow rate of less than 15 ml/min can achieve effective dialysis (see below).

Start, frequency and duration and speed of dialysis

From reasoning detailed above one can deduce that dialysis should be started before the BUN reaches 100 to 120 mg/dl (36 to 43 mmol/l) and used every or every other day as necessary to keep the BUN from exceeding these values. The first few dialyses in a patient are ordinarily associated with more side effects than later ones (157). The early part of each dialysis is also associated with more dialysis complications. For this reason, dialysis should be started slowly, and blood flow should be limited for the first 30 min. Most adult patients tolerate blood flow through a dialyzer that results in urea clearance of 150 to 200 ml/min. In a normal sized adult, this means a dialyzer urea clearance of 2.5 to 3 ml/kg/min. Such clearance should be uniformly used on all patients. Thus, in a newborn 3 kg baby, one wishes to achieve a urea clearance of only approximately 10 ml/min, but in a 100 kg adult, a urea clearance of approximately 250 to 300 ml/min should be achieved to lower blood urea nitrogen levels effectively. Because urea distributes in total body water, a correction should be made for excessive fat.

Acutely uremic patients should be dialyzed slowly if severely uremic, with a urea clearance of only 1 to 2 ml/kg/min for the first one to four dialyses, by restricting dialyzer size or flow rates or both. A urea clearance of 3 ml/kg/min should then not be used until the third to fifth dialysis, if the patient is severely hyperosmolar. The subsequent frequency and efficiency of the dialyses can then be gauged empirically, based on clinical response, blood nitrogen levels and the need for other therapeutic and diagnostic interventions. In hypercatabolic patients, this rule cannot be strictly followed, because such a regimen may not be sufficient to control uremia.

In addition to slowing the dialysis rate during each dialysis, symptoms can further be decreased by infusing mannitol (1.0 g/kg during the first two dialysis and 0.5 g/kg during the subsequent two dialysis). Other therapeutic measures, such as a higher dextrose or sodium concentration in the dialysis solution to avoid disequilibrium syndrome and hypotension will be discussed below.

With dialysis equipment, including ultrafiltration-volume control, higher dialysate Na and HCO_3, chronic patients tolerate higher efficiency dialysis well. This technique should be studied carefully in those needing dialysis for acute renal failure. Until then, it appears unwise to use hyperefficient dialysis in the seriously ill acute patient.

Anticoagulation

Dialysis patients are routinely anticoagulated with heparin. The usual bolus dosage of heparin is not suitable for most patients with acute renal failure, where many are at risk of bleeding. Heparin should be given by constant infusion. For a 60 to 70 kg patient, approximately 4,000 units of heparin will suffice with modern hollow fiber or parallel plate dialyzers during a 5 h dialysis.

In actively bleeding patients or those where bleeding would be particularly hazardous, an even more cautious approach must be utilized. The old method of neutralizing the heparin at the outlet of the dialyzer, by the simultaneous infusion of protamine, is very complicated, requiring two synchronized pumps. Furthermore, once dialysis is over, protamine is metabolized faster than the heparin and a rebound increase in clotting time with bleeding may occur. Hence, it is preferable to use low-dose heparin infused into the arterial line and let the patient neutralize it. During such treatment, much smaller doses of heparin are infused into the arterial line. The clotting time should be kept below twice normal. It is not necessary to exceed 1,500 to 2,500 units of heparin per dialysis in most patients. Some patients with clotting abnormalities may require much less heparin. No rebound phenomenon occurs with this method and even actively bleeding patients can safely be treated if managed by personnel, skilled in this method (158–160). Drip chambers tend to clot much more easily than the dialyzer. Once the dialysis ends, protamine, calculated to neutralize half of the infused heparin, may be given intravenously to the patients. More sophisticated supervision with activated clotting times and determination of individual heparin requirements, may further decrease the already low risk of bleeding with the use of low dose heparin (160). In a study, comparing regional heparinization with protamine to low dose heparin, the incidence of bleeding was twice as common with heparin-protamine and the incidence of dialyzer clotting not improved (159–161).

Several other methods of anticoagulation have been described. They include citrate (162, 163), prostacyclin (164), ticlopidine (165), gabexate mesilate (166) and low molecular weight heparinoids (167, 168). There is no controlled comparison to heparin and no extensive clinical experience with these anticoagulants. Important indications may be for the occasional patient, who cannot tolerate heparin. A major improvement would be the development of dialyzers requiring *no* anticoagulation (169).

Some patients at risk for bleeding, can be dialyzed without anticoagulation. Cellulose acetate dialyzers are thought to be particularly suited for this purpose, although here are no controlled studies. This method requires a blood flow rate over 300 ml/min. The dialyzer must be rinsed with 200 ml physiologic saline solution, rapidly infused into the arterial blood line every 20 min (170, 171).

Dialyzers and dialysis machines

There is no great difference in efficiency or priming volumes between plate and hollow fiber dialyzers. Hollow fiber dialyzers tend to cause less thrombocytopenia; dialysis with plate dialyzers requires less heparin (122). Coil dialyzers tend to contain somewhat more blood and also have a higher compliance. It is difficult to use hollow fiber dialyzers with the single needle technique because of the very low compliance; special high compliance drip-chambers are then necessary.

Cuprophane is less biocompatible than polycarbonate, polymethylmetacrylate and cellulose acetate and much less biocompatible than polyacrylonitrile, polyamide and polysulfone. With the latter membranes there is less complement activation, hypoxemia and neutropenia (172). Theoretically the last three membranes ought to be best. However, the use of such membranes in chronic dialysis patients has not lessened the incidence of clinical side effects of dialysis (173, 174).

All in all, the choice between the different dialyzers and membranes is at present somewhat arbitrary except in very small children where special small volume dialyzers must be used. A dialyzer and its blood lines should not contain more than 10% of the patient's blood volume. For a newborn child weighing 3.5 or 4 kg, the whole system should not contain much more than 30 to 40 ml (See Chapters 5 and 32). Dialysis machines that control ultrafiltration, allow the use of bicarbonate and a variable sodium dialysate are theoretically advantageous, although clinical studies of sodium gradient have been disappointing (175).

Dialysis solution

The composition of the dialysis fluid should be adjusted to the patient's individual needs. Routine standard dialysis fluid, such as that used for patients with chronic renal failure, is not suitable for the acutely ill patient.

Sodium

Sodium concentration of the dialysis solution should be 140 mmol/l. A lower sodium concentration, as is used in treating hypertension in chronic uremic patients, is unsuitable for patients with acute renal failure. Every study comparing a lower to a more normal concentration of sodium in the dialysis solution shows that the lower sodium concentration is associated with a much higher incidence of hypotension, disequilibrium and other complications (176–179). A method of slowly decreasing the sodium concentration in the dialysis fluid during a dialysis session has recently been described. It results in more stable dialysis but is difficult to achieve with currently available equipment (175–179). If a patient has had hypernatremia for more than one day before dialysis, it is probably best to use a higher than normal dialysate sodium concentration. A concentration of sodium in the dialysis fluid approximately half way between that of the patient's plasma sodium concentration and the normal value is appropriate for the first one or two dialyses. When plasma sodium concentration is reduced too quickly, the patient develops cerebral edema because the brain accumulates idiogenic osmoles to compensate for hypernatremia and these are removed slowly (180).

Potassium

It is often necessary to use dialysis fluid with a low potassium concentration particularly for traumatized and hypercatabolic patients who can rapidly develop hyperkalemia. A low concentration of potassium in dialysis fluid must not be used in the digitalized patient, because severe digitalis intoxication can result if the plasma potassium level is decreased too quickly. Furthermore, the rapid correction of acidosis by dialysis may cause very sudden and marked shifts of potassium from the extra- to the intracellular space that may result in severe or even fatal hypokalemia (181, 182).

Calcium

The most appropriate concentration in dialysate is probably identical to or slightly higher than that of normal plasma ionized calcium, i.e. 2.5 to 3.5 mEq/l (1.5 to 1.75 mmol/l or 5 to 7 mg/dl). Some patients with hypercalcemia must be dialyzed against a dialysis fluid containing no calcium (183). Patients with marked hyperphosphatemia should also have a lower than normal calcium concentration in the dialysis fluid until the plasma phosphorus concentration has been reduced to nearly normal levels. This situation may be particularly common in patients who developed tubular necrosis complicating rhabdomyolysis, lymphoma or leukemia. A higher calcium concentration has been recommended in selected instances to maintain a higher blood pressure during dialysis (139, 184).

Magnesium

It is customary to use a dialysis fluid with a magnesium concentration close to the normal plasma value, i.e. 1.5 to 1.7 mEq/l (0.75 to 0.85 mmol/l, 1.8 to 2.04 mg/dl) although a small fraction of plasma magnesium is protein bound. Patients with alcoholism and successfully hyperalimented patients may be hypomagnesemic and need higher concentrations. Magnesium intoxicated patients, usually resulting from errors in management, may need dialysis against a solution containing no magnesium.

Bicarbonate or acetate

Acetate is widely used instead of bicarbonate in the dialysate. It is technically much easier to use as it does not precipitate with calcium and magnesium unlike bicarbonate. It is also less expensive to prepare. Its buffering action occurs as it consumes a hydrogen ion, when metabolized to acetyl-coenzyme A. Several problems may be associated with the usage of acetate. Some patients with chronic renal failure do not metabolize acetate at a normal rate. The acetate infusion rate from dialysis fluid, even during standard flux dialysis, may temporarily aggravate the metabolic acidosis in such patients. This abnormality may also occur in some patients with acute renal failure. The removal of large amounts of bicarbonate by dialysis could be catastrophic should the patient metabolize acetate slowly.

Some studies suggest that the use of acetate causes more dialysis hypoxemia than occurs with bicarbonate. Acetate decreases peripheral resistance more than bicarbonate does. In some patients this may be beneficial because of decreasing afterload and preload. In septic patients with dilated vasculature and borderline blood pressure, however, such an occurrence could lead to further catastrophic falls in blood pressure.

Many clinical studies have compared acetate to bicarbonate dialysis in patients with acute renal failure. Some concluded that more mannitol and albumin infusions were necessary to maintain blood pressure during acetate than during bicarbonate dialysis, others that there is no difference (185, 186). In a study with a double-blind, cross-over format in 120 dialyses of 30 acute patients, no difference was found between acetate and bicarbonate dialysis solution in blood pressure maintenance or other clinical dialysis problems (187). In this study, a dialysis solution sodium concentration of 140 mmol/l, as well as slow dialysis and mannitol infusion were used. Wehle et al (188), found that blood pressure fell more during acetate than during bicarbonate dialysis only when a low sodium concentration (133 mmol/l) was used. It did not occur when a sodium concentration of 145 mmol/l was used in the dialysis solution.

An empirical approach seems reasonable. Bicarbonate dialysis should be used for the most critically ill patients or those who appear to have trouble with acetate dialysis.

Dextrose

Some dextrose should be used in the dialysis fluid. When dextrose-free dialysis is used, negative nitrogen balance occurs during the dialysis, suggesting gluconeogenesis (189). Furthermore, there are more subjective complaints and more episodes of hypotension when patients undergo dialysis without dextrose in the bath fluid (190). The minimum dextrose level in the dialysis solution should be 100 mg/dl (5.6 mmol/l). A much higher dextrose level (approximately 700 mg/dl [39 mmol/l]) during the initial dialysis may prevent disequilibrium. Slightly increased dextrose concentrations, such as 250 mg/dl (14 mmol/l), will supply some calories and still not raise plasma glucose levels more than 20 to 30 mg/dl, i.e. 1.1 to 1.7 mmol/l (191).

Phosphorus

Most patients with acute renal failure have hyperphosphatemia. Certain disorders such as heat stroke and some burns are associated with hypophosphatemia (192, 193). Hypophosphatemia may also be the result of successful hyperalimentation as illustrated in Figure 11. In these cases, phosphorus in normal physiologic concentration, approximately 4 mg/dl (1.3 mmol/l) should be added to the dialysis solution. To avoid precipitation, it must not be added to the concentrate but must be diluted before mixing with the dialysis solution, which contains calcium.

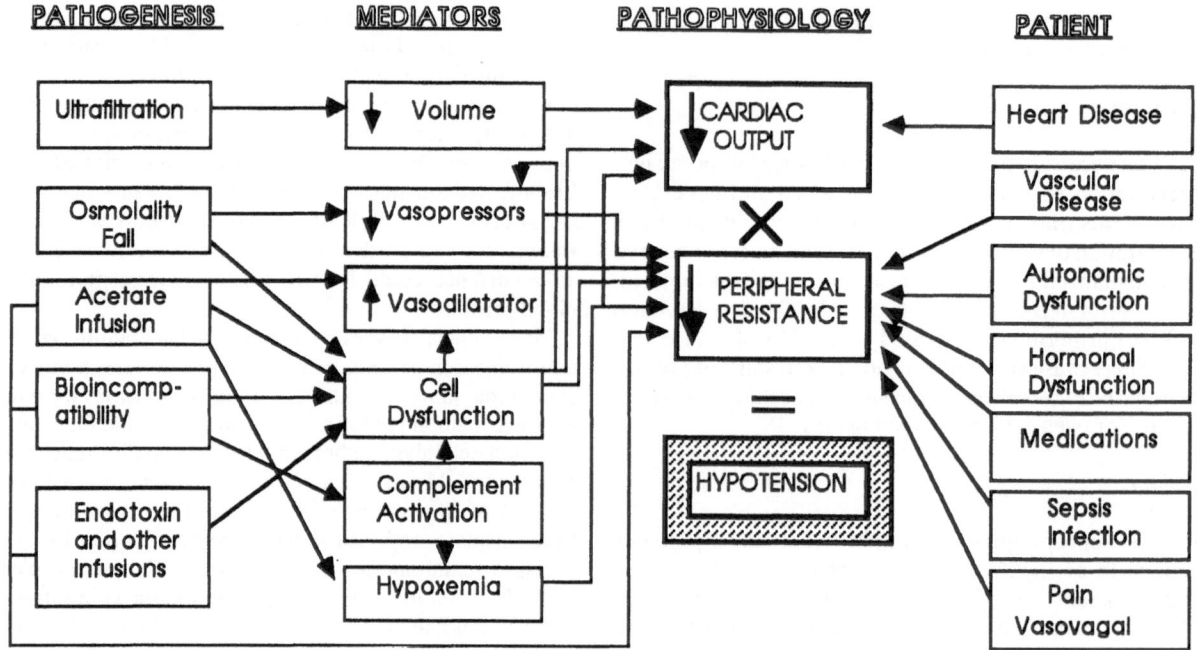

Figure 12. Scheme of the mechanisms underlying dialysis-induced hypotension. Many pathogenic factors may operate during dialysis. They activate mediators that, directly or through other mediators in turn, will decrease cardiac output, peripheral resistance or both. Factors in patients may interfere with the defense against the dialysis-induced decrease in cardiac output or peripheral resistance.

Chloride

Chloride concentration simply makes up the difference between cation and anions in dialysis fluid. In some patients with profound metabolic alkalosis, usually secondary to nasogastric drainage, a lower than normal acetate or bicarbonate and a higher than normal chloride concentration may be beneficial (194).

Complications and their treatment

Blood pressure problems

The most common and dangerous problem occurring during hemodialysis is acute hypotension. Figure 12 outlines factors contributing to or causing hypotension and Table 4 the various treatments and preventions of dialysis hypotension. Hypotension (a blood pressure fall exceeding 25%) occurs in approximately 20 to 50% or all acute dialyses (157, 187, 195, 196). The pathogenesis is multifactorial, poorly understood and thus a source of controversy. Some confusion is semantic from failing to differentiate between pathogenesis, mediators, pathophysiology and underlying pathology.

Ultrafiltration alone rarely causes hypotension because the body's defense mechanisms to compensate for sudden volume reduction, function efficiently unless dialysis is also performed simultaneously (197–199). In markedly fluid overloaded patients with labile blood pressure, isolated ultrafiltration can, therefore, be used. During ultrafiltration, potassium and hydrogen ion removal is inhibited, and be-

cause of the Donnan equilibrium acidosis and hyperkalemia may worsen. The use of *sequential* ultrafiltration-dialysis seems to be of limited use in patients with acute renal failure. During this treatment, the first half of an artificial kidney treatment is spent ultrafiltering the patient's blood without any dialysis fluid perfusing the dialyzer. Thereafter, the hydrostatic and osmotic pressures are equalized across the dialysis membrane and no fluid is removed while dialysis fluid flows promoting diffusion.

There is no difference in the decrement in plasma volume at the end of simultaneous compared to sequential dialysis-ultrafiltration in dogs (200). Large clinical trials have shown that hypotension during the dialysis period of sequential ultrafiltration-dialysis is equal to that of simultaneous dialysis-ultrafiltration (201–203). In patients with acute renal failure it may be preferable to perform ultrafiltration one day and dialysis the next, rather than using sequencing. The induced hypovolemia can also be combated by infusion of colloid solutions, or if much fluid removal is needed, by concentrated colloid such as 25% albumin solution. Theoretically, such a solution mobilizes fluid from the extracapillary, extracellular space into the intravascular space but the exact role of hyperoncotic albumin remains controversial (204).

The acute decrease in plasma osmolality that occurs during dialysis contributes importantly to the pathogenesis of hypotension (205–207). All studies to date, comparing dialysis solutions of varied sodium concentrations, have shown a decreased incidence and severity of hypotension with higher than normal sodium concentrations (176–178). The infusion of mannitol also attenuates the decrease in plasma osmolality and hypotension as, to a lesser extent, does the addition of dextrose to the dialysis solution (190, 205–207). Glycerol infusion has also been used for this purpose (208). The mechanism whereby the decrease in plasma osmolality causes hypotension is multifactorial; the cellular edema associated with decreased plasma osmolality interferes with the release of vasoactive amines. Other explanations include enhanced prostaglandin release, decrease of plasma antidiuretic hormone activity and loss of vasoactive amines through the dialysis membrane (208–220).

Interactions of blood components with the dialyzer membrane, e.g. complement activation resulting in leukocyte adherence and sequestration of leukocytes in the lungs, decrease PaO$_2$, potentially contributing to hypotension. Hypoxia occurring in patients dialyzed for acute renal failure should be treated with an increased oxygen content in the inspired air. The non-cellulosic membranes are more biocompatible and cause less hypoxemia (172–174, 221).

Underlying pathology in severely ill acute renal failure patients may prevent them from compensating for dialysis induced hypotension. Autonomic dysfunction is sometimes present in uremic patients and vasoactive amines are infused

empirically to prevent or treat dialysis induced hypotension (222–225).

In some patients, notably the elderly and those with prior cardiac surgery or heart disease, myocardial dysfunction may impair their ability to increase cardiac output in response to the fall of peripheral resistance that occurs during dialysis. β-agonists may be useful in such patients.

It should be kept in mind that patients may use antihypertensive agents or other drugs that cause hypotension. Such drugs (e.g. β-blockers, methyldopa, phenothiazines) should be discontinued (226).

Patients with sepsis are also more susceptible to blood pressure problems, as are those under vasovagal stimulation by severe pain. Antimicrobials or analgesics may stabilize hemodynamics in such patients.

The many therapies used for dialysis hypotension are outlined in Table 4.

Cardiac arrhythmias

In the acutely ill patient, underlying cardiac problems may contribute to the genesis of arrhythmias, as may the marked electrolyte shifts that often occur during dialysis. As noted above, patients taking digitalis should not undergo dialysis against lower than normal potassium concentration in the dialysis fluid, unless exceptional circumstances exist. Constant cardiac monitoring must then be employed. When arrythmias occur, they should be treated, remembering that certain drugs may have more prolonged effects in patients with renal failure.

Electrolyte abnormalities

In acute renal failure electrolyte disturbances are common. During dialysis numerous changes occur depending on the composition of the dialysis fluid and associated non-dialytic management. These aspects are discussed in the section on compositon of dialysis fluid.

Disequilibrium

Dialysis almost invariably causes some degree of cerebral edema because of intracellular water migration into brain cells. This is most pronounced during the early phase of dialysis, accompanying a pronounced fall in plasma osmolality. It can be combated and avoided as mentioned above by higher sodium and dextrose concentrations in the dialysis fluid or by mannitol or glycerol infusion. Small children, those with previous brain damage and older patients are most susceptible to cerebral edema during dialysis. Children and patients with brain damage tend to convulse; older patients frequently develop psychosis. Families should be alerted to the possibility of transient psychosis during dialysis. Because disequilibrium occurs most frequently when starting dialysis in patients with advanced uremia, initiation of dialysis should not be delayed until the patient is severely uremic. The patient's BUN ordinarily should not be allowed to exceed 100 mg/dl (35.7 mmol/l of urea). However, pa-

Table 4. Treatment of dialysis hypotension.

	Treatment
Pathogenic factors	
Ultrafiltration	Frequent, short dialysis
	Continuous methods
	Constant ultrafiltration
	Separate dialysis and ultrafiltration
Osmolality fall	Slow dialysis efficiency
	Frequent short dialysis
	Higher Na-dialysate
	Infuse: Na, mannitol, other osmolar agents
Bio-incompatibility	New membranes
Acetate infusion	Bicarbonate dialysis
Endotoxin infusion	Clean dialysate
	Tighter membranes
Mediators	
Volume	Smaller dialysers
	Osmolar agents
	Hyperoncotic albumin
Vasopressors	Vasoactive amines
Vasodilatators	Dialysate temperature
	Prostaglandin inhibition
	Higher dialysate calcium
Patient factors	
Heart disease	Beta-agonists
Medications	Discontinue
Vascular disease	?
Autonomic dysfunction	Vasoactive amines
Hormonal dysfunction	Steroids
Infection	Cure
Pain	Ameliorate
Vasovagal	Atropine

tients are frequently severely uremic with very high BUN levels when first admitted. As previously discussed treatment should then start with short dialyses with low clearance technique, which should be repeated daily until uremia has been partly corrected. Infusions of osmotically active substances such as mannitol or concentrated sodium decrease the cerebral edema.

Cell destruction

Hemodialysis influences the formed blood elements. Ten to 15 min after the start of dialysis, the leukocyte count falls to very low values (172–174, 221, 227–230). The leukopenia is attributed to increased leukocyte margination and sequestration in the pulmonary capillaries mediated by complement activation. This theory, however, has been challenged because some membranes markedly activate complement but do not cause leukopenia, whereas the reverse is true for other membranes (230). There is presently no entirely satisfactory explanation for the leukopenia. An adverse effect of the leukopenia is the associated hypoxemia, which should be treated with supplemental oxygen.

Platelets also decrease during dialysis. A mean decrement of 15% can be expected, but catastrophic falls can occur for unexplained reasons. Plate dialyzers may cause more thrombocytopenia than hollow fiber dialyzers, although this observation remains unconfirmed. The cause of the thrombocytopenia is unknown (122).

Patients should not show any evidence of hemolysis during dialysis (231). Marked hemolysis should alert the physician to errors in the dialysis procedure. Such errors include grossly aberrant composition or dialysis fluid contamination with zinc, copper, chloramine or formaldehyde or overheating of the dialysis solution (see also Chapter 33).

Hypoxemia

During hemodialysis, PaO_2 will fall 10 to 20 mm Hg. In a patient with normal oxygen tension before dialysis, this is of no consequence as it changes the blood oxygen saturation very little. However, in a seriously ill patient with a low initial PaO_2, this may be catastrophic. These patients should be given supplemental oxygen.

The decrease in PaO_2 is multifactorial, partly hypoxemia is due to complement activation and complement-mediated leukostasis in the pulmonary capillaries (221, 227–230, 232). However, complement activation, leukopenia and decreases in PaO_2 can be disassociated. Some of the decrease in PaO_2 is due to the removal of CO_2 during dialysis. The resultant decrease of the respiratory drive, lowers PaO_2. Bubbling of CO_2 through the dialysis solution can greatly ameliorate the fall in PaO_2. Finally, the metabolism of acetate into acetyl-coenzyme A requires CO_2 and oxygen consumption may be increased during acetate dialysis. However, there is no difference in oxygen consumption between acetate and bicarbonate dialyses (233). The decreased arterial oxygen tension during dialysis is thus multifactorial. Whatever the ultimate cause, it is clear that critically ill

patients with acute renal failure should receive oxygen supplementation during hemodialysis.

PERITONEAL DIALYSIS

Peritoneal dialysis is discussed in detail in chapters 22 to 25.

There is no difference in the mortality rate of acute renal failure whether the patient is treated with peritoneal or hemodialysis (87–89, 107). Certain patients, such as those with head trauma, marked cardiovascular instability and contaminated abdominal cavities should preferentially be treated by peritoneal dialysis (84, 234, 235). Patients with a stoma or contamination in or near the abdominal wall, hypercatabolic patients and those who need to be treated quickly to allow time for other therapeutic or diagnostic procedures should undergo hemodialysis. Peritoneal dialysis also cannot be used in patients with a large disruption of the peritoneal space such as occurs after surgery for an aortic aneurysm. It should be avoided in patients who have had recent intestinal surgery, as a catheter close to the bowel suture lines impairs healing (236).

Continuous slow peritoneal dialysis may be particularly beneficial for critically ill patients with acute renal failure, correction of body chemistries proceeds smoothly with time for the body's compensatory mechanisms to adjust. It avoids cycling of plasma chemistry and osmolality and needs no anticoagulation (237).

Access to the peritoneum

Peritoneal access can be obtained either with a stiff Teflon or soft Silastic catheter. Either can be placed by a percutaneous puncture technique or through a mini-laparotomy. The soft Silastic catheter, because of its longer subcutaneous tunnel, decreases the incidence of peritonitis caused by bacterial migration along the catheter. This catheter is tolerated better and seems to allow more efficient drainage of dialysate than the stiff catheter. A mini-laparotomy avoids bowel perforation, a possible complication of the percutaneous technique in these patients, who frequently have paralytic ileus or a mechanically distended bowel.

Choice of fluids and additives

Presently available commercial peritoneal dialysis solutions contain electrolytes in their usual extracellular concentrations. Exceptions are potassium, which is usually not added and lactate, which is used instead of bicarbonate. The dextrose monohydrate concentration is varied between 1.5 and 4.25 g/dl (76 to 215 mmol/l).

Because of the slow nature of peritoneal dialysis, there is less need for individual adjustment of the electrolyte composition of the dialysis solution. Potassium is added as indicated depending on the patient's plasma potassium level. A dextrose monohydrate concentration of 1.5 g/dl (76 mmol/l) usually induces little net fluid removal from a patient. The more concentrated solution (4.25 g/dl

[215 mmol/l]) removes 250 to 500 ml of fluid per hour depending on cycling techniques (see Chapters 23 and 24). Heparin is no longer added routinely to the dialysis solution. Some will use heparin for the first few exchanges in a concentration of 500 to 1,000 units per liter of dialysis fluid. Heparin is added to the dialysis fluid, however, in patients with peritonitis to prevent obstruction of the catheter by fibrinous exudate. In the patient with an intact peritoneum, there is usually negligible absorption of heparin from the dialysate. If high doses are used, cathastrophic bleeding may occur.

Antibiotics are of no value prophylactically. They should be added to the dialysate and also used systematically, however, in patients with pre-existing peritonitis or those who develop peritonitis. Peritoneal lavage with antibiotics improves survival in patients with peritonitis. Antibiotics are added to the dialysis fluid to achieve a level equal to the desired plasma water concentration. Once the patient has received a loading dose there is often no need to give more systemic antibiotics. Plasma levels obviously should be measured.

A number of vasodilating pharmacological agents can be added to peritoneal dialysis fluid to increase the efficiency of the procedure. They include dopamine, glucagon, isopropterenol, tolazoline, nitroprusside, dipyridamole, prostaglandins and prostaglandin precursors (see Chapter 24). Moderate increases in dialysis efficiency can be achieved but none have been widely used clinically. The most frequently used agent for this purpose is probably nitroprusside, in a

Table 5. Complications of peritoneal dialysis.

I.	Mechanical:	Pain
		Hemorrhage
		Puncture of intraabdominal organ
		Leakage
		Inadequate drainage
		Dissection of fluid
		Wound/bowel suture problems
		Intraperitoneal catheter loss
II.	Metabolic:	Hypo/hyperglycemia
		Hypo/hypernatremia
		Hypo/hyperkalemia
		Acidosis/alkalosis
		Protein/amino acid loss
III.	Cardiovascular/ pulmonary:	Fluid overload/pulmonary edema
		Hypotension
		Hypertension
		Arrythmia/cardiac arrest
		Atelectasis
		Pneumonia
		Aspiration
		Hydrothorax
IV.	Infectious complications:	Abscess at puncture site
		Bacterial/fungal peritonitis
		(Sterile peritonitis)

See text (and Chapter 24) for details.

dialysis fluid concentration of 4 to 5 μg/l (15 to 19 mmol/l). It has little or no systemic effect when used in this fashion (238).

Complications of peritoneal dialysis

The complications of peritoneal dialysis are outlined in Table 5. They have been described by several authors and are discussed in detail in Chapter 24. They will be only briefly discussed here.

Technical problems

The first technical problems of peritoneal dialysis include perforation of the intestine or bladder. Most authors suggest that when the intestine is perforated, the catheter should be replaced. Peritoneal dialysis with antibiotics added to the dialysis solution should then be instituted as it augments cleaning of the abdominal cavity and decreases the risk of peritonitis. Most such puncture wounds of the intestine heal spontaneously (239, 240).

Drainage problems during peritoneal dialysis are ordinarily due to dislodging or plugging of the catheter. Sometimes the problem can be solved by the use of a Fogarty embolectomy catheter to remove a fibrin plug from the peritoneal catheter. Changing the patient's position sometimes improves drainage. Often, the catheter needs to be replaced.

Metabolic complications

Hyperglycemia can occur with any form of peritoneal dialysis as large amounts (100 to 200 g/day) of dextrose are absorbed from the solution. This is a greater problem if the patient also receives hyperalimentation. Frequent glucose determinations are then necessary. The addition of small amounts of insulin to the peritoneal dialysis solution (such as 20 units to the 1.5% solution and two to three times that amount to the 4.25% solution) may stabilize the glucose levels even in the diabetic patients (240–242).

Hypernatremia may occur during osmotic ultrafiltration because water traverses the peritoneum more easily than sodium (see Chapters 23 and 24). The addition of furosemide to the dialysate has been suggested to increase sodium transport (243). Hyponatremia is a rare complication of dialysis usually due to inappropriate composition of dialysis solution.

Hypokalemia may occur because of potassium removal or a shift intracellularly, resulting from correction of acidosis and dextrose infusion.

Some patients with lactic acidosis cannot be dialyzed using solutions containing lactate as they do not metabolize it rapidly enough to correct their acidosis. Special solutions containing bicarbonate must be used in such patients (244).

Large amounts of protein and amino acids may be lost in the dialysate, particularly when peritonitis exists. Plasma concentrations of these substances should be monitored and repletion intravenously is often necessary (245, 246).

Cardiovascular and pulmonary complications

Arrhythmias and hypotension can occur during the instillation of the dialysis solution. This should be avoided by slowing the inflow rate or decreasing the infusion volume. Atelectasis and hypostatic pneumonia may complicate peritoneal dialysis, but can be partially counteracted by physical therapy. Hydrothorax occurs in 5 to 10% of patients with acute renal failure treated by peritoneal dialysis. It can obviously be a disastrous complication in an acutely ill patient.

Infectious complications

The most common complication of any form of peritoneal dialysis is peritonitis. The incidence should decrease when a long subcutaneous tunnel with a soft peritoneal dialysis catheter and a closed system of dialysis fluid delivery are used. Peritonitis can be diagnosed promptly by inspecting the dialysate for turbidity and by daily microscopic examination. More than 500 leukocytes/μl signifies peritonitis. A test-strip for leukocytes has also been used. When peritonitis is suspected, antibiotics should be added to the dialysate after fluid has been sent for culture. Sometimes parenteral administration of antibiotics is also necessary. Daily cultures of peritoneal fluid in such patients may detect an infection early (247, 248).

SLOW CONTINUOUS HEMOFILTRATION
(see also Chapter 15)

Slow continuous arterio-venous hemofiltration is technically simple because there is no requirement for a blood pump or monitoring equipment. Only an arteriovenous shunt, blood lines, filter, heparin infusion pump and a warmer for the intravenous replacement fluid are needed. It is desirable to have a device that compares the ultrafiltration rate to intravenous fluid administration (146, 147, 249–256). The hemofilter is connected directly to an arteriovenous shunt. The arterial pressure and venous resistance produce a transmembrane pressure (TMP) that usually results in an ultrafiltrate of 10 to 15 ml/min (147, 249–253). If a low blood pressure or low venous resistance cause a low filtration rate, this can be enhanced by decreasing the pressure on the filtrate side of the filter, by connecting it to a negative pressure outlet. Predilution also enhances the clearance of the filter (257). Different brands of filters show marked differences in molecular rejection (251). However, for molecules, smaller than 1,000 to 2,000 daltons (urea, creatinine, uric acid), with membrane rejections of nearly zero the clearance equals the ultrafiltration rate. Protein-coating causes large variations in the rejection of larger molecules (251). The membranes used for hemofiltration have a high degree of biocompatability. Thus, complement is not activated and leukopenia and hypoxemia do not occur (144, 145, 147). There is usually also a high degree of cardiovascular stability. At least in the beginning of therapy, blood pressure

and pulse rate do not change (145, 254). Hyper- and superalimentation is easy to perform by adding calories and amino acids to the substitution fluids.

Disadvantages of the therapy are the need for continuous heparin, the changing fluid balance and changes in heart rate and blood pressure that may occur late in the treatment. Together these problems lead to the requirement of large commitment of nursing staff time (147, 258).

Several reports of clinical results have now appeared (146, 147, 249–258). Early, there was a high mortality rate, 79%, but in the later studies 45% of acute patients survived, the same survival as reported for intermittent hemodialysis (256).

Access

An arteriovenous connection is needed through a Scribner shunt. Indwelling catheters in the femoral artery and femoral vein have been advocated but thrombosis of both vessels has also been described and this routine is best avoided (144, 145, 151, 255). A blood pump is necessary if a vein-to-vein approach is used. Pressure meters and air detectors are then required and this defeats the technical simplicity of the procedure.

Filter

Many filters have been tested clinically. Presently most widely used are the Amicon and Gambro filters (147, 251, 253). All use highly biocompatible membranes, but there are marked variations in protein coating (251). This probably has no clinical relevance.

Anticoagulation

Continuous hemofiltration requires continuous anticoagulation. Bleeding complications have been reported frequently. (144, 145, 147, 249, 252, 256, 258). In some patients continuous filtration has been performed without any anticoagulation (259). The need for continuous anticoagulation makes this method unsafe in patients at high risk for bleeding.

Complications

The main clinical problem of slow continuous arteriovenous hemofiltration is bleeding. During the initial phase, there are few cardiovascular symptoms, but these sometimes increase if filtration is used for an extended time. In one crossover study comparing slow continuous hemofiltration to intermittent hemodialysis in patients with acute renal failure, there was less hypotension and tachyarrhythmia per time unit on slow continuous hemofiltration. However, when complications were normalized to achieved BUN clearance, there were twice as many hypotensive and four times as many tacharrhythmic episodes on slow continuous hemofiltration (147, 258). These may have been caused by excessive ultrafiltration, due to the technique or may have been the usual problems occurring early with any technical procedures. Some patients are difficult to treat because they rapidly clot the filters in spite of adequate anticoagulation.

OTHER DIALYSIS METHODS

Slow continuous hemodialysis, intermittent and continuous hemodiafiltration and pleural dialysis have been used in acute renal failure, but there is no large clinical body of experience or information obtained with thse procedures (260–262).

IMPROVING SURVIVAL

It is clear that the mortality of acute renal failure depends mainly on the underlying disease. Thus, in patients dialyzed acutely for primary kidney disease, the mortality is only 24%, whereas in acute tubular necrosis, a complication of various medical and surgical insults, it approaches 70%. The mortality rate of tubular necrosis correlates with the primary disease. In obstetric-gynecologic cases, the mortality is usually only between 10 and 20%, whereas when tubular necrosis follows major cardiovascular or gastrointestinal surgery it can rise to 80% (Table 2). Improved survival rates, therefore, must depend mostly on improved management of the underlying disease. Aggressive surgery and a high index of suspicion for surgical complications are necessary. Because infectious complications are so commonly the proximate cause of death for these patients, improved antibiotic treatment based on frequent cultures and sensitivity tests to guide the choice of antibiotics and dosage adjustment and use of some of the newer antibiotics also may help decrease mortality. Antibiotic barrage, such as suggested for immunosuppressed patients with cancer has not been studied in patients with acute renal failure and should be. Increasing usage and an increased understanding of hyperalimentation could also contribute to a decrease in mortality rate by improving recovery from surgery and immune defense.

Many attempts have been made to improve the dialysis treatment itself. Earlier start, more frequent and more efficient dialysis have all been suggested as means of improving survival for patients with acute renal failure. Results have been contradictory except when comparing very early to very late dialysis. Most centers now utilize dialysis before the BUN reaches 100 to 110 mg/dl (36 to 39 mmol/l of urea) and use almost daily- or every other day dialysis. In the study by Gillum et al (86), there was no difference in either survival or complications between daily and every other day dialysis. This, coupled with the report by Mentzer et al (85), that dialysis requiring acute renal failure following cadaver transplantation, was inconsequential for survival, suggest that acute dialysis has reached a high degree of safety and perfection. Conversely, it is unlikely that any technical changes in the procedure of acute blood purification is going to have a measurable impact on survival. Patients do not die because of dialysis problems. They die because we cannot

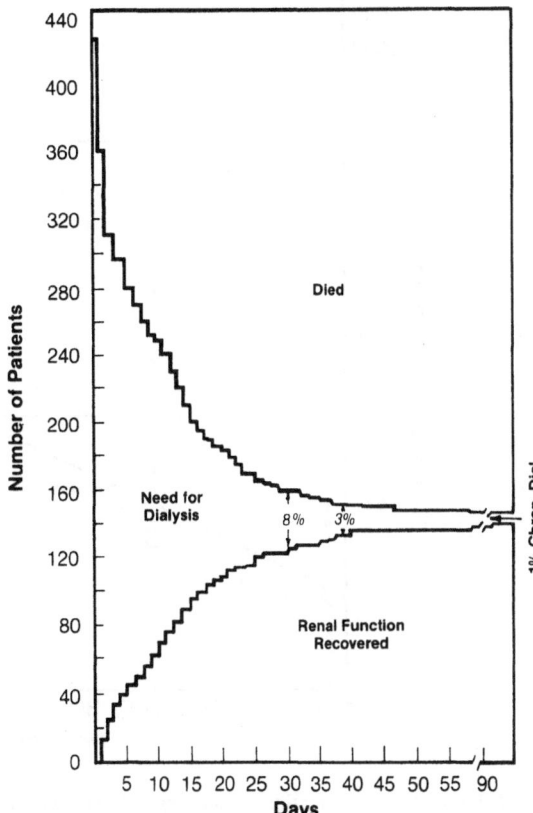

Figure 13. Clinical course of 432 patients with acute tubular necrosis who needed dialysis. The median time for patients who recovered renal function is approximately 12 days, for those who die, 5 days. By 30 days, 92% of the patients recovered renal function or died. At 40 days, only 3% of the patients remain on dialysis. Ultimately, only 1% of the patients started on dialysis (4% of those who survive) need chronic dialysis. (From [10], reproduced with permission of the American Society for Artificial Organs).

yet cure their basic disease, underlying pathology or their complicating infections.

RECOVERY OF RENAL FUNCTION; NEED FOR CONTINUED DIALYSIS

The clinical course of acute tubular necrosis is rapid. This is illustrated in Figure 13. In patients dialyzed for acute renal failure at the University of Minnesota, the median interval between initiation of dialysis and recovery of renal function of the survivors was 12 days. The median time between start of dialysis and death was 5 days. By 1 month 92% and by $1\frac{1}{2}$ months 97% of the patients had either regained renal function or had died. After 45 days of acute renal failure $\frac{1}{3}$ of the remaining patients died. $\frac{1}{3}$ recovered renal function and $\frac{1}{3}$ needed regular dialysis. The longest time a patient was

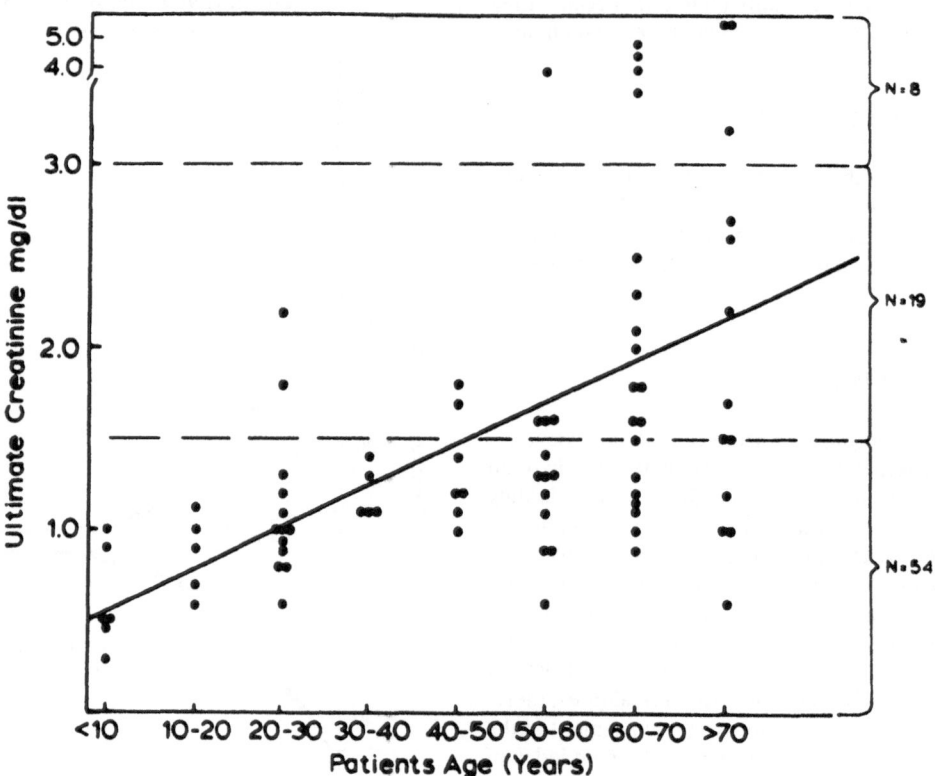

Figure 14. Ultimate serum creatinine versus age of patients who needed dialysis for acute tubular necrosis. There is a direct relation of ultimate serum creatinine level to age. Severe chronic renal failure occurs only in patients over the age of 50 years. (From [10], reproduced with permission of the American Society for Artificial Internal Organs).

dialyzed and recovered renal function was 88 days (10).

These data are similar to those from comparable groups of patients during the past few decades. Thus, Alwall (4) reported that in the early years of dialysis patients with acute tubular necrosis needed dialysis for an average of 15 days. One patient in his series did not recover renal function until 65 days after initiation of dialysis. In the Glasgow experience between 1959 and 1970, the mean duration of dialysis for acute renal failure was 11 days and the longest time to recovery of kidney function was 42 days (8). Obviously, these figures have not changed over the years. Thus, these patients have a swift clinical course and although they require an enormous investment in care and equipment, few patients require dialysis and intensive care for more than 4 weeks. Renal function usually continues to improve for approximately one month after the last dialysis. Approximately one-third of the patients are left with moderate renal dysfunction (plasma creatinine level 1.5 to 3 mg/dl [133 to 265 μmol/l]) and 10% have residual chronic renal failure with plasma creatinine concentration exceeding 3 mg/dl (265 μmol/l) (10, 260, 263–268). The duration of dialysis for acute tubular necrosis does not correlate with the ultimate plasma creatinine concentration. Thus, patients who were dialyzed only once eventually had the same plasma cre-

atinine concentration (more than 1 month after the last dialysis) as those who needed dialysis for more than 1 month (10). One patient needed dialysis for almost 3 months but ultimately reached a serum creatinine level of 1.2 mg/dl (106 μmol/l). Age, however, is directly related to the final serum creatinine concentration (Figure 14). Older patients progress to chronic renal failure, more often than younger patients do. Patients with severe urinary tract infections complicating acute tubular necrosis, also have less recovery of PAH and inulin clearance and urinary concentrating ability (268). Isolated cases of severe irreversible renal failure have been reported (269–271).

Six among approximately 500 patients have remained on chronic hemodialysis after they developed what was thought to be acute tubular necrosis. Three of them sustained acute renal failure after operations for aortic aneurysms. Cholesterol embolization, a known cause of chronic renal failure, may have contributed to their need for chronic hemodialysis. One patient had undergone methoxyflurane anesthesia, also a known cause of irreversible renal failure. In two patients, however, no known cause of chronic renal failure complicating the acute tubular necrosis could be identified (10, 269). Bilateral renal cortical necrosis also begins acutely and results in irreversible renal failure requiring chronic dialysis.

Thus, of the patients who come to dialysis for acute tubular necrosis, approximately two-thirds will die, usually quite fast. Of the one-third who survive, almost 65% have complete return of renal function. Approximately 25% will be left with moderate renal insufficiency (creatinine <3 mg/dl). 10% will have severe chronic renal failure (creatinine >3 mg/dl [265 μmol/l]), and 5% will need chronic dialysis (10).

CONCLUSIONS

Most patients with acute renal failure suffer from acute tubular necrosis. The mortality rate in these patients remains between 20 and 80% and has not improved with time. This is probably due to improvement in conservative management that leaves more severely ill patients in need of acute dialysis than before. Acute hemodialysis remains the main stay of treatment for these patients. New developments include continuous peritoneal dialysis and continuous hemofiltration. Improved treatment of the basic disease, causing acute tubular necrosis and of infections, seem to offer the best chances for improving survival. Technical modifications of the dialysis procedure are unlikely to have a great impact.

The patients with acute tubular necrosis have a very rapid clinical course. Moderate, clinically insignificant renal dysfunction is not an uncommon sequel. Severe chronic renal failure is unusual and the persistent need for maintenance hemodialysis is rare.

REFERENCES

1. Kolff WJ: First clinical experience with the artificial kidney. *Ann Intern Med* 62: 608, 1965
2. Alwall N: On the artificial kidney. I. Apparatus for dialysis of the blood in vivo. *Acta Med Scand* 128: 317, 1947
3. Murray G: Development of an artificial kidney; experimental and clinical experiences. *Arch Surg* 55: 505, 1947
4. Alwall N: *Therapeutic and Diagnostic Problems in Severe Renal Failure.* Copenhagen, Munksgaard, 1963
5. Merrill JP, Smith S, Callahan EJ, Thorn GW: Use of artificial kidney: clinical experience. *J Clin Invest* 29: 425, 1950
6. Teschan PE, Post RS, Smith LH, Abernathy RS, Davis JH, Gray DM, Howard JM, Johnson KE, Klopp E, Mundy RL, O'Meara MP, Rush BF: Post-traumatic renal insufficiency in military casualties. I. Clinical characteristics. *Am J Med* 18: 172, 1955
7. Balslov JT, Jorgensen HE: A survey of 499 patients with acute anuric renal insufficiency, causes, treatment, complications and mortality. *Am J Med* 34: 753, 1963
8. Kennedy AC, Burton JA, Luke RG, Briggs JD, Lindsay RM, Allison MEM, Edward N, Dargie HJ: Factors affecting the prognosis in acute renal failure, A survey of 251 cases. *Q J Med* 42: 73, 1973
9. Kirkland K, Edwards KDG, Whyte HM: Oliguric renal failure: A report of 400 cases including classification, survival and response to dialysis. *Australas Ann Med* 14: 275, 1965
10. Kjellstrand CM, Ebben J, Davin T: Time of death, recovery of renal function, development of chronic renal failure and need for chronic hemodialysis in patients with acute tubular necrosis. *Trans Am Soc Artif Intern Organs* 27: 45, 1981
11. Teschan PE, Baxter CR, O'Brien TF, Freuhof JN, Hall WH: Prophylactic hemodialysis in the treatment of acute renal failure. *Ann Intern Med* 53: 992, 1960
12. Lundberg M: Dialysbehandling vid akut njurinsufficiens. (Dialysis treatment for acute renal insufficiency) *Läkartidningen* 67: 487, 1970
13. Eliahou HA, Boichis H, Bott-Kanner G, Barell V, Bar-Noach N, Modan B: An epidemiologic study of renal failure. II. Acute renal failure. *Am J Epidemiol* 101: 281, 1975
14. Karatso A, Juhasz I, Koves S, Balogh F: Estimated frequency of acute and chronic renal insufficiencies in a transdanubian region of Hungary. *Int Urol Nephrol* 7: 321, 1975
15. Lachhein L, Kielstein R, Sauer K, Reinschke P, Muller V, Krumhaar I, Falkenhagen D, Schmidt R, Klinkmann H: Evaluation of 433 cases of acute renal failure. *Proc Eur Dial Transplant Assoc* 14: 628, 1977
16. Wing AJ, Broyer M, Brunner FP, Brynger H, Challa S, Donckerwolke RA, Gretz N, Jacobs C, Kramer P, Selwood NH: Combined report on regular dialysis and transplantation in Europe, XIII, 1982. *Proc Eur Dial Transplant Assoc* 20: 5, 1983
17. Hou S, Bushinsky DA, Wish H, Cohen JJ, Harrington JT: Hospital-acquired renal insufficiency: A prospective study. *Am J Med* 74: 243, 1983
18. Porter GA, Bennett WM: Nephrotoxin-induced acute renal failure. in: *Acute Renal Failure,* edited by Brenner BM, Stein JH, New York, Churchill, Livingstone, 1980
19. Hermreck AS, Ruiz-Ocana FM, Proberts KS, Meisel RL, Crawford DG: Mechanisms for oliguria in acute renal failure. *Surgery* 82: 141, 1977
20. Levinsky NG: Pathophysiology of acute renal failure. *N Engl J Med* 296: 1453, 1977
21. Solez K, Morel-Maroger L, Sraer JD: The morphology of 'acute tubular necrosis' in man: Analysis of 57 renal biopsies and a comparison with the glycerol model. *Medicine* 58: 362, 1979
22. Myers BD, Carrie BJ, Yee RR, Hilberman M, Michaels AS: Pathophysiology of hemodynamically mediated acute renal failure in man. *Kidney Int* 18: 110, 1980
23. Olbricht CHJ: Experimental models of acute renal failure. *Contrib Nephrol* 19: 110, 1980
24. Conger JD, Schrier RW: Renal hemodynamics in acute renal failure. *Annu Rev Physiol* 42: 603, 1980
25. Richmond JM, Walker JF, Avila A, Petrakis A, Finley RJ, Sibbald WJ, Linton AL: Renal and cardiovascular response to nonhypotensive sepsis in a large animal model with peritonitis. *Surgery* 97: 205, 1985
26. Zager RA, Sharma HM, Johannes GA: Gentamicin increases renal susceptibility to an acute ischemic insult. *J Lab Clin Med* 101: 670, 1983
27. Fink MP, MacVittie TJ, Casey LC: Effects of nonsteroidal anti-inflammatory drugs on renal function in septic dogs. *J Surg Res* 36: 516, 1984
28. Harkonen S, Kjellstrand C: Contrast nephropathy. *Am J Nephrol* 1: 69, 1981
29. Rasmussen HH, Lloyd SI: Acute renal failure. *Am J Med* 73: 211, 1984
30. Miller PD, Krebs RA, Neal BJ, McIntyre DO: Polyuric prerenal failure. *Arch Intern Med* 140: 907, 1980
31. Ellenbogen P, Schieble F, Talner L: Sensitivity of gray scale ultrasound in detecting urinary tract obstruction. *Am J Roentgenol* 130: 731, 1978

32. Rascoff JH, Golden RA, Spinowitz BS, Charytan C: Non-dilated obstructive nephropathy. *Arch Intern Med* 143: 696, 1983

33. Mc Clennan B: Current approaches to the azotemic patient. *Radiol Clin North Am* 17: 314, 1979

34. Wilson DR: Renal function during and following obstruction. *Annu Rev Med* 28: 329, 1977

35. Pru C, Kjellstrand CM: Indices and urinary chemistries in the differential diagnosis of pre-renal failure and acute tubular necrosis. *Semin Nephrol* 5: 224, 1985

36. Ransohoff DF, Feinstein AR: Problems of spectrum and bias in evaluating the efficacy of diagnostic tests. *N Engl J Med* 299: 926, 1978

37. Brown R, Babcock R, Tablert J, Gruenberg J, Czurak C, Campbell M: Renal function in critically ill postoperative patients: sequential assessment of creatinine, osmolar and free water clearance. *Crit Care Med* 8: 68, 1980

38. Levinsky NG, Bernard DB, Johnsson PA: Enhancement of recovery of acute renal failure: effects of mannitol and diuretics. in *Acute Renal Failure,* edited by Brenner BM, Stein JH, New York, Churchill Livingstone, 1980, p 163

39. Mann HJ, Fuhs DW, Hemstrom CA: Acute renal failure. *Drug Intell Clin Pharm* 20: 421, 1986

40. Henderson IS, Beattie TJ, Kennedy AC: Dopamine hydrochloride in oliguric states. *Lancet* 2: 827, 1980

41. Neiberger RE, Passmore JC: Effects of dopamine on canine intrarenal blood flow distribution during hemorrhage. *Kidney Int* 15: 219, 1979

42. Lindner A: Synergism of dopamine and furosemide in diuretic-resistant, oliguric acute renal failure. *Nephron* 33: 121, 1983

43. Schafferhans K, Heidbreder E, Grimm D, Heidland A: Norepinephrine-induced acute renal failure: Beneficial effects of atrial natriuretic factor. *Nephron* 44: 240, 1986

44. Paller MS: Free radical scavengers in mercuric chloride-induced acute renal failure in the rat. *J Lab Clin Med* 105: 459, 1985

45. Paller MS, Hoidal JR, Ferris TF: Oxygen free radicals in ischemic acute renal failure in the rat. *J Clin Invest* 74: 1156, 1984

46. Siegel NJ, Glazier WB, Chaudry IH, Gaudio KM, Lytton B, Baue AE, Kashgarian M: Enhanced recovery from acute renal failure by the postischemic infusion of adenine nucleotides and magnesium chloride in rats. *Kidney Int* 7: 338, 1980

47. Sumpio BE, Chaudry IH, Baue AE: Reduction of the drug-induced nephrotoxicity by ATP- $MgCl_2$. 1. Effects on the cis-diamminedicholoroplatinum-treated isolated perfused kidneys. *J Surg Res* 38: 429, 1985

48. Oken DE, Sprinke FM, Kirschbaum BB, Landwehr DM: Amino acid therapy in the treatment of experimental acute renal failure in the rat. *Kidney Int* 17: 14, 1980

49. Loutzenhiser R, Epstein M: Calcium antagonists and the kidney. Hospital Practice Jan 15; 63, 1987

50. Wagner K, Albrecht S, Neumayer H-H: Prevention of delayed graft function in cadaveric kidney transplantation by a calcium antagonist. Preliminary results of two prospective randomized trials. *Transplant Proc* 18: 510, 1986

51. Wagner K, Schultze G, Molzahn M, Neumayer H-H: The influence of long-term infusion of the calcium antagonist diltiazem on postischemic acute renal failure in conscious dogs. *Klin Wochenschr* 64: 135, 1986

52. Abel RM, Beck CH, Abbott WM, Ryan JA, Barnett GO, Fisher JE: Improved survival from acute renal failure after with intravenous essential L-amino acids and glucose. *N Engl J Med* 288: 695, 1973

53. Baek SM, Makabali GG, Bryan-Brown CW, Kusek J, Shoemaker WC: The influence of parenteral nutrition on the course of acute renal failure. *Surg Gynecol Obstet* 141: 405, 1975

54. Asbach HW, Stoeckel H, Schuler HW, Conradi R, Wiedemann K, Mohring K, Rohl L: The treatment of hypercatabolic acute renal failure by adequate nutrition and haemodialysis. *Acta Anaesthesiol Scand* 18: 255, 1974

55. Leonard CD, Luke RG, Siegel RR: Parenteral essential amino acids in acute renal failure. *Urology* 6: 154, 1975

56. Borges H, Hocks J, Kjellstrand C: Mannitol intoxication in patients with renal failure. *Arch Intern Med* 142: 63, 1982

57. Smith JH, Merrell RC, Raffin TA: Reversal of postoperative anuria by decompressive celiotomy. *Arch Intern Med* 145: 553, 1985

58. Gehrig JJ: Oliguria and increased intra-abdominal pressure. *JAMA* 253: 39, 1985

59. Chugh KS: Clinicopathological spectrum of acute renal failure in India. *Proc First Asian Pacific Congr Nephrol Hihol Univ, Dept of Med, Tokyo* 1979, p 133

60. Chugh KS, Pal Y, Chakravarty RN, Datta DB, Mehta R, Sakhuja V, Mandal AK, Sommers SC: Acute renal failure following poisonous snakebite. *Am J Kidney Dis* 4: 30, 1984

61. Sitprija V: The kidney in acute tropical disease. *Abstacts 8th Int Congress Nephrol* 8: 279, 1981

62. Lordon RE, Burton JR: Post-traumatic renal failure in military personnel in Southeast Asia: experience at Clark USAF Hospital. Republic of the Philippines. *Am J Med* 53; 137, 1972

63. Fischer RP: High mortality of post-traumatic renal insufficiency in Vietnam: a review of 96 cases. *Am Surg* 40: 172, 1974

64. Stone WJ, Knepshield JH: Post-traumatic acute renal insufficiency in Vietnam. *Clin Nephrol* 2: 186, 1974

65. Barsoum RS, Rihan ZEB, Baligh OK, Hozayen A, El-Ghonaimy EHG, Ramzy MF, Ibrahuim AS: Acute renal failure in the 1973 Middle East War: experience of a specialized base hospital: effect of the site of injury. *J Trauma* 20: 303, 1980

66. Bullock ML, Umen AJ, Finkelstein M, Keane WF: The assessment of risk factors in 462 patients with acute renal failure. *Am J Kidney Dis* 5: 97, 1985

67. Plough AL, Salem S: Social and contextual factors in the analysis of mortality in end-stage renal disease patients: implications for health policy. *Am J Public Health* 7: 1293, 1982

68. Avram MM, Pahilan A, Altman E, Gan A, Iancu M: A 15-year experience with intradialytic treatment mortality. *Abstracts Am Soc Artif Intern Organs* 11: 41, 1982

69. Friedman EA, Manis T, Delano BG, Rao TKS, Levits CS, Lundin AP III: Extraordinary safety of hemodialysis. *Abstracts Am Soc Artif Intern Organs* 11: 48, 1982

70. McMurray SD, Luft FC, Maxwell DR, Hamburger RJ, Futty D, Swed JJ, Lavelle KJ, Kleit SA: Prevailing patterns and predictor variables in patients with acute tubular necrosis. *Arch Intern Med* 138: 950, 1978

71. Gornick CC Jr, Kjellstrand CM: Acute renal failure complicating aortic aneurysm surgery. *Nephron* 35: 145, 1983

72. Wheeler DC, Feehally J, Walls J: High risk acute renal failure. *Q J Med* 61: 977, 1986

73. Abreo K, Vishnu Moorthy A, Osborne M: Changing patterns and outcome of acute renal failure requiring hemodialysis. *Arch Intern Med* 146: 1338, 1986

74. Rasmussen HH, Pitt EA, Ibels LS, McNeil DR: Prediction of outcome in acute renal failure by discriminant analysis of clinical variables. *Arch Intern Med* 145: 2015, 1985

75. Lien J, Chan V: Risk factors influencing survival in acute renal failure treated by hemodialysis. *Arch Intern Med* 145: 2067, 1985

76. Anderson RJ, Linas SL, Berns AS, Henrich WL, Miller TR, Gabow PA, Schrier RW: Nonoliguric acute renal failure. *New Engl J Med* 296: 1134, 1977

77. Kunz A, Glinz W, Keusch G, Binswanger U: Akutes Nierenversagen bei polytraumatisierten Patienten. (Acute renal failure in multiply traumatized patients.) *Schweiz Med Wochenschr* 114: 876, 1984

78. Wagner DP, Knaus WA, Draper EA: Physiologic abnormalities and outcome from acute disease. *Arch Intern Med* 146: 1389, 1986

79. Corwin HL, Teplick RS, Schreiber MJ, Fang LST, Bonventre JV, Coggins CH: Prediction of outcome in acute renal failure. *Am J Nephrol* 7: 8, 1987

80. Bell RC, Coalson JJ, Smith JD, Johannson WG: Multiple organ system failure and infection in adult respiratory distress syndrome. *Ann Intern Med* 99: 293, 1983

81. Cioffi WG, Ashikaga T, Gamelli RL: Probability of surviving postoperative acute renal failure. *Ann Surg* 2: 205, 1984

82. Polk HC Jr, Shields CL: Remote organ failure: A valid sign of occult intra-abdominal infection. *Surgery* 81: 310, 1977

83. Fry DE, Pearlstein L, Fulton RL, Polk HC Jr: Multiple system organ failure. *Arch Surg* 115: 136, 1980

84. Matas AJ, Payne WD, Simmons RL, Buselmeier TJ, Kjellstrand CM: Acute renal failure following blunt civilian trauma. *Ann Surg* 185: 301, 1977

85. Mentzer SJ, Fryd DS, Kjellstrand CM: Why do patients with postsurgical acute tubular necrosis die? *Arch Surg* 120: 907, 1985

86. Gillum DM, Dixon BS, Yanover MJ, Kelleher SP, Shapiro MD, Benedetti RG, Dillingham MA, Paller MS, Goldberg JP, Tomford RC, Gordon JA, Conger JD: The role of intensive dialysis in acute renal failure. *Clin Nephrol* 5: 249, 1986

87. Kleinknecht D, Junger P, Chanard J, Barbanel C, Ganeval D: Uremic and non-uremic complications in acute renal failure: evaluation of early and frequent dialysis on prognosis. *Kidney Int* 1: 190, 1972

88. Marshall VC: Acute renal failure in surgical patients. *Br J Surg* 58: 17, 1971

89. Stott RB, Ogg CS, Cameron JS, Bewick M: Why the persistently high mortality in acute renal failure? *Lancet* 2: 75, 1972

90. Zimmerman JE: Respiratory failure complicating posttraumatic acute renal failure: etiology, clinical features and management. *Ann Surg* 174: 12, 1971

91. Lucas CE, Ledgerwood AM, Shier MR, Bradley VE: The renal factor in the post-traumatic 'fluid overload' syndrome. *J Trauma* 17: 667, 1977

92. Kjellstrand CM, Davin TJ, Matas AJ, Buselmeier TJ: Postoperative acute renal failure: diagnosis, etiologic and symptomatic treatment and prognosis. in: *Clinical Surgical Care*, edited by Najarian JS, Delaney JP, New York, Stratton Intercontinental Med Book Corp, 1977, p 309

93. Kohen JA, Opsahl JA, Kjellstrand CM: Deceptive patterns of uremic pulmonary edema. *Am J Kidney Dis* 7:456, 1986

94. Bland R, Shoemaker WC, Shabot MM: Physiologic monitoring goals for the critically ill patient. *Surg Gynecol Obstet* 147: 833, 1978

95. Holliday RL, Doris PJ: Monitoring the critically ill surgical patient. *Can Med Assoc J* 121: 931, 1979

96. Anderson CC, Shahvari MBG, Zimmerman JE: The treatment of pulmonary edema in the absence of renal function – a role for sorbitol and furosemide. *JAMA* 241: 1008, 1979

97. Bercovitch DD, Davidman M, Lichter M: Hyperkalemia provoked by acute hepatic necrosis. *Am J Nephrol* 6: 296, 1986

98. Galler M, Folkert VW, Schlondorff D: Reversible acute renal insufficiency and hyperkalemia following indomethacin therapy. *JAMA* 246: 155, 1981

99. Hylander B: Survival of extreme hyperkalemia. *Acta Med Scand* 221: 121, 1987

100. Montoliu J, Lenz XM, Revert L: Potassium-lowering effect of albuterol for hyperkalemia in renal failure. *Arch Intern Med* 147: 713, 1987

101. Wolk PJ, Apicella MA: The effect of renal function on the febrile response to bacteremia. *Arch Intern Med* 138: 1084, 1978

102. Goldblum SE, Reed WP: Host defenses and immunologic alterations associated with chronic hemodialysis. *Ann Intern Med* 93: 597, 1980

103. Peresecerschi G, Blum M, Aviram A, Spirer ZH: Impaired neutrophil response to acute bacterial infection in dialyzed patients. *Arch Intern Med* 141: 1301, 1981

104. Burke JP, Garibaldi RA, Britt MR, Jacobson JA, Conti M, Alling DW: Prevention of catheter-associated urinary tract infections. *Am J Med* 70: 655, 1981

105. Turck M, Stamm W: Nosocomial infection of the urinary tract. *Am J Med* 70: 651, 1981

106. Rowley KM, Clubb KS, Walker Smith GJ, Cabin HS: Right-sided infective endocarditis as a consequence of flow-directed pulmonary-artery catheterization. *N Engl J Med* 311: 1152, 1984

107. Marshall V: Secondary surgical intervention in acute renal failure. *Aust NZ J Surg* 44: 96, 1974

108. Kornhall S: Acute renal failure in surgical disease with special regard to neglected complications. *Acta Chir Scand* 419: 3, 1971

109. Sinanan M, Maier RV, Carrico CJ: Laparotomy for intra-abdominal sepsis in patients in an Intensive Care Unit. *Arch Surg* 119: 652, 1984

110. Feinsten EI, Blumenkrantz MJ, Healy M: Clinical and metabolic response to parenteral nutrition in acute renal failure. A controlled double blind study. *Medicine* 60: 124, 1981

111. Daly JM, Dudrick SJ, Copeland EM: Intravenous hyperalimentation: effect on delayed cutaneous hypersensitivity in cancer patients. *Ann Surg* 192: 587, 1980

112. Dionigi R, Zonta A, Dominioni L, Gnes F, Ballabio A: The effects of total parenteral nutrition on immunodepression due to malnutrition. *Ann Surg* 185: 467, 1977

113. Mullen JL, Buzby GP, Matthews DC, Smale BF, Rosato EF: Reduction of operative morbidity and mortality by combined preoperative and postoperative nutritional support. *Ann Surg* 192: 604, 1980

114. Michel L, Serrano A, Malt RA: Nutritional support of hospitalized patients. *N Engl J Med* 304: 1147, 1981

115. Editorial: Current status of peripheral alimentation. *Ann Intern Med* 95: 114, 1981

116. Padberg FT, Ruggiero J, Blackburn GL, Bistrian BR: Central venous catheterization of parenteral nutrition. *Ann Surg* 193: 264, 1981

117. Abel RM: Acute renal failure, role of parenteral nutrition. *Contemp Surg* 13: 21, 1978

118. Sargent JA, Gotch FA: Nutrition and treatment of the acutely ill patient using urea kinetics. *Dial Transplant* 10: 314, 1981

119. Blagg CR, Parsons FM: Earlier dialysis and anabolic steroids in acute renal failure. *Am Heart J* 61: 287, 1961

120. Cerra FB: Hypermetabolism, organ failure, and metabolic support. *Surgery* 1: 1, 1987

121. Kopple JD, Gordon SI, Wang M, Swendseid ME: Factors affecting serum and urinary guanidinosuccinic acid levels in normal and uremic subjects. *J Lab Clin Med* 90: 303, 1977

122. Lynch RE, Bosl RH, Streifel AJ, Ebben JP, Ehlers SM, Kjellstrand CM: Dialysis thrombocytopenia: parallel plate vs hollow fiber dialyzers. *Trans Am Soc Artif Intern Organs* 24: 704, 1978

123. Vicks SL, Gross ML, Schmitt GW: Massive hemorrhage due to hemodialysis-associated thrombocytopenia. *Am J Nephrol* 3: 30, 1983

124. Janson PA, Jubelirer S, Weinsten M, Deykin D: Treatment of the bleeding tendency in uremia with cryoprecipitate. *New Engl J Med* 303: 1318, 1980

125. Mannucci PM, Remuzzi G, Pusineri F, Lombardi R, Valsecchi C, Mecca G, Zimmerman TS: Deamino-8-arginine vasopressin shortens bleeding in uremia. *N Engl J Med* 308: 8, 1983

126. Liu YK, Kosfeld RE, Marcum SG: Treatment of uraemic bleeding with conjugated oestrogen. *Lancet* 2: 887, 1984

127. Czer LSC, Shoemaker WC: Optimal hematocrit value in critically ill postoperative patients. *Surg Gynecol Obstet* 147: 363, 1978

128. Livio M, Marchesi D, Remuzzi G, Gotti E, Mecca G, Gaetano G: Uraemic bleeding: role of anaemia and beneficial effect of red cell transfusions. *Lancet* 2: 1013, 1982

129. Remuzzi G, Marchesi D, Cavenaghi AE, Livio M, Donati MB, de Gaetano G, Mecca G: Bleeding in renal failure: a possible role of vascular prostacyclin (PGI$_2$). *Clin Nephrol* 12: 127, 1979

130. Shuman RB, Schuster DP, Zuckerman GR: Prophylactic therapy for stress ulcer bleeding: A reappraisal. *Ann Intern Med* 106: 562, 1987

131. Ardaillou R, Beaufils M, Nivez M-P, Isaac R, Mayaud C, Sraer J-D: Increased plasma calcitonin in early acute renal failure. *Clin Sci Mol Med* 49: 301, 1975

132. Weinstein RS, Hudson JB: Parathyroid hormone and 25-hydroxycholecalciferol levels in hypercalcemia of acute renal failure. *Arch Intern Med* 140: 410, 1980

133. Arieff AI, Massry SG: Calcium metabolism of brain in acute renal failure: effects of uremia, hemodialysis and parathyroid hormone. *J Clin Invest* 53: 387, 1974

134. de Torrente A, Berl T, Cohn PD, Kawamoto E, Hertz P, Schrier RW: Hypercalcemia of acute renal failure; clinical significance and pathogenesis. *Am J Med* 61: 119, 1976

135. Feinstein EI, Akmal M, Telfer N, Massry SG: Delayed hypercalcemia with acute renal failure associated with nontraumatic rhabdomyolysis. *Arch Intern Med* 141: 753, 1981

136. Chugh KS, Nath IVS, Ubroi HS, Singhal PC, Pareek SK, Sarkar AK: Acute renal failure due to non-traumatic rhabdomyolysis. *Postgrad Med J* 55: 386, 1979

137. Schiller WR, Long CL, Blakemore WS: Creatinine and nitrogen excretion in seriously ill and injured patients. *Surg Gynecol Obstet* 149: 561, 1979

138. Kjellstrand CM, Campbell DC, von Hartizsch B, Buselmeier TJ: Hyperuricemic acute renal failure. *Arch Intern Med* 133: 349, 1974

139. Zawada ET, Bennett EP, Steinson JB, Ramirez G: Serum calcium in blood pressure regulation during hemodialysis. *Arch Intern Med* 141: 657, 1981

140. Kelton J, Kelley WN, Holmes EW: A rapid method for the diagnosis of acute uric acid nephropathy. *Arch Intern Med* 138: 612, 1978

141. Zaloga GP, Chernow B: Hypocalcemia in critical illness. *JAMA* 10: 1924, 1986

142. Zaloga GP, Rainey TG: Hypocalcemia in the critically ill: When to suspect and what to do. *J Crit Illness*, 1(4): 12, 1986

143. Reed Jr WE, Sabatini S: The use of drugs in renal failure. *Semin Nephrol* 6: 259, 1986

144. Olbricht C, Mueller C, Schurek HJ: Treatment of acute renal failure in patients with multiple organ failure by continuous spontaneous hemofiltration. *Trans Am Soc Artif Intern Organs* 28: 33, 1982

145. Kramer P, Bohler J, Kehr A, Gröne HJ, Schrader J, Matthaei D, Scheler F: Intensive care potential of continuous arteriovenous hemofiltration. *Trans Am Soc Artif Intern Organs* 28: 28, 1982

146. Frisch J, Kindler J, Schmitter H, Glöckner WM, Sieberth H-G. Performance of CAVH in ARF therapy. in *CAVH*, edited by La Greca G, Fabris A, Ronco C, Milan, Wichtig Editore, 1986, p 283

147. Kohen JA, Whitley KY, Kjellstrand CM: Continuous arteriovenous hemofiltration: A comparison with hemodialysis in acute renal failure. *Trans Am Soc Artif Intern Organs* 31: 169, 1985

148. Fischer RP, Griffen WO, Clark DS: Early dialysis in the treatment of acute renal failure. *Surgery* 123: 1019, 1966

149. Gotch FA: Kinetics of hemodialysis. *Artif Organs* 4: 272, 1986

150. Buselmeier TJ, Rynasiewicz JJ, Howard RH, Sutherland DE, Davin TD, Lynch RE, Hodson EH, Simmons RL, Najarian JS, Kjellstrand CM: Fistulization of shunt vasculature: A unique approach to fistula development. *Br J Med* 2: 933, 1977

151. Kjellstrand CM, Merino GE, Mauer SM, Casali R, Buselmeier TJ: Complications of percutaneous femoral vein catheterizations for hemodialysis. *Clin Nephrol* 4: 37, 1975

152. Hansbrough JF, Narrod JA, Stiegman GV: Cardiac perforation and tamponade from a malpositioned subclavian dialysis catheter. *Nephron* 32: 363, 1982

153. Tapson JS, Uldall PR: Delayed onset of hemothorax: and unusual complication of subclavian access for hemodialysis. *Nephron* 40: 495, 1985

154. El-Nachef, Rashed F, Ricanati ES: Occlusion of the subclavian vein: a complication of indwelling subclavian venous catheters for hemodialysis. *Clin Nephrol* 24: 42, 1985

155. Erben J, Kvasnicka J, Bastecky J, Groh J, Zahradnik J, Rozsival V, Bastecka D, Fixa P, Kozak J, Herout V: Longterm experience with the technique of subclavian and femoral vein cannulation in hemodialysis. *Artif Organs* 3: 241, 1979

156. Sherertz RJ, Falk RJ, Huffman KA, Thoman CA, Mattern WD: Infections associated with subclavian Uldall catheters. *Arch Intern Med* 143: 52, 1983

157. Rosa AA, Fryd DS, Kjellstrand CM: Dialysis symptoms and stabilization in long-term dialysis, practical application of the CUSUM plot. *Arch Intern Med* 140: 804, 1980

158. Kjellstrand CM, Buselmeier TJ: A simple method for anticoagulation during pre- and postoperative hemodialysis, avoiding rebound phenomenon. *Surgery* 72: 630, 1972

159. Swartz RD, Port FK: Preventing hemorrhage in high-risk hemodialysis: Regional versus low-dose heparin. *Kidney Int* 16: 513, 1979

160. Shapiro WB, Faubert PF, Porush JG, Chou S: Low-dose heparin in routine hemodialysis monitored by activated partial thromboplastin time. *Artif Organs* 3: 73, 1979

161. Farrell PC, Ward RA, Schindhelm K, Gotch FA: Precise anticoagulation for routine hemodialysis. *J Lab Clin Med* 92: 164, 1978

162. Hocken AG, Hurst PL: Citrate regional anticoagulation in hemodialysis. *Nephron* 46: 1, 1987

163. Ashouri OS: Regional sodium citrate anticoagulation in patients with active bleeding undergoing hemodialysis. *Uremia Invest* 9: 45, 1985–6

164. Turney JH, Williams LC, Fewell MR, Parsons V, Weston MJ: Platelet protection and heparin sparing with prostacyclin during regular dialysis therapy. *Lancet* 2: 219, 1980

165. Gross ML, Bush H, Weinger R, Hamburger RJ, Flamenbaum W: A comparison of ticlopidine and heparin on hemodialysis in dogs. *J Lab Clin Med* 100: 887, 1982

166. Taenaka O, Shimada Y, Hirata T, Nishijima A, Yoshiya I: New Approach to regional anticoagulation in hemodialysis using gabexate mesilate (FOY). *Crit Care Med* 10: 773, 1982

167. Schrader J, Valentin R, Tönnis H-J, Hildebrand U, Stibbe W, Armstrong VW, Kandt M, Köstering H, Quellhorst E: Low molecular weight heparin in hemodialysis and hemofiltration patients. *Kidney Int* 28: 823, 1985

168. Ljungberg B, Blombäck M, Johnsson H, Lins L-E: A single dose of a low molecular weight heparin fragment for anticoagulation during hemodialysis. *Clin Nephrol* 1: 31, 1986

169. Arnander C, Hjelte MB, Lins LE, Larm O, Larsson R, Olsson P: Blood compatibility of a hollow-fiber dialyzer with a new coating of covalently bound heparin. *Proc Eur Soc Artif Organs* 9: 312, 1982

170. Casati S, Moia M, Graziani G, Cantaluppi A, Citterio A, Mannucci PM, Ponticelli C: Hemodialysis without anticoagulants: efficiency and hemostatic aspects. *Clin Nephrol* 21: 102, 1984

171. Ivanovich P, Xu CG, Kwaan HC, Hathiwala S: Studies of coagulation and platelet functions I, heparin-free hemodialysis. *Nephron* 33: 116, 1983

172. Hoenich NA, Levett D, Fawcett S, Woffindin C, Kerr DNS: Biocompatibility of haemodialysis membranes. *J Biomed Eng* 8: 3, 1986

173. Shaldon S, Deschodt G, Branger B, Granolleras C, Baldamus CA, Koch KM, Lysaght MJ, Dinarello CA: Haemodialysis hypotension: The interleukin hypothesis restated. *Proc Eur Dial Transplant Assoc Eur Ren Assoc* 22: 229, 1985

174. Branger B, Deschodt G, Oulès R, Granolleras C, Alsabadani N, Baudin G, Balducchi J-P, Fourcade J, Shaldon S: Can vascular stability be improved with short acetate hemodialysis if biocompatible membranes are used? *Proc Int Symp Trondheim*, Basel, Karger AG, 1985, p 214

175. Daugirdas JT, Al-Kadusi RR, Ing TS, Norusis MJ: A double-blind evaluation of sodium gradient hemodialysis. *Am J Nephrol* 5: 163, 1985

176. Levine J, Falk B, Henriquez M, Raja RM, Dramer MS, Rosenbaum JL: Effects of varying dialysate sodium using large surface area dialyzers. *Trans Am Soc Artif Intern Organs* 24: 139, 1978

177. Boquin E, Parnell S, Grondin G, Wollard C, Leonard D, Michaels R, Levin NW: Crossover study of the effects of different dialysate sodium concentrations in large surface area, short-term dialysis. *Proc Clin Dial Transplant Forum* 7: 48, 1977

178. Ogden DA: A double blind crossover comparison of high and low sodium dialysis. *Proc Clin Dial Transplant Forum* 8: 157, 1978

179. Chen WT, Ing TS, Daugirdas JT, Humayun HM, Brescia DJ, Gandhi VC, Hano JE, Kheirbek O: Hydrostatic ultrafiltration during hemodialysis using decreasing sodium dialysate. *Artif Organs* 4: 187, 1980

180. Feig PU, McCurdy DK: The hypertonic state. *N Engl J Med* 294: 1444, 1977

181. Wiegand CF, Davin TD, Raij L, Kjellstrand CM: Severe hypokalemia induced by hemodialysis. *Arch Intern Med* 141: 167, 1981

182. Sherman RA, Hwang ER, Bernholc AS, Eisinger RP: Variability in potassium removal by hemodialysis. *Am J Nephrol* 6: 284, 1986

183. Eisenberg E, Gotch FA: Normocalcemic hyperparathyroidism culminating in hypercalcemic crisis, treatment with hemodialysis. *Arch Intern Med* 122: 258, 1968

184. Maynar JC, Cruz C, Kleerekoper M, Levin NW: Blood pressure response to changes in serum ionized calcium during hemodialysis. *Ann Intern Med* 104: 358, 1986

185. Leunissen KML, Hoorntje SJ, Fiers HA, Dekkers WT, Mulder AW: Acetate versus bicarbonate hemodialysis in critically ill patients. *Nephron* 42: 146, 1986

186. Mansell MA, Morgan SH, Moore R, Kong CH, Laker MF, Wing JA: Cardiovascular and acid-base effects of acetate and bicarbonate haemodialysis. *Nephrol Dial Transplant* 1: 229, 1987

187. Borges HF, Fryd DS, Rosa AA, Kjellstrand CM: Hypotension during acetate and bicarbonate dialysis in patients with acute renal failure. *Am J Nephrol* 1: 24, 1981

188. Wehle B, Asaba H, Castenfors J, Fürst P, Grahn A, Gunnarsson B, Shaldon S, Bergström J: The influence of dialysis fluid composition on the blood pressure response during dialysis. *Clin Nephrol* 12: 62, 1978

189. Wathen R, Keshaviah P, Hommeyer P, Cadwell K, Comty C: Role of dialysate glucose in preventing gluconeogenesis during hemodialysis. *Trans Am Soc Artif Intern Organs* 23: 393, 1977

190. Leski M, Niethammer T, Wyss T: Glucose-enriched dialysate and tolerance to maintenance hemodialysis. *Nephron* 24: 271, 1979

191. Rodrigo R, Shideman J, McHugh R, Buselmeier T, Kjellstrand CM: Osmolality changes during hemodialysis. Natural history, clinical correlations, and influence of dialysate glucose and intravenous mannitol. *Ann Intern Med* 86: 554, 1977

192. Nordstrom H, Lennquist S, Lindell B, Sjöberg HE: Hypophosphataemia in severe burns. *Acta Chir Scand* 143: 395, 1977

193. Knochel JP, Caksey JH: The mechanism of hypophosphatemia in acute heat stroke. *JAMA* 238: 425, 1977

194. Ayus JC, Olivero JJ, Adrogue HJ: Alkalemia associated with renal failure. *Arch Intern Med* 140: 513, 1980

195. Degoulet P, Roulx J-P, Aime F, Berger C, Bloch P, Goupy F, Legrain M: Programme dialyse-informatique III. Données epidémiologiques stratégies de dialyse et résultats biologiques (Dialysis program information. Epidemiological data of different dialysis strategies and biological results). *J Urol Nephrol* (Paris) 82: 1001, 1976 (in French)

196. Kjellstrand CM: Can hypotension during dialysis be avoided? *Controv Nephrol* 2: 12, 1980

197. Ing TS, Ashbach DL, Kanter A, Oyama JH, Armbruster KFW, Merkel FK: Fluid removal with negative-pressure hydrostatic ultrafiltration using a partial vacuum. *Nephron* 14: 451, 1975

198. Bergström J, Asaba H, Fürst P, Oules R: Dialysis, ultrafiltration, and blood pressure. *Proc Eur Dial Transplant Assoc* 13: 293, 1976

199. Gerhardt RE, Abdulla AM, Mach SJ, Hudson JB: Isolated ultrafiltration in the treatment of fluid overload in cardiogenic shock. *Arch Intern Med* 139: 358, 1979

200. Keshaviah P, Ilstrup K, Constantini E, Berkseth R, Shapiro F: The influence of ultrafiltration and diffusion on cardiovascular parameters. *Trans Am Soc Artif Intern Organs* 26: 328, 1980

201. Pierides AM, Kurts SB, Johnson WJ: Ultrafiltration followed by hemodialysis. A longterm trial and acute studies. *J Dial* 2: 325, 1978

202. Jones EO, Ward MK, Hoenich NA, Kerr DNS: Separation of dialysis and ultrafiltration – does it really help? *Proc Eur Dial Transplant Assoc* 14: 160, 1977

203. Glabman S, Geronemus R, von Albertini B, Kahn T, Moutoussis G, Bosch JP: Clinical trial of maintenance sequential ultrafiltration and dialysis. *Trans Am Soc Artif Intern Organs* 25: 394, 1979

204. Marty AT: Hyperoncotic albumin therapy. *Surg Gynecol Obstet* 139: 105, 1974

205. Rosa AA, Shideman J, McHugh R, Duncan D, Kjellstrand CM: The importance of osmolality fall and ultrafiltration rate on hemodialysis side effects. *Nephron* 27: 134, 1981

206. Kjellstrand CM, Rosa AA, Shideman JR: Hypotension during hemodialysis: osmolality fall is an important pathogenic factor. *asaio J* 3: 11, 1980

207. Henrich WL, Woodard TD, Blachley JD, Gomez-Sanchez C, Pettinger W, Cronin RE: Role of osmolality in blood pressure stability after dialysis and ultrafiltration. *Kidney Int* 18: 480, 1980

208. Van Stone JC, Carey J, Meyer R, Murrin C: Hemodialysis with glycerol containing dialysate. *asaio J* 2: 119, 1979

209. Leithner C, Sinzinger H, Stummvoll HK, Klein K, Silberbauer K, Peskar BA: Enhanced 6-OXO-PGF levels in plasma during hemodialysis. *Prostaglandins Med* 5: 425, 1980

210. Borges H, Shideman J, Kjellstrand CM: Hypotension during chronic hemodialysis: on the effects of prostaglandin inhibition. *Nephron* 42: 120, 1986

211. Vaziri ND, Skowsky R, Warner A: Effect of isoosmolar volume reduction during hemofiltration on plasma antidiuretic hormone in patients with chronic renal failure. *Int J Artif Organs* 3: 322, 1980

212. Nord E, Danovitch GM: Vasopressin response in hemodialysis patients. *Kidney Int* 16: 234, 1979

213. Arieff AI, Lazarowitz VC, Guisado R: Experimental dialysis disequilibrium syndrome: prevention with glycerol. *Kidney Int* 14: 270, 1978

214. Korchik WP, Brown DC, DeMaster EG: Hemodialysis induced hypotension. *Int J Artif Organs* 1: 151, 1978

215. Korchick WP, DeMaster EG, Brown DC: Plasma norepinephrine and hemodialysis. *Kidney Int* 12: 484, 1977

216. Ksiqzek A: Dopamine-beta-hydroxylase activity and catecholamine levels in the plasma of patients with renal failure. *Nephron* 24: 170, 1979

217. Zuccelli P, Catizone L, Esposti ED, Fusaroli M, Ligabue A, Zuccala A: Influence of ultrafiltration on plasma renin activity and adrenergic system. *Nephron* 21: 317, 1978

218. Cannella G, Picotti GB, Mioni G, Cristinelli L, Maiorca R: Blood pressure behaviors during dialysis and ultrafiltration. A pathogenic hypothesis on hemodialysis-induced hypotension. *Int J Artif Organs* 1: 69, 1978

219. Brecht HM, Ernest W, Koch KM: Plasma noradrenaline levels in regular hemodialysis patients. *Proc Eur Dial Transplant Assoc* 12: 281, 1976

220. Schultze G, Maiga M, Neumayer H, Wagner K, Keller F, Molzahn M, Nigam S: Prostaglandin E₂ promotes hypotension on low-sodium hemodialysis. *Nephron* 37: 250, 1984

221. Craddock PR, Fehr J, Daimasso AP, Brigham KL, Jacob HS: Hemodialysis leukopenia: pulmonary vascular leukostasis resulting from complement activation by dialyzer cellophane membranes. *J Clin Invest* 59: 879, 1977

222. McGrath BP, Tiller DJ, Bune A, Chalmers JP, Horner PI, Uther JB: Autonomic blockade and the Valsalva maneuver in patients on maintenance hemodialysis: a hemodynamic study. *Kidney Int* 12: 294, 1977

223. Ewing DJ, Winney R: Autonomic function in patients with chronic renal failure on intermittent haemodialysis. *Nephron* 15: 424, 1975

224. Nies AS, Robertson D, Stone WJ: Hemodialysis hypotension is not the result of uremic peripheral autonomic neuropathy. *J Lab Clin Med* 94: 395, 1979

225. Kersh ES, Kronfield SJ, Unger A, Opooer RW, Cantor S, Cohn K: Autonomic insufficiency in uremia as a cause of hemodialysis-induced hypotension. *N Engl J Med* 290: 650, 1974

226. DeFremont JF, Coevert B, Andrejak M, Makdassi R, Quichaud J, Lambrey G, Gueris J, Caillens C, Harichaux P, Alexandre JM, Fournier A: Effects of antihypertensive drugs on dialysis-resistant hypertension, plasma renin and dopamine betahydroxylase activities, metabolic risk factors and calcium phosphate homeostasis: Comparison of metoprolol, alphamethyldopa and clonidine in a cross-over trial. *Clin Nephrol* 12: 198, 1979

227. MacGrigor RR: Granulocyte adherence changes induced by hemodialysis, endotoxin, epinephrine, and glucocorticoids. *Ann Intern Med* 86: 35, 1977

228. Craddock PR, Fehr J, Brigham KL, Kronenberg RS, Jacob HS: Complement and leukocyte-mediated pulmonary dysfunction in hemodialysis. *N Engl J Med* 296: 769, 1977

229. Agar JW, Hull JD, Kaplan M, Pletka PG: Acute cardiopulmonary decompensation and complement activation during hemodialysis. *Ann Intern Med* 94: 792, 1981

230. Aljama P, Bire PAE, Ward MK, Feest TG, Walker W, Tanboga H, Sussman M, Kerr DNS: Haemodialysis-induced leucopenia and activation of complement: effects of different membranes. *Proc Eur Dial Transplant Assoc* 15: 144, 1978

231. von Hartitzsch B, Carr D, Kjellstrand CM, Kerr DNS: Normal red cell survival in well dialyzed patients. *Trans Am Soc Artif Intern Organs* 19: 471, 1973

232. Aurigemma NM, Feldman NT, Gottlieb M, Ingran RH, Lazarus JM, Lowrie EG: Arterial oxygenation during hemodialysis. *N Engl J Med* 297: 871, 1977

233. Mault JR, Dechert RE, Bartlett RH, Swartz RD, Ferguson SK: Oxygen consumption during hemodialysis for acute renal failure. *Trans Am Soc Artif Intern Organs* 28: 510, 1982

234. Casali R, Simmons RL, Najarian JS, von Hartitzsch B, Buselmeier TJ, Kjellstrand CM: Acute renal insufficiency complicating major cardiovascular surgery. *Ann Surg* 181: 370, 1975

235. Sipkins JH, Kjellstrand CM: Severe head trauma and acute renal failure. *Nephron* 28: 36, 1981

236. Tolhurst Cleaver CL, Hopkins AD, Kee Kwong KC NG, Rafiery AT: The effect of postoperative peritoneal lavage on survival, peritoneal wound healing and adhesion formation following fecal peritonitis: an experimental study in the rat. *Br J Surg* 61: 601, 1974

237. Posen GA, Luiselto J: Continuous equilibration peritoneal dialysis in the treatment of acute and chronic renal failure. *Proc Clin Dial Transplant Forum* 9: 50, 1979

238. Nolph KD, Ghods AJ, Van Stone J, Brown PA: The effects of intraperitoneal vasodilators on peritoneal clearances. *Trans Am Soc Artif Intern Organs* 22: 586, 1976

239. Rubin J, Oreopoulos DG, Lio TT, Mathews R, de Veber GA: Management of peritonitis and bowel perforation during chronic peritoneal dialysis. *Nephron* 16: 220, 1976

240. Simkin EP, Wright FK: Perforating injuries of the bowel complicating peritoneal catheter insertion. *Lancet* 1: 64, 1968

241. Grodstein GP, Blumenkrantz MJ, Kopple JD, Moran JK, Coburn JW: Glucose absorption during continuous ambulatory peritoneal dialysis. *Kidney Int* 19: 564, 1981

242. Crossley K, Kjellstrand CM: Intraperitoneal insulin for control of blood sugar in diabetic patients during peritoneal dialysis. *Br Med J* 1: 269, 1971

243. Maher JF, Hohnadel DC, Shea C, DiSanzo F, Cassetta M: Effect of intraperitoneal diuretics on solute transport during hypertonic dialysis. *Clin Nephrol* 7: 96, 1977

244. Vaziri ND, Ness R, Wellikson L, Barton C, Greep N: Bicarbonate buffered peritoneal dialysis an effective adjunct in the treatment of lactic acidosis. *Am J Med* 67: 392, 1979

245. Blumenkrantz MJ, Gahl GM, Kopple JD, Kamdar AV, Jones MR, Kessel M, Coburn JW: Protein losses during peritoneal dialysis. *Kidney Int* 19: 593, 1981

246. Rubin J, McFarland S, Hellems EW, Bower JD: Peritoneal dialysis during peritonitis. *Kidney Int* 19: 460, 1981

247. Hurley RM, Muogbo D, Wilson GW, Ali MAM: Peritoneal effluent cellularity: predictor of bacterial peritonitis. *Kidney Int* 8: 427, 1975

248. Chan LK, Oliver DO: Simple method for early detection of peritonitis in patients on continuous ambulatory peritoneal dialysis. *Lancet* 2: 1336, 1979

249. Kramer P, Kaufhold G, Grone HJ, Wigger W, Rieger J: Management of anuric intensive-care patients with arteriovenous hemofiltration. *Int J Artif Intern Organs* 3: 225, 1980

250. Kramer P, Wigger W, Rieger J, Mattaei D, Scheler F: Arteriovenous haemofiltration: a new and simple method for treatment of over-hydrated patients resistant to diuretics. *Klin Wochenschr* 55: 1121, 1977

251. Feldhoff P, Turnham T, Klein E: Effect of plasma proteins on the sieving spectra of hemofilters. *Artif Organs* 8: 186, 1984

252. Kaplan A, Longnecker RE, Folkert VW: Continuous arteriovenous hemofiltration. *Ann Intern Med* 100: 358, 1984

253. Lauer A, Saccaggi A, Ronco C, Belledone M, Glabman S, Bosch JP: Continuous arteriovenous hemofiltration in the critically ill patient. *Ann Intern Med* 99: 455, 1983

254. Paganini EP, Fouad F, Tarazi RC, Bravo EL, Nakamoto S: Hemodynamics of isolated ultrafiltration in chronic hemodialysis patients. *Trans Am Soc Artif Intern Organs* 25: 422, 1979

255. Höfliger N, Keusch G, Baumann PC, Geroulanos S, Glinz W, Largiader J, Binswanger U: Die kontinuierliche arterio-venöse Haemofiltration zur Behandlung des akuten Nierenversagens. (Continuous arteriovenous hemofiltration for treatment of acute renal failure.) *Schweiz Med Wochenschr* 115: 242, 1985

256. Weiss LG, Wikström B, Danielsson BG, Fellström B, Tufvesson G: Clinical experience and outcome of 100 patients treated with CAVH for acute renal failure. in *CAVH* edited by La Greca G, Fabris A, Ronco C, Milan, Wichtig Editore, 1986, p 277

257. Kaplan A: Enhanced efficiency during continuous arteriovenous hemofiltration: the use of predilution. *Int J Artif Organs* 3: 139, 1986

258. Dodd NJ, O'Donovan RM, Bennett-Jones DN, Brylance PB, Bewick M, Parsons V, Weston MJ: Arteriovenous haemofiltration: a recent advance in the management of renal failure. *Br Med J* 287: 1008, 1983

259. Eisele G, Paganini EP: Heparin-free continuous acute renal replacement therapy. *Artif Organs* 14: 46, 1985

260. Ing TS, Daugirdas JT, Bregman H, Leehey DJ: Continuous arteriovenous hemodialysis. *Int J Artif Organs* 3: 117, 1985

261. Lindholm T: Pleural dialysis in a case of acute renal failure. *Acta Med Scand* 165: 239, 1959

262. Sheth KJ, Glichlich M: Pleural dialysis in acute renal failure. *Clin Nephrol* 6: 370, 1976

263. Finkenstaedt JT, Merrill JP: Renal function after recovery from acute renal failure. *N Engl J Med* 254: 1023, 1956

264. Price JDE, Palmer RA: A functional and morphological follow-up study of acute renal failure. *Arch Intern Med* 105: 90, 1960

265. Briggs JD, Kennedy AC, Young LN, Luke RG, Gray M: Renal function after acute tubular necrosis. *Br J Med* 3: 513, 1967

266. Hall JW, Johnson WJ: Maher FT, Hunt JC: Immediate and long-term prognosis in acute renal failure. *Ann Intern Med* 73: 515, 1970

267. Lewers DT, Mathew TH, Maher JF, Schreiner GE: Long-term follow-up of renal function and histology after acute tubular necrosis. *Ann Intern Med* 73: 523, 1970

268. Fuchs HJ, Thelen M, Wibrandt R: Die Nierenfunktion nach akutem Nierenversagen – Eine Langzeitstudie an 70 Patienten (Renal function after acute renal failure – a long-term study). *Dtsch Med Wochenschr* 99: 1641, 1974 (in German)

269. Merino GE, Buselmeier TJ, Kjellstrand CM: Postoperative chronic renal failure: a new syndrome? *Ann Surg* 182: 37, 1975

270. Levin ML, Simon NM, Herdson PB, del Greco F: Acute renal failure followed by protracted, slowly resolving chronic uremia. *J Chron Dis* 25: 645, 1972

271. Siegler RL, Bloomer HA: Acute renal failure with prolonged oliguria: an account of five cases. *JAMA* 225: 133, 1973

PLANNING, DEVELOPING AND OPERATING A DIALYSIS PROGRAMME

ROWAN G. WALKER and ANTHONY J.F. d'APICE

INTRODUCTION

The emergence of nephrology as a major clinical sub-speciality of internal medicine occurred during the 1960's, coinciding with the development of dialysis and transplantation, procedures which at that time were hazardous and complicated in the highly selected patients. In the 1980's, however, nephrologists offer a wide range of treatment modalities to virtually all patients with end-stage renal disease (ESRD) and 'dialysis' encompasses several different but readily available procedures that can be easily performed by the patients themselves in almost any location (1–4).

As dialysis procedures have become increasingly successful in the past two decades, there has been an ever increasing number of patients undergoing dialysis and an even greater increase in the cost of managing them. Figure 1 shows the steadily increasing number of patients treated by dialysis in Australia and although the number and distribution of patients differs from that in other regions, the incremental rate is similar to that in most developed countries.

Two important elements determining the number of patients treated by dialysis are the rate of entry or acceptance, which reflects predominantly the regional economy and health policy and secondly the rate of exit, which comprises the rates of transplantation and mortality. It is likely that the number of patients on dialysis programmes will continue to increase because restriction of entry based on age, primary renal disease or other medical disease is now generally considered unacceptable. Furthermore, despite increased graft survival rate, the actual rate of transplantation remains well below the level required to reduce the dialysis population (Figure 1).

The reduction in the cost of dialysis has been a major determinant of trends in dialysis care in the 1980's. Today a high proportion of patients in many countries dialyse at home, or in self-care/limited care centres and fewer in the high cost hospital based dialysis centres. This chapter discusses the emphasis on development of decentralized dialysis in an overview of dialysis planning, development and operation.

BASIC DATA REQUIRED FOR PLANNING

Funding

Central information in planning the programme is the level of funding and its future security because these determine the number of patients that can ultimately be treated and consequently whether restrictions must be imposed on entry (Figure 2).

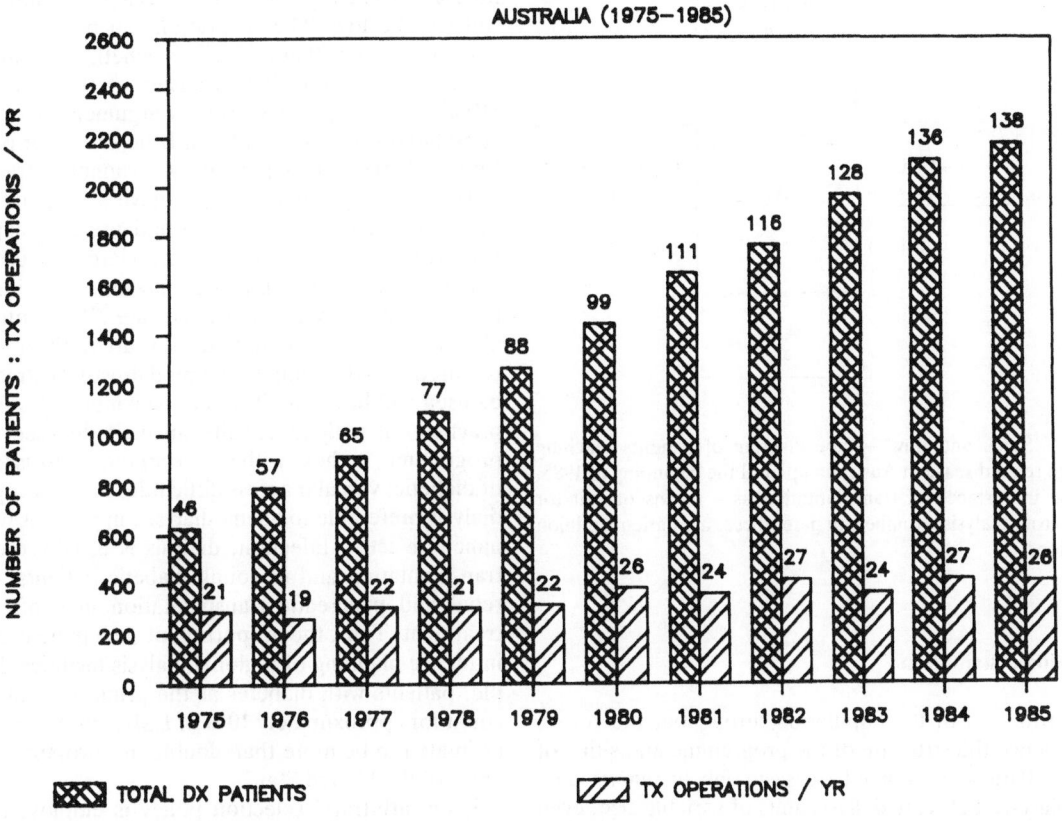

Figure 1. Diagram showing the increasing number of patients treated by maintenance dialysis (Dx) in Australia over the past decade. Numerals at top of the bars indicate number of patients/million of population. Note comparison with transplantation (Tx) rate which has been very constant over the same period. Despite transplantation, the number of dialysis patients increases. Numerals above Tx operation bars equal the number of Tx operations/million population/year.

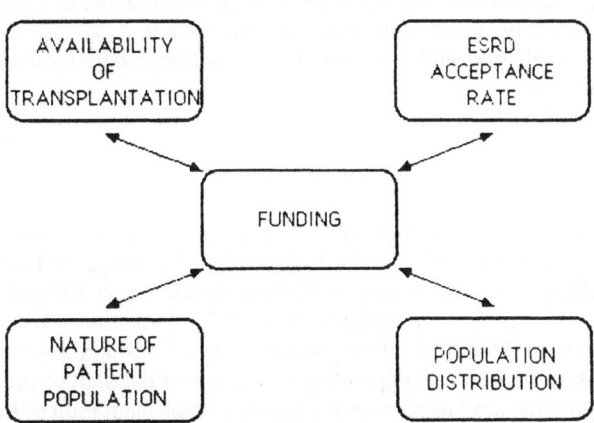

Figure 2. Diagrammatic representation of basic data required for planning a dialysis programme with funding as the central component.

Patient acceptance rate

In the absence of financial restrictions most developed countries accept 30 to 50 patients/million population/year for treatment of ESRD. Predictions of population size can be obtained from the Government Statistician.

When financial restrictions limit the number of new patients with renal failure that can be treated, it is probably best to design and accept 'arbitrary' criteria so that the input rate is appropriate to the situation and also constant. Because such arbitrary criteria are largely necessitated by politics, they should be formally endorsed by the funding (usually Government) authority. The other source of patients is re-entry after failed transplantation a rate dependent on the size of the transplantation programme and its success rate. Despite an improving graft survival rate in recent years, the re-entry rate in Australia in 1984 remained at approximately 35% of the annual transplant rate or 8% of total number of transplant patients (Figure 3).

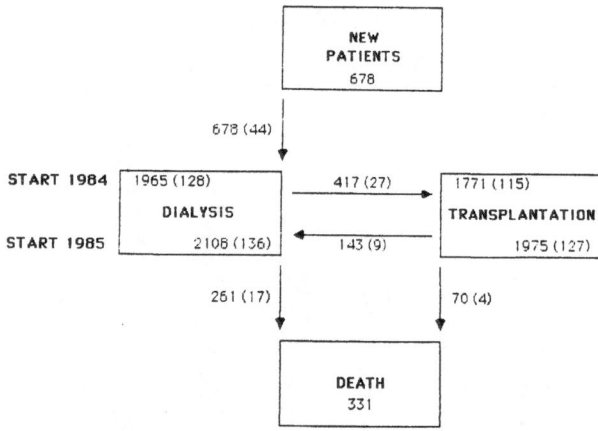

Figure 3. 'Stock and flow' – type diagram of patients reaching end-stage renal disease in Australia up until the beginning of 1985. Note the importance of transplantation as a means of exit for patients from dialysis. Numbers in parentheses are patients/million population.

Population distribution

The distribution of the population throughout the region will influence the structure of the programme and siting of facilities. Patients in isolated areas can only be managed by home dialysis. Self-care dialysis units of variable size, even single patient units, can be established in community health centres, country hospitals and limited care facilities. Larger self-care units can be sited throughout the suburban areas of large cities to reduce the travelling time of patients. The location of major centre dialysis units is essentially dependent on existing hospitals and the population distribution may well have changed since they were built.

Nature of patient population

Paediatric patients present special problems. They are ideally dialysed at home. However, unless the population of the region is very large, the number of paediatric patients will be too few to justify a separate core dialysis service. The referral rate of paediatric patients (<15 years of age) with renal failure is approximately 1.0 to 1.5 patients/million population/year in most countries.

Hepatitis-B antigen (HBsAg) positive patients are another special group. Attitudes about how to manage this problem vary from taking virtually no precautions, particularly in an area with a high HBsAg carriage rate, to complete isolation of all HBsAg positive patients.

Many compromise 'solutions' have arisen largely for pragmatic reasons. The opportunity to manage the problem optimally presents when planning a new regional dialysis programme and it is the authors' view that total separation of HBsAg antigen positive and negative patients should be

achieved. This is particularly important in countries where the HBsAg carriage rate is low, because the immunity rate will also be low. The separation can be most effectively made by testing all new referrals, whether as ward or clinic patients, with immediate transfer of those found to be HBsAg antigen positive. Similar arguments should now be considered for non-A and non-B hepatitis but particularly for HTLV III positive patients who cannot be transplanted.

Technically, all patients who have severe uraemia, can now be treated regardless of age and intercurrent problems. Elderly patients with severe atherosclerosis, those with malignancy, with active infection or with severe immunologically mediated systemic diseases are all potentially treatable. In a situation of unlimited resources, the only decision required is to determine what modality of treatment should be used and how long it should be continued. Although in practice, all patients require an individualised treatment programme, in those with severe atherosclerosis (idiopathic or diabetic) vascular access difficulties may make peritoneal dialysis preferable to haemodialysis, in patients with malignancy or active infection, dialysis is usually preferred to transplantation and in young diabetic patients, combined renal and pancreatic transplantation may offer optimal treatment. Thus, the proportion of such patient groups will influence planning of regional dialysis facilities. For example, patients with diabetes as the primary renal lesion account for approximately 10% of ESRD in Australia but are estimated to be more than double this proportion in many areas of the United States.

If an 'arbitrary' selection policy is employed for fiscal reasons, one can expect that the dialysis patient population will be younger and healthier. This will of course influence the relative proportions that will be best managed by different dialysis modalities and at different sites. The main effect will be a reduction in the numbers of patients who can only be managed by hospital based centre dialysis. Conversely, even in the presence of a restrictive selection policy, the passage of time will generate an increasing number of aging and/or medically unfit patients, who cannot reasonably be transplanted and who will require hospital based centre dialysis.

Availability of transplantation

Figure 3 is a flow chart of entry and exit to and from dialysis and transplantation in Australia in 1984. The only exits from dialysis are death or transplantation. The annual dialysis death rate is approximately 30 to 40% of the annual entry rate or 10 to 12% of all patients dialysed during the year. Both figures vary depending on the age of the dialysis programme (and its patients). The rate of transplantation is the only adjustable factor other than the entry rate. The flow chart shows that the number of dialysis patients in Australia increased by 7% during 1984. Without transplantation, it would have increased by about 25%. Obviously the availability of a transplantation programme and its level of activity are critical components of the equation.

PHILOSOPHY AND POLICY

Every dialysis programme has a basic philosophy. It is usually not so well developed, however, as to be more than a series of policies which reflect an unstated and often unformed philosophy. In the main, the philosophy depends on the personalities of the dominant staff and the pressures exerted by the patient load and financial considerations.

Planning and developing a new regional dialysis programme offers the opportunity to develop a philosophy and put it into practice through a series of policies. The final product will inevitably be a compromise between what is felt to be ideal and what can practically be offered as a result of various restrictions. Probably the most difficult area, which will influence the programme to the greatest extent is the selection of patients.

Dialysis options and relationship with transplantation

Despite the marked variations in practice, the authors feel strongly that successful transplantation should be the ultimate aim for virtually all patients. Clearly, the decision about transplantation will have major implications for the dialysis programme, particularly in relation to the number of patients that have to be managed and the rate of growth of programme. The relationship between dialysis and transplantation can either be an association between physically distinct, separately staffed programmes or a fully integrated programme.

A major advantage of a fully integrated programme, is the integration of the staff, so that patients are cared for by the same staff and in the same place from presentation for the

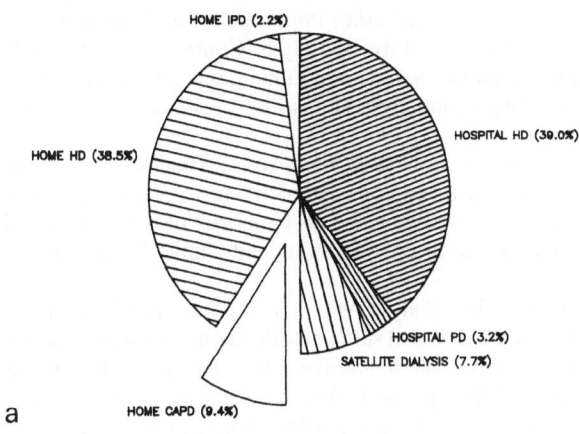

a

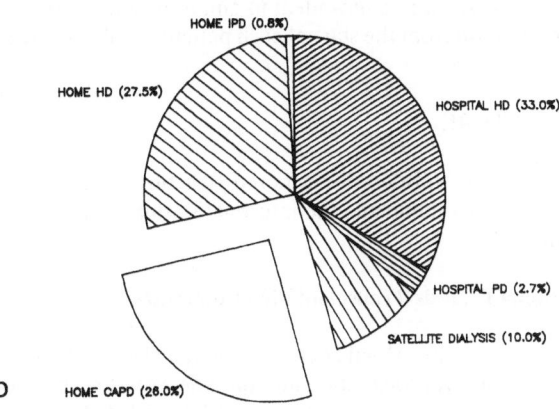

b

Figures 5a and b. Diagram of relative importance of treatment modalities comparing 1980 with 1984. Note increasing proportion of patients in self-care forms of dialysis in 1984 (64.3%) compared with 1980 (57.8%) and the emphasis on CAPD. Note the marked increase in CAPD to being a major form of self-care dialysis by the beginning of 1985.

rest of their lives. At a practical level, integration assists in optimal preparation for transplantation. Probably the only circumstance where a definite policy not to transplant any patients should be pursued, would be when the mortality rate or success rate of the particular transplant service are unacceptable. A regional dialysis and transplantation service should offer, or have available, all currently employed modes of dialysis and transplantation (Figure 4).

Self-help as a dialysis option

The increasing number of dialysis patients makes it impossible to provide dialysis exclusively in hospital centre dialysis units. The role of the hospital dialysis centre is changing quickly from the site where most patients are managed to

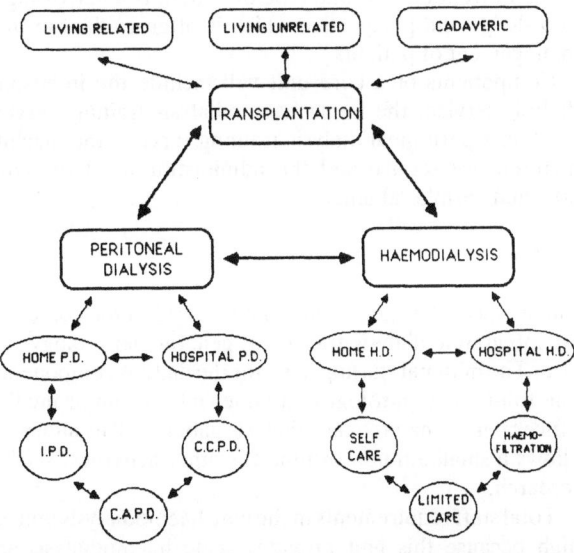

Figure 4. Diagram indicating the various treatment modalities which should be offered in a fully integrated regional dialysis programme. H.D. = haemodialysis, P.D. = peritoneal dialysis, IPD = intermittent peritoneal dialysis, CAPD = continuous ambulatory peritoneal dialysis, CCPD = combination of IPD and CAPD.

the back-up system for a large home and self-care based programme. In this respect, continuous ambulatory peritoneal dialysis (CAPD), the major form of peritoneal dialysis, is becoming of increasing importance, but haemodialysis remains the major form of dialysis. Consequently, in developing a regional dialysis programme, one is concerned with providing haemodialysis at a variety of sites (Figure 5A and 5B).

Dialysis (peritoneal or haemo-) is virtually always commenced as an in-hospital form of therapy. After stabilisation and training, however, the vast majority of patients should move to the home environment of into limited care/self care facilities.

Historically, dialysis was a procedure which medical, nursing and technical staff performed on patients who had a purely passive role themselves. The changes in the sites at which dialysis is performed have been necessarily accompanied by increased patient participation in their own dialysis. The level of patient participation can vary from complete self-dialysis at home to none in a hospital based unit. Because of the need for patient mobility between the various sites of dialysis, it is now ideal to aim at maximum patient participation from the start of each patient's dialysis career.

STRUCTURE

This section will describe a tiered structure of a regional dialysis programme and the interrelationship of its components.

National Dialysis-Transplantation Committee

Such a committee should define broad policies in relation to dialysis and transplantation and provide expert opinion on problem areas: A major role is as a lobbyist with government authorities. A National Dialysis-Transplantation Registry, as described later, is a natural component.

A National Dialysis-Transplantation Committee should represent a medical viewpoint. Hence, its membership should represent the medical personnel involved in dialysis and transplantation in each of the regions of the country. In Australia, this committee is formed under the auspices of the Australian Kidney Foundation and Australian Nephrology Society. Examples of areas of activity of a National Dialysis-Transplantation Committee are inter-regional organ sharing schemes, organ retrieval programmes, publication of educational material, and interaction with National Standards Associations in relation to standards for dialysis equipment and water purification policy.

Regions

The formation of regions within a country will usually be decided by pre-existing political or other organisational boundaries. Hence, they will often differ markedly in size. In Australia, the geopolitical boundaries of the six states define the regions whose populations vary from 0.25 to 6 million. Each region contains a variable number of major dialysis or dialysis-transplantation facilities – core units – based on major teaching and university affiliated hospitals. The core units are independent and relate to one another and to regional funding authorities through Regional Dialysis-Transplantation Committees. The population drainage areas of each core unit may be fixed by the health authority or be more flexible as in Australia, allowing some degree of competition between core units.

Core units

Dialysis should not be viewed in isolation from nephrology or transplantation. Consequently, core dialysis units and transplantation units should be integral parts of general nephrology services. Yet, hospital based dialysis should not be the basic method providing dialysis. The core unit should rather function only as a new patient entry point, acute dialysis service and support system for both transplantation and a decentralised maintenance dialysis service.

Organisation

The core unit should be the smallest part of the dialysis service but control the activities of all the physically or numerically larger peripheral units.

Probably the most important organisational aspect is designing the staff structure so that medical, nursing and paramedical staff have a broad exposure to all aspects of nephrology, including transplantation, while having their major responsibility in a particular component. This can be achieved by dual responsibility and (or) rotation of staff. A disadvantage of having staff permanently committed to one mode of treatment or one type of patient is a narrowing of knowledge and perspective which is often evident in their management of patients.

Components of a core unit will include the in-hospital dialysis service, the home haemodialysis training service, the home peritoneal dialysis training service, the machine maintenance service and the administration of the core-attached peripheral units.

Staffing

The medical staff needs should be viewed in the context of an integrated dialysis-transplant-general nephrology service. The minimal staffing need for the dialysis component is one full-time nephrologist and one (intern) junior medical officer per 50 maintenance dialysis patients. This allocation allows a small amount of time for other activities, such as research.

Total staff requirements in the core haemodialysis unit are high because this unit provides acute haemodialysis and dialysis of new patients and those who are unable to self-dialyse or have superimposed acute medical problems. The patient-to-staff ratio should not exceed 2 : 1. This ratio does not include staff used for administration, record keeping and staff training.

Technical staff requirements vary depending on the type of machinery e.g. central delivery systems and single patient units. The technical staff will cover the whole dialysis service including home dialysis and self-care units. Two maintenance technicians can manage the machinery of up to 120 dialysis patients.

Hospitals and health authorities are notoriously reluctant to provide adequate administrative assistance to dialysis services. Despite this reluctance, dialysis has a large business component because of the large staff number and high cost of the technology. A dialysis service maintaining 100 patients requires one senior administrator and two clerks. This staffing level is cost efficient because of savings that can be made in purchasing and stock control.

Facilities

The dialysis programme should be able to offer the modalities of treatment outlined in Figure 4. The role of the core unit is largely in dialysis of new patients, acute renal failure, problem patients and providing the medical management, administration, staff training, paramedical services and technical services for the whole programme. Special facilities of the core unit include a machine workshop and vehicles for visiting home dialysis patients and peripheral units. Ideally, a central computer for patient records and programme administration should be available. Such a facility can also be used to collect and transmit data to central registry areas and for research purposes.

Size and number of core units

Various factors influence the size of a regional dialysis programme and have been discussed previously. The size of the individual core units will depend on their number and distribution and on whether their drainage areas are regulated. In the authors' view, the upper limit for maximal efficiency of an individual dialysis programme within a region is approximately 250 patients.

However, it is probably unwise to allow one programme to reach this size because subsequently it tends to stagnate. In any dialysis programme there are always a proportion of patients who by passage of time or by the ravages of failed transplantation become untransplantable or hospital dialysis dependent or both. The number of these dependent patients increases progressively with time. Once a core unit stops growing, the proportion of dependent patients will increase markedly, the transplant rate will tend to fall and finally the programme will collapse onto its base, the in-hospital dialysis unit. It can be better to develop two or more units simultaneously or only a few years apart so that the growth of each is less rapid.

The initial planning of the region should decide the number of core units and the timing of their commencement. The size of the core dialysis units should be designed initially to suit the final need and not the immediate requirement only. Expansion of a hospital-based facility is often impossible after the original structure has been designed. Generous allocation of space is essential to allow future growth. The initial plans need not include all the plumbing and water purification plant necessary at some future date, but should not prohibit expansion or modification of the basic technology.

A core unit haemodialysis facility should allow space for 10 to 12 haemodialysis chairs (stations). Allowing three dialyses per patient per week and two shifts per day, this facility will cope with 40 to 48 patients. The size of the core unit haemodialysis facility determines the size of the total dialysis population that can be supported in peripheral facilities and at home. A 10 station centre unit can support about 250 patients in toto. It is worth re-emphasising that as a dialysis programme ages, it generates a steadily increasing number of dependent patients and consequently the size of the dialysis population outside the hospital centre cannot be expanded beyond its capacity to support them.

The relation of the size of the hospital centre to the total dialysis population is also affected by the balance of the various modalities by which the non-hospital patients are managed. For example, CAPD is an attractive method of managing a large number of patients without need for expensive facilities. However, an epidemic of antibiotic resistant peritonitis can quickly produce a sudden influx of patients to hospital-based haemodialysis. At present, the optimal proportional size of a peritoneal dialysis programme would appear to be approximately one-third to one-half of the total dialysis population of the core unit.

Patient management

Unless there are virtually unlimited resources or affiliated private hospital dialysis facilities or both, new patients who are acceptable candidates for entry into the programme must understand that there are a few ground rules, the observance of which are essential for their entry and continued treatment.

Unfortunately, it is sometimes necessary to insist that patients follow these rules because their failure to do so can jeopardise the management of others or waste valuable resources such as donor kidneys. Thus, it is essential to educate patients about the way the system works.

The day-to-day management of the patients is best conducted by the dialysis staff with medical staff intervening only when problems develop. The aim should be to make dialysis a self-care procedure, with nursing or technical assistance if necessary and medical management by out-patient visits only, except in urgent situations.

Peripheral units

The majority of patients will be dialysed outside the hospital after a short period of adjustment to dialysis. Several possible sites and levels of staffing are possible.

Satellite dialysis

This type of dialysis service is a small scale or geographically remote replica of a hospital dialysis unit. The necessity for such units depends on the geographic distribution of core units and the total dialysis population. For example, a city with a population of 100,000 situated 100 miles (approximately 160 km) from the nearest core unit, would not warrant a full dialysis-transplant service, but may require a small, fully-staffed dialysis service. This type of unit is not a low staff/patient ratio service and can be optimally used by siting it in a general hospital where it can provide acute dialysis and can also function as a home dialysis training facility. Such units should be under the control of a core unit rather than function fully independently. This can be achieved by medical staff joint appointments and rotation of staff in both directions, even if only for short periods, to allow continuing education. Transplantation should be performed at the core unit.

Limited-care dialysis

This type of dialysis service may or may not be geographically remote from the core dialysis unit. The main role for such a service is to accommodate patients who would otherwise be at home or at self-care centres but who for social, medical, haemodialysis access or other reasons are unable to be accommodated that way. An example would be the single patient who has limited eyesight and inability to self-needle. The limited-care unit is a relatively low staff/patient ratio service and can be operated optimally by locating it in a position, separate from the main core unit but perhaps geographically close. The amount of staffing required for a 10 station (40 patient) unit of this type is three per shift and should include nursing as well as technical staff. Staff should rotate between this unit and the core in-hospital unit.

Self-care dialysis

This form of self-help dialysis is particularly appropriate for those for whom home dialysis is difficult or impossible for social reasons such as an unsatisfactory home environment of lack of an assistant. The aim is to provide a place where patients can dialyse themselves with virtually no assistance and/or supervision. As in home dialysis, responsibility for the dialysis resides primarily with the patient. These units have an optimal size of 10 stations (40 patients) and can be managed very easily by two staff per shift. This staff level is necessary for industrial reasons, patient confidence and mutual support, but may exceed that dictated by the work load alone. This allows patient training to be conducted at the self-care centres. These centres are able to be 'personalised' and made much more attractive and less clinical than a hospital dialysis unit and are popular with patients. The amount of patient time per dialysis and the capital and maintenance cost can be reduced by using a central delivery system.

The cost of self-care dialysis is comparable to that of home dialysis and is much less expensive than hospital based dialysis. These units can be sited in relation to patient demography and the facilities can be shared by several core units.

The management should be shared through the core unit to which it primarily relates and the staff should rotate through the parent unit. Smaller self-care units of one, two or up to eight stations are suitable for medium to large sized towns and can be staffed by part-time workers who are trained in the core unit and regularly return there for a few weeks. The capital cost of such mini-units is usually no more than that involved in establishing a single patient on home dialysis because they can be sited in existing district hospitals or community centres.

Private dialysis

Depending on a particular country's National Health Scheme, it may be possible to manage some patients in satellite units as private patients. This has the advantage of shifting some of the burden of cost from the State to the Private Health Funds.

The authors deem it desirable, if possible, to have all private dialysis units 'linked' with existing core units. This ensures that medical personnel involved in private dialysis are subject to quality assurance peer review, and that all patients have equal access to all modalities of ESRD therapy, especially renal transplantation.

Home dialysis

The majority of patients on dialysis can be managed either by home dialysis or in self-care centres. The popularity of home dialysis varies geographically and seems to relate inversely to the financial reward for institutional dialysis. As is often emphasised by its opponents, home dialysis can place some stress on domestic relationships, but is most often satisfactory, provided there is adequate space and family support. The peripheral unit to which home dialysis patients relate is the home dialysis training centre. This may be physically associated with the hospital centre, a self-care unit, or totally separate. A large home training facility can provide its service to several core units but final management should remain with one core unit. In designing a home dialysis training unit, provision should be made for several two bedroom apartments in which patients who live a long distance away can be accommodated during training.

Holiday dialysis

Advantageously transplantation enables patients to go on holidays. The provision of holiday dialysis facilities extends this advantage to dialysis patients. The authors' patients have used the Redy (Sorb)-system dialysis machine, CAPD and caravans equipped with dialysis machines in addition to visitor status dialysis, to enable them to have a holiday. Dialysis holiday homes, established by patient interest groups, provide excellent holiday facilities for the patient and his whole family. Service clubs are often willing to sponsor the establishment of those facilities. In Australia, most units are happy to accept visitors for dialysis provided they are HBsAg and HTLV III negative. One potential disadvantage of international travel is that holiday dialysis often comes at a higher price in foreign countries and may not be covered by the home country health insurance.

Hepatitis B/HTLV III positive unit

The management of HBsAg positive patients varies depending on the prevalence of antigenaemia in the population. In most developed countries, hepatitis B antigenaemia is uncommon (<1% of the population), and consequently the level of immunity is low. The major concern is accidental infection of staff. One satisfactory approach is to transfer all antigen positive patients to a special hepatitis unit. This should be supported by a high level of awareness, in the core units of the region.

It is our practice to test all new nephrology patients for hepatitis B antigenaemia at their first visit whether this involves hospital admission or a clinic visit. All staff, including domestic staff, and all dialysis patients are tested monthly. HBsAg positive staff are not employed in the dialysis area, and any patient found to be positive is transferred to a special unit which serves seven core units. These patients are only returned to the core units when they are HBs antibody positive of persistently antigen negative. Transplantation of antigen positive patients is performed at the special unit. Staff from positive units should not rotate through core units.

Recently, effective anti-hepatitis B vaccins have become available. Most nephrology staff members have agreed to be vaccinated. The desirability of attempting to vaccinate all dialysis patients remains controversial.

The last 5 years has seen the rapid spread of AIDS (acquired immune deficiency syndrome) and the finding of occasional patients with HTLV III (or I & IV) antibodies on screening of dialysis populations. It is our practice to identify high risk dialysis patients by questionnaire and to screen all dialysis patients for the HTLV III antibody. HTLV III positive patients are transferred to the same unit which manages HBsAg positive patients. High risk patients and HTLV III positive patients are not transplanted.

Paediatric unit

Opinion varies as to whether children (<15 years) should be managed in essentially adult dialysis transplant services or paediatric services. The argument arises because of the relatively small number of children reaching end-stage renal failure. In Australia, the whole paediatric ESRD load is approximately 15 to 20 new patients per year. This would be only sufficient to justify a single free standing paediatric service for the whole country, something which is quite impractical geographically. Conversely, a series of very small paediatric services would likely lead to a lower quality of care because of insufficient patients at any one centre to provide continuing experience and activity for staff. Relatively small or intermediate sized paediatric populations (<20 new patients/year) can be optimally managed in conjunction with an adult service. Joint medical staff appoint-

ments between paediatric and adult institutions (units) are essential to provide specialized paediatric (medical, surgical, anaesthetic, psychological and para-medical) support for children being nursed in predominantly an adult situation. The authors have found such a scheme outstandingly successful and very cost-effective.

Interrelationships

Regions

Major interactions between regional dialysis programmes relate to organ sharing schemes, patient transfers and holiday dialysis. The value of a National Dialysis-Transplant Committee in policy definition and interaction with government has been discussed.

Core units

Within a regional programme, close cooperation between core units is highly desirable. Such cooperation should be sought at all levels. A regional dialysis-transplant committee representing each core unit facilitates the coordination of all components such as the HBsAg positive units, paediatric services and home dialysis training units. In most cases these should be under the control of one core unit with access available to other units. Standardisation of dialysis machinery and disposables throughout a region is desirable and facilitates patient transfer. It is also particularly useful in price negotiations for supply of consumables, such as dialysers, lines, and dialysis fluid concentrate, which can be put up for tender to supply the whole region.

Sharing of experience should also be encouraged by regular inter-unit meetings at a nursing and technical level. Such meetings can result in standardisation of dialysis techniques throughout the region without authoritative imposition.

Each unit should develop an area of particular interest and expertise. Coordination of these special interests results in a valuable broad range of expertise being available in the region. Brief rotation of selected senior nursing and technical staff through other core units may also be of value.

Peripheral units

The desirability of rotation of staff of peripheral units through the core unit has been discussed. This prevents the staff and patients in peripheral units from becoming isolated and allows continuing staff education. Patient movement between dialysis facilities should be flexible. It is often valuable to allow home dialysis patients several weeks of dialysis in a self-care centre each year to give their helper a holiday from duty.

Medical management

Dialysis patients and sometimes their whole families tend to use the dialysis medical staff for all their medical needs. This can be unwittingly fostered by both the family practitioners and the nephrologists. Adequate communication usually overcomes the problem, particularly if the family doctor, who has probably never seen a dialysis patient before, is given a clear understanding of the process and is asked to contact the nephrologist whenever the patient is seen, particularly if any change in therapy is contemplated. The major role must remain with the nephrologist, who should see the patient, even if long distances are involved, at least once every 3 months.

Ancillary services

Each patient requires the services of a variable number of councillors, dieticians, social workers, psychiatrists and clergy. In most cases the need for these services for an individual patient must be perceived by the nephrologist who should initiate and coordinate their involvement. Local community social workers and welfare agencies can often be of considerable assistance and their activities are most easily coordinated by the family practitioner in consultation with the nephrologist. Often a valuable local support system can be established and is particularly necessary when the patient is dialysing at home and is a long distance from the core unit.

EDUCATION

Staff

The quality of any dialysis service ultimately depends on the quality of the staff training. The key person is the Staff Educator who must be a practical rather than a theoretical educator. Ideally, new nursing staff should be fully trained as nephrology nurses before commencing special dialysis training. Dialysis training should include rotation through various peripheral units including the home dialysis training centre and a self-care dialysis unit. The bulk of the training should be practical and the trainees should be supernumerary during most of the training period.

Compulsory refresher courses, particularly for peripheral unit staff rotating through the core unit, should be run at regular intervals. In addition, the Staff Educator should monitor all staff at their work at least annually.

Patients

Patient education should begin well before commencement of dialysis. Self help, self control and cooperation are the main lessons which patients find difficult to accept. From the patients' point of view, learning about their illness, its implications and how to cope with their fear of dialysis and the unknown, are the most important areas.

Patient education should be structured towards self dialysis, which can usually be achieved within a few months. Education, started before dialysis began, should be repeated after commencement and stabilisation. The education should stress that dialysis is only one phase of management of their illness and that for most patients successful transplantation is the ultimate aim.

Patient and staff dialysis societies

Both patients and staff should be encouraged to form regional or national societies. Patient dialysis associations provide considerable support and education for their members and can overcome many problems which the patient accepts as insoluble or does not discuss with the medical and nursing staff. It is desirable that patient associations should have an interested 'medical adviser', who can often clear up common misconceptions thereby preventing these societies becoming counter-productive.

Dialysis nurses and technicians should be encouraged to form a scientific society and form links with the National Nephrology Society. These societies play an important role in continuing education just as medical scientific societies do.

Community

Education of the community is mainly concerned with preventive medical aspects (e.g. the dangers of analgesic abuse) and the value of kidney transplantation. A high level of community awareness about transplantation lowers the refusal rate when relatives are approached for permission for cadaveric renal donation. Regional transplantation coordinators can be utilized in this regard, not only for educating the community but also for increasing the awareness of medical staff in isolated regions to the overall community value of identifying potential organ donors.

RESEARCH

In planning, research should be regarded as an integral part of the regional dialysis programme. Each core unit should develop and maintain an active research programme in its area of special interest and expertise. Dialysis is often viewed as purely a business or service commitment. However, the quality of the service will depend in part on the academic interest and activity in the scientific aspects of chronic renal failure and its management.

In planning the programme, research should be given a high priority. This should be implemented by employing sufficient medical, nursing and technical staff and allocating sufficient space to enable research to be conducted. However, the most important aspect is to make proven research ability a high priority when selecting the medical staff, particularly the directors of core units. A closely cooperating group of core units within a National or Regional Dialysis Programme can undertake collaborative controlled trials that would be impossible or unduly prolonged in single units.

QUALITY CONTROL AND RECORD KEEPING

These aspects of a dialysis programme are closely linked. Units which have poor records usually have poor quality control and are likely to have poor results – if these could be assessed.

Medical records are one of the neglected areas of many hospitals. Indeed, the very large, often massive amount of data generated by a nephrology-dialysis-transplant service overwhelms their systems. Unless the hospital's medical record system is exceptional, it is worthwhile establishing partially independent record systems in each core unit. These should include all patients in the dialysis-transplant programme. In planning a new programme, proper record keeping with a rapid retrieval, integration and analysis system should be given a high priority. These specifications can only be met by computerisation. When the costs of computerisation are related to the cost of dialysing one patient for one year, they are not overwhelming. Peripheral units should link to the core unit computer system, otherwise much of the important data will never be recorded. Adequate, accessible, analysable records form the basis of any quality control system. Each core unit should regularly analyse its results and subject them to peer review.

Each country should have a National Dialysis and Transplant Registry and health funding authorities should insist on complete data returns as a condition of funding, if co-operation cannot be obtained on a voluntary basis. The Australian-New Zealand Dialysis Transplant Registry is an outstanding example with complete registration and data return on all patients who have ever entered dialysis-transplant programmes. This body of data is thus unique in being unselected. It provides a firm data base for predictions of future needs, quality control and peer review and answers to many scientific questions. New questions should be asked prospectively to examine new areas of interest because retrospective returns may be inaccurate or incomplete. It should be feasible to link by computer all core units in all regions to the National Registry.

COST AND FUNDING OF DIALYSIS

The cost of management of ESRD, particularly by dialysis, has been mentioned in different contexts in previous sections of this chapter. Most doctors avoid thinking about medical costs and most health administrators seem to think of nothing else.

The rapid escalation of the costs of health care and of social welfare during the last two decades have resulted in these two areas of government spending being particular targets for Treasury inspired pruning or no growth policies in most developed countries. The health administrators are given a static or shrinking budget to administer. Concurrently, there has been a trend toward favourable treatment of community based and low technology programmes. This is obviously at the expense of high technology programmes of which dialysis is an outstanding example.

Dialysis is progressively expanding and consequently increasing in cost. The attack of health administrators is to minimise this growth and given the incentive they will undoubtedly succeed. Eventually, the cost issue must be faced by both doctors and patients. The alternatives are limited; either reduce the cost per dialysis so that more patients can be dialysed for the same total cost or continue the status quo in which most patients are receiving high cost institutional dialysis and restrict entry to dialysis by arbitrary criteria. Both approaches, either separately or together, are now being taken in different countries. With the view that all medically suitable patients should be accepted for dialysis, the future trend in the management of ESRD will be toward the least expensive treatment modalities. The approach to planning a new regional dialysis programme outlined in this chapter is based on the belief that high quality management can be provided by the programme which is based on the less expensive forms of treatment, namely transplantation and home and self-care dialysis.

Comparative costing

Table 1 shows the approximate relative costs of various methods of managing end-stage renal failure.

The actual costs vary considerably from country to country and with time, although the relative costs appear to remain fairly constant. It is obvious that hospital based haemodialysis and peritoneal dialysis are expensive ways of managing ESRD compared to transplantation and home and self-care haemodialysis or CAPD.

SUMMARY

The major current and future problem in providing management for ESRD is one of escalating numbers of patients and cost. Consequently, both currently established and new regional dialysis programmes must be modified or planned to provide the service economically and be capable of expansion. Both of these requirements are best met by a programme in which the majority of patients are managed by transplantation and limited care, self-care or home dialysis.

Table 1. Approximate comparative annual maintenance cost of different methods of managing end-stage renal disease (Australia 1985).

Type of treatment	Relative cost $
Hospital HD	1.00
Hospital PD	1.00
Home HD	0.35
Self-care HD	0.35
Limited-care HD	0.50
CAPD	0.30
CCPD	0.55
Cadaveric transplantation – 1st year	0.70
Cadaveric transplantation – subsequent years	0.25

Cadaveric transplantation assumes Cyclosporin-A as one of the maintenance immunosuppressive drugs. Approximate cost of a single patient on maintenance Hospital HD in Australia is approximately A$ 30,000/year.

Hospital based facilities should remain reserved for new patients' induction and management of problem patients.

Thus, most patients will dialyse themselves, decreasing cost by reducing staff requirements, and at the same time increasing the patients benefit by greater independence. The effective management of such a decentralised dialysis programme requires a high level of communication and clearly defined relationship between the various components of the programme.

It should be emphasised that, without a plan or organisation of centralised management, situations may arise wherein optimal treatment is not provided to patients. For instance, personal biases and economic incentives among uncontrolled competing physicians can cause inequities in patient care with limited options favouring institutional dialysis, imbalance of facilities, higher expenditures and impediments to cooperative clinical research.

REFERENCES

1. Brunner FP, Broyer M, Brynger H, Challah S, Fassbinder W, Oules R, Rizzoni G, Selwood NH, Wing AJ: Combined report on regular dialysis and transplantation in Europe, IV, 1984 (and preceding years). *Proc Eur Dial Transplant Assoc* 22: 3, 1985
2. Broyer M, Rizzoni G, Brunner FRP, Brynger H, Challah S, Fassbinder W, Oules R, Selwood NH, Wing AJ: Combined report on regular dialysis and transplantation of children in Europe, XIV, 1984 (and preceding years). *Proc Eur Dial Transplant Assoc* 22: 55, 1985
3. Mathew TH: Dialysis 1984. *Med J Aust* 142: 301, 1985
4. Disney AP: Ninth Report of the Australia and New Zealand Combined Dialysis and Transplant Registry (ANZDATA), August, 1986 (and preceding years)

PATIENT SELECTION AND INTEGRATION OF RENAL REPLACEMENT THERAPY

TIMOTHY H. MATHEW

INTRODUCTION

The selection policy used for patients presenting for treatment in a renal replacement program is based on multiple factors which include medical and social aspects and the availability of facilities. Where facilities are not a restricting factor, only a small percentage of patients referred for treatment need be refused (1). Few countries, however, have demonstrated a capacity or willingness to put unrestricted resources at the disposal of nephrologists. Thus, from the outset attention has been paid to the efficient utilisation of available facilities. In Australia on cost grounds, an early decision was taken to promote transplantation actively. It soon became apparent that for optimal therapy to be offered to all patients a combination or 'integration' of dialysis and transplantation was necessary (2) and that this could be based on an attempt to find a successful transplant for all medically suitable candidates (1). This approach, now practiced widely in many countries is believed to make maximum use of resources while providing patients with the best possible quality of life.

SELECTION OF PATIENTS

The problem of selection of patients is easily dismissed as a non issue in those countries where adequate facilities exist and refusal for treatment need be made only on medical grounds. It is cogent to remember though that only in USA, Canada, Australia, Japan and in some parts of Europe, are more than 20 patients/million/year accepted for active treatment. In large parts of Africa, Asia, South East Asia and South America, dialysis and transplantation facilities continue to be either non-existent or very restricted in their availability. In those countries with a reduced acceptance rate, ability to pay and age are the greatest discriminants (3).

The original criteria used by the Seattle Medical Advisory Committee appear 25 years later, to provide a reasonable basis for selection on medical grounds when some selection is necessary. These criteria selected stable adults under the age of 45 with no irreversible cardiovascular disease who cooperate well with treatment. Undoubtedly criteria similar to these are still in use in many countries. The Seattle plan of having a second committee consisting of lay members, to rank priority for treatment among those deemed medically suitable was initially followed in many units but was progressively abandoned in the late 1960's (4). The view has been advanced (5) that if selection is necessary, a 'first come, first served' lottery method is the one most ethically feasible and in practice it is the method mostly followed by physicians who are forced to act as 'gatekeepers'.

Selection for renal replacement treatment usually means selection for dialysis treatment as it is seldom possible and is

Table 1. Factors influencing acceptance onto treatment programme.

Adequate facilities available	Inadequate facilities
Quality of life anticipated	Quality of life anticipated
Age	Age
Compliance (e.g. psychosis)	Compliance (e.g. psychosis)
	Vascular Status
	Ability to self dialyse
	– home/satellite
	Likelihood of transplant
	– live donor source
	– cadaver donor source

usually undesirable on medical grounds to transplant a patient without prior dialysis. An exception to this is when a living donor is available and treatment (which may include short term dialysis) can be aimed at a finite date. However, as there are no absolute contraindications to long term dialysis and as dialysis is the backbone of a treatment program, selection for the program is primarily a selection onto dialysis. Once on dialysis, decisions must be made regarding the type of dialysis, the option of transplantation and the source of kidney donor. As hospital dialysis space is frequently the major restriction, patients who can be seen as transient in this role may be favoured. Even where adequate facilities exist to dialyse all comers, a recommendation not to commence dialysis is sometimes in the best overall interest of the patient. Specific factors influencing the selection process are summarised in Table 1.

Factors applying when adequate dialysis facilities are available

Expected quality of life

The predicted quality of life on the renal replacement program is the overriding consideration in any medically based decision to refuse acceptance onto a program. All factors, physical and mental affect the quality of life achievable by an individual. Assessment is sometimes easy. The 78 year old widow immobilised by a stroke and dependent for existence on nursing support would be accepted onto very few programs and in fact may not even be referred to a nephrologist despite advanced renal failure. Conversely, assessment may be very difficult as in the case of a 55 year old single epileptic man with no family support and with a record of non-compliance, alcoholism and depression. Experience has shown such patients tend to do poorly but this is not wholly predictable. Here the reasonable decision is to commence a trial of dialysis and to assess progress. It is not easy to withdraw therapy but it must be considered in the event that dialysis is only prolonging misery. Withdrawal of therapy has been reported to occur in up to 9% of patients commencing dialysis and to be a more common occurrence in the aged, in diabetic patients and in those dependent on nursing home care for basic support. Only 50% of patients withdrawn from dialysis were said to be mentally competent. This experience is clearly an outcome of acceptance onto dialysis of all comers and underlines the fact that a trial of dialysis with the option of later withdrawal is feasible (6).

In countries with a reduced acceptance rate one factor operating is the phenomenon of under-referral from primary care physicians. A comparison of attitudes to selection onto dialysis was recently reported from the United Kingdom and clearly showed a greater reluctance on the part of non nephrologists (compared to nephrologists) to recommend dialysis in patients with social and medical problems (7).

Despite some evidence to the contrary (8) the majority of patients maintained on dialysis experience a reasonable quality of life. In Australia, less than 20% of patients maintained on dialysis are classified as medically unfit for work (9).

Age

As in most medical conditions the risk of treatment by dialysis or transplantation rises with increasing age. This has been clearly established by the European (3), Australian (10), and Canadian (11) Registries. (Table 2). The marked decrease in survival seen in those over the age of 60 years has led to a general reluctance to accept patients of this age for transplantation. However, recent experience in the cyclosporin era has seen improved results (12).

There is no absolute age limit to acceptance onto a dialysis program. In countries with no apparent limit to available facilities there has been a tendency to offer dialysis to all candidates including the bedridden aged. The expected quality of life and apparent age should weigh more heavily than the calendar age though in most countries it is rare for patients over 70 years to be accepted. However, in most Canadian provinces over 200 new patients per million of population over 65 (age adjusted) were started on dialysis in 1985 (10). A policy of accepting all comers is unlikely to be seen in the long term as justifiable utilisation of the health dollar and can be criticised in human terms as well. Dialysis should not differ from other areas in medicine in this regard. The real danger is that if physicians are not seen to be using appropriate discretion in treatment decisions then funds will be reduced arbitrarily and young patients who are medically fit may have to be refused active treatment.

Age, therefore, has already been shown to be a major discriminant of success in both dialysis and transplantation. It may be used either as an absolute contra-indication for the 70 year plus group or as a means of selection in the presence of restricted facilities.

Anticipated compliance

Occasionally patients who are manifestly psychotic or have a past history of psychosis present with chronic renal failure. They pose a difficult problem and are often deemed unsuitable for either dialysis or transplantation. The overriding consideration is whether they will comply with the restrictions and therapies needed to make both dialysis and

Table 2. Effect of age on patient survival.

Age years	Percent survival at 3 years	
	Transplant	Dialysis
0–19	93	88
20–39	88	81
40–59	74	69
60+	61	55

All patients on dialysis (n = 5,042 patients) and transplantation (n = 1,285) 1978–1983 ANZDATA Registry.

transplantation successful. Endogenous depression (particularly if previously severe enough to necessitate hospitalisation) in our experience predicts the likelihood of a poor outcome particularly if complications should occur during treatment. Adrenal corticosteroids post-transplantation also may accentuate an otherwise compensated or latent psychosis and this must be considered before committment to transplantation occurs.

Additional factors applying when dialysis facility availability is restricted

Vascular status

Atherosclerosis with occlusion of major arteries poses technical difficulties for both haemodialysis and transplantation procedures. Atherosclerosis is common in patients (particularly diabetics) presenting for treatment and there may be a past history of myocardial infarction or stroke (13). It is seldom necessary to refuse treatment to a patient on vascular grounds alone unless organ damage secondary to ischaemia is severe and incapacitating. Vascular access for haemodialysis can almost always be obtained. If necessary a graft (e.g. umbilical vein) can be performed from a large artery to a large vein. In the difficult case, peritoneal dialysis provides a reasonable alternative.

Atheroma of the pelvic vessels may provide difficulties to the transplant surgeon but in practice it is usually possible to establish blood flow to a transplanted kidney even if operative disobliteration of the iliac vessels prior to transplant insertion is necessary.

With restricted facilities, established vascular disease at presentation may well be used as a discriminating factor. Atherosclerotic complications are the major cause of death on a renal replacement program particularly with dialysis (7). However, it is common experience that patients, even when there are gross atheromata at multiple sites, may continue satisfactorily on dialysis for up to 10 years with no new major vascular events. Accordingly, refusal of the individual patient on the grounds of atheroma is fraught with possible injustice.

Ability to self dialyse

In the face of restricted hospital based facilities the ability of patients to self dialyse makes possible out of hospital self care dialysis in a home or satellite (limited care) unit. The two advantages of this are the lower cost (estimated at $^1/_2$ the cost of hospital dialysis) and the avoidance of overcrowding in the hospital unit which will always have a finite limit of space (14).

The percentage of patients capable of home dialysis is at least 50% (7) and up to an additional 20 to 30% can cope with limited assistance in a satellite centre or with CAPD. This leaves only a small number of patients ultimately dependent long term on a hospital unit. Although hospital units can theoretically be run on a low staff:patient ratio through practicing self care, in practice this is virtually impossible to achieve. With the ready availability of medical staff, the mixture of sick and well patients and the accumulated hard core of dependent patients all mitigating against self-care, those patients who can self dialyse feel penalised for doing so and motivation to put in the extra effort needed will soon diminish.

In the Australian experience the ability and motivation to home dialyse is found more commonly in the educated and upper income groups. This relates to suitable space in the family home and the availability of a partner who has the time to assist in the procedure. An important aspect of the success of home dialysis in Australia has been the provision by the Government of all hardware and disposables free of charge to all patients and the fact that no renal physician depends for his basic income on fees generated through attending the dialysis. Accordingly neither patients nor physicians contend with any financial barrier in deciding whether to do dialysis at home.

Geographical isolation of distant country patients has been another factor encouraging patients in Australia to dialyse at home. When faced with the alternative of moving house and job to a remote city the majority of patients find the motivation to embark on home dialysis.

The willingness or ability to self dialyse thus can be an important factor in the selection of patients onto programs with restricted space. However, if as in Australia where over 80% of all patients, if offered the right circumstances, can self dialyse, this criterion alone should not frequently result in refusal.

Likelihood of transplantation

Apart from non hospital dialysis or death, transplantation offers the only exit from hospital based dialysis. Greater experience has increased our ability to assess transplantation likelihood. The Australian Registry has examined this in recent years and Table 3 summarizes the findings. Some of the restrictions such as recent diagnosis of malignancy are absolute but others such as age are relative. In a competitive situation with inadequate dialysis facilities even the relative contraindications may be used as a reason for exclusion from

Table 3. Likelihood of cadaver transplantation.*

	Percent
No restriction	34
Restriction	
Serological	10
Medical	15
– coronary artery disease	7
– lung disease	2
– malignancy	4
– technical	2
Age deemed too high	21
Patient disinclination	10
Other reasons	10

* Data from ANZDATA Registry (9).

a program based on cadaveric transplantation. Patients with a high degree of sensitization to HLA are extremely hard to transplant successfully and may become effectively untransplantable. This state of sensitization is not always apparent prior to starting dialysis and may in fact be induced whilst dialysis dependent consequent upon blood transfusion. With the wide acceptance of deliberate transfusion as a means of increasing the graft success rate, increasing numbers of these highly sensitized patients have accumulated and occupy available dialysis facilities.

The waiting time for a cadaveric transplant depends on the pool size and the cadaver donor procurement rate. In Australia the median wait for a first cadaver graft had increased from 6 months in 1973 to over 18 months in 1982, this representing a relatively short wait by world standards (15). In one series with cadaver transplantation being actively promoted, 85% of patients were maintained on a functioning graft 4 years from commencement on the program (1).

There is hope that in the future we can select from a given group of medically fit patients, those with a high chance of graft success. At the moment advantage is gained by good matching at the HLA, B and DR loci (7). The future may see refinements to matching technique and better means of early testing of intrinsic immune reactivity. As the case is strong to use the scarce resource of cadaver kidneys in those patients with a higher chance of success it is possible that an early accurate assessment of the likelihood of graft success could be made and a significant selection barrier for transplantation created.

Regional, national and international organ swapping schemes already exist in order to achieve better tissue matching. The future is likely to see even more well matched kidneys exchanged as the benefit of matching (particularly on the B and DR locus) becomes more apparent and as storage techniques are improved and simplified. The availability of cyclosporin has not blunted this advantage of matching in the Australian experience (7).

In the selection of patients to maximise graft success rates, due regard must be paid to the risk run by the patient. Mortality rates have declined in recent years but are still significant. It is in this area that great discretion and judgement is needed. The temptation to attempt transplantation in the hope that a successful graft will cure underlying problems is not conducive to achieving a maximum graft success rate. Similarly pressure to use a kidney locally 'to build up the numbers' or because 'it is ours as we procured it' often means the best recipient is not offered the kidney and consequently the overall graft success rate will suffer.

The availability of a live related donor over-rides these considerations. This was the major factor determining acceptance for end stage renal failure treatment in USA in the early 1970's and in many parts of the world living donation offers the only chance of surviving end-stage renal failure. In Australia and United Kingdom, 11% and 9%, respectively, of all transplants in 1984 were from a living related source. It is believed unlikely that this rate of live donation can rise substantially if one haplotype matching or better is demanded. However, where significant cadaver donation is impos-

sible due to cultural and religious difficulties (e.g. Asia and Middle East) live donation has been extended to include extended family donors with no matching. Donor specific transfusion and cyclosporin have contributed to excellent success rates in this situation.

Factors mitigating against a successful transplant include a previous history of early graft rejection and the diagnosis of 'malignant' focal glomerulosclerosis as the original cause of kidney failure. Focal glomerulosclerosis frequently recurs in a graft and may cause early graft failure (10). In both these situations the reduced chance of graft success provides a relative contraindication to future grafting.

If transplant likelihood is assessed as low or negative, long term dialysis becomes the only available therapy and in this situation the pressure on a patient to dialyse in a non-hospital based setting will likely be even more intense.

Practical problems related to selection

The right to reject

A philosophy has developed in some areas that dialysis physicians have no right to reject any patient asking for dialysis. It is suggested that the situation should be no different with dialysis treatment than it is with other areas of medical therapy. Physicians do have the right and indeed the responsibility to offer therapy only when it is indicated and when in their judgement it is in the best interests of the patient (16). Cancer surgery is not offered to patients with wide spread malignancy. Dialysis therapy should not be offered to patients in whom therapy will prolong misery and suffering and indeed may create an extra burden. Failure to exhibit reasonable responsibility in these matters runs the risk of adversely affecting the attitude of the community to the provision of dialysis facilities. Either guidelines will be set up for physicians to follow or more likely there will be an overall financial cut-back which will force dialysis physicians to make these judgements.

Who makes the decision to refuse dialysis?

The responsibility for refusal rests on the shoulders of the caring physician. This responsibility may be delegated to others, such as a special selection committee, but this seldom happens in recent times. When definite medical contraindications to acceptance onto dialysis exist, this decision must be communicated and explained in a conventional manner. If the refusal in the case of a medically suitable person is because of lack of dialysis facilities then this should be clearly explained to all involved including the hospital administration. If the refusal is based on a mixture of medical and social reasons then the whole caring team should be consulted, a second opinion sought if necessary, and the patient and his family involved in the decision making process. The final decision should be seen to rest with the physician because when the relatives are made to feel it was their decision it is difficult to avoid later feelings of guilt and anxiety.

Patient involvement in decision making

The attitudes of the previous generation, which regarded medical decisions as law and recognized little need or right for the patient to be involved in any decisions, have largely been replaced. Consumerism first came to the USA but is now being felt in all countries to a variable degree. There is now no question that patients should always be involved in decisions affecting their own treatment particularly those of a negative kind which may involve their own life and death. It is up to the medical profession to accommodate itself to this approach.

While an occasional patient refuses to accept the idea of treatment by dialysis or transplantation, it is remarkable how few patients maintain their negative stance when the chips are finally down. Quite frequently the 'not for me' attitude will be exhibited for many months. This form of denial is effective in allowing a temporary escape from the reality of impending treatment and should not be mistaken by the caring team as a definitive decision. Only rarely in our experience will the refusal persist, and in those patients depression is usually so severe that their mental state would preclude successful treatment.

It is rare, as noted above, for the decision not to proceed with active therapy to be a point of disagreement between the patient or his relatives and the doctor. If the decision is made due to restricted facilities in a medically suitable candidate then the doctor must make this clear and in doing so remove himself from any position of blame for the situation. If disagreement about medical suitability does arise, then a second opinion should be sought. If doubt continues, a trial of therapy would usually be commenced with a definite time scale announced. To deny dialysis therapy on medical grounds where reasonable doubt exists is not different to denying other types of medical care. In the process a doctor may well place himself in legal jeopardy.

The Australian experience in the last decade, where there was no meaningful restriction on dialysis space, has been such, that in the small number of cases justifying refusal on medical grounds, the relatives and patient usually understand the medical logic and agree with the suggested course of action.

The option of no active treatment

In some patients a trial of dialysis will have been undertaken and after some time has elapsed it will be evident that continuation of dialysis is not in the patient's best interest. An example of this may be the patient with peripheral vascular disease who is having severe rest pain necessitating narcotic analgesia and who is so confused with cerebrovascular disease that life is vegetative. Similarly when a transplant has failed (usually after some years of function) it may be deemed unwise by both patient and doctor for dialysis to be reinstituted. In these situations involving cessation of therapy it is crucial for the whole team to be aware of the decision and for any dissenting views to be discussed and resolved. The full support and understanding of the caring team is needed through these times. It takes only one dissenting voice to create in the relatives a great amount of anxiety and doubt with later feelings of guilt and anger.

Death from uremia usually involves increasing confusion and a gradual lapse into unconsciousness. From this point of view uremia is not an unpleasant way to die and usually involves no pain. It is however, important to assiduously avoid fluid overload with the consequent unpleasantness of pulmonary oedema.

Decision making, the ideal versus the practical

As in most areas of medicine the final decision will often be a compromise of the ideal and the practical. For example it may be necessary to perform peritoneal dialysis as a holding manouvre until blood vessel access develops to a useable stage. It may be necessary to use hospital based dialysis for some weeks waiting for a place in the home training queue. One area where experience has proved there to be no room for compromise is that of performing transplantation to get out of dialysis complications. Transplantation results will only be good when patients are optimally fit at the time of transplantation and all factors are operating in the favour of the patient. To rush into a transplant because of transient difficulties with dialysis brings with it a lower transplant success rate and this can throw the transplant program into disrepute. It is extraordinarily seldom for a dialysis patient in a competent dialysis program genuinely to need an urgent transplant. Further sites for access are always available and perhaps apart from dialysis dementia or neuropathy all problems on dialysis are helped by more dialysis and time. Thus, transplanting out of trouble should be a rare event and arguably should not be allowed to occur.

Decision making, the individual versus the group

In the complex matter of caring for chronic renal failure patients, it must constantly be borne in mind that any decision is very visible and potentially has a long lasting result. The wrong decision will easily put fuel on the fire of those mounting a case against widespread availability of dialysis and it is easy in the process to do the overall group a grave disadvantage. It is our belief that the majority of patients are advantaged and the overall quality of life improved when the organization allows a well integrated program of dialysis and transplantation. Very few patients will have to be refused from such a program which, if based on active cadaver transplantation, will provide the best and cheapest result for most people. The major block in such a program will be in hospital based dialysis space which is finite. However, in Australia as adequate self care satellite facilities (with reduced staffing numbers and consequently operating on a low cost basis) are made available and with the open ended option of CAPD the problem of limited hospital facilities has not been a major restriction.

Local versus regional policies

It is easy for various hospitals within a city or region to develop different beliefs and philosophies regarding dialysis and transplantation. In this situation patients may be referred or find their own way to other units if they are displeased with the decisions of the first unit. Whilst recognizing the desirability of competition in order to avoid a monopoly situation it is, however, meaningless if such policies cannot be enforced on a regional basis. Otherwise the outcome is that one hospital puts more patients on dialysis than the next. It, therefore, seems highly desirable for hospitals within a region to resolve policy differences and apply them uniformly. The same can be argued at a national level for the mobile population of America, Europe and Australia soon find their way to the point of least resistance if that is necessary for their perceived advantage.

INTEGRATION OF DIALYSIS AND TRANSPLANTATION

Integration of dialysis and transplant programs was first reported in the early 1970's and was put into practice in many areas soon thereafter (1, 2). By integration it is meant that the two treatments, dialysis and transplantation, are regarded to be complementary and not competitive, with patients progressing from one treatment to the other and back as medically indicated from time to time.

For integration to be applied successfully it is necessary to have both modalities of treatment readily available and for the caring physician to feel a committment to both treatments. This occurs most easily where the dialysis physician is involved in the transplant program. If the transplant program is run by a surgical team and nephrology (dialysis) physicians are excluded from any meaningful involvement, barriers develop and attitudes are created against transplantation. This can lead to a dichotomy with the path which patients follow being determined by the initial referral and having nothing necessarily to do with the real needs of the patient. This division is accentuated if some patients are returned to a dialysis physician's care post graft failure in a weakened wasted condition (as is sometimes difficult to avoid) and all the patients grafted successfully are never seen again except by the surgical team (15).

In all Australian cities integrated programs exist and in most of these a nephrologist effectively controls both treatments. This does not necessarily impinge on or weaken the traditional surgical role and responsibility. It is a team event with various degrees of involvement for physicians and surgeons. The crucial point is that the physician is not excluded from significant interaction with the transplant team. This makes it easier for the physician to maintain a positive attitude regarding transplantations and to reflect this to the dialysis patients.

One essential feature in running a successful integrated program is to have available all modalities and locations of dialysis so that the optimal dialysis regime can be tailored for each patient. This allows the best preparation for transplantation. The transplant program must have a reasonable availability of cadaver kidneys – if the average wait for a cadaver transplant is 5 years it is difficult to sustain meaningful integration.

The integrated approach provides flexibility in management and should allow both therapies to be practiced successfully to the benefit of the patients. Transplantation can be offered when the patient is ready and fit and the return to dialysis can occur at an optimal time if the graft is failing. To time these events to the patient's greatest advantage requires all options to be freely available and for the right judgements to be made. The flexibility allows either medical or social pressures to be accommodated. In Australia the decision by a patient to stay on dialysis and to refuse transplantation would usually bring with it firm pressure to dialyse out of hospital.

It can be seen that the integrated approach allows better tailoring of the ideal program for the individual but it also has advantage for the community. As integration tends to maximise the rate of transplantation (through increased motivation of physicians and their patients) and as the cost of transplantation is significantly lower than dialysis, there accrues a large cost benefit. Another advantage is the significant increase in rehabilitation rate experienced by patients post transplant with a consequent increased contribution to society.

The cadaver donor procurement rate is also affected by an integrated approach. If a transplant program is well supported by all nephrologists and is successful, non-renal physicians and surgeons in charge of potential donors are much more likely to initiate appropriate action than if the reverse is true. This will lead to an increased referral of donors and a consequent improvement in the supply of kidneys.

Whilst integration is most easily achieved within one institution there is no reason why an integrated program cannot accommodate several dialysis units feeding one transplant unit. In this situation good communications are paramount with regular contact occurring with all physicians so that there is a definite feeling of involvement. The essential point is that all dialysis physicians must have a meaningful involvement in the transplant program.

Patients must be aware of this integration of therapies and will usually find it plausible and reassuring. This is particularly so if continuity of care occurs and the patient is not made to feel like the meat in the sandwich. With an integrated program the decisions can be taken with only one aim in mind, that which is best for the individual patient.

In summary an integrated approach to dialysis and transplantation allows patients to access the treatment option which is best for them at any point in time. It prevents the isolation of dialysis from transplantation which if it exists may adversely affect both areas with consequent reduction in the quality of patient care. Further integration by maximising transplantation allows a greater number of patients to be treated at a lower and more acceptable cost to the community.

QUALITY OF LIFE

The quality of life of the chronic dialysis patients is reviewed elsewhere in this book, but it is appropriate at this point to make mention of it because it affects the selection of patients and organization of a combined program of dialysis and transplantation. Brief mention was made above of quality of life as an issue which should be considered in the selection of all patients.

Experience through the years has revealed the remarkable adaptability of patients to their various burdens and difficulties. In most people the instinct for survival is strong and lifestyles, ambitions and ideas are all capable of great modification given sufficient stress. Frequently, patients will say they do not want to continue with treatment unless 'life can be lived to the fullest'. Yet, only a few months later, they will accept a lifestyle which has many restrictions. When dialysis facilities have been available without restriction there is a tendency for physicians to avoid denying therapy and to leave such decisions in the hands of patients. This may result in the continuation of dialysis in situations where, by any criteria, life can only be said to be miserable for the patient and all those around him. The instinct for survival is so strong that seldom will a patient or his family initiate what amounts to public suicide or the voluntary suggestion of treatment withdrawal. Here, the dialysis physician should exhibit his responsibility and the right to intervene. As noted above the patient and family seldom disagree with decisions made by experienced dialysis personnel and which are explained fully to them. There can come a point where continuation of dialysis is unwarranted and the identification of this by the dialysis physician and his assistance to the family at this time is usually seen as positive. In between the two ends of the spectrum there is a grey zone and here much difficulty may ensue unless a trial of dialysis is offered.

Objective assessment of the quality of life is extraordinarily difficult and superficial questionnaires particularly involving assessments made by others may be quite misleading. Despite these difficulties the Australia and New Zealand Dialysis and Transplant (ANZDATA) Registry has for some years asked physicians to rank rehabilitation and to score quality of life for all patients on dialysis and transplantation. The rehabilitation pattern in Australia through the last decade has been a consistent one and is shown in Table 4.

This assessment has been criticized for being work orientated but it continues to provide health administrators, politicians and the community with a tangible measure as to the success of the programs. The data shown in Table 4 are similar to European data (3). A substantially better rehabilitation rate in patients on a functioning transplant (88% classified able to work) is achieved compared to patients on dialysis (72% classified able to work). Over twice as many patients on dialysis are classified medically unfit to work. These figures do not take account of the difference in mean ages between the groups and as with all figures comparing dialysis and transplantation suffer from the bias which usually results in the transplantation of fitter patients away from dialysis. Despite these precautions the data confirm the strong clinical impression that the general degree of rehabilitation post-transplant tends to exceed that on dialysis. This overall degree of rehabilitation is highly desirable to justify the large expenditure of public money on renal replacement programs. Both the European and Australian data show a better rehabilitation rate for home dialysis compared to hospital dialysis, but to a degree this reflects the younger and fitter patient population dialysed at home. In the European experience there is very little difference between the home dialysis patient potential for employment and that of transplanted patients.

It must be remembered that the best available measures of the quality of life at this time are subjective and it is therefore desirable to use great caution in making any judgements on this basis. Predicting adjustment to dialysis and quality of life obtainable is fraught with difficulty. Many patients who create initial concern to the caring team about their ability to cope and achieve a reasonable quality of life on dialysis, survive happily and with a positive life many years later. While there is no correct figure an appropriate patient rejection rate for the 1980's in a situation where dialysis facilities are not restricted should be somewhere between 1 and 10%. If any unit is refusing more than 10% of patients offered to it for dialysis then the guidelines being used should be carefully reassessed. Confirmation that one is making right judgements may come from having the occasional failure. If all patients started on dialysis do well then it seems likely that some patients are being refused unnecessarily. The occasional failure and necessity to withdraw therapy will show one's judgement (while not perfect) is erring on the preferred side of giving patients the benefit of doubt.

Table 4. Rehabilitation of patients on dialysis and transplantation.

	On dialysis Percent	On function Tx Percent
Fulltime work	34	68
Part time work	22	11
Able to work but unemployed	3	4
Able to work but retired (>60 yrs)	13	5
Total able to work	72	88
Unwilling to work	6	5
Medically unfit to work	19	7
Dialysis schedule precludes work	3	–
Total unable or unwilling to work	28	12

Assessment of 2,174 Dialysis patients and 2,167 patients on a functioning transplant at 31/10/85 from ANZDATA Registry (9).

REFERENCES

1. Mathew TH, Marshall VC, Vikraman P, Hill AVL, Johnson W, McOmish D, Morris PJ, Kincaid-Smith P: Integrated programme of dialysis and renal transplantation. *Lancet* 2: 137, 1975

2. Clunie GJA, Hartley LCJ, Ribush NT, Emmerson BT, Morgan TO: An integrated service for the treatment of irreversible renal failure. *Med J Aust* 2: 403, 1971

3. Brynger H, Brunner FP, Chantler C, Donckerwolcke RA, Jacobs C, Kramer P, Selwood NH, Wing AJ: Combined report on regular dialysis and transplantation in Europe, X, 1979. *Proc Eur Dial Transplant Assoc* 17: 3, 1980

4. Katz AH, Proctor DM: Social psychological characteristics of patients receiving haemodialysis in treatment for chronic renal failure. *Public Health Service, Kidney Disease Control Program.* July 1969

5. Abrams HS: Psychiatry and prolongation of life. in *Proceedings of the Conference on Emerging. Medical, Moral and Legal Concerns.* edited by Siemsen A, Griefer I, Honolulu, St. Francis Hospital, 1976, p 63

6. Neu S, Kjellstrand CM: Stopping long term dialysis. An empirical study of withdrawal of life supporting treatment. *N Engl J Med* 314: 14, 1986

7. Challah S, Wing AJ, Bauer R, Morris RW, Schroeder SA: Negative selection of patients for dialysis and transplantation in the United Kingdom. *Br Med J* 288: 1119, 1984

8. Gutman TA, Stead WW, Robinson RR: Physical activity and employment status of patients on maintenance dialysis. *N Engl J Med* 304: 309, 1981

9. *Ninth Report of ANZDATA Registry.* edited by Disney AP, Adelaide, The Queen Elizabeth Hospital Publ, 1986, p 30

10. Disney APS, Correll R: Report of the Australia and New Zealand Combined Dialysis and Transplant Registry. *Med J Aust* 1: 117, 1981

11. Canadian Renal Failure Register. Ottowa, Kidney Foundation of Canada, 1985, p 130

12. Wombolt D, Goldberg M, Hurwitz R: Efficacy of renal transplantation in the elderly. *Kidney Int* 31: 471, 1987

13. Lindner A, Charra B, Sherrard DJ, Scribner BH: Accelerated atherosclerosis in prolonged maintenance dialysis. *N Engl J Med* 290: 697, 1974

14. Mahony J: Cost analysis of dialysis alternatives. in *Peritoneal Dialysis* edited by Atkins RC, Thomson NM, Farrell PC, Edinburgh, London, Churchill-Livingstone, 1981, p 418

15. *Seventh Annual Report of the ANZDATA Registry,* edited by Disney AP, Adelaide, Queen Elizabeth Hospital, 1980, p 24

16. Inglefinger RJ: Arrogance. *New Eng J Med* 303: 1507, 1980

17. De Palma J: Guest Editorial. *Dial Transplant* 4 (5): 6, 1975

REGULAR DIALYSIS TREATMENT

BARBARA G. DELANO

INTRODUCTION

Chronic hemodialysis has been a reality for close to 30 years. This procedure, originally limited to a few highly selected and carefully followed patients, is now performed on more than 250,000 people worldwide. Dialysis professionals were also a small, select group, but the tremendous growth of this therapy has made it imperative for all health care workers to become familiar with the care of the dialysis patient. Extensive technical information on selection of equipment and solutions as well as monitoring and managing patient complications is discussed elsewhere in this book. This chapter deals with some of the practical aspects of hemodialysis. It covers such areas as initiation and termination of regular dialysis therapy, selecting a dialysis schedule and special considerations in offering hemodialysis to high risk groups of patients; a brief outline for the routine monitoring of the hemodialysis patient is also presented.

INITIATION OF MAINTENANCE HEMODIALYSIS

When

There is no difficulty in deciding to begin dialysis in a severely symptomatic uremic patient. The asymptomatic patient, inexorably deteriorating in terms of measured renal function, does create a problem, however, as to when to abandon conservative therapy in favor of dialysis. Controversy still exists over the optimal time to initiate regular dialysis therapy.

The staunchest advocates of early initiation of maintenance hemodialysis have been Bonomini and coworkers (1). In 1975, they stated that patients begun on therapy at creatinine clearances of 15 to 21 ml/min had an excellent 4 year survival, (85%). Bonomini (2) explained these results by suggesting that in patients whose endogenous creatinine clearances are 5 ml/min or less, uremic complications are more pronounced and will irreversibly progress despite maintenance hemodialysis. Indeed, he suggests that by starting hemodialysis at a higher creatinine clearance, the harmful effects of protein depletion can be eliminated, and renal and extrarenal hormone equilibrium may be better preserved (3).

Scribner (4) points out that Bonomini's patients may not be representative of general selection criteria. Survival of Bonomini's patients with a creatinine clearance of 0 to 5 ml/min, who were dialyzed two to three times per week for 5 to 10 h, was inexplicably poor (only 40% were alive after 4 years). Depending on age and coexisting systemic diseases, annual mortality in regularly dialyzed patients ranges from 5 to 10% in most large centers around the world. Poor survival together with deterioration of motor nerve conduction velocities in Bonomini's patients were interpreted by Scribner as evidence of inadequate dialysis, thereby invalidating the conclusions as to efficacy of the 'early' treatment schedule.

Bonomini (5), subsequently looking at longer survival, (10 years) reported an 88% 10 year survival in patients began on therapy at a creatinine clearance of 10 ml/min, compared to a 55%, 10 year survival for patients started late, i.e. at a creatinine clearance of 2 to 4 ml/min. In addition, 'early' patients spent less time in the hospital (5 days/year/patient) versus 14 days/year/patient) for late starters. Indeed, in one study that looked at the comparative cost to benefit, including cost for dialysis sessions, hospitalization, and wages earned, analysis of early versus late dialysis over 5 years, revealed a 20% savings for a group of early starting patients over late starters (6).

Substantial clinical experience indicates that for most patients maintenance hemodialysis is best initiated when the patients' creatinine clearance is approximately 5 ml/min. As residual renal function falls below this level, the patient becomes catabolic, loses weight and develops such complications as motor neuropathy and pericarditis.

Ratcliffe, Phillips, and Oliver (7) compared two groups of patients initiating hemodialysis at creatinine clearances of either above or below 6 ml/min. Serious complications, which prolonged the hospital stay at the beginning of dialysis, were present in 9% of the early referred group and 70% of the late referred group.

Maher (8) found that, depending on diagnosis, renal diseases progress at differing rates; occasionally, patients survive without dialysis for as long as 3 years after reaching a serum creatinine concentration of 10 mg/dl (884 μmol/l). By contrast accelerated deterioration in renal function over weeks to months is common in systemic sclerosis, malignant hypertension and rapidly progressive glomerulonephritis.

While at our institution we have generally subscribed to the 5 ml/min starting point for maintenance hemodialysis, the patient's clinical condition is more important than laboratory measurements of glomerular filtration rate. We occasionally see patients with uremic symptoms (i.e. nausea, vomiting, lassitude) at a serum creatinine concentration of 5 mg/dl (442 μmol/l) (creatinine clearance of approximately 10 ml/min) who subjectively feel much improved after a dialysis. Usually, these patients have diabetes mellitus, or other systemic illness. In such cases, a trial of dialysis may be warranted and if the patient feels better, it may be wise to begin maintenance dialysis at that time.

Time to plan

Ideally, with early recognition of irreversible renal disease, there is adequate opportunity to plan for the smooth initiation of long term hemodialysis. As soon as it becomes clear that a patient has progressive renal failure, the patient, family and medical advisors should review the probable rate of deterioration and the types of treatment available. The suitability of hemodialysis, peritoneal dialysis or transplantation may vary according to the patient's age, diagnosis and preference. In our program every new patient meets with both the transplant surgeon and the nephrologist. Whenever

possible and appropriate, the new patient should also meet someone who is leading an active life after many years of dialysis. Hurdling the barriers of psychological adjustment to regular dialysis is made easier by full and frank disclosure of all facts to the patient.

At the outset, management of renal failure should begin with providing vascular access well in advance of its need, in order to allow the arteriovenous fistula to 'mature'. Elderly, obese and diabetic patients may require 2 to 4 months before a fistula is ready for use. The Cimino-Brescia arteriovenous fistula (9) is the access of choice for most patients. In patients with small or thrombosed veins, (e.g. diabetics) A PTFE or bovine carotid heterograft may be the procedure of choice (10).

We usually perform vascular access surgery when the creatinine clearance has fallen to approximately 10 ml/min. Patients who can be anticipated to have a 'slow access maturation', such as diabetic patients, should have surgery earlier (15 to 20 ml/min). In those individuals with slowly progressive diseases (e.g. polycystic kidney disease) we may delay vascular access until their clearance has fallen to 6 to 8 ml/min (which may take months to years).

No time to plan

Unfortunately, all too frequently patients present with far advanced uremia requiring immediate dialysis. These patients may be handled in the following ways:

1. Permanent access (a fistula or artery heterograft) is placed in the non-dominant arm (to permit self-puncture of the fistula if the patient is going to be on home or limited care dialysis). For immediate use a Scribner shunt is temporarily placed in the dominant arm. In older or diabetic patients two arteriovenous anastomoses, however, may lead to high-output cardiac failure (11, 12). Further drawbacks are that vessels used for the shunt are permanently destroyed and shunts have a recognized propensity for thrombosis and infection.

2. Permanent access may be placed in the non-dominant arm, and repetitive peritoneal dialysis performed until the access is mature. Occasionally, in patients with polycystic kidneys, pyelonephritis, obstructive uropathy, high urine volume, urinary tract infection, or extracellular dehydration, an occasional peritoneal dialysis may delay the need for maintenance hemodialysis for a long time (a delay of 4 years has been observed after one peritoneal dialysis [13]). Intermittent peritoneal dialysis or continuous ambulatory peritoneal dialysis is also an acceptable mode of long term therapy.

3. Permanent access is placed in the non-dominant arm and the patient sustained by repeated subclavian vein canulation (14), or by the placement of a semi-permanent double lumen subclavian line (15). Here, complications include infection, superior vena cava thromboses, pneumothorax, and retained catheter (16).

4. The plan we have found most useful, is to create permanent access in the non-dominant arm while sustaining the patient with hemodialysis via percutaneous femoral ve-

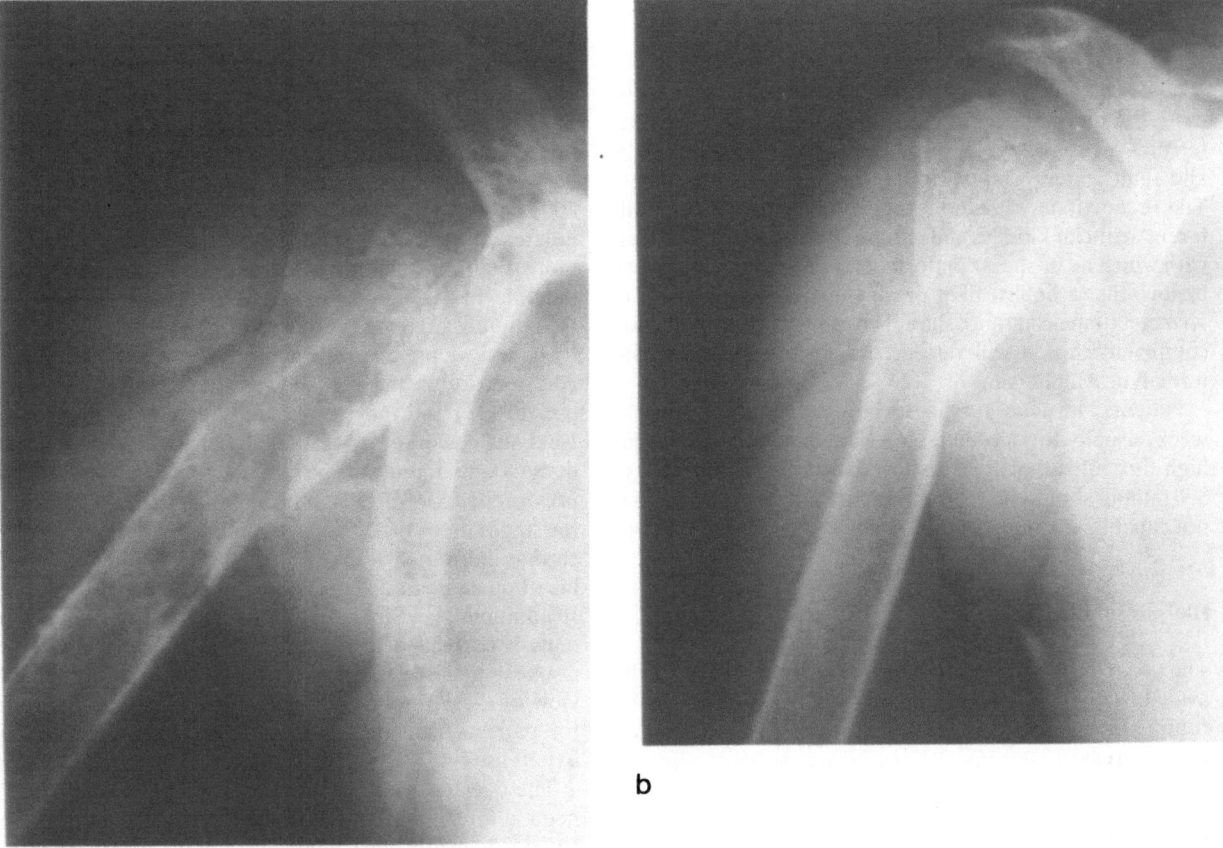

Figure 1. Radiographs of the right humerus in a patient with biopsy proven aluminum associated osteomalacia: A – Non-healing fracture; B – Callus formation 15 months after 1500 mg deferoxamine infusion during each dialysis.

nous catheters until the fistula matures (17, 18). Our experience has been described previously (19). Repeated femoral catheter dialysis can be successfully performed over many months. We have found the procedure to be simple, safe and easily performed by selected members of our nursing staff after suitable instruction. Femoral catheter dialysis is associated with infrequent but appreciable complications. These include bleeding at the catheter site, iliofemoral vein thrombosis with pulmonary embolism and perforation of the inferior vena cava (20).

TERMINATION OF DIALYSIS

Recently, Neu and Kjellstrand have focused attention on the practice of stopping long term dialysis (21). In their study of 1766 patients who started hemodialysis between January 1966 and July 1983, dialysis was discontinued in 155, accounting for an astonishing 22% of all deaths. One half of

the patients were competent when the decision was made. Although dialysis was stopped most frequently in diabetic patients, the demented and patients who were blind or who had suffered a stroke, in 17% of the patients there were no associated complications. This report has opened up a Pandora's box and resulted in a symposium offering opposing physician's and philosopher's views (22). The interest generated has clearly pointed out the need to discuss these issues further. Until some guidelines are available, each physician must make his or her own decision in these matters.

A much easier problem is when to discontinue dialysis because of the return of sufficient renal function to allow the patient to live without the machine. This has been reported in patients with malignant hypertension (23, 24), gout (25), scleroderma (26), systemic lupus erythematosus (27) and myeloma kidney (28). A pre-dialysis serum creatinine concentration equal to or lower than the previous post-dialysis creatinine concentration, and an increase in the patient's urine volume are important clues suggesting the return of renal function.

START OF MAINTENANCE HEMODIALYSIS

Dialysis prescription

When a patient begins hemodialysis, the physician must write the dialysis 'prescription'. Individual patient characteristics such as body size, age, residual creatinine clearance and fluid volume status will determine the choices made. The practitioner should become familiar with several different artificial kidneys and choose from among the models with which he or she is comfortable. For an adult patient we believe that a hollow fiber or plate dialyzer with a high *in vivo* creatinine clearance should be used. The ultrafiltration coefficient chosen will vary according to the patient's interdialytic weight gain.

Patients, in general, should be dialyzed three times a week, usually for 4 h, unless special equipment is used for high flux, ultrashort dialysis (see below). A blood flow of 300 ml/min should be the goal, unless the vascular access is not capable of supplying this amount.

Dialysis solution

There is considerable variation in the composition of the available dialysis fluid formulas that can be used for the routine dialysis patient. Attention must be paid to the following areas:

Potassium

For the standard dialysis patient, a dialysis fluid potassium concentration of 2 mEq/l is routine. If the patient is very catabolic, or tends to have an excessive dietary intake of potassium, a zero or 1 mEq/l bath may be ideal. In a patient with heart disease, receiving cardiac glycosides, the potassium concentration should be raised to 3 mEq/l to prevent cardiac arrhythmias.

Sodium

Sodium is the major determinant of osmolality in the dialysis solution. Early dialyses regimes favored a 'low sodium bath', i.e., 130 mEq/l. The rational was that a post dialysis sodium concentration in that range would control thirst and blood pressure. This level of sodium unfortunately is frequently associated with hypotension and cramping during the dialysis treatment. For this reason, plus the introduction of newer technologies which permit better fluid removal, the recent trend is to use 'high' sodium i.e. 140 to 145 mEq/l. Some patients do complain of excessive thirst on this bath. Another possible strategy is to vary the sodium concentration during the dialysis. One can dialyze against a 'high' sodium concentration for 3 to 3.5 h to prevent cramping and then switch to a lower sodium bath during the last 0.5 to 1 h. Thus, the patient's post dialysis serum sodium concentration is in the low normal range.

Acetate vs bicarbonate

Because of the propensity of bicarbonate to combine with calcium in the dialysis solution concentrate and form a precipitate of calcium carbonate, acetate has been used as the major element to correct acidosis in dialysis patients. Acetate is metabolized to CO_2 and H_2O in peripheral tissues (29). The maximum rate of metabolism is approximately 300 mmol/h (30). With the recent use of larger dialyzers and greater blood flows, some investigators have found that more than 300 mmol/h of acetate may be transferred to patients during dialysis (31).

Sodium acetate has been shown, at least experimentally, to have a depressive effect on the myocardium (32). In addition, acetate has a greater vasodilatory effect than bicarbonate (33) and may lower the patient's blood pressure. Iseki and coworkers (34) studied six patients during acetate dialysis and found an average decrease in mean arterial pressure (MAP) of 15%, a mean fall in the total peripheral resistance index of 31%, and a compensatory increase in the cardiac index of 28%. When these same patients underwent bicarbonate hemodialysis none of these changes were seen. In addition, Van Stone (35) found that a bicarbonate hemodialysis corrects acidosis faster than acetate dialysis. This also resulted in better arterial oxygenation for the patient. In view of these findings, bicarbonate dialysate is preferable for patients with unstable cardiovascular systems and or hypotension (36).

The question as to whether or not a bicarbonate bath is needed for the 'usual' chronic patient is not yet answered. Brezin, Schwartz and Chinitz (37) studied 104 patients using a cross-over design, and found less fall in blood pressure but more muscle cramping with a bicarbonate bath. They defined a group of patients who were 'acetate intolerant', that is, had a blood pressure drop of greater than 10 mm Hg. Vinay and co-workers (38) believe it is possible to identify those patients unable to metabolize the acetate load properly by formulating an individual index of acetate metabolism for each patient. This can be estimated by examining the net gain or loss of bicarbonate per dialysis as a function of the initial plasma bicarbonate level. In their study they found that 10% of patients, mostly females, cannot be satisfactorily dialyzed using acetate and should be placed on bicarbonate.

Other variables in the dialysis solution include calcium, magnesium and glucose.

Initiating dialysis

The initial dialysis, particularly if a patient is very uremic, may result in dialysis disequilibrium (39). This occurs towards the end of dialysis, after rapid lowering of the blood urea nitrogen concentration (40), and consists clinically of a syndrome of headache, nausea, vomiting, blurred vision, seizures and rarely, coma and death.

The most consistent finding in patients with dialysis disequilibrium is an elevated cerebrospinal fluid (CSF) pressure and cerebral edema. The exact cause of the cerebral edema is not known. One explanation is that urea is cleared more rapidly from the blood than from the CSF. Indeed, the urea concentration in the CSF is 14 to 19 mmol/l (84 to 114 mg/dl) higher than in plasma, causing an appreciably higher osmolality. Presumably this 'draws' fluid in and the CSF pressure rises (41, 42), although it should be noted, CSF pressure generally rises whether dialysis is slow or rapid, with or without the presence of the disequilibrium syndrome (43). Animal studies, however, have shown that the rate of clearance of urea from the CSF is the same as from the plasma (44).

Other possible causes of dialysis disequilibrium are hypoglycemia (45), hyponatremia (46) and acidosis (47). Arieff and Massry (48) have experimentally demonstrated a fall in the CSF pH while arterial pH returned towards normal during rapid hemodialysis. A fall in the intracellular pH of the cerebral cortex and a rise in brain water content have also been demonstrated (49).

The solute that contributes to the observed rise of brain intracellular osmolality has not been identified. Changes in the measured solutes in the brain cannot account for the rise in osmolality (48). The fall in bicarbonate concentration of both cerebrospinal fluid and brain suggest the appearance of organic acids which could be the by-products of protein or polypeptide metabolism (50). These unidentified solutes have been termed idiogenic osmols (48).

In an attempt to minimize the disequilibrium syndrome, dialysis can be initiated with short frequent treatments: We dialyze for 2 h on day one, 2 to 4 h on day two, no dialysis on day three, 4 h on day four, and then proceed with routine thrice weekly 4 h treatments.

Other methods of avoiding or reducing the disequilibrium syndrome have been suggested (51–53). These include adding such osmotically active solutes as dextrose, glycerol or mannitol to the dialysate or substituting bicarbonate for acetate in order to minimize rapid alterations in plasma osmolality or bicarbonate concentration during dialysis.

If the dialysis disequilibrium syndrome does occur, intravenous injection of 50 ml of 50% dextrose or mannitol may improve the situation transiently, particularly if given within minutes of the onset of headache. These injections may be repeated two or three times over the next 2 h. Dialysis should be discontinued, at least temporarily, if patient discomfort is severe.

HEMODIALYSIS SCHEDULES

Adequacy of dialysis

Because dialysis is time consuming and expensive, there is great interest in shortening the duration of the procedure. To accomplish this requires evaluation of differing dialysis protocols, but always in light of effective treatment or so-called adequacy of dialysis. Obviously, any worthwhile innovation in dialysis scheduling must assure that the patient will fare no worse and, hopefully, will actually be benefited. As Blagg (54) has recently elaborated 'adequate dialysis'

has still not been satisfactorily defined even after all these years. Certainly, patient 'well-being' is a measure of adequate dialysis but depends on many variables including the patient's size, diet, personality and home situation. Many nephrologists, therefore would like dialysis adequacy to be based on some objective, quantitative measures of what such treatments actually do (55).

Statistical methods of assessing the adequacy of hemodialysis began with the dialysis index of Babb and Scribner (56, 57). Gotch and Sargent (58) have suggested mathematical modeling. Keshaviah and Collins (59), in order to assess the efficiency of dialysis, recently popularized the use of an index, $(K\tau/V)$ where K = urea clearance (ml/min), τ = treatment duration (min) and V = volume of urea distribution.

They believe that a $(K\tau/V)$ of 1 to 1.4 constitutes adequate dialysis, and a value <0.8 is inadequate. Farrell (60) supports the use of kinetic modeling, particularly using urea, and states that while a $(K\tau/V)$ index of greater than 1.0 does not guarantee adequate dialysis, an index less than this does alert the staff to the potential for under dialysis. Other workers continue to rely on such quantifiable tests as changes in the EEG (55), measurement of the vibration sensitive threshold (61), and peripheral nerve function testing (62). Still other physicians view adequacy of dialysis in more general terms. Kopple and Swenseid (63), for example, stipulate that adequate dialysis must permit good nutrition, particularly the intake of protein and amino acids. Desforges (64) states that adequate dialysis improves but does not correct the anemia of uremia, but good dialysis reverses the bleeding tendency and may improve leukocyte function. Parker (65) believes adequate dialysis is that in which the resting muscle membrane potential returns to and remains normal. The status of the patients' bones (66) and cardiovascular system (67, 68) must also be considered in formulating an assessment of sufficient dialysis therapy. The defination of adequate dialysis by DePalma (69), though perhaps imprecise, is nevertheless still useful until a specific quantifiable substitute is found. It is: 'Adequate dialysis is that which permits the patient to be rehabilitated, eat a reasonable diet, make blood, maintain a near normal blood pressure, and prevent the development or progression of neuropathy'.

Adequacy of a single dialysis

The biochemical changes that occur during a single dialysis depend on several factors: At any point during a stable dialysis the concentration of a substance (e.g., urea) depends on its rate of generation, its volume of distribution, the patients' residual renal function, the hemodialyzer clearance and the elapsed dialysis time (70).

Hemodialysis clearance depends on the type of membrane, the total dialyzer surface area and the flow rates of blood and dialysis fluid. A 50 to 60% reduction in serum creatinine and urea concentrations is desirable during a single hemodialysis. If this is not obtained, the following questions must be asked:

1. Is the kidney surface area and creatinine clearance adequate? A big muscular man obviously needs a 'larger' dialyzer than a small woman.
2. Is the blood flow adequate? In patients without heart disease and with good vascular access, blood flows of 275 to 300 ml/min may be maintained with impunity.
3. Are the hours of dialysis adequate? Most dialyses in our unit are 4 h in duration (see below).
4. Is blood recirculation occurring? At our institution, recirculation of blood has caused recurrent uremic symptoms with dialysis time periods that had previously been adequate (71). Recirculation can occur in the presence of normal venous pressure and good blood flow, although increasing venous pressure may be a clue to a failing access. The percentage of recirculation is calculated in the following way: the BUN is determined in the blood going to the dialyzer (C_a), in the blood from the dialyzer (C_v) and in peripheral blood (C_p). Samples should be taken simultaneously and the following formula is used:

$$\frac{C_p - C_a}{C_p - C_v} \times 100 = \% \text{ recirculation.}$$

If more than 20% of the blood is found to be recirculating, an angiogram and corrective access surgery should be strongly considered. Recirculation is a well recognized risk in single needle dialysis

Short dialysis

In the early days of Kiil dialysis, patients routinely spent 28 to 36 h per week on the machine. Coils and the hollow fiber configuration, as well as improvement in dialysis membranes led to the fairly standard 4 h, 3 times a week regimen for the usual patient.

Economic considerations, patient preference and newer technology have now led to a proliferation of units offering 'rapid, high efficiency dialysis'.

The definition of short dialysis varies from between 4.5 to 12 h per week. For example, Raja and co-workers (72) recently reported the results of a group of 69 patients who had been dialyzed for more than 10 years on a schedule of 8 to 12 h/week. They report a 30% patient survival at 14 years. In analyzing their data, young age, female sex, black race and absence of hypertension where correlated with good survival. This study used fairly standard dialysis equipment, and would hardly be classified as 'short time' by today's standards.

Keshaviah and Collins (59) have treated 250 patients from 2.5 to 3.5 h/treatment (mean time 2.75 h) with a high efficiency dialyzer (Travenol CH 170), A bicarbonate bath, and a mean blood flow of 353 ml/min. In this large study, there was no increased hospitalizations or symptoms compared to 'standard' dialysis. Their patients had a 2 year cummulative survival of 79%.

Rotellar et al (73) devised a large surface hemodialyzer (5 m²), increased blood flow to 500 ml/min and dialysate flow to 1000 ml/min and dialyzed patients for 6 h/week using a bicarbonate bath. With this system, they obtained a dialyz-er clearance of 345 ml/min vs. 175 ml/min, and an ultrafiltration rate of 98 ml/min compared to 45 ml/min for their standard equipment. Muscle cramping and mild disequilibrium necessitated using a bath with a higher concentration of potassium and glucose than is usual. They successfully treated 25 patients for more than 1 year with no change in serum chemistries, bone status or nerve conduction.

Rubin, Friedmann and Berlyne (74) successfully dialyzed 12 patients on a Hospal 3000S (high flux) dialyzer using volumetrically controlled monitors at a blood flow rate of 400 ml/min for 3 h, twice weekly. In this study, a high sodium (145 mEq/l) acetate bath was used as the buffer.

To summarize, one can quote Keshaviah and co-workers (59) who state that significant reductions in treatment time are possible using high blood flows, higher efficiency dialyzers, ultrafiltration control systems and bicarbonate as a buffer source – but adequacy of dialysis must be preserved. In addition, these high-efficiency therapies are technically complex and must be simplified if widespread usage is to follow.

Infrequent dialysis

In addition to experimentation with the number of hours per dialysis treatment, there have been trials of decreased numbers of treatments per week. Most centers dialyze patients three times per week. In a comparative study, we demonstrated that patients dialyzed three times per week, rather than the same number of hours twice a week, had higher hematocrits, lower pre-dialysis serum creatinine and urea concentrations, and a greater sense of well-being (75).

Dyck and co-workers (76) studied the effects of dialyzing a group of 11 patients once per week (8 h for men, 6 h for women) while maintaining them on a stringent diet. This was a crossover study and the same group of patients were dialyzed three times per week (8 h for men, 6 h for women) while on a more liberal diet. Only 5 of 11 patients completed the study, among the dropouts were three deaths, two transplants and one withdrawal. All patients disliked the restricted protein diet and noticed an increase in weakness and fatigue; but, between the two study periods there was no significant difference in cutaneous sensation, motor nerve conduction, or electromyograms. By contrast, Friedman and co-workers (77) were unsuccessful in an attempt to reduce dialysis frequency to once per week by giving patients intestinal sorbents (oxystarch and charcoal) although a severely restricted protein intake was not a part of the regimen.

Another interesting direction in seeking optimal dialysis was pursued first by Snyder and co-workers (78) and then by Manohar et al (79). They increased the frequency of dialysis to five 2 h treatments per week. A single needle system was used for access. A group of ten patients treated in this way for an average of 21 months had no significant difference from a control group of conventionally treated patients in terms of hematocrit, creatinine concentration and parathyroid hormone levels. Motor nerve conduction velocities remained normal. They also had no hospitalizations, access failures or other complications during the study period. By increasing the frequency of dialysis, it has been postulated that there is a reduction in the magnitude of the metabolic and physiologic changes produced during each period of dialysis (80).

Caution must be used in evaluating these studies because different types and sizes of dialyzers were used. Strict crossover studies were not followed nor was residual renal function clearly compared in various groups. At the moment, we feel that any attempt to reduce the frequency of dialysis to less than three times per week in the absence of significant residual renal function is fraught with danger. The number of hours per treatment will be based on the dialyzer selected, patient size, blood flow and residual renal function. For a patient with a creatinine clearance less than 1.0 ml/min, each treatment should last 4 h unless special equipment and membranes are used.

THE PORTABLE SUITCASE KIDNEY

One way of making dialysis schedules less onerous is to facilitate travel. Our increasing experience with the use of the portable suitcase kidney, shows that our early enthusiasm was warranted (81). This easily carried machine, which requires only a tap water source and standard electric current, has been used on approximately 100 vacations and trips by patients from our center. Australia-antigen (HBsAg) positive patients may travel freely. The use of the suitcase kidney is, of course, limited to those patients trained in self-dialysis.

ROUTINE MONITORING OF MEDICAL PROBLEMS

Table 1. Routine tests.

At initiation of dialysis and at annual physical examination.
1. Bloods:
   Serum electrolytes, urea nitrogen (BUN), glucose, creatinine, Mg, lipids, Ca, PO_4, parathyroid hormone, ferritin, uric acid, complete blood count (CBC), liver function tests, serologic tests for hepatitis, syphilis
2. Electrocardiogram, ? Echocardiogram
3. X-rays:
   Chest and hand films.
4. Miscellaneous:
   Tine test for tuberculosis, stool guaiac.

Monthly Bloods
   Pre- and postdialysis BUN, serum creatinine, electrolytes, glucose.
Predialysis sample, liver profile, Ca, PO_4, hepatitis screen hematocrit

---

Note: Other testing, of course, should be done as clinically indicated.

Detailed discussions of the common medical problems of dialysis patients are covered in other sections of this book.

We would like, however, to include a 'worksheet' tabular approach that serves as a general guide to dealing with some of these problems. In addition, we will give our schedule for laboratory and other testing of chronic dialysis patients.

Anemia (82)

Table 2. Evaluation and treatment plan for anemia in dialysis patients.

I. *Diagnostic tests*
   a) Hematocrit, hemoglobin, leukocyte count, hemoglobin electrophoresis, serum folate, vitamin B_{12} and histidine levels
   b) Serum zinc, nickel and manganese levels, serum iron, iron binding capacity, ferritin level. If low:
      1. Check stool for guaiac positive material
      2. Check frequency of blood tests
      3. Check amount of blood left in dialyzer
   c) Red blood cell indices
      If evidence of hemolysis, eliminate possible causes such as copper, nitrate or chloramine toxicity, improperly mixed dialysate or drugs and hypophosphatemia
   d) Bone marrow

II. *Treatment*
   a) If serum folate low, give folic acid 1 mg/day
   b) If vitamin B_{12} low, give vitamin B_{12}, 1000 mg
   c) If histidine low, give histidine 10 mg/day
   d) If iron low:
      1. Ferrous sulfate 600 mg at bedtime without phosphate binders (84)
      2. If no response in 2 months then intravenous or intramuscular Imferon 2 ml once per week for 4 weeks, then once every 2 weeks for 2 months and finally once per month
   e) If anemia persists prescribe androgens Nandrolone decanoate 3 mg/kg (85) or testosterone enanthate 4 mg/kg once per week until a response is elicited, and then 200 mg per month thereafter
   f) Daily moderate exercise (86)
   g) If hyperparathyroidism found consider parathyroidectomy (87)
   h) Transfuse only:
      1. If the patient is symptomatic from anemia
      2. In the elderly or patients with atherosclerotic heart disease and hematocrit of less than 25%
      3. If the hematocrit is less than 15% for one month
   i) Erthyropoietin

The anemia of renal disease may soon be a non-existent problem because of the availability of erthyropoietin. Eschbach et al (83) have demonstrated a rise in the hematocrit and depletion of high serum ferritin levels in 18 of 25 patients treated with this medication. While the appropriate dose and administration of this drug is being worked out we must not forget other causes of anemia in dialysis patients. These causes include decreased red cell survival, blood loss (from mucosal irritation and iatrogenic blood testing) and increased hemolysis. Effective hemodialysis alone will improve the hematocrit in some patients.

Renal osteodystrophy (88)

Table 3. Evaluation and management of renal osteodystrophy.

I. *Initial Evaluation*
1. *Biochemical*
   a) Calcium
      If high: search for other explanations including multiple myeloma, solid tumor, vitamin D toxicity, sarcoid, immobilization
      If low: check serum albumin concentration, adjust dialysate Ca level (at least 3 mEq/l [1.5 mmol/l]), 1,25 dihydroxycholicalciferol 0.25 to 1.5 μg day (89), Ca supplements (90)
   b) Phosphorus
      If high: phosphorus binders i.e., amphogel with meals (91) (may lead to osteomalacia see below), low phosphate diet, calcium carbonate (92), 1 to 3 g with each meal (observe carefully for hypercalcemia [93]), magnesium salts (94)
      If low: diminish amount phosphorus binders
   c) Alkaline phosphatase
      If high: fractionate alkaline phosphatase to eliminate liver function abnormalities.
   d) Serum parathormone level
      if normal or slightly high consider bone biopsy.
2. *X-Rays*
   Metabolic bone survey, hand films best (95), skull, pelvis, hands, long bones, chest.
3. Bone biopsy and labelling with tetracycline (96).

II. *Management*
1. Control phosphate (pre-dialysis 4 to 6 mg) as above
2. Use dialysis fluid with calcium of 3 to 4 mEq/l
3. 1,25 vitamin D 0.25 to 1.5 μg/day (97) or 1 alpha vitamin D (98)
4. Calcium supplements
5. If parathyroid hormone remains high, intravenous administration of 1,25 dihydroxycholecalciferol (99)
6. Parathyroidectomy with re-implant of gland in forearm
7. If aluminum bone toxicity present, deferoxamine infusion 1.5 g 1 to 2 times/week at end of dialysis (100) (See Figure 1).

Renal osteodystrophy continues to be a major complication of uremia and may become more apparent and severe as hemodialysis prolongs life. In addition, the long standing practice of prescribing aluminum containing phosphorus binders may lead to aluminum accumulation in bone and another severe bone disease (usually osteomalacia). Nonetheless, with our current understanding of vitamin D metabolism and parathyroid hormone regulation it is now possible to control and treat bone disease in many patients.

Hypertension

More than 80% of patients starting hemodialysis have hypertension (101). The major etiological factor is salt and

Table 4. Characterization and treatment of hypertension in renal failure.

I. *Mild* (70% patients)
   a) *Definition*
      1. Predialysis diastolic blood pressure 100 mm Hg or less
      2. Controllable by volume removal during dialysis
      3. Plasma renin activity (PRA) usually normal
   b) *Treatment*
      1. Ultrafiltration
      2. Dietary salt and fluid control

II. *Moderate* (20%)
   a) *Definition*
      1. Predialysis diastolic blood pressure of 110 to 120 mm Hg
      2. Blood pressure easily controlled with medication
      3. PRA higher than Group I, but usually normal
   b) *Treatment*
      1. Dietary salt and fluid control
      2. Ultrafiltration during dialysis
      3. Medications (first try drugs on non-dialysis days and then every day if needed)
      4. Clonidine hydrochloride to 2.4 mg daily (central acting may cause drowsiness [104])
      5. Prazosin, no dose adjustment needed
      6. Beta adrenergic blocking drugs (103)
      7. Calcium channel blockers e.g., nifedepine 10–20 mg orally (105) or sublinguil nifedepine (106)

III. *Severe high blood pressure* (10%)
   a) *Definition*
      1. Diastolic blood pressure of 120 to 140 mm Hg or more (may be associated with visual problems, cachexia and ascites)
      2. PRA usually high
      3. Dopamine β-hydroxylase (DBH) may be high
      4. Failure of above drug regimens to control blood pressure
   b) *Treatment*
      1. Ultrafiltration
      2. Salt and fluid dietary control
      3. Minoxidil 2.5 mg orally daily (to total of 40 mg daily) (107) (may have to add diuretic)
      4. Captopril 100 mg bid (108) (check K$^+$ carefully) (109)
      5. Hemofiltration (particularly if DBH level exceeds 50 IU (110) or if blood pressure not controlled, or side effects intolerable)
      6. Bilateral nephrectomy (rarely if ever needed since introduction of minoxidil and captopril)

water retention leading to an increased extra-cellular volume. Thus adequate salt and water removal will control blood pressure in 70 to 75% of the patients. Other factors implicated in causing hypertension in this patient group are the renin-angiotension system, the sympathetic nervous system, and prostaglandins (102). Plasma renin is inappropriately elevated in about 25 to 30% of patients with end stage renal disease (103).

Many drugs are available to treat these patients and a

'step-care' approach is preferable. The aim should be to maintain blood pressure at below 150/90 mm/Hg.

Heart disease

Table 5. Evaluation and treatment of heart disease.

A. *Pericarditis* (111)
  I. *Evaluation*
      a) History and physical examination (chest pain, friction rub, fever, etc)
          1. For signs of cardiac tamponade do immediate pericardiocentesis
      b) Electrocardiogram (EKG): ST-segment elevation, electrical alterans, low voltage
      c) X-ray: Rapid change in heart size and shape with normal lungs
      d) Echocardiogram
      e) Bacterial, viral, fungal studies
  II. *Treatment*
      a) Daily dialysis (111) with regional or 'tight' heparinization. If no response in 2 weeks,
      b) Indomethacin 50 mg orally four times a day (112). If no response in one week,
      c) Pericardiocentesis with or without intrapericardial steroid instillation, triamcinolone hexacetonide (113)
      d) Pericardectomy (114)

B. *Congestive heart failure*
  I. *Evaluation*
      a) History and physical examination (blood pressure, shortness of breath, rales, gallop)
      b) EKG, chest x-ray
      c) Echocardiogram
      d) Check serum triglycerides, lipoproteins and cholesterol
  II. *Treatment*
      a) If fluid overload: improve ultrafiltration, restrict dietary salt, control hypertension and look for vascular or myocardial calcification from hyperparathyroidism
      b) If cardiac output high: improve anemia (115), measure blood flow through arteriovenous fistula. If 20 percent or more of cardiac output goes through the fistula, occlude temporarily. If there is improvement, surgically decrease size of fistula (116), and enalapril (2.5 to 40 mg daily (117)
      c) If cardiac output low: intensive dialysis (118), digoxin – normal digitalizing dose, $1/2$ to $1/3$ maintenance dose (check serum levels frequently), use dialysis solution with 3 mEq K^+/l, enalapril and consider CAPD
      d) For cardiac arrhythymia: holter monitor during dialysis (119), check potassium and quinidine 400 mg orally before dialysis (120)

C. *Bacterial endocarditis* (121)
  I. *Evaluation*
      a) History and physical examination, history of drug abuse
      b) Blood cultures (minimum of six)
      c) Examine access site for infection
  II. *Treatment*
      a) Appropriate antibiotics (4 to 6 weeks)
      b) Remove infected angioaccess
      c) If necessary, valve replacement (open heart surgery)

As the dialysis population has become less selected and older, the incidence of heart disease has increased. Cardiovascular disease is the major cause of death of dialysis patients. We include an evaluation and treatment plan for some of the more common types of cardiac problems encountered.

REGULAR HEMODIALYSIS TREATMENT FOR HIGH RISK PATIENTS

With increasing dialysis facilities and experience, regular dialysis treatment has been extended to groups of patients who in previous years were excluded. Reported below are some guidelines to follow in dialyzing high risk or unusual patients.

Diabetes mellitus

Diabetes mellitus accounts for approximately one quarter of all new cases of end stage renal disease in the United States (122). At our institution and others, transplantation is thought to be the treatment of choice: unfortunately, many diabetic patients are not suitable candidates for this therapy because of age or associated medical problems. Thus, the great majority of uremic diabetic patients are treated by hemodialysis.

Early survival of diabetics on hemodialysis was dismal (123), but is improving. Legrain et al (124) reported a 4 year dialysis survival of insulin dependent diabetic patients of 55%. Similarly, Whitley and Shapiro (125) found a three year survival of diabetic patients on dialysis of 55%.

The problems associated with delivering dialyses to these patients have been nicely reviewed by Kjellstrand and colleagues (126). Vascular access should be placed early (serum creatinine level 4 to 5 mg/dl [354 to 442 μmol/l]) in diabetic patients and renal replacement therapy initiated when the creatinine reaches 8 or 9 mg/dl (708 or 796 μmol/l). The patients' veins may have been previously damaged from intravenous lines and thus a bovine or PTFE graft may have to be created.

The actual performance of hemodialysis is usually far from routine. Diabetic patients have 20% more instances of hypotension and 50% more problems with hypertension than non-diabetic patients (126). The high prevalence of autonomic neuropathy makes it difficult for their cardiovascular system to compensate for dialysis induced volume changes.

Diabetic patients have more gastroparesis and more nausea and vomiting than their euglycemic counterparts. This and other factors lead to a high degree of malnutrition. A high protein intake (1.5 g/kg) should be encouraged. Some glucose should be included in the dialysis solution, lest glucose removal, glucogenesis and malnutrition result (127). Insulin requirements change with the initiation of hemodialysis and frequently increase. Careful blood glucose monitoring, particularly in the early stage of hemodialysis is important.

The deterioration of vision in diabetic patients on hemodialysis previously was abysmal, leading to a 35% yearly loss of vision due to progression of retinopathy or occular hemorrhage (128). The possible role of heparin in this was the basis for some authors to recommended peritoneal dialysis for these patients. However, a recent comparison of hemodialysis and peritoneal dialysis in 112 diabetic patients found that in both groups of patients better blood pressure control was associated with stabilization of eyesight, and no significant changes in vision could be attributed to the dialysis modality or systemic heparinization (129). Amputation of digits and extremities remains a major problem for diabetic patients; diabetes accounts for 50 to 70% of all non-traumatic amputations (125). However, once a patient starts hemodialysis, the incidence of amputation is less. This may be due to decreased capillary endothelial aggregation of platelets in uremia (130).

Vascular disease remains the most common cause of demise in diabetics on hemodialysis. It accounts for 75% of the deaths in the first 18 months. Sepsis and withdrawal from dialysis are also important later causes (124).

The elderly

Older patients, frequently excluded from early dialysis programs, may now enter with ease, at least in the United States. According to Medicare data for 1985, a startling 67% of the patients on dialysis were 50 years of age or older (131). In some other countries, advanced age continues to be a barrier to receipt of treatment (132).

Rotellar and co-workers (133) studied 26 patients who began hemodialysis at ages 65 to 85 (mean 74 years) and compared them to an equal number of patients who began dialysis at a mean age of 45 (range 40 to 55). While more of the elderly died during the first year of treatment, their mortality was similar to an equivalently aged, non-dialysis population. When compared to the younger patients, there was no difference in vascular access survival or hematocrit, although the older group had more frequent episodes of hypotension and did not tolerate overhydration as well. Similarly, Taube, et al (134) found a 5 year survival of 61.5% in 64 patients beginning dialysis at ages 55 to 72. In addition only 12.5% of that group were greatly disabled. Rathaus and Beinheim (135) also found that elderly patients did as well as younger ones. Conversely, Chester and co-workers (136), found twice as many medical problems, (more gastrointestinal bleeding, a higher transfusion requirement and more heart disease) in an older dialysis population. Of interest is the fact that older patients may be more compliant with their diet.

When dialyzing the elderly, it is advisable to maintain the hematocrit above 25% to minimize myocardial anoxia. Patients on digoxin will require a higher potassium concentration in the bath and their vascular access must be carefully observed to make sure that it is not an excessive strain on cardiac output.

In addition, a bicarbonate bath may be advisable if the older patient is found to be 'acetate intolerant'.

Atherosclerotic heart disease

Patients with severe atherosclerotic heart disease (ASHD) may present difficult problems for the hemodialyzer: the majority of deaths in chronic hemodialysis programs are attributed to cardiovascular disease (120). Although Lundin et al (137) have reported that patients without significant risk factors or underlying heart disease have a low probability of developing subsequent atherosclerotic complications, Rostand (138) reported that those patients with ischemic heart disease prior to the onset of hemodialysis had a poor prognosis. He also notes that only 39 of 320 patients without evidence of prior heart disease developed it during a 7 year follow-up period, and these patients were older, had a higher blood pressure and higher triglyceride levels.

In patients who have congestive failure, hemodialysis may improve cardiac function by preload and after-load reduction (117). The anemia of uremia, hypertension, fluid overload and vascular access may all aggravate ASHD.

Delano and co-workers (115) have shown that correction of anemia can result in normalization of cardiac output in dialysis patients. Therefore, in dialyzing patients with atherosclerotic heart disease, we recommend maintaining the hematocrit above 25%.

Patients taking digoxin, when studied by Holter monitoring, have a high rate (39%) of serious arrhythmias during dialysis (119). Such patients should be dialyzed against a bath containing 3.0 to 3.5 mEq/l of K$^+$ and should receive quinidine sulfate 400 mg orally 45 min prior to dialysis (139).

Many patients develop angina during dialysis. If this cannot be easily controlled with drug therapy, one should consider transferring the patients to peritoneal dialysis.

Cardiac surgery in dialysis patients

Cardiac disease continues to be a major cause of death in long term dialysis patients. So it is not surprising that the numbers of dialysis patients undergoing coronary artery bypass (CABP) and other cardiac surgery is rapidly increasing.

Marshall and co-workers (140) performed bypass surgery on 12 long-term dialysis patients. They found only a slight increase in morbidity and mortality compared to non uremic patients. Among the techniques used to optimize survival were the following: They transfused the patients to keep the hematocrit between 20 and 25%. The mean arterial pressure (MAP) was kept at 60 to 90 mm Hg postoperatively. They used radial artery systemic pressure and Swan Ganz monitoring. Dialysis was performed on the day prior to and 2 days after surgery.

Pavie et al (141) also described their operative technique in 20 dialysis patients undergoing cardiac surgery. Twelve patients had valvular heart surgery and eight had CABP. All patients were operated on immediately following a session of dialysis. During anesthesia and cardiopulmonary bypass every effort was made to preserve the peripheral arterial and venous vessels for eventual arteriovenous fistulae. This was done by using the jugular vein and dorsalis pedis arteries for monitoring. Arterial blood pressure was maintained above 60 mm Hg and large doses of heparin were used to protect the arteriovenous shunts.

Zawada, Stinson and Done (142) performed concurrent hemodialysis during bypass in one patient. The need for postoperative dialysis was thus delayed for 72 h. Laws and co-workers (143) also successfully performed cardiac surgery on ten long term hemodialysis patients. Their management of these patients includes the following:

1. The patients had a dialysis immediately before and after the diagnostic catheterization and cineangiogram. A limited amount of dye was used.
2. Hemodialysis was performed at some time during the 24 h prior to surgery.
3. The patients were transfused to a hematocrit of 25% and careful attention was paid to control of serum potassium levels.
4. Intravenous fluids were kept to a minimum during surgery.
5. The patients' fistulas were protected by padding; blood pressures and venipunctures were not done in the access arm.
6. The timing of the post operative hemodialyses depended on the patients' status.

In three patients, intra-operative peritoneal dialysis was started and maintained for one week postoperatively. This greatly simplified fluid and potassium management.

In summary, cardiac surgery is now possible for the chronic dialysis patient, as long as careful attention is paid to the fluid and electrolyte status and care is taken to protect the vascular access.

Sickle cell anemia

Renal failure, though uncommon in patients with sickle cell anemia, occasionally leads to the necessity for dialysis and transplantation (144, 145).

Gonzalez-Carrillo and co-workers (146) maintained a patient with sickle cell anemia by dialysis for 10 months prior to transplantation. Among the strategies they used for a successful, comfortable treatment was the use of frequent blood transfusions to maintain the sickle hemoglobin level at less than 20%. They also gave the patient 40% oxygen by face mask throughout dialysis to keep his PO_2 at 95 to 125 mm Hg, since hypoxia is a known stimulus to crises. Szwed, Yum and Hogan (147) reported on a fascinating patient: This 25 year old man required a unit of blood approximately every 5 weeks before beginning hemodialysis. After 8 months of dialysis his transfusion requirements increased to the point where one unit/week was needed to maintain a hematocrit of 16%. At that time a palpable spleen was first detected. The patient underwent splenectomy and has done well for 4 years requiring only one unit of blood every 3 to 4 months. Thus a careful search for hypersplenism, although unlikely, should be done in patients with sickle cell disease on dialysis.

Our own experience in dialyzing six such patients, re-

vealed high blood requirements (1.5 to 2.0 units/month) (148). All our patients had limited cardiac reserve and one had a thrombotic intracranial stroke.

In an interesting related topic, non-uremic sickle cell disease patients have undergone extracorporeal carbamylation with cyanate in an attempt to prevent sickling, using an arteriovenous fistula (149).

Systemic lupus erythematosus

Although early reports of dialysis in patients with lupus erythrematosus were discouraging (150), more recent experience has suggested that such patients may do quite well. Because many of the early deaths in uremic lupus patients were infectious complications of steroids one approach suggested by Coplon et al (151) is 'early dialysis' accompanied by marked steroid reduction to control only the extrarenal manifestations. The return of sufficient renal function to permit the patient a rather prolonged dialysis free interval, though rare, is possible.

Kimberly and coworkers (27) have maintained 39 patients on dialysis for periods ranging from 4 months to 9 years. The majority of their patients, 24, were serologically or clinically quiescent despite the withdrawal of immunosuppressive therapy.

Coplon and coworkers subsequent series (152) of dialysis in 28 patients only found three with mildly active extra-renal lupus. Pahl et al (153, 154), followed 12 patients for an average of 31 months (range 6 to 72), and also found that with the onset of dialysis there was partial improvement in extra-renal manifestations seen in all but two patients. Their series only included one early death, a cardiopulmonary arrest within one week of beginning dialysis, and one unrelated late death.

Although we also had a poor early experience with lupus patients on dialysis (155), our more recent patients do as well as the other patients in the same age range. One woman in her 4th year of dialysis has bilateral aseptic necrosis of the hips from prior steroid therapy.

Heroin addicts and AIDS patients

Renal failure due to heroin abuse is common in certain urban centers. At one of our hospitals, Kings County, approximately 20% of the 470 new patients who started hemodialysis during the past 5 years were intravenous drug abusers (156).

The associated medical problems we have most often seen are: difficulty in establishing vascular access because the patients' veins have been destroyed previously by self-administered drugs, Staphyloccocal sepsis and bacterial endocarditis. Disruptive behavior in the dialysis unit and frequent absence from treatment are also common.

Eighteen of our drug addict patients have developed the acquired immune deficiency syndrome (AIDS) (157). Our experience in dialyzing them, as well as 31 other patients with AIDS who developed end stage renal failure, is that only two patients survived more than 6 months, and none lived longer than 9 months. Most patients died of severe cachexia and or infection.

Originally, the dialyses on AIDS patients was performed with strict isolation techniques. We used separate machines, the staff was gowned, gloved, masked and wore goggles. More recently the CDC guidelines (158) for dialysis of AIDS patients have been adopted by our unit. These are basically the same guidelines for dialysis of hepatitis antigen positive patients.

However, extreme caution in the canulation of AIDS patients, the handling of their blood, and disposal of needles used on them must be observed. At the present time it is not known if any dialysis patient who is not in a 'high risk group' has developed HIV infection.

Multiple myeloma

Renal insufficiency occurs in 55% of patients with myeloma, and is usually associated with a poor prognosis. Some success has been reported in dialyzing myeloma patients and occasionally renal function improves sufficiently to stop treatment after prolonged periods of dialysis (159).

Johnson et al (160) reported 11 patients who survived from 2 to 64 months although only two patients lived longer than one year. More recently, Cosio and coworkers (161) reported on 34 patients who required dialysis because of myeloma. They had a 53% one-year survival. In four of their cases, dialysis was discontinued because of intractable bone pain.

Lazarus et al (162) studied eight patients with myeloma and renal failure who required dialysis. All patients had at least one severe infection and all were markedly anemic. Of interest is the fact that there were three long term survivals and one as long as 7 years. No mention was made of any technical problems during the dialyses. On the other hand, Coward, Mallick and Delmore (163) had bad experiences with three myeloma patients who required 'long term' dialysis: In one patient, dialysis was discontinued at 2 months because of extensive amyloid polyneuropathy and in another at 3 months because of 'severe technical problems'. The third patient died of a myocardial infarction at 2 months. In our experience with myeloma patients, no special problems in the delivery of dialysis therapy was noted.

Randall and coworkers (164) dialyzing two patients with light chain disease found that these patients deposited the light chains in their heart, liver and other organs. They suggest that in such patients, peritoneal dialysis may be the procedure of choice. They believe that the light chains were deposited in the organs because they were not removed by hemodialysis, whereas light chains may traverse the peritoneal membrane.

Scleroderma

The renin angiotension system probably plays an important role in the severe hypertension and rapid renal deterioration seen in scleroderma. The oral angiotension converting enzyme inhibitor, captopril, has therefore been used in these patients. Waeber et al (165) obtained good blood pressure control in three hypertensive patients with scleroderma. Despite this, renal function deteriorated and hemodialysis was started. There was also no substantial improvement in the skin lesions in contradistinction to earlier reports (166). The three patients all died of respiratory failure within one month of starting treatment.

On the other hand, Zawada et al (167) was able to avoid hemodialysis in three of four patients treated with captopril. Most patients with this disease have associated cardiac, pulmonary and vascular problems that limit survival on dialysis, although Simon, et al (168) collected 40 patients with scleroderma, 13 of whom survived for periods of up to 3 years. Difficulty in maintaining a patent vascular access is frequently reported (169, 170). The use of warfarin was able to restore sufficient renal function to discontinue hemodialysis in two reported cases (171).

Amyloidosis

Ari et al (172) found very few differences in dialyzing ten patients with amyloidosis compared to ten control patients. Average shunt life, serum albumin concentration and hematocrit were the same in both groups, and they reported no difficulty in the hemodialysis procedure.

In addition, amelioration of the symptoms of familial Mediterranean fever in those patients with amyloidosis has been reported during dialysis (173). Both Shapiro et al (174), and Avram and co-workers (175) reported difficulties in hemodialyzing patients with amyloidosis and nephrotic syndrome, including edema that was resistant to removal because of hypoalbuminemia, hypovolemia leading to early clotting of arteriovenous fistulae and frequent episodes of hypotension during dialysis. Both groups infused large amounts of albumin (150 g/week to 600 g/2 weeks) without benefit. Only bilateral surgical nephrectomy (174) or 'medical nephrectomy' (destruction of residual renal function by nephrotoxic metallic salts (175) permitted the serum albumin to rise to a level where dialysis was no longer a problem.

Suzuki et al (176), were able to maintain a patient with amyloidosis on hemodialysis for 5 years, despite frequent clotting of the vascular access. Stone and co-workers (177) believe that patients with amyloidosis are not desirable candidates for hemodialysis for the following reasons. Hearts with amyloid involvement may be unable to tolerate hemodynamic stresses and the hemodialysis membranes are impermeable to the amyloid fibril precursors, the immunoglobulin light chains. They suggest that peritoneal dialysis is preferable to hemodialysis in these patients because the paraprotein may be removed by this route.

Of concern, are the reports of amyloid deposits developing in long term dialysis patients. This may present as carpal tunnel syndrome (178), synovial (179) and bone deposits (180).

Pregnancy

In pregnant women who develop acute renal failure, dialysis may successfully maintain the fetus until delivery (181, 182). In addition, the occurrence of ovulation in some patients with chronic renal failure (183) makes pregnancy possible in this group of women as well. The need for birth control in sexually active young women must, therefore, be considered. While most chronic dialysis patients who do become pregnant usually abort, either spontaneously or therapeutically, 18 such patients have had successful births (184).

If a woman on dialysis becomes pregnant, certain manipulations will increase her chances of having a healthy infant. The frequency and total hours of dialysis should be increased in an attempt to keep the BUN less than 70 to 84 mg/dl (25 to 30 mmol/l) (185). The increased frequency of dialysis will also permit a high protein (greater than 80 g), calcium rich diet.

The blood pressure should be rigorously controlled, and hypotension with its attendent placental ischemia avoided. A hematocrit of approximately 30% should be maintained, and 'tight', or regional heparinization is desirable.

The onset of labor has averaged 34 weeks, and the birth weight of the infants is low (186).

Liver disease

In patients who have liver disease, particularly with ascites, hemodialysis can be difficult.

Ellis and Avner (187) were able to achieve effective dialysis in only four of 13 patients in a series of 133 children who developed renal failure in the perioperative period of liver transplantation. The remaining dialyses were marked by moderate to severe hypotension requiring large volumes of 25% salt poor albumin, mannitol or saline. In addition, two patients died of severe hemorrhage while receiving low dose heparin. Similar problems were seen in an adult series of 84 dialysis patients with liver disease (188).

To optimize hemodialysis one should use bicarbonate as the buffer because it does not require hepatic metabolism, and is associated with less of a fall in blood pressure. The use of a parallel plate dialyzer will minimize the heparin required. Blood, salt poor albumin and fresh frozen plasma may be used liberally, but vasopressors may still be required to maintain blood pressure.

Dialysis related ascites is an entity that develops in some patients once they are on hemodialysis. In some cases this is associated with severe hypertension and cachexia (189). Etiologies are varied, and include previous peritoneal dialysis, cirrhosis, tuberculosis, overhydration, infections, peritonitis, hemosiderosis, hepatitis, Hodgkins disease, portal hypertension (due to polycystic liver) and nephrotic syndrome (190, 191).

Dialysis ascites can occasionally be controlled by peritoneo-venous shunting (192, 193) or water immersion (194).

REFERENCES

1. Bonomini V: On optimal dialysis. *Kidney Int* 7 (Suppl 3): S365, 1975
2. Bonomini V, Albertazzi A, Vangelista A, Botorotti GC, Stefoni S, Scolari MP: Residual renal function and effective rehabilitation in chronic dialysis. *Nephron* 16: 89, 1976
3. Bonomini V: Long term early dialysis. *3rd Int Conf Uremia Capri* (Abstracts) 7, 1980
4. Scribner BH: A critical comment. *Nephron* 16: 100, 1976
5. Bonomini V: Early dialysis up-dated. *In J Artif Organs* 4: 54, 1981
6. Bonomini V, Baldrati L, Stefoni S: Comparative cost/benefit analysis in early and late dialysis. *Nephron* 33: 1, 1983
7. Ratcliffe PJ, Phillips RE, Oliver DV: Late referral for maintenance dialysis. *Br Med J* 288: 441, 1983
8. Maher JF: When should maintenance dialysis be initiated? *Nephron* 16: 83, 1976
9. Brescia MJ, Cimino JE, Appel K, Hurwich BJ: Chronic hemodialysis using venipuncture and a surgically created arteriovenous fistula. *N Eng J Med* 275: 1089, 1966
10. Butt KMH, Rao TKS, Maki T, Mashimo S, Manis T, Delano BG, Kountz SL, Friedman EA: Bovine heterograft as a preferential hemodialysis access. *Trans Am Soc Artif Intern Organs* 20: 339, 1974
11. Bergrem H, Flatmark A, Simonsen S: Dialysis fistulas and cardiac failure. *Acta Med Scand* 204: 191, 1978
12. Ahearn DJ, Maher JF: Heart failure as a complication of hemodialysis arteriovenous fistula. *Ann Intern Med* 77: 201, 1972
13. Maher JF, Ahern DJ, Bryan CW, Nolph KD: Prognosis of chronic renal failure. III. Survival after one peritoneal dialysis. *Nephron* 15: 8, 1975
14. Davis D, Peterson J, Feldman R, Cho C, Stevick CA: Subclavian venous stenosis. A complication of subclavian dialysis. *JAMA* 252: 3404, 1984
15. Tapson JS, Hoenich NA, Ward MK, Wilkinson R: Evaluation of the Shiley dual lumen subclavian hemodialysis catheter. *Trans Am Soc Artif Intern Organs* 16: 140, 1985
16. Cheung AK, Gregory MC: Subclavian vein thrombosis in hemodialysis patients. *Trans Am Soc Artif Intern Organs* 16: 131, 1985
17. Arana VA: Percutaneous femoral vein catheterization in patients requiring hemodialysis. *J Urol* 106: 492, 1971
18. Shaldon S, Silva H, Pomeroy J, Rao AI, Rosen SM: Percutaneous femoral venous catheterization and reusable dialyzer in the treatment of acute renal failure. *Trans Am Soc Artif Intern Organs* 10: 133, 1964
19. Pascua LJ: Vascular access update. *Trans Am Soc Artif Intern Organs* 25: 526, 1979
20. Kjellstrand CM, Merino GE, Mauer SM, Casal R, Buselmeier TJ: Complications of percutaneous femoral vein catheterization for hemodialysis. *Clin Nephrol* 4: 37, 1975
21. Neu S, Kjellstrand CM: Stopping long term dialysis. An empirical study of withdrawal of life supporting treatment. *N Eng J Med* 314: 14, 1986
22. Kjellstrand CM, Dolan JM, Rachels J, Epstein FH: Is one allowed to stop artificial organs, allowing patients to die? *Trans Am Soc Artif Intern Organs* 32: 671, 1986
23. Bacon BR, Ricanati ES: Severe and prolonged renal insufficiency. Reversal in a patient with malignant hypertension. *JAMA* 239: 1159, 1978
24. Mitchell HC, Graham RM, Pettinger WA: Renal function during long term treatment of hypertension with minoxidil. *Ann Intern Med* 93: 676, 1980

25. Maxey RW, Rao TKS, Manis T, Delano BG, Friedman EA: Return of renal function after commencing maintenance hemodialysis. *Proc Clin Dial Transplant Forum* 5: 12, 1975

26. Kohorst WR, Bay WH: Reversal of end stage kidney failure in two scleroderma patients treated with anticoagulants. *Am J Kidney Dis* 2: 347, 1982

27. Kimberly RP, Lockshin MD, Sherman RL, Beary JR, Mowiadian J, Cheich J: End stage lupus nephritis clinical course to and outcome on dialysis. *Medicine* 60: 277, 1981

28. Barton CH, Vaziri ND: Dialysis and transplantation in multiple myeloma. *Int J Artif Organs* 7: 317, 1984

29. Lundquist F, Tygstrup N, Winkler KI: Ethanol metabolism and free acetate in the human liver. *J Clin Invest* 41: 955, 1962

30. Lundquist F: Production and utilization of free acetate in man. *Nature* 193: 579, 1962

31. Lewis EJ, Tolchin N, Roberts JL: High mass transfer hemodialysis and acetate metabolism. *Proc Ren Physicians Assoc* 1: 10, 1977

32. Graefe U, Milutanovic J, Follete WE: Less dialysis morbidity and vascular irritability with bicarbonate in dialysate. *Ann Intern Med* 88: 331, 1978

33. Aizaiva Y, Ohmoii T, Imai K: Depressant action of acetate upon the human cardiovascular system. *Clin Nephrol* 8: 477, 1977

34. Iseki K, Onoyama K, Maeda T: Comparison of hemodynamics induced by conventional acetate hemodialysis, bicarbonate hemodialysis and hemofiltration. *Clin Nephrol* 14: 294, 1980

35. Van Stone JC: The effect of bicarbonate in stable chronic hemodialysis patients. *Dial Transplant* 8: 703, 1979

36. Scribner BH: Indication for bicarbonate – containing dialysate in the care of the critically ill patient. *Proc Ren Physicians Assoc* 1: 25, 1977

37. Brezin JH, Schwartz AB, Chinitz JL: Switch from acetate to bicarbonate dialysis. Better dialysis tolerance but failure to improve acidosis and hypertriglyceridemia. *Trans Am Soc Artif Intern Organs* 31: 343, 1985

38. Vinay P, Prudhomme J, Vinet B, Cournoyer G, DeGoulet P, Levillem, Gougoux A, St Louis G, Lapierre L, Piette Y: Acetate metabolism and bicarbonate generation during hemodialysis; 10 years of observation. *Kidney Int* 31: 1194, 1987

39. Arieff A: Neurological manifestations of uremia. in *The Kidney*, edited by Brenner BM, Rector FC Jr, Philadelphia, WB Saunders, Co 1986, 1731

40. Kennedy AC, Linton AL, Eaton JC: Urea levels in cerebrospinal fluid after haemodialysis. *Lancet* 1: 410, 1962

41. Rosen SM, O'Connor K, Shaldon S: Haemodialysis disequilibrium. *Br Med J* 2: 672, 1964

42. Hampers CL, Doak PB, Callaghan MN, Tyler HR, Merrill JP: The electroencephalogram and spinal fluid during hemodialysis. I. *Arch Intern Med* 118: 340, 1966

43. Mahoney CA, Arieff AI: Central and peripheral nervous system effects of chronic renal failure. *Kidney Int* 24: 170, 1983

44. Arieff AI, Massry SG, Barrientos A, Kleeman CR: Brain, water, and electrolyte metabolism in uremia: Effects of slow and rapid hemodialysis. *Kidney Int* 4: 177, 1973

45. Riggs GA, Bereu BA: Hypoglycemia. A complication of hemodialysis. *N Eng J Med* 277: 1139, 1967

46. Wakim KG: Predominance of hyponatremia over hypoosmolality in simulation of the dialysis disequilibrium syndrome. *Mayo Clin Proc* 44: 433, 1969

47. Cowie J, Lambie AT, Robson JS: The influence of extracorporeal dialysis on the acid base composition of blood and cerebrospinal fluid. *Clin Sci* 23: 397, 1962

48. Arieff AI, Massry SG: Dialysis disequilibrium syndrome. in *Clinical Aspects of Uremia and Dialysis,* edited by Massry SG, Sellers AL, Springfield IL, CC Thomas, 1976, p 36

49. Arieff AI, Guisado R, Massry SG, Lazarowitz VC: Central nervous system pH in uremia and the effects of hemodialysis. *J Clin Invest* 58: 306, 1976

50. Bito LA, Myers RE: On the physiological response of the cerebral cortex to acute stress. *J Physiol (London)* 221: 349, 1972

51. Rodrigo F, Shideman J, McHuch R, Buselmeier T, Kjellstrand C: Osmolality changes during hemodialysis. *Ann Intern Med* 86: 554, 1977

52. Scribner BH: Less-dialysis-induced morbidity and vascular instability with bicarbonate dialysis. *Ann Intern Med* 88: 332, 1978

53. Rosen RA, Lazarowitz VC, Arieff AI: Dialysis disequilibrium syndrome prevention with glycerol. *Kidney Int* 14: 683, 1978

54. Blagg CR: Adequacy of dialysis. *Am J Kidney Dis* 4: 218, 1984

55. Teschan PE: Clinical estimates of treatment adequacy: *Artif Organs* 10: 201, 1986

56. Babb AL, Scribner BH: Quantitative description of dialysis treatment I: A dialysis Index. *Kidney Int* 7 (Suppl 2): S23, 1975

57. Ahmad S, Babb AL, Milutinovic J, Scribner BH: Effect of residual renal function on minimal dialysis requirements. *Proc Eur Dial Transplant Assoc* 16: 107, 1979

58. Gotch FA, Sargent JA, Peters JH: Studies on the molecular etiology of uremia. *Kidney Int* 7: (Suppl 2): S276, 1975

59. Keshaviah P, Collins A: Rapid high efficiency bicarbonate hemodialysis. *Trans Am Soc Artif Intern Organs* 32: 17, 1986

60. Farrell PC: Adequacy of dialysis: Marker molecules and kinetic modeling. *Artif Organs* 10: 195, 1986

61. Read DJ, Feest TG, Holman RH: Vibration sensory threshold: A guide to adequacy of dialysis. *Proc Eur Dial Transplant Assoc* 19: 253, 1983

62. Dyck PJ, Johnson WJ, Lambert EH, O'Brian PC, Daube JR, Oviatt KF: Comparison of symptoms, chemistries and nerve function to access adequacy of dialysis. *Neurology* 29: 1361, 1979

63. Kopple JD, Swendseid ME: Protein and amino acid metabolism in uremia patients undergoing maintenance hemodialysis. *Kidney Int* 7 (Suppl 2): S64, 1975

64. Desforges JR: A review of the effects of hemodialysis on the blood in uremia. *Kidney Int* 7 (Suppl 2): S123, 1975

65. Parker TF: Study of trans-membrane potential as an assessment of the adequacy of dialysis. *Proc 12th Annu Contractors Conf Artif Kidney Program, NIAMDD*, edited by Mackey BB, NIH Publ No 81–1979, 1981, p 226

66. Slatopolsky E: Recommendations for treatment of renal osteodystrophy in dialysis patient. *Kidney Int* 7 (Suppl 2): S253, 1975

67. Lazarus JM, Lowrie EG, Hampers CL, Merrill JP: Cardiovascular disease in uremic patients on hemodialysis. *Kidney Int* 7 (Suppl 2): S167, 1975

68. DelGreco F, Simon NM, Davies W: Hypertension in chronic renal failure. The role of sodium volume homeostasis and the renal pressor system. *Kidney Int* 7 (Suppl 2): S176, 1975

69. DePalma JR: Adequate hemodialysis schedule. *N Eng J Med* 285: 353, 1972

70. Colton CK, Lowrie EG: Hemodialysis: Physical principles and technical considerations. in *The Kidney* edited by Brenner BM, Rector FC, Philadelphia PA, WB Saunders Co, 1981, p 2425

71. Seidman MS, Lundin AP, Brown CD, Friedman EA, Berlyne GM: Extent of blood recirculation during two needle hemo-

dialysis . *Abstracts Am Soc Artif Intern Organs* 8: 56, 1979

72. Raja R, Kramer M, Goldstein S, Caruane R, Lerner A: Short hemodialysis – 10 year follow-up. *Trans Am Soc Artif Intern Organs* 32: 374, 1986

73. Rotellar E, Martinez E, Soniso JM, Barrios J, Simo R, Mulero JR, Perez D, Bandres S, Pinol J: Why dialyze more than 6 hours a week? *Proc Eur Dial Transplant Assoc* 22: 312, 1985

74. Rubin JE, Friedmann P, Berlyne GM: Rapid blood flow short dialysis does not adversely affect clinical, biochemical, or nutritional status of patients. *Trans Am Soc Artif Intern Organs* 32: 377, 1986

75. Delano BG, Goodwin NJ: Patient transfer from center to home hemodialysis. *Abstracts Am Soc Nephrol* 4: 19, 1970

76. Dyck PJ, Johnson WJ, Lambert EH, Nelson RA, O'Brien RC: Uremic neuropathy-controlled study of restricted protein and fluid diet and infrequent hemodialysis versus conventional hemodialysis treatment. *Mayo Clinic Proc* 50: 641, 1975

77. Friedman EA, Saltzman MJ, Delano BG, Frank WM, Hirsch SR, Beyer MM, Galonsky RS: Clinical efficacy of oxidized starch in uremia. *Proc 10th Annu Contractors' Conf Chronic Uremia Program of NIAMDD*, edited by Mackey BB, DHEW Publ no (NIH) 77–1442, 1977, p 112

78. Snyder D, Louis BM, Gorfien P, Mordujovich J: Clinical experience with long term brief 'daily' haemodialysis. *Proc Eur Dial Transplant Assoc* 11: 128, 1975

79. Manohar ND, Louis BM, Gorfien P, Lipner HI: Success of frequent short hemodialysis. *Trans Am Soc Artif Intern Organs* 27: 604, 1981

80. Kjellstrand CM, Evans RL, Peterson RJ, Shideman JR, Von Hartitzsch B, Buselmeier TJ: The 'unphysiology' of dialysis: A major cause of dialysis side effects? *Kidney Int* 7 (Suppl 2): S30, 1975

81. Briefel GR, Hutchisson JT, Galonsky RS, Hessert RL, Friedman EA: Compact travel hemodialysis system. *Proc Clin Dial Transplant Forum* 5: 61, 1975

82. Norris SH, Kurtzman NA: Minimizing anemia in the chronic hemodialysis patient. *Int J Artif Organs* 9: 199, 1986

83. Eschbach J, Egrie JC, Downing R, Browne JK, Adamson JW: Correction of the anemia of end stage renal disease with recombinant human erythropoietin: *N Eng J Med* 316: 73, 1987

84. Parker PA, Izard MW, Maher JF: Therapy of iron deficiency anemia in patients on maintenance hemodialysis. *Nephron* 23: 181, 1979

85. Neff MS, Goldberg J, Slifkin RF, Eiser AR: A comparison of androgens for anemia in patients on hemodialysis. *N Engl J Med* 304: 871, 1981

86. Goldberg AP, Hagberg JM, Delmez JA, Haynes ME: Metabolic effects of exercise training in hemodialysis patients. *Kidney Int* 18: 754, 1980

87. Barbour GL: Effect of parathyroidectomy on anemia in chronic renal failure. *Arch Intern Med* 139: 889, 1979

88. Sherrard DJ, Oh SM, Maloney NA, Andess D, Coburn JW: Uremic osteodystrophy. in *Proc Symp Clin Disorders Bone Mineral Metab*, edited by Frame B, Potts JT, Amsterdam, Excerpta Medica 1984, p 254

89. Kumar R: The metabolism and mechanism of action of 1,25 – dihydroxyivitamin D_3. *Kidney Int* 30: 793, 1986

90. Oettinger CW, Merrill R, Blanton T, Briggs W: Reduced calcium absorption after nephrectomy in uremic patients. *New Engl J Med* 291, 458, 1974

91. Delmez JA, Fallon MD, Harter HR, Hruska KA, Slatopolsky E, Teitelbaum SL: Does strict phosphorus control prevent osteomalacia? *J Clin Endocrinol Metab* 62: 747, 1986

92. Slatopolsky E, Weerts C, Lopez-Hilker S, Norwood K, Zink M, Wintus D, Delmez JA: Calcium carbonate as a phosphate binder in patients with chronic renal failure undergoing dialysis. *N Eng J Med* 315, 175, 1986

93. Stein HD, Yudis M, Sirota RA: Calcium carbonate as a phosphate binder (Letter): *N Eng J Med* 316: 109, 1987

94. O'Donovan R, Baldwin D, Hammer M, Moniz C, Parsons V: Substitution of aluminum salts by magnesium salts in control of dialysis hyperphosphatemia. *Lancet* 1: 880, 1986

95. Sundaram M, Joyce PF, Shields JB, Riaz MA, Sagar S: Terminal phalangeal tufts: earliest site of renal osteodystrophy findings in hemodialysis patients. *Am J Roentgenol* 133: 25, 1979

96. Maloney NA, Ott SM, Alfrey AC, Miller NG, Coburn JW, Sherrard DJ: Histological quantification of aluminum in iliac bone from patients with renal failure. *J Lab Clin Med* 99: 206, 1982

97. Delmez JA, Dougan S, Gearing BK, Rothstein M, Windus DW, Rapg N, Slatopolsky E: The effects of intraperitoneal calcitriol on calcium and parathyroid hormone. *Kidney Int* 31: 795, 1987

98. Fournier A, Bordier P, Gueris J, Sebert JL, Marie P, Ferriere C, Bedrossian J, Deluca HF: Comparison of 1 alpha-hydroxy-cholecalciferol and 25-hydroxycholecalciferol in the treatment of bone mineralization. Greater effect of 25-hydroxy-cholecalciferol on bone mineralization. *Kidney Int* 15: 196, 1979

99. Slatopolsky E, Weerts C, Thielan J, Horst R, Harter H, Martin KJ: Marked suppression of 1,25-dihydroxcholecalciferol in uremic patients. *J Clin Invest* 74: 2146, 1984

100. Phelps KR, Einhorn TA, Vigorita VJ, Lundin AP, Friedman EA: Fracture healing with deferoxamine therapy in a patient with aluminum – associated osteomalacia. *Trans Am Soc Artif Intern Organs* 32: 198, 1986

101. Bauer JH, Reams GP: Antihypertensive treatment in patients with renal disease. *The Kidney* (National Kidney Foundation) 19: 11, 1986

102. Diamond SM, Henrich WL: Hypertension in dialysis patients. *Int J Artif Organs* 9: 213, 1986

103. Lindner A, Douglas SW, Adamson JW: Propranol effects in long term hemodialysis patient with renin-dependent hypertension. *Ann Intern Med* 88: 457, 1978

104. Sullivan J, Johnson JB: The management of hypertension in patients with renal insufficiency. *Semin Nephrol* 3: 40, 1983

105. Moreira J, Barata JD, Olias J: Antihypertensive action of calcium blockade in hypertensive patients with chronic renal disease. *Nephron* 41: 314, 1985

106. Hannedovcke T, Josse S, Godia M, Fillastre JP: Efficacy of nifedipine in the acute treatment of hypertension in hemodialysis patients. *Curr Ther Res* 38: 383, 1985

107. Bennett WM, Golper TA, Muther RS, McCarron DA: Efficacy of minoxidil in treatment of severe hypertension in systemic disorders. *J Cardiovasc Pharmacol* 2 (Suppl 2): S142, 1980

108. Bazilinski N: CEI inhibitors in hemodialysis. *Int J Artif Organs* 6: 62, 1983

109. Papadimitriou M, Zamboulis C, Alexopoulos E, Liamos H, Sakellariou G, Memmos D, Metaxis P: Alarming hyperkalemia during captopril administration in patients on regular hemodialysis. *Dial Transplant* 14: 473, 1985

110. Henderson LW: Hemofiltration for the treatment of hypertension associated with end stage renal failure. *Artif Organs* 4: 103, 1980

111. DePace NL, Nestico PF, Schwartz AB, Mintz GS, Schwartz JS, Kotler MN, Swartz C: Predicting success in intensive dialysis in the treatment of uremic pericarditis: *Am J Med* 76: 38, 1984

112. Minuth ANW, Nottebohm GA, Eknoyan G, Suki NW: Indomethacin treatment of pericarditis in chronic hemodialysis patients: *Arch Intern Med* 135: 807, 1975

113. Quigg RJ: Local steroids in dialysis associated pericardial effusion. A single i.p. administration of triamincinolone. *Arch Intern Med* 145: 2249, 1985

114. Lornoy W, DeBroe M, Hilderson J, Boghaert A, Cuvelier J, Derom F, Ringoir S: Uremic pericarditis in chronic hemodialysis patients. Treatment by surgical pericardiostomy. *Acta Clin Belg* 32: 230, 1977

115. Delano BG, Nacht R, Friedman EA, Krasnow N: Myocardial anaerobiosis in anemia in uremic man. *Am J Cardiol* 29: 39, 1972

116. Anderson CB: Cardiac failure and upper arteriovenous dialysis fistula. *Arch Intern Med* 136: 292, 1976

117. The Consensus Trial Study Group Effects of Enalapril on Mortality in Severe Congestive Heart Failure. *N Engl J Med* 316: 1429, 1987

118. Blaustein AS, Schmitt G, Foster MC, Hayes RV, Bronstein S: Serial effects on left ventricular load and contraction during hemodialysis. *Am Heart J* 111: 340, 1986

119. Ramirez G, Brueggemeyer CD, Newton JL: Cardiac arrhythmia on hemodialysis in chronic renal failure patients. *Nephron* 36: 212, 1984

120. Rostand SG, Kirk KA, Rutsky EA: Dialysis-associated heart disease! Insights from coronary angiography. *Kidney Int* 25: 653, 1984

121. King K, Harkness J: Infective endocarditis in the 1980's. Aetiology and diagnosis. *Med J Aust* 144: 536, 1986

122. Kjellstrand CM: A comparison of dialysis and transplantation in patients with end stage renal failure of diabetes. in *Diabetic Renal-Retinal Syndrome* edited by Friedman EA, L'Esperance FA, New York, Grune & Stratton, 1986, p 333

123. Ghavamian M, Gutch CF, Kopp KF, Kolff WJ: The sad truth about hemodialysis in diabetics. *JAMA* 222: 1386, 1972

124. Legrain M, Rottembourg J, Bentchikson N, Porgnet JL, Issad B, Barthelemy A, Strippoli P, Gahl GM, DeGroc F: Dialysis treatment of insulin dependent diabetic patients. 10 years experience. *Clin Nephrol* 21: 72, 1984

125. Whitley KY, Shapiro FL: Hemodialysis for end-stage diabetic nephropathy. in *Diabetic – Renal Retinal Syndrome*, edited by Friedman EA, L'Esperance FA, New York, Grune & Stratton, 1986, p 349

126. Kjellstrand CM, Whitley K, Comty CM, Shapiro FL: Dialysis in patients with diabetes mellitus. *Diabetic Nephropathy* 2: 5, 1983

127. Wathen RL, Keshaviah P, Hommeyer P, Cadwell K, Comty CM: The metabolic effects of hemodialysis with and without glucose in the dialysate. *Am J Clin Nutr* 31: 1870, 1978

128. Blagg CR: Visual and vascular problems in dialyzed diabetic patients. *Kidney Int* 6 (Suppl 1): S27, 1974

129. Diaz-Buxo JA, Burges NP, Greenman M, Chandeir JT, Farmer CP, Walker PJ: Visual function in diabetic patients undergoing dialysis. Comparison of peritoneal and hemodialysis. *Int J Artif Organs* 7: 257, 1984

130. Wautier JL, Paton RC, Wautier MP, Pintgmy D, Abadie E, Passa P, Caen PJ: Increased adhesions of erythrocytes to endothelial cells in diabetes mellitus and its relation to vascular complications. *N Eng J Med* 305: 237, 1981

131. End Stage Renal Disease. Patient Profile Tables 1985. *Contemp Dial Nephrol* 8: 34, 1987

132. Berylne GM: Over 50 and uremic = death. The failure of the British National Health Service to provide adequate dialysis facilities. *Nephron* 31: 189, 1982

133. Rotellar E, Lubelza RA, Rotellar C, Martinez-Camps E, Alia MV, Valls R: Must patients over 65 be hemodialyzed? *Nephron* 41: 152, 1985

134. Taube DA, Winder EA, Ogg CS, Bewick M, Cameron JS, Rudge CJ, Williams DG: Successful treatment of middle aged and elderly patients with end stage renal disease. *Br Med J* 286: 2018, 1983

135. Rathaus M, Bernheim JL: Are your elderly patients good candidates for dialysis. *Geriatrics* 33: 56, 1978

136. Chester AC, Rakowski TA, Argy WP Jr, Giacalone A, Schreiner GE: Hemodialysis in the eighth and ninth decades of life. *Arch Intern Med* 139: 1001, 1979

137. Lundin AP, Adler AJ, Feinroth MV, Berlyne GM, Friedman EA: Maintenance hemodialysis – survival beyond the first decade. *JAMA* 244: 38, 1980

138. Rostand SG: Ischemic heart disease in patients undergoing maintenance hemodialysis. *Kidney Int* 16: 600, 1979

139. Blumberg A, Hausermann M, Strub B, Jenzer HR: Cardiac arrhythmias in patients on maintenance hemodialysis. *Nephron* 33: 91, 1983

140. Marshall WG, Rossi WP, Meng RL, Wedige RL, Stechen T: Coronary artery bypass in dialysis patients. *Ann Thorac Surg* 46: 512, 1986

141. Pavie A, Mussat T, Valle D, Rottembourg J, Barthebemy A, Gandbakhch I, Legrain M, Carbol C: Open heart cardiac surgery in severe renal insufficiency and dialysis patients. *Arch Mal Couer* 78: 242, 1985

142. Zawada ET Jr, Stinson JB, Done G: New perspectives on coronary artery disease in hemodialysis patients. *South Med J* 75: 694, 1982

143. Laws KH, Merrill WH, Aammon JW Jr, Prager RL, Bender HW: Cardiac surgery in patients with chronic renal disease. *Ann Thorac Surg* 42: 152, 1986

144. Chattarjee SN: National study on the natural history of renal allografts in sickle cell disease or trait. *Nephron* 25: 199, 1980

145. Elberg AJ, Baker R, Kock K, Gorman H, Wenger AJ, Strauss J: Transfusion required in patients with sickle cell disease on hemodialysis (Letter). *N Eng J Med* 294: 44, 1976

146. Gonzalez-Carrillo M, Rudge CJ, Parsons V, Bewick M, White JM: Renal transplantation in sickle cell disease. *Clin Nephrol* 18: 209, 1982

147. Szwed JJ, Yum MN, Hogan R: A beneficial effect of splenectomy in sickle cell anemia and chronic renal failure. *Am J Med Sci* 279: 169, 1980

148. Manis T, Friedman EA: Sickle hemoglobinopathy and the kidney. *Contr Nephrol* 7: 211, 1977

149. Lee MY, Uvelli DA, Agodoa LC, Scribner BH, Finch CA, Babb AL: Clinical studies of a continuous extracorporeal cyanate treatment system for patients with sickle cell anemia. *J Lab Clin Med* 100: 344, 1982

150. Gral T, Schroth P, Rosen V, Sellers A, Maxwell MH: Is chronic hemodialysis indicated in the treatment of terminal lupus nephritis. *Am Soc Nephrol* (Abst) 4: 31, 1970

151. Coplon NS, Siegel R, Fries J: Hemodialysis in end stage renal lupus nephritis. *Trans Amer Soc Artif Organs* 19: 302, 1973

152. Coplon NS, Diskin CJ, Petersen J, Swenson RS: The long term clinical course of systemic lupus erythematosus in end-stage renal disease. *N Eng J Med* 308: 186, 1983

153. Pahl MV, Vaziri ND: Maintenance hemodialysis in end stage lupus nephritis. *Int J Art Organs* 7: 243, 1984

154. Pahl MV, Vaziri ND, Saiki JK, Upham Q, Ness R: Chronic hemodialysis in end stage lupus nephritis changes of clinical and serological activity. *Artif Organs* 8: 423, 1984

155. Delano BG, Feinroth MV, Feinroth M, Friedman EA: Home

and medical center hemodialysis: Dollar comparison and pay-back period. *JAMA* 246: 230, 1981

156. Rao TKS, Friedman EA, Nicastri AD: The types of renal disease in the acquired immunodeficiency syndrome. *New Engl J Med* 316: 1062, 1987

157. Rao TKS, Manis T, Friedman EA: Dismal prognosis despite maintenance hemodialysis in AIDS nephropathy and chronic uremia. *Trans Am Soc Artif Organs* 31: 160, 1985

158. Recommendations for Providing Dialysis Treatment to Patients Infected with Human T-Lymphotiopic Virus Type III/Lymphadenopathy: *Associated Virus, MMWR* 35: 376, 1986

159. Barton CH, Vaziri ND: Dialysis and transplantation in multiple myeloma. *Int J Artif Organs* 7: 317, 1984

160. Johnson WJ, Kyle RA, Dahlberg PJ: Dialysis in the treatment of multiple myeloma. *Mayo Clin Proc* 55: 65, 1980

161. Cosio FG, Pence TV, Shapiro FL, Kjellstrand CM: Severe renal failure in multiple myeloma. *Clin Nephrol* 15: 206, 1981

162. Lazarus HM, Adelstein DJ, Herzig RH, Smith MC: Long term survival of patients with multiple myeloma and acute renal failure at presentation. *Am J Kidney Dis* 2: 521, 1983

163. Coward RA, Mallick NP, Delmore IW: Should patients with renal failure associated with myeloma be dialyzed? *Br Med J* 287: 1575, 1983

164. Randall RE, Williamson WC, Mullinax F, Tung MF, Still JS: Manifestations of systemic light chain deposition. *Am J Med* 60: 293, 1976

165. Waeber B, Schaller MD, Wauters JP, Brunner HR: Deterioration of renal function in hypertensive patients with scleroderma despite blood pressure normalization with captopril. *Klin Wochenschr* 84: 728, 1984

166. Barker DJ, Farr MJ: Resolution of cutaneous manifestations of systemic sclerosis after haemodialysis. *Br Med J* 1: 501, 1976

167. Zawada ET Jr, Clements PJ, Furst DA, Bloomer HA, Paulie HE, Maxwell MH: Clinical course of patients with scleroderma renal crises treated with captopril. *Nephron* 27: 74, 1981

168. Simon NM, Graham MB, Kyser FA, Gashti EN: Resolution of renal failure with malignant hypertension in scleroderma. Case report and review of the literature. *Am J Med* 67: 533, 1979

169. Javier P, Dumler F, Levin NW: Renal scleroderma. Comparison of different modalities of treatment. *South Med J* 73: 657, 1980

170. Leroy ED, Fleischmann RM: The management of renal scleroderma. Experience with dialysis nephrectomy and transplantation. *Am J Med* 64: 974, 1978

171. Kohorst WR, Bay WH: Reversal of end stage kidney failure in two scleroderma patients treated with anticoagulation. *Am J Kidney Dis* 2: 347, 1982

172. Ari JB, Zlotnik M, Oren A, Berlyne GM: Dialysis in renal failure caused by amyloidosis of familial Mediterranean fever. *Arch Intern Med* 136: 449, 1976

173. Rubinger D, Friedlaender MM, Popovtzer MM: Amelioration of familial Mediterranean fever during hemodialysis. *N Engl J Med* 301: 142, 1979

174. Shapiro W, Chou SY, Porush JC: Nephrectomy for intractable proteinuria secondary to severe nephrotic syndrome. *Abstracts Am Soc Nephrol* 8: 24, 1975

175. Avram MM, Lapinid N, Lipner H: Medical Nephrectomy.

The use of metallic salts in uncontrollable massive nephrotic syndrome. *Trans Am Soc Artif Intern Organs* 22: 431, 1976

176. Suzuki H, Konishi K, Izumi Y, Saruta T, Ozawa Y, Kato E: Long-term hemodialysis in a patient with primary amyloidosis, renal failure and avascular necrosis of the femoral head. *South Med J* 1982 75: 1018, 1982

177. Stone WJ, Latos DL, Lankford PG, Baker AS: Chronic peritoneal dialysis in a patient with primary amyloidosis, renal failure and factor X deficiency. *South Med J* 71: 764, 1978

178. Zamora JL, Rose JE, Rosario V, Noon GP: Hemodialysis associated carpal tunnel syndrome. A clinical review. *Nephron* 41: 70, 1985

179. Cary N: Synovial amyloid deposits and chronic haemodialysis (Letter). *Ann Rheum Dis* 45: 438, 1986

180. DiRaimondo CR, Casey TT, DiRaimondo CV, Stone WJ: Pathologic fractures associated with idiopathic amyloidosis of bone in chronic hemodialysis patients. *Nephron* 434, 22, 1986

181. Nemoto R, Sugiyama Y, Kuwahara M, Kato T, Tsuchida S: Successful delivery of a patient on hemodialysis for acute renal failure. A case report and review of the literature. *J Urol* 118: 673, 1977

182. Naik RB, Clark AC, Warren DJ: Acute proliferative glomerulonephritis with crescents and renal failure in pregnancy successfully managed by intermittent haemodialysis. Case report. *Br J Obstet Gynaecol* 86: 819, 1979

183. Lim VS: Reproductive function in patients with renal insufficiency. *Am J Kidney Dis* 9: 363, 1987

184. Roxe DM, McLoughlin MM: Reproductive capacity in female patients on chronic hemodialysis. *Int J Artif Organs* 7: 249, 1984

185. Sheriff MH, Hardman, M, Lamont CA, Shepherd R, Warren DJ: Successful pregnancy in a 44-year-old haemodialysis patient. *Br J Obstet Gynaecol* 85: 386, 1978

186. Hou S: Pregnancy in women requiring dialysis for renal failure. *Am J Kidney Dis* 9: 368, 1987

187. Ellis D, Avner ED: Renal failure and dialysis therapy in children with hepatic failure in the perioperative period of orthotopic liver transplant. *Clin Nephrol* 25: 295, 1986

188. Wilkinson SP, Weston MJ, Parsons V, Williams R: Dialysis in the treatment of renal failure in patients with liver disease. *Clin Nephrol* 8: 287, 1977

189. Hobar PC, Turner WW Jr, Valentine RJ: Successful use of the Denver peritoneovenous shunt in patients with nephrogenic ascites. *Surgery* 101: 161, 1987

190. Gotloib L, Servadis C: Ascites in patients undergoing maintenance hemodialysis. *Am J Med* 61: 65, 1976

191. Arismendi GS, Izard MW, Hampton WR, Maher JF: The clinical spectrum of ascites associated with maintenance dialysis. *Am J Med* 60: 46, 1976

192. Kearns PJ, Polhemus RJ, Oakes D, Rabkin R: Hepatorenal syndrome managed with hemodialysis, then reversed by peritoneovenous shunting. *J Clin Gastroenterol* 7: 341, 1985

193. Gandhi VC, Leehey DJ, Stanley MM, Nemchausky BA, Daugirdas JT, Greenlee HB, Jablokow VR, Ing TS: Peritoneovenous shunting in patients with cirrhotic ascites and end-stage renal failure. *Am J Kidney Dis* 6: 185, 1985

194. Ponce P, Moreira P: Water immersion in an anuric cirrhotic patient. *Nephron* 43: 144, 1986

HOME HEMODIALYSIS

GIUSEPPE D'AMICO and CLAUDIO BAZZI

CHOICE OF MODALITY (AN HISTORICAL REVIEW. FACTORS BEHIND THE GEOGRAPHICAL DIFFERENCES IN THE SPREAD OF HOME HEMODIALYSIS)

Historical review (a changing setting)

Programs to teach patients to hemodialyze themselves at home were developed, mainly because of the high cost of in-center maintenance dialysis and the shortage of hospital facilities, first in Boston in 1964 (1) and subsequently in Seattle (2) and in London (3) in 1965. Both in the USA and in the UK the percentage of patients treated at home increased rapidly thereafter, with a peak of 40% of all patients on regular dialysis treatment in the USA treated by home hemodialysis (HHD) at the end of 1971 (4) and of 62% in the UK by the end of 1980 (5). Experience with this new modality of dialysis treatment extended to Australia, where more than 50% of patients were treated at home by the end of 1977 (6), to Canada where 25% of all dialysis patients underwent HHD by the end of 1977 (7) and to many countries in Europe, where around 20% were reached by the end of 1980 in Denmark, Sweden, Switzerland, Ireland, the Federal Republic of Germany and France (5). Those nephrologists and nurses who developed programs of HHD in their own centers agreed unanimously that this modality, when properly accepted by the staff and correctly presented to a selected group of potential candidates, represented the best treatment for a large percentage of uremic patients, in terms of well being, survival, independence, rehabilitation and cost. However, the expansion of HHD was not distributed equally in different countries or even in different geographical locations within single countries. In some centers, and sometimes in extended geographical areas, it was virtually ignored. Furthermore, in those countries and areas in which the acceptance had been good at the beginning, the use of HHD became progressively less regular and not so widespread through the years. In the USA the percentage of patients with end-stage renal disease (ESRD) treated by HHD, after reaching the peak of 40% in 1971, started to decrease in 1972, had already declined to 12% in 1978 (8) and was only 5.2% by end of 1984, according to data from the Health Care Financial Administration. In Europe the decline started more recently. In the 5 year period from the end of 1980 to the end of 1985 the percentage of all patients with ESRD treated by HHD had decreased from 62% to

30% in the UK and from 20% to less than 10% in the Federal Republic of Germany (9). In our unit, where an HHD program was started in 1970, the total number of patients treated with this dialysis modality progressively increased to a maximum of 87 (49% of the entire population on dialysis treatment) during 1982 (Figure 1), subsequently decreasing to 58 (35.5% of the entire population) at the end of 1986.

It is thus obvious that the diffusion of this modality of regular dialysis treatment (RDT) has been conditioned by many factors that have very little to do with its clinical efficacy and economic advantages.

Factors that favored the spread of HHD

The 'go home or die' situation

This modality was initially developed to offer an acceptable form of regular dialysis treatment when there was a shortage of dialysis facilities in the hospitals. This 'go home or die' situation remained the major factor favoring the diffusion of HHD, even after it became evident that this treatment was neither harmful nor complicated and offered such results in survival and rehabilitation as to make it an optimal form of dialysis treatment. In the late 1960s, before Medicare began financing treatment for kidney failure, this pressure to send patients home was given added impetus by enacted regulations and by the limited financial facilities and hospital beds in the USA. In the UK the pressure produced by the shortage of hospital facilities still exists, the more recent decrease in the number of HHD patients in that country being due to the availability of alternative modalities of out-center self-dialysis treatment, mainly CAPD.

The example set by patients already dialyzing at home

Another important factor that favors acceptance of HHD, in those centers with established successful programs that provide all the other more recently developed alternative modalities of dialysis (self-dialysis stations, limited-care dialysis units, CAPD programs), is the belief on the part of clinicians and nurses that HHD is the optimal form of treatment for a selected group of patients. This conviction still plays an important part in general strategy of dialysis treatment and helps to relieve the burden placed on hospital facilities, of which there is always a chronic scarcity.

A determined staff is essential for convincing new patients that treatment at home is possible. Such a staff encourages the contact of new candidates for HHD and their partners with patients who are already successfully trained and their families. This contact can be very helpful in breaking down their obvious resistance and in overcoming their reluctance to engage in such a binding enterprise.

Factors that hampered the diffusion of HHD

Governmental regulations and economic factors

Without any doubt, the regulations and the availability of economic resources for direct or indirect payment for dialysis treatment are the most important determinants in favoring or inhibiting the diffusion of HHD (10). In the USA in July 1973, legislation (public Law 92–603) eliminated the heavy financial burden facing patients being treated for ESRD, but favored the private institutions performing exclusively out-patient dialysis in hospital or satellite units with reimbursement for services. The sharp and rapid decrease in patients being dialyzed at home was a logical consequence of such imperfect regulation, which has not subsequently been corrected (due to pressure from proprietary dialysis corporations?). A method of financing dialysis that would encourage home dialysis and simultaneously substantially reduce the enormous financial burden on the Medicare ESRD Program needs to be developed. In 1983, Schmidt et al (11) observed in the USA that the 25% of the states with the highest prevalence of home dialysis patients also had the highest percentage of patients being dialyzed in nonprofit facilities. Similar data have been reported by Gardner (12). Thus, it would appear that the facilities caring for patients under Medicare reimbursement may be faced with a serious economic disincentive and when operating for profit may be disinclined or unable to provide home dialysis.

A similar mechanism operates even in Italy. Since the reimbursement fees from the Regional Administrations favor the private facilities offering in-center dialysis, in the regions of the Southern part of the country, with a high number of such private units, the percentage of home patients (including HHD and CAPD) was less than 1% at the end of 1985, versus 28.3% (12.4% in HHD and 15.9% in CAPD) in the Northern region, Lombardia, in which the number of private profit-making facilities has been kept at very low levels by a policy favoring the development of public hospital facilities (13).

Another country in which legal constraint hinders the diffusion of HHD is Japan. There, hemodialysis is totally reimbursable by the Federal government only when a doctor is present. Furthermore, another law specifically prohibits the self-administration of drugs in the home. The result is that only 120 patients were on HHD in Japan in 1982 (14).

Development of other modalities of self-dialysis (CAPD, self-dialysis in out-patient facilities)

Many centers operating HHD programs concurrently began programs of self-dialysis within out-patient facilities in order to treat patients trained comparably to those in the HHD program, but who did not have partners or a suitable place in the home. In our self-dialysis facility a nurse acts as a common partner to many patients carrying out their treatments autonomously. Since its institution in 1979, it has been the proper location for treating some patients who have personal or family difficulties that are impediments to training and who would have been sent home with some risk of failure in the absence of such an alternative. But the alternative modality of self dialysis that has diverted many potentially suitable patients from HHD programs is continuous ambulatory peritoneal dialysis (CAPD). Almost everywhere the avail-

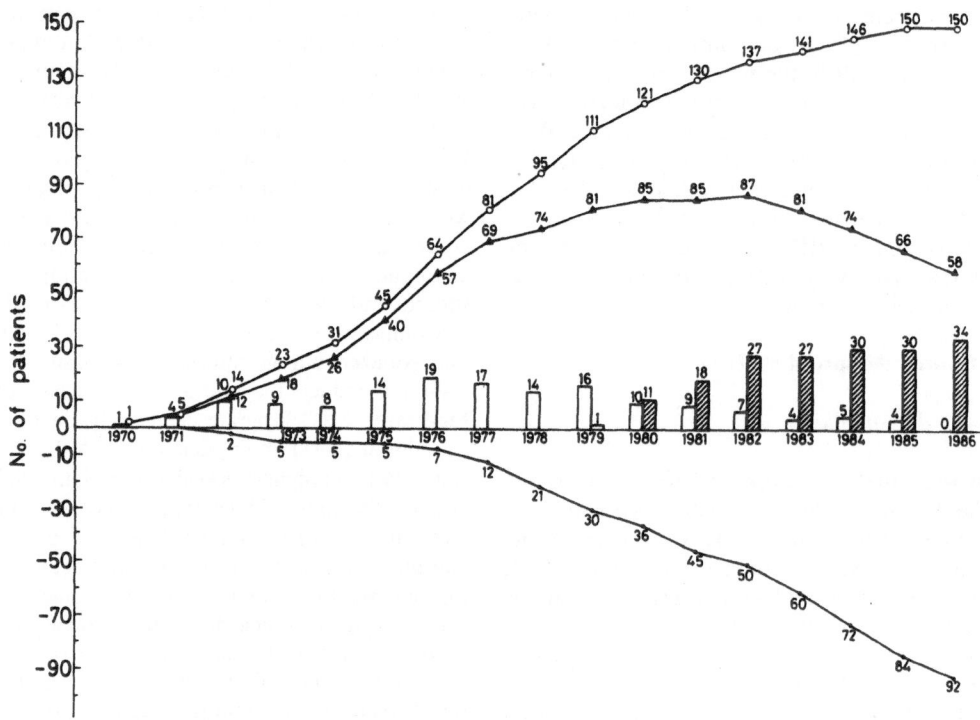

Figure 1. Patients on home hemodialysis and on CAPD at the end of each year at the St Carlo Hospital in Milan: (□) patients who started HHD during the year; (—○—) total number of patients having entered the HHD program at the end of the year; (—●—) total number of patients having stopped HHD at the end of the year; (—▲—) total number of patients still on HHD at the end of each year; (▨) total number of patients on CAPD at the end of each year.

ability of a CAPD program has caused and still produces a decline in the number of patients treated at home by hemodialysis. In the UK, while the percentage of HHD patients decreased from more than 50% of all dialysis patients at the end of 1980 to 30% at the end of 1985, the percentage of patients on CAPD increased from less than 20% to nearly 40% (9). In our own program, the recent decrease in the number of new patients starting HHD annually coincides with the start of a concomitant CAPD program (Figure 1).

Distrust of the staff for the HHD

The success of a HHD program depends highly on the conviction and enthusiasm of the staff in general, and in particular of those that are especially dedicated to it. In the absence of other economic motivating factors, the lack of such a program in a center is due to distrust by the staff, who refuse additional organizing efforts, are not motivated to acquire new competence and fear new responsibilities. In some cases, this attitude pervades a large geographical area and acts as an impediment to fighting for modification of governmental regulations that deter HHD programs. This appears to be the situation in Japan (14).

CHOOSING SUITABLE PATIENTS

Although in a recent survey of the preferences of 49 nephrologists among the different ESRD treatment options HHD was the dialysis modality chosen by the majority (15), different clinicians dealing with HHD programs tended to give divergent estimates about the percentage of patients suitable for such treatment on the basis of their personal experience. Estimates have ranged from 20 to 80% (16–18). The percentage of 65% of all dialysis patients treated by HHD reached in the UK, when no other form of home treatment was available, demonstrates that a very high rate of successful training can be achieved even on a national basis. CAPD is now a recognized and increasingly accepted technique for home dialysis and since the population of patients suitable for HHD and that for CAPD overlap somewhat, we believe that HHD can be fairly estimated to still be the treatment of choice for about 30 to 35% of all patients referred to a center that can offer all the different types of dialysis treatment including CAPD, self-dialysis in an outpatient facility and limited-care treatment in satellite units. As Figure 2 shows, frequent transfers from one modality to another occur in a setting organized in this way.

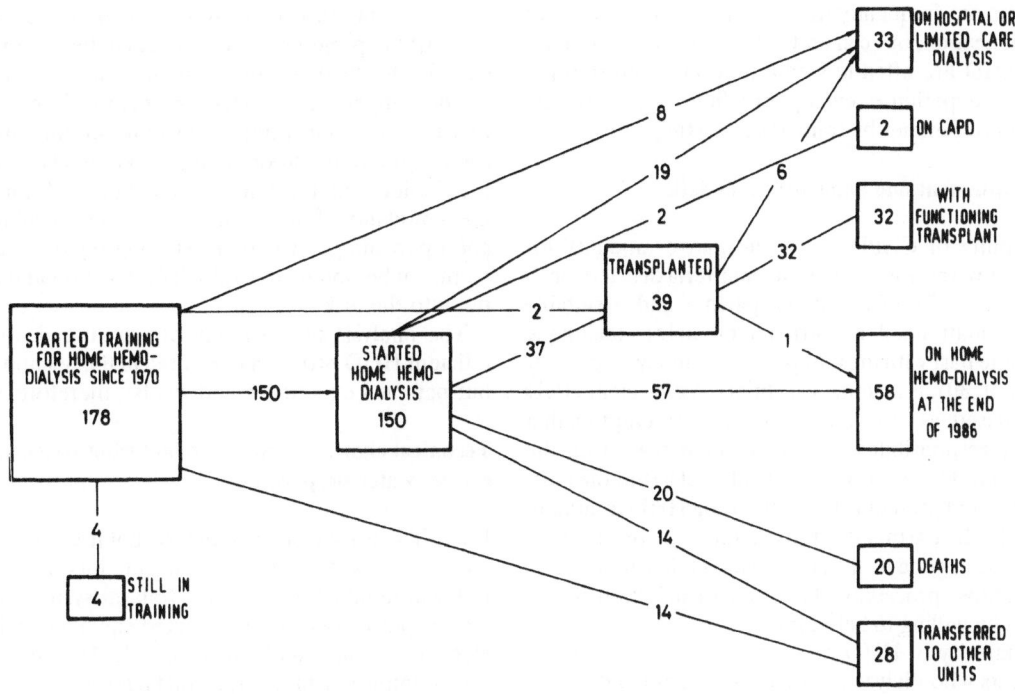

Figure 2. Home hemodialysis program at the St Carlo Hospital in Milan. Changes in the modality of treatment before the end of 1986.

Age and clinical conditions

The availability of CAPD has limited the range of clinical conditions in which HHD is used. In the past, very elderly patients, patients with severe cardiovascular diseases or with concomitant systemic diseases (diabetes, collagen diseases) were frequently included in the HHD program, with fairly good results (19–23). Since other strategies of treatment have become available, we and other nephrologists prefer CAPD for those high risk patients who can be treated at home, while we still propose HHD as the best modality in patients with rather good general clinical condition.

Advanced chronological age is not considered an absolute contraindication for HHD (20, 21, 24, 25). Some very elderly patients who are in good clinical condition, mentally stable and willing to cooperate can cope with HHD even better than the younger patients can. We avoid including in our HHD program patients older than 70 years when the only available partner is an aged husband or wife. In our experience such a partner may himself frequently have complicating diseases which will interrupt the home treatment. Many nephrologists prefer CAPD for elderly patients. Children are also a special problem. They benefit from home treatment because they can enjoy the continuity of home life. However, they may thrive at the expense of anxiety in the parents (26). In our opinion, CAPD is usually indicated for children, since it frees the young patients and their parents from the anxiety and fear experienced during the hemodialysis procedure and permits a more liberal diet.

Psychological and educational conditions

It is accepted that psychological problems can interfere with successful adjustment to hemodialysis, particularly HHD, and may also contribute to self-destructive behavior (27). A recent analysis of the psychological factors associated with an increased probability of failure when a patient enters HHD indicates that patients who fail have higher levels of depression and self-depreciation and higher levels of stress associated with fear of death, pain during dialysis and blood clotting (28). Denial, a psychological defense mechanism, considered by some to exist in all dialysis patients, was significantly present in patients over 45 years who continued HHD successfully (28). Patients with a tendency to despair, hopelessness and helplessness, who feel unable to cope and who sense loss of environmental support, are more likely to fail in a HHD program. Unfortunately, the psychological profile of a candidate for HHD is determined in end-stage renal failure before the start of hemodialysis treatment, when severe uremic intoxication and the inherent anxiety produced by the introduction of the new complex procedure of hemodialysis, potentially reversible phenomena, may hinder appropriate evaluation.

In our experience, another psychological characteristic which must be evaluated in a candidate for HHD is willingness to cooperate and to follow strictly the instructions given during training. Independent patients who tend to have personal interpretations and to modify the rules that they have been instructed to follow are poor candidates. Since such patients are frequently those with the highest level of academic education, one can understand why the best candidates for HHD are often less educated but motivated patients. In our experience, even poorly literate patients and partners can sometimes be trained successfully.

Family environment and home accommodation

The availability of CAPD as an alternative modality for home dialysis permits us to use stricter criteria of selection in terms of availability of a suitable partner and a suitable house. The 'unattended' nocturnal hemodialysis technique adopted in the past with the pumpless Kiil kidney, especially in the UK (29, 30), is no longer justified. An efficient HHD program is based, as we will see later, on the assumption that the primary responsibility for treatment is placed on the patient himself. However, the availability of a suitable partner is an essential prerequisite for choosing HHD treatment for a patient. The partner must live in the same residence as the patient, be in good health, have enough time to dedicate to the repetitive procedure, have ties of affection to the patient and be willing to help him.

In the majority of HHD programs it is possible to find some patients who dialyze at home with a paid and impersonal partner, usually a nurse expert in dialysis techniques. Such an arrangement should be an exception. To permit home treatment, the house of the patient must be sufficiently large and clean. An extra room for the dialysis procedure is not necessary and is used only by a minority of patients (8.8% of home patients in Bazzato and Onesti's series [23], 10% in our series). In the majority of cases, a bedroom or a livingroom is adapted for the treatment, and a deionizer is installed in the bathroom. The complicated readaptations of the house or the relocation of the family to new homes sometimes used in the UK in the past (31, 32) are not necessary nowadays. Other modalities, including CAPD or self-dialysis in an outpatient facility, can be chosen when the house is too small, or overcrowded or not clean enough.

ORGANIZATION OF A HOME HEMODIALYSIS PROGRAM

During the last 20 years we have visited many centers that conduct programs of HHD in different countries throughout the world, to compare operational aspects and results. We have always been struck by the tremendous differences among the different centers in the way they perform HHD, and even more by the fact that, in spite of these differences, especially in the modality of training the patients, the majority of the programs appeared to work well and give comparable results.

There are obviously many reasons for the differences: 1) the health organization and legislation of the country, 2) the local socio-economical environment, 3) some logistic and organizational characteristics of the centers (availability of separate spaces and dedicated staff), 4) the numbers and types of uremic patients referred to the center, 5) the current availability of other different modalities of out-center dialy-

sis treatment. In each center the experience in the initial stage of the program tends to become the standard and the stimulus for further improvement in the system is reduced.

The comparison of such different modalities convinced us that the single most important requisite for running a successful program and obtaining good quality training is the firm belief of all the components of the staff that HHD is a good modality of treatment and that successful training of a good percentage of patients starting regular dialysis treatment can be obtained if sufficient devotion and attention is put into the task.

The analysis of the many organizational aspects of an efficient HHD program presented in this section is based on our personal experience and will be, therefore, subjective.

Technical choice (machines, monitoring systems, blood access, water preparation)

It is still controversial whether or not it is more convenient and safe to perform HHD with simplified machines with a reduced number of automated alarm systems or with the most sophisticated new automated equipment with multiple electronic gadgets and safety controls. The supporters of the use of simple machines argue that it is easier and safer for the patients and their partners to learn to manage them correctly (33). In the first few years of our experience, up to 1972–1973, we used simple tank machines with only a few fundamental electronic monitoring circuits. Subsequently, we shifted to the more sophisticated machines that technology has made available in these last 15 years. The conversion to the new systems, which required new training of the old patients in the hospital, usually for limited periods of time, was easy and smooth in all cases. All patients and partners, no matter how educated they are, can learn without major difficulties or risk to operate the modern automated equipment with proportioning pumps for water preparation and electronically guided fixed programs requiring minimal manual attention. With such new equipment there are fewer mistakes in the operation and any breakdowns that may occur are easily and quickly repaired if the manufacturing companies provide good emergency technical assistance. Since the number of alarms in such sophisticated equipments is increased, the patients must be educated to avoid the habit of disconnecting some alarms to eliminate irritating noises or pulsing lights.

We think that, in spite of their higher cost, the disposable dialyzers are preferable at home to the cheaper Kiil dialyzers, which some units in the UK and in France still use. The reuse of such disposable dialyzers is safer in the home than in the hospital center, since there is no possibility of mixing up other patients dialysers and blood lines.

Water preparation is mandatory in HHD, even though it increases the cost of the treatment. It requires small deionizers or reverse osmosis units to be installed at home. The proportioning pumps incorporated in the modern monitoring equipment provide the optimal mixing of such water with the saline concentrate to produce the necessary amounts of dialysis fluid. Finally, we want to stress that establishment of a satisfactory vascular access, which can be repeatedly punctured by the patient himself or by the partner, is the principal factor for the success or failure of HHD. An internal arterovenous fistula suitable for easy self venipuncture should be made ready some time before training for HHD starts. The patient should have multiple choices of sites for inserting the needles.

Training of the patient and the partner

We will express our personal view in answering to the following questions:

Who must be trained?

In spite of the conviction we have already expressed that today the existence of a suitable, collaborative partner is a 'conditio sine qua non' before starting the training of a patient, we are absolutely convinced that HHD can and must be carried out safely and effectively by the patient himself. The correct role of the partner is that of helper who gives psychological support and can intervene if the patient becomes temporarily incapacitated physically and unable to control his dialysis (profound hypotension, cramps) and is, therefore, in danger of making errors. This approach has two fundamental advantages over that which gives major responsibilities to the partner: 1) it markedly reduces the anxiety and psychological dependence of the patient on the partner (with the consequent agressive behavior), since it allows the patient to acquire the theoretical knowledge and skills and therefore to be active in performing the treatment and dealing with the machinery; 2) it markedly reduces the emotional involvement of the partner, the stress deriving from the predominant responsibility in the care of somebody else and the burden of the necessity to be both present physically and continuously alert during all phases of the treatment.

It is obvious that the policy of teaching the patients independent self dialysis and allowing them to make the choice of involving others in their treatment produces different results in different familial situations. These depend mainly on such factors as dominance, distribution of work, decision making and dependency amongst married partners. Some of our patients prefer to do everything for themselves, while others require help from the family, either in preparing for dialysis and cleaning the equipment or as assistance during the treatment.

We start the training for the patient alone, as many others do. Only after some weeks, when the patient has already learned self-dialysis, do we start to train the partner, teaching him the same principles that the patient has already learned independently. If at the end of the training the partner appears to be insufficiently reliable or refuses to assume the responsibility of helping the patient at home, the trained patient can then be sent to our self-dialysis facility.

When should training be started?

We agree with Blagg and Peterson (34) that the best time to encourage patients to opt for HHD is before they start dialysis treatment or, for those patients for whom there is no opportunity for such discussions prior to starting treatment, during the first few weeks of such treatment, once they have recovered from acute complications and become medically stable. This is often a time of shock and denial, a time when the patient is not quite ready to face the enormous change in lifestyle that ESRD entails and is therefore easy to influence. The beliefs of the nephrologist and his team about the different modalities of treatment are then of paramount importance in conditioning the final decision by the patient. On the contrary, if the patient has been dialyzed as an outpatient for a significant period of time and has become dependent on the center and its staff, it is more difficult to convince him of the advantages offered by home treatment. In our experience, the discussion of treatment options must include a visit by the patient to the home dialysis training unit and talks with patients who already successfully perform HHD.

Who will supervise the training and where will it be done?

Assigned specialized nurses and a designated area are, in our opinion, essential factors for the success of a HHD program. The assigned team is useful since it permits us to choose from the nurses working in the dialysis unit those who are best suited for the teaching. In fact, not everybody has the special ability to transfer knowledge, regardless of the diverse capacities of the pupils and to establish correct psychological rapport with them, in order to obtain the necessary confidence and trust. The assigned team is also useful because it makes available for referral a small number of experienced and proven nurses for any kind of problem once the patients have started dialysis at home.

We also give the responsibility for our HHD program to a restricted number of physicians, with partial yearly turnover, so that the entire medical staff is aware of the problems of all home patients and can take the necessary measures in case of emergency calls.

Both nurses and doctors share the responsibility for training, but without any doubt the nurses are more directly and deeply involved; the success of a HHD program depends mainly on their skills, enthusiasm and sensitivity to the pupil's needs, which allow them to adjust their teaching methods appropriately.

The team should, if possible, work in a training area separate from the hospital dialysis area (20, 35, 36), separating trainees from the other dialysis patients who may be very ill and psychologically dependent and may have a negative attitude toward home dialysis. In this quiet area the patient and his partner can learn better and can be left alone to perform the last few dialysis sessions at the end of the training period without any help or supervision.

What is the best way to train a patient?

There are no definite rules that apply in all units to all patients. On the contrary, we are convinced that the training team that achieves the best results has found its way to communicate correctly with the trainee, using individualized techniques for different pupils. Many teaching aids have been developed for generalized or local use. They include slides, tapes, films and instruction manuals. However, all these aids can not be of general use in a single training unit if the correct approach of adjusting the teaching methods to the different needs of the different pupils is to be adopted. None of them 'can replace the infinite flexibility of the human voice to describe and emphasise the subject being taught' (31). Flexibility is necessary because of the different educational level and intelligence of the trainees, but also because of their different psychological reactions. The approach can not be the same for a patient or partner who is very frightened and needs reassurance and for another who is not sufficiently aware that something can go wrong and may, therefore, be careless.

After 20 years of experience with our HHD program we still do not feel it is necessary to develop or utilize audio-visual systems, and only very simple instruction manuals are currently used by us as teaching aids, to illustrate the main concepts and procedures which are listed in Tables 1 and 2. We use particular care to teach the trainees all the clinical and pathogenetic aspects of uremia and their modifications by the dialytic treatment and also the specific technical terminology which will allow the patients and their partners to converse intelligently from home over the telephone with the center's staff.

How much time is required for correct training?

As we have said, there are so many differences in the types of trainee and their capacity for learning differs widely for many reasons. Hence, a precise duration of the training is difficult to forecast. We, as well as others, have sent some

patients home after only 6 weeks, while for others more than 6 months were necessary for adequate training. In an analysis of 1,063 patients trained for HHD in the United States (37), the mean training time was 69 days. Patients successfully trained in less than 70 days had a significantly higher cumulative survival than those trained for more than 70 days (37). Our experience confirms that patients who are more easily trained manage dialysis better afterwards.

In our unit, the decision that the patient is ready to go home is made collectively by the training team, and a written certification of qualification is signed by some members of the team and by the physician in charge of the dialysis unit, as required by the regional administration that will financially support the subsequent home treatment.

Once the training has been completed and some sessions of treatment have taken place in the training area without any help from the staff, we like others (31, 38) facilitate transfer of the patients by sending a home dialysis nurse to the home. She inspects the home to be sure that everything is ready for comfortable treatment and is present for the first dialysis at home, giving psychological reassurance and practical help. A visit by the same nurse is usually repeated every 2 or 3 years, to check that the procedure followed is still correct and to assess the confidence of the patients and their family members.

Medical follow-up

When training has been performed correctly the subsequent home treatment is usually so safe that no emergency or regular visits to the home by the physicians are necessary. If some clinical or technical complication occurs during a dialysis session, we prefer to ask the patient to halt dialysis and come immediately to our center. Obviously, the clinical conditions of all patients must be checked regularly at the unit.

We see the patients every 4 to 6 weeks (or more frequently, when necessary) in a special out-patient clinic run by the staff of the HHD unit. The patients bring to the clinic all the special records that they have been instructed to fill for each dialysis session. Laboratory analyses are performed at each out-patient visit.

There must be a special direct phone line into the dialysis unit that can be used day and night by all patients on home treatment who may need to ask urgently for clinical or

Table 1. Home hemodialysis training check list.

Measurement of blood pressure, pulse, temperature, body weight
Cleaning and care of cannulae and fistulae
Venipuncture and treatment of possible complications
Water deionising techniques and water testing
Heparin preparation and administration
Blood and heparin pumps
Machine structure and monitor's control of blood pressure,
    dialysis fluid osmolarity, temperature and flux
Connections, dialyser priming and starting
Assisting the patient during dialysis: ultrafiltration,
    administration of fluid, blood and medications
Finishing
Rinsing and sterilizing
Collecting blood samples
Collecting dialysate samples
Filling in home charts

Table 2. Handling of emergencies of home hemodialysis.

Electricity failure
Water failure
Deioniser failure, hard water danger and symptoms
Lines disconnection and rupture; blood leak
Coagulation and changing of bubble catcher
Pyrogen reaction
Arterial hypotension and shock
Hypertensive crisis
Cramps
Returning blood to patient under gravity

---

technical advice and information. It is a rather general opinion among the physicians in charge of HHD programs that the role of the local family doctor in case of clinical complications is, unfortunately, of necessity very limited because of insufficient knowledge of the medical aspects of dialysis.

Technical assistance and supplies of materials

An important factor in the success of the HHD program is a good and prompt technical assistance for all the equipment installed at home. Such assistance is sometimes provided by the technicians of the dialysis center, while in other circumstances a regular maintenance service is signed with the manufacturing industries, which requires them to provide quick, on site repairs within a few hours in case of any technical trouble. In the great majority of cases a temporary technical drawback should cause only a short delay in starting the dialysis session at home, avoiding changing in the location of treatment from home to the hospital center.

Reliable, regular delivery of supplies to the patient's house is necessary. For large centers this task is usually contracted out to a commercial firm. Obviously, the staff must accurately control the type and numbers of all items delivered to the home.

Legal problems

The legal implications of HHD, thoroughly analyzed by Bailey et al (21) in 1970, were a matter of concern in the late 1960s when the new modality of dialysis was still in an experimental phase. In particular, the questions of whether or not a partner in home dialysis might be considered to be practicing medicine without a professional license and the problem of the responsibility of the physicians for home treatment have been debated. In these last 15 years, home treatment has been universally accepted as a valid modality of dialysis by the Public Health Service Administrations of almost all countries, and special national or regional laws have regulated the matter, reducing the risk of serious medicolegal problems. In many countries an 'informed consent' form is signed by the patient and the partner and a 'certification of qualification' for performing the treatment at home is signed for both by the staff at the end of the training.

Cost

In spite of the claim by proprietary dialysis corporations in the USA that the cost of home dialysis is equal to or exceeds that of out-patient dialysis (39), the great majority of nephrologists and public administrations in all parts of the world, using different ways of evaluating costs, have concluded that HHD is the cheapest modality of dialysis treatment, even cheaper than CAPD, with the cost about half that of treatment in a center (40–42). This is due mainly to the fact that assistance by the partner is cost free. Payment for HHD aides has been proposed in the USA as a means of inducing a shift from in-center hemodialysis. It is obvious that such additional payments would reduce the financial advantages of HHD.

CLINICAL RESULTS OF HHD

Survival

Comparing the different modalities of dialysis treatment and transplantation in terms of the survival rate is complicated by at least two sets of problems: 1) many patients who start a particular therapy become 'lost to observation' because they change to another therapy, 2) the subpopulations of patients treated by the different modalities are always selected and not randomly assigned.

There is no doubt that this second bias, selection of patients, favors HHD treatment, since patients assigned to this modality of dialysis are often younger, in better clinical condition and willing to cooperate. It can, at least in part, explain why the survival rate of HHD patients, calculated by all the models of analysis proposed, has always exceeded that of patients dialyzed in-center (43–53). The actual survival rates vary greatly in the different units (37). The EDTA registry reported in 1984 a 5 year survival of HHD patients in France of 80% versus 55% of patients on in-hospital dialysis (46). For our selected population of 150 patients, we have a survival rate of 72% after 10 years. For an unselected group of 109 patients treated at Downstate Medical Center in Brooklin by Delano et al (49), the overall survival after 10 years was 77%. However, they stressed the fact that survival was definitely less for the subgroup of patients with severe systemic diseases, mainly diabetes mellitus (49).

Better survival of HHD patients less than 50 years of age than of those over 50 has also been reported (47, 54). However, it has been sufficiently proven that even after adjusting the life-table analysis for age and other clinical risk factors, survival on HHD is at least as good as that on in-center HD and CAPD (44, 47, 48).

Quality of life and rehabilitation

In comparison with patients on in-center dialysis, HHD patients enjoy some advantages that favor a better quality of life and social rehabilitation. These are:

More personal freedom and less infringement on work time

This is because of the possibility to choose the most suitable time for the dialysis session and to avoid travelling to a hospital center, which usually requires more time than that spent to prepare dialysis at home. The integration of dialysis into the life of the patient gives him a better opportunity for employment. This type of advantage is greater for HHD patients than for CAPD patients (55), since the latter must lose some time during the working hours of the day for changing bags.

Avoiding stressful contact with the hospital milieu

Avoidance of the stressful continuous contact with the hospital environment and with other severely ill dialysis patients is considered so advantageous and important by the majority of HHD patients that it is very difficult to convince them to transfer the treatment temporarily to the hospital when some clinical complication or technical trouble occurs.

Advantages of self-treatment and possibility of a better 'tailoring' of dialysis treatment

The greater knowledge the patient acquires about treatment and the greater flexibility in duration of a single dialysis session and in the number of sessions per week, with well-regulated loss of fluid and optimal depuration, result in a more efficient and better tolerated treatment and an increased sense of well being. This better quality of treatment is very frequently reported to the doctors by patients who have successfully moved from in-center HD to home HD.

Lesser exposure to infection

This advantage has been especially significant for hepatitis, but applies to all hospital-acquired infections.

Better rehabilitation of HHD patients no matter what the criteria used to evaluated it (employment opportunities, quality of private life), has been reported by all nephrologists running HHD programs, based on their personal experience. It has been confirmed by the EDTA survey, covering Europe (56). Of our HHD patients 81% are able to work full or part-time. A comparison in Canada between the two modalities of home dialysis, HHD and CAPD, by an 'employment adaptation index' demonstrated better rehabilitation of HHD patients (55). It is obvious that the criteria of selection for patients allocated to the different modalities of treatment may affect the degree of rehabilitation.

Medical complications

The medical and surgical complications of HHD patients, including those that cause death, are not different from those of in center patients, and are described elsewhere in this book. However, as a consequence of the selection of patients treated at home, not only is survival better, as we have already reported, but all other complications requiring hospitalization have been reported to be fewer than those of in-center patients (39, 57, 58).

Twenty of the 150 patients who entered our HHD program since 1971 died before the end of 1986. Cardiovascular complications including myocardial infarction (seven cases) and cerebrovascular accidents (six cases) were the most frequent causes of death. Malignancy was responsible for two deaths and severe infections for two others.

As for clinical complications requiring hospitalization, it must be emphasized that no hospitalization whatsoever for medical troubles has been necessary up to now for nearly half of our HHD patients and no more than two periods of hospitalization during the entire duration of treatment have been required for another 30% of them.

Acute medical emergencies in the home are rare. In our experience, they can be managed with the rapid transfer of the patient to the center, after a telephone consultation and discontinuation of the dialysis session.

An increase in the necessity of dialysis in the center must be seriously expected as the population of HHD patients increases. It can be estimated that one hospital bed (and appropriate dialysis facilities) must be available for each 10 to 15 patients dialyzed at home (59).

Technical complications

These are no different from those that can occur in hospital dialysis, but have a lower incidence, because of the better maintenance of the equipment and the greater attention to correct execution of technical maneuvers. The most frequent mishaps are indicated in Table 2, since the possibility of their occurrence is stressed in the training and sometimes simulated during it. As stated above technical complications can usually be managed without any transfer of the treatment to in-center if good maintenance servicing is provided.

Discontinuation of HHD treatment

A certain number of patients fail to go on with home treatment after variable periods of time, even after selection of candidates and of partners and the evaluation of the adequacy of family environment and home accomodation has indicated they should be sufficient and the training has been successfully completed. The only alternative treatment in the 1960s was a return to hospital. Transfer to a limited care facility became possible in the 1970s. A shift to another modality of home treatment, CAPD, has become available since the beginning of the 1980s. The current possibility of multiple choices has not only reduced the number of patients enrolled in a HHD program in the most recent years, but has also increased the number of HHD patients who ask for and obtain changes in the modality of their dialysis treatments. In our unit, failure of HHD was very rare until the mid 1970s probably because we were not in a position to offer other alternative modalities except hospital dialysis and it was very difficult to find places in our in-center dialysis program. In the last 10 years, patients have moved to our self-care facility or to hospital dialysis after variable periods of HHD treatment, and a few of them have preferred CAPD (Figure 2).

Let us analyze the most frequent causes for HHD failure.

Increased risk due to clinical complications

Especially when the criteria of selection, including age as well as comorbid clinical conditions, are not very strict the risk of having some old or very ill patients in HHD treatment increases with the increase in the duration of the dialysis treatment, and many patients must return to in-center dialysis. This problem is a serious one in those geographical areas, such as the UK, in which HHD has been offered for many years to the majority of patients as the only modality of dialysis treatment. In our unit, deterioration of the clinical condition, usually after many years of treatment with this modality, has been the most frequent cause of removal from the HHD program. Eight patients have returned to hospital dialysis and 11 have been transferred to our self-service facility (Figure 2).

Unavailability of the partner. Family stress and strain

We consider these two situations together, because the latter is one of the most important causes, even though not the only one, of unavailability of the partner.

The preliminary evaluation of the familial environment and good training, which should prevent unnecessary anxiety, are not always sufficient to avoid a situation of increasing stress and fear in the partner once home treatment is started. Without question, assisting with HHD requires a significant commitment of time from the partner and the establishment or maintenance of a stable relationship between the partner and the patient (60). According to Bryan's recent survey of 469 individuals participating in the Renal Dialysis Study in the USA (201 home patients and 268 facility patients) anxiety of the partner is not always a major problem. When it does exist, it is especially related to the possibility that the patient might die while undergoing treatment (60, 61). Even the long-lasting impact on the every day activities of the family is usually well tolerated. The most critical problem is the possible distortion of the proper relationship between the patient and the partner, probably favored by preexisting conditions of instability and aggravated by a difficult adjustment of the patient to dialysis (excessive dependence, aggressive behavior, depression), creating an excessive burden of responsibility for the partner. The results of the survey of Bryan (61) indicated that the psychosocial problems among the HHD patients and their families were in general well managed, and that a fair adjustment to them was usually achieved. As Bryan stated, 'the consequences of dialysis-related tensions and stresses do not result in an increased incidence of severe problems, in particular those which would be of such a nature as to promote divorce' (61). However, in another accurate Canadian study of the psychological factors influencing the success of 136 patients on HHD, 'inability of the spouse to cope' or 'other familial problems' were the major (28/35) causes of failure of the treatment (28). Among such familial problems, other causes of unavailability of the trained partner, such as death, chronic disease, new work activity or the necessity to move to another less suitable house must be considered.

CONCLUDING REMARKS

In conclusion, we believe that HHD is still a valid modality of treatment for ESRD. Even when the renal unit can provide a choice between many alternative strategies of treatment, such as hospital dialysis, limited care dialysis, self-service in-center dialysis, CAPD and CCPD, for as many as 30 to 35% of patients HHD is the preferable treatment, the one that gives the best clinical results with the maximal psycho-social freedom and rehabilitation and with the lowest cost for society.

The principal factor required for a good HHD program is a determined team of nephrologists and nurses who believe in the role of this dialysis strategy, are dedicated to it and are able to convince the potential candidates and their partners.

Young, moderately well-educated and cooperative adult patients with a cohabiting partner, (usually the spouse, the parents or a son) with suitable familial environment and a suitable house, are the ideal candidates for HHD, but children and elderly patients can also be successfully treated with HHD. The training must be primarily addressed to the patient, giving the patient an active role in performing the treatment and reducing psychological dependence on the partner, whose emotional involvement and responsibility are thus markedly less.

When selection and the training have been carried out correctly, clinical emergencies and serious technical mishaps at home are easily managed. Failure of HHD treatment due to familial stress of inability of the partner to cope are rather uncommon events. The major cause of definitive discontinuation of this form of treatment, usually after many years, is the development of severe clinical complications, increasing the risk of home treatment.

REFERENCES

1. Merrill JP, Schupak E, Cameron E, Hampers CL: Hemodialysis in the home. *JAMA* 190: 468, 1964
2. Curtis FK, Cole JJ, Fellow BJ, Tyler LL, Scribner BH: Hemodialysis in the home. *Trans Am Soc Artif Intern Organs* 11: 7, 1965
3. Baillod RA, Comty C, Ilahi M, Konotey-Ahulu FID, Sevitt L, Shaldon S: Overnight hemodialysis in the home. *Proc Eur Dial Transplant Assoc* 2: 99, 1965
4. Jenkins PG, Gutmann FD, Rieselbach RE: Self-hemodialysis. The optimal mode of dialytic therapy. *Arch Intern Med* 136: 357, 1976
5. Jacobs C, Broyer M, Brunner FP, Brynger H, Donckerwolcke RA, Kramer P, Selwood NH, Wing AJ, Blake PH: Combined report on regular dialysis and transplantation in Europe. *Proc Eur Dial Transplant Assoc* 18: 4, 1981
6. Editorial: Dialysis and Transplantation. *Med J Aust* 1: 102, 1981
7. Shimizu A: Dialysis in Canada today. *Int J Artif Organs* 4: 41, 1981
8. Department of Health, Education, and Welfare, ESRD Facility Survey System, Dec 31, 1978
9. Combined report on regular dialysis and transplantation in Europe, XVI, 1985. Presented at the 23rd Congress of the European Dialysis and Transplant Association, European Renal Association. Budapest, June 29, 1986
10. Rennie D, Rettig RA, Wing AJ: Limited resources and the treatment of end-stage renal failure in Britain and the United States. *Q J Med* 56: 321, 1985
11. Schmidt RW, Blumenkrantz M, Wiegmann TB: The dilemmas of patients treatment for end-stage renal disease. *Am J Kidney Dis* 3: 37, 1983
12. Gardner K: Profit and the end-stage renal disease program. *N Engl J Med* 305: 401, 1981
13. D'Amico G: Treating end-stage renal failure in Italy. in *Renal Failure. Who Cares?* edited by Parsons FM, Ogg CS: Lancaster, MTP Press Ltd, 1983, p 89
14. Robin-Tani M: Worldwide renal care. *Contemp Dial* (11): 50, 1983

15. Dunhan C, Mattern WD, McGaghie WC: Preferences of nephrologists among end-stage renal disease treatment options. *Am J Nephrol* 5: 470, 1985

16. Blagg CR, De Palma J, Jacobberger P: Home dialysis. *Dial Transplant* 2: 10, 1973

17. Deber R, Blidner L, Barnsley J, Uldall R: Choice of treatment: what factors are important? *Dial Transplant* 11: 1053, 1982

18. Smith M, Hong B, Michelman J, Robson A: Treatment bias in the management of end-stage renal disease. *Am J Kidney Dis* 3: 21, 1983

19. Baillod RA, Comty CM, Crockett R, Shaldon S: Experience with regular hemodialysis in the home. *Proc Eur Dial Transplant Assoc* 3: 126, 1967

20. Blagg CR, Daly SM, Rosenquist BJ, Jensen WM, Eschbach JW: The importance of patient training in home hemodialysis. *Ann Intern Med* 73: 841, 1970

21. Bailey GL, Hampers CL, Merrill JP, Paine PA: The artificial kidney at home: A look five years later. *JAMA* 212: 1850, 1970

22. Shapiro FL: Comprehensive regional approach to the chronic renal failure problem. *Perspect Biol* 13: 597, 1970

23. Bazzato G, Onesti G: *Hemodialysis in the Home*. Springfield, IL, CC Thomas Co 1975

24. Mion C, Issautier R: L'hémodialyse de suppléance à domicile: Un an d'expérience en Languedoc-Rousillon. (Hemodialysis conducted at home: an experience in Languedoc-Rousillon.) *J Urol Nephrol* 76: 358, 1970

25. Ackad A, Haimov M, Hering A, Schupak E: Subcutaneous arterial-venous fistula in home hemodialysis. *Trans Am Soc Artif Intern Organs* 16: 280, 1970

26. Wass VJ, Barratt TM, Howarth RV, Marshall WA, Chantler C, Ogg CS, Cameron JS, Baillod RA, Moorhead JF: Home hemodialysis in children. *Lancet* 1: 242, 1977

27. Levy NB: Psychological factors affecting long term survivorship on hemodialysis. *Dial Transplant* 8: 880, 1979

28. Richmond JM, Lindsay RM, Burton HJ, Conley J, Wai L: Psychological and physiological factors predicting the outcome on home hemodialysis. *Clin Nephrol* 17: 109, 1982

29. Shaldon S: Independence in maintenance hemodialysis. *Lancet* 1: 520, 1968

30. Baillod RA, Comty C, Ilahi M, Konotey-Ahulu FID, Sevitt L, Shaldon S: Overnight hemodialysis in the home. *Proc Eur Dial Transplant Assoc* 2: 99, 1965

31. Baillod RA: Home dialysis. in *Replacement of Renal Function by Dialysis*, edited by Drukker W, Parsons FM, Maher JF, 2nd edition, The Hague, Martinus Nijhoff, 1983, p 493

32. Philips SG: Adaptation of houses for home dialysis. *Br Med J* 1: 770, 1971

33. Kaye M, McDade D, Comty C: An appraisal of equipment for hemodialysis in the home. *Proc Eur Dial Transplant Assoc* 7: 56, 1969

34. Blagg CR, Peterson L: When is the best time to encourage patients for home hemodialysis and how do you deal with reluctance on their part? *Dial Transplant* 12: 759, 1983

35. Blagg CR, Daly SM, Rosenquist BJ, Jensen WM, Eschbach JW: The importance of patient training in home hemodialysis. *Ann Intern Med* 73: 841, 1970

36. Blagg CR: Home hemodialysis. *Am J Med Sci* 264: 169, 1972

37. Roberts JL: Analysis and outcome of 1063 patients trained for home hemodialysis. *Kidney Int* 9: 363, 1976

38. Roberts CM, Pavitt L: The value of a home dialysis nurse to a renal unit. *Proc Eur Dial Transplant Nurses Ass* 5: 27, 1977

39. Hampers CL, Hager EB: The delivery of dialysis services on a nationwide basis: can we afford the nonprofit system? *Dial Transplant* 8: 417, 1979

40. Blagg CR: Home dialysis costs less than outpatient dialysis. *N Engl J Med* 308: 431, 1983

41. Wing AJ: Choosing a dialysis therapy: narrative summary of a panel discussion. *Am J Kidney Dis* 4: 256, 1984

42. Rozenbaum EA, Pliskin JS, Barnoon S, Chaimovitz C: Comparative study of costs and quality of life of chronic ambulatory peritoneal dialysis and hemodialysis patients in Israel. *Isr J Med Sci* 21: 335, 1985

43. Wing AJ: Survival on integrated therapies. What assumptions shall we make? *Am J Kidney Dis* 4: 224, 1984

44. Capelli JP, Carniscioli TC, Vallorani RD, Bobeck JD: Comparative analysis of survival on home hemodialysis, in center hemodialysis and chronic peritoneal dialysis (CAPD-IPD) therapies. *Dial Transplant* 14: 38, 1985

45. Frascino JA: A comparison of self-care dialysis modalities. Home hemodialysis, continuous ambulatory peritoneal dialysis, in-center self-care dialysis. *Dial Transplant* 14: 13, 1985

46. Kramer P, Broyer M, Brunner FP, Brynger H, Challah S, Oulés R, Rizzoni G, Selwood NH, Wing AJ, Bolàa EA: Combined report of regular dialysis and transplantation in Europe. *Proc Eur Dial Transplant Assoc* 21: 2, 1984

47. Weller JM, Port FK, Swartz RD, Ferguson CW, Williams GW, Jacobs JF: Analysis of survival of end-stage renal disease patients. *Kidney Int* 21: 78, 1982

48. Williams GW, Weller JW, Ferguson CW, Forsythe SB, Wu S: Survival of endstage renal disease patients: age-adjusted differences in treatment outcome. *Kidney Int* 24: 691, 1983

49. Delano BG, Feiuroth MV, Feiuroth M, Friedman EA: Home and medical center hemodialysis. Dollar comparison and payback period. *JAMA* 246: 230, 1981

50. Remmers AR, Lindley JD, Cotton DL: Home dialysis a six year experience with 107 consecutive patients. *Trans Am Soc Artif Intern Organs* 20: 184, 1974

51. Walker PJ, Grim HE, Johnson K: Long term hemodialysis for patients over 50. *Geriatrics* 31: 55, 1976

52. Cestero RVM, Jacobs MO, Freeman RB: A regional end-stage renal disease program: twelve years experience. *Ann Intern Med* 93: 494, 1980

53. Baillod RA, Varghese Z, Fernando ON, Moorhead JF: Review of 71 patients receiving renal replacement for greater than 10 years, in *Uremia-Pathobiology of Patients Treated for 10 Years or More*, edited by Giordano C, Friedman EA, Milan, Wichtig Editore, 1981, p 35

54. Gross JB, Keane WF, McDonald AK: Survival and rehabilitation of patients on home hemodialysis a five year experience. *Ann Intern Med* 78: 341, 1973

55. Lindsay RM, Richmond J, Burton H, Conley J, Clark WF, Linton AL: Is home dialysis too stressful? *Controv Nephrol* 3: 395, 1981

56. Gurland HJ, Brunner FP, Dehn H, Härlen H, Parsons FM, Schärer K: Combined report on regular dialysis and transplantation in Europe. *Proc Eur Dial Transplant Assoc* 10: 15, 1973

57. Burton BT, Kruger KK, Bryan FA Jr: National Registry of long-term dialysis patients. *JAMA* 218: 718, 1971

58. Johnson WJ, Hathaway DS, Anderson CF, Carlson RA: Hemodialysis: Comparison of treatment in the medical center, community hospital, and home. *Arch Intern Med* 125: 462, 1970

59. Smith EKM, Curtis JR, McDonald SJ, de Wardener HE: Hemodialysis in the home: Problems and frustrations. *Lancet* 1: 614, 1969

60. Bryan FA Jr, Evans RW: Hemodialysis partners. *Kidney Int* 17: 250, 1980

61. Bryan FA Jr: The patient and family in home dialysis. *Controv Nephrol* 3: 406, 1981

INTERNATIONAL REVIEW OF RENAL REPLACEMENT THERAPY: STRATEGIES AND RESULTS

FELIX P. BRUNNER, ANTONY J. WING, SHEILA R. DYKES, HANS O.A. BRYNGER,
WINFRED FASSBINDER and NEVILLE H. SELWOOD

RENAL RECPLACEMENT THERAPY WORLDWIDE

Previous editions of this chapter have charted the expansion of renal replacement therapy (RRT). In 1976, we estimated that the global total of patients who owed their lives to an artificial kidney machine was 64,000 (1). By the close of 1980, there were approximately 150,000 patients alive on regular haemodialysis therapy, 37% of them in the USA, 33% in Europe, 24% in Japan and 6% in other countries. Functioning renal transplants gave life to approximately 37,000 patients, 49% of whom were in the USA, 35% in Europe and 16% in other countries. Continuous ambulatory peritoneal dialysis (CAPD), a treatment modality not available in 1976 supported around 7,000 patients by the end of 1980 (2).

Data have been drawn from various registries and personal commnications in order to assemble the best available information on the demography of RRT for this chapter. Achievements in 37 countries are known through centralised registries which record individual patients. The Australian Kidney Foundation sponsors a combined dialysis and transplant Registry for Australia and New Zealand (3). The Kidney Foundation of Canada runs the Canadian Renal Failure Register (4) and there is also a South African Dialysis and Transplant Registry (5). All these registries have adopted methodology based on that of the Registry of the European Dialysis and Transplant Association – European Renal Association (EDTA Registry) which has for 22 years published data from 32 countries in both Western and Eastern Europe and including territories around the Mediterra-

nean littoral (6). The Japanese Society for Dialysis Therapy now reports 88.4% of patients individually registered (7). Unfortunately, comparable demographic information is not available from the USA, but reports of the Health Care Financing Administration (HCFA) are thought to include around 80% of American dialysis patients (8), lacking patients treated in the Veterans Administration system, the military hospitals, the 7 to 10% who are not entitled to Medicare benefits and those who expired before the 3 month waiting period for Medicare entitlement. The proposed US Patient Registry should rectify this situation and provide a wealth of demographic and clinical information. Some preliminary data have been collected in South America but nothing is published about activity in Russia and, not surprisingly, there is very little RRT practiced in the third world.

By the close of 1986, the numbers of patients recorded by the registries plus an extrapolation from HCFA data for the USA amounted to some 330,000 patients on RRT worldwide, of whom 70% were on haemodialysis, 9% on peritoneal dialysis and 21% had functioning grafts. Of this total, the largest proportion, 37%, was in USA while Europe had 33%, Japan, 21% and the remainder, 9% (Table 1). It is unlikely that there are more than a few thousand patients treated in Russia and in the third world. By 1988, one may predict that almost half a million patients worldwide will be alive on RRT.

The rate of acceptance of new patients was highest in Japan at 117 patients per million population (pmp) with the USA HCFA sample representing 112 patients pmp. Rates in

Western Europe were little more than half these numbers (Table 2). There were seven European countries which accepted over 60 new patients pmp in 1986. Tranplantation rates were much below the rates for acceptance of new patients and exceeded 30 pmp in only ten countries and 40 pmp in just three Nordic countries.

EVOLUTION OF NATIONAL PROGRAMMES

Japan

Japan had 604 patients on dialysis per million of the total population of 121.7 million on 31 December 1986, the largest per capita number in any country; of these 73,537 patients, 97% were on haemodialysis (only 154 patients at home); the remainder on peritoneal dialysis (PD) (7). Numbers of Japanese dialysis patients increased by 10.9% in the year, and 9,735 had been on treatment for more than 10 years, of

Table 1. Numbers of patients alive on treatment per million population (pmp) 31 December 1986 (or 1985). Some figures were estimated (*) and those for Australia and New Zealand are at 31 October. Population figures are taken from the most recent World Bank Atlas (16).

Country	Patients pmp							
	Haemodialysis		Peritoneal dialysis		Functioning graft		Total live patients	
	1986	(1985)	1986	(1985)	1986	(1985)	1986	(1985)
Japan	587		17		NA		604	
USA	321		59		170		550	
Switzerland	187		43		176		405	
Belgium	243		18		129		392	
Luxembourg	274		3		107		384	
Israel	223		72		86		381	
France	225		20		100		345	
Canada	115		61		165		341	
Fed Rep Germany	274		10		55		339	
Spain	239		20		78		337	
Sweden	118		30		180		328	
Netherlands	147		32		140		319	
Italy	240		27		37		304	
Cyprus	212		0		87		299	
Australia	104		40		150		294	
Austria	200		6		86		292	
Portugal	245		3		23		271	
Finland	60		41		169		270	
Denmark	108		46		113		267	
Norway	49		9		203		261	
New Zealand	70		51		128		250	
United Kingdom	71		51		118		240	
Ireland	70		18		107		195	
Greece	140		20		35		195	
Yugoslavia	166		6		20		192	
Iceland	29		50		79		158	
German Dem Rep	113		1		36		150	
Bulgaria	124		< 1		4		128	
Uruguay		(116)		NA		NA		
Czechoslovakia	75		< 1		31		107	
Hungary	48		5		17		70	
Brazil	55*		7*		8*		70*	
South Africa	23		11		36		70	
Tunisia	59		3		2		64	
Poland	30		2		15		47	
Libya	24		0		6		30	
Turkey	18		1		8		26	
Egypt	21		1		4		26	
Algeria	16		2		4		22	
Morocco	15		< 1		1		16	

whom three patients had survived for over 20 years and a further 632 for over 15 years. Centralised records of transplantation in Japan are not available but activity is small despite the vast number of patients on dialysis.

Figure 1 shows how the unrelenting expansion of hospital haemodialysis has been made possible by the growth of facilities with almost one station for every two patients. At the close of 1986, there were 1,745 centres in Japan (14.3 pmp), this representing an increase of 10% on the previous year's figure. Over 34,000 staff were involved with the care of these patients: 6,218 doctors (of which 23% worked whole time in dialysis), 14,984 nurses (78% whole

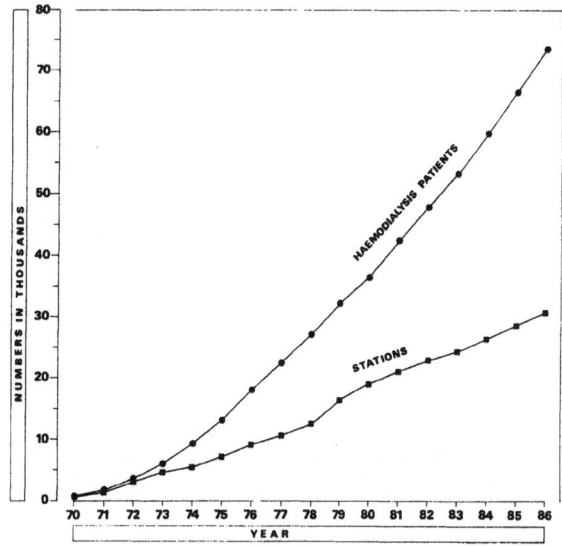

Figure 1. Numbers of chronic dialysis patients and of stations in Japan, 1970 to 1986. Data of the Japanese Society for Dialysis Therapy.

time), 2,884 technicians (17% whole time), 2,308 nurse assistants (72% whole time), 3,310 dialysis technicians (82% whole time), 2,264 dietitians (20% whole time), 547 social workers (14% whole time) and 1,565 others (73% whole time) (7).

United States of America

The contribution of the different methods of dialysis to the US end-stage renal disease (ESRD) programme is shown in Figure 2, derived from HCFA data (8). In-unit haemodialysis was still the fastest growing method of therapy although home peritoneal dialysis (90% CAPD) was making an increasing contribution.

Home haemodialysis declined steadily from its early popularity (40% of all haemodialysis patients) prior to commencement of the Medicare ESRD programme in July 1973 to 12% in 1978. Despite enactment of Public Law 95-292 on 1 October 1978 which removed perceived disincentives to home dialysis the proportion on home haemodialysis continued to fall and was less than 6% of the total in 1985.

The extension of Medicare benefits had other effects on the demography of the patient population in the USA. Age distribution shifted so that the proportion of patients aged over 55 increased from 7% in 1967 to 45% in 1978 (9) and by 1986 patients aged over 60 comprised 52% of new enrolments under the HCFA. The proportion of blacks increased progressively and accounted for 26% of 26,654 newly enrolled HCFA patients in 1986 compared to 11% of the general population. Thus Medicare has brought about important advances in access to medical services, although treatment has never been equally distributed throughout the USA (10).

Total Medicare reimbursements amounted to US $1,876

Table 2. Numbers of new patients and of transplant operations per million population (pmp) during 1986 (or 1985). Countries listed according to the rank order of Table 1.

Country	New patients pmp		Transplants pmp	
	1986	(1985)	1986	(1985)
Japan	117		NA	
USA	112		38	
Luxembourg	85		14	
Belgium	74		30	
Austria	70		36	
Canada	66		34	
Fed Rep Germany	66		27	
Switzerland	65		40	
Cyprus	62		0	
Sweden	60		42	
Norway	59		41	
Israel	58		22	
Denmark	56		44	
Greece	54		6	
Uruguay		(53)	NA	
Spain	51		23	
Portugal	50		9	
Italy	49		4	
Netherlands	48		30	
United Kingdom	47		29	
France	44		24	
Australia	44		27	
Finland	44		29	
New Zealand	38		31	
Yugoslavia	37		6	
Iceland	37		0	
Bulgaria	37		< 1	
German Dem Rep	35		10	
Ireland	33		28	
Czechoslovakia	27		10	
Tunisia	19		1	
Hungary	16		5	
Algeria	15		< 1	
Poland	13		7	
Egypt	12		2	
South Africa	11		11	
Turkey	9		3	
Libya	6		0	
Morocco	5		< 1	

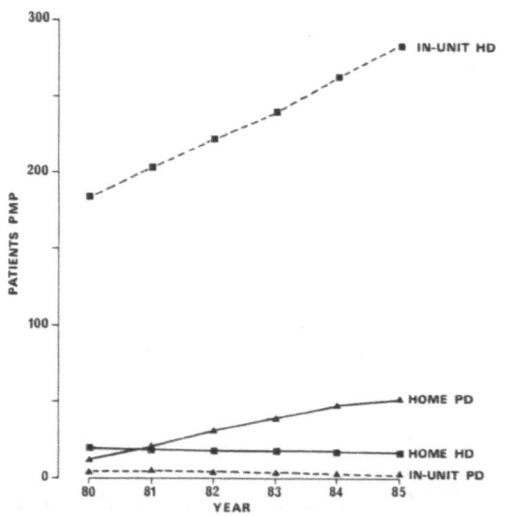

Figure 2. Contribution of different modes of dialysis to ESRD programme in USA, 1980 to 1985. HCFA Medicare programme data.

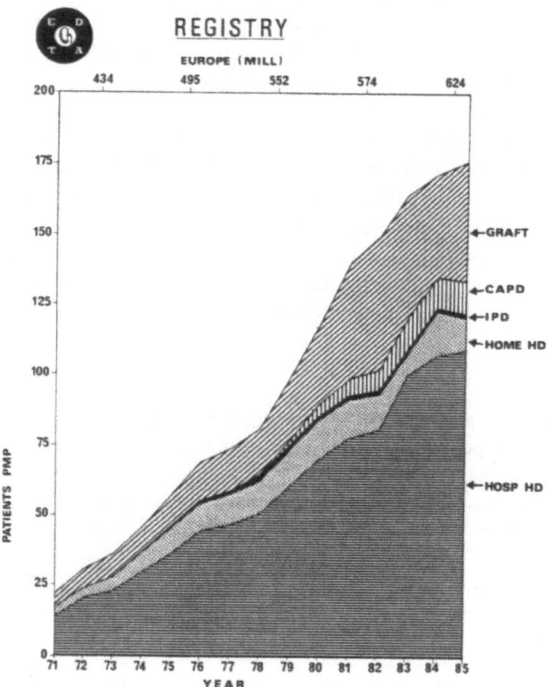

Figure 3. The EDTA Registry: Growth in numbers of live patients per million population on 31 December 1971 to 1985, according to their method of therapy.

million in 1985 for 103,997 enrolled patients but the annual rate of growth in expenditure which had been 58% in the first year of Medicare funding slowed to 14% between 1982 and 1983 and, according to preliminary figures, showed little increase thereafter. Per capita expenditure was relatively stable problably due to the original rates being set too high and to the introduction of dialyser re-use and lower cost equipment (11). The steady numerical increase in transplants performed in the Medicare population has also helped to restrain the per capita reimbursements (12).

Transplantation has made a large contribution in USA, and grafting reported to HCFA reached 32 and 38 pmp in 1985 and 1986 respectively. In 1986, 21% of the grafts were from live donors. Black patients were under-represented, accounting for only 20% of transplanted patients in 1986, and 75% of all transplants were done in whites. By the close of 1985, 9,354 patients were on the waiting list for a cadaver graft, equivalent to 11% of dialysis patients and the annual percentage change from 1980 to 1985 was +13.1%. Of 8,574 cadaver kidneys harvested in 1985, 5% were not used. A total of approximately 85,000 renal transplant operations had been performed in the USA by the end of 1985 and some 35,000 patients were alive with functioning grafts at that time.

Europe

The EDTA Registry has been collecting data from European centres since 1965. Included in this survey are 33 countries with a total population of 624 million (6). The largest proportion of patients has been treated by hospital haemodialysis; the contribution of home haemodialysis is waning and those of CAPD and of renal transplantation are becoming increasingly important (Figure 3).

Different patterns have emerged in different countries and six contrasting programmes are shown in Figure 4. Belgium had accumulated 392 live patients pmp by the close of 1986 using hospital haemodialysis provided in 6.0 centres pmp backed up by very little home haemodialysis or CAPD but on which a successful transplant programme has been based.

In the Federal Republic of Germany (FRG) and France there has been a similar expansion of haemodialysis which, in both cases, has included a significant but declining input from home haemodialysis. In the FRG, home haemodialysis, used for 21% of haemodialysis patients in 1979, has been largely replaced by economically efficient minimal care centres; only 6% of patients were dialysing at home in 1986. In France 17% of haemodialysis patients treated themselves at home in 1979, 16% in 1986. There were 5.4 centres pmp in FRG and 3.9 pmp in France. France had the more active CAPD programme; this modality has not proved popular in the FRG. In both these countries transplantation, previously restricted to a limited number of centres is becoming more widely available and in the FRG 20% of dialysis patients were on a waiting list for a cadaver graft on 31 December 1986 and in France 16%.

The German Democratic Republic (GDR) with a population of 16.7 million has the most advanced programme in Eastern Europe with 3.2 centres pmp providing basically two modes of therapy, hospital haemodialysis and renal transplantation. The parallel increase in patients on these

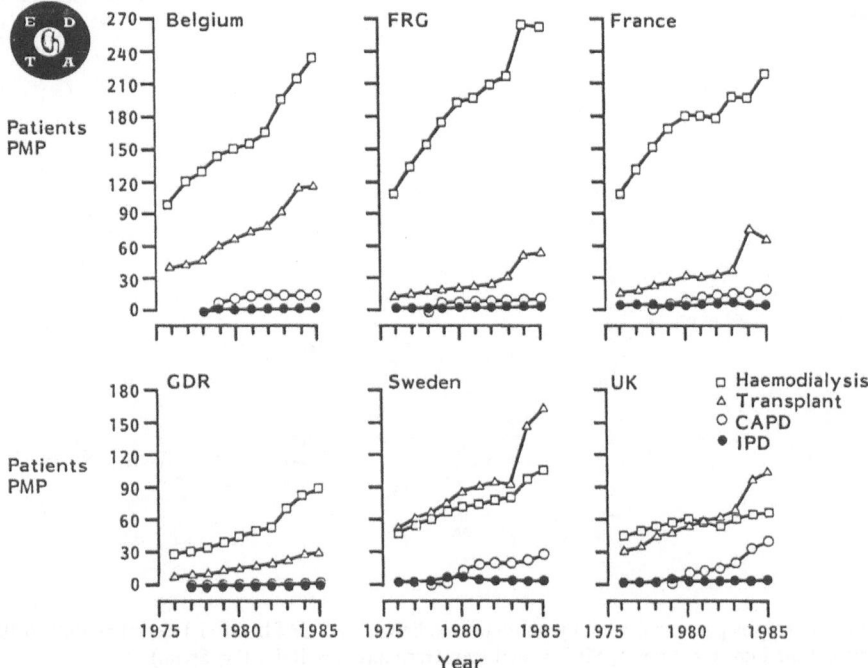

Figure 4. Patterns of development of treatment programmes in six European countries. Numbers of patients on haemodialysis, IPD, CAPD and with a functioning transplant per million population are shown for 31 December 1975 to 1985.

two treatments suggests that they were geared together and that most patients commencing dialysis were selected as also being suitable for renal transplantation. However, only 28% of GDR dialysis patients were on a cadaver graft waiting list, although in all other Eastern European countries the proportion was larger.

Sweden, like Denmark, Norway and Finland, has had an objective of early transplantation of patients since the early years and in all these countries the numbers of patients alive with a functioning graft were greater than those on any other form of therapy. In Sweden 29%, in Denmark 23%, in Norway 39% and in Finland 32% of dialysis patients were on a cadaver graft waiting list. The Scandinavian countries now regularly achieve an annual transplant rate of 40 pmp. Finland and Denmark used almost exclusively cadaveric kidneys while the proportions of living donors were 20% in Sweden and 45% in Norway in 1986.

Treatment in the United Kingdom (UK) has been constrained by the small number of centres which reached only 1.2 pmp in 1986. Thus, firstly home haemodialysis and, secondly CAPD found favour as modes of independent dialysis which relieve pressure on the overfull centres. During the 1970s two thirds of UK haemodialysis patients treated themselves at home. This has decreased since the advent of CAPD (Figure 5) and was down to 47% by the close of 1986. Meanwhile CAPD has soared ahead to 40% of all dialysis patients, becoming first choice therapy particularly for older patients and for those with diabetes or cardiovascular diseases (13). Transplantation remains the single most impor-

tant mode of therapy in the British Isles and Ireland and 45% of dialysis patients in UK and 55% in Ireland were on a waiting list for a cadaver graft on 31 December 1986. Because patients are selected for suitability for transplantation and independent dialysis, there has been a tendency to exclude the elderly from treatment in UK (Figure 6).

Australia and New Zealand

The well documented programmes in these two countries with small widely scattered populations are of particular interest. In 1985 to 1986 the numbers of patients kept alive by functioning transplants in both of these countries overtook the numbers of patients on all forms of dialysis combined (Figure 7). This has been achieved because of early implementation of a transplant orientated programme and with transplantation rates of 27 pmp in Australia and 31 pmp in New Zealand supporting a new patient acceptance rate of 44 pmp and 38 pmp respectively.

Central and South America

There were 131 centres serving a population of 130 million in Brazil in 1983 (14). Representatives of the Brazilian Society of Nephrology estimated the total number of patients on dialysis at 8,000 at the close of 1986 and, although approximately 2,500 renal transplants had been performed over 20 years, the number of patients alive with functioning grafts could only be guessed.

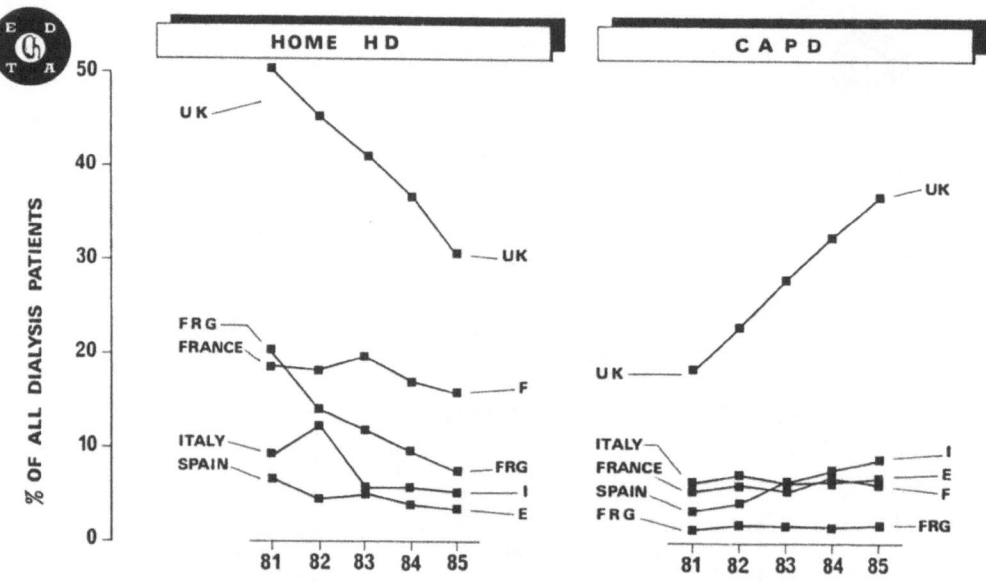

Figure 5. Proportion of all dialysis patients treated by home haemodialysis and CAPD on 31 December 1981 to 1985 in five European countries (UK = United Kingdom, F = France, FRG = Fed Rep Germany, I = Italy, E = Spain).

Uruguay has the most advanced programme in South America with a total of 350 patients on haemodialysis (116 pmp) in 1985 and a new patient acceptance rate of 53 pmp for the population of 3 million.

In Cuba a cumulative total of 744 renal transplants had been reported from five centres by 1985 with 259 added in the last 5 years, and 230 stations were available for dialysis to serve the population of 10 million.

South Africa

There were 34 centres in South Africa and Namibia in 1985 which achieved a new patient acceptance rate of 12 pmp, comprising rates of 34 pmp in South African caucasoids, 26 pmp in Cape Coloureds, 20 pmp in Asiatics and 5 pmp in South African Negroes (5). Total living patients amounted to 812 on dialysis (32% on PD) and 713 alive with functioning grafts.

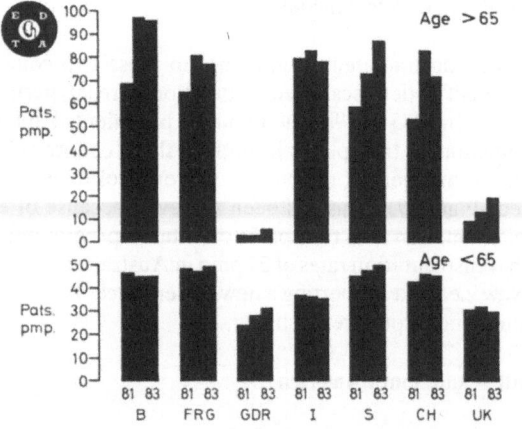

Figure 6. Age specific acceptance rate of new patients aged more than 65 (upper panel) and less than 65 (lower panel) in relation to population age structure in seven countries, 1981 to 1983 (B = Belgium, FRG = Fed Rep Germany, GDR = German Dem Rep, I = Italy, S = Sweden, CH = Switzerland, UK = United Kingdom).

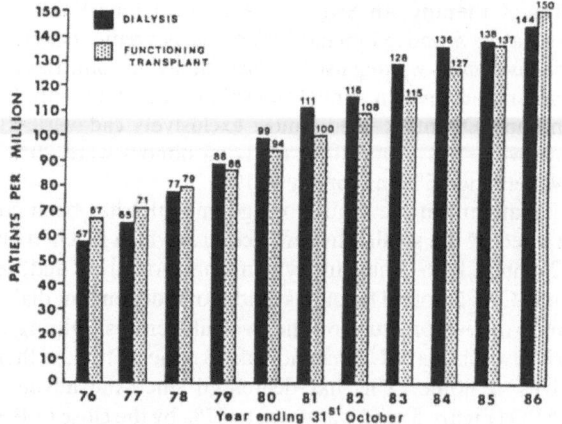

Figure 7. Numbers of patients per million population treated by dialysis and by functioning transplants in Australia on 31 October 1976 to 1986. ANZ data.

TREATMENT STRATEGIES

Two countries with contrasting treatment strategies are compared in Figure 8, FRG (upper panel) and UK (lower panel). Within each country the cohort of patients who commenced RRT in 1977 is compared with the 1982 cohort. Each patient was entered in the analysis at the date of his first treatment. Patient survival, shown at the top of each panel, was calculated for RRT irrespective of any transitions between therapies. The proportional contribution of the different methods of treatment was approximated by con-

structing the areas from 3-monthly analyses. In other words, the areas illustrate the probability of a single patient in the cohort being on any one of the different methods of treatment (15).

Strategy in the FRG is dominated by in-centre haemodialysis and the probability of a patient changing to home haemodialysis was smaller for the 1982 cohort than for the 1977 cohort. A small contribution was made by CAPD to the treatment of the 1982 cohort, and the probability of a patient being transplanted was small. In the UK, 29% of the 1977 cohort began with intermittent peritoneal dialysis

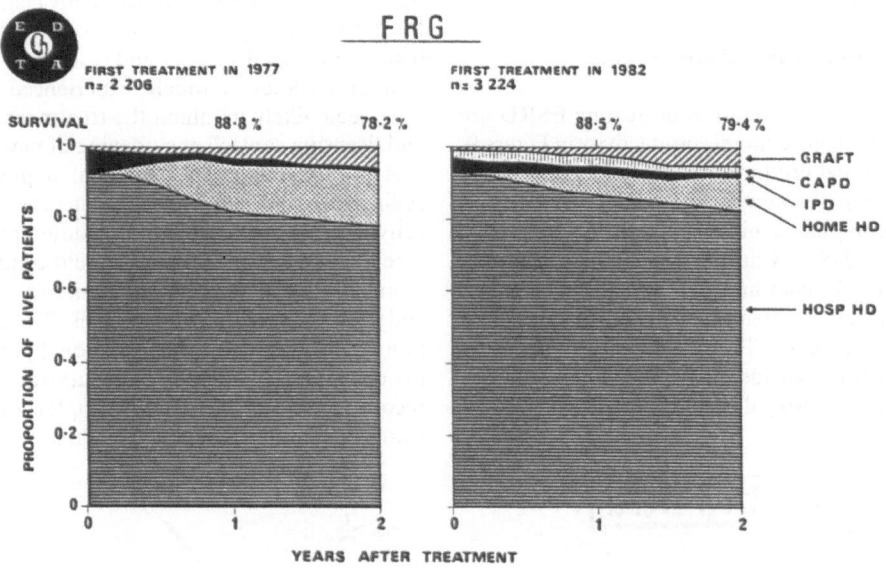

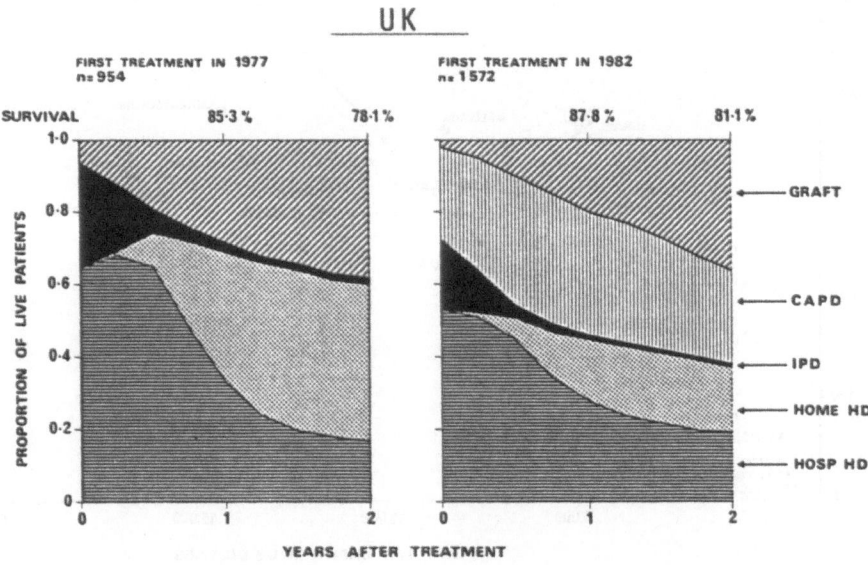

Figure 8. Proportional contribution of different modes of therapy to overall survival in patients who commenced RRT in 1977 and 1982 in Fed Rep Germany (upper panel) and United Kingdom (lower panel). (See text for full description of method of calculation).

(IPD) and over 45% of the 1982 cohort began with IPD or CAPD. By 2 years after first treatment 43% of the 1977 cohort were on home haemodialysis but only 18% of the 1982 cohort. Less than 10% of either cohort started with a transplant but 38% of the 1977 cohort and 35% of the 1982 cohort were grafted by the end of their first 2 years RRT. Overall patient survival on the two strategies was similar for the two 1977 cohorts and also for the two 1982 cohorts, but the selection of patients for treatment was not likely to be the same and therefore the contribution of high risk patients to the two programmes was probably not equal. Since maintenance of a renal transplant in the less expensive mode of therapy, the cost per patient per year works out lower in UK than in FRG (15).

Economic constraints on national programmes

Achievements of different countries in treating ESRD are shown in relation to their economic productivity in Figure 9. Data on gross national products (GNP) were provided by the World Bank (16). The numbers of patients surviving on RRT (Table 1) correlate significantly with the per capita GNP expressed in US $. Canada, Switzerland, Sweden, Denmark, Norway, Iceland and Libya treated below one standard deviation fewer patients than their respective GNP would seem able to support. This could indicate that these countries have a lower incidence of ESRD than Japan, Israel, Cyprus, Spain, Portugal and Yugoslavia which treat-

ed over one standard deviation more patients than would be predicted from their GNP. The intercept of the regression line, at US $1,661, suggests that it is difficult, or possibly even inappropriate for countries with a GNP lower than this to put many patients on treatment. None of the countries included in Table 1 has a per capita GNP of $400 or less, but more than half of the world's population lives in countries whose economic productivity is below this level (16), and there is every reason to believe that the incidence of ESRD is higher in these poorer countries of the South.

RRT is expensive life preserving therapy; a patient's opportunity of survival depends on the economic status of the country into which he is born. Developing countries have other medical priorities which rightly claim their resources. Most countries appear to be uncomfortably aware of the high cost of renal services and restriction of further expansion of facilities is widely experienced. Reimbursement rates seem likely to inhibit the treatment of high risk cases and licensing controls the opening of new facilities.

Arbitrary limitations of patient numbers or of budget ceilings are alternative mechanisms for containing clinical activity which are available under different systems of health care. The resulting pressures should conduce to more economic choices in the sphere of equipment and staffing ratios and of overall treatment strategies. The more transplantation contributes to a local or national programme, the less the cost of each patient-year of survival. It is interesting to record in the statistics in this chapter a growing trend towards increased transplantation rates.

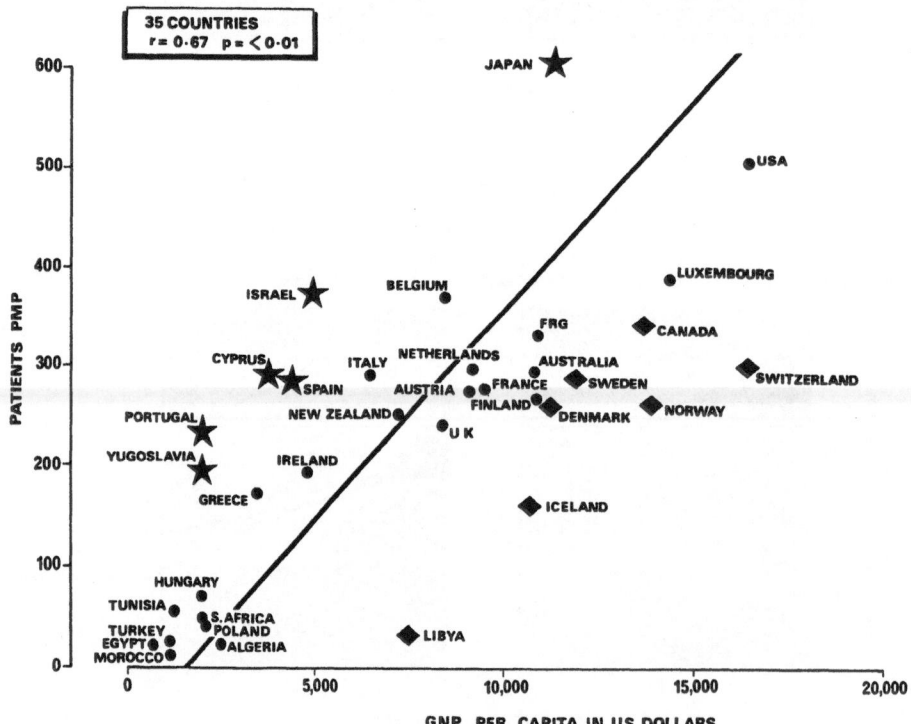

Figure 9. Correlation between number of patients alive on treatment of ESRD (Table 1) and GNP using data provided by the World Bank (16).

Haemodialysis strategies

Progressive shortening of haemodialysis treatment occurred during the 1970s and by 1980 three 4-h sessions had become the norm in most centres. The EDTA Registry recorded this change in practice and related it to the following factors: time of dialysis, frequency of dialysis, country of treatment, choice of haemodialyser, residual renal function and body weight (17).

The most important factor in reducing dialysis hours was the introduction of the arteriovenous fistula bringing with it pumped haemodialysis which ensured good blood flow and therefore efficient dialysis throughout the session. Staffing convenience accelerated the demise of long overnight treatments. In most countries clinicians appear to have been persuaded that three times a week treatment is superior to twice a week. As Figure 10 shows many patients who dialysed twice a week received only 8 h dialysis per week. This figure also suggests that 4-h or 5-h sessions were chosen for convenience and that a physician may prescribe shorter dialysis hours not by shortening the thrice weekly sessions but by changing to twice weekly treatments. By 1984 only 13% of patients dialysed twice a week and 63% of these were on treatment in a small group of countries: Netherlands, France, UK, Egypt and Eastern European countries.

There were also distinct national differences in dialyser preferences. Kiil-type of non-disposable dialysers have almost disappeared (Figure 11) but were still used by 2% of French and British patients. Parallel flow disposable dialysers were used by 28% of European patients but by over 40% of those in Denmark, Finland, Iceland, Ireland, Italy, Libya and UK. Coil dialysers have declined in popularity since the late 1970s but were still used by over 60% of patients in Czechoslovakia, Lebanon, Poland and Turkey. Capillary (hollow fibre) dialysers now hold the greatest share of the market. There were 260 different capillary dialysers appearing under 23 brand names in Europe in 1986. In Japan, 97% of 900,382 dialysers used in December 1986 were hollow fibre type (7). Despite the current interest in dialyser re-use

in the USA only 12% of European centres practiced this in 1985 and only in Bulgaria, Poland and UK did more than one third of centres report this practice.

We have observed a trend for some patient variables to affect dialysis schedules. In 1979 we studied the effect of residual renal function (gauged by residual urine volume) and found in pooled European data that the mean dialysis time in anuric patients was just over 2h/week more than in those with a daily urine volume over 1,000 ml. Analysis of the relationship between dialysis time and patients' body weight in pooled data showed very little adjustment except when patients at the extremes of body weight (1 to 39 kg versus 90 to 129 kg) were compared.

More striking differences emerged when national practices were compared (Figure 12). Twice weekly dialysis (upper panel) was very likely to result in less than 10 h of dialysis per week in FRG, Italy and Spain but French and British pa-

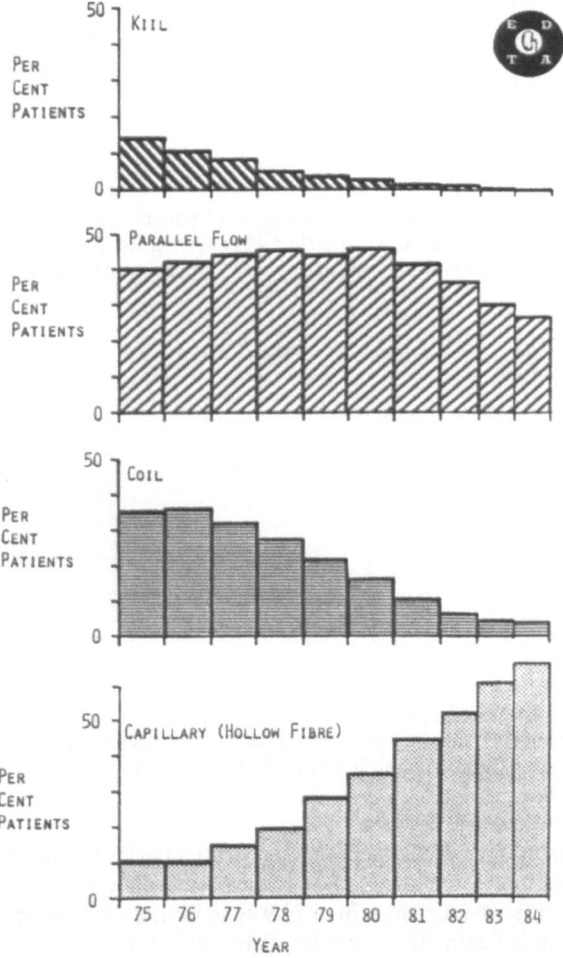

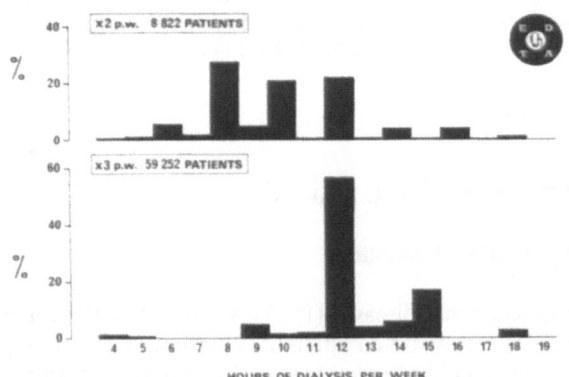

Figure 10. Frequency of distribution (%) of hours per week hospital haemodialysis in patients who dialysed twice per week and thrice per week in 1984.

Figure 11. Proportion (%) of patients using each of four main types of dialyser, 1975 to 1984. Data was obtained by asking for the dialyser most commonly used for each patient during each year.

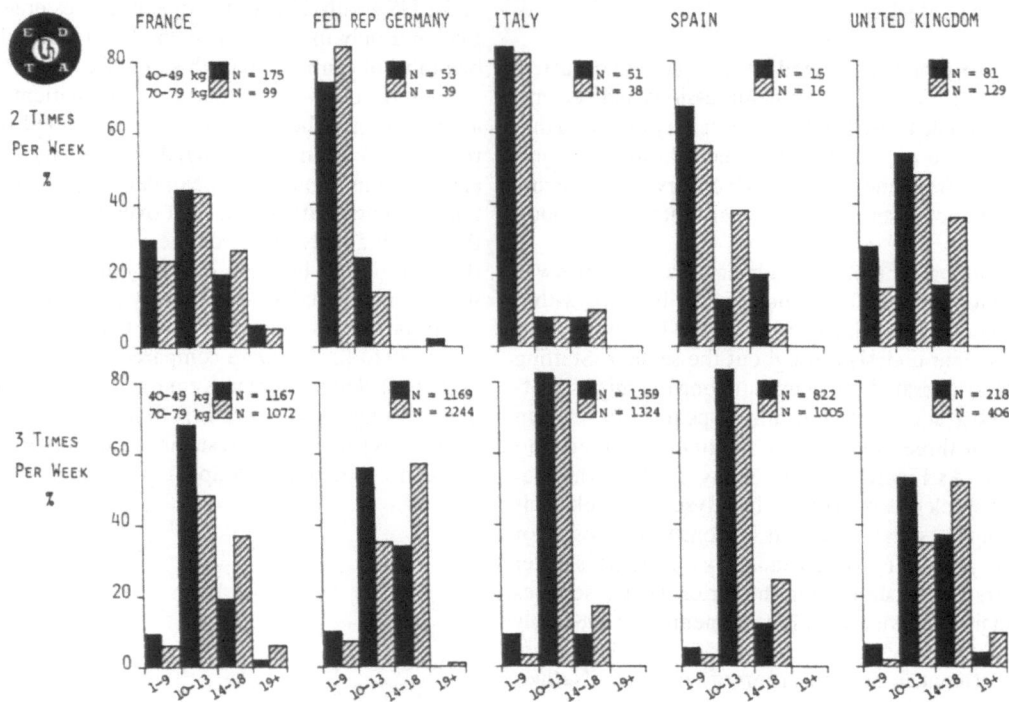

Figure 12. Proportional distribution of patients according to weekly duration of haemodialysis (hospital or home) in five European countries. Patients who weighed 40 to 49.9 kg are compared with those who weighed 70 to 79.9 kg and the numbers of patients in each of these cohorts is shown in each panel. Upper row of panels is patients dialysed twice, and lower row, those dialysed three times per week.

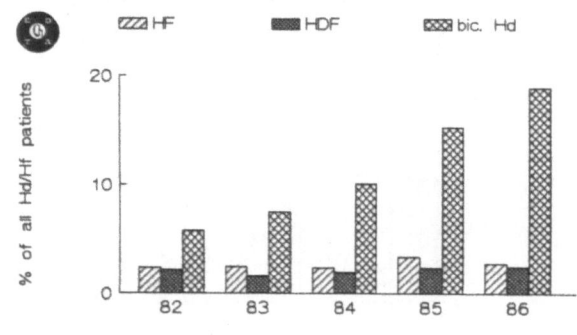

Figure 13. Proportion (%) of all haemodialyses/haemofiltration patients treated by haemofiltration, haemodiafiltration and bicarbonate haemodialysis in Europe in 1982 to 1986.

tients received longer treatment. Patients who weighed 40 to 49.9 kg were more likely to receive fewer dialysis hours than those who weighed 70 to 79.9 kg in France and Britain but not in Spain. Thrice weekly dialysis (lower panel) appeared to consist mostly of three 4-h sessions especially in Italy and Spain and to a lesser extent in France. In FRG and UK a greater proportion received upwards of 14 h per week and in these two countries hours were more likely to be adjusted according to the patients' weight (the distribution of heavier

patients is shifted to the right in Figure 12 compared to the distribution of lighter patients).

We conclude that selection of patients for different haemodialysis schedules is influenced not only by patient variables but also by such considerations as staffing convenience and local fashions (17).

Of the newer techniques of blood purification, haemofiltration and haemodiafiltration have not become fashionable in Europe, but bicarbonate haemodialysis has increased over the past 5 years and up to 19% of patients were treated by this method in 1986 (Figure 13). In Japan 57.6% of 73,537 dialysis patients received bicarbonate haemodialysis in 1986 (7).

PRIMARY RENAL DISEASE

Geographical variations

Primary renal diseases (PRD) diagnosed as the cause of ESRD vary between different countries. However, apparent geographical variations must be interpreted with caution.

First, the range of diagnostic possibilities on the registration documents is not strictly comparable. HCFA enrolment offers six main classifications and 10% of patients have no diagnosis recorded (8). The Japanese Registry has 21 PRD (7) and there is no opportunity for the clinician to admit his ignorance and record an equivalent of 'chronic renal failure, aetiology uncertain' which is selected as the working diagnosis for an increasing percentage of patients on the EDTA Registry, and for a much larger percentage of elderly cases (Table 3 and Figure 14). These and other detailed differences make it difficult to compare the reports

Table 3. Primary renal diseases in new patients commencing treatment in 1985 according to two age categories, 15 to 64 and 65 and over. EDTA Registry data.

Causes of end-stage renal failure	Age at start of renal replacement therapy, 1985 (%)	
	15-64	*65 and over*
Chronic renal failure, aetiology uncertain	14.0	21.2
Glomerulonephritis		
– histologically not examined	16.5	9.3
– histologically examined	10.7	3.7
Pyelo – interstitial nephritis		
– cause not specified	9.4	12.1
– associated with neurogenic bladder	0.4	0.1
– due to congenital obstructive uropathy with of without vesico-ureteric reflux	1.5	0.3
– due to acquired obstructive uropathy	1.3	3.1
– due to vesico-ureteric reflux without obstruction	1.4	0.2
– due to urolithiasis	2.6	3.3
– due to other cause	0.5	0.3
Nephropathy		
– caused by drugs or nephrotoxins – cause not specified	0.1	0.3
– due to analgesic drugs	2.4	4.3
Cystic kidney disease – type unspecified	2.0	1.3
Polycystic kidneys		
– adult type	6.8	4.3
– infantile and juvenile types	0.1	0
Medullary cystic disease, including nephronophthisis	0.2	0
Hereditary/familial nephropathy	1.6	0.3
Hereditary nephritis with nerve deafness (Alport's syndrome)	0.6	0.1
Cystinosis	< 0.1	0
Oxalosis	0.1	< 0.1
Renal vascular disease		
– type unspecified	1.9	6.2
– malignant hypertension (no primary renal disease)	1.8	0.8
– hypertension (no primary renal disease)	4.1	8.1
– polyarteritis	0.3	0.5
Wegener's granulomatosis	0.2	0.2
Diabetes		
– insulin dependent (type I)	8.6	6.5
– non-insulin dependent (type II)	2.4	4.9
Myelomatosis	0.7	2.1
Amyloid	1.6	1.8
Lupus erythematosus	1.0	0.2
Henoch-Schönlein purpura	0.3	0.1
Goodpasture's syndrome	0.4	0.2
Scleroderma	0.2	0.3
Haemolytic uraemic syndrome (Moschcowitz syndrome)	0.2	< 0.1
Multi-system disease – other	0.3	0.4
Cortical or tubular necrosis	0.3	0.3
Tuberculosis	0.7	0.9
Gout	0.6	0.7
Nephrocalcinosis and hypercalcaemic nephropathy	0.2	0.2
Balkan nephropathy	0.6	0.2
Kidney tumour	0.3	0.5
Traumatic or surgical loss of kidney	0.2	0.2
Other identified renal disorders	0.6	0.5
Total patients with diagnosis available	15,877	4,594

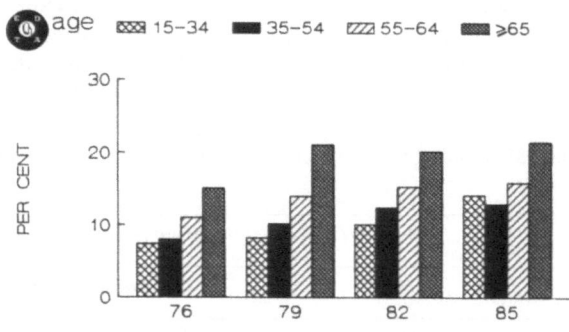

Figure 14. Proportion (%) of new patients commencing RRT in 1976, 1979, 1982 and 1985 who were diagnosed als having 'chronic renal failure, aetiology uncertain' according to age ranges 15 to 34, 35 to 54, 55 to 64 and 65 or over.

of the large registries. Furthermore, all registries bear a heavy responsibility for forcing their correspondents into a mould of nosology which may not be flexible enough to accommodate developing clinical insights.

Second, patients accepted for treatment do not represent the incidence of all the causes of ESRD because of selection. Probably all patiens who wish it are treated in the USA and Japan but in Europe lower acceptance rates (Table 2) imply variation in selection. This is immediately obvious when the age specific selection rates are compared (Figure 6), but it is also possible that patients with certain diseases are preferentially excluded; for example, diabetic patients or those with severe cardiovascular problems because of medical contraindications and those with analgesic nephropathy because of psychological unsuitability.

Thirdly, bias may be introduced by local diagnostic fashions. The diagnosis of chronic pyelonephritis (or interstitial nephritis) is probably made on different clinical criteria in different European countries but it still accounts for 15 to 25% of cases (Table 3). However, in Australia only 1% of patients were diagnosed as pyelonephritis whereas reflux and analgesic nephropathies together accounted for 18 to 28% of new patients in the years 1982 to 1985 (3).

Age of treated population

Increasingly liberal policies for selection of patients for RRT result in a change in the proportional contributions of causes of ESRD to the population accepted for treatment. More patients with diabetes and hypertension and even with malignant disease such as myeloma have been included in recent years (Table 3).

In Japan the average age of 12,565 new patients in 1986 was 55.1 years and 55% were diagnosed as having chronic glomerulonephritis (average age 52.9 years) and 21% as diabetes (average age 58.8 years) leaving small proportions allocated to other diseases with, for example, only 3% said to have cystic kidney disease (7).

New HCFA enrolments in 1986 numbered 26,654 and

7,664 of these (29%) had diabetes mellitus with other complications; 26% of the diabetic patients were black and 30% were aged 60 to 69. The second largest group comprised patients with hypertension with heart and renal diseases (24%) and 38% of these were black and 41% were aged over 70 (70% over 60) (8). Only 31% of Medicare ESRD patients were aged less than 50, 52% were aged over 60.

The Canadian Renal Failure Register has documented that the growth in patient numbers in recent years is due chiefly to an increased acceptance of elderly cases (4). The age specific acceptance rate of patients aged 45 to 64 increased from 106.1 to 126.8 pmp from 1981 to 1986 whereas the rates for 65 to 74 year olds and for over 75 year olds rose from 151.1 to 238.2 pmp and from 84.7 to 138.4 pmp respectively over the same 5 year period. During this period the proportional contribution of glomerulonephritis diminished slightly whereas those of renal vascular diseases and of diabetes increased, comprising 14% and 20% respectively of new patients starting treatment in 1986. More than half of the patients aged over 65 had renal vascular diseases.

Amongst 700 patients who commenced treatment in Australia between 1 November 1985 and 31 October 1986 (44 pmp) 42% were aged less than 50 and 30% over 60 (3). There were lower frequencies of hypertension (9%) and diabetes (6%) than included in North American and Japanese patient intakes, but analgesic nephropathy (19%) and polycystic kidney disease (9%) figured prominently. These differences reflect not only the high incidence of analgesic nephropathy in Australia but also the effect of a transplant orientated policy on non-selection of elderly patients with vascular disease and diabetes.

Causes of ESRD in Europe

European data on PRD has been used to show (Table 3) the more detailed breakdown of clinical diagnoses available on the EDTA Registry and the different proportional contributions in young adults (15 to 55) and elderly (over 65) patients. Geographical variations have been demonstrated in analgesic nephropathy which is still frequent in Switzerland and Belgium, in Balkan nephropathy and in diabetes in Nordic countries.

It is characteristic of analgesic nephropathy that it occurs in local pockets of high incidence, often close alongside areas of relative freedom from the disease. Figure 15 compares the age specific acceptance rates for females during the 3 years 1981 to 1983 in Belgium and France. Each 10 year age cohort is considered separately and the contribution of new patients with analgesic nephropathy is shown in black. Higher take-on rates in Belgium compared to France in each age group are accounted for by patients suffering the results of analgesic abuse. The low rate of recognition of analgesic nephropathy in France does not seem to be due to a failure of diagnosis and it is probable that the French habit of using a higher proportion of single compound analgesics is safer than the mixed compounds found across the border and over the counter in the market places of Belgium.

Nordic countries report a higher incidence of ESRD due

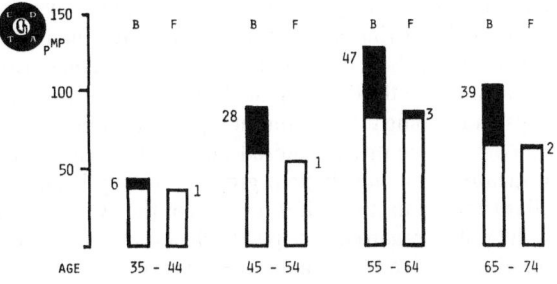

Figure 15. Analgesic nephropathy: age specific acceptance for RRT in females 1981 to 1983 in Belgium (B) and France (F) showing the increment due to analgesic nephropathy shaded black on top of the rates for all other diseases in four age groups, 35 to 44, 45 to 54, 55 to 64 and 65 to 74.

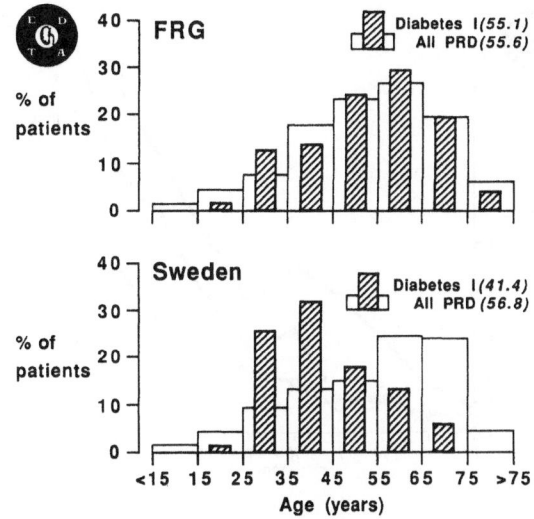

Figure 16. Diabetes: age distribution and median age of patients who commenced RRT in 1983 to 1985 in Fed Rep Germany and Sweden to compare age distribution of insulin dependent diabetes (type I) and all PRD in these two countries.

to diabetes in young patients than is found in the rest of Europe. Figure 16 compares the age distribution of insulin dependent (type I) diabetes in the FRG and Sweden. In the FRG the distribution follows the pattern for all PRD with a peak incidence between 55 and 65 (median age 55.1) but in Sweden it is shifted to the left with a peak incidence between 35 and 45 (median age 41.4). The explanation does not appear to lie in any difference in selection practice or in the nomenclature of disease. It appears that there is some genetically or environmentally determined factor which renders Nordic patients more likely to develop the serious long-term consequences of type I diabetes at an earlier age than patients in other countries do.

In Europe, as in North America the increased acceptance of elderly patients includes a growing proportion with hypertensive and vascular diseases. This is illustrated by Figure 17 which shows the age specific acceptance rate from 1974 to 1983 for patients aged over 65 in Belgium, Italy and FRG. These patients represent high risk cases for whom survival expectations are limited and who cannot look forward to the prospect of transplantation without considerable hazard.

COMPARATIVE SURVIVAL STATISTICS

The life-table method for calculation of patient survival rates was first used in American cancer research programmes (18–21). The method was applied to dialysis and transplanted patients in 1969 (22) and used to compare dialysed and transplanted patients in 1970 (23). Since then innumerable studies have been published on groups of patients from single or multiple centres and comparing a wide variety of factors which might influence survival. Unfortunately, the life-table method has often been used uncritically and applied to unallowably small patient samples. If results are to be meaningful from an actuarial point of view, the group from which survival rates are calculated must include at least 20 deaths and cumulated survival statistics must not be extended beyond the time interval with the last death. The advantage of survival calculations based on a single centre is that patient selection criteria are likely to be

more uniform than in a combined study. However, not only patient selection criteria but also bias regarding a wide variety of factors, may be more uniform. What would appear to be right for one centre may be wrong for others. The so-called 'centre effect' was studied in the United Kingdom where delivery of health care through its National Health Service can be assumed to be more uniform and consistent than in other countries. Nevertheless, death rates for patients on any form of therapy varied more than three-fold between centres, and first cadaveric graft survival at 2 years ranged from 82% in the 'best' to 20% in the 'worst' centre (24).

For these reasons the following discussion has been restricted mainly to survival calculations of the EDTA Registry which continues to be the largest international venture of collecting and providing data on patients with end-stage renal failure on combined treatment programmes by any form of dialysis and renal transplantation. Table 4 summarizes survival on any single or combination of modes of renal replacement therapy for all patients recorded by the EDTA Registry who started treatment in 1980 to 1984 and 1970 to 1984 (25). It should be noted that many patients with end-stage renal disease who have survived beyond the 15 year mark, have benefited from integrated treatment of dialysis and transplantation. At the end of 1985 there were more than 2,000 patients on the files of the EDTA Registry who had lived longer than 15 years on renal replacement therapy. Of these, 34% were treated by in-centre haemodialysis, 11% by home haemodialysis, 2% by continuous peritoneal dialysis and 52% had a functioning graft. This percentage of transplanted patients is probably an underestimate of the true proportion of patients with long-lasting functioning transplants, since some of the largest European transplant centres have failed to report their patients to the EDTA

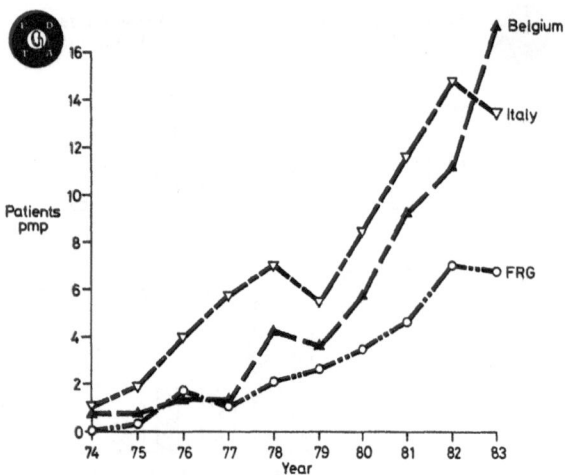

Figure 17. Hypertensive/vascular disease: age specific acceptance rate for patients aged over 65 with hypertensive/vascular diseases as the cause of ESRD in Belgium, Italy and Fed Rep Germany, 1974 to 1983.

Registry. It can be safely assumed, therefore, that the percentage of patients with a fuctioning graft 15 or more years after starting renal replacement therapy was between 70 and 100% in Northern European countries, UK and Ireland, Benelux countries, Switzerland and Austria.

Some of the factors that determine patient survival are discussed below. The major factor is age at start of treatment. Of some importance are primary renal disease and method of treatment. Sex has little, if any, influence on survival on renal replacement therapy.

Survival as related to age at start of treatment

Age at start of treatment plays a decisive role in determining survival on all forms of dialysis as well as for living donor and cadaver transplantation (Table 4) (25). The best survival rates have been achieved in paediatric patients aged 10 to 14. Younger children have higher death rates and only 70% of the 0 to 4 year cohort as compared to 85% of the 10 to 14 cohort starting renal replacement therapy in the early 1980s survived for 5 years or more.

After childhood there is a steady decrease in survival rates with increasing age. Thus, in the early 1980s 5 year survival decreased from 80% or above in patients below 35 years, to barely 50% in the 55 to 64 year age group, and less than a third of those aged over 65 survived the 5 year mark. Of those commencing renal replacement therapy in the early 1970s there remained almost 50% of the young adults but less than 10% of the 55 to 64 cohort who survived up to 15 years.

Survival as related to the method of treatment

Survival for patients on home haemodialysis has usually been superior to survival on hospital haemodialysis and survival with a living donor transplant better than with a cadaveric transplant (1, 23). However, such comparisons must be unfair to the different methods, because the patient groups undergoing these different types of treatment are far from comparable or randomised nor do they carry similar risk factors for dying. Patient groups on dialysis and with similar transplants may differ because of the availability of, and the policy regarding recipient selection for renal transplantation. Active transplantation of low risk patients may remove good risk patients from the haemodialysis group leaving the poor risk patients on dialysis. Conversely, there may be selection of poor risk patients for the transplanted group if transplantation is used as a way of no return for patients doing extremely poorly on dialysis.

Selection of patients partly explains better results observed in the home dialysed group. Clinical selection criteria include absence of 'high risk' medical complications, good nutrition and social conditions plus, usually, a well motivated partner. Further selection occurs because of the mortality of the early months of dialysis in the hospital required for stabilising and training before patients commence home dialysis. Deaths during this period count as death on hospital dialysis and effectively select out some high risk patients from entering home dialysis programmes. Social, psychological or medical reasons compelling home patients to return to hospital dialysis might also select out a group at higher risk of dying. Furthermore, home haemodialysis is barely available or non-existent in some countries and the proportional contribution of home haemodialysis may vary considerably among centres and regions in other countries. For all of these reasons, no seperate survival figures are shown for patients on home haemodialysis. Rather, periods of home haemodialysis were included in the calculation of survival of the first haemodialysis shown in Table 4. With the vast majority of patients on renal replacement therapy having undergone treatment by haemodialysis, it comes as no surprise to find very similar survival rates on the first haemodialysis as observed after start of any form of renal replacement therapy.

Until the late 1970s, peritoneal dialysis had been used as a definitive treatment for a small number of patients only, the majority of them concentrated in a few centres with specialised interest in this form of treatment. With the advent of CAPD a dramatic increase in the use of the peritoneum as dialysis membrane has occurred. One group of Canadian authors have proposed that up to 50% of patients with end-stage renal failure might be suitable for CAPD (26), and in the early 1980s the majority of young diabetic patients have been started on CAPD in many European centres (27). Little can be said about patient survival on CAPD as compared to other methods of treatment. Selection of patients for either haemodialysis or CAPD has not been randomised. Local preference, availability of facilities, anticipated complications with vascular access or diabetes mellitus often determined whether a patient was started on CAPD rather than haemodialysis. Conditions which might have been associated with definite differences is mortality were thus likely to be distributed unevenly between patients on CAPD as compared to haemodialysis (13). In fact, a much higher proportion of diabetic patients have been treated with CAPD which was the first method of renal replacement therapy in over 50% of Finnish, British and Swiss patients with end-stage renal failure due to diabetes, who commenced renal replacement therapy in 1983 to 1985 (27). Furthermore, many patients who started renal replacement therapy with CAPD were subsequently transplanted (Great Britain and Nordic countries) or changed over to haemodialysis, which resulted in rapidly decreasing numbers of live patients at risk. Nevertheless, survival rates on CAPD were quite satisfactory as shown in Table 4 (25).

For renal transplantation, survival calculations must distinguish between patient and graft survival. Patient survival is defined as the period beginning with the day of the transplant operation until either the day of the death of the patient or the conclusion of the period of observation. This may include periods of dialysis or re-transplant after the first transplant has ceased to function. Graft survival is defined as the period beginning with the day of the transplant until either transplant failure (including death with functioning transplant) or the conclusion of the period of observation.

Patient and graft survival rates have improved between the early 1970s and the 1980s regarding both cadaveric and living donor transplantation. The improvement is particularly striking for patient survival after cadaveric transplantation (Table 4). This is not only due to the tremendous decline in the risk of dying during the early post-operative period but also results from a lower mortality at any time beyond the first months after grafting (25). It should be stressed again that this mortality includes all deaths, also those occurring at any time after graft failure, i.e. on dialysis after a failed graft or after regrafting. Taking all these deaths

Table 4. Patient survival on renal replacement therapy for patients commencing treatment in 1980 to 1984 compared to those starting 1970 to 1974. An asterisk (*) denotes less than 30 patients at risk.

Methods of treatment Age groups	Starting 1980–84			Starting 1970–74			
	n	2 yr %	5 yr %	n	5 yr %	10 yr %	15 yr %
All treatments combined							
0– 4	297	80	70	34	*	*	*
5– 9	676	87	82	182	51	43	*
10–14	1,404	91	85	570	69	58	52
15–34	18,972	88	80	9,404	65	54	48
35–44	15,048	84	70	7,073	55	41	28
45–54	21,866	81	61	7,160	48	28	16
55–64	21,885	74	49	3,251	37	14	*
65+	16,562	61	31	584	25	7	*
On first haemodialysis (including haemofiltration, home haemodialysis)							
0–14	1.894	91	82	733	69	60	*
15–34	16,858	89	80	9,060	68	58	51
35–44	13.252	86	71	6,843	59	45	31
45–54	19,507	83	63	6,907	52	31	17
55–64	18,919	77	53	3,099	39	15	*
65+	13,217	65	35	549	27	7	*
After CAD first graft							
0–14	911	91	86	191	67	57	*
15–44	12,794	91	83	4,396	61	49	39
45–64	6,161	81	67	1,837	40	24	15
65+	173	71	53	7	*	*	*
After LD first graft							
0–14	268	95	92	77	78	69	*
15–44	1,913	93	87	766	75	65	56
45+	229	83	72	88	63	47	*

On first CAPD (including CCPD) starting 1981–84	n	2 yr %	4 yr %
0–14	452	90	*
15–44	3,082	88	74
45–64	5,399	74	54
65+	2,403	57	30

into account, patient survival rates in all age groups have, nevertheless, risen above those of the never grafted dialysis population as a whole. Several explanations are conceivable. Some lethal complications encountered in dialysed patients might no longer occur with a successful transplant, or conversely, transplantation might be performed in a selected physically fitter dialysis population that would have a better survival despite transplantation. The latter might be particularly pertinent to explain the excellent survival rate of graft recipients above the age of 65.

The age dependence of survival on renal replacement therapy in general is also apparent in patient and graft survival after cadaveric as well as living donor transplantation. However, the impact of recipient age on graft survival has become much smaller in recent years (25) compared to the early 1970s (28). In the early 1980s average graft survival rates at one year for first cadaver grafts were 69% for recipients below 45 compared to 67% for those above 45, and 51% for the younger compared to 46% for the older age group at 5 years. The number of grafts lost due to rejection was earlier shown to be similar in all age groups (28). It was the frequency of non-immunological complications including death with a functioning graft, that increased in parallel with rising age. The decreasing impact of age on graft survival in recent years may be due, in part, to the lower steroid regimens prescribed and in part to selection policies which include more high risk patients amongst the young and fewer high risk patients amongst the elderly.

The best survival rates have traditionally been achieved in patients who were lucky enough to receive a graft from a living related donor. More than half of those transplanted in the early 1970s have survived to the 15 year mark and in more than a third of them this first living donor graft was still functioning (25). In the early 1980s paediatric recipients of living donor first grafts had a 5 year graft survival of 61% despite the fact that no more than 5% of grafts came from HLA-identical siblings whilst 94% were donated by their parents. The proportion of parent donors obviously cannot but decrease with rising age of the recipients and was 58% in the 15 to 44 and 20% in the older than 45 cohort. HLA-identical sibling donors accounted for 29% and 53% of the 15 to 44 and 45+ cohort respectively. Living related donors other than identical or haploidentical were used rarely and accounted for some 2% of grafts performed in 1980 to 1984 on the EDTA Registry's files (25).

Patient survival after second grafts is quite comparable to that found after first grafting (25), whilst average graft survival rates for cadaveric second transplants (but not for living related donor second grafts (25)) have usually been found to be slightly lower than for first transplants and drastically reduced for third and fourth grafts (25, 28–30). Cadaveric third grafts performed between 1980 and 1984 had an immediate failure of 10% and graft survival was no higher thant 52% at one and 47% at 2 years (25). Bad prognostic signs for re-transplants are early loss by rejection of the previous graft (25, 30–33) and the formation of cytotoxic antibodies after a failed graft (30, 32). However, excellent graft survival has been obtained in second grafts when the first graft functioned for more than one year (25, 30–33), and also in third grafts when the second graft functioned for more than one year (34).

Renal transplantation has come a long way and patient survival rates not only for living related but also for cadaveric transplantation have reached a quite satisfactory level. It no longer seems true that the prospect of a better quality of life with a functioning transplant would have to be balanced against a markedly increased risk of an early death after transplantation. Long-term survival in end stage renal failure appears to be improved not only by living related donor, but also by cadaveric transplantation.

Survival as related to primary renal disease

Little difference in patient survival was recorded when groups with the common primary renal diseases such as glomerulonephritis or pyelonephritis were compared in the early 1970s (35). This has not changed in recent years as shown in Table 5 regarding patients on the EDTA Registry's files commencing renal replacement therapy in 1980 to 84. Some 80% of patients with glomerulonephritis, pyelone-

Table 5. Patient survival according to primary renal disease in patients commencing RRT in 1980 to 1984.

Primary renal disease Age groups	Male			Female		
	n	2 yr %	5 yr %	n	2 yr %	5 yr %
Glomerulonephritis						
15–44	9,271	89	80	4,342	88	78
45–64	6,640	82	60	2,907	81	62
Pyelo-Interstitial Nephritis						
15–44	2,852	88	79	2,801	90	79
45–64	3,722	78	55	4,372	81	60
Cystic Kidney Diseases						
15–44	961	91	81	710	95	86
45–64	2,621	86	66	2,722	90	73

phritis or interstitial nephritis survived to the 5 year mark in the age group 15 to 44 and 60% in the age group 45 to 64 at start of renal replacement therapy. Patients with polycystic kidney diseases had slightly better survival which was particularly evident in females with polycystic kidney diseases aged 45 to 64.

Systemic diseases (Table 6) including diabetic nephropathy, primary hypertension and malignancies, which cause end stage renal failure, increase the risk of dying on renal replacement therapy in comparison to the common primary renal diseases (25, 29, 36–38). This is particularly true for the large population with diabetic nephropathy, which comprised 8 to 16% of patients commencing renal replacement therapy in 1985 in the majority of European countries and has reached a proportion of 20 to 30% in Sweden and over 30% in Finland. Young diabetic patients succumbed at three times the annual death rate of patients with standard primary renal diseases (chronic renal failure aetiology uncertain, glomerulonephritis, pyelo-interstitial nephritis, toxic nephropathy, cystic kidney diseases) of the same age and no more than 50% survived the 5 year mark (25). Lower survival is also obtained in patients with amyloidosis and with vasculitides which include polyarteritis and Wegener's granulomatosis. The outcome of chronic renal failure in scleroderma remains grim with 43% of 82 patients having died within one year after starting renal replacement therapy in 1980 to 1984. In contrast, patients treated for end stage renal failure due to lupus erythematosus appear to fare quite well: their survival rates were comparable to those of patients with the common primary renal diseases. Cystinosis, and to some extent oxalosis, not infrequently lead to end-stage renal failure in paediatric patients. Survival of patients with cystinosis was similar to that of patients with standard primary renal diseases and graft survival was even better than average with 80% of grafts still functioning at one year, which confirms the earlier finding of diminished immunological responsiveness in cystinotic patients (39). Patients with primary oxalosis aged up to 25 at start of renal replacement therapy in 1980 to 1984 had annual mortality rates

between 10 and 20% and 11 of 18 cadaveric grafts were lost within the first year. However, the outlook for patients with primary oxalosis may soon change for the better with correction of the enzyme defect by liver transplantation.

CAUSES OF DEATH

The EDTA Registry has traditionally asked clinicians to record the 'main cause of death' in patients on renal replacement therapy. The percentage of the most frequently recorded causes of death and some conditions peculiar to patients on certain forms of renal replacement therapy are shown in Table 7 for deaths which have occurred in 1981 to 1985.

Cardiovascular causes of death

Cardiovascular causes have been held responsible for the demise in 52.6% of patients dying whilst undergoing maintenance dialysis and in 36.8% of those dying with a functioning graft. Cardiac arrest (including that due to hyperkalaemia) and cardiac failure (due to hypertension, over-hydration and other causes) were less frequently recorded in grafted patients for obvious reasons. A relatively high proportion of deaths in grafted patients were related to coronary artery disease and pulmonary embolism. The proportions of cardiac causes of death varied markedly according to age (Table 8), whilst most other causes of death were recorded with similar percentages across the age groups. Paediatric patients rarely, if ever, died due to myocardial infarction and ischaemia, but a high percentage succumbed to cardiac failure and cardiac arrest. The proportion of deaths due to coronary artery disease increased with age, whilst that due to cardiac failure and cardiac arrest decreased with rising age.

Myocardial ischaemia and infarction

Coronary artery disease has long been recognised as a leading cause of death in patients on renal replacement therapy. Compared to the general population, coronary deaths were over 100 times more frequent in renal patients aged 15 to 35 and some 10 times more frequent in those aged over 55 (36). Lindner and colleagues (40) suggested that the high death rate due to coronary artery disease would accelerate even further with time on maintenance dialysis. This could not be confirmed by the EDTA Registry at least for the first 5 years after starting haemodialysis or with a functioning cadaveric first graft (36). The worst group regarding coronary artery disease are patients on renal replacement therapy as a result of diabetic nephropathy. In these diabetic patients, the proportion of deaths due to myocardial ischaemia and infarction was 17.6% and did not vary with age. The mortality due to coronary artery disease in young diabetic patients on renal replacement therapy was thus found to be at least 10 times higher than in patients with standard primary renal diseases, if the three times higher annual death rate of

Table 6. Patient survival of those patients with systemic diseases as cause of end stage renal failure and who commenced RRT in 1980 to 1984.

Systemic disease Age groups	Number of patients	2 yr %	5 yr %
Diabetic Nephropathy			
15–44	2,678	66	44
45–64	3,739	57	25
65+	1,240	42	13
Amyloidosis			
15–44	399	71	52
45–64	776	51	25
Lupus erythematosus	830	79	65
Vasculitides	487	65	43

diabetic patients is taken into account.

Excessive interdialytic weight gain was found to raise mortality due to cardiac causes in patients on haemodialysis as shown in Figure 18. This excess mortality did not result from a higher rate of myocardial ischaemia and infarction or cerebrovascular accident. It was mainly due to cardiac failure from over-hydration or hypertension and cardiac arrest due to unknown cause or hyperkalaemia.

Cerebrovascular accident

This has also long been noted as a frequent cause of death in renal patients. We compared the death rate from cerebro-

vascular accident in patients on renal replacement therapy to that of the general population in France, where this cause of death has been recorded at an intermediate rate among the large European countries. Compared to the population of France, patients on renal replacement therapy older than 55 had a death rate from cerebrovascular accident which was some 20 times, those aged 35 to 54 years some 50 times and those aged 15 to 34 some 250 times higher than the general population (36). In 1981 to 1985, the proportion of deaths due to cerebrovascular accident was lower in patients dying with a functioning graft (Table 8). However, it varied little with age and with primary renal disease. Between 10% and 12% of deaths in patients on dialysis were attributed to

Table 7. Proportional distribution (%) of causes of death in patients who died 1981 to 1985 on dialysis or with a functioning graft. Only data for patients with standard primary renal diseases (chronic renal failure aetiology uncertain, glomerulonephritis, pyelo/interstitial nephritis, toxic nephropathy, cystic kidney diseases) have been included.

	On dialysis		With functioning graft	
Myocardial ischaemia and infarction	12.3		16.8	
Cardiac arrest	12.9		4.5	
Cardiac failure	14.1		4.6	
Haemorrhagic pericarditis	1.3		0.1	
Pulmonary embolus	1.1		3.3	
Cerebro-vascular accident	10.9		7.5	
Total cardiovascular causes		52.6		36.8
Septicaemia	6.8		11.8	
Generalised viral infection	0.2		2.2	
Pulmonary infection (bacterial, fungal, viral)	3.4		9.0	
Tuberculosis	0.5		0.7	
Other infection	1.0		1.9	
Total infectious causes (excluding hepatitis)		11.9		25.6
Hepatitis B	0.9		2.1	
Other liver diseases	1.7		4.6	
Pancreatitis	0.6		1.6	
Haemorrhage	4.1		5.6	
Mesenteric infarction	0.5		0.3	
Peritonitis (including perforation of bowel)	2.1		1.4	
Sclerosing (or adhesive) peritoneal disease	0.2		–	
Malignant disease due to immunosuppression	0.3		4.9	
Other malignant disease	4.8		2.7	
Suicide	0.7		1.1	
Therapy ceased	1.9		0.4	
Accident	1.0		0.9	
Other causes	6.4		5.1	
Uncertain/not determined/unknown	9.3		6.9	
Number of deaths	25,904 = 100%		2.172 = 100%	

Table 8. Proportion (%) of cardiac causes of death in ungrafted patients with standard primary renal diseases, 1981 to 1985.

Age at death	Number of deaths	Myocardial ischaemia and infarction	Cardiac arrest	Cardiac failure	Haemorrhagic pericarditis
<15	133	1.5	19.6	28.6	3.8
15–44	3,625	5.8	16.6	20.7	3.0
45–64	12,058	14.1	12.5	13.4	1.4
65+	8,233	13.2	11.8	12.4	0.4

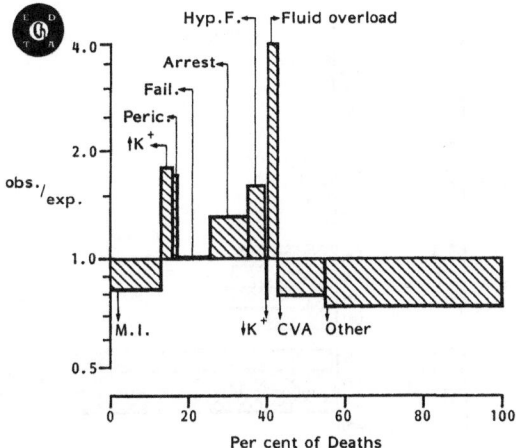

Figure 18. Ratio of observed to expected deaths in 1984 amongst patients reported with excessive interdialytic weight gain in that year. The analysis was based on patients who commenced treatment between 1975 and 1984 with standard primary renal diseases. Cardiac and vascular causes of death are shown as follows: myocardial infarction and ischaemia (MI), hyperkalaemia ($\uparrow K^+$), haemorrhagic pericarditis (Peric.), other causes of cardiac failure (Fail.), cardiac arrest cause unknown (Arrest), hypertensive cardiac failure (Hyp.F.), hypokalaemia ($\downarrow K^+$), fluid overload and cerebrovascular accident (CVA). Other causes of death are grouped together. The figure also shows the frequency distribution of the different causes of death in 1984.

cerebrovascular accident, and this was just as true for the paediatric as for the younger up to the oldest adult groups. The proportion of cerebrovascular deaths in patients with diabetic nephropathy was also 11% and did not differ between young and old diabetics. Although the proportion of cerebrovascular deaths was similar comparing diabetic patients to those with other primary renal diseases, the absolute rate of death due to cerebrovascular accident was at least three times higher in young diabetics, in keeping with the much higher overall mortality in this unfortunate group of patients. As expected for adult polycystic kidney disease, there was a slightly higher proportion (15.3%) of deaths attributed to cerebrovascular accident in polycystic patients on dialysis.

Infectious causes of death

One price to be paid for a successful transplant is an increased susceptibility to infectious complications. It comes as no surprise, therefore, that the proportion of infectious causes of death has been higher in grafted patients (Table 7). This was particularly evident in the early phase after grafting (36). However, the percentage of deaths due to septicaemia and pulmonary infections was no higher in patients who died after their graft had been functioning for more than 2 years compared to patients undergoing maintenance dialysis.

Malignancies

Malignancies possibly induced by immunosuppressive therapy are rare in patients on dialysis but have been the cause of death in almost 5% of the patients with standard primary renal disease who died with a functioning graft in 1981 to 1985 (Table 7). The proportion of deaths due to any other malignancy was higher in patients on dialysis which is easily explained by the higher mean age of the dialysis population and possibly also by non-selection for transplantation of patients with malignancies. Cancer deaths in patients with standard primary renal diseases accounted for 2.1% of total deaths in non-grafted patients below the age of 45 and 5.6% in those dying above the age of 45. Malignancy was given as the cause of 15% of deaths in patients with acquired obstructive pyelonephritis and in 7.5% with analgesic nephropathy. Diabetic patients with their high mortality due to cardiovascular diseases had a low proportion of deaths due to malignancy amounting to 1.0% only.

Sclerosing peritoneal disease

Sclerosing peritoneal disease, although rare, has been a devastating and often lethal complication of peritoneal dialysis (41). Following a report that exposure to chlorhexidine might be responsible (42), the EDTA Registry conducted a retrospective case control study comparing exposure to a large variety of sterilising agents and drugs as well as prevalence of infectious peritonitis (43). Exposure to no other agent or drug but chlorhexidine for sterilising tubing connections was highly significantly associated with the development of this devastating condition. It was suggested that use of chlorhexidine for sterilising the tubing connection should be abandoned. Hopefully, sclerosing peritoneal disease will thus disappear or become extremely rare in the not too distant future.

DISABLING BONE AND JOINT DISEASE

Disabling bone disease (defined as bone pain requiring regular analgesics, fracture(s), major deformity, aseptic necrosis and slipped epiphysis) was found to develop in 10 to 20% of patients after more than 5 years on renal replacement therapy and appeared to be less frequent in patients with a functioning graft (29). Apart from renal osteodystrophy which can be controlled or improved with vitamin D metabolite therapy, phosphate binders and parathyroidectomy, the syndrome of β_2 microglobulin amyloidosis associated bone and articular disease has been recognised recently (44–46). Beta-2-microglobulin amyloidosis appears to develop in the majority of patients on long-term dialysis and was suggested to be related to the low β_2 microglobulin clearance of the artificial kidney. In fact, the commonly used cellulosic membranes do not remove β_2 microglobulin or may even raise its serum level during dialysis. It was hoped that the more permeable polyacrylonitrile or polysulfone dialysers which allow removal of β_2 microglobulin and regularly lower its serum levels were going to prevent or retard the development of β_2 microglobulin amyloidosis (47). The EDTA Registry, therefore, conducted a retrospective case control study comparing dialysis on polyacrylonitrile dialysers to controls on cuprophan. To be included in the study, the cases had to have spent more than 10 years on haemodialysis and to have used polyacrylonitrile dialysers for more than the most recent 5 years at least. Random controls on cuprophan were picked from the files of the Registry at 31 December 1985. Of the cases and controls combined 65% were reported to suffer from joint pain in 1987. Polyacrylonitrile cases seemed to fare slightly better than cuprophan controls. However, no statistically significant differences could be detected between the 51 cases and controls regarding the prevalence of pain, carpal tunnel syndrome, radiological signs such as periarticular bone cysts and erosive polyarthropathy, as well as regarding histological proof of amyloid deposition. Hence, convincing evidence as to whether or not highly permeable polyacrylonitrile or polysulfone membranes are of value in retarding β_2 microglobulin amyloidosis has yet to be provided.

Parathyroidectomy

Control of renal osteodystrophy improves quality of life in patients on RRT. However, conservative measures not infrequently fail, and surgical parathyroidectomy may become necessary in an appreciable proportion of patients not only on maintenance dialysis but also after grafting. Hence, the EDTA Registry analysed the incidence and the prevalence of a first parathyroidectomy (48). In 1983, the overall incidence of a first parathyroidectomy was 12/1,000 patients at risk and the prevalence 42/1,000 patients alive at the end of the year. Parathyroidectomy was much more frequently performed in patients on dialysis as compared to those with a functioning graft. With increasing time on dialysis, the incidence of a first parathyroidectomy rose from some 5/1,000 annually in the first 2 to 3 years on dialysis to over 40/1,000 in patients who had spent 10 years or more on maintenance dialysis. Accordingly, the prevalence of having undergone a first parathyroidectomy rose with increasing time on dialysis from about 5/1,000 at the start of renal replacement therapy (parathyroidectomy performed before initial therapy for end-stage renal failure) to 200 to 250/1,000 after 10 years or more on dialysis. The highest prevalence was noted in Great Britain and in the Nordic countries where about half the patients never grafted had undergone a first parathyroidectomy after 10 or more years on dialysis. Primary renal disease appeared to influence the frequency of this operation to a small extent only. Thus the incidence and the prevalence of a first parathyroidectomy were similar in patients with glomerulonephritis and with pyelonephritis or interstitial nephritis (Figure 19). However, parathyroidectomies were performed much less frequently in patients with diabetic nephropathy as expected from the strikingly lower severity of hyperparathyroid bone disease reported for diabetic patients receiving haemodialysis (49).

The need for parathyroidectomy appeared to decrease

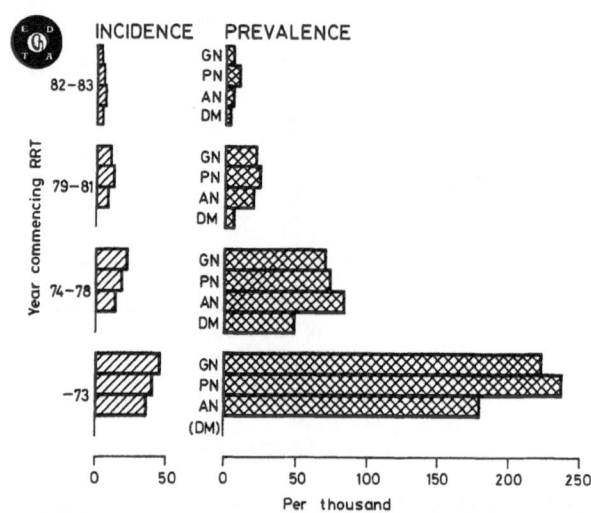

Figure 19. Incidence and prevalence of parathyroidectomy, 1983, according to primary renal disease in patients never grafted. (GN = glomerulonephritis, PN = pyelo/interstitial nephritis, AN = analgesic nephropathy, DM = diabetes mellitus).

markedly after successful transplantation (48). The incidence was still relatively high early after transplantation with 11/1,000 for patients who had received their first cadaveric graft in 1982 or 1983, but declined to less than 4/1,000 patients with a functioning graft performed before 1982. The need for parathyroidectomy after successful grafting seemed to depend also on the time spent on dialysis prior to grafting, which is not surprising in view of the highly increased incidence of parathyroidectomy after long years on dialysis in non-grafted patients as noted above. Thus the recipients of a functioning first cadaveric graft, who had spent less than one year on dialysis prior to grafting, had a prevalence of 22/1,000 in contrast to those with more than one year of dialysis before grafting, whose prevalence of a first parathyroidectomy amounted to 53/1,000.

SUCCESSFUL PREGNANCIES

That pregnancy is possible on renal replacement therapy demonstrates the high quality of life achieved in some patients. However, successful pregnancies are exceedingly rare in patients on haemodialysis (50, 51) or CAPD (52). No more than about 11% of the 490 successful pregnancies recorded by the EDTA Registry up to the end of 1985 occurred in women on hamodialysis and 0.4% in women on CAPD. Although conception and successful pregnancy can occur with significant residual glomerular filtration, most of these mothers had some residual renal function and many children were conceived before their mothers commenced maintenance dialysis (50). Large series of pregnancies in transplanted patients have been published (51, 53, 54). It has been estimated that one out of every 50 women of child-bearing age with a functioning transplant becomes pregnant (55). Rates of spontaneous abortion, stillbirth and ruptured ectopic pregnancy appear to be similar in transplanted patients to the normal population (53). Mean duration of pregnancy was 33 weeks in 32 dialysed and 36 weeks in 265 transplanted mothers. Some 70% of close to 500 pregnancies lasted less than 38 weeks compared to 10% of pregnancies in healthy mothers. Birth weight averaged at 1.8 kg and rarely exceeded 2.5 kg in dialysed mothers. Infants of transplanted mothers weighed 2.6 kg on average and thus had lower birth weights than the general population, too. However, the comparison between birth weight and gestational age showed that most newborns, although premature, were not small for their gestational age. Of these newborns, death within the first month of life was recorded for 1.8%, all of whom, with one exception, weighed less than 1.8 kg at birth. Congenital abnormalities have not been recorded with increased frequency in children born to mothers on renal replacement therapy. The incidence of major congenital defects was lower or identical to that in the general population regarding chromosomal, monogenic and multifactorial congenital defects. Twins and even triplets have been recorded at similar rates in transplanted mothers as in the general population and quite a few women have had more than one healthy baby. Of great concern are changes in transplant function associated with pregnancy. Some 20% of mothers identified by the EDTA Registry before 1979 had evidence of damage to the transplant during pregnancy and some grafts were lost (51). However, most transplants have continued to function normally during and after the pregnancy.

CONCLUSIONS

There is widespread concern to record activity in dialysis and transplantation and this appears to be felt, not only by doctors practising in the field but also by politicians, health care planners, patient activist groups and editors of medical journals. Demographic analyses on pooled data collected by central registries have shown that national programmes are developing along different lines. Economic factors have overriding importance. Many national programmes still rely on haemodialysis as the major form of renal replacement therapy, whilst CAPD has been established as an important and excellent method in its own right in other countries. Renal transplantation activity has risen everywhere and more than 40 transplants per million population per year have been performed in some countries, particularly in Northern Europe.

The age distribution of patients varies and there are apparent differences in the distribution of primary renal diseases, some of which may represent true geographical variations while others may be due to either differences in diagnostic fashions or in the availability of facilities.

Patient survival on dialysis and after grafting has improved recently. Survival on CAPD is definitely not inferior to that on haemodialysis if the high proportion of diabetics treated preferentially with CAPD is taken into account.

Quality of life as measured by rehabilitation to work, prevalence of disabling bone disease or parathyroidectomy and procreative potential is inferior on dialysis as compared to successful grafting.

Haemodialysis in hospital and at home, peritoneal dialysis and transplantation are complementary forms of treatment. The trend is to offer all treatments in an integrated programme (see also Chapter 28). The choice for any particular individual patient will be governed by availability as well as by the results as given in this chapter. Long-term survivors who have been treated for more than 10 years have mostly received mixed treatment and the majority of the European survivors beyond 15 years of renal replacement therapy have a functioning graft. The appropriate mode of treatment for a patient may change with altered medical or domestic circumstances. With increased awareness of the prospects and problems, patiens may be expected to make their own request for changes of treatment.

ACKNOWLEDGEMENTS

We are grateful to the Editors of Reports prepared by non European Registries for permission to quote their data and acknowledge our own indebtedness to the directors and staffs of renal units throughout Europe who have faithfully maintained the data base of the EDTA Registry for 22 years.

We are grateful to the following for permission to republish figures:

A J Davison, Editor, EDTA – ERA Proceedings, Pitman Medical, London and also of Nephrology Dialysis Transplantation, Springer-Verlag, London: Figures 5, 6, 13, 14, 15, 17, 19.

H J Gurland, Editor of Uraemia Therapy: Perspectives for the Next Quarter Century, Springer-Verlag, Heidelberg, 1987: Figure 8.

V Cambi, Editor of Short Dialysis, Martinus Nijhoff, New York, 1987: Figure 12.

Figure 7 comes from the 10th Report of the Australian and New Zealand Registry and is reproduced by kind permission of the Editor, A P S Disney.

REFERENCES

1. Gurland HJ, Wing AJ, Jacobs C, Brunner FP: Comparative review between dialysis and transplantation. In *Replacement of Renal Function by Dialysis*, edited by Drukker W, Parsons FM, Maher JF, The Hague, Boston, London, Martinus Nijhoff, 1978, p 663
2. Wing AJ, Brunner FP, Brynger HOA, Jacobs C, Kramer P: Comparative review between dialysis and transplantation. In *Replacement of Renal Function by Dialysis*, Second Edition, edited by Drukker W, Parsons FM, Maher JF, The Hague, Boston, London, Martinus Nijhoff, 1983, p 850
3. *Tenth Report of ANZ DATA Registry*, edited by Disney APS, Woodville South, South Australia, The Queen Elizabeth Hospital, 1987
4. *Canadian Renal Failure Register. 1985 Report. Kidney Foundation of Canada*, Ottawa, Canada, Ottawa Civic Hospital, 1987
5. *Combined Report on Maintenance Dialysis and Transplantation in the Republic of South Africa – 1985*. du Toit ED, Seggie J, Pascoe M, MacGregor KJ: South African Dialysis and Trans-

plantation Registry, Private Bag 4, Observatory, Cape 7935 South Africa

6. EDTA Registry centre survey, 1985. Report from the European Dialysis and Transplant Association Registry. *Nephrol Dial Transplant* 2: 475, 1987

7. *Present Status in Japan 1986,* edited by Odaka M for the Japanese Society for Dialysis Therapy, Japan, Chiba University, 1987

8. *End-stage Renal Disease Patient Profile Tables.* Baltimore, Maryland, ESRD Information Analysis Branch, Health Care Financing Administration, Department of Health and Human Services, 1986

9. Evans RW, Blagg CR, Bryan FA: Implications for health care policy – a social and demographic profile of hemodialysis patients in the United States. *JAMA* 245: 487, 1981

10. Relman AS, Rennie D: Treatment of end-stage renal disease: free but not equal. *N Engl J Med* 1303: 996, 1980

11. Rosansky SJ, Eggers PW: Trends in the US ESRD population: 1973–1983. *Am J Kidney Dis* 9: 91, 1987

12. Krakauer H, Grauman JS, McMullan MR, Creede CC: The recent US experience in the treatment of end stage renal disease by dialysis and transplantation. *New Engl J Med* 308: 1558, 1983

13. Gokal R, King J, Bogle S, Marsh F, Oliver D, Jakubowski C, Hunt L, Baillod R, Ogg C, Ward M, Wilkinson R: Outcome in patients on continuous ambulatory peritoneal dialysis and haemodialysis : 4 year analysis of a prospective multicentre study. *Lancet* 2: 1105, 1987

14. dia Paula FJ, Lanhez LE, Ancao MS, Draibe SA: Registro Brasileiro de Dialise e Transplante. (Brasilian Registry of Dialysis and Transplantation.) *J Bras Nefrol* 6: 89, 1984

15. Wing AJ, Selwood NH, Brunner FP: Demography of uremia and its treatment. in *Uremia Therapy: Perspectives for the Next Quarter Century,* edited by Gurland HJ, Springer-Verlag, Heidelberg, 1987, p 252

16. World Bank Atlas , Washington DC, World Bank, 1987

17. Wing AJ, Brunner FP, Challah S: Haemodialysis strategies in European countries. in *Short Dialysis,* edited by Cambi V, Boston, Martinus Nijhoff, 1987, p 33

18. Berkson J, Gagie RP: Calculation of survival rates for cancer. *Proc Staff Meet Mayo Clin* 25: 270, 1950

19. Cutler SJ, Ederer F: Maximum utilization of the life table method in analyzing survival. *J Chronic Dis* 8: 699, 1958

20. Ederer F, Axtell LM, Cutler SJ: The relative survival rate: a statistical methodology. *Natl Cancer Inst Monogr* 6: 101, 1961

21. Merrell M, Schulman LE: Determination of prognosis in chronic disease, illustrated by systemic lupus erythematosus. *J Chronic Dis* 1: 12, 1955

22. Lewis EJ, Foster DM, de la Puente J, Scurlock C: Survival data for patients undergoing chronic intermittent hemodialysis. *Ann Intern Med* 70: 311, 1969

23. Gurland HJ, Härlen H, Henze H, Spoek MG: Intermittent dialysis and renal transplantation in Europe: Survival rates. *Proc Eur Dial Transplant Assoc* 7: 20, 1970

24. UK Transplant Service, Southmead, Bristol, UK. *Annual Report* 1980

25. Brunner FP, Broyer M, Challah S, Dykes SR, Brynger H, Fassbinder W, Oulès R, Rizzoni G, Selwood NH, Wing AJ: Survival on renal replacement therapy: Data from the EDTA Registry. Nephrol Dial Transplant 3: 109, 1988

26. Fenton SSA, Cattran DC, Allan AF, Ruthledge P, Ampil M, Dadson J, Locking H, Smith SD, Wilson DR: Initial experience with continuous ambulatory peritoneal dialysis. *Artif Organs* 3: 206, 1979

27. Challah S, Brunner FP, Wing AJ (on behalf of the EDTA Registry): Evolution of the treatment of patients with diabetic nephropathy by renal replacement therapy in Europe over a decade: Data from the EDTA Registry. in *The Kidney and Hypertension in Diabetes,* edited by Mogensen CE, Boston, Martinus·Nijhoff, 1987, p 365

28. Gurland HJ, Brunner FP, Chantler C, Jabobs C, Schärer K, Selwood NH, Spies G, Wing AJ: Combined report on regular dialysis and transplantation in Europe, VI, 1975. *Proc Eur Dial Transplant Assoc* 13: 2, 1976

29. Brynger H, Brunner FP, Chantler C, Donckerwolcke RA, Jacobs C, Kramer P, Selwood NH, Wing AJ: Combined report on regular dialysis and transplantation in Europe, X, 1979. *Proc Eur Dial Transplant Assoc* 17: 2, 1980

30. Opelz G, Terasaki PI: Recipient selection for renal re-transplantation. *Transplantation* 21: 488, 1976

31. Wing AJ, Brunner FP, Brynger H, Chantler C, Donckerwolcke RA, Gurland HJ, Hathway RA, Jacobs C, Selwood NH: Combined report on regular dialysis and transplantation in Europe, VIII, 1977. *Proc Eur Dial Transplant Assoc* 15: 3, 1978

32. Claes G, Gustavsson A, Heidemann M: Outcome of renal re-transplantation. *Proc Eur Dial Transplant Assoc* 13: 152, 1976

33. Casali R, Simmons RL, Ferguson RM, Mauer SM, Kjellstrand CM, Buselmeier TJ, Najarian JS: Factors related to success or failure of second renal transplants. *Ann Surg* 184: 145, 1976

34. Opelz G, Terasaki PI: Absence of immunization effect in human kidney re-transplantation. *N Eng J Med* 299: 369, 1978

35. Roberts JL: Analysis and outcome of 1,063 patients trained for home hemodialysis. *Kidney Int* 9: 363, 1976

36. Brunner FP, Brynger H, Chantler C, Donckerwolcke RA, Hathway RA, Jacobs C, Selwood NH, Wing AJ: Combined report on regular dialysis and transplantation in Europe, IX, 1978. *Proc Eur Dial Transplant Assoc* 16: 3, 1979

37. Held PJ, Pauly MV, Diamond L: Survival analysis of patients undergoing dialysis. *JAMA* 257: 645, 1987

38. Jacobs C, Broyer M, Brunner FP, Brynger H, Donckerwolcke RA, Kramer P, Selwood NH, Wing AJ, Blake PH: Combined report on regular dialysis and transplantation in Europe, XI, 1980. *Proc Eur Dial Transplant Assoc* 18: 2, 1981

39. Broyer M, Donckerwolcke RA, Brunner FP, Brynger H, Jacobs C, Kramer P, Selwood NH, Wing AJ, Blake PH: Combined report on regular dialysis and transplantation of children in Europe, 1980. *Proc Eur Dial Transplant Assoc* 18: 60, 1981

40. Lindner A, Charra B, Sherrard DJ, Scribner BH: Accelerated atherosclerosis in prolonged maintenance hemodialysis. *N Eng J Med* 290: 6, 1974

41. Slingeneyer A, Mion C, Mourad G, Canaud B, Faller B, Béraud JJ: Progressive sclerosing peritonitis: a late and severe complication of maintenance peritoneal dialysis. *Trans Am Soc Artif Intern Organs* 29: 633, 1983

42. Junor BJR, Briggs JD, Forwell MA, Dobbie JW, Henderson I: Sclerosing peritonitis – the contribution of chlorhexidine in alcohol. *Peritoneal Dial Bull* 15: 101, 1985

43. Oulès R, Challah S, Brunner FP: Case control study to determine the cause of sclerosing peritoneal disease. *Nephrol Dial Transplant* 3: 66, 1988

44. Assenat H, Calemard E, Charra B, Laurent G, Terrat JC, Vanel T: Hémodialyse, syndrome du canal carpien et substance amyloide. (Hemodialysis, carpal tunnel syndrome and amyloid.) *Nouv Press Med* 9: 1715, 1980

45. Kachel HG, Altmeyer P, Baldamus CA, Koch KM: Deposition of an amyloid like substance as a possible complication of regular dialysis treatment. *Contr Nephrol* 36: 127, 1983

46. Shirahama T, Skinner M, Cohen AS, Gejyo F, Arakawa M, Suzuki M, Hirasawa Y: Histochemical and immunohistochemical characterisation of amyloid associated with chronic haemodialysis as beta-2-microglobulin. *Lab Invest* 53: 705, 1985

47. Vincent C, Revillard JP, Galland M, Traeger J: Serum beta-2-microglobulin in hemodialyzed patients. *Nephron* 21: 260, 1978

48. Brunner FP, Broyer M, Brynger H, Challah S, Fassbinder W, Oulès R, Rizzoni G, Selwood NH, Wing AJ: Combined report on regular dialysis and transplantation in Europe, XV, 1984. *Proc Eur Dial Transplant Assoc* 22: 5, 1985

49. Vincenti F, Arnaud SB, Recker R, Genant H, Amend WJ, Feduska NJ, Salvatierra O: Parathyroid and bone response of the diabetic patient to uremia. *Kidney Int* 25: 677, 1984

50. Challah S, Wing AJ, Broyer M, Rizzoni G: Successful pregnancies in women on regular dialysis treatment and women with a functioning transplant. in *The Kidney in Pregnancy*, edited by Andreucci VE, The Hague, Martinus Nijhoff, 1986, p 185

51. Registration Committee of the European Dialysis and Transplant Association: Successful pregnancies in women treated by dialysis and kidney transplantation. *Br J Obstet Gynaecol* 87: 839, 1980

52. Cattran DC, Benzie RJ: Pregnancy in a continuous ambulatory peritoneal dialysis patient. *Peritoneal Dial Bull* 3: 13, 1983

53. Rudolph JE, Schweizer RT, Bartus SA: Pregnancy in renal transplant patients. *Transplantation* 26: 27, 1979

54. Davison JM: Pregnancy in renal transplant recipients: clinical perspectives. *Contrib Nephrol* 37: 170, 1984

55. Editorial: Pregnancy after renal transplantation. *Br Med J* 1: 733, 1976

RENAL REPLACEMENT THERAPY IN CHILDREN

MICHEL BROYER, CYRIL CHANTLER, RAYMOND DONCKERWOLCKE and GIANFRANCO RIZZONI

INTRODUCTION

Renal function in infants and children

Successful management of acute renal failure (ARF) in children, particularly infants, requires knowledge of the functional characteristics of the kidney during development and understanding of the metabolic balance of the growing child. The newborn kidney is immature containing only 17% of its adult cellular complement; at 6 months postnatally cell division is complete and further growth is due to an increase in cell size. Nephron formation is complete before birth but superficial cortical nephrons are not functionally mature; at birth the more mature juxtamedullary nephrons contribute a greater proportion of total glomerular filtration than in the adult. There is a proportional increase in juxtamedullary blood flow but total renal blood flow is low because of the high renal vascular resistance. Glomerular filtration rate (GFR) at birth averages about 20 ml/min/1.73 m² body surface area but the rapid postnatal increase in renal blood flow is associated with a rapid rise in GFR to 48 ml/min/1.73 m² at one month and to 80 ml/min/1.73 m² by 6 months of age (1).

It is likely that the low GFR is controlled by the immaturity of tubular function thus preventing over-perfusion of nephrons and wasting of salt and water (2, 3); fractional reabsorption of filtered sodium in the proximal tubule is reduced with greater reabsorption in the distal tubule to maintain sodium balance. Excessive urinary sodium loss is present in very immature infants between 28 and 32 weeks gestation (3) and sodium wasting is also common in infants with obstructive uropathy and distal tubular damage.

The low GFR, the low blood flow, the high renal vascular resistance and the immaturity of the tubules suggest that functional reserve of the neonatal kidney is small and it is not surprising that further impairment of blood flow can lead to acute renal failure. The high haematocrit at birth also reduces renal blood flow and anoxia from birth asphyxia is common. Hence, minor degrees of renal impairment occur in the newborn and acute renal failure occurs more frequently than at any other time during childhood (Table 1).

Metabolic and fluid balance

Water requirement is directly proportional to energy expenditure and it is fortuitously convenient that the expenditure of one kilocalorie requires the consumption of one millilitre (ml) of water. Basal metabolic rate is about $1,000 \, \text{kcal/m}^2$ body surface area, thus the basal water requirement is $1,000 \, \text{ml/m}^2$. Conditions in hospital, increase energy consumption by 50%. Therefore, the normal water intake is about $1,500 \, \text{ml/m}^2$ of which $400 \, \text{ml/m}^2$ is utilised by insensible losses. The water requirement increases by $12\%/1°\text{C}$ that body temperature exceeds $37°\text{C}$.

Metabolic rate and energy requirement correlate closely with body surface area (4). Thus both the energy intake and water requirement can be calculated from the child's surface area. In the anuric child the daily water requirement may be taken as $400 \, \text{ml/m}^2$ plus measured losses.

Infants and to a lesser extent children have a much higher metabolic rate in relation to body mass than adults (4) and, given the relation between body surface area and metabolic rate, the ratio of surface area to weight is increased. Thus, the energy requirement per kilogram body weight of an infant is 3 to 4 times higher than for an adult. Expressed per unit body weight the energy requirement may be calculated as $100 \, \text{kcal/kg}$ up to $10 \, \text{kg}$ bodyweight plus $50 \, \text{kcal/kg}$ between 10 and $20 \, \text{kg}$ plus $20 \, \text{kcal/kg}$ for weights exceeding $20 \, \text{kg}$. Babies between 5 and $10 \, \text{kg}$ require $120 \, \text{kcal/kg}$ and those between 2.5 and $5 \, \text{kg}$ need $150 \, \text{kcal/kg}$. Insensible water loss and water turnover in relation to body weight is five times higher in an infant compared to an adult. Conse-

quently, serious derangements of fluid and electrolyte metabolism such as acidosis, uraemia and hyperkalaemia occur rapidly in infants with acute renal failure. The problem is compounded by the absence of normal thirst control because a baby is unable to make known his need for more water when depleted of fluid or overloaded with sodium.

GFR per surface area is comparable in children and adults from the age of one year and food intake is, as noted, roughly comparable when related to body surface area but not to weight. The intake of nutrients such as protein, or salts, is determined by the amount of food consumed which, in turn, depends on the energy intake. These other nutrients are all consumed in excess of need and this excess is excreted in the urine. The relationship between GFR and surface area means that GFR is higher in relation to body mass in a child which helps to preserve body composition. Obviously this advantage is lost in renal failure emphasising the importance of careful management of the intake of energy and other nutrients. These considerations also affect the amount of dialysis required by an anuric child and the size of the dialyser which can be used, as will be discussed later.

Blood pressure rises steadily throughout childhood from an upper limit of 100/65 at birth to 130/80 mm Hg at 13 years. Care must be taken to use a blood pressure cuff of sufficient size to avoid erroneously high readings; the inflatable bladder should be centred over the brachial artery encircling at least three quarters of the circumference of the arm and the width of the cuff should be at least two-thirds of the length of the upper arm. Stiff cuffs fastened with velcro should be avoided.

ACUTE RENAL FAILURE IN INFANCY AND CHILDHOOD

Aetiology

The incidence and causes of acute renal failure (Table 2) vary in different countries depending on the general quality of health care and environmental conditions. Table 1 shows the diagnosis in 42 children referred to Guy's Hospital over one year; 30% were less than 4 weeks old. Poor renal perfusion accounted for nearly half of all referrals; the cause

Table 1. Causes of acute renal failure related to age in 42 children seen at Guy's Hospital in 1983.

Cause	Neonates (birth to 4 wk)	Infants (5 wk to 1 yr)	Children (1 yr to 14 yr)
Pre-renal			3
Poor renal perfusion	12	4	7
Infection	1		
Hemolytic-uraemic syndrome			3
Glomerular nephritis			6
Acute on chronic	1		1
Other	1		2
Total	15	4	23

is usually obvious and includes gastroenteritis, pyloric stenosis, cardiac failure, post-surgery especially after cardiovascular operations (5), burns and renal vascular catastrophies in the newborn. Sudden relapse of nephrotic syndrome is commonly associated with hypovolaemia due to the rapid loss of salt and water into the extracellular space as the plasma albumin concentration falls. This occasionally leads to ARF and may also be associated with circulatory collapse or, in association with the hypercoagulability state of nephrotic syndrome, with vascular thrombosis. The best test to detect haemoconcentration is the haemoglobin concentration because pulse and blood pressure may be surprisingly well maintained by peripheral vasoconstriction which is reflected by a wide gap between the rectal and peripheral temperature.

As previously noted, the newborn kidney is especially susceptible to vascular damage. Medullary or papillary necrosis may accompany severe acute tubular necrosis. Hyperosmolar solutions used for contrast renal radiology may cause medullary damage. Cortical necrosis occurs after severe fluid loss, birth asphyxia, haemorrhage, or burns; focal necrotising lesions in other organs are common. Renal venous thrombosis is expecially common in infants; 70% of cases present in the first month of life (6, 7). Antecedent events include shock, perinatal asphyxia, cyanotic heart disease and hyperosmolar dehydration and frequently disseminated intravascular coagulation is found.

Urinary tract infection in the newborn is often complicated by septicaemia perhaps because of the low concentration of circulating immunoglobulin at this age; accordingly, it may present with generalised symptoms and signs such as vomiting, lethargy and jaundice. Congenital obstructive uropathy is complicated by inability to concentrate the urine and by sodium wasting due to distal nephron damage. Hence, these infants may present severely fluid depleted. ARF following extensive and complicated surgery is now less common perhaps because of improved anaesthesia and awareness of fluid and electrolyte requirements. But, it is still frequent after prolonged cardiopulmonary bypass (8) or following vascular surgery in the neonate (5). More careful attention to the need to maintain or restore circulatory blood volume with more liberal use of plasma expanders and physiological saline, rather than dextrose in water, during and after surgery is likely to reduce the incidence further (9).

Pathogenesis

The pathophysiology of ARF has bene recently reviewed (8, 10). Injury to the tubules is central to the oliguria though the mechanisms by which tubular damage reduces urine flow are not entirely clear. Back leak of filtrate through damaged tubules, and tubular obstruction from necrotic cell debris may occur. Increased solute delivery to the macula densa because of reduced reabsorption by damaged tubules is thought to stimulate renin release in the juxtaglomerular apparatus, which by increasing the intrarenal production of angiotensin II constricts the afferent arteriole thus reducing GFR (2). This prevents overperfusion of damaged nephrons and the considerable loss of salt and water that would occur.

As already noted, the mature neonate despite tubular immaturity has a well developed capacity to conserve sodium suggesting that the low GFR results from suppression of superficial nephron filtration by tubular glomerular feedback. Thus even a small further impairment of tubular function might lead to suppression of glomerular filtration and ARF; simply stated, the neonate is born halfway to ARF.

Nonoliguric ARF now occurs more commonly. Many measures used to ameliorate ARF in experimental animals such as plasma volume expansion, inotropic stimulation of cardiac output vasodilator therapy and particularly the use of dopamine hydrochloride which causes renal vasodilation and inhibits proximal sodium reabsorption contribute to the maintenance of glomerular filtrate and urine flow. Mannitol increases renal blood flow and induces osmotic diuresis thus clearing cellular debris from the tubular lumen. Frusemide also appears to reduce afferent arteriolar resistance restoring the transcapillary pressure gradient across the glomerular capillary wall. Hence, nonoliguric renal failure probably often represents an attenuated form of tubular necrosis. The ARF associated with tubular toxins may be nonoliguric; we have observed this pattern with ARF complicating gentamicin toxicity in the newborn. The maintenance of urine flow under such circumstances may confuse and delay diagnosis.

Table 2. Causes of acute renal failure.

Glomerulonephritis
  Acute postinfectious glomerulonephritis
  Henoch Schonlein nephritis
  Systemic lupus erythematosus
  Goodpasture disease
  Others
Interstitial nephritis
  Acute pyelonephritis
  Drug induced (methicillin, diuretics)
  Post viral
  Idiopathic
Acute tubular necrosis
  Anoxia, ischaemia, hypovolaemia, hypotension
  Septicaemia
  Nephrotoxins, mercury, nonsteroidal anti-inflammatory drugs, myoglobin, aminoglycosides, cis-platinum
  Combinations of above (burns, trauma, surgery)
Vascular disorders
  Hemolytic uraemic syndrome
  Cortical necrosis
  Renal venous thrombosis
  Disseminated intravascular coagulation
Crystalluria
  Uric acid (following anti tumour therapy)
  Sulphonamides
  Oxalic acid (ingestion of polyethylene glycol)
Acute on chronic
  e.g. infection with obstructive uropathy
  dehydration with 1 gA nephropathy
Miscellaneous (rare) cases

Assessment and initial therapy

Children, especially infants, with ARF are usually dangerously ill and for the reasons outlined the metabolic derangements are rapid in onset and severe. Therefore, treatment and investigation must proceed simultaneously. Whilst the indications for dialysis are similar to those for adults, the increased metabolism and energy demands necessitate more frequent dialysis for it is difficult to manage an anuric catabolic infant conservatively. The initial assessment includes clinical evaluation of the degree of fluid loss, blood pressure measurement, if necessary using Doppler ultrasound (11), central and peripheral temperature measurement to gauge tissue perfusion (9), haemoglobin and plasma and urine electrolytes. Urine sodium and urea concentrations are especially useful to determine the adequacy of renal perfusion; fractional excretion of sodium is less than 2% with pre-renal failure (12). From these determinations the amount of intravenous fluid required to restore extracellular volume can be calculated, but careful continuous monitoring is essential to prevent overload. The blood volume of a child can be calculated as 80 ml/kg. Thus, an initial transfusion 20 ml/kg of whole blood or plasma in a shocked child is usually safe. An obviously saline-depleted infant will have lost about 10% of body weight as water, so the rapid infusion of 20 ml/kg of physiological saline can be given whilst more precise calculations are being undertaken. If peripheral circulation is not restored by adequate fluid replacement, even though blood pressure and venous pressure are normal, then the use of a peripheral vasodilator (hydralazine, or chlorpromazine 0.1 mg/kg intravenously [IV]) often restores urine flow. Hypernatraemia should be corrected only slowly over 48 h to avoid neurological damage; the calculated water deficit being supplied by sodium solutions of 25 to 40 mmol/l providing not more than 100 ml/kg of *free* water per 24 h. Hypertension usually responds to IV or intramuscular (IM) hydralazine 0.5 to 1.0 mg/kg or to the infusion of labetolol 1 to 3 mg/kg/h. Hyperkalaemia, if life-threatening, should be treated with 2.5% calcium gluconate 2 ml/kg. Acidosis should be corrected and calcium-potassium exchange resin (1 g/kg orally and rectally) can be administered. Recently the intravenous infusion of salbutomol (0.5 mg/15 min) has been shown to lower plasma potassium significantly in adults with hyperkalaemia complicating renal failure (13). Hypocalcaemia in the neonate presents with jittery movements or convulsions and should be treated with IV calcium gluconate. Hypoglycaemia requires IV dextrose (1 g/kg). Metabolic acidosis can be corrected with 8.4% sodium bicarbonate (1 mmol/ml) diluted before use; 2 mmol/kg will raise plasma bicarbonate by about 6 mmol/l in the infant. It is not advisable to correct the acidosis completely because of the risk of hypokalaemia, decrease of ionized calcaemia, and the sodium load involved in the treatment. Intensive treatment of possible septicaemia should be undertaken after blood cultures have been obtained. Care must be exercised when drugs whose excretion depends on renal function are used; the dose should be reduced accordingly and the plasma concentration measured at intervals.

Traumatic investigations involving renal radiology, or renal biopsy should only be undertaken when the condition of the child has been stabilised if necessary by dialysis. Nonetheless, urgency is imperative because an obstructed infected urinary tract may require immediate surgery to establish adequate drainage. The most useful investigation is sonography of the kidneys and urinary tract undertaken by a skilled operator (14). Not only can this demonstrate obstruction but the patency of the renal vasculature can often be confirmed. If however the child is anuric the obstructed urinary tract may not be dilated and the dilation will only become apparent when urine flow recommences (15). The next most useful investigation in an emergency is micturating cystography to determine the presence of vesico-ureteric reflux and to exclude obstruction of bladder outflow.

Conservative management

Whilst dialysis is usually resorted to at an early stage, careful control of fluid, electrolyte and nutritional intake is required. After the fluid deficit has been corrected, intake should be reduced to the level of insensible loss plus an allowance for pyrexia, abnormal losses, urine output and loss by ultrafiltration during dialysis. Electrolyte requirements are difficult to estimate and intake should be kept as low as possible with sodium and potassium intake not exceeding 2 mmol/kg/24 h unless the child receives dialysis. An adequate calcium intake of 500 mg/24 h should be ensured, if necessary by feeding supplements. The high energy intake of infants has been mentioned and at least 150 kcals/kg/day is required at birth. About 2 g/kg of first class protein should be provided at birth falling to 1 g/kg at 1 year and thereafter. Suitable oral feeds which take account of all these requirements can be made by using low solute or humanised cows milk preparations (SMA, S_{26}, Ostermilk new, Cow and Gate baby milk plus) but unmodified cows milk or evaporated milk is not suitable. Extra energy can be provided with double cream (4 kcals/ml), or arachis oil emulsion (Prosparol) and with a glucose polymer such as caloreen or calonutrin. A high energy low water feed can be made up using energy supplements (Table 3). Alkali can be added as sodium bicarbonate (1 to 2 mmol/kg/24 h). The osmolality of the feed should be measured and the concentration slowly increased to prevent diarrhoea and vomiting. With older children the help of an experienced dietician is essential so that account can be taken of the child's taste preferences. The important point is to ensure that the diet prescribed is actually eaten and this can only be done with the child's co-

Table 3. Composition of energy feed for renal failure

Glucose polymer	200 g
Arachis oil emulsion	130 ml
Water	400 ml

Flavour to taste with chocolate or milk shake flavourings. Provides 1385 kcal in 464 ml water, protein as clinifeed (Laboratories Sopharga Puteaux France) may be added.

operation. Alternatively, an adequate intake can be ensured by nasogastric tube feeding.

Maintaining adequate nutrition in infants with renal failure who cannot be maintained on an oral intake is extremely difficult and even with the most concentrated IV feeding regimes frequent dialysis is essential to remove the excess water involved. Continuous arteriovenous haemofiltration is especially valuable in the management of ARF allowing much better control of fluid balance than peritoneal dialysis (see below).

Renal replacement therapy in acute renal failure

Indications for the treatment of acute renal failure by renal replacement therapy are: fluid overload refractory to diuretics and associated with hypertension or congestive heart failure, a hypercatabolic state, or the requirement of large amounts of fluids for parenteral malnutrition or for sustaining systemic circulation. Also patients with prolonged oliguria require dialysis.

In ARF due to primary kidney disease either peritoneal or haemodialysis may be used. In newborns and infants peritoneal dialysis is the treatment of choice, because of its simplicity, availability, relative safety and effectiveness. Children weighing more than 20 kg with a prolonged oliguria are often treated with haemodialysis after one or two peritoneal dialyses. Available facilities and expertise often determine the choice between peritoneal dialysis and haemodialysis in older children. There is no evidence that outcome is better with either technique. For critically ill patients when ARF complicates severe infections or major operations, either mode of dialysis is often inadequate. Continuous arteriovenous ultrafiltration allows considerable fluid intake for administration of nutrients and drugs without the danger of fluid overload and therefore may provide a safer alternative in these patients.

Peritoneal dialysis in acute renal failure

The technique and equipment used for acute dialysis are similar to those used for chronic intermittent peritoneal dialysis in children. If dialysis has to be performed urgently a plastic disposable peritoneal catheter may be inserted at the bedside instead of the surgical insertion of a Silastic catheter requiring a laparotomy. In critically ill newborns or infants it is generally recommended to control respiratory movements by a respirator with endotracheal intubation before inserting a peritoneal catheter.

Procedure of catheter insertion
Premedication with diazepam (0.25 mg/kg IV) chlorpromazine (0.5 mg/kg IM) or chloral hydrate (30 mg/kg rectally) is recommended in an anxious child. After local anaesthesia with procaine, the abdomen should be primed with 20 ml dialysis solution/kg through a small bore needle or cannula prior to inserting the peritoneal catheter. This is necessary to avoid the catheter penetrating an intra-abdominal organ

such as the inferior vena cava for the small infant is unable to tense the abdominal muscles when the catheter is inserted. A special paediatric plastic peritoneal catheter (available from McGaw, Vygon, Wallace) with stylet is then inserted through a small skin incision, a few centimeters below the umbilicus in the midline; when the peritoneum is entered, the stylet is removed and the catheter advanced to the left side of the pelvis. When midline insertion is not possible, the catheter can be inserted in the flank, outside the line of the inferior epigastric artery. After insertion, it is better to dialyse for a few days and then remove the catheter, allowing a period on conservative management before reinsertion than to leave the same catheter in place indefinitely. If prolonged peritoneal dialysis is envisaged a cuffed Silastic cannula can be inserted with a long skin tunnel after initial conventional peritoneal dialysis.

Complications related to insertion of stylet catheters
These include catheter malfunction perforation of a viscus and bleeding. Obstruction of the catheter may be caused by omental fat, fibrin or blood clots. Extravasation of fluid into the abdominal wall frequently complicates peritoneal dialysis in children. The use of a suitable catheter, which should be correctly inserted with all perforations inside the peritoneal cavity will avoid this problem. The cannula must be removed when any leakage occurs in the abdominal wall. Perforation of a viscus (bowel or bladder) is a rare complication. The catheter should be removed and reinserted; usually the perforation closes spontaneously. Bleeding after insertion of the catheter, continuing during the first cycles, is not uncommon. Exceptionally the haemorrhage is considerable, leading to hypotension and shock.

Haemodialysis in acute renal failure

Vascular access
For emergency haemodialysis a simple immediately usable vascular access is required. Methods for cannulation of the superior and inferior vena cava have been developed. Superior vena cava catheterisation is effected through the subclavian or jugular vein (see vascular access chronic haemodialysis). Acute haemodialysis using one or two percutaneous femoral vein catheters is possible even in small children and a single needle device allows dialysis through a single femoral vein catheter. When two catheters are to be inserted in small children, it is easier to catheterise each femoral vein instead of insertion of both catheters on the same side. Femoral catheterisation is useful when only a few dialyses are necessary but for prolonged treatment subclavian cannulation is preferred.

Technique of haemodialysis
The technique of haemodialysis in acute renal failure does not differ from that in chronic renal failure. However, patients with ARF often have an unstable cardiovascular system, making dialysis more hazardous.

In acute dialysis vigorous ultrafiltration is often required. To avoid circulatory collapse, a dialyzer allowing careful regulation of ultrafiltration and without compliance during application of negative pressure for ultrafiltration is preferred.

Using a dialyzer with restricted efficiency (urea clearance less than 1.5 ml/kg/min), bicarbonate containing dialysate and infusion of mannitol during dialysis may enhance haemodynamic stability.

Continuous arteriovenous haemofiltration

Continuous arteriovenous haemofiltration (CAVH) is an extracorporeal blood treatment in which fluid and non-protein plasma solutes are removed in a continuous process. The system consists of a small haemofilter connected to an artery and a vein. Systemic blood pressure achieves blood flow through the circuit. The pressure gradient across the membrane filters plasma water and dissolved solutes, into a collection bag. This gradient is determined by the mean arterial blood pressure (opposed by the oncotic pressure from the plasma proteins) and the negative filtrate pressure resulting from the difference in height between the filter and the collection bag (16, 17). If large volumes of uremic ultrafiltrate are removed and substitution fluids administered, the procedure can be used as a renal replacement therapy. Slow continuous ultrafiltration (SCUF) without fluid substitution can be used to remove excess fluid. Both methods are applicable in newborns, infants and children.

Indications
CAVH is indicated whenever haemodialysis or peritoneal dialysis is precluded, because of technical problems or because of the unstable clinical condition of the patient. It is ideally suited for critically ill patients with ARF who have multiple organ failure or are haemodynamically unstable. This may be the case in patients who develop ARF following septic shock or after cardiopulmonary bypass surgery. It also may be used in patients with life-threatening edema resistent to diuretic therapy or peritoneal dialysis (18).

Technical aspects
As the driving force for blood flow in CAVH is the gradient between arterial and venous pressures, cannulation of an artery as well as a vein is required. This can be obtained with catheters or an arteriovenous shunt.

During the first days of life catheterisation of the umbilical vessels may provide an efficient access. In infants and children catheters are placed in femoral or brachial arteries as arterial access, while jugular or femoral veins are used for the return of blood (19). Peripheral cannulation should be avoided because of the high risk of thrombosis due to haemoconcentration and the infusion of hypertonic replacement solutions. To avoid unnecessary pressure loss, short cannulas (25 to 33 mm) of 18 to 20 gauge should be used. Thereby flood flow rates 15 to 50 ml/min may be achieved. A shunt can be placed either in an arm or a leg. Blood flow is higher when femoral artery cannulation is performed than when a peripheral shunt is used. If blood flow is not sufficient, a pump may be used.

Special short pediatric blood lines with low blood volume (8 ml) are commercially available (Amicon, Gambro). The arterial line has a port for heparin infusion and another for blood sampling. The venous line has a port for the infusion of replacement fluids and a sampling port. At the inlet and outlet of the circuit three way stopcocks are placed allowing lavage of the filter or replacement of the filter after clotting. A long ultrafiltration line connects the ultrafilter and a collection bag. Adaptation of the height between filter and collection bag allows modification of negative pressure within the filter and thereby of transmembrane pressure and ultrafiltrate production. There are commercially available hemofilters suitable for CAVH in infants and children. A polysulfonic hemofilter produced by Amicon is suitable for use in newborns and infants.

This minifilter with a $0.005\,m^2$ surface area containing 25 hollow fibers has a total blood volume of 6 ml. Special characteristics of this filter are the low internal resistance to blood flow, low ultrafiltration rates at spontaneously achieved pressures (0.5 to 2.0 ml/min) and low filtration fractions (5 to 9%) (19). In older children the Gambro hemofilter FH22 may be used. This hollow fiber filter has a $0.16\,m^2$ polyamide membrane and a blood priming volume of 11 ml. At a blood flow of 50 ml/min an ultrafiltration rate of 2 to 5 ml/min, according to transmembrane pressure gradient (60 to 120 mm Hg), is achieved.

Heparinised saline is used to prime the blood lines and filter, but to prevent clotting of the filter, heparinisation must be maintained throughout treatment. A loading dose of heparin (50 U/kg) is administered followed by continuous infusion of heparin at 10 to 15 U/kg/h. Activated clotting time is measured every 3 h and the heparin dose is adjusted accordingly.

Strict control of all intake and output of fluids is required to maintain body fluid balance. When the main objective is to control fluid balance by SCUF the amount of fluid given is determined by the needs for parenteral nutrition and intravenous drug administration. When CAVH is used to prevent uremia, large amounts of ultrafiltrate (more than 15% of body weight) must be removed and replaced by a solution that achieves electrolyte and acid-base balance. Ringer-lactate or normal saline with appropriate additions of calcium and magnesium and separate infusion of bicarbonate may be used (16).

Clinical experience
CAVH or SCUF have been succesfully used in premature babies, in infants and in children for the following clinical indications.
Fluid overload
Precise control of the rate and volume of ultrafiltrate formation made CAVH a safe method of fluid removal in infants and children. Weight losses up to 15% of body weight were well tolerated without side effects (18). Hypotension was noted if the rate of ultrafiltration exceeded 0.5 ml/kg/min; but was not related to the volume of plasma water removed (18).

Renal replacement therapy (19, 20)

Due to the identical composition of ultrafiltrate and plasma water, CAVH is limited in removing uremic waste products by the ultrafiltrate volume. Ultrafiltrate formation and administration of substitution fluids in excess of 15% of body weight are required to obtain sufficient solute clearances (16). In highly catabolic patients with high rates of urea generation, the treatment is insufficient in removing waste products. In those patients CAVH must be used in conjunction with non-ultrafiltrative hemodialysis or substituted by peritoneal dialysis (17).

Parenteral nutrition in acute renal failure

CAVH allows administration of large quantities of fluids in anuric patients without the risk of fluid overload. Besides administration of glucose, lipids and amino acids the intravenous fluids must also compensate for the loss of electrolytes with the ultrafiltrate.

Complications

The complications and cause of death in ARF relate primarily to the underlying cause of renal failure and to the complications of peritoneal dialysis, most of which can be avoided. The incidence of peritonitis can be reduced by scrupulous attention to asepsis and by reducing the duration of dialysis.

Convulsions are common especially in infants and are usually attributed to a combination of factors such as uraemia, hyponatraemia, hypocalcaemia and hypertension, though the primary disorder causing the renal failure e.g. haemolytic uraemic syndrome may be implicated. Again, good management can minimise the risk. Hyperglycaemia is not uncommon especially when peritoneal dialysis solutions with a high dextrose concentration are used for fluid removal. In this respect it is usually not necessary to use a concentration greater than 3 g/dl (3%). The hyperglycaemia is also related to the glucose intolerance associated with the overall catabolic state of uraemia and infection. There is some evidence that extra insulin in these circumstances will reduce net protein catabolism as well as lower the blood glucose. Certainly, blood glucose must be carefully monitored because high levels will increase plasma osmolarity and rapid change will increase the risk of cerebral complications. Careful control of IV hypertonic dextrose infusions is also very important; unfortunately it is often not possible to substitute IV fat emulsions for dextrose as an alternative source of energy because of the reduced clearance of plasma lipids in uraemia.

Conclusion

The prognosis of acute renal failure in childhood is relatively good and a majority of children if properly managed make a full recovery. The services required to achieve this are, however, formidable, requiring skilled paediatric nursing, chemical pathology and haematology, paediatric radiology and nuclear medicine, paediatric dieticians and social workers, nephrologists familiar with paediatric problems, and experienced paediatric urologists as well as the general ne-

phrology and dialysis expertise. Accordingly, such services tend to be concentrated in a few units serving a large population.

CHRONIC RENAL FAILURE IN INFANCY AND CHILDHOOD

Incidence and age of onset

The incidence of end stage renal disease (ESRD) in children less than 15 is now much better known than previously. The annual collection of data by international and national registries gives a good concept of this incidence.

The annual incidence of ESRD (Figure 1) can be estimated by the acceptance rate of new patients reported for the five major European Countries by the European Dialysis and Transplant Association (EDTA) Registry (21) for the years 1976 to 1985; it increased slowly but steadily until the last 2 years and now ranges between 4 and 8 new patients per million child population (below age 15). Because in countries such as France the incidence of ESRD can be overestimated due to the acceptance of patients from abroad, a more realistic figure in the late 1980s is approximately 6 new children per million child population per year. This is confirmed by the data from the Canadian Registry (22) which collects the totality of the paediatric cases in that country. It is difficult to foresee whether the incidence and acceptance rate, and, therefore, the need for renal replacement therapy will further increase in the future or not. The increase in the acceptance of younger children will raise this figure, while the decrease in the natality rate and also a better comprehensive conservative treatment during the predialysis period might decrease it.

The annual acceptance rate, of children less than 5 also increased in the last decade and does not differ much from that observed in older children varying between 2 and 6 per million population under age 5 (23).

The age distribution of children accepted for treatment of ESRD changed during recent years. In a total of 516 new paediatric patients starting renal replacement therapy (RRT) in 1985, 15.3% were under age 5, 29.8% were between 5 and 10 and 54.8 were 10 to 14 years old. The proportion of younger children (between 5 and 10 and less than 5) substantially increased during the last 5 years (21) and will probably increase even more in the future.

Primary renal disease in children

The incidence of different primary renal diseases (PRD) which caused ESRD in 2,368 children aged less than 15 in the period 1981 to 1985 is shown in Table 4.

Glomerulonephritis and pyelonephritis account approximately for 25% each while hereditary/familial nephropathies and congenital hypoplasia-dysplasia represent, altogether, 30% of PRD. Multisystem diseases account for 10% of all PRDs while only 6% of the patients reached ESRD because of uncertain cause. The examination of the in-

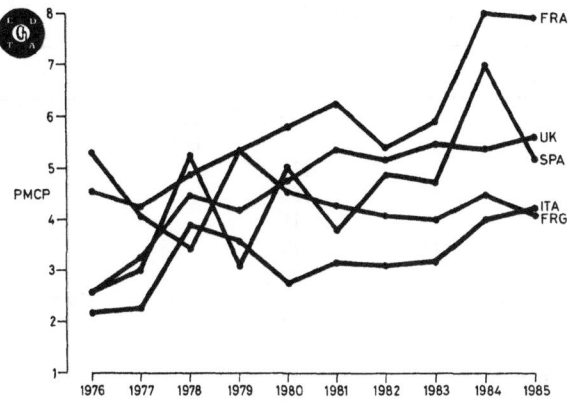

Figure 1. Acceptance rate of new paediatric patients onto renal replacement programmes in the five largest European countries between 1976 and 1985 expressed per million child population (PMCP). (FRA-France, SPA-Spain, UK-United-Kingdom, FRG-Federal Republic of Germany, ITA-Italy). (with permission of ED-TA registry committee).

cidences of different PRD groups from 1981 to 1985 confirms the tendency of GN to decrease as a cause of ESRD while the other groups of PRD, including that of aetiology uncertain, remain rather stable (Table 5).

In the group of glomerulonephritis (GN), steroid resistant nephrotic syndrome with focal glomerulosclerosis (FSGS) accounts for approximately 27%, dense deposits membranoproliferative GN for 7.4% and IgA nephropathy for 3.7% (21). The other main histologically identified glomerulopathies leading to ESRD are membranoproliferative GN type I and endo and extracapillary proliferative GN which, all together, account for a further 40%; 28% of all glomerulopathies are not histologically examined (21).

Organisation of services and facilities required for children

The relatively small number of children starting dialysis each year results in logistics that differ from those in adults. It has been suggested that a limited number of specialised children's centres should be established to cope with the problem rather than treat the occasional child who presents with chronic renal failure in a local adult centre. Treatment of children in adult centres often results in complications due to inappropriate dialysis technique; moreover treatment of children on an adult ward may create additional psychological problems in both categories.

One paediatric centre per million child population per country was considered sufficient to provide treatment for all children with end stage renal disease. But to avoid too long distance travel more centres have been created in some countries. By the end of 1985 there were 97 centres that defined themselves as specialised paediatric centres in the centre questionnaire of the EDTA-ERA. They treated 73% of the 934 patients under age 15 undergoing renal replacement therapy in Europe (24).

Paediatrics units, which should be separated from adult treatment areas, are usually small (two to six dialysis beds) with a relatively high staff to patient ratio. They have to be run by a paediatric nephrologist fully trained in both specialities. Nurses of such units must be experienced with children and dialysis. Several facilities not required for adult patients are needed in a paediatric specialised unit including a full time dietician, social worker, teacher and a psychologist. A dietician is all the more important as dietary prescription is of major interest in children. One out of seven deaths reported in the paediatrics EDTA registry in children on dialysis in the period 1981–1985 was caused by hyperkalaemia and cardio-vascular overload, both complications related to dietary non compliance. A teacher should be attached to the hospital team to provide tutoring during dialysis and to establish a direct liaison between the hospital and the school in order to achieve the best possible educational program for each child. Instruction during dialysis also emphasises the importance of a proper educational programme. The role of social worker and psychologist are obvious for helping families to cope with all the problems generated by dialysis. Paediatric surgery and urology, and the support of a general paediatric unit are also required.

A paediatric specialised unit must be capable of offering all modes of treatmente for ESRD, not only hospital haemodialysis but also continuous ambulatory peritoneal dialysis (CAPD) and home hemodialysis. Above all, a kidney transplantation has to be planned for the child as soon as possible, either in the same hospital or in another. When a specialised paediatric unit is not available in the vicinity for a child with ESRD it is recommended at least to start dialysis in the nearest specialised centre and to continue afterwards a regular clinical assessment in this unit as the child undergoes maintenance dialysis in a non specialised centre.

Medical problems

Growth failure and endocrine disorders

Growth retardation is a common though not an inevitable consequence of chronic renal failure. Many children are already small by the time dialysis is initiated (25). Figure 2 shows the proportion of children with selected primary renal diseases whose height at the start of treatment was lower than 3 SD of normal in the EDTA paediatric registry. In this figure children commencing treatment in 1976 to 1980 are compared with those commencing treatment in 1981 to 1985. Height deficit was less in this last cohort possibly as a result of better conservation treatment before the start of renal replacement therapy (21). Growth after transplantation generally exceeds that on dialysis , which is often poor, though normal growth is sometimes observed (26). This point is emphasized later. Recent experience with careful dietary management of chronic renal failure in prepubertal children, including the prevention of renal osteodystrophy, has demonstrated catch-up growth particularly in infants (27). Prevention of severe growth retardation in children depends on intensive nutritional support prior to ESRD and early transplantation when possible. Long-term dialysis is

Table 4. Distribution of primary renal diseases in Europe leading to ESRD in 1981 to 1985, EDTA Pediatric Registry.

Causes of end-stage renal failure			
Chronic renal failure, aetiology uncertain		135	5.7%
Glomerulonephritis		611	25.8%
histologically not examined	131		
severe nephrotic syndrome with focal sclerosis	161		
* IgA nephropathy (proven by immunofluorescence)	11		
** dense deposit disease (proven by immunofluorescence and/or electron microscopy)	18		
other glomerulonephritis, histologically examined	290		
Pyelonephritis/interstitial nephritis		582	24.6%
cause not specified	77		
associated with neurogenic bladder	31		
due to congenital obstructive uropathy with or without vesico-ureteric reflux	237		
due to acquired obstructive uropathy	19		
due to vesico-ureteric reflux without obstruction	192		
due to urolithiasis	12		
due to other cause	14		
Hereditary/familial nephropathy		370	15.6%
cystic kidney disease – type unspecified	11		
polycystic kidneys, adult type (dominant)	10		
polycystic kidneys, infantile (recessive)	28		
medullary cystic disease, including nephronophthisis	150		
other specified type of cystic kidney disease	9		
hereditary/familial nephropathy – type unspecified	15		
hereditary nephritis with nerve deafness (Alport's Syndrome)	38		
cystinosis	75		
primary oxalosis	22		
other hereditary nephropathy	12		
Congenital hypoplasia/dysplasia		311	13.1%
congenital hypoplasia – type unspecified	137		
oligomeganephrotic hypoplasia	36		
congenital renal dysplasia with of without urinary tract malformation	120		
syndrome of agenesis of abdominal muscles (Prune Belly Syndrome)	18		
Renal vascular disease		37	1.6%
type unspecified	6		
due to malignant hypertension (no primary renal disease)	5		
due to hypertension (no primary renal disease)	14		
due to polyarteritis	4		
Wegener's granulomatosis	1		
other renal vascular disease – classified	7		
Multi-system disease		239	10.1%
diabetes – insulin dependent (Type I)	9		
amyloid	8		
lupus erythematosus	19		
Henoch/Schönlein purpura	56		
Goodpasture's Syndrome	2		
Haemolytic Uraemic Syndrome (Moschcowitz Syndrome)	115		
other multi-stystem disease	30		
Miscellaneous		83	3.5%
nephropathy caused by drugs	10		
cortical or tubular necrosis	19		
nephrocalcinosis and hypercalcaemic nephropathy	14		
kidney tumour	17		
traumatic or surgical loss of kidney	6		
other identified renal disorders	17		

* Introduced in 1983.
** Introduced in 1984.

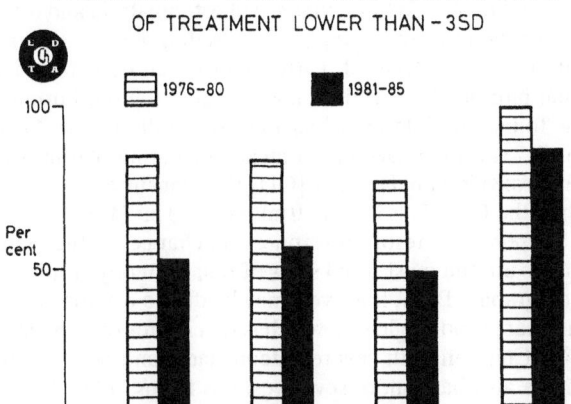

PROPORTION OF CHILDREN WITH HEIGHT AT START
OF TREATMENT LOWER THAN -3SD

Figure 2. Proportion of children, with selected primary renal diseases, whose height at start of treatment was lower than minus 3 SD of normal. Children commencing treatment in 1976 to 1980 are compared with those commencing treatment in 1981 to 1985. Height deficit was less in 1981 to 1985.

not recommended, though it is unavoidable in some cases.

The very greatest attention must be paid to growth in children with renal failure. At present, many reach adult life severely stunted (28) which causes considerable psychological disturbance both to the children and to their parents. Height should be measured accurately using precise apparatus, and both height and weight should be recorded every 3 months (29).

Inadequate nutrition is indicated if the weight is less than expected for the height and correlates with poor growth (30, 31). Measurement of triceps and subscapular skinfold thickness also provide useful indicators of nutritional adequacy. Skeletal maturation is often retarded by at least 2 years and should be assessed regularly (32). Radiographs for bone age should be carefully inspected for evidence of osteomalacia and secondary hyperparathyroidism. Serum parathyroid hormone levels should be measured regularly. Pubertal development is delayed by chronic renal failure and should be charted regularly; pubertal delay correlates with the retardation in bone age (33). The delayed onset of puberty con-

tributes to the emotional disturbances suffered by these children. The delay in bone age is of practical importance because affected individuals continue to grow, albeit slowly, at an age when normal children have ceased to grow and their final height may be better than anticipated. Nutritional and metabolic consequence of chronic renal failure in children have been recently reviewed (34). All nutrients other than energy are normally ingested in excess of requirement and the excess is excreted in the urine. A balance between intake and output is maintained in chronic renal failure, otherwise progressive changes in body composition would occur rapidly leading to death. The severity of chronic renal failure is characterised by the extent ot the changes in body composition that are necessary in order to maintain the balance between intake and output. Dialysis is required when the renal capacity for excretion is so limited that the changes in body composition become incompatible with life. It is obvious that control of intake by altering diet is fundamental in the management of chronic renal failure and in determining the need for dialysis.

Anorexia, which is a frequent characteristic of renal insufficiency, naturally lowers the intake of nutrients such as protein and electrolytes, normally consumed excessively and therefore reduces the alterations in body composition that would otherwise occur. However, the reduced intake frequently leads to energy malnutrition which increases the tendency to catabolism and the risk of intercurrent infection from reduced immune competence. The energy content of the diet should be increased to maintain normal energy intake, whilst reducing the intake of all other nutrients as necessary to limit the changes in body composition.

The reduced energy intake characteristic of chronic renal failure is exacerbated by abnormal energy metabolism, with a reduced peripheral consumption of glucose for energy in spite of secondary hyperinsulinaemia (35). In addition, the pancreatic response to hyperglycaemia is inhibited by secondary hyperparathyroidism (36). Uraemic alterations in energy metabolism necessarily affect protein metabolism. Hence, protein malnutrition occurs despite an adequate dietary intake of protein. Reductions in cell mass, plasma protein concentration, plasma branch chain amino acid concentrations, the protein content of muscle, and protein turnover and muscle protein synthesis have all been observed in patients with chronic renal insufficiency (34). In addition, a

Table 5. Distribution of primary renal diseases in Europe: evolution from 1981 to 1985, EDTA Pediatric Registry.

Causes of end stage renal failure in new patients from 1981 to 1985	1981 (%)	1982 (%)	1983 (%)	1984 (%)	1985 (%)
Chronic renal failure, aetiology uncertain	5.9	5.3	6.0	4.8	6.3
Glomerulonephritis	29.7	23.8	25.9	26.4	23.2
Pyelonephritis/interstitial nephritis	22.8	26.1	22.1	27.9	21.8
Hereditary/familial nephropathy	15.9	12.3	18.4	12.9	18.1
Congenital hypoplasia/dysplasia	12.3	13.7	12.8	12.7	15.5
Renal vascular disease	1.4	1.8	2.0	1.3	1.2
Multi-system disease	9.7	14.4	8.6	11.6	7.1
Other	2.1	2.3	4.0	2.2	6.5

dialysable constituent of uraemic plasma has a direct inhibitory effect on protein synthesis *in vitro* (37). Reduction of nitrogen intake in uraemic children sufficient to maintain the blood urea below 20 mmol/l has improved growth as well as glucose metabolism during hyperglycaemia with a reduction in insulin resistance (38).

Sodium retention with an increase in total body sodium content is common in chronic renal failure, but is not invariable. Some individuals, particularly children with obstructive uropathy or a renal dysplasia, may be salt depleted and in some the syndrome of hyporeninaemic hypoaldosteronism develops and reduces growth (39).

Many disturbances of endocrine function have been described in chronic renal failure but their relation to the metabolic abnormalities of uraemia and in particular to growth retardation are poorly understood (40). Basal levels of growth hormone measured by radioimmunoassay are high though it is not known whether all the measured growth hormone is biologically active or whether there is a normal receptor response. It is also unknown whether supraphysiological doses of growth hormone would improve growth in uraemic children though there is some evidence to suggest an effect in rats. Insulin like growth factor 1 (somatomedin A and C) is believed to mediate the action of growth hormone. Interpretation of the plasma concentration of this substance in chronic renal failure is complicated by the method of assay, whether radioimmunoassay or bioassay, by the uraemic modification of plasma protein binding, and by the possible presence of a low molecular weight inhibitor of activity in uraemia. It is not surprising therefore that results in chronic renal failure have been conflicting. Hyperprolactinaemia occurs in chronic renal failure; levels are unaffected by dialysis but return to normal after renal transplantation. Hyperprolactinaemia may be partly responsible for the delay in pubertal development which characterises chronic renal failure in children. Testosterone levels are normal in prepubertal boys with chronic renal failure but may be reduced after puberty. High basal levels of luteinising hormone with loss of the normal pulsatile pattern of secretion have been demonstrated in men with chronic renal failure. Overnight profile studies in boys with chronic renal failure and growth retardation have shown a blunted response for follicle stimulating hormone.

Plasma cortisol concentrations are normal in children with chronic renal failure (41). Thyroid function is within the low normal range with depressed TSH levels (42) except in children with cystinosis who frequently develop hypothyroidism with increased plasma TSH concentrations (43).

Renal osteodystrophy

Osteodystrophy is common in children with chronic renal failure (44). Its occurrence is probably stimulated by the rapid turnover rate of bone associated with remodelling and growth. In addition to the changes which occur in adults (see Chapter 44) the metaphyseal growth zone is affected and abnormalities similar to nutritional rickets are seen on radiographs. Osteodystrophy is especially common in children

with congenital renal disease leading to renal insufficiency early in life (45). Whilst evidence of osteomalacia and osteitis fibrosa may not be apparent on radiographs until renal failure is well advanced, early changes can be detected in bone biopsies (44). Raised levels of parathyroid hormone are found in children when the GFR falls below 45 ml/min/1.73 m^2 (46). Decreased mean circulating plasma 1,25 dihydroxyvitamin D (1,25 [OH]$_2$D$_3$ concentrations occur when the GFR falls below 50 ml/min/1.73 m^2 (44).

Subperiostial resorption zones and changes at the metaphyses are the most usual signs of renal osteodystrophy on radiography. Both, however, may be due to osteitis fibrosa and there is no single sign which is specific for osteomalacia (44). Children with severe osteomalacia and slipped epiphyses also have more severe osteitis fibrosa (44). Unless recognised early bone deformities can appear with alarming rapidity in the young infant. Soft tissue and vascular calcification are less common though corneal and conjunctival calcification sometimes occur. Epiphyseolysis is a severe complication of renal osteodystrophy in children and is associated with the accumulation of woven bone and fibrous tissue in the radiolucent zone between ossification centres (47). The osteodystrophy should be treated medically before orthopaedic surgery is undertaken to correct any deformity. Attempts to stabilise slipped epiphyses e.g. by screws should be discouraged even though the epiphyses especially in the femoral region, may consolidate outside the normal position (47).

Avascular necrosis of bone, especially in the head of the femur, is a well recognised complication occurring after transplantation but can also occur in children on dialysis. It is undesirable to perform femoral head replacement operations in small children but a femoral osteotomy is often successful in alleviating pain and abolishing the limp in symptomatic children. Early mobilisation after surgery is desirable and the operation is tolerated well as long as it is undertaken after the osteodystrophy has been suppressed medically.

Aluminium accumulation is a major factor in vitamin D refractory osteomalacia in children with renal failure (44). Normal subjects absorb small amounts of aluminium following the oral administration of aluminium hydroxide and this is usually excreted by the kidney but accumulates when renal function is reduced. Young children probably absorb more aluminium from the intestine than adults do when treated with aluminium hydroxide. Serum Ca concentrations tend to be normal or raised and some children develop hypercalcaemia spontaneously or after only small doses of vitamin D or calcium supplements. Serum parathyroid hormone levels tend to be lower but high levels do not exclude aluminium intoxication (44). Plasma Al levels probably reflect recent aluminium intake and do not accurately indicate body aluminium content. A rise in plasma Al concentration is more than 150 μg/l after deferoxamine infusion is a useful though not entirely precise predictor of an increased total bone aluminium content (44, 48).

Serial measurements of serum parathyroid hormone concentrations are useful in monitoring therapy in children with renal osteodystrophy but individual values have to be interpreted with caution because most available assays recognise breakdown fragments of parathyroid hormone which accumulate in chronic renal failure.

Prevention of renal osteodystrophy in children with chronic renal insufficiency should be considered early in the course of the disease. We routinely monitor bone radiographs and parathyroid hormone concentrations when the GFR is below 35 ml/min/1.73 m². Treatment of renal osteodystrophy requires regular supplementation with vitamin D derivatives to heal osteomalacia and suppress hyperparathyroidism and phosphate absorption should be reduced by restricting dietary phosphate intake and using agents that bind phosphate in the intestine.

The preparation of vitamin D used for prophylaxis and treatment depends on availability and compliance (Table 6). We tend to use either 1 alpha(OH)D$_3$ or 1,25(OH)$_2$D$_3$, though preparations of the latter which are suitable for infants are not available. Supplements of vitamin D are only prescribed after the plasma phosphate concentration has been reduced to within the normal range. The plasma Ca concentration is raised to the upper limit of normal but it is vitally important that the level is monitored regularly to prevent hypercalcaemia which can lead to further deterioration in renal function. The plasma phosphate concentration is reduced towards but not below the lower limit of normal by restricting the intake of dairy products particularly milk, cheese and yoghurt.

Phosphate binders are administered with meals as necessary to achieve the desired plasma phosphate concentration. Aluminium hydroxide is used for new patients with high plasma Ca × P products and once the plasma phospate has been lowered calcium carbonate is substituted (49, 50). The Ca × P product is kept below 4.8 (mmol/l x mmol/l).

This regime has suppressed hyperparathyroidism for periods up to 3 years (50) and did not induce a decline in renal function over this period. Since its introduction, parathyroidectomy for uncontrolled hyperparathyroidism has not been necessary. Whilst suppression of hyperparathyroidism was demonstrable both by serum hormone concentrations and bone biopsy the latter revealed less successful remineralisation of bone perhaps because of prior exposure to aluminium.

The dialysate Ca concentration chosen is usually 1.75 mmol/l (7 mg/dl) but this depends on such factors as dietary calcium intake (see below) plasma Ca concentration and vitamin D intake.

Anaemia

Children on regular haemodialysis are usually profoundly anaemic (see also Chapter 40) and require regular transfusions to maintain haemoglobin levels above 5 g/dl; in one study the mean haematocrit in children treated by haemodialysis was 19.3% ± 2.9% (51). Prepubertal children are more anaemic than pubertal children and require more transfusions.

Many factors probably contribute to the severe anaemia in children but the most important is blood loss in the dialyser; as noted previously the volume of the dialyser and the blood lines in relation to blood volume of the patient is greater in a child and therefore the potential blood losses are relatively larger.

Intestinal losses also contribute importantly (52). It is necessary to restrict losses from repeated blood sampling and the blood left in the dialyser and blood lines should be carefully returned to the patient. One of the main advantages of CAPD in children is the less severe anaemia.

Occasionally haemolytic anaemia occurs due to copper, nitrite, or chloramine in the water supply (53). Hypersplenism can occur (54) and persistently low white cell and platelet counts and a palpable spleen (though this is not invariably present) suggest the need for red cell survival and splenic uptake studies; splenectomy can lead to a rise in haemoglobin concentration. Bilateral nephrectomy should be avoided when possible. Iron supplements should not be given routinely to children who are receiving frequent transfusions lest iron overload occur and body iron stores should be monitored by serum ferritin concentrations (55). Severe iron toxicity may be treated with deferoxamine though this is rarely required (56). Treatment with erythropoetin will probably become available during the next few years and there is no doubt that the eradication of anaemia in children on dialysis will considerably improve their lives enabling perhaps more children to be transplanted by preventing the sensitisation that may occur with frequent blood transfusions (57).

Cardiovascular complications

Hypertension in children on regular haemodialysis usually responds to increased salt and water removal by ultrafiltration during dialysis. Inadequate dialysis with dialysers that are too small or too large (leading to hypotension during dialysis and hypertension after washback) is the commonest cause of persistent hypertension in children treated by regular haemodialysis.

Some children persistently develop hypotension during conventional haemodialysis which necessitates saline or plasma infusion to stabilise blood pressure and leads to hypertension after dialysis. Sequential ultrafiltration and dialysis in such patients usually allows sufficient fluid remov-

Table 6. Vitamin D preparations for use in the treatment of renal osteodystrophy in children.

	Dose(μg/day		Half-life
	prophylaxis	treatment	
25(OH)D$_3$	12.5–25	50–150	2 weeks
dihydrotachysterol	120–150	500–2000	weeks
1α(OH)D$_3$	0.25–0.5	1–4	hours
1,25(OH)$_2$D$_3$	0.12–0.25	0.5–2.0	4–6 hours

al during dialysis without hypotension.

A vicious circle of hypertension between dialyses, hypotension on dialysis and therefore inadequate dialysis, high blood urea concentrations, anorexia with poor food intake leading to malnutrition and hypercatabolism can easily develop. This requires extra attention to nutrition using energy supplements and even nasoenteric feeding combined with frequent short dialyses until the patient's condition stabilises. Rapid weight gain between dialysis with hypertension is generally due to excessive sodium intake increasing thirst rather than being due to simply drinking too much water, for these children are rarely hyponatraemic.

In occasional children severe hypertension is due to hyperrenininaemia. This is especially common in children with renal failure due to haemolytic ureamic syndrome or focal glomerular sclerosis. In such children excessive salt and water removal during dialysis does not control blood pressure but results in nausea, anorexia and lethargy. The introduction of angiotensin converting enzyme inhibitors such as captopril or enalapril will usually control the hypertension and improve the child's health, appetite and activity; bilateral nephrectomy is now required only rarely.

Chronic hypertension, uraemia, and malnutrition all contribute to impaired cardiac performance in children on haemodialysis but anaemia and, in some children increased cardiac output caused by large arteriovenous fistulae are of a special importance. Echocardiography may reveal impaired left ventricular performance and a uraemic cardiomyopathy in some children (58). Cardiac arrest and pulmonary oedema are among the causes of death in children on dialysis; frequent cardiac assessment is an important part of management.

Neurological complications

Neurological complications (see Chapter 46) are rare in children in chronic renal failure who are being properly dialysed. Nonetheless neurological development is often below normal in children with severe chronic renal failure dating from infancy. Developmental delay has been detected in over 60% of such cases and particularly affects gross motor and language development (59). There is some evidence that early transplantation may improve development in such children (60). The cause of this developmental delay and the long term prognosis are not yet determined. Malnutrition, poor electrolyte control with wide swings in plasma osmolality in early life, and aluminium toxicity from the ingestion of aluminium hydroxide have been implicated (59, 61).

REGULAR HAEMODIALYSIS IN CHILDREN

The basic principles and procedures of haemodialysis in children are the same as in adults. However, haemodialysis of (small) children is associated with complications such as shunt and fistula failures, hypotension, nausea, vomiting, abdominal pain and encephalopathy during dialysis and hypertension, cardiac failure and pulmonary oedema following dialysis when equipment and methods designed for adults are used. Several modifications in techniques and equipment are required for paediatric purposes.

Vascular access

Angioaccess is a major problem in paediatric patients. Although external arteriovenous cannulae have been used extensively for chronic dialysis in children, the short functional life of shunts and the frequent complications (thrombosis, infections) has led to abandonment of this type of vascular access.

A better temporary vascular access is achieved by a percutaneously placed indwelling catheter in the jugular or subclavian vein. A silicone rubber catheter (Hickman) is positioned into the right atrium and fixed subcutaneously with a Dacron cuff. Depending on the size of the patient catheters with an internal diameter of 1.6 or 2.6 mm can be used. Both double and single lumen catheters are available. After dialysis 3 ml heparinised saline is injected into the catheter and a cap is placed at the external end. Fewer complications and a longer life span are noticed than with Scribner shunts (62, 63).

Brescia-Cimino radiocephalic fistulae at the wrist also have a low complication rate in children. The side (artery) to end (vein) anastomosis should be preferred to the end to end anastomosis because of the better flow through the hand when the distal portion of the artery remains patent. In small children, weighing less than 15 kg, the use of microsurgical techniques or secondary superficialisation of a deep vein or both allows construction of arteriovenous fistulae (64, 65). Shortness of the puncturable part of the vein often requires the use of single needle technique in children. It should be pointed out that this technique reduces dialysis efficiency. Maximizing arterial inflow volume decreases recirculation but requires a compliance chamber in the dialysis circuit to avoid increased hydrostatic pressure and thereby excessive ultrafiltration and increases extracorporeal blood volume (66).

A saphenous vein autograft is an efficient alternative if the forearm vessels are not suitable for fistula creation. Excellent results were obtained in children with autogenous saphenous vein grafts inserted in a loop configuration in the forearm (65, 67). A common complication of these grafts placed between the brachial artery and cephalic vein is the enormous dilatation of the vessel and aneurysm formation after long term use. Moreover, the high blood flow through the fistula may induce congestive heart failure. Polytetrafluoroethylene (PTFE) grafts (Goretex, Impra) may also be used for vascular access in children. When this graft is inserted in the thigh between the superficial femoral artery and the proximal saphenous vein, attention should be given not to place the graft too deeply into the subcutaneous tissue to avoid cannulation problems. Although efficient dialysis with PTFE grafts has been reported, a higher complication rate (thrombosis, infection) was noticed than with Brescia-Cimino fistulas or saphenous vein grafts (68).

Choice of dialyzer and blood lines

The dialyzer should be carefully adapted to the size of the patient. Selection relates to the blood volume of the dialyzer and blood lines and to the efficiency of the dialyzer.

The volume of the extracorporeal blood circuit should never exceed 10% of the patient's blood volume (80 ml/kg body weight). For severely anaemic patients a volume of less than 7% of the patient's blood volume is preferable. Calculation of extracorporeal blood volume should include increases of dialyzer blood volume during application of negative pressure for ultrafiltration. Special paediatric blood lines with volumes varying between 35 and 75 ml are commercially available. Paediatric blood lines with 3 mm internal diameter tubing will restrict blood flow to less than 75 ml/min. If higher blood flows are required special short blood lines with larger inner diameter will reduce extracorporeal blood volume. Although blood flow rates must be individually determined for each patient, general guidelines are proposed based on the patient's weight. Appropriate blood flow rates are calculated using the equation: flow (ml/min) = 2.5 × body weight (kg) + 100. In children weighing less than 10 kg blood flow rates should not exceed 75 ml/min, and in children weighing more than 40 kg rates up to 250 ml/min can be used.

Several disposable hollow fibre and flat plate dialyzers are suitable for the treatment of children. The patient's body weight and surface area and clinical condition should determine the clearance characteristics of the dialyzer to be used (Table 7).

To avoid dialysis disequilibrium it is safer to start treatment with a urea clearance not exceeding 3 ml/min/kg. Subsequently the choice of the dialyzer should be adapted to the individual tolerance of the patient, but dialyzers with urea clearances ranging between 6 and 8 ml/min/kg are required for regular short dialyses.

Fluid removal during haemodialysis is a function of transmembrane hydrostatic pressure and osmotic gradients. The rate of fluid removal depends on the dialyzer membrane surface area and hydraulic permeability. A dialyzer that accurately predicts ultrafiltration is required unless special devices for regulation of ultrafiltration are used.

Management of regular dialysis in children

The dialysis should be adjusted to the individual need of the child as determined not only by the size of the patient but also by individual variations in dialysis tolerance. Therefore, careful observation of the patient during dialysis is necessary. In small children critical changes in vital signs may appear. Regular control of vital signs is extremely important.

Especially in small children careful control of ultrafiltration is mandatory. Special devices for accurate control of ultrafiltration should be used; if not available continuous weight recording is imperative. Weight readings should be unaffected by normal movements of the patient or by the dialysis equipment.

General heparinisation can be effected by administration of a bolus of 50 U heparin/kg body weight at the beginning of dialysis, followed by infusion of 25 U heparin/kg/h.

In patients weighing 10 to 15 kg and without marked fluid retention (less than 2.5% of body weight) between dialysis, the priming fluid is often transfused into the patient at the beginning of the procedure. In very small children, weighing less than 10 kg, transfusion of the priming fluid into the patient is always required. In larger children the priming fluid is discharged unless the patient did not gain weight during the interdialytic period. At the end of dialysis the extracorporeal blood is transfused back to the patient. Only small amounts of saline (less than 100 ml) are used for the dialyzer washback procedure.

Ultrafiltration should be planned carefully and any excessive fluid loss should be replaced throughout dialysis. Ultrafiltration combined with dialysis has to be reduced to less than 5% of body weight in order to avoid severe hypoten-

Table 7. Characteristics of some disposable paediatric dialyzers.

Dialyzers	Membrane		Priming volume (ml)	Ultrafiltration coefficient (ml/h /mm Hg)	Urea clearance at Q_B (ml/min)			
	Nature	Surface area (m²)			75	100	150	200
ASAHI AM 0.3	Cuprammonium	0.30	30	1.4	59	73	93	–
ASAHI AM 0.6	Cuprammonium	0.60	60	2.1	69	88	100	–
ASAHI PAN50P	PAN	0.50	50	7.0*	–	96	–	138
GAMBRO MINI-MINOR	Cuprophane	0.23	20	0.5	37	57	–	–
GAMBRO 10-1N	Cuprophane	0.40	50	1.5	58	65	80	–
NIPRO 0.5	Cellulose acetate	0.50	38	2.5	–	–	–	88
NIPRO 0.7	Cellulose acetate	0.70	51	2.0	–	–	–	112
NIPRO 0.9	Cellulose acetate	0.90	61	3.0	–	–	–	132
BIOSPAL 1200S	PAN	0.50	60	23.0*	70	84	98	99
SORIN	Cuprophane	0.70	63	2.5	–	–	–	150
HEMOFLOW F40	Polysulfone	0.65	45	20.0*	–	100	–	150
SORIN HFT60	Polysulfone	0.80	44		–	–	–	200

* Must be used with an ultrafiltration control device.

sion during dialysis. Treatment of hypotension requires administration of 0.9% saline, 20% mannitol or albumen solution.

The requirement for dialysis is proportional to the metabolic rate, because the intake of all nutrients is proportional to metabolic rate. Metabolic rate is proportional to body surface area (BSA) which for a child is greater in relation to body weight than for an adult. Due to the high need for calories, protein and fluids relative to body weight, the child will accumulate metabolic waste products faster than adults do. Therefore, paediatric patients need more dialysis in relation to their body weight than adults. Children without significant residual kidney function are often dialysed thrice weekly. The duration of dialysis is determined by the time required for adequate fluid and solute removal. In patients with a moderately restricted protein intake (below 1.5 g/kg/day) adequate solute removal is achieved with a 3 to 5 h dialysis three times weekly.

Because most paediatric dialyzers have small ultrafiltration coefficients, dialysis time is often determined by fluid removal requirements. Shortening dialysis time is achieved by the use of dialyzers with highly permeable membranes or by haemodiafiltration.

Complications

Side effects related to the 'unphysiology' of dialysis may develop. These include nausea, vomiting, headache, hypotension and convulsions (disequilibrium syndrome). Convulsions occur in 10% of dialysed children but EEG abnormalities are found more often if continuously registered during dialysis (69). A rapid decline in plasma osmolality with shifting of water into the cells, a reduction of peripheral vascular resistance by acetate, high ultrafiltration rates and blood volume shifts to the dialyzer may contribute to these side effects.

If symptoms persist despite restriction of the efficiency of the dialyzer and avoidance of dialyzers with poor compliance characteristics, other measures must be taken. Dissociation of the dialysis and ultrafiltration procedure will allow ultrafiltration without the development of hypotension. During sequential ultrafiltration and dialysis a period of ultrafiltration precedes or follows standard dialysis, using the same dialyzer. Ultrafiltration is effected by an increase in transmembrane pressure. This is generated by application of a negative pressure across the non-blood side of the dialyzer's membrane or a positive pressure on the blood side of the membrane. During this procedure dialysate bypasses the dialyzer. Transmembrane pressure differences up to 500 mm Hg have to be used (70).

Intravenous infusion of mannitol at 1 g/kg will also reduce the decrease in serum osmolality during dialysis. However, mannitol will accumulate and reach a steady state level within a few dialyses with infusions. At this level an amount equal to that infused will be removed during each dialysis and it will be inefficient in preventing the decrease in osmolality. To avoid accumulation mannitol should be administered only once weekly (71).

The substitution of bicarbonate for acetate has significantly improved dialysis tolerance in children (72, 73). In the absence of a special device for the preparation of bicarbonate dialysate the use of biofiltration may result in a similar improvement in dialysis tolerance (74). Biofiltration is a haemodiafiltration technique performed with a dialysate containing acetate using dialyzers with highly permeable membranes and carefully controlled ultrafiltration. Substitution fluids containing bicarbonate are used (75). In children ultrafiltration rates of $2,000 \text{ ml}/1.73 \text{ m}^2$ per dialysis were achieved. Ultrafiltered fluids in excess of required net ultrafiltrate were replaced by isotonic bicarbonate. Improvement of dialysis tolerance similar to that achieved by bicarbonate dialysis was found (73).

Modification in composition of the dialysate will also affect symptoms associated with dialysis. Improved tolerance to haemodialysis can be obtained using 400 mg/dl dextrose enriched dialysate, which reduces the fall in serum osmolality during dialysis (75). However high dialysate dextrose concentrations increase the risk of bacterial proliferation and endotoxin release. Another way to increase plasma osmolality is to use dialysate with a high sodium concentration (145 mmol/l). High sodium levels may be maintained at a constant level but also a progressive decrease in dialysate sodium concentration throughout dialysis has been used to avoid chronic volume expansion, hypertension and heart failure (76). Excessive ultrafiltration during dialysis will induce intolerance. Accurate assessments of dry weight may be achieved by measurements of inulin distribution volume (IDV). In children developing hypotension during ultrafiltration an IDV less than 22% of body weight was found (77). Hypotension between dialyses sometimes occurs in nephrectomised patients, despite salt and fluid retention (78). The use of hypertonic dialysate may increase blood pressure in these patients. Persistance or increase of hypertension during dialysis, despite adequate ultrafiltration, is occasionally seen. If in those patients hypertension resists treatment with inhibitors of converting enzyme (captopril, enalapril) bilateral nephrectomy may be required. Recurrent pericarditis despite adequate dialysis occasionally occurs in children. These children are mostly hypertensive and usually overhydrated. If clinical assessment of fluid overload is difficult in these patients, IDV determination may be useful. In fluid overloaded patients IDV in excess of 29% of body weight was found (77). Excessive interdialytic weight gain related to dietary non compliance increases mortality rate in dialysed children (79). Hyperkalaemia occurs more frequently in small children than in adults during catabolic states or from high intakes and also represents a vital risk.

Hypersensitivity reactions related to dialysis material (first use syndrome) have been reported in children and may occur at any time after the start of treatment by dialysis (80). Symptoms resembling anaphylaxis start within 1 to 60 min following the onset of the dialysis procedure and range from urticaria to cardiopulmonary collapse. Their severity may require interruption of the dialysis procedure and emergency treatment.

Practical directives for haemodialysis in children

Preparation for dialysis

Before its initiation, dialysis has to be explained to the child by drawings and by attending a dialysis session of other children.

For blood access an arteriovenous fistula is created several months prior to the start of dialysis. Serum creatinine is quantified frequently to determine the time of fistula creation and subsequently the start of dialysis (Table 8). The rate of deterioration or renal function must also be considered when deciding on the time of fistula creation. In children selected for maintenance peritoneal dialysis an arteriovenous fistula is also constructed in order to create an immediately usable vascular access for haemodialysis if peritoneal dialysis fails.

Preparations for home dialysis are initiated at the time of fistula creation if the patient and his family are willing to perform the treatment at home.

Dietary prescriptions and controls for adequate nutrition are essential. Cumulative interdialytic weight gain from excessive fluid intake should be distinguished from real weight gain from an increase of the child's body mass.

The child should have his own responsibility for this interdialytic weight increase. Calorie and protein intakes are assessed by diet surveys recorded during similar interdialytic periods at monthly intervals. Calculation of the urea generation rate can be used to check adherence to the prescribed protein intake (81).

Dialysis technique

Fistula needles of gauge 18 to 14 are required for adequate blood flow. Single needle technique allows adequate dialysis even in small children with only a short vessel area available for needle insertion (2 to 3 cm).

Primary nursing improves the quality of care for paediatric patients. Individual nurse-patient allocation not only provides more efficient technical work, but also improves patient's adaptation to treatment.

The play-leader and teacher have to plan a playing and educational programme for each patient during the time spent on dialysis. Adequate cooperation between home school and the dialysis teaching team is required to obtain optimal schooling.

A basic rule is to adjust each dialysis according to the individual requirement of each child. Estimation of 'dry or ideal' body weight is essential. Percentile cards should be used to determine the ideal weight according to the child's body height and build. If the patient thrives and grows and the muscle mass increases, the ideal body weight also increases.

The choice of the dialyzer should be individually adapted to each patient. A special procedure has to be applied for the first sessions including the use of a less effective dialyzer (urea clearance less than 3 ml/kg), a shorter duration of dialysis (1.5 to 2 h), prophylactic use of diazepam (2 to 5 mg IV) and administration of mannitaol IV during dialysis (1 g/kg). Subsequently the dialyzer and duration of dialysis should be adapted to individual tolerance and requirements. The blood volume of the extracorporeal circuit (volumes of blood lines and dialyzer, including the additional volume due to compliance of the dialyzer) should not exceed 10% of the child's circulation blood volume.

The prescribed amount of ultrafiltration during dialysis depends on the interdialytic weight gain. Excessive weight gain between dialyses is usually due to high sodium intake with secondary excessive water intake; limitation of dietary sodium should be encouraged. Fluid loss by ultrafiltration during dialysis in excess of 5% of body weight will induce symptoms of hypotension. Precise and continuous monitoring and regulation of ultrafiltration is mandatory in paediatric patients. Continuous weight recording is less reliable. Weight changes may be caused by food and fluid intake, fluid loss by vomiting and by shifting of blood into (or out of) the dialyzer, due to volume changes caused by compliance of the membrane. If ultrafiltration in excess of 5% of body weight is required sequential ultrafiltration and dialysis should be applied. Small amounts of saline usually correct hypotension during dialysis.

Individual differences in dialysis tolerance are often observed. To obviate regular recurrence of headache, dizziness, nausea, abdominal pain and vomiting during dialysis the following modifications in treatment may be considered (82): withdrawal of antihypertensive drugs prior to analysis, reconsider the choice of the dialyzer, infusion of mannital (1 g/kg) during the first dialysis of the week, substitution of acetate by bicarbonate as the alkalinising buffer in the dialysate, and sequential hypertonic dialysis (use of decreasing dialysis fluid sodium concentrations during dialysis).

In paediatric patients dialysis twice a week may allow satisfactory rehabilitation but three dialyses a week are recommended allowing a more liberal dietary and fluid intake and reducing the side-effects during dialysis with vigorous ultrafiltration. In young children (< 5 years) the higher metabolic rate and poor compliance to the diet requires three dialyses per week.

Individual determination of total dialysis time per week will prevent overdialysis and may save time for the unit and the patient. Adapting dialysis time to obtain predialysis blood urea values less than 30 mmol/l will usually provide adequate dialysis. In Table 9 the proposed combinations of dialysis time, dialyzer size and blood flow rates according to patient's size are given.

Table 8. Fistula creation and start of dialysis.

age (yr)	Fistula creation at serum creatinine	Start of dialysis at serum creatinine
1– 5	350–550 μmol/l	650–700 μmol/l
5–10	450–650 μmol/l	700–800 μmol/l
10–15	550–700 μmol/l	800–900 μmol/l

Creatinine 100 μmol/l = 1.13 mg/dl

Close supervision of the patient is required during dialysis. Careful observation will reveal agitation, color changes and abdominal pain. These clinical signs often precede hypotension. Regular determination of body weight and blood pressure pre- and postdialysis is required.

Treatment of complications during dialysis

Institution of dialysis often improves hypertension markedly, but many children remain hypertensive despite dialysis with ultrafiltration. Hypertensive emergencies are treated by diazoxide (5 mg/kg IV) or labetalol (0.5 mg/kg IV). For prolonged treatment of hypertension beta-adrenergic blocking agents are preferred to methyldopa because of less frequent adverse reactions. In cases of refractory hypertension the administration of captopril or enalapril is usually effective.

Ultrafiltration with an inappropriate dialyzer is the most common cause of hypotension during dialysis. Saline, mannitol and albumen solutions are commonly used to treat hypotension.

Convulsions during dialysis should be treated by administration of diazepam (5 to 10 mg acccording to body weight). Recurrent convulsions are either due to cerebral abnormalities or inappropriate dialysis technique.

REGULAR PERITONEAL DIALYSIS

Regular peritoneal dialysis has been extensively used in the treatment of ESRD in children and has been shown as effective as regular haemodialysis for control of uremia and its complications. Since the introduction of CAPD an increasing number of paediatric patients have undergone peritoneal dialysis.

In 1985, 24% of all children on regular dialysis in Europe were undergoing CAPD (83).

Types of peritoneal dialysis

There are three types of peritoneal dialysis: intermittent peritoneal dialysis (IPD), continuous ambulatory peritoneal dialysis (CAPD) and continuous cyclic peritoneal dialysis (CCPD).

Intermittent peritoneal dialysis

Technique

IPD is performed through an indwelling Silastic catheter, tailored to the size of the child. The adult size (intraperitoneal portion: 15 cm) is used for children weighing more than 30 kg. The paediatric size (12 cm) for those between 10 and 30 kg and the neonatal size (10 cm) in smaller children. Straight and curled catheters with one or two Dacron cuffs are used.

Catheter placement technique is similar in children and adults. Modifications proposed in children are the insertion of the catheter beneath the body of the rectus muscle instead of a midline entry site in order to have more tissue in which to bury the cuff. Also omentectomy is performed at the time of cannula insertion in small children because they are more susceptible to obstruction of the catheter by omental fringes (84).

After insertion of the catheter, dialysis is started immediately and continued without interruption for 4 to 6 days to avoid early catheter obstruction by fibrin plugs. Dialysis is subsequently performed two or three times per week with a duration of 40 to 60 h/week according to blood chemical concentrations, fluid balance, and residual renal function.

The volume for one exchange is calculated on a body weight basis: 20 to 30 ml/kg at the start progressively increasing to 40 to 50 mg/kg. Automatic or semi-automatic cycling machines performing one cycle every 30 min are used. The availability of low volume cycler machines has made IPD possible even in small children.

Dialysis solution contains sodium (132 to 141 mmol/l), chloride (100 to 110 mmol/l), lactate rather than acetate (30 to 45 mmol/l) and dextrose (76 mmol/l). Potassium is added (2 mmol/l) to the solution if the predialysis serum level is less than 4 mmol/l. A hypertonic solution containing 215 mmol/l of dextrose (4.25%) is used for one or more exchanges if required for adequate extracellular fluid volume control.

Indications

The introduction of CAPD and subsequently CCPD has relegated IPD to a secondary role. However, treatment fatigue often occurs in families of children treated with CAPD. In such instances temporary in-center IPD or home IPD performed overnight two times a week may allow the patient and his familiy a more normal life style.

Table 9. Proposed combinations of dialysis time, dialyzer size and blood flow rates according to patient's size.

patient				dialyzer				
age (yr)	weight (kg)	BSA (m²)	bloodvolume (ml)	DSA (m²)	Extracorporeal blood volume (ml)	blood flow (ml/min)	Cl_{BUN} (ml/min)	time (h) dialysis
2	11	0.50	770	0.37	75	125	44	3–5
4	17	0.75	1190	0.56	115	145	68	3–5
9	28	1.00	1960	0.75	190	170	112	3–5
14	43	1.30	3010	0.98	300	190	172	3–5

Results

Relatively few reports on children treated by IPD are available (85, 86). These data show that IPD and CAPD are equally effective for the treatment of chronic uremia. However patients on IPD have higher BUN and serum creatinine levels than those on CAPD. Plasma proteins usually remain normal, but in small children substantial protein loss leading to moderate hypoalbuminaemia has been noticed. Linear growth, control of hypertension and anaemia seem to be similar on IPD and on CAPD.

Continuous ambulatory peritoneal dialysis

Technique

CAPD is performed through an indwelling catheter surgically inserted as described above for IPD. Immediately following insertion, the patient is dialyzed with an automatic cycling machine for 4 to 6 days, while gradually dwell time (10 min to 4 h) and the volume of dialysate (10 to 50 ml/kg) are increased. Prophylactic antibiotics are administered before surgery (tobramycin 1.5 mg/kg IV and cephalothin 20 mg/kg IV).

During the period of 'break in' heparin (500 IU/l) and cephalothin (250 mg/l) are added to the dialysis solution. Subsequently CAPD is started on the basis of four exchanges per day with 50 ml/kg of dialysis solution. After commencing regular CAPD, the patients and their parents are trained to perform CAPD at home. Children 10 years of age or older are able to learn the technique themselves. Teaching of parents or patients includes such aspects as bag change, dressing change, measurements of blood pressure and recognition of signs of peritonitis. They are advised about correct 'dry weight' and the type of dialysis fluid required to maintain that weight. Once the patient is discharged from the hospital, close contact is maintained by telephone. Regular attendances, at least once a month, at the dialysis centre are required (87).

Indications

The choice to perform CAPD should be a collective decision of the patient, his family and the nephrology team. CAPD may be a better alternative in the treatment of ESRD in infants in whom haemodialysis is difficult to perform, in children living a long distance from the dialysis centre, in patients with no vascular access sites available for haemodialysis and for patients at risk for increased intracranial pressure. Also patients with poor haemodialysis tolerance and children with severe psychological problems related to the haemodialysis should benefit from conversion to CAPD. Children whose parents are afraid or unwilling to accept responsibility to perform the treatment at home, are regarded as unsuitable for CAPD.

Results

Clearances of small and middle molecules with CAPD are higher than with IPD, but BUN and plasma creatinine values are higher than in patients on regular haemodialysis. Patients on CAPD use less phosphate binders and exchange resins that those on haemodialysis. Haematocrits are also higher than in regular haemodialysis patients (88, 89). Normal growth was not different in patients on CAPD compared to those on haemodialysis (90). Rehabilitation of children on CAPD is excellent and fulltime school attendance is frequently achieved. Physical activity could be almost normal, but some limitations, in order to protect the cutaneous exit site of the catheter, are recommended.

Continuous cycling peritoneal dialysis

Technique

CCPD consists of a long diurnal exchange, lasting 12 to 15 h and multiple nocturnal exchanges of variable duration. In children four to five, 2-h exchanges with an automatic cycler delivering up to 50 ml/kg of dialysate are performed during the night. None or only one daytime dwell using a smaller dialysate volume is effected (91).

Indications

Patients who require more than four daily exchanges to control the biochemical abnormalities of uremia or to obtain adequate ultrafiltration, and those who are unable to tolerate the dialysate volume required to achieve adequate dialysis, because of hydrothorax, repeated hernia or dialysate leak, may benefit from conversion to CCPD. CCPD may be primarily chosen over CAPD by parents who are unavailable to perform the daytime exchanges and by patients attending school who are unable to perform the procedure at school (92).

Results

CCPD is as efficient as CAPD in biochemical control of uremia. Procedural difference between CAPD and CCPD may lead to a lower rate of peritonitis with the latter (93). In small children the shorter dwell time of CCPD will increase ultrafiltration.

Clinical management of children on peritoneal dialysis

Peritoneal dialysis prescription

The appropriate peritoneal dialysis prescription in children should be based on analysis of the contribution of residual renal function and the peritoneal dialysis clearance needed to achieve adequate solute removal and on the amount of ultrafiltration required to maintain water balance.

Prescription for CAPD

The aims of CAPD are to maintain stable concentrations of solutes within the body and water balance. Blood urea levels are often used as indicators of uremic toxicity and therefore dialytic therapy is adapted to maintain BUN at 20 mmol/l. Calculations of urea generation rate may be used to determine peritoneal dialysis prescription (94). BUN generation rate is approximately 125 to 150 mg/kg/day. In order to achieve stable BUN values combined peritoneal and renal elimination must equal the urea generation rate. The dialysate volume required to clear generated urea can easily be calculated because at the completion of the long dwell periods used in CAPD, dialysate urea levels equal BUN. The estimated dialysate volume should be reduced by the contribution of residual renal function to urea clearance and by the volume of ultrafiltrate. Also clearances of other solutes may be used to determine adequacy of dialysis. Peritoneal creatinine clearance should exceed 6 ml/min/1.73 m² (95).

The amount of body water that needs to be ultrafiltered should be calculated on the basis of 'dry weight'. Dry weight is determined on clinical symptoms but in hypertensive children measurements of extracellular fluid volume may be required. Ultrafiltrate volumes depend on dextrose concentration of the dialysate, exchange volumes and duration of the exchange. Drainage volumes after a 4 h exchange exceed infused volumes of dialysate containing dextrose monohydrate in concentrations of 1.5% and 4.25% by approximately 15 to 25% and 30 to 40% respectively (94).

It should be noted that in small children ultrafiltrate volumes are usually less; this is probably due to enhanced dextrose absorption. Therefore dialysis and ultrafiltration requirements as well as individual peritoneal membrane characteristics will determine the number of exchanges, dwell time and dextrose concentration used (86).

Nutrition

In addition to the recommendations given later, calculation of energy intake should include glucose uptake (3.75 kcal/g) from the dialysate. In children less than 6 years old glucose absorption (2.74 ± 1.05 g/kg/day) is higher than in older children (1.49 ± 0.72 g/kg/day) (96).

The recommended protein intake for children on CAPD is 1.5 to 2.0 g/kg, whereas in infants 2.5 to 3.0 g/kg is proposed. Also protein loss into the dialysate is higher in younger patients (0.24 ± 0.04 g/kg/day) compared to older children (0.17 ± 0.06 g/kg/day) (97).

In children undergoing CAPD high serum levels of triglycerides and cholesterol were found. The hypertriglyceridemia was related to impaired clearance of triglycerides (96). The uptake of glucose from the dialysate may also increase triglyceride production.

Increases in cholesterol and triglycerides were also more pronounced in younger children, who also had higher protein losses in the dialysate (97). Dietary fat should provide about 50% of dietary energy intake with a ratio of polyunsaturated to saturated fatty acid of 1.5 to 1.0. This fatty acid ratio may reduce serum triglyceride levels.

Mineral metabolism

Despite stable serum Ca levels, worsening of renal osteodystrophy in children treated with CAPD has been reported. During CAPD vitamin D binding protein and 25-hydroxy vitamin D are lost into the dialysate. Using a dialysate with 1.75 mmol/l of calcium, losses of calcium into the dialysate are minimal. Salusky et al (98) reported that higher doses of calcitriol (0.25 to 2.25 ug/day), than those commonly used in hemodialysis patients, should be used to treat secondary hyperparathyroidism.

Complications of peritoneal dialysis

Peritonitis

Peritonitis is a major complication of peritoneal dialysis. The incidence of peritonitis in patients on CAPD is about one episode every 10.5 patient months, but more than 30% of the patients are still peritonitis-free after 24 months of treatment. In the majority of cases peritonitis is caused by failure in technique, but may be associated with exit site infection or tunnel infections. Two thirds of the organisms isolated are gram positive (Staph aureus, Staph epidermidis, Strept viridans) and one third is gram negative. Fungal infections are occasionally found. An incidence of 'culture negative' peritonitis in up to 50% of cases was reported (99).

Abdominal pain, fever and cloudy dialysate are the most consistent clinical signs of peritonitis. Peritonitis with clear fluid and low dialysate cell count (less than 100 cells/μl) is unusual in patients on CAPD but may be found in patients on intermittent peritoneal dialysis.

Treatment of peritonitis

On CAPD the patient or his parents are told to call the hospital if signs of peritonitis occur. Unless they can reach the dialysis unit quickly, they are instructed to start treatment at home. After drainage of the abdominal cavity, the dialysate is saved for gram staining, cell count and culture. Thereafter three rapid exchanges with the usual volumes are performed, and CAPD is then resumed on a 6-h schedule with antibiotics and heparin added to each bag of dialysate. If no result of gram stain is available, a loading dose of 500 mg of cephalothin per liter of dialysate and of 1.7 mg/kg of tobramycin and 500 IU of heparin is added to the first exchange. Thereafter, 250 mg of cephalothin per liter is added to the dialysate. If a gram positive organism is identified, cephalothin treatment alone is continued, while if a gram negative organism is found, tobramycin alone is used (10 mg/l). In the presence of no growth both antibiotics are continued. Treatment is continued for 12 days with repeated cultures on day 5 and 10. Afterwards treatment is prolonged if clinically required. Antibiotic treatment is modified according to bacteriologic examination if dialysate fluid has not become clear after 48 h of treatment (Dosage see Table 10). Heparin is added to the dialysate until the fluid is clear and fibrin clots disappear (87).

With peritonitis, CCPD patients are switched to CAPD for at least one week and treatment is similar to that in patients on CAPD. For patients treated by IPD, after the diagnosis of peritonitis is made, three rapid exchanges are performed. Following these three exchanges, an exchange with a loading dose of 500 mg of cephalothin per liter, tobramycin 1.7 mg/kg and 500 IU of heparin is effected. This exchange is left in the abdomen for 6 h. Continuous peritoneal lavage containing a maintenance dose of antibiotics (cephalothin 100 mg/l and tobramycin 10 mg/l) is initiated for 2 days followed by daily dialysis for 3 days. Antibiotics are added to the dialysis fluid for 2 weeks. Also oral antibiotics are added to the treatment (85)

Outcome of peritonitis

Early treatment results in improvement of symptoms after 24 h. Recurrent or persistent peritonitis may develop despite appropriate antibiotic treatment in patients with skin-exit site or tunnel infection. With persistent bacterial infection for more than 5 days, in the presence of fungal peritonitis and in severe skin-exit or tunnel infections, the peritoneal catheter should be removed.

Hernia

Children may develop inguinal or ventral (incisional) hernias. Commonly these hernias appear within the first months of dialysis and are more frequent in young children. Incisional hernias at the site of catheter insertion are more often found in patients with a midline incision and in those who developed dialysate leak in the postoperative period.

Hydrothorax complicating peritoneal dialysis was also reported in children (100). The use of CCPD with small dialysate volumes may prevent recurrence of hydrothorax. No data regarding adhesion pleurodesis with talc or tetracycline have been reported in children.

Electrolyte abnormalities

Hypernatraemia may occur from more rapid removal of water than sodium and can be caused by dialysis solutions containing high dextrose concentration during treatment with IPD. Treatment consists of prolonging dialysis cycles or the substitution of the dialysis fluid by a solution with a sodium concentration of 130 mmol/l. Hyponatremia has been reported in infants treated with CAPD requiring significant ultrafiltration. In this situation dialysate sodium loss may exceed oral sodium intake. Symptomatic hypotension may complicate such sodium loss (101).

Table 10. Recommended doses of intraperitoneal antibiotics in the treatment of peritonitis in patients on CAPD.

	Loading dose	Maintenance dose
Cephalothin	500 mg/l	250 mg/l
Cephradine	250 mg/l	125 mg/l
Tobramycin	1.7 mg/kg/bag	8 mg/l
Gentamicin	1.5 mg/kg/bag	10 mg/l
Ampicillin	500 mg/l	50 mg/l
Cloxacillin	1000 mg/l	100 mg/l
Vancomycin	10 mg/kg/bag	30 mg/l
Clindamycin	300 mg/l	50 mg/l
Amikacin	250 mg/l	50 mg/l

Changes of Peritoneal Membrane Characteristics

A permanent loss of ultrafiltration associated with increased glucose absorption from the dialysate, while peritoneal clearances remained unaltered, has been noted. During long term peritoneal dialysis these functional alterations were associated with histological alterations of the peritoneal membrane (102). Sclerosing encapsulating peritonitis was found in some patients. In these patients the thickened and sclerotic peritoneal membrane may incarcerate the small bowel and lead to bowel obstruction. Several factors such as peritonitis, dialysate containing acetate buffer, use of chlorhexidine as antiseptic agent during exchanges, and use of beta blockers, have been related to the development of membrane alterations (103).

Peritoneal dialysis in infants

Indications

Indications for CAPD in infants are replacement of renal function for end-stage renal disease or following bilateral nephrectomy. Indications for beginning peritoneal dialysis include fluid and electrolyte abnormalities or failure to thrive despite optimal medical management. Bilateral nephrectomy may be required in infants with massive urinary protein loss due to steroid resistant nephrotic syndrome and in patients with bilateral Wilm's tumor (86).

Technical aspects

The peritoneal membrane of infants is relatively larger and more permeable than that of children and adults. Peritoneal diffusion rates for urea, glucose, middle molecules and protein are higher when related to body size. The rapid absorption of glucose dissipates the osmotic gradient, decreasing ultrafiltration capacity. However, dialysate volume is a major determinant of ultrafiltration, and adequate ultrafiltration may be obtained if dialysate volumes of $1,200 ml/m^2$ are used (101).

The technique of CAPD is similar in infants and larger children. The availability of 250 and 275 ml dialysate containers has made application of CAPD in infants possible. However, to improve ultrafiltration shorter dwell times are often used. In infants at least five exchanges a day are performed. Different modifications in technique were proposed to avoid frequent disconnection procedures required by shorting dwell times. Conley et al (104) used two bags adapted to a Y connector that allowed multiple exchanges a day while entering the system only once. Warady et al (105) used recirculating dialysis with a 2 l dialysate bag. Exchange volumes of 40 ml/kg, determined by weighing the bag of dialysate on a bedside scale, were infused into the peritoneal cavity and after completion of a 1-h dwell the peritoneal effluent drained back into the same bag. Once connected the system was not broken until completion of dialysis (8 h/day) (105).

Nutrition

Energy intake should at least equal recommended dietary allowances (RDA). Protein intake should meet RDA (2.5 to 3 g/kg/day) plus replace protein lost in the dialysate (0.25 g/kg/day). Carbohydrate, fat and protein supplements must be added to the formula, if fluid restriction is required because of anuria (86).

In infants with minimal residual urine production, dialysate sodium losses due to ultrafiltration will exceed intake, requiring oral sodium chloride supplementation (101). These nutritional requirements are often not met with ad lib intake. Frequently intermittent nasogastric or continuous transpyloric tube feedings will be necessary.

Burn-out

Burn-out or treatment fatigue has been reported in both children and parents during CAPD. Behavior patterns indicative of burn-out are: failure to maintain accurate home records, failure to take medications, frequent episodes of infections, neglect of appointments and inability to make decisions (106).

Measures for dealing with burn-out are regular contact and home visits by the nursing staff, contact with other families of children on CAPD, personal attention by one of the team members, retraining, and involving more family members in the treatment (106). Conversion to CCPD has been a major mode of dealing with CAPD burn-out, especially in families of very young children and adolescents (92).

KIDNEY TRANSPLANTATION IN CHILDREN

Kidney transplantation is the treatment of choice for children with end stage renal disease while dialysis is usually considered as a means for awaiting transplant surgery, or an interlude between two grafts after an initial failure.

Although this principle is agreed upon by the majority of nephrologists, transplantation is not always possible when needed, which explains why all children with ESRD do not have a functioning graft. On December 31, 1985, out of 1,641 patients with ESRD less than 15 years of age recorded in the registry of the EDTA, only 744 had a functioning graft, but the proportion of grafted children varied from country to country, reaching for example 87% in Sweden or 58% in UK, but only 33% in Italy (83). Another way of presenting transplantation strategy is to consider the proportion of patients surviving by the means of a graft at different times after starting renal replacement therapy. Using this mode of analysis, more than 50% of children had a functioning graft after one year in Nordic countries, while the 50% mark was reached by 2 years in UK, 3 years in FRG and 4 years in France (83). Thus, the mean waiting time on dialysis is very variable according to country, longer for a cadaver than for a living related graft. Both sources of

kidney are used for transplanting children. In spite of the current controversy about transplanting a kidney from a living donor, all agree to use such donation for paediatric patients. Nevertheless, here again marked differences in policy are noted between countries. In Europe in 1985 out of 384 transplantations, 63 (16%) were performed from living related donors (83). This proportion was much higher in North America reaching 80% of transplantations in some single centre reports.

Some children are transplanted directly without even a short period on dialysis. According to the data of the EDTA registry, 96 out of 2,211 patients starting treatment under age 15 in the years 1981 to 1985 were directly grafted (4.3%); this proportion was as high as 20% in Nordic countries. Another trend is to perform the 2nd graft when the 1st fails without passage again on dialysis.

Preparation of children for transplantation

The preparation protocol may be different according to the center, but for children, several points have to be carefully considered. Blood transfusions continue to be considered as useful preoperatively by many groups. The severity of anaemia of children with ESRD usually will indicate transfusion as well (until recombinant erythropoietin becomes available). The crucial point is to look for cytotoxic antibodies after each transfusion in order to stop administering blood containing sensitising HLA antigens if sensitisation appears with only the use of frozen-thawed or especially with filtered blood. Some centres use the donor specific transfusion protocol before a transplantation with a living related donor. Recent reports do not seem to confirm the need of such a protocol when using cyclosporine after grafting. Evaluation and repair of low urinary tract abnormalities is mandatory. A voiding cystogram is part of the check list before grafting. Massive reflux may be an indication for nephroureterectomy. A small pathological bladder may be enlarged with a segment of gut. Moreover, a Bricker neocystostomy may be performed as a first step in patients without any bladder available e.g. those with spina bifida or neurological bladder.

Immunizations have to be updated, especially those using a living attenuated virus such as varicella and measles, immunization should be performed at least 2 months before grafting.

Severe hypertension caused by native kidneys is usually considered as indication for a left nephrectomy in a first step, in order to excise totally the native kidneys with a right nephrectomy at the time of transplantation. The same approach may be applied for children with persisting nephrotic syndrome and massive proteinurea.

For children who had convulsions and receive phenobarbital or hydantoins, it is recommended to try and switch to other anticonvulsivant drugs such as valproic acid or clonazepam which do not induce hepatic microsomial catabolism of corticosteroid and cyclosporine.

Perioperative management

At the time of transplantation, with a cadaver transplant, the best HLA matching is sought since the best results continue to be observed in well matched grafts, even in patients receiving cyclosporine (107).

An adult kidney can be grafted in a young patient, as was shown in several series (108), but below 10 to 12 kg it would be probably better to use a pediatric cadaver kidney.

Operative and post-operative management have to be very careful in children. Hemodynamic stability must be maintained at the time of declamping the graft renal artery. The best way for succeeding on this point is to check continuously pulmonary artery pressure by means of a Swan Ganz catheter and maintain pressure between 20 and 25 mm Hg. Vital parameters and difference between peripheral and central temperature are also used postoperatively as basic guides for the management (108, 109).

Medical treatment and follow up

The immunosuppressive regimen after grafting is similar in children and in adult patients, except for adapted doses of drugs according to body size. But the incrimination of corticosteroids in growth retardation mandates selection of immunosupressive protocols for children using the lowest corticosteroid dosage as possible.

Immunosuppressive treatment has to be continued indefinitely and part of the follow up is to monitor and encourage compliance to the medical prescription, since noncompliance is a major cause of graft failure in adolescents (110, 111).

The *conventional treatment* consists of azathioprine and prednisone. The dose of azathioprine is usually adjusted to body weight (2 to 3 mg/kg). This is decreased with renal insufficiency down to 1 to 2 mg/kg according to the GFR. Azathioprine is stopped at least briefly in case of viral infection. Some patients develop a cholestatic hepatotoxicity with this drug leading to its termination. Prednisone is progressively tapered down to a daily dose defined by the transplant unit between 5 and 10 mg/m². Many pediatric patients are switched to alternate day therapy receiving twice this dose every other day.

Cyclosporine is becoming the basis of most of the immunosuppressive protocols in children. Patients receiving cyclosporine have a dose generally adjusted at the start according to the blood or plasma trough level; the aim is currently to maintain a blood level between 150 and 400 ng/ml or a plasma level between 50 and 150 ng/ml. This is obtained usually with a dose of 4 to 10 mg/kg. Some authors have recommended administering cyclosporine on the basis of body surface area giving an initial dose of 500 mg/m² (112). There are many different protocols using cyclosporine, with and without corticosteroids, associated with low dose azathioprine (triple therapy) or not, prescribed from the day of grafting or after 1 to 6 weeks, prescribed undefinitely or for some months with secondary conversion to conventional treatment. None of these protocols has definitely proved its superiority; all need a careful follow up of the patient looking for side effects of cyclosporine, mainly nephrotoxicity suspected by an increase of plasma creatinine but sometimes only discovered on systematic transplant biopsy.

Other prescriptions in transplanted children include antihypertensive agents or anticonvulsivants (preferably valproic acid or clonazepam). Prevention of corticosteroid effects on bone is attempted by calcium or vitamin D supplements with a careful follow up of calciuria and calcaemia.

Diagnosis of rejection. The main complication of transplantation remains rejection, consequently the main objective of the follow up is to detect rejection as early as possible. The classical acute rejection crisis includes symptoms as fever, graft tenderness, oliguria and decrease of GFR. In fact after the 1st month such symptoms are rather rare and rejection is only marked by biochemical symptoms such as a slight increase in plasma creatinine, slight proteinuria (of glomerular and tubular origin), acidosis and lower hemoglobin. Echography of the graft may detect obvious findings such as increase in the size of the graft, decreased echogenicity of the renal pyramids, thickening of the renal cortex and nonhomogenous regional loss of cortical echogenicity with overall increase or decrease in cortical thickness. Transplant biopsy is sometimes needed to ascertain the diagnosis and direct treatment. This treatment consists usually in IV high dose methylprednisolone (1 g/1.73 m²) followed or not by a temporary increase of daily prednisone. Rejection crisis may also be treated with success by antilymphocyte or antithymocyte globulins.

Other causes of impairment of GFR and increase of plasma creatinine are also sometimes detected. These include obstruction of the urinary tract by lithiasis or secondary stenosis usually shown by graft echography, stenosis of the renal artery of the graft always associated with severe hypertension and nephrotoxicity of cyclosporine which is the main problem in patients receiving this drug. Nephrotoxicity may be proved by immediate improvement of renal function after stopping cyclosporine for 1 or 2 days; in dubious cases a renal biopsy may be useful.

The follow up of a child with a functioning graft has to cope with two difficulties. On one hand follow up should not interfere too much with the day to day life and especially the school attendance and the planned vacations and on the other hand it is important not to miss any problem at its beginning especially rejection. This follow up is mainly the responsibility of the transplant unit where the graft was performed, but individual solutions may be found involving a local physician or laboratory or both, previously informed to react to any 10 to 20% increase in plasma creatinine concentration and to slight proteinuria. The frequency of biological checkings, at first weekly, can be spaced to every 3 weeks or month after 1 year, and to every 2 months after 3 to 5 years. Any change in the immunosuppressive protocol indicates more frequent monitoring. Regular outpatient consultations are mandatory to check all biological data, to detect any complications related or not to the treatment, to note growth velocity and last but not least to check the drug compliance.

Results and causes of failure

The general results of transplantation in children improved clearly in recent years, probably due to the new immunosuppressive agents. Actuarial first cadaver graft survival in patients transplanted under 15 years of age in the EDTA registry in the years 1981 to 1985 was 75% at 6 months 68% at 1 year and 60% at 2 years. Children transplanted in 1983 to 1985 receiving cyclosporine (n at start = 274) had a better graft survival: 80% at 6 months and 75% at 1 year versus respectively 74% and 68% in others (n at start = 350). Monocentric studies reported higher survival rates, for example 80% at 1 year and 69% at 3 years under conventional treatment (110) while with cyclosporine graft survival was reported as high as 93% at 1 year and 78% at 3 years (112).

Long term results are only known for patients having received conventional immunosuppression; graft survival was 40% at 10 years in a monocentric report (110).

Live related donor (LRD) transplantation, leads to better results. In the EDTA registry of the 267 LRD grafts performed in 1981 to 1985 actuarial graft survival was 87% at 6 months 82% at 1 year and 79% at 2 years. Here again data from monocentric studies are even better.

The major cause of graft failure remains rejection accounting for two thirds of failures in the paediatric EDTA registry (79) but other causes in children include postoperative vascular thrombosis and also recurrence of primary renal diseases such as nephrotic syndrome with focal sclerosis and oxalosis.

Growth after transplantation

Growth is very variable after a kidney graft; a catch up curve is reported in only 20 to 50% of the cases while one third of patients continue to be stunted (113–115).

A number of factors may interfere with growth after transplantation. The most important are renal function of the graft and corticosteroid therapy. Renal function has to be normal or almost normal for catch up growth which was rarely observed in patients with a plasma creatinine above 120 μmol/l, in contrast to observations in patients with chronic renal failure under conservative treatment. Corticosteroids are known to limit growth velocity at doses above 5 or 6 mg/m²/day, and this is the case of most children under conventional treatment. Giving corticosteroids every other day may improve growth velocity and is recommended in children whenever possible especially at puberty (113). New immunosuppressive regimens using cyclosporine are generally associated with less corticosteroids and reportedly allow a better growth rate (116). Children under 7 years were reported to grow better but a catch up curve may also be observed in older patients. There is an inverse relationship between growth velocity after transplantation and statural stunting at the start; the smaller for age the child is, the better the standard deviation score after grafting (113). Bone maturation is also important to follow since a pubertal growth spurt, observed in 1/3 of patients, was reported for a bone age of 11 in girls and of 13 in boys, earlier than in normal subjects, but occurring with a delay of 1 to 5 years considering chronological age (113).

Adult height was analysed in 185 females and 191 males recorded in the EDTA registry as having started RRT under age 15. It was 154.3 cm in females and 161.3 cm in males ranging from 135 to 180 cm in both sexes. Patients grafted under the age of 15 did not have a higher ultimate height, but those who were never grafted were shorter than other patients.

In summary growth after transplantation, already better than under dialysis, will probably improve in the future with new immunosuppressive regimens, allowing a higher ultimate height to be reached.

Complications after transplantation

A number of complications may occur after kidney transplantation. In the post operative period acute tubular necrosis is frequently observed and when severe may lead to a permanent reduction in nephron mass. Thrombosis of the transplant renal artery or vein is a cause of primary anuria, more frequent in young children than in adults, leading to the loss of the graft (79). Surgical complications such as urinary leak also can occur.

Acute rejection crisis, as already mentioned, is the main complication; it is sometimes irreversible, especially in the first weeks after transplantation, but is usually controlled by adequate treatment. Chronic rejection is most often the sequel of an acute crisis but may also develop insidiously. Transplant biopsy is useful for the precise diagnosis of the lesions.

Hypertension is also a major cause of concern in transplanted children with a high risk of encephalopathy and neurological sequelae (117, 118). Blood pressure has to be checked frequently and hypotensive drugs have to be administrated and adjusted as necessary. Transplant angiography must be performed if there is any doubt about a renal artery stenosis.

Infections are also a permanent risk in children under immunosuppression. In the early postoperative period they are especially vulnerable to septicaemia and cytomegalovirus infection. The prognosis of infectious complications depends on early diagnosis and specific treatment.

Complications related to steroids are also possible; gastroduodenal haemorrhage, psychiatric disturbances and diabetes mellitus are quite rare and only observed in the first few weeks post grafting. Aseptic bone necrosis was a major complication of high dose steroid protocols but its prevalence has dramatically decreased in the recent years (110). Osteoporosis may also develop in the long term.

Late surgical complications as urinary lithiasis, secondary stenosis of urinary anastomosis or lymphocoele are quite rare and usually do not affect graft survival.

SURVIVAL AND CAUSES OF DEATH

Survival of patients on renal replacement therapy (RRT)

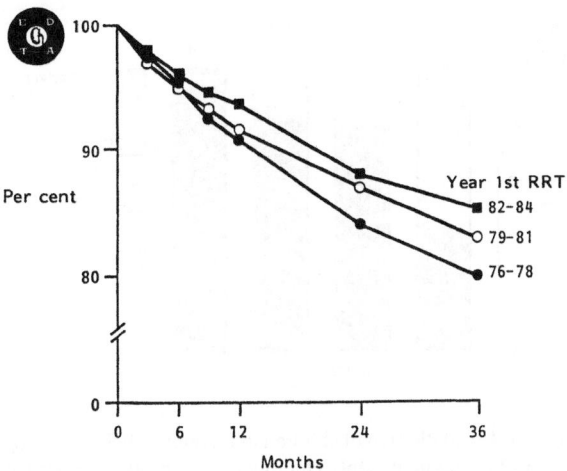

Figure 3. Survival of paediatric patients after first renal replacement therapy shown according to year of first treatment.

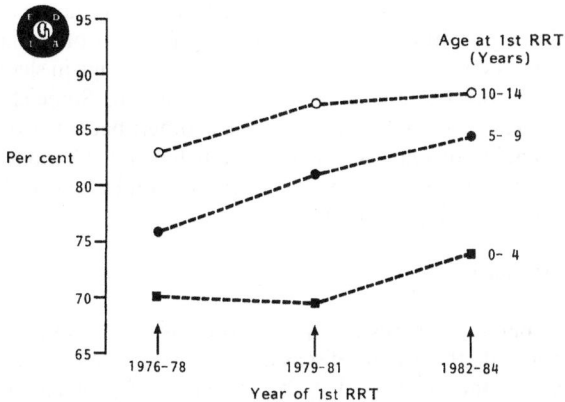

Figure 4. Comparison of 3-year patient survival after first renal replacement therapy for paediatric patients according to year of first treatment and age at first treatment.

has been studied widely, especially based on the experience of individual centres. For this reason the resuslts reported by different authors vary widely, depending not only on the quality of care but also on the selection criteria and, therefore, on the characteristics of children accepted for RRT. Data obtained from the EDTA Registry provide the average survival for children treated in many centres in all European countries. The 3-year survival of children after first RRT increased from 80% in those who started RRT in 1976 to 1978 to 86% in those who reached ESRD in 1982 to 1984 (23) (Figure 3). This improvement with time in the 3-year survival rate is also apparent for each of the age groups 0 to 4, 5 to 9 and 10 to 14. It is noteworthy that younger children (0 to 4 years old) have a worse 3-year survival (73%) than those aged 5 to 9 (83%) and 10 to 14 (84%) respectively (23) (Figure 4).

The comparison of patient survival on different modes of RRT has to be made with caution because the populations are not necessarily comparable but can be selected according to different criteria. Furthermore the patients are assigned to a given group only depending on their last mode of renal replacement therapy. With these limitations, home hemodialysis provides a 5-year survival of 84% compared to 74% for hospital hemodialysis (119).

It is well known that cardiovascular abnormalities are the main causes of death in children on chronic dialysis treatment. A recent survey by the Paediatric Registry of the EDTA on all causes of death occurring from 1981 to 1985 showed that hyperkalaemia accounted for 7.2% of all deaths, hypertensive cardiac failure for 6.0% fluid overload for 9.7% and cerebrovascular accident for 6.9% (83). Excess weight gain, defined as a gain exceeding 8% of body weight at least once a week between 2 hemodialysis sessions, appeared to be a problem in children aged 5 to 10 (79). From that study it appeared very clear that mortality during 1983 was higher among children with excess weight gain (7.5%) than in those without it (2.5%).

The second most frequent group of causes are infections (approximately 17% of all deaths); note also that 4.0% of the deaths were due to malignant diseases (83).

Causes of death on chronic dialysis do not differ substantially in children and in patients over 15, except for myocardial ischemia and infarction which are much more frequent in adults.

PSYCHOSOCIAL PROBLEMS

Optimal functioning of a dialysis programme for children not only requires appropriate medical and technical knowledge but simultaneous attention must also be paid to the emotional and social impact of the treatment on the juvenile patients and their families (120). A team including physicians, nurses, social workers, teachers and a psychologist should be available to cope with the problems relating to the child and his disease as discussed in the section on organisation of services and facilities for treatment of children.

The child and his disease

Even before beginning regular dialysis treatment the behaviour of young patients is influenced by their, longstanding disease. At this stage the children are invariably depressed. Mutilation in conception and representation of their body image frequently prevail. The children are preoccupied with their illness and show evidence of a clear consciousness of death. They resent having their lives full of unpleasant restrictions. The relationships of these children are characterised by withdrawal from social contacts and increasing dependence on their parents. Dialysis adds another important stress to the patient and adaptation at the beginning of treatment is often difficult. Anxiety, that may be either obvious or repressed will influence adaptation to the treatment. When the child's health improves drastic changes in attitudes and behaviour are frequently seen. The child becomes more active and less frightened. However, during the following months frequently recurring patterns of maladjustment emerge characterised by passivity, refuge in sleep, inaccessibility to others, anorexia and vomiting. Some children react with excessive dependence, others become overdemanding or react with aggressive behaviour. Complications and necessary surgical procedures will influence the incidence of these setbacks.

The families

The parents, depressed by the problems of a child with chronic life threatening disease, often put too high expectations on the effect of dialysis. Therefore, if problems increase or even persist important reactions may occur such as aggressive behaviour to the staff, lack of cooperation and unreasonable demands on the medical team. Faced with the problems of repetitive dialysis, the entire family is confronted with a series of stresses and demands that influence the relationships both within and beyond the family. Daily life is disturbed by the demanding programme: dialysis, diet, medication, restrictions of activity and hospitalisations of the child. The stresses and burdens that this situation places upon the family accentuate personal problems of members of the family such as psychosomatic diseases, danger of family breakdown and relational problems of the parents at their work. The other children in the family may experience various degrees of emotional deprivation.

The dialysis team

The dialysis team participates with parents and children in all emotional problems generated during treatment. The demands of meeting the emotional needs of the patients and their families, however, often extend beyond the capacity of the team members. This sometimes leads to reactions of withdrawal into regressive patterns in members of the team and disruption of communications within the group. Assistance by a paediatric psychiatrist will be necessary in crisis situations. Team discussions may be helpful to place problems in perspective and allow team members to support each other at times of stress.

REHABILITATION

The aim of regular dialysis treatment of paediatric patients is not only to prolong life but also to provide a basis for normal, physical, social and intellectuel development.

Rehabilitation should already be initiated during conservative treatment of the youthful chronic renal failure patient. Successful rehabilitation during dialysis largely depends on the previous support, and can only be obtained by a harmonious team as in a specialised paediatric unit. Proper school facilities and arrangements for leisure times and holidays should be provided. A normal school programme should be attained whenever possible. However, the time lost on recurrent dialysis may be a hindrance. In this respect

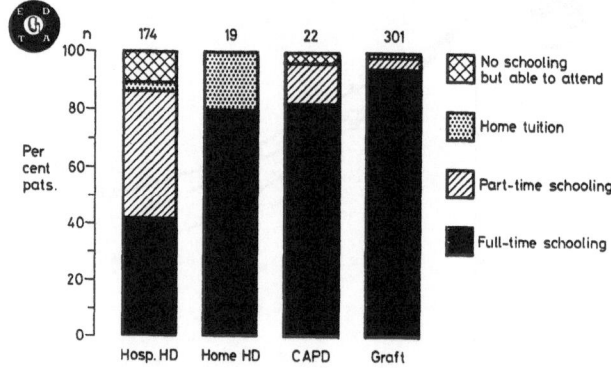

Figure 5. Rehabilitation of children in December 1984 according to method of treatment. Only children continuously on a particular form of renal replacement therapy for the whole of 1984 were included in the analysis.

home dialysis should be encouraged.

Physical activities need not be restricted during leisure time although anaemia may be a limiting factor. Normal leisure times should be encouraged within the child's own possibilities to overcome the natural resistance of overprotective relatives. School attendance has to be assessed regularly. Information on schooling was available in the EDTA registry from the 1984 special pediatric questionnaire. Only patients continuously on a particular mode of treatment for the year were included in the analysis. Type of schooling is shown in Figure 5 according to the mode of therapy in 1984; schooling included attendance at either an ordinary or a special school, part-time schooling included attendance on a regular or irregular basis. Full time schooling as an index of rehabilitation was noted in only 41% of children on hospital hemodialysis while 80% of children on CAPD and home hemodialysis attented school full time. However, the best rehabilitation was achieved in children grafted with 94% reported at school full time in 1984.

The reported long term rehabilitation has also been excellent in young adults who started renal replacement therapy as children and who have been successfully grafted (110, 121, 122). Social failures were especially related to poor school attendance in the primary school period (123), which emphasizes that adequate attention to teaching and education should have high priority and should be undertaken at an early stage.

DIETARY PRESCRIPTION

The high energy requirements relative to body weight in children have been discussed and the impact of uraemia on the nutritional status of a child is more drastic because the energy deficit caused by the anorexia of renal failure is greater (34). It is important to ensure an adequate food intake for children on dialysis. It has been shown the difference in growth between prepubertal children on dialysis in whom weight was normal for height compared with children who were undernourished (31).

Energy intake should at least satisfy the recommended daily allowances for children as set out in Table 11. Energy supplements taken with meals consisting of fat (double cream, polyunsaturated oil emulsions) and carbohydrate (glucose polymer) flavoured to taste are useful to increase total energy intake. This also serves to reduce the intake of other foods containing nutrients, such as protein and electrolytes, normally consumed in excess of need. If anorexia is severe, particularly when associated with catabolic stress from intercurrent infection, then nasoenteric feeding through indwelling soft cannulae can be useful in breaking the vicious circle of anorexia and malnutrition.

Protein intake should be controlled so that the predialysis blood urea concentration does not exceed 25 to 35 mmol/l. Minimum protein requirements should, however, be satisfied (Table 11). If high quality protein is given, the intake can probably be reduced as necessary so that protein supplies not more than 4 to 6% of total calories in the diet. By comparison human milk or human milk substitutes provide about 8% of total calories from protein whereas the normal intake can exceed 12%. Very low protein diets can be supplemented by feeding essential amino or keto acids but this is expensive and rarely required (126–128). Too severe a restriction of protein intake can lead to protein malnutrition and plasma albumin or transferrin levels should be monitored to detect this.

Phosphate intake should be reduced by limiting or removing dairy products in the diet as discussed above. Calcium intake should be maintained, if necessary by feeding calcium supplements, and in this respect calcium from calcium carbonate, given as a phosphate binder, is absorbed. Sodium supplements are rarely required in children on dialysis though they may be necessary in some children with residual renal function, especially in case of nephronophthisis. Similarly, bicarbonate supplements are rarely required in children on dialysis to prevent metabolic acidosis. An adequate intake of all vitamins should be given because of losses in the dialysate and the restricted nutritional intake. Pyridoxine

deficiency occurs in chronic renal failure and supplements of pyridoxine hydrochloride (10 mg dialy) should be provided (129, 130). Folate deficiency can occur even in the presence of normal serum folate acid concentrations owing to alterations in folate metabolism (130), but excessive accumulation of folic acid has been also reported in patients on dialysis (131).

Iron, zinc, copper, manganese, chromium, cobalt, selenium, iodine and fluoride (see also chapter 49) are essential or beneficial to man (132). The accumulation of aluminium and iron has already been mentioned but copper toxicity can also occur and may be associated with anaemia (133). Tissue zinc levels are usually increased (132) but low levels of plasma zinc have been observed (133). A number of abnormalities in patients with renal failure such as anorexia impaired taste acuity and poor growth have been attributed to zinc deficiency.

Children do not respond well to special diets and it is usually better to influence their consumption of normal foods rather than to prescribe special foods; nevertheless low protein noodles or bread may be useful. Above all tension over eating must be avoided otherwise a refusal to eat may develop. An experienced dietician working with the child and family can do much to encourage a good diet in accordance with the child's own preferences.

Food intake should be monitored regularly by the dietician and evaluated in relation to the nutritional status of the child. As well as the usual and regular biochemical determinations plasma lipids should be monitored. A raised plasma cholesterol is an indication to reduce the content of cholesterol and saturated fat in the diet whilst raised plasma triglyceride levels can be treated by reducing the carbohydrate, especially the sucrose content, and increasing the poly-unsaturated fat content of the diet. Fluid intake is usually limited to the level of insensible loss plus urinary volume but excessive weight gain between dialysis is often due to excessive sodium intake rather than primarily due to drinking too much water though this can occur. This excess of weight gain was found to be associated with an excess of mortality rate in children on dailysis (79).

Table 11. Recommended daily allowances for children.

Age (yr)	Height (cm)	Energy (kcal/day)		Minimum protein (g/day)		Calcium (g)
		A	B	A	B	
0.5–1	72	100/kg	100/kg	1.8/kg	1.8 kg	0.6
1–2	81	1100	1170	18/day	21	0.7
2–4	96	1300	1330	22	25	0.8
4–6	110	1600	1800	29	30,5	0.9
6–8	121	2000	2100	29	33	0.9
8–10	131	2200	2460	31	35	1.0
10–12	141	2450	2600	36	41.5	1.2
12–14 (M)	151	2700	2720	40	45	1.4
12–14 (F)	154	2300	2190	34	46	1.3

A: according to the UK Department of Health and Social Security (124).
B: according to National Research Council Food and Nutrition Board (125).

REFERENCES

1. Arant BS: Postnatal development of renal function during the first year of life. *Pediatr Nephrol* 1: 308, 1987
2. Thurau K, Boylan JW: Acute renal success: the unexpected logic of oliguria in acute renal failure. *Am J Med* 61: 308, 1976
3. Al-Dahhan JA, Haycock GB, Chantler C, Stimmler L: Sodium homeostasis in mature and immature neonates I. Renal aspects. *Arch Dis Child* 58: 335, 1983
4. Holliday MA: Body composition, metabolism and growth. in *Pediatric Nephrology* edited by Holliday MA, Barratt TM Verrier R, Baltimore, Williams & Wilkins, 1987, p 3
5. Rigden SPA, Barratt TM, Dillon MG, De Leval M, Stark J: Acute renal failure complicating cardiopulmonary bypass surgery. *Arch Dis Child* 57: 425, 1982
6. Arneil GL, MacDonald AM, Murphy AV, Sweet RM: Renal venous thrombosis. *Clin Nephrol* 1: 119, 1973
7. Clark AGB, Saunders A, Bewick M, Haycock GB, Chantler C: Neonatal inferior vena cava and renal venous thrombosis treated by thrombectomy and nephrectomy. *Arch Dis Child* 60: 1076, 1985
8. Myers BD, Moran SM: Hemodynamically mediated acute renal failure. *N Eng J Med* 314: 97, 1986
9. Judd BA, Haycock GB, Dalton N, Chantler C: Hyponatraemia in premature babies and following surgery in older children. *Acta Paediatr Scand* 76 (in press) 1987
10. Bird JE, Blantz RC: Acute renal failure: the glomerular and tubular connection. *Pediatr Nephrol* 1: 348, 1987
11. Elseed AM, Shinebourne EA, Joseph MC: Assessment of techniques for measurement of blood pressure in infants and children. *Arch Dis Child* 48: 932, 1973
12. Matthew OP, Jones AS, James E, Bland H, Groshong T: Neonatal renal failure; usefulness of diagnostic indices. *Pediatrics* 65: 57, 1980
13. Montoliu J, Lens XM, Cases A, Campistol JM: Treatment of hyperkalaemia in renal failure; salbutamol versus insulin. *Abstracts Int Congr Nephrol* 10: 10, 1987
14. Gordon I, Barratt TM: Imaging the kidneys and urinary tract in the neonate with acute renal failure. *Pediatr Nephrol* 1: 321, 1987
15. Barratt TM, Dillon MJ, Gordon I, Ransley PG: Clinical Quiz, *Pediatr Nephrol* 1: 379, 1987
16. Kramer P, Bohler J, Kehr A, Grone HJ, Schrader J, Matthaei D, Scheler F: Intensive care potential of continuous arteriovenous hemofiltration. *Trans Am Soc Artif Intern Organs* 28: 28, 1982
17. Golper TA: Continuous arteriovenous hemofiltration in acute renal failure. *Am J Kidney Dis* 6: 373, 1985
18. Abitbol CL, Green MA, Grutner PM and Biancaniello TM: Treatment of critical neonatal edema with hemoultrafiltration. *Int J Pediatr Nephrol* 5: 163, 1984
19. Ronco C: Continuous arteriovenous hemofiltration in infants. in *Acute Continuous Renal Replacement Therapy*, edited by Paganini EP, Den Haag, Martinus Nijhoff, 1986, p 201
20. Lieberman KV: Continuous arteriovenous hemofiltration in children. *Pediatr Nephrol* 1: 330, 1987
21. Broyer M, Brunner FP, Brynger H, Fassbinder W, Guillou PJ, Oules R, Rizzoni G, Selwood NH, Wing AJ: Combined report on regular dialysis and transplantation of children in Europe, XVII, 1986. (personal communication)
22. Arbus GS. 1985 report on pediatric patients. in *Canadian Renal Failure Register*. Kidney foundation of Canada 1986
23. Rizzoni G, Broyer M, Brunner FP, Brynger H, Challah S, Fassbinder W, Guillou PJ, Oules R, Selwood NH, Wing AJ:

Combined report on regular dialysis and transplantation of children in Europe, XVI, 1985. (personal communication)
24. EDTA Registry centre survey 1985. *Nephrol Dial Transplant* 2: 475, 1987
25. Schärer K, Chantler C, Brunner FP, Gurland HJ, Jacobs C, Parsons FM, Seyffart G, Wing AJ: Combined report on regular dialysis and transplantation of children in Europe 1974. *Proc Eur Dial Transplant Assoc* 12: 65, 1975
26. Broyer M, Rizzoni G, Brunner FP, Brynger H, Challah S, Fassbinder W, Oules R, Selwood NH, Wing AJ: Combined report on regular dialysis and transplantation of children in Europe XV, *Proc Eur Dial Transplant Assoc – Eur Ren Assoc* 22: 55, 1985
27. Rees L, Rigden SPA, Chantler C, Haycock GB: Growth and methods of improving growth in chronic renal failure managed conservatively. in *Karger Symposium on Endocrine Abnormalities in Chronic Renal Failure* edited by Schärer K in press 1987.
28. Chantler C, Broyer M, Donckerwolcke RA, Brynger H, Brunner FB, Jacobs C, Kremer P, Selwood NH, Wing AJ: Growth and rehabilitation of long term survivors of treatment for end stage renal failure in childhood. *Proc Eur Dial Transplant Assoc* 18: 329, 1981
29. Barratt TM, Broyer M, Chantler C, Gilli G, Guest G, Marti Henneburg C, Preece MA, Rigden SPA: Assessment of growth. *Am J Kidney Dis* 7: 340, 1986
30. Jones RWA, Rigden S, Barratt TM, Chantler C: The effects of chronic renal failure in infancy on growth nutritional status and body composition. *Pediatr Res* 16: 784, 1982
31. Donckerwolcke RA, Chantler C, Brunner FP, Brynger H, Gurland HJ, Hathway RA, Jacobs C, Selwood NH, Wing AJ: Combined report on regular dialysis and transplantation of children in Europe 1977. *Proc Eur Dial Transplant Assoc* 15: 77, 1978
32. Tanner JM, Whitehouse RH, Marshall WA, Healy MJR, Goldstern H: *Assessment of Skeletal Maturity and Prediction of Adult Height TW2 Method*, London, Academic Press, 1975
33. Broyer M, Kleinknecht C, Loirat C, Marti-Henneberg C, Roy MP: Maturation osseuse et développement pubertaire chez l'enfant et l'adolescent en dialyse chronique. (Osseous maturation and pubertal development in infants and children on chronic dialysis.) *Proc Eur Dial Transplant Assoc* 9: 181, 1972
34. Chantler C, and Holliday MA: Chronic renal insufficiency. in *Pediatric Nephrology* edited by Holliday MA, Barratt TM, Vernier R, Baltimore, Williams & Wilkins, 1987
35. Mak RHK, Turner C, Thompson T, Haycock GB, Chantler C: Glucose metabolism in children with uremia; effect of dietary phosphate and protein. *Kidney Int* 32 (Supp 22) 206, 1987
36. Mak RHK, Haycock GB, Thompson T, Turner C, Chantler C: The role of secondary hyperparathyroidism in the glucose intolerance of chronic renal failure. *J Clin Endocrinol Metab* 60: 229, 1985
37. Delaporte C, Gros F, Anagnostopoulos T: Inhibitory effects of plasma dialysate on protein synthesis in vitro, influence of dialysis and transplantation. *Am J Clin Nutr* 33: 1407, 1980
38. Mak RHK, Turner C, Thompson T, Haycock GB, Chantler C: The effects of a low protein diet with amino/keto acid supplements on glucose metabolism in children with uraemia *J Clin Endocrinology Metab* 63: 985, 1986
39. Rodriguez-Soriano J, Arant BS, Brodehl J, Norman ME: Fluid and electrolyte imbalances in children with chronic renal failure. *Am J Kidney Dis* 7: 268, 1968
40. Rees L, Chantler C: Hormonal alterations that may affect

growth in chronic renal disease. in *Nephrology (Proc Xth Int Congr Nephrol)* edited by Davison A, London, Bailliére Tyndall, 1988, vol 2, p 989

41. Betts PR, House PM, Morris R, Rayner PHW: Serum cortisol concentration in children with chronic renal insufficiency *Arch Dis Child* 50: 245, 1975

42. Czernichow P, Danzet MC, Broyer M, Rappaport R: Abnormal TSH, PRL and GH response to TSH releasing factor in chronic renal failure. *J Clin Endocrinol Metab* 43: 630, 1976

43. Burke J, El-Bishti M, Maisy MN, Chantler C: Hypothyroidism in children with cystinosis. *Arch Dis Child* 53: 947, 1978

44. Mehls O, Salusky IB: Recent advances and controversies in childhood renal osteodystrophy. *Pediatr Nephrol* 1: 212, 1987

45. Broyer M. Chronic renal failure. in *Paediatric Nephrology* edited by Royer P, Habib R, Mathieu H, Broyer M, Philadelphia, WB Saunders Co, 1974, p 358

46. Norman ME, Mazin AT, Borden S, Gruskin A, Anast C, Baren R, Rasmussen H: Early diagnosis of renal osteodystrophy. *J Pediatr* 97: 226, 1980

47. Mehls O, Ritz E, Krempien B, Gilli G, Lush K, Wulich E, Schärer K: Slipped epiphyses in renal osteodystrophy. *Arch Dis Child* 50: 545, 1975

48. Milliner DS, Ottsin Nebeker HG, Andress DL, Sherrard DJ, Alfrey AC, Slatopolsky E, Coburn JW: Deferoxamine infusion test for the diagnosis of aluminium related osteodystrophy. *Ann Intern Med* 101: 775, 1984

49. Turner C, Compson J, Mak RHK, Vedi S, Haycock GB, Chantler C: Reduction in bone turnover and elevation of 1 : 25 dihydroxy cholecalciferol during treatment with high dose phosphate binders in uraemic children. (submitted).

50. Tamanaha K, Mak RHK, Rigden SPA, Turner C, Start KM, Haycock GB, Chantler C: Longterm suppression of hyperparathyroidism by phosphate binders in uraemic children. *Pediatr Nephrol* 1: 145, 1987

51. Wass VJ, Barratt TM, Howarth RV, Marshall WA, Chantler C, Ogg GS, Cameron JS, Baillod RA, Moorhead JF: Home haemodialysis in children. *Lancet* 1: 242, 1977

52. Muller-Wiezel D, Sinn H, Gilli G, Schärer K: Hemodialysis and blood loss in children with chronic renal failure. *Clin Nephrol* 8: 481, 1977

53. Kjellstrand CM, Eaton JW, Yawata Y, Swofford H, Kolpin C, Buselmeier TJ, Von Hartitzsch B, Jacobs HS: Haemolysis in dialysed patients caused by chloramines. *Nephron* 13: 427, 1974

54. Erslev AJ. Management of anaemia of chronic renal failure. *Clin Nephrol* 2: 174, 1974

55. Bell JD, Kincaid WR, Morgan RG, Bunce H, Alperin JB, Sarles HE, Remmers AR: Serum ferritin assay and bone marrow iron stores in patients on maintenance hemodialysis. *Kidney Int* 17: 237, 1980

56. Schärer K, Muller-Wiefel D: Complications of renal failure: haematological complications. in *Pediatric Nephrology* edited by Holliday MA, Barratt TM, Vernier R, Baltimore, Williams & Wilkins, 1987, p 880

57. Winearls CG, Oliver DO, Pipparel MJ, Reid C, Downing MR, Cotes PM: Effect of human erythropoietin derived from recombinant DNA on the anaemia of patients maintained by chronic haemodialysis. *Lancet* 2: 1175, 1986

58. Ullmer HE, Greiner H, Schuler HW, Schärer K: Cardiovascular impairment and physical working capacity in children with chronic renal failure. *Acta Paediatr Scand* 67: 43, 1978

59. Polinsky MS, Kaiser RA, Stover JB, Frankenfield M, Baluarte HJ: Neurologic development of children with severe chronic renal failure from infancy. *Pediatr Nephrol* : 157, 1987

60. Nevins TE: Transplantation in infants less than 1 year of age. *Pediatr Nephrol* 1: 154, 1987

61. Wright D, Rigden SPA, Baird G, Chantler C, Haycock GB, Smith R, Ward GM: Developmental progress of children with chronic renal failure presenting in infancy. (submitted)

62. Mahan ID, Mauer SM, Nevins T: The Hickman catheter: a new hemodialysis device for infants and small children. *Kidney Int* 24: 694, 1983

63. Weiss M, Sutherland DE: Percutaneous subclavian catheterization for hemodialysis in small children. *Surgery* 95: 353, 1984

64. Bourquelot P, Wolfeler L, Lamy L: Microsurgery for hemodialysis distal arteriovenous fistulae in children weighing less than 10 kg. *Int J Microsurg* 3: 187, 1981

65. Gagnadoux MF, Pascal B, Bronstein M, Bourquelot P, Broyer M: Arteriovenous fistulae in small children. *Dial Transplant* 9: 318, 1980

66. Blumenthal SS, Ortiz MA, Kleinman JC, Piering WF: Inflow time and recirculation in single needle hemodialysis. *Am J Kidney Dis* 8: 202, 1986

67. D'Apuzzo VC, Gruskin CM, Brennan CP, Stiles GR, Fine RN: Saphenous vein autograft arteriovenous fistula for extended hemodialysis in children. *Acta Paediatr Scand* 62: 28, 1973

68. Applebaum K, Shaskikumar VL, Somers LA, Baluarte HJ, Gruskin AB, Grossman M, Mc Garvey MJ, Weintraub WK: Improved hemodialysis access in children. *J Pediatr Surg* 15: 764, 1980

69. Ford DM, Portman RJ, Hurst DL, Lum GM: Unsuspected seizures during hemodialysis = effect of dialysate prescription. *Pediatr Nephrol* 1, 1987

70. Ing IS, Vilbar RM, Skin RD: Predialytic isolated ultrafiltration. *Dial Transplant* 7: 557, 1978

71. Swamy AP, Cestero RVM: Mannitol and maintenance hemodialysis. *Artif Organs* 3: 116, 1979

72. Chantler C, Trompeter R, Rigden S, Dalton N, Haycock G: Vascular stability during haemodialysis. in *Paediatric Nephrology* edited by Brodehl J, Ehrich JHH, Berlin, Springer Verlag, 1984, p 96

73. Broyer M, Antignac C: Advances in dialysis treatment in children – an overview. in *Recent Advances in Pediatric Nephrology*, edited by Murakami K, Kitagawa T, Yabuta K, Sakai T, Amsterdam, Elsevier, 1987, p 175

74. Panzetta G, Tissitore N, Valvo E, Lupo A, Loschiavo G, Fabris A, Oldrizzi L, Gammaro L, Rugin C, Bellotti Z, Maschio G: Biofiltration in the treatment of patients with acetate intolerance. *Clin Nephrol* 26: 33, 1986

75. Nevins TE, Kjellstrand CM: Hemodialysis for children: a review. *Int J Pediatr Nephrol* 4: 155, 1983

76. Martin Malo A, Perez R, Gomez J, Burdiel LG, Andres E, Castillo D, Moreno E, Aljano P: Sequential hypertonic dialysis. *Nephron* 40: 458, 1985

77. Leroy M, Dechaux M, Guest G: Extracellular volume and blood pressure in 82 hemodialysed children. *Proc Eur Dial Transplant Assoc – Eur Ren Assoc* 22: 847, 1985

78. Broyer M, Gagnadoux MF, Bacri JL, Laborde K: Problems of long term dialysis in children. in *Pediatric Nephrology*, edited by Gruskin AB, Norman ME, The Hague, Martinus Nijhoff, 1981, p 185

79. Rizzoni G, Broyer M, Brunner FP, Brynger H, Challah S, Kramer P, Oules RE, Selwood NH, Wing AJ, Balas EA: Combined report on regular dialysis and transplantation of children in Europe, XIV, 1983. *Proc Eur Dial Transplant Assoc – Eur Ren Assoc* 21: 69, 1984

80. Villaroel F. Incidence of hypersensitivity in hemodialysis. *Artif Organs* 8: 278, 1984

81. Harmon WE, Spinozzi N, Meyer A, Grupe WE: The use of protein catabolic rate to monitor pediatric hemodialysis. *Dial Transplant* 10: 324, 1981

82. Henrich WL: Hemodynamic instability during hemodialysis. *Kidney Int* 30: 605, 1985

83. Demography of dialysis and transplantation in children in Europe 1985. Report from the European Dialysis and Transplant Association Registry. *Nephrol Dial Transplant* 3: 235, 1988

84. Alexander SR, Tank ES, Corneil AT: Five year's experience with CAPD/CCPD catheters in infants and children. in *CAPD in Children*, edited by Fine RN, Schärer K, Mehls O, Berlin, Springer Verlag, 1985, p 174

85. Jorge Baluarte: Intermittent peritoneal dialysis: Technical and clinical aspects. in *End Stage Renal Disease in Children*, edited by Fine RN, Gruskin AB, Philadelphia, WB Saunders Co, 1984, p 118

86. Gruskin AB, Alexander SR, Baluarte HF, Grupe WE, Harmon W, Potter DE, Salusky IB: Issues in pediatric dialysis. *Am J Kidney Dis* 7: 306, 1986

87. Balfe JW, Stefanidis CJ, Steele BI, Hewitt IK: Continuous ambulatory peritoneal dialysis: clinical aspects. in *End Stage Renal Disease in Children*, edited by Fine RN, Gruskin AB, Philadelphia, WB Saunders Co, 1984, p 135

88. Muller-Wiefel DE, Bonzel KE, Wartha R, Mehls O, Schärer K: Renal anemia in children on CAPD. in *CAPD in Children*, edited by Fine RN, Schärer K, Mehls O, Berlin, Springer Verlag, 1985, p 150

89. Salusky IB, Lucullo L, Nelson P, Fine RN: Continuous ambulatory peritoneal dialysis in children. *Pediatr Clin North Am* 29: 1005, 1982

90. Kohaut EC: Growth of children with end stage renal disease treated with CAPD for at least one year. *Peritoneal Dial Bull* 2: 159, 1982

91. Fine RN: Indications for CAPD and CCPD in children. in *CAPD in Children*, edited by Fine RN, Schärer K, Mehls O, Berlin, Springer Verlag, 1985, p 41

92. Salusky IB, Davidson D, Hall T, Fine RN: Indications for CCPD in the child. *Persp Peritoneal Dial* 3: 48, 1985

93. Diaz-Buxo JA: Incidence of peritonitis with CCPD. *Persp Peritoneal Dial* 3: 49, 1985

94. Gruskin AB: The peritoneal dialysis prescription in children. *Persp Peritoneal Dial* 3: 42, 1985

95. Balfe JW: Peritoneal dialysis. in *Pediatric Nephrology* 2nd edition, edited by Holliday MA, Barratt IM, Vernier RC, Baltimore, Williams & Wilkins, 1987, p 814

96. Salusky IB, Fine RN: Nutritional recommendations for children undergoing continuous peritoneal dialysis. *Persp Peritoneal Dial* 2: 18, 1984

97. Drachman R, Niaudet P, Dartois AM, Broyer M: Protein losses during peritoneal dialysis in children. in *CAPD in Children*, edited by Fine RN, Schärer K, Mehls O, Berlin, Springer Verlag, 1985, p 78

98. Salusky IB, Paunier L, Coburn JW, Kangarloo H, Slatopolsky E, Fine RN. in *CAPD in Children*, edited by Fine RN, Schärer K, Mehls O, Berlin, Springer Verlag, 1985, p 144

99. Leichter HE, Salusky IB, Davidson M, Wilson M, Hall T, Fine RN: Peritonitis in children undergoing CAPD versus CCPD. in *CAPD in Children*, edited by Fine RN, Schärer K, Mehls O, Berlin, Springer Verlag, 1985, p 190

100. Lorentz WB: Acute hydrothorax during peritoneal dialysis. *J Pediatr* 94: 417, 1979

101. Kohaut EC, Alexander SR, Mehls O: The management of the infant on CAPD. in *CAPD in Children*, edited by Fine RN, Schärer K, Mehls O, Berlin, Springer Verlag, 1985, p 97

102. Niaudet P, Drachman R, Gubler MC, Broyer M: Loss of ultrafiltration and peritoneal membrane alterations on CAPD. in *CAPD in Children*, edited by Fine RN, Schärer K, Mehls O, Berlin, Springer Verlag, 1985, p 158

103. Niaudet P, Berard E, Revillon Y, Lothon M, Broyer M: Sclerosing encapsulating peritonitis in children. in *Peritonitis in CAPD, Contribution to Nephrology*. Karger (in press)

104. Conley SB, Brewer ED, Grady S: Normal growth in very small children on peritoneal dialysis. *Abstracts Natl Kidney Found* 12: 8A, 1982

105. Warady BA, Stall C, Paulsen J, Johnson CB, Sedman A, Lum GM: A unique approach to peritoneal dialysis in infants. *Am J Kidney Dis* 7: 235, 1985

106. Hall IL, Wilson M, Davidson D, Foley J: The importance of the CAPD nurse in dealing with patient/family burnout. in *CAPD in Children*, edited by Fine RN, Schärer K, Mehls O, Berlin, Springer Verlag, 1985, p 207

107. Opelz G. Effect of HLA matching in 10,000 cyclosporine treated cadaver kidney transplantation. *Transplant Proc* 19: 641, 1987

108. Broyer M, Gagnadoux MF, Beurton D, Pascal B, Louville J: Transplantation in children: technical aspects drug therapy and problems related to primary renal disease. *Proc Eur Dial Transplant Assoc* 18: 313, 1981

109. Haycock GB: Intra-operative and immediate post-operative care in the management of the paediatric transplant recipient. in *Paediatric Nephrology*, edited by Brodehl J, Ehrich JHH, Berlin, Heidelberg, Springer Verlag, 1984, p 146

110. Broyer M, Gagnadoux MF, Guest G, Beurton D, Niaudet P, Habib R, Busson M: Kidney transplantation in children. Results of 383 grafts performed at Enfants Malades Hospital from 1973 to 1984. *Adv Nephrol* 16: 307, 1987

111. Korsch B, Fine RN, Negrette VR: Non compliance in children with renal transplant. *Pediatrics* 61: 872, 1978.

112. Offner G, Hoyer PF, Brodehl J, Pichlmayr R: Cyclosporin A in paediatric kidney transplantation. *Pediatr Nephrol* 1: 125, 1987

113. Broyer M, Guest G: Croissance après transplantation rénale. in *Journées Parisiennes de Pédiatrie*, Paris, Flammarion Medicine Sciences, 1987, p 135

114. Van Diemen Steenwoorde R, Donckerwolcke R, Brackel H, Wolff ED, De Jong JW: Growth and bone maturation in children after kidney transplantation. *J Pediatr* 110: 351, 1987

115. Fennell RS, Love JT, Carter RL, Hudson TM, Pfaff WW, Howard RJ, Van Densen W, Garin EH, Iravani A, Walker RD, Richard OA: Statistical analysis of statural growth following transplantation. *Eur J Pediatr* 145: 377, 1986

116. Brodehl J, Offner G, Hoyer PF: Cyclosporine in pediatric kidney transplantation. *Adv Nephrol* 16: 335, 1987

117. Broyer M, Guest G, Gagnadoux MF, Beurton D: Hypertension following renal transplantation in children. *Pediatr Nephrol* 1: 16, 1987

118. Tejani A. Post transplant hypertension and hypertensive encephalopathy in renal allograft recipient. *Nephron* 34: 73, 1983

119. Broyer M, Donckerwolcke RA, Brunner FP, Brynger H, Challah S, Gretz N, Jacobs C, Kramer P, Selwood NH, Wing AJ: Combined report on regular dialysis and transplantation of children in Europe, XIII, 1982. *Proc Eur Dial Transplant Assoc – Eur Ren Assoc* 20: 79, 1983

120. Korsch B. Current issues in comprehensive care for children

with chronic illness. in *Paediatric Nephrology*, edited by Brodehl J, Ehrich JHH, Berlin, Heidelberg, Springer Verlag, 1984, p 179

121. Chantler C, Broyer M, Donckerwolcke R, Brynger H, Brunner FP, Jacobs C, Kramer P, Selwood NH, Wing A. Growth and rehabilitation of the long term survivous of treatment for end stage renal failure in childhood. *Proc Eur Dial Transplant Assoc* 18: 329, 1981

122. Ettenger RB, Korsch BM, Main ME, Fine RN: Social rehabilitation of children and adolescents with end stage renal disease. in *Rehabilitation in Chronic Renal Failure*, edited by Chyatte SB, Baltimore, Williams & Wilkins, 1979, p 115

123. Andre JL, Picon G: Aspects psychosociaux du traitement de l'insuffisance rénale terminale. (Psychosocial aspects of treatment of terminal renal insufficiency.) in *26e congrés des pédiatres de langue Française*, edited by Regnier, Toulouse, Fournié, 1981, p 611

124. Dept of Helath and Social Security: Recommended intakes of nutrients for the United Kingdom. *Reports of Public Health and Medical Subjects*, London, N° 120 HM Stationery Office, 1969

125. *National Research Council, Food and Nutrition Board. Recommended Dietary Allowances*, 9th edition Washington DC, National Academy of Sciences, 1980

126. Jones RWA, Dalton N, Start K, El Bishti M, Chantler C: Oral essential amino acid supplements in children with advanced chronic renal failure. *Am J Clin Nutr* 33: 1696, 1980

127. Counahan R, El Bishti M, Chantler C: Oral essential amino acids in children on regular haemodialysis. *Clin Nephrol* 9: 11, 1978

128. Jones RWA, Dalton N, Turner C, Start K, Haycock GB, Chantler C: Oral essential amino acid and keto acid supplements in children with chronic renal failure. *Kidney Int* 24: 95, 1983

129. Kopple JD: Abnormal amino acid and protein metabolism in uremia. *Kidney Int* 14: 340, 1978

130. Kopple JD, Swendseid ME: Vitamin nutrition in patients undergoing maintenance hemodialysis. *Kidney Int* 7 (Suppl 2): S-79, 1975

131. Leung AC, Henderson IS, Maharai D, Thomson G: Excessive accumulation of folic acid in uremic patients on dialysis. *Dial Transplant* 14: 575, 1985

132. Sandstead HH: Trace elements in uremia and hemodialysis. *Am J Clin Nutr* 33: 1501, 1980

133. Tsukamoto Y, Iwanami S, Marumano F: Disturbances of trace element concentrations in plasma of patients in chronic renal failure. *Nephron* 26: 274, 1980

ACUTE COMPLICATIONS ASSOCIATED WITH HEMODIALYSIS

CHRISTOPHER R. BLAGG

INTRODUCTION

In the 27 years since maintenance hemodialysis was first introduced in Seattle, this treatment has been revolutionized. In 1960 maintenance hemodialysis for chronic renal failure was a 14-h experimental procedure, performed on a few highly selected patients by a team of physicians and other staff who were uncertain of the complications which might ensue, both during the dialysis and as a result of the prolongation of life by this new treatment. Now there are more than 300,000 patients treated by maintenance dialysis throughout the world, and almost all of them have their treatment supervised by nurses or by technicians. There are also thousands of patients who perform their own hemodialysis treatment at home.

Hemodialysis has proved to be a remarkably safe procedure, and the major complications occurring in association with it have been documented carefully. Despite development of more biocompatible membranes and newer techniques such as hemofiltration and hemodiafiltration, it seems unlikely that significant new acute complications of hemodialysis will be described in the future. Nevertheless, new complications association with long-term dialysis continue to be described. For example, the previous edition of this book included carpal tunnel syndrome as a recognized complication in dialysis patients, but its possible relationship to beta-2 microglobulin production and amyloidosis had not yet been recognized.

This chapter briefly reviews the major complications associated with hemodialysis and, in particular, those not dealt with at length elsewhere in this book. In general, it excludes complications occurring in the dialysis patient that do not relate directly to the procedure. The topics discussed are not an exhaustive list of all the complications that have been recorded as occurring or that relate to hemodialysis, but rather those considered most important or interesting. Similarly, when therapy is described, the emphasis is generally on treatment which is felt the most appropriate in the light of personal experience.

Dialysis patients may develop the same emergency and semi-emergency situations that can occur in any other type of patient, and treatment may be identical with that in the nondialysis patient or may be modified because of concurrent renal failure and dialysis treatment. In addition, certain complications are specific to the patient undergoing hemodialysis. For an exhaustive discussion of the risks and hazards associated with the dialysis equipment, the reader is referred to the report by Keshaviah and co-workers (1) and to Chapter 12.

SUDDEN DEATH IN HEMODIALYSIS PATIENTS

Death in hemodialysis patients is most commonly related to cardiovascular disease and its complications. Sudden death and death due to hemorrhage may occur at any time during hemodialysis itself or between dialyses (2). Deaths related to dialysis but occurring between dialyses are most comonly due to pericardial tamponade from pericardial effusion or result from suicide (3). Suicide may be by deliberate exsanguination or by electrolyte imbalance because of dietary indiscretion involving salt and water or potassium, as well as the more usual forms of suicide. The frequency of suicide in dialysis patients is greater than in the general population, but information is not available as to whether suicide is more common in dialysis patients than in patients with other life-threatening chronic diseases.

Sudden death occurring during hemodialysis is an unusual event (4). The usual causes, many of which are discussed below, include brain herniation; air embolism; acute hemorrhage which may also result from machine malfunction or disconnection; electrocution; cardiac arrhythmias, primarily related to potassium abnormalities; complications of subclavian intravenous catheter insertion; cardiac conduction defects; and other technical problems related to the dialysis procedure.

HYPOTENSION, DISEQUILIBRIUM, AND RELATED SYMPTOMS

The most frequently encountered problems in dialysis patients relate to hypotension occurring during dialysis, nonspecific symptoms during and after dialysis apparently un-related to hypotension or disequilibrium, and the dialysis disequilibrium syndrome. The latter remains a potential problem in patients with acute renal failure and in patients first starting treatment by maintenance dialysis.

Hypotension

Episodes of hypotension occur in 20% to 30% of all hemodialyses (5, 6), and relate to various factors affecting cardiac output and systemic vascular resistance (7, 8). Cardiac output depends on myocardial contractility and filling volume, which in turn relates to vascular volume and heart rate, the increase of which may be limited in dialysis patients. Systemic vascular resistance is controlled through the autonomic nervous system and the presence of various vasoactive substances, and inability to increase vascular resistance is important in the development of dialysis hypotension. When not the result of a specific cause such as septicemia, arrhythmia, myocardial infarction, or another cardiac problem, hypotension in hemodialysis generally is secondary to acute reduction in blood volume due either to excessive ultrafiltration or to acute hemorrhage. Symptoms are similar, whatever the cause, and may include unexplained anxiety, nausea and pallor, possibly vomiting which may result in temporary relief, headache and cramps. On sitting up, the patient becomes dizzy, develops tachycardia, and may become unconscious.

Hypovolemia decreases cardiac refilling pressure and stroke volume which, with reduced or absent vasoconstriction, results in hypotension if cardiac output is not maintained by increasing the heart rate (8).

Hypotension associated with sodium and fluid depletion

Hypotension as a result of sodium and fluid depletion may occur at any time during or shortly after dialysis, and the time of onset may give a clue to the cause. Predialysis blood volume is less in patients who suffer from hypotensive episodes during hemodialysis (9), and this may be aggravated by previous vomiting, diarrhea, fever, or reduced dietary sodium intake. In such patients the predialysis weight is low. Many patients have mild symptoms of hypotension on connection to the dialyzer during their early dialyses, but generally this problem does not persist.

Hypotension occurring during the course of dialysis usually is due to excessive ultrafiltration which results in hypovolemia and a decrease in stroke volume (10). Excessive ultrafiltration may result from too short a dialysis with consequent rapid ultrafiltration, an incorrect estimate of the ultrafiltration rate required to remove accumulated fluid, or venous obstruction with consequent increased pressure in the dialyzer and excessive ultrafiltration. Hypotension during dialysis also may be an early indication of a pericardial effusion. Hypovolemia is particularly likely to occur with use of a lower dialysis fluid sodium concentration (11), and hypotension is less frequent when dialysate sodium is higher (12).

Occasionally, hypotension may occur shortly after dialysis. The most likely cause is excessive ultrafiltration, symptoms appearing when the patient becomes active following the end of dialysis.

Other factors related to dialysis hypotension

Autonomic dysfunction also may play a significant role in toleration of hypovolemia during hemodialysis. Reduced baroceptor sensitivity has been demonstrated by abnormal responses to the Valsalva maneuver and the amyl nitrite test, and may relate to the existence of autonomic neuropathy in many dialysis patients (13). However, recent studies have shown that while cardiac efferent parasympathetic pathways may be affected, adrenergic responses are normal (14, 15).

Left ventricular function is also important, and dialysis patients generally have increased cardiac output related to anemia and the presence of an arteriovenous fistula. Abnormal left ventricular function in keeping with a uremic cardiomyopathy has been shown (16), and hemodynamic changes during dialysis correlate with predialysis left ventricular function (17).

Other factors which may be associated with hypotensive episodes during dialysis include the occurrence of myocardial infarction, pulmonary embolism, hemorrhage, sepsis, and the excessive use of antihypertensive medications.

The role of acetate and hypoxemia

With development of automated single-pass dialysis equipment in the 1960s, acetate became the standard anion in dialysate, replacing bicarbonate because of the need to prevent precipitation of calcium and magnesium (18). Acetate is readily metabolized in the body, resulting in the regeneration of bicarbonate from carbon dioxide (19).

More recently, with larger surface area dialyzers and more rapid dialysis, transport of acetate into blood can occur at a rate exceeding the capacity of the body to metabolize it, and this is associated with hypotension (20, 21). Acetate ion is a vasodilator (22), and during dialysis the drop in systemic vascular resistance correlates with the plasma acetate level (23). This effect is greatest at the start of dialysis when the blood acetate level increases rapidly (24). The usual effect of acetate on the heart is to increase heart rate and improve left ventricular function and cardiac output, thus tending to compensate for the drop in vascular resistance (25). A cardiodepressant effect of acetate on dialysis patients has been described (26), but a recent study failed to confirm a direct myocardial depressant effect (27).

Acetate metabolism also results in hypoxemia (28) and decreased carbon dioxide consumption (29), and there is also a loss of CO_2 through the dialyzer (30). Hypoxemia also may result from blood-membrane interaction, and this effect is greater with cellulosic membranes than with newer synthetic membranes (31). Activation of the complement cascade following exposure of blood to the cellophane membrane (32) causes white-cell aggregation in the pulmonary vascular bed. This results in transient leukopenia early in dialysis, associated with hypoxemia which correlates with the severity of the leukopenia (33). The incidence and severity of hypotensive and other symptoms during dialysis can be ameliorated by the administration of oxygen (34), but this does not affect the vasodilatory effects of acetate (35).

Dialysis hypotension and vasoactive substances

Decreasing dialysate flow rate and less efficient dialysis has been shown to reduce the incidence of hypotensive episodes during dialysis. This could be the result of slower intercompartmental fluid shifts, but also might relate to increased depletion of vasoactive substances such as epinephrine and norepinephrine which may be removed through the dialysis membrane (36). However, the concentration of epinephrine and norepinephrine in blood does not necessarily correlate with their concentration at the vessel walls, and hypotension more likely results from imparied vasoconstrictor response due to autonomic dysfunction (37). Use of cooled dialysate has also been shown to reduce the incidence of hypotension (38), perhaps because of increased norepinephrine release as a result of the cooling (39).

Other dialyzer-related effects on blood pressure

Hypotension and a syndrome resembling anaphylaxis may occur at the onset of dialysis in some patients (40), particularly with the first use of a cuprophan dialyzer (41). Symptoms disappear when dialysis is discontinued without return of blood to the patient, but may recur with use of the same membrane. These reactions may be related to either bacterial endotoxins (42) or hypersensitivity to ethylene oxide used in sterilization of the dialyzer (43). This hypersensitivity may be associated with eosinophilia and elevated plasma IgG levels (44).

While full blown anaphylaxis is rare, on occasion this may be fatal (45). More frequently, hypotension and related symptoms develop during the first 30 min of dialysis with a new dialyzer, usually in association with use of a cuprophan membrane. This 'first-use syndrome' may be related to complement activation and is much less frequent with other synthetic membranes (46). Dialyzer reuse more or less removes the complement-activating potential of the membrane (47), and this provides a rationale for multiple reuse of dialyzers in patients with symptoms occurring early during dialysis. The association of first-use syndrome with complement activation also suggests that the complement-activating potential of a dialysis membrane is a useful index of its biocompatability (48).

Prevention and treatment

Prevention of hypotension during hemodialysis requires accurate assessment of the patient's dry weight, monitoring of dietary sodium intake, knowledge of whether the patient is taking antihypertensive medications, and consideration of the type of dialyzer and the dialysate composition.

Increasing the dialysis fluid sodium concentration from

126 to 140 mmol/l reduces the number of hypotensive episodes (12), and at least one study has shown that raising the dialysate sodium level higher than 137 mmol/l does not produce further improvement (49). The higher dialysate sodium concentration induces tachycardia which compensates for hypovolemia (50), reduces the blood pressure drop resulting when the carotid sinus is stimulated (51), and produces a lesser increase in the plasma level of prostaglandin E_2 than does use of hypotonic dialysis fluid (52). However, use of such dialysate may increase weight gain between dialyses and so require increased ultrafiltration during dialysis. Sequential ultrafiltration has also been used to reduce the incidence of hypotensive episodes.

The use of dialysis fluid containing bicarbonate rather than acetate also reduces the severity of side effects, even with the use of high sodium dialysis fluid (53), but does not significantly reduce the frequency of hypotensive episodes (45). The long-term use of bicarbonate dialysis solution eventually increases predialysis plasma bicarbonate concentration (55). This suggests better correction of metabolic acidosis (56). It also results in better control of serum phosphate levels (57).

The treatment of hypotension occurring during dialysis includes lying the patient flat, and reducing negative dialysate compartment pressure to zero to prevent further ultrafiltration. Other possible causes of hypotension, particularly cardiac complications, pericardial effusion, or septicemia, must be excluded. With mild symptoms, intake of a salty food such as soup or potato chips may be all that is required. If hypotension persists or becomes more severe, an appropriate volume of a saline must be administered via the venous blood line. The volume and rate of infusion must be based on the response of symptoms and blood pressure (58).

Disequilibrium symdrome

Clinical manifestations

Dialysis disequilibrium syndrome is now seen most commonly during hemodialysis of severely uremic patients with acute renal failure and occasionally in patients with chronic renal failure who are commencing maintenance hemodialysis, particularly when using large-surface-area or high-flux dialyzers and shorter dialysis times.

Mild disequilibrium may present only as restlessness and headache during dialysis, sometimes associated with nausea, vomiting, blurring of vision, and muscle twitching. Blood pressure may be raised, and there may be disorientation and tremor. Seizures occur in more severe cases and occasionally may be accompanied by cardiac arrhythmias (59). Both grand mal and petit mal seizures may occur, but focal signs are more often associated with preexisting neurologic disease (60). With current dialysis techniques, seizures, coma and death are uncommon occurrences.

Pathogenesis

Cerebral edema is regarded as the major cause of disequilib-

rium because of the consistent occurrence of an associated elevated cerebrospinal fluid (CSF) pressure and also the finding of cerebral edema in patients dying with this syndrome. During hemodialysis the urea concentration and osmolality in the CSF fall more slowly than in blood, and a concomitant rise in CSF pressure occurs, the so-called reverse urea shift (61,62). After rapid hemodialysis in uremic dogs, the urea concentration is only marginally higher in the brain than in plasma (63). Consequently, the rate of urea clearance from the brain more or less parallels that from plasma, and there is a delay in clearance of urea from CSF during dialysis. This is associated with a paradoxical acidosis in the CSF and a fall in CSF pH during dialysis, despite correction of systemic metabolic acidosis and rise in arterial pH (59). The alteration in CSF pH may impair mentation, and the intracellular acidosis in the brain can increase intracellular osmolality by altering osmotic activity of intracellular cations, resulting in brain edema.

The paradoxical CSF acidosis during correction of metabolic acidosis depends on more rapid diffusion of carbon dioxide than bicarbonate across the blood-brain barrier, so that during hemodialysis CSF pCO_2 is rapidly corrected, while bicarbonate concentration remains low. However, in maintenance dialysis arterial pCO_2 does not increase at the end of dialysis or shortly thereafter (64); and in rapidly hemodialyzed patients, no difference is found in pCO_2 or bicarbonate concentration in plasma or lumbar CSF, whether disequilibrium occurs or not (65).

Hypoglycemia (66) and hyponatremia (67) have also been suggested as causes for disequilibrium, but there is little evidence that hypoglycemia plays any significant role in this, although the mild hyponatremia associated with use of dialysate of low sodium concentration may play a minor role.

Brain edema causing disequilibrium also may result from generation of idiogenic osmoles in the brain during dialysis (68,69). This theory is based on experiments in uremic dogs showing a significant osmotic gradient between brain and blood during dialysis not due to changes in concentrations of sodium, potassium, chloride, calcium, magnesium, or urea in the brain. The nature of these idiogenic osmoles remains unclear, but their genesis may relate to changes in intracellular binding of sodium and potassium caused by their replacement by ammonium ions resulting from the equilibrium between glutamine and glutamic acid. Thus, an increase in glutamic acid concentration in the brain could cause a fall in intracellular pH, loss of hydrogen ion into the CSF, and a fall of CSF pH and rise in brain osmolality due to accumulation of acid osmoles.

Diagnosis

The characteristic electroencephalogram (EEG) findings of disequilibrium are an increase of slow wave activity with increased spike wave activity and bursts of delta waves, and with loss of normal alpha rhythm (68). However, more recently it has been shown that the EEG is normal and disequilibrium does not occur with the use of bicarbonate dialysate (70, 71). The CSF pressure is normal in the uncomplicated nondialyzed uremic patient, but generally rises during dialysis whether disequilibrium occurs or not. This does not necessarily indicate brain edema, but could be due to an increase in CSF volume or cerebral blood flow. However, autopsies of patients who died during dialysis have shown brain swelling, often with tentorial herniation; and early studies of brain density using computerized tomographic (CT) scanning and densitometric analysis showed that brain density falls significantly during and after hemodialysis. These changes are in keeping with a postdialysis gain in cerebral water, and were particularly marked in the region of the basal ganglia (72). More recent studies in stable hemodialysis patients have shown no postdialysis EEG deterioration or change in brain density and ventricular size (73).

The differential diagnosis of disequilibrium includes a number of conditions discussed elsewhere. These include hypotension, nonspecific malaise associated with rapid dialysis, subdural hematoma, cerebrovascular accident ,the uremic syndrome, hypertensive encephalopathy, dialysis dementia, cardiac arrhythmias, hyponatremia, hypernatremia, hypoglycemia, copper intoxication, and other conditions.

Prevention and treatment

Prevention of disequilibrium was originally achieved by adding osmotically active solute to the dialysate. This prevents the fall in plasma osmolality resulting from urea removal by passage of osmotically active solute from dialysate to plasma, so reducing the brain-plasma osmolality gradient. Solutes used have included urea (74), dextrose (75), fructose (61), mannitol (76), sodium chloride (77), and glycerol (78), but results generally have not been impressive. Because disequilibrium occurs most commonly during rapid hemodialysis, the simplest preventive measure is to slow the rate of biochemical change by shorter and more frequent dialyses, with or without reduction in blood flow. This approach is useful in patients with acute renal failure and in the initial phase of maintenance dialysis, particularly in patients with severe overhydration, severe metabolic acidosis, or very high BUN levels. Alternatively, peritoneal dialysis with resulting slower biochemical changes may be effective, although disequilibrium has also been described with this technique.

While shorter, more frequent hemodialysis is preferable, anticonvulsant drugs may be used in both the prevention and treatment of disequilibrium, although they have no effect on cerebral edema. In extremely uremic patients first starting dialysis, phenytoin may be useful in prevention as a loading dose of 1,000 mg (4 mmol) at least one day before commencing dialysis, followed by a maintenance dose of 300 to 400 mg daily until the patient is stable and uremia is controlled. Phenytoin is of little value during seizure activity as, although it enters the brain rapidly, the brain level also declines very rapidly unless there is continued administration. Intravenous diazepam (Valium) produces high brain levels within minutes and is one of the most effective agents for suppression of acute seizure activity. The effect of in-

travenous injection lasts 30 to 60 min, and respiratory depression is less than with barbiturates (79). Short-acting barbiturates, such as thiopental or pentobarbital, also are effective within minutes, but are more dangerous because of the greater respiratory depression.

COMPLICATIONS ASSOCIATED WITH BIOCHEMICAL CHANGES

Incorrect proportioning in the preparation of dialysis solution may occur as a result of both technical and human errors, the most important consequences being the development of acute hyponatremia or hypernatremia, depending upon the error. Both of these conditions may result in confusion, lethargy, muscle weakness, myoclonus, seizures, coma, and death (80).

Hyponatremia

Hyponatremia occurs when plasma is allowed to equilibrate with hypotonic dialysis fluid. With batch-mix dialysis equipment, hyponatremia and hypoosmolality can occur at the start of dialysis or following a bath change as a result of failure to add concentrate, failure to test dialysate prior to use, or use of the wrong quantity of concentrate or water. In proportioning systems, failure to connect to the concentrate container and to note or set the conductivity limits or both (and failure to follow the checklist for initiation of dialysis) will produce hyponatremia at the start of dialysis. Hyponatremia can also occur during the course of dialysis with a proportioning system if the concentrate container runs dry and the conductivity limits have not been set appropriately (see also remarks on monitoring of conductivity in Chapter 12).

Acute hypoosmolality causes the abrupt onset of hemolysis (81) with transient marked hyperkalemia which, assuming the patient survives the acute episode, rapidly subsides as potassium distributes throughout the body compartments. In addition, any residual renal function may be jeopardized if acute renal failure develops. At the same time as acute hemolysis occurs, the massive infusion of water from the hypotonic dialysate results in hypervolemia, hemodilution of all plasma constituents, acute water intoxication, and cerebral edema (82).

Symptoms include pain in the vein receiving the hypotonic hemolyzed blood from the dialyzer, anxiety, restlessness and headache. Pulse rate decreases initially, then increases, and the patient develops precordial pain, cold and clammy skin, and distended neck veins, the latter associated with myocardial dysfunction. Severe lumbar pain and abdominal cramps also may occur, perhaps due to ischemia.

Treatment consists of clamping the blood lines; the hemolyzed blood must not be returned from the dialyzer to the patient. When clinically indicated, 100% oxygen should be administered and the patient placed on a cardiac monitor with a defibrillator available. In the event of seizures, intravenous diazepam should be given. Blood should be obtained for baseline hematocrit, plasma hemoglobin, serum electrolytes, crossmatching, and serum enzyme levels. At the same time, a further batch of dialysate should be prepared, or in the case of a proportioning system, this could remain in bypass with appropriate concentrate until the dialysate composition is up to normal levels. Dialysis then should be restarted without delay, using a new dialyzer. Once dialysis has recommenced, a high transmembrane pressure is necessary to remove water excess, and it may be necessary to infuse saline, colloid, or blood to maintain blood pressure. Following dialysis, the hematocrit, serum hemoglobin and electrolyte concentrations should be remeasured, and the patient hospitalized for 24 to 48 h for serial enzyme studies and observation for possible myocardial damage.

Prevention of acute hyponatremia and hypoosmolality depends on meticulous attention to detail in preparing for dialysis. The final step before connecting dialyzer and patient should be checking of the dialysate in a batch system, or checking the conductivity meter and its setting with a proportioning system.

Hypernatremia

Hypernatremia and hyperosmolality due to use of inappropriate dialysate (83) may occur inadvertently with a batch-mix system if the wrong concentrate or wrong volume of concentrate or water is used and no check of the dialysate is made prior to dialysis. It may also occur when water and concentrate are incompletely mixed. With a proportioning system, this problem can only occur if the conductivity meter malfunctions or the alarm points are not set appropriately and the proportioning system is maladjusted; if the water treatment equipment malfunctions (84); or in a hydraulically driven proportioning system, if the concentrate source is elevated, so providing a head of pressure to the system.

The effects of hypernatremia include transfer of water from the intracellular to the extracellular space, causing intracellular water depletion and hyperosmolality. Depending upon the rapidity of the shifts of sodium and water, the extracellular volume may be increased or decreased; in any event, the extracellular fluid is hyperosmolar and cell volume is contracted. Symptoms include headache, nausea and vomiting, profound thirst, convulsions, coma, and death (80, 82).

Hyperkalemia

Serious hyperkalemia is an uncommon problem in patients on maintenance dialysis except in those who are markedly underdialyzed or following significant dietary indiscretion. In patients using single-needle dialysis, hyperkalemia may develop if recirculation occurs. This can be recognized by a disparity between the urea concentration of blood from the dialyzer and that from a peripheral vessel. The concentration of potassium in dialysate, usually between 1.0 and 3.0 mmol/l, results in net removal of potassium during dialy-

sis. Potassium-free dialysis solution can be used, but usually causes subnormal postdialysis plasma potassium levels which may contribute to postdialysis fatigue. Consequently, most patients are dialyzed with a dialysis fluid potassium concentration of at least 1.0 mmol/l.

Nevertheless, hyperkalemia may develop in association with hemolysis, as described elsewhere in this chapter. Hyperkalemia has also occurred in association with severe hyperglycemia in diabetic dialysis patients. This was ascribed to passive transfer of potassium from the intracellular space as a result of hyperosmolality of the extracellular fluid because of the severe hyperglycemia; insulin deficiency also may have played a role. Thus, in dialyzed diabetic patients, adequate blood glucose control is essential.

For patients receiving digitalis and related drugs, and particularly patients with left ventricular hypertrophy, rapid lowering of the serum potassium level during dialysis is a well-recognized cause of cardiac arrhythmias (85). Consequently, it is usual to dialyze such patients with a dialysis fluid potassium concentration of between 2.0 and 3.5 mmol/l, depending on the patient's serum potassium level. Ventricular extrasystoles, sinus tachycardia, atrial fibrillation, and other arrhythmias may occur and can cause sudden death. Electrocardiographic monitoring should be used if problems are anticipated during dialysis of a digitalized patient. The occurrence of potentially lethal hyperkalemia in patients on relatively small maintenance doses of digoxin has been described (86).

Hypokalemia

Hypokalemia is not generally severe in patients with chronic renal failure, but may result from prolonged potassium loss secondary to nausea, vomiting, diarrhea, nasogastric suction, or diuretic therapy. Hypokalemia during dialysis usually is not a significant problem, but sometimes may be life-threatening when associated with marked predialysis acidosis. In these circumstances, dialysis with rapid correction of the acidosis results in a major transcompartmental shift of potassium at a rate exceeding the capacity for transfer of potassium across the dialysis membrane; as a result, severe hypokalemia may develop (87). Patients likely to suffer from this problem have a history suggestive of potassium loss and a low or low-normal predialysis serum potassium level together with a low serum bicarbonate level and severe acidosis. Use of a high potassium dialysate should be considered in such patients, and serum potassium levels should be monitored during dialysis.

Hypercalcemia and hypermagnesemia

In the early days of hemodialysis, dialysis fluid was prepared using untreated tap water. However, it became obvious that in locations where the water contained high concentrations of calcium or magnesium, and particularly when these levels fluctuated appreciably, water for dialysis solution required treatment prior to use. All water used for dialysis fluid preparation must be treated by deionization, reverse osmosis, or a combination of these processes (1, 88) in order to control the levels of divalent cations and also to remove aluminium, fluoride, and other trace minerals that may be present. In some areas the mineral content of the water is so high that considerable water treatment is necessary (see Chapter 12).

The 'hard water syndrome' is an acute syndrome occurring during dialysis, precipitated by hypercalcemia and hypermagnesemia, and associated with failure of the water treatment process (89). Nausea and vomiting occur after the first hour of dialysis, and may persist throughout the treatment. Hypertension accompanies the vomiting, even if there is significant weight loss due to ultrafiltration during dialysis, and the rise in systolic pressure is greater than that of the diastolic pressure. This increase in blood pressure is attributed to the acute hypercalcemia, which may also cause acute pancreatitis (90). Lethargy, muscular weakness, headache, and an acute central nervous syndrome similar to dialysis dementia and associated with disorientation, dysarthria, seizures, myoclonic jerks, hallucinations, irritability, confusion, memory and judgment defects, and bizarre behavior have been described (91). If there is hypermagnesemia, burning sensations in the skin also may occur.

If the hard water syndrome develops, dialysis should be stopped and restarted as soon as possible using appropriately treated water for dialysis fluid preparation. Prevention depends upon regular maintenance and servicing of water treatment equipment.

Hypercalcemia in hemodialysis patients is a well recognized manifestation of secondary hyperparathyroidism. It has also been described in association with hyperthyroidism (92), as a manifestation of vitamin A toxicity due to excessive use of multivitamin preparations containing this vitamin (93), and in patients with tuberculosis, resulting from extrarenal production of calcitriol (94).

Hypermagnesemia may occur in dialysis patients, but is unlikely to be sufficient to cause symptoms unless the patient is taking magnesium containing phosphate binders (95). Although not an acute problem, use of a dialysate magnesium concentration of 0.5 mmol/l (1.0 mEq/l or a 1.2 mg/dl) induces slight hypermagnesemia and an elevated bone magnesium content. It has also been shown that a rise in plasma magnesium concentration in dialysis patients reduces circulating plasma parathyroid hormone levels (96).

Conversely, studies with magnesium-free dialysate and dialysis fluid containing only 0.25 mmol/l (0.5 mEq/l or 0.6 mg/dl) of magnesium have shown this may stimulate parathyroid hormone production, so increasing 1,25-dihydroxycholecalciferol production, intestinal calcium absorption, and bone mineralization (97). Hypomagnesemia may also cause arrhythmias in dialysis patients, especially in those receiving digitalis (98).

Miscellaneous dialysis fluid-related problems

Acute copper intoxication and hemolysis secondary to leaching of copper from copper tubing in a dialysis fluid supply system in association with a fall in pH following deionizer exhaustion has been reported (99). Chronic copper poisoning can also occur when dialysis solution is made from untreated water supplied through copper pipes (101, 101).

Intoxication with other metals such as zinc (102, 103), lead (104), and nickel (105) may occur, and other trace elements such as fluoride may accumulate in dialysis patients. These problems are discussed in detail in Chapter 49. Hemolysis associated with nitrates (106) and with chloramines (107) in the water used for dialysate has also been reported.

Dialysis fluid concentrate errors can cause serious acid-base abnormalities (108). It is possible to dialyze using acid concentrate in place of acetate, and the proportioning equipment can dilute this to the appropriate conductivity, resulting in severe metabolic acidosis. Similarly, the wrong acid and bicarbonate concentration can be used in the wrong equipment. Consequently, it is important to take considerable care in preparation for dialysis.

FEVER AND ENDOTOXEMIA

Infections and pyrogen reactions

Febrile reactions during dialysis usually are associated with endotoxemia causing a 'pyrogen' reaction. Less commonly they are due to infection, and rarely they result from failure of temperature control of the dialysis equipment.

Fever due to infection is most likely to occur at the start of dialysis or shortly after its end, while fever and chills developing during the course of dialysis are much more apt to be due to a pyrogen reaction in association with endotoxemia (109, 110).

Fever at the start of dialysis usually is due to contaminated equipment, and may be more likely to occur with a dialyzer which has been stored and reused if procedures are not followed carefully (see also Chapter 18). In the event of fever developing at the start of dialysis, treatment should be stopped, appropriate measures taken for investigation and treatment of infection, and dialysis restarted using fresh equipment.

Fever developing within an hour or so of the termination of dialysis suggests infection has occurred during the coming-off procedure. The risks of contamination and air embolism are reasons to prefer saline rinsing rather than air rinsing to return blood from the dialyzer at the end of dialysis. The patient should be investigated and treated for possible infection.

Fever developing during the course of dialysis generally is due to a pyrogen reaction secondary to endotoxemia. Usually the fever is associated with chills and nausea, and sometimes hypotension. The severity of the episode varies from very mild to very severe, but in general responds promptly to treatment with antipyretics. Circulating endotoxins or endotoxin-like activity have been shown in blood taken from patients during febrile episodes, and endotoxin has been demonstrated in dialysate (109) and in hollow fiber dialyzers (111). Endotoxin may be introduced from the dialysate, and high titers of antibodies against bacterial endotoxins have been found in dialysis patients (112). Although theoretically the pore size of cellulosic membranes is too small to allow passage of a molecule the size of endotoxin, small isolated defects could permit passage of sufficient endotoxin to cause a pyrogen reaction. With increasing use of more porous membranes, it is essential to insure sterility and nonpyrogenicity of the dialysate (113). Pyrogen reactions occurring with hollow fiber dialyzers containing a cellulosic membrane may be associated with endotoxins in the linters remaining in the dialyzer following manufacture, while in contrast, extracts of cuprammonium-derived hollow fibers do not show Limulus amebocyte lysate reactivity (111).

Treatment of a pyrogen reaction occurring during dialysis is with antipyretic agents. The possibility of infection should always be considered (114), but most febrile reactions occurring during dialysis are associated with contamination by pyrogens.

Prevention of pyrogen reactions requires effective cleaning and disinfection of dialysis equipment, as microbial contamination of the water used for dialysis is frequent (115). This may be particularly important for home dialysis patients, an appreciable number of whom have been found to use inadequately cleaned equipment (116). With high-efficiency dialysis using more porous synthetic membranes, it becomes essential to use effective water treatment to insure nonpyrogenicity of the dialysate (113). In addition, liquid bicarbonate concentrate can support rapid bacterial growth and endotoxin production and so should not be stored for prolonged periods of time, and bacteriological monitoring should be carried out before use and at least weekly. If concentrate is prepared from powder, this should be done immediately prior to dialysis, and all containers should be rinsed and disinfected daily (117). Pyrogen reactions have also been reported with use of a heparinized saline solution which was contaminated (118). Despite repeated patient concerns, dialyzer reuse generally has not been associated with an increase in the incidence of pyrogen reactions (119).

Overheated dialysate

Failure of the thermostat in the dialysate temperature monitoring system may result in overheating of the dialysate. This can cause immediate severe hemolysis and lethal hyperkalemia, or, if less severe, milder hemolysis may develop gradually. Thermostat failure causes a gradual rise in dialysate temperature, noted by the conscious patient as an increasing sensation of warmth. If undetected, heat-induced red cell damage may occur (120); but if the patient is not obtunded, overheating will be detected before the temperature rise is extreme.

If the dialysate temperature rises above 51°C, immediate and massive hemolysis can occur and may result in death from acute hyperkalemia (121). If the dialysate overheats to temperatures between 47°C and 51°C, the onset of hemolysis may be delayed for up to 48 h (122.123).

Prevention of this rare complication requires setting the high-temperature monitor on the dialysis equipment to

alarm so as to prevent temperatures in excess of 42°C.

In the event of a dialysate temperature rise to 51°C, dialysis must be stopped immediately, and the blood in the system should not be returned to the patient. The patient should be monitored closely for development of hyperkalemia, transfused if necessary, and have a further dialysis with fresh equipment as soon as possible.

AIR EMBOLISM

Air embolism is an ever-present risk during hemodialysis because of the combination of a blood pump and the extended extracorporeal blood circuit (124). The frequency of significant air embolism during hemodialysis is uncertain, and cases generally go unreported. Nevertheless, with present-day equipment, the frequency is likely to be small.

Causes

Many causes of air embolism have been recognized (1). Air leakage may occur into the portion of the extracorporeal blood circuit which is under subatmospheric pressure, i.e. the prepump segment during fistula dialysis. Leakage can occur around the fistula needle or needle hub, as a result of arterial disconnection, through the heparin syringe at the connection to the tubing, between barrel and plunger, or through a crack in the barrel wall, at the arterial monitor line connection, in the arterial monitor, at a defective arterial drip chamber, through a split pump segment, or through a vented intravenous bottle. Air also can pass in large quantities from dialysate to blood in the dialyzer. Refrigerated dialysate, as once used, could contain a large amount of dissolved air likely to come out of solution when the dialysate was warmed by blood in the dialyzer. This may still be seen when water used to prepare the dialysis fluid is very cold, so allowing more air to be dissolved than the deaerating capacity of the equipment. A similar problem may be seen if the deaerater is defective. Air embolism is also a possible complication with the use of subclavian vein access (125). Finally, air embolism may occur as a result of an error in the procedure for returning blood to the patient at the end of dialysis.

Signs and symptoms of air embolism

Death is said to have occurred with as little as 5 ml of air, although this must be extremely uncommon and would require very selective placement of the air. The amount of air necessary to produce symptoms depends on several factors. For example, more air can be tolerated as microbubbles infused at a slow rate, thus allowing time for the air to dissolve in the blood. Arterial introduction of air can cause death by occlusion of a major cerebral or coronary artery. During hemodialysis, air usually enters the body through the venous end of the extracorporeal blood circuit, although air can be infused into an artery during a cannulation procedure.

The signs and symptoms of air embolism depend in large part upon position. If the patient is sitting or the head is elevated, air entering an arm vein will travel through the axillary and subclavian veins, then in retrograde fashion up the jugular vein to the cerebral venous system where it obstructs the venules in the brain, resulting in cell damage. Death may ensue if a critical area of the brain is affected. Classically, the patient is said to cry out in alarm because of the sound of air rushing through the venous system to the brain, then, depending on the volume of air infused, convulse, lose consciousness, and possibly die.

When the patient is lying flat, air passes to the right atrium and right ventricle where it forms a foam, so interfering with the pumping ability of the heart. Especially if the patient is lying on his right side, air may pass through the pulmonary arteries to block the pulmonary capillary bed and cause acute pulmonary hypertension. Some air may pass through the lungs to the left ventricle and systemic circulation, resulting in arterial embolization and possibly cardiac arrhythmias and neurological defects. In these circumstances, the patient develops acute dyspnea, cough, and tightness in the chest, gasps for breath, becomes agitated and cyanosed, and may lapse into unconsciousness. Depending on the volume of air, respiratory arrest may occur. Upon examination, pulse and blood pressure may be unobtainable, and auscultation may reveal a churning sound caused by foaming of blood within the heart.

If the patient is in the Trendelenburg position because of hypotension at the time that air embolism occurs, air will pass to the lower extremities and cause patchy cyanosis associated with partial blockage of the circulation. If infusion of air is stopped in time and the patient is kept in position so that the air remains trapped in the leg veins, there may be no serious sequelae.

Treatment

When air embolism is detected, the venous blood lines must be clamped *immediately,* before any other action is taken. The patient should be positioned with chest and head down, turned on the left side. If the patient is dialyzing on a bed, they should be pulled off, leaving hips and legs on the bed. The bed can then be put in the Trendelenburg position and the patient slid back on to it, remaining on his left side throughout. If air embolism occurs while dialyzing in a chair, the patient can be pulled off so that the left shoulder is on the floor and the hips are still elevated. The patient should remain in this position in the ambulance en route to the hospital. This position traps air at the apex of the right ventricle, away from the pulmonary valve, so that the right ventricle acts as a bubble trap. Blood can continue to flow to the pulmonary arteries and lungs through the more dependent portion of the right ventricle.

If the patient is conscious, 100% oxygen by mask should be given. If unconscious, an airway or endotracheal tube should be placed and assisted respiration using 100% oxygen started.

If the patient is in cardiopulmonary distress and examination reveals foam in the right heart, percutaneous aspiration of foam may be necessary using an intracardiac needle and large syringe. Cardiac massage should not be commenced until foam has been removed from the right ventricle, so as to avoid passage of air into the pulmonary bed and left heart, so compounding the problem with arterial embolization. The use of 100% oxygen helps to supply oxygen to those parts of the lungs still being adequately perfused, and also increases the gas pressure gradient for nitrogen from bubbles to blood, so increasing diffusion. Other measures include intravenous adminstration of corticosteroids to reduce cerebral edema, and infusion of heparin and low molecular weight dextran to increase microcirculation (124). If available, consideration should be given to putting the patient in a compression chamber so as to drive the embolized air into solution. The patient can then go through decompression at a rate which will allow air to be expired through the lungs without coming out of solution (126).

Prevention of air embolism

Because air embolism is a life-threatening complication of hemodialysis, and treatment is difficult, often with poor results, prevention is of paramount importance. All intravenous fluids administered into the extracorporeal blood circuit should come only from collapsible plastic bags, as these can withstand pressures of at least 150 mmHg without withdrawing air. This is particularly important if fluid is administered into the subatmospheric pressure area of the prepump segment of the blood circuit. Preferably, intravenous fluids should be administered through the venous drip chamber as rapidly as possible, with the blood pump turned off, and this also avoids puncturing the arterial drip chamber or blood line sleeve. Care should always be taken whenever intravenous fluid is being administered during dialysis.

Heparin should be infused into the extracorporeal blood circuit at a point beyond the blood pump, i.e. against a positive pressure gradient. All needle-blood line connections must be tight, as must all arterial or prepump monitor line connections. An infusion sleeve on the prepump segment should not be used unless absolutely necessary. An air detector with a blood line clamp must be used on the venous blood line. Photocell air detectors may not detect very fine microbubbles unless the detector sensitivity is set so as to give frequent false alarms, and clot on the wall of the drip chamber may mask the photocell, so permitting the bubble trap to empty undetected. Conductance type air detectors are preferable and depend on change in capacitance across the drip chamber when it empties to actuate a blood line clamp (see also Chapter 12).

Perhaps the greatest risk of air embolism occurs if an air rinse is used to empty the dialyzer of blood at the end of dialysis. While air, or air and saline rinsing is said to be the most effective means to empty the extracorporeal circuit, the potential risk is such that saline rinsing should generally be used. In the event air is used, the proper procedure must be followed scrupulously. Both patient and attendant should have hemostats placed across the venous blood line so that either can clamp the tubing at the end of the rinse, and the complete attention of both must be focused on the procedure. If the dialyzer is being emptied using air pumped through the blood pump, the attendant must keep one hand on the blood pump switch at all times. If blood is being returned using a hand-squeezed pump, enough pressure must be used to keep blood flowing freely into the venous drip chamber. If possible, the air detector and line clamp on the venous line should remain in the 'active' mode during the rinse procedure.

HEMORRHAGE

An increased incidence of spontaneous bleeding episodes occurs in hemodialysis patients. These include gastrointestinal bleeding, subdural hematoma, uremic hemopericardium, retroperitoneal hematoma, hemorrhagic pleural effusion, spontaneous bleeding into the anterior chamber of the eye, subcapsular hematoma of the liver, and bleeding into the skin and other sites. Such bleeding is related to several factors, including heparinization during dialysis, ongoing anticoagulant therapy, and the functional platelet abnormalities of uremia (127, 128). Platelet-membrane interactions cause platelet adhesion on the dialyzer membrane, formation of platelet factor 4, beta-thromboglobulin and thromboxane (129, 130), defects in platelet aggregation (131), and thrombocytopenia (132, 133). These interactions may be dependent on the characteristics of the dialysis membrane (134). The abnormalities in platelet function and prostacyclin activity are not always corrected by dialysis (135, 136). Thus the dialysis patient is always at some risk of bleeding. Petechial hemorrhages, blood blisters in the skin, and bruising around fistula punctures are common, and usually have no significance except as a reminder of the potential risk of bleeding. The possibility of internal bleeding always must be considered in any instance of unexplained hypotension during or after dialysis.

Gastrointestinal bleeding

The causes of gastrointestinal bleeding in maintenance hemodialysis patients generally are similar to those in nonuremic patients, including peptic ulceration, aspirin ingestion, hiatal hernia, and colon ulcers (137). In general, serum gastrin levels are higher than normal in dialysis patients, and some, particularly the elderly, have associated gastric hyposecretion; these patients have the highest incidence of gastrointestinal hemorrhage. Chronic gastritis is also relatively common in chronic renal failure patients, and may be responsible for much of the morbidity from gastrointestinal complications during hemodialysis (138). Gastrointestinal bleeding is an indication for the use of regional heparinization, low-dose or no heparin during dialysis (139) or peritoneal dialysis. Otherwise, the treatment of gastrointestinal bleeding in dialysis patients is straightforward, apart from the need to coordinate surgery with the dialysis schedule.

Subdural hematoma

Subdural hematoma occurs in up to 3% of hemodialysis patients (140, 141), and should be suspected in any patient with headache or neurologic symptoms resembling disequilibrium but which are not readily explained by this or other causes. Contributory factors include head trauma, anticoagulation, excessive ultrafiltration, hypertension, and the increased cerebrospinal fluid pressure and brain swelling which may occur during dialysis. Frequent episodes of access-site infection or cannula clotting are said to be common in such patients.

The symptoms and signs of subdudral hematoma may be nonspecific and are often confused with disequilibrium. However, the latter is unusual with maintenance dialysis except in new patients. The symptoms of disequilibrium usually do not fluctuate as much as those of subdural hematoma, and although headache is common with disequilibrium, it usually disappears shortly after dialysis. A diagnosis of subdural hematoma should always be considered when a previously stable dialysis patient presents with unexplained symptoms suggestive of disequilibrium. Headaches usually are severe, persisting through subsequent dialyses, and there may be focal or multifocal neurologic signs which may fluctuate. Neurologic signs are usually of little value in localizing the site of the intracranial bleeding.

Lumbar puncture and electroencephalography are of little help in diagnosis, as abnormalities of both can occur with disequilibrium, and radioisotope scanning produces an appreciable percentage of false negative results. The most useful investigations include cerebral arteriography (142), echoencephalography, and computerized tomography of the brain.

When subdural hematoma is a serious possibility, it may be preferable to use peritoneal dialysis until the diagnosis is confirmed or rejected (143). Treatment is by surgical exploration and removal of clot, but the results are disappointing, with a reported patient survival of less than 50% (144, 145). This is comparable to the results of treatment of acute subdural hematoma in nonuremic patients, where mortality is approximately 75% (146).

Uremic hemopericardium

Pericarditis is not uncommon in dialysis patients, and may occur early in the course of treatment or at any time after the patient becomes stabilized on dialysis (147). While the former is commonly uremic in origin, pericarditis in a stable dialysis patient is more likely to be associated with cytomegalic or other virus infection, and has also been described in patients receiving minoxidil for refractory hypertension (148). Pericardial effusion appears to be more common in patients on hemodialysis than in those treated by peritoneal dialysis (149). Pericarditis without effusion is an indication for more frequent dialysis, preferably with regional heparinization or low-dose heparin, or for peritoneal dialysis to avoid the use of anticoagulants.

An obvious pericardial effusion may develop in a small number of patients and may be associated with bleeding into the pericardial sac. While relatively uncommon, this is important to diagnose because of the potential risk of tamponade, which may escape early recognition. Such patients often give a history of preceding upper respiratory infection, and have symptoms of chest pain, respiratory distress, hypotension, and evidence of fluid overload. This is usually associated with fever and symptoms suggestive of a mild upper respiratory or gastrointestinal viral infection. In patients developing signs and symptoms suggestive of pericardial effusion, the diagnosis should be confirmed by X ray, sonography, isotope scanning, or other means. Initial treatment, particularly for smaller effusions, should be repeated pericardiocentesis with installation of a nonabsorbable steriod into the pericardial sac (150). If this fails, pericardectomy or pericardial fenestration usually is required (151). An enlarging effusion despite repeated pericardiocentesis requires prompt surgical drainage before hypotension or tamponade occur.

Retroperitoneal hematoma

Spontaneous retroperitoneal hemorrhage with a resultant hematoma is an uncommon complication of hemodialysis, occurring in less than 1% of patients (152). Diagnosis may be difficult in the absence of a history of trauma. There may be massive bleeding into the retroperitoneal space requiring transfusion of a large volume of blood, or the onset may be more insidious. Predisposing factors include minor trauma and anticoagulation, although spontaneous retroperitoneal bleeding is a rare complication in nonuremic patients receiving anticoagulants. An iatrogenic retroperitoneal hematoma can result afrom perforation of the iliac vein during insertion of a catheter via the femoral vein by the Seldinger technique.

Retroperitoneal bleeding presents with abdominal and flank or back pain, frequently associated with a distended abdomen and hypoactive or absent bowel sounds. An abdominal mass may be palpable. X-ray of the abdomen may show a soft tissue density and absence of the psoas shadow, and a barium contrast meal may show a nonspecific ileitis. Fever can occur after significant bleeding without evidence of simultaneous infection. Bleeding around the pancreas can cause pancreatic injury and an increase in the serum levels of pancreatic enzymes. Neuropathy due to retroperitoneal bleeding and hemorrhage around the femoral nerve has also been described. Selective renal angiography may be helpful in diagnosing perirenal hemorrhage (153), and sonography is also useful.

Treatment is usually conservative, with replacement of blood loss and hemodialysis using minimal or no heparin or peritoneal dialysis. Anticoagulant therapy should be stopped and the patient kept at rest. Surgical exploration usually is unnecessary. Spontaneous retroperitoneal bleeding should be considered in any hemodialysis patient with unexplained acute abdominal distress and a falling hematocrit without obvious external blood loss.

Hemorrhagic pleural effusion

Pleuritis is a complication of uremia (154), and hemorrhagic pleural effusion occasionally occurs in dialysis patients (155), probably related to anticoagulation in a patient with a fibrinous pleuritis. Treatment includes hemodialysis with low dose or no heparin, peritoneal dialysis, pleurocentesis, and use of a nonabsorbable steroid as in the treatment of pericarditis. The possible development of pulmonary constriction must be borne in mind in the patient who has had recurrent hemorrhagic pleuritis. A hemorrhagic pleural effusion should always suggest the need to exclude the possibility of coexisting cancer or tuberculosis.

Subcapsular liver hematoma

Spontaneous subcapsular liver hematoma may occur in dialysis patients and should be considered if such a patient presents with right upper quadrant pain, a rising alkaline phosphatase level, and falling hematocrit, without evidenced of external blood loss (156, 157). Radioisotope scanning can provide supporting evidence. Management depends upon the extent and location of the liver injury and may require evacuation or partial hepatectomy.

Epidural spinal hematoma

Epidural spinal hematoma occurs occasionally in dialysis patients, presumably as a result of anticoagulation. Symptoms of cord compression develop, with rapid onset of bilateral leg weakness and sensory loss, resulting in paraparesis and paraplegia. The development of spinal cord signs in a dialysis patient is an indication for urgent treatment, as permanent paraplegia may result unless there is early surgical evacuation of the compressing hematoma.

Hemorrhages into the skin

Petechial hemorrhages and an increased frequency of blood blisters and bruising around fistula punctures are not uncommon in dialysis patients. Typical subungual splinter hemorrhages, identical with those of bacterial endocarditis, also may occur (158).

MISCELLANEOUS PROBLEMS ASSOCIATED WITH DIALYSIS

Restlessness and insomnia are frequent symptoms in patients with severe uremia, particularly in the months immediately prior to starting dialysis. Usually these symptoms are relieved within a few weeks of starting treatment.

When these symptoms develop in a stable patient on maintenance hemodialysis, causes such as anxiety are most likely, but the possibility of inadequate dialysis should always be considered. Consequently, predialysis blood chemistry should be reviewed in any dialysis patient developing insomnia and restlessness. Treatment is symptomatic. In a home hemodialysis patient suffering from insomnia, medication should be avoided in the period shortly before dialysis.

Restless legs

The restless leg syndrome is an irresistable compulsion to move the legs, occurring particularly when the patient is at rest, and often worse at night. It may be associated with paresthesiae, pruritus, and dull aches in the legs. It occurs in 40% of patients with chronic renal failure (159) and may be an early manifestation of neuropathy. The pathogenesis is obscure, and no abnormalities of nerves or muscles have been shown (160). Restlessness causes insomnia and may also be associated with nocturnal myoclonus. The syndrome causes embarrassment and can affect job performance, yet patients may not volunteer information on this problem except on direct questioning. Relief may occur with institution of dialysis or with the use of mild tranquilizers (161) or Levodopa (162).

Hypoglycemia due to beta-blocking agents

Beta adrenergic-blocking agents are used in the treatment of the hypertension of chronic renal failure, for treatment of persistent hypertension in dialysis patients, and for control of angina and arrhythmias. Severe acute hypoglycemia with beta-blocking agents was first described in association with the use of glucose-free dialysate in a single-pass system for patients who had fasted for more than 18 h (163). Episodes of profound hypoglycemia have been reported in nondiabetic dialysis patients receiving propranolol for hypertension and who were not fasting (164). The effect of beta-blocking drugs on glucose metabolism is complex, and may result in either hypoglycemia or hyperglycemia (165). Hypoglycemia is presumably the result of the effects on hepatic glycogenolysis, glucagon release, and lipolysis (166), and other possible contributory factors include poor nutritional intake with decreased glycogen stores and other causes of liver dysfunction. Hypoglycemia has also been reported in dialysis patients undergoing hyperalimentation with solutions of high dextrose content, presumably due to rapid passage of glucose from blood to dialysate (167).

Symptoms and signs of hypoglycemia include a sharp rise of blood pressure, presumably due to release of catecholamines, vomiting, and unconsciousness occurring early in dialysis. Hypoglycemia should be ruled out whenever such symptoms develop in any dialysis patient receiving beta-blocking agents.

Because beta-blocking agents are in common use, many dialysis patients, especially with those with diabetes, liver dysfunction, or poor nutrition, may have transient episodes of hypoglycemia without autonomic symptoms because these are prevented by the beta blocker. Since use of a glucose-free dialysate may contribute to development of hypoglycemia, glucose-containing dialysate should always be used for patients receiving beta blockers. Alternatively, frequent blood sugar determinations may be made on main-

tenance hemodialysis patients taking beta blockers.

Dermatological abnormalities associated with hemodialysis

Xerosis, pruritus, skin infections, and disorders of pigmentation occur in patients with chronic renal failure and in dialysis patients (168–170). Among the other dermatological problems reported in such patients are lesions resembling erythema multiforme, bullous dermatosis, and porphyria cutanea tarda. Bullous dermatosis is characterized by the occurrence of moderately painful bullae on the dorsa of the hands and feet, unassociated with trauma (171, 172). The cause is unknown, and the condition is not related to medication, although there is a suggestion sunlight may be a causative factor.

Porphyria cutanea tarda

Porphyria cutanea tarda has been reported in dialysis patients (173, 174), presumably due to insufficient removal of porphyrins by dialysis. This results in high levels of plasma porphyrins and severe, potentially mutilating skin lesions. Iron overload may be a precipitating factor (175), as this catalyzes production of activated oxygen species which can cause oxidative damage to the erythrocytes (176). Treatment is very difficult because chloroquine is ineffective (175), and venesection is not usually practical because of anemia. A recent case report described dramatic improvement in one patient during treatment with deferoxamine for iron overload (177).

Pruritus

Pruritus frequently complicates end-stage renal disease, occurring in 50% to 75% of patients (178), and a survey found that 37% of hemodialysis patients had bothersome itching, and an additional 41% had experienced this in the past (179). In two thirds of the patients who had experienced pruritus, discomfort was most severe or only occurred during or soon after dialysis. Local topical emollients and orally administered antipruritic agents were relatively ineffective, providing relief in only about 18% of patients. While somewhat less of a problem with adequate dialysis, pruritus remains a distressing problem for many patients.

The etiology of pruritus remains unclear, although various changes have been found in the skin of dialysis patients. Dermal mast cells are increased, and pruritus might result from release of histamine as a result of extracorporeal circulation (178), and ketotifen, a putative mast cell stabilizer, has been shown to relieve itching (180). Biopsies have shown elevated skin contents of calcium, magnesium and phosphorus in patients with pruritus; and following successful treatment with ultraviolet B (UVB), the skin phosphorus level was reduced to values comparable with nonpruritic uremic patients, suggesting increased divalent ion content precipitating microdeposits of calcium or magnesium phosphate in the skin may be responsible for pruritus (181). Microangiopathy has also been described in skin from uremic and dialysis patients, changes which regressed following transplantation (182), and pruritus associated with hypercalcemia and secondary hyperparathyroidism shows a dramatic response to subtotal parathyroidectomy (183).

In a double-blind study, 100 mg (427 mmol) of lidocaine intravenously relieved pruritus completely in some patients and had a marked effect in others (184). Unfortunately, relief lasted only for one day following infusion, pruritus always recurring by the next day. Blood levels of lidocaine achieved were no greater than those used in treating cardiac arrhythmias; and if the drug was given at a rate no greater than 7 mg (13 mmol/min), no adverse effects were noted other than occasional episodes of hypotension. In patients with chronic renal failure, lidocaine has a normal plasma half-life, suggesting that persistence of relief into the day after administration is due either to a metabolite normally excreted by the kidney being active as an antipruritic agent, or lidocaine is acting in a kinetic compartment from which the drug has a very slow rate of egress.

Administration of the nonabsorbable anion-exchange resin, cholestyramine, has also met with some success in the treatment of uremic pruritus, 5 g twice daily in juice producing partial relief in most patients in a randomized, four-week, double-blind study (185). Cholestyramine has the ability to bind organic acids, which may be a clue to a chemical cause for pruritus. It also relieves the itching of obstructive jaundice, possibly by binding bile acids, and reduces the itching of polycythemia vera. However, another study failed to show relief of uremic pruritus by cholestyramine (186), and this drug may induce or aggravate metabolic acidosis (187) and is very difficult to present in a palatable form.

Relief of uremic pruritus with oral charcoal, 6 g daily, has been reported in an eight-week double-blind cross-over study (188). Charcoal is presumed to act as a sorbent of numerous organic and inorganic compounds. Heparin infusion has also been described as relieving pruritus (189), as has reduction of the dialysate magnesium concentration to 2.0 mmol/l (0.48 mg/dl) and consequent lowering of the predialysis serum magnesium concentration (190). Modified acupuncture technique using electrical needle stimulation has also been shown to provide relief in a controlled but not blinded study (191).

In 1977 relief of uremic pruritus with the use of phototherapy was reported (192), and sunburn-spectrum ultraviolet (UVB) phototherapy using slightly below-minimum erythemal doses of ultraviolet B radiation has been shown to be beneficial (193). When patients were treated by applying UVB phototherapy to one-half of the body and placebo phototherapy to the other half, there was generalized improvement of itching without localization of benefit to the treated side, suggesting a systemic effect of UVB phototherapy. Remissions of up to several months were obtained, and a more rapid response occurred with more intensive schedules of treatment and with a second course of phototherapy (194). Possible explanations for the response to UVB phototherapy include inactivation of circulating substance(s) present in uremia and responsible for pruritus, a

photoproduct with a long half-life may relieve pruritus without directly affecting the cause, or an effect of the reduction of skin phosphorus to levels comparable to those in nonpruritic uremic patients and healthy volunteers (181). Ultraviolet A (UVA) light also was reported to relieve pruritus in dialysis patients (195), but a placebo-controlled trial failed to confirm this (196).

As is usual in medicine, the wide range of measures available to treat uremic pruritus suggests that none is universally effective, and that a better understanding of the cause of itching is required. Meanwhile, general measures should not be neglected, including the use of antihistamines, tranquilizers, and sedatives (197), and the wearing of light clothing and few bedclothes. Tepid baths or showers may help the patient who has difficulty in sleeping due to itching, and may give sufficient though temporary relief to allow sleep. Cooling of the skin can be achieved by application of a lotion such as calamine, but local anesthetic or antihistamine creams should be avoided because of the risk of allergic contact sensitization.

Muscle cramps

Painful muscle cramps are common in nondialyzed and dialyzed uremic patients, both during and between dialyses, particularly in the elderly. While not life-threatening, cramps may interfere seriously with patient well-being and rehabilitation.

Cramps occur in more than 20% of hemodialysis patients (198) and appear to relate to acute contraction of plasma and extracellular volumes due to rapid fluid removal or hypoosmolality. They tend to occur late during dialysis, more frequently in the legs, typically last about 10 min, taking 3 min to develop and 7 min to dissipate fully, and more frequent in patients who manifest a high degree of anxiety (199). In patients who develop muscle cramps, tonic electromyogram (EMG) activity increases during the latter part of dialysis, and this appears to be a useful predictor of the onset of cramps during dialysis (200).

Quinine sulfate has been used empirically for relief of cramps for many years. Its effectiveness has been confirmed by a double-blind study which showed that 320 mg (1.0 mmol) of quinine sulfate prior to each dialysis was effective in reducing both the frequency and severity of cramps, without hematologic, auditory, or visual side effects (201).

Relief or reduction in the frequency of cramps also has been described with use of a higher dialysis fluid sodium concentration (140 mmol/l) (12), administration of sodium chloride by mouth (202), or with a bolus intravenous injection of hypertonic dextrose or hypertonic saline. Injection of 20 ml of hypertonic (17.5%) (3 mmol/l) saline (203), a solution that must be appropriately labeled to avoid inadvertent use, reduces the effect of ultrafiltration in normalizing the patient's extracellular volume, and consequently hypertonic dextrose may be preferable. Double-blind studies have shown significant relief without complications using hypertonic (50%) dextrose injected intravenously (204, 205). This results in an acute rise of the plasma glucose level which returns to normal within one hour. A double-blind study comparing hypertonic saline, hypertonic dextrose, and 5% dextrose showed no difference between hypertonic dextrose and hypertonic saline, although both were superior to 5% dextrose (206).

The frequency of muscle cramps during dialysis is also related to the dialysis technique, is influenced by the dialysate sodium concentration, and is less frequent with bicarbonate dialysis (207) and with sequential ultrafiltration (208). More recently, development of such techniques as hemofiltration (209) and automatic ultrafiltration control has also reduced the frequency of muscle cramps during treatment.

Priapism

Priapism has been reported to occur at some time in as many as 2.5% of male hemodialysis patients between the ages of 14 and 42 (210, 211). However, a recent multicenter survey in the United States found the considerably lower occurrence rate of only 1 in 196 patients. This difference might relate to the duration of dialysis and associated heparinization which was 6 to 8 h in the 1970's, but at the time of the more recent study was only 3.5 to 5.5 h (212). In most cases, priapism develops during or within a few hours after dialysis, suggesting a cause-and-effect relationship. It is not generally related to sexual activity, and patients may be sleeping when awakened by a painful erection. Erections are known to occur during rapid-eye-movement sleep, irrespective of dream content, and this may be a precipitating factor.

Most incidents of priapism develop while heparinized on hemodialysis, do not occur with peritoneal dialysis, and are not associated with generalized clotting problems or long-term anticoagulation. Priapism is known to occur in patients heparinized following myocardial infarction, pulmonary embolism, and thrombophlebitis (213), and heparin may increase blood viscosity by causing precipitation of fibrin degradation products, enhance thrombin generation, and cause abnormal spontaneous platelet aggregation. A relatively high hematocrit and hypovolemia as a result of ultrafiltration increase blood viscosity and may be precipitating factors, and heparinized blood clots more readily in the presence of acidosis. Androgen therapy has also been thought important in the genesis of priapism in some patients (214), and androgens should be discontinued in male patients with hematocrits greater than 25 so as to avoid an increased frequency of erections. The future availability of recombinant human erythropoietin should eliminate the need for androgens in dialysis patients.

The prognosis for return of sexual function after priapism is very poor in dialysis patients, despite venous bypass surgery. Following such surgery, only a small number of patients retain the capacity to sustain erection. Other treatments used have included spinal anesthesia and a variety of drugs such as phenothiazines, atropine, and Ancrod. The development of safe and effective penile prostheses have made these the most effective treatment for impotence following priapism.

Membrane biocomptability

Transient and marked leukopenia during the first 30 min of hemodialysis, recognized for many years (215), is associated with transient sequestration of neutrophils in the dialyzer and in the pulmonary capillary bed and the release of free radicals (216). The intitiating mechanism is activation of complement through contact of blood with the dialysis membrane, and this is responsible for increased margination and sequestration of neutrophils in the pulmonary capillaries (217). Trapping of microaggregates of leukocytes leads to hypoxia, and free radicals may also play a role in this (216). White cell studies and pulmonary function tests in patients before, during, and after hemodialysis have shown significant leukopenia and a fall in CO diffusing capacity within 15 min of the start of hemodialysis, and development of hypoxia within 30 min. The white cell count returns to baseline within 1 h, but pO_2 and CO diffusing capacity remain low throughout dialysis, and the level of these is directly related to the initial fall in white cell count (218). This persistence of hypoxia, together with the fact that hypoxia can also occur with dialyzers that do not cause leukopenia (218) has led to considerable investigation of the biocompatibility of various membranes in recent years.

Blood-membrane interactions include complement activation, activation of the coagulation and kallikrein pathways (219), prostaglandin activation (220), activation of monocytes leading to the release of interleukin-1 (221), platelet interactions (133), and absorption of various substances on the membranes (222).

Anaphylactic reactions

An anaphylactic reaction occurring at the start of dialysis is a rare but serious complication of hemodialysis, occurring in 4 of every 100,000 dialyses(45). This appears to be the result of hypersensitivity to ethylene oxide used in sterilizing the dialyzer (223), and antibodies to ethylene oxide have been found in some dialysis patients. The incidence of such antibodies is higher with hemodialysis than in peritoneal dialysis patients (224), and the incidence of hypersensitivity reactions is lower in patients using dialyzers not sterilized with ethylene oxide. The potting compound in the dialyzer may trap ethylene oxide and release this into the circulation at the start of dialysis (225), where it combines with proteins to form a hapten which binds to basophils and mast cells with release of histamine and other vasoactive compounds. This causes acute bronchoconstriction, vasodilatation, and the symptoms of anaphylaxis.

First-use syndrome

Much more common than an anaphylactic reaction is the first-use syndrome which occurs shortly after starting dialysis with a new dialyzer, and results in acute discomfort, with pruritus, back pain, hypotension, and hypoxia. This occurs on first use of a dialyzer with a cuprophane or other cellulosic membrane, but does not occur with synthetic membranes such as polyacrylonitrile. Symptoms decrease or disappear with reuse of cellulosic dialyzers. The syndrome is due to activation of the complement pathway by the membrane, and patients who are more likely to suffer from the first-use syndrome activate complement more vigorously and more quickly than other patients (48).

Usually these reactions are mild and self-limiting, although they may require the use of analgesics, antihistamines, or epinephrine (226). Adequate rinsing of new dialyzers with saline should eliminate this problem.

Postdialysis syndrome

Many patients experience feelings of fatigue and lack of energy immediately following dialysis, and it has been suggested that interleukin-1, synthesized by activated monocytes, may account for these symptoms. This remains to be proven.

Dialyzer reuse and morbidity

Chest and back pain occur with dialysis from time to time, and a double-blind crossover study has shown this is particularly associated with the use of a new dialyzer with a cuprophane membrane (227). A decreased frequency of symptoms has been shown with reused dialyzers and with dialyzers with polyacrylonitrile membranes (228, 229). Despite frequently expressed patient concerns about the safety of dialyzer reuse, there seem to be theoretical reasons for this to be beneficial, and patients using reused dialyzers have fewer dialysis-related days of hospitalization than do patients who do not reuse (230). A recent 5-year study in 4,000 patients of the variables associated with mortality found dialyzer reuse to be associated with a lower death rate (231).

Joint and tendon abnormalities associated with hemodialysis

Hemodialysis patients have long been known to be prone to acute episodes of arthritis or periarthritis, and the appearance of soft tissue calcification in periarticular tissues. More recently, the carpal tunnel syndrome and periarticular pains, particularly around the shoulder and hip girdles in patients on dialysis for many years, have been shown to be associated with beta-2 microglobulin production and the deposition of amyloid in bones, joints, tendons and periarticular structures. These problems are discussed further in Chapter 31.

Spontaneous tendon rupture

Spontaneous tendon rupture in dialysis patients usually affects the quadriceps and the hand. The cause is unclear. Chronic acidosis may lead to degeneration of tendons with changes in their tensile characteristics (232), but pathologic changes at the tendo-osseous junction associated with secondary hyperparathyroidism may be more important (233). The latter view is supported by the association of quadriceps tendon rupture with X-ray evidence of hyperparathyroidism

(234). Tendon rupture occurs after years on dialysis, and in young patients. Finger tendon ruptures usually are ignored by the patient because they are not significantly disabling. Quadriceps tendon rupture is treated by immobilization, physiotherapy, and frequently by parathyroidectomy.

Uremic bursitis

In uremic patients, bursitis with or without effusion, is a manifestation of uremic polyserositis. Most commonly, this presents as an olecranon bursal effusion resulting from trauma, and associated with increased pressure in bursal vessels related to an arteriovenous fistula, together with the anticoagulant effect of heparin. In one report, as many as 6% of hemodialysis patients developed bursitis (235), and all had an arteriovenous fistula and used a cushion under their elbow for support. Bursitis usually occurred over the olecranon on the side of the vascular access, although effusions involving the trochanteric and Achilles bursae also occurred. Treatment consists of aspiration and injection of nonabsorbable steroids. Although aspiration usually is sterile, septic bursitis may also occur.

Septic arthritis

Septic arthritis is a much more common complication in dialysis patients than in the general population (236). Because joint pain is not uncommon in dialysis patients, the possibility of septic arthritis always should be borne in mind. The most common causative organism is a *Staphylococcus*, and the same microorganism is often cultured simultaneously from joint, blood, and/or arteriovenous fistula, suggesting hematogenous spread. Unlike nonuremic septic arthritis, in addition to the usual joints such as knee, elbow, hip and shoulder, other joints involved in dialysis patients include the sternoclavicular, sacroiliac, and acromioclavicular joint, and the arthritis is more frequently multiarticular. Early diagnosis is mandatory in order to minimize the risk of disabling joint disease. Unfortunately, the diagnosis is not always easy because other types of acute arthritis are frequent in dialysis patients, but acute attacks of pseudogout are not usually associated with other systemic complaints. Consequently, septic arthritis should always be considered when a dialysis patient develops arthritis, expecially if associated with fever or infection elsewhere, and an infectious cause must always be excluded by joint aspiration. Once septic arthritis is identified, prompt and early treatment is essential to prevent crippling joint damage.

Tuberculous arthritis

Extrapulmonary tuberculosis is more common in dialysis patients than in the general population (237) and has recently been reported as one cause of acute arthritis in dialysis patients (238). Because of its resemblance to acute septic arthritis, joint aspiration and synovial fluid culture should be considered in any dialysis patient presenting with monoarthritis.

Hearing loss

Hearing loss associated with dialysis may involve both vestibular and cochlear mechanisms and may be due to bleeding in the inner ear space as a consequence of heparinization or result from cellular injury in the hair cells of the cochlea as a result of edema (239). However, the frequent use of ototoxic drugs in dialysis patients making hearing loss difficult to evaluate, and there are contradictory reports as to whether or not most patients with chronic renal failure show evidence of hearing loss on audiometric examination (240, 241).

Visual loss

Occasionally, dialysis patients develop acute visual loss (uremic amaurosis) which can occur rapidly over minutes to hours. Loss of vision is complete, and pupillary reactions and fundoscopic examination are normal. Recovery usually occurs within 2 weeks (242).

Anterior ischemic optic neuropathy resulting in a sudden painless loss of vision has recently been reported in association with hemodialysis-associated hypotension. Presentation is with sudden painless loss of vision during an episode of hypotension on dialysis (243).

Hepatic friction rub

A hepatic friction rub is an auscultatory finding most commonly associated with malignant neoplasm of the liver, but also described in two hemodialysis patients (244). Presumably, such a rub is the equivalent of a uremic pericardial or pleural friction rub, and theoretically should disappear with increased dialysis, although this did not occur.

Mesenteric ischemia

Acute mesenteric ischemia occurs in dialysis patients, generally in association with severe episodes of hypotension and hypovolemia during dialysis. This may or may not result in bowel infarction. Characteristically, there is leukocytosis, and occult blood can be demonstrated in the stools. The diagnosis is suggested by the development of nonspecific abdominal symptoms and leukocytosis following hypotension during dialysis (245).

Bowel infarction

Nonocclusive bowel infarction has been described as a complication occurring in dialysis patients after a large weight loss secondary to vomiting, diarrhea, or ultrafiltration. Frequent and severe hypotension during dialysis occurred more commonly in patients who developed this problem. Death occurred in 9 of 12 patients (246).

Recurrent abdominal pain associated with digoxin

Severe recurrent central abdominal pain, brought on by exertion, occurring shortly after dialysis and especially after ultrafiltration, has been described in an elderly male dialysis patient (247). This was thought to be due to intestinal angina resulting from intestinal ischemia from reduced cardiac output or local vasoconstriction following intravascular volume depletion. Symptoms were relieved by discontinuing digoxin, probably because it is a mesenteric vasoconstrictor. This syndrome may occur in dialysis patients with calcified aortas who undergo rapid ultrafiltration and are taking digoxin. It should be considered as a possible cause of obscure abdominal pain in such patients.

Cecal necrosis

Necrosis of the cecum may be associated with reduced blood flow. Spontaneous perforation of the left side of the colon and cecum has been reported in dialysis patients and those with uremia and was considered secondary to distention from constipation. However, it has been suggested the cecum is more susceptible to ischemia than the remainder of the colon, and maximal distention develops at this point which, in association with impaired blood flow resulting from hypotension, may cause necrosis. A diagnosis of cecal necrosis and perforation should be considered in any dialysis patient who develops acute abdominal symptoms. Early exploration may be necessary (248).

Leachables

Because dialyzer tubing sets are made from plastic, there is always the likelihood of leaching polyvinyl chloride or plasticizer such as di-(2-ethylhexyl) phthalate (DEHP) into the blood (249). The latter probably is not very toxic, although it may affect various enzyme systems (250), but de-esterification produces the biologically active compounds mono-(2-ethylhexyl) phthalate and phthalic acid (251). Polyvinyl chloride has been associated with recurrent episodes of cutaneous necrotizing dermatitis in a dialysis patient (252), probably resulting from an immunologic process. The association between these and other chemicals leached from plastics and the occurrence of such effects as eosinophilia and itching during dialysis has not been clearly established, but substantial exposure does occur in dialysis patients (251). The occasional occurrence of immediate reactions resembling IgE-mediated anaphylaxis in dialysis patients has also been recorded and related to development of antibodies to phthalic anhydride, diphenylmethane diisocyanate (253), and other isocyanates derived from potting compounds (254).

COMMENT

Acute complications occurring during hemodialysis range from the trivial and merely transient to the catastrophic and fatal. Nevertheless, the great majority of dialyses are uneventful, and each year more than 30 million hemodialyses are performed around the world, many of these in patients' homes. Because most dialyses are uneventful, it is important that nursing and technical staff, as well as patients, learn of the acute complications of hemodialysis, their recognition, and the appropriate responses. Patient well-being, whether dialyzing in a center or at home, demands confidence in the treatment and its safety. This can only come from the example of staff who are themselves familiar with the acute complications of hemodialysis and are experienced in their management.

REFERENCES

1. Keshaviah PR, Luehmann D, Shapiro FL, Comty CM: *Investigation of the Risks and Hazards Associated with Hemodialysis Devices.* Technical report, Silver Spring, MD, US Dept Health, Education and Welfare, Food and Drug Administration, 1980.

2. Cohle SD, Graham MA: Sudden death in hemodialysis patients. *J Forensic Sci* 30: 158, 1985

3. Stewart RS: Psychiatric issues in renal dialysis and transplantation. *Hosp Community Psychiatry* 34: 623, 1983

4. Friedman EA: Controversy in renal disease. Dialysis-induced hypotension. *Am J Kidney Dis* 2: 289, 1982

5. Rubin LJ, Gutman RA: Hypotension during hemodialysis. *The Kidney.* 11: 21, 1978

6. Degoulet P, Reach I, Di Giulio S, De Vries C, Rouby JJ, Aime F, Vonlauthen M: Epidemiology of dialysis induced hypotension. *Proc Eur Dial Transplant Assoc* 18: 133, 1981

7. Zucchelli P: Hemodialysis-induced symptomatic hypotension. A review of pathophysiological mechanisms. *Int J Artif Organs* 10: 139, 1987

8. Petitclerc T, Drüeke T, Man NK, Funck-Brentano JL: Cardiovascular stability on hemodialysis. *Adv Nephrol* 16: 351, 1987

9. Kim KE, Neff M, Cohen B, Somerstein M, Chinitz J, Onesti G, Swartz C: Blood volume changes and hypotension during hemodialysis. *Trans Am Soc Artif Intern Organs* 16: 508, 1970

10. Hampl H, Paeprer H, Unger V, Fischer C, Resa I, Kessel M: Hemodynamic changes during hemodialysis, sequential ultrafiltration, and hemofiltration. *Kidney Int* 18: S83, 1980

11. Falls WF Jr., Stacy WK, Bears ES, Haden HT: Dialysis-induced change of extracellular fluid volume in man. *Proc Clin Dial Transplant Forum* 2: 155, 1972

12. Ogden DA: A double blind crossover comparison of high and low sodium dialysis. *Proc Clin Dial Transplant Forum* 8: 157, 1978

13. Heidbreder E, Schafferhans K, Heidland A: Autonomic neuropathy in chronic renal insufficiency: Comparative analysis of diabetic and nondiabetic patients. *Nephron* 41: 50, 1985

14. Nakashima Y, Fouad FM, Nakamoto S, Textor SC, Bravo EL, Tarazi RC: Localization of autonomic nervous system dysfunction in dialysis patients. *Am J Nephrol* 7: 375, 1987

15. Faber MD, Dumler F, Zasuwa GA, Levin NW: Relationship between sympathetic dysfunctcion and hemodialysis instability. *Trans Am Soc Artif Intern Organs* 33: 280, 1987

16. Drüeke T, Le Pailleur C, Meihac B, Koutoudis C, Zingraff J, Di Matteo J, Crosnier J: Congestive cardiomyopathy in ureamic patients on long term haemodialysis. *Br med J* 1: 350, 1977

17. Madsen BR, Alpert MA, Whittins RB, Van Stone J, Ahmad M, Kelly DL: Effect of hemodialysis on left ventricular performance. Analysis of echocardiographic subsets. *Am J Nephrol* 4: 86, 1984

18. Mion CM, Hegstrom RM, Boen ST, Scribner BH: Substitution of sodium acetate for sodium bicarbonate in the bath fluid for hemodialysis. *Trans Am Soc Artif Intern Organs* 10:110, 1964

19. Vinay P, Cardoso M, Tejedor A, Prud'homme M, Levelillae M, Vinet B, Courteau M, Gougoux A, Rengel M, Lapierre L, Piette Y: Acetate metabolism during hemodialysis: metabolic considerations. *Am J Nephrol* 7: 337, 1987

20. Novello A, Kelsch RC, Easterling RE: Acetate intolerance during hemodialysis. *Clin Nephrol* 5: 29, 1976

21. Keshaviah PR: The role of acetate in the etiology of symptomatic hypotension. *Artif Organs* 6: 378, 1982

22. Frohlich ED: Vascular effects of the Krebs intermediate metabolites. *Am J Physiol* 208: 149, 1965

23. Schohn DC, Klein S, Mitsuishi YH, Jahn HA: Correlation between plasma sodium acetate concentration and systemic vascular resistances. *Proc Eur Dial Transplant Assoc* 18: 160, 1981

24. Keshaviah P, Shapiro FL: A critical examination of dialysis-induced hypotension. *Am J Kidney Dis* 2: 290, 1982

25. **Wehle B, Asaba H, Castenfors J, Gunnarsson B, Bergström J: Influence of dialysate composition on cardiovascular function in isovolemic haemodialysis. *Proc Eur Dial Transplant Assoc* 18: 153, 1981**

26. Vincent JL, Vanherweghem JL, Degaute JP, Berre J, Dufaye P, Kahn RJ: Acetate-induced myocardial depression during hemodialysis for acute renal failure. *Kidney Int* 22: 653, 1982

27. Anderson LE, Nixon JV, Henrich WL: Effects of acetate and bicarbonate dialysate on left ventricular performance. *Am J Kidney Dis* 10: 350, 1987

28. Eiser AR, Jayamann D, Kokseng C, Che H, Slivkin RF, Neff MS: Contrasting alterations in pulmonary gas exchange during acetate and bicarbonate dialysis. *Am J Neprhol* 2: 123, 1982

29. Oh MS, Uribarri JV, Del Monte ML, Friedman EA, Carroll HJ: Consumption of CO_2 in metabolism of acetate as an explanation for hypoventilation and hypoxemia during hemodialysis. *Proc Clin Dial Transplant Forum* 9: 226, 1979

30. Igarashi I, Kioi S, Gejyo F, Arakawa M: Physiologic approach to dialysis-induced hypoxemia. Effects of dialyzer material and dialysate composition. *Nephron* 41: 62, 1985

31. Francos GC, Besarab A, Burke JF Jr, Tahamout MV, Gee MH, Flynn JT, Gzesh D: Dialysis-induced hypoxemia: membrane dependent and membrane independent causes. *Am J Kidney Dis* 5: 191, 1985

32. Craddock PR, Fehr J, Brigham KL, Kronenberg RS, Jacob HS: Complement and leukocyte-mediated pulmonary dysfunction in hemodialysis. *N Engl J Med* 296: 769, 1977

33. Hakim RM, Lowrie EG: Hemodialysis-associated neutropenia and hypoxemia: the effect of dialyzer membrane materials. *Nephron* 32: 32, 1982

34. Ahmad S, Pagel M, Shen F, Vizzo J, Scribner BH: The role of hypoxemia in the expression of acetate intolerance. *Kidney Int* 19: 140, 1981

35. Keshaviah P, Carlson L, Constantini E, Shapiro F: Dialysis-induced hypoxemia and hypotension are not causally related. *Trans Am Soc Artif Intern Organs* 30: 159, 1984

36. Ksiazek A: Dopamine-beta-hydroxylase activity and catecholamine levels in the plasma of patients with renal failure. *Nephron* 24: 170, 1979

37. Wehle B, Bevegard S, Castenfors J, Davidsson S, Lindblad LE: Carotid baroreflexes during hemodialysis. *Clin Nephrol* 19: 236, 1983

38. Sherman RA, Rubin MP, Cody RP, Eisinger RP: Ameliora-

tion of hemodialysis-associated hypotension by the use of cool dialysate. *Am J Kidney Dis* 5: 124, 1985

39. Mahida BH, Dumler F, Zasuwa G, Fleig G, Levin NW: Effect of cooled dialysate on serum catecholamines and blood pressure stability. *Trans Am Soc Artif Intern Organs* 29: 384, 1983

40. Nicholls AJ, Platts MM: Anaphylactoid reactions due to haemodialysis, haemofiltration, or membrane plasma seperation. *Br Med J* 285: 1607, 1982

41. Stephens GW, Bernard DB, Idelson BA: Anaphylaxis: an unusual complication of hemodialysis. *Clin Nephrol* 24: 99, 1985

42. Bernick JJ, Port FK, Favero MS: In vivo studies of dialysis-related endotoxemia and bacteremia. *Nephron* 27: 312, 1981

43. Caruana RJ, Hamilton RW, Pearson FC: Dialyzer hypersensitivity syndrome: possible role of allergy to ethylene oxide. Report of 4 cases and review of the literature. *Am J Nephrol* 5: 271, 1985

44. Novello AC, Port FK: Hemodialysis eosinophilia. *Int J Artif Organs* 5: 5, 1982

45. Villarroel F: Incidence of hypersensitivity in hemodialysis. *Artif Organs* 8: 278, 1984

46. Chenoweth DE, Cheung AK, Henderson LW: Anaphylatoxin formation during hemodialysis: effects of different dialyzer membranes. *Kidney Int* 24: 764, 1983

47. Chenoweth DE, Cheung AK, Ward DM, Henderson LW: Anaphylatoxin formation during hemodialysis: comparison of new and re-used dialyzers. *Kidney Int* 24: 770, 1983

48. Hakim RM, Breillatt J, Lazarus JM, Port FK: Complement activation and hypersensitivity reactions to dialysis membranes. *N Engl J Med* 311: 878, 1984

49. Van Stone JC, Cook J: Decreased postdialysis fatigue with increased dialysate sodium concentration. *Proc Clin Dial Transplant Forum* 8: 162, 1978

50. Wehle B, Asaba H, Castenfors J, Fürst P, Gunnarsson B, Shaldon S, Bergström J: Hemodynamic changes during sequential ultrafiltration and dialysis. *Kidney Int* 15: 411, 1979

51. Wehle B, Bevegård S, Castenfors J, Davidsson S, Lindblad LE: Carotid baroreflexes during hemodialysis. *Clin Nephrol* 19: 236, 1983

52. Schultze G, Maiga M, Neumayer HH, Wagner K, Keller F, Molzahn M, Nigam S: Prostaglandin E$_2$ promotes hypotension on low-sodium hemodialysis. *Nephron* 37: 250, 1984

53. Graefe U, Milutinovich J, Follette WC, Vizzo JE, Babb AL, Scribner BH: Less dialysis-induced morbidity and vascular instability with bicarbonate in dialysate. *Ann Intern Med* 88: 332, 1978

54. Wehle B, Asaba H, Castenfors J, Grahn A, Gunnarsson B, Shaldon S, Bergström J: The influence of dialysis fluid composition on the blood pressure response during dialysis. *Clin Nephrol* 10: 62, 1978

55. Fournier G, Gaillard JL, Man MK: Control of acid-base status and phosphatemia with bicarbonate-containing dialysate: A long-term study. in *Progress in Artificial Organs, 1983,* edited by Atsumi K, Maekawa M, Ota K, Cleveland, ISAO Press, 1984, p 470

56. Ahmad S, Pagel M, Vizzo J, Scribner BH: Effect of the normalizaiton of acid-base balance on postdialysis plasma bicarbonate. *Trans Am Soc Artif Intern Organs* 26: 318, 1980

57. Albright R, Kram B, White RP: Postassium and phosphate removal with bicarbonate hemodialysis. *Kidney Int* 23: 141, 1983

58. Ivanovich P, Chenoweth DE, Schmidt R, Klinkmann H, Boxer LA, Jacob HS, Hammerschmidt DE: Symptoms and activation of granulocytes and complement with two dialysis membranes. *Kidney Int* 24: 758, 1983

59. Arieff AI: Dialysis disequilibrium syndrome: Current concepts on pathogenesis. *Controv Nephrol* 4: 367, 1982

60. Tyler HR: Neurologic disorders in renal failure. *Am J Med* 44: 734, 1968

61. Kennedy AC, Linton AL, Eaton JC: Urea levels in cerebrospinal fluid after haemodialysis. *Lancet* 1: 410, 1962

62. Funder J, Wieth JO: Changes in cerebrospinal fluid composition following hemodialysis. *Scand J Clin Lab Invest* 19: 301, 1967

63. Arieff AI, Massry SG, Barrientos A, Kleeman CR: Brain water and electrolyte metabolism in uremia: effects of slow and rapid hemodialysis. *Kidney Int* 4: 177, 1973

64. Rosenbaum BJ, Coburn JW, Shinaberger JH, Massry, SG: Acid-base status during the interdialytic period in patients maintained with chronic hemodialysis.

65. Hampers CL, Doak PB, Callaghan MN, Tyler HR, Merrill JP: The electroencephalogram and spinal fluid during hemodialysis. *Arch Intern Med* 118: 340, 1966

66. Rigg GA, Bercu BA: Hypoglycemia--a complication of hemodialysis. *N Engl J Med* 277: 1139, 1967

67. Wakim KG: Predominance of hypnatremia or hypo-osmolality in simulation of the dialysis disequilibrium syndrome. *Mayo Clin Proc* 44: 433, 1969

68. Arieff AI, Massry SG: Dialysis disequilibrium syndrome. in *Clinical Aspects of Uremia and Dialysis,* edited by Massry SG, Sellers AL, Springfield IL, Charles C. Thomas, 1976, p 34

69. Arieff AI, Lazarowitz VC, Guisado R: Experimental dialysis disequilibrium syndrome: prevention with glycerol. *Kidney Int* 14: 270, 1978

70. Kiley JE, Woodruff MW, Pratt KI: Evaluation of encephalopathy by EEG frequency analysis in chronic dialysis patients. *Clin Nephrol* 5: 245, 1976

71. Hampl H, Klopp HW, Michaels N, Mahiout A, Schilling H, Wolfgruber M, Schiller R, Handfeld F, Kessel M: Electroencephalographic investigations of the disequilibrium syndrome during bicarbonate and acetate dialysis. *Proc Eur Dial Transplant Assoc* 19: 351, 1982

72. La Greca G, Biasioli S, Chiaramonte S, Dettori P, Fabris A, Feriani M, Pina V, Pisani E, Ronco C: Studies on brain density in hemodialysis and peritoneal dialysis. *Nephron* 31: 146, 1982

73. Basile C, Miller JD, Koles ZJ, Grace M, Ulan RA: The effects of dialysis on brain water and EEG in stable chronic uremia. *Am J Kidney Dis* 9: 462, 1987

74. Johnson WJ, Hagge WW, Wagoner RD, Dinapoli RP, Rosevear JW: Effects of urea loading in patients with far-advanced renal failure. *Mayo Clin Proc* 47: 21, 1972

75. Gutman RA, Hickman RO, Chatrian GE, Scribner BH: Failure of high dialysis-fluid glucose to prevent the disequilibrium syndrome. *Lancet* 1: 295, 1967

76. Kjellstrand C, Shideman JR, Santiago EA, Mauer M, Simmons RL, Buselmeier TJ: Technical advances in hemodialysis of very small pediatric patients. *Proc Clin Dial Transplant Forum* 1: 124, 1971

77. Stewart WK, Fleming LW, Manuel MA: Benefits obtained by the use of high sodium dialysate during maintenance haemodialysis. *Proc Eur Dial Transplant Assoc* 9: 111, 1972

78. Guisado R, Arieff AI, Massry SG: Dialysis disequilibrium syndrome: prevention by use of glycerol in the dialysate. *Clin Res* 22: 207A, 1974

79. Mattson RH: The benzodiazepines. in: *Antiepileptic Drugs,* edited by Woodbury DM, Penry KG, Schmidt RP, New York, Raven Press, 1972, p 497

80. Weiner MW, Epstein FH: Signs and symptoms of electrolyte disorders. in *Clinical Disorders of Fluid and Electrolyte Metabolism,* edited by Maxwell MH, Kleman CR, 2nd edition, New York, McGraw-Hill Book Company, 1972, p 629

81. Said R, Quintanilla A, Levin N, Ivanovich P: Acute hemolysis due to profound hypo-osmolality. A complicatoin of hemodialysis. *J Dial* 1: 447, 1977

82. Arieff AI, Guisado R: Effects on the central nervous system of hypernatremic and hyponatremic states. *Kidney Int* 10: 104, 1976

83. Lindner A, Moskovtchenko JF, Traeger J: Accidental mass hypernatremia during hemodialysis. Simultaneous observation in six cases. *Nephron* 9: 99, 1972

84. Nickey WA, Chinitz VL, Kim KE, Onesti G, Swartz C: Hypernatremia from water softener malfunction during home dialysis. *JAMA* 214: 915, 1970

85. Morrison G, Michelson EL, Brown S, Morganroth J: Mechanism and prevention of cardiac arrhythmias in chronic hemodialysis patients. *Kidney Int* 17: 811, 1980

86. Papadakis MA, Wexman MP, Fraser C, Sedlacek SM: Hyperkalemia complicating digoxin toxicity in a patient with renal failure. *Am J Kidney Dis* 5: 64, 1985

87. Wiegand CF, Davin TD, Raij L, Kjellstrand CM: Severe hypokalemia induced by hemodialysis. *Arch Intern Med* 141: 167, 1981

88. Easterling RE: Water treatment for in-center hemodialysis including verification of water quality and disinfection. in *Dialysis Therapy,* edited by Nissenson AR, Fine RN, Philadelphia, Hanley and Belfus, Inc, 1986, p 19

89. Freeman RM, Lawton RL, Chamberlain MA: Hard-water syndrome. *N Engl J Med* 276: 1113, 1967

90. Evans DB, Slapak M: Pancreatitis in the hard water syndrome. *Br Med J* 3: 748, 1975

91. Rivera-Vazquez AB, Noriega-Sanchez A, Ramirez-Gonzalez R, Martinez-Maldonado M: Acute hypercalcemia in hemodialysis patients: distinction from 'dialysis dementia.' *Nephron* 25: 243, 1980

92. Foley RJ, Hamner RW: Hyperthyroidism in end-stage renal disease. *Am J. Nephrol* 5: 292, 1985

93. Farrington K, Miller P, Varghese Z, Baillod RA, Moorhead JF: Vitamin A toxicity and hypercalcaemia in chronic renal failure. *Br Med J* 282: 1999, 1981

94. Felsenfeld AJ, Drezner MK, Llach F: Hypercalcemia and elevated calcitriol in a maintenance dialysis patient with tuberculosis. *Arch Intern Med* 146: 1941, 1986

95. Govan JR, Porter CA, Cook JG, Dixon B, Traffor JA: Acute magnesium poisoning as a complication of chronic intermittent haemodialysis. *Br Med J* 2: 278, 1968

96. McGonigle RJ, Weston MJ, Keenan J, Jackson DB, Parsons V: Effect of hypermagnesemia on circulating plasma parathyroid hormone in patients on regular hemodialysis therapy. *Magnesium* 3: 1, 1984

97. Nilsson P, Johansson SG, Danielson BG: Magnesium studies in hemodialysis patients before and after treatment with low dialysate magnesium. *Nephron* 37: 25, 1984

98. Chachati A, El-Allaf D, Cornet G, Carlier J, Kulbertus H, Gordon JP: Importance of dialysate magnesium in the pathogenesis of cardiac arrhythmias in chronic dialysis patients. *Abstracts, Xth Int Congr Nephrol* 1987, p 130

99. Klein WJ, Jr., Metz EN, Price AR: Acute copper intoxication. A hazard of hemodialysis. *Arch Intern Med* 129: 578, 1972

100. Blomfield J, Dixon SR, McCredie DA: Potential hepatotoxicity of copper in recurrent hemodialysis. *Arch Intern Med* 128: 555, 1971

101. Lyle WH, Payton JE, Hui M: Haemodialysis and copper fever. *Lancet* 1: 1324, 1976

102. Mansouri K, Halsted JA, Gombos EA: Zinc, copper, magnesium and calcium in dialyzed and nondialyzed uremic patients. *Arch Intern Med* 125: 88, 1970

103. Gallery ED, Blomfield J, Dixon SR: Acute zinc toxicity in haemodialysis. *Br Med J* 4: 331, 1972

104. Beattie AD, Moore MR, Devenay WT, Miller AR, Goldberg A: Environmental lead pollution in an urban soft-water area. *Br Med J* 2: 491, 1972

105. Webster JD, Parker TF, Alfrey AC, Smythe WR, Kubo H, Neal G, Hull AR: Acute nickel intoxication by dialysis. *Ann Intern Med* 92: 631, 1980

106. Carlson DJ, Shapiro FL: Methemoglobinemia from well water nitrates: a complication of home dialysis. *Ann Intern Med* 73: 757, 1970

107. Eaton JW, Kolpin CF, Swofford HS, Kjellstrand CM, Jacob HS: Chlorinated urban water: a cause of dialysis-induced hemolytic anemia. *Science* 181: 463, 1973

108. Brueggemeyer CD, Ramirez G: Dialysate concentrate: a potential source for lethal complications. *Nephron* 46: 397, 1987

109. Raij L, Shapiro FL, Michael AF: Endotoxemia in febrile reactions during hemodialysis. *Kidney Int* 4: 57, 1973

110. Peterson MJ, Boyer KM, Carson LA, Favero MS: Pyrogenic reactions from inadequate disinfection of a dialysis fluid distribution system. *Dial Transplant* 7: 52, 1978

111. Pearson FC, Bohon J, Lee W, Bruszer G, Sagona M, Dawe R, Jakuboswki G, Morrison D, Dinarello C: Comparison of chemical analyses of hollow-fiber dialyzer extracts. *Artif Organs* 8: 291, 1984

112. Gazenfield-Gazit E, Eliahou HE: Endotoxin antibodies in patients on maintenance hemodialysis. *Israel J Med Sci* 5: 1032, 1969

113. Keshaviah P, Leuhmann D, Ilstrup K, Collins A: Technical requirements for rapid high-efficiency therapies. *Artif Organs* 10: 189, 1986

114. Kolmos HJ, Moller S: The epidemiology of febrile reactions in haemodialysis. *Acta Med Scand* 203: 345, 1978

115. Blagg CR, Tenckhoff H: Microbial contamination of water used for hemodialysis. *Nephron* 15: 81, 1975

116. Favero MS, Carson LA, Bond WW, Petersen NJ: Factors that influence microbial contamination of fluids associated with hemodialysis machines. *Appl Microbiol* 28: 822, 1974

117. Bland LA, Ridgeway MR, Aguero SM, Carson LA, Favero MS: Potential bacteriologic and endotoxin hazards associated with liquid bicarbonate concentrate. *Trans Am Soc Artif Intern Organs* 33: 542, 1987

118. Kantor RJ, Carson LA, Graham DR, Petersen NJ, Favero MS: Outbreak of pyrogenic reactions at a dialysis center. Association with infusion of heparinized saline solution. *Am J Med* 74: 449, 1983

119. Bland L, Alter M, Favero M, Carson L, Cusick L: Hemodialyzer reuse: practices in the United States and implication for infection control. *Trans Am Soc Artif Intern Organs* 31: 556, 1985

120. Ham TH, Shen SC, Fleming FM, Castle WB: Studies on the destruction of red blood cells, IV. *Blood* 3: 373, 1948

121. Fortner RW, Nowakowski A, Carter CG, King LH Jr., Knepshield JH: Death due to overheated dialysate during dialysis. *Ann Intern Med* 73: 443, 1970

122. Berkes SL, Kahn SI, Chazan JA, Garella S: Prolonged hemolysis from overheated dialysate. *Ann Intern Med* 83: 363, 1975

123. Lynn KL, Boots MA, Mitchell TR: Hemolytic anaemia caused by overheated dialysate *Br Med J* 1: 306, 1979

124. Ward MK, Shadforth M, Hill AV, Kerr DN: Air embolism during haemodialysis. *Br Med J* 3: 74, 1971

125. Canaud B, Beraud JJ, Joyeux H, Mion C: Internal jugular vein cannulation using 2 silastic catheters. A new, simple and safe long-term vascular access for extracorporeal treatment. *Nephron* 43: 133, 1986

126. Baskin SE, Wozniak RF: Hyperbaric oxygenation in the treatment of hemodialysis-associated air embolism. *N Engl J Med* 393: 184, 1975

127. Lindsay RM, Moorthy AV, Koens F, Linton AL; Platelet funciton in dialyzed and non-dialyzed patients with chronic renal failure. *Clin Nephrol* 4: 52, 1975

128. Di Minno G, Martinez J, McKean M, De La Rosa J, Burke JF, Murphy S: Platelet dysfunction in uremia. Multifaceted defect partially corrected by dialysis. *Am J Med* 79: 552, 1985

129. Adler AJ, Berlyne GM: Beta-thromboglobulin and platelet factor 4 levels during hemodialysis. *asaio J* 4: 100, 1981

130. Remuzzi G, Marchesi D, Cavenaghi AE, Livio M, Donati MB, de Gaetano G, Mecca G: Bleeding and renal failure: a possible role of vascular prostacyclin (PGI$_2$). *Clin Nephrol* 12: 127, 1979

131. Pavlopoulus G, Perzahowski C, Hakim RM, Lazarus JM: Platelet aggregation studies during dialysis. *Kidney Int* 29: 221, 1986

132. Vicks SL, Gross ML, Schmitt GW: Massive hemorrhage due to hemodialysis-associated thrombocytopenia. *Am J Nephrol* 3: 30, 1983

133. Hakim RM, Schafer AI: Hemodialysis associated platelet activation and thrombocytopenia. *Am J Med* 78: 575, 1985

134. Himmelfarb J, Lazarus JM, Hakim RM: Increased expression of glycoprotein GP IIb/IIa detected by flow cytometry on platelets during hemodialysis. *Kidney Int* 31: 234, 1987

135. Harker LA, Slichter SJ: Bleeding time as a swelling test for evolution platelet function. *N Engl J Med* 287: 155, 1972

136. Remuzzi G, Marchiaro G, Mecca G, DeGatano G: Bleeding and renal failure: altered platelet function in chronic uremia only partially corrected by hemodialysis. *Nephron* 22: 347, 1978

137. Mills B, Zuckerman G, Sicard G: Discrete colon ulcers as a cause of lower gastrointestinal bleeding and perforation in end-stage renal disease. *Surgery* 89: 548, 1981

138. Gold CH, Morley JE, Viljoen M, Tim Lo, de Fomseca M, Kalk WJ: Gastric acid secretion and serum gastrin levels in patients with chronic renal failure on regular hemodialysis. *Nephron* 125: 92, 1980

139. Shapiro WB, Faubert PF, Chou S-Y, Porush JG: Low-dose heparin in the high-risk bleeding hemodialysis patient monitored by activated partial thromboplastin time. *Dial Transplant* 9: 322, 1980

140. Leonard CD, Weil E, Scribner BH: Subdural hematoma in patients undergoing haemodialysis. *Lancet* 2: 239, 1969

141. Leonard A, Shapiro FL: Subdural hematoma in regularly hemodialyzed patients. *Ann Intern Med* 82: 650, 1975

142. Iaiadinso OA: Early diagnosis of subdural hematoma in hemodialysis patients: use of carotid arteriography. *Angiology* 27: 491, 1976

143. Tietjen DP, Moore J Jr, Gouge SF: Hemodialysis-associated acute subdural hematoma: interim management with peritoneal dialysis. *Am J Nephrol* 7: 478, 1987

144. Talalla A, Halbrook H, Barbour BH, Kurze T: Subdural hematoma associated with long-term hemodialysis for chronic renal disease. *JAMA* 212: 1847, 1970

145. Bechar M, Lakke JP, Hem GK van der, Beks JW, Penning L: Subdural hematoma during long-term hemodialysis. *Arch*

Neurol 26: 513, 1972

146. Richards T, Hoff J: Factors affecting survival from acute subdural hematoma. *Surgery* 75: 253, 1974

147. Marini PV, Hull AR: Uremic pericarditis: a review of incidence and management. *Kidney Int* 7 (Suppl 2): 163, 1975

148. Zarate A, Gelfand MC, Horton JD, Winchester JF, Gottlieb MJ, Lazarus JM, Schreiner GE: Pericardial effusion associated with minoxidil therapy in dialyzed patients. *Int J Artif Organs* 3: 15, 1980

149. Alpert MA, Van Stone J, Twardowski ZJ, Ruder MA, Whiting RB, Velly DL, Madsen BR: Comparative cardiac effects of hemodialysis and continuous ambulatory peritoneal dialysis. *Clin Cardiol* 9: 52, 1986

150. Quigg RJ, Jr, Idelson BA, Yoburn DC, Hymes JL, Schick EC, Bernard DB: Local steroids in dialysis-associated pericardial effusion. A single intrapericardial administration of triamcinolone. *Arch Intern Med* 145: 2249, 1985

151. Ghavamian M, Gutch CF, Hughes RK, Kopp KF, Kolff WJ: Pericardial tamponade in chronic-hemodialysis patients treatment by pericardectomy. *Arch Intern Med* 131: 249, 1973

152. Bhasin HK, Dana CL: Spontaneous retroperitoneal hemorrhage in chronically hemodialyzed patients. *Nephron* 22: 322, 1978

153. Tsai SY, Shimizu AG: Spontaneous perirenal hemorrhage in patients on hemodialysis. *Urology* 5: 523, 1975

154. Nidus BD, Matalon R, Cantacuzino D: Uremic pleuritis--a clinicopathologic entity. *N Engl J Med* 281: 255, 1960

155. Galen MA, Steinberg SM, Lowrie EG, Lazarus JM, Hampers CL, Merrill JP: Hemorrhagic pleural effusion in patients undergoing chronic hemodialysis. *Ann Intern Med* 82: 359, 1975

156. Borra S, Kleinfeld M: Subcapsular liver hematomas in a patient on chronic hemodialysis. *Ann Intern Med* 93: 574, 1980

157. Smetana SS, David E, Pelet D, Bar-Khayim Y: Subcapsular liver hematoma in a patient on chronic hemodialysis. *Nephron* 45: 323, 1987

158. Blum M, Aviram A: Splinter hemorrhages in patients receiving regular hemodialysis. *JAMA* 239: 47, 1978

159. Nielsen VK: The peripheral nerve function in chronic renal failure: a survey. *Acta Med Scand (Suppl)* 573: 1, 1974

160. Harriman DGF, Taverner D, Wolfal AL: Ekbom's syndrome and burning paresthesiae. *Brain* 93: 393, 1970

161. Telstad W, Sorensen O, Larsen S, Lillevold PE, Nyberg-Hansen R, Stensrud P: Treatment of the restless leg syndrome with carbamazepine: a double-blind study. *Br Med J* 288: 444, 1984

162. Van Scheele C: Levodopa in restless legs. *Lancet* 2: 426, 1986

163. Samii K, Ciancioni C, Rottenbourg J, Bisseliches F, Jacobs C: Severe hypoglycemia due to beta-blocking drugs in haemodialysis patients. *Lancet* 1: 545, 1976

164. Grajower MM, Walter L, Albin J: Hypoglycemia in chronic hemodialysis patients: association with propranolol use. *Nephron* 26: 126, 1980

165. Holland OB, Kaplan NM: Propranolol in the treatment of hypertension. *N Engl J Med* 294: 930, 1976

166. Zarate A, Gelfand M, Novello A, Knepshield J, Preuss HG: Propranolol-associated hypoglycemia in patients on maintenance hemodialysis. *Int J Artif Organs* 4: 130, 1981

167. Miller JD, Broom J, Smith G: Severe hypoglycemia due to combined use of parenteral nutrition and renal dialysis. *Br Med J* 285: 9, 1982

168. Youg AW Jr, Sweeney EW, David DS, Cheigh J, Hochaglerenl EL, Sakai S, Stenzel KH, Rubin AL: Dermatologic evaluation of pruritus in patients on hemodialysis. *NY State J Med* 73: 2670, 1973

169. Bencini PL, Montagnino G, Citterio A, Graziani G, Crosti C, Ponticelli C: Cutaneous abnormalities in uremic patients. *Nephron* 40: 316, 1985

170. Kint A, Bussels L, Fernandes M, Ringoir S: Skin and nail disorders in relation to chronic renal failure. *Acta Derm Venereol (Stockh)* 54: 137, 1974

171. Gilchrest B, Rowe JW, Mihm, MC Jr: Bullous dermatosis of hemodialysis. *Ann Intern Med* 83: 480, 1975

172. Webster SB, Dahlberg PJ: Bullous dermatosis of hemodialysis: case report and review of the dermatologic changes in chronic renal failure. *Cutis* 25: 322, 1980

173. Brivet F, Drüeke T, Guillemette J, Zingraff J, Crosnier J: Porphyria cutanea tarda-like syndrome in hemodialyzed patients. *Nephron* 20: 258, 1978

174. Harlan SL, Winkelmann RK: Porphyria cutanea tarda and chronic renal failure. *Mayo Clin Proc* 58: 467, 1983

175. Carcia Parilla J, Ortega R, Pena ML, Rodicio JL, De Salamanca RE, Olmos A, Elder GH: Porphyria cutanea tarda during maintenance haemodialysis. *Br Med J* 2: 1358, 1980

176. Giardini O, Tacoone-Gallucci M, Lubrano R, Recciardi-Tenore G, Bandino D, Silvi I, Ruberto U, Casciani CU: Evidence of red blood cell membrane lipid peroxidation in haemodialysis patients. *Nephron* 36: 235, 1984

177. Praga M, Enriquez de Salamanca R, Andres A, Nieto J, Oliet A, Perpina J, Morales JM: Treatment of hemodialysis-related porphyria cutanea tarda with deferoxamine. *N Engl J Med* 316: 547, 1987

178. Matsumoto M, Ichimaru K, Horie A: Pruritus and mast cell proliferation of the skin in end-stage renal failure. *Clin Nephrol* 23: 285, 1985

179. Gilchrest BA, Stern RS, Steinman TI, Brown RS, Arndt KA, Anderson WW: Clinical features of pruritus among patients undergoing maintenance hemodialysis. *Arch Dermatol* 118: 154, 1982

180. Burke JF, Besarab A, Goyal S, Gitteen S, Schulman E, Francos GF: Elevated histamine levels in uremia: effects of ketotifen on pruritus. *Abstracts, Xth Int Congr Nephrol* 1987, p 128

181. Blachley JD, Blankenship DM, Menter A, Parker TF 3rd, Knochel JP: Uremic pruritus: skin divalent ion content and response to ultraviolet phototherapy. *Am J Kidney Dis* 5: 237, 1985

182. Gilchrest BA, Roxe JW, Mihm MC Jr: Clinical and histological skin changes in chronic renal failure: evidence for a dialysis-resistant, transplant-responsive microangiopathy. *Lancet* 2: 1271, 1980

183. Hampers CL, Katz AI, Wilson RE, Merrill JP: Disappearance of 'uremic' itching after subtotal parthyroidectomy. *N Engl J Med* 279: 695, 1968

184. Tapia L, Cheigh JS, David DS, Sullivan JF, Saal S, Reidenberg MM, Stenzel KH, Rubin AL: Pruritus in dialysis patients treated with parenteral lidocaine. *N Eng J Med* 296: 261, 1977

185. Silverberg DS, Iaina A, Reisin E, Rotzak R, Eliahou HE: Chlolestyramine in uraemic pruritus. *Br Med J* 1: 752, 1977

186. van Leusen R, Kutsch Lojenga JC, Ruben AT: Is cholestyramine helpful in uraemic pruritus? *Br Med J* 1: 918, 1978

187. Wrong OM: Cholestyramine in uraemic pruritus. *Br Med J* 1: 1662, 1977

188. Pederson JA, Matter BJ, Czerwinski AW, Llach F: Relief of idiopathic generalized pruritus in dialysis patients treated with activated oral charcoal. *Ann Intern Med* 93: 446, 1980

189. Yatzidis H, Digenis P, Tountas C: Heparin treatment of uremic itching. *JAMA* 222: 1183, 1972

190. Graf H, Kovarik J, Stummvoll HK, Wolf A: Disappearance of uraemic pruritus after lowering dialysate magnesium concentration. *Br Med J* 2: 1478, 1979

191. Duo LJ: Electrical needle therapy of uremic pruritus. *Nephron* 47: 179, 1987

192. Gilchrest BA, Rowe JW, Brown RS, Steinman TI, Arndt KA: Relief of uremic pruritus with ultraviolet phototherapy. *N Engl J Med* 297: 136, 1977

193. Schultz BC, Roenigk HH Jr: Uremic pruritus treated with the ultraviolet light. *JAMA* 243: 1836, 1980

194. Gilchrest BA, Rowe JW, Brown RS, Steinman TI, Arndt KA: Ultraviolet phototherapy of uremic pruritus. Long-term results and possible mechanism of action. *Ann Intern Med* 91: 17, 1979

195. Hindson C, Taylor A, Martin A, Downey A: UVA light for relief of uraemic pruritus. *Lancet* 1: 215, 1981

196. Taylor R, Taylor AE, Diffey BL, Hindson TC: A placebo-controlled trial of UV-A phototherapy for the treatment of uraemic pruritus. *Nephron* 33: 14, 1983

197. Tapia L: Pruritus on hemodialysis. *Int J Dermatol* 18: 217, 1979

198. Chou CT, Wasserstein A, Schumacher HR, Jr., Fernandez P: Musculoskeletal manifestations in hemodialysis patients. *J. Rheumatol* 12: 1149, 1985

199. Parker KP: Anxiety and complications in patients on hemodialysis. *Nurs Res* 30: 334, 1981

200. Howe RC, Wombolt DG, Michie DD: Analysis of tonic muscle activity and muscle cramps during hemodialysis. *J Dial* 2: 85, 1978

201. Kaji DM, Ackad A, Nottage WG, Stein RM: Prevention of muscle cramps in haemodialysis patients by quinine sulphate. *Lancet* 2: 66, 1976

202. Catto GR, Smith FW, MacLeod M: Treatment of muscle cramps during maintenance haemodialysis. *Br Med J* 3: 389, 1973

203. Jenkins P, Dreher WH: Dialysis-induced muscle cramps: treatment with hypertonic saline and theory as to etiology. *Trans Am Soc Artif Intern Organs* 21: 479, 1975

204. Milutinovich J, Graefe U, Follette WC, Scribner BH: Effect of hypertonic glucose on the muscular cramps of hemodialysis. *Ann Intern Med* 90: 926, 1979

205. Neal CR, Resnikoff E, Unger AM: Treatment of dialysis-related muscle cramps with hypertonic dextrose. *Arch Intern Med* 2: 171, 1981

206. Sherman RA, Goodling KA, Eisinger RP: Acute therapy of hemodialysis-related muscle cramps. *Am J Kidney Dis* 2: 287, 1982

207. Man NK, Fournier G, Thireau P, Gaillard JL, Funck-Brentano JL: Effect of bicarbonate-containing dialysate on chronic hemodialysis patients: a comparative study. *Artif Organs* 6: 421, 1982

208. Bergström J, Asaba H, Fürst P, Oulès R: Dialysis, ultrafiltration, and blood pressure. *Proc Eur Dial Transpl Assoc* 13: 293, 1976

209. Kramer P, Wigger W, Matthai D, Langescheid C, Rieger J, Fuchs C, Rumpf KW, Scheler F: Clinical experience with continuously monitored fluid balance in automatic hemofiltration. *Artif Organs* 2: 147, 1978

210. Sale D, Cameron JS: Priapism during regular dialysis. *Lancet* 2: 1567, 1974

211. Port FK, Fiegel P, Hecking E, Kohler H, Distler A: Priapism during regular haemodialysis. *Lancet* 2: 1287, 1974

212. Singhal PC, Lynn RI, Scharschmidt LA: Priapism and dialysis. *Am J Nephrol* 6: 358, 1986

213. Grace DA, Winter CC: Priapism: an appraisal of manage-

ment of twenty-three patients. *J Urol* 99: 301, 1968

214. Fassbinder W, Frei U, Issantier R, Koch KM, Mion C, Shaldon S, Slingeneyer A: Factors predisposing to priapism in haemodialysis patients. *Proc Eur Dial Transplant Assoc* 12: 380, 1976

215. Kaplow LS, Goffinet JA: Profound neutropenia during the early phase of hemodialysis. *JAMA* 203: 1135, 1968

216. Maher ER, Wickens DG, Griffin JFA, Kyle P, Curtis JR, Dormandy TL: Increased free-radical activity during haemodialysis? *Nephrol Dial Transplant* 2: 169, 1987

217. Mahajan S, Gardiner H, DeTar B, Desai S, Muller B, Johnson N, Briggs W, McDonald F: Relationship between pulmonary functions and hemodialysis-induced leukopenia. *Trans Am Soc Artif Intern Organs* 23: 411, 1977

218. Bogue BA, Butruille Y, Ebert C, Gagneux SA, Strom J: Absence of cardiopulmonary dysfunction using AN–69 as compared with cellulosic membranes. *Proc Clin Dial Transpl Forum* 7: 170, 1977

219. Mahiout A, Jorres A, Meinhold H, Kessel M: Prostaglandin production and extracorporeal complement activation by dialyzer membranes. *Trans Am Soc Artif Intern Organs* 32: 88, 1986

220. Perkowski SZ, Havill AM, Flynn JT, Gee MH: Role of intrapulmonary release of eicosanoids and superoxide anion as mediators of pulmonary dysfunction and endothelial injury in sheep with intermittent complement activation. *Circ Res* 53: 574, 1983

221. Shaldon S, Deschodt G, Branger B, Granolleras C, Baldamus CA, Koch KM, Lysaght MJ, Dinarello CA: Haemodialysis hypotension: The interleukin hypothesis restated. *Proc Eur Dial Transplant Assoc* 22: 229, 1985

222. Schulman G, Cooperberg C, Mason R, Holmes T, Arrias R, Hakim RM, Arbeit LA: The biocompatibility of polyacrylonitrile is dependent on its ability to bind vasoactive substances. *Kidney Int* 31: 245, 1987

223. Dolovich J, Marshall CP, Smith EK, Shimizu A, Pearson FC, Sugona MA, Lee W: Allergy to ethylene oxide in chronic hemodialysis patients. *Artif Organs* 8: 334, 1984

224. Bommer J, Wilhelms OH, Barth HP, Schindele H, Ritz E: Anaphylactoid reactions in dialysis patients: role of ethylene oxide. *Lancet* 2: 1382, 1985

225. Dolovich J, Bell B: Allergy to a product(s) of ethylene oxide gas: demonstration of IgE and IgG antibodies and hapten specificity. *J Allergy Clin Immunol* 62: 30, 1978

226. Ogden DA: New-dialyzer syndrome. *N Engl J Med:* 302: 1262, 1980

227. Bok DV, Pascual L, Herberger C, Sawyer R, Levin NW: Effect of multiple use of dialyzers on intradialytic symptoms. *Proc Clin Dial Transplant Forum* 10: 92, 1980

228. Robson MD, Charoenpanich R, Kant KS, Peterson DW, Flynn J, Cathey M, Pollack V: Effect of first and subsequent use of hemodialyzers on patient well-being. *Am J Nephrol* 6: 101, 1986

229. Chanard J, Brunois JP, Melin JP, Lavaud S, Toupance O: Long-term results of dialysis therapy with a highly permeable membrane. *Artif Organs* 6: 261, 1982

230. Kant KS, Pollak VE, Cathey M, Goetz D, Berlin R: Multiple use of dialyzers: safety and efficacy: *Kidney Int* 19: 728, 1981

231. Held PJ, Pauly MV, Diamond L: Survival analysis of patients undergoing dialysis. *JAMA* 257: 645, 1987

232. Lotem M, Robson MD, Rosenfeld JB: Spontaneous rupture of the quadriceps tendon in patients on chronic haemodialysis. *Ann Rheum Dis* 33: 428, 1974

233. Cirincione RJ, Baker BE: Tendon ruptures with secondary hyperparathyroidism. *J Bone Joint Surg [AM]* 57: 852, 1975

234. Morein G, Goldschmidt Z, Pauker M, Seelenfreund M, Rosenfeld JB, Fried A: Spontaneous tendon ruptures in patients treated by chronic hemodialysis. *Clin Orthop* 124: 209, 1977

235. Handa SP: Uremic bursitis. *Ann Intern Med* 82: 723, 1978

236. Mathews M, Shen FH, Lindner A, Sherrard DJ: Septic arthritis in hemodialyzed patients. *Nephron* 25: 87, 1980

237. Belcon MC, Smith EKM, Kahana LM, Shimizu AG: Tuberculosis in dialysis patients. *Clin Nephrol* 17: 14, 1982

238. Haskell LP, Tannenberg AM: Tuberculosis arthritis in a hemodialysis patient. *Am J Nephrol* 7: 404, 1987

239. Rizvi SS, Holmes RH: Hearing loss from hemodialysis. *Arch Otolaryngol* 160: 751, 1980

240. Charachon R, Moreno-Ribes V, Cordonnier D: Deafness due to renal failure. Clinicopathological study. *Ann Otolaryngol Chir Cervicofac* 95: 179, 1978

241. Mirahmadi MK, Vaziri ND: Hearing loss in end-stage renal disease-effect of dialysis. *J Dial* 4: 159, 1980

242. Tyler HR, Tyler KL: Neurologic complications. in *The Systemic Consequences of Renal Failure*, edited by Eknoyan G, Knochel JP, Orlando FL, Grune & Stratton, 1984, p 311

243. Servilla KS, Groggel GC: Anterior ischemic optic neuropathy as a complication of hemodialysis. *Am J Kidney Dis* 8: 61, 1986

244. Kothari T, Swamy A, Mangla JC, Cestero RV: Hepatic friction rub in uremia. *Arch Intern Med* 140: 419, 1980

245. Dahlberg PJ, Kisken WA, Newcomer KL, Yutuc WR: Mesenteric ischemia in chronic dialysis patients. *Am J Nephrol* 5: 327, 1985

246. Diamond SM, Emmett M, Henrich WL: Bowel infarction as a cause of death in dialysis patients. *JAMA* 256: 2545, 1986

247. Feinroth M, Feinroth MV, Lundin AP, Friedman EA, Berlyne GM: Recurrent abdominal pain associated with digoxin in a patient undergoing maintenance haemodialysis. *Br Med J* 281: 838, 1980

248. Friedell ML: Cecal necrosis in the dialysis-dependent patient. *Am Surg* 51: 621, 1985

249. Nassberger L, Arbin A, Ostelius J: Exposure of patients to phthalates from polyvinyl chloride tubes and bags during dialysis. *Nephron* 45: 286, 1987

250. Lewis LM, Flechtner TW, Kerkay J, Pearson KH, Nakamoto S: Bis (2-ethylhexyl)phthalate concentrations in the serum of hemodialysis patients. *Clin Chem* 24: 741, 1978

251. Pollard GM, Buchanan JF, Slaughter RL, Kohl RK, Shen DD: Circulating concentrations of di (2-ethylhexyl) phthalate and its de-esterified phthalic acid products following plasticizer exposure in patients receiving hemodialysis. *Topical Appl Pharmacol* 79: 257, 1985

252. Bommer J, Ritz E, Andrassy K: Necrotizing dermatitis resulting from hemodialysis with polyvinyl chloride tubing. *Ann Intern Med* 91: 869, 1979

253. Patterson R, Zeiss CR, Roxe D, Pruzansky JJ, Roberts M, Harris KE; Antibodies in hemodialysis patients against hapten-protein and hapten-erythrocytes. *J Lab Clin Med* 96: 347, 1980

254. Chanard J, Lavaud S, Lavaud F, Toupance O, Kochman S: IgE antibodies to isocyanates in hemodialysis patients. *Trans Am Soc Artif Intern Organs* 33: 551, 1987

BLOOD PRESSURE CONTROL IN CHRONIC DIALYSIS PATIENTS

ROBERT J. HEYKA and EMIL P. PAGANINI

PREVALENCE AND SIGNIFICANCE OF HYPERTENSION

In patients undergoing dialysis, hypertension is a common problem that exerts a significant influence on morbidity and mortality. Close to 80% of patients entering a dialysis program have hypertension (1, 2) defined as systolic pressure greater than 150 mm Hg or diastolic pressure greater than 90 mm Hg. In addition, once dialysis is begun, control of hypertension may be less than optimal. A recent study of cardiac risk factors in dialysis patients (3) found 65% of nondiabetic patients and 87% of diabetic patients on dialysis had inadequate control of blood pressure. The prevalance of hypertension in the dialysis population varies with different etiologies of renal failure. Patients with tubulointerstitial disease have the lowest incidence of hypertension. In contrast, those with glomerulonephritis, primary vascular disease (nephrosclerosis, systemic sclerosis, hemolytic uremic syndrome) or diabetic nephropathy have hypertension at rates approaching 90 to 100% (4). This latter population is also more likely to have resistant hypertension once on dialysis.

In 1964 the one-year survival rate for patients undergoing dialysis was 50%; in 1979 despite a higher mean age and the more frequent occurrence of associated systemic disease the one-year survival had risen to 86% (5). With improved survival and a growing population of patients come new problems. Atherosclerosis with its cardiovascular complica-

tions remains the most common cause of death in the dialysis population (6), and hypertension remains the single most important risk factor. A study of dialysis patients with moderate to severe atherosclerosis (as determined by evaluation of iliac vasculature at time of renal transplantation) showed that 90% had hypertension (7). In patients younger than 40 years atherosclerosis was found only in those having a history of hypertension. Not surprisingly, long-term survival while on dialysis is determined in large part by control of hypertension (8). This is especially worrisome in light of the above-mentioned low percentage of dialysis patients whose hypertension is well controlled. Other risk factors for cardiovascular disease in the dialysis population have recently been reviewed (9).

ETIOLOGY AND PATHOGENESIS OF HYPERTENSION

Pathophysiologic considerations

The hypertension arising in chronic renal disease and end stage renal disease (ESRD) does not present a uniform pathophysiologic picture. This is in part due to the multiplicity of the renal diseases that can lead to ESRD, but also reflects the multifactorial nature of the hypertensive process itself. Hypertension is a hemodynamic abnormality that results from the interplay of many factors. These same factors (volume, humoral, neural, cardiac or vascular) are found, albeit in different proportions, in all major forms of hypertension whatever the etiology. The hypertension encountered in different conditions is distinguished not so much by special mechanisms as by the way in which these general pressor mechanisms interact with each other. For example, the 'volume-dependent hypertension' frequently seen in dialysis patients is not peculiar to hypertension seen with renal parenchymal disease. Rather it is a 'pathophysiologic type' in which variations in extracellular fluid volume (ECF) are closely associated with variations in arterial pressure. This very pattern of volume dependency of pressure implies a complex abnormality in circulatory homeostasis. It can occur with renoprivic hypertension and in ESRD, but is also found in such conditions as steroid-induced hypertension, hypervolemic essential hypertension, or hypertension treated with vasodilators or neuro-blocking agents (10). This concept of hypertension as the dynamic interplay of several basic factors has been referred to as a 'mosaic' or 'multifactorial' theory of disease. Since hypertension is multifactorial in its origin, evolution and response to treatment, it is not a static disease characterized by a set pattern but evolves with time and treatment, and treatment may have to be adjusted over time.

Hemodynamics

The two factors most extensively examined and most directly responsible for blood pressure are the cardiac output (CO) and total peripheral resistance (TPR) (11). Studies of the hemodynamics of hypertension in ESRD have shown a persistently elevated TPR. Kim et al (12) compared the hemodynamics of normal controls with hemodialysis patients who were normotensive or hypertensive. The uremic patients as a group had an elevated cardiac index (CI), heart rate, and mean arterial pressure (MAP) but no change in stroke index or difference in TPR. In addition all uremic patients were anemic, with an average hematocrit of 23%. When hypertensive and normotensive uremic patients with equivalent degrees of anemia were compared the only significant difference was an increased TPR in the hypertensive group. CI was elevated in both groups when compared with controls but showed no relation to blood pressure elevation. The normotensive dialysis patients had decreased TPR so that MAP was not elevated. Thus, the hemodynamic differences in hypertensive vs normotensive ESRD patients were related to an inappropriately increased TPR. Six of these ESRD patients were transfused to a hematocrit of at least 40% (13). Their diastolic blood pressure and TPR increased even as CI fell. There was no significant change in body weight or blood volume. The increase in TPR was thought to be related to better oxygen delivery leading to lessening of hypoxic vasodilation, and the fall in CI to an increased blood viscosity with a decrease in venous return and cardiac preload. This hemodynamic response to correction of anemia is very similar to that seen in nonuremic patients with chronic anemia who are subsequently treated (14). Recently our group found in preliminary studies that correction of anemia with human recombinant erythropoietin (r-HuEPO) may

have different hemodynamic effects from those found by Neff and his colleagues (13) in their patients after transfusion. These confusing results demonstrate the complexity of this situation and the need for more complete data.

Sodium–water–volume

As the ability to maintain salt and water balance decreases certain characteristic changes occur in body water and electrolyte composition. There is an increase in plasma volume (PV), ECF volume, total exchangable sodium (Na_E), and total body water (TBH_2O) with a decrease in intracellular water (15–17). Some authors have found a direct relationship between these salt-volume alterations and hypertension in dialysis patients, while others (15,18) have found no (or at best weak) correlations and suggested other pathogenic factors must also be considered. Increased intracellular sodium levels, first described by Welt et al (19) in erythrocytes have also been found in other cells and probably reflect a generalized alteration in transmembrane transport processes. The major question remains: What is the pathophysiologic link between these observed imbalances in salt and water status and the presence of hypertension in this population? Beginning with Starling and later Borst (20) a concept gradually evolved based on the work of many investigators, especially Guyton, Coleman, and their collaborators (21). The relationship of ECF volume expansion to hypertension was described as a series of inescapable steps. Increased ECF and blood volume resulting from renal dysfunction were held responsible for the development of a high cardiac output and the initial rise in blood pressure. Autoregulatory processes set in motion by the increased flow were then postulated as a mechanism to return cardiac output to normal, while hypertension was maintained by increased total peripheral resistance. Examples of this temporal progression in hemodynamic patterns were reported in various types of experimental renal hypertension (22) and in the observations of Coleman et al (23) in nephrectomized patients. However, the sequence of events, from increased ECF to increased TPR through hypervolemia and a rise in cardiac output, was not always observed by others either experimentally (24) or clinically. In a study of anephric dialyzed patients (25) who were normotensive prior to nephrectomy and then underwent salt and water loading there was increased total exchangeable sodium and hypervolemia but no hypertension. A study of 10 dialysis patients, four of whom were anephric, found four patterns of response to salt and water loading (26). There was no increase in blood pressure in two previously normotensive patients (one anephric). Among patients with prior hypertension the majority had an increase blood pressure with simultaneous increase in TPR and no change in CO. Only one of 10 patients studied followed the suggested classic pattern of 'whole body autoregulation'.

The cumulative effect of these observations is to question whether the links between sodium overload and increased TPR must necessarily go through volume expansion, increased cardiac output, and 'whole body autoregulation'

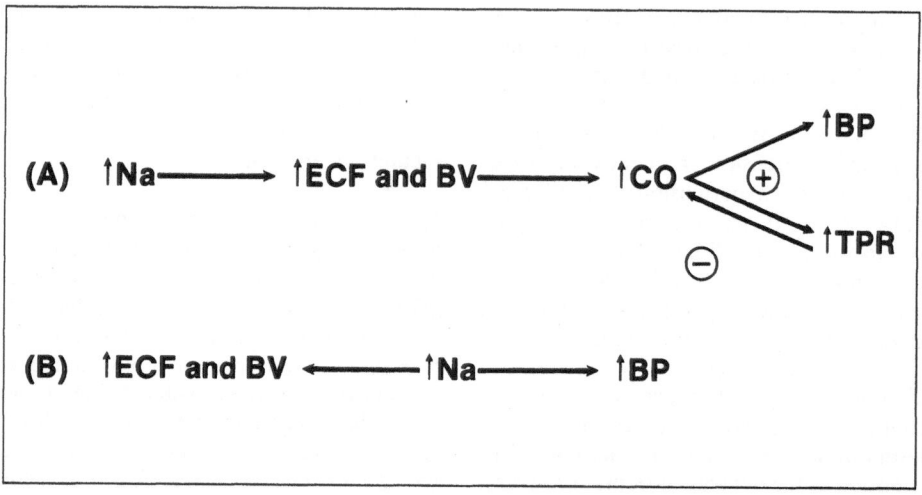

Figure 1. An increase in sodium loading (↑ Na) could conceivably lead to hypertension in two ways: (1) through expansion of extracellular fluid volume (ECF) and hypervolemia leading to a high cardiac output (CO), and subsequent increase in total peripheral resistance (TPR), or (2) the increase in sodium load could lead to hypertension by non-volume-mediated mechanisms (see text), in which case the increased extracellular fluid volume and blood volume (BV) could be an index of the sodium load but not the main mechanism by which hypertension occurs (11).

(Figure 1 Part A). A second possibility (Figure 1 Part B) is that the increased blood or ECF volume may be an index of the sodium load but not necessarily the primary mechanism by which hypertension occurs. Several 'nonvolume' mechanisms have been proposed to link relative or absolute sodium excess and hypertension. These will be discussed and include alterations in vascular reactivity or changes in the architecture of the blood vessel walls (27); increased renin-angiotensin-aldosterone activity; reflex alterations in the sympathetic tone or responsiveness mediated by cardiopulmonary receptors; or decreased ouabain-sensitive sodium-potassium pump function related to a circulating natriuretic hormone with partial cell depolarization (28) or altered sodium exchange (29) leading to increased intracellular calcium and smooth muscle tone. Reduction in arterial pressure by fluid and salt removal may be quantitatively related to volume reduction, but is not necessarily always dependent on it.

Renin-angiotensin-aldosterone axis

Details of the physiology of the renin-angiotensin-aldosterone (RAA) axis have been reviewed elsewhere and will not be repeated here (30). That the RAA axis continues to function even with the destruction of renal parenchymal tissue is apparent. Responsiveness to dehydration, salt restriction and orthostasis, although blunted, is maintained (4). The elevated plasma renin activity (PRA) seen in some dialysis patients with hypertension (31) and the prompt reduction in that hypertension with the angiotensin II receptor antagonist, saralasin (32) or the converting enzyme inhibitor, captopril (33) also demonstrate the continued importance of this system despite decreased renal mass and function.

Aldosterone appears to function as expected in the dialysis patient as well. The main stimuli remain angiotensin-II (A II) and plasma potassium. Secretion is also increased with orthostatic changes or ACTH administration (34). Heparin does not interfere with this control mechanism and aldosterone does not seem to affect blood pressure independently in oliguric patients (34).

Early studies found that hypertension was not controlled by maintenance of dry weight in a minority of ESRD patients (35). These patients with resistant hypertension all had markedly elevated PRA levels. The improved efficiency of hemodialysis made bilateral nephrectomy possible (36) and most patients with resistant hypertension ultimately required this procedure. A study (37) of patients undergoing bilateral nephrectomy found 79% of hypertensive patients had improved control of blood pressure post nephrectomy. Those with increased PRA levels pre-nephrectomy most frequently improved, patients with normal PRA levels having less predictable responses. Post-nephrectomy PRA and angiotensin II (A II) concentrations fell rapidly to nondetectable levels. From studies such as these came the pathophysiologic classificaiton of hypertensive dialysis patients into 'volume-dependent' or 'renin-dependent' categories.

There is however a wide range in PRA values with only about 30% of dialysis patients having PRA values greater than 5 ng/ml/h (38). It is now known that the RAA axis may contribute to hypertension even when PRA levels are not elevated (4). There are several hypotheses, not all mutually exclusive, for the role that renin may play in these patients (39). Renin could cause an initial increase in blood pressure while hypertension is maintained by structural abnormalities in the vessel walls (27). There may be a slow, prolonged effect of A II possibly via increased receptor sensitivity (upregulation) to otherwise 'normal' concentrations of A II

(40). Indirect additive effects of A II, especially on the sympathetic nervous system, may further enhance its vasopressive activity (41). Increased enzymatic activity of plasma renin in uremia has been noted. Studies have shown that a low molecular weight lipid fraction (LMF) of plasma from uremic patients produced less renin suppression than the same LMF from patients without renal failure (42). Perhaps a circulating lipid that modulates renin activity in normal plasma is deficient in uremic patients. The best characterized observation is that 'normal' renin levels are, in fact, inappropriately elevated for the degree of exchangable sodium (Na_E) and water expansion (15,16). Hypertensive dialysis patients were found to have up to two-fold higher mean PRA values for any level of Na_E or blood volume (BV) when compared to normotensive dialysis patients. No significant correlation between MAP and PRA, BV or Na_E existed when each was considered individually. Only when MAP was related to the product of renin · Na_E or renin · BV was there a consistent correlation. Some alteration ('resetting') in the sodium-renin feedback system was thought to be responsible. There remained however, a percentage of patients who were either normotensive with abnormal Na_E · renin products or hypertensive (some severe) with normal Na_E · renin products. It has also been recently demonstrated that many tissues including vascular smooth muscle (43) can produce angiotensinogen and renin and generate A II. Thus it is possible that there are two pathways for A II production – a circulatory system which could respond to acute changes and a tissue system which might control more chronic changes in blood pressure and vascular tone. The tissue renin system could act directly through A II production or indirectly through an effect on the sympathetic nervous system (44).

Sympathetic nervous system

Abnormalities in the autonomic nervous system (ANS) are frequent in ESRD patients, are more prominent in predialysis patients and tend to improve with hemodialysis (45). However the role these abnormalities play in the hypertensive patient is still unclear. The most consistent finding is a defect in either the high-pressure baroreceptors or afferent limb of the autonomic reflex arc (46). Increased levels of plasma catecholamines (CA), most often norepinephrine (NE) and dopamine (DA), have been described, especially in predialysis patients (47). Whether the elevated CA levels represent increased release or decreased re-uptake, metabolism and renal excretion is debated. Occasionally, circulating norepinephrine and dopamine levels return to normal with regular hemodialysis although more often levels are increased predialysis and fall throughout the procedure (48). The exact pathologic relationship between elevations in catecholamine levels and hypertension is still unknown. In one recent study four of five patients with the highest NE levels had no elevations in blood pressure (49). Both increased (50) and decreased (51) vascular responsiveness to circulating catecholamines has been found in several uremia models. A contribution of PTH (possibly via vasodilatory

prostaglandins) to the ANS dysfunction of uremia has recently been proposed (52). Pressor responses, which were diminished, returned to normal post-parathyroidectomy when normal serum calcium levels were maintained. This effect could be blunted with indomethacin. In a study of hypertensive patients on dialysis, there was a close relationship between PRA and NE levels (31). It is known that A II can influence peripheral adrenergic release and re-uptake as well as central activity and that adrenergic activity affects renin release in response to appropriate (or inappropriate?) stimuli. Needless to say, the interactions of the autonomic nervous system with salt, volume, hormonal and vascular factors are complex and the contribution of each in hypertension will vary among patients.

The strongest evidence for a role of the ANS in the hypertension of dialysis patients is the effect of blockade of the system. Total autonomic blockade (53) produces a persistent improvement in hypertension. Selective NE inhibition with the postganglionic blocker debrisoquine also results in a significant blood pressure decrease in hypertensive and, to a lesser extent, normotensive dialysis patients (54).

Calcium-extracellular and intracellular

Alterations in serum calcium

It is known that acute infusions of calcium gluconate raise blood pressure secondary to increased TPR without changes in heart rate or CI (55). The increase in TPR is a direct action of calcium on vascular smooth muscle, which can be blunted with calcium channel blockade (56). Effects on PTH, antidiuretic hormone (ADH), A II, or NE activity have also been postulated (57) but not observed in the above-mentioned studies. Raising the dialysate calcium concentration can lessen the incidence of hemodialysis-related hypotension (58). Conversely, acute hypocalcemia is associated with rapid falls in blood pressure (59).

Intracellular calcium

Cytosolic free calcium
Free cytosolic calcium (Ca_i) may be most important as the 'final common pathway' in the generation and maintenance of hypertension. Several recent reviews discuss this topic in greater detail (60,61). Free Ca_i is necessary for cardiac conduction and contractility, phasic and tonic smooth muscle contraction, and stimulation-secretion coupled reactions in nonmotile cells (62). In arterial and venous vascular smooth muscle cells both resting tonic and active phasic contractions are controlled by free cytosolic Ca_i via its binding to calmodulin (60). Maintenance of Ca_i above the excitation-contraction threshold increases smooth muscle tone and, therefore, TPR.

Natriuretic hormone
Early studies showed that some factor in the serum (and urine) of uremic patients markedly increased natriuresis when infused into rats (63). This as yet poorly characterized

substance has been termed 'natriuretic hormone'. The ouabain-like Na-K pump inhibition produced by natriuretic hormone would normally act to decrease renal tubular absorption of sodium and thereby promote natriuresis. It is distinct from atrial natriuretic factor (ANF) but may be identical to a substance possessing digoxin-like immunoreactivity in the plasma of uremic patients (64). Natriuretic hormone is thought to be produced in the hypothalamus or controlled by hypothalamic products. Lesions in the anterioventral third ventricle (AV3V) have decreased the natriuresis seen with volume expansion in rats (65). The exact role of this substance in the hypertension of chronic renal failure and ESRD is still unclear (66).

Role in hypertension of uremia

Blaustein and Hamlyn (61) proposed a critical link between altered sodium metabolism, sarcolemmal sodium-calcium exchange, and increased Ca_i-the 'natriuretic hormone/Na-Ca exchange/hypertension hypothesis'. In uremic patients this could lead to hypertension through the following sequence of events: Impaired renal sodium excretion and/or increased dietary sodium intake would expand ECF and Na_E and thus stimulate secretion of natriuretic hormone. When the normal renal effects of natriuretic hormone were blunted (CRF) or absent (anephric patients) accumulation would result in an ouabain-like effect on the Na-K pump transport in all cells including neuronal and vascular smooth muscle cells. This and possibly increased passive Na^+ influx would lead to an increased Na_i and by interference with Na-Ca exchange or by increased passive calcium influx would lead to increased Ca_i. The effects on vascular smooth muscle cells would be twofold, an increase in resting tone and an increased vascular reactivity to any stimulus or agonist like A II or NE. In addition, the inhibition of the Na-K pump at synaptic neuronal clefts would lead to decreased Na^+-NE cotransport with increased release and decreased reuptake of NE. Abnormalities in other sarcolemmal transport systems, including Na-K cotransport and Na-Li countertransport, have also been described in essential hypertension (67) and uremia (68). The role of these altered transport processes in hypertension is being actively investigated. The 'natriuretic hormone/Na-Ca exchange/hypertension hypothesis' might represent a unifying hypothesis to explain the long observed relation between abnormalities in salt and water status on the one hand and altered renin and sympathetic nervous system activity on the other.

TREATMENT

Dietary restriction and exercise

Virtually all patients approaching ESRD will need some dietary restriction of sodium and water. In general, barring the obligate sodium wasters, ESRD patients on dialysis need to be restricted to a 2 g sodium diet and a 800 to 1,200 ml fluid intake daily. This strict dietary regimen is unfortunately not followed by a considerable portion of any dialytic population. Excess thirst from elevated plasma renin levels, hyperparathyroidism, diabetes mellitus or use of high dialysate sodium may also make fluid control difficult. In addition, psychological denial of renal disease may play a role in dietary noncompliance.

A study of six male hypertensive patients on hemodialysis who underwent exercise training found that all patients requiring antihypertensive medications were able to decrease the doses and the number of medications required (69). In addition patients with diastolic blood pressure greater than 90 mm Hg on initiation of exercise had reduction to the normal range (74 ± 5 mgHg). This occurred without significant change in body composition. Hemoglobin and hematocrit levels also rose significantly. Given the potential independent beneficial effects of exercise on cardiovascular risk factors, attempts at endurance exercise training certainly seem warranted in dialysis patients. However, other studies have found that only 31 of 100 consecutive male hemodialysis patients could perform within two standard deviations of a control group in a bicycle exercise test (70). This poor exercise tolerance was associated with impaired left ventricular function by echocardiogram, poor employment prospects, and an increased risk of cardiovascular death. A significant percent of patients, and precisely those who need the most aggressive treatment to decrease their risk of cardiovascular disease, may be unable to participate in any exercise program.

Extracorporeal techniques

Concept of dry weight

Vertes et al (35) could control hypertension in 35 of 40 unselected hypertensive dialysis patients with attainment and maintenance of dry weight. This concept is crucial to adequate control of hypertension. Dry weight is defined as that weight below which a normoalbuminemic patient on dialysis will become hypotensive with fluid removal, and above which the same patient will either be hypertensive or show subtle signs of fluid expansion (1). Different studies have shown control of blood pressure in 65 to 80% of dialysis patients with adequate dialysis and maintenance of dry weight. Initial attainment of dry weight should be achieved slowly over approximately 2 months and is the first line of therapy for control of hypertension (Figure 2). Efforts may be hampered by antihypertensive drugs if initially required and by the anatomic presence or absence of kidneys. Overenthusiastic use of medications may induce intradialytic hypotensive events and lead to overestimation of dry weight. It is best to omit the predialysis antihypertensive drug dose. In some instances drugs taken 24 to 36 hr predialysis may still have significant effects. It is therefore prudent to use antihypertensive medications at lower doses with longer intervals between doses and continually reevaluate the antihypertensive regimen as the initial weight is gradually reduced by dialysis. Anephric patients pose similar problems. Onesti et al (25) noted the almost total dependence of arterial pressure on volume in these patients. Frequent intradia-

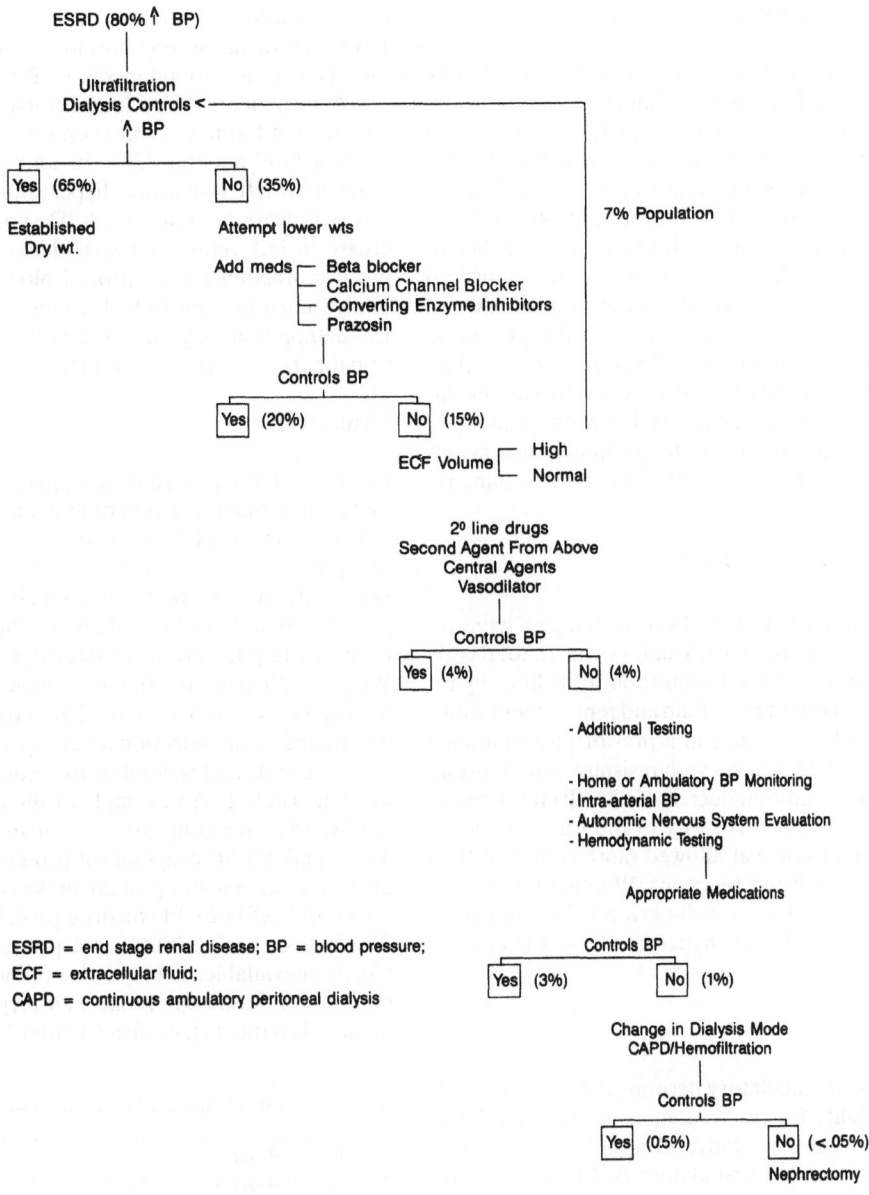

Scheme for approach to blood pressure control in ESRD-dialysis patients.

Figure 2. (Adapted from ref. 1).

lytic hypotensive episodes have been described, and these may also lead to overestimation of true dry weight. An actual determination of ECF volume using radionuclide assays may be necessary at times.

Ultrafiltration/dialysis

Ultrafiltration during dialysis is accomplished by the use of either an osmotic gradient as in peritoneal dialysis or a hydrostatic pressure gradient as in hemodialysis, with these gradients applied across whatever membrane (peritoneal or artificial) is used. For the large majority of patients one can accomplish fluid removal during diffusion dialysis treatment. Once dry weight has been established these techniques can then be adjusted so as to remove only the amount gained by the patient during the preceding interdialytic period. This technique will be sufficient in the vast majority of patients on dialysis for control of hypertension.

Isolated ultrafiltration and sequential dialysis

There is a population of hemodialysis patients who despite expanded volume and increased sodium still become hypotensive during attempts at fluid removal by dialysis. Hypertension that resists standard dialysis techniques requires isolated ultrafiltration for fluid removal. Isosmotic fluid removal can then be followed by diffusion dialysis with no ultrafiltration. This technique leads to a remarkable hemodynamic stability, which is generally ascrcibed to a lack of important osmolar changes during ultrafiltration (71). In our experience the hemodynamic effects of this procedure are characterized by venoconstriction in response to fluid loss instead of the venodilation often associated with regular hemodialysis (72). The result is a stable cardiopulmonary volume and hence a constant cardiac output, which avoids the hypotension of dialysis and allows effective volume removal.

Hemofiltration and other methods

Some patients resistant to the above techniques have responded to hemofiltration (HF). This is in effect a total body water exhange and carries ultrafiltration to its limit by removal of large amounts of body fluid and replacement with a smaller amount of fluid either in a pre- or post-dilutional mode. In a study of 22 patients with resistant hypertension, all but three had a significant decrease in MAP after 6 weeks of HF (73). The increased stability of the vascular system with isosmotic fluid removal allowed more complete fluid removal with fewer adverse reactions. Whether HF offers a significant improvement over well-performed hemodialysis in the control of interdialytic hypertension still is open to debate (74).

CAPD/CCPD

The introduction of ambulatory peritoneal dialysis has added another modality for the treatment of hypertension in ESRD patients. The slow, daily, adjustable ultrafiltration achieved with continuous ambulatory (CAPD) or continuous cyclic (CCPD) peritoneal dialysis allows a smooth attainment of dry weight. There need be less concern with salt and fluid intake as daily sodium losses are greater (75). Levels of Na_E, PRA or aldosterone in CAPD patients are no different when compared to hemodialysis patients (76). Although there does not appear to be any correlation between hypertension and Na_E, PRA or aldosterone when each factor is considered independently (just as with hemodialysis patients) (76) evaluation of various derived products, sympathetic nervous system activity, or transcellular ionic fluxes has not been reported. Water distribution in CAPD patients is different than in HD patients. Values for TBW are normal with an increased ICF and a decreased ECF (77). The explanation and significance of this finding remain to be determined. As mentioned previously, the increased salt (and protein) losses in CAPD patients allow more liberal intake than in HD patients. Whether there is associated loss of vasopressor substances including components of the RAA axis or natriuretic hormone(s) is unknown although most sudies have found increased PRA and renin substrate in CAPD patients (78). Clinical studies indicate that CAPD patients tend to have better control of blood pressure than hemodialysis patients (38). In addition hypertensive patients with left ventricular hypertrophy by echocardiography who were started on CAPD showed a significant decrease in left ventricular wall thickness, improvement in ejection fraction and control of blood pressure (79). Certainly, much remains to be learned about the hemodynamics, pathophysiology, and proper pharmacologic approach to patients on CAPD or CCPD.

Medications

Even with optimal dietary compliance and dialytic therapy there still remains a group of patients who require medication for control of their blood pressure (Figure 2). This group accounts for 20 to 35% of the dialysis population in various studies. As the dialysis population ages and as older patients are accepted into dialysis programs the prevalence of preexisting hypertensive disease will certainly increase. We can anticipate that the percentage of patients requiring medication will also increase. Numerous factors need to be considered in the selection and proper use of an antihypertensive agent, and several of the more important ones are listed in Table 1. An example of the complexity of proper antihypertensive drug use is seen in patients on CAPD. These patients have significant protein loss into the peritoneum and thus greater protein intake is allowed. Data on the effects of CAPD/CCPD on drug-protein binding, volume of distribution, dialyzability, and proper timing of doses is mostly unavailable. Table 2 is an outline of current pharmacologic information on available antihypertensive drugs used in dialysis patients (see also Chapter 51).

Table 1. Factors in choice of antihypertensive medications.

I. *Drug related*
  a) Absorption: gastroparesis, binding to aluminum hydroxide
  b) Pharmacokinetics: volume of distribution, protein binding, half-life, site of metabolism, activity and metabolism of metabolites.
  c) Mechanism(s) of action.
  d) Dialyzability
  e) Interactions with other medications.
  f) Effects on concurrent diseases: diabetes mellitus, arrhythmias, cardiac risk factors (including lipids), atherosclerotic coronary artery disease.
  g) Effectiveness.

II. *Patient related*
  1) Side effects
  2) Compliance
  3) Associated diseases
  4) Cost
  5) Cardiovascular stability on dialysis

Diuretics

Most diuretics should be used cautiously in dialysis patients. Even in patients with some urine output (>500 ml/day) the risks for otologic or nephrotoxicity are increased with the high doses necessary to produce a response. Of the currently available diuretics, the thiazides are generally not effective and if a diuretic is indicated a loop diuretic (either furose-

Table 2. Pharmacokinetics of commonly used antihypertensive drugs.

	Elim. metab.	(L/kg) Volume of distribution	$t^{1/2}$ (hrs) NML/ ESRD[1]	Plasma prot. binding (%)	Dosing	Supplement with dialysis[2]	Miscellaneous
Diuretics							
Thiazides/chlorthalidone	RA				Avoid		
Spironolactone	R				Avoid		K+ Sparing
Triamterene	H(R)				Avoid		Risk of hyperkalemia (All)
Amiloride	R				Avoid		Accumulates in uremia (All)
Acetazolamide	R				Avoid		May potentiate acidosis
Loop agents							
Furosemide	R(H)	0.07–0.21	0.5–1.1/2.4	95	Dosing requirements variable; may be useful in high doses	No	Ototoxicity (All) May augment aminoglycoside toxicity (All)
Ethacrynic A+	H(R)	0.1	2–4/?	90	Avoid		
Bumetanide	R(H)	0.2–0.5	1.2–1.5/1.5	96	May be useful in high doses	?	
Metolazone	R				May be useful in high doses	No	
β-Blockers							
Acebutolol	H	1.2	8–11/7–21	25	25–50% of nml dose[3]	No	Active metab accum
Atenolol	R	0.7	6–9/15–35	<5	25–50% of nml dose[3]	Yes	Active metab accum
Labetalol	H		t–8/6–8		?	?	Metab accum Activity unknown
Metoprolol	H	5–6	2.5–4.5/2.5–4.5	12	50% of nml dose[3]	No	Active metab accum Metab removed with HD
Nadolol	R	2.0	14–24/25–45	25–30	50% of nml dose[3]	Yes	No active metab
Pindolol	H(R)	2.0	3–4/3–4	40–50	Normal	No	No active metab
Propranolol	H	3–4	3.5/2.3	90–96	Sl. reduction	No	Spurious ↑ bili Massive metab accum Activity unknown
Timolol	H	2–4	3–4/4	10	Sl. reduction	No	Active metab accum
Central agonists							
Methyldopa	R(H)	?	1.4–5.8/3–16	<20	Dosing interval 12–24 hrs	Yes (HD/PD)	Active metab accum Prolonged ↓ BP
Clonidine	R	3–6	6–23/39–42	20–30	25–50% of nml dose	No	Risk of rebound HTN No active metab Possible therapeutic window
Converting enzyme Inhibitors							
Captopril	R(H)	0.7	1.9/–	25–30	25–50% of nml dose	Unknown	Active metab accum
Enalapril	R(H)	–	11/unknown	60	25–50% of nml dose	Unknown	Parent drug accum
Calcium channel blockers							
Verapamil	H	3–6	3–7/?	87–93	Normal	No	Metab accum Activity + toxicity unknown
Diltiazem	H	3–5	2–8/–?	80–86	Normal	?	↑ Risk of headache, flushing, dizziness (All)
Nifedipine	H	?	4–5/?	92–98	Normal	?	Effective for acute and chronic control of HTN (No active metab)
Vasodilators							
Diazoxide	R(H)	0.2–0.3	17–31/20–53	87–77	Normal	Yes (HD/PD)	Signif. ↓ in prot. binding Smaller doses or slow infusion to avoid ↓ BP
Hydralazine	H(NR)	0.5–0.9	2–4.5/7–16	87	Dosing interval prolonged 12–24 hrs	No (HD/PD)	Induction of lupus-like syndrome Very prolonged activity, esp. in slow acetylators
Minoxidil	H	2–3	2.8–4.2/3–4	0	Cautious titration	Yes (HD/PD)	Active metab accum Prolonged ↓ BP ↑ Risk of pericardial effusions?
Prazosin	H(R)	1.2–1.7	2–3/?	–	Normal	No (HD/PD)	First dose effect No effect on lipid profile
Nitroprusside	NR	?	<10 min/same	?	Titrate per BP	Yes	Toxic accum thiocyanate Monitor levels

R – Renal   Metab – Metabolites
H – Hepatic   Accum – Accumulate
NR – Nonrenal   ↓ BP – Hypotension
NML – Normal
Adapted from rep. 80, 81, 82.

[1] Includes parent drug and active metabolites.
[2] Information on CAPD/CCPD where available.
[3] Some patients may require dose only after each dialysis.

mide or bumetanide) or metolazone are the drugs of choice. Ethacrynic acid should probably be avoided as there may be a greater risk of toxicity with this agent.

Beta blockers

These drugs have multiple effects on the cardiovascular system, decrease renin release and central adrenergic activity. The fact that beta blockers are also indicated for treatment of angina, various cardiac arrhythmias, or cardioprotection after myocardial infarction makes them attractive medications in the dialysis population. Most beta blockers have been available in the United States and Europe for several years and clinical experience is widespread. Differences among beta blockers relate to their site of metabolism, lipophilicity, cardio-selectivity, intrinsic sympathomimetic activity, and accumulation and activity of metabolites. Table 2 lists the pertinent pharmacokinetics and suggested doses for these drugs. Use of long-acting beta blockers may allow postdialysis administration two to three times per week with adequate control of blood pressure (83). Additional restrictions in the consideration of any beta blocker for therapy are those applicable to the population in general. Bronchospasm, negative inotropic and chronotropic effects, worsening of hyperglycemia, masking of hypoglycemic symptoms, and worsening of peripheral arterial insufficiency are all potential complications.

Central symptholytic agents

Clonidine also has a renin suppressive effect. Although 60% of the drug is normally removed by the kidney only 5 to 10% is removed with dialysis so dosage reduction is required. A major consideration with clonidine is whether a therapeutic window exists such that doses above that window (or long-term accumulation) actcually stimulate peripheral alpha receptors and increase blood pressure (84). In addition, the typical side effects of any central agonist must be considered. These include dry mouth, drowsiness, orthostatic hypotension, impotence, and rebound hypertension with discontinuation or removal of the drug if dialyzable. Alpha methyldopa is eliminated by the kidney and accumulation of metabolites has been noted in dialysis patients (85). It is dialyzable and dosing posthemodialysis is recommended. Side effects similar to those seen with clonidine can be troublesome. In addition, the hypotensive effects of both these agents is markedly potentiated by fluid withdrawal. There is the potential for severe intradialytic hypotension in patients taking either of these drugs. Other drugs with a principally depressive action on the sympathetic nervous system such as reserpine or guanethidine are best avoided, as they may cause severe orthostatic hypotension.

Converting enzyme inhibitors

The converting enzyme inhibiors act via direct interference with the renin-angiotensin-aldosterone axis (86). Additional effects on the kinin or prostaglandin systems have been postulated, particularly for captopril (87). Of the two currently available converting enzyme inhibitors (CEI), captopril and enalapril, the former has been used more extensively in dialysis patients. Captopril used alone or combined with vigorous ultrafiltration controls a large majority of patients with otherwise resistant hypertension (88). Although patients with higher PRA levels have had more consistent reductions in blood pressure even patients with 'normal' PRA levels may respond (89). This is probably related to the pathogenic factors discussed above. Captopril is readily dialyzable and its elimination is similar to that of methyldopa (90). Thus the well known side effects of captopril therapy could be more frequent in dialysis patients. Neutropenia, rash, pruritus, dysgeusia, hyperkalemia, and persistent cough have all been reported. However, the effect of dialysis on the disulfide metabolites is unknown. Enalapril has the potential advantages of longer half-life and fewer side effects due to the absence of the sulfhydryl group present in captopril, but there is less clinical experience with this agent in the dialysis population (91). Enalapril is converted in the liver to its active parent diacid – enalaprilat. There is no further metabolism and excretion is renal (92). Enalaprilat is dialyzable. The role this agent will play in the treatment of dialysis hypertension and its proper dosing remain to be determined.

Calcium channel blockers

Use of the calcium channel blockers (CCB) as antihypertensive agents parallels the previously mentioned interest in intracellular calcium in many forms of hypertension. These agents act primarily as blockers of the voltage-dependent calcium channels in cardiac muscle, smooth muscle, and other excitable cells. They appear to modulate the cycling of sarcolemmal calcium gates and exhibit no actual steric blockade (93). There does not seem to be any effect on intracellular calcium sequestration or release cycles. The avialable agents, verapamil, diltiazem, and nifedipine are remarkably heterogenous, with verapamil being a more potent blocker of cardiac channels, and nifedipine a much more potent blocker of smooth muscle channels.

In the dialysis population a potentially important property of these drugs is that the degree of pressure reduction is proportional to the initial blood pressure and there is lack of 'overshoot' hypotension (60). There are clinical situations where calcium channel blockers may serve additional functions, such as treatment of angina and tachyarrythmias or prophylaxis for vascular headaches. Potential side effects vary with the different CCB. Verapamil is more likely to cause problems with constipation and we have seen patients develop severe constipation when verapamil is combined with aluminum-containing antacids. The negative inotropic and chronotropic effects of this agent can be problematic in patients with left ventricular dysfunction or higher degrees of heart block. Dizziness, lightheadedness, peripheral edema, flushing and headache are more likely to occur with nifedipine and are related to its more potent vasodilation. Information on the altered pharmacokinetics of these drugs in dialysis patients, particularly the accumulation and activity of metabolites, is still incomplete.

The agent most widely studied in dialysis populations is nifedipine. A study with Dahl salt-sensitive hypertensive rats having normal renal function showed nifedipine to be equally potent with minoxidil and more potent than hydralazine (94). Nifedipine has been shown to be effective for both acute and chronic control of blood pressure in dialysis patients. A study of patients with acute blood pressure elevation during hemodialysis found a significant decrease in MAP and TPR that occurred within 15 minutes of oral nifedipine administration and had a maximal effect at 30 minutes (95). There was an increase in the CI and heart rate that was not statistically significant. This could however be problematic in patients with underlying myocardial disease. A recent study (96) found that 'bite and swallow' dosing in acute situations actually led to more rapid rise in plasma concentrations than the more commonly used sublingual administration. Long-term studies (97) have shown no pseudotolerance, edema, or change in weight or heart rate.

Vasodilators

Although converting enzyme inhibitors and calcium channel blockers can be considered vasodilators the more traditional vasodilators are grouped in Table 1. We currently use these agents (Figure 2) as second line drugs for resistant hypertension or for accelerated or malignant hypertension.

Prazosin

This peripheral alpha-1 blocker has been used extensively in dialysis patients. It remains the first choice of several investigators (98). Elimination is hepatic without accumulation of metabolites and supplemental dosing post-hemodialysis is not necessary (99). Significant hypotension (first dose effect) may limit its usefulness in patients with autonomic neuropathy. Despite these caveats the drug is well tolerated in certain patients and provides good control of blood pressure. There are no deleterious effects on plasma lipids with prazosin, which is another potential advantage in decreasing the risk of accelerated atherosclerosis (100).

Hydralazine

This agent undergoes acetylation in the liver and has a longer duration of action in dialysis patients. It often requires the concomitant use of a sympatholytic agent to blunt reflex tachycardia (as with the other vasodilators). It is not removed with hemodialysis so no post-dialysis supplementation is necessary. There is no increase in lupus-like reactions among the uremic population compared with nonuremics on similar dosage schedules. Hydralazine has the advantage of being active by oral, intramuscular, or intravenous administration. This makes the drug attractive for acute treatment of pre- or intradialytic hypertension although its potency in one model of salt-sensitive hypertension is less than that of either minoxidil or nifedipine (94). Response is also less predictable than with other available agents and use in treatment of hypertensive emergencies has declined.

Minoxidil

Historically the use of this potent agent made bilateral nephrectomy unnecessary in the vast majority of patients with CRF and uncontrolled hypertension (101). It is equally effective in the dialysis population. The drug is metabolized in the liver and only about 10 to 12% is excreted unchanged in the urine. Rapid clearance occurs by dialysis secondary to minimal protein binding so supplementation after hemodialysis is necessary. Cautious titration is necessary as prolonged hypotension and myocardial ischemia have been reported (102). The risks of pericardial effusion may be increased in the dialysis population (103). Hirsutism is to be expected and limits the acceptance of this medication, particularly in children and female patients.

Labetalol

Labetalol is a combined alpha and beta blocking agent which has produced prompt reduction in blood pressure and systemic vascular resistance without reflex tachycardia or change in cardiac output (104). Any contraindication to the use of a beta blocker applies equally to this drug. One study has shown labetalol to be effective in about 70% of acute hypertensive episodes in dialysis patients (vs 75% effectiveness of diazoxide) (105). The use of more frequent and smaller boluses of 20 to 50 mg IV push every 15 min has been shown to be equally effective and to decrease the risk of prolonged hypotension (104). Little is known of the pharmacokinetics or effectiveness of labetalol as a chronic oral antihypertensive agent in hemodialysis patients.

Diazoxide

Diazoxide is a direct acting arterial dilator with a rapid onset of action. There is decreased protein binding with uremia and a greater risk of overshoot or prolonged hypotension. Because of this concern two alternate methods of delivery have been used: either minibolus injection of 50 to 100 mg at 10 to 15 minute intervals or slow continuous infusion at 15 mg/minute (106). Both methods have produced a more controlled reduction in blood pressure. Use of diazoxide is not recommended in several acute situations including cerebral and coronary insufficiency (106).

Nitroprusside

Nitroprusside offers the advantage of potent and predictable reduction in blood pressure regardless of the etiology. Close continuous monitoring of blood pressure is required to prevent overshoot. Because it is converted *in vivo* to thiocyanate, which accumulates in renal failure, toxicity can be problematic. In general, use should be limited to less than 48 h and plasma concentrations of thiocyanate should be monitored to avoid levels greater than 10 mg/dl.

Investigation of resistant hypertension

Patients with persistent hypertension despite volume control and first line (or possible a second line) antihypertensive drug therapy need to be reevaluated (Figure 2). There are four general areas of concern: 1) inaccurate blood pressure readings – including pseudohypertension secondary to atherosclerotic peripheral vascular disease (107); 2) patient compliance; 3) drug dosing and effectiveness – including dose frequency, drug-drug interactions, and compensatory reactions to current medications, and 4) secondary hypertension with renal artery stenosis, hyperthyroidism, hyperparathyroidism, and autonomic dysfunction being major considerations. The precise timing of any investigations will vary depending on individual circumstances. The goal is the rational choice of therapy based on firm data rather than on impressions.

The approach to resistant hypertension ought to be systematic and inclusive (108). Appropriate studies can range from rechecking the accuracy of blood pressure readings, to 24-h blood pressure monitoring for significant diurnal patterns of hypertension, to more complete evaluation of volume, hemodynamic, neural, and hormonal factors. Autonomic nervous system dysfunction has been discussed above. The net result is often a markedly fluctuating blood pressure with supine hypertension and orthostatic hypotension. If sympathetic hyperactivity is demonstrated, alpha-1 blockers such as prazosin or central alpha-2 agonists such as alpha methyldopa or clonidine may be appropriate choices. Evaluation of the renin component of hypertension can be obtained from determinations of plasma renin activity or of the blood pressure response to oral captopril. Recent studies (33, 88) of patients with resistant hypertension have shown wide ranges in PRA values, and low PRA levels do not necessarily preclude effective use of a CEI. Hemodynamic studies are frequently of great value in determining the mechanisms responsible for resistance to blood pressure control and in choosing the next line of treatment. They can now be obtained noninvasively by radionuclide and echocardiographic techniques and hence can be used in the follow-up of patients with difficult problems. More accurate assessment of cardiac performance, loading conditions of the heart, distribution of blood volume, and estimates of arterial compliance help draw a more comprehensive view of the problems involved. Hemodynamic studies can also illuminate the problem of 'pseudo-tolerance' or define the cardiac consequences of treatment. Simply stated, it is necessary to determine the status of each individual patient rather than to depend solely on general principles.

Hypertensive urgencies and emergencies

Definition

Hypertensive emergencies are situations wherein blood pressure must be lowered within one hour to reduce patient risk. This usually requires hospitalization and parenteral medications. Urgencies are situations in which blood pressure elevation is not causing immediate end organ damage but should be controlled within 24 h to reduce potential risks. These situations can usually be treated with oral agents and may or may not require hospitalization (109). The clinical situations that are considered hypertensive emergencies and their appropriate management have been

discussed in detail recently (106, 110). Among the various hypertensive emergencies, malignant hypertension can be especially problematic. As expected malignant hypertension is not a uniform process. Especially in dialysis patients, there is enormous variation in the pathogenesis, hemodynamics and optimal therapy (111).

Treatment

The agents used for treatment of hypertensive urgencies and emergencies in dialysis patients are the same drugs effective in the non-dialysis population. They include nifedipine, captopril, hydralazine, labetalol, diazoxide and nitroprusside. They are discussed above and presented in Table 2. The latter three parenteral agents offer the most predictable effects especially in hypertensive emergencies although the appropriate choice will vary depending on the clinical situation (106, 110).

Nephrectomy

As previously mentioned the current armamentarium of drugs available for treatment of hypertension has dramatically reduced the need for nephrectomy in control of resistant blood pressure. In the recent past we have not had to perform a nephrectomy for uncontrolled hypertension in any of our dialysis patients. In addition nephrectomy is not without its problems. The hematocrit can drop substantially, probably secondary to a lack of erythropoietin production. This increases the requirement for blood transfusions and the risk of hepatitis. Calcium absorption is decreased in the anephric state because of the loss of 1,25-dihydroxyvitamin D-3 production by the kidney. Anephric patients are exquisitely sensitive to volume changes, which makes hemodialysis associated hypotension a significant clinical problem. In addition rigid fluid restrictions are needed in patients whose kidneys previously might have been helpful in eliminating some fluid. Finally, morbidity and mortality associated with the surgery itself are important considerations.

HEMODYNAMIC INSTABILITY WITH HEMODIALYSIS

Hemodynamic patterns

One of the most frequently encountered problems in the dialysis process continues to be dialysis related hypotension. Several studies have found this to occur in up to 25 to 50% of dialysis treatments (112). Common symptoms include headache, cramps, nausea, vomiting, and malaise. However, hypotensive episodes may be asymptomatic, so definitions that rely on symptoms will lead to underestimation of the frequency of this problem. Dialysis related hypotension can be defined as a drop in the MAP of at least 30 mm Hg below predialysis values, or a drop of systolic blood pressure below 90 mm Hg (113). Several recent reviews have also discussed the pathophysiology and treatment of this syndrome in more detail (114, 115). Kinet et al (116) invasively studied 14 patients undergoing hemodialysis. They found the following sequence of events in patients who experienced hypotension: 1) hypovolemia secondary to ultrafiltration (UF); 2) decrease in plasma osmolality with delayed plasma refill rate (PRR) and shift of fluid from the interstitial space (ISV) to the intracellular space (ICV); 3) decreased left ventricular filling pressure with disequilibrium between systolic and diastolic filling of the ventricles; 4) fall in stroke volume (SV) and cardiac output (CO); 5) absence of the appropriate responses, either increased heart rate (HR) or total peripheral resistance (TPR), adequate to maintain blood pressure. Thus the two major factors in the pathogenesis of dialysis related hypotension are: 1) the rate of volume reduction and compensatory transcapillary fluid shift from the ISV to blood volume (BV) and; 2) the inadequacy of the neuro-effector responses to that hypovolemia marked by absence of reflex tachycardia and increased TPR. In addition, membrane related reactions may lead to acute hypotension. Table 3 is a summary of the many factors that may predispose a patient to dialysis related hypotension.

Plasma refill rate and hypovolema

The degree of hypovolemia is ultimately related to the difference between the total fluid loss and the plasma volume loss per unit time, that is, the plasma refill rate (PRR). The PRR in turn depends on several factcors including total plasma osmolality, colloid osmotic pressure (COP), and tissue hydration state. A decrease in plasma osmolality hinders mobilization of fluid from the ISV and in fact favors fluid shifts to the ICV (117). Increases in plasma osmolality using high sodium dialysate (118), or mannitol infusions (119) have been found to preserve BV and decrease the incidence of hypotension. Similarly the isosmotic removal of plasma water with UF (72) has been shown to allow greater volume removal with less instability. Perhaps even more important is colloid osmotic pressure (COP) – the contribution to total osmolality made by the plasma protein concentration plus the resultant Gibbs-Donnan equilibrium (120). Rodriguez et al (121) found a similar PRR in patients under-

Table 3. Factors in hemodynamic instability of dialysis.

I. *Generation of hypovolemia*
    A. Plasma refill rate
    B. Vascular tone
    C. Distribution of venous blood

II. *Indequate compensation*
    A. Composition of dialysate
    B. Loss of vasoactive substances
    D. Autonomic dysfunction
    E. Effects of antihypertensive medications
    F. Other medical problems

III. *Membrane related reactions*

going 2 h of hemodialysis or UF despite a fall in plasma osmolality with hemodialysis. This was related to the maintenance of COP, which occurred despite a decline in total plasma osmolality. PRR is faster in patients with a high tissue hydration state. Patients initially overhydrated (with increased total tissue compliance) have more rapid and complete refilling of BV and no evidence of BV contraction or hypotension. However patients near normovolemia (with low tissue compliance) are more likely to have incomplete plasma refilling and a greater incidence of hypotension (122). Redistribution of BV in the peripheral venous capacitance vessels can also decrease central return and thus preload (117). The exact location and extent of this redistribution and the mechanisms responsible await further studies.

Neuro-effector responses

Once hypovolemia secondary to decreased PRR and redistribution of venous volume away from the heart leads to decreased stroke volume and cardiac output, certain neuro-effector responses should be activated to maintain MAP. There are many putative etiologic factors in the inadequate response to hypovolemia, and the contribution of any single factor will vary among patients (Table 3). Acetate has been found by several investigators to have deleterious effects in the hemodialysis population. Vasodilation, decreased cardiac contractility, hypoxemia, and acid-base abnormalities all have been described, any one of which might contribute to hypotension. However, the direct role of acetate in the generation of these complications is still controversial (123). Loss of vasoactive substances such as norepinephrine, A II or vasopressin in the dialysate may be important in the failure of neurogenic response. Reduced baroreceptor sensitivity as determined by response to bolus intravenous phenylephrine has been found in hypotensive prone patients (124). Certain patients exhibit another possible marker of autonomic dysfunctcion, namely failure to increase PRA secondary to blunted NE release (31). Any underlying impairment of cardiac funciton including cardiomyopathy, arrhythmias, pericardial disease or coronary artery disease can preclude an adequate response to decreased stroke volume. Associated medical illnesses such as myocardial infarction, pulmonary embolism, sepsis, or hemorrhage can lead to hypotension independent of any aspect of the hemodialysis procedure and should always be considered. Membrane related reactions can lead to hypotension. The 'first use' phenomenon seen with cupraammonium (cuprophan) cellulose dialyzers can cause severe and sudden hypotension (125). This may be related to production of interleukin-1 (endogenous pyrogen) (126), anaphylatoxin activation (127), exposure to other membrane materials, or to chemicals used in sterilization including ethylene oxide (125). There are thus multiple factors that may influence blood pressure during dialysis. Consequently the prevention of dialysis related hypotension must take into consideration not only the absolute volume removed but also the distribution of the remaining volume; not only receptor or afferent autonomic insufficiency but also effector organ responses;

not only baseline hormonal and cardiac activity but also the ability of these effectors to adapt rapidly and adequately in response to the stresses of dialysis.

Treatment

Altered pharmocokinetics of antihypertensive drugs in dialysis patients may predispose a patient to hemodialysis related hypotension. The potential for this problem is increased in patients taking medications that have long half-lives, are not dialyzable or that have active metabolites which tend to accumulate. Cardiac status should be evaluated for presence of cardiomyopathy of diverse etiologies or for atherosclerotic heart disease. Improvement in left ventricular function after successful coronary artery bypass grafting may mitigate the symptoms of hemodialysis related hypotension. Associated non-dialysis related medical problems should be investigated. Evidence for autonomic dysfunction, especially in the baroreceptor reflexes, should be evaluated and adjustments in treatment protocol made although treatment is usually difficult and unrewarding (114).

Of the dialysis related factors, maintenance of COP and plasma osmolality are problably the most important. Increase in the dialysis fluid sodium concentration to 140 to 142 mEq/l has been shown effective in long-term studies for the prevention of hypotension (128). Acutely, boluses of hypertonic saline or mannitol can be used with the same effect. The risks with the use of these agents to stabilize plasma osmolality are increased hypertension, increased intradialytic weight gain secondary to increased thirst, and congestive heart failure (129). A recent study has shown stabilization of patients prone to hypotension with increased dialysis fluid calcium concentrations (58). However the long-term risks and benefits of this therapy remain to be determined. There have been studies showing improved hemodialysis stability with bicarbonate dialysate (130). This is especially evident in patients who are also treated with a low sodium dialysis fluid. A study (131) of stable patients with or without autonomic neuropathy showed greater stability with bicarbonate than acetate dialysate when dialysis fluid Na^+ was 130 mEq/l. However with the use of a high sodium dialysis solution (141 mEq/l) there was still a difference in stability between patients with autonomic neuropathy and those without neuropathy, but the benefits of a bicarbonate dialysate over an acetate dialysate were no longer evident. Lazarus et al (132) have also shown that the more important factor may be the dialysis fluid sodium concentration. Since the incidence of hypovolemia depends on the rate of plasma water removal a switch from high efficiency rapid dialysis to standard dialysis or to sequential isolated ultrafiltration followed by hemodialysis without further weight loss may lessen instability in some patients. A change in modality to hemofiltration or CAPD may also be necessary in some patients with continued hemodynamic instability.

Hypertension during and following hemodialysis

Dialysis induced hypertension is a poorly described but relatively common entity, defined as the dramatic increase in blood pressure during dialysis. Hypertension can occur either in patients who are hypertensive and receiving treatment or untreated patients who are normotensive at the initiation of dialysis. As dialysis proceeds the blood pressure rises markedly, achieving dramatic values typically during the second half of the procedure. In some cases this phenomenon can be explained by the dialyzability of some antihypertensive drugs and represents a kind of 'rebound' hypertension. In other patients hypertension might represent an enhanced hormonal response to volume or salt depletion, but the exact hemodynamics of this process are still under investigation. Patients prone to hypertensive crises during dialysis were treated with captopril 50 mg PO at the initiation of ultrafiltration (133). Captopril was effective in all patients in preventing elevation of blood pressure during ultrafiltration. Although most patients had PRA levels higher than normal there was no close correlation between these levels and the incidence of hypertensive crises or the prediction of responsiveness to captopril therapy. An additional hemodynamic study performed in two patients found that both patients had a markedly elevated TPR during ultrafiltration. In this small group of patients it appeared that oral captopril at the beginning of ultrafiltration was effective in preventing severe elevations of blood pressure during the procedure and that the hypertension that developed without captopril was hemodynamically characterized by elevated TPR.

REFERENCES

1. Paganini EP, Fouad FM, Tarazi RC: Systemic hypertension in chronic renal failure, in *The Heart and Renal Disease,* edited by O'Rourke RA, Brenner BM, Stein JH, New York, Churchill Livingstone, 1984, p 127
2. Weidmann P, Carlo Beretta-Piccoli C: Chronic renal failure and hypertension, in *Handbook of Hypertension, Vol. 2: Clinical Aspects of Secondary Hypertension,* edited by Robertson JIS, Amsterdam, Elsevier Science Publishers B.V., 1983, p 80
3. Ritz E, Strumpf C, Katz F, Wing AJ, Quellhorst E: Hypertension and cardiovascular risk factors in hemodialyzed diabetic patients. *Hypertension* 7 (suppl II): 118, 1985
4. Weidmann P, Maxwell MH: The renin-angiotensin-aldosterone system in terminal renal failure. *Kidney Int* 8 (suppl 5): S 219, 1975
5. Paganini EP, Tarazi RC: Hypertension in the dialytic population. In *Arterial Hypertension, Pathogenesis, Diagnosis, and Therapy,* edited by Rosenthal J, New York, Springer-Verlag, 1984, p 504
6. Lindner A, Charra B, Sherrard DJ, Scribner BH: Accelerated atherosclerosis in prolonged maintenance hemodialysis. *N Engl J Med* 290: 697, 1974
7. Vincenti F, Amend WJ, Abele J, Feduska NJ, Salvatierra O: The role of hypertension in hemodialysis-associated atherosclerosis. *Am J Med* 68: 363, 1980
8. Charra B, Calemard E, Cuche M, Laurent G: Control of

hypertension and prolonged survival on maintenance hemodialysis. *Nephron* 33: 96, 1983

9. Green D, Stone NJ, Krumlovsky FA: Putative atherogenic factors in patients with chronic renal failure. *Prog Cardiovasc Dis* 26: 133, 1983

10. Tarazi RC, Gifford RW Jr.: Systemic arterial pressure, in *Pathologic Physiology,* edited by Sodeman WA, Sodeman WA Jr., Philadelphia, W.B. Saunders Co, 1979, p 198

11. Tarazi RC: Pathophysiology of essential hypertension. *Am J Med* 75 (suppl 4A): 2, 1983

12. Kim KE, Onesti G, Schwartz AB, Chinitz JL, Swartz C: Hemodynamics of hypertension in chronic end-stage renal disease. *Circulation* 46: 456, 1972

13. Neff MS, Kim KE, Persoff M, Onesti G, Swartz C: Hemodynamics of uremic anemia. *Circulation* 43: 876, 1971

14. Duke M, Abelmann WH: The hemodynamic response to chronic anemia. *Circulation* 39: 503, 1969

15. Weidmann P, Beretta-Piccoli B, Steffin F, Blumberg A, Reubi FC: Hypertension in terminal renal failure. *Kidney Int* 9: 294, 1976

16. Schalekamp MA, Beevers DG, Briggs JD, Brown JJ, Davies DL, Fraser R, Lebel M, Lever AF, Medina A, Morton JJ, Robertson JIS, Tree M: Hypertension in chronic renal failure an abnormal relation between sodium and the renin-angiotensin system. *Am J Med* 55: 379, 1973

17. Brennan BL, Yasumura S, Letteri JM, Cohn SH: Total body electrolyte composition and distribution of body water in uremia. *Kidney Int* 17: 364, 1980

18. McGrath BP, Ledingham JGG: Renin, blood volume and response to saralasin in patients on chronic hemodialysis: evidence against volume and renin 'dependent' hypertension. *Clin Sci Mol Med* 54: 305, 1978

19. Welt LG, Sachs JR, McManus TJ: An ion transport defect in erythrocytes from uremic patients. *Trans Assoc Am Physicians* 77: 169, 1964

20. Borst JG: Hypertension explained by Starling's theory of circulation homeostasis. *Lancet* 1: 677, 1963

21. Guyton AC, Coleman TG: Quantitative analysis of the pathophysiology of hypertension. *Circ Res* 24 (suppl I): 1, 1969

22. Ferrario CM: Contribution of cardiac output and peripheral resistance to experimental renal hypertension. *Am J Physiol* 226: 711, 1974

23. Coleman TG, Bower JD, Langford HG, Guyton AC: Regulation of arterial pressure in the anephric state. *Circulation* 42: 509, 1970

24. Onoyama K, Bravo EL, Tarazi RC: Sodium, extracellular fluid volume, and cardiac output changes in the genesis of mineralocorticoid hypertension in the intact dog. *Hypertension* 1: 331, 1979

25. Onesti G, Kim KE, Greco JA, del Guerico ET, Fernandes M, Swartz C: Blood pressure regulation in end-stage renal disease and anephric man. *Cir Res* 36 (suppl I): 145, 1975

26. Kim KE, Onesti G, DelGuerico ET, Greco J, Fernandes M, Eidelson B, Swartz C: Sequential hemodynamic changes in end-stage renal disease and the anephric state during volume expansion. *Hypertension* 2: 102, 1980

27. Folkow B, Hallback M, Lundgren Y, Sivertsson R, Weiss L: Importance of adaptive changes in vascular design for establishment of primary hypertension, studied in man and in spontaneously hypertensive rats. *Circ Res* 32 (suppl 1): 2, 1973

28. Haddy FJ, Pamnani MB, Clough DL: Humoral factors and the sodium-potassium pump in volume expanded hypertension. *Life Sci* 24: 2105, 1979

29. Blaustein MP: Sodium ions, calcium ions, blood pressure

regulation, and hypertension: a reassessment and a hypothesis. *Am J Physiol* 232: C165, 1977

30. Haber E: The renin-angiotensin system and hypertension. *Kidney Int* 15: 427, 1979

31. Textor SC, Gavras H, Tifft CP, Bernard DB, Idelson B, Brunner HR: Norepinephrine and renin activity in chronic renal failure. Evidence for interacting roles in hemodialysis hypertension. *Hypertension* 3: 294, 1981

32. Mimron A, Shaldon S, Barjon P, Mion C: The effect of an angiotensin antagonist (saralasin) on arterial pressure and plasma aldosterone in hemodialysis-resistant hypertensive patients. *Clin Nephrol* 9: 63, 1978

33. Vaughan ED, Carey RM, Ayers CR, Peach MJ: Hemodialysis-resistant hypertension: Control with an orally active inhibitor of angiotensin-converting enzyme. *J Clin Endocrinol Metab* 48: 869, 1979

34. Weidmann P, Maxwell MH, DeLima J, Hirsch D, Franklin SS: Control of aldosterone responsiveness in terminal renal failure. *Kidney Int* 7: 351, 1975

35. Vertes V, Cangiano JL, Berman LB, Gould A: Hypertension in end-stage renal disease. *N Engl J Med* 280: 978, 1969

36. Kolff WJ, Nakamoto S, Poutasse EF, Straffon RA, Figueroa JE: Effect of bilateral nephrectomy and kidney transplantation on hypertension in man. *Circulation* 29: II-23, 1964

37. Del Greco F, Davies WA, Simon NM, Huang C, Krumlovsky FA: Hypertension of chronic renal failure: Role of sodium and the renal pressor system. *Kidney Int* 7 (suppl 2): S176, 1975

38. Acosta JH: Hypertension in chronic renal disease. *Kidney Int* 22: 703, 1982

39. Swales JD: Arterial wall or plasma renin in hypertension. *Clin Sci* 56: 293, 1979

40. Dickinson CJ, Lawrence JR: A slowly developing pressor response to small concentrations of antiotensin. Its bearing on the pathogenesis of chronic renal hypertension. *Lancet* 1: 1354, 1963

41. Fujii AM, Vatner SF: Direct versus indirect pressor and vasoconstrictor actions of angiotensin in conscious dogs. *Hypertension* 7: 253, 1985

42. Kotchen TA, Talwalkar R, Kaul K: Identification of renin inhibitors in normal and uremic plasma. *J Lab Clin Med* 105: 286, 1985

43. Re R, Fallon JT, Dzau V, Ouay SC, Haber E: Renin synthesis by canine aortic smooth muscle cells in culture. *Life Sci* 30: 99, 1982

44. Dzau VJ: Significance of the vascular renin-angiotensin pathway. *Hypertension* 8: 543, 1986

45. Campese VM, Romoff MS, Levitan D, Lane K, Massry SG: Mechanisms of autonomic nervous system dysfunction in uremia. *Kidney Int* 20: 246, 1981

46. Zucchelli P, Sturani A, Zuccala A, Santoro A, Esposti EG, Chiarini C: Dysfunction of the autonomic nervous system in patients with end-stage renal failure. *Contr Nephrol* 45: 69, 1985

47. Elias AN, Vaziri ND, Maksy M: Plasma norepinephrine, epinephrine, and dopamine levels in end-stage renal disease. *Arch Intern Med* 145: 1013, 1985

48. Frewin DB, Bartholomeusz FDL, Cummings MF, Clarkson AR, Barry LA, Furber B, De Lorenzo C, Jonsson JR, Taylor WB: Changes in plasma catecholamine levels during hemodialysis. *Aust NZ J Med* 14: 31, 1984

49. Cuche JL, Prinseau J, Selz F, Ruget G, Baglin A: Plasma free sulf- and glucuro-conjugated catecholamines in uremic patients. *Kidney Int* 30: 566, 1986

50. Zimlichman RR, Chaimovitz C, Chaichenco Y, Goligorsky M, Rapoport J, Kaplansky J: Vascular hypersensitivity to noradrenaline: a possible mechanism of hypertension in rats with chronic uremia. *Clin Sci* 67: 161, 1984

51. Rascher W, Schomig A, Kreye VA, Ritz E: Diminished vascular response to noradrenaline in experimental chronic uremia. *Kidney Int* 21: 20, 1982

52. Iseki K, Massry SG, Campese VM: Evidence for a role of PTH in the reduced pressor response to norepineprhine in chronic renal failure. *Kidney Int* 28: 11, 1985

53. McGrath BP, Tiller DJ, Bune A, Chalmers JP, Korner PI, Uther JB: Autonomic blockade and the Valsalva maneuver in patients on maintenance hemodialysis: A hemodynamic study: *Kidney Int* 12: 294, 1977

54. Schohn D, Weidmann P, Jahn H, Beretta-Piccoli C: Norepinephrine-related mechanism in hypertension accompanying renal failure. *Kidney Int* 28: 814, 1985

55. Marone C, Beretta-Piccoli C, Weidmann P: Acute hypercalcemic hypertension in man: Role of hemodynamics, catecholamines, and renin. *Kidney Int* 20: 92, 1980

56. Levi M, Ellis M, Chaimovitz C, Berl T: Mechanism of acute hypercalcemic hypertension in the conscious rat: Role of vasoactive hormones and calcium (abstract). *Kidney Int* 25: 203, 1984

57. Sica DA, Harford AM, Zawada ET: Hypercalcemic hypertension in hemodialysis. *Clin Nephrol* 22: 102, 1984

58. Maynard JC, Cruz C, Kleerkoper M, Levin NW: Blood pressure response to changes in serum ionized calcium during hemodialysis. *Ann Intern Med* 104: 358, 1986

59. Llach F, Weidmann P, Reinhart R, Maxwell MH, Coburn JW, Massry SG: Effect of acute and long-standing hypocalcemia on blood pressure and plasma renin activity in man. *J Clin Endocrinol Metab* 38: 841, 1974

60. Braunwald E: Mechanism of action of calcium-channel-blocking agents. *N Engl J Med* 307: 1618, 1982

61. Blaustein MP, Hamlyn JM: Sodium transport inhibition, cell calcium, and hypertension. The Natiuretic hormone/Na$^+$-Ca^{2+} exchange/hypertension hypothesis. *Am J Med* 77 (suppl 4A): 45, 1984

62. Katz AM, Hager WD, Messineo FC, Pappano AJ: Cellular actions and pharmacology of the calcium channel blocking drugs. *Am J Med* 79 (suppl 4A): 2, 1985

63. Bourgoignie JJ, Hwang KH, Espineai C, Klahr S, Bricker NS: A natriuretic factor in the serum of patients with chronic uremia. *J Clin Invest* 51: 1514, 1972

64. Ahmad S, Kenny M, Scribner BH: Hypertension and a digoxin-like substance in the plasma of dialysis patients: Possible marker for a natriuretic hormone . . . *Clin Physiol Biochem* 4: 210, 1986

65. Bealer SL, Haywood JR, Gruber KA, Buckalew VM, Fink GD, Brody MJ, Johnson AK: Preoptic-hypothalamic periventricular lesions reduce natriuresis to volume expansion. *Am J Physiol* 244: R51, 1983

66. Kelly RA, O'Hara DS, Mitch WE, Steinman TI, Goldszer RC, Solomon HS, Smith TW: Endogenous digitalis-like factors in hypertension and chronic renal insufficiency. *Kidney Int* 30: 723, 1986

67. Hilton PJ: Cellular sodium transport in essential hypertension. *N Engl J Med* 314: 222, 1986

68. Corry DB, Tuck ML, Brickman AS, Yanagawa N, Lee DB: Sodium transport in red blood cells from dialyzed uremic patients. *Kidney Int* 29: 1197, 1986

69. Hagberg JM, Goldberg AP, Ehsani AA, Heath GW, Delmez JA, Harter HR: Exercise training improves hypertension in hemodialysis patients. *Am J Nephrol* 3: 209, 1983

70. Heaton A, Amer H, Bullock RE, Ward MK, Hall RJC, Kerr DNS: Importance of impaired exercise tolerance in patients on renal replacement therapy. *Contr Nephrol* 41: 272, 1984

71. Bergström J: Ultrafiltration without dialysis for removal of fluid and solutes in uremia. *Clin Nephrol* 9: 156, 1978

72. Paganini EP, Fouad F, Tarazi RC, Bravo EL, Nakamoto S: Hemodynamics of isolated ultrafiltration in chronic hemodialysis patients. *Trans Am Soc Artif Intern Organs* 25: 422, 1979

73. Quellhorst E, Schuenemann B, Hildebrand U, Neumann W: Hypertension and hemofiltration. *Contr Nephrol* 32: 46, 1982

74. Ritz E, Bosch J, Henderson LW, Kishimoto T, Koch KM, Pierides A, Shaldon S, Streicher E: Hemofiltration and vascular stability. *Contr Nephrol* 32: 200, 1982

75. Mactier RA, Khanna R: Control of blood pressure on CAPD. (In press)

76. Youmbissi J, Sellars L, Shore AC, Poon T, Wilkinson R: Blood pressure on CAPD: Relationship to sodium status, renin, and aldosterone, compared with hemodialysis. In *Frontiers in Peritoneal Dialysis*, edited by Maher JF, Winchester JF, New York, Field, Rich and Associates, 1986, p 450

77. Panzetta G, Guerra U, D'Angelo A, Sandrsini S, Terzi A, Oldrizzi L, Maiorca R: Body fluid spaces in patients on CAPD. *Int J Artif Organs* 7: 89, 1984

78. Glasson P, Favre H, Vallottton MB: Response of blood pressure and the renin-angiotensin-aldosterone system to chronic ambulatory peritoneal dialysis in hypertensive end-stage renal disease. *Clin Sci* 63: 207s, 1982

79. Leenen FHH, Smith DL, Khanna R, Oreopoulos DG: Changes in left ventricular hypertrophy and function in hypertensive patients started on continuous ambulatory peritoneal dialysis. *Am Heart J* 110: 102, 1985

80. Brater DC, Chennavasin P: *Drug Use in Renal Disease.* Sydney, Australia, Adis Health Science Press, 1983: 135

81. Bennett WM, Aronoff GR, Morrison G, Golper TA, Pulliam J, Wolfson M, Singer I: Drug prescribing in renal failure: Dosing guidelines for adults. *Am J Kidney Dis* 3: 155, 1983

82. McMahon FG: *Management of Essential Hypetension The New Low Dose Era,* 2nd Edition, New York, Futura Publishing Company, 1984

83. Michaels RS, Duchin KL, Akbar S, Meister J, Levin NW: Nadolol in hypertensive patients maintained on long-term hemodialysis. *Am Heart J* 108: 1091, 1984

84. Lowenthal DT, Affrine MB, Meyer A, Kinn KE, Falkner B, Sharif K: Pharmacokinetics and pharmacodynamics of clonidine in varying states of renal function. *Chest* 83 (suppl): 386, 1983

85. Myhre E, Brodwall EK, Stenbaek O, Hansen T: Plasma turnover of methyldopa in advanced renal failure. *Acta Med Scand* 191: 343, 1972

86. Vidt DG, Bravo EL, Fouad FM: Captopril. *N Engl J Med* 306: 214, 1982

87. Zusman RM: Renin and non-renin-mediated antihypertensive actions of converting enzyme inhibitors. *Kidney Int* 25: 969, 1984

88. Wauters JP, Waeber B, Brunner HR, Guignard JP, Turini GA, Gavras H: Uncontrollable hypertension in patients on hemodialysis: long-term treatment with captopril and salt subtraction. *Clin Nephrol* 16: 86, 1981

89. Brunner HR, Waeber B, Wauters JP, Turini G, McKinstry D, Gavras H: Inappropriate renin secretion unmasked by captopril in hypertension of chronic renal failure. *Lancet* 2: 704, 1978

90. Hirakata H, Onoyama K, Iaeki K, Omae T, Fumimi S, Yawahara Y: Captopril clearance during hemodialysis treatment. *Clin Nephrol* 16: 321, 1981

91. Bazlinski N: Converting enzyme inhibitors in hemodialysis. *Int J Artif Organs* 6: 62, 1983

92. Kelly J, Doyle G, Donohoe J, Laher M, Vandenburg MJ, Currie WJC, Cooper WD: The pharmacokinetic profile of enalaprilat in normal subjects and patients with renal impairment. *Br J Clin Pharmacol* 18: 274P, 1984

93. Katz AM: Pharmacology and mechanisms of action of calcium-channel blockers. *J Clin Hypertens* 3: 28S, 1986

94. Garthoff B, Kazda S, Knorr A, Gunter T: Factors involved in the antihypertensive action of calcium antagonists. *Hypertension* 5 (suppl II): 34, 1983

95. Kubo K, Shiraishi K, Muto H, Suzuki T, Sugino N: Treatment of hypertension in hemodialysis patients with nifedipine. *Hypertension* 5 (suppl II): 109, 1983

96. McAllister RG: Kinetics and dynamics of nifedipine after oral and sublingual doses. *Am J Med* 81 (suppl 6A): 2, 1986

97. Ambroso GC, Como G, Scalamogna A, Citterio A, Casati S, Ponticelli: Treatment of arterial hypertension with nifedipine in patients with chronic renal insufficiency. *Clin Nephrol* 23: 41, 1985

98. White RP, Rubin AL: Blood pressure control in chronic dialysis patients. In *Replacement of Renal Function by Dialysis*, edited by Drukker W, Parsons FM, Maher JF, 2nd Edition, The Hague, Martinus Nijhoff, 1983, p. 575

99. Lowenthal DT, Hobbs D, Affrime MB, Twomey TM, Martinez EW, Onesti G: Prazosin kinetics and effectiveness in renal failure. *Clin Pharm Ther* 27: 779, 1980

100. Meltzer VN, Goldberg AP, Tindira CA, Naumovich AD, Harter HR: Effects of prazosin and propranolol on blood pressure and plasma lipids in patients undergoing chronic hemodialysis. *Am J Cardiol* 53: 40A, 1984

101. Pettinger WA, Mitchell HC: Minoxidil – An alternative to nephrectomy for refractory hypertension. *N Engl J Med* 289: 167, 1973

102. Campese VM: Minoxidil: A review of its pharmacological properties and therapeutic use. *Drugs* 22: 257, 1981

103. Zarate A, Gelfand MC, Horton JD, Winchester JF, Gottlieb MJ, Lazarus JM, Schreiner GE: Pericardial effusion associated with minoxidil therapy in dialyzed patients. *Int J Artif Organs* 3: 15, 1980

104. Cressman MD, Vidt DG, Giffor RW Jr, Moore WS, Wilson DJ: Intravenous labetalol in the management of severe hypertension and hypertensive emergencies. *Am Heart J* 107: 980, 1984

105. Keusch G, Schiffl H, Binswanger U: Diazoxide and labetalol in acute hypertension during hemodialysis. *Eur J Clin Pharmacol* 25: 523, 1983

106. Vidt DG, Gifford, RW Jr: A compendium for the treatment of hypertensive emergencies. *Cleve Clin Q* 51: 421, 1984

107. Messerli FH, Ventura HO, Amodeo C: Osler's maneuver and pseudohypertension. *N Engl J Med* 312: 1548, 1985

108. Gifford RW Jr, Tarazi RC: Resistant hypertension: Diagnosis and management. *Ann Intern Med* 88: 661, 1978

109. Joint National Committee on Detection, Evaluation, and Treatment of High Blood Pressure: The 1984 Report of the Joint National Committee on Detection, Evaluation, and Treatment of High Blood Pressure. *Arch Intern Med* 144: 1045, 1984

110. Ferguson RK, Vlasses PH: Hypertensive emergencies and urgencies. *JAMA* 255: 1607, 1986

111. Schohn DC, Schmitt RL, Jahn HA: Malignant hypertension in end-stage renal failure: Hemodynamic and hormone status. *Contr Nephrol* 49: 185, 1985

112. Rosa AA, Fryd DS, Kjellstrand CM: Dialysis symptoms and stabilization in long-term dialysis. Practical application of the CUSUM plot. *Arch Intern Med* 140: 804, 1980

113. Azancot I, Degoulet P, Juillet Y, Rottenbourg J, Legrain M: Hemodynamic evaluation of hypotension during chronic hemodialysis. *Clin Nephrol* 8: 213, 1977

114. Henrich WL: Hemodynamic instability during hemodialysis. *Kidney Int* 30: 605, 1986

115. Petticlerc T, Drüecke T, Man NK, Funck-Brentano JL: Cardiovascular stability on hemodialysis. *Adv Nephrol* 16: 351, 1987

116. Kinet JP, Soyeur D, Balland N, Saint-Remy M, Collignon P, Godon JP: Hemodynamic study of hypotension during hemodialysis. *Kidney Int* 21: 868, 1982

117. Chaignon M, Chen WT, Tarazi RC, Bravo EL, Nakamoto S: Effect of hemodialysis on blood volume distribution and cardiac output. *Hypertension* 3: 327, 1981

118. Van Stone JC, Bauer J, Carey J: The effect of dialysate sodium concentration on body fluid distribution during hemodialysis. *Trans Am Soc Artif Intern Organs* 26: 383, 1980

119. Henrich WL, Woodard TD, Blachley JD, Gomez-Sanchez C, Pettinger W, Cronin RE: Role of osmolality in blood pressure stability after dialysis and ultrafiltration. *Kidney Int* 18: 480, 1980

120. Hays RM: Dynamics of body water and electrolytes. In *Clinical Disorders of Fluid and Electrolyte Metabolism*, edited by Maxwell H, Kleeman CR, New York, McGraw-Hill, 1980, p 1

121. Rodriguez M, Pederson JA, Llach F: Effect of dialysis and ultrafiltration on osmolality, colloid osmotic pressure, and vascular refilling. *Kidney Int* 28: 808, 1985

122. Koomans HA, Geers AB, Mees EJD: Plasma volume recovery after ultrafiltration in patients with chronic renal afailure. *Kidney Int* 26: 848, 1984

123. Diamond SM, Henrich WL: Acetate dialysate versus bicarbonate dialysate: A continuing controversy. *Am J Kidney Dis* 9: 3, 1987

124. Nies AS, Robertson D, Stone WJ: Hemodialysis hypotension is not the result of uremic peripheral autonomic neuropathy. *J Lab Clin Med* 94: 395, 1979

125. Ing TS, Daugirdas JT, Popi S, Gandhi VC: First-use syndrome with cuprammonium cellulose dialyzers. *Int J Artif Organs* t: 235, 1983

126. Henderson LW, Koch KM, Dinarello CA, Shaldon S: Hemodialysis hypotension: The interleukin hypothesis. *Blood Purif* 1: 3, 1983

127. Chenoweth DE, Cheung AK, Henderson LW: Anaphylatoxin formation during hemodialysis: Effects of different dialyzer membranes. *Kidney Int* 24: 764, 1983

128. Henrich WL, Woodard TD, McPhaul JJ: The chronic efficacy and safety of high sodium dialysate: Double-blind, crossover study. *Am J Kidney Dis* 2: 349, 1982

129. Wilkinson R, Barber SG, Robson V: Cramps, thirst and hypertension in hemodialysis patients – the influence of dialyzate sodium concentration. *Clin Neprhol* 7: 101, 1977

130. Graefe U, Milutinovich J, Follette WC, Vizzo JE, Babb AL, Scribner BH: Less dialysis-induced morbidity and vascular instability with bicarbonate in dialysate. *Ann Intern Med* 88: 332, 1978

131. Velez RL, Woodard TD, Henrich WL: Acetate and bicarbonate hemodialysis in patients with and without autonomic dysfunction. *Kidney Int* 26: 59, 1984

132. Lazarus JM, Henderson LW, Kjellstrand CM, Weiner MW, Henrich WL, Hakim RM: Cardiovascular instability during hemodialysis. *Trans Am Soc Artif Intern Organs* 28: 656, 1982

133. Bazzato G, Coli U, Landini S, Lucatello S, Fracasso A, Morachiello P, Righetto F. Scanferla A: Prevention of intra- and postdialytic hypertensive crises by captopril. *Contr Nephrol* 41: 292, 1984.

CARDIAC COMPLICATIONS OF UREMIA AND DIALYSIS

JOHN F. MAHER

INTRODUCTION

Before the availability of dialysis treatment, pericarditis was frequently seen in uremic patients, particularly in the terminal stages (1). It was a reliable predictor of impending death and frequently caused death by hemorrhagic effusion, tamponade, or other mechanisms. Cardiomyopathy was a less distinctive abnormality usually attributed to underlying collagen vascular or metabolic disease, or electrolyte abnormalities. Some authors considered that an underlying specific uremic cardiomyopathy also existed but its pathogenesis was uncertain. The frequent observation of heart failure in the uremic population was considered an epiphenomenon related to prior hypertension, atherosclerosis, and extracellular volume expansion.

With the advent of dialysis it became possible to control extracellular fluid volume and hypertension much more effectively, and pericarditis was shown to be a reversible complication of uremia. Cardiac abnormalities became less frequent and were given lower priority than such complications as infection, osteodystrophy and neuropathy. Early reports of series of patients treated by regular dialysis, however, revealed an appreciable percentage of deaths attributed to cardiovascular occlusive disease and heart failure (2–5). These abnormalities accounted for 30% to 40% of deaths of dialysis patients. In 1974, Linder et al (6) reported that 60% of deaths of dialysis patients in Seattle were due to cardiovascular disease, even athough this pioneer patient population was chosen in part because of their absence of underlying vascular dialysis and their young age. They suggested that renal failure treated by dialysis was associated with accelerated atherosclerosis.

In the large cohort of patients included in the European Dialysis and Transplant Registry, 41.5% of deaths have been caused by cardiac events and an additional 11.2% by cerebrovascular accidents (7). Using these data, the major causes of death are illustrated in Figure 1. Cardiovascular disease accounts for more than 54% of all deaths while infection, the second leading cause of death, represents 19% of the group. Even in the 15 to 34 year age group, cardiovascular disease accounts for more than half of all deaths in both the most recent year analyzed, 1979, and among the total registry.

PERICARDITIS

In patients with renal failure pericarditis is a frequent abnormality. Bright (8) recognized aseptic pericarditis and pleuritis in a high fraction of the patients that he examined, and serositis has generally been viewed as one of the distinctive manifestations of uremia. Despite modern treatment pericarditis occurs in about 15% of patients with severe renal failure and accounts for about 2.5% of deaths in uremic patients. With acute renal failure the incidence of pericarditis has decreased from about 50% to about 15% coincident with the earlier and more effective use of dialysis and despite increased diagnostic sensitivity with the use of echocardiography (9).

Pathogenesis

Although pericarditis has characteristically complicated severe renal failure, some patients manifest that complication at BUN concentrations below 100 mg/dl (35.7 mmol/l). Moreover, although the frequency of pericarditis correlates with urea concentrations in plasma, it correlates equally well with plasma creatinine and uric acid concentrations, and even better with plasma phosphorus concentrations (1). Like many other uremic manifestations it has been difficult

TREATED RENAL FAILURE: CAUSE OF DEATH

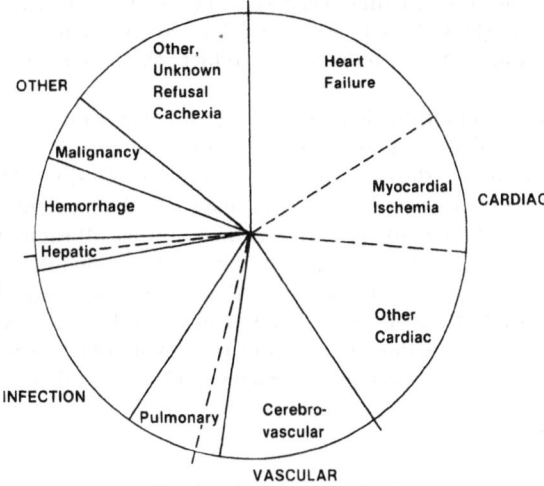

Figure 1. The cause of death of patients with chronic renal failure treated by dialysis is shown. Cardiovascular causes account for more than half of the deaths.

to incriminate a single toxin to account for pericarditis. Factors such as a hyperdynamic left ventricle may contribute to its development, by mechanical irritation superimposed on chemical toxicity. Begström and Fürst (10) have detected increased concentrations of the peptide designated 7C in patients with renal failure when they develop pericarditis. It is not clear, however, that this peptide is causative rather than being released from injured tissue. Pericarditis has also been associated with severe secondary hyperparathyroidism (9, 11), but this case has not been made definitively yet either. The correlation of uremic serositis with accumulation of immune complexes in the plasma despite dialysis is an intriguing observation but is not reconciled with the frequent reversal of the lesion on initiating dialysis treatment. It is also of interest that pericarditis sometimes became manifest after a single dialysis, suggesting that an inflammatory process initiated by peak toxin concentration continued to evolve despite removal of the toxin. The contribution of increased capillary permeability in uremia causing an exudative response to injury has not been adequately assessed. Moreover, platelet dysfunction and the use of heparin can induce a hemorrhagic fluid response to irritant injury. Curiously, pericarditis seems to complicate peritoneal dialysis less frequently than it does hemodialysis, possibly because of the higher permeability of the peritoneum or the avoidance of heparin. The impaired host responses to infection make patients with renal failure more susceptible to pericarditis complicating tuberculosis and viral illness of various types. Coxsackie viruses, echoviruses and influenza viruses have been detected most frequently (12). It is not clear how often undetected viral infection precipitates pericarditis in uremic patients. spontaneous bacterial contamination of pericardial fluid is distinctly rare, however. Finally, some of the diseases that precipitate renal failure can

induce pericarditis directly. Systemic lupus erythematosus is the most notorious example of an illness causing pericarditis and renal failure. Etiologic factors pertinent to uremic pericarditis are listed in Table 1.

Pericarditis complicating renal failure can be classified into two types depending on the time of presentation (13). The first occurs before or at initiation of dialysis treatment and has the characteristics of that observed decades ago. Unless related to the underlying cause of renal disease, it correlates with the degree of azotemia and with left ventricular dysfunction. The second type occurs later in the course of treatment and can be precipitated by viral infection or result from severe hyperparathyroidism reflecting inadequate treatment and sometimes manifesting calcific deposits. The pathology is similar because of the underlying abnormalities in capillary permeability and coagulation.

Pathology

An aseptic inflammation of both layers of the pericardium usually generalized but occasionally beginning in a segment, e.g. posteriorly, characterizes uremic pericarditis (14). The membranes become thick, granulated and coated with a fibrinous exudate. Increased vascularity accompanies the membranous thickening. A serofibrinous exudative effusion frequently complicates uremic pericarditis and may be a marked abnormality even when inflammatory changes are only modest. The effusion may be loculated with fibrous bands fastening the visceral and parietal pericardium. Serosanguinous pericardial effusion is frequent. Although most pericardial effusions are of modest size, fluid accumulation may be severe and lead to cardiac tamponade. Much less frequently, cardiac constriction results from chronic pericardial thickening and fibrous adhesions. Massive intrapericardial hemorrhage occurs infrequently, often in association with heparin therapy.

Clinical features

A characteristic constellation of features in patients with uremic pericarditis includes chest pain, a friction rub, fever,

Table 1. Etiological factors pertinent to uremic pericarditis.

Nitrogenous metabolite retention
    Urea, creatinine, uric acid
        Peptide 7-C
Phosphate
Parathyroid hormone
Hyperdynamic ventricle
    Hypertension, anemia, arteriovenous fistula, fluid overload
Underlying systemic disease
    Lupus erythematosus, polyarteritis
Infection
    Viral, tuberculosis
Anticoagulation
    Platelet dysfunction, heparin
Minoxidil therapy

hypotension, jugular venous distention and cardiac enlargement (9, 11, 13, 15). The clinical features of uremic pericarditis are outlined in Table 2.

The chest pain is similar to that of myocardial infarction except that it is usually localized to the chest and may be aggravated by positional changes. Some patients never experience pain, either because of uremic narcosis or because the inflammatory changes are minimal and effusion occurs early, separating the irritated layers of the pericardium. In the majority of patients, however, chest pain draws attention to the pericardium.

The pericardial friction rub is characteristically a two component or even three component raspy, grating sound timed with the cardiac cycle. It is heard in the vast majority of cases when auscultation is careful and repeated frequently. It is often evanescent, but can also persist for several days. Because pleuritis accompanies pericarditis frequently, a pleural rub which may be more persistent can sometimes help confirm the diagnosis in patients with such features as chest pain and hypotension.

Fever, usually of only modest degree, accompanies pericarditis in virtually all patients. It typically precedes other signs of pericarditis, but severe azotemia blunts the febrile response. Hence, fever may only become apparent after dialysis. Leukocytosis often accompanies the febrile response.

Hypotension is a frequent presenting sign of pericarditis. It may be manifest as mental confusion or disorientation indicative of poor cerebral perfusion, as a decline in residual renal function with features of renal ischemia, as intolerance to ultrafiltration, or as clotting of an angioaccess reflecting stasis of flowing blood. Similar findings may result from decreased cardiac output of other causes. The decreased arterial blood pressure and volume lead to thirst. Hence, inordinate weight gain may occur in an otherwise stable patient.

Because of underlying myocarditis, cardiac arrhythmias are frequent, occuring in about one-fourth of patients with

Table 2. Clinical findings in pericarditis complicating renal failure.

Chest Pain
Pericardial friction rub
Fever
Leukocytosis
Pericardial effusion
  Echocardiogram
  Water bottle radiographic cardiomegaly
  Low voltage electrocardiogram
Arrhythmia
Hypotension, low cardiac output
  Thirst
  Rapid weight gain
  Mental confusion
  Loss of residual renal function
  Intolerance to ultrafiltration
Venous hypertension
Associated pleural rub, effusion

---

uremic pericarditis. Atrial fibrillation or flutter are recognized most frequently. Usually, however the electrocardiogram shows ST elevations and T wave inversions in the precordial leads with decreased voltage when a large effusion is present.

Radiographically demonstrable cardiomegaly may occur because of heart failure but more often in patients with uremic pericarditis is indicative of a large effusion. The characteristic water bottle heart usually signals an extensive effusion. Echocardiography can detect small effusions in patients without other signs (16). When used frequently, the diagnosis of pericarditis complicating renal failure is made more often by echocardiography than when dependent on clinical signs. Although many of these asymptomatic cases resolve spontaneously, they demand close observation.

Complications

Most patients with uremic pericarditis have pericardial effusion demonstrable by echocardiography, but not so frequently by less sensitive techniques. Cardiac tamponade is a potential complication that results when the pressure of the effusion is sufficient to obstruct the inflow of blood to the heart. It relates not only to the volume of pericardial fluid but also to the rate of accumulation which correlates inversely with the distensibility of parietal pericardium. Tamponade is characterized by arterial hypotension, venous hypertension and paradoxical pulse in the patient with an enlarged cardiac silhouette. Symptoms may be precipitated by reduction in blood volume during ultrafiltration dialysis, reducing filling pressure, and will not respond to restoration of volume, only to emergency pericardiocentesis. This complication mimics congestive heart failure which may coexist with pericarditis, except that the lung fields may be clear because of greater compression of the right side of the heart.

Although serosanguinous pericardial effusions are frequent, extensive hemopericardium occurs in only a minority of cases of uremic pericarditis. It may be lethal by virtue of blood loss or by inducing tamponade. Hemopericardium is a major risk of heparin use with hemodialysis in patients with uremic pericarditis and potentially complicates pericardiocentesis.

Myocarditis underlies visceral pericarditis frequently but often is of no consequence. Occasionally such myocarditis causes serious arrhythmias or intractable heart failure. It responds poorly to digitalis and other routine treatment of heart failure, as well as to drainage of pericardial fluid and anti-inflammatory agents. A syndrome of reversible cardiomyopathy with marked cardiomegaly, arrhythmias, pericarditis and hypotension has been described in malnourished, protein-restricted uremic patients (17). It reverses with appropriate nutritional management and control of uremia.

Cardiac arrhythmias frequently occur with uremic pericarditis and may complicate pericardiocentesis. Their cause is multifactorial including intrinsic myocardial disease, ischemia related to cardiac compression and underlying electrolyte abnormalities.

Subacute and chronic constrictive pericarditis may follow

resolution of the acute phase. It leads to manifestations of intractable heart failure from which it must be distinguished. Increasing peripheral edema, hepatomegaly, ascites and hypotension are the hallmarks of this complication. Typically the heart is not enlarged and a pericardial friction rub is more likely absent than present. Chest pain and fever are unusual. Other causes of chronic pericarditis such as tuberculosis should be excluded. Cardiac catheterization can verify the diagnosis.

Treatment

Management of uremic pericarditis includes medical and surgical treatment. Appropriate therapy depends on the clinical setting, the symptoms and the complications. Treatment is outlined in Table 3.

When pericarditis occurs in intreated uremic patients, it is an indication to initiate hemodialysis because it correlates with more severe azotemia (16). Virtually all such patients respond to dialysis (9) and pericarditis occurring early in the course of dialysis treatment or in association with inadequate dialysis is expected to respond to intensification of dialysis, usually increasing to daily treatment. The 10% who fail to respond and the 15% who recur despite intensive dialysis should be evaluated for other possible causes. Hemodialysis should be carried out with low dose or regional heparization, and peritoneal dialysis may be preferable to avoid heparin, achieve high middle molecular weight solute clearance and accomplish ultrafiltration slowly. Patients must be observed carefully, especially during dialysis for signs of arterial hypotension, increasing venous hypertension and paradoxical pulse which should call for surgical decompression of the pericardium. Similarly, in patients with residual renal function, potent diuretics may relieve

Table 3. Management of uremic pericarditis.

1. Clinical monitoring
    Arterial and venous blood pressures
    Serial echocardiograms
2. Treatment of left ventricular function
    Rest, adequate diet
    Judicious salt and water restriction
    Careful ultrafiltration
3. Intensification of dialysis
    Low dose or regional heparinization
    Peritoneal dialysis
4. Non steroidal anti-inflammatory drugs
5. Search for other etiologies
6. Prednisone
    High dose, systemic, short course
    Intrapericardial triamcinolone
7. Surgical treatment
    Needle aspiration, tube drainage
        (diagnostic or emergency)
    Pericardial window
    Pericardectomy (preferable)
        Anterior
        Total

fluid retention but can precipitate cardiac compression.

Anti-inflammatory drugs have good rationale for treatment of pericarditis and have been successful in about half of the uremic patients so treated (18). Although the experience is most abundant with indomethacin, other nonsteroidals may prove equally effective. Side effects of nonsteroidal anti-inflammatory drugs such as bleeding and hyperkalemia may limit their use.

In limited trials prednisone has had a pronounced anti-inflammatory effect on uremic pericarditis, reducing pain, fever and effusion (11, 19). Treatment should be high dose (40 mg/day or more) but should be tapered rapidly to avoid serious side effects. Preliminary experience suggests that the local instillation of the nonabsorbable steroid, triamcinolone, in a high dose (in the range of 5 to 10 mg/kg) after pericardiocentesis, decreases pain, fluid reaccumulation and the need for surgical drainage (13). Absorption of the instilled fluid and a systemic effect cannot be excluded.

Other supportive measures include adequate nutrition, rest, maintenance of fluid balance by control of intake, and when indicated for control of associated arrhythmias or heart failure, the judicious use of digitalis in restricted dosage.

Surgical drainage of pericardial fluid can be accomplished by needle paracentesis, but the complication rate is inordinately high and includes serious arrhythmias and lacerations (9, 18, 20, 21). When available, paracentesis should be performed with echocardiographic or computerized tomographic guidance, and with electrocardiographic and hemodynamic monitoring to improve safety. The risks of pericardiocentesis are less when the effusion is large. Fluid reaccumulation is likely. Despite its hazards, needle paracentesis is indicated as an emergency procedure in patients with cardiac tamponade and as a diagnostic procedure when other causes such as tuberculosis are reasonably suspected. When used therapeutically, it is probably advisable in most instances to carry out tube drainage. Nevertheless, a definitive surgical procedure is often required within 48 h. Definitive surgical drainage of the pericardium usually requires total pericardectomy or anterior pericardectomy (21, 22). Small pericardial windows easily close allowing reaccumulation of fluid and requiring additional surgery. Subxiphoid windows should, therefore, probably be restrictded to only the poorest risk patients.

It is not clear how aggressive therapy should be for patients who are incidentally found to have pericardial effusion by echocardiography, especially when performed for other indications and when asymptomatic. These patients merit close observation, especially of arterial and venous pressure and by sequential echocardiograms. Effusions that are resolving promptly can be left alone, stable effusions may merit nonsteroidal anti-inflammatory drugs, and expanding effusions probably should be approached aggressively with elective surgical drainage.

HYPERTROPHIC CARDIOMYOPATHY

Although a specific uremic cardiomyopathy has been suspected for many years (1, 23), its existence has been doubted and difficult to identify amid the many potential causes of cardiac dysfunction in patients with renal failure. Recent echocardiografphic studies of patients undergoing long term dialysis reveal a high prevalence of concentric myocardial hypertrophy and asymmetric septal hypertrophy unaccounted for by hypertension or atherosclerosis (24–27). In addition to hypertension, risk factors for myocardial hypertrophy in uremic patients appear to be uncontrolled azotemia, a large arteriovenous fistula, anemia, hyperparathyroidism, circulatory overload, β adrenergic stimuli and excess catecholamines. The uremic myocardium shows decreased chronotropic and inotropic responses to vagal and cervical sympathetic stimuli (28), as seen in other forms of congestive heart failure. This presynaptic and postsynaptic inhibition could be interpreted as indicating a high basal level of catecholamine stimulation but could also reflect a decreased energy level of the myocardium. Interestingly, it has been concluded that the left ventricular posterior wall thickness correlates inversely with plasma immunoreactive parathyroid hormone levels, and the extent of hypertrophy is actually inadequate for the stress on the ventricle (29). This is reflected by an increase in the ratio left ventricular radius/ posterior wall thickness. Left ventricular end diastolic dimensions correlate with the severity of anemia and the size of the arteriovenous fistula. The role of autonomic neuropathy in the pathogenesis of uremic cardiomyopathy and left ventricular dysfunction is not clear. Evidence for such neuropathy includes reduced beat-to-beat variation (R-R interval) consistent with loss of vagal tone, an abnormality that correlates with volume unresponsive hypotension, and one that is corrected by renal transplantation (30). Autonomic dysfunction may relate to resistance to the action of catecholamines. At a 50% maximal oxygen consumption exercise, there is an exaggerated norepinephrine (but not epinephrine) response but a blunted rise in heart rate and systolic blood pressure (31).

Clinical effects of uremic cardiomyopathy include an imparied response to fluid overload precipitating congestive heart failure, an increased incidence of ventricular arrhythmias induced by hemodialysis, more frequent episodes of dialysis hypotension and decreased myocardial contractility (23, 32, 33).

Until the pathogenesis of uremic cardiomyopathy is understood better its prevention can only depend on general measures to improve control of azotemia and nutrition. Control of secondary hyperparathyroidism seems particularly important. For patients with cardiomyopathy, management of salt and water balance and of anemia and restriction of arteriovenous fistula flow are pertinent.

LEFT VENTRICULAR DYSFUNCTION

Although cardiac output and cardiac index are often normal, the values are elevated in a high percentage of patients with renal failure and mean values of dialysis patients are typically increased (9, 34, 35). Major pathogenetic factors

for these changes and for the high left ventricular stroke work index are the pressure and volume loads and the anemia. Impaired contractility is indicated by declining stroke volume and ejection fraction, along with rising left ventricular end systolic and end diastolic volumes. In uremic patients contractility indices decrease with ejection volume and ejection fraction declining, while left ventricular end systolic volume and end diastolic volume increase (34, 36, 37). These cardiac abnormalities appear to begin relatively early during the course of chronic renal failure but are tolerated while at rest. The low left ventricular ejection fraction correlates with impaired exercise tolerance, which in turn is associated with unemployment. Hence, cardiac abnormalities are a major impediment to rehabilitation in patients undergoing dialysis. The impaired ventricular ejection relates to decreased fractional shortening of myocardial fibers and a decreased velocity of circumferential fiber shortening. These abnormalities may reflect impaired energy metabolism of the myocardium.

Acute effects of hemodialysis on left ventricular function

Numerous factors changed by dialysis affect cardiac performance. Among these are blood pressure, extracellular fluid volume, pH, acetate loading, and serum concentrations of calcium and potassium. Hence, depending on the presence or absence of underlying cardiovascular disease and the particulars of the dialysis technique the acute effects of hemodialysis on myocardial performance may vary.

Hemodialysis accelerates the velocity of circumferential fiber shortening, the velocity of posterior wall movement and the velocity of movement of the intraventricular septum increasing the speed of left ventricular ejection, raising stroke volume and lowering end diastolic volume (38). In patients with marked circulatory overload the changes may be more pronounced, while underlying myocardial disease may blunt these responses. During isolated ultrafiltration as extracellular fluid volume decreases blood pressure remains constant; cardiac output may decrease while peripheral resistance rises (39). During hemodialysis without ultrafiltration, the strength and rapidity of myocardial contractility increase raising the left ventricular ejection fraction, stroke volume, heart rate and cardiac output (39). Blood pressure rises although peripheral resistance does not change. The increase in myocardial contractility and cardiac output occurring during isolated hemodialysis can reduce myocardial oxygen balance associated with increased utilization of oxygen leading to transitory underperfusion of the myocardium (40). Acetate loading depresses myocardial function and lowers peripheral resistance. Hence, unless bicarbonate dialysis is used, improved myocardial contractility may not be recognized at least until about an hour afterward. After dialysis, not only is baseline ejection time faster but the ejection fraction also increases with exercise in patients with underlying ventricular dysfunction (41). Before dialysis, exercise does not raise the ejection fractoin in such patients and may even lower it. Patients undergoing continuous ambulatory peritoneal dialysis (CAPD) have cardiodynamic indices that resemble those post hemodialysis with a reasonably rapid velocity of circumferential fiber shortening and a lower cardiac index and heart rate than is observed in uremic patients awaiting treatment (42). Possible explanations for more normal values in the CAPD population include lower extracellular fluid volume, less anemia and lower concentrations of toxic middle molecules.

HEART FAILURE

Despite the salutary effects of dialysis, heart failure is a leading cause of death among dialysis patients (7, 43). Hypertension accounts for more than one-third of the cases of congestive heart failure which is often precipitated by fluid overload. The pathogenesis of cardiac failure in patients undergoing dialysis is often multifactorial, however (44). Pathogenetic factors are outlined in Table 4. Hypertension is the most important underlying factor, not only because it complicates about 80% of patients with chronic renal failure but also because it is correctable in the majority of patients. Yet, chronic hypertension, when not accelerated, usually is associated with left ventricular hypertrophy but compensated myocardial function. Salt and water excess, inadequately controlled by dietary restriction and dialysis, is frequently the precipitant of congestive heart failure (41). In this regard enhanced sodium removal by CAPD with good tolerance may reduce the incidence of congestive heart failure. Anemia with hematocrit values below 30% is often associated with a high cardiac output. The added blood flow of a large arteriovenous fistula also demands an increased cardiac output which may precipitate heart failure (45). These factcors are also correctable by management of anemia with blood transfusion, erythropoietin therapy, when available, and such treatments as iron repletion or by banding or revising an oversized angioaccess. The damaged myocardium or the inelastic hypertrophied ventricle may be unable to increase cardiac output sufficiently for these stresses or eject forcefully enough during tachyarrhythmias or adapt to increased metabolic demands provoked, for example by infection, and thus may fail. In addition to hypertension, the major cause of myocardial damage in uremic patients are coronary atherosclerosis and cardiomyopathy. Subpopulations of uremic patients may be more vulnerable to cardiac failure because

the underlying disease that precipitated renal failure also involves the heart. Examples include diabetic vasculopathy, collagen vascular diseases, amyloidosis and oxalosis. Others may incur myocardial damage by accumulation of oxalate or other calcium salts or iron in the heart muscle.

Management of heart failure

The principles underlying the prevention and treatment of heart failure in uremic patients are those that apply to other populations with some important modifications. Prevention begins with control of blood pressure and extracellular fluid volume.

Typically, dialysis patients have very high plasma levels of immunoreactive atrial natriuretic peptide (e.g. 184 pmol/l vs control values of 11 pmol/l) exceeding the levels usually seen with heart failure (46). Rapid decrements with isolated ultrafiltration, more rapid than those with dialysis, are consistent with nonrenal elimination of this peptide and physiological responsiveness in uremic patients, suggesting its value as a marker of fluid excess.

Prevention of volume overload is a very high priority. This hinges on dietary sodium and water restriction and on ultrafiltration during dialysis. For most uremic patients, renal failure is so severe that diuretics are ineffective and their impaired elimination induces cumulative toxicity. After reduction of extracellular fluid volume, many patients with renal failure benefit from antihypertensive drugs with appropriate dosage modification.

Dialysis also prevents heart failure by controlling metabolite concentrations that may inhibit myocardial function and aggravate anemia. Control of anemia by reducing blood loss, adequate nutrition, iron repletion and anabolic steroids is also prophylaxis for myocardial failure. Monitoring and managing lipid abnormalities should have long term benefit in controlling atherosclerosis. Renal failure should not preempt the need for exercise programs, which have been shown to be beneficial in patients undergoing hemodialysis (31).

Echocardiografphy and radionuclide left ventriculography may be used to assess valvular function and the effects of vasodilator therapy, while coronary angiography may be performed to evaluate myocardial perfusion (33, 47). Despite the risks, patients with renal failure should be considered condidates for prophylactic cardiovascular surgery when indicated (48).

Treatment of heart failure in dialyzed patients includes bed rest and adequate oxygenation. Excess fluid should be removed by ultrafiltration; massive excesses require prolonging treatment rather than accelerating it. When removal of volume excess does not achieve adequate improvement, digitalization is warranted with appropriate adjustment of dosage and monitoring of plasma levels. Precipitating causes of heart failure such as tachyarrhythmias, systemic infection, endocarditis, pneumonia or pulmonary embolism should be corrected as necessary. Aminophylline is usually well tolerated and vasodilators for afterload reduction or vasopressor therapy may be indicated in selected patients.

Table 4. Pathogenesis of heart failure associated with renal failure

---

Hypertension: increased peripheral resistance, left ventricular
      hypertrophy
Fluid overload: ventricular dilatation
Anemia: high cardiac output
Coronary atherosclerosis: ischemic myocardial damage,
      dysfunction
Uremic cardiomyopathy: ventricular dysfunction, arrhythmias
Arteriovenous fistula: high cardiac output
Malnutrition: decreased myocardial energy, high output (beri-beri)
Associated systemic diseases: vasculitis, amyloid, oxalosis

With high output heart failure consideration should be given to reducing the fistula flow rate, especially if Branham's sign is present, and to raising the hematocrit by transfusion.

CORONARY ATHEROSCLEROSIS

After Lindner et al (6) emphasized the high prevalence of atherosclerosis in patients treated by maintenance dialysis, several reports (7,43) have confirmed that coronary atherosclerosis is a major contributor to their mortality, accounting directly for death in about 10% of the group. Most of the factors predisposing to atherosclerosis antedate initiation of dialysis treatment and the high prevalence of the disease may relate in part to the patient's survival despite the comorbidity of uremia (49, 50). Controlled for the presence of risk factors, there does not appear to be an increased incidence of atherosclerosis (51) and it is not established that dialysis, per se, as opposed to renal failure, augments these predispositions.

The predisposing risk factors for coronary disease in patients treated by dialysis include hypertension, smoking, diabetes mellites, male sex, hyperlipidemia, hyperparathyroidism, glucose intolerance, hyperuricemia, platelet activation and adherence, somatomedin A and polyamine retention (52–54). In some studies, however, hyperlipemia and hyperuricemia are less critical determinants (51, 55). Exercise lowers the risk. In addition to hypertension an unfavorable VLDL/HDL cholesterol ratio at the onset of dialysis treatment is a poor prognostic sign (56) but a long duration of dialysis therapy does not increase the incidence of coronary atherosclerosis. Indeed, the prevalence of coronary artery disease in long term survivors on dialysis is low. It has been recognized, however, that prolonged dietary protein restriction in lieu of initiating early hemodialysis aggravates the clinical and metabolic problems of atherosclerosis (57).

Although atherosclerosis may induce intermittent claudication or transient cerebral ischemia or stroke, morbidity more frequently derives from angina, arrhythmia and myocardial infarction. Ischemic electrocardiographic abnormalities induced by exercise occur in about 25% of dialysis patients and impede rehabilitation (37). Fluid volume overload is poorly tolerated in patients with depressed myocardial function secondary to coronary artery disease and may contribute to symptoms. Moreover, in patients treated by maintenance hemodialysis, disabling angina pectoris may occur despite angiographically normal coronary arteries (58). In view of underlying cardiomyopathy, anemia, severe hypertension and the arteriovenous fistula, increased myocardial oxygen consumption is not surprising in these patients. Thallium[201] studies of myocardial perfusion reveal such abnormalities as areas of spotty uptake consistent with infarction, or severe ischemia in more than half of the patients studied (59). Although many of these patients were asymptomatic at the time of study, these abnormalities carried a poor prognosis for one year survival. Hemodialysis itself by increasing cardiac output and decreasing myocardial oxygen balance may induce transitory underperfusion of the myocardium (40).

Treatment of angina pectoris in uremic patients does not differ from that of patients with normal renal function except for the emphasis on extracellular fluid volume control and control of anemia and other potential precipitating factors. Nitroglycerin, isosorbide dinitrate, calcium channel blockers and propranolol are tolerated as well as in nonuremic patients.

The acute management of myocardial infarction is similar to that in nonuremic patients. Emphasis should be placed on relief of pain and anxiety, prevention and control of arrhythmias, heart failure and thromboembolism. Fluid restriction should be rigidly conducted. Rapid ultrafiltration-dialysis should be avoided for the first few days to maintain hemodynamic stability and avoid electrolyte imbalance potentially inducing arrhythmias. Digitalis should be used only if strongly indicated and following pharmacokinetic principles. Anticoagulants may be beneficial and are prescribed as for nonuremic patients.

Long term management of myocardial infarction is similar to treatment of those with normal renal function, with emphasis placed on control of hypertension, anemia and fluid overload to reduce the cardiac workload.

Arrhythmias may require long term prophylaxis. Vasodilators such as nitrates, β adrenergic blockers or calcium channel blockers can be beneficial. Long term use of antiplatelet agents such as dipyridamole or aspirin is also well tolerated. The long term use of eicosapentaenoic acid to lower cholesterol has not been studied specifically in uremic patients, although in the short term it significantly reduces serum triglycerides, cholesterol and phospholipids (60). The use of clofibrate can be hazardous in patients with renal failure. Coronary angiography is of value, as in nonuremic patients, to determine whether coronary revascularization is indicated (61). Because of the dangers of iodide toxicity to residual renal function the use of angiography should be selective, the iodide dose kept minimal and hydration maintained.

BACTERIAL ENDOCARDITIS

The clinical course of renal failure is complicated by bacterial endocarditis in about 5% of patients (62–64). This complication is potentially devastating and requires aggressive treatment.

The patients are predisposed to infective endocarditis because of their propensity to infection and because of the presence of endothelial or endocardial abnormalities or both. Susceptibility to infection relates to the effect of uremia itself, to such immunosuppressive drugs as adrenal corticosteroids and to the frequent exposure to invasive procedures including dialysis, often associated with indwelling external conduits. The internal arteriovenous fistula or prosthesis induces intimal injury by causing turbulent blood flow, thereby creating a nidus for infection to occur and decreasing the clearance of pathogenic organisms from the circulation (65). Chronic bacteremia predisposes the patient to infection of the heart valve. Abnormal heart valves, as occur with congenital or rheumatic heart disease, are more vulnerable to infection. Up to 9% of patients with renal failure have aortic diastolic murmurs related to hypertension and to their high cardiac output and systolic flow murmurs are even more frequent. Valvular abnormalities demonstrated echocardiographically occur in about 10% of patients; these involve the mitral or aortic valve, usually are calcific and correlate with phosphate retention and hyperparathyroidism (66–68).

The diagnosis of bacterial endocarditis is often difficult, but more so in uremic patients, causing delays in appropriate treatment. Fever may be blunted by uremia but is usually obvious in well dialyzed patients but easily incorrectly attributed to other causes such as pyrogenic reactions. Prolonged or recurrent fever should always raise the suspicion of endocarditis. Similarly, petechiae, malaise and neurological changes are readily misinterpreted as part of the uremic syndrome. The index of suspicion of endocarditis should be high and blood cultures obtained whenever fever is unexplained or persists. *Staphylococcus aureus* is the most frequent organism identified, although *Streptococcus viridans*, *Enterococcus* and *Listeria monocytogenes* infections also occur. Frequent careful auscultation, echocardiography and detection of regurgitant jets by the Doppler technique may aid in the diagnosis.

Treatment consists of a 6-week course of parenteral antibiotics chosen according to the organism identified and following pharmacokinetic principles. Often, valvular replacement is required (69). Complications of endocarditis in these patients include septic emboli, valvular perforation and heart failure.

CARDIOVASCULAR SURGERY

When indicated, patients should not be denied the benefits of cardiovascular surgery; renal failure does not add prohibitively to the risk. The surgical mortality of pericardectomy has been reduced to below 3% (9). Coronary artery bypass grafts and cardiac valvuloplasty have acceptable mortality rates, not worse than those for patients with normal renal function, although the morbidity may be higher (48, 69). Endocarditis is the most frequent reason for the requirement of valve replacement. Coronary revascularization is usually indicated by angina that is unresponsive to control of hypertension and fluid excess and to drug therapy. Dialysis should precede and follow cardiac surgery in order to control hyperkalemia and fluid overload, and thereby reduce the risks associated with the procedure. Severe coronary artery disease should be corrected before renal transplantation is undertaken. Although a salutary effect of coronary revascularization on the survival rate of dialysis patients has not been clearly established, the improvement in patient morbidity achieved by the procedure has been more convincing. Angina is usually relieved and exercise tolerance improves (61).

ARRHYTHMIAS

Numerous factors increase the vulnerability of uremic patients to arrhythmias as enumerated in Table 5. Underlying heart disease is often present leading to focal areas of myocardial injury and ischemia. Arteriosclerotic coronary artery disease or pericarditis may precipitate arrhythmias by inducing ischemic myocardial damage. Frequently, acute arrhythmias correlate with disturbances in electrolyte concentrations and distribution. Hyperkalemia decreases myocardial conduction leading toward cardiac arrest unless arrhythmias supervene which may culminate in ventricular fibrillation. It is presumed that a high fraction of the approximately 10% of deaths of patients treated by dialysis which are attributed to cardiac arrest (43) are accounted for by hyperkalemia. Cardiotoxicity of potassium is more likely when associated with hyponatremia, hypocalcemia, acidosis, a high extracellular:intracellular concentration ratio and a rapid rate of extracellular increase (70). Uremic patients often have intracellular potassium depletion associated with hyperkalemia that rapidly accelerates between dialyses in association with acidosis and fluid retention diluting extracellular sodium. Hypokalemia can also lead to myocardial necrosis and arrhythmias, expecially in hypercalcemic patients or those treated with digitalis. Hemodialysis may rapidly precipitate digitalis intoxication by altering pH and electrolyte balance. Caution should be taken whenever it is deemed necessary to lower dialysis fluid potassium below 2.0 mEq/l, monitoring cardiac rhythm in this circumstance.

Both hypocalcemia and hypercalcemia are associated with a high incidence of arrhythmia, the latter a particular risk in patients treated aggressively with calcitriol.

When patients are monitored for arrhythmia, however, serious arrhythmias are infrequent except for those with underlying heart disease (71, 72). In patients without heart disease, hemodialysis is not associated with an increased risk of ectopic myocardial activity. In those with underlying cardiopathy as evidenced by echocardiography, monitoring reveals an incidence of arrhythmias including premature ventricular contractions that approaches 50%, more than double that of the control population (32, 72). Hemodialysis induces more serious arrhythmias in about 25% of these patients characterized by couplets or salvos of ectopic ven-

Table 5. Risk factors for arrhythmia in dialyzed patients.

1.	Uremic cardiomyopathy
2.	Ischemic heart disease
3.	Pericarditis
4.	Systemic diseases, e.g., amyloidosis
5.	Potassium imbalance
6.	Calcium disorders
7.	Magnesium imbalance
8.	Acid-base abnormalities
9.	Hypocapnia
10.	Hypoxia
11.	Drug intoxication

tricular activity, ventricular tachycardia or atrial fibrillation, often late in the course of the procedure (73, 74). Patients treated with digitalis who undergo dialysis are especially at risk for serious arrhythmias. In view of the high death rate attributed to cardiac arrest and other causes that may present lethal arrhythmias, the identification of patients vulnerable to this complication because of underlying heart disease is mandatory. Careful control of electrolyte balance, cardiac monitoring and antiarrhythmic prophylaxis with procainamide or lidocaine is warranted in such patients.

ACKNOWLEDGEMENT

The opinions and assertions contained herein are the private views of the author and should not be construed as official or as necessarily reflecting the views of the Uniformed Services University of the Health Sciences or the Department of Defense. There is no objection to publication. The secretarial assistance of Mrs Barbara Fitzgerald is greatly appreciated.

REFERENCES

1. Schreiner GE, Maher JF: *Uremia; Biochemistry, Pathogenesis and Treatment.* Springfield, Charles C. Thomas Co, 1961
2. Drukker W, Alberts C, Ode A, Roosendaal KJ, Wilmink JM: Report on regular dialysis treatment in Europe. *Proc Eur Dial Transplant Assoc* 3: 90, 1966
3. Drukker W, Haagsma-Schouten WAG, Alberts C, Spoek MG: Report on regular dialysis treatment in Europe. *Proc Eur Dial Transplant Assoc* 7: 3, 1970
4. Brunner FP, Gurland HJ, Härlen H, Schärer K, Parsons FM: Combined report on regular dialysis and transplantation in Europe. *Proc Eur Dial Transplant Assoc* 9: 3, 1972
5. Bryan F Jr: National Dialysis Registry report. *Proc 6th Annu Contractors Conf, Artif Kidney Program*, NIAMDD, DHEW Publ No (NIH) 74–248: 201, 1973
6. Lindner A, Charra B, Sherrard DJ, Scribner BH: Accelerated atherosclerosis in prolonged maintenance hemodialysis. *N Engl J Med* 290: 697, 1974
7. Brynger H, Brunner FP, Chantler C, Donckerwolcke RA, Jacobs C, Kramer P, Selwood NH, Wing AJ: Combined report on regular dialysis and transplantation in Europe X 1979. *Proc Eur Dial Transplant Assoc* 17: 2, 1980
8. Bright R: Tabular view of the morbid appearance of 100 cases connected with albuminous urine; with observations. *Guy Hosp Rep* 1: 338, 1836
9. Drüeke T, Le Pailleur C, Zingraff J, Jungers P: Uremic cardiomyopathy and pericarditis. *Adv Nephrol* 9: 33, 1980
10. Bergström J, Fürst P: Uremic middle molecules. *Clin Nephrol* 5: 143, 1976
11. Comty CM, Wathen R, Shapiro FL: Pericarditis in chronic uremia and its sequels. *Ann Intern Med* 75: 173, 1973
12. Osanloo E, Shalhoub RJ, Cioffi RF, Parker RH: Viral pericarditis in patients receiving hemodialysis. *Arch Intern Med* 139: 309, 1979
13. Renfrew R, Buselmeier TJ, Kjellstrand CM: Pericarditis and renal failure. *Annu Rev Med* 31: 345, 1980
14. Langendorf R, Pirani CL: The heart in uremia; an electrocardiographic and pathologic study. *Am Heart J* 33: 282, 1974
15. Wacker W, Merrill JP: Uremic pericarditis in acute and chronic renal failure. *JAMA* 156: 754, 1954
16. Luft FC, Gilman JK, Weyman AE: Pericarditis in the patient with uremia: clinical and echocardiographic evaluation. *Nephron* 25: 160, 1980
17. Bailey GL, Hampers CL, Merrill JP: Reversible cardiomyopathy in uremia. *Trans Am Soc Artif Intern Organs* 13: 263, 1967
18. Minuth ANW, Nottebohm GA, Eknoyan G, Suki WN: Indomethacin treatment of pericarditis in chronic hemodialysis patients. *Arch Intern Med* 135: 807, 1975
19. Eliasson G, Murphy FF: Steroid therapy in uremic patients: A report of three cases. *JAMA* 229: 1634, 1974
20. Silverberg S, Oreopoulos DG, Wise DJ, Uden DE, Meindok H, Jones M, Rapoport A, Deveber GA: Pericarditis in patients undergoing long-term hemodialysis and peritoneal dialysis. Incidence complications and management. *Am J Med* 63: 874, 1977
21. Frame JR, Lucas SK, Pederson JA, Elkins RC: Surgical treatment of pericarditis in the dialysis patient. *Am J Surg* 146: 800, 1983
22. Ghavamian M, Gutch CF, Hughes RK, Kopp KF, Kolff WJ: Pericardial tamponade in chronic hemodialysis patients; treatment by pericardectomy. *Arch Intern Med* 131: 249, 1983
23. Raab W: Cardiotoxic substances in the blood and heart muscle in uremia (their nature and action). *J Lab Clin Med* 29: 715, 1944
24. Klein J, McLeish K, Hodsden J, Lordon R: Hypertrophic cardiomyopathy: an acquired disorder of end-stage renal disease. *Trans Am Soc Artif Intern Organs* 29: 120, 1983
25. Lai KN, Ng J, Whitford J, Buttfield I, Fossett RG, Mathew TH: Left ventricular function in uremia: echocardiographic and radionuclide assessment in patients on maintenance hemodialysis. *Clin Nephrol* 23: 125, 1985
26. Renger A, Müller M, Jutzler GA, Bette L: Echocardiographic evaluation of left ventricular dimensions and function in chronic hemodialysis patients with cardiomegaly. *Clin Nephrol* 21: 164, 1984
27. Bernardi D, Bernini L, Cini G, Ghioni S, Benechi I: Asymmetric septal hypertrophy and sympathetic overactivity in normotensive hemodialyzed patients. *Am Heart J* 109: 539, 1985
28. Yates MS, Critchley MA, Askey EA, Bowmer CJ: Cardiac reactivity in rats with acute renal failure. *J Pharm Pharmacol* 37: 175, 1985
29. London GM, Fabiani F, Marchais SJ, de Vernejoul MC, Guerin AP, Safar ME, Metivier F, Llach F: Uremic cardiomyopathy: an inadequate left ventricular hypertrophy. *Kidney Int* 31: 973, 1987
30. Endre ZH, Perl SI, Krager EW, Charlesworth JA, MacDonald GJ: Reduced cardiac beat-to-beat variation in chronic renal failure: A ubiquitous marker of autonomic neuropathy. *Clin Sci* 62: 561, 1982
31. Kettner A, Goldberg A, Harter H: Endurance exercise in hemodialysis patients. Effects on the sympathetic nervous system and serum glucose regulation. *Contrib Nephrol* 41: 269, 1984
32. Quereda C, Orte L, Martesanz R, Ortuña J: Ventricular ectopic activity in hemodialysis. *Nephron* 42: 181, 1986
33. Hung J, Harris PJ, Uren RF, Tiller DJ, Kelly DT: Uremic cardiomyopathy – effect of hemodialysis on left ventricular function in end-stage renal failure. *N Engl J Med* 302: 547, 1980
34. Hampl H, Schäfer GE, Kessel M: Hemodynamic state in severe chronic renal failure. Pathophysiological aspects of cardiovascular function and the importance of bicarbonate dialysis. *Ne-*

phron 39: 102, 1985

35. Ikram H, Lynn KL, Bailey RR, Little PJ: Cardiovascular changes in chronic hemodialysis patients. *Kidney Int* 24: 371, 1983

36. Drüeke T, Le Pailleur C, Sigal-Saglier M, Zingraff J, Crosnier J, Di Matteo J: Left ventricular function in hemodialyzed patients with cardiomegaly. *Nephron* 28: 80, 1981

37. Bullock RE, Amer HA, Simpson I, Ward MK, Hall RJC: Cardiac abnormalities and exercise tolerance in patients receiving renal replacement therapy. *Br Med J* 289: 1479, 1984

38. Gilmartin JJ, Duffy BS, Finnegan P, McCready N: Non invasive study of left ventricular function in chronic renal failure before and after hemodialysis. *Clin Nephrol* 20: 55, 1983

39. Cini G, Camici M, Pentimore F, Palla R: Echocardiographic hemodynamic study during ultrafiltration sequential dialysis. *Nephron* 30: 124, 1982

40. Pedersen T, Rasmussen K, Cleemann-Rasmussen K: Effects of hemodialysis on cardiac performance and transmural myocardial perfusion. *Clin Nephrol* 19: 31, 1983

41. Wizemann V, Kramer W, Thormann J, Kindler M: Exercise-induced ventricular dysfunction: reversible by hemodialysis. *Trans Am Soc Artif Intern Organs* 30: 567, 1984

42. Alpert MA, Van Stone J, Twardowski ZJ, Ruder MA, Whiting RB, Kelly DL, Madsen BR: Comparative cardiac effects of hemodialysis and continuous ambulatory peritoneal dialysis. *Clin Cardiol* 9: 52, 1986

43. Wing AJ, Brunner FP, Brynger H, Jacobs C, Kramer P, Selwood NH, Gretz N: Cardiovascular-related causes of death and the fate of patients with renovascular disease. *Contrib Nephrol* 41: 306, 1984

44. Comty CM, Shapiro FL: Cardiac complications of regular dialysis therapy. in *Replacemetn of Renal Function by Dialysis*, edited by Drukker W, Parsons FM, Maher JF, 2nd edition, The Hague, Martinus Nijhoff, 1983, p 595

45. Ahearn DJ, Maher JF: Heart failure as a complication of hemodialysis arteriovenous fistula. *Ann Intern Med* 77: 201, 1972

46. Wilkins MR, Wood JA, Adu D, Late CJ, Kendall MJ, Michael J: Changes in plasma immunoreactive atrial natriuretic peptide during sequential ultrafiltration and haemodialysis. *Clin Sci* 71: 157, 1986

47. Schott CR, Le Sar JF, Kotler NM, Parry WR, Segal BL: The spectrum of echocardiographic findings in chronic renal failure. *Cardiovasc Med* 3: 217, 1978

48. Rottenbourg J, Mussat T, Gandjbaklch I, Barthelemy A, Toledano D, Gahl GM, Cabrol C: Open heart surgery in patients with end-stage renal disease. *Proc Eur Dial Transplant Assoc Eur Ren Assoc* 20: 169, 1983

49. Burke JF Jr, Francos GC, Moore LL, Cho SY, Lasker N: Accelerated atherosclerosis in chronic dialysis patients – another look. *Nephron* 21: 181, 1978

50. Nichols AJ, Catto GRD, Edward N, Engeset J, Macleod M: Accelerated atherosclerosis in long term dialysis and renal-transplant patients: fact of fiction. *Lancet* 1: 276, 1980

51. Rostand SG, Gretes JC, Kirk KA, Rutsky EA, Andreoli TE: Ischemic heart disease in patients with uremia undergoing maintenance hemodialysis. *Kidney Int* 16: 600, 1979

52. Bagdade JD: Accelerated atherosclerosis in patients on maintenance dialysis. *Adv Nephrol* 9: 7, 1980

53. Hahn R, Oette K, Mondorf H, Funke K, Sieberth HG: Analysis of cardiovascular risk factors in chronic hemodialysis patients with special attention to the hyperlipoproteinemias. *Atherosclerosis* 48: 279, 1983

54. Green D, Stone NJ, Krumlovsky FA: Putative atherogenic factors in patients with chronic renal failure. *Prog Cardiovasc Dis* 26: 133, 1983

55. Degoulet P, Legrain M, Réach I, Aimé F, Devriès C, Rojas P, Jabobs C: Mortality risk factors in patients treated by chronic hemodialysis. Report of the Diaphen collaborative study. *Nephron* 31: 103, 1982

56. Kindler J, Sieberth HG, Hahn R, Glöckner WM, Vlako M, Pelzer R: Does atherosclerosis caused by dialysis limit this treatment. *Proc Eur Dial Transplant Assoc* 19: 168, 1982

57. Bonomini V, Feletti C, Scolari MP, Stefoni S, Vangelista SA: Atherosclerosis in uremia: a longitudinal study. *Am J Clin Nutr* 33: 1493, 1980

58. Roig E, Betriu A, Castoñer A, Magrina J, Sanz G, Navarro-Lopez F: Disabling angina pectoris with normal coronary arteries in patients undergoing long-term hemodialysis. *Am J Med* 71: 431, 1981

59. Dudczak R, Fridrich L, Derfler K, Kletter K, Frischauf H, Marosi L, Schmidt P, Zazgornik J: Myocardial studies in haemodialysis patients. *Proc Eur Dial Transplant Assoc* 21:251, 1984

60. Hamazaki T, Nakazawa R, Tateno S, Shishido H, Isoda K, Hattori Y, Yoshida T, Fujita T, Yano S, Kumagi A: Effects of fish oil rich in eicosapentaenoic acid on serum lipid in hyperlipidemic hemodialysis patients. *Kidney Int* 26: 81, 1984

61. Francis GS, Sharma BIM, Collins AJ, Helseth HK, Comty CM: Coronary artery surgery in patients with end-stage renal disease. *Ann Intern Med* 92: 499, 1980

62. Leonard A, Raij L, Shapiro FL: Bacterial endocarditis in regularly dialyzed patients. *Kidney Int* 4: 407, 1973

63. Ayus JC, Frommer JP, Young JB: Cardiovascular complications of uremia and dialysis. in *Therapy of Renal Diseases and Related Disorders*, edited by Suki WN, Massry SG, The Hague, Martinus Nijhoff, 1984, p 483

64. Cross AS, Steigbigel RT: Infective endocarditis and access site infections in patients on hemodialysis. *Medicine* 55: 453, 1976

65. Lillehei CW, Bobb JRR, Visscher MB: Occurrence of endocarditis with valvular deformities in dogs with arteriovenous fistulae. *Proc Soc Exp Biol Med* 75: 9, 1950

66. Forman MB, Virmani R, Robertson RM, Stone WJ: Mitral annular calcification in chronic renal failure. *Chest* 85: 367, 1984

67. Maher ER, Curtis JR: Calcific aortic stenosis in chronic renal failure. *Lancet* 2: 1007, 1985

68. Scharf S, Wexler J, Longnecker RE, Blaufox MD: Cardiovascular disease in patients on chronic hemodialytic therapy. *Progr Cardiovasc Dis* 22: 343, 1980

69. Laws KH, Merrill WH, Harman JW, Prager RL, Bender HW Jr: Cardiac surgery in patients with chronic renal disease. *Ann Thorac Surg* 42: 152, 1986

70. Merrill JP: *The Treatment of Renal Failure: Therapeutic Principles in the Management of Acute and Chronic Uremia*. New York, Grune & Stratton, 1955, p 238

71. Wizemann V, Kramer W, Funke T, Schutterle G: Dialysis-induced cardiac arrhythmias: fact or fiction. Importance of preexisting cardiac disease in the inducction of arrhythmias during renal replacement therapy. *Nephron* 39: 356, 1985

72. Blumberg A, Hausermann M, Strub B, Jenzer HR: Cardiac arrhythmias in patients on maintenance hemodialysis. *Nephron* 33: 91, 1983

73. Niwa A, Taniguchi K, Ito H, Nagawa S, Takeuchi J, Sasaoka T, Kanayama M: Echocardiographic and Holter findings in 321 uremic patients on maintenance hemodialysis. *Jpn Heart J* 26: 403, 1985

74. Ramirez G, Brueggemeyer CD, Newton JL: Cardiac arrhythmias on hemodialysis in chronic renal failure patients. *Nephron* 36: 212, 1984

HYPERLIPIDAEMIA AND ATHEROSCLEROSIS IN CHRONIC DIALYSIS PATIENTS

DAVID C. WHEELER, PAUL SWENY, ZACHARIAH VARGHESE and
JOHN F. MOORHEAD

INTRODUCTION

The association between hyperlipidaemia and kidney disease was first noted in 1827 by Bright who described lactescent serum in patients with the nephrotic syndrome. The advent of dialysis and renal transplantation has allowed more detailed study of lipoprotein metabolism in chronic renal failure and accumulating evidence of accelerated atherosclerosis in these patients has renewed interest in uraemic hyperlipidaemia. This chapter will document the lipid and lipoprotein abnormalities observed in dialysis patients, will outline the possible mechanisms involved in their aetiology and will discuss how such abnormalities may represent risk factors in the pathogenesis of atherosclerosis.

Many studies have demonstrated that lipid abnormalities occur in patients with chronic renal failure before and after institution of dialysis therapy (1). The most common lipid abnormality observed is hypertriglyceridaemia and corresponds to type IV of the Frederickson classification. The reported incidence of this abnormality in dialysis patients has varied between 28 and 100% (2). Comparison of peritoneal and haemodialysis patients shows a similar frequency in both groups (3). A 5 year follow-up study of 220 haemodialysis patients showed that triglyceride levels did not rise with time (4).

There is now considerable evidence that patients on renal replacement therapy experience an increased risk of death from ischaemic heart disease. Hyperlipidaemia is likely to be an important risk factor in the development of premature atherosclerosis in such patients, but the serum triglyceride levels observed do not adequately explain the increased incidence of myocardial infarction and it is possible that subtle changes in lipoprotein particles may increase their atherogenicity (5). In addition, many patients with chronic renal failure have abnormal lipids for several years prior to initiation of renal replacement therapy. Lipoprotein patterns during this period may differ from those observed in the dialysis population, particularly in nephrotic patients, and may represent a more significant risk factor for the development of atherosclerosis.

Although renal transplantation is outside the scope of this book it is important to appreciate that hyperlipidaemia continues to affect many renal allograft recipients even when graft function is normal. Following transplantation, cholesterol levels tend to rise and HDL cholesterol may return to normal. Transplant patients continue to experience an increased incidence of death from ischaemic heart disease when compared with the normal population (6) and lipid abnormalities likewise constitute an important risk factor in these patients.

HYPERLIPIDAEMIA

Normal lipoprotein metabolism

Before discussing the abnormalities observed in uraemia, normal lipoprotein metabolism will be described (Figure 1). Cholesterol and triglyceride are virtually insoluble in water and circulate in the bloodstream associated with proteins in lipoprotein particles. These particles are composed of a core containing cholesterol esters and triglyceride surrounded by an outer coating of phospholipids, unesterified cholesterol and apoproteins. Differences in protein and lipid composition allow classification of particles into five major groups which can be roughly separated by ultracentrifugation. The properties of these five groups, chylomicrons (CM), very low density lipoproteins (VLDL), intermediate density lipoproteins (IDL) low density lipoproteins (LDL) and high density lipoproteins (HDL) are outlined in Table 1. This

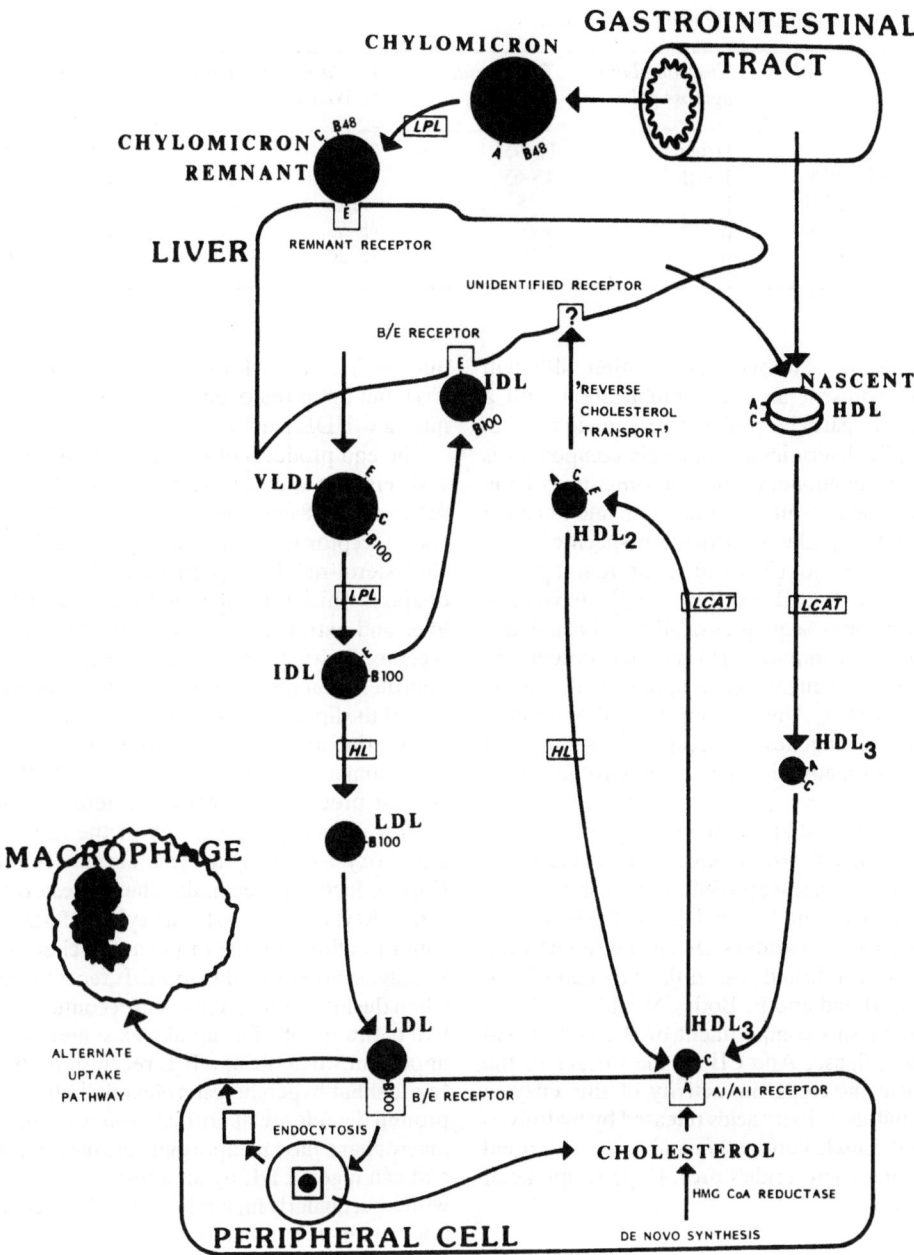

Figure 1. Normal lipoprotein metabolism. Chylomicrons are synthesised in the gut from dietary lipids and hydrolysed by lipoprotein lipase (LPL) leaving remnants which are taken up by the liver via a specific receptor. Very low density lipoprotein (VLDL) is synthesised and secreted by the liver and hydrolysed by LPL and hepatic lipase (HL) to intermediate density lipoprotein (IDL) and low density lipoprotein (LDL). LDL delivers cholesterol to peripheral tissues by binding to the apo B/E receptor. Internalisation of bound lipoprotein supresses cellular cholesterol synthesis by inhibiting 3-hydroxy-3-methylglutaryl coenzyme A reductase (HMG CoA reductase). Nascent high density lipoprotein (HDL) is synthesised by the gut and liver and accepts cholesterol from overladen cells. Scavanged cholesterol is subsequently hydrolysed by lecithin-cholesterol acyltransferase (LCAT) and the mature HDL particle is probably taken up by the liver via an unidentified receptor.

Table 1. Physicochemical properties of human lipoproteins.

Class	Density g/ml	Electromobility agarose-gel	Triglyceride % Weight	Esterified cholesterol % Weight	Major apoproteins
Chylomicrons	>0.95	Origin	80–95	2–4	AI, B48, C1, CII, E
VLDL	0.95–1.006	Pre-β	45–65	16–22	B100, CI, CII, CIII, E
IDL	1.006–1.019	β	~35	~25	B100, E
LDL	1.019–1.063	β	4–8	45–50	B100
HDL	1.063–1.210	α	2–7	15–20	AI, AII, CI, CII, CIII, E

separation is not absolute and such classification, although convenient, may represent an over simplification with a complete spectrum of particles probably existing in circulation. The genetically determined apoprotein component is vitally important in maintaining the conformation of the particle, in influencing enzymatic degradation and in acting as a ligand for cellular uptake of particles by specific receptors (7). At least eight major classes of apoprotein (apo AI, AII, B48, B100, C1, CII, CIII and E [Table 2]), have been identified and the primary sequences of all have been determined. The apoprotein composition of each lipoprotein subclass is well defined although several apoproteins can exchange between particles. The identification of abnormalities of apoproteins, their genes and receptors has improved our understanding of many disorders of lipoprotein metablolism (8).

Chylomicrons, the largest lipoproteins, are synthesised in the intestine from dietary triglycerides and cholesterol. These particles initially possess apo B48, apo A1 and AII but acquire apo CI, CII, CIII and E from HDL in the lymphatic system. VLDL particles are synthesised and secreted by the liver, are rich in triglyceride and possess the larger apo B100, apo CI, CII and CIII and apo E. Both CM and VLDL are hydrolyzed in the plasma compartment by the endothelial enzyme lipoprotein lipase. Apo CII on the surface of the lipoprotein particle increases the activity of this enzyme whilst apo CIII inhibits it. Fatty acids released by hydrolysis provide energy for muscle contraction and are re-esterified in adipocytes to form triglyceride stores. Hepatic uptake of

Table 2. Molecular mass and functions of human apoproteins.

Class	Molecular mass Daltons	Functions
AI	28,000	Activation LCAT
AII	17,000	–
B48	264,000	–
B100	549,000	Ligand for LDL receptor
C1	6,500	Activation LCAT
CII	8,800	Activation lipoprotein lipase
CIII	8,750	Inhibition lipoprotein lipase
E	~ 36,000	Ligand for LDL receptor

intermediate particles is inhibited by the presence of apo CIII, but this is removed along with apo A and incorporated into new HDL particles.

The end products of CM and VLDL metabolism are the CM remnant and LDL respectively. The CM remnant possesses apo B48 and apo E and is avidly taken up by the liver via a receptor which appears to be specific for apo E. The cholesterol-rich LDL particles each have a single molecule of apo B which is recognised by the apo B/E receptor of the liver and extrahepatic tissues. Binding to this cell surface receptor is followed by internalization of the receptor/lipoprotein complex, recycling of the receptor and degradation of the lipoprotein by lysosomal enzymes thus delivering triglyceride and cholesterol to the cell. To maintain cholesterol homeostasis, internalization of LDL regulates three cellular processes. Firstly cholesterol synthesis by the cell itself is slowed by supression of the rate-limiting enzyme, 3-hydroxy-3-methylglutaryl coenzyme A reductase (HMG CoA reductase). Secondly, the cholesterol-esterifying enzyme, Acyl CoA cholesterol acyltransferase (ACAT) is activated to allow storage of incoming cholesterol in the cell. Finally, synthesis of the apo B/E receptor itself is inhibited when the intracellular cholesterol content rises (9). Alternative pathways of LDL uptake exist and may be particularly important when the apo B/E receptor is absent or defective (eg familial hypercholesterolaemia [10]), or when the apoprotein ligands are abnormal as may occur in uraemia. The macrophage has an important role in scavanging cholesterol and can ingest LDL by an alternative receptor mechanism with a particularly high affinity for the acetylated form of the lipoprotein (11). Macrophages that have taken up large amounts of cholesterol becoming laden with cholesterol-ester droplets (foam cells) are found in atheromatous plaques and this back-up pathway of cholesterol metabolism may contribute to lipid deposition in the atheromatous plaque.

High density lipoproteins, a group of small heterogeneous particles, are synthesized by the liver and intestine and secreted as discoid precursors possessing apo AI, AII and C. These precursors are converted to mature spherical particles by the enzyme lecithin-cholesterol acyltransferase (LCAT) which catalyses the esterification of cholesterol. During maturation, HDL accepts lipids from the triglyceride-rich lipoproteins and from cell membranes. Cholesterol laden cells bind HDL, possibly via a receptor, promoting efflux of lipid stores (12). This process, termed reverse cholesterol

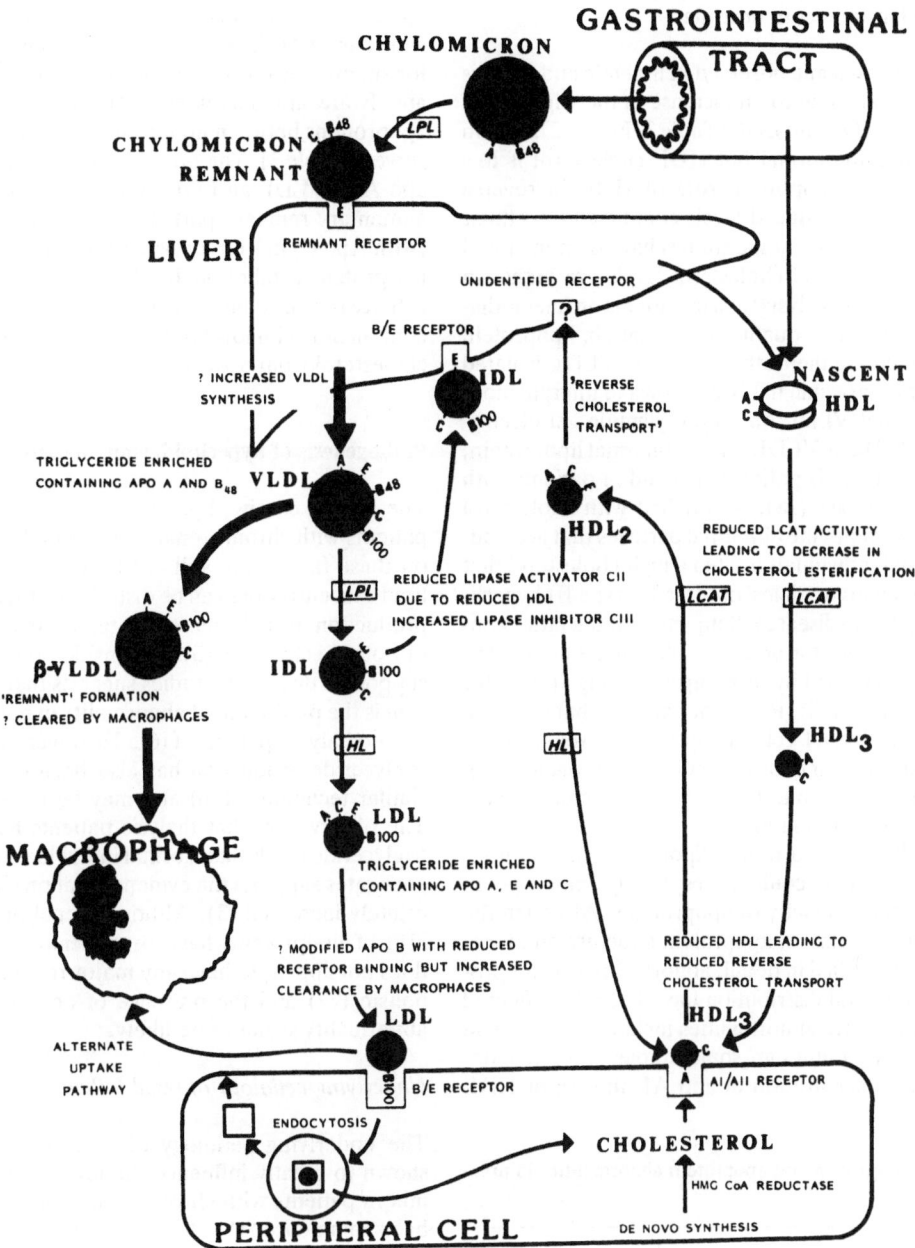

Figure 2. Abnormalities of lipoprotein metabolism in uraemia. Hepatic VLDL synthesis may be increased and catabolism is impaired due to deficient lipoprotein and hepatic lipase activity. VLDL remnants which are not cleared efficiently by the apo B/E receptor are taken up by macrophages via the alternative pathway. LDL particles are enriched with triglyceride and possess an abnormal complement of apoproteins which uraemic toxins may modify. Receptor binding of this particle is probably also reduced and it may also be cleared by macrophages. Reduced HDL levels and LCAT activity impair reverse cholesterol transport and lead to cellular cholesterol accumulation.

transport, may explain the negative correlation between HDL cholesterol and accelerated vascular disease (13). During maturation the apoprotein content of HDL is also modified. Apo E orginating from VLDL and CM displaces apo AI to become predominant, apo AI circulating back to newly formed HDL particles. The fate of mature HDL remains uncertain. It may be taken up by peripheral tissues in the same way as LDL via the apo B/E receptor but hepatic uptake is important if excess cholesterol is to be excreted via the biliary tract. The nature of the hepatic HDL receptor remains uncertain but appears to be distinct from both the chylomicron remnant and apo B/E receptors.

Lipoprotein abnormalities in uraemia

The hypertriglyceridaemia observed in uraemic and dialysis patients is essentially due to an increase in the triglyceride content of VLDL, IDL and LDL (Table 3, Figure 2). Serum cholesterol is usually normal but HDL cholesterol is low (14). Because of the important role of HDL in reverse cholesterol transport, reduced levels could lead to cellular cholesterol accumulation. Some studies have demonstrated that both triglyceride and cholesterol levels are higher in patients on peritoneal dialysis than in patients on haemodialysis (15, 16). In addition qualitative changes in lipoprotein particles may increase their atherogenicity. VLDL isolated from patients with uraemia has been shown to migrate more slowly than normal VLDL on polyacrylamide gel electrophoresis (so called beta-VLDL). This abnormal lipoprotein, found in 58% of dialysis patients (17) and in patients with coronary artery disease (18), is enriched with cholesterol and apo E. It resembles the abnormal particles that accumulate when normal individuals are fed a high-cholesterol diet (19) and the 'remnant particles' observed in type III hyperlipidaemia (broad beta disease). Subjects with the latter condition are homozygous for an apo E phenotype designated E2 which is characterised by its reduced binding affinity for the apo B/E receptor (20). Remnant particles that circulate as a result of decreased cellular uptake are removed by macrophages and appear to be particularly atherogenic (19). The incidence of ischaemic heart disease is considerably increased in this condition (20).

Because of their central role in lipoprotein metabolism, changes in apoproteins could be especially important in increasing the atherogenicity of lipoproteins. Although the effects of uraemic toxins on apoprotein structure and function has not been studied in detail, abnormalities of apoprotein concentration and distribution have been documented (Table 3). Quantitative abnormalities include a decrease in total apo A levels, (although some studies have demonstrated that the concentration of apo AI, the major HDL apoprotein, is normal [21]). Apo CII levels are decreased whilst apo CIII increased, creating an unfavourable activator/suppressor ratio for lipoprotein lipase (2, 22). Levels of apo B are also increased (23). Abnormal distribution of apoproteins between lipoprotein particles has also been observed (Table 3). The presence of apo B48 in VLDL and of apo A in VLDL an LDL suggest a greater contribution of alimentary remnant particles (24). The presence of apo E (with Apo C) in LDL provides further evidence of defective lipoprotein catabolism by lipoprotein lipase (24). LCAT activity is also reduced in uraemic patients (25) and this, in conjunction with low HDL levels may impair the removal of cholesterol from tissues.

Pathogenesis of hyperlipidaemia in dialysis patients

The factors causing lipid and lipoprotein abnormalities in patients with chronic renal failure and the effects of dialysis on these factors are still not fully understood (1). Plasma lipid concentrations can be disturbed either by an increase in production, by a decrease in catabolism or by a combination of both mechanisms (3). A considerable body of evidence supported by kinetic studies suggests that defective catabolism is the predominant abnormality in both peritoneal- and haemodialysis patients (16). However, increased hepatic triglyceride production has also been demonstrated using similar techniques (26) and may be a contributing factor. The observation that dialysis patients have higher serum triglyceride levels than normal individuals with similar clearance rates supports the evidence that production is inappropriately increased (3). Although renal uptake and catabolism of lipoproteins have been demonstrated, the kidney does not appear to have any major role in lipoprotein catabolism (27) and the presence of an extrarenal metabolic abnormality seems more likely.

Underlying aetiology of renal failure

The underlying aetiology of renal disease has not been shown to greatly influence the level of hypertriglyceridaemia in patients with chronic renal failure once dialysis has been commenced (5). A lower total serum cholesterol level has been demonstrated in patients with glomerulonephritis. This contrasts with the high cholesterol levels in patients with glomerular disease and the nephrotic syndrome with relatively well preserved renal function (28).

Insulin resistance

Increased hepatic lipoprotein production appears to be important in the hyperlipidaemia associated with the nephrotic syndrome and relates to a generalized increase in hepatic protein synthesis to 'compensate' for urinary protein loss (29). In the absence of proteinuria, any increase in hepatic synthesis has to be explained by some other mechanism. The correlation between fasting insulin and triglyceride levels led to the hypothesis that peripheral insulin resistance caus-

Table 3. Serum lipoprotein and apoprotein abnormalities in uraemia.

Lipoprotein	Triglyceride	Cholesterol
VLDL	Increased	Increased
IDL	Increased	–
LDL	Increased	–
HDL	Increased	Decreased

Apoprotein	Total concentration	Distribution
AI	Decreased	–
AIV	Increased	Present in LDL
B48/100	Increased	APO B48 in VLDL
CII	Drecreased	Present in LDL
CIII	Increased	Present in LDL
E	–	Present in LDL

es hyperinsulinaemia which stimulates hepatic VLDL secretion (30). Although insulin resistance has been demonstrated in uraemia (31), insulin does not appear to enhance triglyceride production in the rat liver *in vitro* (32). Hence, there is little evidence to support the theory that insulin resistance is important in dialysis hyperlipidaemia.

Lipase deficiency

Impaired catabolism of lipoproteins in peritoneal- and haemodialysis patients has been well documented, both by the estimation of intralipid clearance (33, 34) and by kinetic studies using radiolabelled glycerol (16). Intralipid clearance correlates negatively with serum triglyceride levels (3) and positively with lipoprotein and hepatic lipase function (35). Enzyme activity measured after intravenous heparin is decreased in haemodialysis patients. Hepatic lipase may be particularly important in clearing remnant particles and a selective deficiency of this enzyme has been observed (36). Circulating enzyme inhibitors have also been demonstrated (37). The concentration of inhibitor does not appear to be reduced by haemodialysis although haemofiltration may be beneficial (38). The inbalance of apoprotein co-factors comprising a reduction of apo C2 and elevation of apo C3 levels probably contributes to reduced lipoprotein lipase activity (39). HDL is an important reservoir of apo C2 and reduced HDL concentration may explain the inverse correlation between HDL cholesterol and total triglyceride (1).

Haemodialysis itself does not appear to reduce lipase activity although repeated heparin administration can deplete enzyme stores (40). Patients treated by peritoneal dialysis also demonstrate similar triglyceride clearance defects (3) and heparin-free haemodialysis does not seem to improve lipolytic enzyme activities (41). A sequential study of six uraemic predialysis patients showed reduced post-heparin lipase activity which did not change significantly after regular haemodialysis was instituted (42).

Carnitine deficiency

Carnitine is a naturally occuring quaternary amine that carries long-chain fatty acids across the inner mitochondrial membrane to the site of oxidation in the mitochondrial matrix. A deficiency of carnitine may result in a decrease in mitochondrial fatty acid oxidation. Increased delivery of fatty acids to the liver may increase triglyceride synthesis contributing to hypertriglyceridaemia. Carnitine is derived from dietary intake but is also synthesized in the liver and the kidney. Carnitine deficiency has been demonstrated in haemo- but not in peritoneal dialysis patients (43). Although loss of carnitine in dialysate exceeds normal urinary excretion, it appears that decreased synthesis also occurs due to deficiency of the precursor, lysine (44). This amino acid is removed by dialysis and low serum concentrations have been noted in dialysis patients (45). In some studies treatment with carnitine has improved lipid abnormalities (45). Others have not substantiated these findings and have noted different response patterns with a paradoxical increase in serum triglyceride in some patients and inconsistent responses to two different doses in others (46).

Dialysis fluid

Sugars derived from dialysis fluid constitute a source of calories but there is little evidence to suggest that they contribute significantly to hypertriglyceridaemia. Longer dwell times and higher glucose concentrations of dialysis fluid would theoretically render patients on continuous ambulatory peritoneal dialysis at greater risk. Haemodialysis using glucose-free dialysis fluid does not appear to have any beneficial effect on lipid abnormalities (47) and glucose-free fluid for peritoneal dialysis is currently under assessment. Acetate loads from dialysis fluid probably also make a small contribution to hypertriglyceridaemia in some patients (48).

Treatment of lipid abnormalities in dialysis patients

Dietary fat intake has been shown to influence lipoprotein composition. High-fat, high-cholesterol diets can lead to production of atherogenic lipoproteins, some of which resemble the remnant particles observed in patients treated by dialysis (19). National dietary recommendations aim to reduce total and saturated fat and similar principles should be applied when modifying the diets of dialysis patients. Historically, protein restriction in renal patients has been balanced by an increase in fat derived largely from dairy products and resulting in high saturated to polyunsaturated fat ratios. Such diets should be avoided and attention paid to increasing unsaturated fats when replacing calories usually provided by protein.

Specific dietary treatment of lipid abnormalities associated with dialysis has been successful. A low cholesterol diet with high polyunsaturated/saturated fat ratio has been shown to reduce total and LDL cholesterol but not to increase HDL cholesterol (49). An increase in polyunsaturated fatty acids alone normalises triglyceride and HDL cholesterol in some predialysis uraemic patients (50).

Increasing efficiency of dialysis appears to have a small beneficial effect on triglyceride metabolism as measured by triglyceride turnover (16). Improvements of lipid abnormalities using haemofiltration have also been achieved (38) but such beneficial effects are not confirmed by all studies. Clofibrate is commonly used in the treatment of hypertriglyceridaemia. It acts by increasing lipoprotein lipase activity in adipose tissue and normalises high triglyceride and low HDL cholesterol levels (51). Clofibric acid, the active metabolite, undergoes renal elimination and the drug should be used with caution in dialysis patients to avoid myo- and hepatotoxicity. The usual recommended dose of 1 to 2g/week may still cause mild elevations of creatine phosphokinase.

Fish oil supplements rich in marine polyunsaturated fatty acids may prove to be an effective, safe alternative and are currently being assessed.

ATHEROSCLEROSIS

Evidence for accelerated atherosclerosis

An increased incidence of cardiovascular disease in dialysis patients was first reported in 1974 (52). In this retrospective study of 39 haemodialysis patients followed for between 1 and 13 years there were 14 death attributed to atherosclerosis, an incidence comparable with that found in type II hyperlipidaemia. This initial report was not fully substantiated by subsequent studies, the association was questioned and the importance of other risk factors emphasized (53, 54). However, study of larger populations has confirmed that patients on dialysis experience a substantially increased risk of atherosclerosis. In 1981 the risk of death from myocardial infarction in a haemodialysis population aged 35 to 54 was 20 times greater than that of an age-matched population. For patients over the age of 55 years the risk was nine times greater (55). This risk also extends to the transplant population. Cardiovascular disease remains the most common causes of death in patients on renal replacement therapy (56).

Pathogenesis of atherosclerosis

The normal arterial intima is composed of a thin layer of endothelial cells immediately adjacent to the lumen and forming a barrier between the blood and the vessel wall. These cells are attached to a thin basement membrane deep to which lies loose connective tissue containing a few smooth muscle cells and separated from the adjacent media by the internal elastic lamina. The underlying media, in contrast consists of tightly packed smooth muscle cells arranged in concentric layers. In the development of an atherosclerotic plaque, the intima becomes thickened by proliferation of smooth muscle cells and macrophages, lipid is deposited and connective tissue content is increased.

The pathogenesis of atherosclerosis is not fully understood and several theories have been put forward to explain the intimal changes observed (57). Although animal models have been useful in defining the role of lipids, macrophages, smooth muscle cells, platelets and cell-derived growth factors in atherosclerosis, it has proved difficult to determine the sequence of events that lead to the formation of the atheromatous plaque in humans (Figure 3). In particular, the role of endothelial injury remains unclear (58).

Endothelial damage may occur at an early stage due to mechanical, chemical or viral injury. By exposing the underlying intima, it leads to infiltration by lipid and monocytes and the formation of platelet thrombi. Conversely, such endothelial damage may occur secondary to accumulation of lipid and cells within the intima.

There is little doubt that lipids play an important role in the formation of the atheromatous plaque. Lipoproteins, notably LDL, have been demonstrated in intimal lesions (59). Fatty streaks, which may be the precursors of atheromatous plaques, are composed of almost entirely of lipid in association with macrophages and lymphocytes and may

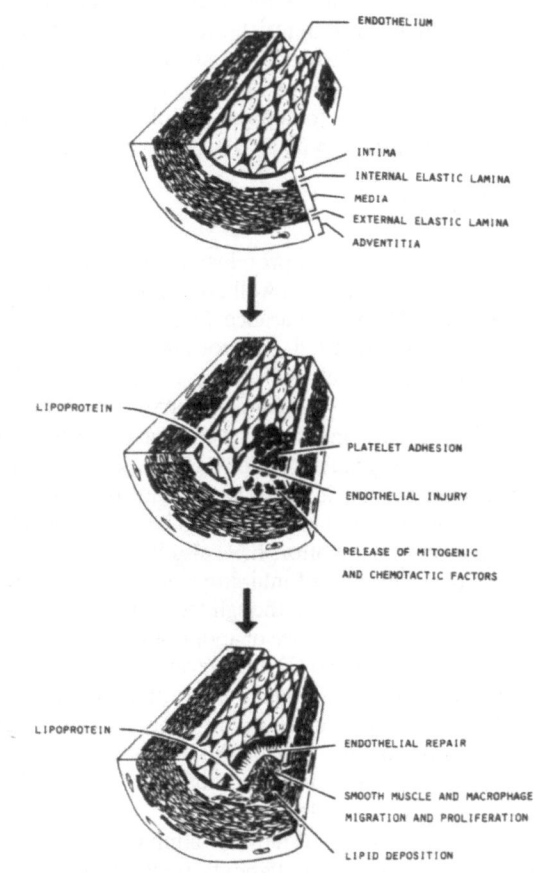

Figure 3. Pathogenesis of atherosclerosis. Endothelial injury, which may occur secondary to deposition of lipid, exposes the underlying intima and leads to attachment of platelets and monocytes. Growth factors secreted by these adherent cells and by the damaged endothelium itself stimulate migration and proliferation of smooth muscle cells from the adjacent media and eventually convert the fatty streak to the fibrous plaque. Smooth muscle cells, along with macrophages derived from invading monocytes, engulf deposited lipid and become foam cells.

represent an inflammatory response to lipid deposition in the intima. Binding of negatively charged glycosaminoglycans to positively charged apo B may lead to trapping of this lipoprotein and disturbed intimal glycosaminoglycan composition could explain the accumulation of lipid in diseased areas (60). Lipid deposition may stimulate smooth muscle proliferation causing migration of smooth muscle cells into the intima from the neighbouring media. In conjunction with invading macrophages, these cells remove the foreign substance by phagocytosis. Although these cells attempt to hydrolyse engulfed lipid, intracellular accumulation of esterified cholesterol occurs giving rise to the characteristic foam cell (11).

Chemoattractants and growth factors appear to be important in intimal proliferation (61). One such substance, platelet-derived growth factor, is released when platelet thrombi form at sites of endothelial damage and stimulates migration of vascular smooth muscle cells from the adjacent intima. Proliferation and matrix secretion by these cells is also increased. Similar substances derived from macrophages, damaged endothelium and smooth muscle cells themselves may also be important in plaque formation (61).

The development of recombinant DNA technology has allowed investigation of genetic markers of atherosclerosis. Because apoproteins play a central role in lipoprotein metabolism the genes coding for these proteins are currently being studied in detail. Associations between apo A1 and B genotypes and coronary artery disease have been demonstrated and further investigation will lead to an improved understanding of the genetics markers of atherosclerosis (62).

Environmental factors are also important. Associations between atherosclerosis and smoking are well established but the role of dietary fat intake is less well understood. Diets rich in cholesterol have been shown to induce formation of abnormal lipoproteins that resemble the remnant particles observed in type III hyperlipidaemia (beta VLDL) (19). Clearance of these particles by macrophages via the alternative pathway that removes excess LDL may contribute to cholesterol accumulation in these cells. Cholesterol feeding also leads to formation of an abnormal HDL which is rich in apo E (HDLc). This particle has a high affinity for the apo B/E receptor and may thus deliver cholesterol to the cell (19).

Risk Factors for atherosclerosis in dialysis patients

Smoking and hypertension

Several factors have been implicated in contributing to accelerated atherosclerosis in dialysis patients (Figure 4). Smoking and hypertension are correctable and may be more important than lipoprotein abnormalities (63).

Uraemic toxins

Toxins accumulating in uraemia may cause endothelial injury or damage the underlying intima once this has been exposed. Serum from patients on dialysis has been shown to stimulate proliferation of cultured smooth muscle cells *in vitro* (64). This mitogenic action is lost when polyamines are selectively removed. These naturally occurring substances, which are important for normal growth, are excreted by the kidney and accumulate in renal failure. Their precursor amino acid, methionine also accumulates in homocysteinuria and high polyamine concentrations may explain the increased incidence of atherosclerosis associated with this inborn error of metabolism. Other possible factors which may contribute to endothelial or intimal injury include hormones, particularly parathyroid hormone, and free oxygen radicles.

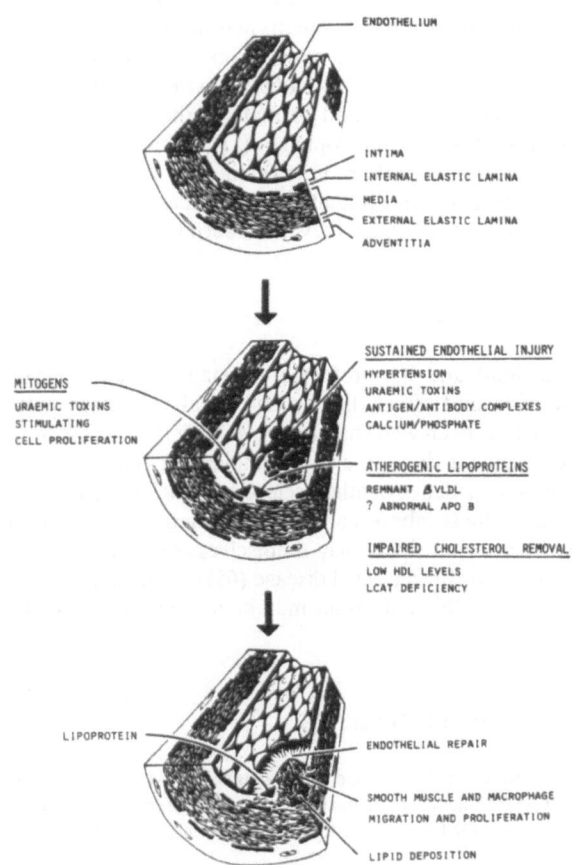

Figure 4. Factors that may accelerate atherosclerosis in uraemia. Hypertension and uraemic toxins may cause or potentiate endothelial injury. Uraemic toxins may also stimulate cell proliferation in the exposed intima. Abnormal 'remnant' VLDL and possibly LDL with chemically modified apo B readily deposit within the vessel wall. Reduced HDL levels and LCAT activity impair the return of excess cholesterol to the liver.

Lipid abnormalities

The major lipid abnormalities associated with uraemia are likely to contribute to accelerated atherosclerosis in these patients. Hypertriglyceridaemia has been shown to be an independent risk factor in the development of atherosclerosis in univariate analysis. In multivariate analysis, however, HDL cholesterol is a far more powerful predictor of coronary artery disease (13). Low HDL cholesterol concentrations and LCAT deficiency would be expected to impair the process of reverse cholesterol transport and thus contribute to tissue cholesterol accumulation in dialysis patients. The remnant particles found in dialysis patients and in patients with type III hyperlipidaemia appear to be particularly atherogenic. These cholesterol-rich particles are taken up by a specific macrophage receptor that is only partially suppressed by intracellular cholesterol content and lead to cellular cholesterol accumulation (19). Characterisation of apoproteins in uraemic patients may improve current understanding of the pathogenesis of lipoprotein abnormalities and the increased incidence of atherosclerosis. Just as acetylated LDL does not bind normally to the apo B/E receptor but is removed by macrophages (11), *in vivo* chemical modification of apoproteins in uraemia may alter their binding characteristics and potentiate the atherogenicity of the lipoproteins with which they are associated.

CONCLUSIONS

The lipid and lipoprotein abnormalities that complicate uraemia and affect dialysis and renal transplant patients have now been well characterised. With the success of renal replacement therapy and accumulating evidence of an increased incidence of atherosclerosis in such patients, correction of these abnormalities has gained new importance. Evidence that lipids may themselves contribute to kidney damage in chronic renal disease (65) has further stimulated interest in this important metabolic consequence of uraemia.

ACKNOWLEDGEMENTS

The authors acknowledge the assistance of Mrs Anne Freuchen (bibliographic research and retrieval), Mr Nazeem Nanjee (illustrations) and Dr Premod Mistry (criticism of manuscript).

REFERENCES

1. Chan MK, Varghese Z, Moorhead JF: Lipid abnormalities in uremia, dialysis and transplantation, *Kidney Int* 19: 625, 1981
2. Ponticelli C, Barbi G, Cantaluppi A, Donati C, Annoni G, Brancaccio D: Lipid abnormalities in maintenance dialysis patients and renal transplant recipients. *Kidney Int* 13 (Suppl. 8): S72, 1978
3. Chan MK, Varghese Z, Persaud JW, Baillod RA, Moorhead JF: Hyperlipidemia in patients on maintenance hemo- and peritoneal dialysis: the relative pathogenetic role of triglyceride production and triglyceride removal. *Clin Nephrol* 17: 183, 1982
4. Haas LB, Wahl PW, Sherrard DJ: A Longitudinal study of lipid abnormalities in renal failure. *Nephron* 33: 145, 1983
5. Somer JB, Aitken JM, Abbott LK, Charlesworth JA, MacDonald G, Blacket RB: Lipoprotein lipids in chronic renal failure and hemodialysis: The influence of etiology and implications for atherogenesis. *Atherosclerosis* 34: 353, 1979
6. Brunner FP, Brynger H, Chantler C, Donckerwolcke RA, Hathway RA, Jacobs C, Selwood NH, Wing AJ: Combined report on regular dialysis and transplantation in Europe, IX, 1978. *Proc Eur Dial Transplant Assoc* 16: 2, 1979
7. Mahley RW, Innerarity TL, Rall SC, Weisgraber KH: Plasma lipoproteins: apolipoprotein structure and function. *J Lipid Res* 25: 1277, 1984
8. Rees A: DNA markers in the hyperlipidaemias and atherosclerosis. *J R Coll Physicians* (London) 21: 51, 1987
9. Brown MS, Goldstein JL: A receptor-mediated pathway for cholesterol homeostasis. *Science* 232: 34, 1986
10. Tolleshaug H, Hobgood KK, Brown MS, Goldstein JL: The LDL receptor locus in familial hypercholesterolemia: Multiple mutations disrupt transport and processing of a membrane receptor. *Cell* 32: 941, 1983
11. Brown MS, Goldstein JL: Lipoprotein metabolism in the macrophage: Implications for cholesterol deposition in atherosclerosis. *Annu Rev Biochem* 52: 223, 1983
12. Fidge NH, Nestel PJ: Identification of apolipoproteins involved in the interaction of human high density lipoprotein 3 with receptors on cultured cells. *J Biol Chem* 260: 3570, 1985
13. Gordon T, Castelli WP, Hjortland MC, Kannel WB, Dawber TR: High density lipoprotein as a protective factor against coronary heart disease. The Framingham study. *Am J Med* 62: 707, 1977
14. Bagdade JD, Albers JJ: Plasma high-density lipoprotein concentrations in chronic hemodialysis and renal transplant patients. *N Engl J Med* 296: 1436, 1977
15. Chan MK, Yeung CK: Lipid metabolism in 31 Chinese patients on three 2-L exchanges of CAPD. *Peritoneal Dial Bull* 6: 12, 1986
16. Cattran DC, Fenton SSA, Wilson DR, Steiner G: Defective triglyceride removal in lipemia associated with peritoneal dialysis and haemodialysis. *Ann Intern Med* 85: 29, 1976
17. Minamisono T, Wada M, Akamatsu A, Okabe M, Handa Y, Morita T, Asagami C, Naito HK, Nakamoto S, Lewis LA, Mise J: Dyslipoproteinemia (a remnant lipoprotein disease) in uremic patients on hemodialysis. *Clin Chim Acta* 84: 163, 1978
18. Papadopoulos NM, Bedynek JL: Serum lipoprotein patterns in patients with coronary atherosclerosis. *Clin Chim Acta* 44: 153, 1973
19. Mahley RW: Atherogenic hyperlipoproteinemia. *Med Clin North Am* 66: 375, 1982
20. Mahley RW, Angelin B: Type III hyperlipoproteinemia: Recent insights into the genetic defect of familial dysbetalipoproteinemia. *Adv Intern Med* 29: 385, 1984
21. Brunzell JD, Albers JJ, Hass LB, Goldberg AP, Agadoa L, Sherrard DJ: Prevalence of serum lipid abnormalities in chronic hemodialysis. *Metabolism* 26: 903, 1977
22. Staprans I, Felts JM, Zacherle B: Apoprotein composition of plasma lipoproteins in uremic patients on hemodialysis. *Clin Chim Acta* 93: 135, 1979
23. Drüeke T, Lacour B, Roullet J, Funck-Brentano J: Recent advances in factors that alter lipid metabolism in chronic renal failure. *Kidney Int* 24 (Suppl 16): S134, 1983
24. Nestel PJ, Fidge NH, Tan MH: Increased lipoprotein remnant formation in chronic renal failure. *N Engl J Med* 307: 329, 1982
25. Chan MK, Ramdial L, Varghese Z, Persaud JW, Baillod RA, Moorhead JF: Plasma lecithin-cholesterol acyltransferase activities in uraemic patients. *Clin Chim Acta* 119: 65, 1982
26. Cramp DG, Tickner TR, Beale DJ, Moorhead JF, Wills MR: Plasma triglyceride secretion and metabolism in chronic renal failure. *Clin Chim Acta* 76: 237, 1977
27. Shore VG, Forte T, Licht H, Lewis SB: Serum and urinary lipoproteins in the human nephrotic syndrome: Evidence for renal catabolism of lipoproteins. *Metabolism* 31: 258, 1982
28. Newmark SR, Anderson CF, Donadio JV, Ellefson RD: Lipoprotein profiles in adult nephrotics. *Mayo Clinic Proc* 50: 359, 1975
29. Marsh JB, Drabkin DL, Braun GA, Parks JS: Factors in the stimulation of protein synthesis by subcellular preparations from rat liver. *J Biol Chem* 241: 4168, 1966
30. Bagdade JD, Porte D, Bierman EL: Hypertriglyceridemia: A metabolic consequence of chronic renal failure. *N Engl J Med* 279: 181, 1968

31. Westervelt FB: Insulin effect in uremia. *J Lab Clin Med* 74: 79, 1969

32. Rubenstein B, Rubinstein D: The effect of fasting on esterification of palmitate by rat liver in vitro. *Can J Biochem* 44: 129, 1966

33. Russell GI, Davies TG, Walls J: Evaluation of the intravenous fat tolerance test in chronic renal disease. *Clin Nephrol* 13: 282, 1980

34. Turgan C, Feehally J, Bennett S, Davies TJ, Walls J: Accelerated hypertriglyceridemia in patients on continuous ambulatory peritoneal dialysis-a preventable abnormality. *Int J Artif Organs* 4: 158, 1981

35. Chan MK, Persaud JW, Varghese Z, Moorhead JF: Postheparin hepatic and lipoprotein lipase activities in nephrotic syndrome. *Aust NZ J Med* 14: 841, 1984

36. Mordasini R, Frey F, Flury W, Klose G, Greten H: Selective deficiency of hepatic triglyceride lipase in uremic patients. *N Engl J Med* 297: 1362, 1977

37. Murase T, Cattran DC, Rubenstein B, Steiner G: Inhibition of lipoprotein lipase by uremic plasma. A possible cause of hypertriglyceridemia. *Metabolism* 24: 1279, 1975

38. Di Giulio S, Lacour B, Man NK, Martinez-Natera F, Faguer P, Drüeke T, Funck-Brentano JL: Post heparin lipolytic activity in uremic patients treated by hemofiltration. *Contrib Nephrol* 29: 143, 1982

39. Rapoport J, Aviram M, Chaimovitz C, Brook JG: Defective high-density lipoprotein composition in patients on chronic hemodialysis: A possible mechanism for atherosclerosis. *N Engl J Med* 299: 1326, 1978

40. Ibels LS, Reardon MF, Nestel PJ: Plasma post-heparin lipolytic activity and triglyceride clearance in uremic and hemodialysis patients and renal allograft recipients. *J Lab Clin Med* 87: 648, 1976

41. Matsui N, Nakamura Y, Shinoda T, Iwamoto H, Yoshiyama N, Nakagawa S, Takeuchi J, Teraoka J: The effect of heparin-free dialysis on abnormal lipid metabolism in patients on regular dialysis treatment. *Proc Eur Dial Transplant Assoc* 17: 253, 1980

42. Huttunen JK, Pasternack A, Vänttinen T, Ehnholm C, Nikkilä EA: Lipoprotein metabolism in patients with chronic uremia. *Acta Med Scand* 204: 211, 1978

43. Leschke M, Rumpf KW, Eisenhauer T, Fuchs C, Becker K, Köthe U, Scheler F: Quantitative assessment of carnitine loss during hemodialysis and hemofiltration. *Kidney Int* 24 (Suppl 16): S143, 1983

44. Gulyassy PF, Aviram A, Peters JH: Evaluation of amino acid and protein requirements in chronic uremia. *Arch Intern Med* 126: 855, 1970

45. Lacour B, Di Giulio S, Chanard J, Ciancioni C, Haguet M, Lebkiri B, Basile C, Drüeke T, Assan R, Funck-Brentano JL: Carnitine improves lipid anomalies in haemodialysis patients. *Lancet* ii: 763, 1980

46. Chan MK, Persaud JW, Varghese Z, Baillod RA, Moorhead JF: Response patterns to DL-carnitine in patients on maintenance haemodialysis. *Nephron* 30: 240, 1982

47. Swamy AP, Cestero RVM, Campbell RG, Freeman RB: Long-term effect of dialysate glucose on the lipid levels of maintenance hemodialysis patients. *Trans Am Soc Artif Intern Organs* 21: 54, 1976

48. Giorcelli G, Dalmasso F, Bruno M, Pellegrino S, Tondolo M, Sirkka M, Vacha G: RDT with acetate-free bicarbonate buffered dialysis fluid: Long-term effects on lipid pattern, acid-base balance and oxygen delivery. *Proc Eur Dial Transplant Assoc* 16: 115, 1979

49. Wass VJ, Jarrett RJ, Meilton V, Start MK, Mattock M, Ogg CS, Cameron JS: Effect of a long-term fat-modified diet on serum lipoprotein levels of cholesterol and triglyceride in patients on home haemodialysis. *Clin Sci* 60: 81, 1981

50. Tsukamoto Y, Okubo M, Yoneda T, Marumo F, Nakamura H: Effect of a polyunsaturated fatty acid-rich diet on serum lipids in patients with chronic renal failure. *Nephron* 31: 236, 1982

51. Bagdade JD, Shantharam VV, Sollek M, Albers JJ: Effect of clofibrate on plasma lipids and high density lipoprotein levels in renal allograft recipients. *Clin Nephrol* 12: 83, 1979

52. Lindner A, Charra B, Sherrard DJ, Scribner BH: Accelerated atherosclerosis in prolonged maintenance hemodialysis. *N Engl J Med* 290: 697, 1974

53. Nicholls AJ, Catto GRD, Edward N, Engeset J, Macleod M: Accelerated atherosclerosis in long-term dialysis and renal transplant patients: Fact or fiction? *Lancet* i: 276, 1980

54. Burke JF, Francos GC, Moore LL, Cho SY, Lasker N: Accelerated atherosclerosis in chronic dialysis patients – Another look. *Nephron* 21: 181, 1978

55. Kramer P, Broyer M, Brunner FP, Brynger H, Donckerwolcke RA, Jacobs C, Selwood NH, Wing AJ: Combined report on regular dialysis and transplantation in Europe, XII, 1981. *Proc Eur Dial Transplant Assoc* 19: 4, 1982

56. Broyer M, Brunner FP, Brynger H, Fassbinder W, Guillou PJ, Oulès R, Rizzoni G, Selwood NH, Wing AJ, Challah S, Dykes SR: Demography of dialysis and transplantation in Europe, 1984. *Nephrol Dial Transplant* 1: 1, 1986

57. Ross R, Glomset JA: The pathogenesis of atherosclerosis. *New Engl J Med* 295: 369 and 420, 1976

58. Moore S: Pathogenesis of atherosclerosis *Metabolism* 34: 13, 1985

59. Wissler RW: The emerging cellular pathobiology of atherosclerosis. *Artery* 5: 409, 1979

60. Iverius P: The interaction between human plasma lipoproteins and connective tissue glycosaminoglycans. *J Biol Chem* 247: 2607, 1972

61. Ross R: The pathogenesis of atherosclerosis - An update. *N Engl J Med* 314: 488, 1986

62. Zannis VI, Breslow JL: Genetic mutations affecting human lipoprotein metabolism. *Adv Hum Genet* 14: 125, 1984

63. Haire H, Sherrard D, Scardapane D, Curtis FK, Brunzell JD: Smoking, hypertension and mortality in a maintenance dialysis population. *Cardiovasc Med* 3: 1163, 1978

64. Bagdade JD: Chronic renal failure and atherogenesis: serum factors stimulate the proliferation of human arterial smooth muscle cells. *Atherosclerosis* 34: 243, 1979

65. Moorhead JF, Chan MK, El-Nahas M, Varghese Z: Lipid nephrotoxicity in chronic progressive glomerular and tubulo-interstitial disease. *Lancet* ii: 1309, 1982

ACID-BASE HOMEOSTASIS IN CLINICAL DIALYSIS

GIUSEPPE LA GRECA, ALDO FABRIS, MARIANO FERIANI, STEFANO CHIARAMONTE and
CLAUDIO RONCO

INTRODUCTION

Since the earliest experiences with hemodialysis, the correction of uremic acidosis has represented a complex problem still not completely resolved.

Kolff in 1943 (1), and later Scribner et al (2), used a dialysis solution with 27 mmol/l of bicarbonate as a buffer. Bicarbonate containing dialysate was prepared in large containers before the dialysis session thus creating problems related to calcium and magnesium precipitation, to easy bacterial contamination and finally to the rate of delivery, limited to 500 ml/min.

In 1964, in Seattle, Mion et al (3) introduced the use of acetate as alkaline equivalent in the dialysis fluid. Acetate containing solutions were easily prepared, chemically stable and microbiologically safe. Rapidly, acetate solutions became widely applied in clinical dialysis, being used world wide for more than 20 years. The low cost, the equimolar conversion to bicarbonate in the body and the bacteriostatic effect in the solution, made acetate a first choice substrate for the correction of acid-base derangements in hemodialysis. Acetate solutions rendered hemodialysis more simple thus stimulating the proliferation of renal replacement therapy, as shown by more than 200,000 patients on regular dialysis treatment at the end of 1985.

In the late 1970's, new dialytic strategies, based on more efficient dialyzers and highly permeable membranes, that increased dialysis efficiency and shortened treatment time uncovered technical and clinical limitations imposed by acetate. Hence, the use of bicarbonate in clinical dialysis has been reintroduced recently, supported by new procedures of dialysate preparation, mixing and delivery. The high clinical tolerance and new technological advances now make bicarbonate dialysis more popular suggesting its future replacement of acetate dialysis.

ACID BASE BALANCE IN CLINICAL DIALYSIS

Mechanism of acid-base correction

Correction of metabolic acidosis in the uremic patients represents one of the fundamental aims of dialysis. In patients on maintenance hemodialysis, the physiologic restoration of body buffer content normally accomplished by the kidneys, should be replaced by the buffer administration through the dialysis membrane. Base gain during dialysis simulates the bicarbonate regeneration process by the normal kidneys.

Diet and metabolism are potential source of fixed non volatile acids. Sulfur of the sulfuric containing amino acids is oxidized to sulfuric acid; phosphate of proteins and phospholipids is metabolized to phosphoric acid and, finally, organic acids can be produced in excess of the metabolic elimination capacity.

Because these acids can not exist as free dissociated ions in the body fluids, they are instantaneously buffered, mostly by bicarbonate with consequent production of the corresponding sodium salts and carbonic acid. Carbonic acid is then transformed into H_2O and CO_2, the latter being excreted by the lungs. By this buffering, the net loss of one alkaline equivalent occurs for each hydrogen ion neutralized.

In patients without renal function the maintenance of acid base balance will only be achieved when the dialytic base gain equals the patient's metabolic acid production.

Acid production and removal

Endogenous acid production in uremic patients ranges between 0.7 and 1.2 mmol/kg/24 h. These values, mostly depending on diet and metabolism, appear similar to those observed in normal subjects. However the precise evaluation of the daily acid production in a single patient, would require metabolic balance studies. Since this procedure may be extremely complex, easier methods of calculation have to be used clinically. It has been pointed out by Gotch et al (4) that in normal subjects the ratio between net acid excretion in the urine and protein catabolic rate is constant and equal to 0.77. The normal daily acid production is, therefore, calculated as

$$H^+G_{24h} = PCR \times 0.77. \qquad [1]$$

Assuming a similar rate of production in hemodialysis patients without residual renal function (4), the hydrogen ion accumulation between two dialysis sessions can be calculated as:

$$H^+G_x = PCR \times 0.77 \times N \qquad [2]$$

where H^+ Gx is the interdialytic hydrogen ion generation (mmol), PCR is the protein catabolic rate (g/kg/24 h), and N is the number of days between two dialysis sessions.

Furthermore, besides bicarbonate, other alkaline equivalents lost through dialysis must be considered, as an additional source of acids (H^+ Gd) (5).

The overall weekly acid production in hemodialysis patients without residual renal function can therefore be calculated as:

$$H^+G_w = (PCR \times 0.77 \times 7) + (H^+G_d \times n) \qquad [3]$$

where H^+ Gw is the weekly acid generation in the body, H^+ Gd represents the amount of acid equivalents generated in the body during each dialysis session due to bicarbonate and other alkali losses in the dialysate. n is the number of dialysis sessions in a week.

Hemodialysis cannot remove large quantities of free hydrogen ion because of its low concentration in the blood. As hydrogen ions are produced, they are rapidly buffered by plasma bicarbonate and other body buffers thus remaining at very low concentration in plasma water (4).

In hemodialysis, therefore, H^+ removal from the blood is mainly achieved by the flux of alkaline equivalents from dialysate into the blood, with replacement of the depleted buffers. Hence, during dialysis fixed acids are converted to volatile acids.

To achieve adequate correction of metabolic acidosis the amount of buffers administered with dialysis should at least equal overall acid production in the patient. Base transfer across the dialysis membrane, is generally achieved in clinical dialysis by using acetate or bicarbonate containing dialysate.

Once acetate has entered the body, it is rapidly metabolized in the Krebs cycle and almost totally converted into bicarbonate. Of this bicarbonate 20% repletes body stores while 80% is lost across the membrane in the dialysate (6).

According to the formula:

$$CO_2 + H_2O \rightleftharpoons H_2CO_3 \rightleftharpoons H^+ + HCO_3^- \qquad [4]$$

the bicarbonate loss during dialysis causes a significant CO_2 removal by a shift to the right of the equilibrium.

Not only is CO_2 removed as bicarbonate, but also as a dissolved gas. However since plasma CO_2 concentration as a dissolved gas is very low (about 1 mmol/l) the losses under this form are small (0.2 to 0.3 mmol/min). Furthermore, while dissolved CO_2 is neutral and does not affect the acid base balance, CO_2 losses as bicarbonate influence acid base balance considerably creating an equimolar accumulation of H^+ in the body (7).

Hence, in acetate dialysis, the overall dialytic mass transfer rate of CO_2, averages 3 mmol/min and takes place in two ways: a) transport of dissolved CO_2 as a neutral gas, and b) transport of CO_2 as bicarbonate. These two forms represent respectively 2% and 24% of the overall CO_2 metabolic production (11 ± 3 mmol/min) (7).

In the dialytic transport of CO_2 the participation of red blood cells has also been postulated.

Bosch et al (8) demonstrated that the amount of total CO_2 found in the dialysate exceeds the amount calculated to have left the blood in the same period. They suggested that CO_2 may be generated in the red cells during passage through the dialyzer. As CO_2 is lost in the dialysate, a concentration gradient is created between red cells and plasma. This gradient operates as a diffusive driving force for CO_2 through the red cell wall.

Since CO_2 diffuses faster than bicarbonate, intracellular pH increases stimulating the pentose phosphate pathway which leads to further intracellular CO_2 production. As a consequence, the total CO_2 appearing in the dialysate may exceed the amount that has left the blood. Of course, such a phenomenon influences total CO_2 mass balance calculations.

During dialysis there is additional source of acid generation caused by the flux across the membrane of anions of organic acids such as lactate, β-hydroxybutyrate and acetoacetate. Under normal conditions these substances and their relative acids are neutralized by oxidation to CO_2 and H_2O. If the anions are removed by dialysis, the oxidation does not take place with a consequent net accumulation of hydrogen ions (9). A similar phenomenon occurs when other Krebs cycle intermediates, such as fumarate, succinate and glutarate, are lost in the dialysate, although the amount of these compounds lost across the membrane is very low.

A significant increase in blood levels of intermediates such as aceto-acetate and β-hydroxybutyrate and therefore an increased loss in the dialysate is observed when glucose free dialysis solutions are used. Under these conditions glucose is also lost in the dialysate and its plasma level falls causing a parallel decrease of insulin concentration. Low plasma levels of insulin may limit the rate of acetate metabo-

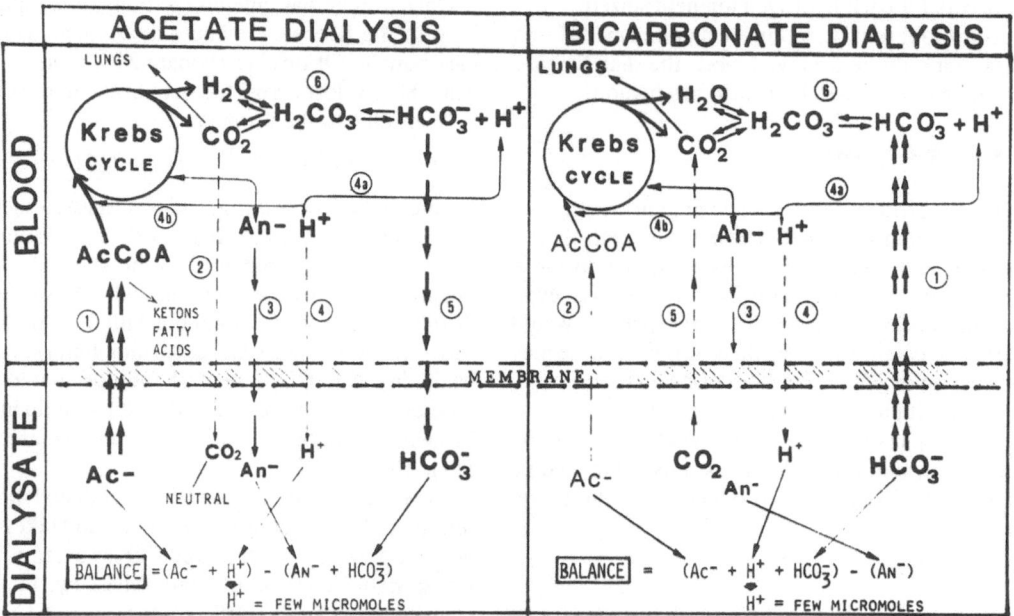

Figure 1. Mechanisms of acid-base correction in acetate and bicarbonate hemodialysis.
Acetate dialysis: the final balance depends on the base gain (acetate infused in the blood and hydrogen ions lost in the dialysate) minus the base loss (anions of organic acids and bicarbonate).
Bicarbonate dialysis: the final balance depends on the base gain (bicarbonate + small amounts of acetate and the hydrogen ions lost in the dialysate) minus the base loss (anions of organic acids). (See text).

lism in the Krebs cycle, increasing metabolic intermediates, or ketoacids and fatty acids via alternative pathways (10).

When dialysis fluid containing bicarbonate is used, bicarbonate losses do not occur; base losses are mostly due to the flux of organic anions in the dialysate. Under these conditions, however, organic anion loss in the dialysate is less than in acetate dialysis because of their lower production. The final bicarbonate balance will mainly depend on the dialysate/plasma concentration gradient. Bicarbonate containing solutions generally have a very high pCO_2; this may depend on the CO_2 insufflation in a closed system or on the chemical reaction with small quantities of acetic acid. Both these processes are utilized to maintain the dialysis solution chemically stable. Because of the difference in pCO_2 between plasma and dialysate, some dissolved CO_2 is administered to the patient during dialysis. However since dissolved CO_2 is neutral this does not interfere with acid base balance, and the excess CO_2 is finally excreted by the lungs (Figure 1).

Buffer balance

Vreman et al (11) measured a total infusion of acetate per dialysis of $1,165 \pm 49$ mmol, using dialyzers with surface areas varying between 1 and 2.5 m^2. Tolchin et al (12) reported total acetate infusion per dialysis varying from 788 ± 45 to $1,048 \pm 100$ mmol. These results were obtained with 2.5 m^2 dialyzers and two different dialysis solutions containing 30 and 40 mmol/l of acetate, respectively. Gotch et al (4)

found an average acetate infusion of 780 ± 61 mmol/dialysis utilizing dialyzers of 1.3 and 1.8 m^2. Kishimoto (13) observed a total infusion of acetate per dialysis of 819 ± 125 mmol with 1.1 m^2 dialyzers. In those studies bicarbonate losses varied from 550 to 900 mmol/dialysis. The additional loss of alkaline equivalents such as lactate and β-hydroxybutyrate ranged from 50 to 100 mmol/dialysis (4). Some of these authors calculated weekly net base balances slightly positive or at least near zero. This, however, contrasts with the frequent observation of patients undergoing chronic acetate dialysis with a pre-dialytic plasma bicarbonate ranging from 14 to 18 mmol/l (14).

The buffer balance in bicarbonate dialysis has not yet been studied extensively. Gotch et al (4) have reported a weekly balance in eight patients undergoing bicarbonate dialysis with 1.3 to 1.8 m^2 dialyzers, blood flow of 200 ml/min, dialysate flow of 400 ml/min and 36 mmol/l of bicarbonate in the dialysate. In this study the net base gain was calculated taking into account other factors such as ultrafiltration, net H$^+$ generation and lactate and β-hydroxybutyrate losses during dialysis. The average weekly H$^+$ generation was 352 mmol; β-hydroxybutyrate and lactate losses were 37 and 55 mmol/week, respectively. Bicarbonate mass transfer was 618 mmol/week (206 mmol/dialysis). The final net base gain was +175 mmol/week. Such a positive balance might even be higher considering the patients uptake of acetate derived from the acid part of the dialysis concentrate. In case of body buffer depletion this positive balance may help restore the acid-base equilibrium and to replenish the buffer stores. However when the acid-base status is near normal only small amounts of base are required and excessive base administration can cause alkalosis.

Controlled studies of patients treated with bicarbonate dialysis for more than 12 weeks demonstrated the high risk of postdialytic alkalosis with plasma bicarbonate levels exceeding 30 mmol/l and blood pH higher than 7.55. This acute alkalosis may cause encephalopathy, nausea, vomiting and lethargy and such chronic effects as calcium deposition in soft tissues. On the basis of these observations Ward et al (15) suggest progressive reduction of dialysate bicarbonate concentration over time. On the other hand, studies carried out with dialysis solutions containing 31 mmol/l of bicarbonate and 5 mmol/l of acetate, have shown insufficient correction of metabolic acidosis and no significant differences from the results achieved with acetate dialysis (14).

Considerable variability among different balance studies can be observed. It is likely that several parameters not considered in these studies may play important roles in the final calculations. Different dialyzers, blood and dialysate flows and buffer concentrations make the studies not comparable. Accurate balance studies taking into account all possible variables would be required to identify the real acid-base balance in hemodialysis.

Oral base supplements

Although several studies of dialysis patients demonstrate that the net weekly base influx may compensate for daily H^+ production (4), before each dialysis metabolic acidosis is characteristic.

For this reason some authors (15) have suggested the use of oral alkaline supplements in the interdialytic period.

However, although these substances generally correct uremic acidosis, their participation in the final acid-base status is not easy to evaluate because of many variants. Among these, the most important are the individual differences on intestinal absorption, the volume of total body water, which relates to the interdialytic weight gain, and the possible interference with other drugs.

All these factors must be taken into account to assess the acid-base balance of the individual patient which does not depend only on the dialytic base gain.

FACTORS AFFECTING BUFFER BALANCE IN CLINICAL DIALYSIS

Mass transfer of buffers across dialysis membranes is achieved as for other solutes via diffusive or convective transport or both. However, the rapid conversion into other metabolites and the equilibration in a wide distribution space make mass balance calculations for these substances more complex and difficult.

Diffusive transport

The amount of acetate that diffuses across the membrane is a function of the concentration gradient between dialysate and blood and the membrane surface area. Other factors influencing acetate mass transfer are the temperature and a constant, defined as diffusivity, which depends on the membrane material and its interface with the solute and solvent under consideration. Since the latter factors are fairly stable in clinical dialysis, the concentration gradient and the surface area of the membrane are the major determinants of acetate transport. Once the surface area of the dialyzer has been established, acetate mass transfer rate (AcMTR) will depend on acetate dialysance (AcD) and on its average concentration gradient between dialysate and plasma during dialysis $(Cd_i - Cp_i)$: Since Dialysance = $MTR/(Cd_i - Cp_i)$, therefore MTR = $D(C_{di} - C_{pi})$. A simplified weekly mass balance calculation

$$H^+G_w = AcMTR \times n \times dt = D(Cd_i - Cp_i) \times n \times dt \quad [5]$$

where $H+Gw$ is the weekly acid production, n is the number of dialysis sessions in a week, and dt is the duration of the dialysis session, would define the exact amount of buffer to administer in a week to balance the overall acid production:

$$H^+G_w - NBG_w = 0 \quad [6]$$

where NBG_w is the net base gain during the week.

This amount of buffer could be achieved varying the dialysate concentration of acetate, the blood flow, the dialyzer surface area, the number of dialyses per week or the duration of each session. From equation [5] it would be theoretically possible to predict the dialysate concentration of acetate adequate for this purpose. The average concentration of acetate in dialysis solutions is 35 to 38 mmol/l while the blood acetate concentration at the beginning of the session is only 0.1 mmol/l. This gradient is the driving force moving acetate across the membrane. With 1 m² dialyzers a countercurrent blood/dialysate flow ratio of 250/500 guarantees an average acetate clearance of 125 ml/min, i.e. an average mass transfer rate of 4.75 mmol/min. Several techniques have been used to increase the acetate MTR during dialysis. Increasing blood flow results in a parallel increase in acetate dialysance until the curve reaches a plateau which is determined by the limiting effect of the membrane permeability and surface area (Figure 2). Higher mass transfer rates were achieved by Bjaeldager et al (16) by increasing acetate concentration in the bath from 32.6 to 38.2 mmol/l. Mansell et al (17) however, demonstrated that significant variations of blood acetate levels in patients undergoing acetate dialysis do not result in parallel changes of acetate fluxes across the membrane. As patients passed from 2.4 to 4.5 mmol/l of acetatemia during dialysis the acetate flux changed from 202 to 191 mmol/h/1.73 m² while in patients passing from 5.5 to 15.6 mmol/l the acetate flux changed from 195 to 229 mmol/h/1.73 m². It is still controversial whether small variations in the dialysate/blood concentration gradient may influence significantly the rate of acetate transport. Furthermore, the rate of acetate transport is lower than one would predict by

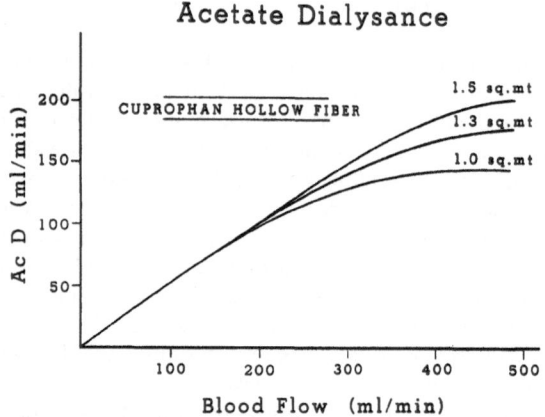

Figure 2. Acetate dialysance versus blood flow with cuprophan hollow fiber dialyzers of different surface area.

its molecular weight. The negative charges and the large hydration mantle of the molecule may in fact reduce the final diffusivity coefficient.

The rate of conversion of acetate into bicarbonate has been demonstrated to vary from 2.5 to 5.5 mmol/min with a mean value of 5 mmol/min in normals and 3 mmol/min in the uremic population. This conversion prevents dissipation of the gradient between dialysate and blood that would take place with accumulation of infused acetate. Accumulation may occur, however, as demonstrated by Tolchin et al (12), when high blood flows and large surface areas are utilized, and highly efficient treatments are performed. Under those conditions the high mass transfer of acetate across the membrane may exceed the maximal metabolic capacity (18–21). In this situation the plasma concentration of acetate may reach values above 10 mmol/l, which are considered dangerous and life threatening. Since clearances of acetate and urea are linked, it appears that urea clearance cannot be increased in acetate dialysis over a certain limit lest dangerously high mass transfer of acetate occur. In highly efficient treatments, another limitation derives from the high total CO_2 clearance and the consequent bicarbonate losses which may even be greater than the amount of acetate administered and may worsen the metabolic acidosis (22).

When bicarbonate containing dialysate is used a concentration gradient of 6 to 20 mmol/l between dialysate and blood is the driving force moving the buffer across the membrane. This gradient must be adequate to generate a bicarbonate flux into the blood sufficient to restore the body buffer stores without inducing alkalosis at the end of dialysis. A bicarbonate concentration in the dialysate varying from 30 to 38 mmol/l may generate in 240 min a mass transfer of buffer ranging from 150 to 250 mmol depending on predialysis serum bicarbonate concentration. Sargent and Gotch (7) found that bicarbonate flux across the membrane is a function of the inlet concentration gradient (Cdi − Cpi). For a gradient between 18 and 23 mmol they reported a bicarbonate MTR of 2.0 to 2.7 mmol/min with an average

dialysance of 118 ml/min. These results, however, are highly influenced by the blood and dialysate flows and by the geometry of the dialyzer and cannot be assumed as constant values. The bicarbonate concentrations now used clinically were not derived from kinetic studies but came mostly from empirical evaluations of their clinical adequacy. However, since the individual requirement of buffer administration varies among patients, it is difficult to propose a universally adequate fixed concentration; the personalization of the dialysis bath would be useful in answering the individual needs. The bicarbonate concentration should be also adapted to the state of body buffer depletion; when a full restoration of the body stores is required, higher concentrations of bicarbonate may be required to achieve a remarkably positive base balance, while lower concentrations (30 mmol/l) may be enough to maintain serum levels under adequate control after repletion is achieved. Ward and Wathen (23) have also recommended varying the concentration of bicarbonate in the dialysate during the dialysis session to avoid postdialytic alkalaemia.

Furthermore, other substances move through the membrane governed by concentration gradients and affect the final 'net base gain'. In bicarbonate dialysis small amounts of acetic acid are in the dialysate (3 to 5 mmol/l) creating a flux of acetate into the blood ranging from 0.2 to 0.8 mmol/min. Because of its conversion to bicarbonate, acetate can produce a further base gain during bicarbonate dialysis varying from 50 to 200 mmol/session. Finally the mass transfer rate of organic anions generally ranges between 0.2 and 0.5 mmol/min while only a few micromoles of free hydrogen ions cross the membrane in response to very low concentration gradients.

Convective transport

Base transfer across the dialysis membrane can also be achieved by convection. While the reciprocal influence of diffusion and convection is a complex process, extremely difficult to evaluate, the kinetics of buffers in exclusively convective therapies such as hemofiltration or ultrafiltration is quite easily understood. During standard hemodialysis dry weight is achieved via ultrafiltration of plasma water. This process leads to a certain bicarbonate loss that cannot be precisely evaluated because of the continuous interference of diffusion. In this condition, convective transport is present but it is not a pure and separate process. Its influence on the final bicarbonate balance can more precisely be evaluated by collecting the total spent dialysate and measuring the bicarbonate concentration (24).

The base balance in mixed diffusive-convective treatments, such as hemodiafiltration, is further complicated by the reinfusion of replacement solutions. Large amounts of bicarbonate are lost by convection in the ultrafiltrate and again the precise evaluation can only be made by collecting the entire pool of dialysate. The reinfusion of commercially prepared buffer containing solutions allows substitution of the bases lost via ultrafiltration and increases plasma bicarbonate concentration.

FACTORS AFFECTING DIALYTIC ACID–BASE BALANCE

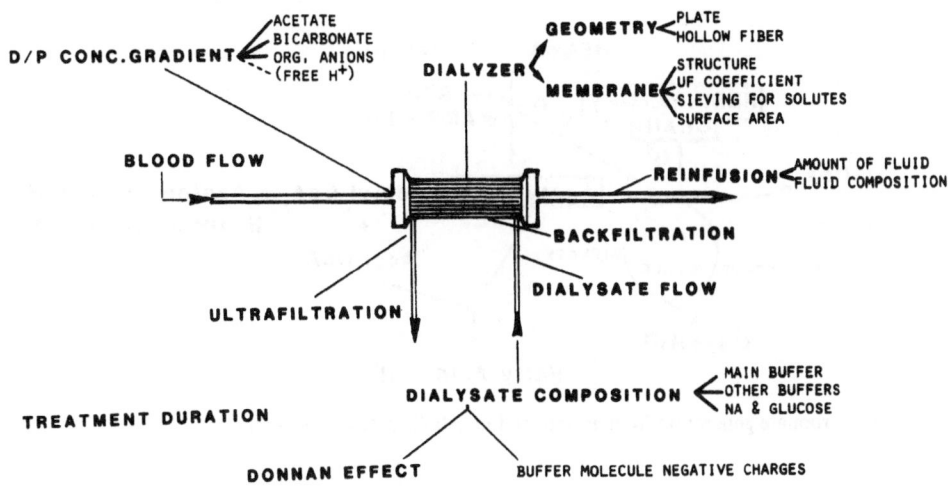

Figure 3. Factors affecting acid-base balance in clinical dialysis (see text).

The average buffer concentration in the replacement solutions (acetate, lactate or bicarbonate) varies from 35 to 60 mmol/l. This amount of alkaline equivalents infused directly helps to restore the body buffer content and offsets the base losses via ultrafiltration. In these treatments the final balance therefore depends on the same diffusive parameters as in hemodialysis plus the convective component which is linked to the number of liters of fluid exchanged per session.

The base balance calculation is easier in hemofiltration where a pure convective mechanism operates and solute transport is mostly governed by the permeability of the membrane (25–27). Since non diffusable anions, such as proteins, are present on one side of the membrane, the concentration of bicarbonate in the ultrafiltrate will be determined by the Donnan equilibrium which will provide for the electroneutrality on both sides of membrane. Therefore, the bicarbonate concentration in the ultrafiltrate is generally higher than in plasma water and sieving values ranges between 1.10 and 1.15 depending on the plasma protein concentration at the inlet of the filter and the filtration fraction. In this case, the product of the bicarbonate concentration in the ultrafiltrate times the volume of ultrafiltrate produced will equal the amount of base losses in a session. The buffers infused via replacement solution will balance these losses and will also give the excess amount of alkaline equivalents necessary to balance the metabolic acid production.

The net base balance in different types of substitutive therapy therefore depends on several factors that may affect the kinetics of buffers during the treatment (Figure 3).

BUFFER CHEMISTRY

Sodium salts of metabolizable organic acids can generate alkaline equivalents according to the formula:

$$NaOA + H_2CO_3 \rightarrow HOA + NaHCO_3 \qquad [7]$$

This process takes place only when the anion is completely metabolized to a neutral compound or decarboxylated to CO_2 and H_2O. Although several substrates have been proposed in the past (28, 29) as potential alkaline equivalents in humans e.g., succinate, fumarate and ketoglutarate, serious side effects discouraged their use and only acetate or lactate are utilized in clinical dialysis.

Acetate

Sodium acetate, originally proposed by Mudge (30), has a molecular weight of 136 daltons. It is almost completely dissociated in the body fluids because of its low pK (4.7). Acetate is mostly metabolized in peripheral tissues (31), although in the past, the liver was considered the main site of metabolism (32).

Acetate thiokinase activates the reaction between acetate and CoA to form AcetylCoA and one hydrogen ion is captured in this process. AcetylCoA may enter different metabolic pathways such as decarboxylation in the Krebs cycle, condensation to ketone bodies or fatty acids and glucose generation via gluconeogenesis (Figure 4).

The buffering effect is concluded and the hydrogen ion is transferred to the respiratory chain only when AcetylCoA is decarboxylated. When alternative pathways are entered or the decarboxylation process is incomplete, the buffering effect is delayed until the intermediate products are completely decarboxylated.

Several attempts have been made to quantify the amount of acetate infused during dialysis that is immediately oxidized in the Krebs cycle. Tolchin et al (12), by measuring the rate of conversion into bicarbonate, found approximate values of 93% while Davidson et al (33) and Morin et al (34)

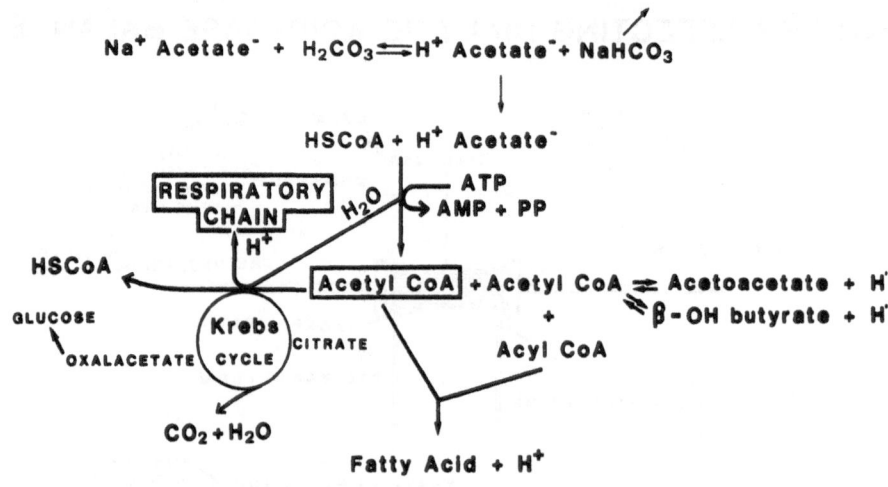

Figure 4. Mechanism of bicarbonate generation from acetate and metabolic pathways of acetate.

have shown values of 70% using ^{14}C acetate. Recently Stutke et al (35), using a sophisticated radioisotopic method, demonstrated that only 54% of the infused acetate is immediately oxidized during dialysis while 46% enters alternative pathways. This low rate of oxidation might be explained by the fact that acetate is not a usual major metabolic fuel and differences may arise in the way the Krebs cycle handles acetate as compared to pyruvate (Figure 5). In pyruvate metabolism only 3-carbon moieties are concerned when oxaloacetate is transformed into citrate (Krebs cycle), compared to 2-carbon moieties for acetate (10). The significance of this difference remains to be established.

During dialysis, acetate is the main source of AcCoA representing about 65% of the energy requirement (35). As a consequence the β-oxydation of long chain fatty acids is spared and trigliceryde synthesis is favored (36). This fact may explain the potential lipogenic action of acetate.

When glucose free dialysate is used, a remarkable increase of free fatty acids, ketone bodies and gluconeogenesis precursors can be noted (37). Concurrently serum insulin levels fall suggesting a possible role of this hormone in acetate metabolism. High levels of acetoacetate and β-hydroxybutyrate can also be found in highly efficient dialysis treatments, probably depending on the large acetate load (11). These metabolites commonly dissociate in body fluids, and release hydrogen ions, so their previous buffering effect vanishes. However, when not lost in the dialysate, they can still operate as buffers being reconverted to AcCoA. Acetate metabolism depends on an intact oxidative phosphorylation system; since Krebs cycle activity is regulated by the ATP/ADP ratio, when ATP concentration increases acetate metabolism is slowed (10).

Lundquist (31) estimated at 5 mmol/min the maximal rate of acetate metabolism in normal subjects. Such a rate seems to be lower in dialysis patients (3 to 4 mmol/min) because of a possible impairment of the Krebs cycle activity. In fact Yamakawa et al (38) have found that malate and citrate increase during acetate dialysis and isocitrate becomes detectable in the blood when acetate levels exceed 7 mmol/l.

The complete decarboxylation of 1 mol of acetate, leads to the production of 2 mol of CO_2 and consumes 2 mol of O_2. Since 1 mol of CO_2 is consumed in the acetate → acetic acid reaction, the final CO_2/O_2 ratio is 1/2 (39).

$$CO_2 \text{ (consumed)} + H_2O + CH_3COONa \rightarrow NaHCO_3 + CH_3COOH \quad [8]$$
$$CH_3COOH + 2O_2 \text{ (consumed)} = 2CO_2 \text{ (produced)} + 2H_2O \quad [8a]$$

Therefore, if the buffer was the main source of energy, the RQ should be reduced, but several factors may interfere with the final value of this ratio.

Lactate

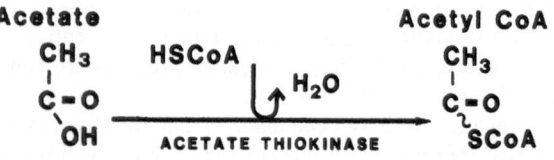

Figure 5. Mechanism of acetyl CoA generation from pyruvate and acetate.

Lactate, introduced by Hartmann in 1930 (40) as an alkalinizing substrate, has a molecular weight of 112 daltons and a

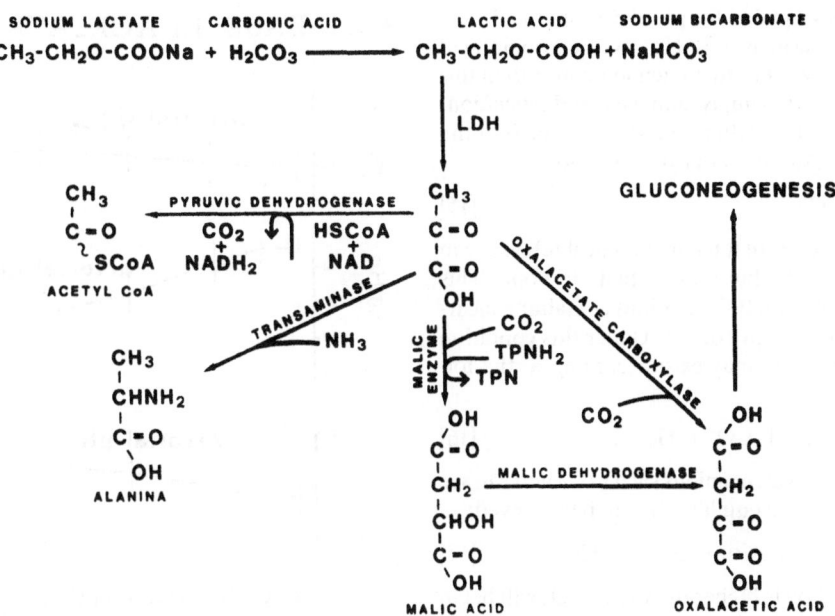

Figure 6. Metabolic pathways of lactate.

pK of 3.7 in the body fluids. While it has never been routinely used in hemodialysis, lactate is mainly utilized as a buffer for peritoneal dialysis and hemofiltration substitution fluids. In nature two stereoisomeric forms of lactate exist: D- and L-lactate. In humans small quantities of D-lactate are normally generated in the methylglyoxal pathway, while the predominant form is L-lactate.

D-lactate is slowly metabolized by a nonspecific enzyme (D-2-hydroxyacid-dehydrogenase), NAD independent. L-lactate, on the contrary, is easily metabolized to pyruvate by lactic dehydrogenase, NAD dependent. The metabolic pathways of lactate are reported in Figure 6. The buffering effect of lactate is accomplished by its complete metabolism via the Krebs cycle as for acetate, or via gluconeogenesis. The final results of these two pathways are:

1) OXIDATION: $CH_3 - CH(OH) - COO^- + 3O_2 \rightarrow 3CO_2 + 3H_2O$ [9]

2) GLUCONEOGENESIS: $2CH_3 - CH(OH) - COO^- + 2H^+ \rightarrow C_6H_{12}O_6$ [10]

With incomplete metabolism of lactate, the buffering effect does not take place. Searle and Cavalieri (41) demonstrated that 80 to 85% of the lactate produced in the normal metabolism is oxidized in the Krebs cycle, and only 15 to 20% is converted to glucose. While the oxidation takes place in all the cells with aerobic metabolism, gluconeogenesis is confined to the liver and renal cortex. Lactate turnover in normal subjects ranges from 0.77 to 0.87 mmol/Kg/h (41). In patients with hepatic disease the metabolic rate may be lower with a consequent increase of serum levels. In CAPD patients the lactate infusion is about 0.19 mmol/Kg/h, that is 25% of endogenous metabolic production (42). This lactate load does not represent a metabolic problem in patients with

normal hepatic function as some studies report normal values of intermediate metabolites (43,44).

Bicarbonate

Bicarbonate is the physiologic buffer in the body fluids. It has a molecular weight of 61 daltons and a pK of 6.305 at 37°C. Bicarbonate is part of a complex system including carbonic acid, carbonate and carbon dioxide:

$CO_2 + H_2O \leftrightharpoons H_2CO_3 \leftrightharpoons H^+ + HCO_3^- \leftrightharpoons 2H^+ + CO_3^=$ [11]

When acid is added or dissolved CO_2 leaves the system, the reaction speedily shifts to the left, while the reaction to the right is slow in the absence of carbonic anhydrase (45, 46). However, since this enzyme is almost ubiquitous (47), the carbonic acid concentration in body fluids is proportional to the dissolved CO_2 concentration. At the temperature and ionic strenght of the body fluids, the equilibrium

$H_2O + CO_2 \leftrightharpoons H_2CO_3$ [12]

is greatly towards CO_2 formation with a H_2CO_3/CO_2 ratio of 1/340. The concentration of dissolved CO_2 is proportional, according to Henry's law, to the partial pressure of CO_2 gas or:

$dCO_2 = \alpha pCO_2$ [13]

where α is the CO_2 solubility coefficient which in the blood is 0.0301 mmol/l/mm Hg.

The first dissociation of carbonic acid

$H_2CO_3 \leftrightharpoons H^+ + HCO_3^-$ [14]

occurs instantaneously and equilibrium would be reached

when the pH becomes equal to the pK of carbonic acid. The true pK of carbonic acid is 3.8. However carbonic acid appears to be a much weaker hydrogen ion donor than this dissociation constant would imply, and the first dissociation, called 'first apparent dissociation', has a pK of 6.10 in the blood. The second dissociation of carbonic acid

$$HCO_3^- \leftrightarrows H^+ + CO_3^= \qquad [15]$$

has a pK of 9.8 and therefore it has no practical relevance in body fluids except for the buffering activity in bone. This however, is important in dialysis solutions containing bicarbonate which may reach a pH of 8.4. Under this condition bicarbonate and carbonate may exist according to the following equilibrium:

$$Na^+ + HCO_3^- \leftrightarrows Na^+ + CO_3^= + H^+ \qquad [16]$$

Since in the dialysate, divalent anions such as Ca and Mg are also present, the following equilibrium will be achieved:

$$NaHCO_3 + CaCl_2 \leftrightarrows CaCo_3 + NaCl + HCl \qquad [17]$$

When pH of the solution is higher than 7, $CaCO_3$ will begin to precipitate thus reducing the bicarbonate concentration. A high CO_2 content may avoid this precipitation shifting to the left the following reaction:

$$Ca(HCO_3)_2 \leftrightarrows CaCO_3 + H_2O + CO_2 \qquad [18]$$

forming a soluble salt of calcium.

Since CO_2 is volatile, the CO_2 content of the solution tends to be reduced over a prolonged period of time facilitating $CaCO_3$ formation. This problem has been solved by the separation of Ca and bicarbonate in two containers and mixing them just before the filter. Meanwhile by the formula:

$$NaHCO_3 + CH_3COOH \leftrightarrows CH_3COONa + H_2O + CO_2 \qquad [19]$$

small amounts of acetic acid in the solution containing calcium, permit the achievement of a high CO_2 content in the final mixed dialysate.

ACETATE DIALYSIS

The use of acetate in dialysis may influence the patient's clinical conditions both during treatment and in the interdialytic period. Specific effects on acid-base equilibrium (EAB), ventilation, cardiovascular activity and endogenous metabolism can be observed.

Effects on acid base

Acetate dialysis is characterized by a flux of acetate into the blood and concurrent losses of bicarbonate in the dialysate.

In the first 30 min of dialysis acetate metabolism may not be fast enough to balance bicarbonate losses and a fall of HCO_3 and pH can be observed. This effect may even worsen the metabolic acidosis in this period (20). Subsequently, the rate of acetate utilization increases counterbalancing bicar-

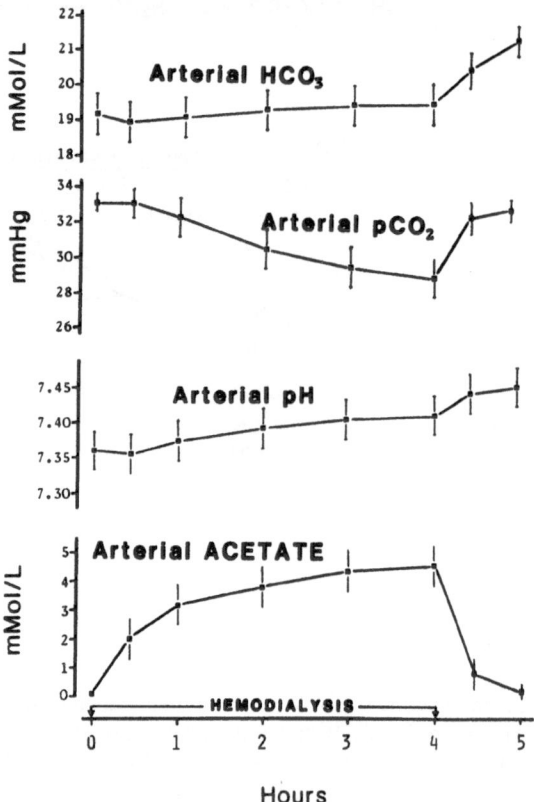

ACID-BASE in ACETATE DIALYSIS

Figure 7. Blood gases and acid-base behavior during acetate dialysis.

bonate losses; patients therefore show a progressive decrease of pCO_2, an increase of blood pH and a relative stability of plasma bicarbonate (Figure 7). Plasma acetate levels rise during the session reaching at the end an average value of 5 mmol/l (11,21). After dialysis has ceased pH and HCO_3 rapidly increase while pCO_2 returns to predialytic values (11). These effects depend on the sudden decrease of bicarbonate losses through the dialyzer and on the complete metabolism of acetate accumulated in the body. These observations are typical of a standard dialysis session carried out with blood flow of 250 ml/min, dialysate flow of 500 ml/min and cuprophan dialyzers for 240 min. When high surface area dialyzers are utilized (12, 48) acetate and bicarbonate fluxes across the membrane are greater and the consequent effects on acid-base equilibrium are more considerable. In these conditions the maximal acetate metabolic rate is frequently exceeded with a consequent accumulation of the buffer in the blood. This substantially decreases plasma bicarbonate and pCO_2, while variations of pH are either slight (48) or towards alkalemia (12). At the end of the session a remarkable increase of pH, pCO_2 and bicarbonate is observed leading to metabolic alkalosis (48). These observations suggest the possible limitations imposed by acetate dialysis in increasing the efficiency of the treatment and reducing treatment time.

In between two dialysis sessions, blood pH and bicarbonate progressively decrease in accord with the metabolic acid production and its accumulation in the body.

In a 60 kg patient, with a theoretical HCO_3 distribution space of 35 l, plasma bicarbonate should decrease by about 2 mmol/24 h when daily acid production is about 70 mmol and it is completely buffered by the bicarbonate system. Based on these calculations, one could predict the plasma bicarbonate concentration at the beginning of the subsequent session, to be 4 to 6 mmol lower than that observed at the end of the previous dialysis. However, the calculation is only theoretical and an extreme variability of the pre-dialytic bicarbonate concentrations can be noted in patients on regular dialysis treatment. This variability may depend on the intervention of buffers other than bicarbonate, on different daily acid productions and on variations of the interdialytic weight gain.

Effects on ventilation

Acetate dialysis significantly decreases arterial pO_2 during the entire duration of the treatment. This fall of pO_2 occurs in about 90% of patients ranging between 5 and 35 mm Hg (average value 14 mm Hg) (49). After the treatment, pO_2 values return to the pre-dialytic values within 1 or 2 h. Some authors have suggested that this dialysis induced hypoxemia might be important in the genesis of some intradialytic symptoms especially hypotension particularly evident in patients with compromised cardio-pulmonary function.

This hypoxemia has a multifactorial origin and its pathophysiology has not yet been totally clarified.

Dialytic hypoxemia has been ascribed to a possible Bohr effect (51). The pH increase during dialysis might lead to a parallel increase in hemoglobin affinity for O_2. In this setting, although a stable pO_2 and blood oxygen content are maintained, the O_2 delivery to the tissues decreases significantly. However, it has been pointed out by Hirszel et al (52) that the variations of blood pH and 2,3 diphosphoglycerate inside the red cells, as well as other intracellular phosphates, are not sufficient to explain completely the dialysis induced hypoxemia.

Bischel et al (53), have suggested that hypoxia may depend on a microembolisation in the lungs due to circulating micro-aggregates of platelets, leukocytes or fibrin deriving from the blood/membrane interaction. In other studies, however (54), the microfiltration of venous blood was not able to prevent hypoxemia during dialysis. Craddock et al (55) have suggested that the blood interaction with cuprophan membranes may activate complement via the alternative pathway with a consequent leukocyte agglutination and pulmonary trapping of the microaggregates and a final effect of neutropenia. This might lead to an impairment of gas diffusion in the lungs and consequent hypoxia.

Two observations, however, are in contrast with this hypothesis:

1) hypoxemia also occurs with more biocompatible membranes such as polyacrylonitrile or polysulphone in which complement activation does not take place and neutropenia is blunted (56);

2) during isolated ultrafiltration with cellulosic membranes the neutropenic effect is present but hypoxemia does not occur (57).

Sherlock et al (58) and Aurigemma (54) have proposed that the CO_2 losses across dialysis membrane could be the main cause of hypoventilation and hypoxemia. The reduced CO_2 excretion with increased O_2 consumption, without any alteration of A-a O_2 gradient, determines a significant fall of RQ. RQ, however, is in the normal range when its calcula-

Table 1.

Ref.	Year	Author	Hypotension	Nausea	Vomiting	Headache	Cramps
(67)	1977	Aizawa	−	0	0	0	0
(48)	1978	Graefe	+	0	+	+	+
(90)	1978	Whele (Na 145)	−	0	0	0	0
	1978	Whele (Na 135)	+	0	0	0	0
(87)	1980	Van Stone	−	0	0	0	0
(89)	1980	Iseki	+	0	0	0	0
(86)	1981	Borges	−	−	−	−	−
(91)	1983	Chen	+	0	0	0	0
(14)	1987	La Greca	+	−	−	−	−
(92)	1982	Hampl	+	0	0	0	0
(93)	1984	Vanholder	−	+	+	−	−
(84)	1985	Hakim	+	−	−	0	−
(98)	1987	Mansell	−	0	0	0	0
(99)	1984	Velez (Na 141)	−	0	0	0	0
(94)	1982	Pagel	+	+	−	−	0

+ = Significantly better with bicarbonate.
− = No difference with acetate.
0 = Not studied.

tion takes into account CO_2 losses through the dialyzer. As a further proof of this hypothesis, these authors demonstrated that hypoventilation and hypoxemia can be avoided by bubbling CO_2 in the dialysate. Dolan et al (59) have recently demonstrated the occurrence of hypoventilation-hypoxemia in acetate but not in bicarbonate dialysis where CO_2 losses do not take place. The importance of hypoventilation in inducing hypoxemia during dialysis has also been confirmed by Bouffard et al (60). These authors have demonstrated that hypoxemia does not take place in patients with acute renal failure dialyzed with mechanical ventilatory support.

A different approach to the problem has been proposed by Oh et al (39). They suggest that acetate metabolism may be the main cause of increased O_2 consumption and decreased CO_2 production with a consequent RQ reduction. This reduction will be proportional to the amount of acetate administered to the patient as observed by Raja et al (61) who noted more hypoxemia during dialysis carried out with higher acetate concentration in the dialysate. In conclusion (62) dialysis induced hypoxemia appears to be a multifactorial phenomenon and, although it has not yet been completely clarified, two major determinants are generally considered: acetate infusion and metabolism, and CO_2 losses through the dialyzer. An important contribution of the latter process already pointed out in the early seventies (63), is supported by the occurrence of hypoxemia in bicarbonate dialysis without bubling CO_2 in the dialysate (61) and by the absence of hypoxemia when CO_2 is bubbled in the dialysate both in acetate dialysis (64), and in bicarbonate dialysis (58).

Cardiovascular effects

When cardiovascular effects of acetate dialysis are considered, it is important to distinguish the specific effects determined by acetate from the general effects generated by dialysis treatment.

It is well known that acetate infusion in man has a vasodilatory effect (65, 66). It has, therefore, been suggested that in some patients acetate could be the main cause of hypotension and other cardiovascular effects recorded during dialysis. Kirkendol et al (28), studying the effects of an intravenous bolus of acetate in anesthetized dogs, concluded that acetate produces a dose-dependent reduction of the myocardial performance and of arterial blood pressure thus suggesting a cardiodepressant action of the buffer. The same finding was reported by Aizawa et al (67). However, in a subsequent study carried out at a constant rate of acetate infusion, Kirkendol et al (68) found an increase in cardiac output and a decrease of total peripheral resistance and mean arterial pressure. These effects on cardiac output were later confirmed by Chen et al (69) using echocardiography. Studies carried out in normal anesthetized dogs infused with increasing doses of acetate (70) showed an increase of cardiac output, heart rate, stroke volume and a decrease of peripheral resistance suggesting that acetate has a positive inotropic effect on the myocardium. Metha et al (71) later confirmed these findings excluding a myocardio-depressant action of acetate in patients undergoing dialysis therapy.

Finally in a recent study carried out in healthy volunteers treated with isovolemic acetate dialysis, Danielsson et al (72) demonstrated with invasive techniques that a systemic vasodilation is produced during dialysis, compensated by a heart rate dependent increase of cardiac output. Thus, it has been widely demonstrated that acetate has a direct vasodilatory effect although its pathogenesis is not clear. A possible interaction of acetate with ionized calcium necessary for the contraction of the vascular musculature (66) or a direct vasodilatory effect induced by acetate metabolites such as adenosine or adenine nucleotides (70) have been suggested. The myocardial response to this vasodilation is an increase in cardiac output in the attempt to maintain a stable blood pressure. This response, however, may be altered during dialysis because of a remarkable autonomic nerve dysfunction or a borderline cardiomyopathy.

Hence, dialysis induced hypotension is probably due to different mechanisms and several factors. One of them could be an insufficient increase in cardiac output in response of the vasodilation induced by acetate. Hypoxemia, altered serum osmolality, ultrafiltration and hypovolemia with a consequent reduction of the vascular filling pressure may also contribute to this pathologic event during acetate dialysis (73).

Metabolic effects

Acetate represents an important substrate for different metabolic pathways. During its metabolism via AcCoA, acetate can be partially shifted to lipids synthesis probably contributing to the hyperlipidemia and accelerated atherosclerosis of patients on regular dialysis treatment. However, Rorke et al (74) demonstrated, using labelled acetate on dialyzed dogs, that only 1% or less of the infused acetate is incorporated in the plasma lipids. This amount represents the regular metabolic turnover and it does not imply increased lipid production or deposition in the tissues. Other studies carried out in humans on acetate dialysis and in animals fed an atherogenic diet supplemented with acetate or bicarbonate (75), have also concluded that there is no evidence for a significant lipidogenic effect of acetate. Morin et al (76) in a crossover study on patients on acetate and bicarbonate dialysis, could not detect significant differences between the two dialysis treatment periods; hyperlipidemia of dialyzed patients depends more on reduced lipid removal than on increased production. Acetate therefore is not an important source of lipids and this metabolic pathway might only become critical when other lipogenic factors coexist.

Although acetate represents the main caloric substrate during dialysis, it is not a relevant caloric source overall, generating only 200 Cal/mol (12). Since the total amount of acetate given per session is about 1 mol, the caloric load from acetate metabolism represents less than 5% of the weekly caloric intake in a standard patient.

Effects on bone

The effects of metabolic acidosis on uremic oesteodystrophy

are still unclear. Acidosis can contribute to the pathogenesis of bone disease in uremia and may cause progressive loss of acid-soluble calcium carbonate from bone and a negative calcium balance (77). The involvement of the bone in buffering an acid load has been demonstrated both in humans (78) and in animal experimental models (79).

Lemann et al in 1966 (78) demonstrated that after an ammonium chloride load, mineral bone may participate in the overall buffering process. With chronic acidosis, different buffer systems are activated in the following sequence: 1) extracellular buffers, 2) extracellular and intracellular buffers, 3) intracellular and bone buffers and 4) bone buffers alone. When an acid load ceases, extracellular and intracellular buffers are completely repleted while the calcium lost from the bone is not completely restored and the amount of acid given is not completely excreted. Lemann et al suggested that this observation may demonstrate the interaction between bone calcium and hydrogen ions when chronic acidosis is present.

In patients on acetate dialysis, the participation of extracellular, intracellular and bone buffers should depend on the weekly acid-base balances of the patient and on their long term effects. When negative base balances occur devastating effects on bone mineralization would be expected in the long run. On the contrary, when base balance is near zero without a progressive accumulation of hydrogen ions in the body and a mild stable metabolic acidosis is present, severe bone disease should be less likely. The latter condition would mimic, as suggested by Gennari (80), the clinical setting of proximal renal tubular acidosis where a resetting of plasma bicarbonate at a lower level is present and no bone disease is observed.

However in acetate dialysis the base balance may frequently be negative and a continuous administration of oral alkaline supplementations may be required (81).

Accordingly, a continuous loss of bone mineral in patients dialyzed with acetate has been reported (78). This observation does not clarify whether dialysis may induce osteodystrophy by such pathogenetic factors as hyperparathyroidism, vitamin D deficiency and aluminum intoxication, or by maintaining a constant degree of acidosis. The final effect of uremic acidosis, per se, on the bone composition, therefore, remains difficult to clarify.

Control studies on dialyzed patients in whom a stable correction of acidosis is achieved are not available today. Such a population would represent in the future an interesting group to explore the effects of acidosis as an isolated factor on bone metabolism.

BICARBONATE DIALYSIS

The mechanism of correction of metabolic acidosis operating in bicarbonate dialysis differs from that of acetate dialysis (Figure 1). This results in different effects on acid-base balance, ventilation, cardiovascular function and metabolism.

Effects on acid-base status

In bicarbonate dialysis, blood pH and plasma bicarbonate progressively increase throughout the session while pCO_2 shows stable values (82, 83) or a moderate increase (48). At the end of dialysis a moderate metabolic alkalosis can be observed; its degree depends on the total bicarbonate balance and on the pre-dialytic acid-base status. Thereafter, blood pH and plasma bicarbonate progressively decrease until the subsequent dialysis. This behavior contrasts with acetate dialysis where the rapid metabolism of the infused acetate in the absence of bicarbonate losses temporarily increases pH and plasma bicarbonate. Patients treated by bicarbonate dialysis generally present for subsequent dialyses with an acid-base status close to normal, but some have an acidotic status similar to that observed in acetate dialysis (84), despite a positive buffer balance (4). Despite a slightly positive base balance in bicarbonate dialysis, it is still controversial whether acid-base correction with this treatment is more effective than with acetate.

Effects on ventilation

The effects of bicarbonate dialysis on ventilation and in particular on the possible occurrence of dialysis induced hypoxemia are still controversial. Some authors (85, 86) have observed no differences in patients treated alternatively with bicarbonate and acetate dialysis. Others (12, 83, 87) could observe hypoxemia in patients undergoing bicarbonate dialysis. The observation of dialysis induced hypoxemia in some patients treated with bicarbonate dialysis might depend on the bicarbonate concentration in the dialysate. In fact, dialysate concentrations of bicarbonate higher than 37 mmol/l might be responsible for a rapid alkalinization of the patient with a consequent compensatory hypoventilation (88).

Cardiovascular effects

Several studies report a better clinical tolerance of bicarbonate dialysis in terms of incidence of hypotensive episodes and intradialytic symptomatology such as nausea, vomiting, encephalopathy and cramps (48, 87, 89). Unanimous agreement on this point has not yet been reached, however (Table 1).

Patients on bicarbonate hemodialysis respond hemodynamically quite differently from those on acetate dialysis. Under similar conditions of ultrafiltration, bicarbonate dialysis achieves better stability of mean arterial pressure due to the maintenance of systemic vascular resistance, cardiac output and heart rate within adequate ranges (89). This hemodynamic response observed in bicarbonate dialysis, may be explained by the absence of the vasodilatory effect of acetate, or a favorable effect of alkalosis on vascular reactivity (95). Furthermore, myocardial contractility and left ventricular function may be improved in this condition (96), despite a possible reduction in myocardial reactivity due to variations of ionized calcium related to alkalosis (97). Recently, Mansell et al (98), comparing acetate and bicarbonate dialysis, showed a significant increase of heart rate only with acetate, while blood pressure and peripheral resistance were similar. They attributed the beneficial effects of bicarbonate dialysis more to a steadiness of the arterial pO_2 during the treatment, than to the absence of adverse cardiovascular effects of acetate. Furthermore, when high sodium dialysis solutions are used, the differences in vascular stability between acetate and bicarbonate dialysis seem to be cancelled. Comparative studies could not show significant advantages of bicarbonate versus acetate dialysis when high sodium dialysis fluid was used (99). Moreover, Henrich et al (100) reported similar hemodynamic responses with acetate and bicarbonate dialysis when dialysis fluid with higher osmolality was used, although with bicarbonate dialysis the number of therapeutic interventions was significantly less. But the constant use of high sodium concentrations in the dialysis fluid may increase the incidence of hypertension, thirst and excessive interdialytic weight gain. Hence, it is still controversial whether bicarbonate dialysis may directly benefit vascular stability during dialysis; although the vasodilatory effects of acetate are avoided bicarbonate dialysis cannot really eliminate other causes of hypotension such as ultrafiltration and preload reduction with a consequent reduction of the vascular filling pressure.

Effects on metabolism and bone

Bicarbonate has no significant metabolic effects, per se, and therefore does not interfere with biochemical processes such as gluconeogenesis or lipid synthesis. Morin et al (76) have demonstrated that no significant differences in cholesterol, triglycerydes, LDL, VLDL and HDL can be noted between acetate and bicarbonate dialysis. No long term osteomorphometric studies in patients treated with bicarbonate dialysis are available. But bicarbonate dialysis, by correcting metabolic acidosis more effectively should have a beneficial effect on the mineral bone by reducing the buffer requirements from this compartment.

HEMOFILTRATION

Few acid base studies have been carried out in patients treated by hemofiltration (HF). The net base balance in post dilutional HF is obtained by the difference between the base losses in the ultrafiltrate (HCO_3, organic anions and part of the buffer infused intravenously) and the amount of base administered to the patient via the substitution fluid. The buffers utilized in the replacement solutions are acetate and lactate at an average concentration of 40 mmol/l. Only experimental studies have been carried out with bicarbonate containing solutions (101); this buffer is not used clinically. Comparative studies have demonstrated that in HF pO_2, pCO_2, pH and bicarbonate have a behavior similar to that observed in acetate dialysis (102). Specifically, pO_2 shows a moderate decrease, pCO_2 remains stable and pH and bicarbonate progressively increase during the session. However,

pCO_2 and plasma bicarbonate concentrations are significantly higher in HF. Comparing the two techniques in the long run, HF appears to correct acid base status better than acetate dialysis does.

Similar results have been achieved by Schaefer et al (103), who compared acetate dialysis with hemofiltration using lactate as the substitution fluid buffer. HF patients showed less alterations in pO_2, a stability of pCO_2 which is slightly higher than with acetate dialysis and a significantly higher bicarbonate concentration when the session was stopped. In both groups pH increased, but more so in the HF patients after the end of the treatment; however HF patients experienced a significant initial drop of pH accompanied by a decrease in HCO_3 concentration, probably related to accumulation of lactate in plasma at this time.

Better control of pH in HF has been observed by Kishimoto et al (13). In studies comparing HF and acetate dialysis they noted that although the net load of acetate was comparable with HF and hemodialysis (660 vs 819 mmol respectively); acetate conversion into bicarbonate was significantly greater in HF.

Several schedules of hemofiltration have been proposed. They mainly differ in the number of liters exchanged per session and in the composition of substitution fluid. On line production of replacement fluid has also been proposed to avoid the problems related to the wide variability of the commercially prepared solutions in Europe. All these new treatments present different buffer balances and the final acid-base status therefore relates to the technique used.

HEMODIAFILTRATION AND RAPID DIALYSIS

Since blood purification in hemodiafiltration (HDF) is achieved with a mixed diffusive-convective transport, base balance calculations are extremely complex. However, one focal point in HDF, is the large amount of bicarbonate lost in the dialysate due to the high ultrafiltration rates and to the use of highly efficient dialyzers (24, 104).

The classic HDF proposed by Leber et al in 1978 (105), utilized a dialysis fluid containing acetate as a buffer and 9 l of substitution fluid containing lactate at a concentration of 40 mmol/l. Some authors (106, 107) later reported a better cardiovascular stability in HDF when bicarbonate replaces acetate in the dialysis solution. Others (104) suggested that bicarbonate substitution fluid may maintain a satisfactory acid-base status in patients on chronic HDF.

These preliminary observations suggest that bicarbonate should be preferred in HDF both for dialysis solution and replacement solutions. The use of acetate containing dialysis fluid may promote bicarbonate loss and induce an acetate load greater than the maximal metabolic capacity. On the other hand, substitution fluid containing lactate might progressively increase plasma lactate concentrations with consequent metabolic problems.

A recent study on base balance in HDF using bicarbonate both in the dialysis solution (31 mmol/l) and in the substitution fluid (41 mmol/l) (107) suggested that bicarbonate losses correlate with the amount of ultrafiltrate produced during the treatment. But, the amount of buffer administered via substitution fluid is generally sufficient to maintain an adequate base balance. Bicarbonate losses during an HDF session carried out exchanging 9 l of fluid averages 300 mmol. Under these conditions, the reinfusion of 9 l of substitution fluid containing 41 mmol/l of HCO₃ allows for a slightly positive HCO₃ balance with a total acid-base balance near zero when other substances influencing the final balance are considered. Furthermore, blood gases remain fairly stable during treatment with a general steadiness of cardiovascular function and ventilation.

The recent clinical introduction of highly permeable membranes and equipments with ultrafiltration control systems has stimulated new interest in HDF and several new techniques have been developed. In Europe HDF is carried out utilizing variable amounts of substitution fluid. Hence, the buffer concentration must be adapted to the amount of fluid exchanged per session. When low volumes of fluid are utilized and a lower convective component is present as in biofiltration (3 l/session), higher buffer concentrations are used in the substitution fluid (60 to 100 mmol/l) (24). Even higher quantities of bicarbonate are reinfused when acetate is completely eliminated from dialysate such as in Acetate-Free-Biofiltration. Finally, the replacement process is not always carried out utilizing commercially prepared solutions. New techniques have been proposed (22) in which the replacement of fluid lost via ultrafiltration is achieved by backfiltration of sterile dialysate through the hemodiafilter.

In all these new techniques the acid-base balance has not yet been studied even though a satisfactory correction of metabolic acidosis is frequently achieved. A final problem to be clarified concerns the use of highly efficient treatments that allow for a marked reduction of dialysis treatment time. While it is clear that bicarbonate is the only possible buffer for highly efficient treatments, it is still controversial whether acid-base balance can be maintained within acceptable ranges with these rapid techniques.

SORBENTS AND RECIRCULATING DIALYSIS

Recirculating dialysis is a depuration system utilizing a low dialysate volume which recirculates in a closed circuit being regenerated continuously by a regenerating cartridge. In USA the system originally named REDY (now Sorb System) is the most popular. It utilizes 5.5 l of dialysate and the cartridge holds urease, cation and anion exchangers and activated carbon (108).

In Europe and expecially in Italy, the procedure is known as short recirculating dialysis and utilizes either 20 or 40 l of dialysate and the cartridge contains only activated carbon and aluminum silicate (109).

Both acetate and bicarbonate are used as buffer. The overall acid base balance is the result of three events: the transfer of buffer from dialysate to the patient, the additional generation of bicarbonate by urea breakdown and the progressive reduction of bicarbonate losses across the dia-

lyzer membrane, as blood and dialysate concentrations tend to equilibrate during treatment.

Moreover, when bicarbonate buffer is utilized, the high dialysate PCO₂ counteracts the CO₂ loss across the dialyzer membrane with consequent reduced intradialytic hypocapnia, hypoventilation and hypoxemia.

On the basis of these principles, recirculating dialysis allows a good intradialytic vascular stability and a satisfactory correction of acidosis (110).

LACTIC ACIDOSIS

Lactic acidosis is an acid base disorder characterized by a plasma lactate concentration higher than 5 mEq/l and blood pH lower than 7.2. The prognosis is poor, expecially when severe hypotension is present.

Etiologically two types of lactic acidosis can be distinguished. Type A results from tissue hypoxia (reduced tissue perfusion or reduced arterial O₂ content) and type B is secondary to a metabolic derangement (generalized disease such as diabetes mellitus, liver failure or sepsis, increased peripheral O₂ demand, drug intoxications or congenital metabolic disorders). The identification and the treatment of the underlying cause represent the first and most important step for therapy of lactic acidosis.

Bicarbonate administration is advised when acidosis is severe. The rationale for such a therapy is the need to expand extracellular volume and to counteract hemodynamic effects of acidosis.

Recently, the use of bicarbonate has been criticized strongly on the basis of experimental studies in animals showing that alkalinizing therapy can increase gut lactate production and decrease liver and erythrocyte intracellular pH, cardiac output and blood pressure (111). In spite of that, the use of bicarbonate, as symptomatic therapy, to restore pH to a hemodynamically safe value seems to be reasonable (112).

As the individual dose requirement is not easy to determine, the administration of large amounts of bicarbonate can lead to hypernatremia, hyperosmolarity and volume overload.

Forced diuresis by a potent loop diuretic may prevent these complications. Alternatively, peritoneal dialysis, hemodialysis and hemofiltration can be used in patients with both normal and impaired renal function to prevent or to treat fluid-electrolyte overload and to supply buffers. Obviously the use of lactate buffer must be avoided and acetate must be reserved for patients without severe hypotension. Bicarbonate should be the ideal buffer for these patients as it ensures a physiological alkali provision and avoids acetate induced hypoxemia. As a confirmation, it has been employed successfully in peritoneal dialysis and in hemodialysis (113, 114).

ACID-BASE IN PERITONEAL DIALYSIS

Although intermittent peritoneal dialysis (IPD) has been for years an alternative treatment in patients with end-stage renal disease, this type of treatment has now been almost abandoned and continuous ambulatory peritoneal dialysis (CAPD) represents the most common intracorporeal dialysis treatment.

One of the major results achieved with CAPD is the good correction of metabolic acidosis and the maintenance of a satisfactory acid-base status. This is confirmed by an average plasma bicarbonate concentration in patients on CAPD ranging between 22 and 25 mmol/l (44). This result appears to be stable over time and acid-base fluctuation typical of intermittent treatments are not observed. The steadiness of acid-base status probably depends on the continuous infusion of buffers in the absence of significant losses of bicarbonate and permits a certain stability of blood gases and ventilation.

Lactate is the commonly used buffer in CAPD. Acetate has also been used in the past but it has been subsequently abandoned when suspected to be responsible for long term side effects such as ultrafiltration loss, severe anatomical alterations of peritoneal membrane and sclerosing peritonitis (115, 116). Furthermore it has been pointed out that acetate levels in the blood may reach dangerously high concentrations with consequent undesired effects (42). Bicarbonate has been recently proposed as the buffer for CAPD but few experimental studies have been carried out until now (117).

Weekly buffer balance in patients on CAPD can be calculated as follows:

$$NBGw = n [Binf - (HCO_3 + OA)lost - TAd] - H^+ Gw$$

where NBGw is net base gain per week; n is number of exchanges in a week; Binf is Buffer infused in each exchange; $(HCO_3 + OA)$lost = bicarbonate and organic acid anions lost in the dialysate in each exchange; TAd is titratable acidity of the inlet dialysis solution (118); $H^+ Gw$ is weekly metabolic acid production.

In CAPD, long dwell times, permit an almost complete transfer of the buffer from the dialysis solution into the blood. As shown in Figure 8, the buffer disappearance rate is maximal in the first few minutes of the exchange while it subsequently approaches zero. This behavior is important because it also permits an adequate buffer transfer when rapid exchanges are scheduled. Since in CAPD the buffer diffuses almost completely from dialysate, the major determinants of net base gain are the concentration of the buffer in the inlet dialysis solution and dwell time.

Figure 9 reports the significant correlation between the daily buffer gain and the concentration of the buffer in the dialysis solution. Accordingly, it would be possible to predict the daily buffer gain in a given patient on the basis of the buffer concentration in the dialysis solution. It must be noted that D-lactate and L-lactate may have different rates of transport. Rubin et al (119) demonstrated that the peritoneal membrane can operate a stereospecific selection in the process of lactate transport. L-lactate has an higher mass transfer rate (MTR) and it is rapidly metabolized in the

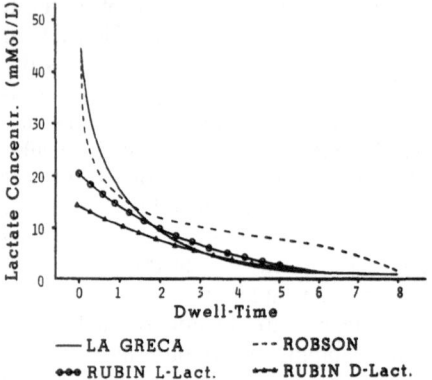

LACTATE DISAPPEARANCE FROM DIALYSATE

Figure 8. Disappearance of lactate from dialysate (42,119,120). When higher concentrations of lactate are used, the rate of transport of the buffer is maximal in the first minutes of each exchange while it approaches zero asymptotically in the following hours. This explains why a satisfactory buffer transfer can be achieved also on intermittent peritoneal dialysis with rapid exchanges and why the buffer disappears almost completely in long dwell time exchanges.

body. D-lactate is metabolized more slowly, but the very low MTR permits complete metabolism of this stereoisomeric compound as well.

During dialysis, bicarbonate back diffuses in the dialysate. However, bicarbonate losses in peritoneal dialysis are not easy to quantify because of specific problems related to ultrafiltration, plasma HCO_3 concentration and methodology of measurement of HCO_3 in the dialysate.

Ultrafiltration is the major determinant of bicarbonate losses in the dialysate. It is evident that when dialysate/plasma equilibration takes place, an increase in drainage volume due to ultrafiltration, causes a greater loss of bicarbonate. The same effect is determined by higher HCO_3 plasma concentrations although several studies suggest a possible feed back mechanism between plasma bicarbonate concentration and amount of bicarbonate lost in the dialysate (117, 120). An increased plasma bicarbonate level causes a parallel increase of bicarbonate losses until the dialysate/plasma equilibration is reached and no more bicarbonate diffuses. It may also be argued that a Donnan equilibrium could cause bicarbonate losses greater than expected from the plasma concentration because of the presence of non diffusable anions such as plasma proteins in the blood compartment, but this phenomenon is too small for any clinical relevance.

A further problem concerns the method of measurement of the carbonic acid/bicarbonate system in the peritoneal dialysis solution. It does not have the same pK as in blood so the measurements cannot be correctly done with the commonly used analyzers.

Finally we must consider the losses in the dialysate of metabolizable anions of organic acids. These substances represent effective alkaline equivalents since their metabolism produces bicarbonate. Among these substrates, only

LACTATE MASS TRANSFER IN CAPD

DAILY GAIN VERSUS DIALYSATE CONCENTRATION

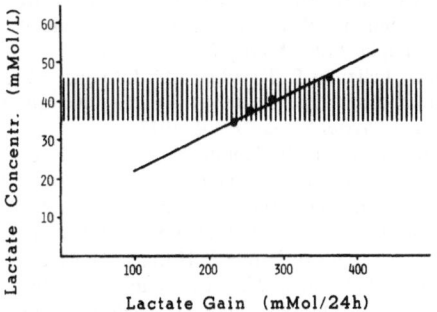

Figure 9. Mass transfer of lactate in CAPD in relation with lactate concentration in the dialysis solution (42,43,119,120).

acetoacetate and β-hydroxybutyrate have quantitative relevance. Teehan et al (43) have reported daily losses in the dialysate of 1.0 ± 0.3 mmol of acetoacetate and 4.1 ± 1.9 of β-hydroxybutyrate. Other substances are lost in the dialysate such as tricarboxylic anions although they have never been quantified. Yet a significant anion gap (36 ± 17 mmol/24 h) is observed in the effluent dialysate (43).

For all these reasons a remarkable difference among the various acid-base balance studies can be noted, although there is a general agreement that CAPD corrects metabolic acidosis very well (42, 44, 120). The different results of acid-balance studies depend on the several variables mentioned above. But the major determinant of the net base gain is the concentration of the buffer in the dialysis solution.

FINAL REMARKS

Review of the literature and clinical experience confirm that correction of metabolic acidosis in uremic patients with dialysis is not yet optimized and still presents many controversies. The progressive substitution of standard acetate dialysis with bicarbonate dialysis appears to be supported by several observations. Bicarbonate is the physiologic buffer, it does not require metabolic conversion and it does not cause any known side effect except for possible alkalosis deriving from excessive administration. Technological problems concerning dialysis equipment and solutions have been overcome and treatment costs are not significantly higher using bicarbonate dialysate. Finally, the excellent clinical tolerance of bicarbonate dialysis, makes this treatment a first choice therapy today.

This trend assumes more and more importance in relation to the widening application in clinical practice of highly efficient treatments with a consistent reduction of dialysis treatment time. Bicarbonate in fact becomes mandatory as a buffer for hemodialysis when high surface area dialyzers and highly permeable membranes are utilized in conjunction with high blood and dialysate flows.

A satisfactory correction of uremic acidosis is certainly possible as shown by the acid-base status achieved in CAPD patients. Acid-base homeostasis in CAPD patients demonstrates that limiting bicarbonate losses during treatment is a key point of this puzzling problem.

A final consideration concerns the necessity to achieve a good acid base status in dialysis patients and the need to make great efforts at metabolic correction with dialysis treatment. Some authors suggest that this is a negligible problem which does not cause any long term clinical effects (80). We believe that all possible efforts must be made to achieve, together with an adequate blood purification, the best possible correction of metabolic acidosis in uremic patients. This concept derives from the conviction that acidosis may interfere with several functions of the body such as ventilation, cardiovascular activity, gastrointestinal and skeletal metabolism and finally chemical and enzymatic reactions.

REFERENCES

1. Kolff WJ: Le rein artificiel: un dialyseur a grande surface. (The artificial kidney: a large surface dialyzer.) *Presse Med* 52: 103, 1944
2. Scribner BH, Caner JEZ, Buri R: The technique of continuous hemodialysis. *Trans Am Soc Artif Intern Organs* 6: 88, 1960
3. Mion CM, Hegstrom RM, Boen ST: Substitution of sodium acetate for sodium bicarbonate in the bath fluid for hemodialysis. *Trans Am Soc Artif Intern Organs* 10: 110, 1964
4. Gotch FA, Sargent JA, Keen ML: Hydrogen ion balance in dialysis therapy. *Artif Organs* 6: 388, 1982
5. Assomull VM, Vreman HJ, Weiner MW: Mass balance of base equivalents during hemodialysis: Importance of organic acid anions. *Proc Clin Dial Transplant Forum* 8: 137, 1978
6. Mioni G, Gropuzzo M, Farazza A, Messa P, Montanaro D, Adorati M, Paviotti G, Messa M, Lo Greco P: La reazione di attivazione dell 'acetato nel trattamento emodialitico. (The reason for activation of acetate during hemodialysis treatment.) *Minerva Nefrol* 29: 137, 1982
7. Sargent JA, Gotch FA: Bicarbonate and carbon dioxide transport during hemodialysis. *asaio J* 2: 61, 1979
8. Bosch JP, Glabman S. Moutoussis G, Belledonne M, von Albertini B, Kahn T: Carbon dioxide removal in acetate hemodialysis: Effects on acid base balance. *Kidney Int* 25: 830, 1984
9. Christensen HN: General concepts of neutrality regulation *Am J Surg* 103: 286, 1962
10. Wathen RL, Ward RA: Disturbances in fluid, electrolyte, and acid base in the dialysis patient, in *Textbook of Nephrology* Vol 2, edited by Massry SG, Glassock RJ, Baltimore, Williams & Wilkins, 1983, p 7.98
11. Vreman HJ, Assomull VM, Kaiser BA, Blaschke TF, Weiner MW: Acetate metabolism and acid-base homeostasis during hemodialysis: Influence of dialyzer efficiency and rate of acetate metabolism. *Kidney Int* 18 (Suppl 10): 62, 1980
12. Tolchin N, Roberts JL, Hayashi J, Lewis EJ: Metabolic consequences of high mass-transfer hemodialysis. *Kidney Int* 11: 366, 1977
13. Kishimoto T, Yamamoto T, Yamamoto K, Yamagami S, Nishitani H, Mizutani Y, Yamakawa M, Maekawa M: Ace-

tate kinetics during hemodialysis and hemofiltration. *Blood Purif* 2: 81, 1984

14. La Greca G, Feriani M, Bragantini L, Petrosino L, Santoro A, Altieri P: Effects of acetate and bicarbonate dialysate on vascular stability: a prospective multicentric study. *Int J Artif Organs* 10: 15, 1987

15. Ward RA, Wathen RL, Williams TE: Effects of long-term bicarbonate hemodialysis (BHD) on acid-base status. *Trans Am Soc Artif Intern Organs* 28: 295, 1982

16. Bjældager PAL, Christiansen E, Jensen HÆ, Paulev PEK: Improved effect of hemodialysis on acidemic patients from an acetate concentration of 38 mMol/L. *Nephron* 27: 142, 1981

17. Mansell MA, Nunan TO, Laker MF, Boon NA, Wing AJ: Incidence and significance of rising blood acetate levels during hemodialysis. *Clin Nephrol* 12: 22, 1979

18. Richards RH, Vreman HJ, Zager Ph, Feldman C, Blaschke T, Weiner MW: Acetate metabolism in normal human subject. *Am J Kidney Dis* 2: 47, 1982

19. Lewis EJ, Tolchin N, Roberts JL: Estimation of the metabolic conversion of acetate to bicarbonate during hemodialysis. *Kidney Int* 18 (Suppl 10): 51, 1980

20. Kveim M, Nesbakken R: Utilisation of exogenous acetate during hemodialysis. *Trans Am Soc Artif Intern Organs* 21: 138, 1975

21. Kaiser BA, Potter DE, Bryant RE, Vreman HJ, Weiner MW: Acid-base changes and acetate metabolism during routine and high efficiency hemodialysis in children. *Kidney Int* 19: 70, 1981

22. von Albertini B, Miller JH, Gardner PW, Shinaberger JH: High-flux hemodiafiltration: under six hours/week treatment. *Trans Am Soc Artif Intern Organs* 30: 227, 1984

23. Ward RA, Wathen RL: Utilization of bicarbonate for base repletion in hemodialysis. *Artif Organs* 6: 369, 1982

24. Feriani M, Bragantini L, Dell'Aquila R, Chiaramonte S, Fabris A, Biasioli S, Ronco C, Brendolan A, La Greca G: Buffer kinetics in biofiltration. *Int J Artif Organs* 9 (S-3): 1, 1986

25. Sprenger KBG, Kratz W, Lewis AE, Stadtmüller U: Kinetic modeling of hemodialysis, hemofiltration, and hemodiafiltration. *Kidney Int* 24: 143, 1983

26. Colton CK, Henderson LW, Ford CA, Lysaght MJ: Kinetics of hemodiafiltration. I. In vitro transport characteristics of a hollow-fiber blood ultrafilter. *J Lab Clin Med* 85: 355, 1975

27. Henderson LW, Colton CK, Ford CA: Kinetics of hemodiafiltration. II. Clinical characterization of a blood cleansing modality. *J Lab Clin Med* 85: 372, 1975

28. Kirkendol PL, Devia CJ, Bower JD, Holbert RD: A comparison of the cardiovascular effects of sodium acetate, sodium bicarbonate and other potential sources of fixed base in hemodialysate solutions. *Trans Am Soc Artif Intern Organs* 23: 399, 1977

29. Wathen RL, Ward RA, Harding GB, Meyer LC: Acid-base and metabolic responses to anion infusion in the anesthetized dog. *Kidney Int* 21: 592, 1982

30. Mudge GH, Manning JA, Gilman A: Sodium acetate as a source of fixed base. *Proc Soc Exp Biol Med* 71: 136, 1949

31. Lundquist F: Production and utilization of free acetate in man. *Nature* 193: 579, 1962

32. Harper PV, Neal WB, Hlavacek GR: Acetate utilization in dog. *Metabolism* 2: 62, 1953

33. Davidson WD, Morin RJ, Srikantaiah M, Basset L: The role of acetate in dialysate for hemodialysis. *11th Annu Contractor's Conf Artif Kidney Program, NIAMDD* edited by Mackey BB, DHEW Publ No (NIH) 79-1448, 1978, p 75

34- Morin RJ, Guo LSS, Rorke SJ, Davidson WD: Lipid metabo-

lism in non-uremic dogs during and after hemodialysis with acetate. *J Dial* 2: 113, 1978

35. Skutches CL, Sigler MH, Teehan BP, Cooper JH, Reichard GA: Contribution of dialysate acetate to energy metabolism: Metabolic implications. *Kidney Int* 23: 57, 1983

36. Karlsson N, Fellenius E, Kiessling KH: Influence of acetate on the metabolism of palmitate in the perfuse hindquarter of the rat. *Acta Physiol Scand* 99: 156, 1977

37. Wathen RL, Keshaviah P, Hommeyer P, Cadwell K, Comty CM: The metabolic effects of hemodialysis with and without glucose in the dialysate. *Am J Clin Nutr* 31: 1870, 1978

38. Yamakawa M, Yamamoto T, Kishimoto T, Mizutani J, Yatsuboshi M, Nishitani H, Hirata S, Horiuchi N, Maekawa M: Serum levels of acetate and TCA cycle intermediates during hemodialysis in relation to symptoms. *Nephron* 32: 155, 1982

39. Oh MS, Uribarri J, Del Monte ML, Friedman EA, Carroll HJ: Consumption of CO_2 in metabolism of acetate as an explanation for hypoventilation and hypoxemia during hemodialysis. *Proc Clin Dial Transplant Forum* 9: 226, 1979

40. Hartmann AF, Senn MJE: Studies in the metabolism of sodium lactate. *J Clin Invest* 11: 327, 1932

41. Searle GL, Cavalieri RR: Determination of lactate kinetics in the human analysis of data from single injection. *Proc Soc Exp Biol Med* 139: 1002, 1972

42. La Greca G, Biasioli S, Chiaramonte S, Davi M, Fabris A, Feriani M, Pisani E, Ronco C, Zen F: Acid-base balance on peritoneal dialysis. *Clin Nephrol* 16: 1, 1981

43. Teehan BP, Schleifer CR, Reichard GA, Cupit MC, Sigler MH, Haff AC: Acid-base studies in CAPD. in: *CAPD Update,* edited by Moncrief JW, Popovich RP, New York, Masson Publ Inc, 1981, p 95

44. Fabris A, Biasioli S, Chiaramonte S, Feriani M, Pisani E, Ronco C, Cantarella G, La Greca G: Buffer metabolism in CAPD: Relationship with respiratory dynamics. *Trans Am Soc Artif Intern Organs* 28: 270, 1982

45. Gibbson BH, Edsall JT: Rate of hydration of carbon dioxide and dehydration at 25° C. *J Biol Chem* 238: 3501, 1963

46. Gray BA: The rate of approach to equilibrium in uncatalyzed CO_2 hydration reactions: the theoretical effect of buffering capacity. *Respir Physiol* 11: 223, 1971

47. Maren TH: Carbonic anhydrase: chemistry, physiology and inhibition. *Physiol Rev* 47: 595, 1967

48. Graefe U, Milutinovich J, Follette WC, Vizzo JE, Babb AL, Scribner BH: Less dialysis-induced morbidity and vascular instability with bicarbonate in dialysate. *Ann Intern Med* 88: 332, 1978

49. Nissenson AR, Kraut JA, Shinaberger JH: Dialysis-associated hypoxemia: Pathogenesis and prevention. *asaio J* 7: 1, 1984

50. Keshaviah P, Carlson L, Costantini E, Shapiro F: Dialysis induced hypoxemia and hypotension are not causally related. *Trans Am Soc Artif Intern Organs* 30: 159, 1984

51. Wathen RL, Ferris FZ, Nagar D, Keshaviah P: An alternative explanation for dialysis-induced arterial hypoxemia (Abstract) *Kidney Int* 14: 689, 1978

52. Hirszel P, Maher JF, Tempel GE, Mengel CE: Effect of hemodialysis on factors influencing oxygen transport. *J Lab Clin Med* 85: 978, 1975

53. Bischel MD, Scoles BG, Mohler JG: Evidence for pulmonary microembolization during hemodialysis. *Chest* 67: 335, 1975

54. Aurigemma NM, Feldman NT, Gottlieb M, Ingram RH, Lazarus JM, Lowrie EG: Arterial oxygenation during hemodialysis. *N Engl J Med* 297: 871, 1977

55. Craddock PR, Fehr J, Brigham KL, Kronenberg RS, Jacob

HS: Complement and leukocyte-mediated pulmonary dysfunction in hemodialysis. *N Engl J Med* 296: 770, 1977

56. Jacob AI, Gavellas G, Zarco R, Perez G, Bourgoignie JJ: Leucopenia, hypoxia and complement function with different hemodialysis membranes. *Kidney Int* 18: 105, 1980

57. Brautbar N, Shinaberger JH, Miller JH, Nachman M: Hemodialysis hypoxemia: evaluation of mechanism utilizing sequential ultrafiltration-dialysis. *Nephron* 26: 96, 1980

58. Sherlock J, Ledwith J, Letteri J: Hypoventilation and hypoxemia during hemodialysis: reflex response to removal of CO₂ across the dialyzer. *Trans Am Soc Artif Intern Organs* 23: 406, 1977

59. Dolan MJ, Whipp BJ, Davidson WD, Weitzman RE, Wasserman K: Hypopnea associated with acetate hemodialysis: carbon dioxide flow-dependent ventilation. *N Engl J Med* 305: 72, 1981

60. Bouffard Y, Viale JP, Annat G, Guillaume C, Percival C, Bertrand O, Motin J: Pulmonary gas exchange during hemodialysis. *Kidney Int* 30: 920, 1986

61. Raja RM, Kramer MS, Rosenbaum R, Bolisay CG, Krug MJ: Hemodialysis associated hypoxemia. Role of acetate and pH in etiology. *Trans Am Soc Artif Intern Organs* 27: 180, 1981

62. Garella S, Chang BS: Hemodialysis-associated hypoxemia. *Am J Nephrol* 4: 273, 1984

63. Graziani G, Ponticelli C, Di Filippo G, Radaelli B: Acid-base changes in hemodialysis. *Br Med J* 3: 163, 1970

64. Romaldini H, Stabile C, Faro S, Lopes Dos Santos M, Ramos OL, Ribeiro Ratto O: Pulmonary ventilation during hemodialysis. *Nephron* 32: 131, 1982

65. Bauer W, Richards JW: A vasodilator action of acetate. *J Physiol* (London) 66: 371, 1928

66. Frohlich ED: Vascular effects of the Krebs intermediate metabolites. *Am J Physiol* 208: 149, 1965

67. Aizawa Y, Ohmori T, Imai K, Nara Y, Matsuoka M, Hirakawa Y: Depressant action of acetate upon the human cardiovascular system. *Clin Nephrol* 8: 477, 1977

68. Kirkendol PL, Robie NW, Gonzalez FM, Devia CJ: Cardiac and vascular effects of infused sodium acetate in dogs. *Trans Am Soc Artif Intern Organs* 24: 714, 1978

69. Chen TS, Friedman HS, Del Monte M, Smith AJ: Hemodynamic changes during dialysis. *Proc Clin Dial Transplant Forum* 9: 66, 1979

70. Liang CS, Lowenstein JM: Metabolic control of the circulation effects of acetate and pyruvate. *J Clin Invest* 62: 1029, 1978

71. Metha BR, Fischer D, Ahmad M, Dubose TD Jr: Effects of acetate and bicarbonate hemodialysis on cardiac function in chronic dialysis patients. *Kidney Int* 24: 782, 1983

72. Danielsson A, Freyschuss U, Bergström J: Cardiovascular function and alveolar gas exchange during isovolemic hemodialysis with acetate in healthy man. *Blood Purif* 5: 41, 1987

73. Kinet JP, Soyeur D, Balland N, Saint-Remy M, Collignon P, Godon JP: Hemodynamic study of hypotension during hemodialysis. *Kidney Int* 21: 868, 1982

74. Rorke SJ, Davidson WD, Guo SS, Morin RJ: Metabolic fate of C-Acetate during dialysis. *Proc Eur Dial Transplant Assoc* 13: 394, 1976

75. Assomull VM, Vreman HJ, Weiner MW: Evidence that acetate in dialysate does not stimulate lipid synthesis. *Proc Clin Dial Transplant Forum* 9: 73, 1979

76. Morin RJ, Srikanraiah MV, Woodley Z, Davidson WD: Effect of acetate vs bicarbonate on plasma lipid and lipoprotein levels in uremic patients. *J Dial* 4: 9, 1980

77. Massry SG: Divalent ion metabolism and renal osteodystrophy. in *Textbook of Nephrology* Vol 2. edited by Massry SG, Glassock RJ, Baltimore, Williams & Wilkins, 1983, p 7, 104

78. Lemann J Jr, Litzow JR, Lennon EJ: The effects of chronic acid loads in normal man: Further evidence for the participation of bone mineral in the defense against chronic metabolic acidosis. *J Clin Invest* 45: 1608, 1966

79. Barzel US, Jowsey J: The effects of chronic acid and alkalai administration on bone turnover in adult rat. *Clin Sci* 36: 517, 1969

80. Gennari FJ: Acid-base balance in dialysis patients. *Kidney Int* 28: 678, 1985

81. Van Stone JC: Oral base replacement in patients on hemodialysis. *Ann Intern Med* 101: 199, 1984

82. Man NK, Fournier G, Thireau P, Gaillard JL, Funck-Brentano JL: Effect of bicarbonate-containing dialysate on chronic hemodialysis patients: A comparative study. *Artif Organs* 6: 421, 1982

83. Nissenson AR: Prevention of dialysis-induced hypoxemia by bicarbonate dialysis. *Trans Am Soc Artif Intern Organs* 26: 339, 1980

84. Hakim RM, Pontzer MA, Tilton D, Lazarus JM, Gottlieb MN: Effects of acetate and bicarbonate dialysis in stable chronic dialysis patients. *Kidney Int* 28: 535, 1985

85. Abu-Hamdan DK, Mahajan SK, Desai S, Choi CW, Mueller B, Briggs WA, McDonald FD: Hypoxemia during bicarbonate dialysis *Abstracts Am Soc Nephrol* 13: 33A, 1980

86. Borges H, Fryd DS, Rosa AA, Kjellstrand CM: Hypotension during acetate and bicarbonate dialysis in patients with acute renal failure. *Am J Nephrol* 1: 24, 1981

87. Van Stone JC: A clinical comparison of bicarbonate and acetate dialysates. *Cont Dial* (9): 25, 1980

88. Eiser AR, Jayammane D, Kokseng C, Che H, Slifkin RF, Neff MS: Contrasting alterations in pulmonary gas exchange during acetate and bicarbonate hemodialysis. *Am J Nephrol* 2: 123, 1982

89. Iseki K, Onoyama K, Maeda T, Shimamatsu K, Harada A, Fujimi S, Omae T: Comparison of hemodynamics induced by conventional acetate hemodialysis, bicarbonate hemodialysis and ultrafiltration. *Clin Nephrol* 14: 294, 1980

90. Whele B, Asaba H, Casterfors J, Fürst P, Grahn A, Gunnarson B, Shaldon S, Bergström J: The influence of dialysis fluid composition on the blood pressure response during dialysis. *Clin Nephrol* 10: 62, 1978

91. Chen T, Friedman H, Smith A, Del Monte M: Hemodynamic changes during hemodialysis role of dialysate. *Clin Nephrol* 20: 190, 1983

92. Hampl H, Wolfquiler M, Pustelruk A, Schiller R, Hanefeld F, Kessel M: Advantage of bicarbonate hemodialysis. *Artif Organs* 6: 410, 1982

93. Vanholder R, Piron M, Ringoir S: Absence of a beneficial haemodynamic effect of bicarbonate vs acetate haemodialysis. *Proc Eur Dial Transplant Assoc* 21: 195, 1984

94. Pagel MD, Ahmad S, Vizzo JE, Scribner BH: Acetate and bicarbonate fluctuations and acetate intolerance during dialysis. *Kidney Int* 21: 513, 1982

95. Mitchell J, Wildenthal K, Johnson R: The effects of acid-base disturbances on cardiovascular and pulmonary function. *Kidney Int* 1: 375, 1972

96. Ruder MA, Alpert MA, Van Stone J, Selmon MR, Kelly DL, Haynie JD, Perkins SK: Comparative effects of acetate and bicarbonate hemodialysis on left ventricular function. *Kidney Int* 27: 768, 1985

97. Henrich W, Hunt J, Nixon J: Increased ionized calcium and left ventricular contractility during hemodialysis. *N Engl J Med* 310: 19, 1983

98. Mansell MA, Morgan SH, Moore R, Kong KH, Laker MF, Wing AJ: Cardiovascular and acid-base effects of acetate and bicarbonate hemodialysis. *Dial Transplant* 1: 229, 1987

99. Velez RL, Woodard TD, Henrich WL: Acetate and bicarbonate hemodialysis in patients with and without autonomic dysfunction. *Kidney Int* 26: 59, 1984

100. Henrich WL, Woodard TD, Meyer BD, Chappell TR, Rubin LJ: High sodium bicarbonate and acetate hemodialysis: Double-blind crossover comparison of hemodynamic and ventilatory effects. *Kidney Int* 24: 240, 1983

101. Feriani M, Biasioli S, Fabris A, Chiaramonte S, Ronco C, Bragantini L, Brendolan A, Dell'Aquila R, La Greca G: Calcium and bicarbonate containing solutions for peritoneal dialysis and hemofiltration in *Progress in Artif Organs* edited by Nose Y, Kjellstrand C, Ivanovich P, Cleveland, ISAO Press, 1986, p. 277

102. Bosch JP, Lauer A: Acid-base balance in hemofiltration in *Hemofiltration* edited by Henderson LW, Quellhorst EA, Baldamus CA, Lysaght MJ, Berlin, Springer Verlag, 1986, p. 147

103. Schaefer K, Ryzlewicz T, Sandri M, von Bernewitz S, von Herrath D: Effect of hemofiltration on acid-base status and ventilation. *Contr Nephrol* 32: 69, 1982

104. Arisi L, Calderini C, David S, Manari A, Mancuso S, Cambi V: Acid base balance in hypertonic hemodiafiltration. in *Uremic Acidosis,* edited by Petrella E, Milan Wichtig Editore, 1983, p 71

105. Leber HW, Wizemann V, Goubeand G, Rawer P, Schütterle G: Simultaneous hemofiltration/hemodialysis: an effective alternative to hemofiltration and conventional hemodialysis in the treatment of uremic patients. *Clin Nephrol* 9: 115, 1978

106. Scheider H, Liornin E, Streicher E: Haemodynamic studies of diffusive and convective procedures using a polysulphone membrane. *Contrib Nephrol* 46: 134, 1985

107. Feriani M, Biasioli S, Bragantini L, Dell'Aquila R, Fabris A, Ronco C, Chiaramonte S, Brendolan A, Milan M, La Greca G: Buffer balance in bicarbonate hemodiafiltration. *Trans Am Soc Artif Intern Organs* 32: 422, 1986

108. Gordon A, Greembaum MA, Marantz LB, McArthur MJ, Maxwell MH: A sorbent-based low volume dialysate system. *Trans Am Soc Artif Intern Organs* 15: 347, 1969

109. Bigi L, Orlandini GC, Cappelli G, Savazzi A, Lusvarghi E, Petrella E, Cambi V: Long term use of a stable bicarbonate containing dialysate. *J Dial* 3: 119, 1979

110. Salvadeo A, Piazza W, Galli F, Segagni S, Villa G, Bovio G, Poggio F, Picardi L: Vascular stability in bicarbonate recirculating dialysis in *Uremic Acidosis* edited by Petrella E, Milan, Wichtig Editore 1981, p 135

111. Stacpole PW: Lactic acidosis: The case against bicarbonate therapy. *Ann Intern Med* 105: 276, 1986

112. Madias NE: Lactic acidosis. *Kidney Int* 29: 752, 1986

113. Vaziri ND, Ness R, Wellikson L, Barton C, Greep N: Bicarbonate buffered peritoneal dialysis: An effective adjunct in the treatment of lactic acidosis. *Am J Med* 67: 392, 1979

114. Chalopin JM, Tanger Y, Besancenot JF, Cabanne JF, Rifle G: Treatment of metformin associated lactic acidosis with closed recirculation bicarbonate buffered hemodialysis. *Arch Intern Med* 144: 203, 1984

115. Faller B, Marichal JF: Loss of ultrafiltration in CAPD; a role for acetate. *Peritoneal Dial Bull* 4: 10, 1984

116. Slingeneyer A, Mion C, Mourad G, Canaud B, Faller B, Beraud JJ: Progressive sclerosing peritonitis. A late and severe complication of maintenance peritoneal dialysis. *Trans Am Soc Artif Intern Organs* 29: 633, 1983

117. Feriani M, Biasioli S, Borin D, Bragantini L, Brendolan A, Chiaramonte S, Dell'Aquila R, Fabris A, Ronco C, La Greca G: Bicarbonate buffer for CAPD solution. *Trans Am Soc Artif Intern Organs* 31: 668, 1985

118. Pedersen FB, Ryttof N, Deleuran P, Dragsholt C, Kildeberg P: Acetate vs lactate in peritoneal dialysis solutions. *Nephron* 39: 55, 1985

119. Rubin J, Adair C, Johnson B, Bower JD: Stereospecific lactate absorption during peritoneal dialysis. *Nephron* 31: 224, 1982.

120. Robson MD, Faivoseviz A, Malmoud H: Physiological transfer of acid base, in *Continuous Ambulatory Peritoneal Dialysis, Proc Int Symposium* edited by Legrain M, Amsterdam, Excerpta Medica, 1980, p 194

PULMONARY ASPECTS OF DIALYSIS PATIENTS

MARC E. DE BROE, ROBERT R. LINS and WILFRIED A. DE BACKER

INTRODUCTION

Patients with acute or end-stage chronic renal failure, whether treated by dialysis or not, frequently develop pulmonary complications such as edema, pleural effusion and infection. In addition, hemodialysis treatment is always accompanied with a variable degree of hypoxemia at the start or towards the end of the treatment session. Respiratory failure secondary to hyperkalemia is a life threatening, fortunately rare complication, in chronic hemodialysis.

UREMIC LUNG

Radiologists first described the characteristic butterfly or batwing appearance in anteroposterior X-rays of the lung. The periphery of the lung remains normally translucent, while more central areas are opaque and display a waist-like constriction of the shadow. As this entity frequently complicates end-stage renal failure it was referred to as 'uremic lung'. Later on, it was also recognized in other conditions as in acute rheumatic fever and chronic left ventricular failure. In patients with chronic renal failure, the pressure forces in the Starling equation often favor secondary pulmonary edema. Hydrostatic pressures in the central circulation may be high because of increased intravascular volume or congestive heart failure or both.

Intravascular oncotic pressure may also be low because of hypoproteinemia, predisposing to pulmonary edema at lower hydrostatic pressures (1). For these reasons alone, butterfly infiltrates of pulmonary edema on chest radiograph would be expected. Uremic lung thus is a form of pulmonary edema which can eventually result in fibrotic interstitial changes.

In the early phase the alveoli contain fibrinous edema fluid and the interlobular septa are very edematous and swollen. Usually the edema fluid is completely absorbed, but in more chronic persistent cases the exudate organizes and fibrotic changes occur in the interstitium.

The characteristic distribution of the edematous exudate found in 'uremic lung' is largely explained by diversion of flow to more central parts of the lung which are supplied by the shortest arterial pathway. Indeed, the raised pulmonary venous pressure due to left ventricular failure causes reflex vasoconstriction in the pulmonary arteries especially of the longer arterial pathways resulting in diversion of the blood flow through more central parts of the lung.

It is now generally agreed that uremic lung is a forms of pulmonary edema caused primarily by left ventricular failure and pulmonary engorgement, but in which in addition a local capillary toxic factor and possibly deficient fibrinolysis also play a part. This toxic factor, still unknown and most probably the same as mentioned in the occurrence of uremic pleuritis, increases the permeability of alveolar capillaries resulting in leakage of macromolecular proteins and even red blood cells.

The most important cause of lung edema in dialysis patients is noncompliance with fluid restriction, a rather frequent condition especially in patients with no or negligible residual diuresis. Patients with acute renal failure are also highly susceptible to pulmonary edema. Indeed, they frequently have decreased plasma oncotic pressure, an increased hydrostatic pressure in pulmonary capillaries because of fluid overload and changes in alveolar capillaries due to their uremic state. Severe fluid overload in patients with acute renal failure not responding to high doses of loop diuretics, is a classical indication for emergency dialysis with ultrafiltration or continuous slow ultrafiltration.

PLEURAL EFFUSION IN DIALYSIS

Richard Bright noted that in patients who died of nephritis 'of all the membranes the pleura has decidedly been most often diseased' (2). Uremic patients have an increased susceptibility to many causes of transudative or exudative pleural effusion such as congestive heart failure, nephrotic syndrome, salt and water retention and infection (3). In addition there exists an idiopathic uremic pleural effusion.

Furthermore, dialysis patients may develop pleural effusion directly related to their type of treatment such as a catheter related superior vena cava obstruction or subclavian venous catheter leak (4). With peritoneal dialysis a leakage of dialysate through a small, often congenital diaphragmatic defect may result in a small pleural effusion relieved by erect posture, up to a massive usually right-sided hydrothorax within hours to days after starting this type of treatment.

Idiopathic pleural involvement in uremia and in dialysis patients results from necrotizing fibrinous inflammation and often results in a serous serosanguineous or even hemorrhagic effusion (5, 6). This type of pleural reaction may occur without concomitant overhydration and without apparent cause; gradual spontaneous resolution often occurs sometimes followed by recurrences (5). One should search carefully for evidence of coexisting pericardial effusion in these cases. A few patients have progressive disease wherein the pleural fluid becomes gelatinuous and a thick fibrous peel develops (7, 8). Fibrous uremic pleuritis causes progressive restriction of pulmonary function with restricted lung volumes and disabling dyspnea of increasing severity until relieved by surgical decortication (7).

The etiology and/or pathogenesis of uremic pleuritis remains unknown and has been the subject of numerous speculations (3). It must be emphasized that the finding of bloody pleural effusion in an uremic patient (dialyzed or not) requires the exclusion of all causes of hemorrhagic pleural effusion before it is concluded to be due to uremia.

DIALYSIS ASSOCIATED HYPOXEMIA

The dialysis patient, being treated intermittently on a three times weekly schedule, is exposed during the short dialysis period (4 h) to abrupt changes in the internal milieu.

The patient slowly accumulates H^+ ions during the 44 h interdialytic period and is in a respiratory compensated (hyperventilation) metabolic acidosis at the start of dialysis. Indeed, a HCO_3^- level between 17 and 23 mEq/l and a rather low $PaCO_2$ of 33 to 36 mm Hg is observed. Four hours

later, using a biocompatible (polyacrylonitrile, PAN) or bioincompatible membrane (cuprophane, CP) and a bicarbonate or acetate dialysis bath, he ends up with a slight degree of metabolic alkalosis, mild to moderate hypoventilation, with or without breathing irregularities (Figure 1 A,B). Defined in another way: the dialysis patient is an acid accumulator for 44 h followed by a 4 h efficient period of retitration which is accompanied by a variable degree of hypoxemia.

The latter phenomenon has been the subject of numerous investigations during the last 10 years (for review see 9-12). As happens with complex biological processes the conclusions reached by different investigators are conflicting depending on their viewpoint and the variables they examined. Since Sherlock and colleagues in 1977 (13) showed that patients dialyzed with an acetate containing dialysate developed hypoxemia and attributed it to the hypoventilation following CO_2 losses through the dialyzer a number of other mechanisms have been proposed, defended by some, questioned by others. The various proposed mechanisms will be critically evaluated and the respective role of the two most important ones i.e. 'CO_2 unloading' and the 'complement activation – hypoxemia' cascade will be defined.

Pulmonary microembolization

Bishel et al (14) suggested that microemboli of particulate material (platelets, leukocytes, fibrin) originating from the interaction between blood and the extracorporeal circuit might be responsible for decrease in arterial oxygen tension (PaO_2). This hypothesis could not be confirmed by others (15) since hypoxemia occurred despite microfiltration of venous blood.

Changes in oxygen transport and ventilation due to correction of acidosis (Bohr effect, metabolic alkalosis)

The small increase in pH which is usually observed in the course of hemodialysis (16, Figure 1B) could theoretically lead to hypoxemia on the basis of an alkalosis-induced central respiratory center depression, or the alkalinization of the blood can result in greater oxygen-hemoglobin affinities (Bohr effect) (17).

Dialysis induced hypoxemia however can be temporally dissociated from the change in systemic pH (18). Hemodialysis with bicarbonate-containing dialysate can be performed in the absence of clear changes in ventilation and PaO_2 despite a systemic alkalosis. On the other hand dialysis hypoxemia has been shown to occur even in the absence of changes in systemic pH (19, 20). Such discordant responses suggest a minor role for the correction of acidosis observed in the course of hemodialysis and indicate that additional factors dependent on the dialysate composition or the membrane used or both account for the dialysis hypoxemia.

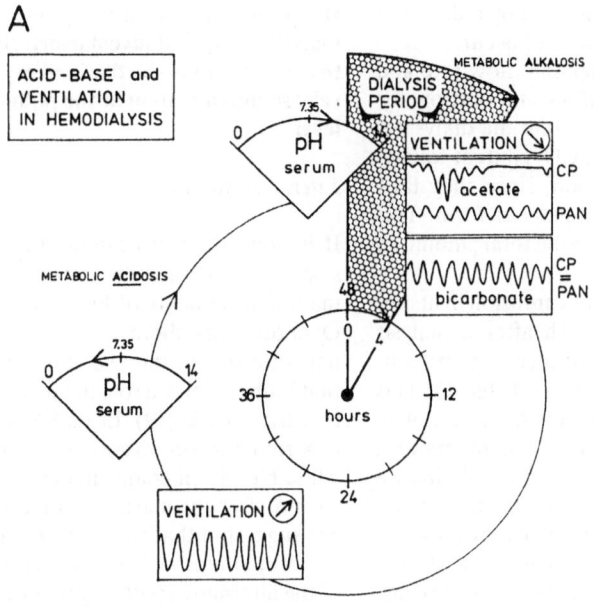

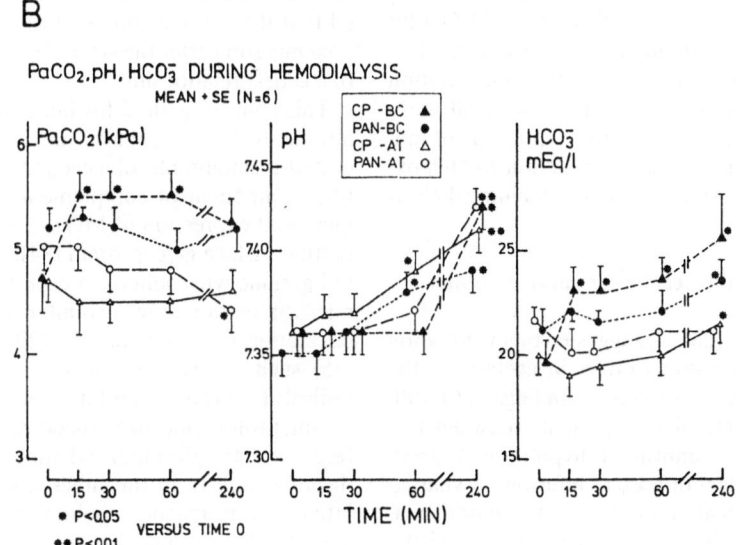

Figure 1. (A) Acid base, ventilation, (B) $PaCO_2$, systemic pH, and arterial HCO_3^- during hemodialysis. Abbreviations: CP, cuprophane membrane; PAN, polyacrylonitrile membrane; AT, acetate-containing dialysate; BC, bicarbonate containing dialysate; $PaCO_2$, arterial carbon dioxide tension. ⩗⩗⩗ = regular, ⩗⩗⩗ = irregular breathing pattern. Figure 1B reprinted from (19) with permission.

Hypoventilation from lower respiratory quotient during acetate metabolism

Another possible explanation for the observed decreased ventilation during hemodialysis has been sought in the metabolism of acetate gained (3 to 4 mmol/min) during a dialysis session using dialysis fluid containing acetate (21). As proposed the metabolism of acetate results in a higher oxygen consumption (VO_2) and a decreased CO_2 production

(VCO_2), leading to a substantial reduction in respiratory quotient (RQ), therefore resulting in hypoventilation and consequently hypoxemia (22, 23). Although this explanation seems attractive, some arguments weaken this possibility. Firstly, Romaldini et al (24, 25) showed no hypoxemia and decrease in RQ in the course of dialysis with an acetate containing dialysate in which CO_2 was bubbled. If the metabolism of acetate plays an important role in the hemodialysis-induced hypoxemia, the bubbling of CO_2 into the bath should not affect this mechanism. Consequently a decrease in RQ due to acetate metabolism would still occur.

Secondly, Oh et al (23) used the dialysate flow rate and PCO_2 difference between dialysate inflow and outflow for the estimation of HCO_3^- and CO_2 losses into the dialysate. They were unable to calculate the total CO_2 content following the Henderson-Hasselbalch equation, since they take into account only the dissolved CO_2 in gaseous form. This leads to a substantial underestimation of the total amount of CO_2 lost into the dialysate.

Thirdly, we could show (26) that acetate infusion in hemodialysis patients (4 mmol/min) given 24 h after a dialysis session (a non-dialysis day) has no significant effect on ventilation, blood gases and breathing patterns (Table 1). This contrasts with previous observations by Oh et al (23), who studied the effect of acetate metabolism in volunteers with normal renal function. The small decrease in ventilation we observed can totally be accounted for by the abrupt increase in pH resulting in metabolic alkalosis (26). The respiratory center is known to be very sensitive to changes in H^+ ion concentration and this marked increase in systemic pH causes come decrease in alveolar ventilation and sometimes a small fall in PaO_2.

The metabolism of acetate resulted in a decreased VCO_2 production and an unchanged or slightly increased VO_2 (20) and a low RQ. Despite acetate metabolism as indicated by the steadily increase in plasma bicarbonate concentration and in pH hypoxemia did not occur. In view of all these arguments, it is difficult to maintain the hypothesis of metabolism of acetate as a cause of hypoventilation and hypoxemia during hemodialysis with an acetate containing dialysis solution.

Direct effect of acetate on the central respiratory center

Nissenson (27) and others (28, 29) suggested that ventilation decreases secondarily to a direct effect of acetate on the central respiratory center. Our recent findings (26) with acetate infusion in chronic dialysis patients between two dialysis sessions, could not confirm this hypothesis. Indeed, we could not find any effect of acetate infusion on ventilation, blood gases and breathing patterns, the latter measured using respiratory inductance plethysmography (30).

Hypoventilation from 'CO₂ unloading' during acetate dialysis; increased alveolar-arterial oxygen gradient due to complement activation-leukocyte trapping-mediator release-inflammation at the pulmonary microcirculatory level

Literature survey

It is appropriate to discuss these two mechanisms in the same section since they are strongly interrelated and the main determinants of hemodialysis associated hypoxemia. Over the years, there have been strong supporters and opponents for one of the two concepts. It turned out, however, that both can play a role in the development of the hemodialysis hypoxemia (19). In 1968 Kaplow and Goffinet (31) first reported the occurrence of a significant decrease in the white blood cell count, mainly granulocytes between 2 and 15 min after the start of hemodialysis. Craddock et al (32, 33) suggested that this transient granulocytopenia was due to intrapulmonary leukostasis resulting from the activation of the alternative pathway of the complement system. These authors found a decrease in PaO_2 soon after the start of hemodialysis and an increase in the calculated alveolar-arterial oxygen tension difference ($AaDO_2$). They suggested that the parallel course of the early leukopenia and hypoxemia soon after the start of hemodialysis were indicative of a causal relationship.

This concept gained further support by reports that the interaction between plasma and the dialyzer membrane generated a small-molecular-weight cleavage fragment of the fifth component of complement, i.e. C5a, modulating an increased expression of MO1, a granulocyte adhesion promoting surface glycoprotein (34). These aggregated activated granulocytes adhere to each other and also to the first microcirculation they encounter, i.e. the pulmonary microcirculation (8, 20) where they liberate lysosomal enzymes (35) such as elastase, vasoactive mediators, and oxygen radicals (36) causing endothelial damage releasing into the serum, proteins localized specifically at this microcirculation (e.g. human placental alkaline phosphatase (37)) and thromboxane from the lungs (38). This results in a local inflammatory reaction, pulmonary hypertension and some degree of hypoxemia. The transience of this phenomenon is due to selective down-regulation of the cellular response to

Table 1. Gas exchange during acetate infusion.

	Before	*15 min*	*30 min*	*60 min*
pH	7.37 ± 0.02	7.40 ± 0.02	7.43** ± 0.02	7.47** ± 0.01
PaO_2 (mm Hg)	92.6 ± 6.0	87.2 ± 4.6	91.4 ± 8.2	86.4 ± 9.2
$PaCO_2$ (mm Hg)	38.4 ± 1.7	39.0 ± 1.3	39.2 ± 1.3	40.2 ± 1.3
HCO_3 (mmol/l)	22.6 ± 1.6	24.6* ± 0.9	26.2** ± 1.3	29.6** ± 1.4
RQ	0.78 ± 0.05	0.72* ± 0.04	0.71.** ± 0.05	0.63** ± 0.04
VO_2 (ml/min)	264 ± 30	248 ± 19	271 ± 24	272 ± 30
VCO_2 (ml/min)	217 ± 41	180 ± 22	197 ± 27	175 ± 30

pH, arterial oxygen tension (PaO_2), arterial carbon dioxide tension ($PaCO_2$), arterial bicarbonate concentration (HCO_3^-), respiratory exchange ratio (RQ), oxygen consumption (VO_2), carbon dioxide production (VCO_2), expressed as mean ± SEM of five patients before and during acetate infusion. Symbols are: *p>0.05; **p>0.01, both p values are versus values obtained before the start of the infusion.

C5a, which limits the deleterious effect of adherent granulocytes on the endothelium (16). Alternatively Sherlock et al (13), Aurigemma et al (15) and Dumler and Levin (39) attributed the major cause of hypoxemia to alveolar hypoventilation subsequent to the loss of carbon dioxide in the dialysate (CO_2-unloading, Table 2). This was supported by their finding that no hypoxemia occurred if the drecrease of PCO_2 in the dialysate was prevented. These results were only partially confirmed by Tolchin et al (40), since in their 'constant PCO_2 dialysate' set-up they still found a small decrease in PaO_2.

Recently, Dolan et al (20) proposed once more that hypoventilation secondary to CO_2 losses through the dialyzer is the most important mechanism of hypoxemia observed with acetate dialysis. In this well-designed and controlled set of experiments, hypoxemia developed when acetate-containing dialysate was used; the fall in PaO_2 was accompanied by decreased ventilation and maintenance of normal $PaCO_2$. By contrast, neither hypoxemia nor decreased ventilation were seen when bicarbonate-containing dialysate (with CO_2 bubbling) was used.

Whereas the respiratory quotient remained unchanged in the course of bicarbonate dialysis, it dropped from approximately 0.80 to approximately 0.64 in the course of acetate dialysis; these values were calculated from the amounts of CO_2 excreted and of oxygen taken up by the lungs. Brautbar et al (41) showed that improved hemodynamic function and removal of excess interstitial fluid during ultrafiltration must be taken into account in the interpretation of hemodialysis hypoxemia. The absence of hypoxemia during bioincompatible membrane dialysis using prostacyclin can also be interpreted in this context (42).

Respective role of CO_2 unloading and complement activation-pulmonary inflammation in dialysis associated hypoxemia

To unravel the respective roles of the two main proposed mechanisms of dialysis associated hypoxemia we studied the same group of patients, selected to be clinically stable and having comparable predialysis PaO_2 values, submitted in a randomized order to a dialysis session using a biocompatible (polyacrylonitrile, PAN) or bioincompatible (cuprophane, CP) membrane, and acetate (AT) of bicarbonate (BC, $PCO_2 = 35$ mm Hg) in the dialysate.

We found (Figure 2 ABC) that the worst pair of experimental conditions was CP membrane and AT containing dialysate. Indeed both complement activation-leukopenia and subsequent increase in $AaDO_2$ together with reduction in alveolar PO_2, respiratory quotient (RQ) and mean inspiratory flow resulting in the most striking decrease in PaO_2 was observed.

The best combination without any effect on leukocytes, PAO_2, RQ, ventilation and PaO_2 was dialysis with a biocompatible membrane (PAN) and BC in the dialysate. When a CP membrane and BC in the dialysate was used. leukopenia together with an early reversible increase in $AaDO_2$ and decrease in PaO_2 was observed. With a PAN membrane and AT in the dialysate a delayed sustained decrease in PAO_2 RQ and PaO_2 was seen, $AaDO_2$ remained unchanged. It is striking to note that the increase in $AaDO_2$ with CP membrane dialysis was sustained or transient depending respectively on AT or BC in the dialysate. The 'scavenger' function of BC offers a possible explanation for this intriguing observation.

In summary the two types of membranes have a markedly different effect upon leukocyte count, $AaDO_2$ and PaO_2 shortly after the start of hemodialysis. Furthermore, independent of the type of membrane used, dialysis solution containing acetate always induces a sustained striking decrease in alveolar PO_2 (hypoventilation) RQ and PaO_2.

It was concluded that both mechanisms may occur separately or simultaneously depending on the dialysis set-up.

Intrapulmonary leukostasis with mediator release and inflammation at the level of the pulmonary microcirculation is an early event depending upon the biocompatibility of the dialyser membrane used and has a measurable but rather limited effect upon the PaO_2.

Alveolar hypoventilation depends upon the CO_2 unloading capacity of the hemodialysis set-up, is independent of the dialyzer membrane and can have an important effect on PaO_2. This hypoventilation can be due to extracoporeal losses of CO_2 or (and) due to changes in the endogenous production of carbon dioxide ($\dot{V}CO_2$) and consumption of oxygen ($\dot{V}O_2$) secondary to the metabolism of acetate (the latter mechanism was discussed earlier in the text). To us it seems most likely that the loss of CO_2 into the dialysate with PCO_2 in the blood returning to the patient decreasing to as low as 10 to 15 mm Hg causes alveolar hypoventilation and hypoxemia. The observed hypoventilation, unaccompanied

Table 2. Mass transport of CO_2 during hemodialysis. Acetate containing dialysate single pass.

	Before (afferent)	Dialyser	After (efferent)
pH	7.31 ± 0.01		7.33 ± 0.01
PCO_2 (mm Hg)	36.8 ± 0.05		14.0 ± 0.8
HCO_3^- (mEq/l)	20.5 ± 0.5		9.2 ± 0.5
Dissolved CO_2 (ml/dl)	2.66 ± 0.03		1.07 ± 0.06
Total CO_2 content (ml/dl)	42.7 ± 1.0		17.1 ± 1.2

CO_2 loss at blood flow of 200–300 ml/min = $50 - 75$ ml/min.
Metabolic production of CO_2 at rest = 200–300 ml/min.

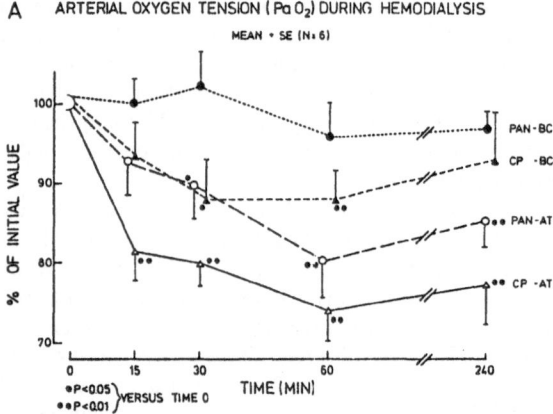

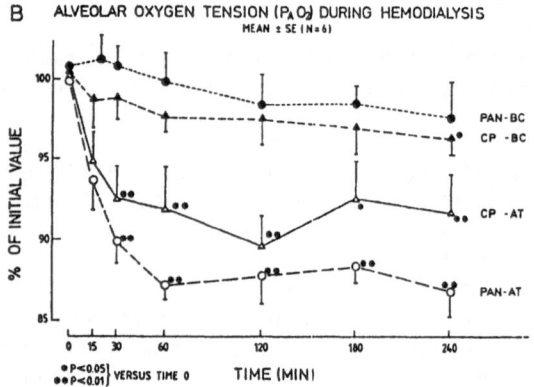

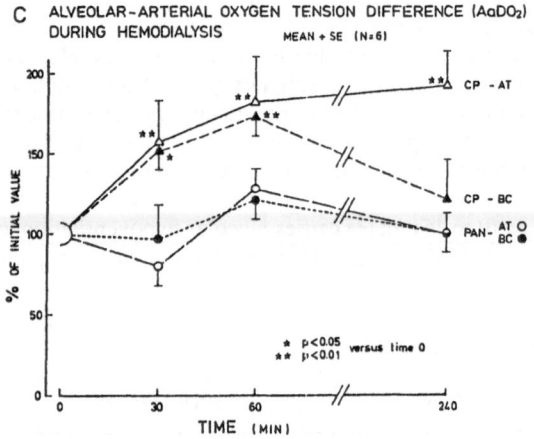

Figure 2. Arterial oxygen tension (PaO₂) (A), alveolar oxygen tension (PaO₂) (B) and alveolar-arterial oxygen tension difference during hemodialysis (AaDO₂) (C) using a bioincompatible (CP) and biocompatible (PAN) membrane and an acetate (AT) or bicarbonate (BC) dialysate in six patients. *p>0.05 − **p>0.01; both values are versus time 0. Figure 2 AB, reprinted from (19) with permission.

by CO_2-retention, resulting in a rather small decrease in $PaCO_2$ (see Figure 1B), is characterized by a decreased respiratory drive (decrease in $\dot{V}T/Ti$). Phillipson, Duffin and Cooper (43) have demonstrated the critical dependence of respiratory drive and rhythmicity on the metabolic carbon dioxide load by causing complete cessation of breathing at normal arterial blood gases in adult sheep, when CO_2 was removed from the blood at a rate equal to its metabolic production. The suggestion that this hypoventilation could be mediated through slowly adapting chemoreceptors in the venous circulation or in the lungs reacting to a low venous PCO_2 (Table 2) is an attractive possibility (44) necessitating however, pulmonary venous blood sampling in strictly controlled condition. Recently, more experimental evidence has been presented for the presence in dogs and cats of CO_2 sensitive pulmonary chemoreceptors that interact with the nonpulmonary chemoreceptors in the control of minute ventilation (45, 46). Wasserman et al (47) demonstrated in dogs that when venous CO_2 is artificially increased, ventilation increased proportionally providing additional evidence for the existence of pre- or pulmonary chemoreceptors sensitive to PCO_2.

Role of the early-limited-complement-activation-induced hypoxemia in the generation of irregular breathing

As mentioned earlier, intrapulmonary leukostasis, mediator release and inflammation at the level of the pulmonary microcirculation are early dialyzer membrane dependent effects with a measurable but rather limited influence on the PaO_2. On the other hand, the CO_2 unloading results in alveolar hypoventilation and may have an important effect on PaO_2. To gain more insight into the mechanism of this alveolar hypoventilation, ventilation and breathing patterns were studied using respiratory inductance plethysmography (RIP). This method indeed allows (30) both qualitative and quantitative measurements and avoids the important artefacts caused by breathing through a mouthpiece (48).

As in our previous studies, we used a biocompatible (PAN) or bioincompatible (CP) dialyzer membrane in combination with an acetate (AT) or bicarbonate (BC) bath. Comparable results to our previous studies (19) were obtained for the different ventilation parameters. However, we were surprised by the marked irregularities in the breathing pattern during CP-AT dialysis. Whereas in the three other dialysis modes, an almost regular breathing pattern was observed (Figure 30) in the CP-AT mode important variation in the tidal volume from breath to breath (Figure 3A), apneas exceeding 10 sec (Figure 30, Figure 4) and real periodic breathing were observed (Figure 3C).

The intriguing observation here was that the important irregular breathing pattern observed in the CP-AT dialysis was not, or almost not, seen in the other dialysis modes especially the PAN-AT mode which is also accompanied by an important CO_2 unloading. This suggested strongly the important role of the early 'complement activated' hypoxemia, being the most striking difference between the CP-AT and PAN-AT dialysis, in the generation of the irregular breathing patterns.

Breathing patterns during hemodialysis

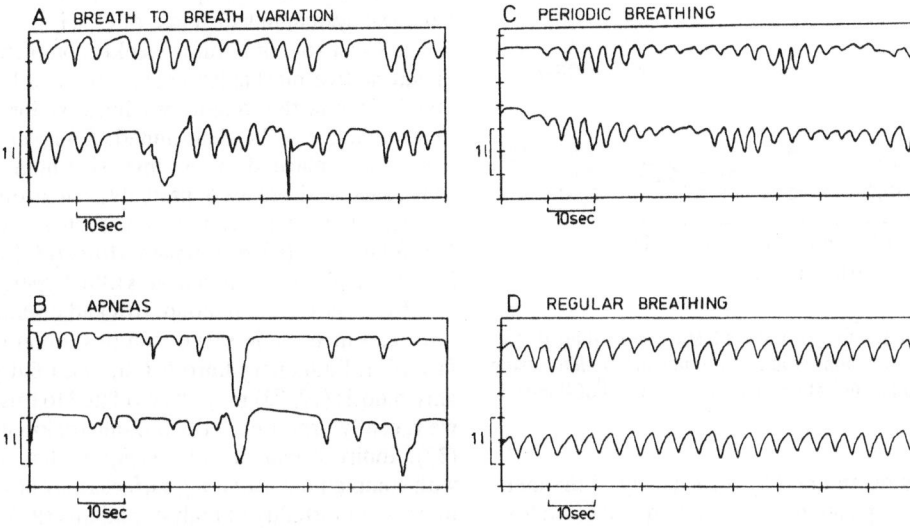

Figure 3. Breathing patterns obtained during different dialysis modes. A, B, C, were seen during the CP-AT dialysis. During PAN-BC, PAN-AT, CP-BC dialysis, an almost constant regular breathing pattern was observed (D). For abbreviation see legend of Figure 1. Reprinted from (54) with permission.

A number of our recent observations and some reported data support our concept that hypoxemia is necessary in the pathogenesis of irregular breathing seen during extracorporeal CO_2 unloading.

Firstly, in some patients dialyzed with the CP-AT set up with negligible leukopenia and subsequently no hypoxemia due to very limited complement activation, as has been described also by others (49), no irregular breathing was observed.

Secondly, administration of oxygen to patients presenting abnormal breathing patterns during CP-AT dialysis almost immediately turned this irregular breathing into a regular one without changes in the minute ventilation (50). Thirdly, using the biofiltration technique (51) which allows a gradual progressive controlled CO_2 unloading, we observed irregular breathing only when CO_2 unloading was accompanied by a certain degree of hypoxemia induced by the use of a bioincompatible membrane.

Finally, the observed irregularities in breathing during bioincompatible hemodialysis with CO_2 unloading can be compared to those observed at high altitude. At high altitude, lowlanders hyperventilate to compensate for the decreased inspiratory oxygen tension. This hyperventilation, however, does not prevent hypoxemia at extreme altitudes and at the same time makes the lowlanders hypocapnic. In this situation irregular breathing and especially periodic breathing is observed (52). Oxygen breathing again promptly eliminates this periodic breathing.

Several mechanisms can account for the observed breathing irregularities. Correction of acidosis is highly unlikely since during the first hour no significant differences in pH were observed during CP-AT dialysis although irregular breathing is already present.

It could be argued that the patients were sleeping. In such a clinical setting the controlling role of the cortex is diminished rendering ventilation mediated by the peripheral chemical control systems and resulting in irregular breathing patterns (53). We could rule out this sleeping hypothesis by measuring body movements using 'Actigraphy' (54).

The direct effect of acetate as a cause of irregular breathing was also excluded by our observation in dialysis patients infused with acetate outside a dialysis session (26).

The CO_2 unloading combined with mild hypoxemia itself thus clearly seems to be the most obvious cause of the breathing irregularities during CP-AT dialysis. The values of $PaCO_2$ of approximately 33 mm Hg found in AT bath dialysis is the one known to be the critical point for switch-off of central CO_2 chemoreceptors (27, 43).

When this point is reached in hypoxic conditions, ventilation became at least partly dependent on the output of the peripheral chemoreceptors which are stimulated by hypoxemia (55, 56) In other words in hypoxic conditions the peripheral chemoreceptors react briskly to changes in $PaCO_2$ which is immediately reflected in the breathing pattern.

Without hypoxemia CO_2 unloading itself, such as seen during PAN-AT, does not result in irregular breathing. The observed rather important hypoventilation in this setting could be mediated through slowly adapting chemoreceptors in the venous circulation or in the lungs reacting to a low PCO_2 in the blood returning to the patient. Several experimental observations fit with this hypothesis (24, 44, 46, 47).

In summary (Table 3), the pathophysiology of the hemodialysis associated hypoxemia depends highly on the dialysate composition as well as on the type of membrane used.

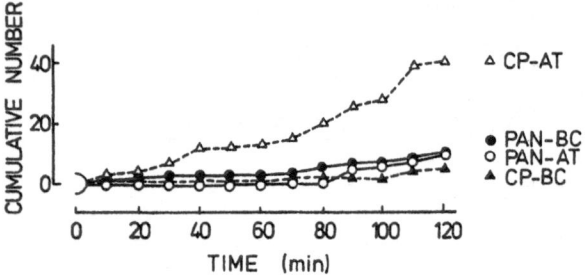

Figure 4. Cumulative number of apneas lasting more than 10 seconds expressed as a total number at a given time in 5 patients using different dialysis modes. For abbreviations see legend of Figure 1.

The latter effect is determined by the capacity of the membrane to activate complement with its subsequent cascade of biological events.

During PAN-BC, CP-BC dialysis the decrease in alveolar ventilation in the absence or negligible decrease in PaO_2 is due to the sensitivity of the central respiratory center to the increased systemic pH and HCO_3^-; during PAN-AT dialysis an important CO_2 unloading occurs (low PCO_2 in the blood returning to the patient) which added to the previous effects results in a more pronounced decrease in $\dot{V}E$ and $\dot{V}T$; during CP-AT dialysis the complement activation induced early hypoxemia superimposed on the CO_2 unloading results in hypoventilation and irregular breathing.

Clinical implication of dialysis associated hypoxemia

The clinical implication of this dialysis-induced hypoxemia is of immediate importance to those dialyzed patients with an already compromised cardiopulmonary function. They represent 10 to 15% of an average dialysis population who have predialysis PaO_2 values below 80 mm Hg. The additional 25% decrease of PaO_2 after the start of dialysis using a bioincompatible membrane and acetate in the dialysis solu-

tion results in desaturation (57). These patients should be dialysed with a non-complement-activating membrane and a dialysis system in which loss of CO_2 is prevented.

The exact role of a thrice weekly complement activation or alternative mechanisms (58, 59) using bioincompatible membranes in the long-term clinical status of dialysis patients remains to be determined. Complement activation has been implicated in an impressive number of observations, such as decrease of predialysis neutrophil count (60); polymorphonuclear dysfunction, such as chemotaxis (61, 62); adherence (63–65); phagocytosis (66); increase in oxidative metabolism of leukocytes (36); hypersensitivity reaction (67); activation of monocytes and interleukin-1 release (68); and increase in expression of C3b on neutrophil surface (69). Pulmonary fibrosis (70, 71), joint problems, and amyloidosis (72, 73) may all be related to this mechanism as we recently proposed for beta-2-microglobulin amyloidosis (37). Indirect evidence also suggests that chronic dialysis with complement activating surfaces may be associated with increased morbidity of dialysis patients (9, 74–77)

THE LUNG IN THE CHRONICALLY DIALYZED PATIENT

Changes in lung mechanics and lung hemodynamics occur even without overt signs or symptoms in patients with end-stage chronic renal failure. Lee and Stretton (71) studied the pulmonary function of 55 patients with chronic renal failure, 10 of them undergoing chronic dialysis treatment. These patients had no clinical nor radiographic evidence of lung disease.

They found a defect in gas transfer (decrease in carbon monoxide diffusing capacity [DLCO]) due to a reduction in the diffusing capacity across the alveolar capillary membrane, vital capacities were decreased indicative of mild restriction, while forced vital capacity and the ratio of the forced vital capacity in the first second to the vital capacity ruled out obstructive disease.

In a study dealing with the long term survival of regular dialysis treatment patients, over 10 years on dialysis, Avram

Table 3. Summary of the important events and mechanisms related to the hemodialysis associated hypoxemia (see also text). Meanings of the abbreviations are in the legend to Figure 1.

	Early hypoxemia	CO_2 Unloading	Hypoventilation	Irregular breathing	Mechanisms	
PAN-BC	–	–	+/–	–	pH ↑ , HCO_3^- ↑ centr. respir. depression	
CP-BC	+	–	+/–	–	pH ↑ , HCO_3^- ↑ centr. respir. depression	
PAN-AT	–	++	++	–	pH ↑ , HCO_3^- ↑ centr. respir. depression	+ Co_2 unloading: pulm. CO_2 chemoreceptors ? $\dot{V}E$ ↓ $\dot{V}T$ ↓
CP-AT	+	++	++	++	pH ↑ , HCO_3^- ↑ centr. respir. depression	+CO_2 unloading: pulm. CO_2 chemoreceptors ? $\dot{V}E$ ↓ $\dot{V}T$ ↓ \ + hypoxemia: apneas period. breath.

(78) found that eight out of 11 of these patients had severe restrictive lung function. The effects of hemodialysis on pulmonary function appear attributable to changes in fluid volume. Dialysis causes an increase in the diffusing capacity (79), decrease in closing capacity (80), increased ventilation to basilar areas of the lung (79), and in patients with edema an increase in vital capacity (81). All these changes can be explained by a decrease in lung water content (82).

In addition to these limited observations concerning the functional pulmonary changes in end-stage renal failure (with or without dialysis) patients, there are also some important pathological observations. Soft tissue calcification was identified in 79% of dialysis patients and 44% in nondialysis patients with chronic renal failure (70, 83). Lesions were severe in 36% of the dialysis population and were most frequently found in heart, lungs and stomach. Serum calcium levels were slightly higher in patients with calcifications, but there was no measurable association with the duration of dialysis, serum phosphorus concentration, calcium × phosphorus product, serum bicarbonate level or arterial pH. A critical assessment of the role of parathyroid hormone in the pathogenisis of this pulmonary calcifications is still required. Pulmonary clinical symptoms were scarce, X-ray findings were absent except in a single patient.

The calcific lesion consists in deposits occurring as linear bands occasionally as granular humps in alveolar septal walls. Varying degree of thickening and fibrosis of the alveolar walls accompanying the deposits. Calcium was found frequently located within the walls of pulmonary vessels and smaller bronchi. In general vascular calcifications in the lungs paralleled those of the pulmonary parenchyma. By X-ray diffraction a whitlockite crystal pattern $(CaMg)_3$ $(PO_4)_2$ was found predominantly, with calcium pyrophosphate in these pulmonary calcifications.

Pulmonary function tests showed a close relation between changes in vital capacity, DLCO and the severity of lung calcifications. However, the limitation of significant abnormalities of vital capacity and diffusion to those with the severest histopathological changes suggests that the degree of septal thickening and fibrosis rather than the mere presence of calcium deposits determined the magnitude of the functional changes.

The available biochemical data are not sufficient to evaluate adequately either the cause or pathogenisis of these metabolic calcifications, fibrosis and alveolar septal thickening.

Several hypotheses (70) have been put forth but none of these would explain all aspects of this disorder(s), although the variable degree of secondary hyperparathyroidism present in almost all patients with severe renal failure, whether treated by dialysis or not has to be taken into account. It remains speculative to link the thrice weekly complement activation, observed in the majority of patients dialysed with bioincompatible membranes, accompanied by an acute inflammatory reaction at the level of the pulmonary microcirculation, with the morphological lung lesions observed in the majority of the chronically hemodialyzed subjects.

PULMONARY FUNCTION DURING PERITONEAL DIALYSIS

Peritoneal dialysis has been associated with significant alterations, in pulmonary functions and gas exchange (84–86).

Atelectasis, pneumonia, purulent bronchitis, chronic pleural effusion and acute hydrothorax are among the various complications which may occur during peritoneal dialysis (84, 87). At least atelectasis of the basal segments of the lung is considered as the consequence of the upward displacement of the diaphragm following overdistention of the peritoneal cavity with dialysate. During continuous ambulatory peritoneal dialysis (CAPD) the time allowed for drainout is as short as possible and may not be long enough to permit the atelectic segment to re-expand; hence, continued dialysis may decrease the vital capacity. Transient, mild, statistically significant, reductions in functional residual capacity, residual volume and total lung capacity were observed during peritoneal dialysis (86). Others found in addition a fall in arterial PO_2 of 3 to 35 mm Hg when the abdomen is distended with 2 l of dialysis fluid (85, 88). The PaO_2 returns to normal when the dialysate is drained out. These changes could only be confirmed at the beginning of CAPD and they are small and clinically irrelevant (89). When the values prior to infusion were measured in the sitting position and those obtained after infusion in the supine position, a drop of 11.5 mm Hg of PaO_2 without any change in vital capacity was observed. This was due to a further decrease in functional residual capacity (FRC) leading to airways closure at FRC, impaired ventilation to dependent lung zones and increased venous admixture. With time these changes in lung function associated with CAPD seem to become less evident, perhaps because of adaptive mechanisms. However during periods of peritonitis, a 25 to 30% drop in vital capacity and a 11.7 mm Hg drop in PaO_2 was observed (89). The most likely explanation is altered mobility of the diaphragm because of pain. Recently a great number of respiratory parameters were studied in CAPD patients, including spirometry, resistance, conductance and thoracic gas volumes. No statistically significant differences in the results were found in stable patients between studies when dialysis fluid was infused and drained out (90). In a severely ill patient the level of consciousness may be diminished, causing impaired cough reflex. Bronchial secretions may pool in the basal atelectic segments predisposing to purulent bronchitis or pneumonia or both (87). Pleural effusions mostly right-sided, are also a well-known complication of CAPD and rarely massive hydrothorax may occur. In most instances of this complication, peritoneal dialysis has to be discontinued. In a few cases successful pleurodesis has been described (91).

In view of these considerations, extracorporeal dialysis seems to be preferable to peritoneal dialysis in the presence of acute and chronic respiratory insufficiency.

CONTRIBUTION OF HEMODIALYSIS TO BASIC LUNG PHYSIOLOGY

Pulmonary gas exchange

Activation of the alternative pathway of the complement system and subsequent inflammatory processes have been thought to be involved in the pathogenisis of several pulmonary diseases. One of them is the Adult Respiratory Distress Syndrome (ARDS) which remains a problem without effective treatment. This is partly due to the lack of good models in the human.

We felt that the phenomena occurring in hemodialysis patients may at least partly mimic the pathogenetic pathway of ARDS. Indeed, it could be well demonstrated that the activation of the alternative pathway of the complement system by some dialysis membranes results in leuko-aggregation, trapping of the activated leukocytes in the first microcirculation they encounter, i.e. the pulmonary microcirculation, releasing mediators and inducing acute inflammation, increasing the alveolar-arterial oxygen gradient and subsequent hypoxemia. Furthermore, the use of bicarbonate in the dialysis solution showed a modulating effect on this inflammatory reaction suggesting a scavenger effect of bicarbonate. In dialysis with membranes considered to be biocompatible (i.e. not activating complement) disturbances in pulmonary gas exchanges are absent. These observations can be considered as a clinical proof of the local pulmonary inflammation in humans during extracorporeal circulation. In addition some preliminary data obtained in the well controllable hemodialysis model with prostacyclin give some hope for the development of pharmacological inhibition of these phenomena.

Ventilation during venous CO_2-unloading

The study of the chemical control of ventilation in humans has been faced with several problems. One of them is the ventilatory adaptation during CO_2-unloading. Until now only studies dealing with 'ventilatory-unloading' due to induced hyperventilation have been available. They have the disadvantage that measurements can only be performed during a very short period of time and simultaneous control of the inspiratory oxygen concentration is difficult to obtain. Hemodialysis and biofiltration allows us to study in humans the ventilatory adaptations to controllable degrees of venous CO_2-unloading.

Although ventilation decreases due to the correction of the acidosis it could be demonstrated that the CO_2 unloading in itself is associated with a degree of hypoventilation that cannot be accounted for by the acid-base changes. In addition to the overall decrease in ventilation, the breathing pattern in hypoxic patients undergoing CO_2-unloading becomes irregular with episodes of apnea. We believe that this is due to a dysrhythmogenic effect of the stimulated peripheral chemoreceptors since oxygen breathing eliminates the irregularities in breathing.

Nevertheless, the decrease in ventilation does not prevent a small but very reproducible and significant decrease in $PaCO_2$. This observation seems to be the first indication in humans for a weaker interdependence between ventilation and $PaCO_2$ in the hypocapnic range of the ventilatory-PCO_2 response curve. It is a first argument to accept that also in man the CO_2 response curve becomes shaped as a dog-leg in this hypocapnic area, in other words that ventilation became less dependent on changes in $PaCO_2$.

Further studies with biofiltration will allow us to detect more accurately the cut-off value of $PaCO_2$ where the CO_2 response curve becomes alinear (or dog-leg shaped). We believe that these observations will add to our understanding of the ventilatory adaptations in man in situations where chemical control is important such as at high altitude and during sleep.

CONCLUSION

The lung is the target organ predisposed to suffer from the important disturbances in the water and electrolyte balance characteristic for the patient with end stage renal failure.

Dialysis associated hypoxemia is multifactorial in origin. Part of this hypoxemia is determined by biocompatibility of the membrane used, part is due to CO_2 unloading and its consequent hypoventilation. Correction of acidosis (increase of systemic pH) goes along with a depression of the central respiratory center contributing to a limited extent to the dialysis-associated hypoxemia.

The long term effect of thrice weekly complement activation on pulmonary function is not known. It is striking to note that the literature does not contain a prospective study of the lung function during chronic hemo- or peritoneal dialysis. Based on present knowledge it is recommended that elderly patients, those with compromised cardiopulmonary function, patients who have experienced hypersensitivity to cellulose based membranes, and those with acute renal failure, should be dialyzed with a biocompatible membrane and bicarbonate-containing dialysate.

ACKNOWLEDGEMENT

We are thankful to R.M. Heyrman, M.D. for help during the preparation of part of this manuscript. This study was partly supported by grants of the Belgian National Fund for Scientific Medical Research (FGWO, FRSM) grant 3.0069.82 (MEDB) and by the Scientific Planning of the Belgian Government, contract 82-87/47.MEDB. The secreterial work of Erik Snelders is once more greatly appreciated.

REFERENCES

1. Guyton A, Linsey A: Effect of elevated left atrial pressure and decreased plasma protein concentration on the development of pulmonary edema. *Circ Res* 7: 649, 1959
2. Bright R: Tabular view of the morbid appearance in 100 cases connected with albuminous urine, with observations. *Guys Hosp Rep* 1: 380, 1836

3. Maher JF: Uremic pleuritis. *Am J Kidney Dis* 10: 19, 1987

4. Cradio A, Mena A, Figuerdo R, Reige E, Avello F: Late perforation of superior vena cava and effusion caused by central venous catheter. *Anaesth Intensive Care* 9: 286, 1981

5. Berger HW, Rammohan G, Neff MS, Buhain WJ: Uremic pleural effusion. A study in 14 patients on chronic dialysis. *Ann Intern Med* 82: 363, 1975

6. Galen MA, Steinberg SM, Lowrie FG, Lazarus JM, Hampers CL, Merrill JP: Hemorrhagic pleural effusion in patients undergoing chronic hemodialysis. *Ann Intern Med* 82: 359, 1975

7. Rodelas R, Rakowski TA, Argy WP, Schreiner GE: Fibrosing uremic pleuritis during hemodialysis. *JAMA* 243: 2424, 1980

8. Brown CM, Sloan DF, Berns AS, Kanter A: Fibrosing uremic pleuritis during hemodialysis. *JAMA* 245: 705, 1981

9. Cheung AK, Henderson LW: Effects of complement activation by hemodialysis membranes. *Am J Nephrol* 6: 81, 1986

10. Duarte R: Blood pressure, ventilation and lipid imbalance during hemodialysis: effect of dialysate composition. *Blood Purif* 3: 199, 1985

11. Eiser A: Pulmonary gas exchange during hemodialysis and peritoneal dialysis: interaction between respiration and metabolism. *Am J Kidney Dis* 6: 131, 1985

12. Garella S, Chang BS: Hemodialysis-associated hypoxemia. *Am J Nephrol* 4: 273, 1984

13. Sherlock J, Ledwith JK, Letteri J: Hypoventilation and hypoxemia during hemodialysis: reflex response to removal of CO_2 across the dialyzer. *Trans Am Soc Artif Intern Organs* 23: 406, 1977

14. Bischel MD, Scoles BG, Mohler JG: Evidence for pulmonary microembolization during hemodialysis. *Chest* 67: 335, 1976

15. Aurigemma NM, Feldman NT, Gottlieb M, Ingram RH, Lazarus JM, Lowrie FG, Arterial oxygenation during hemodialysis. *N Engl J Med* 297: 871, 1977

16. Skubitz KM, Craddock PR: Reversal of hemodialysis granulocytopenia and pulmonary leukostasis. A clinical manifestation of selective downregulation of granulocyte response to C5a desarg. *J Clin Invest* 67: 1383, 1981

17. Wathen RL, Ferris FZ, Nagar D, Keshaviah P: An alternative explanation for dialysis-induced arterial hypoxemia. *Kidney Int* 14: 689, 1978

18. Hampl H, Paeper H, Unger V, Fischer CH, Resa I, Kessel M: Hemodynamic changes during hemodialysis, sequential ultrafiltration and hemofiltration. *Kidney Int* 18: S83, 1980

19. De Backer WA, Verpooten GA, Borgonjon DA, Vermeire PA, Lins RR, De Broe ME: Hypoxemia during hemodialysis: effects of different membranes and dialysate compositions. *Kidney Int* 23: 738, 1983

20. Dolan MJ, Whipp BJ, Davidson WD, Weitzman RE, Wasserman K: Hypopnea associated with acetate hemodialysis: carbon dioxide-flow dependent ventilation. *N Engl J Med* 305: 72, 1981

21. Ikeda T, Hirasawa Y, Aizawa Y, Shibita A, Gejyo F, Ei K: Effect of acetate upon arterial gases. *J Dial* 3: 135, 1979

22. Eiser AR, Jahamanne D, Kokseng C, Che H, Slifkin RF, Neff MS: Contrasting alterations in pulmonary gas exchange during acetate and bicarbonate hemodialysis. *Am J Nephrol* 2: 123, 1982

23. Oh MS, Uribarri J, Del Monte MI, Heneghan WF, Kee CS, Friedman EA, Carroll HJ: A mechanism of hypoxemia during hemodialysis: consumption of CO_2 in metabolism of acetate. *Am J Nephrol* 5: 366, 1985

24. Romaldini H, Rodriguez-Roisin R, Lopez FA, Ziegler TW, Bencowitz HZ, Wagner PD: The mechanism of arterial hypoxemia during hemodialysis. *Am Rev Respir Dis* 129: 780, 1984

25. Romaldini H, Stabile C, Faro S, Lopes Dos Santos M, Ramos OL, Ribeiro Ratto O: Pulmonary ventilation during hemodialysis. *Nephron* 32: 131, 1982

26. Heyrman RM, De Backer WA, Van Waeleghem JP, Wittesaele WM, De Broe ME: The effect of acetate on ventilation in hemodialysis patients. *Nephron* 1988 (submitted)

27. Nissenson A: Prevention of dialysis induced hypoxemia by bicarbonate dialysis. *Trans Am Soc Artif Intern Organs* 26: 339, 1980

28. Raja R, Kramer M, Rosenbaum JL, Bolisay C, Krug M: Prevention of hypotension during isoosmolar hemodialysis with bicarbonate dialysate. *Trans Am Soc Artif Intern Organs* 26: 375, 1980

29. Van Stone J, Bauer J, Carey J: The effect of dialysate sodium concentration on body fluid distribution during hemodialysis. *Trans Am Soc Artif Intern Organs* 26: 283, 1980

30. Cohn MA, Rao AS, Broudy M, Birch S, Watson H, Atkins N: The respiratory inductive plethysmograph: a new non-invasive monitor of respiration. *Bull Eur Physiopathol Resp* 18: 643, 1983

31. Kaplow LS, Goffinet JA: Profound neutropenia during the early phase of hemodialysis. *JAMA* 203: 1135, 1968

32. Craddock PR, Fehr J, Brigham KL, Kronenberg R, Jacobs HS: Complement and leukocyte-medicated pulmonary dysfunction in hemodialysis. *N Engl J Med* 296: 769, 1977

33. Craddock PR, Fehr J, Dalmasso AP, Brigham KL, Jacobs HS: Hemodialysis leucopenia: pulmonary vascular leucostasis resulting from complement activation by dialyzer cellophane membranes. *J Clin Invest* 59: 879, 1977

34. Amin Arnaout M, Hakim RM, Todd RF, Dana N, Colten HR: Increased expression of an adhesion-promoting surface glycoprotein in the granulocytopenia of hemodialysis. *N Engl J Med* 312: 457, 1985

35. Horl WH, Jochum M, Heidland A, Fritz H: Release of granulocyte proteinases during hemodialysis. *Am J Nephrol* 3: 213, 1983

36. Ritchey EE, Wallin JD, Shah SV: Chemiluminescence and superoxide anion production by leukocytes from chronic hemodialysis patients. *Kidney Int* 19: 359, 1981

37. De Broe ME, Nouwen EJ, Van Waeleghem JP: On the mechanism and site of production of B2 microglobulin during hemodialysis. *Nephrol Dial Transplant* 2: 124, 1987

38. Cheung AK, Baranowski RL, Wayman AL: The role of thromboxane in cuprophan-induced pulmonary hypertension. *Kidney Int* 31: 1072, 1987

39. Dumler F, Levin NW: Leucopenia and hypoxia, unrelated effects of hemodialysis, *Arch Intern Med* 139: 1103, 1979

40. Tolchin N, Roberts JL, Lewis EJ: Respiratory gas exchange by high efficiency hemodialyzer. *Nephron* 21: 137, 1978

41. Brautbar N, Shinaberger JH, Miller JH, Nachman M: Hemodialysis hypoxemia: evaluation of mechanisms utilizing sequential ultrafiltration dialysis. *Nephron* 26: 96, 1980

42. De Broe ME, De Backer WA, Verpooten GA, Vermeire PA, Van Waeleghem JP, Herman AG: Leucopenia and hypoxemia during hemodialysis with different types of membranes: effect of prostacyclin. *Contr Nephrol* 36: 26, 1983

43. Phillipson EA, Duffin J, Cooper JD: Critical dependence of respiratory rhythmicity on metabolic CO_2 load. *J Appl Physiol* 50: 45, 1981

44. Kolobow T, Gattonini L, Tomlinson TA, Pierce JE: Control of breathing using an extracorporeal membrane lung. *Anesthesiology* 46: 138, 1977

45. Ponte J, Purves MJ: CO_2 and venous return and their interaction as stimuli to ventilation in the cat. *J Physiol* 274: 455, 1978

46. Sheldon ML, Green JF: Evidence for pulmonary CO2 chemosensitivity: effects on ventilation. *J Appl Physiol* 52: 1192, 1982

47. Wasserman K, Whipp BJ, Casaburi R, Hutsman DJ, Dastagna J, Lugliani R: Regulation of arterial PCO2 during intravenous CO2 loading. *J Appl Physiol* 38: 651, 1975

48. Rodenstein DO, Mercenier C, Stanescu DC: Influence of the respiratory route on the resting breathing pattern in humans. *Am Rev Respir Dis* 131: 163, 1985

49. Abu-Hamdan DK, Desai SG, Mahajan SK, Muller BF, Briggs WA, Lynne-Davies P, McDonald FD: Hypoxemia during hemodialysis using acetate versus bicarbonate dialysate. *Am J Nephrol* 4: 248, 1984

50. Heyrman RM, De Backer WA, Van Waeleghem JP, Willemen MJ, Vermeire PA, De Broe ME: Effect of oxygen administration on the breathing pattern during hemodialysis in man. *Eur Resp J* (in press)

51. Panzetta G, Tessitore N, Valvo E, Lupo A, Loschiavo C, Fabris A, Oldrizzi L, Gammaro L, Rugiu C, Bellotti Z, Maschio G: Biofiltration in the treatment of patients with acetate dialysis intolerance. *Clin Nephrol* 26: 33, 1986

52. West, JB: Man at extreme altitude. *J Appl Physiol* 52: 1399, 1982

53. Berssenbrugge A, Dempsey J, Iber C, Skatrud J, Wilson P: Mechanisms of hypoxia-induced periodic breathing during sleep in humans. *J Physiol (Lond)* 343: 507, 1983

54. De Backer WA, Heyrman RM, Wittesale WM, Waeleghem JP, Vermeire PA, De Broe ME: Ventilation and breathing patterns during hemodialysis induced carbon dioxide unloading. *Am Rev Respir Dis* 136: 406, 1987

55. Berkenbosch A, Van Beek JHGM, Olievier CN, De Goede J, Quanjer PH: Central respiratory CO2, sensitivity at extreme hypoxapnia. *Respir Physiol* 55: 95, 1984

56. Lahiri S, Hsiao C, Zhng R, Mokashi A, Nishino T: Peripheral chemoreceptors in respiratory oscillations. *I Appl Physiol* 58: 1901, 1985

57. Peres-Serrano A, Fernandeze-Vega F, Alvarez-Grande J: Hypoxemia during hemodialysis in patients with impairment in pulmonary function. *Nephron* 42: 14, 1986

58. Camussi G, Segolini G, Rotunno M, Vercellone A: Mechanism involved in acute granulocytopenia in hemodialysis: Cell-membrane direct interactions. *Int J Artif Organs* 1: 123, 1978

59. Danielson BG, Hallgren R, Benge P: Neutrophil and eosinophil degranulation by hemodialysis membrane. *Contrib Nephrol* 37: 83, 1984

60. Hakim RM, Fearon DAT, Lazarus JM, Perzanowski CS: Biocompatibility of dialysis membranes: effect of chronic complement activation. *Kidney Int* 26: 194, 1984

61. Greene WH, Casann RS, Mauer M, Quie P: The effect of hemodialysis on neutrophil chemotactic responsiveness. *J Lab Clin Med* 88: 971, 1976

62. Henderson LW, Miller ME, Hamilton RW, Norman ME: Hemodialysis leukopenia and polymorph random mobility – a possible correlation. *J Lab Clin Med* 85: 191, 1975

63. Chenoweth PE, Cheung AK, Henderson LW: Anaphylatoxin formation during hemodialysis: effects of different dialyzer membranes. *Kidney Int* 24: 764, 1983

64. Lespier-Dexter LE, Guerra C, Ojeda W, Martinez-Maldonado M: Granulocyte adherence in uremia and hemodialysis. *Nephron* 24: 64, 1979

65. McGregor RR: Granulocyte adherence changes induced by hemodialysis, endotoxin, epinephrine, and glucocorticoids. *Ann Intern Med* 86: 35, 1977

66. Hallgren R, Fjellstrom KE, Hakansson L, Venge P: Kinetic studies of phagocytosis. II. The serum-independent uptake of IgG-coated particles by polymorphonuclear leukocytes from uremic patients on regular dialysis treatment. *J Lab Clin Med* 94: 277, 1979

67. Hakim RM, Breillatt J, Lazarus JM, Port RK, Complement activation and hypersensitivity reaction to dialysis membranes. *N Engl J Med* 311: 878, 1984

68. Dinarello CA: The biology of interleukin-1 and its relevance to hemodialysis. *Blood Purif* 1: 197, 1983

69. Lee J, Hakim RM, Fearon DT: Increased expression of the C3b receptor by neutrophils and complement activation during hemodialysis. *Clin Exp Immunol* 56: 205, 1984

70. Conger JD, Hammond WS, Alfrey AC, Contiguglia SR, Stanford RE, Huffer WE: Pulmonary calcification in chronic dialysis patients. *Ann Intern Med* 83: 330, 1975

71. Lee HY, Stretton TB, Barnes AM: The lungs in renal failure. *Thorax* 30: 46, 1975

72. Schwarz A, Keller F, Seyfert S, Poll W, Molzahn M, Distler A: Carpal tunnel syndrome, a late complication in chronic hemodialysis. *Deutsch Med Wochenschr* 109: 285, 1984

73. Allieu Y, Asencio G, Mailhe D, Baldet P, Mion C: Carpal tunnel syndrome in chronic hemodialysis patients. *Rev Chir Orthop* 69: 233, 1983

74. Bok DU, Pascular L, Herberger C, Sawyer R, Levin NW: Effect of multiple use of dialyzers on intradialytic symptoms. *Proc Clin Dial Transplant Forum* 10: 92, 1980

75. Kant KS, Pollak VE, Cathey M, Goetz D, Berlin R: Multiple use of dialyzers: safety and efficacy. *Kidney Int* 19: 728, 1981

76. Man NK, Fournier G, Thireau P, Gaillard JL, Funck Brentano JL: The effect of bicarbonate containing dialysate on chronic hemodialysis patients: A comparative study. *Artif Organs* 6: 421, 1982

77. Chanard J, Brunois JP, Melin JP, Lavaud S, Toupance O: Long-term results of dialysis therapy with a highly permeable membrane. *Artif Organs* 6: 261, 1982

78. Avram MM: The Long Island College Hospital experience with the decade or longer hemodialysis patient. in *Prevention of Kidney Disease and Long-term Suvival* edited by Avram MM, New York, London, Plenum Publ Co, 1982, p 165

79. Zidulka A, Despas PJ, Milic-Emili J, Anthonisen NR: Pulmonary function with acute loss of excess lung water by hemodialysis in patients with chronic uremia. *Am J Med* 55: 134, 1973

80. Craig DB, Wahba WM, Don HF, Couture JG, Becklake MB: Closing volume and its relationship to gas exchange in seated and supine positions. *J Appl Physiol* 31: 717, 1971

81. Robson M, Levin A, Ravid M: Serial measurement of vital capacity in patients on chronic hemodialysis. *Nephron* 19: 60, 1977

82. Brigham KL, Bernard G: Pulmonary complications of chronic renal failure. *Semin Nephrol* 1: 188, 1981

83. Kuzela DC, Huffer WE, Conger JD, Winter SD, Hammond WS: Soft tissue calcification in chronic dialysis patients. *Am J Pathol* 86: 403, 1977

84. Berlyne GM, Lee HA, Ralston AJ, Woodlock JA: Pulmonary complications of peritoneal dialysis. *Lancet* 2: 75, 1966

85. Goggin MJ, Joekes AM: Pulmonary gas exchange during peritoneal dialysis. *Br Med J* 2: 247, 1971

86. Ahluwalia M, Ishikawa S, Gellman M, Shah T, Sekar T, MacDonnel KF: Pulmonary functions during peritoneal dialysis. *Clin Nephrol* 18: 251, 1982

87. Khanna R, Oreopoulos DG: Complications of peritoneal dialysis other than peritonitis. in *Peritoneal Dialysis*, edited by Nolph KD, The Hague, Martinus Nijhoff, 1985, p 441

88. Freedman S, Maberly DJ: Pulmonary gas exchange during dialysis. *Br Med J* 3: 48, 1971

89. Taveira Da Silva AM, Davis WB, Winchester JF, Coleman DE, Wei CW: Peritonitis, dialysate infusion and lung function in continuous ambulatory peritoneal (CAPD) *Clin Nephrol* 24: 79, 1985

90. O'Brien AAJ, Power J, O'Brien L, Clancy L, Keogh JAB: The effect of 2 L dialysate on respiratory function. *Peritoneal Dial*

Bull 7: S57, 1987

91. Scheldewaert R, Bogaerts Y, Pauwels R, Van der Straeten M, Ringoir S, Lameire N: Management of a massive hydrothorax in a CAPD patient: a case report and a review of the literature. *Peritoneal Dial Bull* 2: 69, 1982

GASTROINTESTINAL COMPLICATIONS OF RENAL FAILURE

MICHAEL ADLER and CHARLES TOUSSAINT

INTRODUCTION

Renal failure may lead to changes in structure and function of virtually every segment of the digestive tract. As extensive papers devoted to gastrointestinal abnormalities in uraemic patients have been published (1–4), the aim of this chapter is to vitalise the topic by reviewing recent literature and referring to personal experiences resulting from collaborative studies between nephrologists and gastroenterologists at our institution.

The following guidelines were applied as regularly as feasible for each section of this chapter : 1) physiopathology in the uraemic state; 2) description of clinical entities with emphasis on pathology, aetiopathogenesis, diagnosis and management. Readers interested in physiology of the normal digestive tract should consult the last edition of Johnson's Gastrointestinal Physiology (5).

ORAL CAVITY AND OESOPHAGUS

Parotitis

Parotitis which used to be an ominous complication of end-stage renal failure, is no longer observed in uraemic patients. While Dahlberg et al (6) found no evidence of salivary glands dysfunction in haemodialysis patients, Van Der Lichte et al (7) observed extremely low salivary sodium concentration associated with profoundly decreased flowrate in such patients.

Stomatitis

Uraemic stomatitis is characterized by coated tongue, painful ulcerations of mucous membranes, and by a metallic taste (2).

Uraemic breath

Described as 'fishy', uraemic breath is usually considered as a consequence of an increased salivary ammonia concentration secondary to bacterial urea hydrolysis. It has also been related to high concentrations of secondary and tertiary amines (2) and to poor oral hygiene.

Oesophagitis

Oesophagitis was the most common oesophageal lesion found at autopsy in haemodialysis patients (8). An increased incidence of hiatal hernia was decribed in end-stage renal failure patients, particularly in those with polycystic kidneys (9).

STOMACH AND DUODENUM

Psysiopathology in uremia

Gastric secretion

Conflicting data regarding gastric secretion in uraemia have been reported. Some showed hyperchlorhydria (10, 11) while others demonstrated low acid output (12, 13). Those discrepancies may be due to the mixing of dialysed and not dialysed patients, as discussed below. Large variability in the serum concentration of gastrointestinal hormones will probably yield different rates of gastric secretion in individual patients. Usually no correlation is observed, however, between the gastric secretion rate and the serum gastrin level (10, 14, 15). From studies on dialysed and undialysed patients, Taylor et al (16) concluded that basal serum gastrin concentrations were higher than in normal control subjects, without a difference between these categories of uraemic patients. In that study, maximal acid output correlated inversely with serum gastrin level.

It now appears well-established that chronic uraemic patients not treated by dialysis secrete less acid than normal individuals, both in the basal state (17) and after pentagastrin stimulation (18, 19). This relative hypochlorhydria could be explained by high intraluminal concentration of ammonium ions with ensuing neutralization of hydrochloric acid (20), and by enhanced back-diffusion of protons by the gastric mucosa (21). Atrophic gastritis with decreased parietal cell sensitivity to gastrin is frequently observed in uraemic patients (17, 22), and could readily explain the low gastric secretion rate, but this oversimplification has been refuted (18).

Serum gastrin levels are usually increased in undialysed uraemic patients (19, 23). Reasons for this include: 1) hypo- or achlorhydria which is a well-known stimulus of gastrin release (24) 2) G cell hyperplasia (22) and 3) inadequate renal gastrin inactivation (25). In dialysed uraemic patients, gastric acid secretion is increased in comparison with undialysed patients (16, 26), suggesting that some inhibitor of gastric acid secretion is removed by haemodialysis. Increased acid secretion in dialysis patients could thus be explained by a decreased level of gastric inhibitory peptide (GIP), a well-known inhibitor of acid secretion which is removed by haemodialysis (27). Hypercalcaemia during haemodialysis could also stimulate gastric acid secretion (28).

Hypergastrinaemia is probably not responsible for increased gastric acid secretion in haemodialysed patients for the following reasons: 1) only insignificant increases (18, 23) or decreases (16) in serum gastrin levels have been recorded during haemodialysis and 2) only big gastrin G34, and not little gastrin G17, which has a potency six times greater than big gastrin G34 in stimulating acid secretion, has been shown to be eliminated more slowly by the kidney in chronic renal failure (16, 17).

Gastric emptying

Few investigations have concerned gastric motility in the uraemic state. Normal fluid and solid gastric emptying rates have been found in haemodialysed patients (29, 30). In one study, delayed gastric emptying was observed in uraemic patients not undergoing haemodialysis (29).

Erosive gastroduodenitis

In 1934, Jaffe and Laing (31) reported on gastrointestinal autopsy findings in 136 patients who had died in uraemia. In the majority of cases, diffuse haemorrhagic or pseudomembranous lesions were found. Since the introduction of haemodialysis in the treatment of end-stage renal failure, the nature and distribution of the lesions have profoundly changed.

However, in comparison with the normal population, chronic dialysis patients seem to show an increased incidence of mucosal lesions in the upper digestive tract. Pathologic evidence of gastritis was present in 10 to 44% of patients in a large series (8, 32), and this was confirmed by Mitchell et al (33). Furthermore the incidence of atrophic gastritis also seems to be increased in uraemic patients (17, 33, 34).

It is, however, difficult to establish on a morphological basis the true incidence of gastric mucosal lesions in uraemic patients in comparison to the general population because adequate epidemiological studies and morphometric evaluations are lacking. Furthermore, assessment of the true incidence of duodenitis would be an impossible task since mild changes, usually in patchy distribution, were observed in about 30% of healthy volunteers (35).

Aetiopathogenesis of gastroduodenitis in uraemia is probably multifactorial. Uraemia itself (33), biliary reflux (33), acid hypersecretion (10) and hypergastrinaemia (34) have been implicated. Some authors, however, claim that hypochlorhydria is associated with an increased incidence of bleeding from erosive gastroduodenitis or peptic ulcer (36).

Diagnosis

The endoscopic appearance of the mucosal lesions (37) consists of oedematous, erythematous and friable, usually nodular folds (Figure 1). Nodular appearance (Figure 2) is particularly frequent in the duodenum (38) where it is observed in 34% of patients in end-stage renal failure, compared to 4% in the general population. Duodenal pseudomelanosis is also observed in chronic renal failure (39).

Management

Superficial gastroduodenitis is usually successfully managed by antacid supplementation. This has also been advocated to prevent severe post-transplant ulcerations, but effectiveness of this policy has not been demonstrated. In critically ill patients, antacid titration was found superior to cimetidine for preventing upper gastrointestinal tract bleeding (40).

Gastroduodenal mucosal erosions bleed only uncommonly, but they can do so if associated with haemostatic abnormalities such as platelet dysfunction, often seen in uraemia (41, 42). In case of bleeding, for example with peptic ulcer, peritoneal dialysis may be preferred to haemodialysis or haemodialysis may be conducted under citrate of heparin regional anticoagulation (59).

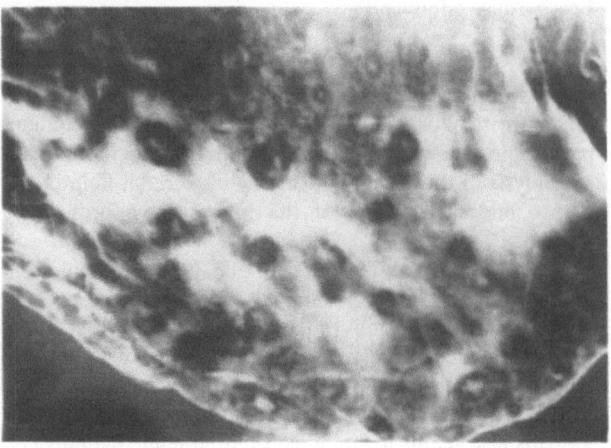

Figure 1. Nodular appearance of gastric mucosa with ulcerations, in a case of uraemic erosive gastritis with severe bleeding (courtesy of Dr L. Engelholm).

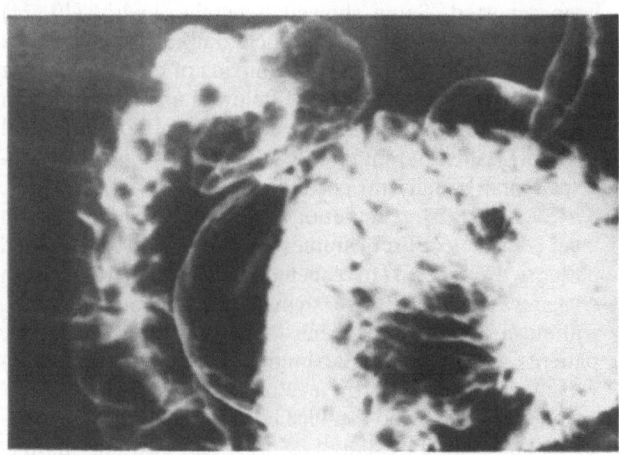

Figure 2. Nodular duodenal folds in the same patient as in **Figure 1** (courtesy of Dr L. Engelholm).

Peptic ulcer disease (PUD)

According to a recent report based on autopsy material, PUD was observed in 24% of haemodialysed patients versus 10% in the general population (8). Other reports, based on endoscopy, showed a prevalence of 11% of PUD in haemodialysis patients, compared to 15% in control individuals (43). Discrepancies in PUD prevalence in various series could be due to differences in sampling, antacid administration, and doses of antacids used.

The high incidence of PUD in chronic haemodialysis patients and the acid hypersecretion frequently observed in them, together with the high morbidity rate of gastroduodenal bleeding or perforation or both (35 to 75%) have led some groups to advocate prophylactic surgery of PUD prior to transplantation (44). Such a radical policy seems unwarranted for, as mentioned before, antacid therapy alone may constitute good prophylaxis. On the other hand, the use of cimetidine or ranitidine for prophylaxis of PUD is controversial. Furthermore, the receptor antagonists may enhance delayed hypersensitivity (45), with the theoretical consequence of increasing the risk of rejection. These drugs also increase serum creatinine levels in cyclosporine – treated kidney recipients (46). In conclusion, antacid therapy should be preferred to the receptor antagonists or to surgery in candidates for kidney transplantation. Routine endoscopy and radiology should be advocated prior to transplantation. If active PUD is detected, transplant surgery should be postponed and vigourous therapy initiated. In view of their absence of side-effects, particularly their lack of influence on cytochrome P450 and on the basis of a possible lower recurrence rate of PUD, sucralfate (48) or bismuth subcitrate (48) may be preferred in this setting.

Upper gastrointestinal bleeding

Upper gastrointestinal bleeding occurring in uraemic patients may be due to *haemorragic gastritis* or *duodenitis* or both or to a *peptic ulcer.* The haemostatic abnormalities observed in renal failure (41, 42) could explain the higher rates of recurrent bleeding (49), of morbidity (such patients need twice as many transfusions), and of mortality (3 to 7% [10]) in patients with chronic renal failure in comparison to the general population.

Endoscopy offers the best yield for determining the cause of bleeding. Recent reports emphasize the high incidence of *vascular ectasiae* as sources of bleeding in uraemic patients (49, 50). The aetiopathogenesis of those acquired vascular lesions is not readily apparent. An unidentified factor accumulating in uraemia could act on the vasculature (51). Arterial hypertension may contribute to dilatation of submucosal venules (52). Aluminium hydroxide gels in common use in these patients have been incriminated on the basis that they can cause skin telangiectasiae (53). Vascular calcinosis in the setting of secondary hyperparathyroidism has also been incriminated (54). Finally, telangiectasiae could also bleed because of underlying haemostatic abnormalities (41, 42).

Bleeding vascular lesions can be successfully treated at endoscopy by electrocoagulation, laser or heater probe (55), together with the eventual correction of underlying clotting abnormalities, using cryoprecipitate or agents such as de-amino-d-arginine-vasopressin (DDAVP) (56), oestrogens or a combination of oestrogens and progesterone (57, 58). If the patient has to be dialysed during active bleeding, haemodialysis should be conducted under regional anti-coagulation, using heparin or citrate (59) or peritoneal dialysis may be preferred. Endoscopic instrumentations should be preferably performed on the day after haemodialysis, especially when they include biopsy.

SMALL INTESTINE

Physiopathology in uraemia

The main functions of the small instestine are to digest nutritients and absorb them from the lumen into the circulation and to transport the residue into the colon. Abnormalities in the migrating motor complex may be associated with bacterial overgrowth, intestinal stasis and pseudo-obstructive syndromes which all can occur in the setting of kidney failure.

Malabsorption

Morphological and functional changes of the small intestine have been reported in uraemia (60, 61). Impaired absorption of calcium (60), fat (62), folate, amino acids, sugars, vitamin D and iron have been observed in renal failure (63, 64). Those abnormalities could be explained by intestinal ischaemia, uraemic toxins, bacterial overgrowth or vitamin D deficency alone or in combination (60).

Ischaemic enteropathy

Patients with renal failure are at higher risk of developing ischaemic enteropathy (65), both of the occlusive type (due to accelerated atheromatosis) and of the non-occlusive type (due to microangiopathy).

This will be discussed in more detail in the section concerning the colon and rectum.

Mesenteric ischaemia can produce a broad spectrum of syndromes, from abdominal colicky pain to massive infarction of the bowel and intestinal perforation. The syndrome frequently occurs after a period of hypovolaemia in the course of a haemodialysis session. Pre-existing vascular lesions could constitute an important predisposing factor (66).

COLON AND RECTUM

No systematic studies have been performed concerning colonic function in uraemia, although diarrhoea constitutes a commonly reported symptom in chronic renal failure. Well characterized clinical entities, however, are observed in this setting.

Diarrhoea and colitis

As in non-uraemic patients, diarrhoea occurring in uraemia is most frequently due to inflammatory disease of the colon caused by infection of bacterial, viral or parasitic origin, or it may be of the ischaemic type (67). Colicky abdominal pain, bloody or bloodless diarrhoea, fever and leucocytosis are the usual presenting symptoms.

Bacterial colitis may be due to toxins which either provoke the mucosa to secrete salt and water (enterotoxins), or act by causing tissue damage (cytotoxins). Both pathogenic mechanisms are usually operating for the commonly encountered bacteria : *E. coli, Campylobacter, Yersinia, Salmonella, Shigella* and *C. difficile.*

Infectious colitis is commonly observed in haemodialysis patients, due to possible cross-infection in the unit (68), and also to the frequent administration of antibiotics to those patients, leading to growth of abnormal colonic bacterial flora. Due to depressed immunity, infectious colitis is not unfrequently complicated by septicaemia in uraemic patients (69).

Ischaemic disease of the colon is frequently observed in haemodialysis patients (8). It may be caused by one or several of the following factors : accelerated atherosclerosis, arterial hypertension, hyperlipaemia, antithrombin III deficiency (65), and perdialytic hypotensive episodes. Ischaemic colitis can be favoured by vessel occlusion (70); most often large vessels are patent, but a microangiopathy similar to that seen in diabetes can be observed (71).

Diagnosis of colitis in uraemic patients includes stool culture, direct examination of faeces for ova, parasites and leucocytes, blood serology when indicated (viruses, *Amoebae Yersinia enterocolitica*, etc), and colonoscopy with biopsy. Biopsy specimens should be evaluated both by histology, with special stains for bacteria, viruses and fungi, as indicated, and by microbiology, with bacterial and viral cultures. Owing to the high incidence of *Clostridium difficile* colitis in uraemic patients (72), search for its specific toxin should be performed. The endoscopic yellowish pseudomembranous appearance of *Clostridium difficile* colitis may be lacking, and this type of colitis may occur long after the interruption of antibiotic administration and even in patients who have not received those drugs.

Management of infectious colitis includes the administration of appropriate antibiotics or antiparasitic drugs. *Clostridium difficile* colitis should be treated with oral vancomycin; in case of recurrence, which is observed in 14 to 20% of cases (73), metronidazole, bacitracin or lactulose may be tried.

Ischaemic colitis without gangrene and perforation is best managed by parenteral alimentation which, owing to the large volumes infused, usually necessitates daily haemodialysis with ultrafiltration.

Intestinal pseudo-obstruction and colonic perforation

In 1948, Ogilvie (74) described in uraemic patients a syndrome consisting of chronic abdominal pain and non-obstructive dilatation of the colon. Although pseudo-obstruction usually involves the small bowel in diabetic neuropathy, amyloidosis and scleroderma, uraemic pseudo-obstruction is typically located in the colon, as originally described (74).

The usual symptoms are chronic constipation and abdominal pain and distension. Colonic perforation occurs in 30 to 50% of the cases (75), particularly when the caecal diameter exceeds 12 cm.

Several factors may contribute to the development of this syndrome: aluminium gels, fluid and electrolyte disturbances, autonomic neuropathy and drugs impairing bowel motility (76).

The diagnosis is suggested by clinical data and confirmed by plain film of the abdomen. The differential diagnosis includes mechanical obstruction due to volvulus or adhesions, old ischaemic colitis, carcinoma or faecal or antacid impaction.

When the diagnosis of colonic perforation is established in an uraemic patient, it can be the consequence of undiagnosed colonic pseudo-obstruction, but also of stercoral ulceration, most often located in the sigmoid, of idiopathic caecal ulcer (77), of ischaemic colitis or of diverticulitis. The mortality rate of colonic perforation is 70 to 80% in uraemic patients (78), as compared to 36 to 49% in the general population (79).

Idiopathic ulcers of the caecum can also present with bleeding, and they can be solitary or multiple. Fibrin thrombi and necrotic infarcts secondary to localized ischaemia are frequently observed in their close vicinity (80).

Management of colonic pseudo-obstruction includes nasogastric aspiration and parenteral fluid administration. Deflation via the colonoscope or via a long Faucher tube introduced under radioscopic monitoring (81) constitutes the best form of therapy (Figure 3). In case of failure of those measures, surgical alternatives are subtotal colectomy or tube caecostomy.

Faecal or antacid impaction should be treated energetically either manually or with the use of laxatives as well as various enemas, including gastrografin.

In order to prevent colonic psuedo-obstruction or impaction, chronic constipation should be avoided in uraemic patients, aluminium hydroxide should be replaced by calcium carbonate as a phosphorus-chelating agent (82), and lubricants along with a fiber-enriched diet should be used.

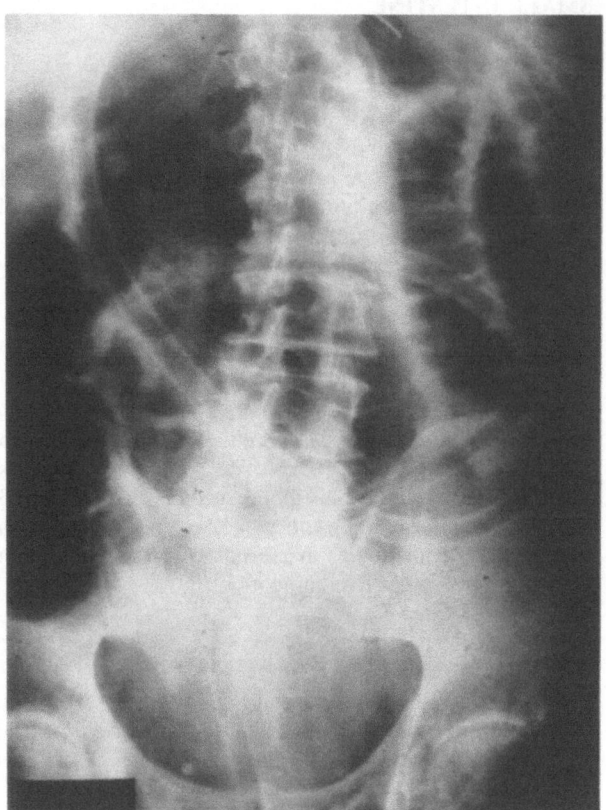

Figure 3. Colonic desinflation via a Faucher tube in a case of colonic pseudo-obstruction (courtesy of Dr L. Engelholm).

Diverticulitis

Colonic diverticula may be present in up to 49% of patients with chronic renal failure, but this incidence may not differ from that of an age-matched control population without renal disease (83).

Diverticulitis, however, would occur at an earlier age in the uraemic population, carrying high morbidity (88%) and mortality (28%) rates, due to the high incidence of perforation (85). Diverticulosis seems to be particularly frequent in polycystic kidney disease, with an incidence of 10/12 patients, compared to 1/31 patients with other types of chronic renal failure (83).

Management of patients with diverticulosis consists of high fiber diet with avoidance of constipation. In case of diverticulitis, early surgery is mandatory, using preferentially the Hartmann procedure.

Haemochezia (rectal bleeding)

Severe haemochezia can be caused by peptic ulcer with arterial bleeding or, very unfrequently, by ruptured oesophageal varices, but its cause is to be found most commonly in the colon. In uraemic patients, colonic bleeding may be due to diverticula, most often right-sided, angiodysplasia (85),

idiopathic caecal (86) or rectal (87) ulcers, or ischaemic colitis. Haemostatic disturbances, such as platelet dysfunction (41, 42), thrombocytopenia, or the use of heparin for haemodialysis or of warfarin, sometimes used for maintaining arteriovenous shunt patency, may increase the incidence and severity of all types of bleeding in uraemia.

In our experience (88), the yield of diagnosis the aetiology of haemochezia is greater with coloscopy than with arteriography or radio-isotope studies. Barium enema has no place in this setting.

Therapeutic endoscopy, using bipolar electrocoagulation or a heater probe can be applied to bleeding angiodysplasia or rectal and colonic ulcer. Intraarterial vasopressin (for right-sided lesions) and correction of haemostatic abnormalities, using cryoprecipitate or DDAVP (56) or oestrogen or an oestrogen-progesterone combination (57, 58) may sometimes be helpful.

Surgery must be considered in case of failure of conservative management, and is the therapy of choice in case of diverticular bleeding.

PANCREAS

Exocrine pancreatic function seems to be frequently impaired in chronic renal failure. Normal pancreatic function was found in only 28% of chronic uraemic patients studied by the secretin-pancreozymin test (89). With the use of a similar method, amylase and lipase outputs were found decreased in duodenal aspirates, and steatorrhea was observed in 50% of the investigated patients (90). Decreased pancreatic bicarbonate secretion in response to secretory stimulation has also been reported (89).

On the other hand, Owyang et al (91) observed an enhanced trypsin (but not lipase) secretion following intraduodenal mannitol and intravenous cholecystokinin pancreozymin (CCK-PZ) infusions. Those findings were ascribed to increased levels of fasting stimulatory hormones, such as CCK-PZ, in chronic renal failure, with sustained pancreatic stimulation. It should be stressed that the latter results contradict those obtained with the secretin-pancreozymin test descirbed above. Studies evaluating modifications of the pure pancreatic juice in uraemic patients treated by haemodialysis confirm higher volumes and higher protein output compared to subjects free of any organic disease (92).

Pancreatitis

A high prevalence of pancreatic disease has been reported in chronic renal failure (93, 94). Pathologic changes in the pancreas, mostly those of chronic pancreatitis, were observed at autopsy in 57% of chronic haemodialysis patients (94). Chronic pancreatitis frequently impairs digestion and may be responsible for malnutrition and for the wasting syndrome sometimes observed in patients with end-stage renal failure (90).

Acute pancreatitis also occurs more frequently in uraemic (2.3%) than in non-uraemic (0.5%) patients (95). The risk is greater in patients treated by peritoneal dialysis than in those maintained on haemodialysis (96).

Pancreatic changes occurring in uraemia have been ascribed to hyperparathyroidism (97), hypertriglyceridaemia, accelerated atherosclerosis, hepatitis, chemical peritonitis in peritoneal dialysis (96), drug toxicity or to commoner causes of pancreatitis such as alcohol and biliary conditions. It may also follow splenectomy or left nephrectomy.

The diagnosis of chronic pancreatitis can be established by detection of steatorrhoea (24 h stool collection or ^{14}C-triolein breath test), by endoscopic pancreatography, or by analysis of duodenal aspirate or of pure pancreatic secretion.

Frequently the diagnosis of acute pancreatitis is difficult, due to nonspecificity of clinical signs and of amylase, lipase and trypsin determinations in uraemic patients. CT scan evaluation of the pancreas is promising (98), but its sensitivity is still difficult to appraise.

Management of acute pancreatitis in uraemia includes parenteral nutrition with daily dialysis.

Hyperamylasaemia

Interpretation of hyperamylasaemia in patients with renal failure may be difficult. Total serum amylase is usually

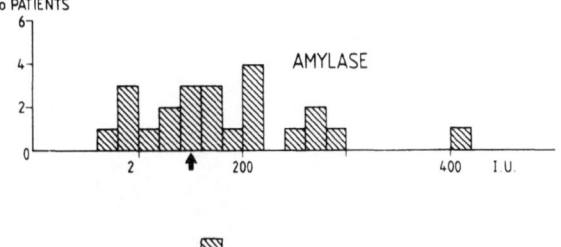
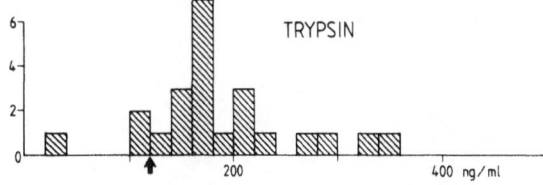
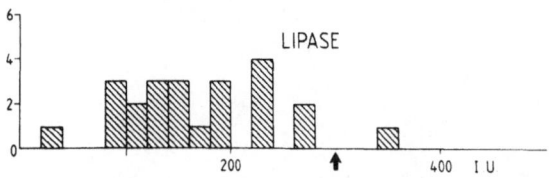

Figure 4. Histograms representing simultaneous determinations of serum amylase, trypsin and lipase levels in 23 end-stage renal patients treated by haemodialysis. Arrows indicate upper values obtained in control normal subjects. While amylase and trypsin concentrations are increased in the majority of patients, lipase concentrations are normal in 22 of the 23 patients (courtesy of Dr H. Ooms).

raised up to 2 to 3 times the normal value due to retention of both pancreatic and salivary isoenzymes (99). Liver dysfunction and hyperparathyroidism (100) can also play a role.

In our experience, lipase is less influenced by renal insufficiency than serum amylase and trypsin levels (Figure 4), and could thus be more useful in the diagnosis of acute pancreatitis in uraemic patients. Our data confirm previous reports from the literature (101, 102).

LIVER

Physiopathology in uraemia

Several abnormalities in hepatic metabolism have been described in renal failure. They concern carbohydrate (103), triglyceride (104) and protein (105) metabolisms.

Alterations in drug metabolism by the liver have not been extensively assessed. In rabbits, no significant effect of chronic renal failure on hepatic morphology was observed (106). Furthermore, no changes were noted in antipyrine clearance (evaluating microsomal oxidative drug metabolism) and in galactose elimination capacity (evaluating cytosolic hepatocyte function), suggesting the lack of significant alterations in liver function induced by uraemia. In man,

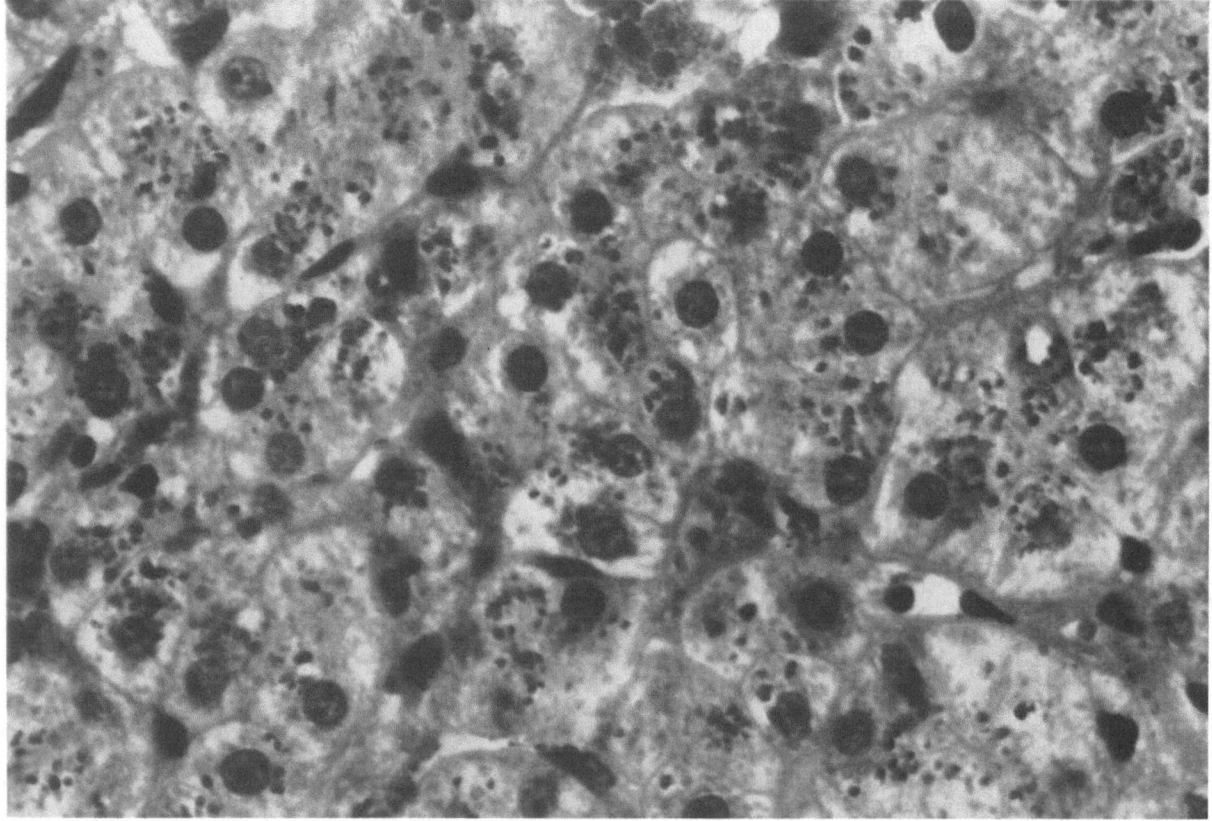

Figure 5. Heavy deposits of lipofuscin in a case of chronic phenacetin abuse (Schmorl stain, x 1000, courtesy of Dr P. Ketelbant).

however, impaired metabolic clearance of some drugs can be expected owing to a reduced microsomal content of cytochrome P450 observed in uraemia (107).

Alterations in liver function tests

Increases in serum enzymes, of short or long duration, often with recurrences, are frequently observed in haemodialysis patients. They could be the consequence of viral infections, pigment accumulation, drug-induced liver diseases, congestion, steatosis or biliary pathology (108).

Viral diseases of the liver occurring so commonly in those patients are described in Chapter 42.

Pigment accumulation in the liver includes iron (109) or phenacetin. We observed a 49 year old woman on dialysis for end-stage renal failure due to phenacetin abuse who presented with hepatomegaly, abnormal liver tests and increased serum iron and ferritin serum levels. Liver biopsy (Figure 5) showed massive deposition of lipofuscin, as demonstrated by the Schmorl stain.

The leaking of plasticizers such as diethylhexylphtalate, which are added to polyvinyl chloride tubings and containers used for haemodialysis, has been shown to produce biochemical as well as morphological abnormalities in the liver of sub-human primates (110). Silicone, used some years ago in blood pumps, may be responsible for hepatic fibrosis and granulomatosis, leading to chronic hepatitis (111).

Drug-induced liver diseases (Table 1) should constitute frequent causes of liver test abnormalities in haemodialysis patients, particularly in older patients, although this point has not been extensively investigated (112). Liver histology may disclose acute or chronic, even active, hepatitis, cirrhosis, vascular lesions, or neoplasms.

While hepatic cysts, which are present in 50% of patients with polycystic kidney disease, lead only extremely rarely to any complication, a few cases of severe bacterial infections with Gram negative septicaemia have occurred in liver cysts in some long-term dialysed (113) and kidney transplant (114) patients. As renal cyst infection is far more common, diagnosis of liver cyst infection can be better suggested in nephrectomised patients. Gallium or labeled leucocyte scintigraphy may help to locate the infectious process within the liver while CT scan does not seem to be very helpful (114). Cyst puncture under ultrasonographic guidance may establish the diagnosis.

Establishing the cause of liver dysfunction in patients with renal failure may be quite difficult. The following blood analysis should be performed : ferritin, viral serology, tissue

Table 1. Drug-induced liver diseases.

A. Parenchymatous	II. *Chronic*	B. *Phospholipidosis*	F. *Vascular lesions*
I. *Acute*	1. *Fibrosis*	Amiodarone	I. *Hepatic veins*
1. *Cytotoxic*	Methotrexate	C. *Pigment storage*	Immunosuppressive and
a. Necrosis	2. *Active chronic hepatitis*	I. *Lipofuscin*	antineoplastic drugs
Halothane	(antinuclear antibody	Phenacetin	Oral contraceptives
Paracetamol	frequently present)	Phenothiazine	II. *Sinusoids*
Isoniazid	Alpha methyl dopa	Cascara	Oral contraceptives
b. Steatosis	Nitrofurantoin	II. *Iron*	Azathioprine
Tetracyclines	Paracetamol	Blood transfusions	Anabolic agents
Corticosteroids	Isoniazid	Portocaval shunt	Vitamin A
2. *Cholestatic*	3. *Posthepatitis cirrhosis*	D. *Granuloma*	III. *Portal vein*
Oral contraceptives	Same agents	Talc	Vitamin A
Chlorpromazine	4. *Steatocirrhosis*	Silicone	Azathioprine
Erythromicyn	Methotrexate	Allopurinol	Oral contraceptives
3. *Mixed*	5. *Biliary cirrhosis*	Sulfonamides	IV. *Hepatic artery*
Sulfonamides	Chlorpromazine	Quinidine	Oral contraceptives
	Tolbutamide	Phenylbutazone	Amphetamines
	Ajmaline	E. *Tumours*	
	Thiabendazole	I. *Angiosarcoma*	
		Anabolic drugs	
		Vinyl chloride	
		II. *Adenoma*	
		Oral contraceptives	
		Anabolic drugs	
		III. *Hepatoma*	
		Oral contraceptives	

antibodies, alpha-foetoprotein, along with liver function tests such as ^{14}C-aminopyrine-breath test and serum bile acids level. Ultrasonography and liver biopsy may be extremely helpful.

In patients who are candidates for kidney transplantation, biopsy of the liver should be done in every case where the aetiology of hepatic dysfunction could not be established by non-invasive procedures. The important value of biopsy in cases with viral hepatitis is discussed in Chapter 42.

REFERENCES

1. Jacobs E: Le retentissement digestif de l'insuffisance rénale. (Digestive consequences of renal insufficiency) *Acta Med Belg* 20: 349, 1957
2. Gilbert R, Goyal RK: The gastrointestinal system, in *The Systemic Consequences of Renal Failure,* edited by Eknoyan G, Knochel JP, New York, Grune and Stratton 1984, p 133
3. Mujais SK, Sabatini S, Kurtzman NA: Pathophysiology of the uremic syndrome. in *The Kidney,* edited by Brenner BM, Rector FC Jr, Philadelphia, W.B. Saunders Company, 1986, p 1587
4. Dewayne Andrews M, Papper S: The kidneys and the urinary tract, in *Bockus Gatroenterology,* edited by Berk JE, Philadelphia, W.B. Saunders Company, 1985, p 4613
5. Johnson LR: *Gastrointestinal Physiology,* St Louis, The CV Mosby Company, 1985
6. Dahlberg WH, Sreebny LM, King B: Studies of parotid saliva and blood in hemodialysis patients. *J Appl Physiol* 23: 100, 1967
7. Van Der Lichte JL, Mulder AW, Michels LFE: Parotid gland

dysfunction in hemodialysis patients. *Neth J Med* 26: 39, 1983
8. Vaziri ND, Dure-Smith B, Miller R, Mirahmad MK: Pathology of gastrointestinal tract in chronic hemodialysis patients : an autopsy study of 78 cases. *Am J Gastroenterol* 80: 608, 1985
9. Bailey GL, Griffiths H, Locke JP: Gastrointestinal abnormalities in uremia. *Abstracts Am Soc Nephrol* 5: 5, 1971
10. Sullivan SN, Tustanoff E, Slaughter DN: Hypergastrinemia and gastric acid hypersecretion in uremia. *Clin Nephrol* 5: 25, 1976
11. Shepherd AMM, Stewart WK, Wormsley KG: Peptic ulceration in chronic renal failure. *Lancet,* 1: 1957, 1973
12. Korman MG, Laver MC, Hansky J: Hypergastrinaemia in chronic renal failure. *Br Med J* 1: 209, 1972
13. Reisman TN, Derez GO, Rogers AI: Gastric secretory function in patients with chronic renal failure undergoing maintenance hemodialysis. *Am J Dig Dis* 21: 1044, 1976
14. Gedde-Dahl G: Serum gastrin responses to food stimulation in male azotemic patients. *Scand J Gastroenterol* 10: 683, 1975
15. Hansky J, King RW, Holdsworth S: Serum gastrin in chronic renal failure, in *Gastrointestinal Hormones,* edited by Thompson JC, Austin, University of Texas Press, p 111
16. Taylor IL, Sells, RA, Mc Connell RB, Dockrav GJ: Serum gastrin in patients with chronic renal failure. *Gut* 21: 1062, 1980
17. Muto S, Murayama N, Asano Y, Hosoda S, Miyata M: Hypergastrinemia and achlorhydria in chronic renal failure. *Nephron,* 40: 143, 1985
18. Paimela H: Persistence of gastric hypoacidity in uremic patients after renal transplantation. *Scand J Gastroenterol* 20: 873, 1985
19. El Ghonaimy E, Barsoum R, Soliman M, El Fikky A, Rashwan S, El Rouby O, Haddad S, El Khashab O, Abouzeid M, Hassaballah N, Hassaballah A: Serum gastrin in chronic renal failure. *Nephron* 39: 86, 1985

20. Fleshler B, Gabuzda GJ: Effect of ammonium chloride and urea infusions on ammonium levels and acidity of gastric juice. *Gut* 6: 349, 1965

21. Shapira N, Skillman JJ, Steinman TI, Silen W: Gastric mucosal permeability and gastric acid secretion before and after hemodialysis patients with chronic renal failure. *Surgery* 83: 528, 1978

22. Carlei F, Caruso V, Lezoche E, Ruscitto G, Lackie P, Casciani U, Speranza V, Polak JM: Hyperplasia of antral G cells in uremic patients *Digestion* 29: 26, 1984

23. Sirinek KR, Oidorisio TM, Gaskill HV, Levine BA: Chronic renal failure: effect of hemodialysis on gastrointestinal hormones *Am J Surg* 148: 732, 1984

24. Walsh JH, Grossman M: Gastrin. *N Engl J Med* 297: 1324, 1975

25. Clendinnen BG, Davidson WD, Reeder DD, Jackson BM, Thompson JC: Renal uptake and excretion of gastrin in the dog. *Surg Gyn Obstet* 132: 1039, 1971

26. Dinoso VP, Murthy SNS, Saris AL, Clearrfield HR, Lyons P, Nickey W, Simonian S: Gastric and pancreatic function in patients with end-stage renal disease. *J Clin Gastroenterol* 4: 321, 1982

27. Owyang C, Miller LJ, Dimagno EP, Brennan LA, Go VLW: Gastrointestinal hormone profile in renal insufficiency. *Mayo Clin Proc* 54: 769, 1979

28. Goldstein H, Murphy D, Sokol A, Rubini ME: Gastric acid secretion in patients undergoing chronic dialysis. *Arch Intern Med* 120: 645, 1967

29. Mc Namee PT, Moore GW, Mc Geown MG, Doherty CC: Gastric emptying in chronic renal failure. *Br Med J* 291: 310, 1985

30. Wright RA, Clemente R, Watchen R: Gastric emptying in patients with chronic renal failure receiving hemodialysis. *Arch Intern Med* 144: 495, 1984

31. Jaffe RM, Laing DR: Changes of the digestive tract in uremia: a pathologic anatomic study. *Arch Intern Med* 53: 851, 1934

32. Franzin G, Musola R, Mencarelli R: Morphological changes of the gastroduodenal mucosa in regular dialysis uremic patients. *Histopathology* 6: 429, 1982

33. Mitchell CJ, Jewell DP, Lewin RM, Mc Laughin JE, Moorhead JF: Gastric function and histology in chronic renal failure. *J Clin Path* 32: 208, 1979

34. Milito G, Taccone-Gallucci M, Brancaleone C, Nardi F, Filingeri V, Cesca D, Casciani CU: Assessment of the upper gastrointestinal tract in hemodialysis patients awaiting renal transplantation. *Am J Gastroenterol* 78: 328, 1983

35. Kreuning J, Bosman FT, Kuiper G, Van Der Wal AM, Lindeman J: Gastric and duodenal mucosa in 'healthy' individuals. *J Clin Path* 31: 69, 1978

36. Gold CH, Morley JE, Viljoen M, Ou Tim L, Defonseca M, Kalk WJ: Gastric acid secretion and serum gastrin levels in patients with chronic renal failure on regular hemodialysis. *Nephron* 25: 92, 1980.

37. Margolis DM, Saylor JL, Geisse G, Deschryver-Kecskemeti K, Harter HR, Zuckerman GR: Upper gastrointestinal disease in chronic renal failure. *Arch Intern Med* 138: 1214, 1978

38. Zuckerman GR, Mills BA, Koehler RE, Siegel A, Harter HR, Descryver-Kecskemeti K: Nodular duodenitis. Pathologic and clinical characteristics in patients with end-stage renal disease. *Dig Dis Sc* 28: 1018, 1983

39. Gupta TD, Weinstock JV: Duodenal pseudomelanosis associated with chronic renal failure. *Gastrointest Endosc* 32: 358, 1986

40. Priebe HJ, Skillman JJ, Bushnell LS, Long PC, Silen W: Antacid versus cimetidine in preventing acute gastrointestinal bleeding. *N Engl J Med* 302: 426, 1980

41. Andrassy K: Uremia as a cause of bleeding. *Am J Nephrol* 5: 313, 1985

42. Carvalho ACA: Bleeding in uremia – a clinical challenge. *N Engl J Med* 308: 38, 1983

43. Andriulli A, Malfi B, Recchia S, Ponti V, Triolo G, Segoloni G: Patients with chronic renal failure are not a risk of developing chronic peptic ulcers. *Clin Nephrol* 23: 245, 1985

44. Linder MM, Kösters W, Rethel R: Prophylactic gastric operations in uremic patients prior to renal transplantation. *World J Surg* 3: 501, 1979

45. Jorizzo JL, Sams WM Jr, Jegasothy BV, Olansky J: Cimetidine as an immunomodulator : chronic mucocutaneous candidasis as a model. *Ann Intern Med* 92: 192, 1980

46. Jarowenko MV, Van Buren CT, Kramer WG, Lorber MI, Flechner SM, Kahan BD: Ranitidine, cimetidine and the cyclosporine – treated recipient. *Transplantation* 42: 311, 1986

47. Behar J, Roufail W, Thomas E, Keller F, Deinback W, Tesler M: Efficacy of sucralfate in the prevention and recurrence of duodenal ulcer. *Gastroenterology* 90: 1343, 1986 (abstract)

48. Hamilton I, O'Conner HJ, Wood NC, Bradbury I, Akon ATR: Healing and recurrence of duodenal ulcer after treatment with tripotassium; dicitrato-bismuthate tablets or cimetidine. *Gut* 27: 106, 1986

49. Zuckerman GR, Cornette GL, Clouse RE, Harter HR: Upper gastrointestinal bleeding in patients with chronic renal failure. *Ann Intern Med* 102: 588, 1985

50. Dave PB, Romeu J, Antonelli A, Eiser AR: Gastrointestinal telangiectasias. *Arch Intern Med* 144: 1781, 1984

51. Cunningham JT: Gastric telangiectasias in chronic hemodialysis patients : a report of six cases. *Gastroenterology* 81: 1131, 1981

52. Boley SJ, Sammartano R, Adams A, Dibase A, Kleinhaus S, Sprayregen S: On the nature and etiology of vascular ectasias of the colon: degenerative lesions of aging. *Gastroenterology* 72: 650, 1977

53. Therialut G, Cordier S, Harvey R: Skin telangiectasias in workers at an aluminum plant. *N Engl J Med* 303: 1278, 1980

54. Lindner A, Charra B, Sherrard DJ, Scribner BH: Accelerated atherosclerosis in prolonged maintenance hemodialysis. *N Engl J Med* 290: 617, 1974

55. Fleischer D: Endoscopic therapy of upper gastrointestinal bleeding in humans. *Gastroenterology* 90: 217, 1986

56. Mannucci PM, Remuzzi G, Pusineri F, Lombardi R, Valsecchi C, Mecca G, Zimmerman TS: Deamino-8-d-arginine vasopressin shortens the bleeding time in uremia. *N Engl J Med* 308: 8, 1983

57. Bronner MH, Pate MB, Cunningham JT, Marsh WH: Estrogen-progesterone therapy for bleeding gastrointestinal telangiectasias in chronic renal failure. *Ann Intern Med* 105: 371, 1986

58. Liu YK, Kosfeld RE, Marcum SG: Treatment of uraemic bleeding with conjugated oestrogen. *Lancet* 2: 887, 1984

59. Pinnick RV, Wiegmann TB, Diederich DA: Regional citrate anticoagulation for hemodialysis in the patient at high risk for bleeding. *N Engl J Med* 308: 258, 1983

60. Goldstein DA, Horowitz RE, Petit S, Haldimann B, Massry SG: The duodenal mucosa in patients with renal failure : response to 1,25 $(OH)_2D_3$. *Kidney Int* 19: 324, 1981

61. Wizemann V, Ludwig D, Kuhl R, Bargmann I: Digestive-absorptive function of the intestinal brush border in uremia. *Am J Clin Nutr* 31: 1642, 1978

62. Drukker A, Levy E, Bronza N, Stankiewicz H, Goldstein R:

Impaired intestinal fat absorption in chronic renal failure, *Nephron* 30: 154, 1982

63. Said HM, Vaziri ND, Kariger RH, Hollander ND: Intestinal absorption of 5-methyltetrahydrofolate in experimental uremia. *Acta Vitaminol Enzymol* 6: 339, 1984

64. Delano BG, Manis JG, Manis T: Iron absorption in experimental uremia. *Nephron* 19: 26, 1977

65. Dahlberg PJ, Kisken WA, Newcomer KL, Yutuc WR: Mesenteric ischemia in chronic dialysis patients. *Am J Nephrol* 5: 327, 1985

66. Lindner A, Charra B, Sherrard DJ, Scribner BH: Accelerated atherosclerosis in prolonged maintenance hemodialysis. *N Engl J Med* 290: 697, 1974

67. Margolis MD, Etheredge EE, Garza-Garza R, Hruska K, Anderson BC: Ischemic bowel disease following bilateral nephrectomy or renal transplant. *Surgery* 82: 667, 1977

68. Lockyer WA, Feinfeld DA, Cherubin CE, Carvounis GC, Iancu M, Avram MM: An outbreak of Salmonella enteritis and septicemia in a population of uremic patients. *Arch Intern Med* 140: 943, 1980

69. Goldblum SE, Reed WP: Host defenses and immunologic alterations associated with chronic hemodialysis. *Ann Intern Med* 93: 597, 1980

70. Marston A: Ischemic colitis, in *Intestinal Ischemia*, edited by Arnold E, Frome and London Butler and Tanner Ltd, 1977, p143

71. Ahonen RE, Makitie J, Kock B: Striated muscle capillaries in uremic patients and in renal transplant recipients. *Arch Intern Med* 141: 867, 1981

72. Leung AC, Orange G, Mc Lay A, Henderson IS: Clostridium difficile-associated colitis in uremic patients. *Clin Nephrol* 24: 242, 1985

73. Bartlett JG, Taylor NS, Chang TW, Dzink J: Clinical and laboratory observations in Clostridium difficile colitis. *Am J Clin Nutr* 33: 2521, 1980

74. Ogilvie H: Large intestine colic due to sympathetic deprivation : new clinical syndrome. *Br Med J* 2: 671, 1948

75. Nanni G, Garbini A, Luchetti P, Nanni G, Ronconi P, Casagneto M: Ogilvie's syndrome (acute colonic pseudoobstuction). *Dis Colon Rectum* 136: 66, 1982

76. Adams DL, Rutsky EA, Rostand SG, Han SY: Lower gastrointestinal tract dysfunction in patients receiving long-term hemodialysis. *Arch Intern Med* 142: 303, 1982

77. Freidman MHW, Mac Kenzie WC: Simple ulcers of the colon. Report of four cases. *Can J Surg* 2: 287, 1959

78. Bailey GL, Griffiths H, Lock PJ: Gastrointestinal abnormalities in uremia. *Abstracts Am Soc Nephrol* 5: 5, 1971

79. Wood CD: Acute perforations of the colon. *Dis Colon Rectum* 20: 126, 1977

80. Bischel MD, Reese T, Engel J: Spontaneous perforation of the colon in a hemodialysis patient. *Am J Gastroenterol* 74: 182, 1980

81. Jabbour G, Panzer JM, Adler M, Van Gossum A, Cemachovic I, Cremer M: Endoscopic management of Ogilvie's syndrome. *Acta Gastroenter Belg* 50: 411, 1987

82. Welch JP, Schweizer RT, Bartus SA: Management of antacid impactions in hemodialysis and renal transplant patients. *Am J Surg* 139: 561, 1980

83. Scheff RJ, Zuckerman G, Harter H, Delmez J, Koehler R: Diverticular disease in patients with chronic renal failure due to polycystic kidney disease. *Ann Intern Med* 92: 202, 1980

84. Starnes HF, Lazarus JM, Vineyard G: Surgery for diverticulitis in renal failure. *Dis Colon Rectum* 28: 827, 1985

85. Flynn CT, Chandran PKG: Renal failure and angiodysplasia

of the colon. *Ann Intern Med* 103: 154, 1985

86. Mills B, Zuckerman G, Sicard G: Discrete colon ulcers as a cause of lower gastrointestinal bleeding and perforation in end-stage renal disease. *Surgery* 89: 548, 1981

87. Goldberg M, Hoffman GC, Wonbolt DG: Massive hemorrhage from rectal ulcers in chronic renal failure. *Ann Intern Med* 100: 397, 1984

88. Desmarez B, Adler M, Buset M, Ansay J, Delcour C, Jeanmart J, Finne R, Cremer M: The value of colonoscopy in the diagnosis and management of severe hematochezia. *Mt Sinai J Med* 53: 478, 1986

89. Bartos B, Melichar J, Erben J: The function of the exocrine pancreas in chronic renal disease. *Digestion* 3: 33, 1970

90. Sachs EF, Hurwitz FJ, Bloch HM, Milne FJ: Pancreatic exocrine hypofunction in the wasting syndrome of end-stage renal disease. *Am J Gastoenterol* 78: 170, 1983

91. Owyang C, Miller LJ, Dimagno EP, Mitchell JC, Go VLW: Pancreatic exocrine function in severe human chronic renal failure. *Gut* 23: 357, 1982

92. Frayssine TR, Sahel J, Multinger L, Saingra A, Murisasco A, Sarler H: Modifications de la secrétion pancréatique pure chez les patients atteints d'insuffisance rénale chronique traités par hémodialyse. (modifications of pancreatic secretion in patients affected with chronic renal insufficiency treated by hemodialysis.) *Néphrologie* 2: 158, 1981

93. Baggenstoss AH: The pancreas in uremia : a histopathologic study. *Am J Path* 24: 1033, 1948

94. Avram MM: High prevalence of pancreatic disease in chronic renal failure. *Nephron* 18: 68, 1977

95. Rutsky EA, Robards M, Van Dyke A, Rostand SG: Acute pancreatitis in patients with end-stage renal disease without transplantation. *Arch Intern Med* 146: 1741, 1986

96. Carvana RJ, Wolfman NT, Karstaedt N, Wilson DJ: Pancreatitis : an important cause of abdominal symptoms in patients on peritoneal dialysis. *Am J Kidney Dis* 7: 135, 1986

97. Avram RM, Iancu M: Pancreatic disease in uremia and parathyroid hormone excess. *Nephron* 32: 60, 1982

98. Van Dyke JA, Rutsky EA, Stanley RJ: Acute pancreatitis associated with end-stage renal disease. *Radiology* 160: 403, 1986

99. Levitt MD, Ellis C: Serum isoamylase measurements in pancreatitis complicating chronic renal failure. *J Lab Clin Med* 93: 71, 1979

100. Stepan JJ, Skrma J, Havranek T, Lachmanova J, Hazuka V, Tomasek R: Role of secondary hyperparathyroidism and liver function in hyperamylasemia in chronic renal failure. *Digestion* 33: 168, 1986

101. Fahrenkrug J, Staun-Olsen P, Magid E: Immunoreactive trypsin and pancreatic isoamylase activity in serum of patients with chronic renal failure or hepatic cirrhosis. *Clin Chem* 27: 1655, 1981

102. Lott JA, Patel ST, Sawhney AK, Kazmierczak S, Love JE: Assays of serum lipase : analytical and clinical considerations, *Clin Chem* 32: 1290, 1986

103. Brissot P, Simon P, Meyrier A: Uremia and the liver. Hepatic metabolism of carbohydrates, lipids and proteins. *Nephron* 29: 14, 1981

104. Ibels LS, Simons LA, King JO, Williams PF, Neale FC, Stewart JH: Studies on the nature and causes of hyperlipidaemia in uraemia, maintenance haemodialysis and renal transplantation. *Q J Med* 76: 601, 1975

105. Grossman SB, Shafritz DA: Influence of chronic renal failure on protein synthesis and albumin metabolism in rat liver. *J Clin Invest* 59: 869, 1977

106. Tvedegaard E, Enghusen V, Poulsen Vilstrup H, Klemthomsen H: Functional status of the liver during chronic renal failure : an experimental study in the rabbit. *Liver 5*: 183, 1985

107. Quintanilla AP: Liver dysfunction in dialysis patients. *Int J Artif Organs 9*: 1, 1986

108. Pahl MW, Vaziri ND, Dure-Smith B, Miller R, Mirabmodi MK: Hepatobiliary pathology in hemodialysis patients : an autopsy study of 78 cases. *Am J Gastroenterol 81*: 783, 1986

109. Gokal R, Millard PR, Watherall DJ, Callender STE, Ledingham JGG, Oliver DO: Iron metabolism in haemodialysis patients. *Q J Med 8*: 369, 1979

110. Neergaard J, Nielsen B, Faurby V: Plasticizers in PVC and the occurrence of hepatitis in a hemodialysis unit. *Scand J Urol Nephrol 5*: 141, 1971

111. Leon G, As Y: Silicone : a possible iatrogenic cause of hepatic dysfunction in hemodialysis patients. *Pathology 15*: 193, 1983

112. Adler M, Ros P, Cremer M, Quiriny M, Henry JP, Lecocq E: Lésions hépatiques induites par les médicaments. (Hepatic lesions induced by drugs.) *Rev med Brux 7*: 81, 1986

113. Grünfeld JP, Albouze G, Jungers P, Landois P, Dana A, Droz D, Moynot A, Lafforgue B, Bousztyn E, Franco D: Liver changes and complications in adult polycystic kidney disease. *Adv Nephrol 14*: 1, 1984

114. Bourgeois N, Kinnaert P, Vereerstraeten P, Schoutens A, Toussaint C: Infection of hepatic cysts following kidney transplantation in polycystic disease. *World J Surg 7*: 629, 1983

HEMATOLOGICAL PROBLEMS OF DIALYSIS PATIENTS

JOSEPH W. ESCHBACH

INTRODUCTION

Recently, there have been numerous significant advances in our knowledge about the pathophysiology and management of the anemia of chronic renal failure. Aluminum, which dialysis patients receive as phosphate binders, can interfere with erythropoiesis (1, 2); significant evidence has been presented to suggest that uremic inhibitors play a minor, if any, role in the causation of the anemia (3, 4); an uremic, anemic sheep model corrected the anemia with infusions of plasma-rich sheep erythropoietin (Epo) and no *in vivo* nor *in vitro* erythroid marrow inhibition could be demonstrated (5, 6); and finally, recombinant human erythropoietin (rHuEpo) has been reproduced by recombinant genetic technology methods and has been shown in clinical trials to be effective in eliminating the anemia in almost all hemodialysis patients to which it has been given (7, 8). The measurement of Epo in plasma is now easier and more reliable with the use of radioimmunoassays to either human urinary or recombinant human Epo.

PATHOPHYSIOLOGY OF THE ANEMIA

The hematologic findings in most new dialysis patients are consistent with a hypoproliferative anemia; the blood smear morphology shows normochromic and normocytic red cells, which frequently will show 'burr' (9) or helmet cells. The reticulocyte count, when corrected for the degree of anemia, is usually less than twice normal (10), and the bone marrow morphology depicts an erythroid:granulocyte ratio that is slightly decreased or normal. The serum iron concentration, transferrin level, transferrin saturation, and serum ferritin levels are usually normal, but a coexisting inflammatory state will decrease both the serum iron and transferrin while elevating the serum ferritin.

The pathogenesis of the anemia is primarily due to decreased Epo production by the diseased kidney. Ninety percent of Epo is synthesized normally in the kidney from secretory cells within either the renal proximal tubular area (11) or the interstitium (12), whereas 10% is produced in the liver (13). Serum RIA Epo levels are in the 'normal' range (13 to 21 mU/ml) (14, 15), but are approximately 1/10 to 1/100 of what they should be, since subjects with normal kidney function who develop an acute anemia of similar magnitude (i.e., from bleeding) will produce serum Epo levels of 100 to 1000 mU/ml (15). The use of Epo totally corrects the anemia either in a uremic animal model or in hemodialysis patients. A number of animal models have been developed and some (16–18), but not all (19), indicate that exogenous Epo is effective in the uremic environment. However, the only system using homologous Epo was a sheep model in which Epo-rich plasma corrected the anemia of mild and severely uremic sheep, the latter requiring intermittent hemodialysis (5). The Epo-rich plasma was just as effective in uremic as in normal sheep as determined by ferrokinetic and reticulocyte responses. The biological clearance of Epo was similar in both study conditions (20). Preliminary trials in hemodialysis patients using rHuEpo indicate that the uncomplicated hypoproliferative anemia can be corrected despite the persistence of the 'uremic' milieu.

However, despite the above evidence that the anemia may be primarily an endocrine deficiency, the role of uremic inhibitors must still be considered for the following reasons. There have been isolated examples of elevated serum Epo levels in dialysis patients (21, 22), especially when a concentrated bioassay was employed (23). If 'inhibitors' were present, they would explain the persistent anemia despite elevated Epo levels. However, no concomitant measurements of erythropoiesis were done to rule out a transient erythroid stimulus from the elevated Epo levels. Although no inhibitors could be detected in the uremic, anemic sheep model (6), an animal model is not necessarily analogous to the human state. Moreover, although rHuEpo is effective in hemodialysis patients, Epo has yet to be infused into normal humans to quantitate its erythropoietic effect as compared to its effect in dialysis patients. When this is studied, the effect of uremic solutes on erythroid function will be conclusively determined.

Inhibitors to erythroid marrow function have been postulated for years. Initially clinicians thought that the anemia was due to the uremia (24), but when Epo was found to be produced by the kidney in the 1950s (25), the role of uremic inhibitors was thought to be of less importance. However, since the late 1950s, various *in vitro* tests have shown that uremic serum contains one or more substances that suppress erythroid cell growth (26, 27). Many investigators consistently found that if uremic sera was added to erythroid progenitor cells (erythroid colony forming units or CFU-E), and incubated with nutrient media and Epo, CFU-E proliferation was inhibited when compared to the addition of identical quantities of normal sera (28, 29). Several compounds have even been suggested to be the specific erythroid inhibitor. These include spermine (30) parathyroid hormone (31) and ribonuclease (32). All these studies have been marred by the lack of proper controls and an inability to correlate to clinical reality.

Most *in vitro* studies using CFU-E have employed mouse, rat or dog erythroid marrow cells. Using this system, it has now been shown that the uremic inhibition of CFU-E is non-specific; that is, there is also inhibition of the granulocyte/macrocyte (CFU-GM) and megakaryocyte cell lines by uremic sera (4), yet no such inhibition of leukocyte or platelet production exists in vivo, and leukocyte and platelet concentrations in the blood of patients with renal failure are usually normal. Spermine inhibits CFU-GM as well as CFU-E, suggesting it is not a specific erythroid inhibitor

(20). Spermine levels have not even been found to be elevated in dialysis patients (33). Whereas the crude extract of the parathyroid gland is inhibitory to both BFU-E (erythroid burst forming unit, and earlier progenitor cell line than CFU-E) and CFU-GM, and to heme synthesis (34), but not to CFU-E (30), the biologically active N-terminal fragment (amino acids 1–34) and the pure intact molecule (1–84) fail to inhibit significantly *in vitro* hematopoiesis (35, 36). Ribonuclease does not inhibit BFU-E, and the amount required to inhibit CFU-E *in vitro* far exceeds the levels found in dialysis patients (31). While there appears to be a substance in serum of human dialysis patients that inhibits various hematologic progenitor cells of other species, such inhibition cannot be demonstrated when an entirely autologous in-vitro system is employed (37). Therefore, uremic inhibitors of erythroid function may be *in vitro* artifacts, and probably of little or no physiological significance.

Red cell survival, usually 120 days, is shortened by the time advanced renal failure develops. This mild hemolysis develops only when the blood urea nitrogen level exceeds 80 mg/dl (23,6 mmol/l) during progressive renal insufficiency (38); therefore, the pathogenesis is thought to be due to some uremic factor (39), but hemodialysis or various forms of peritoneal dialysis fail to correct the hemolysis completely. Of interest though is that when red cell survival was quantitated using ^{51}Cr labelling in hemodialysis patients in 1986, the mean half-life was 23 days (normal 28–32), which is significantly longer than when similar studies were done 10 to 20 years earlier. This degree of hemolysis should not cause anemia, if Epo production were normal.

Blood loss is an additional mechanism occasionally contributing to the anemia even before maintenance dialysis is required (40). This may occur because of the uremic-induced platelet dysfunction which allows for easier bleeding (41).

EFFECTS OF DIALYSIS

Improvements

Anemia may improve with dialysis treatment because of favorable effects on coagulation, red cell survival or erythropoiesis or a combination of these.

Most forms of bleeding, such as ecchymoses, epistaxis, and pericardial and gastrointestinal bleeding, when associated with severe uremia, can be reduced or eliminated by the initiation of regular dialysis therapy. Hemodialysis and peritoneal dialysis will improve, but not necessarily reverse, platelet dysfunction, accounting for the decrease in bleeding (42–44), which in turn may lessen the severity of the anemia.

Red cell survival may improve with initiation of hemodialysis (45), but usually not to normal levels (46).

Erythropoiesis may improve with either hemodialysis or continuous ambulatory peritoneal dialysis (CAPD), but if it occurs, may be more marked and occur sooner with the latter therapy. While ferrokinetic studies indicate that erythropoiesis improves within the first 6 to 12 months of hemodialysis (47), the rise in the hematocrit may not be great, whereas a number of reports indicate that there may be a dramatic increase in the hematocrit when CAPD is initiated (48–50). The mechanism for the improved hematocrit with CAPD is not well understood, but it has been postulated that the more permeable peritoneal membrane allows for better solute clearance so that patients with higher levels of Epo have better erythropoiesis (48), or else improved Epo production occurs (51). However, such mechanisms do not explain why only some CAPD patients achieve significant hematocrit increases. The hematocrit also increases with time in a number of hemodialysis patients. About 3% have normal hematocrit levels (52), and an even higher percent will eventually increase their hematocrit values from the 20s to the 30s. Since red cell survival does not increase significantly with time on dialysis (53–55), there has to be an increase in erythropoiesis to explain these changes. A subtle increase in erythropoiesis may not be associated with measureable increases in serum Epo levels. One explanation has been the associated development of acquired cystic renal disease which may be associated with increased Epo secretion (56). However, acquired cystic renal disease is seen in 30% of dialysis patients (57) and is not consistently related to higher hematocrit levels (58).

Complications of the dialysis procedure

Bleeding

Both *acute bleeding* and *chronic blood loss* may be associated with the dialysis procedure. Acute bleeding from vascular access puncture sites either before or after dialysis occurs relatively frequently but rarely is of such magnitude to lower the hematocrit (hemoglobin) level. Chronic blood loss, on the other hand, is characteristic of the hemodialysis patient because of the repetitious dialyzer blood loss associated with each dialysis. The blood loss varies in amount depending on the dialyzer, adequacy of heparinization, and the blood-return rinsing technique. Isotope studies have quantitated this blood loss to vary between 4 and 50 ml of whole blood per dialysis (59). If there was an average loss of 20 ml of whole blood per dialysis, associated with an average hematocrit of 25%, and a milliliter of red blood cells contains 1.0 mg of iron, then thrice-weekly dialysis results in approximately 780 mg of iron lost per year by dialyzer blood residual alone. In addition, blood loss from periodic laboratory tests, the occasional clotting of blood in the dialyzer, and/or membrane ruptures and accidental losses of whole blood from cannulas or fistulas at the initiation or termination of each hemodialysis, may double this amount. Since mobilizable body iron stores are between 1200 and 1500 mg (60), iron deficiency can easily develop unless periodic iron repletion occurs.

Iron deficiency

Because of these losses, iron deficiency is a very common complication for the hemodialysis patient and can develop within 6 months to 2 years even in the absence of overt bleeding. The primary effect of iron deficiency is to decrease erythropoiesis, because iron is necessary for new red cell formation. Body iron stores can be estimated by bone marrow evaluation of reticuloendothelial iron granules (61), but quantitation is now also possible by measuring the serum ferritin levels. A radioimmunoassay of serum ferritin (62) is reliable, much less expensive than a bone marrow procedure, and simpler to repeat. The serum ferritin is an assay of iron stores, since intracellular reticuloendothelial iron is complexed in the ferritin molecule and this is in equilibration with the relatively small amount of intravascular ferritin (63), and repeatedly has been shown to be the easiest way to diagnose iron deficiency (64). Serum iron levels and transferrin saturation are usually unreliable indicators of iron deficiency in anemic dialysis patients (65). Since the advent of rHuEpo therapy, a functional state of iron deficiency may occur, especially during large, initial doses of rHuEpo (8). In this situation, the serum iron and transferrin saturation may fall to below 50 ng/ml and 20%, respectively, while the serum ferritin concentration is still within the normal range or is elevated. It has been postulated that the iron uptake of the rHuEpo-stimulated erythroid cell exceeds the rate the reticuloendothelial cell can release storage iron (8).

Folate deficiency

Should dialyzer losses of folic acid exceed dietary intake folate deficiency may occur. Serum levels of folic acid decrease during hemodialysis (66), but not after peritoneal dialysis (67), and megaloblastic marrow changes characteristic of folate deficiency have been described in hemodialysis patients (68). Most studies, however, suggest that folate deficiency rarely develops in patients consuming 60 to 80 g of dietary protein daily (67, 69), a diet which contains enough folic acid to replace easily that which is lost via dialysis. If serum folate levels are to be measured, it is best to use the Lactobacillus casei assay, a heat-extract radioassay, since the elevated unsaturated serum folate-binding protein, commonly observed in chronic renal failure, falsely lowers the more routine folate radioassay (70). Because it takes over 4 months of a dietary intake of less than the minimum daily requirement of 50 μg to lead to megaloblastic marrow changes and macrocytic peripheral red cells, red cell levels, in contrast to serum levels, of folic acid correlate better with functional folate deficiency. Therefore, patients whose dietary protein intake is chronically low, or who consume folate antagonists such as diphenylhydantoin (phenytoin) are prone to develop a macrocytic anemia superimposed on their existing anemia of chronic renal failure. Macrocytosis, though, can also be observed with iron overload (71), especially in the iron overloaded patient receiving rHuEpo therapy (7).

Acute hemolysis

During dialysis acute hemolysis rarely occurs, but if not

recognized and treated quickly, it can be fatal. Technical complications can lead to at least five mechanisms of red cell injury; 1) oxidant red cell destruction after exposure to dialysate containing copper (72–74), chloramine (75, 76), or nitrate (77); 2) inhibition of red cell glycolysis from dialysate containing formaldehyde (78); 3) thermal red cell injury from overheated dialysate (79); 4) mechanical red cell trauma from a malfunctioning or improper blood pump or partial obstruction within the extracorporeal circuit (80); and 5) osmolar trauma from hypo- or hypertonic dialysate (81). Hemolysis can be suspected by noting a bright red appearance to the blood returning to the patient from the dialyzer. Nausea, vomiting, hypotension, hyperkalemia and cardiac arrest may quickly follow. If the patient has been exposed to hypotonic dialysate, acute water intoxication may be more serious than the hemolysis; acute swelling of the brain will occur leading to encephalopathy and seizures. Treatment of these conditions requires discontinuing dialysis immediately once the complication is recognized. If acute water intoxication is suspected, however, dialysis should be resumed with normotonic dialysate. Proper monitoring of the dialysis procedure and appropriate response to alarm conditions should prevent or minimize these complications.

Aluminum excess

Aluminum toxicity, resulting in microcytosis, was initially noted in hemodialysis patients using dialysis water supplies contaminated with high concentrations of aluminum (82, 83). Removal of the aluminum from the water supply by reverse osmosis corrects the microcytosis and may improve the anemia (84). (However, the major cause of aluminum-induced microcytosis is now iatrogenic, see below.)

FACTORS AFFECTING THE ANEMIA

Hemolysis

Dialysis patients are vulnerable to both acute and chronic hemolysis.

Acute hemolysis

Whenever the hematocrit suddenly falls in the absence of other, more common complications, acute hemolysis should be considered, especially if the patient has an underlying systemic disease such as systemic lupus erythmatosis, a vasculitis or sickle cell disease, or if a new medication has been initiated such as a penicillin, an antimalarial, or a cephalosporin-related compound. Acute hemolysis, unrelated to the dialysis procedure, is unusual, however. Anti-N-like cold agglutinins develop in many hemodialysis patients after dialyzer reuse and sterilization with formaldehyde (85). Acute hemolytic episodes may occur and remit spontaneously in these circumstances (86). However, not all dialysis patients similarly exposed to dialyzer reuse and formaldehyde develop these antibodies (87).

Chronic hemolysis

Either hypersplenism or severe hypophosphatemia may induce chronic hemolysis. *Hypersplenism* should be suspected in patients with a palpable spleen, leukopenia, thrombocytopenia and increasing transfusion requirements. Splenomegaly should be confirmed with an isotopic scan, and hemolysis confirmed by isotopic red cell survival studies. ^{51}Chromium labelled red cell studies usually disclose a half-life of less than one-fourth of normal (in contrast to the usual half-life of one-third to two-thirds of normal in dialysis patients). Functional splenomegaly should then be confirmed with a simultaneous ^{51}Chromium-labelled red cell sequestration study in which a 2 : 1 or greater uptake by the spleen in comparison to the heart or liver is documented (88). The causes of this complication are probably multifactorial and include chronic hepatitis (89), transfusion-induced hemosiderosis (90), severe marrow fibrosis (91), silicone (92) and other causes of acute hemolysis (93). Splenectomy is beneficial if the above functional derangements are demonstrated. However, since some patients are able to maintain stable hematocrits despite the increased hemolysis because of marrow compensation (94), the advent of erythropoietin therapy may eliminate the need for splenectomy in the future.

Hypophosphatemia occasionally occurs from severe dietary protein restriction or the overzealous ingestion of aluminum containing phosphate-binding gels. If the serum level falls below 1 mg/dl (0.32 mmol/l), a failure-to-thrive syndrome occurs from poor tissue oxygenation because of depletion in red cell ADP and probably red cell 2,3-DPG levels (95).

Decreased erythropoiesis

Red cell production is reduced in chronic renal failure because of relative Epo deficiency, but can be further reduced as the result of the following situations: bilateral nephrectomy, transfusions, aluminum toxicity, iron deficiency, folate deficiency, inflammation, osteitis fibrosis, and possibly histidine deficiency.

Bilateral nephrectomy

Surgical creation of the *anephric* state leads to a further decrease in the hematocrit, with levels decreasing from a mean of 25% to 15% (96). After bilateral nephrectomy, plasma erythropoietin levels may decrease five fold (23, 97), leading to a three-fold decrement in erythropoiesis as shown by ferrokinetic measurements (98). This indicates that even though there may be little or no excretory function in remnant, native kidneys, the endocrine function may continue to contribute to erythropoiesis.

Transfusions

Although useful for temporarily relieving the hypoxic symptoms of anemia, transfusions may suppress erythropoiesis.

There is a feedback mechanism between the kidney and erythroid marrow governed by hypoxia or hyperoxia. When polycythemia is induced by transfusion, Epo production and erythropoiesis are suppressed. However, it is not necessary to produce polycythemia to demonstrate transfusion-induced erythroid marrow suppression, since a change in hemoglobin from 4 to 7 g/dl in a subject with normal renal function is enough to decrease urinary and plasma Epo levels (99). There is also evidence that this feedback mechanism persists in chronic renal failure and dialysis patients. Erythropoiesis decreased in hypertransfused, anemic, uremic sheep (100), and in hemodialysis patients whose hematocrits were artificially raised from 20 to 30% (47) as documented by ferrokinetics. The percent of marrow normoblasts was also found to decrease in seven anephric patients who were transfused from a hematocrit of 24 to 33% (101), and plasma levels of radioimmunoassayed Epo fell from 25.0 to 16.4 mU/ml in 16 hemodialysis patients transfused with two units of red blood cells (hematocrit 16.9 to 24.8) (102). In this latter study, reticulocytes were also suppressed. Hence, erythroid suppression by transfusion of at least two units of red cells has been documented by changes in four different criteria: erythroid morphology, reticulocytes (corrected for the anemia), plasma Epo levels, and ferrokinetics.

Aluminum toxicity

Aluminum can be toxic to erythroid function (2, 82–84). A microcytosis, unexplained by iron deficiency or other causes such as thalassemia or lead poisoning, is the clue to erythropoietic aluminum toxicity, which is confirmed by the demonstration of significant aluminum tissue stores by deferoxamine-induced mobilization. Toxicity is due to excessive deposition of aluminum from oral intake of aluminum hydroxide consumed to bind dietary phosphates. However, many patients with a long history of aluminum ingestion do not exhibit microcytosis. It is not clear at this time what other factors might predispose the dialysis patient to aluminum-induced microcytosis, which usually precedes the onset of aluminum-induced dementia (82). Although the mechanism by which aluminum suppresses erythropoiesis is not fully understood, two observations attest to the fact that erythroid function is impaired. 1) Deferoxamine, a chelating agent known to bind and remove aluminum from tissue storage sites by subsequent removal by dialysis, if given intravenously at least weekly, will restore normocytosis within several months of therapy and eventually (within 3 to 12 months), restore the hematocrit to higher levels (2), and/or show improved erythropoiesis by ferrokinetics (103). 2) The presence of an aluminum-induced microcytosis has also been shown to blunt the erythroid marrow stimulation that usually occurs with recombinant human erythropoietin (104). The development of microcytosis implies that the developing erythroid cell cannot incorporate enough iron, hence the cell becomes smaller than normal. Although it has been stated that aluminum is bound to transferrin (105), it is unlikely that such binding explains the inability of transfer-

rin to transport iron into the erythroid cell. If aluminum competition for the two iron binding sites on transferrin was the pathogenesis of the microcytosis, then in the presence of iron overload iron saturation of transferrin would not be observed. Iron excess appears to be unrelated to aluminum excess.

Iron deficiency

The non-transfused, hemodialysis patient is vulnerable to iron deficiency, because of the repetitive blood losses associated with the dialysis procedure (see above). With the advent of rHuEpo therapy, relative, or functional iron deficiency has emerged as one of the causes of inadequate Epo responsiveness (8, 104). Characteristically, patients without iron overload, when initially stimulated with relatively large amounts of rHuEpo, require more iron for erythroid synthesis than the reticuloendothelial cells can release to circulating transferrin for subsequent delivery to the erythroid marrow. Hence, a functional state of iron deficiency may develop in which the transferrin iron saturation falls below 20% and the serum iron falls below 50 ug/ml, while the serum ferritin remains above 100 ng/ml. Reticulocytosis may decrease and the rate of rise of the hematocrit will slow, until extra iron is provided.

Folate deficiency

When dialyzer folate losses exceed dietary intake folate deficiency can occur (see above), which may retard erythropoiesis, particularly in the non-Epo stimulated state. In this setting, dialysis patients receiving phenytoin are prone to folate deficiency.

Inflammation

Although inflammation has always been known to interfere with erythropoiesis, it has been hard to evaluate its significance until the advent of rHuEpo therapy. The inflammatory state associated with surgery or medical conditions, e.g. pericarditis, is enough to blunt the effect of rHuEpo as indicated by a reduction in the usual level of reticulocytosis and (depending on the extent of the involved tissue trauma) the hematocrit achieved (104, 106). This effect may last from 1 to 6 weeks despite optimal rHuEpo therapy. The mechanism for this decreased erythropoiesis is a reticuloendothelial blockade that prevents iron from being released to circulating transferrin for subsequent heme synthesis.

Osteitis fibrosa

Frequently, osteitis fibrosis secondary to hyperparathyroidism complicates long-standing renal failure; it often accentuates the hypoproliferative anemia of chronic renal failure. While some studies have suggested that parathyroid hormone may directly inhibit erythropoiesis (31), studies employing purified PTH failed to inhibit erythropoiesis *in vitro* (35). Several observations attest to the suppression of erythropoiesis *in vivo* by severe hyperparathyroidism: 1) a significant number of dialysis patients improve their anemia after subtotal parathyroidectomy (107–109); 2) severe hyperparathyroidism, as judged by elevated amino-terminal PTH and alkaline phosphatase levels, can blunt the effectiveness of rHuEpo (104). Because it is marrow fibrosis, as judged by bone biopsy, and not elevated PTH levels (109, 110), that most accurately predicts those that may improve their anemia after subtotal parathyroidectomy, erythropoiesis is not inhibited by PTH directly, but rather it is the marrow fibrosis that probably prevents erythroid marrow expansion.

Histidine deficiency

Theoretically, histidine deficiency can accentuate the anemia of dialysis patients. Histidine is an essential amino acid (111), and is one of the amino acids that links iron to the globin molecule. Histidine deficiency may result in a significant reduction of the hemoglobin concentration in both normal subjects and chronic uremic patients (111), but on the other hand, raising low levels of plasma histidine with dietary histidine supplementation does not necessarily improve the hematocrit (112, 113). Only those patients restricting protein intake are prone to low histidine blood levels; therefore histidine supplementation is necessary only for those on a low protein diet. Yet, consuming extra histidine does not ensure improved erythropoiesis.

Inhibitors

Inhibition of erythropoiesis by uremic solutes has been postulated for many years. The uremic environment impairs cell proliferation, including the lymphocyte response to mitogens (114), and *in vitro* erythropoiesis (115). However, subsequent studies suggest that if inhibition of erythropoiesis occurs, it is minimal and easily overcome by rHuEpo. (See earlier section for more details.)

MANAGEMENT OF ANEMIA

Erythropoietin

The uncomplicated, normochromic, normocytic anemia of chronic renal failure is now correctable with the renal hormone, erythropoietin, now produced with recombinant genetic techniques (116). At present rHuEpo is undergoing extensive investigational, clinical trials. Hopefully, in the very near future, pending FDA approval, it will be available for routine use, and will then be the primary treatment for the anemia. Recombinant human erythropoietin, in doses of 50 or more Units/kg, three times a week intravenously, will eventually correct the anemia and eliminate transfusion requirements (7, 8). The rate of rise in the hematocrit varies according to the rHuEpo dose. The packed red cell volume increases by 1.0 ml/dl (1.0%) per week with 50 U/kg, 1.75 ml/dl per week with 150 U/kg, 3.0 ml/dl per week with 300 U/kg, and 3.3 ml/dl per week with 500 U/kg. Once a hematocrit of 35 is achieved, the dose should be adjusted to maintain the hematocrit between 33 and 38. Preliminary experience indicates that most patients require 37.5 to 100 U/kg, three times a week, to maintain such a hematocrit, whereas a minority will require much larger amounts (104). Pharmacokinetic studies of rHuEpo indicate that the half-life is 9.3 ± 3.2 h (117), so it is appropriate to dose three times a week, intravenously, which can coincide with hemodialysis treatments. However, rHuEpo can also be given subcutaneously or intramuscularly, and blood levels, although not of the magnitude seen with comparable doses intravenously, are maintained at elevated levels for at least a week (117). This provides the theoretical basis for weekly subcutaneous injection of rHuEpo for continuous ambulatory peritoneal dialysis patients.

Iron

Replacement iron therapy will be more essential when rHuEpo therapy is routine, particularly for patients not iron overloaded. Increased stimulation of the erythroid marrow by Epo requires more iron for hemoglobin production, hence the need for more exogenous iron. During the acute stimulation with relatively high amounts of rHuEpo (>100 U/kg), parenteral iron may be required to replete iron stores rapidly, whereas during maintenance therapy with ≤100 U/kg, oral iron may be adequate. The serum ferritin concentration remains the best non-invasive means to quantitate iron stores, and should be obtained at least every month during acute rHuEpo stimulation, at least every 2 to 3 months during maintenance rHuEpo therapy and every 6 months in non-rHuEpo treated patients. In contrast to previous observations that there was a lack of correlation of serum iron and percent transferrin-iron saturations to iron deficiency in dialysis patients (65), these measurements may be low despite an elevated serum ferritin level. We interpret this as a relative state of iron deficiency because the rHuEpo-stimulated erythroid cells require iron from transferrin receptors in excess of the ability of the reticuloendothelial cells to release iron to transferrin.

In patients not requiring or unable to receive rHuEpo, iron balance is determined by the responsiveness of the erythroid marrow. Patients with poor erythroid function often require transfusions, leading to iron overload, whereas those with more active erythropoiesis require more iron for hemoglobin synthesis and also lose iron-containing red cells in the dialyzer, hence are prone to become iron deficient.

Iron stores are best quantitated by the serum ferritin level (63), which relates inversely to iron absorption (65), a physiologic feed-back mechanism altered only in primary hemochromatosis (118). Iron absorption is physiologic in dialysis patients (65, 119). Early studies suggesting that iron absorption was abnormal failed to correlate absorption to the level of iron stores as reflected by the serum ferritin level. Iron deficiency occurs with serum ferritin levels of less than 50 ng/ml (119) or 30 ng/ml (65). In the hemodialysis patient with a non-stimulated, hypoproliferative erythroid marrow, iron deficiency may not develop from chronic dialyzer blood loss for up to 6 to 24 months, unless there are unanticipated acute blood losses. Once iron deficiency is diagnosed, oral iron usually can correct it (120, 121), but optimal absorption occurs between meals dissociated from the ingestion of phosphate binders. Recommended agents include iron sulfate and iron gluconate, 300 mg, three times a day. Parenteral iron, in the form of Imferon®, because of its relatively high incidence (11%) of anaphylactoid reactions (122), should be reserved for the individual unable to tolerate oral iron. If Imferon® is used, a total of 0.5 to 1.0 g is needed. The total non-erythroid iron stores rarely exceeds 1.5 g (60).

Folic acid

Folic acid, multivitamins, pyridoxine, histidine and occasionally other amino acid supplements are often given to dialysis patients to replace either suspected dietary deficiencies or extra losses due to dialysis. Generally an adequate dietary protein intake provides more than enough of these substances to compensate for dialyzer losses. In the past, patients with poor appetites were in need of these substances but in those patients responding to rHuEpo, appetites increase so that these dietary supplements are probably unnecessary.

Androgens

Androgens, previously the only drugs able to stimulate red cell production, will no longer be needed when rHuEpo is available for routine use. Until then, androgens, either as nandrolone deconate or fluoxymesterone, may be of value in raising the packed red blood cell volume by as much as 5 ml/dl. Since nandrolone deconate therapy has been shown to be superior to fluoxymesterone (123), it should be the primary drug and used for at least 6 months at 3 mg/kg/week, intramuscularly. If there is no response after 6 to 9 months of therapy, oral fluoxymesterone, 10 to 30 mg dialy, should be employed for at least 4 to 6 months. Anephric patients generally do not have an erythroid response to androgens, though exceptions have been reported (124–126). The mechanism of action of these anabolic agents primarily involves the stimulation of remnant renal erythropoietin and secondarily direct erythroid marrow stimulation (127). Hepatic synthesis of Epo probably occurs as well, particularly from fluoxymesterone, which can affect hepatic cellular function. Both drugs have side effects (occurring in up to 25% [123]). These include myalgias secondary to elevated creatine phosphokinase levels, chipmunk-like facies, and warfarin enhancement associated with fluoxymesterone (128) and hirsute features in females, priapism in males, and injection site hematomas observed with nandrolone deconate (129). These drugs should be discontinued once a maximal response occurs, since elevated hematocrit levels may persist despite drug withdrawal.

Transfusions

Red cell transfusions for anemic dialysis patients will soon be unnecessary once rHuEpo becomes routinely available. There may be some exceptions, such as a patient undergoing major surgery associated with much blood loss (e.g. hip replacement), severe infections and severe aluminum intoxication. If rHuEpo is not available, judicious use of transfusion may be necessary if androgen therapy is ineffective. Only one unit, as packed red cells, should be given at a time in order to prevent volume overload and to minimize erythroid marrow suppression. Several studies have indicated that the erythroid marrow of anemic dialysis patients can be suppressed by relative hypertransfusion (47, 102). Other risks of transfusions include sensitization leading to the development of cytotoxic antibodies against a future kidney transplant, and infectious illnesses such as hepatitis. Therefore, if transfusion is needed to reduce symptoms of severe hypoxia, one unit is enough to improve transiently tissue oxygenation, unless there is marked blood loss.

Other factors

Exercise, when done as part of a routine exercise program, can result in a significant hematocrit rise in selected individuals (130). *Cobaltous chloride* will stimulate erythropoiesis (131), but it is too toxic for routine use (132). Although some nephrologists think that *improved dialysis clearance* of small and middle molecules will improve the anemia, there are few data to support this hypothesis. An early study (47) indicated that changing from biweekly to triweekly dialysis improved erythropoiesis as documented by ferrokinetics, but simultaneous to this change, transfusions were discontinued or reduced significantly, thus reducing the transfusion-induced erythroid suppression. The National Cooperative Dialysis Study indicated that hematocrit levels were higher in patients with lower BUN values (133), but actual BUN levels were not reported, and there were marked variations between cooperating centers. A prospective study of 6 months of reduced hemodialysis hours, three times a week, in which middle and small molecular clearances were decreased, disclosed no change in hematocrit levels (134). *Nutritional factors* are of little value in stimulating erythropoiesis other than iron and folic acid, when deficiencies of these factors exist. Although an anemia has been associated with malnutrition (135), no evidence exists in dialysis patients that the undernourished are more anemic. Of interest is that nutrition improves in rHuEpo-treated patients as the anemia is reversed, suggesting that the anemia results in poor nutrition, and not the converse. The routine use of multivitamins for treatment of the anemia is unnecessary, particularly in the patient receiving rHuEpo.

IRON OVERLOAD

Non-erythroid iron stores normally vary between 1200 and 1500 mg (60). Iron balance is generally maintained by a delicate inverse feedback mechanism between iron stores and iron absorption, with iron stores now being easily quantitated by measuring the serum ferritin level, which is in equilibrium with tissue iron stores (63). A serum ferritin exceeding 300 ng/ml indicates iron excess, or iron overload. Iron overload in dialysis patients develops either because of inappropriate, routine use of parenteral iron (used to 'prevent' iron deficiency from dialyzer blood loss) not monitored by serial serum ferritin levels, or because of the routine use of red blood cell transfusions. Since one unit of red cells contains approximately 200 mg of iron (1.0 mg/ml of red cells), iron excess can easily develop from multiple transfusions in the absence of significant blood loss. There is an increase in serum ferritin of 60 ng/ml for every unit of blood transfused (136). Iron is initially stored in the reticuloendothelial cells of the liver, marrow and other organs and eventually leads to tissue hemosiderosis in which iron is also deposited within parenchymal cells. Finally, iron may eventually interfere with cellular function, which indicates secondary hemochromatosis. Unfortunately, few data are available indicating at what level of iron stores cellular dysfunction can occur. The histological presence of iron within a hepatocyte or myocardial cell does not necessarily indicate tissue dysfunction. However, the transfusion of two to three units of red cells per month for 4 years to non-uremic anemic patients resulted in evidence of cardiac, liver and pancreatic dysfunction (137). Serum ferritin levels were as high as 5000 ng/ml, levels frequently observed in heavily transfused dialysis patients without evidence of dysfunction of these organ systems. However, primary hemochromatosis, in which there is an inappropriate increased intestinal absorption of iron, is also associated with these organ dysfunctions. Proximal muscle myopathy has also been observed in iron overloaded dialysis patients whose serum ferritin levels exceed 1000 ng/ml (138), but this observation has not been confirmed (139), and non-cardiac myopathy is an unusual complication of secondary hemochromatosis (137), and is not observed in primary hemochromatosis.

Regardless of the difficulties in knowing whether tissue dysfunction is occurring from iron overload, the potential is present. Until the avialability of rHuEpo, the elimination of iron overload has been very difficult because deferoxamine, the only practical chelating agent available to remove tissue iron, cannot bind enough iron to result in a net negative iron balance if red cell transfusions are continued (140). Iron overload can now be prevented and eventually eliminated by the use of rHuEpo, which improves erythropoiesis and eliminates the need for red cell transfusions. Serum ferritin levels have been shown to decrease significantly correlating with the duration of rHuEpo therapy (8). This is due to the shift of reticuloendothelial iron into newly formed red cells, and to the simultaneous loss of red cell iron via the dialyzer. As the hematocrit rises, there is more iron loss per milliliter of whole blood dialyzer residual. Iron removal could even be enhanced, if necessary, by periodic phlebotomy since the dose of rHuEpo could be increased to adjust for the increased blood loss.

Within 5 years of the routine use of rHuEpo, iron overload should no longer be a clinical entity in dialysis patients, except in the rare patient who may be refractory to rHuEpo.

BLEEDING ABNORMALITIES

Pathophysiology

Bleeding frequently complicates chronic renal failure; it can be reduced or aggravated by dialysis. A qualitative defect in platelet function is the major abnormality caused probably by one or more uremic toxins. The exact identity of these is unknown, although the dialyzable phenolic compounds and guanidinosuccinic acid present in uremic sera inhibit platelet function *in vitro* (141, 142).

Platelets function by adhering initially to any traumatized endothelial subsurface. Platelet adhesion depends on the presence of Von Willebrand factor. After adhesion, the hemostatic plug grows by the aggregation of more platelets to each other. Aggregation is promoted by the platelet-binding of the agonists thrombin, epinephrine, collagen, ADP, and by the release of the membrane phospholipid, platelet factor 3. Platelet aggregation leads to release of various membrane proteins, such as platelet factor 4 (PF4) and β-thromboglobulin, as well as the activation of enzymatic processes that enhance the conversion of prothrombin to thrombin on the platelet surface, in turn allowing fibrinogen to be converted to fibrin. Platelet physiology has been reviewed in detail recently (42, 143, 144).

The major clinical abnormality in uremia is a bleeding time prolonged greater than three times normal (145). The exact cause of this is not known, but the following abnormalities may contribute: a defect in platelet adhesion, as shown in vitro (146, 147); defective platelet aggregation in response to ADP, epinephrine and collagen induced by uremic plasma and guanidinosuccinic acid (142, 144); decreased platelet production of thromboxane A_2 (148); decreased in vitro release of platelet factor 3 in the presence of phenol compounds (149); severe anemia (150); and elevated serum levels of PGI_2 (prostacyclin) (151). PTH, initially thought to inhibit platelet function (152), probably plays little role in this defect (153). Many of these hemostatic abnormalities have recently been reviewed (154).

Beneficial effects of regular dialysis therapy

The bleeding time, normally less than 8 min, usually exceeds 20 to 30 min in untreated uremic patients, and shortens to within the normal range with repeated peritoneal dialysis (155) and usually, though not necessarily, with conventional hemodialysis (44, 155). In vitro tests of platelet function disclose that platelet adhesiveness decreases when the plasma creatinine rises above 6 mg/dl and improves only slightly with twice-weekly hemodialysis (156) and peritoneal dialysis (157). Platelet aggregation improves only slightly with twice-weekly hemodialysis but returns to normal with peritoneal dialysis (157) and thrice-weekly hemodialysis that provides the same total hours ($12 \, m^2 \cdot h$) per week as twice-weekly hemodialysis (158). Others have shown normalization in platelet adhesiveness and aggregation by hemodialysis (159). The significance of normalization of these in vitro tests is not clear as bleeding times were not done. In one study of well hemodialyzed patients ($18 m^2 \cdot h/wk$), bleeding times were normal despite depressed in vitro platelet aggregation (160). Yet the clinical impression is that uremic bleeding is greatly reduced by repetitive hemo- or peritoneal dialysis.

Complications of the dialysis procedure

The only bleeding complication associated with peritoneal dialysis might be bleeding occurring during the insertion of the peritoneal catheter. This is most unusual and usually ceases spontaneously (161). The hemodialysis procedure may alter the platelet count, its function, and therefore coagulation. Dialysis membranes such as cuprophan, but not polyacrylonitrile (162, 163), when exposed to blood platelets, induce complement activation with C_3a desArg, significant transient thrombocytopenia and platelet activation with the release of thromboxane B_2. These effects occur within 30 to 60 min of beginning hemodialysis, even with heparinization, or normalize within 3 to 4 h of dialysis. Not only do platelet counts decrease transiently during dialysis because of platelet consumption (164), PF_4 and β-thromboglobulin levels also increase due to platelet release (165). PF_4 possesses antiheparin activity, referred to as heparin neutralizing activity (HNA). Although heparinization during hemodialysis may reduce some of the above platelet-membrane reactions, it does not prevent them, and variable amounts of HNA secreted by the reacting platelets may account for the variable heparin requirements needed to prevent thrombosis during dialysis (166, 167). Prostacyclin (PGI_2), an inhibitor of platelet activation secreted by vascular endothelium, may prevent the normal platelet-membrane aggregation reaction, as indicated by normalization of platelet and β-thromboglobulin levels with prostacyclin infusion during heparin-free hemodialysis (168, 169). However, PGI_2 is not appropriate for routine clinical use since severe hypotension may occur, especially with acetate dialysis (170). Although thrombocytopenia is common during hemodialysis with cuprophan membranes, it is unusual for it to be sustained. Marked post-dialysis thrombocytopenia has been observed after the use of vancomycin (171), deferoxamine (172), and spontaneously (173), but in this latter case, vancomycin may have contributed. Any cause of splenomegaly (see page 854) can lead to thrombocytopenia as well.

Treatment of the coagulation disorders

The platelet dysfunction is reversed by adequate hemo- or peritoneal dialysis, suggesting that a dialyzable toxin is responsible for the abnormality. However, raising the hematocrit to above 30, either by transfusion (148, 150) or by rHuEpo (174), will also markedly improve bleeding times. Deamino-8-D-arginine vasopressin (175) and cryoprecipitate (176), if infused into non-dialyzed uremic patients will shorten the prolonged bleeding times making it possible to perform surgery safely if necessary.

Thromboses may increase within the vascular access of dialysis patients and various antithrombotic agents have been used with varying success. Warfarin compounds help retard thrombotic episodes but increase the risk of bleeding because of their effects on the intrinsic clotting mechanism. Low doses of aspirin can reduce dialyzer-membrane thrombus formation (177), as well as arteriovenous cannula thrombosis (178). Platelet cyclo-oxygenase, an enzyme that activates thromboxane A_2 formation which converts to the more stable thromboxane B_2, one of the platelet aggregation mechanisms, is irreversibly inhibited for 4 to 10 days by a single 200 mg dose of aspirin (143). Sulfinpyrazone has also reduced arteriovenous shunt thromboses (200 mg tid). Although this drug also inhibits platelet cyclo-oxygenase and decreases platelet aggregation in vitro, its in-vivo mechanism is unknown, since it does not impair platelet function in vivo and no bleeding tendency is seen in patients taking this drug (143).

LEUKOCYTE CHANGES

Chronic renal failure is also depicted as an immunodeficient state that results in an increased incidence of infection. Cellular and functional abnormalities in leukocytes, as well as the alterations that occur with either hemo- or peritoneal dialysis, may explain at least some or all of the reasons for the immunodepressed state.

Cellular changes

Total leukocyte counts are often normal, but of the five types of leukocytes, only the circulating lymphocyte count is reduced (179–181). Both T_4 and T_8 lymphocyte subsets are reduced by almost 50% (180). B cells are also decreased in number (181, 182).

Functional changes

T lymphocytes from patients with chronic renal failure have a decreased proliferative response when stimulated (by concanavalin A, phytohemagglutinin and pokeweed mitogen) and produce less interleukin 2 (IL-2) (180). The cause of these changes is not necessarily due to inhibitory substances (180), and prior red cell transfusions may contribute to the suppression noted (183). Neutrophils of dialysis patients exhibit decreased in-vitro chemotactic response, decreased numbers of C5a receptors (also observed with monocytes), and decreased oxidative metabolic response to chemotatic stimuli such as C5a (184). (See Chapter 41 for more detail.)

Changes during hemodialysis

The most profound and rapid onset of neutropenia and monocytopenia in humans occurs within the first 15 min of hemodialysis if cellulose membranes are used (185–188). Within 2 to 3 h there is a rebound resulting in higher post-dialysis neutrophil and monocyte levels than pre-dialysis. This reaction is minimal with noncellulose membranes. It is now well known that contact of blood with the cellulose membranes activates the alternative pathway of complement to generate C5a. Neutrophils and monocytes are then aggregated by C5a, leading to increased adherence of these cells to capillary endothelial surfaces. The first capillary bed exposed to blood returning from the hemodialyzer is the pulmonary bed. This results in pulmonary sequestration of these white cell aggregates (189). The recovery of peripheral blood neutrophil and monocyte levels is either due to the return of these leukocytes from the lung or the premature release of immature neutrophils from the bone marrow or both. (187). Reuse of a dialyzer ablates the complement activation (190), presumably because fibrin interferes with blood contacting cellulose directly.

Despite the marked changes noted above, it is not clear whether these lead to acute or long-term detrimental clinical effects. It has been postulated that the chemotactic unresponsiveness of neutrophils may be due to the C5a generated during hemodialysis in the presence of decreased availability of C5a receptors (188). However, in-vitro studies indicate that there is not a decrease in C5a binding by neutrophils during hemodialysis and that some adaptive mechanism develops to modulate the effects of excessive C5a generation from cellulosic membranes (188).

Changes during peritoneal dialysis

In addition to the functional leukocyte defects noted earlier in patients with chronic renal failure, peritoneal dialysis compounds these defects by depleting the peritoneum of phagocytic cells, and diluting existing opsonins (184). This may contribute to the high incidence of peritonitis in patients treated with continuous ambulatory peritoneal dialysis.

REFERENCES

1. Kaiser L, Schwartz KA: Aluminum-induced anemia. *Am J Kidney Dis* 6: 348, 1985
2. Schwartz KA, Dombrouski J, Burnatowska-Hledin M, Mayor G: Microcytic anemia in dialysis patients: Reversible marker of aluminum toxicity. *Am J Kidney Dis* 9: 217, 1987
3. Eschbach J, Adamson J: Anemia of end-stage renal disease (ESRD). *Kidney Int* 28: 1, 1985
4. Delwiche F, Segal G, Eschbach J, Adamson J: Hematopoietic inhibitors in chronic failure: Lack of in vitro specificity. *Kidney Int* 29: 641, 1986
5. Eschbach J, Mladenovic J, Garcia JF, Wahl PW, Adamson JW: The anemia of chronic renal failure in sheep: Response to erythropoietin-rich plasma in vivo. *J Clin Invest* 74: 434, 1984
6. Mladenovic J, Eschbach JW, Garcia JF, Adamson JW: The anaemia of chronic renal failure in sheep: studies *in vitro*. *Br J Haematol* 58: 491, 1984
7. Winearls CG, Oliver DO, Pippard MJ, Reid C, Downing MR, Cotes PM: Effect of human erythropoietin derived from recombinant DNA on the anaemia of patients maintained by chronic haemodialysis. *Lancet* 2: 1175, 1986
8. Eschbach JW, Egrie JC, Downing MR, Browne JK, Adamson JW: Correction of the anemia of end-stage renal disease with recombinant human erythropoietin. *N Engl J Med* 316: 73, 1987
9. Aherne WA: The 'burr' red cell and azotemia. *J Clin Path* 10: 252, 1957
10. Shaw AB, Scholes MC: Reticulocytosis in renal failure. *Lancet* 1: 799, 1967
11. Caro J, Erslev AJ: Biologic and immunologic erythropoietin in extracts from hypoxic whole rat kidneys and in their tubular and glomerular fractions. *J Lab Clin Med* 103: 922, 1984
12. Besareb A, Caro J, Erslev A: Eruthropoietin synthesis in the isolated perfused kidneys. *Abstracts Int Congr Nephrol* 10: 257, 1987
13. Fried W: The liver as a source of extrarenal erythropoietin production. *Blood* 40: 671, 1973
14. Cotes PM: Immunoreactive erythropoietin in serum. I. Evidence for the validity of the assay method and the physiological relevance of estimates. *Br J Haematol* 50: 427, 1982
15. Garcia JF, Ebbe SN, Hollander L, Cutting HO, Miller ME, Cronkite EP: Radioimmunoassay of erythropoietin: Circulating levels in normal and polycythemic human beings. *J Lab Clin Med* 99: 624, 1982
16. Van Stone JC, Max P: Effect of erythropoietin on anemia of peritoneally dialyzed anephric rats. *Kidney Int* 15: 370, 1979
17. Anagnostou A, Barone J, Kedo A, Fried W: Effect of erythropoietin therapy on the red cell volume of uremic and non-uremic rats. *Br J Haematol* 37: 85, 1977
18. Caro J, Erslev AJ: Erythropoiesis and response to erythropoietin in rats with chronic uremia. *Blood* 50 (Suppl 1): 123, 1979
19. Reissmann KR, Nomura T, Gunn RW, Brosius F: Erythropoietic response to anemia of erythropoietin injection in uremic rats with or without functioning renal tissue. *Blood* 16: 1411, 1960
20. Mladenovic J, Eschbach JW, Koup JR, Garcia JF, Adamson JW: Erythropoietin kinetics in normal and uremic sheep. *J Lab Clin Med* 105: 659, 1985
21. Radtke HW, Frei U, Erbes PM, Schoeppe W, Koch KM: Improving anemia by hemodialysis: Effect on serum erythropoietin. *Kidney Int* 17: 382, 1980
22. McGonigle RJS, Husserl F, Wallin JD, Fisher JW: Hemodialysis and continuous ambulatory peritoneal dialysis effects on erythropoiesis in renal failure. *Kidney Int* 25: 430, 1984
23. Caro J, Brown S, Miller O, Murray T, Erslev AJ: Erythropoietin levels in uremic nephric and anephric patients. *J Lab Clin Med* 93: 449, 1979
24. Callen IR, Limari LR: Blood and bone marrow studies in renal disease. *Am J Clin Path* 20: 3, 1950
25. Erslev AJ: Humoral regulation of red cell production. *Blood* 8: 349, 1953
26. Markson JL, Rennie JB: The anemia of chronic renal insufficiency. *Scott Med J* 1: 320, 1956
27. McDermott FT, Galbraigh AH, Corlett RJ: Inhibition of cell proliferation in renal failure and its significance to the uraemic syndrome: A review. *Scot Med J* 20: 317, 1975
28. Moriyama J, Saito H, Kinoshita Y: Erythropoietin inhibition in the plasma from patients with chronic renal failure. *Haematologia* 4: 15, 1970
29. Fisher JW: Mechanism of the anemia of chronic renal failure. Editorial review. *Nephron* 25: 106, 1980
30. Radtke HW, Rege AB, LaMarche MB, Bartos D, Campbell RA, Fisher JW: Identification of spermine as an inhibitor of erythropoiesis in patients with chronic renal failure. *J Clin Invest* 67: 1623, 1981
31. Meytes D, Bogin E, Ma A, Dukes PP, Massry SG: Effects on parathyroid hormone on erythropoiesis. *J Clin Invest* 67: 1263, 1981

32. Freedman MH, Saunders EF, Cattran DC, Rabin EZ: Ribonuclease inhibition of erythropoiesis in anemia of uremia. *Am J Kidney Dis* 2: 530, 1983

33. Spragg BP, Bentley DP, Coles GA: Anaemia of chronic renal failure. Polyamines are not raised in uraemic serum. *Nephron* 38: 65, 1984

34. Dunn CDR, Trent D: The effect of parathyroid hormone on erythropoiesis in serum-free cultures of fetal mouse liver cells (41108). *Proc Soc Exp Biol Med* 166: 556, 1981

35. Delwiche F, Garrity MJ, Powel JS, Robertson RP, Adamson JW: High levels of the circulating form of parathyroid hormone do not inhibit *in vitro* erythropoiesis. *J Lab Clin Med* 102: 613, 1983

36. McGonigle RJS, Keogh AM, Weston JM, Parsons V, Crofts MAJ: Iron status in chronic hemodialysis patients – treatment of transfusional iron overload with desferrioxamine. *Dial Transplant* 13: 214, 1984

37. Segal GM, Eschbach JW, Egrie JC, Stueve T, Adamson JW: The anemia of end-stage renal disease: Progenitor cell response. *Kidney Int* 33: 983, 1988

38. Adamson JW, Eschbach JW, Finch CA: The kidney and erythropoiesis. *Am J Med* 44: 725, 1968

39. Chaplin H, Mollison PL: Red cell life-span in nephritis and in hepatic cirrhosis. *Clin Sci* 12: 351, 1953

40. Loge JP, Lange RD, Moore CV: Characterization of the anemia associated with chronic renal insufficiency. *Am J Med* 24: 4, 1958

41. Lewis JH, Zucker MB, Ferguson JH: Bleeding tendency in uremia. *Blood* 11: 1073, 1956

42. Deykin D: Uremic bleeding. *Kidney Int* 24: 698, 1983

43. Lindsay RM, Moorthy AV, Koens F, Linton AL: Platelet function in dialyzed and non-dialyzed patients with chronic renal failure. *Clin Nephrol* 4: 50, 1975

44. Remuzzi G, Livio M, Marchiaro G, Mecca G, de Gaetano G: Bleeding in renal failure: Altered platelet function in chronic uraemia only partially corrected by haemodialysis. *Nephron* 22: 347, 1978

45. Koch KM, Patyna WD, Shaldon S, Werner E: Anemia of the regular hemodialysis patient and its treatment. *Nephron* 12: 405, 1974

46. Eschbach JW, Korn D, Finch CA: ^{14}C cyanate as a tag for red cell survival in normal and uremic man. *J Lab Clin Med* 89: 823, 1977

47. Eschbach JW, Adamson JW, Cook JD: Disorders of red blood cell production in uremia. *Arch Intern Med* 126: 812, 1970

48. Zappacosta AR, Caro J, Erslev A: Normalization of hematocrit in patients with end-stage renal disease on continuous ambulatory peritoneal dialysis. *Am J Med* 72: 53, 1982

49. De Paepe MBJ, Schelstraete KHG, Ringoir SMG, Lameire NH: Influence of continuous ambulatory peritoneal dialysis on the anemia of endstage renal disease. *Kidney Int* 23: 744, 1983

50. Mehta BR, Mogridge C, Bell JD: Changes in red cell mass, plasma volume and hematocrit in patients on CAPD. *Trans Am Soc Artif Intern Organs* 24: 50, 1983

51. Chandra M, Clemons G, McVicar M, Bluestone P, Mailloux L: Serum immunoreactive erythropoietin (Ep) levels in patients on continuous ambulatory peritoneal dialysis (CAPD). *Kidney Int* 27: 178, 1985

52. Charles G, Lundin AP III, Delano BG, Brown C, Friedman EA: Absence of anemia in maintenance hemodialysis. *Int J Artif Organs* 4: 277, 1981

53. Blumberg A, Marti HR: Red cell metabolism and haemolysis in patients on dialysis. *Proc Eur Dial Transplant Assoc* 9: 91, 1972

54. Eschbach JW, Funk D, Adamson JW, Kuhn I, Scribner BH, Finch CA: Erythropoiesis in patients with renal failure undergoing chronic dialysis. *N Engl J Med* 276: 653, 1967

55. Kominami N, Lowrie EG, Iahez LE, Sharken A, Hampers CL, Merrill JP, Lange RD: The effect of total nephrectomy on hematopoiesis in patients undergoing chronic hemodialysis. *J Lab Clin Med* 78: 524, 1971

56. Shalhoub RJ, Rajan U, Kim VV, Goldwasser E, Kark JA, Antoniou LD: Erythrocytosis in patients on long-term hemodialysis. *Ann Intern Med* 97: 686, 1982

57. Gardner KD: Acquired renal cystic disease and renal adenocarcinoma in patients on long-term hemodialysis. *N Engl J Med* 310: 390, 1984

58. Levine E, Grantham JJ, Slusher SL, Greathouse JL, Krohn BP: CT of acquired cystic kidney disease and renal tumors in long-term dialysis patients. *Am J Radiol* 142: 125, 1984

59. Lindsay RM, Burton JA, Dargie HJ, Prentice CRM, Kennedy AC: Dialyzer blood loss. *Clin Nephrol* 1: 24, 1973

60. Haskins D, Stevens AR Jr, Finch S, Finch CA: Iron metabolism. Iron stores in man as measured by phlebotomy. *J Clin Invest* 31: 543, 1952

61. Fong TP, Smith EC, Thomas W Jr, Westerman MP: Diagnostic significance of bone marrow biopsy in chronic renal disease. *Nephron* 12: 81, 1974

62. Miles LEM, Lipschitz DA, Bieber CP, Cook JD: Measurement of serum ferritin by a 2-site immunoradiometric assay. *Anal Biochem* 61: 209, 1974

63. Jacobs A, Path FRC, Worwood M: Ferritin in serum: Clinical and biological implications. *Med Progr* 292: 951, 1975

64. Mirahamadi KS, Wellington LP, Winer RL, Dabir-Vaziri N, Byer B, Gorman JT, Rosen SM: Serum ferritin level. Determinant of iron requirement in hemodialysis patients. *JAMA* 238: 601, 1977

65. Eschbach JW, Cook JD, Scribner BH, Finch CA: Iron balance in hemodialysis patients. *Ann Intern Med* 87: 710, 1977

66. Whitehead VM, Comty CH, Posen GA, Kaye M: Homeostasis of folic acid in patients undergoing maintenance hemodialysis. *N Engl J Med* 279: 970, 1980

67. Hemmeloff Andersen KE: Folic acid status of patients with chronic renal failure maintained by dialysis. *Clin Nephrol* 8: 510, 1977

68. Hampers CL, Streiff R, Nathan DG, Snyder D, Merrill JP: Megaloblastic hematopoiesis in uremia and in patients on long-term dialysis. *N Engl J Med* 276: 551, 1967

69. Cunningham J, Sharman VL, Goodwin FJ, Marsh FP: Do patients receiving haemodialysis need folic acid supplements? *Br Med J* 282: 1582, 1981

70. Eichner ER, Paine CJ, Dickson VL, Hargrove MD Jr: Clinical and laboratory observations on serum folate-binding protein. *Blood* 46: 599, 1975

71. Gokal R, Weatherall DJ, Bunch C: Iron induced increase in red cell size in haemodialysis patients. *Q J Med* 48: 393, 1979

72. Matter BJ, Pederson J, Psimenos G, Lindeman RD: Lethal copper intoxication in hemodialysis. *Trans Am Soc Artif Intern Organs* 15: 309, 1969

73. Ivanovich P, Manzler A, Drake R: Acute hemolysis following hemodialysis. *Trans Am Soc Artif Intern Organs* 15: 316, 1969

74. Manzler AD, Schreiner AW: Copper-induced acute hemolytic anemia. A new complication of hemodialysis. *Ann Intern Med* 73: 409, 1970

75. Higgins MR, Gace M, Ulan RA, Silverberg DS, Bettcher KB, Dossetor JB: Anemia in hemodialysis patients. *Arch Intern Med* 137: 172, 1977

76. Yawata Y, Howe R, Jacob HS: Abnormal red cell metabolism causing hemolysis in uremia. A defect potentiated by tap water hemodialysis. *Ann Intern Med* 79: 362, 1973

77. Carlson DJ, Shapiro FL: Methemoglobinemia from well water nitrates: A complication of home dialysis. *Ann Intern Med* 73: 757, 1970

78. Pun KK, Yeung CK, Chan TK: Acute intravascular hemolysis due to accidental formalin intoxication during hemodialysis. *Clin Nephrol* 21: 188, 1984

79. Berkes SL, Kahn SI, Chazan JA, Garella S: Prolonged hemolysis from overheated dialysate. *Ann Intern Med* 83: 363, 1975

80. Francos GC, Burke Jr JF, Besarb A, Martinez J, Kirkwood RG, Hummel LA: An unsuspected cause of acute hemolysis during hemodialysis. *Trans Am Soc Artif Intern Organs* 24: 140, 1983

81. Said R, Quintanilla A, Levin H, Ivanovich P: Acute hemolysis due to profound hypo-osmolality. A complication of hemodialysis. *J Dial* 1: 447, 1977

82. Short AIK, Winney RJ, Robson JS: Reversible microcytic hypochromic anaemia in dialysis patients due to aluminum intoxication. *Proc Eur Dial Transplant Assoc* 17: 226, 1980

83. Wills MR, Savory J: Aluminum poisoning: Dialysis encephalophathy, osteomalacia, and anaemia. *Lancet* I: 29, 1983

84. Swartz RD: Deferoxamine and aluminum removal. *Am J Kidney Dis* 6: 358, 1985

85. Kaehny WD, Miller GE, White WL: Relationship between dialyzer reuse and the presence of anti-N-like antibodies in chronic hemodialysis patients. *Kidney Int* 12: 59, 1977

86. Crosson JT, Moulds J, Comty CM, Polesky HF: A clinical study of anti-N_{DP} in the sera of patients in a large repetitive hemodialysis program. *Kidney Int* 10: 463, 1976

87. Fassbinder W, Pilar J, Scheuermann E, Koch M: Formaldehyde and the occurrence of anti-N-like cold agglutinins in RDT patients. *Proc Eur Dial Transplant Assoc* 13: 333, 1976

88. Asaba H, Bergström J, Lundgren G, Sorbo B, Tranaeus A, Zachrisson L: Hypersequestration of ^{51}Cr-labelled erythrocytes as a criterion for splenectomy in regular hemodialysis patients. *Clin Nephrol* 8: 304, 1977

89. Bischel MD, Neiman RS, Berne TV, Telfer N, Lukes RJ, Barbour BH: Hypersplenism in the uremic hemodialyzed patient. *Nephron* 9: 146, 1972

90. Hartley LCJ, Morgan TO, Innis MD, Clunie CJA: Splenectomy for anaemia in patients on regular haemodialysis. *Lancet* 2: 1343, 1971

91. Weinberg SG, Lubin A, Wiener S, Deoras MP, Ghose MK, Kopelman RC: Myelofibrosis and renal osteodystrophy. *Am J Med* 63: 755, 1977

92. Bommer J, Ritz E, Waldherr R: Silicone-induced splenomegaly. *N Engl J Med* 305, 1077, 1981

93. Rosenmund A, Binswanger U, Straub PW: Oxidative injury to erythrocytes, cell rigidity, and splenic hemolysis in hemodialyzed uremic patients. *Ann Intern Med* 82: 460, 1975

94. Morgan T, Innes M, Ribush N: The management of the anaemia of patients on chronic haemodialysis. *Med J Aust* 1: 848, 1972

95. Lichtman MA, Miller DR, Freeman RB: Erythrocyte adenosine triphosphate depletion during hypophosphatemia in a uremic subject. *N Engl J Med* 280: 240, 1969

96. Stenzel KH, Cheigh JS, Sullivan JF, Tapia L, Riggio RR, Rubin AL: Clinical effects of bilateral nephrectromy. *Am J Med* 58: 69, 1975

97. DeKlerk G, Wilmink JM, Rosengarten PCJ, Vet RJWM, Goudsmit R: Serum erythropoietin (ESF) titers in anemia of chronic renal failure. *J Lab Clin Med* 100: 720, 1982

98. Eschbach JW: Iron kinetics in healthy individuals and in chronic renal insufficiency. *Contr Nephrol* 38: 129, 1983

99. Gurney CW, Jacobson LO, Goldwasser E: The physiologic and clinical significance of erythropoietin. *Ann Intern Med* 49: 363, 1958

100. Eschbach JW, Detter JC, Adamson JW: Physiologic studies in normal and uremic sheep. II. Changes in erythropoiesis and oxygen transport. *Kidney Int* 18: 732, 1980

101. Van Ypersele de Strihou, Stragier A: Effect of bilateral nephrectomy on transfusion requirements of patients undergoing chronic dialysis. *Lancet* 2: 705, 1969

102. Walle AJ, Wong GY, Clemons GK, Garcia JF, Niedermayer W: Erythropoietin-hematocrit feedback in the anemia of end-stage renal disease. *Kidney Int* 31: 1205, 1987

103. Eschbach JW, unpublished observations.

104. Eschbach JW, Adamson JW: Recombinant human erythropoietin: implications for nephrology. *Am J Kidney Dis* 11: 203, 1988

105. Trapp GA: Plasma aluminum is bound to transferrin. *Life Sci* 33: 3111, 1983

106. Winearls CG: personal observation.

107. Shasha SM, Better OS, Winaver J, Chaimovitz C, Barzilai A, Erlik D: Improvement in the anemia of hemodialyzed patients following subtotal parathyroidectomy. *Israel J Med Sci* 14: 328, 1978

108. Zingraff J, Drüeke T, Marie P, Man NK, Jungers P, Bordier P: Anemia and secondary hyperparathyroidism. *Arch Intern Med* 138: 1650, 1978

109. Potasman I, Better OS: The role of secondary hyperparathyroidism in the anemia of chronic renal failure. *Nephron* 33: 229, 1983

110. Barbour GL: Effect of parathyroidectomy on anemia in chronic renal failure. *Arch Intern Med* 139: 889, 1979

111. Kopple JD, Swendseid ME: Evidence that histidine is an essential amino acid in normal and chronically uremic man. *J Clin Invest* 55: 881, 1975

112. Jontofsohn R, Heinze V, Katz N, Stuber U, Wilke H, Kluthe R: Histidine and iron supplementation in dialysis and predialysis patients. *Proc Eur Dial Transplant Assoc* 11: 391, 1974

113. Reeves RD, Barbour GL, Robertson CS, Crumb CK: Failure of histidine supplementation to improve anemia in chronic dialysis patients. *Am J Clin Nutr* 30: 579, 1977

114. Kasakura S, Lowenstein L: The effect of uremic blood on mixed leukocyte reaction and cultures of leukocytes with PHA. *Transplantation* 2: 283, 1967

115. Wallner SF, Ward HP, Vautrin R, Alfrey AC, Mishell J: The anemia of chronic renal failure: *In vitro* response of bone marrow to erythropoietin (38931). *Proc Soc Exp Biol Med* 149: 939, 1975

116. Lin F-K, Suggs S, Lin C-H, Browne JK, Smalling R, Egrie JC, Chen KK, Fox GM, Martin F, Stabinsky Z: Cloning and expression of the human erythropoietin gene. *Proc Natl Acad Sci USA* 82: 7580, 1985

117. Egrie JC, Eschbach JW, Adamson JW: Pharmacokinetics of recombinant human erythropoietin (r-HuEpo) administered to hemodialysis patients. *Kidney Int* 33: 262, 1988

118. Finch CA: The detection of iron overload. *N Engl J Med* 307: 1702, 1982

119. Gokal R, Millard PR, Weatherall DJ, Callender STE, Ledingham JGG, Oliver DO: Iron metabolism in haemodialysis patients. *Q J Med* 48: 369, 1979

120. Strickland ID, Chaput de Saintonge DM, Boulton FE, Francis B, Roubikova J, Waters JI: The therapeutic equivalence of oral and intravenous iron in renal dialysis patients. *Clin Nephrol* 7: 55, 1977

121. Parker PA, Izard MW, Maher JF: Therapy of iron deficiency anemia in patients on maintenance dialysis. *Nephron* 23: 181, 1979

122. Hamstra RD, Block MH, Schocket AL: Intravenous iron dextran in clinical medicine. *JAMA* 243: 1726, 1980

123. Neff MS, Goldberg J, Slifkin RF, Eiser AR, Calamia V, Kaplan M, Baez A, Gupta S, Mattoo N: A comparison of androgens for anemia in patients on hemodialysis. *N Engl J Med* 304: 871, 1981

124. Eschbach JW, Adamson JW: Improvement in the anemia of chronic renal failure with fluoxymesterone. *Ann Intern Med* 78: 527, 1973

125. Radtke HW, Erbes PM, Schippers E, Koch KM: Serum erythropoietin concentration in anephric patients. *Nephron* 2: 361, 1978

126. Shaldon S, Koch KM, Opperman F, Patyna WD: Testosterone therapy for anaemia in maintenance dialysis. *Br Med J* 3: 212, 1971

127. Singer JW, Adamson JW: Steroids and hematopoiesis. II. The effect of steroids on *in vitro* erythroid colony growth: Evidence for different target cells for different classes of steroids. *J Cell Physiol* 88: 135, 1976

128. Ahmad S, Goodman W, Pagel M, Shen F: Accelerated creatinine generation and elevated CPK due to androgens. *Proc Clin Dial Transplant Forum* 10: 174, 1980

129. Editorial. Androgens in the anaemia of chronic renal failure. *Br Med J* 2: 417, 1977

130. Goldberg AP, Hagberg JM, Delmez JA, Haynes ME, Harter HR: Metabolic effects of exercise training in hemodialysis patients. *Kidney Int* 18: 754, 1980

131. Curtis JR, Goode GC, Herrington J, Urdaneta LE: Possible cobalt toxicity in maintenance hemodialysis patients after treatment with cobaltous chloride: A study of blood and tissue cobalt concentrations in normal subjects and patients with terminal renal failure. *Clin Nephrol* 5: 61, 1976

132. Editorial: Cobalt in severe renal failure. *Lancet* 2: 26, 1976

133. Santiago GC, Rao TKS, Laird NM: Effect of dialysis therapy on the hematopoietic system: The National Cooperative Dialysis Study. *Kidney Int* 23 (Suppl 13): S95, 1983

134. Teschan PE, Ginn HE, Bourne JR, Ward JR, Schaffer JD: A prospective study of renal dialysis. *Trans Am Soc Artif Intern Organs J* 3: 108, 1983

135. Stefanidis CJ, Papadakis JT, Patrikarea A, Christodoulidou Ch, Ziroyannis PN, Papadoyannakis NJ: The effect of nutrition on anemia of patients on hemodialysis. *Kidney Int* (Abstract) 31: 870, 1987

136. Hegsted DM: The correlation of serum ferritin and body iron stores. *Nutr Rev* 33: 11, 1975

137. Schafer AI, Cheron RG, Dluhy R, Cooper B, Gleason RE, Soeldner JS, Bunn HF: Clinical consequences of acquired transfusional iron overload in adults. *N Engl J Med* 304: 319, 1981

138. Bregman H, Winchester JF, Knepshield JH, Gelfand MC, Manz HJ, Schreiner GE: Iron-overload-associated myopathy in patients on maintenance haemodialysis: A histocompatibility-linked disorder. *Lancet* 2: 882, 1980

139. Simon P, Brissot P: Hemosiderosis and hemochromatosis in maintenance hemodialysis patients: Diagnosis and treatment by desferoxamine. *Kidney Int* 20: 311, 1981

140. McGonigle RJS, Keogh AM, Weston JM, Parsons V, Crofts MAJ: Iron status in chronic hemodialysis patients – treatment of transfusional iron overload with desferrioxamine. *Dial Transplant* 13: 214, 1984

141. Horowitz HI, Stein IM, Cohen BD, White JG: Further studies on the platelet-inhibitory effect of guanidinosuccinic acid and its role in uremic bleeding. *Am J Med* 49: 336, 1970

142. Rabiner SF, Molinas F: The role of phenol and phenolic acids on the thrombocytopathy and defective platelet aggregation of patients with renal failure. *Am J Med* 49: 346, 1970

143. Huebsch LB, Harker LA: Disorders of platelet function. *West J Med* 134: 109, 1981

144. Shattil SJ, Bennett JS: Platelets and their membranes in hemostasis: Physiology and pathophysiology. *Ann Intern Med* 94: 108, 1981

145. Castaldi PA, Rozenberg MC, Stewart JH: The bleeding disorder or uraemia. A qualitative platelet defect. *Lancet* 2: 66, 1966

146. Nenci GG, Berrettini M, Agnelli G, Parise P, Buoncristiani U, Ballatori E: Effect of peritoneal dialysis, haemodialysis and kidney transplantation on blood platelet function. I. Platelet aggregation by ADP and epinephrine. *Nephron* 23: 287, 1979

147. Salzman EW, Neri LL: Adhesiveness of blood platelets in uremia. *Thromb Diath Haemorrh* 15: 84, 1966

148. Remuzzi G: Abnormalities of platelet and coagulation function in renal failure. *Kidney Int* 27: 101, 1985

149. Horowitz HI: Uremic toxins and platelet function. *Arch Intern Med* 126: 823, 1970

150. Livio M, Marchesi D, Remizzu G, Gotti E, Mecca G, de Gaetano G: Uraemic bleeding: Role of anaemia and beneficial effect of red cell transfusions. *Lancet* 2: 1013, 1982

151. Remuzzi G, Marchesi D, Cavenaghi AE, Livio M, Donati MB, de Gaetano G, Mecca G: Bleeding in renal failure: A possible role of vascular prostacyclin (PGI$_2$). *Clin Nephrol* 12: 127, 1979

152. Remuzzi G, Dodesini P, Livio M, Mecca G, Benigni A, Schieppati A, Poletti E, de Gaetano G: Parathyroid hormone inhibits human platelet function. *Lancet* 2: 1321, 1981

153. Docci D, Turci F, Delvecchio C, Gollini C, Baldrati L, Pistocchi E: Lack of evidence for the role of secondary hyperparathyroidism in the pathogenesis of uremic thrombocytopathy. *Nephron* 43: 28, 1986

154. Jubelirer SJ: Hemostatic abnormalities in renal disease. *Am J Kidney Dis* 5: 219, 1985

155. Harker LA, Slichter SJ: The bleeding time as a screening test for evaluation of platelet function. *N Engl J Med* 287: 155, 1972

156. Lindsay RM, Moorthy AV, Koens F, Linton AL: Platelet function in dialyzed and non-dialyzed patient with chronic renal failure. *Clin Nephrol* 4: 52, 1975

157. Lindsay RM, Friesen M, Koens F, Linton AL, Oreopoulos D, de Veber G: Platelet function in patients on long term peritoneal dialysis. *Clin Nephrol* 6: 335, 1976

158. Lindsay RM, Friesen M, Aronstam A, Andrus F, Clark WF, Linton AL: Improvement of platelet function by increased frequency of hemodialysis. *Clin Nephrol* 10: 67, 1978

159. Jorgenson KA, Ingeberg S: Platelets and platelet function in patients with chronic uremia on maintenance hemodialysis. *Nephron* 23: 233, 1979

160. Wathen R, Smith M, Keshaviah P, Comty C, Shapiro F: Depressed in vitro aggregation of platelets of chronic hemodialysis patients: A role for cyclic AMP. *Trans Am Soc Artif Intern Organs* 21: 320, 1975

161. Tenckhoff H: *Chronic Peritoneal Dialysis Manual*, Seattle, University of Washington, 1974

162. Docci D, Turci F, Del Vecchio C, Bilancioni R, Cenciotti L, Pretolani E: Hemodialysis-associated platelet loss: Study of the relative contribution of dialyzer membrane composition

and geometry. *Int J Artif Organs* 7: 337, 1984

163. Hakim RM, Schaefer AI: Hemodialysis-associated platelet activation and thrombocytopenia. *Am J Med* 78: 575, 1985

164. Lindsay RM, Prentice CRM, Davidson JF, Burton JA, McNicol GP: Haemostatic changes during dialysis associated with thrombus formation on dialysis membranes. *Br Med J* 2: 454, 1972

165. Rucinski B, Niewiarowski S, James P, Walz DA, Budzynski AZ: Antiheparin proteins secreted by human platelets. Purification, characterization, and radioimmunoassay. *Blood* 53: 47, 1969

166. Aronstam A, Dennis B, Friesen MJ, Clark WF, Linton AL, Lindsay RM: Heparin neutralizing activity in patients with renal disease on maintenance hemodialysis. *Thromb Haemost* 39: 695, 1978

167. Lindsay RM: Variable heparin requirements during hemodialysis – Why? Commentary. *Trans Am Soc Artif Intern Organs* 3: 81, 1980

168. Turney JH, Fewell MR, Williams LC, Parsons V, Weston MJ: Platelet protection and heparin sparing with prostacyclin during regular dialysis therapy. *Lancet* 2: 219, 1980

169. Smith MC, Danviriyasup K, Crow JW, Cato AE, Park GD, Hassid A, Dunn MJ: Prostacyclin substitution for heparin in long-term hemodialysis. *Am J Med* 73: 669, 1982

170. Zusman RM, Rubin RH, Cato AE, Cocchetto DM, Crow JW, Tolkoff-Rubin N: Hemodialysis using prostacyclin instead of heparin as the sole antithrombotic agent. *N Engl J Med* 304: 934, 1981

171. Walker RW, Heaton A: Thrombocytopenia due to vancomycin. *Lancet* 1: 932, 1985

172. Walker JA, Sherman RA, Eisinger RP: Thrombocytopenia associated with intravenous desferrioxamine. *Am J Kidney Dis* 4: 254, 1985

173. Vicks SL, Gross ML, Schmitt GW: Massive hemorrhage due to hemodialysis-associated thrombocytopenia. *Am J Nephrol* 3: 30, 1983

174. Casati S, Passerini P, Graziani G, Moia M, Della Valle P, Mannucci PM, Ponticelli C: Human recombinant erythropoietin corrects anemia and bleeding tendency in hemodialysis patients. *Abstracts Int Congr Nephrol* 10: 129, 1987

175. Mannucci PM, Remuzzi G, Pusineri F, Lombardi R, Valsecchi C, Mecca G, Zimmerman TS: Deamino-8-d-arginine vasopressin shortens the bleeding time in uremia. *N Engl J Med* 308: 8, 1983

176. Janson PA, Jubeliere SJ, Weinstein MJ, Deykin D: Treatment of the bleeding tendency in uremia with cryoprecipitate. *N Engl J Med* 303: 1318, 1980

177. Lindsay RM, Ferguson D, Prentice CRM, Burton JA, McNicol GP: Reduction of thrombus formation on dialyser membranes by aspirin and RA 233. *Lancet* 2: 1287, 1972

178. Harter HR, Burch JW, Majerus PW, Stanford N, Delmez JA, Anderson CB, Weerts C: Prevention of thrombosis in patients on hemodialysis by low-dose aspirin. *N Engl J Med* 301: 577, 1979

179. Hoy WE, Cestero RVM, Freeman RB: Deficiency of T and B lymphocytes in uremic subjects and partial improvement with maintenance hemodialysis. *Nephron* 20: 182, 1978

180. Kurz P, Kohler H, Meuer S, Hutterroth T, Meyer zum Buschenfelde K-H: Impaired cellular immune responses in chronic renal failure: Evidence for a T cell defect. *Kidney Int* 29: 1209, 1986

181. Raska K Jr, Raskova J, Shea SM, Frankel RM, Wood RH, Lifter J, Ghobrial I, Eisinger RP, Homer L: T cell subsets and cellular immunity in end-stage renal disease. *Am J Med* 75: 734, 1983

182. Raskova J, Ghobrial I, Shea SM, Eisinger RP, Raska K Jr: Suppressor cells in end-stage renal disease. *Am J Med* 76: 847, 1984

183. Smith MD, Hardy G, Williams JD, Coles GA: Suppressor cell numbers and activity in non-transfused renal dialysis patients. *Clin Nephrol* 20: 130, 1983

184. Lewis SL, Van Epps DE: Neutrophil and monocyte alterations in chronic dialysis patients. *Am J Kidney Dis* 9: 381, 1987

185. Kaplow LS, Goffinet JA: Profound neutropenia during the early phase of hemodialysis. *JAMA* 203: 1135, 1968

186. Gral T, Schroth P, DePalma JR, Gordon A: Leukocyte dynamics with three types of hemodialyzers. *Trans Am Soc Artif Intern Organs* 15: 45, 1969

187. Brubaker LH, Nolph KD: Mechanisms of recovery from neutropenia induced by hemodialysis. *Blood* 38: 623, 1971

188. Lewis SL, Van Epps DE, Chenoweth DE: Leukocyte C5a receptor modulation during hemodialysis. *Kidney Int* 31: 112, 1987

189. Craddock PR, Fehr J, Brigham KL, Kronenberg RS, Jacob HS: Complement and leukocyte-mediated pulmonary dysfunction in hemodialysis. *N Engl J Med* 296: 769, 1977

190. Savdie E, Bruce L, Vincent PC: Modified neutropenic response to re-used dialyzers in patients with chronic renal failure. *Clin Nephrol* 8: 422, 1977

HOST DEFENSES AND INFECTIOUS COMPLICATIONS IN MAINTENANCE HEMODIALYSIS PATIENTS

WILLIAM F. KEANE and MICHAEL F. MADDY

INTRODUCTION

Prior to the advent of chronic hemodialysis, infection was a frequent terminal or pre-terminal event in patients with end-stage renal disease (ESRD). With the development of chronic hemodialysis therapy, infectious complications still result in significant morbidity and mortality, with up to one-third of deaths being attributable to infections (1–5). Despite improvement in dialysis and medical therapies, infection continues to account for a significant proportion (15 to 20%) of deaths in the chronic dialysis population (6–8). While this increased risk of infection is due in part to the necessity of blood access, there are abnormalities of the immune system in ESRD patients which may contribute to their predilection for infectious complications. In this chapter, we will review the incidence and types of infectious complications which occur in patients undergoing chronic hemodialysis, as well as outline our current understanding of the immune status of the dialysis patient. It is important to emphasize that the vast majority of infections are due to commonly occurring organisms, not opportunistic or unusual organisms, and that repetitive exposure to infectious risk factors has a major influence on the types of infections observed.

UREMIA AS AN IMMUNOCOMPROMISED STATE

Several historic and more recent observations serve to outline the variety of immunologic perturbations of uremia. A delay in the rejection of both renal and skin allografts has been demonstrated in human as well as experimental uremic models (9–13). Clinically, an abnormal response to the hepatitis B virus, as evidenced by a milder but more prolonged infection and a higher incidence of chronic hepatitis, is well documented (14–17). A purported increase in the incidence of malignancy in ESRD patients has also been attributed to decreased immune system surveillance (18–21).

Lastly, amelioration of the clinical manifestations of systemic lupus erythematosis in uremic and chronic hemodialysis patients suggests an alteration in immune system function (22). In addition to these clinical observations, numerous *in vivo* and *in vitro* tests have characterized the nature of the underlying mechanisms of these phenomena. Table 1 summarizes the results of the various studies used to define the alterations observed in the immunologic responsiveness of the uremic patient.

Humoral immunity

Serum levels of immunoglobulins A, G and M have generally been reported as normal (23–25), despite a consistently observed decrease in the B-lymphocyte cell population (23, 26, 27). This decline in B cell numbers may correct with initiation of dialysis (25, 26). An increased incidence of autoantibodies has been reported in dialysis patients, suggesting an intact humoral immune system (24, 28). In some cases, these autoantibodies are thought be secondary to the hemodialysis procedure, such as anti-N-like antibodies from formaldehyde exposure or antinuclear antigen antibodies, presumably secondary to repetitive exposure to nuclear material entrapped on the dialysis membrane (29–32). However, they are also present in the peritoneal dialysis population (28).

Although early studies of vaccination responses using tetanus or diptheria toxoid suggested near normal antibody responses (33, 34), recent experience indicates that the uremic patient is less humorally responsive. Antibody levels after typhoid toxin or keyhole limpet hemocyanin are reduced (35–38). Antibody responses to influenza vaccine are generally comparable to controls (39–41), although one report showed a reduced response with severe uremia (42). After standard pneumococcal vaccination, antibody responses can be detected in the majority of ESRD patients, but in lower titers than observed in normals (43, 44). These titers are not as long-lasting in ESRD patients receiving dialysis therapy and antibody titers fall to unprotective levels more quickly (45, 46). In spite of recommendations to the contrary from the Center for Disease Control (47), some groups are recommending re-vaccination against pneumococci and have reported a low incidence of adverse reactions to re-vaccination (48). Hepatitis B vaccination has also resulted in an antibody response which is less than that seen in normal subjects (49–51). However, with the use of more potent vaccine, more frequent dosing schedules, or additional doses, higher rates of antibody response can be achieved (52–54). Here again antibody titers are not sustained (55, 56). Potentially underlying these abnormal responses, a decrease in IgG production by B lymphocytes from both uremic and hemodialyzed patients has been demonstrated *in vitro* (25, 26, 57–59).

In summary, humoral responses in dialysis patients are less than those observed in nonuremic subjects, both clinically and experimentally. Although the mechanism for this diminished response is not known, a decreased production of immunoglobulin by uremic B cells to specific stimuli may be a pivotal defect in observed abnormal immune responses.

Lymphocyte function

Delayed hypersensitivity as evaluated by skin testing is decreased to a variety of antigens in both dialyzed and uremic patients (24, 35, 37, 38, 60, 61). Patients with cutaneous anergy may have a normal cellular *in vitro* response to these antigens, indicating that the lack of reactivity is not due to an absence of antigen specificity (61).

A moderate decline in lymphocyte numbers involving both the B cell and T cell lines has generally been observed in ESRD patients (23–26, 61, 62). The mechanism of this lymphopenia is unclear, but with maintenance dialysis the lymphopenia may improve (27). The presence of lymphopenia has led to the suggestion that the defect in cell-mediated immunity is secondary to a decrease in cell numbers (35, 63). However, under conditions of equal cell numbers, the blastogenic response of uremic lymphocytes in autologous plasma to mitogen stimulation (e.g., concanavalin-A or phytohemaglutinin) or to mixed lymphocyte culture has generally been observed to be decreased compared to nonuremic controls (60, 62, 64–66). In the majority of studies, uremic plasma suppresses normal T cell responses when tested *in vitro* (23, 66–69), and uremic cells function abnormally even when cultured in nonuremic plasma (23, 25, 52, 58, 64, 70). Improvement of responses after dialysis or transplantation suggests that these changes are due to the uremic milieu (25, 38, 60, 62, 68). In this regard, middle molecules, such as guanidine derivatives, have been shown to suppress T cell function *in vitro* (71–74). Suppressive plasma factors, such as a very low density lipoprotein, have also been identified in experimental models of uremia (75–77). Thus, evidence supports both an inhibitory effect of uremic plasma and an intrinsic cellular defect as being responsible for the T cell dysfunction observed.

The presence of adherent cells in isolated lymphocyte preparations from rat models first suggested that abnormalities of immunologic cell/cell interaction may account for decreased lymphocyte responsiveness (78–80). However, use of monoclonal antibodies to identify T cell subtypes has generally shown no change in helper/suppressor T cell ratios despite a decreased absolute number of helper cells in ESRD patients (81–84). Therefore, it has been suggested that the suppressor cells may be more active, and this has been demonstrated *in vitro* for hemodialyzed patients (85–86). The precise nature of this suppressor cell, however, remains unclear. The removal of suppressor T cells using OKT8 monoclonal antibodies improved lymphocyte mitogen response (85). Alternatively, depletion of monocyte/

Table 1. Immunology of uremia.

	Result
Humoral immunity	
Immunoglobulin levels	N
Vaccination response	N, ↓
In vitro B cell response	↓
Lymphocyte function	
Lymphocyte number	↓
Blastogenic response	N, ↓
Cutaneous hypersensitivity	N, ↓
Cytokine production	↓
Helper/Suppressor ratios	N
Suppressor cell activity	N, ↑
Killer cell activity	N, ↓
Macrophage function	
Macrophage number	N, ↓
Phagocytosis	N, ↓
Mobility	N, ↓
Antigen presentation	↓
Suppressor activity	↑, ↓
Polymorphonuclear cell function	
PMN number	N
Chemotaxis	N, ↓
Adherence	↓
Phagocytosis	N, ↓
Intracellular killing	N, ↓

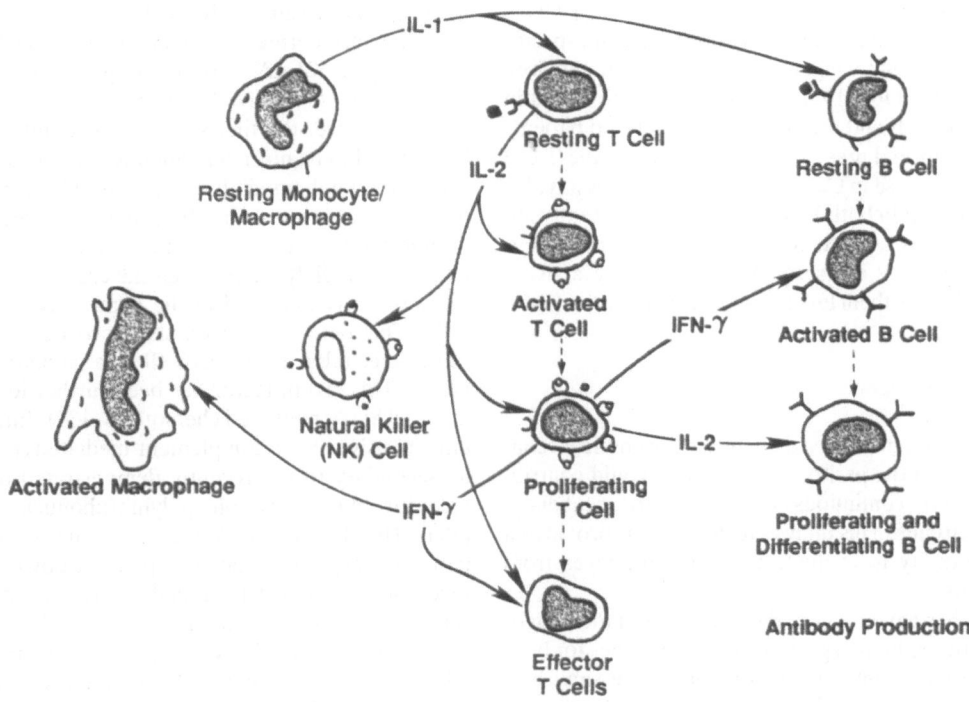

Figure 1. Cytokine pathways for immunomodulation. (IL = interleukin, IFN = interferon). From Fauci AS, Rosenberg SA, Sherwin SA, Dinarello CA, Longo DL, Lane HC: Immunomodulators in clinical medicine. *Ann Intern Med* 106: 421, 1987, with permission.

macrophage cells from cultures has also improved lymphocyte responses (59, 87, 88). Arachidonic acid metabolites play a role in macrophage/lymphocyte immunomodulation, and inhibition of prostaglandin production with indomethacin has altered lymphocyte blastogenic responses *in vitro* (87, 89). This supports the premise that the macrophage may be a key factor in suppressing lymphocyte function in ESRD patients. This is of even greater interest as the number of macrophages in end-stage renal disease patients is frequently increased (81, 82, 90).

Biochemical signaling between cells of the immune system is known to play an important role in their regulation (Figure 1). Production of these crucial cytokines appears to be altered in the uremic state. Interferon, necessary for optimal activation of macrophages, B lymphocytes and cytotoxic T cells, is produced in reduced amounts *in vitro* by lymphocytes from both uremic and hemodialyzed patients (91, 92). The production of interleukin-2, which serves to activate B cell antibody production, T cell differentiation, and natural killer cells, has also been found to be low in mitogen stimulated lymphocytes from hemodialyzed individuals (84). Lastly, it has recently been demonstrated that levels of the monokine interleukin-1 (IL-1) are elevated in hemodialysis patients (93). Whether this is due to increased production or a decreased degradation has not been ascertained, but it has been shown that interaction with endotoxin, dialysis membranes and acetate can stimulate IL-1 production from monocytes (94–96). What impact this may

have on immune responses is unclear, but given the importance of IL-1 to the enhancement of B and T lymphocyte function, further study is essential.

The final arm of the lymphocyte network is the natural killer cell, which is believed to be important for tumor surveillance and antiviral immunity. Few studies have been done to characterize natural killer cell activity in ESRD patients, but when natural killer cells from hemodialyzed patients have been studied in normal serum, their function has been normal (82, 90, 97).

Thus, considerable evidence attests to functional abnormalities of lymphocytes in ESRD patients. These abnormalities appear to relate not only to intrinsic cellular defects due to the uremic milieu, but also to abnormal intercellular interactions and altered production of various cytokines.

Mononuclear phagocytic system function

The mononuclear phagocytic system, which includes circulating monocytes, activated macrophages, and resident macrophages of the reticuloendothelial system, has not been extensively studied in uremic or chronic hemodialysis patients. The mononuclear cell has a pivotal role in the immune system cascade, as it is responsible for antigen presentation to the lymphocyte, phagocytic activity, and immunomodulation. The phagocytic activity of macrophages from hemodialyzed patients is depressed as measured by the Rebuck window technique (98, 99). Ingestion of IgG coated red cells *in vitro* has been found to be decreased (100). Incubation of normal macrophages in uremic serum, specifically its high molecular weight fraction, results in impaired phagocytic activity (101, 102). It has also been reported in experimental models and recently in hemodialyzed patients that there is abnormal presentation of antigen to the T cell (103, 104). A decrease in C_{5a} binding by monocytes has also been demonstrated in both hemodialysis and peritoneal dialysis patients. This suggests that chronic complement activation (evidenced by elevated plasma C_{3a}) may activate these cells and make them less responsive to infection (105).

Peritoneal macrophages

Recently, attention has focused on the pathogenetic mechanisms operative in the peritoneal cavity that could contribute to peritonitis in continuous ambulatory peritoneal dialysis (CAPD) patients. This dialysis technique has provided a unique opportunity to evaluate tissue macrophages from uremic patients.

In vitro studies have suggested that in general the phagocytic capabilities of human peritoneal macrophages for both gram-positive and gram-negative organisms are similar to those of normal human polymorphonuclear leukocytes or monocytes (106–108). However, there are several factors that might compromise the function of these cells *in vivo*. Since IgG levels in the local peritoneal environment of CAPD patients are extremely low, and this is the principal opsonin for gram-positive organisms, peritoneal macrophages may not phagocytize these organisms. Likewise, due to low levels of C_3, opsonic recognition of gram-negative bacteria may be impeded (C_{3b}, the opsonic fragment of C_3, is a key opsonin for gram-negative bacteria). The low pH and high osmolality of dialysis solutions may also temporarily impair phagocytic cell function (109). In addition to these deficits in opsonization, experimental data have also suggested that the ability of the peritoneal macrophage to kill certain strains of *Staphylococcus aureus, S. epidermidis,* as well as fungal organisms, such as *Candida albicans,* may be impaired (110–114). These combined deficits of opsonic molecules, as well as altered intracellular killing of these microorganisms, has recently been prospectively correlated with an increased incidence of clinical peritonitis in CAPD patients (115, 116).

Polymorphonuclear cell function

Neutrophil numbers in chronic renal failure and hemodialysis are generally reported to be normal to slightly elevated, in spite of the demonstration of an inhibitor of granulopoiesis in the serum of uremic patients (117–119). This contrasts with the profound complement-mediated leukopenia demonstrated immediately after the initiation of hemodialysis (120). In addition, leukocyte response to acute infection may be blunted, and *in vivo* studies of neutrophil response are mixed, with a normal neutrophil inflammatory response

being observed using the Rebuck window technique, but not with the intradermal or subcutaneous injection of urate crystals (99, 121–123). *In vitro,* polymorphonuclear cell functions are generally observed to be abnormal. Granulocyte adherance, the first step in neutrophil migration, has been found to be normal in undialyzed uremic patients, but is abnormal in hemodialysis patients (124, 125). Decreased neutrophil chemotaxis has been demonstrated in untreated uremic patients, as well as in those treated by either peritoneal or hemodialysis, although the chemotactic response is more severely impaired in the hemodialyzed group (126–129). This defect has been shown to be due to both an intrinsic cellular defect, as well as a circulating inhibitory factor. This serum factor has been further identified to be directed at C_{5a} mediated chemotaxis (130). Intrinsic cellular unresponsiveness to complement-mediated chemotaxis may be secondary to the recently demonstrated decreased C_{5a} receptor avialability on polymorphonuclear leukocytes (105). This decrease in C_{5a} receptors is noted even in CAPD patients, suggesting that the apparent down-regulation of receptors is not just hemodialysis associated but may be related to the uremic state as well.

Studies of the phagocytic capacity of neutrophils in uremia have been conflicting. Normal and depressed phagocytic activity have been seen in neutrophils from either uremic or hemodialyzed patients *in vitro* when studied either in uremic or in normal serum (23, 97, 124, 126, 131, 132). In one study, decreased phagocytic activity correlated with elevated serum phosphorus levels, and the abnormality corrected with lowering of the phosphorus level to normal (131). Several studies have also demonstrated that generation of reactive oxygen intermediates may be reduced, a defect that could lead to reduced intracellular killing of bacteria (133–135). The precise role that these neutrophil abnormalities may have in the clinical response to infection in ESRD patients has not been defined.

Effects of nutrition

Protein calorie malnutrition has been demonstrated to produce lymphopenia, decreased lymphocyte function, and abnormal neutrophil function, and the prevalence of protein calorie malnutrition is increased in the dialysis population (136–139). This has been attributed to amino acid losses during dialysis, as well as decreased overall dietary intake (140, 141). Indeed, the immune abnormalities of uremia bear a striking resemblance to those of malnutrition (141, 142). Clinically, malnutrition has been linked to increased infection-related hospitalization of dialysis patients and decreased lymphocyte function (143, 144). Finally, the reversal of skin test anergy and lymphopenia was demonstrated in two patients after 3 months of protein and calorie supplementation (145).

Other nutritional factors have also been studied. Vitamin B_6 deficiencies have been associated with an impairment of immune function, and low levels have been found in hemodialysis patients. Improvements in polymorphonuclear phagocytic activity and improved lymphocyte response to mitogens have been demonstrated with B_6 supplementation (146). Severe zinc deficiency can widely impair immune system function, and improvements in delayed hypersensitivity, mitogen-induced lymphocyte blastogenesis, and granulocyte mobility have been seen with zinc therapy in hemodialysis patients (147–149). Thus, nutritional abnormalities related to uremia and hemodialysis may contribute to abnormalities of immune function, but their relative contribution has not been clearly defined.

Effects of transfusion

Improved allograft survival has been reported in patients who have received multiple transfusions (150–151). Improved graft survival in multiply transfused patients suggests a defect in cell mediated immunity secondary to transfusion. A comparison of previously transfused to nontransfused hemodialysis patients demonstrated a significant difference in the degree of lymphopenia, with the transfused patients showing the most marked lymphopenia (152). Lymphocytes from multiply transfused patients show a reduced mixed lymphocyte culture reactivity and a decreased phytohemagglutinin response, and a decline in mixed lymphocyte culture response has been demonstrated immediately after transfusion in ESRD patients (153, 154). Individuals with greater than five transfusions compared to those with less than five blood transfusions demonstrated a significant difference in response to a battery of tests including spontaneous blastogenesis, mixed lymphocyte culture (MLC) and delayed cutaneous hypersensitivity (155). Importantly, this correlated significantly with graft survival.

The nature of this suppressive effect appears to be multifactorial. Anti-HLA antibodies produced by the nonspecific stimulation of B cells in lymphocyte preparations could interfere with stimulated responses, and depletion of B cells from mixed lymphocyte cultures restores MLC reactivity to the normal range (153). This suggests that nonspecific production of anti-HLA antibodies could have an immunosuppressive effect. Induction of suppressor cell activity has also been observed after blood transfusions in hemodialysis patients (155–158). Helper/suppressor ratios are also decreased in multi-transfused dialysis patients (152–155). Monocytes from patients with multiple transfusions demonstrate enhanced lymphocyte-suppressive activity, and treatment of cell preparations with indomethacin or radiation reduces transfusion induced suppression, further suggesting monocyte involvement in the induced suppression (155, 159, 160).

It is, therefore, intriguing to speculate whether many of the abnormalities of the ESRD patient's immune system are, in part, secondary to the transfusions they receive. This, coupled with the interactions of nutritional factors, uremic toxins, and differing dialysis techniques may account for the tremendous heterogeneity observed in the immune responses of ESRD patients.

REVIEW OF INFECTIOUS COMPLICATIONS IN HEMODIALYSIS PATIENTS

Patient population

In a previous study, infectious complications over a 42 month period between 1972 to 1975 were reviewed (161). In this study, 455 patients with a total of 8,105 treatment months were evaluated. This included 7,202 treatment months in nondiabetic patients and 903 in patients with diabetes. This retrospective analysis included all patients accepted for chronic hemodialysis who received this therapy for a minimum of one month. Using similar study criteria, we retrospectively reviewed our experience for a 36 month period from 1982 to 1985 (162). This study includes 851 patients and a total of 15,486 treatment months; 569 nondiabetic and 282 diabetic hemodialysis patients with 10,729 and 4,757 treatment months, respectively. These two data bases therefore provide a relative comparative index of the importance of infections and their complications over a decade of experience in maintenance hemodialysis patients.

Mortality

It is well established that infection accounts for a significant proportion of deaths in hemodialysis patients. Early studies reported that between 12 to 38% of deaths were infection related, and this frequency has remained relatively unchanged in recent reports (1–8). Previously, we reported 111 deaths during a 42 month period, with 22 (19.8%) directly attributable to infection (161). Our more recent experience indicates little change in the incidence of infection-related death, with 32 of the 201 (15.9%) deaths seen from 1982 to 85 primarily caused by infection (162). Thus, a rate of 2.1 deaths/1,000 treatment months was observed in the 1980's series, lower, but not dramatically different than an incidence of 2.7/1,000 treatment months in the 1970's series.

Two notable risk factors for infectious death are indicated by our data. In both studies, there is an increased incidence of death by infection in diabetic hemodialysis patients. In the 1970's and 1980's studies, diabetic infection-related deaths were 4.4 and 2.7 deaths/1,000 treatment months, respectively. In comparison, infection-related deaths in nondiabetic patients were 2.5 and 0.9 deaths/1,000 treatment months. Thus, infection-related deaths are two to three-fold more likely in diabetic patients. Age is also an important factor. Over 60% of the patients dying from infection in the 1972 to 1975 study were over 60 years of age, and 78% of those who died primarily from infectious complications during 1982 to 1985 were over 60 years of age.

There is little change in the most common sources of infectious deaths over the last decade (Table 2). Access-related infection, pulmonary and intra-abdominal sepsis predominated in both series. Documented bacteremia was present in approximately half of the cases in both series. The average length of time from the initiation of dialysis to infection-related death was 25 months in the earlier study, and 42 months in the recent review.

Bacteremia

Incidence

Bacteremia has been reported to occur with a prevalence of 9.5 to 20% in chronic hemodialysis patients (1, 161, 163, 164). In our experience, bacteremia was defined as one or more positive blood cultures not felt to be a contaminant on the basis of corresponding clinical evidence of infection, such as fever, rigors, elevated white count or localizing symptoms. Using these criteria, our 1972 to 1975 study revealed 124 episodes of bacteremia in 91 patients over a 42 month period (161). This represents an incidence of 15.3 episodes of bacteremia per 1000 treatment months, and a prevalence of 20%. A similar incidence of 12.5 episodes/1,000 treatment months was reported by others (163). In comparison, the 36 month period in the 1980's demonstrated 97 episodes of bacteremia in 67 patients (162). This represents an incidence of 6.3/1,000 treatment months, and a prevalence of 7.8%. Thus, there appears to be a reduction in the incidence of bacteremia in our center over the course of the last 10 years.

In our 1970's experience, diabetic patients developed bacteremia more often with 32.1 episodes/1,000 treatment months versus only 13.2/1,000 treatment months in non-diabetic patients (161). In our more recent experience, minimal differences were found between diabetic and non-diabetic hemodialysis patients; indeed, diabetics had 4.6 episodes of bacteremia/1,000 treatment months while 6.0/1,000 treatment months were observed in non-diabetic patients (162). This may reflect the fact that in the earlier study, diabetics made up only 11% of the treatment months recorded, while they now represent 31% of the treatment months, as well as approximately one-third of the patients.

Infecting organisms

The organisms isolated from bacteremic episodes in both of our reviews are listed for comparison in Table 3. As can be seen in both studies, gram-positive organisms predominate, although this preponderance is not as dramatic in the later study. While they made up 74% of isolates previously, a decade later they only represent 53%. In comparison, gram-positive organisms have been reported to account for 62 and 73% of isolates in studies from other centers covering the early 1970's (163–164).

Bacteremia secondary to access infection

Access infection has been reported to account for from 48 to 72% of all bacteremic episodes in hemodialysis patients (161–164). In our experience, access infections were associated with 56 and 48% of bacteremic episodes (Table 3). Although access infections accounted for the largest proportion of total bacteremias, the incidence of access-related bacteremia has declined in the decade between our two studies. In the early 1970's, access-related bacteremia accounted for 8.5 episodes/1,000 treatment months, while in the 1980's it accounted for only 3 episodes/1,000 treatment months (161, 162). This, in part, is explained by the decreased use of the cannula as a blood access device. In the 1970's, cannulas contributed to 75% of the access-related bacteremias. In contrast, they were only responsible for six bacteremias in our most recent review.

While gram-negative infections accounted for 20% of access-related bacteremias in our 1970's experience, they made up 34% of isolates in the 1982 of 1985 period. This can be explained in part by recurrent gram-negative infections in the Hemasite blood access device which was evaluated at our center during that later period. Importantly, they accounted for 43% of access-related bacteremias, and 14 of the 16 gram-negative organisms isolated.

Bacteremia not associated with access infection

This category includes two groups, one in which no definite source of bacteria could be found, and the other where a source other than the access site was demonstrated. In the early 1970's, non-access related bacteria accounted for 45% of the overall bacteremias, 35 episodes from non-access sites and 20 episodes from unknown sources (161). Among the bacteremias from unknown sources, gram-positive organisms accounted for 18 of the 20 episodes, suggesting occult access infection as the major cause. Among those episodes where a source other than the access could be demonstrated, gram-positive organisms still predominated (Table 3). In this category, the gastrointestinal tract was the most common source (Table 4).

In the 1980's, access unrelated bacteremias made up a majority (52%) of bacteremic episodes (162). This included 22 episodes where no source was clearly identified and in 28 episodes where a non-access source could be found. Sources of infection in this latter group were quite similar to our

Table 2. Assocation between primary site of infection and death.

Source	Blood access device	Pulmonary	Intra-abdominal	Genito-urinary	Endo-carditis*	Meningitis	Skin	Other
1972–75 (n = 22)	5	5	5	4	1	2	0	0
1982–85 (n = 32)	8	7	7	2	2	0	2	4
total (54)	13	12	12	6	3	2	2	4
(%)	(24.1)	(22.2)	(22.2)	(11.1)	(5.6)	(3.7)	(3.7)	(7.4)

* Does not include cases where endocarditis was felt to be secondary to another primary source such as access.

previous experience (Table 4). Of note in our 1980's study is that gram-negative organisms made up a majority of the organisms isolated (55%). Interestingly, in the 1972 to 1975 series, there were 4.3 episodes/1,000 treatment months of bacteremias from sources identified other than the access, while in the 1980's series, these had decreased to only 1.8/1,000 treatment months.

Mortality

The overall mortality from bacteremic episodes in the 1970's series was 19 (15%) of 120 episodes (161). In comparison, in the 1980's study, there were 14 deaths (14%) in 97 episodes (162). Thus, it appears that although overall incidence of

bacteremia is lower, the mortality with any given episode remains the same. This continued relatively low mortality from bacteremia is of interest given the increasing prevalence of gram-negative organisms in bacteremic episodes. Mortality from access-related infections also remains low; it was 10% in the 1970's study and 8.5% in 1980's study.

Bacteriology

The majority of the isolates in both bacteremia series were gram-positive organisms (Table 3). Non unexpectedly, *Staphylococcus aureus* was the most predominant isolate. Sixty percent of hemodialysis patients have been shown to have *S. aureus* colonization, a three-fold higher incidence than

Table 3. Relationship between bacteriology and site of infection; comparison of 1972–75 and 1982–85.

	1972–75 (124 episodes)			1982–85 (97 episodes)		
	Access related	Other or unknown	Total*	Access related	Other or unknown	Total*
Gram-positive organisms	58	37	95	29	24	53
Staphylococcus aureus	35	5	40	20	4	24
S. epidermidis	20	10	30	4	3	7
Pneumococcal	–	5	5	–	5	5
Enterococcus	1	6	7	2	7	9
Streptococcus sp	2	2	4	3	3	6
Listeria monocytes	–	2	2	–	1	1
Clostridium perfringes	–	1	1	–	1	1
Other gram-positive**	–	6	6	–	–	0
Anaerobes						
Bacteroides fragilis	–	–	0	2	–	2
Gram-negative organisms	14	18	32	16	29	45
Escherichia coli	4	12	16	2	16	18
Serratia sp	4	2	6	4	1	5
Pseudomonas sp	1	–	1	3	4	7
Klebsiella-Enterobacter	3	3	6	–	5	5
Proteus sp	1	1	2	5	1	6
Hemophilus sp	–	–	0	1	1	2
Other gram-negative***	1	$	1	1	1	2

* Totals exceed number of episodes due to polymicrobial bacteremias.
** Other gram-positive includes Bacillas species and Diphtheroids.
*** Other gram-negatives includes other Eikenella corrodens, Achromobacter sp and Citrobacter freundii.

Table 4. Source of infection in access unrelated bacteremias.

	Gastrointestinal tract	Genitourinary tract	Respiratory tract	Miscellaneous (skin, sinus, etc.)
1972–75 (n = 35)	12	7	7	9
1982–85 (n = 28)	6	10	7	5
Total (63) (%)	18 (29%)	17 (27%)	14 (22%)	14 (22%)

chronic renal failure patients not on dialysis (165). This appears to be specific to the dialyzing patient, since the dialysis staff in the same unit have a colonization rate of only 30%, which is also several times higher than a normal healthy population. This high rate of staphylococcal carriage in hemodialysis patients is not present at the initiation of dialysis, but is acquired over the first several months (165). This increased incidence of colonization, especially in terms of nasal carriage, has further been associated with an increased risk of acquiring staphylococcal bacteremia (166). Methods aimed at decreasing this colonization, particularly the intermittent use of rifampin, have been shown to decrease shunt infections and bacteremia secondary to staphylococcal organisms (167).

Complications of bacteremia

Several complications of bacteremia and access infection are well recognized in hemodialysis patients: bacterial endocarditis, osteomyelitis, septic arthritis and septic pulmonary emboli (161, 168–170). The potentially prolonged bacteremic state unique to access infections may contribute to the prevalence of these otherwise unusual complications. In addition, the increased metabolic demands and catabolism of the septic state may have profound effects, especially if superimposed on a marginal nutritional status. Sepsis-related hypotension may further complicate the dialysis procedure itself at a time when dialysis requirements may be increased. The frequent onset of pericarditis after infection or surgery suggests that routine dialysis regimens may be inadequate during these hypermetabolic periods (171–172).

Bacterial endocarditis

Bacterial endocarditis in regularly dialyzed patients has been the subject of a number of studies. Early studies demonstrated a prevalence of 2.7 to 4.4% (173–176). *S. aureus* has been the predominant organism and access infection the most common source of the organism. Overall mortality for this complication has been approximately 50% (177). In our 1970's study, nine episodes of bacterial endocarditis were recorded, a rate of 1.2/1,000 treatment months and a prevalence of 2.0% (161). *S. aureus* was the infecting organism in six of the cases, and the aortic valve was involved in eight of the nine. Six of the nine survived, with the other three dying as a consequence of acute cerebral embolic events. Successful valve replacement was accomplished in two of these patients.

In our recent review, only four episodes of endocarditis were documented during the study period, an incidence of 0.26/1,000 treatment months and a prevalence of only 0.5% (162). However, three of the four patients died; two with *S. aureus* infection, and one with *E. coli*. The surviving patient had enterococcal mitral valve endocarditis which resolved with antibiotic therapy alone. Thus, while the incidence of endocarditis appears to be declining, the mortality associated with this complication remains high.

Osteomyelitis and septic arthritis

Metastatic infection of bones and joints is a well recognized complication of infection in hemodialyzed patients (168, 170, 178–180). In our 1970's study, 11 patients were found who had eight episodes of osteomyelitis and six episodes of septic arthritis, an overall incidence of 1.7 episodes/1,000 treatment months (161). These complications were observed in the diabetic patients at an eight-fold higher incidence than in a non-diabetic counterpart (7.8 vs 1.0 episodes/1,000 treatment months). This predeliction for the diabetic patient continues, as in our recent experience, six cases of osteomyelitis were observed, five of them in diabetics (162). In the 1970's review, blood access device was the origin of infection in eight cases (57)%, and *S. aureus* was isolated in 10 of the episodes (161). Other organisms found included *S. epidermidis* in three *Serratia marcescens* in two, and *Clostridium perfringens*, *Klebsiella enterobacter* and *E. coli* in one each. In some patients with osteomyelitis, more than one organism was isolated from the culture of the bony lesion.

The diagnosis of osteomyelitis still presents considerable difficulty. Nonspecific symptoms such as a low grade fever, malaise and weight loss may dominate the clinical picture. The frequent lack of radiographic changes often delays diagnosis. In early studies, osteomyelitis was more common in vertebral bodies and in ribs (180), while in both our 1970's and 1980's experience, the distal upper and lower extremities were the most frequent sites for infection (161, 162). Therapeutically, long-term antibiotics, combined with early debridement of the osteomyelitic lesion was usually successful. However, in diabetic patients, amputation of the affected limb was frequently necessary.

In the 1972 to 1975 study, septic arthritis most commonly involved the joints, wrist and *S. aureus* was the most frequent infecting organism (161). This experience is not dissimilar to that reported by others (178). In our 1982 to 1985 bacteremia review, three patients were found to have metastatic joint infections, all of them with *S. aureus* (162). These included two in the shoulder joint and one in acromioclavicular joint. As in our previous experience, all of the patients responded to systemic antimicrobial therapy without late sequela.

Septic pulmonary emboli

In dialysis patients with chronic underlying cannulas or subcutaneous fistulas subjected to repetitive venipuncture, the development of an infected thrombophlebitis or endarteritis associated with septic pulmonary emboli should not be unexpected (163, 164, 181–183). However, given the frequency of blood access device infections, this is clinically a rather uncommon complication. It occurred at a rate of 0.7 episodes/1,000 treatment months in the 1972 to 1975 series (161). However, we were unable to document septic pulmonary emboli as a complication of access infection in our 1980's study. The reason for this is unclear, but again could relate to reduced use of the cannula at our centers.

The diagnosis of septic pulmonary emboli should be considered if fever, cough and pleuritic chest pain develop during a dialysis treatment, especially in the setting of an underlying access infection. While previous reports have emphasized that septic pulmonary emboli may develop in the absence of obvious access infection (181, 182), in our experience, evidence for an associated infection of blood access device was present in all episodes, five of them in cannulas, and two in bovine carotid fistulas. The infecting organism in these cases was *S. aureus* in three, *S. epidermidis* in two, and one each of *S. marcescens* and *E. coli*. Antibiotic therapy has been reported as successful treatment of septic pulmonary emboli, even without the removal of the blood access device (163, 164). However, our usual approach has been to remove the access immediately while treating the infection with appropriate antimicrobial therapy. With this combination of systemic antimicrobial therapy and the removal of the access device, all of the above cases were treated successfully.

Access infections

Infection of vascular access has always been a vexing problem and a cause of significant morbidity and mortality in the hemodialysis population. Access infections are consistently the leading cause of bacteremia in hemodialysis patients (161–164), and one of the leading causes of access failure (184–186). Infection of a blood access device is defined by the presence of a local inflammatory reaction and positive cultures obtained from the suppurative area. Overall, access infections occurred at a rate of 73 episodes/1,000 treatment months in our 1970's review (161). This rate has most probably declined in the 1980's with a reduced utilization of external Silastic catheters which accounted for the majority of infections in the 1970's (Table 4). In our 1970's experience, cannula infections occurred at a rate of 150/1000 treatment months (161). Comparable rates of infection in cannulas ranging from 35 to 145 episodes/1,000 treatment months have been reported by others (187, 188). The superiority of internal access devices as compared to external Silastic catheters is quite clear from the 1970's series (Table 5). The development of the Brescia-Cimino fistula has had as one of its major benefits a dramatically decreased incidence of infection (189). The incidence of infection with this form of access varies from 8 to 20 episodes/1,000 treatment months with a prevalence of less than 1% up to 5% of all such fistulae (184, 186, 188, 190, 191). Bovine carotid artery heterografts (BCAH) and polytetrafluorethylene grafts (PTFE) also have significantly lower rates of infection than do cannulas, but are several times more susceptible to infection than simple fistulas. Infection with BCAH and PTFE occurs in 6 to 25% of grafts and accounts for 10 to 30% of graft losses with BCAH or PTFE (184, 186, 191–195). Carbon coated needle free access devices such as Biocarbon® or Hemasite® are also associated with frequent infections. They occur with a prevalence of approximately 25% at a rate as high as 45 episodes/1,000 treatment months (186, 197). As noted above, many of these devices were infected with gram-negative bacteria and resulted in a high incidence of bacteremia.

Bacteriology and treatment

The preponderance of gram-positive organisms isolated from access infections is demonstrated in Table 6. Most access infections in our 1970 series were treated on an outpatient basis with systemic antibiotic therapy stressing good gram-positive coverage. However, 19.2% of these infections were severe enough to warrant hospitalization, with two-thirds of these patients demonstrating bacteremia. Among the hospitalized group, 60% required removal of the access device, most frequently external Silastic catheters. Ligation or removal of an access site felt to be the source of bacteremia is not routine in our institution for internal fistulae, but surgical intervention is performed for drainage of an abscess or resection of an aneurysmal dilatation to avoid potential graft erosion. This conservative approach is not universally accepted, and management of infected access grafts is variable (186, 188, 191, 193, 195–197, 200).

The effectiveness of long-term prophylactic antibiotics to reduce the frequency of access infections is controversial. Due to the wide spectrum of organisms which may be seen in access infections, it is improbable that any one antibiotic would be effective against all organisms. In addition, the possibility of the induction of resistant strains must be considered. Prophylactic vancomycin was used in one uncontrolled study of 25 patients where it was demonstrated that

Table 5. Summary of blood access device experience during 42 months (1972–1975).

Type of access	Number inserted (%)	Months of access utilization[a]	Mean access survival time (months)	Number of episodes of infections	Number of infections/month of access utilization
Cannula	397(54.4)	3105	7.8	464	0.15
Simple fistula	180(24.7)	2423	13.5	52	0.02
Bovine carotid fistula	128(17.6)	2044	16.0	68	0.03
Other[b]	23(3.2)	478	NA	2	NA
Totals	728	8050	–	586	–

[a] This represents actual number of months the access device was utilized for hemodialysis.

[b] This group includes saphenous vein fistulas, Sparks-mandril fistulas and other access devices not regularly used in the authors' center.

S. aureus infections were reduced, but there was an increase in infections caused by organisms from the *Klebsiella enterobacter* group (201). Recently, there is evidence that intermittent use of rifampin prophylactically may decrease the incidence of staphylococcal access infections and bacteremia (167). In addition, short term antibiotic prophylaxis may be of value during procedures associated with transient bacteremias.

Systemic infections

Respiratory infection

A number of factors which may predispose hemodialysis patients to an increased risk of acquiring pulmonary infection have been identified. The permissive role of pathologic changes associated with uremic pulmonary edema, such as thick, tenacious mucous in the upper airways, the presence of hyaline-like membranes and alveolar fibrinous exudates could interfere with clearance of potential pathogens (202–205). A decreased pulmonary clearance for coagulase-positive staphylococci has been seen in experimental uremic models using mice (206). In addition, altered nasalpharyngeal flora seen in chronically ill and hospitalized patients may predispose the hemodialysis patient to the development of pulmonary infections (207).

In our 1970 experience, there were 40 episodes of pulmonary infections in 35 patients, an incidence of 5.7/1,000 treatment months (161). *Streptococcus pneumoniae* was isolated in 50% of the patients who were admitted with a primary diagnosis of pneumonia. In contrast, gram-negative organisms were frequently isolated in patients who developed pneumonias while in the hospital. There was no difference in the frequency of this infection between diabetic and non-diabetic patients. Death occurred in 12% of those patients who were admitted with a diagnosis of pneumonia while 57% of those patients with hospital-acquired pneumonia eventually died. Chronic obstructive pulmonary disease and cardiac decompensation were common associated conditions in patients with respiratory infections. In comparison, an incidence of pulmonary infections as high as 51% has

Table 6. Bacteriology of blood access device infections, 1972–1975.

Gram positive organisms	480	(81.9%)
Staphylococcus epidermidis	195	(33.3%)
Staphylococcus aureus	191	(32.6%)
Streptococcus species	46	(7.8%)
Diphtheroids	46	(7.8%)
Bacillus species	2	(0.3%)
Gram negative organisms	106	(18.1%)
Klebsiella-enterobacter	36	(6.1%)
Escherichia coli	23	(3.9%)
Pseudomonas aeurginosa	20	(3.4%)
Serratia marcescens	8	(1.4%)
Other	19	(3.2%)

been reported by others with a mortality of approximately 50% (1).

Urinary tract infections

With a decrease in urine output accompanying the development of renal failure, the subsequent stasis of urine flow might be expected to predispose the hemodialysis patient to an increased risk of urinary tract infection. In fact, bacteriuria has been reported in 28 to 58% of chronic hemodialysis patients (208, 209). The significance of this bacteriuria is unclear. We previously documented 19 episodes of symptomatic urinary tract infections in 16 patients in our 1970 series (161). This is an incidence of 2.3/1,000 treatment months. Polycystic kidney disease was the underlying diagnosis in eight of these 16 patients (50%). In five of them, the clinical course was complicated by the development of a perinephric abscess refractory to systemic antibiotic therapy necessitating surgical nephrectomy. Three of these patients died postoperatively. This experience is similar to that of others, where an incidence of symptomatic urinary tract infection of 11.6% has been shown and where four of the 11 patients so diagnosed had polycystic kidney disease as a cause of their renal failure (210). The treatment of urinary tract infections in hemodialysis patients may be difficult because in the absence of urinary flow, normal mechanisms for concentrating antibiotics at the site of infection may not be operative. However, it has been shown that significant levels of antibiotics can be obtained in the urine using ampicillin or trimethoprim/sulfamethoxazole in patients with severe end-stage disease (211).

Unusual infections

The purported high incidence of mycobacterial infection may be presumptive evidence of the presence of defects in the immune system of hemodialysis patients. Rates of tuberculosis have been reported at 10 to 15 times those found in the normal population, and they may account for approximately 1% of deaths of hemodialysis patients (212–218). Mortality from tubercular infection in hemodialyzed patients ranges from 0 to 75%, and the diagnosis is frequently made at autopsy. Indeed, the nonspecific symptoms of fever, anorexia and weight loss, plus the tendency for extrapulmonary disease make the diagnosis exceedingly difficult. Routine cultures and skin tests are frequently negative and the diagnosis is often delayed. The most reliable results for obtaining the diagnosis are found with culture of tissue biopsies of appropriate sources, and, when the diagnosis is made, the response to therapy is usually good.

Another unusual pathogen which has been reported in hemodialysis patients is *Listeria monocytogenes*. This organism is an unusual human pathogen and occasionally leads to clinical infections in renal transplant recipients or other immunosuppressed individuals. It has been reported as causing bacteremia and endocarditis in a number of ESRD patients (173, 219, 220)., and appeared as a cause of bacteremia in both of our bacteremia reviews (Table 3). Recently, it has been suggested that iron overload may be an etiologic factor in the development of listerosis in the hemodialysis group (221).

SUMMARY

Infection in patients with ESRD receiving maintenance hemodialysis therapy remains a common cause of morbidity and mortality. The frequent and repetitive exposure of hemodialysis patients to potential risk factors during the normal course of their therapy is a unique medical situation which contributes to this increased susceptibility. However, with the greater use of subcutaneous blood access devices rather than external Silastic catheters, the contribution of blood access to infectious complications appears to be decreasing. In addition, the enhanced susceptibility to infection secondary to alterations in immune response induced by the uremic state *per se,* or by contributing factors, such as nutritional deficiencies, transfusions, and interactions with the hemodialysis process itself, appear to play an important role in determining the type, incidence and outcome of these infectious complications.

REFERENCES

1. Montgomerie JZ, Kalmanson GM, Guze LB: Renal failure and infection. *Medicine* 47: 1, 1968
2. Blagg CR, Hickman RO, Eschbach JW, Scribner BH: Home hemodialysis: Six years experience. *N Engl J Med* 283: 1126, 1970
3. Burton BT, Krueger KK, Bryan FA Jr: National registry of long-term dialysis patients. *JAMA* 218: 718, 1971
4. Gurland HJ, Brunner FP, v Dehn H, Harlen H, Parsons FM, Schärer K: Combined report on regular dialysis and transplantation in Europe III, 1972. *Proc Eur Dial Transplant Assoc* 10: XVII, 1973
5. Lowrie EG, Lazarus JM, Mogelin AJ, Baily FL, Hampers CL, Wilson RE, Merrill JP: Survival of patients undergoing chronic hemodialysis and renal transplantation. *N Engl J Med* 288: 863, 1973
6. Johnson WJ, Kurtz SB, Anderson CF, Mitchell JC III, Zincke H, O'Fallon WM: Results of treatment of renal fialure by means of home hemodialysis. *Mayo Clin Proc* 59: 663, 1984
7. Johnson WJ, Kurtz SB, Mitchell JC III, VanDenBerg CJ, Wochos DN, O'Fallon WM, Sterioff S: Results of treatment of center hemodialysis patients. *Mayo Clin Proc* 59: 669, 1984
8. Santiago A, Chazan JA: Factors associated with mortality among 405 chronic hemodialysis patients who died between 1973 and 1985. *Kidney Int* 31: 245, 1987
9. Hume DM, Merrill JP, Miller BF, Thorn GW: Experiences with renal homotransplantation in humans. Report of nine cases. *J Clin Invest* 32: 327, 1955
10. Mannick JA, Powers JH, Mithoefer J, Ferrebee JW: Renal transplantation in azotemic dogs. *Surgery* 47: 340, 1960
11. Dammin GJ, Couch NP, Murray JE: Prolonged survival of skin homografts in uremia patients. *Ann NY Acad Sci* 64: 967, 1957
12. Smiddy FG, Burwell NG, Parsons FM: The effect of acute uraemia upon the survival of skin homografts. *Br J Surg* 48: 328, 1960
13. Morrison AB, Maness K, Tawes R: Skin homograft survival in chronic renal insufficiency. *Arch Pathol* 75: 139, 1963
14. London WT, DiFiglia M, Sutnick AI, Blumberg BS: An epidemic of hepatitis in a chronic hemodialysis unit: Australia antigen and differences in host response. *N Engl J Med* 281: 571, 1969
15. London WT, Drew JS, Lustbader ED, Werner BG, Blumberg BS: Host responses to hepatitis B infection in patients in a chronic hemodialysis unit. *Kidney Int* 12: 51, 1977
16. Ribot S, Rothstein M, Goldblatt M, Grasso M: Duration of hepatitis B surface antigenemia (HBsAg) in hemodialysis patients. *Arch Intern Med* 139: 178, 1979
17. Szmuness W, Prince AM, Grady GF, Mann MK, Levine RW, Friedman EA, Jacobs MJ, Josephson A, Ribot S, Shapiro FL, Stenzel KH, Suki WN, Vyas G: Hepatitis B infection. A point-prevalance study in 15 U.S. hemodialysis centers. *JAMA* 227: 901, 1974
18. Matas AJ, Simmons RL, Kjellstrand CM, Buselmeier TJ, Najarian JS: Increased incidence of malignancy during chronic renal failure. *Lancet* 1: 883, 1975
19. Sutherland GA, Glass J, Gabriel R: Increased incidence of malignancy in chronic renal failure. *Nephron* 18: 182, 1977
20. Lindner A, Farewell YJ, Sherrard DJ: High incidence of neoplasia in uremic patients receiving long-term dialysis. *Nephron* 27: 292, 1981
21. Degaauet P, Reach J, Jacobs C: Cancer in patients on hemodialysis. *N Engl J Med* 300: 1279, 1979
22. Coplon NS, Diskin CJ, Peterson J, Sivenson RS: The long-term clinical course of systemic lupus erythematosus in end-stage renal disease. *N Engl J Med* 308: 186, 1983
23. Hosking CS, Atkins RC, Scott DR, Holdsworth SR, Fitzgerald MG, Shelton MJ: Immune and phagocytic functions in patients on maintenance hemodialysis and posttransplantation. *Clin Nephrol* 6: 501, 1976
24. Casciani CU, DeSimone C, Bonini S: Immunological aspects of chronic uremia. *Kidney Int* 13 (Suppl 8): S49, 1978
25. Raskova J, Ghobrial I, Czerwinski DK, Shea SM, Gisinger RP, Raska K Jr: B-cell activation and immunoregulation in end-stage renal disease patients receiving hemodialysis. *Arch Intern Med* 147: 89, 1987
26. Quadracci LJ, Ringden O, Krzymanski M: The effect of uremia and transplantation on lymphocyte subpopulations. *Kidney Int* 10: 179, 1976
27. Hoy WE, Cestero RVM, Freeman RB: Deficiency of T and B lymphocytes in uremic subjects and partial improvement with maintenance hemodialysis. *Nephron* 20: 182, 1978
28. Gagnon RF, Shuster J, Kaye M: Auto-immunity in patients with end-stage renal disease maintained on hemodialysis and continuous ambulatory peritoneal dialysis. *J Clin Lab Immunol* 11: 155, 1983
29. Howell ED, Perkins HA: Anti-N-like antibodies in the sera of patients undergoing chronic hemodialysis. *Vox Sang* 23: 291, 1972
30. Crosson JT, Moulds J, Comty CM, Polesky HF: A clinical study of anti N-$_{DP}$ in the sera of patients in a large repetive hemodialysis program. *Kidney Int* 10: 463, 1976
31. Kaehny WD, Miller GE, White WL: Relationship between dialyzer reuse and the presence of anti-N-like antibodies in chronic hemodialysis patients. *Kidney Int* 12: 59, 1977
32. Nolph KD, Husted FC, Sharp GC, Siemsen AW: Antibodies to nuclear antigens in patients undergoing long-term hemodialysis. *Am J Med* 60: 673, 1976
33. Balch HH: The effect of severe battle injury and post-traumatic renal failure on resistance to infection. *Ann Surg* 142: 145, 1955

34. Stoloff IL, Stout R, Myerson RM, Havens WP Jr: Production of antibody in patients with uremia. *N Engl J Med* 259: 320, 1958

35. Wilson WEC, Kirkpatrick CH, Talmage DW: Suppression of immunologic reponsiveness in uremia. *Ann Intern Med* 61: 1, 1965

36. Boulton-Jones JM, Vick R, Cameron JS, Block PH: Immune responses in uremia. *Clin Nephrol* 1: 351, 1973

37. Byron PR, Mallick NP, Taylor G: Immune potential in human uraemia. I. Relationship of glomerular filtration rate to depression of immune potential. *J Clin Path* 29: 765, 1976

38. Byron PR, Mallick NP, Taylor G: Immune potential in human uremia. 2. Changes after regular hemodialysis therapy. *J Clin Path* 29: 770, 1976

39. Jordan MC, Rousseau WE, Tegtmeier GE, Noble GR, Muth RG, Chin TDY: Immunogenicity of inactivated influenza virus vaccine in chronic renal failure. *Ann Intern Med* 79: 790, 1973

40. Ortbals DW, Marks ES, Liebhaber H: Influenza immunization in patients with chronic renal disease. *JAMA* 239: 2562, 1978

41. Osanloo EA, Berlin BS, Popli S, Ing TS, Cummings JE, Ghandi VC, Geis WP, Hano JE: Antibody response to influenza vaccination in patients with chronic renal failure. *Kidney Int* 14: 209, 1978

42. Pabico RC, Douglas RG, Betts RF, McKenna BA, Freeman RB: Influenza vaccination of patients with glomerular diseases. *Ann Intern Med* 81: 171, 1974

43. Simberkoff MS, Schiffman G, Katz LA, Spicehandler JR, Moldover NH, Rahal JJ Jr: Pneumococcal capsular polysaccharide vaccination in adult chronic hemodialysis patients. *J Lab Clin Med* 96: 363, 1980

44. Linnemann CC Jr, First MR, Schiffman G: Response to pneumococcal vaccine in renal transplant and hemodialysis patients. *Arch Intern Med* 141: 1637, 1981

45. Nikoskelainen J, Koskela M, Forsström J, Kasanen A, Leinonen M: Persistence of antibodies to pneumococcal vaccine in patients with chronic renal failure. *Kidney Int* 28: 672, 1985

46. Rytel MW, Dailey MP, Schiffman G, Hoffman RG, Piering WF: Pneumococcal vaccine immunization of patients with renal impairment. *Proc Soc Exp Biol Med* 182: 468, 1986

47. Immunization Practices Advisory Committee: Update! Pneumococcal polysaccharide vaccine usage – United States. Recommendations of the immunization practices advisory committee. *Ann Intern Med* 101: 348, 1984

48. Linnemann CC, First MR, Schiffman G: Revaccination of renal transplant and hemodialysis recipients with pneumococcal vaccine. *Arch Intern Med* 146: 1554, 1986

49. Stevens CE, Szmuness W, Goodman AI, Weseley SA, Fotino M: Hepatitis B vaccine: Immune responses in haemodialysis patients. *Lancet* 2: 1211, 1980

50. Crosnier J, Jungers P, Courouce AM, Laplanche A, Benhamou E, Degos F, Lacour B, Prunet P, Cerisier Y, Guesry P: Randomized placebo-controlled trial of hepatitis B surface antigen vaccine in French haemodialysis units: II, haemodialysis patients. *Lancet* 1: 797, 1981

51. Stevens CE, Alter HJ, Taylor PE, Zang EA, Harley EJ, Szmuness W, and the dialysis vaccine trial study group: Hepatitis B vaccine in patients receiving hemodialysis. Immunogenecity and efficacy. *N Engl J Med* 311: 496, 1984

52. Desmyter J, Colaert J, DeGroote G, Reynders M, Reerink-Brongers EE, Lelie PN, Dees PJ, Reesink HW, and the Leuver renal transplantation collaborative group: Efficacy of heat-inactivated hepatitis B vaccine in haemodialysis patients and staff. *Lancet* 2: 1323, 1983

53. Benhamou E, Courouce AM, Jungers P, Laplanche A, Degos F, Brangier J, Crosnier J: Hepatitis B vaccine: Randomized trial of immunogenecity in hemodialysis patients. *Clin Nephrol* 21: 143, 1984

54. Kohler H, Arnold W, Renschin G, Dormeyer HH, Zum Buschenfelde KHM: Active hepatitis B vaccination of dialysis patients and medical staff. *Kidney Int* 25: 124, 1984

55. de Graeff PA, Dankert J, de Zeeuw D, Gips CH, van der Hem GK: Immune reponse to two different hepatitis B vaccines in haemodialysis patients: a 2 year follow-up. *Nephron* 40: 155, 1985

56. Benhamou E, Courouce A-M, Laplanche A, Jungers P, Tron JF, Crosnier J: Longterm results of hepatitis B vaccination in patients on dialysis. *N Engl J Med* 314: 1710, 1986

57. Kunori T, Fehrman I, Ringden O, Moller E: *In vitro* characterization of immunological responsiveness of uremic patients. *Nephron* 26: 234, 1980

58. Kurz P, Kohler H, Meuer S, Hutteroth T, Zum Buschenfelde K-H M: Impaired cellular immune responses in chronic renal failure: Evidence for a T cell defect. *Kidney Int* 29: 1209, 1986

59. Osaki K, Otsuka H, Uomizu K, Harada R, Otsuji Y, Hashimoto S: Monocyte-mediated suppression of mitogen responses of lymphocytes in uremic patients. *Nephron* 34: 87, 1983

60. Huber H, Pastner D, Dittrich P, Braunsteiner H: *In vitro* reactivity of huyman leukocytes in uraemia – a comparison with the impairment of delayed hypersensitivity. *Clin Exp Immunol* 5: 75, 1969

61. Selroos O, Pasternack A, Virolainen M: Skin test sensitivity and antigen-induced lymphocyte transformation in uraemia. *Clin Exp Immunol* 14: 365, 1973

62. Elves MW, Israels MCG, Collinge M: An assessment of the mixed leucocyte reaction in renal failure. *Lancet* 1: 682, 1966

63. Sengar DPS, Hyslop DB, Rashid A, Harris JC: T-rosettes in hemodialysis patients and renal allograft recipients. *Cell Immunol* 20: 92, 1975

64. Kauffman CA, Manzler AD, Phair JP: Cell-mediated immunity in patients on long-term haemodialysis. *Clin Exp Immunol* 22: 54, 1975

65. Kamata K, Okubo M, Sada M: Immunosuppresive factors in uraemic sera are composed of both dialysable and non-dialysable components. *Clin Exp Immunol* 54: 277, 1983

66. Holdsworth SR, Fitzgerald MG, Hosking CS, Atkins RC: The effect of maintenance dialysis on lymphocyte function. I. Haemodialysis. *Clin Exp Immunol* 33: 95, 1978

67. Silk MR: The effect of uremic plasma on lymphocyte transformation. *Invest Urol* 5: 195, 1967

68. Newberry WM, Sanford JP: Defective cellular immunity in renal failure: Depression of reactivity of lymphocytes to phytohemagglutinin by renal failure serum. *J Clin Invest* 50: 1262, 1971

69. Sengar DPS, Rashid A, Harris JE: *In vitro* reactivity of lymphocytes obtained from uraemic patients maintained on hemodialysis. *Clin Exp Immunol* 21: 298, 1975

70. Nakhla LS, Goggin MJ: Lymphocyte transformation in chronic renal failure. *Immunology* 24: 229, 1973

71. Fehrman I, Ringden O, Bergström J: MLC-blocking factors in uremic sera. *Clin Nephrol* 14: 183, 1980

72. Slavin RG, Fitch CD: Inhibition of lymphocyte transformation by guanido succinic acid, a surplus metabolite in uremia. *Experimentai* (Basel) 27: 1340, 1971

73. Hanicki Z, Cichocki T, Sarwecka-Keller M, Klein A, Komorowska Z: Influence of middle-sized molecule aggregates from dialysate of uremic patients on lymphocyte transformation *in vitro*. *Nephron* 17: 73, 1976

74. Harris JE, Page D, Posen G, Stewart T: Supression of *in vitro* lymphocyte function by uremic toxins. *J Urol* 108: 312, 1972

75. Raska K Jr, Morrison AB, Raskova J: Humoral inhibitors of the immune response in uremia. III. The immunosuppressive factor of uremic rat serum is a very low density lipoprotein. *Lab Invest* 42: 636, 1980

76. Stewart E, Miller TE: Host immune status in uraemia. II. Serum factors and lymphocyte transformation. *Clin Exp Immunol* 41: 123, 1980

77. Mezzano S, Pesce AJ, Pollak VE, Michael JG: Analysis of humoral and cellular factors that contribute to impaired immune responsiveness in experimental uremia. *Nephron* 36: 15, 1984

78. Raskova J, Morrison AB: A decrease in cell-mediated immunity in uremia associated with an increase in activity of suppressor cells. *Am J Pathol* 84: 1, 1976

79. Alevy YG, Slavin RG, Hutcheson P: Immune response in experimentally induced uremia. I. Suppression in mitogen responses by adherent cells in chronic uremia. *Clin Immun Immunpath* 19: 8, 1981

80. Raskova J, Raska K: Humoral inhibitors of the immune response in uremia. V. Induction of suppressor cells *in vitro* by uremic serum. *Am J Pathol* 111: 149, 1983

81. Lortran JE, Kiepiela P, Coovadia HM, Seedat YK: Suppressor cells assayed by numerical and functional tests in chronic renal failure. *Kidney Int* 22: 192, 1982

82. Raska K, Raskova J, Shea SM, Frankel RM, Wood RH, Lifter J, Ghobrial I, Eisinger RP, Homer L: T cell subsets and cellular immunity in end-stage renal disease. *Am J Med* 75: 734, 1983

83. Chida Y, Sakurai S, Yoshiyama N: The effect of hemodialysis on lymphocyte subsets during dialysis. *Clin Nephrol* 25: 159, 1986

84. Chatenoud L, Dugas B, Beaurain G, Touam M, Drüeke T, Vasquez A, Galaraud P, Back J-F, DelFraissy J-F: Presence of reactivated T cells in hemodialyzed patients. Their possible role in altered immunity. *Proc Natl Acad Sci* 83: 7457, 1986

85. Raskova J, Ghobrial I, Shea SM, Eisinger RP, Raska K: Suppressor cells in end-stage renal disease. Functional assays and monoclonal antibody analysis. *Am J Med* 76: 847, 1984

86. Guillon PJ, Woodhouse LF, Davison AM, Giles GR: Suppressor cell activity of peripheral mononuclear cells from patients undergoing chronic hemodialysis. *Biomedicine* 32: 11, 1980

87. Ruddy MC, Rubin AL, Novogrodsky A, Stenzel K: Decreased macrophage-mediated suppression of lymphocyte activation in chronic renal failure. *Am J Med* 75: 571, 1983

88. Tsakolos ND, Theoharides TC, Herdler ED, Guffinet J, Dwyer JM, Whisler HL, Askenase PW: Immune defects in chronic renal impairment: evidence for defective regulation of lymphocyte response by macrophages from patients with chronic renal impairment on haemodialysis. *Clin Exp Immunol* 63: 218, 1986

89. Kleiman KS, Zoschke DC: Suppression of human lymphocyte responses in chronic renal failure mediated by adherent cells: analysis in serum-free media. *J Lab Clin Med* 106: 262, 1985

90. Walter WC, Bachvaroff RJ, Raisbeck AP, Egelandsdal B, Pullis C, Shen L, Rapaport FT: Immunologic monitoring in patients with end-stage renal disease. *J Clin Immunol* 4: 364, 1984

91. Sanders LS, Luby JP, Sanford JP, Hull AR: Suppression of interferon response in lymphocytes from patients with uremia. *J Lab Clin Med* 77: 768, 1971

92. Gal G, Toth M, Toth S: Interferon production by leukocytes of dialysed chronic uraemic patients. *Proc Eur Transplant Assoc* 18: 188, 1981

93. Luger A, Kovarik J, Stummvoll H-K, Urbanska A, Luger TA: Blood-membrane interaction in hemodialysis leads to increased cytokine production. *Kidney Int* 32: 84, 1987

94. Bingel M, Lonnemann G, Shaldon S, Koch KM, Dinarello CA: Human interleukin-1 production during hemodialysis. *Nephron* 43: 161, 1986

95. Lonneman G, Koch KM, Shaldon S: Induction of interleukin-1 (IL-1) from human monocytes adhering to hemodialysis (HD) membranes. *Kidney Int* 31: 238, 1987

96. Shaldon S, Bingel M, Lonneman G, Dinarello CA, Koch KM: Human interleukin-1 (IL-1) production is enhanced by sodium acetate. *Abstracts Am Soc Artif Intern Organs* 16: 33, 1987

97. Charpentier B, Lang P, Martin B, Noury J, Mathieu D, Fries D: Depressed polymorphonuclear leukocyte functions associated with normal cytotoxic functions of T and natural killer cells during chronic hemodialysis. *Clin Nephrol* 19: 288, 1983

98. Ringoir S, VanLooy L, Van de Heyning P, Lerous-Roels G: Impairment of phagocytic activity of macrophages as studied by the skin window test in patients on regular hemodialysis treatment. *Clin Nephrol* 4: 234, 1975

99. Hanicki Z, Cichocki T, Komorowska Z, Sulowicz W, Smolenski O: Some aspects of cellular immunity in untreated and maintenance hemodialysis patients. *Nephron* 23: 273, 1979

100. Urbanitz D, Sieberth HG: Impaired phagocytic activity of human monocytes in respect to reduced antibacterial resistance in uremia. *Clin Nephrol* 4: 13, 1975

101. Jorstad S, Viken KE: Inhibitory effects of plasma from uraemic patients on human mononuclear phagocytes cultures *in vitro*. *Acta Pathol Microbiol Scand* (C) 85: 169, 1977

102. Jorstad S, Kvernes S: Uraemic toxins of high molecular weight inhibiting human mononuclear phagocytes cultures *in vitro*. *Acta Pathol Microbiol Scand* (C) 86: 221, 1978

103. Alevy YG, Mueller KR, Slavin RG: Immune response in experimentally induced uremia. VI. Uremic macrophages are defective in their ability to present antigen to T cells. *Clin Immunol Immune Pathol* 29: 433, 1983

104. Gibbons R, Martinez O, Lim V, Garovoy MR: Defective antigen presentation in uremia: a monocyte defect. *Kidney Int* 31: 232, 1987

105. Lewis SL, Van Epps DE, Chenoweth DE: C5a receptor modulation on neutrophils and monocytes from chronic hemodialysis and peritoneal dialysis patients. *Clin Nephrol* 26: 37, 1986

106. Keane WF, Comty CM, Verbrugh HA, Peterson PK: Opsonic deficiency of peritoneal dialysis effluent in continuous ambulatory peritoneal dialysis. *Kidney Int* 25: 539, 1984

107. Keane WF, Peterson PK: Host defense mechanisms of the peritoneal cavity and continuous ambulatory peritoneal dialysis. *Peritoneal Dial Bull* 4: 122, 1984

108. Goldstein CS, Bomalaski JS, Zurier RB, Neilson EG, Douglas SD: Analysis of peritoneal macrophages in continuous peritoneal dialysis patients. *Kidney Int* 26: 733, 1984

109. Duwea K, Vas SI, Weatherhead JW: The effect of the composition of peritoneal dialysis fluid on chemiluminescence phagocytosis and bactericidal activity *in vitro*. *Infect Immunity* 33: 130, 1981

110. Peterson PK, Gaziano E, Devalon M, Peterson LA, Keane WF: Antimicrobial activities of dialysis elicited and resident human peritoneal macrophages. *Infect Immunity* 49: 212, 1985

111. Peterson PK, Lee D, Suh HJ, Devalon M, Nelson RD, Keane WF: Intracellular survival of *Candida albicans* in peritoneal macrophages from chronic peritoneal dialysis patients. *Am J Kidney Dis* 7: 146, 1986

112. Kleinman MF, Doehring RO, Furman KI, Koornhof GJ: Importance of intracellular organisms in CAPD. In: *Frontiers in Peritoneal Dialysis,* edited by Maher JF, Winchester JF, New York, Field, Rich and Assoc, 1986, p 546

113. Verbrugh HA, Van Bronswizk H, Lien P: The fate of phagocytized *Staphylococcus epidermidis:* Survival and growth in human mononuclear phagocytes as a potential pathogenic mechanism. In: *Pathogenicity and Clinical Significance of Coagulase-negative Staphylococci,* edited by Pulvaer G, Quie PG, Peters G, Stuttgart, New York, Gustav Fischer Verlag, 1987, p 55

114. Buggy BP, Schaberg DR, Swartz RD: Intraleukocyte sequestration as a cause of persistent *Staphylococcus aureus* peritonitis in continuous ambulatory peritoneal dialysis. *Am J Med* 76: 1035, 1984

115. Lamperi S, Carozzi S: Defective opsonic activity of peritoneal effluent during continuous ambulatory peritoneal dialysis (CAPD): Importance and prevention. *Peritoneal Dial Bull* 6: 87, 1986

116. Lamperi S, Carozzi S: Suppressor resident peritoneal macrophages and peritonitis incidence in continous ambulatory peritoneal dialysis. *Nephron* 44: 219, 1986

117. Jensson O: Observations on the blood leucocyte picture in acute uraemia. *Br J Haematol* 4: 422, 1958

118. Riis P, Stougaard J: The peripheral blood leukocytes in chronic renal insufficiency. *Dan Med Bull* 6: 85, 1959

119. Vincent PC, Sutherland R, Morris TCM, Chapman GV: Inhibitor of *in vitro* granulopoiesis in plasma of patients with renal failure. *Lancet* 2: 864, 1978

120. Craddock PR, Fehr J, Dalmasso AP, Brigham KL, Jacob HS: Hemodialysis leukopenia. Pulmonary vascular leukostasis resulting from complement activation by dialyzer cellophane membranes. *J Clin Invest* 59: 879, 1977

121. Peresecenschi G, Blum M, Aviram A, Spirer ZH: Impaired neutrophil response to acute bacterial infection in dialyzed patients. *Arch Intern Med* 191: 1301, 1981

122. Brayton RG, Stokes PE, Schwartz MS, Louria DB: Effect of alcohol and various diseases on leukocyte mobilization, phagocytosis and intracellular bacterial killing. *N Engl J Med* 282: 123, 1970

123. Buchanan WW, Klinenberg JR, Seegmiller JE: The inflammatory response to injected microcrystalline monosodium urate in normal hyperuremic, gouty and uremic subjects. *Arthritis Rheum* 8: 361, 1968

124. Abrutyn E, Solomons NW, St. Clair L, MacGregor RR, Root RK: Granulocyte function in patients with chronic renal failure: Surface adherence, phagocytosis and bacteriocidal activity *in vitro. J Infect Dis* 135: 1, 1977

125. Lespier-Dexter LE, Guerra C, Ojeda W, Martinez-Maldonado M: Granulocyte adherence in uremia and hemodialysis. *Nephron* 24: 64, 1979

126. Salant DJ, Glover A-M, Anderson R, Meyers AM, Rabkin R, Myburgh JA, Rabson AR: Depressed neutrophil chemotaxis in patients with chronic renal failure and after renal transplantation. *J Lab Clin Med* 88: 536, 1976

127. Siriwatratananonta P, Sinsakul V, Stern K, Slavin RG: Defective chemotaxis in uremia. *J Lab Clin Med* 92: 402, 1978

128. Greene WH, Ray C, Mauer SM, Quie PG: The effect of hemodialysis on neutrophil chemotactic responsiveness. *J Lab Clin Med* 88: 971, 1976

129. Bjorksten B, Mauer SM, Mills EL, Quie PG: The effect of hemodialysis on neutrophil chemotactic responsiveness. *Acta Med Scand* 203: 67, 1978

130. Goldblum SE, Van Epps DE, Reed WP: Serum inhibitor of C5 fragment-mediated polymorphonuclear leukocyte chemotaxis associated with chronic hemodialysis. *J Clin Invest* 64: 255, 1979

131. Hallgren R, Fjellstrom K-E, Hakansson L, Venge P: The serum-independent uptake of IgG-coated particles by polymorphonuclear leukocytes from uremic patients on regular dialysis treatment. *J Lab Clin Med* 94: 277, 1979

132. Montgomery JZ, Kalmanson GM, Guze LB: Leukocyte phagocytosis and serum bactericidal activity in chronic renal failure. *Am J Med Sci* 264: 385, 1972

133. Ritchey EE, Wallin JD, Shah SV: Chemiluminescence and superoxide anion production by leukocytes from chronic hemodialysis patients. *Kidney Int* 19: 349, 1981

134. Cohen MS, Elliot DM, Chaplinski T, Pike MM, Niedel JE: A defect in the oxidative metabolism of human polymorphonuclear leukocytes that remain in circulation early in hemodialysis. *Blood* 60: 1283, 1982

135. Briggs WA, Sillix DH, Mahajan S, McDonald FD: Leukocyute metabolism and function in uremia. *Kidney Int* 24 (Suppl 16): 593, 1983

136. Chandra RK: Rosette-forming T lymphocytes and cell-mediated immunity in malnutrition. *Br Med J* 3: 608, 1974

137. Schopfer K, Douglas SD: Neutrophil function in children with kwashiorkor. *J Lab Clin Med* 88: 450, 1976

138. Thunberg BJ, Swamy AP, Cestero RVM: Cross-sectional and longitudinal nutritional measurements in maintenance hemodialysis patients. *Am J Clin Nutr* 34: 2005, 1980

139. Guarnier G, Ranieri F, Lipartiti T, Spangaro F, Giuntini D, Faccini L, Toigo G, Legnani F, Raimandi A, Campanacci L: Protein-calorie malnutrition in hemodialysis patients. *Int J Artif Organs* 3: 143, 1980

140. Comty CM, Wathen RL, Shapiro F: Protein metabolism in renal failure. *Urology* 1: 528, 1973

141. Mattern WD, Hak LJ, Lamanna RW, Tensley KM, Laffell MS: Malnutrition, altered immune function, and the risk of infection in maintenance hemodialysis patients. *Am J Kidney Dis* 1: 206, 1982

142. Glassock RJ: Nutrition, immunology, and renal disease. *Kidney Int* 74 (Suppl 16): S194, 1983

143. Acchiardo SR, Moore LW, Latour PA: Malnutrition as the main factor in morbidity and mortality of hemodialysis patients. *Kidney Int* 24 (Suppl 16): S199, 1983

144. Wolfsun M, Strong CJ, Minturn D, Gray DK, Kopple JD: Nutritional status and lymphocyte function in maintenance hemodialysis patients. *Am J Clin Nutr* 39: 547, 1984

145. Hak LJ, Lefell MS, Lamanna RW, Teasley KM, Bazzarre CH, Mattern WD: Reversal of skin test anergy during maintenance hemodialysis by protein and caloric supplementation *Am J Clin Nutr* 36: 1089, 1982

146. Casciato DA, McAdam LP, Kopple JD, Bluestone R, Goldberg LS, Clements PJ, Knutson DW: Immunologic abnormalities in hemodialysis patients: improvement after pyridoxine therapy. *Nephron* 38: 9, 1984

147. Antoniou LD, Shalhoub RJ, Schechter GP: The effect of zinc on cellular immunity in chronic uremia. *Am J Clin Nutr* 34: 1912, 1981

148. Antoniou LD, Shalhoub RJ: Zinc-induced enhancement of lymphocyte function and viability in chronic uremia. *Nephron* 40: 13, 1985

149. Briggs WA, Pederson MM, Mahajan SK, Sillix DH, Prasad AS, McDonald FD: Lymphocyte and granulocyte function in zinc-treated and zinc-deficient hemodialysis patients. *Kidney Int* 21: 827, 1982

150. Opelz G, Sengar DPS, Mickey MR, Terasaki PI: Effect of

blood transfusions on subsequent kidney transplants. *Transplant Proc* 5: 523, 1973

151. Opelz G, Terasaki PI; Improvement of kidney-graft survival with increased numbers of blood transfusions. *N Engl J Med* 299: 799, 1978

152. Bender BS, Curtis JL, Nagel JE, Chrest FJ, Kraus ES, Briefel GR, Adler WH: Analysis of immune status of hemodialyzed adults: Association with prior transfusion. *Kidney Int* 26: 436, 1984

153. Fehrman I, Ringden O, Moller E, Lundgren G, Groth C-G: Is cell-mediated immunity in the uremic patient affected by blood transfusion? *Transplant Proc* 13: 164, 1981

154. Klatzmann D, Gluckman JC, Foucault C, Bensussan A, Assobga U, Duboust A: Suppression of lymphocyte reactivity by blood transfusions in uremic patients. *Transplantation* 35: 332, 1983

155. Kerman RH, Van Buren CT, Payne W, Flechner S, Agostino G, Conley S, Brewer E, Kahan BD: The influence of pretransplant blood transfusions from random donors on immune parameters affecting cadaveric allograft survival. *Transplantation* 36: 50, 1983

156. Smith MD, Hardy G, Williams JD, Coles GA: Suppressor cell numbers and activity in non-transfused renal dialysis patients. *Clin Nephrol* 20: 130, 1983

157. Smith MD, Williams JD, Coles GA, Salaman JR: The effect of blood transfusion on T-suppressor cells in renal dialysis patients. *Transplant Proc* 13: 181, 1981

158. Smith MD, Williams JD, Coles GA, Salaman JR: Blood transfusions, suppressor T cells, and renal transplant survival. *Transplantation* 36: 647, 1983

159. Klatzmann D, Bensussan A, Gluckman JC, Foucault C, Dansset J, Sasportes M: Blood transfusions suppress lymphocyte reactivity in uremic patients. II. Evidence for soluble suppressor factors. *Transplantation* 36: 337, 1983

160. Roy R, Lachance J-G, Noel R, Grose JH, Beaudoin R: Improved renal allograft function and survival following nonspecific blood transfusions. I. Induction of soluble suppressor factors inhibiting the mitogenic response. *Transplantation* 41: 640, 1986

161. Keane WF, Shapiro FL, Raij L: Incidence and type of infections occurring in 445 chronic hemodialysis patients. *Trans Am Soc Artif Intern Organs* 23: 41, 1977

162. Maddy M, Keane WF: Unpublished observations.

163. Dobkin JF, Miller MH, Steigbigel NH: Septicemia in patients on chronic hemodialysis. *Ann Intern Med* 88: 28, 1978

164. Nsouli KA, Lazarus M, Schoenbaum SC, Gottlieb MN, Lowrie EG, Shocair M: Bacteremic infection in hemodialysis. *Arch Intern Med* 139: 1255, 1979

165. Kirmani N, Tuazon CU, Murray HW, Parrish AE, Sheagren JN: *Staphylococcus aureus* carriage rate of patients receiving long-term hemodialysis. *Arch Intern Med* 138: 1657, 1978

166. Goldblum SE, Ulrich JA, Goldman RS, Reed WP: Nasal and cutaneous flora among hemodialysis patients and personnel: Quantitative and qualitative characterization and patterns of *Staphylococcal* carriage. *Am J Kidney Dis* 2: 281, 1982

167. Yu VL, Goetz A, Wagener M, Smith PB, Rihs JD, Hanchett J, Zuravleff JJ; *Staphylococcus aureus* nasal carriage and infection in patients on hemodialysis. Efficacy of antibiotic prophylaxis. *N Engl J Med* 315: 91, 1986

168. Latos DL, Stone WJ, Alford RH: *Staphylococcus aureus* bacteremia in hemodialysis patients. *J Dial* 1: 399, 1977

169. Francioli P, Masur H: Complications of *Staphylococcus aureus* bacteremia. Occurrence in patients undergoing long-term hemodialysis. *Arch Intern Med* 142: 1655, 1982

170. Quarles LD, Rutsky EA, Rostard SG: *Staphylococcus aureus* bacteremia in patients on chronic hemodialysis. *Am J Kidney Dis* 6: 412, 1985

171. Comty CM, Cohen SL, Shapiro FL: Pericarditis in chronic uremia and its sequels. *Ann Intern Med* 75: 173, 1971

172. Bailey GI, Hampers CL, Hager EB, Merrill JP: Uremic pericarditis: Clinical features and management. *Circulation* 38: 582, 1968

173. Leonard A, Raij L, Shapiro FL: Bacterial endocarditis in regularly dialyzed patients. *Kidney Int* 4: 401, 1973

174. Goodman JS, Crews HD, Ginn HE, Koenig MG: Bacterial endocarditis as a possible complication of chronic hemodialysis. *N Engl J Med* 280: 876, 1969

175. King LH Jr, Bradley KP, Shires DL Jr, Donohue JP, Glover JL: Bacterial endocarditis in chronic hemodialysis patients: a complication more common than previously suspected. *Surgery* 69: 554, 1971

176. Ribot S, Rothfeld D, Frankel HJ: Infectious endocarditis in maintenance hemodialysis patients. *Am J Med Sci* 264: 183, 1972

177. Keane WF, Raij LR: Host defenses and infectious complications in maintenance hemodialysis patients. In: *Replacement of Renal Function by Dialysis*, edited by Drukker W, Parsons FM, Maher JF, Second Edition, The Hague. Martinus Nijhoff, 1983, p 646

178. Matthews M, Shen F-H, Lindner A, Sherrard DJ: Septic arthritis in hemodialyzed patients. *Nephron* 25: 87, 1980

179. Parker MA, Tuazon CU: Cervical osteomyelitis. Infection due to *Staphylococcus epidermidis* in hemodialysis patients. *JAMA* 240: 50, 1978

180. Leonard A, Comty CM, Shapiro FL, Raij L: Osteomyelitis in hemodialysis patients. *Ann Intern Med* 78: 651, 1973

181. Goodwin NJ, Castronuovo JJ, Friedman EA: Recurrent septic pulmonary embolization complicating maintenance hemodialysis. *Ann Intern Med* 71: 29, 1969

182. Levi J, Robson M, Rosenfeld JB: Septicemia and pulmonary embolism complicating use of arteriovenous fistula in maintenance haemodialysis. *Lancet* 2: 288, 1970

183. Shapiro FL, Messner RP, Smith UT: Satellite hemodialysis. *Ann Intern Med* 69: 673, 1968

184. Aman LC, Levin NW, Smith DW: Hemodialysis access site morbidity. *Proc Clin Dial Transplant Forum* 10: 277, 1980

185. Porter JA, Sharp WV, Walsh EJ: Complications of vascular access in a dialysis population. *Current Surgery* 42: 298, 1985

186. Winsett OE, Wolma FJ: Complications of vascular access for hemodialysis. *South Med J* 78: 513, 1985

187. Kaslow RA, Zellner SR: Infection in patients on hemodialysis. *Lancet* 2: 117, 1972

188. Ralston AJ, Harlow GR, Jones DM, Davis P: Infections of Scribner and Brescia arteriovenous shunts. *Br Med J* 3: 408, 1971

189. Brescia MJ, Cimino JE, Appel K, Hurwich BJ: Chronic hemodialysis using venipuncture and a surgically created arteriovenous fistula. *N Engl J Med* 275: 1089, 1966

190. Kinnaert P, Vereerstraeten P, Toussaint C, Van Geertrayden J: Nine year's experience with internal arteriovenous fistulas for haemodialysis. *Br J Surg* 64: 242, 1977

191. Palder SB, Kirkman RL, Whittemore AD, Hakim RM, La Zarns IM, Tilney NL: Vascular access for hemodialysis. *Ann Surg* 202: 235, 1985

192. Vanderwerf BA, Rattazzi LC, Katzma KA, Schild AF: Three year experience with bovine graft arteriovenous (A-V) fistulas in 100 patients. *Trans Am Soc Artif Intern Organs* 21: 296, 1975

193. Yokoyama T, Bower R, Chinitz J, Schwartz A, Swartz C: Experience with 100 bovine arteriografts for maintenance hemodialysis. *Trans Am Soc Artif Intern Organs* 20: 328, 1974

194. Merickel JH, Anderson RC, Knutson R, Lipshultz ML, Hitchcock CR: Bovine carotid artery shunts in vascular access surgery. *Arch Surg* 109: 245, 1974

195. Lilly L, Ngheim D, Mendez-Picon G, Lee HM: Comparison between bovine heterograft and expanded PTFE grafts for dialysis access. *Am J Surg* 46: 694, 1980

196. Bhat DJ, Tellis VA, Kohlberg WI, Driscoll B, Veith FJ: Management of sepsis involving expanded polyterafluoroethylene grafts for hemodialysis access. *Surgery* 87: 445, 1980

197. Savanayagam P, Schwartz AB, Soricelli RR, Lyons R, Chinitz J: A comparative study of 402 bovine heterografts and 225 reinforced expanded PTFE grafts as AVF in the ESRD patients. *Trans Am Soc Artif Intern Organs* 26: 88, 1980

198. Nissenson AR: The bioCARBON vascular access system (bVAS)* no-needle hemodialysis. *Trans Am Soc Artif Intern Organs* 29: 784, 1983

199. Collins AJ, Ilstrup K, Keshaviah P, Shapiro F: Multicenter clinical experience with the Hemasite® blood access device. *Trans Am Soc Artif Intern Organs* 29: 789, 1983

200. Ngheim DD, Schulak JA, Corry RJ: Management of the infected hemodialysis access grafts. *Trans Am Soc Artif Intern Organs* 29: 360, 1983

201. Morris AJ, Bilinsky RT: Prevention of staphylococcal shunt infections by continuous vancomycin prophylaxis. *Am J Med Sci* 261: 88, 1971

202. Bass HE, Singer E: Pulmonary changes in uremia. *JAMA* 144: 819, 1950

203. Bass HE, Greenberg D, Singer E: Pulmonary changes in uremia. *JAMA* 148: 724, 1952

204. Hopps HC, Wissler RW: Uremic pneumonitis. *Am J Pathol* 31: 261, 1955

205. Rackow EL, Fein IA, Sprung C, Grodman RS: Uremic pulmonary edema. *Am J Med* 64: 1084, 1978

206. Goldstein E, Green GM: The effect of acute renal failure on the bacterial clearance mechanisms of the lung. *J Lab Clin Med* 68: 531, 1966

207. Johanson WG, Pierce AK, Sanford JP: Changing pharyngeal bacterial flora of hospitalized patients. *N Engl J Med* 281: 1137, 1969

208. Jadav SK, Sant SM, Acharya VN: Bacteriology of urinary tract infection in patients of renal failure undergoing dialysis. *J Postgrad Med* 23: 10, 1977

209. Saitoh H, Nakamura K, Hida M, Satoh T: Urinary tract infection in oliguric patients with chronic renal failure. *J Urol* 133: 990, 1985

210. Rault R: Symptomatic urinary tract infection in patients on maintenance hemodialysis. *Nephron* 37: 82, 1989

211. Bennett WM, Craven R: Urinary tract infections in patients with severe renal disease. *JAMA* 236: 946, 1976

212. Pradham RP, Katz LA, Nidus BD, Matalon R, Eisinger RP: Tuberculosis in dialyzed patients. *JAMA* 229: 798, 1974

213. Papadimitriou M, Memmos D, Metaxas P: Tuberculosis in patients on regular hemodialysis. *Nephron* 24: 53, 1979

214. Andrew OT, Schoenfeld P, Hopewell PC, Humphreys M: Tuberculosis in patients with end-stage renal disease. *Am J Med* 68: 59, 1980

215. Lundin AP, Adler AJ, Berlyne GM, Friedman EA: Tuberculosis in patients undergoing maintenance hemodialysis. *Am J Med* 67: 597, 1979

216. Rutsky EA, Rostand SG: Mycobacteriosis in patients with chronic renal failure. *Arch Intern Med* 140: 57, 1980

217. Sasaki S, Akiba T, Suenaga M, Tomura S, Yoshiyama N, Nakagawa S, Shoji T, Sasaoka T, Takeuchi J: Ten years' survey of dialysis-associated tuberculosis. *Nephron* 24: 141, 1979

218. Belcon MC, Smith EKM, Kahana LM, Shimizu AG: Tuberculosis in dialysis patients. *Clin Nephrol* 17: 14, 1982

219. Zeitlin J, Carvounis CP, Murphy RG, Tortora GT: Graft infection and bacteremia with *Listeria monocytogenes* in a patient receiving hemodialysis. *Arch Intern Med* 142: 2191, 1982

220. Woolridge TD, Cox JW: Graft infection and bacteremia. *Arch Intern Med* 143: 1070, 1983

221. Mossey RT, Sondheimer J: Listerosis in patients with long-term hemodialysis and transfusional iron overload. *Am J Med* 79: 393, 1985

DIALYSIS ASSOCIATED HEPATITIS

JEAN CROSNIER, FRANÇOISE DEGOS and PAUL JUNGERS

INTRODUCTION

Viral hepatitis, especially type B hepatitis, is a major problem in dialysis units throughout the world. Due to the deficient immune status of uremic subjects, which renders them unable to eliminate the virus, infected patients acting as virus reservoirs transmit the infection to other patients, to dialysis unit staff, to other categories of hospital personnel, and to their own families.

Until 1982, despite all efforts directed towards detection and isolation of infected patients, prevention of cross-infection and passive immunotherapy, an alarming increase in the number of infected patients and staff was observed in most countries, and hepatitis B was responsible for considerable morbidity and mortality.

Only since the start of active immunization by hepatitis B vaccine in 1982 has a decline in the incidence of infection been observed. Thus, the development of safe and efficient vaccines against hepatitis B virus was an important therapeutic advance. At the present time, thanks to extensive vaccination, eradication of hepatitis B from dialysis units and protection of all health care workers is becoming an attainable goal.

FREQUENCY AND SEVERITY OF VIRAL HEPATITIS IN DIALYSIS UNITS

Pre-serologic period

An abnormally high incidence of hepatitis in hemodialysis units, among both patients and staff, has been noted from the very beginning of hemodialysis treatment, in Europe (1–6) and in the United States (7–10). The outbreaks were often epidemic, and several fatal cases were reported among staff and patients (11). The annual statistical reports of the European Dialysis and Transplant Association clearly reflected a rapid spread of hepatitis in hemodialysis units. A center was considered contaminated when at least two persons, either patients or staff, had contracted clinically apparent hepatitis. In 1967, 23% of the 81 European units reporting were contaminated. During that year, 45 dialysis patients and 26 staff members had become infected (12). Four years later, 43% of the 367 European centers were contaminated, with 583 patients and 402 staff members having contracted the disease (13). The fatality rate in Europe in 1972 was 2.4% among staff and 0.2% among dialysis patients; hepatitis accounted for about 2% of all deaths in these patients (14). The situation was no better in the U.S.A., where a survey of 65 centers between 1967 and 1970 showed that, on the basis of clinically apparent jaundice or elevation of transaminases, 55 centers (82%) were contaminated (15).

Virus B hepatitis

After 1970, when serologic detection of the surface antigen of hepatitis B virus (HBsAg), initially termed 'Australia antigen', became routinely available (16, 17), the incidence of hepatitis B infection could be accurately evaluated. It became evident that, since HBV infection is often clinically asymptomatic in dialysis patients (9), its actual spread was greater than supposed.

On the basis of HBs antigenemia, 48% of the 702 units in Europe were contaminated in 1973 (18). Of a total number of 16,237 patients treated, of whom 11,014 were regularly screened for HBsAg, 1,095 (10%) contracted HBsAg-positive hepatitis during the year and 1,150 (10.4%) were chronic carriers of the antigen; during the same year 604 staff members became infected, and three of these cases were fatal. A point-prevalence study in 15 dialysis units in the United States in 1973 indicated a similarly high contamination rate, with HBsAg positivity in 16% of patients and 2% of staff, and a further 34% of patients and 31% of staff having serologic evidence of past infection (19). Moreover, more than half of the home contacts of carrier patients, particularly the spouse, were infected, and HBV infection rapidly gained among other hospital staff members, especially laboratory personnel and transplant teams.

In some countries, especially in the United Kingdom and Scandinavia, prophylactic measures against cross infection and for early detection and isolation of infected patients had effectively prevented the spread of virus B hepatitis. However, the disease remained highly endemic in dialysis units in most other countries. At the beginning of the 1980s, despite partial protection by specific immunoglobulins, contamination among patients and staff reached its highest rates. The total number of new cases in Europe attained nearly 1,800 per year in patients and 500 in staff in 1979 and 1980 (20, 21). From 1982 to 1985, with the beginning of vaccination programs in France and Belgium (22), followed by other countries, the annual incidence decreased in Europe as a whole. This decline was especially evident in staff (23–26) and was less in dialysis patients, in whom a mean of about 1,400 new cases per year was recorded during the same period.

Virus A hepatitis

At the same time, with the development of specific serologic markers for type A hepatitis virus (HAV) (27, 28), it became apparent that some cases of hepatitis were due to HAV. However, the incidence of HAV hepatitis in dialysis units was considerably lower than that of HBV. In the United States, a study in 15 dialysis units revealed a prevalence rate of serologic markers for HAV in patients and staff identical to that observed in socioeconomically comparable blood donors of similar age range (29). In Europe, the EDTA reports indicate an incidence of new cases of type A hepatitis of about 50 per year in dialysis patients and about 20 per year

in staff during the past 6 years (21–26). As no fatality was observed, and as HAV does not appear to be associated with a chronic carrier state (29) or to induce chronic liver disease (30), type A hepatitis does not represent a major problem in dialysis units.

Non-A, non-B hepatitis

By contrast, after the development of serologic techniques for the identification of type A and type B hepatitis, another type of serum-transmitted hepatitis was recognized by exclusion. It could not be ascribed to HAV or HBV, or to cytomagalovirus (CMV) or Epstein-Barr virus (EBV), and was termed non-A, non-B (NANB) hepatitis virus (31). This type of hepatitis is transmitted parenterally, mainly by blood transfusions (32–34) because the lack of specific serologic markers precludes screening of donor blood for the NANB virus. Even the exclusion of blood donors with high alanine-aminotransferase (ALT) activity (35) does not completely protect against the risk of NANB transmission, and dialysis patients have thus been infected through blood transfusions. Reports of NANB hepatitis in dialysis units are few, probably because in units with widespread HBV infection, NANB may pass unnoticed. In HBV-free units, on the other hand, clusters of patients with abnormal ALT levels have been reported (36–39). These reports mention a frequent tendency to progression toward chronic hepatitis, as in other transfused patients (40–42). Since 1980 the EDTA reports have analytically distinguished among the annual incidence of HBV, HAV and NANB hepatitis in European dialysis units (22–26). In the year 1980, the proportion of NANB hepatitis was 17% of 2,235 cases of hepatitis in patients and 9% of 566 cases in staff (21). During the subsequent 5 years, as shown in Table 1, the progressive decrease of HBV infection in dialysis units, due to extensive vaccination programs in several European countries, has been offset by a growing number of cases of NANB hepatitis, with a mean incidence of more than 700 new cases per year. This figure represents more than 30% of all cases of hepatitis in patients. Among staff members both the absolute annual number and the proportion of NANB to other types of hepatitis remained quite unchanged (22–26).

Hepatitis in transplant recipients

In transplanted patients, a high incidence of HBV infection was noted long ago (6, 43) since in most patients, antigenemia was present during maintenance dialysis treatment. Once infected, transplanted patients usually remained chronic carriers, thus contributing to the spread of HBV infection among hospital staff.

The incidence of HBV infection was evaluated as low in the first studies on liver disorders in kidney transplant recipients. However, the laboratory tests used in the early 1970s are now considered to have been poorly sensitive, and this early evaluation may therefore have underestimated the incidence (44–46). Nevertheless, the prevalence of HBV infection reported for North American and French transplant recipients is clearly different. This discrepancy may be due to different means of selecting patients for renal transplantation, as well as to the treatment in French units of a large number of patients from the Mediterranean region, where the prevalence of HBV infection is high. Before vaccination the incidence of HBV infection in renal transplantation units was 3% in North America (47) and 45% in our French center (48). Since the introduction of vaccination, three series in North America reported similar low incidences of 1%, 10% and 6% (49–51) while a higher incidence of 17% was found in South Africa (52). In our French center the prevalence of documented HBV infection since 1981, after the introduction of HBV vaccination, is 15.8% (53).

HEPATITIS IN HEMODIALYZED PATIENTS AND DIALYSIS STAFF

Since the epidemiology and clinical aspects of NANB infection are very similar to those of HBV, they can be described in the same chapter. However, since there is unfortunately still no reliable marker for non-A, non-B virus, epidemiologic studies can only be made by exclusion, and the relationships between non-A, non-B and HBV or HBV-related viruses will be discussed below.

Virus B hepatitis

Acute hepatitis due to hepatitis B virus

The clinical course of HBV infection in hemodialysis patients is known to be remarkably asymptomatic, without jaundice, and with its major risk being a tendency to chronic progression. This tendency has been attributed to immunodepression due to chronic renal failure. A study of dialysis patients showed that both persistent HBs carriers and patients without evidence of past or present HBV infection

had a significant decrease in both absolute number of lymphocytes and in functional T lymphocytes. There was no significant difference between the number of T lymphocytes in dialysis patients who had made a normal recovery from HBV infection as compared with healthy normal subjects (54), suggesting that the response to HBV infection may depend on the severity of immunodepression. However, host factors influence the outcome, e.g. males are more likely than females to develop chronic carriage (9), and differences in the major histocompatibility system have also been described (55).

HBV infection, defined as the presence of HBsAg in the serum, can be divided into several phases. Among patients with detectable HBsAg in the serum, viral replication, that is *the* active form of the disease, can be detected using either serological markers, i.e., the HBe/anti-HBe system, or molecular markers of viral replication, namely the detection of DNA polymerase activity, the enzyme involved in viral replication (56) or better, the detection of HBV DNA in serum. This stage is associated with the presence of free viral DNA in the liver and in this case viral replication can be ascertained (57, 58).

Typically, in patients with normal renal function, HBsAg appears in the serum 8 weeks after exposure, simultaneously with HBe (59) (Figure 1). Two weeks later anti-HBc can be detected in the serum. The first serological sign of improvement is the disappearance of HBeAg and the appearance of anti-HBe at the fourth week. Then HBsAg disappears and anti-HBs appears by 12 weeks. In dialysis patients, the evolution of these serological markers is greatly delayed and the usual time interval of 6 months used to predict the course and resolution of acute viral hepatitis must be increased to 12 months. Moreover, the risk of developing HBs chronic carriage, evaluated as approximately 5% of the patients with acute hepatitis in Europe and North America, is much higher, approximately 30% of hemodialysis patients (60, 61).

Table 1. Annual incidence of new cases of B, A and NANB hepatitis in dialysis units in Europe between 1980 and 1985.

Type of hepatitis	1980	1981	1982	1983	1984	1985
Patients						
B	1801	1614	1360	1473	1402	1384
A	52	63	71	85	41	54
NANB	382 (17%)*	541 (24%)	566 (28%)	728 (32%)	731 (34%)	744 (34%)
Total	2235	2218	1997	2286	2174	2182
Staff						
B	493 (11)**	460 (19)	315 (5)	275 (0)	251 (1)	263 (0)
A	22	23	12	29	13	11
NANB	51 (9%)*	41 (8%)	52 (7%)	24 (7%)	96 (26%)	38 (13%)
Total	566	524	379	328	360	285

* In brackets: % of NANB hepatitis vs. total number of viral hepatitis.
** In brackets: number of fatal cases.

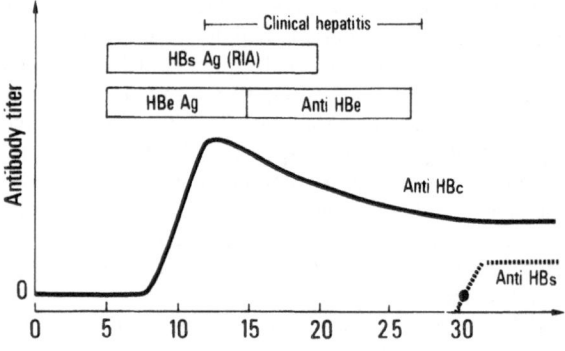

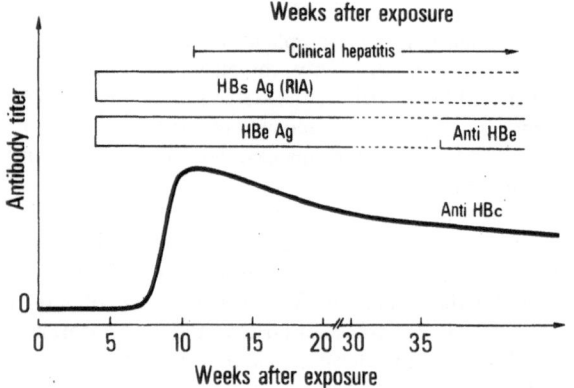

Figure 1. Comparative course of HBV markers in non-uremic patients with acute viral hepatitis (top) and in hemodialyzed patients infected with HBV (bottom).

Hepatitis B virus chronic infection

Infection with HBV can be observed either during the phase of viral replication with detectable serological markers such as HBeAg, DNA polymerase or HBV DNA, and of course HBsAg, or at the later phase of infection when viral replication has disappeared and the virus is integrated in the host genome. At this later period, HBsAg is still present but the serological markers of replication have disappeared and anti-HBe can be detected (62). This virological status is not directly related to the histological lesions and serological and biochemical abnormalities cannot be considered as reflecting (and therefore not predictive of) the histological status of the liver (63).

In general more than half of the infected patients in dialysis units become persistent symptomless HBsAg carriers without biochemical evidence of hepatitis. However, in these patients markers of high infectivity, i.e., HBeAg, HBV DNA and/or high levels of DNA polymerase activity are found in the serum (62). In the others, biochemical abnormalities may persist longer than one year, and a liver biopsy is indicated to detect the possibility of chronic liver disease.

In a group of 111 hemodialyzed patients studied between 1972 and 1980 (64), 71 patients became HBsAg positive at some time during follow-up. The interval between initiation of dialysis and detection of HBsAg ranged from 1 to 29 months (mean 7.3 months). Fifty-one patients remained persistently HBsAg positive (72%) and 20 reverted to HBsAg negative with or without detectable anti-HBs (28%). In this latter group, the duration of HBs antigenemia ranged from 1 to 48 months (mean 11.4 months) with only 80% reverting to anti-HBs within 6 months. The patients can therefore be divided into three groups according to HBV markers: chronic HBV carriers (HBsAg positive with or without viral replication), patients with transient and resolved HBV infection (anti-HBs and/or anti-HBc positive) and patients without any obvious marker of present or past HBV infection (no HBV marker). (Currently, the use of HBV vaccination in these patients would provide a fourth group, those who have developed active anti-HBs antibodies.)

Two points can be made on the basis of the above observations:

1) The extended duration of HBs antigenemia in hemodialyzed patients suggests that a patient must be followed-up for 12 months after occurrence of HBV infection before being considered as a chronic HBV carrier.

2) The ability of hemodialyzed patients to develop anti-HBs can be evaluated as approximately 28 to 30%. This event, which is of major importance in the course of HBV infection, is virtually never observed after transplantation; among 1,000 patients in the literature, only two cases have been reported (47, 53).

Histological lesions

With regard to the histological lesions observed in such patients, a current problem is to determine whether they should be taken into account in the selection of candidates for renal transplantation. Very few studies are available on this question, however. The risk involved in performing transparietal liver biopsy in hemodialysis patients is certainly higher than in other patients; all teams have experienced severe complications such as hemoperitonitis or intrahepatic hematomas. In our experience such events were rare and never fatal. Disorders of primary hemostasis, most of which are undectectable on usual tests, even the measurement of Ivy bleeding time, are probably responsible for such complications in these patients, who receive heparin at each hemodialysis session. We have therefore decided to perform all needle biopsies in hemodialysis patients by the transjugular venous approach which appears safe and gives liver samples of sufficient size when performed in specialized centers (65). Given the safety of this method, it is our opinion that liver biopsy should be performed to evaluate the histological liver status of all hemodialysis patients who have biochemical liver abnormalities for over 12 months.

In any case, the histological lesions observed at the time of renal transplantation can be considered the consequence of the previous period of treatment by hemodialysis.

The severity of histological lesions is usually evaluated according to the international classification (66) in healthy carriers, i.e., chronic persistent hepatitis and chronic active hepatitis with or without cirrhosis. However, in these immunocompromised patients the distinction between chronic persistent and chronic active hepatitis appears arbitrary since the inflammatory process usually does not respect the limiting plate and necrosis is generally absent or mild. Therefore, the tendency at the present time is to distinguish between patients with normal liver and patients with chronic hepatitis, with or without cirrhosis (52).

The histological status of the 111 hemodialysis patients in the series described above was studied. The incidence of HBV infection has of course decreased in France since that time, due to large-scale vaccination programs and the institution of HBV-free centers. Nevertheless, this study was informative with regard to HBV-related events in patients receiving regular hemodialysis treatment. Among the 111 patients studied, 61 underwent liver biopsy because of a suspected liver disease, and in 50 the biopsy was performed during abdominal surgery (nephrectomy or splenectomy). Among the 111 patients, histological examination showed normal liver in 39 and chronic hepatitis in 72. The liver lesions were studied in relation to HBV markers. Of the 51 HBsAg carriers, only eight had normal liver, whereas among the patients with antibodies to HBV or without any HBV markers, 31/60 (50%) had normal liver. Severe chronic hepatitis was observed in 21 patients, all of them HBsAg positive (Table 2).

Among the 51 HBsAg carriers, viral replication evaluated by the presence of HBeAg was present in 30. Such replication was associated with severe histologic features since 9/11 patients with chronic active hepatitis with or without cirrhosis had viral replication detectable by HBeAg or by more direct means which detect molecular signs of multiplication such as DNA polymerase activity, or HBV DNA detection by molecular hybridization in the serum.

Histological follow-up

The progression of liver lesions during the hemodialysis period, compared with the evolutive risk when renal failure is treated by transplantation, remains the main question. This study did not yield sufficient information on this point since only 14 hemodialysis patients, 10 of them HBsAg carriers, had a second liver biopsy. However, among the 10 HBsAg carriers, four already had chronic active hepatitis and further deterioration of liver status was observed in these four. Another series in the literature reports the hepatologic course in 10 patients who were chronic HBsAg carriers treated by regular hemodialysis. Clearance of HBsAg was observed in 4/10, and over a 5-year follow-up, only one patient was considered to have chronic active hepatitis (67).

Delta virus

The Delta virus, a defective RNA virus, occurs only in the presence of HBs antigen (68). Infection with Delta virus may occur simultaneously with HBV infection (called a co-infection), or as a superinfection in an HBV chronic carrier. Superinfection with Delta virus has not been described in the literature in hemodialysis patients. It is a very rare event in renal transplant recipients; two cases of superinfection in association with fulminant liver failure were recently reported (69).

Hepatitis in HBsAg negative patients

Since the first studies on hepatitis in hemodialyzed patients and in kidney transplant recipients, acute and chronic hepatitis in non-HBs carriers have been documented (70, 71).

Hepatitis A virus and viruses of the herpes group

Hepatitis A virus (HAV) does not represent a major problem in dialysis units (29). Its prevalence varies according to geographic area. Other hepatitis observed in this particular group of patients was attributed to various viruses such as herpes simplex virus (72–75) or cytomegalovirus, especially in renal transplant recipients, but mainly to non-A, non-B virus (76, 77).

The so-called non-A non-B infections

In the absence of a reliable marker for non-A, non-B infection, its possible role cannot be confirmed. However, the clinical entity of NANB infection is obvious to all physicians, and differences between B and NANB infection can be described (78). This clinical description, however, might subsequently be subdivided when more precise virological

Table 2. Relationship between liver lesions and HBs antigenemia.

Patients	Normal liver	Lobular hepatitis	Chronic persistent hepatitis	Chronic active hepatitis
51 chronic HBsAg carriers	8	6	16	21
20 transient HBsAg carriers	9	4	7	0
40 HBsAg negative patients	22	5	13	0
Total: 111 hemodialyzed patients	39 (31.5%)	15 (13.5%)	36 (32.4%)	21 (18.9%)

From Degott C et al 1983 (64).

markers become available. The clinical outcome of non-A non-B acute hepatitis was described as different from that of B since the evolution of the disease was more delayed, with the possibility of recurrent episodes of transaminases increase separated by phases without any biochemical abnormalities. Such recurrent phases can be observed over a long period and can resolve spontaneously, raising the problem of the definition of the chronic carrier stage (Figure 2). Unfortunately, attempts so far to describe reproducible serological viral markers have failed, and the diagnosis of non-A, non-B hepatitis can only be one of exclusion. In French centers the high prevalence of HBV infection before the beginning of vaccination may have led to underestimating the importance and frequency of hepatitis not related to HBV. At the present time the decreased incidence of HBV allows observation of chronic liver diseases in the absence of HBsAg (21, 36–39). However, studies concerning the evolution of such liver lesions during chronic hemodialysis and after renal transplantation are not yet available.

New markers of HBV-related infection in HBsAg-negative patients

Two main new markers of B or B-related viruses have been described. They are monoclonal anti-HBs antibodies and the detection by molecular hybridization in the liver of the integrated HBV genome (79). Through the use of these new markers, it has been found that some cases of presumed NANB infection were actually B infections.

Detection of HBV infection by monoclonal anti-HBs antibodies

The detection of HBsAg by polyclonal radioimmunoassays (RIA), which was used in most centers during the past 10 years, now appears obsolete. In a recent large-scale program in Japan (81), the use of monoclonal antibodies to HBsAg, especially in hemodialysis patients, gave informative data. The study was based on the use of both first-generation (polyclonal) and second generation (monoclonal) RIA of HBsAg on a population of 375 patients treated by chronic hemodialysis. The lower limit of detection for hepatitis B surface antigen-associated determinants in the serum was approximately 55 and 15 pg/ml respectively. Fourteen of the 375 chronic hemodialysis patients were positive for HBsAg by both polyclonal and monoclonal assays. However, in addition 17 were identified as harboring hepatitis B virus infection only by the monoclonal radioimmunoassays. It is noteworthy that transaminases were found increased in only 4 out of the 17 patients positive for monoclonal RIA, and that one patient died with hepatocellular carcinoma. Therefore, despite efforts to isolate HBsAg positive patients, a substantial number of hemodialysis patients still acquire HBV infection. This demonstrates the need to improve the sensitivity of current polyclonal assays. Such patients may be able to transmit hepatitis to other patients, as has been shown in a chimpanzee experimental model (81). Hepatitis infection was transmitted to chimpanzees by two serum samples which were reactive only by monoclonal

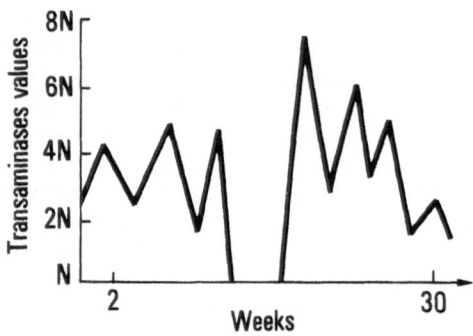

Figure 2. Transaminase activity in a hemodialyzed patient with Non-A Non-B hepatitis.

RIA. The infection was characterized by a long incubation period (>70 days) and produced elevation of transaminases values and histological features of liver injury. Moreover, HBV DNA was detected in the liver with signs of viral replication during the hepatitis phase of the experiment. This finding provided evidence that infection due to HBV or to a closely related virus can occur and be detected by monoclonal HBs RIA together with detection of HBV DNA by molecular hybridization techniques in the liver.

Detection of HBV DNA sequences in the liver of HBsAg negative patients

The presence of HB virus in a liver homogenate is detected by use of a radiolabelled HBV DNA probe and the Southern technique. The virus can either be integrated into the host genome or, when viral replication is present, be detected as free monomeric bands (57). In a large group of patients with HBsAg negative chronic liver disease this technique disclosed the presence of HBV DNA in the liver, suggesting the role of this virus in the genesis of the disease in the absence of usual markers of HBV infection (82). Such techniques must be performed on large liver samples and are not available in hemodialyzed patients. However, results recently obtained during the first 2 months following kidney transplantation, in collaboration with Dr. Brechot and co-workers of the Pasteur Institute in Paris, are informative and might subsequently be extrapolated to hemodialysis pateints (82).

A group of 56 HBsAg negative recently transplanted patients was prospectively studied. Each underwent liver biopsy for assessment of histological status; when the size of the liver sample was adequate (35 patients), the HBV DNA hybridation technique was performed simultaneously with the histological study. Whenever possible, sequential studies of serum HBV DNA were performed. HBV DNA was detected in the serum with a spot test assay and in the liver with the Southern blot technique. The probe was a full-length cloned HBV DNA obtained after separation from the cloning vector. The specificity and sensitivity of the assays were based on the following procedures: (1) the use of a purified insert, (2) highly stringent conditions of hybridization, (3) inclusion of control DNA from subjects with normal liver and with non-HBV related liver diseases, (4) exclusion of bacterial and plasmid contamination of the samples tested by rehybridization of the filter with a probe consisting only of the cloning vector. Among the 56 patients studied, 29 had normal liver and 27 chronic liver disease (i.e., chronic persistent or mild chronic active hepatitis). The existence of liver disease in almost half of the patients who were candidates for renal transplantation is a matter of concern and had not previously been documented. Forty patients were anti-HBs and/or anti-HBc positive (some of them as a consequence of previous vaccination) and 16 had no serological HBV marker (Table 3). None of these patients had detectable HBV DNA in the serum at initial testing. Sequential studies of serum HBV DNA were performed in 35 patients (mean 3.5 sera per patient) and HBV DNA appeared during immunosuppressive therapy in seven patients, reflecting the appearance of viral replication. Twenty-seven patients were tested for HBV DNA in the liver; 12 of them had normal liver and 15 chronic hepatitis. HBV DNA was detected in the liver of 10 patients with chronic hepatitis, including two without any HBV marker, whereas it was detected in only two patients with normal liver. The relationship between the existence of histologic chronic hepatitis and the detection of liver HBV DNA was statistically significant (Table 4). These results suggest that the possibility of HBV infection in this group of patients is not limited to HBsAg positive patients since a high prevalence of liver HBV DNA sequences is found despite HBsAg negativity. Half of the patients without detectable serum HBV DNA had a chronic liver lesion proven by liver biopsy. This high prevalence must be emphasized although no cirrhosis was observed. Thus, given the percentage of patients with HBV DNA in the liver and antibodies to HBV in the serum, the relevance of anti-HBs and anti-HBc detection in these HBsAg negative, immunodepressed patients with histologically proven chronic liver disease might be questioned. The possible pathogenic role of HBV in such cases was already suggested in a large group of patients with chronic hepatitis (83) and has been reported by other groups (84, 85), although with variable frequency. Furthermore, these results are in accordance with the detection of HBV infection in hemodialysis patients as reported above (80). Lastly, the possible role of HBV or HBV-related viruses in the pathogenesis of liver diseases is reinforced by the significantly higher prevalence of liver HBV DNA in patients with chronic hepatitis as compared to the normal liver group.

Classification of the patients

The presence of HBV DNA or the detection of HBsAg by the use of monoclonal antibodies in a new category of patients, previously presumed to have non-A non-B infection, raises the problem of the scope of this infection. These new techniques can probably detect HBV variants. (Such variants have previously been described for other viruses.)

However, even with the use of sophisticated molecular biology, it does not appear that all types of hepatitis can be considered as HBV or HBV-related at the present time. The group of non-A non-B infections is probably heterogenous and constituted in part of these B variant infections. In the small group of transplanted patients presented above, HBV DNA was detected in the liver of 10/15 (2/3) of the patients with chronic hepatitis. Therefore, 1/3 of cases of hepatitis remain unexplained and possibly related to other viruses.

Strategy of screening for liver involvement in hemodialysis units

All these results raise the question of the strategy for detecting liver involvement in hemodialysis patients with or without abnormalities on liver tests, and HBsAg positive or negative. The value of monitoring the serum activity of transaminases as well as HBV markers was assessed in a group of 406 hemodialyzed patients over a 4-year period of two dialysis units in Texas (86). Only 30% of the patients had normal transaminases values on all occasions. Most abnormal values were lower than 1.5 times the upper limit of normal, and were not explained. The prevalence of HBsAg at entry in the unit was 4.4%, and during follow-up 6.6% of the patients acquired HBsAg; 17.7% of the patients had antibodies to HBV at entry, and 3.5% acquired antibodies during the follow-up. False positive anti-HBc reactions were observed in 15 patients (4%) and the authors conclude that: (1) the monitoring of dialysis patients with transaminases is probably reasonable, but minor abnormalities should be interpreted with caution; (2) there is no justification for routine screening of patients with anti-HBc or anti-HBs. Initial screening with HBsAg, anti-HBc and anti-HBs is recommended for everyone entering the units in order to define potential HBV carriers as well as candidates for HBV vaccination; (3) all weak antibody results should be interpreted with great caution, especially if this represents the only marker of HBV infection. In our opinion these data are

Table 3. HBV markers and HBV DNA status in HBsAg negative patients.

Histology	Number of patients	No HBV marker	Anti-HBs+	Anti-HBc+	Anti-HBs+ anti-HBc+	Serum HBV DNA*§	Liver HBV DNA
Normal liver	29	10	9	1	9	6/29	2/12
Chronic hepatitis	27	6	8	3	10	1/27	10/15

* Patients were considered as positive if at least one serum sample was positive during the course of the study.
§ 35/56 patients were tested sequentially.

interesting from the epidemiologic point of view, but the absence of any histological control in these patients known to have asymptomatic liver disease detectable only by liver biopsy examination, would certainly underestimate the prevalence of actual liver involvement in this large series of patients. Therefore we would recommend the use of transvenous liver biopsy when liver disease is suspected in either HBsAg positive or negative patients on a permanent or fluctuant increase of transaminases, the presence of liver disease being of major importance in the transplantation decision.

Is hepatitis B a contraindication to renal transplantation in hemodialysis patients?

Whether related or not to HBV infection, the morbidity and mortality of transplant recipients with liver diseases is a major problem, a very few data on this subject are available (87, 88). In a series of 82 renal transplant patients, hepatic dysfunction was reported in 31, as well as two deaths due to acute liver failure, but the report did not include any pathological examination (71). Subsequently, the incidence of liver dysfunction was evaluated as 10% in a series of 405 patients, with a mortality rate in this latter group of 45% as compared to 16% in the nonhepatitis group (49).

Parfrey et al (50) reported a markedly decreased actuarial survival of patients with chronic liver disease compared to long-surviving transplanted controls. Poor prognosis due to HBV was observed in a group of 22 HBsAg positive renal transplant recipients whose serum transaminases were probably increased for at least one year. Eleven of them died of liver disease, five of hepatic failure, three with hepatocellular carcinoma and three with complications related to portal hypertension.

In the Necker series the presence or absence of HBsAg in the serum allowed distinction between two groups of patients. With a 13 year follow-up, mortality differed significantly in the two groups since 17.5% of the HBsAg positive patients died as compared with 7.6% of the HBsAg negative patients. However, severe hepatic failure was never observed in HBs negative patients, whereas it was the cause of half the deaths in HBs positive patients, and the only reason for increased mortality among these patients. Thus, the presence of HBs antigen appears to expose the renal transplant recipient not only to increased mortality due to hepatic failure (70, 88), whether primary or secondary in a context of a generalized infection (49, 88, 89), but also to a higher

incidence of hepatic involvement. Hence, the increased risk of mortality due to hepatic involvement, which is around 10% in HBs positive patients, is in fact less than it would appear when only HBs positive patients whose transaminases levels have been abnormally high for one year are selected. This variation in approach between the study of Parfrey et al (67) and our study probably also explains the difference in estimated severity of chronic hepatic disease in transplanted patients.

All these results question the indication of kidney transplantation in patients with liver disease. The new approaches to the diagnosis of HBV infection have demonstrated that the detection of HBV in the serum is not totally reliable and that many patients can be considered as having HBV infection in spite of serum HBsAg negativity. Therefore, the selection criteria for transplant candidates cannot be limited to serological data but should also include histological findings; in fact, long-term immunosuppression might be deleterious from the viral point of view for a patient with severe histologically demonstrated liver disease. However, this remains an assumption and requires further studies.

In the opinion of some authors (90, 91), the presence of HBs antigen, considered as a marker of defective immune response, would lead to better graft survival. In our experience, actuarial survival studies of grafts in 495 patients in whom HBV status had been determined did not confirm this hypothesis. In fact, graft survival in HBs positive patients was not significantly better than in HBs negative patients. However, since graft survival involved loss of the transplant through either graft rejection or death of the patient, graft survival in HBs positive patients should have been influenced by the higher mortality rate in such patients. The fact that, contrarily, graft survival was similar in the two groups leads us to conclude that transplant loss was higher in HBs negative patients

Considering histology as probably the most reliable means of patient classification, liver changes were compared to patient survival. Among 43 patients with histologically documented normal liver at the time of transplantation, 15 were HBsAg positive and 28 were HBsAg negative; 14 of the HBs positive patients developed liver lesions within a 57-month mean follow-up, while 11 of the HBs negative patients developed minimal liver disease and only one developed severe chronic active hepatitis. On the other hand, 13 patients were found to have histologically proven cirrhosis (12 of whom were HBsAg positive). It is noteworthy that 4 of these 13 patients died from liver failure. Hepatic disease was detected by liver biopsy studies at the time of transplantation in 60% of HBs positive patients but only in 10% of HBs negative patients. Histologically proven chronic liver disease was demonstrated in 60% of the HBsAg positive patients at the time of transplantation, and this rate rose to 93.3% of the HBsAg positive patients after the seventh year posttransplantation. Alcohol intake is an obvious factor increasing the severity of such liver disease, particularly in HBs positive patients, as it is in non-immunocompromised individuals (92).

Immunosuppression, which is required for both preven-

Table 4. Liver HBV DNA results in HBsAg negative patients.

Histology	HBV DNA in liver	
	Positive	Negative
Normal liver	2	10
Chronic hepatitis	10	5

Statistically different, $p < 0.05$, $Chi^2 = 4.87$.

tion and treatment of graft rejection, potentiates replication of the HB virus (93–95). This replication reactivation, or its persistence when this was studied, was found in almost all our patients (52, 83), whatever their HBe status. In addition, spontaneous disappearance of the HBe antigen is rare in immunosuppressed patients, although we observed such an occurrence in one of our patients.

The oncogenic risk is known to be particularly high in patients receiving immunosuppressive treatment. Hepatocellular carcinoma, which is strongly associated with HBV (96–98), should therefore frequently occur in transplant recipients (99, 100).

It is clear that the precise influence of transplantation on the prevalence and course of chronic hepatic disease is difficult to determine in the absence of randomized studies permitting comparison with nonimmunosuppressed individuals, but especially with patients treated by regular hemodialysis. Unfortunately the lack of a study comparing the survival and the outcome of liver disease in HBsAg positive patients treated either by hemodialysis or by renal transplantation so far precludes a decision as to which may be the better therapy in these cases.

PREVENTION OF HEPATITIS B IN DIALYSIS UNITS

Sources and routes of infection

The key factors explaining the contamination of patients and staff in hemodialysis units are the frequent long-term persistence of antigenemia in infected patients, making them permanent virus reservoirs, and the frequent exposure to blood and serous fluids of these patients, resulting in cross-infection of other patients and staff. Thus, dialysis-associated hepatitis is essentially a cross-infection problem.

Initially, blood transfusions were thought to be the main source of the introduction of the virus into dialysis units (101). Since 1970, only HBsAg-free blood has been used. Thus, blood transfusion certainly is no longer a major route of contamination, particularly in view of the fact that the subtypes of HBsAg most frequently encountered in dialysis patients are very different from those observed in blood donors in the same country (102, 103). Usually, HB virus is introduced into a center by a patient not known to be an antigen carrier because most infected uremic patients are asymptomatic (104). Thereafter, due to the frequent indefinite persistence of antigenemia in uremics, such a patient acts as a highly infective virus reservoir, resulting in the spread of HBV infection throughout the entire dialysis unit, to patients, the unit staff and other hospital personnel (105).

The transmission occurs via percutaneous or permucosal routes and results from blood spray during cannulation of arteriovenous fistulae, splashes or drops of blood (or serum) on skin, clothing or bedding, or from contact with used dialysis material (106, 107). Staff may be infected by accidental needle pricks, contamination of cuts or skin lesions, blood spraying into the eyes or mouth, or even by smoking or eating in the dialysis ward. HBsAg has also been found in the ascitic fluid of positive patients treated by peritoneal dialysis (108). Not only are nurses, physicians and technicians directly working in dialysis units at risk of HBV contamination, but also roentgenologists, surgeons, dentists and all other personnel involved in the care of infected patients, as well as laboratory personnel working in clinical or research laboratories and manipulating blood or serum specimens from infected subjects. Moreover, the presence of the virus has been demonstrated in saliva, vaginal secretions and sperm (109). Thus, spouses or other intimate contacts of infected patients (or staff members) are also at high risk and need protection.

General prophylactic measures in dialysis units

Before passive and active immunization against HBV became available, the only means of preventing and controlling HBV infection in dialysis units was immediate detection and isolation of infected patients combined with strict cross-infection prophylaxis. Recommendations aimed at the prevention of spread of any type of hepatitis infection within dialysis centers were given in detail in the Public Health Laboratory Service (PHLS) report (110) and in the preceding edition of the present chapter by Dr. S. Polakoff. Their principles are: 1) Immediate identification and exclusion from the HBV-free dialysis unit of any patient positive for HBsAg; 2) General hygienic precautions directed against spread of infective agents within the center; 3) Prevention of spread of infection out of the dialysis unit, especially to the patient's family and to other hospital staff. In particular, blood samples from patients positive for HBsAg should carry special labels indicating the risk to laboratory personnel. Any surgeon, roentgenologist or dentist to whom the patient is referred should also be advised of the risk.

These measures are exacting and time-consuming. They remain essential, however, because despite successful immunoprophylaxis against HB virus, they are still the only means of protection against the spread of other infective agents, especially non-A, non-B hepatitis virus.

The earliest and largest experience resulting in successful prevention of hepatitis B infection in dialysis units originated in Great Britain, where a nationwide preventive program was started in 1968 before HBV infection had been introduced into the majority of dialysis units. Within 2 years of the generalized application of the advisory group recommendations, the rising incidence of HBV infection was halted (111–113). By contrast, the epidemiologic situation was much less favorable in most units in Europe and the United States, where such prevention programs were initiated later or less strictly applied, resulting in a continuously growing incidence of HBV infection until the start of large-scale programs of active immunization (18, 19).

Passive immunization

The protective efficacy of specific anti-HBs human immunoglobulin preparations was first demonstrated in a study conducted in an institution for mentally retarded children in whom HBV infection was endemic (114). Standard immunoglobulins (ISG), despite a low anti-HBs content, had also given some protection in a similar population of institutionalized children (115). ISG may act, at least in part, through active immunization, because some batches of ISG contain occult HBsAg which can induce the development of anti-HBs antibodies (116).

Passive immunization with HBIG was used either for post-exposure protection after accidental inoculation in staff, or as regular preventive treatment in both staff and dialysis patients before vaccine was available.

Among patients, three controlled trials demonstrated the protective efficacy of HBIG injections. In the study of Desmyter et al (117) in Belgium, only 2 of 15 dialysis patients who received HBIG injections at 6-month intervals developed transient antigenemia, whereas 10 of 14 patients who received anti-HBs-poor ISG became HBsAg positive, persistently in five. In a large multicentric trial in the USA, dialysis patients receiving high-titer HBIG had a significantly lower attack rate than those receiving intermediate-titer HBIG or anti-HBs-poor ISG, but protection was not absolute in the first group (118). By contrast, in the study of Kleinknecht et al (119) in two highly contaminated units in France, none of the 15 patients who received HBIG at intervals of 5 to 8 weeks became HBsAg positive, whereas in the control group who received no immunoglobulin, antigenemia developed in 10 of 13 patients and persisted in five. The latter study suggests that HBIG are effective in preventing HBV infection provided the interval between two injections is not longer than 2 months, whereas protocols using 3 to 6-month intervals between HBIG injections seem less protective.

The same appears true concerning staff. In the controlled study reported by Prince et al (120) the attack rate in staff members who received high-titer HBIG was lower than in the two groups who received low-titer HBIG or ISG, but the difference was not significant and late cases of hepatitis B occurred some months after the second injection. Similarly, Iwarson et al (121) observed one case of hepatitis B 5 months after the second HBIG injection. By contrast, using repeated injections every 5 weeks during the first 4 months and every 8 weeks thereafter, Couroucé-Pauty et al (122) observed absolute protection in staff members of four highly infected dialysis units in the Paris area. The attack rate declined from 44% to zero and no hepatitis B was observed among 90 staff members protected from 4 to 26 months, whereas among eight subjects who refused or stopped HBIG injections, three developed hepatitis B (122). Retrospective titration of serum samples indicated that no HBV infection occurred in subjects having a residual anti-HBs titer higher than 10 mIU/ml, whereas hepatitis B occurred in subjects having a residual titer below this value.

Single injections of HBIG are used by laboratory or hospital staff after accidental inoculation or transmucosal projection of HBsAg positive material. In 80 laboratory and dialysis staff members having received a single dose of HBIG within 7 days following accidental contamination,

HBsAg positive clinical hepatitis developed in only two, whereas eight developed active anti-HBs (122). Other trials of post-exposure passive immunization also showed a high, although not absolute, protective efficacy (123, 124).

If the use of HBIG after accidental contamination undoubtedly is a simple and efficient means of protection in a staff member not already protected by vaccination, the regular use of HBIG to prevent HBV infection in patients and staff of dialysis units, although effective, has several disadvantages. HBIG doses have to be repeated at short intervals of 6 to 8 weeks in order to maintain protective anti-HBs levels, and such repeated injections often become painful or even may lead to hypersensitivity, obliging termination of prophylaxis (122). Moreover, HBIG preparations are expensive and a shortage of donors rich in anti-HBs antibody is to be anticipated, although anti-HBs titers in human donors may be increased by a booster injection of hepatitis B vaccine (125). Thus, clearly, only active immunization by vaccine could adequately solve the problem of large-scale, long-lasting prophylaxis in high-risk populations.

Active immunization

Principles of plasma-derived vaccine preparation and demonstration of protective efficacy

Active immunization against HBV is based on the production of anti-HBs antibodies in response to the injection of purified particles of the surface antigen of the virus. Due to the impossibility of cultivating HBV in vitro, all first generation vaccines were prepared from an unusual source of viral antigen, i.e., from the plasma of chronic HBsAg carriers.

Krugman and corworkers first demonstrated that a human plasma rich in HBsAg particles and containing complete virions, when heated for 1 min at 98° C, lost infectivity but retained immunogenicity (126). Since that time, several groups have developed improved methods for purifying and inactivating human sera containing HBsAg particles, in order to eliminate all types of viruses or residual proteins from the final vaccine. Stringent recommendations have been formulated by the World Health Organization, including at least two steps of inactivation, in order to guarantee the total safety of the vaccines. The technical solutions adopted for the production of the industrial vaccines differ with regard to the choice of the starting material, purification and inactivation procedures, adsorption of the vaccine and final antigenic concentration (127–129).

More than a dozen plasma-derived vaccines have been developed in various countries, but at the present time only two are licensed. One is the Merck vaccine (Heptavax B), which uses as starting material plasma containing high titers of HBsAg (only of *ad* specificity) and of HBeAg and Dane particles. This vaccine is inactivated by pepsin digestion and urea denaturation followed by formalin 1:4000 in order to eliminate any residual trace of human serum proteins, according to the procedure developed by Hilleman and coworkers (130). The final antigen concentration is either 20 or 40 μg per dose. The drastic inactivation procedure by enzyme digestion may possibly be responsible for a loss in antigenic potency (128). The other vaccine is the French Pasteur vaccine (HEVAC B), prepared according to a procedure initially devised by Maupas and coworkers (131) and further industrially developed by Adamowicz and colleagues (132). The starting material is plasma from healthy donors positive for HBsAg (with both *ad* and *ay* subtypes) but devoid of HBV virions or HBeAg. Purification is obtained by three steps of zonal centrifugation, and inactivation is achieved through two centrifugations in cesium chloride gradient followed by formalin treatment, thus avoiding HBsAg protein denaturing processes such as enzyme treatment. The final antigen concentration is 5 μg per dose. This vaccine appears to retain a high immunogenic potency, which is especially apparent in immunodeficient subjects such as uremic patients. Another plasma-derived vaccine has been developed in the Netherlands Red Cross blood transfusion service, the heat-inactivated (CLB) vaccine. It uses as starting material a plasma rich in HBsAg and HBe particles, inactivated only by heating. The final antigen content is 3 μg per dose, and this vaccine also has a powerful immunogenicity (133).

The absence of infectivity of these three vaccines has been extensively tested on the chimpanzee, the only animal suitable for potency and safety assays of HB vaccines (134). Both the Merck and the Pasteur vaccine were licensed in mid-1982. More than 4 million doses of the latter have been dispensed to date without serious side-effects. The highly sophisticated purifying processes and the final testing on the chimpanzee used by both manufacturers give absolute certitude of non-infectivity of the vaccines, including for the HTLV III/LAV (HIV) virus (135, 136).

The protective efficacy of the Merck vaccine had been initially tested in a placebo-controlled trial which started in November 1978 in male homosexuals in the New York area, a population at high risk of HBV infection (137). The protocol involved two intramuscular injections of 40 μg each one month apart, followed by a booster injection at 6 months (138). The HBV infection rate was significantly lower in vaccine (7.6%) than in placebo recipients (35%, $p < 10^{-4}$) during an observation period of 18 months. Within 3 months of the first injection, 87% of the vaccinees developed anti-HBs antibody, this rate further rising to 96% following the booster injection. Several HBV infections occurred during the first 6 months following the start of vaccination, most limited to an isolated anti-HBc conversion (138, 139). This study first demonstrated that protection is in relation with the development of anti-HBs antibody at a minimum level which corresponds to what subsequently was estimated to be about 10 sample ratio units (SRU) or 10 mIU/ml. In France, a pilot study conducted in 1975 in highly contaminated dialysis units in the Loire Valley had shown a dramatic reduction in the annual incidence of HBV infections in vaccinated staff members and dialysis patients, compared to the preceding period without vaccination (131). However, the first randomized placebo-controlled efficacy trial in healthy hospital staff was made in dialysis units throughout France and was initiated in April 1979 (140).

Vaccination in healthy medical staff

Immunogenicity and protective efficacy of the vaccines in healthy staff

The protective efficacy of hepatitis B vaccines in healthy medical staff of dialysis units has been demonstrated by placebo-controlled trials of the two licensed vaccines.

The French trial involved 367 staff members of 48 high-risk dialysis units and showed a highly significant difference in the number of HBV infections between the group receiving the Pasteur vaccine and the placebo group (6/164 vs. 19/154, $p < 0.005$). No HBV infection was observed in vaccine recipients after three injections given at monthly intervals (139). Anti-HBs antibody developed at a titer of 10 mIU/ml or more in 94% of subjects after the third injection and this proportion rose to 97.5% following a booster injection given 15 months later. The geometric mean titer (GMT) of anti-HBs in responders was 591 mIU/ml after the third injection and rose to 16,600 mIU/ml following booster injection (141).

The American trial involved 865 staff members of 43 hemodialysis units in the United States, using two monthly injections of 20 μg Merck vaccine followed by a booster at 6 months. The incidence of HBV infections was significantly lower in the vaccine group (2.2%) than in the placebo group (9.9%, $p < 0.01$), a protective efficacy of 77%. Anti-HBs antibody developed in 75% of subjects one month after the first injection and in 93% 3 months later, and this proportion rose to 96% following the 6th-month booster. In a sample of 100 subjects, GMT was 50 to 70 mIU/ml after the second dose and 1009 mIU/ml following the booster (142).

In another controlled trial, 152 healthy staff of 18 Belgian dialysis units were given either three doses of the CLB vaccine, 3 μg per dose, or placebo, at monthly intervals (143). Due to the small number of subjects, the protective efficacy of the vaccine could not be statistically demonstrated, but only two HBV infections occurred in the vaccine group whereas six (including five with HBsAg conversion) occurred in the placebo group during a 14-month follow-up. Anti-HBs at a level $\geq$ 10 mIU/ml were found in 94% of vaccinees after the third injection, with a peak GMT of about 700 mIU/ml. The results of these controlled trials agree with those of subsequent studies in hospital health care personnel (144, 145). Taken together, they indicate that with each of the vaccines used, vaccination in healthy staff provides protective levels of anti-HBS (i.e., $\geq$ 10 mIU/ml) in about 95% of subjects. However, acquisition of anti-HBs antibody is more delayed with the Merck vaccine than with the Pasteur or the CLB vaccine, using the corresponding recommended schedules. Also, the peak values of anti-HBs following primary vaccination and the booster were much greater using the two latter vaccines than the former.

Low responses to the vaccine in healthy staff

Nevertheless, about 5% of healthy subjects were non- or weak responders on the standard schedules recommended, and an even higher proportion of vaccine failures were observed in some trials (146–148).

Such unresponsiveness to vaccination has been attributed, in some instances, to inappropriate storage of the vaccine, i.e., inadvertent freezing instead of optimal storage at temperatures of 2 to 8°C (149). Another explanation was that intramuscular injection in the buttocks, the initially recommended route for the Merck vaccine, is less effective than injection in the gluteal region or, better, in the deltoid muscle. In health care workers, Ukena et al (148) observed only 58% of responders among 133 subjects injected into the buttocks, but 87% among 53 others vaccinated by arm injection and, of 20 non-responders following buttock injection, 85% developed antibody after a subsequent course of vaccine in the arm. This was confirmed in other reports. Among 20 hemodialysis centers that vaccinated staff members in the arm, the combined seroconversion rate was 93.9%, as compared with 81% in 23 centers using buttock injection (150). Thus, the anatomical site of injection may be an important factor in vaccine efficacy. Adipose tissue in the gluteal region, especially in females, may alter the vaccine uptake (151). As a matter of fact, poor responders often tend to be older, female or obese (152). Therefore, new recommendations have been formulated for intramuscular vaccine injections in the deltoid (153).

However, disappointingly low seroconversion rates, of the order of 80 or less, have been reported by some authors in healthy hospital staff members, despite adequate vaccine storage and site of injection, without a clear explanation other than an accidentally reduced immunogenic potency of the lots of vaccine used. Such observations may suggest the need for serologic follow-up of highly exposed health care workers in order to ascertain whether they are effectively protected against HBV infection (146, 147).

Finally, even in the series reporting the highest rates of responders following primary vaccination, there is a small percentage of non- or low responders. The reasons for such unresponsiveness in healthy subjects supposed to be immunocompetent are not fully understood. Genetic factors may possibly be involved, since a higher than expected frequency of HLA-DR7 and HLA-DR3 phenotypes was reported in a prospective study of 28 hypo- or low responders (154) selected from 666 vaccinated health care workers participating in the Boston inter-hospital hepatitis B vaccine study (144). Fortunately, it has been shown that nearly half of the persons who did not produce anti-HBs in response to the initial vaccination course developed antibody after one or two additional doses (147, 154).

Passive-active immunization

Whatever the vaccine and the injection schedule used, acquisition of a protective level of antibody never is immediate and usually needs up to 3 months using the Pasteur or CLB vaccine with three injections at monthly intervals, or up to 5 or 6 months following the first two injections of the Merck 20 μg vaccine. Therefore, in subjects exposed to a high risk of HBV infection, immediate protection requires a combination of passive immunization by means of HBIG and of vaccination ('passive-active' immunization). Several groups have prospectively evaluated the safety of this technique by comparing different time schedules of combined injections of HBIG and vaccine to active immunization alone. Szmuness et al. (155), using the Merck vaccine, and Goudeau et al (156), Courouce et al (157) and Mesnier et al (158) using the Pasteur vaccine, afforded the demonstration that passive antibody from HBIG does not interfere with the development of active antibody promoted by the vaccine, even given the same day, provided the HBIG and vaccine are injected at different sites. In these concordant controlled studies, the levels of anti-HBs antibody and the kinetics of the response elicited by passive-active immunization did not differ from those observed following pure active immunization.

Duration of protection

An important concern is the duration of protection afforded by vaccination against HBV infection and, consequently, the need for revaccination and the choice of optimal time for such booster doses. The solution of this problem requires definition of the minimum protective level of actively acquired anti-HBs and knowledge of the time course of anti-HBs decline for each of the vaccines used. In the earlier randomized efficacy trials, a close relationship between protective efficacy and immunogenicity of the vaccines was demonstrated, and the minimal protective level was found to correspond about 10 mIU/ml (138, 140, 159). Longitudinal surveillance of healthy subjects submitted to vaccination provided further information. Using the 20 μg Merck vaccine, Jilg et al (160) in Germany and Grob et al (161) in Switzerland observed a similar rate of decline in anti-HBs levels in all vaccinees, with an initially rapid decrease of about 90% within the first 2 years and then a slower decline of about 50% during the subsequent 2 years. Recently, Hadler and coworkers (149, 162) reported the long-term analysis of the duration of antibody and protection provided by the 20 μg Merck vaccine in 773 male homosexuals who participated in the multicenter efficacy trial started in April 1980 and who were followed for 5 years after the 6-month booster injection. No antibody was detectable 5 years later in 15% of them, and 27% had a residual level below 10 mIU/ml. However, all HBV infections except one manifested only anti-HBc seroconversion together with an increased anti-HBs level, and the only infection with transient HBsAg positivity was asymptomatic. Thus, even low levels of antibody seem to protect against symptomatic hepatitis B and to prevent the development of a chronic carrier state.

Using the Pasteur vaccine, long persistence of a protective level of anti-HBs antibody was observed in an even higher proportion of healthy staff members by Goudeau et al (145) and by our group. Five years after booster injection, 93% retained an anti-HBs titer of no less than 10 mIU/ml, including 85% with titers of 50 mIU/ml or more (163, 164).

Vaccination in subjects positive for HBsAg, anti-HBc or anti-HBs

Another problem is the quality of response and possible side-effects when vaccinating subjects positive for anti-HBc and/or anti-HBs, or those positive for HBsAg. In all randomized placebo-controlled efficacy studies, a number of HBV events, including seroconversion to HBsAg, occurred in the vaccine group during the first months of vaccination at a time when antibody had not yet developed. In most cases, vaccination appeared to prevent persistent antigenemia and to limit viral replication (138, 140). In chronic carriers of the surface antigen, Dienstag et al (165) administered repeated doses of the Merck vaccine at 40 μg in an attempt to eliminate antigenemia. Vaccination was ineffective suppressing HBsAg but appeared to be safe (165). Thus, the vaccine produces neither therapeutic nor adverse effects in subjects acutely or chronically positive for HBsAg.

Naturally acquired anti-HBs antibody alone is found in a substantial proportion of hospital staff, raising the question of whether this represents previous HBV infection with immunity against further exposure or false positivity with non-protective antibody (166). One would expect a rapidly evolving, anamnestic antibody reponse following vaccine injection in the former case and a slower, primary-type response in the latter. Moreover, isolated anti-HBs is usually an IgM antibody, whereas antibody associated with recovery from hepatitis B infection is of the IgG class (167). Werner et al (168) tested 46 health care workers having isolated anti-HBs (usually of low titer) with a single 20 μg dose of the Merck vaccine. Anamnestic responses were observed in only 10 subjects, mainly in those whose basal anti-HBs level was the highest (168). These authors suggest that healthy staff with isolated anti-HBs titers below 40 mIU/ml should receive a full course of vaccination. Goudeau et al (145) gave a single 5 μg dose of Pasteur vaccine to 42 healthy subjects with isolated anti-HBs and the same dose as a routine booster to 42 healthy staff who had responded to the full course of three injections. The proportion of subjects having a marked increase in anti-HBs level was lower in the group with isolated anti-HBs than in responders to the vaccine.

The significance of isolated anti-HBc in healthy staff is also heterogeneous and appears to vary among countries. Among 14 hospital staff members in France, a true anamnestic response was observed in only one (169) whereas in Italy, anamnestic responses were observed in five of nine anti-HBc IgG positive subjects (170) and in Greece, such a response was reported in 8 of 16 anti-HBc (none of IgM class) positive subjects (171). Overall, these data indicate that in populations with moderate or low prevalence of natural immunity, anamnestic responses in persons with isolated anti-HBc or low-titer anti-HBs are rather infrequent. Thus, screening for anti-HBs or anti-HBc is probably not cost-effective and it would appear preferable to vaccinate health care workers prior to professional exposure without screening since the vaccine causes no adverse effects in immune individuals (172, 173).

Vaccination in dialysis patients

Impaired immune responsiveness in dialysis patients
Active immunization of hemodialysis patients is crucial for eradicating HBV infection from dialysis units. However, the development of anti-HBs antibody is inhibited in these subjects by the immunodeficient state that characterizes uremic patients and which is not improved, or even worsened, by maintenance hemodialysis (174). The defects in immune response of uremics are observed at both the humoral and cellular levels (175, 176). Evidence for a T-cell defect has been shown in dialysis patients (177) as well as in uremic patients from the early stages of chronic renal failure (178). Similar impairment in immune responses is also observed in transplanted patients, even with a well functioning graft, due to the long-term use of immunosuppressive agents. Thus, impaired immune response to various vaccines is to be expected in uremic, dialyzed and transplanted patients. As a matter of fact, low antibody titers have been found in response to influenza vaccination (179) and to pneumococcal vaccine (180, 181), in both dialysis patients and kidney transplant recipients. The same is true with regard to hepatitis B vaccines. Maupas et al (182) first mentioned in their pilot study that the proportion of responders was lower in dialysis patients than in healthy staff members, i.e., 62% vs. 94%, following a standard course of three injections of 5 μg vaccine. The same was observed, although to a lesser degree, by Stevens et al (183) after 3 injections of the Merck vaccine at 40 μg, that is, twice the recommended dose for healthy adults, in 79 hemodialysis patients.

Immunogenir·y and protective efficacy of the vaccines in dialysis patients
The efficacy of the Pasteur and CLB vaccines has been demonstrated in dialysis patients. The first placebo-controlled, randomized efficacy trial of hepatitis B vaccine in chronic dialysis ptients involved 31 high-risk dialysis units in France (184). Three 5 μg doses of Pasteur vaccine were given at monthly intervals, as in healthy staff. Protective efficacy was demonstrated by the significantly lower incidence of HBV infections in the vaccine than in the placebo group during a 12-month follow-up (21% vs. 45%, p< 0.02). This study also clearly showed that the proportion of responders was markedly lower in dialysis patients than in healthy staff (60% vs. 96%), and the same was true for peak anti-HBs levels in responders. The adverse influence of age was striking, with 80% of responders in patients under 50 years of age and only 43% in those over 50. This was confirmed in the study of Goudeau et al (145), where older patients had a more delayed and weaker response than younger subjects.

The protective efficacy of the heat-inactivated vaccine was established in 401 dialysis patients in 18 dialysis units in Belgium, who received four doses of 3 μg CLB vaccine at 0, 1, 2 and 5 months, instead of three injections at monthly intervals as was given in staff (143). The HBV attack rate was significantly reduced in vaccinees (4% vs. 17.8%), a protective efficacy rate of 78%. Vaccination induced anti-HBs at a level of 10 mIU/ml or more in 59% of patients following the third injection.

By contrast, in a large prospective placebo-controlled multicentric trial in 1311 patients of 41 dialysis units in the United States, Stevens and coworkers, using the 40 μg

Merck vaccine at 0, 1 and 6 months, failed to demonstrate protective efficacy, as the attack rate was similarly low in both placebo and vaccine groups, 5.4% and 6.4% respectively (185). Of 562 vaccinated patients, 50% responded to full vaccination, and the peak (GMT) anti-HBs level, in a representative sample of 93 responders, was 139 mIU/ml. The influence of age was also striking, with 63.7% of responders under 40 years of age and only 37.3% over sixty.

Subsequent studies in several European countries, mostly using the Merck vaccine, confirmed the poor immune response of dialysis patients both in terms of proportion of responders and of peak antibody titer when using the standard vaccination schedule recommended for healthy staff (186–191).

Reinforced vaccine protocols in dialysis patients

Thus, the question arose whether reinforced protocols could overcome the deficient immunization of dialysis patients, by increasing the dose of antigen, the number of injections, or both. The first comparative, prospective randomized trial was performed in 215 patients in the Paris area (192). When compared to the standard protocol (three doses of $5 \mu g$ Pasteur vaccine at monthly intervals), the two reinforced protocols (three injections of $10 \mu g$, or four injections of $5 \mu g$, the fourth given 2 months later) induced a significantly greater proportion of responders (respectively 75 and 69.4% vs. 45.6%) and higer anti-HBs peak titers 6 months after the first injection (GMT: 192 and 268 vs. 60 mIU/ml) and following booster injection at 1 year (GMT: 1123 and 524 vs. 144 mIU/ml) (193). Although the results obtained with the two reinforced protocols did not differ statistically, the last schedule, using four injections of the $5 \mu g$ dose, had the best cost/efficacy ratio and was thus adopted as the recommended protocol for all uremic patients. A similarly reinforced schedule using the Pasteur vaccine was tested by Goudeau et al (145). The proportion of responders rose from 56% after the third injection to 67% after the fourth, the gain in responders being particularly notable in older patients (145).

Other reinforced protocols using multiple doses of either the Merck vaccine ($40 \mu g$ per dose) (186, 194) or the heat-inactivated CLB vaccine at $27 \mu g$ per dose (189, 191) improved the proportion of responders in dialysis patients up to 80% or more, together with an increase in anti-HBs titers. Thus, dialysis patients seem to be 'slow' responders, who need more intense and more repeated antigenic stimulation to elicit antibody production than healthy subjects. As a matter of fact, the proportion of responders, in a population of aged dialysis patients, rose from 44 to 90% when the number of Pasteur vaccine injections increased from 4 to 14 (195). Thus, a consensus has emerged that reinforced protocols are routinely needed in dialysis patients, whatever the vaccine used.

Passive-active immunization in dialysis patients

As the development of anti-HBs antibody is slower in dialysis patients than in healthy subjects, there is a need for combined passive-active immunization in patients exposed to a high risk of contamination. As for healthy staff, several studies have established that concomitant injection of HBIG does not inhibit the development of vaccine-induced antibody (156–158, 186, 187). Thus, passive-active immunization should be recommended in patients having to start dialysis treatment in a contaminated unit.

Duration of protection in dialysis patients

The duration of protection afforded by vaccination in dialysis patients has been studied by several groups. Protective anti-HBs levels lasted for at least 1 year in all patients who received a fourth injection in the protocol of Goudeau et al (145). Benhamou et al (192, 193) longitudinally studied the time course of anti-HBs in patients participating in the above-mentioned efficacy trial following the booster injection given at 1 year. The rate of decline was parallel in all patients and the slope of the curves was similar to that observed in healthy staff, but the interval before anti-HBs titers fell below 10 mIU/ml was shorter because post-booster peak values were, as a mean, 10 times lower than those observed in healthy subjects. Projection of the curves showed that an anti-HBs level above 10 mIU/ml should be maintained for at least 2 years in patients having peak values of 1,000 mIU/ml or more (196). However, in patients exposed to a high risk of HBV infection, assessment of anti-HBs titer at regular intervals, especially in weak responders, should allow the best prediction of the optimal time for revaccination.

Vaccination in chronic uremic patients prior to dialysis

As the impaired anti-HBs production in dialysis patients is related to the state of uremia, one could expect that vaccination at an early stage of renal failure should obtain a better immune response. Additionally, better prevention of HBV infection in dialysis units could be expected if patients starting dialysis were already protected by a high concentration of anti-HBs antibody. Several trials of vaccination prior to initiation of dialysis have been performed in chronic uremic patients with various degress of renal failure. They have all shown that immune response to hepatitis B vaccine is impaired in uremic patients, as in dialysis patients, even at an early stage of chronic renal failure.

In a comparative study using the $40 \mu g$ Merck vaccine at 0, 1 and 6 months in 29 dialyzed patients and in 12 end-stage uremics, Bommer et al (186) observed similarly low conversion rates (45% and 41% respectively, after booster injection) and peak antibody levels. The same authors further compared the response of 24 patients having moderate chronic renal failure, with plasma creatinine (Pcr) in the range of 1.4 to 3.5 mg/dl (124 to 310 umol/l), and of 43 staff members after three injections of $20 \mu g$ Merck vaccine at 0, 1 and 6 months. Seroconversion rates following booster were significantly lower in uremics than in staff (65% vs. 90%), although mean anti-HBs peaks in responders were similar in both groups (187). Using the same protocol, Kurz et al (178) obtained a proportion of responders of only 54% among 35 uremics with a mean Pcr value of 4.9 mg/dl, compared to

94% in 19 healthy controls. The seroconversion rate was equally low in the 20 patients with moderate renal failure (Pcr in the range of 1.5 to 3.5 mg/dl [133 to 310 umol/l]) and in the 15 who had more advanced uremia (Pcr 3.6 to 9.1 mg/dl [319 to 805 umol/l]). Marked alterations in lymphocyte functions were present at the early stage of renal failure, explaining the weak response to the vaccine observed in these patients (177). Using the Pasteur vaccine, Rottembourg et al (197) observed a proportion of responders of 74.5% following three 5 μg injections at monthly intervals and 84.5% following the booster injection at 1 year in 51 uremic patients with mean Pcr of 632 umol/l. Another trial was started in July 1982 in Necker Hospital. The proportion of responders following three injections of 5 μg Pasteur vaccine was only 60%, with a marked adverse effect of age on the immune response and a slightly better response in patients with Pcr under 400 umol/l (3.5 mg/dl) than above this value (198). This experience was further extended to a total number of 204 patients with various degrees of renal failure (199). Vaccine schedule included three injections of Pasteur vaccine at monthly intervals, followed by a fourth injection 2 months later. This increased the proportion of responders by 42%, in parallel with a four-fold increase in the anti-HBs titer. Five of 11 non-responsive patients did respond after a fifth injection. Similarly, the booster injection at 1 year induced response in 9 of 18 patients who were still nonresponders after the third or fourth injections. Thus, each supplementary injection induced a gain in responders of 40 to 50 percent, with a concomitant rise in anti-HBs titer.

Thus, clinical experience with all vaccines confirms that impairment in the immune response exists in uremic patients to a degree similar to that observed in dialysis patients. However, as in the latter, reinforced protocols using higher doses of vaccine and/or additional injections can overcome this deficient response and elicit a proportion of responders and anti-HBs levels close to that observed in healthy subjects.

Alternatives to plasma-derived vaccines: the second generation vaccines

In the absence of successful replication of HBV in cell cultures, the unique source of antigenic material for vaccine preparation was the plasma of chronic carriers of HBsAg. Due to the increasing utilisation of HB vaccines in exposed populations, a shortage of this source of antigenic material is to be feared. Moreover, the use of plasma-derived material implies sophisticated and expensive procedures to obtain perfect purification and inactivation of surface antigen particles, and costly safety testing on the only susceptible animal, the chimpanzee. Thus, the need for producing large quantities of vaccine at the lowest possible cost and avoiding the use of plasma-derived material stimulated other approaches to the production of HB vaccines. The different means used to develop second-generation vaccines have been recently reviewed (126–128, 200). They include in vitro production of synthetic polypeptides, cell-line derived vaccines and re-

combinant DNA technology.

A variety of peptides which contain the amino acid sequence of the major HBsAg antigenic site have been synthesized, but such synthetic vaccines, due to their small molecular size, are poorly antigenic and need to be prepared as popypeptide micelles (201) or to be attached to larger carrier molecules. None is operational at the present time.

The recent demonstration of the presence of HBV-DNA sequences in the cellular genome of human hepatocellular carcinoma cell lines led several groups to evaluate the possible interest of HBsAg producing cell lines, but the clinical use of such vaccines derived from transformed cancerous cells raises major, still unresolved ethical problems.

At the present time, DNA-recombinant technology appears to offer the most promising approach to the production of safe and highly immunogenic vaccines. The basic principle is to isolate the fraction of the HBV genome coding for selected envelope proteins and to transplant this fraction into a host cell, which can be a bacterium (such as E. Coli or bacillus subtilis), a virus (such as vaccinia virus or simian virus SV40), a yeast (such as Saccharomyces cerevisiae) or a mammalian cell, such as the Chinese hamster ovary (CHO) line. The host cells produce the specific HBV proteins corresponding to the HBV-DNA they have incorporated.

Recent studies have shown that the receptor for polymerized human serum albumin, which plays a major role in the penetration of HBV virions into liver cells, is associated with the peptide coded for by the pre-S region of the HBV genome. This pre-S antigen appears to be of great importance in protecting against the penetration of HB virus into hepatic cells and in neutralizing the virus. Anti-pre-S antibody is the first neutralizing antibody to appear in natural HBV infection. It inhibits attachment of HBV to the surface of liver cells, whereas anti-S antibody lacks this property (202). Therefore, a vaccine incorporating the pre-S determinant might have advantages over the conventional preparations which contain mainly, or only, the S protein (203–205).

The processes for purification differ with respect to the vector used. With the bacterial and yeast recombinant vaccines, HBsAg is incorporated into the cell, and the cellular components have to be removed to obtain purified HBsAg, as yeast cells do not excrete HBsAg particles and have to be disrupted. Technical difficulties in the purification procedures have delayed the development of bacterial recombinant vaccines, but yeast-derived vaccine technology is more advanced. Several yeast-recombinant vaccines have entered the industrial production phase and two are already licensed, one by Merck, Sharp and Dohme (Recombivax), the other by Smith-Kline RIT Laboratories (Engerix B). Both have only S proteins. Clinical trials in healthy adults have shown the immunogenic potency of these vaccines to be similar to that of the Merck plasma-derived vaccine (206–210).

The CHO-derived vaccine under development at Pasteur Institute contains both the S and the pre-S proteins, the latter at a very high concentration. As CHO cells spontaneously excrete HBsAg particles, no cellular disruption is needed and the purification procedure is alleviated. This vaccine induced a greater anti-HBs production in mice than did a vaccine with the same S protein content but devoid of the pre-S protein (203). Only prospective studies, comparing the different DNA-recombinant vaccines to the first generation plasma vaccines in both healthy and immuno-compromised subjects, may confirm or not the expected superior results of the second-generation vaccines in terms of immunogenicity and long-term protective efficacy.

Results of vaccination and organizational problems of hepatitis B prevention in dialysis units

Results of vaccination in dialysis units

The generalized use of vaccination since 1982 has dramatically reduced, in a few years, the high morbidity and mortality due to HBV infection in dialysis units, at least in those European countries where extensive vaccination campaigns were promoted early in patients and staff. The analysis of the annual reports of the European Dialysis and Transplant Association from 1981 to 1985 clearly indicates a drastic reduction in the incidence of new cases of hepatitis B in dialysis units in Austria, Belgium, the Federal Republic of Germany, France, Greece and Switzerland, and more recently in Italy and Spain (22–26). From 1981 to 1985, the total annual number of new cases of virus B hepatitis in the first six countries listed above fell from 755 to 249 in dialysis patients and, even more strikingly, from 163 to 6 in staff.

In Great Britain, the Netherlands and Scandinavia, where the incidence of hepatitis B was already very low due to strict application of measures for prevention of cross-infection, the overall annual incidence remained low during the same period, without vaccination. The decline in the annual incidence of hepatitis B is depicted for Europe as a whole and for some representative European countries in Table 5. By contrast, in the group of other European and North African countries, where no generalized vaccination campaigns were undertaken, hepatitis B infection did not diminish and

even rose during the past 5 years, in proportion to the increasing number of patients beginning dialysis treatment.

The situation in the United States is less clear. Despite financial support given to patients and staff for vaccination, there seems to exist some reluctance to using the vaccine on the part of patients and even staff. This is probably due to an unfounded fear of HTLV III/LAV (HIV) infection (211), despite reassuring evidence as to the safety of plasma-derived vaccines (212, 213). A survey of the Centers for Disease Control bearing on 1,255 dialysis centers throughout the USA in 1983 (the first year the vaccine was available) indicated that whereas 71% of centers declared using the vaccine, only 6% of the estimated eligible patients and 32% of estimated eligible staff had received the complete schedule of inoculation by the end of 1983 (214).

Organizational problems of hepatitis prevention in hospital staff

At the present time the problem of prevention of hepatitis B in dialysis units can no longer be considered separately, but must be included within the wider perspective of protection of health care workers, especially those in hospitals (215). Whereas the incidence of HBV infection has markedly decreased in most dialysis units due to early and active vaccination campaigns, the incidence of HBV infection is growing in other categories of health care personnel. Recent statistics in Great Britain provided evidence of an increasing incidence of HBV infection among hospital staff, especially laboratory personnel, with 25% more new cases recorded in the 1980–1984 period than during the preceding 5 years (216).

The logistical problems with regard to vaccination differ between health care personnel and uremic patients. In healthy staff members, based on cost-effectiveness analysis (217), a consensus has emerged that vaccination without prescreening for HBV serologic markers and without subsequent determination of the peak anti-HBs titer should be recommended for large-scale programs, at least for new

Table 5. Decrease in the annual incidence of new cases of hepatitis B in dialysis patients and in staff of dialysis units in Europe as a whole and in four representative countries from 1981 through 1985.

	1981	*1982*	*1983*	*1984*	*1985*
Dialysis patients					
Europe (total)	1614	1360	1473	1402	1384
France	341	230	159	132	89
West Germany	206	117	117	90	68
Switzerland	26	4	11	3	1
United Kingdom	5	2	6	9	6
Staff					
Europe (total)	460	315	275	251	236
France	73	38	15	10	2
West Germany	55	47	19	9	4
Switzerland	8	4	0	0	0
United Kingdom	2	1	1	1	1

personnel not immediately exposed to a high risk of contamination (172, 173).

Another issue is the need for anti-HBs titration after vaccination and the choice of time schedule for revaccination. Data gained from longitudinal studies in healthy adults indicate that the length of persistence of anti-HBs is directly proportional to the peak level obtained after full vaccination. Thus, ideally, testing anti-HBs after vaccination and giving booster injections at intervals determined by peak antibody response should be the most appropriate procedure. However, such a strategy would be costly and difficult to implement for large-scale vaccination campaigns (218). Moreover, in view of the long-lasting protective efficacy of the vaccines, since even low levels of anti-HBs continue to protect against clinically significant HBV and development of a chronic carrier state, the need for revaccinating as soon as the anti-HBs level has fallen below 10 mIU/ml may be questioned. Thus, in health care workers exposed to a moderate risk of infection, a standard timing of booster injection, based on the average antibody persistence of the vaccine used, may be proposed, such as after 5 years for the Merck vaccine and after 10 years for the Pasteur vaccine. However, in staff working in high-risk units such as contaminated dialysis units, transplant or intensive care units, or for surgeons and laboratory staff, when cost is not an issue, post-vaccination testing should be considered an important ethical question, in view of the few, but unpredictable, cases of no or low response in healthy subjects. Such subjects should either be given additional dose(s) of vaccine in order to promote immune response or be moved to another less exposed unit. Also, those having been subjected to accidental heavy contamination such as a needle prick or mucous blood projection should have their anti-HBs level tested and should receive HBIG together with booster vaccine injection (153).

The problem is different in uremic patients, whether dialyzed or not. Screening for HBV markers is part of the routine surveillance of these patients and, even if costly, significant savings are to be expected from early vaccination. The optimal strategy now appears to be to vaccinate uremic subjects at least one year prior to the anticipated beginning of dialysis, for instance, when plasma creatinine is about 400 to 500 μmol/L. The protocol involves at least four injections (with 40 μg dosage when using Merck vaccine), with anti-HBs titration following the last injection, and additional injection(s) when no (or poor) response is obtained following the fourth injection. Following the booster injection, the peak anti-HBs value may give an indication as to the duration of protection and provide guidance for scheduling subsequent titrations, for instance every 2 or 3 months when peak value is under 500 mIU/ml, or every 4 to 6 months when it is higher, in order to perform the booster injection at the optimal time. Perhaps the new second-generation vaccines will prove to be more immunogenic in these immunodeficient patients. In any case, persistent observance of cross-infection precautions in dialysis units is recommended, in order to avoid transmission of other infective agents such as non-A, non-B virus.

CONCLUSION

In conclusion, the results obtained in a few years by vaccination are very impressive. For the first time, a dramatic reduction in the incidence of hepatitis B infection was observed in both patients and staff of hemodialysis units. Eradication of hepatitis B, which can be expected in the near future, will allow proper evaluation of the incidence and consequences of so-called non-A, non-B hepatitis. Whether or not HBs antigenemia and/or chronic liver lesions may influence indications for renal transplantation in dialysis patients infected by HBV still remains a partially unresolved problem. This constitutes an additional reason, if needed, to make all efforts toward effective prevention of HBV infection in uremic patients.

REFERENCES

1. Jones PO, Goldsmith HJ, Wright FK, Roberts C, Watson DC: Viral hepatitis: a staff hazard in dialysis units. *Lancet* 1: 835, 1967
2. Eastwood JB, Curtis JR, Wing AJ, de Wardener HE: Hepatitis in a maintenance hemodialysis unit. *Ann Intern Med* 69: 59, 1966
3. Ringertz O, Nyström B: Viral hepatitis in connection with hemodialysis and kidney transplantation. *Scand J Urol Nephrol* 1: 192, 1967
4. Ringertz O, Nyström B: Hepatitis B in a haemodialysis unit. *Lancet* 2: 745, 1969
5. Jacobs C, Legrain M: A propos d'une épidémie d'hépatite dans un centre d'hémodialyse chronique (Apropos of an epidemic of hepatitis in a chronic dialysis center.) *J Urol Nephrol* 74: 333, 1968
6. Leski M, Grivaux C, Couroucé-Pauty AM: L'antigène Australie dans un unité d'hémodialyse périodique et de transplantation. (Austrialia antigen in a periodic hemodialysis and renal transplantation unit.) *Presse Méd* 79: 391, 1971
7. Forrest JN Jr, Dismukes WE: Dialysis-associated hepatitis in 108 U.S. hemodialysis units. *Clin Res* 16: 383, 1968
8. Friedman EA, Thomson GE: Hepatitis complicating chronic haemodialysis. *Lancet* 2: 675, 1966
9. London WT, DiFiglia M, Sutnick AI, Blumberg BS: An epidemic of hepatitis in a chronic hemodialysis unit. Australia antigen and differences in host response. *N Engl J Med* 281: 571, 1969
10. Huggins CE, Blumberg BS, Giger K, Grady GF: Hepatitis in hemodialysis units. *N Engl J Med* 263: 657, 1970
11. Bone JM, Tonkin RW, Davison AM, Marmion BP, Robson JS: Outbreak of dialysis-associated hepatitis in Edinburgh, 1969–1970. *Proc Eur Dial Transplant Assoc* 8: 189, 1971
12. Drukker W, Haagsma-Schouten WAG, Albert C, Baarda B: Report on regular dialysis treatment in Europe. *Proc Eur Dial Transplant Assoc* 7: 3, 1970
13. Parsons FM, Brunner FP, Gurland HJ, Härlen H: Combined report on regular dialysis and transplantation in Europe, I, 1970. *Proc Eur Dial Transplant Assoc* 8: 3, 1971
14. Gurland HJ, Brunner FP, Dehn H, Härlen H, Parsons FM, Schärer K: Combined report on regular dialysis and transplantation in Europe, III, 1972. *Proc Eur Dial Transplant Assoc* 8: 17, 1973
15. Garibaldi RA, Forrest JN, Bryan JA, Hanson BF, Dismukes

WWE: Hemodialysis-associated hepatitis. *JAMA* 255: 384, 1973

16. Blumberg BS, Sutnick AI, London WT: Hepatitis and leukemia: their relation to Australia antigen. *Bull NY Acad Med* 44: 1566, 1968
17. Prince AM: An antigen detected in the blood during the incubation of serum hepatitis. *Proc Natl Acad Sci USA* 60: 814, 1968
18. Parsons FM, Brunner FP, Burck HC, Gräser W, Gurland HJ, Härlen H, Schärer K, Spies GW: Statistical report. *Proc Eur Dial Transplant Assoc* 11: 53, 1974
19. Szmuness W, Prince AM, Grady GF, Mann MK, Levine RN, Friedman EA, Jacobs MJ, Josephson A, Ribot S, Shapiro FL, Stenzel KH, Suki WN, Vyas G: Hepatitis B infection: a point-prevalence study in 15 US hemodialysis centers. *JAMA* 227: 901, 1974
20. Brynger H, Brunner FP, Chantler C, Donckerwolcke RA, Jacobs C, Kramer P, Selwood NH, Wing AJ: Combined report on regular dialysis and transplantation in Europe, X, 1979. *Proc Eur Dial Transplant Assoc* 17: 2, 1980
21. Jacobs C, Broyer M, Brunner FP, Brynger H, Donckerwolcke RA, Kramer P, Selwood NJ, Wing AJ, Blake AH: Combined report on regular dialysis and transplantation in Europe, XI, 1980. *Proc Eur Dial Transplant Assoc* 18: 2, 1981
22. Broyer M, Brunner FP, Brynger H, Donckerwolcke RA, Jacobs C, Kramer P, Selwood NH, Wing AJ: Combined report on regular dialysis and transplantation in Europe XII, 1981. *Proc Eur Dial Transplant Assoc* 19: 4, 1982
23. Wing AJ, Broyer M, Brunner FP, Brynger H, Challah S, Donckerwolcke RA, Gretz N, Jacobs C, Kramer P, Selwood NH: Combined report on regular dialysis and transplantation in Europe XIII, 1982. *Proc Eur Dial Transplant Assoc* 20: 5, 1983
24. Kramer P, Broyer M, Brunner FP, Brynger H, Challah S, Oulès R, Rizzoni G, Selwood NH, Wing AJ, Balas EA: Combined report on regular dialysis and transplantation in Europe XIV, 1983. *Proc Eur Dial Transplant Assoc Eur Ren Assoc* 2: 5, 1984
25. Brunner FP, Broyer M, Brynger H, Challah S, Fassbinder W, Oulès R, Rizzoni G, Selwood NH, Wing AJ: Combined report on regular dialysis and transplantation in Europe, XV, 1984. *Proc Eur Dial Transplant Assoc Eur Ren Assoc* 22: 5, 1985
26. Oulès R, Fassbinder W, Broyer M, Brunner FP, Brynger H, Challah S, Guillou PJ, Rizzoni G, Selwood NH, Wing AJ: Combined report on regular dialysis and transplantation in Europe, XVI, 1985
27. Bradley DW, Maynard JE, Hindman SH, Hornbech CL, Fields HA, McCaustland KA, Cook EH: Serodiagnosis of viral hepatitis A by radioimmunoassay. *J Clin Microbiol* 5: 521, 1977
28. Feinstone SM, Purcell RH: New methods for the serodiagnosis of hepatitis A. *Gastroenterology* 78: 1092, 1980
29. Szmuness W, Dienstag JL, Purcell RH, Prince AM, Stevens CE, Levine RW: Hepatitis type A and hemodialysis. *Ann Intern Med* 87: 8, 1977
30. Mathiesen LR, Hardt F, Dietrichson O, Purcell RH, Wong D, Skinhoj P, Nielsen JO, Zoffman H, Iversen K: The Copenhagen hepatitis acuta programme. The role of acute hepatitis A, B and non-A, non-B in the development of chronic active liver disease. *Scand J Gastroenterol* 15: 49, 1980
31. Alter HJ, Holland PV, Purcell RH: The emerging pattern of post-transfusion hepatitis. *Am J Med Sci* 270: 329, 1975
32. Feinstone SM, Kapikian AZ, Purcell RH, Alter HJ, Holland

PV: Transfusion-associated hepatitis not due to viral hepatitis type A or B. *N Engl J Med* 292: 767, 1975
33. Alter HJ, Purcell RH, Holland PV, Feinstone SM, Morrow AG, Moritsugu Y: Clinical and serological analysis of tranfusion-associated hepatitis. *Lancet* 2: 838, 1975
34. Hoofnagle JA, Gerety RJ, Tabor E, Feinstone SM, Barker LF, Purcell RH: Transmission of non-A, non-B hepatitis. *Ann Intern Med* 87: 14, 1977
35. Aach RD, Szmuness W, Mosley JW, Hollinger FB, Kahn R, Stevens CE, Edwards VM, Weich J: Serum alanine aminotransferase of donors in relation to the risk of non-A, non-B hepatitis in recipients. *N Engl J Med* 304: 899, 1981
36. Galbraith RM, Portman B, Eddleston ALWF, Williams R, Gower PE: Chronic liver disease developing after outbreak of HBsAg-negative hepatitis in haemodialysis unit. *Lancet* 2: 886, 1975
37. Avram MM, Feinfeld DA, Gan AC: Non-A, non-B hepatitis: a new syndrome in uraemic patients. *Proc Eur Dial Transplant Assoc* 16: 141, 1979
38. Galbraith RM, Dienstag JL, Purcell RH, Gower PH, Zuckerman AJ, Williams R: Non-A, non-B hepatitis associated with chronic liver disease in a haemodialysis unit. *Lancet* 1: 951, 1979
39. Simon N, Méry JP, Trépo C, Vitvitski L, Couroucé AM: A non-A, non-B hepatitis epidemic in an HB antigen-free hemodialysis unit. Demonstration of serological markers of non-A, non-B virus. *Proc Eur Dial Transplant Assoc* 17: 173, 1980
40. Berman M, Alter HJ, Ishak KG, Purcell RH, Jones EA: The chronic sequelae of non-A, non-B hepatitis. *Ann Intern Med* 91: 1, 1979
41. Knodell RG, Conrak ME, Ishak KG: Development of chronic liver disease after acute non-A, non-B post-transfusion hepatitis. *Gastroenterology* 72: 902, 1977
42. Rakela J, Redeker AG: Chronic liver disease after acute non-A, non-B viral hepatitis. *Gastroenterology* 77: 1200, 1979
43. Nielsen V, Clausen E, Ranek L: Liver impairment during chronic hemodialysis and after renal transplantation. *Acta Med Scand* 197: 229, 1975
44. Reed W, Lucas ZJ, Kempson R, Cohn R: Renal transplantation in patients with Australian antigenemia. *Transplant Proc* 3: 342, 1971
45. Thomas DR, Bogie W, Blainey JD, Robinson BHB, Dawson-Edwards P, Barnes AD: Hepatitis in a renal transplant unit. *Br J Surg* 59: 310, 1972
46. Aronoff A, Gault MH, Haung SH: Hepatitis with Australia antigenemia following renal transplantation. *Canad Med Assoc J* 108: 43, 1973
47. Ware AJ, Luby JP, Hollinger B, Eigenbrodt EH, Cuthbert JA, Atkins CR, Shorey J, Hull AR, Combes B: Etiology of liver disease in renal transplant patients. *Ann Intern Med* 91: 364, 1979
48. Degos F, Degott C, Bedrossian J, Camilieri JP, Barbanel C, Duboust A, Rueff B, Benhamou JP, Kreis H: Is renal transplantation involved in post-transplantation liver disease? A prospective study. *Transplantation* 29: 100, 1980
49. La Quaglia NP, Tolkoff-Rubin NE, Dienstag JL, Cosimi AB, Herrin JT, Kelly M, Rubin RH: Impact of hepatitis on renal transplantation. *Transplantation* 32: 504, 1981
50. Parfrey PS, Forbes RDC, Hutchinson TA, Kenick S, Farge E, Dauphinee WD, Seely JF, Guttman RD: The impact of renal transplantation on the course of hepatitis B liver disease. *Transplantation* 39: 610, 1985
51. Weir MR, Kirkman RL, Strom TB, Tilney NL: Liver disease in recipients of long-functioning renal allografts. *Kidney Int* 28: 839, 1985

52. Dusheiko G, Song E, Bowyer S, Whitcutt M, Maier G, Meyers A, Kew MC: Natural history of hepatitis B virus infection in renal transplant recipients. A fifteen-year follow-up. *Hepatology* 3: 330, 1983

53. Degos F, Debure A, Kreis H: Hepatitis in renal transplant recipients. *Transplantation Rev* 1: 159, 1987

54. Degast GC, Houwen B, Van der Hem GK, The JH: T lymphocyte number and function and the course of hepatitis B in hemodialysis patients. *Infect Immun* 14: 1138, 1976

55. Descamps B, Jungers P, Naret C, Zingraff J, Bach JF: HLA 1 B 8 phenotype association and HBs antigenemia evolution in 440 hemodialyzed patients. *Digestion* 15: 171, 1977

56. Robinson WS: Hepatitis B Dane particle DNA structure and the mechanism of the endogenous DNA polymerase reaction. In: *Viral Hepatitis,* edited by Vyas GN, Cohen JN, Schmid R, Philadelphia, Franklin Institute Press, 1978, p 139

57. Bréchot C, Hadchouel M, Scotto J, Degos F, Charnay P, Trépo C, Tiollais P, Berthelot P: Detection of hepatitis B virus DNA in liver and serum: a direct appraisal of the chronic carrier state. *Lancet* 2: 765, 1981

58. Bonino F, Hoyer B, Ford E, Shih JW, Purcell RH, Gerin JL: Hepatitis B virus DNA in the sera of HBs carriers. *Hepatology* 1: 386, 1981

59. Hoofnagle JH, Seeff LB, Bales ZB, Gerety RJ, Tabor E: Serologic responses in hepatitis B. In: *Viral Hepatitis,* edited by Vyas GN, Cohen SN, Schmid R, Philadelphia, Franklin Institute Press, 1978, p 219

60. Overby LR, Ling CM, Decker RH, Mushahwar IK, Chau K: Serodiagnostic profiles of viral hepatitis. In: *Viral Hepatitis,* edited by Szmuness W, Alter HJ, Maynard JE, Philadelphia, Franklin Institute Press, 1981, p 169

61. Nordenfelt E, Lindholm T, Lofgren B, Moestrup T, Reinicke V: Different categories of chronic HBsAg carriers; a long-term follow up. In: *Viral Hepatitis,* edited by Szmuness W, Alter HJ, Maynard JE, Philadelphia, Franklin Institute Press, 1981, p 237

62. Hoofnagle JH, Alter HJ: Chronic viral hepatitis. In: *Viral Hepatitis and Liver Disease,* edited by Vyas GN, Dienstag JL, Hoofnagle JH, Orlando, Grune and Stratton, 1984, p 97

63. Coughlin GP, Van Deth AG, Disney APS, Hay J, Wangel AG: Liver disease and the e antigen in HBsAg carriers with chronic renal failure. *Gut* 21: 118, 1980

64. Degott C, Degos F, Jungers P, Naret C, Couroucé AM, Potet F, Crosnier J: Relationship between liver histopathological changes and HBsAg in 111 patients treated by long-term hemodialysis. *Liver* 3: 377, 1983

65. Lebrec D, Degott C, Rueff B, Benhamou JP: Transvenous (transjugular) liver biopsy: an experience based on 100 biopsies. *Am J Dig Dis* 23: 302, 1978

66. Scheuer PJ: *Liver Biopsy Interpretation,* 3rd edition, London, Baillière Tindall, 1980

67. Parfrey PS, Forbes RDC, Hutchinson TA, Beaudoin JG, Dauphinee WD, Guttmann RD: The prevalence and progression of liver disease in renal transplant recipients: a histological study. *Transplant Proc* 16: 1103, 1984

68. Rizetto M: The delta agent. *Hepatology* 3: 729, 1983

69. Kharsa G, Degott C, Degos F, Carnot F, Potet F, Kreis H: Fulminant hepatitis in renal transplant recipients: role of delta agent. *Transplantation,* 44: 221, 1987

70. Sopko J, Anuras S: Liver disease in renal transplant recipients. *Am J Med* 64: 139, 1978

71. Ware AJ, Luby JP, Eigenbrodt EM, Long DL, Hull AR: Spectrum of liver disease in renal transplant recipients. *Gastroenterology* 68: 755, 1975

72. Cheeseman SH, Henle W, Rubin RH, Tolkoff-Rubin NE, Cosimi E, Cantell K, Winkle S, Herrin JT, Black PH, Russell PS, Hirsch MS: Epstein-Barr virus infection in renal transplant recipients; effect of antithymocyte globulin and interferon. *Ann Intern Med* 93: 39, 1980

73. Elliott WC, Houghton DC, Bryant RE, Wicklund R, Bany JM, Bennett WM: Herpes simplex type 1 hepatitis in renal transplantation. *Arch Intern Med* 140: 1656, 1968

74. Holdsworth SR, Atkins RC, Scott DF, Hayes K: Systemic herpes simplex infection with fulminant hepatitis post-transplantation. *Aust NZ J Med* 6: 588, 1976

75. Montgomerie JZ, Becroft DMO, Croxson MC, Doak PB, North JDK: Herpes simplex virus infection after renal transplantation. *Lancet* 2: 867, 1969

76. Trépo C, Vitvitski L, Hantz O, Pichoud C, Blancy B, Chevallier P, Trépo D, Babin S, Sepetjan M: Characterization and detection of a virus related to HBV in NANB hepatitis. In: *Viral Hepatitis,* edited by Szmuness W, Alter HJ, Maynard JE, Philadelphia, Franklin Institute Press, 1981, p 339

77. Trépo C, Degos F, Vitvitski L, Calson R, Chossegros P, Pichard C, Hantz D, Chevallier P, Chevré JC, Simon N, Peyrol S, Grimaud JA, Feldman G, Sepetjan M, Wands J: Evidence for a transmissible Non A non B agent inextricably linked with hepatitis B virus. In: *Viral Hepatitis and Liver Disease,* edited by Vyas GN, Dienstag JL, Hoofnagle JH, Orlando, Grune and Stratton 1984, p 355

78. Alter HJ, Hoofnagle JH: Non A non B observations on the first decade. In: *Viral Hepatitis and Liver Disease,* edited by Vyas GN, Dienstag JL, Hoofnagle JH, Orlando, Grune and Stratton 1984, p 345

79. Schafritz DA, Lieberman HM, Isselbacher KJ, Wands JR: Monoclonal radioimmunoassays for hepatitis B surface antigen. Demonstration of hepatitis B virus DNA or related sequences in serum and viral epitopes in immune complexes. *Proc Natl Acad Sci USA* 79: 5675, 1982

80. Fujita YK, Kamata K, Kameda H, Isselbacher KJ, Wands JR: Detection of hepatitis B virus infection in hepatitis B surface antigen negative hemodialysis patients by monoclonal radioimmunoassays. *Gastroenterology* 91: 1457, 1986

81. Wands J, Fujita YK, Isselbacher K, Degott C, Schellekens H, Dazza MC, Thiers V, Tiollais P, Brechot C: Identification and transmission of hepatitis-related variants. *Proc Natl Acad Sci USA* 83: 6608, 1986

82. Bréchot C, Degos F, Lugassy C, Thiers V, Zafrani S, Franco D, Bismuth H, Trépo C, Benhamou JP, Wands J, Isselbacher K, Tiollais P, Berthelot P: Hepatitis B virus DNA in patients with chronic liver disease and negative tests for hepatitis B surface antigen. *N Engl J Med* 312: 270, 1985

83. Degos F, Lugassy C, Degott C, Debure A, Carnot F, Thiers V, Tiollais P, Kreis H, Bréchot C: HBV and HBV related infection in renal transplant recipients. A prospective study of 90 patients. *Gastroenterology* 94: 151, 1988

84. Figus A, Blum HE, Vyas GN, Virgilis S, Cao A, Lippi M, Lai E, Balestrieri A: Hepatitis B nucleotide sequences in non A non B or hepatitis B related chronic liver disease. *Hepatology* 4: 364, 1984

85. Harrison TJ, Anderson MG, Murray Lyon IM, Zuckerman AJ: Hepatitis B virus DNA in the hepatocytes: a series of 160 biopsies. *J Hepatol* 1: 10, 1986

86. Ware AJ, Gorder NL, Gurian LE, Douglas C, Shorey JW, Parker T: Value of screening for markers of hepatitis in dialysis units. *Hepatology* 3: 513, 1983

87. Hillis WD, Hillis A, Walter WG: Hepatitis B surface antigenemia in renal transplant recipients. Increased mortality risk. *JAMA* 243: 329, 1979

88. Kirkman RL, Strom TB, Weir MR, Tilney NL: Late mortality and morbidity in recipients of long-term renal allografts. *Transplantation* 34: 347, 1982

89. Weissberg JI, Andres LL, Smith CI, Weick S, Nichols JE, Garcia G, Robinson WS, Merigan TC, Gregory PB: Survival in chronic hepatitis B. An analysis of 379 patients. *Ann Intern Med* 101: 613, 1984

90. London WT, Drew JS, Blumberg BS, Grossmann PA, Lyons PJ: Association of graft survival with host response to hepatitis B infection in patients with kidney transplants. *N Engl J Med* 296: 241, 1969

91. Pirson Y, Alexandre GPJ, Van Ypersele de Strihou C: Long-term effect of HBs antigenemia on patient survival after renal transplantation. *N Engl J Med* 296: 194, 1977

92. Villa E, Rubbiana L, Barchi T, Ferretti I, Grisendi A, de Palma M, Bellentani S, Manenti F: Susceptibility of chronic symptomless HBsAg carriers to ethanol induced hepatic damage. *Lancet* 2: 1243, 1982

93. Hoofnagle JH, Davis GL, Pappas SC, Hanson RG, Peters M, Arigan MI, Waggoner JG, Jones A, Seeff LB: A short course of prednisolone in chronic type B hepatitis. Report of a randomized, double-blind, placebo-controlled trial. *Ann Intern Med* 104: 12, 1986

94. Lam KC, Lai CL, Trépo C, Wu PC: Deleterious effect of prednisolone in HBsAg positive chronic active hepatitis. *N Engl J Med* 304: 380, 1981

95. Sagnelli E, Piccinino F, Manzillo G, Felaco FM, Filippini P, Maio G, Pasquale G, Izzo C: Effect of immunosuppressive therapy on HBsAg positive chronic active hepatitis in relation to presence or absence of HBeAg and anti-HBe. *Hepatology* 5: 690, 1983

96. Bréchot C, Nalpas B, Couroucé AM, Duhamel G, Callard P, Carnot F, Tiollais P, Berthelot P: Evidence that hepatitis B has a role in liver cell carcinoma in alcoholic liver disease. *N Engl J Med* 306: 1384, 1982

97. Kew MC: The hepatitis B virus and hepatocellular carcinoma. *Semin Liver Disease* 1: 59, 1981

98. Shafritz DA, Shouval JD, Sherman HI, Hadziyannis SJ, Kew MC: Integration of hepatitis B virus DNA into the genome of liver cells in chronic liver disease and hepatocellular carcinoma. *N Engl J Med* 305: 1067, 1981

99. Arbus GS, Hung RH: Hepatocarcinoma and myocardial fibrosis in an 8–3/4 year old renal transplant recipient. *Canad Med Assoc J* 107: 431, 1972

100. Schroeter GPJ, Weill R, Penn I, Speers WC, Waddell WR: Hepatocellular carcinoma assoicated with hepatitis B infection after kidney transplantation. *Lancet* 2: 381, 1982

101. Reinicke V, Dybkjaer E, Poulsen H, Banke O, Lylloff K, Nordenfelt E: A study of Australia-antigen positive blood donors and their recipients with special reference to liver histology. *N Engl J Med* 286: 867, 1972

102. Couroucé-Pauty AM, Soulier JP: Further data on HBs antigen subtypes. Geographical distribution. *Vox Sang* 27: 533, 1974

103. Soulier JP, Jungers P, Zingraff J: Virus B hepatitis in hemodialysis centers. *Adv Nephrol* 6: 383, 1976

104. Polakoff S, Cossart YE, Tillett HE: Hepatitis in dialysis units in the United Kingdom. *Br Med J* 3: 94, 1972

105. Turner GC, Bruce-White GB: SH antigen in haemodialysis-associated hepatitis. *Lancet* 2: 121, 1969

106. Pattison CP, Maynard JE, Berquist KR, Webster HM: Serological and epidemiological studies of hepatitis B in haemodialysis units. *Lancet* 2: 172, 1973

107. Dankert J, Uitentuis J, Houwen B, Tegzess AM, van der Hem GK: Hepatitis B surface antigen in environmental samples from hemodialysis units. *J Infect Dis* 134: 112, 1976

108. Salo RJ, Salo AA, Fahlberg WJ, Ellzey JP: Hepatitis B surface antigen (HBsAg) in peritoneal fluid of HBsAg carriers undergoing peritoneal dialysis. *J Med Virol* 6: 29, 1980

109. Heathcote H, Cameron CH, Dane DS: Hepatitis B antigen in saliva and semen. *Lancet* 1: 71, 1974

110. Public Health Laboratory Service: Infection risks of haemodialysis: some preventive aspects. *Br Med J* 3: 454, 1968

111. Department of Health and Social Security: Report of the Advisory Group on Hepatitis and the Treatment of Chronic Renal Failure 1970–1972. London DHSS, 1972

112. Public Health Laboratory Service Survey: Decrease in the incidence of hepatitis in dialysis units associated with prevention programme. *Br Med J* 4: 751, 1974

113. Public Health Laboratory Service: Hepatitis in retreat from dialysis units in United Kingdom in 1973. *Br Med J* 1: 1579, 1976

114. Krugman S, Giles JP, Hammond J: Viral hepatitis, type B (MS-2 strain): prevention with specific hepatitis B immune serum globulin. *JAMA* 218: 1665, 1971

115. Szmuness W, Prince AM, Goodman M, Ehrlich C, Pick R, Ansari M: Hepatitis B immune serum globulin in prevention of nonparenterally transmitted hepatitis B. *N Engl J Med* 290: 701, 1974

116. Hoofnagle JH, Seeff LB, Bales BZ, Wright EC, Zimmerman HJ, The Veterans Administration Cooperative Study Group: Passive-active immunity from hepatitis B immune globulin. *Ann Intern Med* 91: 813, 1979

117. Desmyter J, Bradburne AF, Vermylen C, Daneels R, Boelaert J: Hepatitis B immunoglobulin in prevention of HBs antigenaemia in haemodialysis patients. *Lancet* 2: 377, 1975

118. Surgenor DMacN, Chalmers TC, Conrad ME, Friedwald WT, Grady GF, Hamilton M, Mosley JW, Prince AM, Stengle JM: Clinical trials of hepatitis B immune globulin. *N Engl J Med* 293: 1060, 1975

119. Kleinknecht D, Couroucé AM, Delons S, Naret C, Adhémar SP, Ciancioni C, Fermanian J: Prevention of hepatitis B in hemodialysis patients using hepatitis B immunoglobulin. *Clin Nephrol* 8: 373, 1977

120. Prince AM, Szmuness W, Mann MK, Vyas GN, Grady GF, Shapiro FL, Suki WN, Friedman EA, Avram MM, Stenkel KH: Hepatitis B immune globulin: Final report of a controlled multicentre trial of efficacy in prevention of dialysis-associated hepatitis. *J Infect Dis* 137: 131, 1978

121. Iwarson S, Ahlmén J, Eriksson E, Hermodsson S, Kjellman H, Ljunggren C, Selander D: Hepatitis B immune globulin in prevention of hepatitis B among hospital staff members. *J Infect Dis* 135: 473, 1977

122. Couroucé-Pauty AM, Delons S, Soulier JP: Attempt to prevent hepatitis by using specific anti-HBs immunoglobulin. *Am J Med Sci* 270: 375, 1975

123. Seeff LB, Wright EC, Zimmerman HJ, Alter HJ, Dietz AA, Felsher BF, Finkelstein JD, Garcia-Pont P, Gerin JL, Greenlee HB Hamilton J, Holland PV, Kaplan PM, Kiernan T, Koff RS, Leevy CM, McAuliffe VJ, Nath N, Purcell RH, Schiff ER, Schwartz CC, Tamburro CH, Vlahcevic Z, Zemel R, Zimmon DS: Type B hepatitis after needlestick exposure: Prevention with hepatitis B immunoglobulin. *Ann Intern Med* 88: 285, 1978

124. Grady GF, Lee VA, Prince AM, Gitnick GL, Fawaz KA, Vyas GN, Levitt MD, Senior JR, Galambos JT, Bynum TE, Singleton JW, Clowdus BF, Akdamar K, Aach RD, Winkleman EI, Schiff GM, Hersch T: Hepatitis B immune globulin

for accidental exposure among medical personnel: final report of a multicentre controlled trial. *J Infect Dis* 138: 625, 1978

125. Couroucé AM, Bouchardeau F, Le Marrec N, Boulard G, Soulier JP: The use of hepatitis B vaccine as booster for donors immune to HBV for the production of hepatitis B immunoblobulin (HBIG). In: *Second WHO/IABS Symposium on Viral Hepatitis*, Basel, S Karger, 1983, p 333

126. Krugman S, Giles JP, Hammond J: Viral hepatitis, type B (MS-2 strain): studies on active immunization. *JAMA* 217: 41, 1971

127. Jungers P, Delagneau JF, Prunet P, Crosnier J: Vaccination against hepatitis B in hemodialysis centers. *Adv Nephrol* 11: 303, 1982

128. Stevens CE, Taylor PE, Tong MJ, Toy PT, Vyas GN: Hepatitis B vaccine: an overview. In: *Viral Hepatitis and Liver Disease,* edited by Vyas GN, Dienstag JL, Hoofnagle JH, Orlando, Grune and Stratton, 1984, p 275

129. Jacobson IM, Dienstag JI: Viral hepatitis vaccines. *Annu Rev Med* 36: 241, 1985

130. Hilleman MR, Buynak EB, Roehm RR, Tytell AA, Bertland AV, Lampson GP: Purified and inactivated human hepatitis B vaccine: Progress report. *Am J Med Sci* 270: 401, 1975

131. Maupas P, Goudeau A, Coursaget P, Drucker J: Immunization against hepatitis B in man. *Lancet* 1: 1367, 1976

132. Adamowicz P, Gerfaux G, Platel A, Muller L, Vacher B, Mazert MC, Prunet P: Large scale production of an hepatitis B vaccine. In: *Hepatitis B Vaccine,* edited by Maupas P, Guesry P, Amsterdam, Elsevier-North Holland, 1981, p 37

133. Brummelhuis HGJ, Wilson-De Stüler LA, Raap AK: Preparation of hepatitis B vaccine by heat inactivation. In: *Hepatitis B Vaccine,* edited by Maupas P, Guesry P, Amsterdam, Elsevier-North Holland, 1981, p 51

134. Purcell RH, Gerin JL: Hepatitis B subunit vaccine: a preliminary report on safety and efficacy tests in chimpanzees. *Am J Med Sci* 270: 395, 1975

135. Hepatitis B vaccine: evidence confirming lack of AIDS transmission. *MMWR* 33: 685, 1984

136. Adamowicz P, Chabanier G, Hyafil F, Lucas G, Prunet P, Reculard P, Vinas R: Elimination of serum proteins and potential virus contaminants during hepatitis B vaccine preparation. *Vaccine* 2: 209, 1984

137. Szmuness W: Large-scale efficacy trials of hepatitis B vaccines in the USA: baseline data and protocols. *J Med Virol* 4: 327, 1979

138. Szmuness W, Stevens CE, Harley EJ, Zang EA, Olesko WR, William DC, Sadovsky R, Morrison JM, Kellnar A: Hepatitis B vaccine. Demonstration of efficacy in controlled clinical trial in a high-risk population in the United States. *N Engl J Med* 303: 833, 1980

139. Szmuness W, Stevens CE, Zang EA, Harley EJ, Kellner A: A controlled clinical trial of the efficacy of the hepatitis B vaccine (Heptavax B): a final report. *Hepatology* 1: 377, 1981

140. Crosnier J, Jungers P, Couroucé AM, Laplanche A, Benhamou E, Degos F, Lacour B, Prunet P, Cerisier Y, Guersy P: Randomised placebo-controlled trial of hepatitis B surface antigen vaccine in French haemodialysis units. I. Medical staff. *Lancet* 1: 455, 1981

141. Laplanche A, Couroucé AM, Benhamou E, Jungers P, Crosnier J: Response to hepatitis B vaccine. *Lancet* 1: 222, 1982

142. Szmuness W, Stevens CE, Harley EJ, Zang EA, Alter JH, Taylor PE, De Vera A, Chen GTS, Kellner A: Hepatitis B vaccine in medical staff of hemodialysis units: efficacy and subtype cross-protection. *N Engl Med* 307: 1481, 1982

143. Desmyter J, Colaert J, De Groote G, Reynders M, Reerink-

Brongers EE, Lelie PN, Dees PJ, Reesink HW: Efficacy of heat-inactivated hepatitis B vaccine in haemodialysis patients and staff. Double-blind placebo-controlled trial. *Lancet* 2: 1323, 1983

144. Dienstag JI, Werner BG, Polk BH, Snydman DR, Craven DE, Platt R, Crumpacker CS, Quellet-Hellstrom R, Grady GF: Hepatitis B vaccine in health care personnel: Safety, immunogenicity and indicators of efficacy. *Ann Intern Med* 101: 34, 1984

145. Goudeau A, Dubois F, Barin F, Dubois MC, Coursaget P: Hepatitis B vaccines: clinical trials in high-risk setting in France (September 1975 – September 1982). In: *Second WHO/IABS Symposium on Viral Hepatitis*, Basel, Karger 1983, p 267

146. Strickler AC, Kibsey PC, Vellend H: Seroconversion rates with hepatitis B vaccine. *Ann Intern Med* 101: 564, 1984

147. Schaaf DM, Lender M, Suedeker P, Graham LA: Hepatitis B vaccine in a hospital. *Ann Intern Med* 101: 720, 1984

148. Ukena T, Esber H, Bessette R, Parks T, Crockers B, Shaw FE: Site of injection and response to hepatitis B vaccine. *N Engl J Med* 313: 579, 1985

149. Francis DP, Hadler SC, Thompson SE, Maynard JE, Ostrow DG, Altman N, Braff EH, O'Malley PM, Hawkins JD, Judson FN, Penley K, Nylund T, Christie G, Meyers F, Moore JN, Gardner A, Doto IL, Miller JH, Reynolds GH, Murphy BL, Schable CA, Clark BT, Curran JW, Redeker AG: The prevention of hepatitis B with vaccine: report of the Centers for Disease Control multi-center efficacy trial among homosexual men. *Ann Intern Med* 97: 362, 1982

150. Centers for Disease Control: Suboptimal response to hepatitis B vaccine given by injection into the buttock *MMWR* 34: 105, 1985

151. Pead PJ, Saeed AA, Hewitt WG, Brownfield RN: Low immune responses to hepatitis B vaccination among healthy subjects. *Lancet* 1: 1152, 1985

152. Weber DJ, Rutala WA, Samsa GP, Santimaw JE, Lemon SM: Obesity as a predictor of poor antibody response to hepatitis B plasma vaccine. *JAMA* 254: 3187, 1985

153. Centers for Disease Control: Recommendations for protection against viral hepatitis. Recommendations of the immunization practices advisory committee. *Ann Intern Med* 103: 391, 1985

154. Craven DE, Awdeh ZL, Kunches LM, Yunis EJ, Dienstag JL, Werner BG, Polk BF, Snydman DR, Platt R, Crumpacker CS, Grady GF, Alper CA: Non responsiveness to hepatitis B vaccine in health care workers. Results of revaccination and genetic typings. *Ann Intern Med* 105: 356, 1986

155. Szmuness W, Stevens CE, Oleszo WR, Godman A: Passive-active immunisation against hepatitis B: immunogenicity studies in adult Americans. *Lancet* 1: 575, 1981

156. Goudeau A, Coursaget P, Barin F, Dubois F, Chiron JP, Denis F, Diop Mar I: Prevention of hepatitis B by active and passive-active immunization. In: *Viral Hepatitis*, edited by Szmuness W, Alter HJ. Maynard JE, Philadelphia, Franklin Institute Press, 1981, p 509

157. Couroucé AM, Naret C, Adhémar JP, Cerisier Y, Bouchardeau F, Masselot JP, Delons S, Guesry P: A study of the switch from passive to active immunization in hemodialysis units. In: *Hepatitis B Vaccine Symposium*, edited by Maupas P, Guesry P, Amsterdam, Elsevier-North Holland, 1981, p 173

158. Mesnier F, Sanchez D, Maurel JP, Moulinier J: Comparative study of active and passive-active immunization in the prevention of hepatitis B infection in high-risk settings. In: *Hepatitis*

B Vaccine Symposium, edited by Maupas P, Guesry P, Amsterdam, Elsevier-North Holland, 1981, p 183

159. Coutinho RA, Lelie N, Albrecht-Van Lent P, Reerink-Brongers EE, Stoutjesdijk L, Dees P, Nivard J, Huisman J, Reesink HIV: Efficacy of a heat inactivated hepatitis B vaccine in male homosexuals: outcome of a placebo controlled double blind trial. *Br Med J* 2: 1305, 1983

160. Jilg W, Schmidt M, Deinhardt F, Zachoval R: Hepatitis B vaccination: how long does protection last? *Lancet* 2: 458, 1984

161. Grob PJ, Dufek A, Joller-Jemelka HI: Hepatitis B Imfung – wann ist eine Booster Injecktion nötig? (Hepatitis B immunization – when is a booster injection necessary?) *Schweiz Med Wschr* 115: 394, 1985

162. Hadler SC, Francis DP, Maynard JE, Thompson SE, Judson FN, Echenberg DF, Ostrow DG, O'Malley PM, Penley KA, Altman NL, Braff E, Shipman GF, Coleman PJ, Mandel EJ: Long-term immunogenicity and efficacy of hepatitis B vaccine in homosexual men. *N Engl J Med* 315: 209, 1986

163. Jungers P, Courroucé AM, Laplanche A, Benhamou E: Hepatitis B vaccine. *N Engl J Med* 316: 47, 1987

164. Jungers P, Courroucé AM, Laplanche A, Benhamou E, Crosnier J: Long-term efficacy and immunogenicity of HEVAC B vaccine in medical staff of hemodialysis units. *Proc Eur Symposium on Hepatitis B Immunization, Evaluation and Perspectives,* Roma, October 1986.

165. Dienstag JL, Stevens CE, Bhan AK, Szmuness W: Hepatitis B vaccine administered to chronic carriers of hepatitis B surface antigen. *Ann Intern Med* 96: 575, 1982

166. Dienstag JL, Ryan DM: Occupational exposure to hepatitis B virus in hospital personnel: infection or immunization? *Am J Epidemiol* 15: 26, 1982

167. Kessler HA, Harris AA, Payne JA, Hudson E, Potkin B, Levin S: Antibodies to hepatitis B surface antigen as the sole hepatitis B marker in hospital personnel. *Ann Intern Med* 103: 21, 1985

168. Werner BG, Dienstag JL, Kuter BJ, Polk BF, Snydman DR, Craven DE, Crumpacker CS, Platt R, Grady GF: Isolated antibody to hepatitis B surface antigen and response to hepatitis B vaccination. *Ann Intern Med* 103: 201, 1985

169. Goudeau A, Dubois F: Immune status of anti-HBc positive individuals. *Lancet* 1: 396, 1984

170. Taliani G, Lece R, Furian C, Nuti M, Bernaschi P, De Bac C: Hepatitis vaccination for a wider diagnostic purpose? *Lancet* 2: 173, 1984

171. Hadziyannis SJ, Hatzakis A: Response to hepatitis B vaccine of anti-HBc positive subject. In: *Hepatitis B Vaccine Symposium (Berne) New Findings and Perspectives,* edited by Tron F, Marnes-la Coquette, Pasteur Vaccins, 1984, p 33

172. Kane MA, Hadler SC, Maynard JE: Antibody to hepatitis B surface antigen and screening before hepatitis vaccination. *Ann Intern Med* 103: 791, 1985

173. Perrillo RP: Screening of health care workers before hepatits B vaccination: more questions than answers. *Ann Intern Med* 103: 793, 1985

174. Goldblum SE, Reed WP: Host defenses and immunologic alterations associated with chronic hemodialysis. *Ann Intern Med* 93: 597, 1980

175. Dobbelstein H: Immune system in uremia. *Nephron* 17: 409, 1976

176. Revillard JP: Immunologic alterations in chronic renal insufficiency. *Adv Nephrol* 8: 365, 1979

177. Kurz P, Köhler H, Meuer S, Hütteroth T, Meyer zum Büschenfelde KH: Impaired cellular immune responses in chronic

renal failure: evidence for a T cell defect. *Kidney Int* 29: 1209, 1986

178. Kurz P, Köhler H, Hütteroth T, Weber M, Meyer zum Büschenfelde KH: Immune defect in the early stage of chronic renal failure. *Proc Eur Dial Transplant Assoc Eur Ren Assoc* 22: 941, 1985

179. Cappel R, Van Beers D, Liesnard C, Dratwa M: Impaired humoral and cell-mediated immune responses in dialyzed patients after influenza vaccination. *Nephron* 33: 21, 1983

180. Linneman CC Jr, First MR, Schiffman G: Response to pneumococcal vaccine in renal transplant and hemodialysis patients. *Arch Intern Med* 141: 1637, 1981

181. Linnemann CC Jr, First MR, Schiffman G: Revaccination of renal transplant and hemodialysis recipients with pneumococcal vaccine. *Arch Intern Med* 146: 1554, 1986

182. Maupas P, Goudeau A, Coursaget P, Drucker J, Bagros P: Hepatitis B vaccine efficacy in high risk settings, a two year study. *Intervirology* 10: 196, 1978

183. Stevens CE, Szmuness W, Goodman AI, Wesely Sa, Fotino M: Hepatitis B vaccine: immune responses in haemodialysis patients. *Lancet* 2: 1211, 1980

184. Crosnier J, Jungers P, Courroucé AM, Laplanche A, Benhamou E, Degos F, Lacour B, Prunet P, Cerisier Y, Guesry P: Randomised placebo-controlled trial of hepatitis B surface antigen vaccine in French haemodialysis units. II. Haemodialysis patients. *Lancet* 1: 797, 1981

185. Stevens CE, Alter HJ, Taylor PE, Zang EA, Harley EJ, Szmuness W: Hepatitis B vaccine in patients receiving hemodialysis. Immunogenicity and efficacy. *N Engl J Med* 311: 496, 1984

186. Bommer J, Ritz E, Andrassy K, Bommer G, Deinhardt F, Jilg W, Daral G: Effect of vaccination schedule and dialysis on hepatitis B vaccination response in uraemic patients. *Proc Eur Dial Transplant Assoc Eur Ren Assoc* 20: 161, 1983

187. Bommer J, Grussendorf M, Jilg W, Deinhardt F, Koch HG, Daral G, Bommer G, Rambause M, Ritz E: Vaccination against hepatitis B in patients with renal insufficiency. *Proc Eur Dial Transplant Assoc Eur Ren Assoc* 21: 300, 1984

188. Köhler H, Arnold W, Renschin G, Dormeyer HH, Meyer zum Büschenfelde KH: Active hepatitis B vaccination of dialysis patients and medical staff. *Kidney Int* 25: 124, 1984

189. De Graff PA, Dankert J, De Zeeuw D, Gips CH, van der Hem GK: Immune response to two different hepatitis B vaccines in haemodialysis patients: a 2-year follow-up. *Nephron* 40: 155, 1985

190. Carreno V, Mora I, Escuin F, Sanchez-Sicilia L, Alvarez V, Casado S, Alcazar JM, Hernando L, Porres JC, Carrasco JL, Lardinois R: Vaccination against hepatits B in renal dialysis units: short or normal vaccination schedule? *Clin Nephrol* 24: 215, 1985

191. Lelie PN, Reesink HW, De Jong-Van Manen S, Dees PJ, Reerink-Brongers EE: Immune response to heat-inactivated hepatitis B vaccine in patients undergoing hemodialysis. Enhancement of the response by increasing the dose of hepatitis B surface antigen from 3 to 27 μg. *Arch Intern Med* 145: 305, 1985

192. Benhamou E, Courroucé AM, Jungers P, Laplanche A, Degos F, Brangier J, Crosnier J: Hepatitis B vaccine: randomized trial of immunogenicity in hemodialysis patients. *Clin Nephrol* 21: 143, 1984

193. Courroucé AM, Jungers P, Benhamou E, Laplanche A, Crosnier J: Hepatitis B in dialysis patients. *N Engl J Med* 311: 1515, 1984

194. Van Geelen JA, Schalm SW, De Visser EM, Heigtink RA:

Immune response to hepatitis B vaccine in hemodialysis patients. *Nephron* 45: 216, 1987

195. Michel P, Janin G, El Yafi S, Chevallier P, Girard P, Laville M, Trépo C: Improvement of immune response in dialysis patients to Hevac B vaccine after multiple injections of vaccine. *Proc Eur Dial Transplant Assoc Eur Ren Assoc* 22: 1077, 1985

196. Benhamou E, Couroucé AM, Laplanche A, Jungers P, Tron F, Crosnier J: Long-term results of hepatitis B vaccination in patients on dialysis. *N Engl J Med* 314: 1710, 1986

197. Rottembourg J, Barthélémy A, Tron F, Laleye B, Boulanger C, Legrain M: Hepatitis B vaccine in uremic patients with end-state renal disease. In: *2nd Hepatitis B Vaccine Symposium (Berne) New Findings and Perspectives*, edited by Tron F, Marnes-la-Coquette Pasteur Vaccins, 1984, p 67

198. Jungers P, Chauveau P, Couroucé AM, Mattlinger B, Crosnier J: Hepatitis B vaccine in non-dialysed uraemic patients: preliminary results. *Proc Eur Dial Transplant Assoc Eur Ren Assoc* 22: 1073, 1985

199. Chauveau P, Loubaris T, Couroucé AM, Mattlinger B, Jungers P: Immune response to hepatitis B vaccine in non-dialysed uremic patients. In preparation

200. Zuckerman AJ: New hepatitis B vaccines. *Br Med J* 1: 492, 1985

201. Skelly J, Howard CR, Zuckerman AJ: Hepatitis B polypeptide vaccine preparation in micelle form. *Nature* 290: 51, 1981

202. Neurath AR, Kent SBH, Strick NS, Taylor P, Stevens CE: Hepatitis B virus contains pre-S gene-encoded domians. *Nature* 315: 154, 1985

203. Coursaget P, Barrès JL, Chriron JP, Adamowicz P: Hepatitis B vaccines with and without polymerised albumin receptors. *Lancet* 1: 152, 1985

204. Milich D, Thornton G, Neurath R, Kent S, Michel ML, Tiollais P, Chisari F: Enhanced immunogenicity of the pre-S region of hepatitis B surface antigen. *Science* 228: 1195, 1985

205. Neurath R, Kent S, Parker K, Prince A, Strick N, Brotman P, Sproul P: Antibodies to a synthetic peptide from pre-S 120-145

region of the hepatitis B virus envelope are virus neutralizing. *Vaccine* 4: 35, 1986

206. Mc Aleer WJ, Buynak EB, Maigetter RZ, Wampler DE, Miller WJ, Hilleman MR: Human hepatitis B vaccine from recombinant yeast. *Nature* 307: 178, 1984

207. Jilg W, Lobeer B, Schmidt M, Wilkse B, Zoulek G, Deinhardt F: Clinical evaluation of a recombinant hepatitis B vaccine. *Lancet* 2: 1174, 1985

208. Scolnick EM, Mc Lean AA, West DJ, Mc Aller WJ, Miller WJ, Buynack EB: Clinical evaluation in healthy adults of a hepatitis B vaccine made by recombinant DNA. *JAMA* 251: 2812, 1984

209. Brown SE, Stanley C, Howard CR, Zuckerman AJ, Steward MW: Antibody responses to recombinant and plasma derived hepatitis B vaccines. *Br Med J* 1: 159, 1986

210. Hollinger FB, Troisi Cl, Pepe PE: Anti-HBs responses to vaccination with a human hepatitis B vaccine made by recombinant DNA technology in yeast. *J Infect Dis* 153: 156, 1986

211. Grady GF: The here and now of hepatitis B immunization. *N Engl J Med* 315: 250, 1986

212. Stevens CE, Taylor PE, Rubinstein P, Ting RCY, Badner AJ, Sarngadharan MG, Gallo RG: Safety of the hepatitis B vaccine. *N Engl J Med* 312: 375, 1985

213. Jacobson IM, Dienstag JL, Zachoval R, Hanrahan BA, Watkins E, Rubin RH: Lack of effect of hepatitis B vaccine on T-cell phenotypes. *N Engl J Med* 311: 1030, 1984

214. Alter MJ, Favero MS, Maynard JE: Hepatitis B vaccine use in chronic hemodialysis centers in the United States. *JAMA* 254: 3200, 1985

215. Finch RG: Time for action on hepatitis immunisation. *Br Med J* 294: 197, 1987

216. Polakoff S: Acute viral hepatitis B: Laboratory reports 1980–84. *Br Med J* 293: 37, 1986

217. Mulley AG, Silverstein MD, Dienstag JL: Indications for use of hepatitis B vaccine, based on cost-effectiveness analysis. *N Engl J Med* 307: 644, 1982

218. Strickler AC: Hepatitis B vaccine. *N Engl J Med* 316: 47, 1987

43

DIALYSIS IN THE ACQUIRED IMMUNODEFICIENCY SYNDROME

T.K. SREEPADA RAO

INTRODUCTION

The Center for Disease Control (CDC) defines acquired immunodeficiency syndrome (AIDS) as a disorder characterized by the development of opportunistic infection(s), and (or) unusual malignancies such as Kaposi's sarcoma, and certain forms of lymphoma in patients without a prior known immunological disorder (1). Risk factors for the development of AIDS include intravenous drug addiction, homosexuality, and exposure to contaminated blood and blood products. In Miami and Brooklyn, there is an increased incidence of AIDS among patients who have recently immigrated from Haiti. The disease is caused by human immunodeficiency virus (HIV), the transmission characteristics of which parallel those of hepatitis B virus. Serological tests are currently available to detect antibodies to the HIV (2). Viral isolation from affected patient's lymphocytes, various body fluids, and organs is also feasible in specialized laboratories. Consequently, it is now possible to establish the diagnosis of AIDS in certain immunocompromized subjects such as renal transplant recipients, and those with autoimmune disorders, who previously were excluded by definition. As of July 1987, over 35,000 cases of AIDS have been reported to the CDC from all parts of the USA. The mortality in AIDS continues to be high, with more than 50% of reported cases dying within 3 to 4 years, primarily from infectious problems.

As the epidemic of AIDS expanded world wide, the spectrum of medical complications seen and reported in these patients also widened. Realizing the scope of multisystem involvement in AIDS, it was inevitable that the nephrologists would soon be involved in identifying, and managing renal problems in such patients.

RENAL INVOLVEMENT IN AIDS

In 1984, approximately 2 years after the initial description of AIDS, a renal syndrome, AIDS associated nephropathy was originally described from our center (3). It is character-

ized by proteinuria greater than 3.5 g/day coupled with glomerular changes of focal and segmental glomerulosclerosis (FSGS), which cause rapid renal functional deterioration resulting in end-stage renal disease (ESRD) within weeks. Subsequently, a similar observation was reported from Miami (4). Others have recorded a variety of renal lesions in AIDS compromising both glomerular and tubular changes, as well as non-specific lesions such as acute tubular necrosis (ATN), nephrocalcinosis, and interstitial nephritis (5–9). Proteinuria, hematuria, leukocyturia, bacteriuria, reduced creatinine clearance, and various electrolyte derangements have also been reported (6). Additional renal perturbations described in AIDS include minimal change nephropathy (8, 9), acute renal failure (ARF) due to the hemolytic uremic syndrome (10), and post infectious immune complex glomerulonephritis (11).

Among the reasons for this apparent increase in reports of

Table 1. Renal failure in patients with AIDS.

I. *Acute renal failure (ARF) incidental to AIDS*
Acute tubular necrosis (ATN) resulting from hypovolemic shock, sepsis, radiocontrast agents or nephrotoxic drugs.
Allergic interstitial nephritis from drugs such as trimethoprim-sulfamethaxazole.
Acute renal insufficiency from nonsteroidal anti-inflammatory drugs (NSAID).
ATN from massive proteinuria and severe hypoalbuminemia
ARF from hemolytic uremic syndrome, and thrombotic thrombocytopenic purpura.
Immune complex glomerulonephritis.

II. *Nephropathy associated with AIDS*
Focal and segmental glomerulosclerosis (AIDS associated nephropathy).

III. *AIDS developing in patients with prior renal disease*
Patients with ESRD from various causes, who develop AIDS while undergoing maintenance dialysis.
AIDS developing in renal transplant recipients.
AIDS as a consequence of renal transplantation.

renal complications in AIDS are that more and more physicians are treating and diagnosing an increasing number of AIDS patients afflicted with problems involving multiple organ systems. Because, during their complicated hospital course, these patients also receive a variety of potentially nephrotoxic drugs and diagnostic agents the incidence of ATN is also on the rise. Moreover, the nephropathy associated with AIDS (3), is now being recognized in many other centers (12). An estimated 5 to 10% of patients with AIDS belonging to certain risk groups may develop a nephropathy leading to irreversible renal failure.

Renal manifestations in patients with AIDS can be classified as shown in Table 1.

This chapter describes briefly these forms of renal disease, and reviews the results of maintenance dialysis in patients with AIDS associated nephropathy, and the clinical course of AIDS in stable dialysis patients. The guidelines proposed in providing dialysis to patients with AIDS are discussed, along with comments on HIV disease and renal transplantation.

AIDS AND ACUTE RENAL FAILURE

The spectrum of ARF seen in patients with AIDS is similar to that observed in other hospitalized patients. The commonest etiology for ARF is renal ischemia due to hypotension and sepsis. Contributing factors include dehydration, sodium depletion, acidosis, varying degrees of respiratory insufficiency, and the use of radiocontrast agents, and nephrotoxic antibiotics. It is not surprising to encounter ARF in sick AIDS patients who are exposed to such ischemic and toxic injuries. What is not evident from our studies and published data is whether or not AIDS patients are more susceptible to acute renal injury than other equally sick patients confined for other reasons. Renal failure may or may not be oliguric and recovery of kidney function can be expected if the patient survives the precipitating event. Some patients receiving drugs such as trimethoprim-sulfamethaxazole develop severe ARF due to hypersensitivity interstitial nephritis. Such ARF is characterized by fever, oligo-anuria, rash with or without eosinophilia and eosinophiluria after drug exposure. With discontinuation of the offending agent, and supportive care including dialysis, recovery is likely, and the prognosis is good. Patients receiving NSAID occasionally develop severe renal failure which is also reversible when the drug is stopped. We have also observed oliguric ARF in two patients with massive proteinuria, and severe hypoalbuminemia; renal function improved after a brief period of hemodialysis. One reported patient with ARF due to the hemolytic uremic syndrome (10), and one of our patients with thrombotic thrombocytopenic purpura and AIDS have died. The course of postinfectious immune complex glomerulonephritis is unknown in AIDS patients.

ARF contributes substantially to the morbidity and mortality in AIDS. In many patients, ARF is a terminal event and death results from sepsis and or respiratory failure. Such patients are hemodynamically so unstable that any form of dialysis therapy is unlikely to be of benefit. Nevertheless, ARF is a potentially reversible and treatable complication in AIDS, and patients should receive supportive dialysis treatments when indicated. In our study, the predisposing factors in 23 patients with ARF included exposure to one or more nephrotoxins, such as radio contrast agents, pentamidine, aminoglycosides, and trimethoprim-sulfamethoxazole, and the nonsteroidal antiinflammatory drug, meclofenamate. Pyrexia, hypotension, dehydration of varying degree superimposed on sepsis, and respiratory insufficiency greatly contributed to their risk of developing ARF. Six of 23 patients with a serum creatinine concentration below 6 mg/dl (531 μmol/l) were managed without dialytic therapy and regained renal function, although one patient died from an overwhelming pneumocystis carinii pneumonia. Among 17 patients with severe azotemia, 11 who were not treated by dialysis primarily because of hemodynamic instability (although three patients regained renal function), died within 3 weeks. The remaining six patients underwent repeated hemodialyses for one to 3 weeks, and five recovered renal function. One patient also died in renal failure from Staphylococcal sepsis despite repeated hemodialysis. The mean duration of survival following recovery of kidney function in four patients was 17 ± 8 months with a range of 10 to 24 months (13).

Similar results have been reported by nephrologists around the country both in our informal surveys (14), and in the phone calls received by us. The ESRD Network 25 data also revealed that of the 68 patients with ARF treated between 1983 and 1985, 52 (76%) died and six (9%) regained kidney function (15). These data indicate that even though ARF in AIDS is associated with a very high mortality rate, a small but appreciable number recover kidney function, and prolonged survival of patients can be expected. Consequently, with ARF, we suggest an approach of both conservative, and aggressive dialytic support for AIDS patients.

NEPHROPATHY ASSOCIATED WITH AIDS

Major groups at risk for developing AIDS include homosexual or bisexual men, intravenous drug addicts, and those who have received contaminated blood or blood products. Among these, only the intravenous drug users have a higher incidence of renal disease and ESRD. Cunningham et al (16, 17) have estimated that the prevalence of sclerosing glomerulonephritis in young black drug addicts between the ages of 18 and 45 is 611 cases per million as compared to 20 per million in the general population. This so called heroin associated nephropathy (HAN) usually presents as nephrotic syndrome in young drug addicts after 2 to 4 years of addiction (18). In about 80% of all reported cases, the predominant renal lesion observed in FSGS (19–26). Generally the renal lesion progresses to total glomerular sclerosis with a progressive rise in serum creatinine concentration along with the development of hypertension leading to ESRD in 4 years. Since intravenous drug addiction is also a major risk factor for developing AIDS, identification of a specific renal syndrome in AIDS requires additional clarification as outlined below.

From our experience over the past 5 years with more than 60 AIDS patients, who manifested proteinuria and or azotemia, and followed subsequently to their demise, we have been able to identify and define the natural history of a syndrome, AIDS associated nephropathy (AAN). AAN is characterized by the nephrotic syndrome (on occasion proteinuria below 2 g/day), accompanied by either normal renal function or azotemia of varying degree in patients with AIDS. Patients are generally young (mean age 33 years) black men (male : female 10 : 1), and approximately 50% are intravenous drug addicts (3, 13). In Miami, and in Brooklyn, about 30 to 40% of patients with AAN are recent immigrants to the USA from Haiti (3, 4, 27). The remaining patients are children with AIDS and gay men. Experience at Miami, and at Brooklyn indicate that 7 to 10% of patients with AIDS develop such a nephropathy (27). From the onset of proteinuria, the course of renal disease is marked by a rapid deterioration to irreversible uremia in 3 to 4 months. The kidney as measured by ultrasonography or at autopsy is enlarged in early stages of the disease, and in those who progress to ESRD, it remains normal in size (27). This is so because the natural history of AAN from the onset of proteinuria or azotemia to development of irreversible uremia is measured in weeks, and there is a disproportionate dilatation of tubules rather than atrophy and replacement with fibrosis. One other prominent feature is that the majority of patients with AAN and uremia continue to be normotensive, while >80% of ESRD patients from other causes of renal failure are hypertensive. Uremia in AAN is associated with an almost universal mortality, and in our unit, no patient has survived beyond one year despite maintenance hemodialysis. Focal and segmental glomerulosclerosis is the predominant histologic finding in biopsied or autopsied patients with AIDS in our experience, as well as in reported studies, although other glomerular lesions have also been described, including 'minimal change disease' (5–9).

The light microscopic and immunofluorescence glomerular findings in AIDS associated FSGS resemble those in heroin associated, idiopathic or other forms of focal sclerosis. The differentiating features in AAN include a greater percent of 'collapsed' glomeruli, and hypertrophy and vacuolization of visceral epithelium (29), more tubular degeneration, and microcystic dilatation of tubules. The ultrastructural lesions regarded as distinctive in AIDS associated FSGS include: many tubuloreticular inclusions in endothelial cells, interstitial cells, and leukocytes, tubular and interstitial cell nuclear bodies, and granular transformation of tubular and interstitial cell chromatin, membranous profiles, test tube and ring shaped forms in nuclei and cytoplasm of different cell types (29). These ultrastructural lesions were found in renal biopsies of two addicts with the nephrotic syndrome, 6 and 22 months before the development of AIDS suggesting that they may be useful markers in predicting the disease (29). The ultrastructural findings resemble those found in blood and a variety of other tissues from AIDS patients (30, 31), and in the germinal centers of lymph nodes from patients with the AIDS related complex (32). Based on these findings, a viral etiology for AAN has been strongly suggested.

DIALYSIS IN AIDS ASSOCIATED NEPHROPATHY

Issues of major concern to nephrologists in dealing with patients with HIV disease, and ESRD are:
1. The results of maintenance hemodialysis for chronic uremia in AIDS patients.
2. The effects of chronic uremia in asymptomatic HIV seropositive patients.
3. Should routine screening of patients and staff be instituted in dialysis patients.
4. The risk to staff members while providing dialysis services.

Studies analyzing the results of maintenance hemodialysis or peritoneal dialysis for ESRD in AAN are very limited. Most reports focus on the renal manifestations of AIDS, and few data are available about the survival of patients treated by dialysis. In this context, it is important to distinguish dialysis patients who meet the CDC definition of AIDS (those who have had at least one documented opportunistic infection, and or Kaposi's sarcoma, or lymphoma), from those who are seropositive for the HIV antibody, but asymptomatic. The prognosis is extremely poor in the former group, while the natural history in the latter is poorly understood. In one prospective study of HIV antibody positive persons without other manifestations, 34.2% of gay men, and 14.9% of intravenous drug addicts developed AIDS when followed over a 3 year period (33). Hence, it is very likely that major urban dialysis units who treat large number of intravenous addicts (in New York, more than 60% of them are HIV antibody positive), will see an increasing number of patients developing AIDS while undergoing maintenance dialysis. Recently, CDC has embarked on a large scale study to determine the prevalence of seropositivity in dialysis units across the country; no data are yet available. On the other hand, an informal survey by CDC revealed that in 1985, among 80,151 patients undergoing maintenance dialysis in 1254 centers in the U.S., there were 244 (0.3%) with HIV disease who were treated in 134 units (34). Additional data are not in hand to draw any conclusions other than to suggest that AIDS is becoming a nationwide problem for dialysis units as well. Follow up of a large number of renal failure patients who are asymptomatic carriers is needed to determine the detrimental (protective?) effects of chronic uremia and abnormal host immune system on the subsequent development of AIDS.

The largest experience of maintenance dialysis in AIDS to date comes from our center and from the Greater New York area (13, 15). In short, the survival of uremic AIDS patients is dismal (35). Between 1982 and June 1987, of the 48 patients with AIDS who progressed to ESRD at our two municipal and state institutions, 12 (28%) were not treated by maintenance hemodialysis either because of their agonal condition or due to family and physician preferences; all died within 4 weeks. Only two of the remaining 36 patients with AAN begun on hemodialysis in a hospital setting under strict isolation guidelines (36) survived for more than 6 months (7 and 9 months respectively), while six lived between 3 and 5 months and 26 for less than 3 months after commencing maintenance treatments. At present, only two patients who have been treated for less than 6 months so far are alive. A similar situation can be appreciated from a recent survey from ESRD Network 25, in which 70 of 79 dialysis facilities in the greater New York area (89%) responded to a questionnaire about their experience with dialysis in AIDS. Of the nine non-responders, seven had not treated any AIDS patients. The 70 responding centers had dialyzed 144 AIDS patients (68 with ARF, and 76 with ESRD) between 1983 and 1985. The number of patients with renal failure had increased from 25 in 1983 to 78 in 1985. In 76 patients with ESRD, 54 (70%) were dead at the time of survey. Among all dialyzed patients, 92% were dead within 6 months, and only two survived beyond 12 months (15). The Network 25 results closely parallel our experience in dialyzing patients with AIDS.

The major clinical problem encountered during maintenance hemodialysis therapy was an unexplained malnutrition and wasting phenomenon in these patients. The clinical course in the dialyzed patients was complicated by severe cachexia without any evidence for an underlying malignancy or an opportunistic infection and which failed to respond to intensive efforts to increase their caloric intake. A variety of nutritional regimens including nasogastric supplementation with commercially available products, parenteral hyperalimentation, lipids, and other agents administered during dialysis and in the intra-dialysis period failed to improve the nutritional status. As a generalization, AIDS associated nephropathy patients during maintenance hemodialysis manifested a 'failure to thrive' syndrome. Only four were able to leave the hospital after the onset of ESRD. Death resulted from a combination of malnutrition with superimposed opportunistic or other intercurrent infections or both.

AIDS IN PATIENTS TREATED BY MAINTENANCE HEMODIALYSIS

With the rapid expansion of the AIDS epidemic in the USA, it was only logical that certain patients with ESRD due to various causes including chronic glomerulonephritis, diabetes mellitus and polycystic kidneys, but belonging to risk groups for AIDS would develop the disease. As predicted, over the past 5 years, 20 intravenous drug addicts have developed AIDS in our center, and sporadic cases have occurred in other facilities. Eighteen of the 20 patients in our study were men, with a mean age of 34 ± 6 years (range 24 to 50) all black, and with a prior history of intravenous drug addiction. They initially presented with a nephrotic syndrome, azotemia and hypertension, and prior to commencing maintenance hemodialysis for a presumed diagnosis of

uremia secondary to HAN, none showed signs or symptoms of AIDS. Their clinical course was stable for 2 to 64 months and equivalent to that of other regular dialysis patients. As is common, in intravenous drug addicts treated by dialysis, establishing and maintaining vascular access was difficult due to repeated infections and clotting, consequent to continued drug abuse. After a mean duration of 16.2 ± 18.9 (median 7, range 2 to 64) months of maintenance dialysis, this subset of patients expressed nonspecific symptoms, retrospectively interpretable as signs of AIDS, such as unexplained weight loss, persistent fever and diarrhea, necessitating hospitalization. The diagnosis of AIDS was established clinically in each patient as per CDC definition when opportunistic infections such as Pneumocystis carinii pneumonia, Mycobacterium avium intracellularae pneumonia, cryptococcal meningitis or esophageal candidiasis was documented. As serial HIV antibody studies were not performed it was impossible to date precisely the onset of AIDS. From the time of onset of constitutional symptoms, there occurred a progressive clinical deterioration marked by severe cachexia and malnutrition in this group of formerly stable uremic patients. Their subsequent course produced a wasting syndrome equivalent to that described above for patients with AIDS associated nephropathy, unresponsive to dialysis and nutritional support. All of them have died from a combination of cachexia and secondary infections within 4 to 12 weeks following the diagnosis of AIDS, with a median survival of one month.

Because of these dismal results, some nephrologists have suggested the use of continuous ambulatory peritoneal dialysis (CAPD) rather than hemodialysis. We have no personal experience, and no studies of CAPD in AIDS patients are available for comment. Theoretically, during CAPD, dialysis staff members will be exposed to peritoneal fluid which may be less infectious than blood.

Our prediction is that the problem of AIDS developing in dialysis patients will increase as the number of treated seropositive (acquired either because of multiple transfusion, or because of high risk life style) subjects increases. There is an urgent need for systematic collection of data from high risk areas to develop future management strategies.

One major observation that needs reemphasis is the fact that no maintenance dialysis patient lacking a known risk factor has developed AIDS either at Brooklyn or other dialysis facilities in the Network 25 area, indicating the low or absent risk of transmission of HIV within a dialysis center.

DIALYSIS IN AIDS

Soon after the description and recognition of AIDS as a disease entity, epidemiologic data indicated that the risk factors for the disease were very similar to those of hepatitis B virus (HBV) infection. Before HIV was indentified as a causative agent, the HBV infection control methods were a model to develop guidelines for dialysis and other health care personnel to follow in caring for patients with AIDS. In the initial years, because of the tremendous media publicity surrounding AIDS, and the reported poor survival of such ptients, there was great concern for the safety of dialysis personnel who were exposed to contaminated blood and peritoneal fluid from infected patients. Extremely conservative precautions including strict isolation of patients, dedicated dialysis machines, and caps, gowns, masks, goggles and booties for medical personnel were employed by us (36) and others initially in providing dialysis treatments for AIDS patients with acute and chronic renal failure. Our understanding of the infective characteristics of HIV increased. It is now known that the AIDS virus is readily inactivated by heating to 56°C for 8 min, or to 60°C for 6 min, and exposure to 70% ethanol or 70% isopropanol, or chlorine (50 mg/l) for 10 to 20 sec, and that the infectivity and concentration of virus in body fluids and blood is very low (37). Current CDC guidelines therefore do not call for such ultraconservative precautions in dialysis units. CDC at present recommends conventional infection control precautions, standard blood and body fluid precautions, and routine disinfection and sterilization strategies commonly employed in dialysis units (38–40). The guidelines do not call for isolation of patients with AIDS or asymptomatic carriers of HIV, or the use of separate machines, or routine testing of staff and patients for HIV antibody. CDC also does not recommend against reuse of dialyzers in known HIV positive patients (40).

A recent report of six persons who acquired HIV infection presumably while caring for HIV infected patients, and who denied other risk factors, has increased the concern for safety in the medical community (41). Four of these cases followed needle stick injuries, and in the other two there was extensive contact with blood or body fluids of the infected patients, and neither observed routine barrier precautions. But in the three ongoing prospective studies assessing the risk of HIV infection in 1,389 health care workers, only one person had seroconverted (41), indicating the very low possibility of transmission of the disease to the staff. On the basis of these observations, CDC reemphasizes the need to implement and enforce strictly the recommended precautions in caring for patients infected with HIV.

We have utilized and recommended the following guidelines in our unit in providing care for such patients.

1. All documented AIDS patients with renal failure whenever possible are isolated for dialysis. Separate machines are preferable to avoid any cross contamination in a busy unit.

2. No reuse of dialyzers or tubing is permitted.

3. The nursing, medical and technical staff should wear protective gloves at all times and extreme care should be taken in the use of disposal of needles. All sharp objects and needles must be deposited without capping immediately after use into nonpenetrable containers.

4. After each use, the exterior of the machine should be cleaned thoroughly with hypochlorite or other commonly used disinfectant solution, and the interior of the machine rinsed with formaldehyde solution.

5. Routine screening of dialysis patients and staff for HIV antibody status is not necessary for infection control. But there is a need for a systematic study to determine the risk of transmission in high risk dialysis units.

6. An ongoing inservice education for staff and patients should be incorporated, and periodic review of infection control procedures should be monitored. This step goes a long way in reducing unnecessary fears among the staff, and in obtaining cooperation in providing a multidisciplinary and compassionate approach to patients with AIDS.

7. It is essential to realize that the infectivity of HIV is very low, and that sterilization can be accomplished easily. Basic precautions followed diligently by dialysis personnel are sufficient to prevent transmission of the disease. Emotional overreactions from the physicians and staff alike must be avoided.

Currently available studies indicate that the prevalence of serological markers of HIV infection in dialysis patients is very low, and the incidence of false positivity is high (42). Peterman et al (43) found that 25 of 520 (4.8%) hemodialysis patients in the Chicago area were seropositive for HIV when tested by enzyme immunoassay, but in only four (0.7%) was the confirmatory Western Blot test positive. In other studies, the incidence of seropositivity has varied from 0.5% to 8% on ELISA, while in only about half of them could the assay be confirmed by Western Blot testing (44–46). The reason for the high false positivity in dialysis patients is probably due to a cross reaction with the HLA antibodies (H9 cell associated antigens) from the many blood transfusions these patients receive (43). In those studies, wherein the dialysis staff members were also tested, the incidence of HIV antibody positivity was either absent or extremely low, indicating once again that the transmission of HIV in dialysis units is very unlikely. Nevertheless, it is imperative that the dialysis staff who are asked to provide care for HIV infected patients, must observe the infection control precautions adequately and take extreme care in disposing of the contaminated materials carefully.

HIV AND RENAL TRANSPLANTATION

Two issues of importance in relation to renal transplantation and HIV disease are:

1. The risk of transmission of HIV to the allograft recipient through an infected donor organ.

2. The risk of renal transplantation and subsequent immunosuppressive drugs in an asymptomatic seropositive renal failure patient.

With reference to the first issue, transmission of HIV through the transplanted kidney was documented in a few instances before the organ donors were routinely tested (47–52). In each of these reports, the donor was a member of the risk group for AIDS, and the seroconversion in previously negative recipients was found 8 to 15 months following transplantation.

Although these recipients evinced leukopenia, lymphopenia, and some infectious complications, none of them yet meet the clinical classification of AIDS. However in one recent study, seropositivity was documented 5 days after a living related donor transplantation, and the recipient subsequently died from AIDS (53). Also interesting in another patient who received a cadaver donor kidney from a HIV positive patient (confirmed retrospectively by ELISA and Western Blot tests), yet remained seronegative 36 months later (54). This dichotomy of observations remains unexplained.

With the ready availability of serologic screening for HIV infection, at present all organ transplantations including the kidneys are performed only after the donor has been tested negative. Very rarely, a recently transfused (infected) donor may be seronegative at the time of organ donation, and may transmit the disease. This event appears to be extremely rare, and may be of some theoretical concern in high risk areas of the country.

The issue of transplantation in asymptomatic HIV carriers is unresolved from current literature. In a report from London (52), one patient who was positive at the time of transplantation, subsequently developed multiple opportunistic infections, thus meeting the criterion for the diagnosis of AIDS. In a large scale study from Houston, none of the patients were confirmed seropositive before transplantation (54). In San Francisco, there were three patients who probably died from AIDS following transplantation (55).

No firm scientific statement can thus be made from these studies about the posttransplant course in seropositive patients. But considering the potential for immunosuppressive agents to predispose patients for infectious complications, it seems prudent at present to avoid transplantation in HIV carriers.

In summary, the spectrum of HIV associated diseases has raised enormous questions for nephrologists and transplant physicians for which scientific answers are few. The ethical and moral issues continue to be major topics of debate. Our own approach has been to individualize a treatment plan for each patient with AIDS and renal failure in consultation with the patient, family, friend and the primary physician (s), taking into consideration the extremely poor prognosis in those with a documented disease, and to discourage positive patients from undergoing transplantation. With a multidisciplinary approach by a well informed staff, compassionate care can be provided to such patients. A better understanding of the wasting syndrome seen in AIDS and ways to treat it may improve the dismal prognosis so far observed. Establishment of a HIV registry in dialysis units may provide more answers about the risks to staff and patients.

REFERENCES

1. Revision of the case definition of acquired immunodeficiency syndrome for national reporting-United States. *MMWR* 34: 373, 1985
2. The impact of routine HTLV-III antibody testing of blood and plasma donors on public health. *JAMA* 256: 1778, 1986
3. Rao TKS, Filippone EJ, Nicastri AD, Landesman SH, Frank E, Chen CK, Friedman EA: Associated focal and segmental glomerulosclerosis in the acquired immunodeficiency syndrome. *N Engl J Med* 310: 669, 1984
4. Pardo V, Aldana M, Colton RM, Fischl MA, Jaffe D, Moskowitz L, Hensley GT, Bourgoignie JJ: Glomerular lesions in the acquired immunodeficiency syndrome. *Ann Intern Med* 101: 429, 1984
5. Gardenswartz MJ, Lerner CW, Seligson GR, Zabetakis PM, Rotterdam H, Tapper ML, Michelis MF, Bruno MS: Renal disease in patients with AIDS: a clinicopathologic study. *Clin Nephrol* 21: 197, 1984
6. Vaziri ND, Barbari A, Licorish K, Cesario T, Gupta S: Spectrum of renal abnormalities in acquired immunedeficiency syndrome. *J Natl Med Assoc* 77: 369, 1985
7. Patrick AL, Roberts LA, Burton EN, Jankey N, Shah DJ: Focal and segmental glomerulosclerosis in the acquired immunodeficiency syndrome. *West Indian Med J* 35: 200, 1986
8. Singer DRJ, Jenkins AP, Gupta S, Evans DJ: Minimal change nephropathy in the acquired immune deficiency syndrome. *Br Med J* 291: 868, 1985
9. Cases A, Montoliu J, Baradad M, Torras A, Castel T, Lens XM, Revert YL: Minimal change renal disease associated to Acquired Immunodeficiency Syndrome. *Med Clin* (Barc) 86: 684, 1986
10. Boccia RV, Gelmann EP, Baker CC, Marti G, Longo DL: A hemolytic-uremic syndrome with the acquired immunodeficiency syndrome. *Ann Intern Med* 101: 716, 1984
11. Dabbs DJ, Kendrick PW, Harris LS: Proliferative glomerulonephritis with immune deposits in the acquired immunodeficiency syndrome. *Kidney Int* 29: 272, 1986
12. Humphreys MH, Schoenfeld PY: Renal complications in patients with the Acquired Immunodeficiency Syndrome (AIDS). *Am J Nephrol* 7: 1, 1987
13. Rao TKS, Friedman EA, Nicastri AD: The types of renal disease in the Acquired Immunodeficiency Syndrome. *N Engl J Med* 316: 1062, 1987
14. Rao TKS, Friedman EA: AIDS associated renal failure: National perspective. *Kidney Int* 29: 201, 1986
15. Dialysis of AIDS patients. Report from End Stage Renal Disease Network 25. May, 1986
16. Cunningham EE, Brentjens OR, Zielezny MA, Andres GA, Venuto RC: Heroin nephropathy a clinicopathologic and epidemiologic study. *Am J Med* 68: 47, 1980
17. Cunningham EE, Zielezny MA, Venuto RC: Heroin associated nephropathy a nationwide problem. *JAMA* 250: 2935, 1983
18. Rao TKS, Nicastri AD, Friedman EA: Natural history of heroin associated nephropathy. *N Engl J Med* 290: 19, 1974
19. Kilcoyne MM, Daly JJ, Gocke DJ, Thomson GE, Meltzer JI, Hsu KC, Tannenbaum M: Nephrotic syndrome in heroin addicts. *Lancet* 1: 17, 1972
20. McGinn JT, McGinn TG, Cherubin CE, Hoffman RS: Nephrotic syndrome in drug addicts. *NY State J Med* 74: 92, 1974
21. Friedman EA, Rao TKS, Nicastri AD: Heroin associated nephropathy. *Nephron* 13: 421, 1974
22. Matalon R, Katz L, Gallo G, Waldo E, Cabaluna C, Eisinger RP: Glomerular sclerosis in adults with nephrotic syndrome. *Ann Intern Med* 80: 488, 1974
23. Treser G, Cherubin C, Lonergan ET, Yoshizawa N, Viswanathan V, Tannenberg AM, Pompa D, Lange K: Renal lesions in narcotic addicts. *Am J Med* 57: 687, 1974
24. Grishman E, Churg J, Porush JG: Glomerular morphology in nephrotic heroin addicts. *Lab Invest* 34: 415, 1976
25. Llach F, Descoeudres C, Massry SG: Heroin associated nephropathy: clinical and histological studies in 19 patients. *Clin Nephrol* 11: 7, 1979
26. Rao TKS, Nicastri AD, Friedman EA: Renal consequences of

narcotic abuse. In: *Nephrology,* edited by Hamburger J, Crosnier J, Grunfeld JP, New York, John Wiley & Sons, 1979, p 843

27. Pardo V, Meneses R, Ossa L, Jaffe DJ, Strauss J, Roth D, Bourgoignie JJ: AIDS related glomerulopathy, occurrence in specific risk groups. *Kidney Int* 31: 1167, 1987

28. D'Agati V, Suh JI, Carbone L, Appel G: HTLV III associated nephropathy: A comparative pathologic study. *Abstracts Am Soc Nephrol* 19: 179A, 1986

29. Chander P, Treser G: Ultrastructural markers of AIDS nephropathy. *Abstracts Am Soc Nephrol* 19: 178A, 1986

30. Bouteille M, Kalifat SR, Delaroue J: Ultrastructural variations of nuclear bodies in human disease. *Ultrastructural Res* 19: 474, 1967

31. Sidhu GS, Stahl RE, El-Sadr W, Cassai ND, Forrester EM, Zolla-Pazner S: The acquired immunodeficiency syndrome: an ultrastructural study. *Human Pathol* 16: 377, 1985

32. Le Tourneau A, Audouin J, Diebold J, Marache C, Tricottet V, Reynes M: LAV-like viral particles in lymph node germinal centers in patients with the persistent lymphdenopathy syndrome and the acquired immunodeficiency syndrome-related complex. *Human Pathol* 17: 1047, 1986

33. Goedert JJ, Biggar RJ, Weiss SH, Eyster ME, Melbye M, Wilson S, Ginsburg HM, Grossman RJ, DiGiola RA, Sanchez WC, Giron JA, Ebbesen P, Gallo RC, Blattner WA: Three-year incidence of AIDS in five cohorts of HTLV-III-infected risk group members. *Science* 231: 992, 1986

34. Favero MS: Personal communication

35. Rao TKS, Manis T, Friedman EA: Dismal prognosis despite maintenance hemodialysis in AIDS nephropathy and chronic uremia. *Trans Am Soc Artif Intern Organs* 31: 160, 1985

36. Rao TKS, Manis T, Friedman EA: Hemodialysis in patients with Acquired Immunodeficiency Syndrome. *Abstracts National Kidney Foundation* p 25, 1983

37. Martin LS, McDougal SJ, Loskoski SL: Disinfection and inactivation of Human T Lymphotropic virus type III/Lymphadenopathy-associated virus. *J Infect Dis* 152: 39, 1985

38. Favero MS: Recommended precautions for patients undergoing hemodialysis who have AIDS or non-A non-B hepatitis. *Infect Control* 6: 301, 1985

39. Summary: Recommendations for preventing transmission of infection with human T-Lymphotropic virus type III/Lymphadenopathy-associated virus in the work place. *MMWR* 34: 681, 1985

40. Recommendations for providing dialysis treatment to patients infected with Human T-Lymphotropic virus TypeIII/Lymphadenopathy-Associated virus. *MMWR* 35: 376, 1986

41. Update: Human immunodeficiency virus infections in Healthcare workers exposed to blood infected patients. *MMWR* 36: 285, 1987

42. Arnow PM, Fellner SK, Harrington R, Leuther M: Assessment of HLTV-III reactivity in hemodialysis patients. *Kidney Int* 31: 227, 1987

43. Peterman TA, Lang GR, Mikos NJ, Solomon SL, Schable CA, Feorino PM, Britz JA, Allen JR: HTLV-III/LAV infection in hemodialysis patients. *JAMA* 255: 2324, 1986

44. Goldman M, Liesnard C, Vanherweghem JL, Dolle N, Toussaint C, Sprecher S, Cogniaux J, Thiry L: Markers of HTLV-III in patients with end stage renal failure treated by hemodialysis. *Br Med J* 293: 161, 1986

45. Fassbinder W, Kuhnl P, Neumayer HH, Offerman G, Seidlund S, Schoeppe W: Prevalenz von antikorpern gegen LAV/HTLV-III bei terminal niereninsuffizienten Patienten unter Hämodialysebehandlung und nach Nierentransplantation. (Prevalence of antibodies against LAV/HTLV III in terminal renal insufficiency patients on hemodialysis and after renal transplantation.) *Dtsch Med Wochenschr* 111: 1087, 1986

46. Schafer K, Asmus G, Hufler M, Von Herrath D: HTLV-III antibodies in hemodialysis patients - a consequence of blood transfusions? *Klin Wochenschr* 64: 621, 1986

47. Cohen J, Winearls C, Oliveira D, Williams G: Opportunistic AIDS. *Lancet* 2: 1209, 1984

48. Prompt CA, Reis MM, Grillo FM, Kopstein J, Kraemer E, Manfro RC, Maia MH, Comiran JB: Transmission of AIDS virus at renal transplantation. *Lancet* 2: 672, 1985

49. L'age-Stehr J, Schwarz A, Offermann G, Langmaack H, Bennhold I, Niedrig M, Koch MA: HTLV-III in kidney transplant recipients. *Lancet* 2: 1361, 1985

50. O'Connell PJ, Mahony JF, Sheil AGR: AIDS after renal transplantation. *Med J Aust* 143: 631, 1985

51. Margreiter R, Fuchs D, Hausen A, Hengster P, Schonitzer D, Spielberger M, Dierich MP, Wachter H: HIV infection in renal allograft recipients. *Lancet* 2: 398, 1986

52. Oliveira DBG, Winearls CG, Cohen J, Ind PW, Williams G: Severe immunosuppression in a renal transplant recipient with HTLV-III antibodies. *Transplantation* 41: 260, 1986

53. Kumar P, Pearson JE, Martin DH, Leech SH, Buisseret PD, Bezbak HC, Gonzalez FM, Royer JR, Streicher HZ, Saxinger C: Transmission of human immunodeficiency virus by transplantation of a renal allograft, with development of the Acquired Immunodeficiency Syndrome. *Ann Intern Med* 106: 244, 1987

54. Kerman RH, Flechner SM, Van Buren CT, Lorber MI, Dawson G, Falk L, Gutierrez R, Hollinger JB, Kahan BD: Investigation of HTLV-3 serology in a renal transplant population. *Transplantation* 43: 244, 1987

55. Feduska NJ, Perkins HA, Melzer MD, Amend WJC, Vincenti F, Tomlanovich S, Garovoy M, Salvatierra O: Observations relating to the incidence of AIDS and other possibly associated conditions in a large population of renal transplant recipients. *Transplant Proc* 19: 2161, 1987

RENAL OSTEODYSTROPHY AND MAINTENANCE DIALYSIS

FRANCISCO LLACH and JACK W. COBURN

INTRODUCTION

In this discussion, the term 'renal osteodystrophy' will be used in a generic sense to include all the clinical syndromes of skeletal disease and altered calcium (Ca) and phosphorus (P) homeostasis resulting from renal failure. The skeletal pathology can include osteitis fibrosa and other features of secondary hyperparathyroidism, osteomalacia, aplastic bone disease, osteoporosis, osteosclerosis, and in children,

retardation of growth. Emphasis will be placed on the manifestations of these syndromes that occur in patients on regular hemodialysis with a consideration of pathogenesis, prevention and management.

Vitamin D

The term, vitamin D, is used to include vitamin D₃ or cholecalciferol, the naturally occurring sterol present in animals,

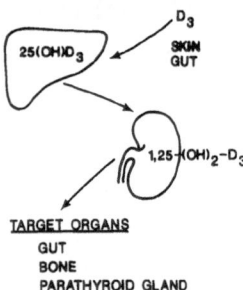

Figure 1. Schema showing the conversion of vitamin D_3 (D_3) to 25-hydroxyvitamin D_3 ($25(OH)D_3$ or calciferol) in the liver and subsequently to 1,25 dihydroxyvitamin D_3 ($1,25(OH)_2D_3$) or calcitriol in the kidney.

and vitamin D_2, or ergocalciferol, a sterol generated through the ultraviolet irradiation of a plant precursor. Vitamin D_3 itself undergoes a two-step metabolism; first, in the liver, where it is converted to 25 hydroxyvitamin D_3 [$25(OH)D_3$] and second in the kidney, where the biologically active form, [$1,25(OH)_2D_3$] is produced (Figure 1). Thus, the kidney plays an important endocrine role by producing $1,25(OH)_2D_3$.

Vitamin D_3 itself is produced in the skin where ultraviolet irradiation converts 7 dehydrotachysterol to pre-vitamin D, which in turn, is converted to vitamin D (1). The latter leaves the skin attached to a specific, high affinity carrier-protein in plasma, an alpha 2 globulin (2). Cholecalciferol is carried to the liver where it is converted to $25(OH)D_3$ (3). This conversion of vitamin D_3 to $25(OH)D_3$ (or calcifediol) is not well regulated. The 25(OH)D which is carried bound to the same vitamin D-binding protein, has a very slow turnover rate, i.e. a half life of 20 to 25 days, and may represent a circulating, 'storage' form of vitamin D (4). The metabolic conversion of $25(OH)D_3$ to $1,25(OH)_2D_3$ (or calcitriol) in the proximal tubular cells is highly regulated; this conversion is controlled by various factors that relate to the need of the organism for Ca and P (5, 6). This conversion is stimulated by parathyroid hormone, hypophosphatemia (or low phosphate diet) and hypocalcemia (7). The metabolic conversion is $1,25(OH)_2D_3$ is also augmented during certain physiologic events such as pregnancy, lactation, and growth, which are associated with increased needs for calcium (8, 9).

Calcitriol, or $1,25(OH)_2D_3$, is also bound to the vitamin D-binding protein but with less affinity than is $25(OH)D_3$; it is carried to several target tissues, including the intestine, bone, kidney, and parathyroid glands (9, 10). Its best known action is on the intestine, where it enhances the active absorption of both Ca and P. It acts in the bone both to mobilize Ca, particularly in the presence of PTH, and to bring about the normal mineralization of osteoid. This may occur through the elevation of serum Ca and P but also through a specific action on collagen metabolism. There are also cellular receptors for calcitriol in the parathyroid glands, pancreas, kidneys, and salivary glands, although its actions in these tissues are uncertain. Recently, calcitriol has been shown to play an important role in the regulation of the

synthesis and secretion of PTH, which is independent of that occurring due to a rise in serum Ca (11, 12). Calcitriol may also have an action on striated muscle, although receptors have not been identified. Most evidence indicates that calcitriol exerts its biological action in a manner similar to other steroid hormones (9, 10). Thus, the sterol is bound to a specific cytosolic receptor and the receptor-hormone complex is transported from the cell cytosol to the nucleus where it induces the synthesis of messenger RNA, which in turn, may stimulate protein synthesis. The synthesis of one or more proteins, one of which may be Ca binding protein, facilitates the entry of Ca into the cell and induces its transepithelial transport. It is presumed that calcitriol may act in a similar manner on other target tissues.

In the absence of vitamin D, there is abnormally low intestinal absorption of Ca and to a lesser extent, of P. This results in hypocalcemia, which leads to secondary hyperparathyroidism and hypophosphatemia. Also, there is impaired mineralization of osteoid (osteomalacia) and proximal myopathy, a prominent feature of vitamin D deficiency, is usually present (13).

Another naturally occurring vitamin D sterol is 24,25 dihydroxyvitamin D_3 [$24,25(OH)_2D_3$]. This sterol is produced in the kidney but perhaps also in the intestine and bone. The absence or very low levels of serum $24,25(OH)_2D_3$ in anephric animals and humans (14) suggests that the kidney is primarily responsible for its generation. The biologic role of $24,25(OH)_2D_3$ is controversial. Some data suggest that when given alone or in combination with calcitriol, it may tend to lower plasma Ca (15) and to stimulate bone mineralization (16); other data suggest it may suppress PTH secretion (17). However, certain mammals may function well without $24,25(OH)_2D_3$ (18). Further studies are needed to clarify the role of $24,25(OH)_2D_3$ in man under natural circumstances and pathologic states.

Parathyroid hormone

Parathyroid hormone (PTH) is a single chain polypeptide of 84 amino acids, which is secreted in response to a fall in blood Ca and to a lesser degree, by changes in the β-adrenergic system. Thus, there is a sigmoidal relationship between serum Ca and PTH, and small changes in blood Ca can influence hormonal secretion. Most changes in PTH occur as serum Ca varies from 7.5 to 10.5 mg/dl (1.88 to 2.63 mmol/l) (19); changes in serum Ca above or below this range have minor effects on PTH secretion (Figure 2). A small but important fraction of PTH secretion is not affected by the blood Ca level, but some basal PTH secretion has been demonstrated in the presence of substantial hypercalcemia (20). The β-adrenergic system, epinephrine and norepinephrine, can augment PTH secretion, and acute hypermagnesemia can suppress PTH secretion, at least transiently (21, 22).

The intact PTH molecule, with a molecular mass of 9,500 daltons, is secreted into the blood; it undergoes rapid cleavage in the liver and kidney with the release of several fragments (23). There are several biologically inactive carboxy-

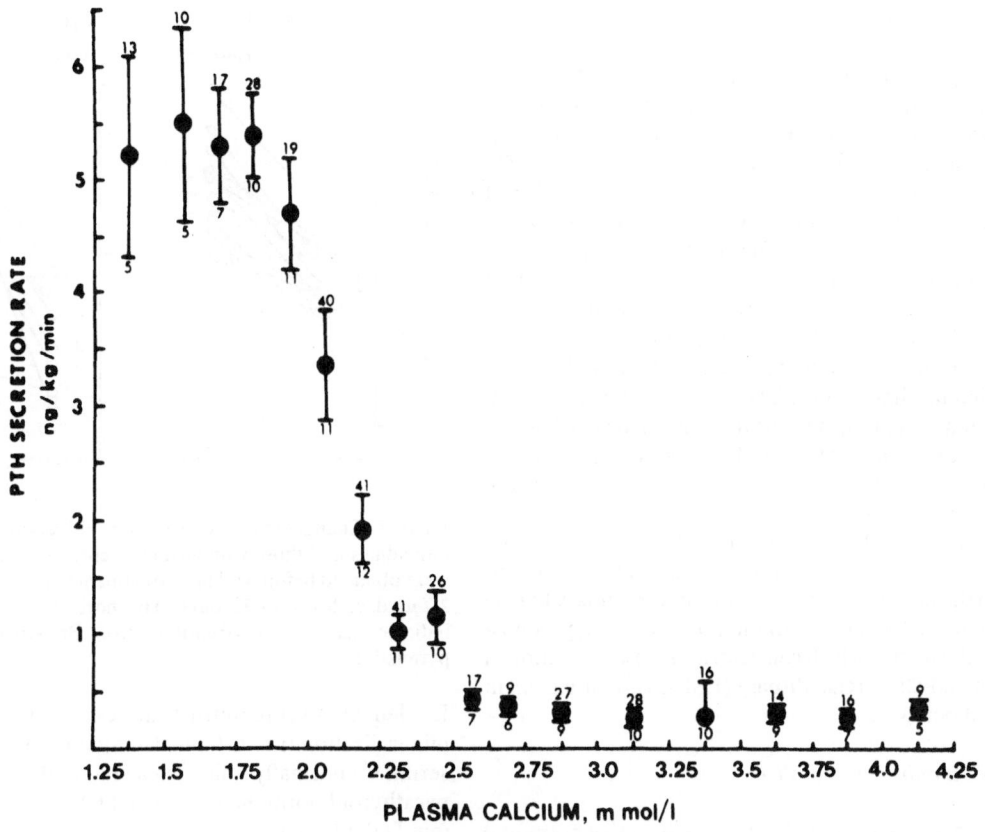

Figure 2. Secretory response of bovine parathyroid gland to changes in plasma Ca. The symbols and vertical bars indicate the secretory rate (mean ± SE). Note the sigmoidal nature of the relationship between secretory rate and plasma calcium concentration. (Modified after Mayer et al [17]).

(Ca: mmoles/l → mg/dl: multiply by 4
Ca: mmoles/l → mEq/l: multiply by 2)

terminal (C-terminal) fragments with molecular weights of approximately 7,000 which have circulating half-lives of 15 to 60 min; the small biologically active amino-terminal (N-terminal) fragment, with a molecular weight of 3,500 to 4,000, has a half life of only 4 to 5 min (24, 25). The C-terminal fragments are removed from the circulation only by the kidney (26): the N-terminal fragment is metabolized primarily by the skeleton (27). The circulating half-life of the C-terminal fragment is much longer than those of either the N-terminal fragment or intact PTH; thus, the blood level of the C-terminal fragment is higher, and more often measured by available radioimmunoassays. Because the kidney is the only organ capable of degrading the C-terminal fragment, patients with renal insufficiency commonly have very high serum levels of PTH as measured by C-terminal assays.

Parathyroid hormone acts on the kidney and bone via activation of the adenylate cyclase system. In the kidney, PTH inhibits the reabsorption of Ca and stimulates the conversion of $25(OH)D_3$ to $1,25(OH)_2D_3$. With end stage renal failure, these biological actions become less important. In bone, PTH increases the conversion of mesenchymal cells to osteoclasts, increases bone resorption and activates osteoblasts. The effect of PTH is to increase bone resorption and formation with an increase in bone turnover.

PATHOGENESIS

The striking skeletal abnormalities observed in advanced uremia are believed to have their origin early in the course of renal disease. Since this chapter emphasizes features of advanced renal disease, these pathogenic events will be discussed briefly (Table 1); please refer elsewhere for detailed reviews (13, 28–31).

Secondary hyperparathyroidism

A decrease in the level of ionized Ca in the blood leads to secretion of PTH and parathyroid gland hyperplasia occurs early in the course of renal insufficiency. As renal disease advances, hypocalcemia and parathyroid hyperplasia may become marked (32). The factors believed to lead to hypocalcemia include: 1) phosphate retention with hyperphosphatemia; 2) abnormal vitamin D metabolism, 3) decreased skeletal response to the calcemic action of PTH, 4) an abnormal set-point for calcium, and 5) a direct modulatory effect of $1,25(OH)_2$ on PTH secretion.

Phosphate retention

It has been proposed that transient and even undetectable elevations in plasma P develop in early renal failure (33, 34). Such transient hyperphosphatemia may lower plasma Ca, thereby stimulating the parathyroid glands to increase PTH secretion. This, in turn, reduces the tubular reabsorption of P, returning plasma P and Ca levels toward normal and a new steady state is achieved. Observations that phosphate ingestion stimulates PTH secretion in normal man (35), that the reduction in P intake in proportion to the decrease in glomerular filtration rate (GFR) can largely prevent secondary hyperparathyroidism in experimental renal failure (34) and the finding that serum PTH correlates positively with plasma P in uremia (36) support this view. However, levels of serum Ca and P may both be reduced in patients with mild renal failure (37, 38), data that are inconsistent with the theory mentioned above.

Overt hyperphosphatemia occurs only when renal function decreases below 25% of normal (32), and then it contributes to the degree of hypocalcemia and secondary hyperparathyroidism. Because of the importance of hyperphosphatemia, the factors which can contribute to an elevation in serum P in end-stage renal disease (ESRD) are discussed in more detail below.

Abnormal vitamin D metabolism

The reduced metabolism of vitamin D to its active hormonal forms may also contribute to the development of hypocalcemia. Several lines of evidence support a view that vitamin D metabolism is abnormal in renal failure: 1) diminished net intestinal absorption of Ca, unresponsive to doses of vitamin

Table 1. Pathogenic factors in uremic bone disease.

A. *Hypocalcemia and secondary hyperparathyroidism*
 1. P retention with hyperparathyroidism
 2. Altered vitamin D metabolism
 3. Skeletal resistance to PTH
 4. Reduced degradation of PTH

B. *Defective skeletal mineralization*
 1. Abnormal collagen synthesis (? vitamin D related)
 2. Abnormal crystal growth and maturation
 3. Skeletal accumulation of aluminum
 4. Accumulation of skeletal Mg
 5. Accumulation of pyrophosphate
 6. Reduced carbonate content

C. *Other factors of uncertain or variable role*
 1. Heparin administration
 2. Acidosis
 3. Phosphate deficiency
 4. Skeletal accumulation of fluoride
 5. Absence of PTH
 6. Modification produced by therapy
  a. anticonvulsants
  b. parathyroidectomy
  c. vitamin D

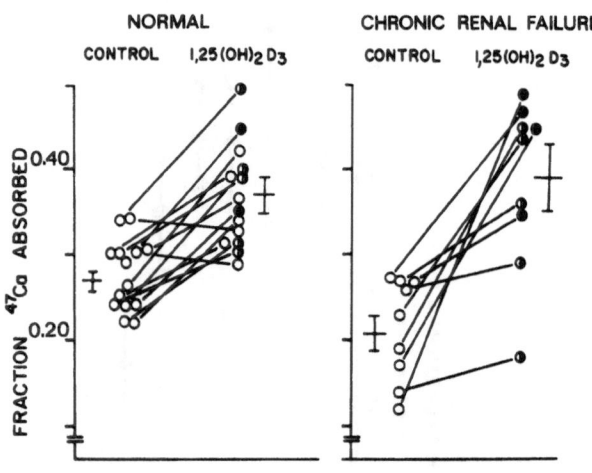

Figure 3. Changes in intestinal calcium absorption (^{47}Ca) in normal individuals and those with advanced chronic renal failure. Values were obtained before and after treatment with $1,25(OH)_2D_3$, 0.6 to 2.7 µg/day, for 7 to 10 days. The horizontal bars and brackets indicate mean ± SEM (Reprinted from Brickman et al [292] with permission).

D adequate to cure nutritional rickets; 2) defective skeletal mineralization (i.e. osteomalacia); and 3) failure to elevate serum Ca normally following a standardized challenge with parathyroid hormone extract (PTE), also a feature of vitamin D deficiency.

The kidney is the only known site of production of $1,25(OH)_2D_3$, the most active hormonal form of vitamin D. Observations in patients with ESRD that plasma levels of calcitriol are low (39), the failure of conversion of radiolabelled $25(OH)D_3$ to $1,25(OH)_2D_3$ (40) and the restoration of intestinal Ca absorption to normal following treatment of calcitriol (Figure 3) support the concept that the renal production of $1,25(OH)_2D_3$ is impaired in advanced renal failure (40, 41).

It is uncertain when in the course of progressive renal impairment, that abnormal vitamin D metabolism develops. Patients with serum creatinine levels below 2.5 mg/dl (220 µmol/l) exhibit normal gut Ca absorption (37), while those with greater azotemia have malabsorption of Ca. As renal disease progresses, this abnormality worsens and intestinal Ca absorption decreases further in dialysis patients after bilateral nephrectomy (42).

Preliminary observations in patients with serum creatinine levels of 1.5 to 3.5 mg/dl (132 to 308 µmmol/l) described normal calcitriol levels (43). However, more recent and detailed observations in children with early renal failure (ERF) (creatinine clearances of 25 to 50 ml/min/1.73 m^2) have described a 40% reduction in calcitriol levels (44). When analyzed over the range covering normal to severely impaired renal function, the PTH values correlated inversely with calcitriol levels. Chesney et al (45) also reported low levels of calcitriol in ERF patients. In addition, they found a significant correlation between the creatinine clearances and the calcitriol levels. Likewise, Juttman et al (46) observed decreased levels of calcitriol in patients with creatinine clearances between 40 and 50 ml/min. Finally, Wilson et al (47) in our laboratory, recently reported low levels of calcitriol in ERF patients with GFR between 50 and 80 ml/min. Thus, the available data suggest that patients with ERF have low-normal or low levels of calcitriol. In addition, in these patients, correction of the hypocalcemia, hypophosphatemia, hypocalciuria and decreased calcemic response to PTH was observed after 6 weeks of therapy with calcitriol 0.25 μg twice a day (46). These data suggest that even in the early stages of renal insufficiency a deficit of calcitriol may have important pathophysiological consequences.

Despite low plasma levels of $1,25(OH)_2D_3$ in most patients with advanced renal failure (39), osteomalacia is not invariably present. The explanation for this is unknown, but hyperphosphatemia may modify or ameliorate the mineralizing defect caused by a deficiency of calcitriol.

What produces a reduction in calcitriol synthesis in these patients is not yet defined. It is possible that calcitriol production by the kidney is related to the functional state of proximal renal tubules and since GFR principally reflects functional renal mass, a decrement in calcitriol may occur slowly and progressively as glomerular filtration declines. In support of this contention is a recent observation in the rat which shows a progressive decrease in renal synthesis of calcitriol following graded nephron mass reduction (48).

Other consequences of vitamin D deficiency which may have important implications in the pathogenesis of uremic bone disease are listed in Table 2 (49). Intestinal P absorption may be reduced in uremia, and calcitriol administration augments net intestinal absorption of P (42). Among the consequences of vitamin D deficiency on the skeleton is an alteration in the development of normal cross-linkage between collagen molecules, which may contribute to altered mineralization (50); a similar phenomenon may occur in uremia (51–53). Presently, there is no agreement whether vitamin D stimulates mineralization directly or by its effect on the extracellular fluid. Bone remineralization following vitamin D treatment when serum Ca and P are unchanged support a direct effect of vitamin D on bone. Impaired P absorption in patients with ESRD may also contribute to the development of osteomalacia.

Table 2. Consequences of lack of active forms of vitamin D.

Intestine
- Reduced Ca absorption
- Reduced P absorption

Skeleton
- Altered collagen synthesis
- Reduced responsiveness of bone to PTH
- Impaired mineralization
- Retarded growth

Parathyroid
- Impaired parathyroid suppression

Muscle
- Proximal myopathy

Decreased calcemic response to PTH

Patients with renal failure exhibit a decreased calcemic response to the calcium-mobilizing action of PTH; such abnormality is an important factor leading to hypocalcemia and secondary hyperparathyroidism in renal failure (54, 55). The infusion of parathyroid extract to patients with mild and advanced renal insufficiency and to those undergoing dialysis fails to elevate serum Ca to normal (55). This increased response to parathyroid extract is unrelated to the magnitude of hyperphosphatemia, hypocalcemia or the preinfusion level of iPTH. Also, a decrease calcemic response to endogenous PTH has been shown (56). The reasons for this PTH resistance are unclear, but high concentrations of uremic metabolites (57), phosphate retention (58) or deficiency of $1,25(OH)_2D_3$ may play a role (54). Recently, Wilson et al (47) have demonstrated in patients with ERF a marked improvement in the calcemic response to PTH following the administration of 0.25 μg of calcitriol twice a day.

Altered renal degradation of PTH

The kidney plays a primary role in the degradation of PTH, particularly the C-terminal fragment (25, 54). Patients with renal insufficiency have impaired degradation of these fragments, with their consequent accumulation in the circulation. Thus, the serum levels of the C-terminal fragments when measured with several currently available radio-immunoassays, are higher in dialysis patients than in those with primary hyperparathyroidism. The metabolic clearance of the intact PTH molecule is also prolonged in dialysis patients, a factor that may prolong the action of PTH, aggravating the renal bone disease (29).

An abnormal set point for Ca may occur in ERF

The secretion of PTH appears to be regulated in a sigmoidal relationship over a narrow range of plasma Ca (19). Recently, it has been shown *in vitro* that isolated parathyroid cells from uremic patients require higher extracellular Ca concentration than normal cells to suppress PTH secretion (59, 60). Thus, the set point for Ca, that is the concentration of Ca required to suppress PTH release by 50% is shifted. An abnormal set point for Ca has recently been demonstrated in dialysis patients by Voigts et al (61). Thus, these patients with overt hyperparathyroidism and biopsy-proven osteitis fibrosa exhibited a marked increase in PTH while hypocalcemia was produced with a zero Ca dialysate. As noted in Figure 4, five of these patients had significant increments in PTH even at moderately decreased serum Ca levels (less than 9 mg/dl [2.25 mmol/l]).

A direct modulatory inhibitory effect of $1,25(OH)_2D$ on PTH secretion

Recently, Lopez et al (62) did not observe a decrease in serum ionized Ca in dogs after a 70% reduction in GFR. On' the contrary, mild hypercalcemia developed, associated

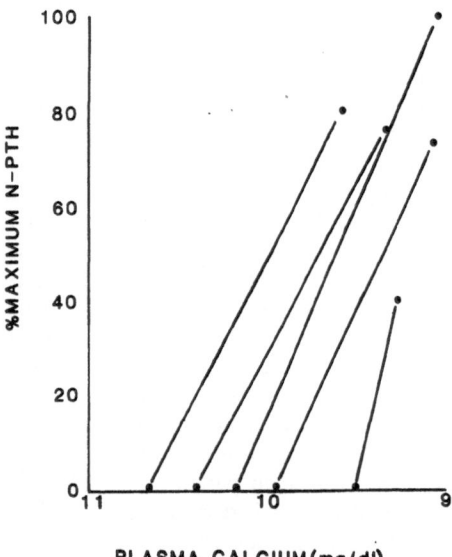

PLASMA CALCIUM(mg/dl)

Figure 4. Response of PTH to changes in plasma calcium concentration induced by a low calcium dialysis in five patients with bone biopsy showing osteitis fibrosa. Note that despite a calcium concentration greater than 9 mg/dl (2.25 mmol/l), all patients responded with a marked increase in PTH. Reproduced from Voigts et al (61) with permission of the publishers.

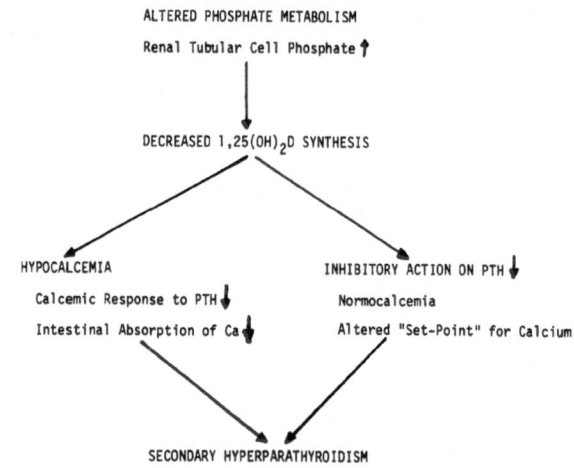

Figure 5. Diagram displaying a hypothetical reference of events leading to secondary hyperparathyroidism in early renal failure.

with low levels of 1,25(OH)$_2$D and high PTH levels. Furthermore, the administration of calcitriol at the time of induction of chronic renal failure (CRF) prevented the development of secondary hyperparathyroidism. These data suggest a direct action of calcitriol on PTH secretion. In addition, Slatopolsky et al (63) recently provided evidence in hemodialysis patients suggestive of a direct suppressive effect of intravenously-administered calcitriol on PTH secretion. This is not surprising because the parathyroid gland possesses abundant specific receptors for 1,25(OH)$_2$D (64) and a Ca binding protein (65). Furthermore, Silver et al (11) recently demonstrated in isolated parathyroid cells a suppressive effect of calcitriol on cytoplasmic mRNA coding for preproparathyroid. Likewise, Cantley et al (12) have recently observed that calcitriol at physiologic concentrations, exerts an important suppressive effect in PTH synthesis and release. Thus, it is conceptually fitting that in view of the complex interrelationship between Ca and PTH, a partial deficiency of calcitriol may ablate the modulatory inhibition of PTH secretion and lead to secondary hyperparathyroidism.

Integration of pathogenic factors leading to secondary hyperparathyroidism

The relative roles of these factors in leading to hypocalcemia and secondary hyperparathyroidism in renal insufficiency are uncertain. As renal failure progresses, reflecting the loss of functioning nephrons, the filtered load of phosphorus per single remaining functional nephron rises increasing the

phosphorus concentration in the proximal tubule. In turn this may increase the intracellular tubular concentration of phosphorus which will inhibit 1-hydroxylation decreasing renal production of calcitriol (47, 66) which, will cause hypocalcemia and/or eliminate the modulatory inhibition of PTH secretion, leading to secondary hyperparathyroidism. Recent observations indicate that dietary P restriction in proportion to the reduction of GFR in patients with mild renal failure can, perhaps by decreasing the filtered load of phosphorus raise the serum level of calcitriol, increase intestinal Ca absorption, reduce serum iPTH, and improve the calcemic response to PTH (67). Furthermore, all of these abnormalities can be corrected with the administration of calcitriol, 0.25 μg twice a day (47). These data support the concept that the concentration of phosphate in the renal tubules may be important in the pathogenesis of secondary hyperparathyroidism. A diagram displaying a hypothetic sequence early in the genesis of secondary hyperparathyroidism is shown in Figure 5. In advanced renal failure, it is likely that hyperphosphatemia, per se, plays an important role in leading to hypocalcemia and aggravating secondary hyperparathyroidism.

Defective mineralization of bone

Defective mineralization or osteomalacia is another pathogenic process affecting bone in patients with advanced renal failure. In contrast to secondary hyperparathyroidism which can be evaluated by measuring the serum levels of PTH, impaired mineralization or osteomalacia is not easy to detect. Moreover, its pathogenesis is not well understood.

Altered vitamin D metabolism

Since plasma levels of calcitriol are markedly depressed in patients with advanced renal failure (68, 69), it is surprising that evidence for impaired mineralization is not observed more frequently in patients with ESRD. Indeed, osteomalacia may be absent even in anephric patients (70). Factors which may explain the seemingly low frequency of osteomalacia may be the hyperphosphatemia and normal levels of other vitamin D sterols such as $25(OH)D_3$ or $24,25(OH)_2D_3$, which may contribute to normal bone mineralization (71, 72). The magnitude of sunlight exposure and supplementation of food with vitamin D in various parts of the world may account for differences in the incidence of osteomalacia observed in the various dialysis units. At present, there is evidence suggesting that aluminum accumulation can impair bone mineralization and lead to osteomalacia. In the United Kingdom, defective skeletal mineralization has been more common than in North America. Eastwood et al (73) suggested that uremic osteomalacia correlates with decreased plasma levels of $25(OH)D_3$. Low plasma levels of $25(OH)D_3$ probably reflect total vitamin D production and intake; relative vitamin D deficiency is more common in Northern Europe than in the United States because of reduced sunlight exposure and less fortification of foods with vitamin D. Low plasma levels of $25(OH)D_3$ are not infrequent in patients with uremia (74) and these levels correlate with the protein content of the diet.

Aluminum accumulation

Convincing data indicate that accumulation of aluminum (Al) can cause osteomalacia, hypercalcemia, encephalopathy, and anemia in patients with chronic renal failure (75, 76). Outbreaks of 'dialysis osteomalacia' were first reported from the United Kingdom and also in areas where encephalopathy was common (77). It was initially suggested that the bone disease arose from fluoride accumulation (78) or was due to phosphate depletion (79). The hypothesis that Al might cause osteomalacia was raised because Al levels were increased in brain tissue of patients who died from dialysis encephalopathy (80, 81); epidemiologic reports demonstrated a correlation between the incidence of osteomalacia and high concentrations of Al in water used for the dialysis solution (82). However, such epidemiologic data did not prove a cause-and-effect relationship. In North America, refractory osteomalacia was observed only sporadically and cases were reported in centers not using water contaminated with Al (83, 84); moreover, encephalopathy was generally absent.

Various reports indicated that the Al levels in bone were increased in dialysis patients, whether measured by neutron activation (85), electron probe (86), atomic absorption spectroscopy (87), or histochemical staining (88). With these techniques, bone Al levels were found to be increased in most dialysis patients and markedly elevated in patients with refractory osteomalacia (87) (Figure 6). The Al content of bone correlated directly with the extent of osteomalacia in these patients; also, both the electron probe and staining method showed that Al was localized along the mineralization front (86, 88–90). Little or no tetracycline was incorporated along areas with heavy Al staining, indicating absent bone formation; Al staining was inversely correlated with bone apposition rate (88).

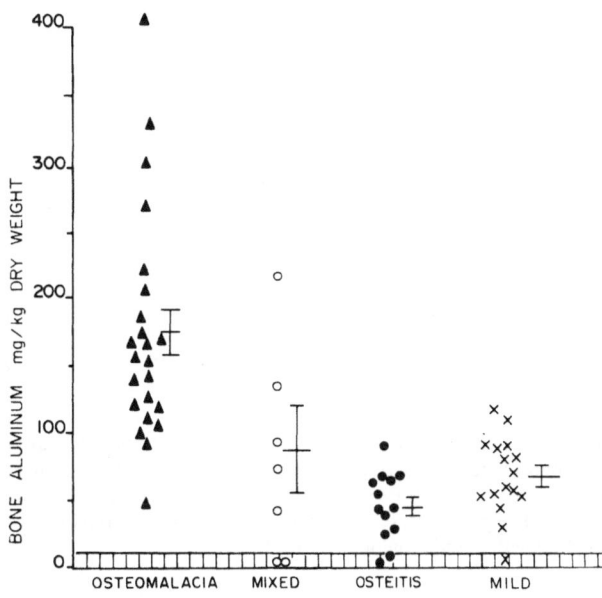

Figure 6. Bone Al content of patients with different types of renal bone disease. Some patients with mild and mixed disease probably had aplastic bone disease. Reproduced from Hodsman et al (87) with permission of the publishers.

In dialysis patients showing bone biopsy features of osteitis fibrosa, mixed features of osteomalacia plus osteitis fibrosa, or mild disease, bone Al content was above normal but the values were generally less than those in patients with osteomalacia (Figure 6) (89, 91). In another subgroup of dialysis patients, bone biopsies showed only mild histologic features; however, these patients often had fractures and bone pain similar to those of patients with osteomalacia (91). In some patients bone biopsies showed patchy areas of wide osteoid, reduced numbers of both osteoblasts and osteoclasts, positive surface staining for Al, and a markedly reduced rate or absence of bone formation, as measured by double tetracycline labeling; this subgroup has been termed aplastic bone disease (91). Serial bone biopsies in some patients have shown the evolution from aplastic bone disease to osteomalacia, suggesting that the aplastic lesion may be a precursor of osteomalacia. Recently, in the experimental animal with Al induced bone disease, Lorenzo et al (92) have suggested that the presence of PTH may be a determining factor in the development of osteomalacia vs aplastic bone disease. Thus, in the parathyroidectomized rat, Al induces aplastic bone disease, rather than osteomalacia.

It is possible that other metals may also produce osteomalacia. Staining for both iron and Al at the mineralization front can be observed in some patients (93). It has also been suggested that silicon and sulfur may accumulate at the mineralization front and cause osteomalacia (94, 95).

Refractoriness to treatment with the active vitamin D sterols is another feature of Al related osteomalacia. When dialysis patients with symptomatic aluminum-related bone

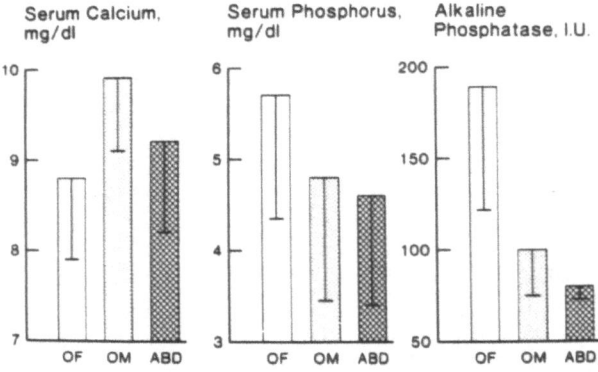

Figure 7a. Serum calcium and phosphorus concentration and alkaline phosphatase activity in dialysis patients with osteitis fibrosa (OF), osteomalacia (OM), and aplastic bone disease (ABD); normal alkaline phosphatase, 30 to 100 IU/l. Reproduced from Llach et al (100) with permission of the publishers.

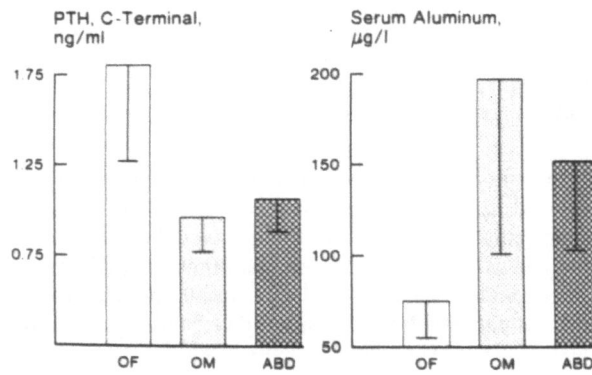

Figure 7b. Parathyroid hormone levels and aluminum concentrations in patients with osteitis fibrosa (OF), osteomalacia (OM), and aplastic bone disease (ABD). Normal range for PTH, 0.1 to 0.3 μg/ml; aluminum 2.3 to 6.4 μg/l. Reproduced from Llach et al (100) with permission of the publishers.

disease were treated with the active vitamin D sterols, they generally had no change in symptoms or improvement of bone disease; however, they often developed hypercalcemia despite administration of only low doses of the vitamin D sterols (79, 84, 96, 97).

The clinical features of this syndrome include axial bone pain, proximal muscle weakness, and fractures of the ribs, vertebrae, pelvis, and hips. Skeletal deformities can be marked (84). Serum Ca levels are usually normal or slightly increased; serum P concentrations do not differ from those observed in other patients with advanced renal failure, and plasma levels of 25(OH)D$_3$ are not depressed. Some patients develop spontaneous hypercalcemia, while in others it occurs during immobilization, treatment with vitamin D or oral Ca supplements, or with the use of high dialysate Ca concentrations (96, 97). Recent data by Rodriguez et al (98)

strongly suggest that the Al-induced hypercalcemia is associated with low ionized Ca levels and high protein bound Ca fraction. Parathyroidectomy has been performed unnecessarily in some patients with hypercalcemia, fractures, and bone pain because of suspected secondary hyperparathyroidism.

Plasma alkaline phosphatase levels have usually been normal in patients from the United Kingdom (99), while elevated levels have been common in patients in the United States (76, 78). Serum levels of calcitriol are low, as expected with end-stage renal disease (21). Serum levels of PTH have generally been lower than usual for dialysis patients (84, 87, 100) and fail to increase normally after the induction of hypocalcemia (101). The biochemical findings of 46 patients with Al induced bone disease as compared with patients with osteitis fibrosa are displayed in Figure 7 (100). The parathyroid gland can accumulate Al preferentially (102); also Al added in vitro inhibits PTH release by parathyroid cells (103). Preliminary data from Diaz et al (104) in a hemodialysis patient, have demonstrated Al accumulation in lysosomes and secretory granules of the parathyroid chief cells (102). Originally it was unclear whether serum PTH levels were low as a result of Al accumulation, per se, or from the mild increase in serum calcium. Furthermore, the low levels of PTH observed in osteomalacic patients responded subnormally when challenged with a hypocalcemic stimulus (101), strongly suggesting that Al toxicity on the parathyroid gland may be the cause of the low levels of PTH (Figure 8). It is likely that Al itself inhibits PTH release, thereby lowering bone turnover and rendering the bone more susceptible to the development of osteomalacia. This is supported by the observation that this bone disease has occurred following parathyroidectomy and after high PTH levels are reduced by treatment with calcitriol (105). There is a different pattern of Al localization in the bones of patients with high PTH levels and osteitis fibrosa as compared to those patients with osteomalacia. In the former, Al is diffusely distributed in bone while in the latter, Al is localized at the mineralization front (90); the localization of Al at the trabecular bone surface may also increase after parathyroidectomy (106). Moreover, the histologic features of aluminum-related osteomalacia can improve substantially after the removal of only modest amounts of Al with infusion of deferoxamine and with only slight increments in serum PTH concentration (107). The mechanism whereby PTH can modify the appearance of osteomalacia is unknown.

A number of experiments in animals have shown that parenteral Al loading can produce osteomalacia. Ellis et al (108) first reported that intraperitoneal injections of Al inhibited mineralization in the epiphyseal cartilage of rats. Other investigators have demonstrated more typical lesions of osteomalacia in trabecular bone of rats and dogs receiving parenteral Al (109–111). Also, a reduction of renal function has been shown to increase susceptibility to osteomalacia, presumably because the kidney is the major route of Al removal (109, 111). Goodman et al (110) observed reduced mineralization of cortical bone without the appearance of

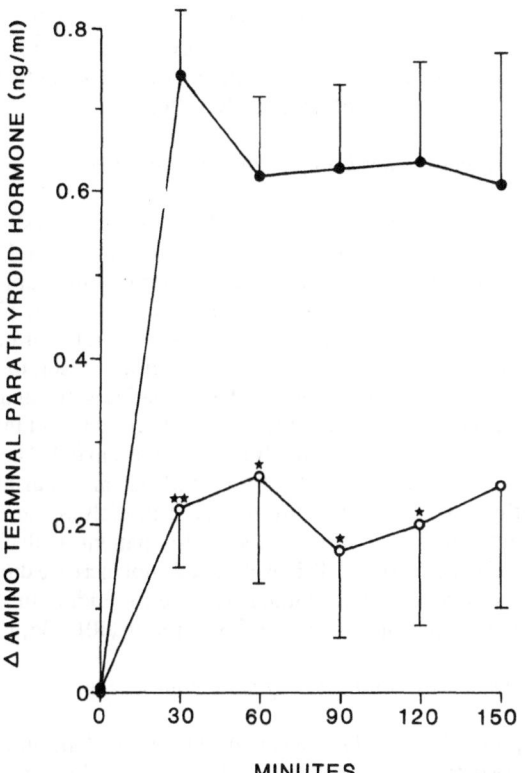

Figure 8. A comparison of PTH response to hypocalcemia in patients with biopsy proven osteomalacia (open circles) and osteitis fibrosa (close circles). Observe the blunted PTH response in patients with osteomalacia. Reproduced from Andress et al (101), with permission of the publisher.

wide osteoid seams in rats after short-term Al loading; such a lesion may be analogous to the 'aplastic' lesion observed in renal failure patients. These observations certainly indicate that parenteral Al loading can induce a bone disease similar to that observed in humans.

Added support for a pathogenic role of Al is supplied by the finding of osteomalacia or 'aplastic' bone disease and Al staining in patients with near-normal renal function who are receiving long-term parenteral nutrition with aluminum-contaminated casein hydrolysate (112).

The first cases of dialysis osteomalacia occurred in dialysis units using water with Al concentrations above 100 μg/l (3.7 μmol/l) (82); however, a high incidence of bone disease has occurred with dialysate Al levels near 50 μg/l (1.9 μmol/l) (113). Since 80 to 90% of Al in plasma is protein-bound, Al is transferred into the patient from the dialysate when the dialysis fluid Al concentration exceeds the level of ultrafilterable Al in blood. Aluminum may arise from other sources: the cartridges used in the past for the regeneration of dialysate (Redy) were found to release Al into dialysate (114); fortunately, this was a transient problem which was solved and has not recurred. Occasionally, some peritoneal dialysate solutions were found to have high concentrations of Al (115), although samples later tested all had Al concen-

trations less than 5 to 7 μg/l (185 to 229 μmol/l) (116). Aluminum has also been found in parenteral albumin solutions (117).

Recently, it has become apparent that the incidence of aluminum-related osteomalacia is higher than previously thought. Llach et al (100) have evaluated the prevalence of the types of bone lesions in a large, unselected dialysis population from a single geographic region; osteitis fibrosis was present in 88 of the 131 patients studied. Osteomalacia was present in 31 patients (23%) and aplastic bone disease was present in 12 (9%). Thus, osteomalacia was observed frequently in patients originally asymptomatic, but over a period of 3 years more than one-third became symptomatic (100). Dialysis was performed with dialysis fluid containing a low concentration of Al, suggesting that the Al burden arose from other sources, most likely aluminum-containing phosphate binders.

It is now quite certain that Al can also accumulate in the body via oral absorption. This was first suggested by Berlyne et al (118) but the findings were largely overlooked. Studies in normal subjects ingesting Al hydroxide indicate that small amounts of Al are absorbed (119); since the kidney is the major route of Al excretion, the absorbed metal can accumulate in patients with renal failure. Aluminum-related bone disease in uremic patients who have never undergone dialysis but who have ingested Al hydroxide clearly indicates that significant amounts of Al can accumulate from oral sources (120–122). Moreover, a close correlation has been noted between plasma Al concentration, which probably indicates recent loading with Al, and the amount of aluminum-containing gels ingested by children undergoing continuous ambulatory peritoneal dialysis (116, 123). In dialysis patients, after use of Al-containing gels is discontinued, plasma Al levels usually fall substantially (124). Further documenting significant oral absorption of Al (Figure 9). Finally, compounds such as citric acid can substantially augment the absorption of Al (125), and the administration of citrate salts combined with aluminum hydroxide may greatly enhance the risk of Al toxicity in renal patients (126).

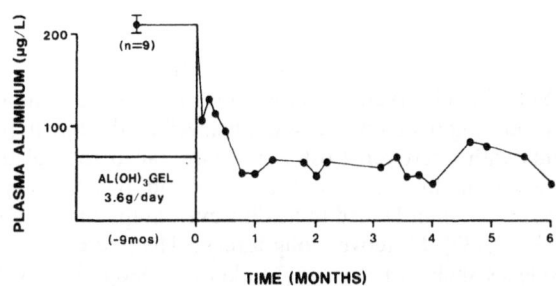

Figure 9. Serial plasma aluminum levels in a patient treated with CAPD and receiving aluminum hydroxide (Al(OH)$_3$ gel), 3.6 g/day for 9 months. At zero time, Al(OH)$_3$ was discontinued and calcium carbonate substituted as the phosphate binder. Reprinted from Hercz et al (124) with permission of the publishers.

Hypophosphatemia

Subnormal levels of serum P can contribute to impaired mineralization of bone; and there is a correlation between osteomalacia and a low serum Ca × P product in patients with advanced renal failure and in those undergoing dialysis (59). On the other hand, such a relationship has not been observed by others, and varying phosphate intake in different parts of the world may be an important factor leading to the differing incidence of osteomalacia. Furthermore, since some of these hypophosphatemic patients were treated with Al containing phosphate binders, the possibility of Al induced osteomalacia was never excluded.

Altered metabolism and synthesis of collagen

The synthesis and maturation of collagen is abnormal in uremia and may contribute to impaired mineralization. Moreover, experimental evidence suggests that vitamin D may improve the maturation of collagen and enhance bone mineralization, observations which suggest that abnormal vitamin D metabolism could contribute to altered collagen metabolism (51, 52).

The role of acidosis

The role of acidosis in contributing to abnormalities in patients with renal failure has yet to be clarified. Observations on the role of bone in buffering the continued acid load in uremia have been derived from analysis of the mineral content of bone obtained at postmortem or biopsy. It has been suggested that hydrogen ion accumulates in bone in association with loss of Ca carbonate from bone (127). However, the existence of crystalline Ca carbonate itself in bone is a matter of controversy. During short-term acid infusion, carbonate is lost from bone in association with sodium rather than Ca. Burnell et al (128) suggested that carbonate and sodium exist in the hydration shell. Although bone may buffer an acid load through the release of carbonate (or bicarbonate), hydrogen ions are accepted in association with bone resorption and apatite dissolution, regardless of the cause of bone resorption. It has been shown that the buffering provided by bone during acidosis is more effective in animals with intact parathyroid glands, presumably because bone turnover is more rapid (129).

Yet other observations point to the minor role of acidosis in producing bone disease in uremia. Alkali therapy in patients with overt renal osteodystrophy failed to heal the bone lesion (130, 131). On the other hand, pharmacologic doses of vitamin D lead to healing even in the presence of acidosis (132). Moreover, long-term acid feeding of animals produces skeletal lesions more akin to osteoporosis, with decreases in both bone mineral content and bone matrix, rather than evidence of secondary hyperparathyroidism (133). Recent observations by Kraut et al (134) have shown that bone resorption is enhanced and bone formation is impaired in the thyroparathyroidectomized rat with metabolic acidosis. However, although these changes may contribute to osteopenia, osteomalacia was not observed. The situation may be more complex in dialysis patients because restoration of body and bone buffer may be incomplete with the use of acetate-containing dialysis fluid.

Reduced plasma levels of parathyroid hormone

One feature of uremic patients with osteomalacia as shown in Figure 7b is the normal or even low levels of serum iPTH (100); moreover, the osteomalacic syndrome may appear following total or sub-total parathyroidectomy (105, 135). The characteristics of this syndrome are low rates of bone apposition and turnover which may occur as a result of the reduced levels of PTH. Thus, in dialysis patients, the magnitude of bone formation at the 'calcification front', an index of bone formation, was directly related to serum iPTH levels (135). Although low levels of serum iPTH can occur after parathyroidectomy, they are observed in dialysis patients without parathyroid surgery (100). Also, patients with osteomalacia have serum iPTH levels that do not increase during an acute hypocalcemic stimulus (Figure 8), adding further evidence of an abnormality in PTH secretion (101, 136, 137).

Oxalate deposits as a cause of renal bone disease

Symptomatic bone disease can arise from the deposition of oxalate in the bone of patients with primary oxalosis, particularly when the original renal failure that occurred due to oxalosis is managed effectively by renal transplantation (138). 'Acquired' oxalosis rarely develops in long-term dialysis patients (139), but when occurring, may be aggravated by the ingestion of large quantities of ascorbic acid (140). Plasma oxalate levels are above normal in patients with renal failure (141), and dialysis patients exhibit an even greater increase of plasma oxalate levels with ascorbic acid ingestion of 500 mg/day (142). In patients with bone disease due to oxalate deposits, bone biopsies disclose typical oxalate crystals, increased osteoid, trabecular fibrosis, and a prominent foreign-body giant cell reaction adjacent to the oxalate crystals. The addition of ascorbic acid to dialysis fluid as an antioxidant could contribute to the increased oxalate levels and predispose to such oxalate deposition. Because the serum of uremic patients is supersaturated with respect to calcium oxalate (143), and because ascorbic acid can raise the serum oxalate even further, large doses of vitamin C should be avoided in patients with renal insufficiency.

HISTOLOGIC FEATURES OF BONE

Techniques for bone biopsy

The study of bone itself has evolved into a clinically useful tool for understanding the pathophysiologic processes involved and as a guide to the management of renal osteodystrophy. Under local anesthesia, a bone biopsy can easily and safely be obtained from the iliac crest. The sample, 5 ×

20 mm, containing trabecular bone and both tables of cortices (144) is fixed in neutral formalin, then transferred to alcohol to prevent Ca loss, and embedded in a hard plastic, such as methacrylate. Thin sections of the undecalcified bone can be cut with a special microtome having a heavy steel blade. Uncalcified osteoid and calcified bone can be readily identified with such methods, unlike the specimen of bone prepared with the usual decalcification.

In addition to the qualitative interpretation of bone histology, quantification of various features and bone dynamics with tetracycline labeling can increase the sensitivity of the method and aid in comparison of biopsy samples. One method utilizes a grid eye-piece placed in the microscope (145); the surfaces of trabecular bone which intersect the grid markings are identified as *forming* (i.e. with osteoblasts and osteoid), *resorbing* (with osteoclasts and Howship's lacunae) or *resting* (bone surface without cellular activity). With another method, the microscopic image of bone is projected on a screen and each specific type of bone surface is traced with an electrical pencil attached to a computer and X-Y plotter (145). Quantitation of the surfaces occupied by active resorption, formation, or by inactive bone can provide static information but they may not provide data on the dynamics of bone formation, mineralization or resorption. Errors in static data may occur if the rate of metabolic activity varies (144); thus, the forming and resorbing surfaces could be twice normal, and yet skeletal dynamics can be normal if the activity of the osteoclasts and osteoblasts is reduced to half of normal. To obviate this problem, tetracycline, a fluorescent marker, which is rapidly incorporated into newly forming bone, is given on two separate occasions; this permits a measure of bone formation rate (146). In practice, the dynamics of trabecular bone are assessed after giving two separate doses of tetracycline, with the 'bone formation rate' quantitated as the distance between the two lines of fluorescence divided by the time between doses.

The dynamics of trabecular bone turnover differ from those of cortical bone, which is organized into units called osteons, which surround a Haversian canal. Cortical bone turnover involves sequential osteoclastic resorption within the Haversian canal; this is followed by osteoblastic formation; also the numerous osteocytes, which are buried within the osteon, can participate in bone resorption through a 'osteocytic osteolysis'.

Osteitis fibrosa

Osteitis fibrosa, which presumably arises due to the high levels of PTH, is characterized by increased bone resorption and formation with a progressive increase in peritrabecular fibrosis (Figure 10A). A greater fraction of trabecular bone surface is occupied by resorption cavities filled with osteoclasts (Howship's lacunae); also, increased numbers of osteoblasts overlie the newly formed unmineralized matrix of bone. As this process becomes severe, the narrow space is filled with fibrous tissue, creating typical 'osteitis fibrosa' (147). Double tetracycline labeling often reveals normal or increased bone turnover in patients with osteitis fibrosa (Figure 10B) (148).

Another feature of osteitis fibrosa is the alignment of collagen strands in an irregular, haphazard 'woven' pattern; this contrasts to the normal parallel alignment of strands of collagen in a lamellar manner. This disorganized structure of collagen in 'woven' bone may lead to defective physical properties of bone in response to stress, and a greater amount of inferior, 'woven bone' may be required to maintain mechanical stability (149). Also, increased mineralization of large quantities of 'woven' bone may contribute to the osteosclerosis seen in uremia.

Osteomalacia

Osteomalacia is characterized by an excess of unmineralized osteoid tissue; this arises from impaired mineralization of the protein matrix of bone. The major feature of osteomalacia is an increase in the width of unmineralized osteoid (Figure 10C). This is also found, to a certain extent, in osteitis fibrosa due to the delay of osteoid mineralization which is formed so rapidly. Therefore, the use of tetracycline labeling to identify impaired mineralization rate is useful in the identification of osteomalacia (Figure 10D). Nonetheless, the criteria employed in the recognition of osteomalacia include: 1) the measurement of the width of osteoid seams; 2) the specific number of osteoid lamellae in these seams; 3) the extent to which bone surface is covered with osteoid; 4) the volume of osteoid expressed as a fraction of total bone surface; and 5) a delayed rate of mineralization by tetracycline labeling (148).

The frequency of osteomalacia appears to have a marked geographic variation. Osteomalacia was initially noted in patients receiving maintenance dialysis (82, 150). Recently, osteomalacia has been observed in patients prior to the initiation of dialysis (120–122). Epidemiologic evidence has implicated the presence of Al in the water since the incidence of osteomalacia is increased greatly in areas of high Al water content (151). Pretreatment of the water with reverse osmosis has decreased the incidence of osteomalacia (152). With the advent of the Maloney stain for Al, it has

Figure 10. A. A representative bone biopsy from a patient with osteitis fibrosa. Distinctive features include large multi-nucleated osteoclasts located in a resorption cavity; osteoid covered with multiple columnar osteoblasts (orange color) and marked endosteal fibrosis (Goldner stain × 200); B. Unstained section of a bone biopsy of a patient with osteitis fibrosa after double tetracycline label. Note the presence of active mineralization and bone formation as evidenced by the uptake of tetracycline and the presence of a double label (yellow bands). The lack of well demarcated label lines demonstrates a disorganized and abnormal mineralization (× 200); C. A representative bone biopsy from a patient with osteomalacia. Characteristic features include broad osteoid seams (red color), lack of cellular activity, irregular scalloped interface between osteoid and mineralized bone (green color) and the absence of marrow fibrosis (Goldner stain × 200); D. Unstained section of a patient with osteomalacia after double tetracycline label. Note the marked decrease in tetracycline uptake evidencing the lack of mineralization. The osteoid seams appear as a lighter shade of green than the mineralized bone (× 200).

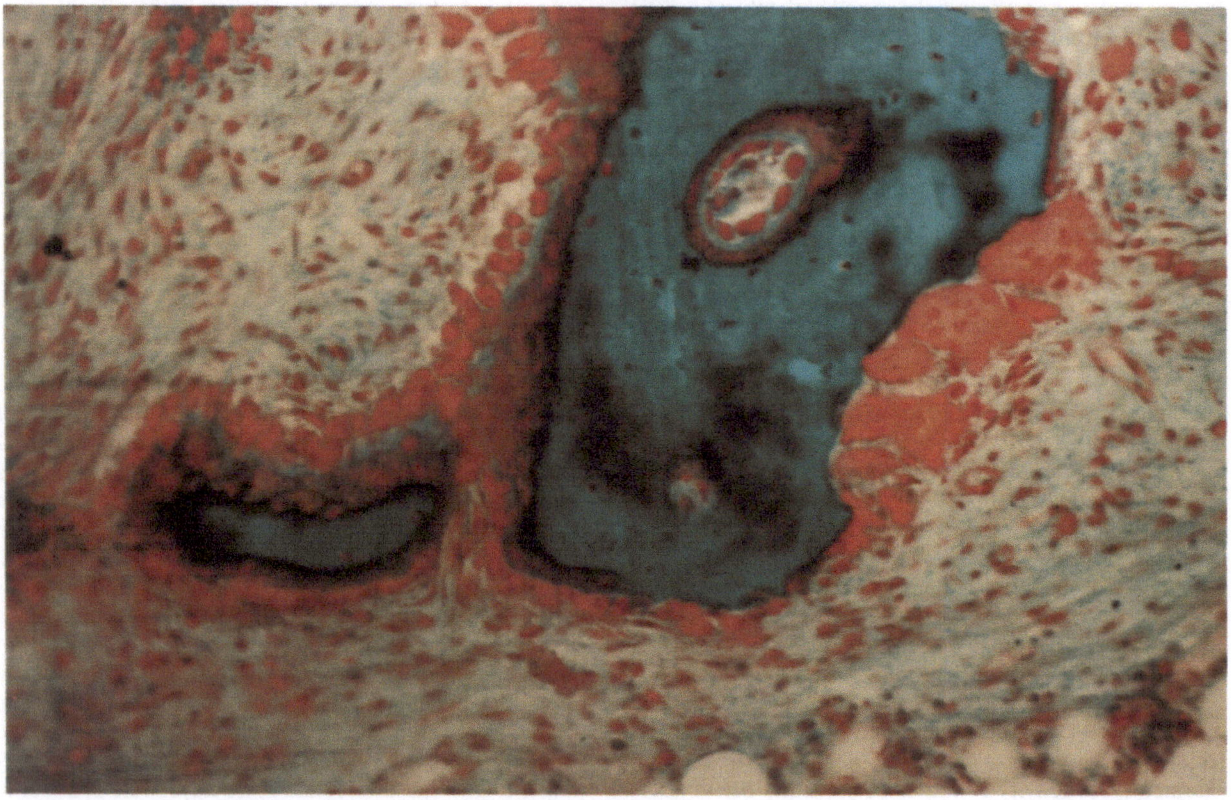

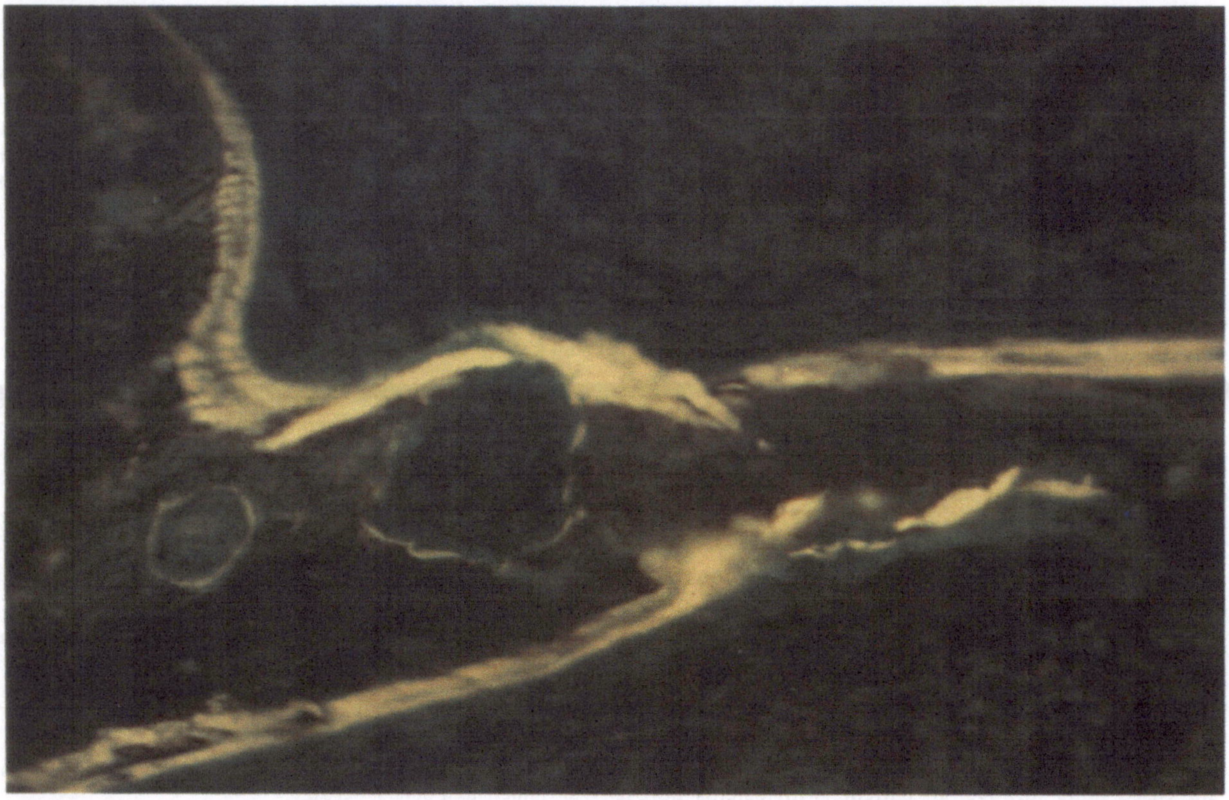

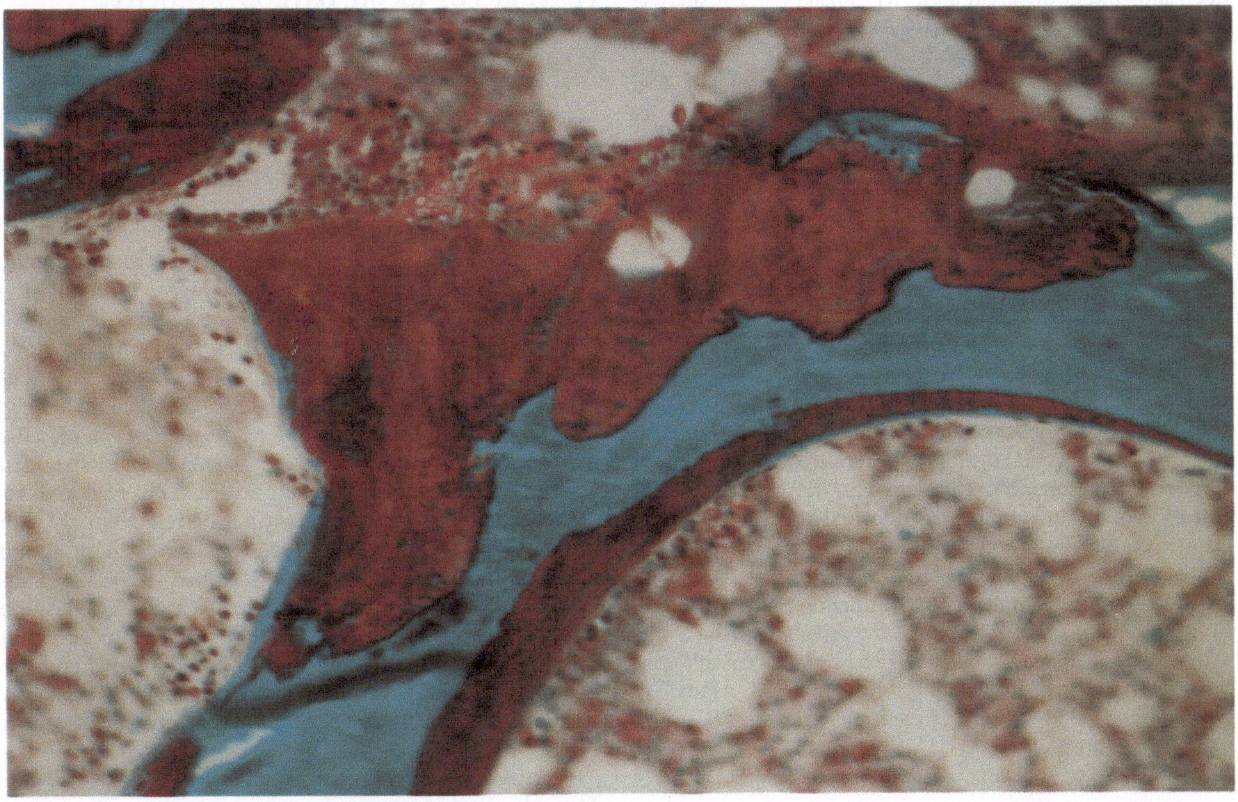

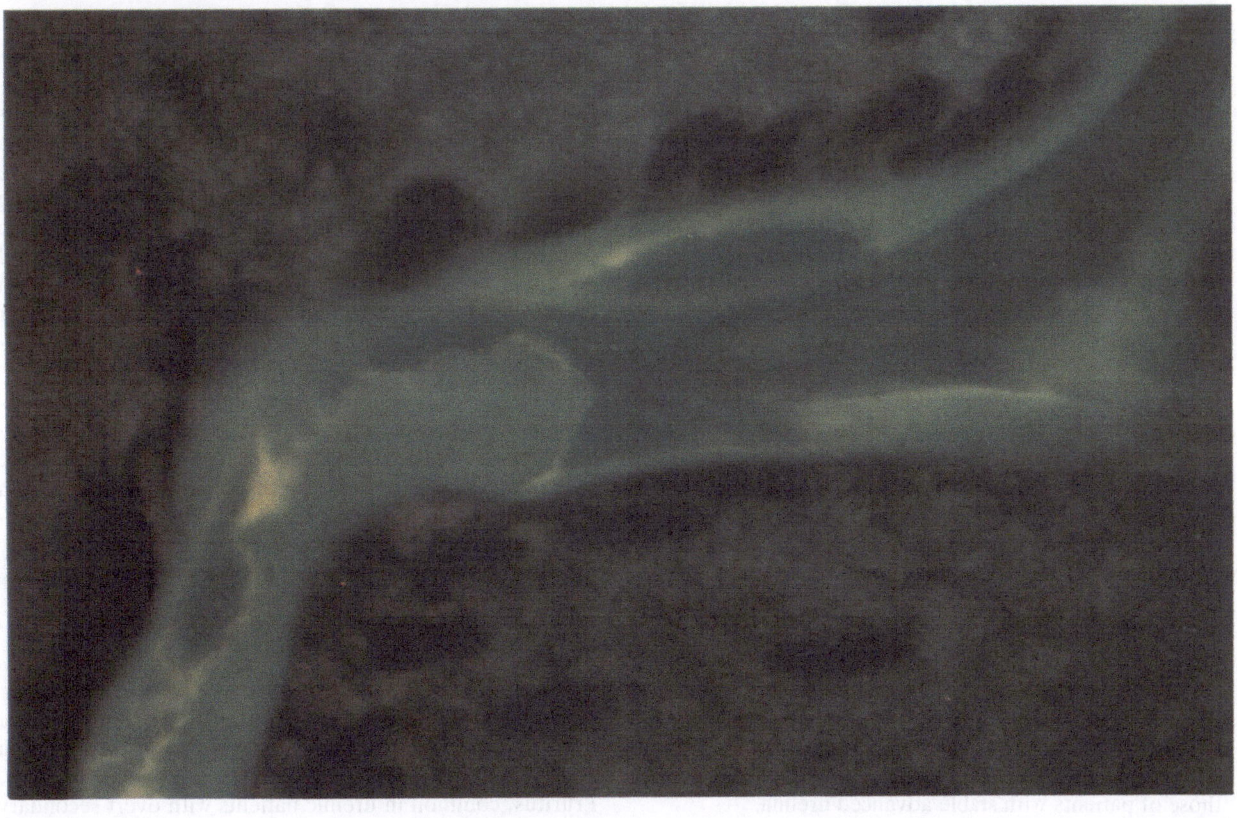

been shown that the great majority of osteomalacic dialysis patients have large deposits of Al in the bone (88). The characteristic pattern is a linear deposition of Al along the interface between trabecular bone and osteoid (89, 98). The degree of osteomalacia has correlated closely with bone Al content, whether analyzed biochemically or histologically (88, 89).

Aplastic bone disease

Another type of bone lesion observed in dialysis patients is aplastic bone disease (92). This entity most likely is the result of Al toxicity. It is characterized by features similar to those of osteomalacia; the major difference is the absence of large osteoid seams. These patients also have a deficiency of cellular activity and absence of endosteal fibrosis; aluminum deposits are present both at the osteoid-bone interface and on the surface of trabecular bone. It seems that Al may be toxic to bone by simultaneously affecting bone formation and remodeling. Thus, aplastic bone disease may be a variant of osteomalacia; both are caused by Al accumulation. As mentioned previously, in the absence of PTH, Al toxicity may be more likely to result in aplastic bone disease rather than osteomalacia (93).

Mixed skeletal lesion

Another sub-group of patients exhibits wide osteoid seams combined with typical features of osteitis fibrosa. Such skeletal lesions are somewhat more common in young patients, in those with hypocalcemia, and in patients who have not undergone dialysis or treatment with vitamin D (149). These histologic features may be characteristic of vitamin D-deficiency itself, with components of both secondary hyperparathyroidism, which commonly occurs with vitamin D deficiency, and osteomalacia. Serum iPTH levels are significantly elevated in these patients (101, 153).

There is disagreement as to whether dialysis treatment can lead to specific qualitative differences in skeletal disease or whether dialysis merely prolongs the lives of patients with end-stage uremia, thereby exposing them to the various pathogenic factors for a longer period of time. Certain incriminating factors unique to dialysis patients are administration of heparin (154), exposure to fluoridated water, exposure to high concentrations of acetate, periodic removal of bicarbonate, exposure to varying concentrations of Ca and Mg in dialysate, and the presence of Al, trace elements, and other substances in dialysate. From their observations on patients studied in Heidelberg, Ritz et al (149) concluded that there are no qualitative differences between the findings in bones of patients undergoing dialysis compared with those of patients with stable advanced uremia.

FEATURES OF RENAL OSTEODYSTROPHY

Symptoms and signs

Some symptoms and signs of renal osteodystrophy are noted in Table 3.

Skeletal pain

Bone pain may develop and progress to become totally disabling, regardless of whether pathology is secondary hyperparathyroidism or osteomalacia, although it is more commonly observed in the latter (100). The pain is generally vague and deep seated and may be in the low back, hips, legs or knees. It may vary in intensity and is often aggravated by gravitational stress and weight bearing; occasionally, the pain is localized about the knee or ankle, and its sudden appearance may suggest an acute arthritis. Physical findings are often absent. Symptoms may not correlate closely with radiographic abnormalities; thus, patients with profound abnormalities on X-ray or bone biopsy may be asymptomatic. In other cases, normally active patients may develop disability over a period of weeks to months to a degree that walking across the room is difficult. Low back pain may arise due to spontaneous vertebral collapse, and chest pain may be the first indication of a rib fracture occurring during a cough or sneeze.

Muscular weakness

Muscle weakness is an important symptom of renal osteodystrophy. The evaluation of muscular strength is difficult, however, when bone pain is present. Weakness characteristically involves the proximal muscles. Initially, patients may note difficulty in climbing stairs or in rising from a sitting position; as the condition progresses, they may have difficulty in walking or in raising from a supine to a sitting position. The gait becomes waddling and resembles that of a penguin. The manifestations may be identical to those of vitamin D deficiency arising from other causes (155). Serum levels of muscle enzymes, such as creatine phosphokinase or aldolase, are generally normal; electromyography may reveal mild abnormalities suggesting a primary myopathy.

Diffuse degeneration of myofibrils characterized by streaming of Z-band material and loss of normal myosin-actin arrangement have been noted (156). A presumed role of vitamin D in producing such myopathy is suggested from the substantial improvement in muscle strength noted within a few days after administration of calcitriol (157) and by the reversal of the ultrastructural abnormalities following treatment with $25(OH)D_3$ (156).

Pruritus

A common symptom in patients with advanced renal failure is pruritus. It may improve or disappear after the initiation of adequate dialysis; however, it persists in some patients. Pruritus, common in uremic patients with overt secondary hyperparathyroidism, may improve or disappear after subtotal parathyroidectomy (158). The mechanism for the pruritus is unknown, but it may relate to a high ionized blood Ca level in patients with overt secondary hyperparathyroidism (158). Pruritus may develop as a consequence of an elevation of blood Ca level from vitamin D overdosage, during a Ca infusion, or with use of a high Ca dialysis solution. Moreover, it may disappear following subtotal parathyroidectomy before there is a change in the skin Ca component. The severe pruritus once frequent in dialysis populations is less commonly observed today with the use of other methods to prevent severe secondary hyperparathyroidism.

Bone deformities and growth retardation

In uremic children, deformities of bone include bowing of the tibia and femur and those due to slipped epiphysis (159) of the distal radius, distal ulna, and proximal femur. Thus, marked ulnar deviation of the hand can occur as a manifestation of a slipped epiphysis. The skeletal pathology associated with a slipped epiphysis is that of secondary hyperparathyroidism, and the radiolucent zone between the epiphyseal ossification center and metaphysis is caused by the accumulation of poorly mineralized woven bone and/or fibrous tissue (159); it does not arise from an excess of cartilage and chondro-osteoid as occurs in vitamin D-deficiency rickets.

Retardation of growth is common in uremic children, but the factors responsible are far from clear. Growth impairment may be partly due to deficient caloric intake (160). Initiation of dialysis and treatment with active forms of vitamin D usually do not result in 'catch-up' growth, although improved growth has followed treatment with calcitriol (161).

Fractures

The syndrome, 'dialysis osteopenia', with fractures has been reported from several centers in the United Kingdom (77, 82) and in North America (84, 100). There is a strong association of this syndrome with the occurrence of dialysis encephalopathy and as many as 30% of dialysis patients may be afflicted in some units (100, 141). A high incidence has been reported in certain centers in North America (100, 150), and a sporadic case may afflict a small fraction of patients (84). Osteomalacia is the primary skeletal lesion in these patients; fractures involving the axial skeleton, i.e., the ribs, vertebral bodies, hips, and even the long bones, are common. These patients may develop scoliosis and substantial loss in height, and may have profound disability.

Periarthritis

Acute pain, redness and swelling of the joints, periarticular structures, and/or tendon sheaths may occur in dialysis patients. This acute monoarticular syndrome may be indistinguishable from an acute arthritis; the joint fluid, if present, is clear without the presence of crystals, which distinguishes this syndrome from acute pseudogout or gouty arthritis. This syndrome probably reflects overt secondary hyperparathyroidism; these patients have higher alkaline phosphatase levels, serum Ca × P products and serum iPTH levels compared to other dialysis patients as is shown in Figure 11 (162).

Occasionally, calcium deposits can be seen radiographically about the affected joints. Synovial tissue biopsy may reveal crystals, which when studied by x-ray defraction are characteristic of hydroxyapatite. In general, this syndrome responds well to treatment with anti-inflammatory agents, such as phenylbutazone or indomethacin; parathyroidectomy may lead to marked improvement.

Tendon rupture

An unusual but troublesome problem noted in dialysis patients is the spontaneous rupture of the tendon in the quadriceps muscle or digits (163). The cause is unclear, but its association with overt secondary hyperparathyroidism and a

---

Table 3. Symptoms and signs of renal osteodystrophy.

A. *Musculoskeletal system*
  1. Bone pain
  2. Fractures
  3. Acute pseudogout
  4. Calcific periarthritis
  5. Skeletal deformities
  6. Proximal myopathy
  7. Spontaneous tendon rupture
  8. Growth retardation
  9. Slipped epiphyses
  10. Tumoral calcification

B. *Cardiopulmonary system*
  1. Congestive heart failure
  2. Heart block
  3. Hypertension

C. *Opthamalogic features*
  1. Corneal calcification (band keratopathy)
  2. Conjuctival calcification: i.e., with 'red' eye or 'white' eye

D. *Dermatologic features*
  1. Pruritus
  2. Cutaneous calcifications

E. *Metabolic, endocrine and hematological features*
  1. Insulin resistance
  2. Hypertriglyceridemia
  3. Impotence
  4. Menstrual abnormalities and/or sterility
  5. Anemia
  6. Pancytopenia

F. *Neurological features*
  1. Dialysis encephalopathy
  2. Peripheral neuropathy
  3. Altered cognitive function (?)
  4. Abnormal EEG (?)

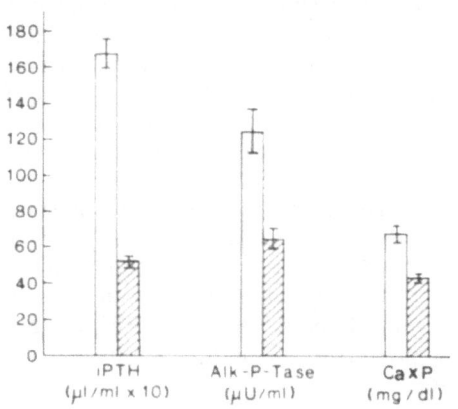

Figure 11. Values of iPTH, serum alkaline phosphatase and Ca × P observed in 12 patients with an acute monoarticular syndrome (open columns) compared with those of the other patients treated by dialysis (hatched columns). (Reproduced from Llach et al [162], with permission).

similar occurrence in primary hyperparathyroidism suggests that high levels of PTH may predispose to this lesion.

Calciphylaxis

This unusual syndrome is characterized by peripheral ischemic necrosis and vascular calcification; it may occur in patients with advanced chronic uremia, in dialysis patients, and in successful renal transplant recipients (164). These lesions are initially characterized by painful, violaceous mottling of the skin, followed by penetrating, progressive gan-grenous ulcerations of the skin of the fingers, toes, and ankles, or fat and muscle of the thighs and/or buttocks (Figure 12). The lesions may fail to heal and can contribute to the patient's death via secondary infection. Extensive calcification commonly involves the media of the arteries; most patients have a history of marked hyperphosphatemia and display bone erosions on X-ray and have elevated plasma iPTH levels. Control of serum P may prevent but not heal those lesions. On the other hand, total healing of the lesions has followed subtotal parathyroidectomy, with striking improvement within 1 to 4 weeks, an observation suggesting that PTH levels may contribute to the pathogenesis of the syndrome (164). The similarity between these lesions and Selye's experimental syndrome, calciphylaxis (165) is striking. Because of the fulminant and even fatal course, subtotal parathyroidectomy should be considered when such lesions first appear.

Miscellaneous symptoms and signs

Certain other symptoms may be common in uremic patients with overt renal osteodystrophy and secondary hyperparathyroidism, although the reasons for these symptoms are unknown. Altered mental or central nervous system function is one such manifestation. Experimental evidence in dogs indicates that acute uremia leads to Ca accumulation within the brain; this depends on high PTH levels and is associated with electroencephalographic abnormalities (166). A clinical counterpart of this experimental syndrome may be suggested by sporadic improvement of encephalopathic symptoms following subtotal parathyroidectomy in a patient with overt secondary hyperparathyroidism (167).

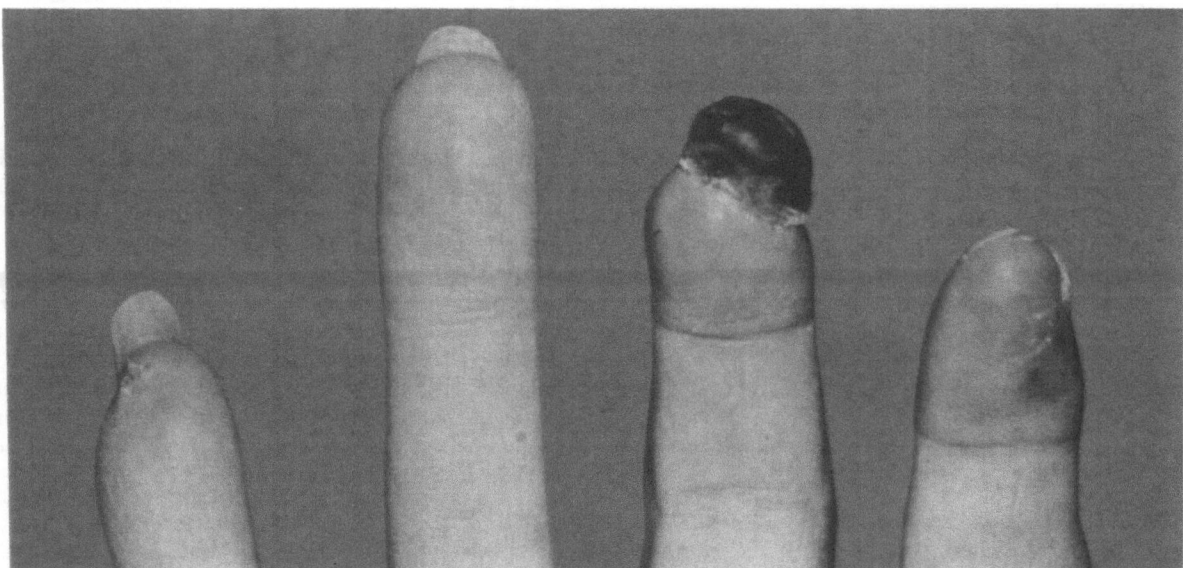

Figure 12. Ischemic necrosis involving the 2nd and 3rd digit of a uremic patient treated with maintenance hemodialysis. There was healing of the lesions following subtotal parathyroidectomy. (Case 3 from Gipstein et al [164]).

Recovery or marked improvement of long-standing impotence has been noted by some patients or their sexual partners after the reversal of secondary hyperparathyroidism (168).

Extensive marrow fibrosis and sclerosis of bone can develop in uremic patients because of secondary hyperparathyroidism; such alterations could contribute to the hematologic abnormalities present in uremia. An association between renal osteodystrophy, myelofibrosis, and abnormal hematopoiesis has been reported by Weinberg et al (169); they noted that patients with leukopenia, thrombocytopenia and severe anemia were more likely to have overt bone disease than other dialysis patients. They suggest that splenomegaly may arise in certain uremic patients to compensate for the replacement of normal erythroid tissue by osteitis fibrosa. Preliminary reports suggest that the hematocrit may increase in uremic patients with secondary hyperparathyroidism following partial parathyroidectomy (170). It seems logical that PTH may suppress erythropoietic function through local factors produced by marrow fibrosis. However, a direct effect of PTH on red blood cells has also been reported (171). Aluminum intoxication may result in hypochromic or normochromic anemia in the absence of iron deficiency (172), which may be reversible upon the cessation of Al loading and/or treatment with the chelating agent, deferoxamine.

Inhibition of platelet function occurs in uremia; Remuzzi et al (173) have demonstrated an inhibitory effect of PTH on platelet aggregation. Elevated blood concentrations of triglycerides have been reported in a substantial fraction of patients with advanced uremia (174). In recently nephrectomized animals, the rapid appearance of secondary hyperparathyroidism is associated with an increase in blood lipids (175). Furthermore, parathyroidectomy partially inhibits the increase in lipids observed after bilateral nephrectomy, while the administration of PTH restores the hyperlipidemia in parathyroidectomized uremic rats (176). Such data support the hypothesis that the hyperlipidemia of uremia may have some relationship to secondary hyperparathyroidism. Other observations suggest that the resistance to insulin action and hyperglycemia observed in uremia may relate to secondary hyperparathyroidism (177).

Uremic patients often have cardiomyopathy. Uremia is associated with an increase in the calcium content of the myocardium; these changes may be due to excess PTH. Recently, London et al (178) by echocardiographic study of the left ventricle in 57 hemodialysis patients have shown that in relation to its stress there is an inadequate left ventricular hypertrophy. This was correlated with the severity of secondary hyperparathyroidism as assessed by PTH levels and bone histomorphometric indices of osteitis fibrosa. Furthermore, Bogin et al (179) examined the in vitro effects of PTH on cultured isolated heart cells. Both PTH fragments caused a significant increase in the number of beats per minute and the cells died earlier than control cells. Moreover, observations of Drüeke et al (180) have shown a marked improvement in the left ventricular function of dialysis patients with secondary hyperparathyroidism after parathyroidectomy.

Biochemical features

The biochemical features of renal osteodystrophy are noted in Table 4.

Hyperphosphatemia

Hyperphosphatemia is prevalent in most dialysis patients. Factors affecting serum P levels in these patients are summarized in Table 5. Of these, the most important are dietary P intake and the ingestion of phosphate-binding gels. As dietary P rises net P absorption increases, although the fractional absorption of P may be slightly below normal in uremia. Results from metabolic balance studies indicate that Al hydroxide gel, 75 to 200 ml/day increases fecal phosphorus by 30 to 144% (181, 182); however, there is little relationship between the amount of Al hydroxide taken and either the net or relative increase in fecal P. When dietary P intake is below 1.0 g/day and Al hydroxide is taken, fecal P often exceeds dietary intake. However, when dietary P is increased to 2.0 g(64 mmol)/day, fecal P is usually below dietary intake despite ingestion of the gels. Thus, a high phosphate diet can offset an effect of treatment with Al hydroxide or carbonate, emphasizing the need for modest dietary P restriction in combination with treatment with phosphate binders. A scheme showing quantitative relationships between dietary and fecal P and the influence of Al hydroxide is given in Figure 13 (183).

Table 4. Biochemical features of renal osteodystrophy.

Hyperphosphatemia	Elevated plasma OH-proline
Hypocalcemia	Elevated plasma cyclic-AMP
Elevated alkaline phosphatase	Hypercalcemia
Hypermagnesemia	Hypophosphatemia
Elevated serum iPTH	Reduced calcitonin
Reduced plasma 1,25(OH)$_2$D	Elevated bone aluminum
Reduced plasma 24.25(OH)$_2$D$_3$	Elevated GLA protein
Increased Ca and Mg content of skin	

Table 5. Factors affecting serum phosphorus in patients undergoing dialysis.

1. Dietary P intake
2. Ingestion of phosphate-binding antacids
3. Skeletal responsiveness to plasma PTH
4. Degree of vitamin D deficiency and treatment with active vitamin D sterols
5. Frequency, duration and efficiency of dialysis
6. Ingestion of carbohydrate (transient effect)
7. Balance between degradation and synthesis of protoplasm
8. Rapid skeletal accretion (i.e., healing of osteomalacia or osteitis fibrosa)
9. Parenteral alimentation
10. Intake of large amounts of oral Ca supplements
11. Phosphate-containing enemas

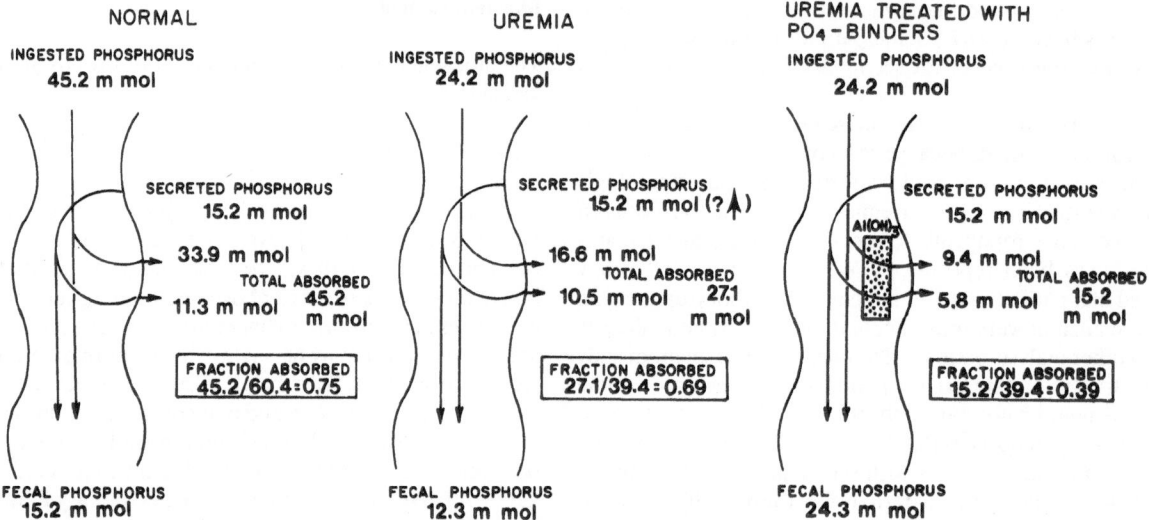

Figure 13. Schema showing approximate amount of phosphorus ingested, its fate in the intestine and the relative contribution of ingested and endogenously secreted phosphorus to total phosphorus lost in the feces. Representative values for a normal man are shown on the left; in the middle are those for a typical uremic patient; the effect of a phosphate-binding gel on phosphorus absorption in uremic patients is shown on the right. (Modified from Coburn et al [183]).
(P [as phosphate] mmol → mg: multiply by 31)

The active forms of vitamin D can increase the net absorption of P (Figure 14) and aggravate the hyperphosphatemia, particularly if the absorbed P remains in the extracellular fluid and is not deposited in bone (48).

Patients with overt secondary hyperparathyroidism may have more hyperphosphatemia than those lacking this syndrome (184); there may also be a more rapid rebound of serum P to high levels during the interdialytic interval in these patients. Presumably, this arises because bone resorption exceeds formation and there is a large pool size for P; a marked fall in serum P often follows subtotal parathyroidectomy or when secondary hyperparathyroidism is suppressed by an active form of vitamin D.

Hypophosphatemia

Occasional dialysis patients exhibit normal or even low plasma P levels despite ingestion of a normal diet and no phosphate-binding gels (185, 186). These patients probably have markedly defective intestinal P transport. Severe hypophosphatemia can also occur during rapid skeletal healing, whether the skeletal disorders is osteomalacia or osteitis fibrosa. In addition, the use of total parenteral nutrition solutions with amino acids and large amounts of glucose can cause hypophosphatemia.

The important pathogenic role of hyperphosphatemia in producing or aggravating secondary hyperparathyroidism has been stressed; however, hypophosphatemia, due to one or more causes, may lead to impaired skeletal mineralization (Table 5). Thus, the severity of features of osteomalacia can correlate inversely with predialysis plasma P levels (Figure 15), an observation that underscores the need to avoid hypophosphatemia and P depletion in dialysis patients.

Hypocalcemia

Reductions in total and ionized serum Ca are common in patients with advanced renal failure; serum Ca levels below the normal range were noted in 40% of uremic patients; some show marked hypocalcemia (32). With the initiation of

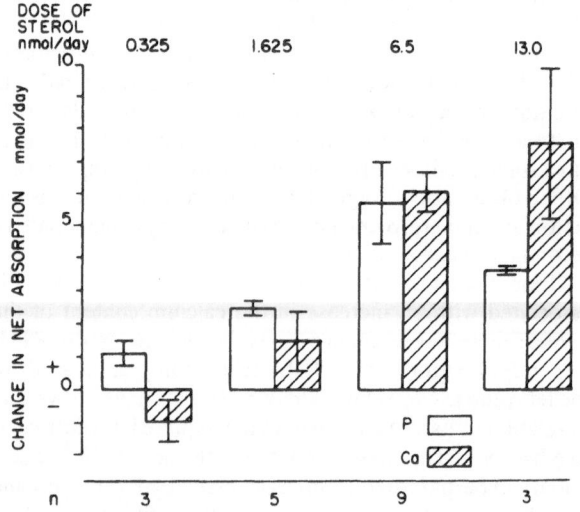

Figure 14. Changes in net absorption of calcium (Ca) and phosphorus (P) after varying daily doses of 1,25(OH)$_2$D$_3$ or 1 alpha (OH)D$_3$. Data in normal subjects and patients with end-stage renal failure are combined (mean ± SEM). The doses of sterol correspond to 0.14, 0.68, 2.7 and 5 μg/day, respectively. (Modified after Coburn et al, with permission of the publisher [294]).
(Ca mmol → mg: multiply by 40.
P [as phosphate] mmol → mg: multiply by 31).

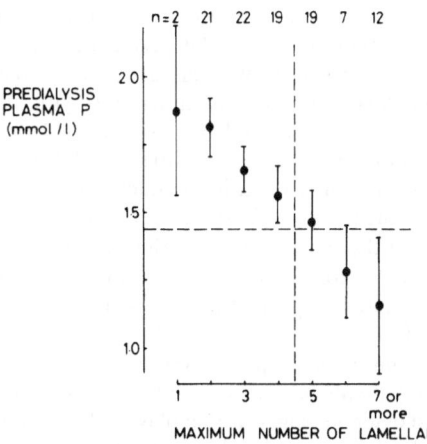

Figure 15. Relationship between mean value of plasma phosphorus (P) immediately prior to hemodialysis (± SEM) and the number of osteoid lamellae identified in bone biopsy in 102 dialysis patients. A horizontal line indicates the upper limit of the normal range. (From Kanis et al [119] slightly modified).
(P mmol/l → mg/dl: multiply by 3.1)

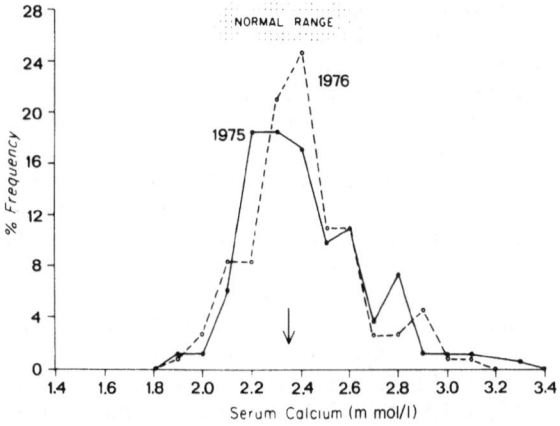

Figure 16. Frequency distribution of serum Ca level for dialysis patients treated at Northwest Kidney Center in Seattle, Washington. Dialysis fluid Mg was 0.5 mmol/l (1.2 mg/dl) in 1975 and 0.25 mmol/l (0.6 mg/dl) in 1976. (Modified after Burnell and Teubner [136])
(Ca mmol/l → mg/dl: multiply by 4)

regular hemodialysis, predialysis serum Ca levels increase and only a small number of patients are hypocalcemic, although the mean values for a group of patients may be below normal. Why serum Ca increases during dialysis is unclear; this can occur despite use of a low dialysis fluid Ca (2.5 mEq/l) and persistent hyperphosphatemia.

Effect of hemodialysis on serum Ca levels

Several factors associated with the dialysis procedure itself influence the level of plasma Ca. These include: the Ca level in dialysate, the rate of Ca movement across the dialyzer; the duration of dialysis; alterations in kinetics of exchange of Ca between various body compartments; changes in the binding of Ca to plasma albumin; and the presence of Ca complexes which are less readily dialyzed than is ionized Ca. The percentage of Ca bound to albumin in dialysis patients is not different from normal; however, dialysis patients often have a higher complexed Ca and a lower ionized Ca (32). With parallel plate dialyzers, the dialysance of Ca, calculated from the non-protein bound fraction in blood, was approximately 60 to 70% of that of urea (187). The total quantity of Ca transferred into a patient from dialysate can reach 700 to 1100 mg over 10 h of dialysis (187) when dialysate Ca level exceeds the plasma diffusible Ca by 1.5 to 2.0 mg/dl (0.375 to 0.5 mmol/l).

Total plasma Ca often increases substantially during hemodialysis. This is due in large part to an increase in plasma albumin induced by ultrafiltration and also to augmented protein-binding of Ca due to an increase in blood pH.

Studies with Ca electrodes show that ionized Ca levels fall even as total Ca increases during dialysis with a dialysis fluid Ca concentration of 2.5 mEq/l (188). The increase in total serum Ca during dialysis with a dialysis solution Ca concentration of 3.0 to 3.5 mEq/l is associated with an acute rise in ionized Ca (188) and fall in plasma PTH (189).

Hypercalcemia

Hypercalcemia may appear spontaneously in patients undergoing hemodialysis; it may occur under at least two circumstances: 1) in conjunction with an overt secondary hyperparathyroidism and 2) with dialysis osteomalacia. The former patients usually have radiographic signs of hyperparathyroidism with markedly elevated levels of serum iPTH (99). Such patients have been classified by some as having 'tertiary' hyperparathyroidism, and it has been implied that there is an autonomous secretion of PTH; however, serum PTH levels usually decrease when serum calcium is elevated. It is possible that marked hyperplasia of the parathyroid glands is responsible for the continued secretion of the PTH excess. Parathyroidectomy is probably the most effective treatment for such patients.

Spontaneous hypercalcemia can also occur in patients with aluminum-induced osteomalacia (100, 161). Recent studies by Rodriguez et al (98) have shown that Al increases Ca binding in the plasma and decreases the concentration of ionized Ca. Thus, as ionized Ca decreases, further movement of Ca from bone and interstitium into the vascular space occurs, resulting in hypercalcemia. Such hypercalcemia may be aggravated by low doses of vitamin D, high Ca intake, or the use of a high concentration of Ca in the dialysis solution (i.e., above 3.25 mEq/l) (190). Parathyroidectomy is contra-indicated in these patients and will rapidly aggravate the condition (105). Hypercalcemia can also develop in dialysis patients in association with treatment with various forms of vitamin D, oral Ca supplements, and the long-term use of dialysis fluid containing Ca of 3.5 mEq/l or above.

Hypermagnesemia

Hypermagnesemia is common in dialysis patients (32). The

kidney plays a major role in regulating plasma Mg and body stores. The intestinal absorption of Mg is normal in patients with advanced renal failure. Thus, the occurrence of hypermagnesemia is not surprising. The dietary intake of Mg in uremic patients ingesting a restricted protein diet is below normal which may prevent hypermagnesemia in many patients. However, abrupt and marked hypermagnesemia can develop when Mg intake is increased by the ingestion of Mg containing laxatives or phosphate binding gels with added Mg oxide (191). The level of Mg in the dialysis solution also influences the plasma Mg levels in patients treated by dialysis. In one other center using a dialysis fluid Mg of 0.5 mEq/l, serum Mg levels ranged from 1.5 to 2.2 mEq/l, while serum levels were 2.5 to 4.5 mEq/l in other patients using a dialysis fluid Mg of 1.5 mEq/l (32). The effect of reducing dialysis fluid Mg from 1.0 mEq/l is shown in Figure 16 (187).

Acute hypermagnesemia can suppress PTH secretion (22), raising the possibility that hypermagnesemia might diminish secondary hyperparathyroidism and, hence, benefit dialysis patients. However, there are no data to indicate that chronic hypermagnesemia has such an effect; this may reflect the fact that mild hypocalcemia is more effective in stimulating PTH secretion than is the suppressive action of hypermagnesemia (22).

Whether chronic hypermagnesemia is harmful in patients with ESRD is not clear. Long term hypermagnesemia may be associated with abnormal bone mineralization in uremia, and skeletal Mg is increased in association with hypermagnesemia (81). Alfrey et al (192, 193) suggested that Mg pyrophosphate, present in excess amounts in bone of uremic patients, may promote abnormal mineral turnover. Moreover, Burnell and Teubner (186) suggested that chemical characteristics of bone improve after dialysate Mg is reduced and hypermagnesemia is prevented. Thus, prolonged and persistent hypermagnesemia may not be desirable in patients undergoing dialysis.

Plasma parathyroid hormone (PTH)

The plasma levels of PTH are commonly elevated in dialysis patients, particularly with the use of antisera directed toward the mid region or the 'C-terminal' fragment. Assays utilizing 'intact' PTH or an 'N-terminal' antisera often show lesser degrees of elevation. Significant correlations between serum PTH and histomorphometric features of osteitis fibrosa have been reported in dialysis patients (194). However, a large number of commercially available radioimmunoassays (RIA) for PTH provide no information about the predictive value of a given serum PTH level with regard to the severity of osteitis fibrosa. Thus, the discrimination between RIA-measured PTH levels in normal subjects from values in patients with primary hyperparathyroidism (195) provides little or no information about the meaning of a PTH level measured in a patient with end-stage renal disease. Unfortunately, only a few assays provide correlative data between serum PTH levels and histologic features of bone disease in uremic patients (194, 196); the interpretation of PTH levels measured by laboratories lacking such information is fraught with difficulty.

A small number of patients with advanced renal failure may have low, normal or even undetectable levels of PTH. Hypomagnesemia can cause low levels on occasions, but low or normal PTH levels are common in patients with 'aluminum induced-osteomalacia' and little or no evidence for osteitis fibrosa (100, 101). Serial levels of serum PTH may be useful to follow the course of patients undergoing long-term dialysis; for a correct interpretation of a PTH assay, it is essential to know the characteristics of the antisera and have information on the correlation between levels of PTH in uremic patients and biologic features of secondary hyperparathyroidism.

In the past, marked hyperplasia and secretion of PTH in certain uremic patients has been considered 'autonomous'; however, most evidence suggests that plasma PTH is subject to feedback regulation and levels do fall during either Ca infusion or dialysis using a high dialysis solution Ca. However, it is often necessary for plasma Ca concentration to be raised to hypercalcemic levels before PTH falls. The contributing factors are massive parathyroid gland hyperplasia and a change in the set point of Ca for PTH secretion. When massive hyperplasia of the parathyroid glands exists, plasma PTH concentration increases as a consequence of the increased parathyroid gland mass for any plasma Ca level since basal secretion of PTH continues despite hypercalcemia (197). Parathyroid hyperplasia, per se, increases this basal secretion in proportion to the increased number of cells. In addition, a change in the set point of calcium for PTH secretion (59), as discussed in the pathogenesis of secondary hyperparathyroidism is another important factor. Thus, dialysis patients with overt secondary hyperparathyroidism have an abnormal set-point for calcium (61) and therapeutically, relative high levels of serum Ca have to be reached in order to suppress secondary hyperparathyroidism (Figure 4).

Alkaline phosphatase, hydroxyproline and cyclic AMP

Although total serum alkaline phosphatase includes isoenzymes arising from liver, intestine, kidney, and bone, its measurement can be a useful indicator of increased osteoblastic activity. An elevated serum alkaline phosphatase may occur with either osteitis fibrosa or osteomalacia, but markedly raised levels may be more common in the former, with higher rates of bone turnover. Plasma alkaline phosphatase may be useful for monitoring therapy of skeletal disease with vitamin D compounds or calcium supplements (see *Management*). Since dialysis patients often have coexisting hepatic abnormalities, liver disease should be excluded as the cause of an elevated alkaline phosphatase. It should be kept in mind that uremic patients can exhibit significant and overt skeletal disease and yet have normal levels of plasma alkaline phosphatase activity.

In studies of large numbers of patients, alkaline phosphatase activity correlates with skeletal histologic features of secondary hyperparathyroidism with percentage of osteoblastic surface and percent of active resorption surface (198). Plasma alkaline phosphatase levels in patients with aluminum-related bone disease (osteomalacia or aplastic bone disease) may not be elevated despite the presence of severe disease (100, 144). Others have reported elevated alkaline phosphatase levels (84, 87); thus, this measurement may not discriminate between Al-related bone disease and osteitis fibrosa.

An elevation of plasma hydroxyproline, both free and peptide bound, may provide an index for increased collagen turnover and bone resorption (199); The hydroxyproline determination is cumbersome and not likely to become widely available. Plasma cyclic AMP is also elevated in uremic patients; however, it does not correlate with the severity of secondary hyperparathyroidism (200).

Bone GLA-protein

Bone GLA-protein (alpha-carboxyglutamic acid), also known as osteocalcin, is an abundant noncollagenous protein synthesized by the osteoblast and appears in the plasma (201). Its concentrations in plasma may reflect bone turnover (202), although plasma levels are also increased when renal function is impaired (203). In a small number of patients undergoing regular dialysis, significant correlations were found between the plasma levels of bone GLA-protein and histologic parameters of bone turnover as well as the degree of peritrabecular fibrosis (204). Recent observations in dialysis patients have shown a good correlation between osteocalcin and alkaline phosphatase, PTH and $25(OH)D_3$ (205). In addition bone GLA-protein is stimulated by calcitriol. Whether this protein may be a noninvasive parameter for the bone evaluation of dialysis patients has not been evaluated; further studies of bone GLA-protein in a large and diverse group of patients with renal osteodystrophy are clearly indicated.

Plasma aluminum levels

Because the kidney is the major organ responsible for the excretion of Al, plasma Al levels are elevated in most patients with ESRD. They are elevated to a greater degree in patients ingesting aluminum-containing gels than in those not taking these drugs; the levels are also markedly elevated in patients undergoing dialysis with dialysate contaminated with Al (152). The plasma level probably reflects a 'recent' aluminum load, and does not correlate well with tissue stores (206). The plasma levels fall slowly over several weeks to months when aluminum intake is discontinued (207). Because of the avid binding of plasma Al to transferrin and albumin, plasma Al levels often increase slightly during a hemodialysis procedure, even when the dialysate is aluminum-free. Plasma Al levels below 40–55 μg/l (1.5 to 2.0 μmol/l) (values in normal individuals range from 2 to 8 μg/l [74 to 296 μmol/l]) generally indicate a low risk of Al accumulation or Al toxicity; the finding of markedly elevated plasma Al levels (i.e. 130 μg/l [4.8 μmol/l]) indicate a high risk of either Al toxicity or its future development unless the Al exposure is reduced. Most patients with Al-related bone disease have markedly elevated plasma Al concentrations

(e.g. >75 to 100 g/l [2.8 to 3.7 μmol/l]). Also, patients with markedly elevated plasma Al levels (e.g. values >150 to 200 μg/l [5.6 to 7.4 μmol/l]) are likely to develop aluminum-related bone disease and/or encephalopathy if the exposure to Al continues (100, 122). There has been some uncertainty about the value of monitoring plasma Al concentrations at regular intervals in dialysis patients. Measuring plasma Al every 3 to 4 months has been recommended (123). Marked elevation of plasma Al levels (e.g. >75 to 100 μg/l [2.8 to 3.7 μmol/l]) in the majority of dialysis patients in one dialysis unit indicates exposure to unacceptably high concentrations of dialysis fluid Al. This could indicate that the water treatment system has malfunctioned at some time in the recent past. Since contamination varies over time, the Al concentration in water or dialysate may be normal at a given moment. Plasma Al levels above 75 to 100 μg/l in the presence of normal dialysis fluid Al concentration may suggest excessive ingestion of aluminum-containing gels (100).

Deferoxamine infusion test

The deferoxamine infusion test was initially proposed as a method to estimate the tissue stores of Al and thereby predict the presence of Al toxicity without the need for a bone biopsy (208). When deferoxamine, 40 mg/kg, is infused over 2 h shortly after the completion of the dialysis procedure, the increment in plasma Al, which reaches a peak and stabilizes after 24 to 36 h post infusion (Figure 17), correlated with the bone content of Al (208). However, not all patients with elevated tissue levels of Al have evidence of

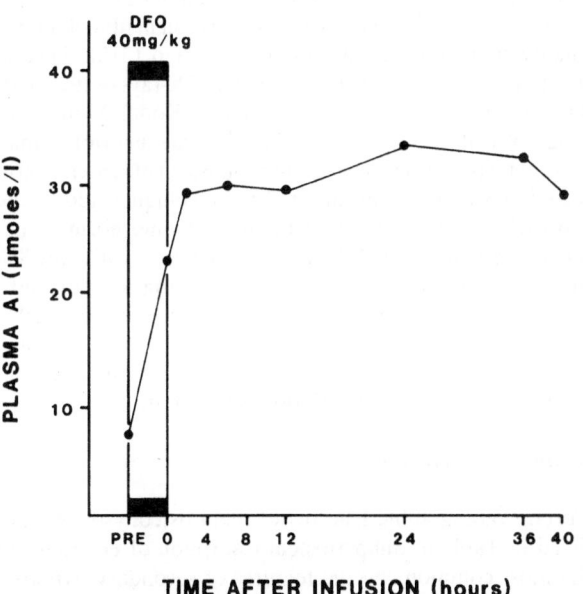

Figure 17. Serial plasma aluminum concentrations after infusion of deferoxamine (DFO), 40 mg/kg in a patient with aluminum related bone disease. The 'DFO infusion' test was done after the completion of a regular hemodialysis (1 μmol/l = 27 μg/l); reproduced from Milliner et al (208) with permission of the publishers.

Al-related bone disease (209). Subsequent studies have shown that many patients with renal failure, including those with osteitis fibrosa, can have substantial tissue Al and yet exhibit no toxic effects of Al (210). When the increment in plasma Al is below 150 to 170 g/l (5.6 to 6.3 μmol/l) the deferoxamine infusion test may help identify patients with little or no risk of Al loading. In contrast, an increment above 400 μg/l (14.8 μmol/l) would indicate a substantial risk of Al accumulation and/or toxicity. When dialysis patients with severe osteitis fibrosa also have marked body accumulation of Al and exhibit a 'positive test', they are at great risk of developing osteomalacia after parathyroidectomy. The finding of a highly abnormal test in such a patient may be an indication to initiate therapy for Al toxicity even before the needed parathyroid surgery. Finally, patients developing Al induced-osteomalacia after parathyroidectomy may have a relatively small increment in serum Al after deferoxamine, despite significant total body Al burden. It appears that the lack of PTH makes Al mobilization more difficult.

Radiographic features

Techniques

The incidence of radiographic abnormalities of the skeleton varies considerably in different dialysis centers. This may reflect true differences related to patient's ages, type of management, and duration of dialysis. However, the radiographic techniques employed, type of X-ray film used, and the interest of the radiologist may also account for differences (211). X-rays of bone, obtained utilizing standard film and developing procedures, result in film of poorer quality than those produced 20 years ago (212). Several techniques can increase the sensitivity of X-rays of the hand. The use of fine grain industrial film (i.e. Kodak M or mammography film), which is developed by manual rather than automatic film processing, and the omission of screen of grid techniques and magnification X-ray techniques add to the sensitivity (213). With conventional viewing, normal phalanges were noted in 67% of uremic patients, with only 8% manifesting marked subperiosteal resorption; with magnification of the same films, only 26% were normal while 29% exhibited substantial resorption (213). However, with such magnification techniques, there is a danger of overreading; familiarity with normal variation is required.

Subperiosteal erosions

Certain radiographic features of renal osteodystrophy are listed in Table 6. Subperiosteal resorption of erosions are the most common specific features of secondary hyperparathyroidism. Erosions may occur in the phalanges, pelvis, distal ends of the clavicles, inferior surfaces of the ribs, femur, mandible and skull. The phalanges are most accessible site for careful radiographic evaluation. If appropriately sensitive techniques are applied, it is uncommon for erosions to be found elsewhere if the hands are normal

(213). In its earliest form, resorption occurs on the radial surfaces of the middle phalanx of the second and/or third digit of the dominant arm (Figure 18). The turf of the terminal phalanx commonly exhibits subperiosteal resorption (213). Meema et al (213) have documented the use and value of magnification of X-ray films particularly of the digits. With the use of careful techniques, subperiosteal resorption may be recognized in 40 to 50% of patients that show increased resorption on bone biopsy (214). Also bone erosions are associated with higher serum iPTH levels in dialysis patients (Figure 19) (215). When Al overload occurs in conjuction with significant subperiosteal erosions, remineralization and normalization of radiographs may not occur when secondary hyperparathyroidism is reversed by treatment with an active vitamin D sterol or by parathyroidectomy (216). Thus, some caution must be exercised in interpreting the presence of subperiosteal erosions as specific radiologic signs of osteitis fibrosa; their presence does not exclude

Table 6. Radiographic and other features of renal osteodystrophy.

Osteopenia (reduced density)
Skeletal features of secondary hyperparathyroidism
   Subperiosteal resorption
   Cortical striations
   Cyst formation (brown tumor)
   Slipped epiphysis
   Mottled ('salt and pepper') skull
   Periosteal new bone formation
Abnormal enchondral ossification
   Rickets-like lesion
   Slipped epiphysis
Osteosclerosis
Pseudofractures (Looser's zones)
Genu valgum
Protrusio acetabuli
Endosteal bone resorption (metacarpal index)
Vertebral collapse (crush fracture)
Spontaneous rib fractures
Osteonecrosis (aseptic necrosis)
Soft tissue calcifications
   Periarticular calcification
   Tumoral calcifications
   Chondrocalcinosis
   Ocular calcification
Cutaneous calcification
   Visceral calcification
      Pulmonary (perfusion-ventilation abnormality)
      Cardiac (conduction defect, congestive heart failure)
   Vascular calcification
      Medial
      Intimal
   Reduced mineral content
      Photon absorptiometry
      Neutron activation
   Abnormal scintiscan
      Increased uptake of 99 mTc polyphosphate
      Symmetrical in osteitis fibrosa
      Identification of fractures (osteomalacia)

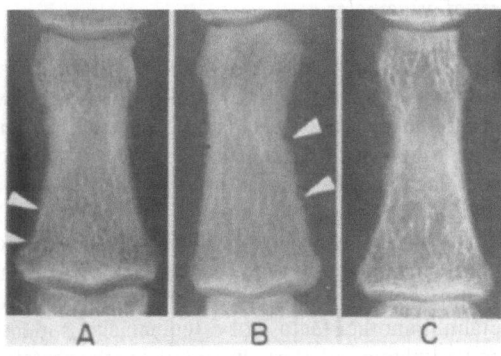

Figure 18. Appearance of subperiosteal erosions in 3 patients with renal osteodystrophy. A. There is an early saucer-shaped lesion with no overlying cortical bone on the lower radial shoulder (arrows). B. Moderately advanced erosion along the radial surface, but without an apparent break in the cortex (arrows). C. There is a cystic honeycomb appearance of the subperiosteal cortex (left). The erosions extend close to the distal interphalangeal joints (Reproduced from Parfitt [211] with permission).

the possibility of Al-induced bone disease.

Cortical striations, resulting from enlarged Haversian canals (Figure 20), occur with secondary hyperparathyroidism and also with increased bone turnover due to other causes, i.e. primary hyperparathyroidism, hyperthyroidism, acromegaly, and during rapid growth (215). They usually occur in association with subperiosteal erosions. Cystic abnormalities of bone (i.e. brown tumors) develop in renal osteodystrophy less often than in primary hyperparathyroidism (217). Such lesions may be painful and when present in the mandible can alter the configuration of the teeth. Almost invariably, subperiosteal erosions accompany cystic lesions. With healing, focal areas of sclerosis may appear.

Abnormalities of the skull

Radiographic alterations of the skull have been divided into four types (218): 1) a diffuse 'ground-glass' appearance, with loss of sharp margins at the vascular grooves and diploic venous channels; 2) a diffuse mottled or granular appearance, which is most frequent and probably represents a network of enlarged resorption spaces within the table of the skull; 3) focal lucent defects, 1 to 3 cm in diameter, which may be present with or without the 'ground-glass' or mottled appearance and 4) focal areas of sclerosis. These abnormalities may disappear completely after appropriate treatment (Figure 21).

Periosteal neostosis

Periosteal new bone formation, termed periosteal neostosis, (219) can appear in 10% of dialysis patients in association with secondary hyperparathyroidism. This appears as a thin external layer of new bone separated from the original periosteum by a clear zone. Subsequently, the cortical bone

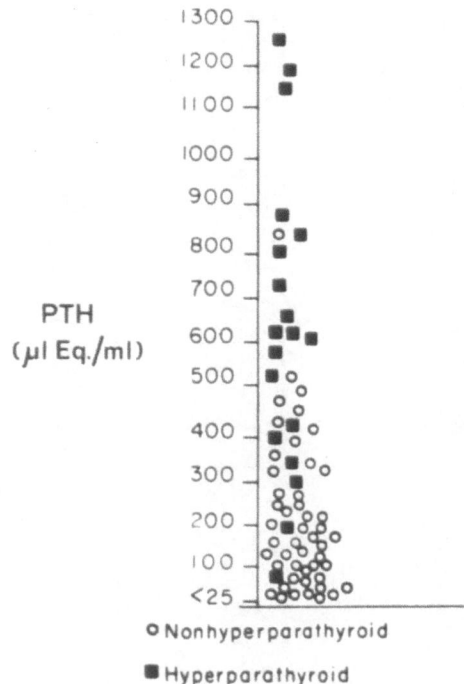

PTH
(μl Eq./ml)

○ Nonhyperparathyroid

■ Hyperparathyroid

Figure 19. Levels of serum immunoreactive parathyroid hormone (PTH) in 71 dialysis patients. Those with clinically apparent secondary hyperparathyroidism (solid symbols) are compared to others lacking overt manifestations. The normal value for PTH is below 46 μl/Eq./ml. (Reproduced from Glassford et al [215] with permission.)

may be thickened as new bone is united with the old. The most frequently involved sites are the metatarsals, pelvis, distal tibia and the hands. This abnormality can be confused with a calcified digital artery and with an artifact produced as a patient moves during radiography (215).

Alterations in growth zone

Abnormalities in the growth zone occur in children with secondary hyperparathyroidism or rickets. It may be difficult to separate true rickets from the 'rickets-like' abnormality of secondary hyperparathyroidism (215). Unlike true rickets, the lesion of hyperparathyroidism exhibits no widening of the physeal zone. and the irregularity of the metaphyseal lucent zone is very severe and extends laterally and blends with superiosteal resorption at the cortex. This lesion is more common in children over 10 years, while true rickets usually occurs before age 5 years. The radiolucent zone is caused by an accumulation of woven bone and/or fibrous tissue in rickets-like lesion, whereas cartilage accumulates in vitamin D-deficiency rickets. The development of a slipped epiphysis is common in the rickets-like lesion; thus, 10% of children with chronic renal failure had this lesion, while it was less common in children undergoing regular dialysis (159). A slipped epiphysis is often associated with pain or

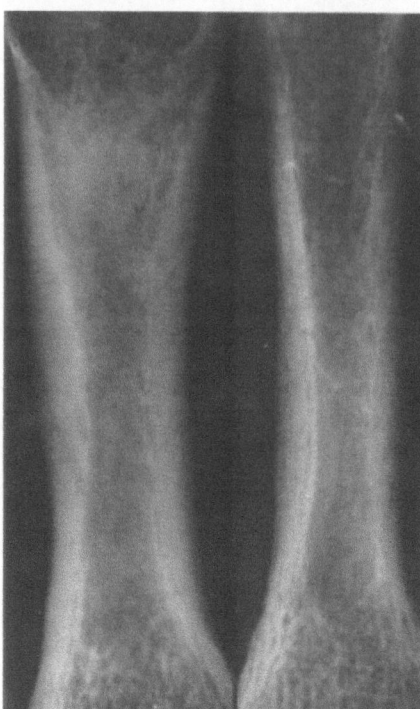

Figure 20. Left: cortical bone appears solid except for nutrient canal in the left cortex. Right: intracortical striations grade 3+ in a 30 year old female patient with end stage renal failure.

abnormal gait; however, some patients are asymptomatic or have referred pain. The rickets-like lesion responds to treatment with vitamin D, probably due to suppression of secondary hyperparathyroidism.

Genu valgum which is the most common cause of adolescent knock knee was observed in over 10% of a series of patients with symptomatic renal osteodystrophy (215). Symptoms include difficulty in walking and pain. Other signs of rickets are often present, but the lesion can complicate secondary hyperparathyroidism. Occasionally, the angulation is so great in weight bearing joints that shearing of physeal plate may occur with partial slipping of the distal femoral epiphysis.

Osteosclerosis

Osteosclerosis, a form of increased density of bone, may occur because of increased thickness and number of trabeculae in spongy bone. The vertebral bodies, pelvis, ribs, skull, and long bone are most commonly involved. It may be more common in young patients. In the spine, this may produce a classic 'rugger jersey' appearance, with dense bands alternating with radiolucent zones. At times, osteosclerosis appears as narrow, dense sclerotic bands sharply demarcated from the rest of the vertebral body.

Features of osteomalacia

Special radiographic features of osteomalacia are rare in uremic patients. Pseudofractures or Looser zones are wide, straight radiolucent bands which abut the cortex perpendicular to the long axis of the bones. These are uncommon in our experience and were noted in less than 2% of dialysis patients in Germany (220), but they occurred in 20% of Australian patients with symptomatic renal osteodystrophy (215). They occur in areas of the pelvis, clavicles, scapulae, and long bones that are subject to mechanical stress. Protrusio acetabuli, another feature of osteomalacia, is identified by a convex bulging with the pelvis overlying the acetabulum (221).

Aseptic necrosis (osteonecrosis) occasionally develops in dialysis patients (222), although it is much more common in renal transplant recipients, and has been attributed to marked secondary hyperparathyroidism.

Osteopenia

A radiographically detected decrease in bone density may be termed osteopenia. This can occur in dialysis patients due to either osteomalacia or osteoporosis. A syndrome termed, 'dialysis osteopenia' is characterized by reduced bone mass, bone pain, and/or fractures, out of proportion to radiographic evidence of osteomalacia or osteitis fibrosa. X-rays showed widened marrow cavities, i.e. increased endosteal resorption. The patients failed to improve after subtotal parathyroidectomy or after large doses of vitamin D; unfortunately, bone histology was not available. The clinical findings in these patients may resemble those of 'dialysis osteomalacia', described above. However, a lack of histological data does not permit classification of these patients (223).

Bone mineral content and metacarpal index

Photon absorptiometry, total body Ca by neutron activation, and scintiscans of the skeleton are other non-invasive methods for evaluating the skeleton. Neutron activation may provide accurate measurement of total bone mineral content (224) but the expense and scarcity of facilities limit its use. Photon absorptiometry measures mineral content by the transmission of gamma rays on photons through bone. It is more accurate than determination of density from X-ray film; however, its use is limited to measurement of cortical bone in the radius, ulna, or phalanges. Bone mineral content can be reduced because of a lower volume of bone tissue, increased intracortical porosity from increased resorption spaces, or replacement of mineralized bone by unmineralized woven bone (215). Photon absorptiometry does not distinguish between the causes of decreased density, and this technique is best combined with detailed radiography.

The metacarpal index is obtained by measuring the dimensions of the cortex of the metacarpal bone on x-ray film. Normal data are available for the second left metacarpal and the 'Metacarpal Index' is the ratio of cortical to total bone

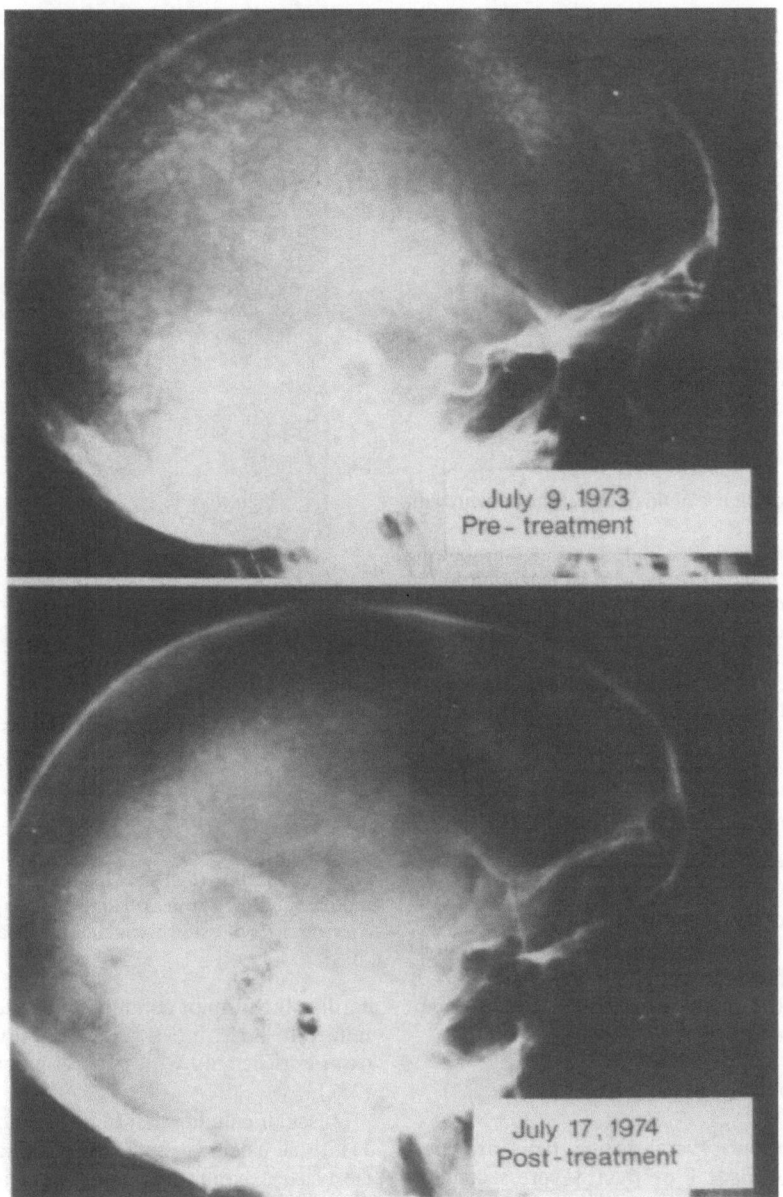

July 9, 1973
Pre-treatment

July 17, 1974
Post-treatment

Figure 21. Radiographs of the skull in a dialysis patient with overt renal osteodystrophy. The upper X-ray was taken before, and the lower after 10 months of treatment with 1,25(OH)$_2$D$_3$.

width. Increased net endosteal resorption has been reported in 28 to 40% of dialysis patients (215, 225). With the use of a dialysis fluid Ca of 2.5 mEq/l, the 'Metacarpal Index' fell 6% in dialysis patients while no change was observed in those utilizing 3.5 mEq/l (226). Other data show neither a correlation between such losses and other evidence of bone disease or between rate of loss and heparin dosage (227).

Scintiscan
Bone scintigraphy, utilizing ^{99m}Tc diphosphonate, can detect

skeletal alterations in dialysis patients and assess their response to treatment. The diphosphonate accumulates in areas of increased bone turnover and increased blood flow (228). The uptake of the diphosphonate may be related to abnormal collagen metabolism (229). Olgaard et al (230) noted abnormal scintigraphy in 90% of their dialysis patients, only 10% of whom had abnormal x-rays, suggesting that this method is more sensitive than radiographs (Figure 22). The symmetrical uptake of diphosphonate throughout the skeleton can be a manifestation of osteitis fibrosa. The

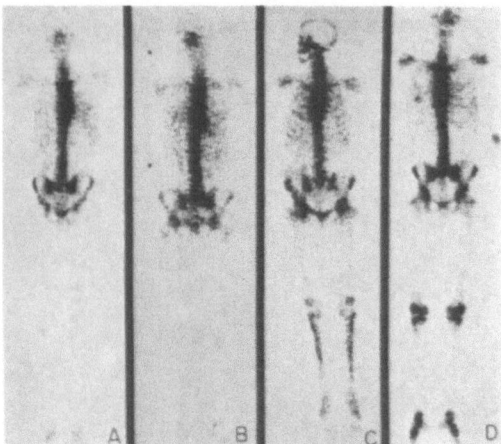

Figure 22. Skeletal scintigrams in a normal subject and patients with renal failure.
A. Grade 0, normal scintigram; B. Grade 1, Scintigram showing abnormal uptake in the femoral heads with an extension to the femoral neck and trochanteric region; C. Grade 2, scintigram showing abnormal uptake in the femoral head and neck and in the proximal half of the tibial shaft; D. Grade 3, scintigram showing extensive uptake in the femoral head and marked uptake in femoral and tibial condyles the tarsus and the proximal part of the metatarsus. (Reproduced from Ølgaard et al [230] with permission of the publisher.)

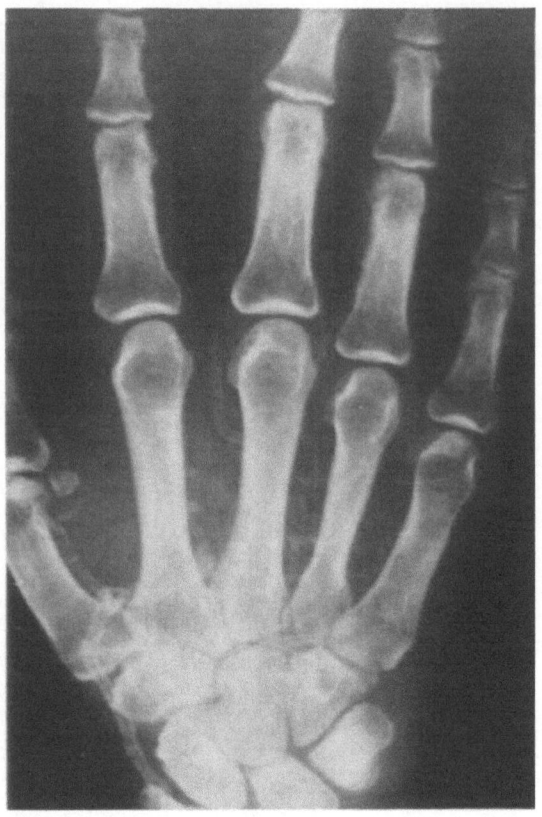

Figure 23. Radiograph showing marked calcification of the digital arteries; although intimal plaques may be present, the appearance is characteristic of extensive media calcification.

scintiscan also may be a sensitive method for detection of multiple fractures, even in the absence of radiographic evidence of such fractures in patients with osteomalacia. Further refinements of the technique involve measurement of kinetics and the plasma clearance of diphosphonate (229). It can be used for the detection of extraskeletal calcification in tissues such as the lung (230).

Soft tissue calcifications

Soft-tissue calcifications of several distinct types are common in ESRD. A high Ca × P product, severe secondary hyperparathyroidism, hypermagnesemia, alkalosis, and local tissue injury each predispose to their development (231, 232). The chemical and crystal composition of visceral calcification was found to differ substantially from that observed in Ca deposits in periarticular, tumoral or vascular sites (233, 234). The first variety is made up of amorphous microcrystals with concentrations of Ca, Mg, and P that resemble those of Ca whitlockite. Calcium deposits localized around the joints may consist of carbonate-containing apatite similar to that in bone; such crystals are more likely to induce inflammation than are amorphous microcrystals.

Calcifications may involve the sclera (band keratopathy), conjunctiva, or skin, where it can present as macular plaques, soft tissue around the joints, and in periarticular sites or within the joint itself (chondrocalcinosis). Visceral calcification of the lungs or heart may cause serious clinical consequences; thus, myocardial calcifications may impair

cardiac function or conduction and lead to congestive heart failure or heart block (235, 236). Pulmonary calcifications can be associated with perfusion-ventilation abnormalities (237).

Vascular calcification can present in two major varieties: 1) intimal calcification, similar to that observed in atherosclerosis, is common in the aorta and large arteries and 2) medial calcification, a form more typical of uremia, involving the media of medium to large size arteries (Figure 23). The lumen of the vessel is often patent but surgery to establish vascular access may be difficult. Because of rigidity of the involved vessel, pulses may be poorly palpable even when circulation is adequate. Medial calcifications may be associated with the syndrome, calciphylaxis, described above.

Soft-tissue calcification is believed to relate to a high Ca × P product. Such calcifications are common with secondary hyperparathyroidism. Parathyroid hormone may be a pathogenic factor, and Ca deposition in certain tissues such as joint, brain and heart may relate directly to high PTH levels (166, 238). Dialysis patients with acute periarthritis have, as a group, higher levels of PTH than other dialysis patients (Figure 11). For unexplained reasons, uremic children rarely develop soft tissue calcification (239).

PREVENTION AND MANAGEMENT

The general objectives of management in dialysis patients are to suppress secondary hyperparathyroidism, produce normal mineralization of osteoid, maintain blood concentrations of Ca, Mg and P near normal, prevent extraosseous calcification, and avoid aluminum toxicity. Therapeutic considerations will be classified as general management, which apply to all dialysis patients, and specific treatment for problems arising in certain patients.

General management

The cornerstone of management includes: 1) prevention of hyperphosphatemia by modest dietary P restriction and administration of P binders; 2) dietary supplements of Ca; 3) and use of an appropriate dialysis fluid Ca concentration. In addition, significant hypermagnesemia should be prevented by avoiding foods or drugs containing excess Mg and by use of an appropriate Mg level in dialysis fluid. Tap water containing fluoride or excess Al should be avoided in the preparation of dialysis solution.

The value of vitamin D as prophylaxis has not yet been clearly established. Most children undergoing dialysis eventually develop overt skeletal disease unless pharmacologic quantities of vitamin D are administered (239); therefore, children should receive treatment with active forms of vitamin D. Indications for parathyroidectomy and treatment of overt disease with specific forms of vitamin D are discussed below.

Control of hyperphosphatemia

Factors which contribute to hyperphosphatemia in dialysis patients are noted in Table 5. In advanced uremia, dietary P intake in excess of 1 to 1.2 g (32 to 39 mmol)/day may lead to hyperphosphatemia despite the intake of substantial amounts of Al hydroxide. With only modest dietary P restriction, the intake can be reduced to 800 to 1000 mg(26 to 32 mmol)/day, facilitating control of serum P with phosphate binders. With such treatment, several weeks may pass before serum P falls, suggesting that P is sequestered in bone and/or soft tissue (240). The reduction of serum P toward normal is often associated with a small increase in serum Ca, a fall in serum PTH, and a reduced incidence of overt secondary hyperparathyroidism (241).

The goal of therapy with phosphate-binding agents is to reduce serum P levels to or near normal. In dialysis patients, predialysis serum P levels are ideally maintained between 4.5 and 6.0 mg/dl (1.44 to 1.92 mmol/l). In patients with advanced renal failure (creatinine clearance <10 ml/min) and in those treated with dialysis, dietary P intake should be restricted to 800 to 1000 mg/day, and P binders should be taken with each meal. Serum Ca and P levels should be monitored at least monthly to permit appropriate dosage adjustment of phosphate-binding compounds. If serum P concentration decreases significantly or remains above the desired range, the number of tablets or capsules should be decreased or increased by 1 to 3 per day.

The available agents for intestinal P binding include the aluminum-containing gels, Ca carbonate and Mg carbonate. The aluminum-containing agents have been most widely used; they include the Al hydroxide and Al carbonate gels which are available as liquid gels, tablets, and capsules. The capsules are less effective than liquid gels in binding P (242); however, patient compliance is usually much better with capsules than with either liquids or tablets. Because of the absorption from these compounds and since Al may accumulate in renal failure, there is the danger of Al toxicity with the use of large doses of Al containing gels. Calcium carbonate is one available alternative to the aluminum-containing compounds (243, 244). Initial reports indicate that 4 to 12 g (40 to 120 mmol) of Ca carbonate taken daily with meals can adequately control serum P concentration. The risks and side effects observed with such therapy have included hypercalcemia and diarrhea (243). When Ca carbonate is given as a phosphate-binding agent, the objective is considerably different than when it is given as a nutritional supplement to enhance Ca absorption (see below). When used as a P binder, it is important that Ca carbonate be given with meals with the dose adjusted to the P content of the individual meal. Under these circumstances, less Ca is absorbed and the risk of hypercalcemia is reduced. Nonetheless, Ca carbonate cannot be taken by all patients and the need still exists for a safe, effective phosphate-binding agent that does not contain Al (243). A major problem with Ca carbonate is the difficulty of concomitant administration of calcitriol which may result in marked hypercalcemia. Recently, O'Donovan et al (245) have used Mg carbonate in 28 patients for 2 years, in substitution for aluminum hydroxide. A significant fall in predialysis Al levels was observed and serum P remained unchanged from previous levels. Since these patients were dialyzed with Mg free dialysate, predialysis Mg concentrations tended to fall toward the normal range. The levels of PTH remained unchanged during the 2 year period. Thus, Mg carbonate may be a useful alternative phosphate binder.

It is equally important to avoid lowering the concentration of serum P to levels below normal to guard against P depletion in uremic patients. Some patients require no phosphate-binding agents, while others require larger doses. Even in patients with renal failure, the overzealous use of P binders can produce hypophosphatemia and P depletion; moreover, worsening of bone disease and osteomalacia may result (246). Also, large doses of aluminum-containing gels increase the risk of Al toxicity, particularly in children with renal failure (116). It was once assumed that Al hydroxide and carbonate were nonabsorbable and totally safe, but evidence now indicates that orally administered Al can be absorbed to a significant extent and may lead to an increased Al content in plasma and various tissues (80, 118).

Secondary hyperparathyroidism may persist or progress in a substantial number of dialysis patients despite prevention of hyperphosphatemia (241).

Calcium concentration in the dialysis fluid

The use of dialysis solution containing Ca, 2.5 to 2.6 mEq/l (1.25 to 1.3 mmol/l), acutely decreases ionized Ca, which should increase PTH secretion; most dialysis centers utilize dialysate with Ca levels of 3.0 to 3.5 mEq/l (1.5 to 1.75 mmol/l). An increase of dialysate Ca from 2.5 to 3.0 mEq/l reduces the incidence of overt skeletal disease (245), but it is not clear whether a further increase in dialysate Ca to 3.5 to 4.0 mEq/l produces any benefit (247). Current evidence indicates no benefit from use of dialysate Ca levels above 3.0 to 3.25 mEq/l, and there may be added risk of extraskeletal Ca deposition (248).

Oral calcium supplements

The diets ingested by dialysis patients often contain enough Ca to prevent negative Ca balance (240, 249), and a daily dietary Ca of 1.5 to 2.0 g(37.5 to 50 mmol)/day can prevent a negative balance. Thus, a therapeutic alternative is dietary Ca supplements with Ca carbonate being the most palatable and least expensive, although other compounds may also be used. The oral administration of large amounts of Ca may suppress secondary hyperparathyroidism and improve bone mineral content (249, 250), although the mineralization may be qualitatively abnormal (251).

Hypercalcemia may develop with use of oral Ca supplements (249, 250). When this occurs in conjunction with a markedly elevated serum PTH and skeletal erosions, overt poorly suppressable hyperparathyroidism is likely, and subtotal parathyroidectomy may be indicated. Dietary Ca can be markedly reduced while an active form of vitamin D (i.e., calcitriol or 1-alpha, $(OH)D_3$) is given; such a regimen may suppress secondary hyperparathyroidism and improve the skeletal disease without aggravating the hypercalcemia.

Dialysis fluid magnesium

The use of dialysate containing Mg, 0.5 mEq/l (0.25 mmol/l), results in predialysis serum Mg levels approaching normal; also, skeletal Mg may also fall in association with an improved chemical composition of bone (186). Medications containing Mg, such as laxatives and Mg-containing antacids, should be avoided, in renal patients not yet on maintenance hemodialysis.

Fluoride-containing water

The effect of using fluoride-containing tap water for preparation of dialysis fluid is controversial (252). Normally excreted by the kidney, fluoride accumulates in the body, particularly in the bone, as kidney function deteriorates. This accumulation is accelerated when fluoride containing water is used for preparing dialysis fluid (253). A correlation between bone fluoride content and the duration of dialysis and both histologic and radiologic evidence of osteodystrophy has been noted (254). Moreover, a high incidence of overt bone disease was reduced after water purification was initiated with removal of fluoride and other substances from the dialysate (255). Others have found that the use of fluoride-containing water does not worsen osteodystrophy provided plasma Ca and P levels are adequately controlled (256). Nonetheless, water treatment for dialysate is recommended when the tap water contains large quantities of fluoride.

Aluminum-containing water

The presence of Al in excess of 10 μg/l (370 μmol/l) in the water utilized for preparing dialysis fluid is associated with a high incidence of osteomalacic bone disease (76–82). With appropriate water-treatment and substantial reduction of its Al content, the incidence of osteomalacia has been markedly reduced (152). Aluminum is a frequent problem primarily in reservoir water of large metropolitan areas where Al silicate is used as flocculent to clear turbidity of the water. The water content of Al in a municipal water supply can vary substantially over a relatively short period of time, and marked increments in the Al concentrations can occur, following the failure of a deionization procedure, with disastrous effects. Regular monitoring of plasma Al levels in all patients in a dialysis center can provide a clue to such a failure of the water purification system. Thus, the findings of elevated plasma Al levels (50 μg/l [1.85 μmol/l]) in all dialysis patients using the water would suggest the failure of water purification, while elevated plasma Al levels in only a fraction of patients would suggest that exposure to excessive quantities of oral Al. When a patient develops fractures and bone histology reveals osteomalacia, the Al levels should be monitored closely in water and dialysate, and appropriate methods of water treatment should be initiated.

Heparin

Large doses of heparin can also impair bone mineralization (257, 258); with shorter duration of dialysis and reduced doses of heparin, the total quantity given to dialysis patients is generally lower than that associated with such demineralization.

Specific treatment

Vitamin D sterols

A considerable number of dialysis patients develop progressive and disabling bone disease despite adherence to phosphate restriction and oral Ca supplementation. Some exhibit symptoms of secondary hyperparathyroidism, while others have either osteomalacia or aplastic bone disease. When the former develops, treatment with various forms of vitamin D, i.e., dihydrotachysterol, 25-hydroxyvitamin D_3, 1-alpha-$(OH)D_3$, or $1,25(OH)_2D_3$ and pharmacologic doses of vitamin D_2 itself may produce clinical improvement, a return of X-rays toward normal, and amelioration of bone pathology (259–262). Also serum levels of alkaline phosphatase and PTH may fall (Figure 24). The decrease in serum

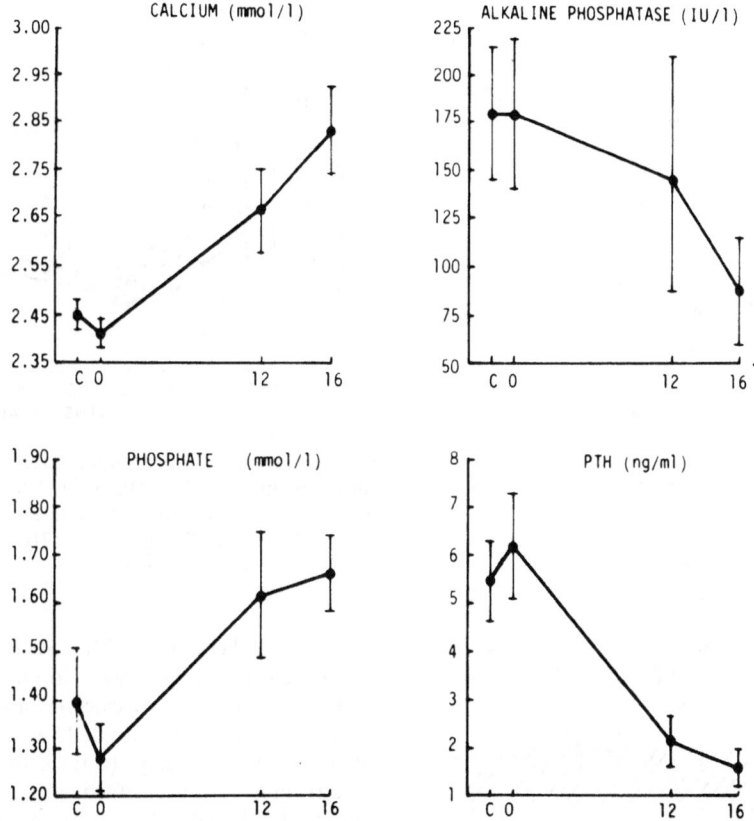

Figure 24. Mean values of plasma Ca, P, alkaline phosphatase, and serum immunoreactive PTH in 10 dialysis patients treated with 1-alpha-(OH)D₃ for 16 months. The initial dose was 1 μg/day, and the dose was adjusted in each patient during the trial. (Modified after Papapoulos et al [268])

(Conversion factors: Ca mmol/l → mg/dl: × 4
P (as phosphate): mmol/l → mg/dl: × 3.1)

iPTH levels to normal during treatment despite only a slight increase in serum Ca suggests that calcitriol directly facilitates the suppression of PTH secretion (Figure 25). Effective forms and doses of vitamin D sterols are summarized in Table 7.

During the first 1 to 2 months of treatment, serum P falls or remains unchanged (Figure 26) despite the increase in P absorption produced by the active forms of vitamin D (49), suggesting skeletal remineralization. Later, as the rate of mineralization slows, continued stimulation of intestinal absorption of Ca and P may produce hypercalcemia and hyperphosphatemia, which readily reverse after discontinuation of the drug or reduction of the dose (Figure 27). Skeletal biopsies usually show reduced fibrous tissues and improved mineralization (261, 263, 264), but bone histology rarely returns to normal.

Other patients treated with other vitamin D sterols, do not improve their skeletal lesions (265). The widened osteoid seams in patients with mixed lesions may improve only slowly during treatment. Although some patients substantially improve their symptoms, particularly those of myopathy, improvement of isolated osteomalacia due to Al

overload is unusual during therapy with 1,25(OH)₂D or 1α(OH)D₃ (84).

Renal osteodystrophy also improves on treatment with 25(OH)D₃ (259); the amount required to stimulate intestinal Ca absorption is three to four fold that needed in normal subjects (266), and a therapeutic benefit is observed only when plasma 25(OH)D₃ levels are two to three times normal (267). Such observations suggest that the effect of 25(OH)D₃ in uremia is pharmacologic rather than physiologic. A major unanswered question is whether 25(OH)D₃ may have effects that differ from those of calcitriol or 1-alpha-(OH)D₃.

Table 7. Forms and approximate doses of vitamin D sterols used for symptomatic renal osteodystrophy.

Vitamin D₂ (ergocalciferol)	0.25–5.0 mg*
Dihydrotachysterol	0.25–4.0 mg
Calcitriol [1,25-hydroxyvitamin D₃; 1,25(OH)₂D₃]	0.20–1.0 μg
1 alpha-hydroxyvitamin D₃ [1 alpha-(OH)D₃]	1.0–2.0 μg
Calcifediol [25-hydroxyvitamin D₃; 25(OH)D₃]	20–50 μg

* Equivalent to 10,000 to 200,000 IU/day (1 IU = 0.025 μg).

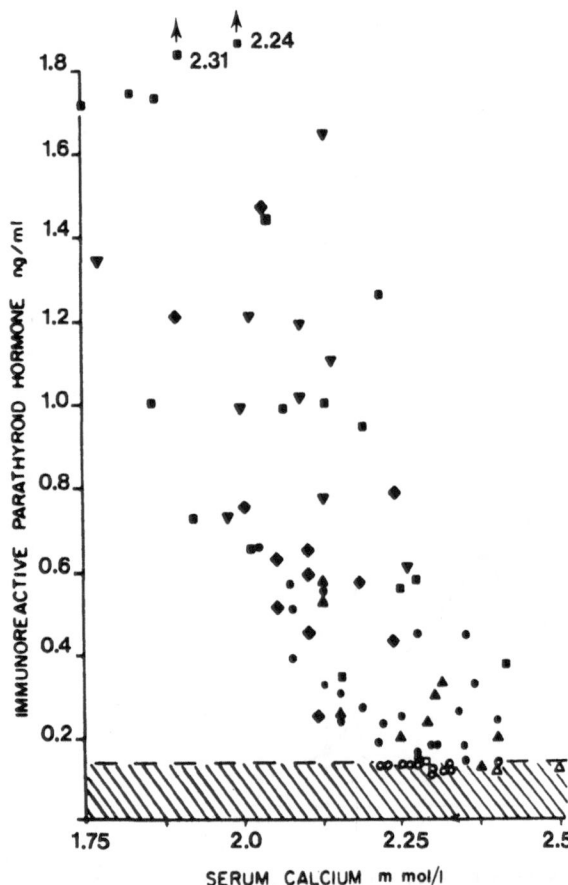

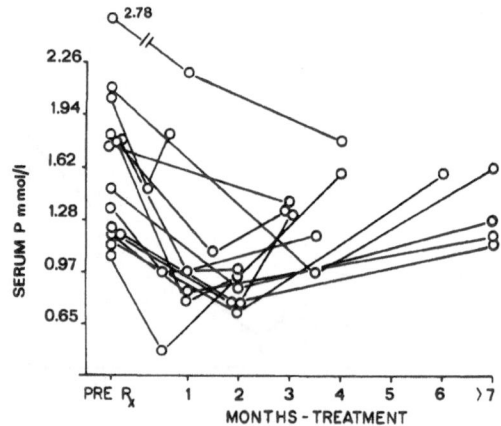

Figure 26. Representative values of serum phosphorus before and during treatment with 1,25(OH)₂D₃. The lowest values usually occurring at 1 to 2 months, and the final value during treatment are shown. (Data from Coburn et al [157]).
(Conversion: P (as phosphate) mmol/l → mg/dl: × 3.1)

or 1-alpha-(OH)D₃ (268, 271). Such patients have marked parathyroid hyperplasia with an increase in the 'set point' for PTH suppression by calcium, and subtotal parathyroidectomy is usually required. In these patients, the use of calcitriol, intravenously, (a form of the drug recently released), may be more effective than the oral form in suppressing PTH (63). Thus, in the future, intravenously ad-

Figure 25. Levels of immunoreactive parathyroid hormone in 4 uremic patients with secondary hyperparathyroidism treated with 1,25(OH)₂D₃. Plasma samples were obtained at intervals of 4 to 7 days. As serum Ca rose, serum iPTH became undetectable even when serum calcium levels were increased from 2 to only 2.5 mmol/l (Modified after Brickman et al [293]).
(Conversion: Ca mmol/l → mg/dl: × 4)

Treatment with 1-alpha-(OH)D₃ produces effects similar to those observed with 1,25(OH)₂D₃ (268, 269). However, the dose required is two to three times larger. Also, there is a slightly slower onset of action and longer duration of effect following the cessation of treatment. Treatment with certain drugs, such as phenytoin or barbiturates, which induce hepatic microsomal enzymes, can reduce the effectiveness of 1α-(OH)D₃ (270). In such patients, treatment with 1,25(OH)₂D₃ may be preferred.

Treatment failure groups

There are patients who show little or no improvement of their skeletal disease when treated with an active form of vitamin D (268). One group of patients exhibits markedly elevated iPTH levels and osteitis fibrosa on bone biopsy. Plasma Ca is either elevated or in the upper normal range before vitamin D treatment, and hypercalcemia can develop within a few weeks of starting treatment with 1,25(OH)₂D₃

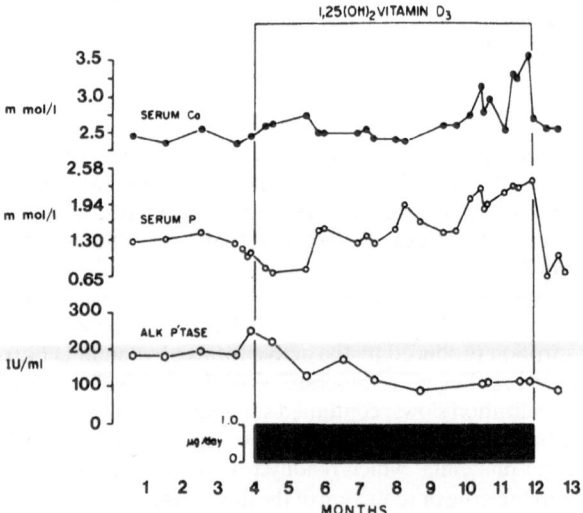

Figure 27. Treatment of renal osteodystrophy with 1,25(OH)₂D₃. Initially a decrease of serum P occurs suggesting remineralization of the skeleton. Later when mineralization slows and stimulation of calcium and phosphate absorption continues, hypercalcemia and hyperphosphatemia may develop. Both however, are rapidly reversed when the drug is discontinued or the dose is reduced. (Adapted from Coburn et al [157])
(Conversion: Ca mmol/l → mg/dl: × 4
P [as Phosphate] mmol/l → mg/dl: × 3.1)

ministered calcitriol may be an effective therapy to achieve 'medical parathyroidectomy'. It is essential that Al toxicity be excluded before parathyroid surgery.

A second group who fail to improve following treatment with $1,25(OH)_2D_3$ or $1\alpha-(OH)_2D_3$ exhibits osteomalacia or aplastic bone; treatment with vitamin D_3 in doses as low as 10,000 IU/day, or calcitriol, 0.1 to 0.25 g/day, can promptly cause hypercalcemia. Bone biopsies disclose aluminum staining along the mineralization front and other evidence of aluminum toxicity may be observed. It is probable that a small number of patients who fail to respond to calcitriol or other vitamin D sterols but who lack evidence of Al accumulation will be found. Other potential causes of such bone diseases include iron, silicon or oxalate toxicity.

Parathyroidectomy

Many manifestations of secondary hyperparathyroidism regress following subtotal parathyroidectomy (164, 272, 273). However, the substantial improvement of patients with overt secondary hyperparathyroidism treated with vitamin D sterols has decreased the need for parathyroid surgery. Nevertheless, indications for parathyroidectomy still exist. Hypercalcemia, if associated with mental symptoms or severe hypertension, for example, can be most quickly reversed following surgical management. However, hypercalcemia alone may not indicate parathyroid hyperplasia; this may occur with Al induced osteomalacia and normal or high PTH levels and during treatment with vitamin D sterols, oral Ca supplements and the use of a high Ca in dialysate. Therefore, evidence for secondary hyperparathyroidism, i.e., bone erosions, markedly elevated levels of serum iPTH, and especially bone biopsy showing osteitis fibrosa should be present before surgery is undertaken. In certain patients, severe osteomalacia may develop following parathyroidectomy (105); thus, the total removal of the parathyroid glands contributes to osteomalacia.

The appearance of ischemic skin ulcerations associated with marked vascular calcifications, i.e. calciphylaxis, is another indication for parathyroidectomy (164). On rare occassions, pruritus may be so severe that surgery should be considered (158), although it is unlikely to produce benefits in the absence of other manifestations of secondary hyperparathyroidism.

Occasionally, progressive extraskeletal calcifications and marked hyperphosphatemia, refractory to therapy, exist and they are indications for parathyroidectomy. Following such surgery, the plasma phosphorus falls and is easier to control. Moreover, radiographs often show substantial improvement of the skeletal lesions after subtotal parathyroidectomy (24).

Two accepted surgical procedures for management of overt secondary hyperparathyroidism are subtotal parathyroidectomy and total parathyroidectomy with parathyroid autotransplantation. Each procedure has its advocates (274); clearly the most important factor is a highly skilled surgeon experienced in parathyroid surgery. Substantial numbers of patients may have recurrence of hyperparathyroidism after subtotal parathyroidectomy; a major advantage of total parathyroidectomy with forearm autotransplantation is avoidance of the high morbidity associated with reexploration of the neck. With either procedure, cryopreservation of parathyroid tissue is of value in case of devascularization of the residual tissue in the neck after subtotal parathyroidectomy or failure of function of implanted tissue in the forearm (275).

During surgery, it is imperative that all the parathyroid glands be identified. The number of glands normally varies from two to six; failure to recognize sites of normal fifth and sixth glands is a common cause of failure of parathyroid surgery (276). When subtotal parathyroidectomy is being performed, it is important that the most suitable gland be identified. Usually the gland that appears least hyperplastic but has an adequate blood supply is the best to resect only partially; 40 to 60 mg of tissue should be left. After visually ascertaining that a satisfactory blood supply is preserved in the parathyroid fraction to remain in place, the surgeon can totally excise the other glands. The residual parathyroid tissue sometimes undergoes hyperplasia, necessitating a second surgical procedure; therefore, it is recommended that the remaining gland be marked by a metal clip and/or a long, black silk suture (277). When only two or three parathyroid glands in the neck or the upper anterior thorax are accessible at the time of neck exploration, the removal of all three glands is recommended under the assumption that the fourth gland is located elsewhere. Tissues should be maintained by cryopreservation should permanent hypoparathyroidism develop (275). This indicates that only two or three glands exist, more commonly the overt hyperparathyroidism is only partially corrected. Good judgment and, even more important, extensive experience of the parathyroid surgeon are clearly important for the identification and management of atypical cases.

For parathyroid transplantation, parathyroid tissue, which has been identified by frozen section, is placed in chilled culture medium, then slices are implanted in multiple pockets in muscle on the lateral aspect of the flexor surface of the forearm of the non-dominant arm (275). Nonabsorbable suture is used to secure the slices in the muscle pockets and to provide a marker for subsequent identification should surgical resection be required. Technical problems during the surgical procedure should be few with blood loss minimal. The patients usually can leave the hospital within a week. A dialysis patient should be dialyzed on the day prior to surgery.

Postoperatively, hypocalcemic tetany and convulsions may occur and lead to serious fractures. The most severe hypocalcemic episode developing during the postoperative period seems to correlate with the extent of osteoclastic activity and alkaline phosphatase level present in the preoperative bone biopsy (278). Such episodes occur with marked reduction of excess bone resorption and improved mineralization of the abnormal bone, i.e., the 'hungry bone' syndrome. Of interest, hypocalcemic seizures may not appear in such patients when serum Ca is the lowest but are observed during the latter hours of hemodialysis or after dialysis.

Total parathyroidectomy is rarely indicated.

To minimize the postoperative hypocalcemia, intravenous infusion of Ca gluconate in doses providing 3.5 mg (88 μmol) Ca/Kg body weight/h, and 0.5 to 1.0 μg/day of calcitriol may be given for 1 to 2 days before surgery and immediately afterwards; also, oral Ca carbonate is given to provide 1,000 to 2,000 mg (25 to 50 mmol) of elemental calcium. Serum P levels usually diminish after surgery as well, although hyperphosphatemia may return and contribute to the decrease in serum Ca concentration.

Tetany may occur postoperatively in these patients; hemodialysis, perhaps by its alkalinizing effect, may predispose to this problem. The quantity of oral Ca needed is often quite large; the Ca dosage can be increased 0.5 to 1.0 g(12.5 to 25 mmol)/day at intervals of 3 to 7 days until the serum Ca concentration begins to increase. If the serum concentration of Ca falls below 7.5 mg/dl (1.88 mmol/l) or if tetany appears, intravenous Ca should be given as well. With such therapy, careful monitoring of serum Ca concentration is mandatory, and administration of phosphate-binding compounds should be adjusted to maintain serum P concentration between 3.5 and 5.0 mg/dl (1.1 and 1.6 mmol/l). Tetany occurring in a uremic patient with severe bone disease is a serious complication. Simultaneous fractures of scapula, clavicle, and/or both femoral necks were reported after an episode of tetany occurred during dialysis (279). Major fractures have been observed (i.e., a spiral fracture of the femur or femoral neck fracture) in three patients after parathyroid surgery; these occurred 1 to 3 weeks after surgery. Interestingly, each occurred late during the hemodialysis procedure itself. In the postoperative management of patients with marked periarticular calcifications, it is advisable to maintain serum Ca levels in the range of 8.0 to 9.0 mg/dl (2.0 to 2.25 mmol/l), until the ectopic calcifications resolve.

In patients with very marked skeletal disease, hypocalcemia may occasionally persist for 2 to 3 months after parathyroidectomy despite treatment with large amounts of oral Ca supplementation and vitamin D or a related sterol. Serum levels of P and Mg concentration may also decrease during this time. If the serum Mg concentration falls below 1.5 mg/dl (1.2 mEq/l), supplemental Mg can be given by mouth. Administration of P salts aggravates hypocalcemia, presenting a dilemma with regard to treatment. If the serum P concentration falls below 2.5 mg/dl (0.8 mmol/l) administration of the P binders should be reduced or stopped, but no effort should be made to increase the P concentration above 3.5 to 4.0 mg/dl (1.1 to 1.3 mmol/l).

Failure of serum Ca concentration to decrease significantly after surgery may indicate that either too much residual parathyroid tissue was left or that the major skeletal pathology in the patient is not severe osteitis fibrosa. Another postoperative complication of total or subtotal parathyroidectomy is the development of aluminum-related osteomalacia (105). The mechanism responsible for this is unclear; most likely, substantial accumulation of Al in bone developed prior to the parathyroidectomy and either high PTH levels or an increased rate of bone turnover had somehow protected the bone from the deleterious effect of Al. After parathyroid surgery, bone turnover decreases markedly and Ca becomes deposited on the mineralization front. The existence of symptomatic osteomalcia after parathyroidectomy indicates that surgery was unneccesary in the presence of hypercalcemia due to pre-existing aluminum-related bone disease.

Insight into the role of vitamin D and its active sterols in the regulation of PTH secretion, combined with better availability may make the management of secondary hyperparathyroidism easier in the end-stage renal disease patient, lessening the need for parathyroid surgery.

Treatment for aluminum-related bone disease

In the presence Al toxicity, the source of Al should be determined and therapy adjusted to prevent further Al loading; this can be done by discontinuing Al-containing gels and properly purifying water for dialysis fluid. Consideration should also be given to therapy with deferoxamine to enhance the removal of Al.

The potential sources of Al, including the water utilized for preparing dialysis fluid, the peritoneal dialysis solution, or other parenteral sources such as albumin, should be evaluated and eliminated. Effort should be made to either discontinue or reduce markedly the intake of the aluminum-containing gels, Al hydroxide and Al carbonate, and assess other sources of Al, such as sucralfate (280). Citric acid or sodium citrate, which can enhance Al absorption (126) should be avoided.

The chelating agent, deferoxamine, has an affinity for Al that is nearly as great as for iron. The aluminum-deferoxamine complex, with a molecular mass of 540 daltons, is slowly but effectively removed by hemodialysis. Deferoxamine has been given regularly to dialysis patients with Al toxicity, and there has been substantial improvement of neurologic and musculoskeletal symptoms of toxicity (210, 281, 282). Clinical improvement occurs within a few weeks and can be dramatic (Figure 28). When the drug is infused into a dialysis patient with Al accumulation, there is a progressive increment in plasma Al over 12 to 24 h to a peak where it remains until the next hemodialysis (Figure 17) (208). The increment in total plasma Al closely parallels the increment of ultrafilterable Al, indicating that the increment occurs as the ultrafilterable aluminum-deferoxamine complex (281). Since Ackrill et al (282) first reported that deferoxamine is useful in the treatment of Al intoxication in dialysis patients, it has been used effectively in several centers (210, 281). The serum biochemical alterations observed during therapy include reductions in serum Ca, transient increments in alkaline phosphatase, and increased serum levels of PTH. Predialysis plasma Al levels slowly decrease over a period of months of prolonged treatment. Bone biopsies have shown a substantial decrease of surface stainable Al, a substantially smaller decrease in total bone Al content, and a marked improvement in bone formation rate (210). Some patients may develop features of osteitis fibrosa. On the other hand, Felsenfeld et al (283) have recently evaluated 18 patients with Al induced osteomalacia before

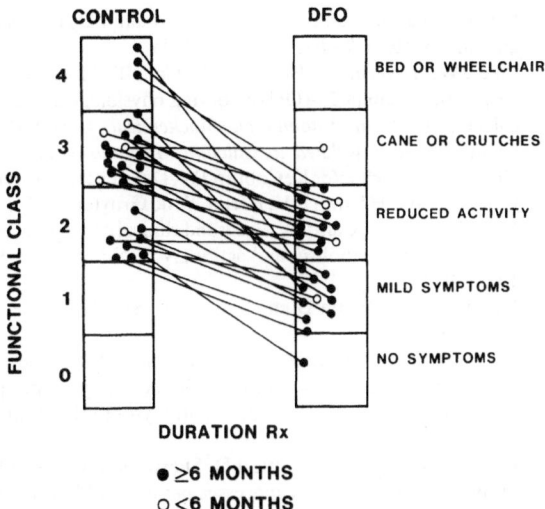

CONTROL   DFO

BED OR WHEELCHAIR

CANE OR CRUTCHES

REDUCED ACTIVITY

MILD SYMPTOMS

NO SYMPTOMS

FUNCTIONAL CLASS

DURATION Rx

● ≥6 MONTHS
○ <6 MONTHS

Figure 28. Changes in the degree of disability of patients with Al related bone disease after treatment with deferoxamine, 1 to 6 g/ week for 3 to 12 months. The degree of musculoskeletal disability was classified according to a modified New York Heart Association classification of heart disease. Reprinted from Nebeker and Coburn (196) with permission of publishers.

and after 1 year therapy with deferoxamine. Bone histology improved only mildly despite substantial clinical improvement and marked removal of stainable bone Al. It should be noted that in the majority of reports describing patients treated with deferoxamine, Al containing phosphate binders were not discontinued. Hence, it is likely that significant Al gut absorption may have contributed to the partial response to deferoxamine observed in some of these studies.

The side effects of deferoxamine therapy include a reduced blood pressure, which can be offset by reducing the infusion rate of deferoxamine, the appearance of allergic skin rashes, and reduced plasma ferritin levels due to the chelation and removal of iron as well as Al; the latter is associated with appearance of iron deficiency. Opthalmic toxicity, including retinal abnormalities and medial opacifications or early cataract formation have also been noted (284, 285). Such toxicity may be more common with deferoxamine in doses above 2.0 g per week. Also, there is evidence that deferoxamine can enhance the pathogenicity of certain bacteria and fungi, including *Yersinia* and the *Rhizopus,* which causes mucormycosis (286). Fatal infections have been noted in dialysis patients receiving the drugs, although the frequency in deferoxamine-treated dialysis patients is unknown.

In patients with documented Al toxicity, aluminum-containing gels should be discontinued, with the substitution of Ca carbonate or Mg carbonate. Treatment with the former is associated with a substantial risk of hypercalcemia in patients with Al toxicity. Thus, Ca carbonate may need to be

withheld until after deferoxamine treatment has been initiated. Another problem encountered has been the appearance of new neurologic symptoms or the worsening of preexisting neurological symptoms early in the course of therapy with deferoxamine. These symptoms may arise due to the relocation of Al within the central nervous system, although their cause is unknown. When this problem arises, it seems most prudent to discontinue deferoxamine therapy; when the symptoms subside, it should be administered more frequently at a lower dose, i.e., 0.5 to 1.0 g during each dialysis.

Aluminum toxicity has responded favorably to renal transplantation, probably because of the slow but continued excretion of Al via the functioning renal allograft. It may be useful to administer deferoxamine to a patient with worsened neurological symptoms after renal transplant. Further studies may clarify the optimal dosage of deferoxamine and the duration of therapy.

Other treatment considerations

Other management considerations, some of which have been referred to earlier, depend on the special circumstances encountered. Loss of skeletal carbonate (or bicarbonate) may be another factor with a deleterious effect on the skeleton; in totally refractory bone disease, a therapeutic trial with bicarbonate-containing dialysate may be reasonable, although there is no evidence to suggest that it is of value. Treatment with a beta-adrenergic blocking drug, such as propranolol, or with cimetidine, has not been proven effective.

It is possible that calcitonin may be useful in certain cases where secondary hyperparathyroidism is inoperable or when it cannot be managed with a vitamin D sterol because of hypercalcemia (287). Calcitonin can act to suppress certain effects of excess PTH, but one report of its short-term administration in uremic patients indicated it had very little overall effect (288).

Finding an appropriate means for managing extraskeletal calcifications which do not respond to control of serum P or parathyroidectomy has been a serious dilemma. Zucchelli et al (289) reported experience with treating nine dialysis patients with the diphosphonate compound sodium EHDP (ethane-1-hydroxyl-1,1-diphosphonate); 7.5 to 10 mg/kg was given for 5 to 9 months to patients who had a well-controlled serum P concentration but persistent ectopic calcification. No change was seen in five patients, but two showed regression of the ectopic calcification and another showed reduced arterial calcification. Bone biopsies after EHDP treatment revealed a significant increase in osteoid volume and osteoid surface without modifying the calcification front. Slight increases in serum alkaline P levels were found in most patients. The EHDP was well-tolerated; however, the patient is at risk of developing osteomalacia with such treatment (290). Its use should therefore be limited to patients with severe extraskeletal calcifications in whom all other therapeutic modalities have failed.

Management of fractures

Rib fractures (probably the most frequent fractures seen in the uremic patient) usually heal slowly over a period of several months. They are usually asymptomatic and require little specific treatment. Traumatic fractures of the long bones and of the femoral neck may have a poor union even after several months. When fractures occur in patients with marked secondary hyperparathyroidism, appropriate surgical repair should be considered, since prolonged immobilization can create even greater complications in such patients. In some patients with fractures due to aluminum-related osteomalacia, slow healing may occur even though Al accumulation has not been specifically treated. In others, non-union of the fracture occurs, but the fracture then heals after initiation of chelation therapy with deferoxamine to remove excess Al.

The successful use of femoral head prosthesis has been reported in patients with end-stage uremia and those on dialysis (291). When secondary hyperparathyroidism exists in a patient with a fracture, it seems preferable to treat the patient with an active form of vitamin D, rather than with parathyroidectomy to decrease the risk of tetany, seizures, and further fractures (279).

ACKNOWLEDGEMENTS

Some of the work described in the present chapter was supported by the Veterans Administration Research Funds from Wadsworth and Oklahoma City Veterans Administration Hospitals.

Figures 10A-10D are reproduced from color photomicrographs kindly provided by A.J. Felsenfeld M.D.

Figure 20 was kindly supplied by H.E. Meema, Toronto Western Hospital.

REFERENCES

1. Holick MF, McNeill SC, MacLaughlin JA, Holick SA, Clark MB, Potts, JT Jr: The physiologic implications of the formation of previtamin D$_3$ in skin. *Trans Assoc Am Physicians* 92: 54, 1979
2. Haddad JG, Walgate J: Radioimmunoassay of the binding protein for vitamin D and its metabolites in human serum. *J Clin Invest* 58: 1217, 1976
3. Ponchon G, DeLuca HF: The role of the liver in the metabolism of vitamin D. *J Clin Invest* 48: 1273, 1969
4. Smith JE, Goodman DS: The turnover and transport of vitamin D and of a polar metabolite with the properties of 25-hydroxycholecalciferol in human plasma. *J Clin Invest* 50: 2159, 1971
5. Gray RW, Omdahl JL, Ghazarian JG, DeLuca HF: 25-hydroxycholecalciferol-1-hydroxylase. *J Biol Chem* 247: 7528, 1972
6. Midgett RJ, Spielvogel AM, Coburn JW, Normal AW: Studies of calciferol metabolism. VII. The renal production of the biologically active form of vitamin D, 1,25-dihydroxycholecalciferol; species, tissue and subcellular distribution. *J Clin Endocrinol* 36: 1153, 1973
7. Hughes MR, Haussler MR, Wergedal J, Baylink DJ: Regulation of plasma 1 alpha,25-dihydroxyvitamin D$_3$ by calcium and phosphate. *Clin Res* 23: 323A, 1975
8. Pike JW, Toverud S, Baass A, McCain T, Haussler MR: Circulating 1 alpha,25-(OH)$_2$D during physiological states of calcium stress. in: *Vitamin D: Biochemical, Chemical and Clinical Aspects Related to Calcium Metabolism*, edited by Norman AW, Schaefer K, Coburn JW, DeLuca HF, Fraser D, Grigoleit HG, Herrath DV, Berlin, W de Gruyter, 1977, p 187
9. Haussler MR, McCain TA: Basic and clinical concepts related to vitamin D metabolism and action. *N Engl J Med* 297: 974, 1041, 1977
10. DeLuca HF: Vitamin D endocrinology. *Ann Intern Med* 85: 367, 1976
11. Silver J, Russell J, Letteri D, Sherwood LM: Vitamin D metabolites suppress cytoplasmic mRNA coding for pre-proparathyroid hormone in isolated parathyroid cells. *Clin Res* 32: 561A, 1984
12. Cantley LK, Russell J, Lettieri D, Sherwood LM: 1,25(OH)$_2$D-dihydroxyvitamin D$_3$ suppresses parathyroid hormone secretion from bovine parathyroid cells in tissue culture. *Endocrinology* 117: 2114, 1985
13. Levine BS, Coburn JW: Physiology of the vitamin D endocrine system and disorders of altered vitamin D metabolism, in: *Hormonal Function and the Kidney*, edited by Brenner BM, Stein JH, New York, Edinburgh and London, Churchill Livingstone, 1979, p 215
14. Horst L, Littledike ET, Gray RW, Napoli JL: Impaired 24,25-dihydroxyvitamin D production in anephric man and pig. *J Clin Invest* 67: 274, 1981
15. Llach F, Brickman AS, Singer FR, Coburn JW: 24,25-dihydroxycholecalciferol, a vitamin D sterol with qualitatively unique effects in uremic man. *Metab Bone Dis and Related Res* 2: 11, 1979
16. Hodsman AB, Wong EGC, Sherrard DJ, Brickman AS, Lee DBN, Singer FR, Norman AW, Coburn JW: Use of 24,25-dihydroxyvitamin D$_3$ in dialysis osteomalacia; preliminary results. in: *Hormonal Control of Calcium Metabolism* edited by Cohn DV, Talmage RV, Mathews JL, Amsterdam, Excerpta Medica, 1981, p 460
17. Henry HL, Taylor AN, Norman AW: Response of chick parathyroid glands to the vitamin D metabolites, 1,25-dihydroxycholecalciferol and 24,25-dihydroxicholecalciferol. *J Nutr* 107: 1918, 1977
18. Tanaka Y, DeLuca HE: Biological activity of 24,25-difluro-25-hydrovitamin D$_3$. *J Biol Chem* 254: 7163, 1979
19. Mayer GP, Hurst JG: Sigmoidal relationship between parathyroid hormone secretion rate and plasma calcium concentration in calves. *Endocrinology* 102: 1036, 1978
20. Mayer GP, Habener JF, Potts JF: Parathyroid hormone secretion in vivo demonstration of a calcium-independent nonsuppressible component of secretion. *J Clin Invest* 57: 678, 1976
21. Mayer GP, Hurst JG, Barto JA, Keaton JA, Moore MP: Effect of epinephrine on parathyroid hormone secretion in calves. *Endocrinology* 104: 1181, 1979
22. Habener JF, Potts JT Jr: Relative effectiveness of magnesium and calcium on the secretion and biosynthesis of parathyroid hormone in vitro. *Endocrinology* 98: 197, 1976
23. Habener JF, Mayer GP, Dee PC, Potts JT Jr: Metabolism of amino- and carboxyl-sequence immunoactive parathyroid hormone in the bovine: Evidence for peripheral cleavage of hormone. *Metabolism* 25: 385, 1976
24. Segre GV, Habener JF, Powell JF, Tregaer JW, Potts JT Jr: Parathyroid hormone in human plasma. Immuno clinical characterization and biological indication. *J Clin Invest* 51: 3163, 1972

25. Segre GV, Mall HD, Habener JF, Potts JT Jr: Metabolism of parathyroid hormone. Pathologic and clinical significance. *Am J Med* 56: 774, 1974

26. Hruska KA, Kopelman R, Rutherford WE, Klahr S, Slatapolsky E: Metabolism of immuno-reactive parathyroid hormone in the dog: The role of kidney and the effect of chronic renal disease. *J Clin Invest* 56: 56, 1975

27. Martin KJ, Hruska K, Freitag JJ, Klahr S, Slatapolsky E: The peripheral metabolism of parathyroid hormone. *N Engl J Med* 301: 1092, 1979

28. Coburn JW and Slatopolsky E: Vitamin D, PTH and renal osteodystrophy. in: *The Kidney,* 2nd Edition, edited by Brenner BM, Rector FG, Philadelphia, WB Saunders Co, 1981, p 2213

29. Parfitt AM: The actions of parathyroid hormone on bone. Relation to bone remodeling and turnover, calcium homeostasis and metabolic bone disease. IV. The state of bones in uremic hyperparathyroidism. The mechanisms of skeletal resistance to PTH in renal failure and pseudo-hypoparathyroidism and the role of PTH in osteoporosis, osteopetrosis and osteofluorosis. *Metabolism* 25: 1157, 1976

30. Slatopolsky E, Hruska K, Martin K, Freitag J: Physiologic and metabolic effects of parathyroid hormone, in: *Hormonal Function and the Kidney,* edited by Brenner BM, Stein JH, New York, Edinburgh, London, Churchill Livingstone, 1979, p 169

31. Ritz E, Malluche HH, Krempien B, Mehls O: Calcium metabolism in renal failure. in: *Disorders of Mineral Metabolism.* Vol III, edited by Bronner F, Coburn JW, New York, Academic Press, 1981, p 152

32. Coburn JR, Popovtzer MM, Massry SG, Kleeman CR: The physiochemical state and renal handling of divalent ions in chronic renal failure. *Arch Intern Med* 124: 302, 1969

33. Slatopolsky E, Caglar S, Pennell DB, Taggart JM, Canterbury J, Reiss E, Bricker NS: On the pathogenesis of hyperparathyroidism in chronic experimental renal insufficiency in the dog. *J Clin Invest* 50: 492, 1971

34. Slatopolsky E, Cagler S, Gradowska L, Canterbury J, Reiss E, Bricker NS: On the prevention of secondary hyperparathyroidism in experimental chronic renal insufficiency using 'proportional reduction' of dietary phosphorus intake. *Kidney Int* 2: 147, 1972

35. Reiss E, Cantebury JM, Bercovitz MA, Kaplin EL: The role of phosphate in the secretion of parathyroid hormone in man. *J Clin Invest* 49: 2146, 1970

36. Fournier AE, Arnaud CD, Johnson WJ, Taylor WF, Goldsmith RS: Etiology of hyperparathyroidism and bone disease during chronic hemodialysis. II. Factors affecting serum immunoreactive parathyroid hormone. *J Clin Invest* 50: 599, 1971

37. Coburn JW, Kopple MH, Brickman AS, Massry SG: Study of intestinal absorption of calcium in patients with renal failure. *Kidney Int* 3: 264, 1973

38. Llach F, Massry SG, Singer FR, Kurokawa K, Kaye JH, Coburn JW: Skeletal resistance of endogenous parathyroid hormone in patients with early renal failure: A possible cause for secondary hyperparathyroidism. *J Clin Endocrinol Metab* 41: 338, 1975

39. Haussler MR, Baylink DJ, Hughes MR, Brumbaugh PF, Wergedal JE, Shen FH, Nielsen RL, Counts SJ, Bursac KM, McCain TA: The assay of 1-alpha-25-dihydroxyvitamin D_3; physiologic and pathologic modulation of circulating hormone levels. *Clin Endocrinol* 5: 151, 1976

40. Mawer EB, Backhouse J, Taylor CM: Failure of formation of 1,25-dihydroxycholecalciferol in chronic renal insufficiency. *Lancet* 1: 626, 1973

41. Brickman AS, Coburn JW, Norman AW: Effect of 1,25-dihydroxycholecalciferol, the active metabolite of vitamin D in uremic man. *N Engl J Med* 287: 891, 1972

42. Oettinger CW, Merrill R, Blanton T, Briggs W: Reduced calcium absorption after nephrectomy in uremic patients. *N Engl J Med* 291: 458, 1975

43. Slatopolsky E, Gray R, Adams ND, Lewis J, Hruska K, Martin K, Klahr S, DeLuca H, Lemann J: Low serum levels of 1,25 dihydroxycholecalciferol are not responsible for the development of secondary hyperparathyroidism in early renal failure. *Kidney Int* 14: 733, 1978

44. Portale AA, Booth EB, Tsai HC, Morris RC: Reduced plasma concentration of 1,25 dihydroxyvitamin D in children with moderate renal insufficiency. *Kidney Int* 21: 627, 1982

45. Chesney RW, Hamstra AJ, Mazess RB, Rose P, DeLuca HF: Circulating vitamin D metabolite concentration in childhood renal disease. *Kidney Int* 21: 65, 1982

46. Juttmann JR, Buurman JC, Dekam E, Visser TJ, Birkenhager JC: Serum concentrations of metabolites of vitamin D in patients with chronic renal failure (CRF). Consequences for the treatment with 1α hydroxy-derivatives. *Clin Endocrinol* 14: 225, 1981

47. Wilson L, Felsenfeld A, Drezner MK, Llach F: Altered divalent ion metabolism in early renal failure: Role of 1,25(OH)$_2$D. *Kidney Int* 27: 565, 1985

48. Kawaguchi Y, Kumura Y, Yakamota M, Inamura N, Tukwi I, Horiwichi N, Swada T, Ogura Y, Oda Y, Miyahara T: Graded mass reduction and synthesis of 1,25 dihydroxyvitamin D_3 in the rat. *Metab Bone Dis Relat Res* 4: 333, 1983

49. Brickman AS, Coburn JW, Massry SG, Norman AW: 1,25-dihydroxyvitamin D_3 in normal man and patients with renal failure. *Ann Intern Med* 80: 161, 1974

50. Brickman AS, Hartenbower DL, Norman AW, Coburn JW: Actions of 1-alpha-hydroxyvitamin D_3 and 1,25-dihydroxyvitamin D_3 on mineral metabolism in man. I. Effects on net absorption of phosphorus. *Am J Clin Nutr* 30: 1064, 1977

51. Mechanic GL, Toverd SU, Ramp WK, Gonnerman WA: The effect of vitamin D on the structural cross links and maturation of chick bone collagen. *Biochem Biophys Acta* 393: 419, 1975

52. Avioli LV: Collagen metabolism, uremia and bone. *Kidney Int* 4: 105, 1973

53. Heidbreder E, Luke F, Heidland A: Kollagenstoffwechsel und Mineralisation des urämischen Knochens – molekularpathologische Aspekte der renal Osteodystrophie. (Collagen metabolism and mineralization of uremic bone-aspects of the molecular pathology of renal osteodystrophy.) *Klin Wochenschr* 54: 341, 1976

54. Massry SG, Stein R, Garty J, Arieff AI, Coburn JW, Norman AW, Friedler RM: A skeletal resistance to the calcemic action of PTH in uremia: role of 1,25(OH)$_2$D$_3$. *Kidney Int* 9: 467, 1976

55. Massry SG, Coburn JW, Lee DBN, Jowsey J, Kleeman CR: Skeletal resistance to parathyroid hormone in renal failure. *Ann Intern Med* 73: 357, 1973

56. Llach F, Massry SG, Singer FR, Kurokawa K, Kaye JH, Coburn JW: Skeletal resistance to endogenous parathyroid hormone in patients with early renal failure: A possible cause for secondary hyperparathyroidism. *J Clin Endocrinol Metab* 41: 338, 1975

57. Willis MR, Jenkins MV: The effect of uraemic metabolites on parathyroid extract induced bone resorption in vitro. *Clin Chim Acta* 73: 121, 1976

58. Somerville PJ, Kaye M: Evidence that resistance to the calcemic action of parathyroid hormone in rats with acute uremia is caused by phosphate retention. *Kidney Int* 16: 552, 1979

59. Brown EM, Wilson RE, Eastman RC, Pallotta J, Marynick SP: Abnormal regulation of parathyroid hormone release by calcium in secondary hyperparathyroidism due to chronic renal failure. *J Clin Endocrinol Metab* 54: 172, 1982

60. Brown E: Set point for calcium: Its role in normal and abnormal secretion. in: *Hormonal Control of Calcium Metabolism*, edited by Cohn DV, Talmage RV, Matthews JL, Amsterdam, Excerpta Medica, 1981, p 35

61. Voigts A, Felsenfeld AJ, Andress J, Llach F: Parathyroid hormone and bone histology: Response to hypocalcemia in osteitis fibrosa. *Kidney Int* 25: 445, 1984

62. Lopez S, Galleran T, Chan W, Rapp N, Martin K, Slatopolsky E: Hypocalcemia may not be the cause of the development of secondary hyperparathyroidism. *Kidney Int* 27: 122, 1985

63. Slatopolsky E, Weerts C, Thielan J, Horst R, Harter H, Martin KJ: Marked suppression of secondary hyperparathyroidism by intravenous administration of 1,25 dihydroxycholecalciferol in uremic patients. *J Clin Invest* 74: 2136, 1984

64. Brumbaugh PF, Hughes MR, Haussler MR: Cytoplasmic and nuclear binding components for 1 alpha, 25 dihydroxyvitamin D_3 in chick parathyroid glands. *Proc Natl Acad Sci USA* 72: 4871, 1975

65. Oldham SB, Fischer JA, Shen LH, Arnaud CD: Isolation and properties of a calcium-binding protein from porcine parathyroid glands. *Biochemistry* 13: 4790, 1974

66. Tanaka Y, DeLuca HF: The control of 25-hydroxyvitamin D metabolism by inorganic phosphorus. *Arch Biochem Biophys* 159: 566, 1973

67. Llach F, Massry SG: On the mechanism of hyperparathyroidism in moderate renal insufficiency. *J Clin Endocrinol Metab* 61: 601, 1985

68. Brumbaugh PF, Haussler DH, Bressler R, Haussler MR: Radioreceptor assay for 1,25-dihydroxyvitamin D_3. *Science* 183: 1089, 1974

69. Eisman JS, Hamstra AJ, Kream BE, DeLuca HF: 1,25-dihydroxyvitamin D in biological fluids; a simplified and sensitive assay. *Science* 193: 1021, 1976

70. Bordier PJ, Tun-Chot S, Eastwood JB, Fornier A, De Warderner HE: Lack of histological evidence of vitamin D abnormality in the bones of anephric patients. *Clin Sci* 44: 33, 1973

71. Bordier P, Rasmussen H, Marie P, Miravet L, Gueris J, Eyckwaert A: Vitamin D metabolites and bone mineralization in man. *J Clin Endocrinol Metab* 46: 284, 1978

72. Malluche HH, Henry H, Meyer-Sabellek W, Sherman D, Massry SG, Norman AW: Effects and interactions of 24,25-dihydroxycholecalciferol and 1,25-dihydroxycholecalciferol on bone. *Am J Physiol* 238: E294, 1980

73. Eastwood JB, Stamp TC, DeWarderner HE, Bordier PJ, Arnaud CD: The effect of 25-hydroxyvitamin D_3 in osteomalacia of chronic renal failure. *Clin Sci Mol Med* 52: 499, 1977

74. Offerman G, von Herrath D, Schaefer K: Serum 25-hydroxycholecalciferol in uremia. *Nephron* 13: 269, 1974

75. Alfrey AC, Hegg A, Crasswell P: Metabolism and toxicity of aluminum in renal failure. *Am J Clin Nutr* 33: 1509, 1980

76. Wills MR, Savory J: Aluminium poisoning: Dialysis encephalopathy, osteomalacia, and anaemia. *Lancet* 2: 29, 1983

77. Ward MK, Feest TG, Willis HA, Parkinson IS, Kerr DNS: Osteomalacic dialysis osteodystrophy: Evidence for a waterborne aetiological agent, probably in aluminium. *Lancet* 1: 841, 1978

78. Siddiqui JY, Simpson SW, Ellis HE, Kerr DNS, Appleton DR, Robinson BH, Hawkins JB, Robertson PW, Taves DR: Fluoride and bone disease in patients on regular haemodialysis. *Proc Eur Dial Transplant Assoc* 8: 149, 1971

79. Pierides AM, Ward MK and Alvarez-Ude F: Long term therapy with 1,25(OH)$_2$D in dialysis bone disease. *Proc Eur Dial Transplant Assoc* 12: 237, 1975

80. Alfrey AC, LeGendre GR, Kaehny WD: Dialysis encephalopathy syndrome: Possible aluminum intoxication. *N Engl J Med* 294: 184, 1976

81. Alfrey AC, Miller NL, Butkus D: Evaluation of body magnesium stores. *J Lab Clin Med* 84: 153, 1974

82. Parkinson IS, Feest TG, Ward MK, Fawcett RWP, Kerr DNS: Fracturing dialysis osteodystrophy and dialysis encephalopathy: An epidemiological survey. *Lancet* 1: 406, 1979

83. Hirooka M, Wako H, Kaneko C, Ishikawa M, Sasaki S: Curative effects of 1-alpha-hydroxycholecalciferol on calcium metabolism and bone disease in patients with chronic renal failure. *J Nutr Sci Vitaminol* 21: 277, 1975

84. Hodsman AB, Sherrard DJ, Wong EGC: Vitamin D-resistant osteomalacia in hemodialysis patients lacking secondary hyperparathyroidism. *Ann Intern Med* 94: 629, 1981

85. Ellis HA: Aluminum and osteomalacia after parathyroidectomy. *Ann Intern Med* 96: 533, 1982

86. Cournot-Witmer J, Plachot JJ, Bourdeau A, Lieberherr M, Jorgetti V, Mendes V, Halpern S, Hemmerle J, Drüeke T, Balsan S: Effect of aluminum on bone and cell localization. *Kidney Int* 29 (Suppl 18): S37, 1986

87. Hodsman AB, Sherrard D, Alfrey A: Bone aluminum and histomorphometric features of renal osteodystrophy. *J Clin Endocrinol Metab* 54: 539, 1982

88. Maloney NA, Ott SM, Alfrey AC, Miller NL, Coburn JW, Sherrard DJ: Histologic quantitation of aluminum in iliac bone from patients with renal failure. *J Lab Clin Med* 99: 206, 1981

89. Ott SM, Maloney NA, Coburn JW, Alfrey AC, Sherrard DJ: The prevalence of bone aluminum deposition in renal osteodystrophy and its relation to the response to calcitriol therapy. *N Engl J Med* 307: 709, 1982

90. Cournot-Witmer G, Zingraff J, Plachot JJ: Aluminum localization in bone from hemodialyzed patients: Relationship to matrix mineralization. *Kidney Int* 20: 375, 1981

91. Sherrard DJ, Ott S, Maloney N, Andress D, Coburn J: Uremic osteodystrophy: Classification, cause and treatment. in: *Proceedings of the Symposium on Clinical Disorders of Bone and Mineral Metabolism.* edited by Frame B, Potts JT Jr, Amsterdam, Excerpta Medica, 1984, p 254

92. Lorenzo V, Rodriguez M, Felsenfeld AJ, Llach F: The effect of parathyroidectomy on aluminum toxicity in the rat (In Press)

93. Pierce-Myli M, Pierides A: Iron and aluminum osteomalacia during hemodialysis. *Kidney Int* 25: 151, 1984

94. Brown DJ, Ham K, Dawborn JK, Xipell JM: D-resistant osteomalacia in dialysis patients: Bone collagen and mineral content and treatment with desferrioxamine and calcitriol. in: *Vitamin D: Chemical, Biochemical and Clinical Endocrinology of Calcium Metabolism.* edited by Norman AW, Schaefer K, Herrath DV, Grigoleit HG, Berlin, Walter de Gruyter, 1982, p 873

95. Brown DJ, Dawborn JK, Ham KN: Treatment of dialysis osteomalacia with desferrioxamine. *Lancet* 1: 343, 1982

96. Boyce BF, Fell GS, Elder HY, Junor BJ, Elliot NL, Beastall G, Fogelman I, Boyle IT: Hypercalcaemic osteomalacia due to aluminium toxicity. *Lancet* 2: 1009, 1982

97. Llach F, Felsenfeld A, Coleman MD, Pederson JA: Prevalence of various types of bone disease in dialysis patients, in: *Nephrology* Vol II edited by Robinson RR, New York, Springer-Verlag, 1984, p 1374

98. Rodriguez M, Felsenfeld AJ, Llach F: The role of aluminum in the development of hypercalcemia in the rat. *Kidney Int* 31: 766, 1987

99. Alvarez-Ude F, Feest TG, Ward MK, Pierides AM, Ellis HA, Peart KM, Simpson W, Weightman D, Kerr DNS: Hemodialysis bone disease: Correlation between chemical, histologic, and other findings. *Kidney Int* 14: 68, 1978

100. Llach F, Felsenfeld AJ, Coleman MD, Keveney JJ, Pederson JA, Medlock TR: The natural course of dialysis osteomalacia. *Kidney Int* 29 (Suppl 18): S74, 1986

101. Andress DL, Felsenfeld AJ, Voigts A, Llach F: Parathyroid hormone response to hypocalcemia in hemodialysis patients with osteomalacia. *Kidney Int* 24: 364, 1983

102. Cann CE, Prussin SG, Gordan GS: Aluminum uptake by the parathyroid glands. *J Clin Endocrinol Metab* 49: 543, 1979

103. Morrissey J, Slatopolsky E: Effect of aluminum on parathyroid hormone secretion. *Kidney Int* 28: 541, 1986

104. Diaz JB, Verbueken AH, Nouwen EJ, D'Haese PC, Lamberts LV, DeBride ME: Aluminum uptake by the parathyroid glands and its subcellular localization in parathyroid cell. *Abstracts Int Congr Nephrol* 10: 4, 1987

105. Felsenfeld AJ, Harrelson JM, Gutman RA, Wells SA, Drezner MK: Osteomalacia after parathyroidectomy in patients with uremia. *Ann Intern Med* 96: 34, 1982

106. Andress DL, Ott SM, Maloney NA, Sherrard DJ: Effect of parathyroidectomy on bone aluminum accumulation in chronic renal failure. *N Engl J Med* 312: 468, 1985

107. Ott SM, Andress DL, Nebeker HG, Milliner DS, Maloney NA, Coburn JW, Sherrard DJ: Desferrioxamine therapy in patients with aluminum-related osteodystrophy. *Kidney Int* 29 (Suppl 18): S108, 1986

108. Ellis HA, McCarthy JH, Herrington J: Bone aluminium in hemodialysed patients and in rats injected with aluminium chloride: Relationship to impaired bone mineralization. *J Clin Pathol* 32: 832, 1979

109. Chan YL, Alfrey AC, Posen S, Lissner D, Hills E, Dunstan CR, Evans RA: Effect of aluminum on normal and uremic rats: tissue distribution, vitamin D metabolites and quantitative bone histology. *Calcif Tissue Int* 35: 344, 1983

110. Goodman WG, Henry DA, Horst R, Nudelman RK, Alfrey AC, Coburn JW: Parenteral aluminum administration in the dog. II. Induction of osteomalacia and effect on vitamin D metabolism. *Kidney Int* 25: 370, 1984

111. Robertson JA, Felsenfeld AJ, Haygood CC, Wilson P, Clarke C, Llach F: Animal model of aluminum induced osteomalacia: Role of chronic renal failure. *Kidney Int* 23: 327, 1983

112. Ott SM, Maloney NA, Klein GL, Alfrey AC, Ament ME, Coburn JW, Sherrard DJ: Aluminum is associated with low bone formation in patients on chronic parenteral nutrition. *Ann Intern Med* 98: 910, 1983

113. Ricanati ES, Ott SM, Klein KL, Alfrey AC, Sherrard DJ, Coburn JW: Evaluation of bone in dialysis patients exposed to aluminum in dialysate. *Kidney Int* 21: 176, 1982

114. Mion C, Branger B, Issautier R, Ellis HA, Rodier M, Shaldon S: Dialysis fracturing osteomalacia without hyperparathyroidism in patients treated with HCO₃ rinsed Redy cartridge. *Trans Am Soc Artif Intern Organs* 27: 634, 1981

115. Cumming AD, Simpson G, Bell D, Cowie JF, Winney RJ: Acute aluminium intoxication in patients on continuous ambulatory peritoneal dialysis. *Lancet* 1: 103, 1982

116. Salusky IB, Coburn JW, Paunier L, Sherrard DJ, Fine RN: Role of aluminum hydroxide in raising serum aluminum levels in children undergoing continuous ambulatory peritoneal dialysis (CAPD). *J Pediatrics* 105: 717, 1984

117. Milliner DS, Shinaberger JH, Shuman P, Coburn JW: Inadvertent aluminum administration during plasma exchange due to aluminum contamination of albumin replacement solutions. *N Engl J Med* 312, 165, 1985

118. Berlyne GM, Ben-Ari J, Pest D, Weinberger J, Stern M, Gilmore, Levine R: Hyperaluminaemia from aluminium resins in renal failure. *Lancet* 2: 494, 1970

119. Kanis JA, Adams ND, Earnshaw M, Heyman G, Ledingham JGG, Oliver DO, Russell RG, Woods CG: Vitamin D, osteomalacia and chronic renal failure. in: *Vitamin D: Biochemical, Chemical, and Clinical Aspects Related to Calcium Metabolism.* edited by Norman AW, Schaefer K, Coburn JW, DeLuca HF, Fraser D, Grigoleit HG, Herrath DV, Berlin, Walter De Gruyter, 1977, p 671

120. Andreoli SP, Bergstein JM, Sherrard DJ: Aluminum intoxication in nondialyzed azotemic children from aluminum containing phosphate binders. *N Engl J Med* 310: 1079, 1984

121. Felsenfeld AJ, Gutman RA, Llach F, Harrelson JM: Osteomalacia in chronic renal failure: A syndrome previously reported only with maintenance dialysis. *Am J Nephrol* 2: 147, 1982

122. Kaye M: Oral aluminum toxicity in non-dialyzed patients with renal failure. *Clin Nephrol* 20: 208, 1983

123. Winney RJ, Cowie JF, Robson JS: The role of plasma aluminum in the detection and prevention of aluminum toxicity. *Kidney Int* 29 (Suppl 18): S91, 1986

124. Herez G, Kraut JA, Andress DA, Howard N, Roberts C, Shinaberger JH, Sherrard DJ, Coburn JW: Use of calcium carbonate as a phosphate binder in dialysis patients. *Miner Electrolyte Metab* 12: 314, 1986

125. Blannina P, Frech W, Ekstrom LG, Loof L, Slorach L: Dietary citric acid enhances absorption of aluminum in antacids. *Clin Chem* 32: 539, 1986

126. Bakir AA, Hryhorczuk DD, Berman E, Dunea G: Acute fatal hyperaluminemic encephalopathy in undialyzed and recently dialyzed uremic patients. *ASAIO Transactions* 32: 171, 1986

127. Pellegrino ED, Biltz RM: The composition of human bone in uremia. *Medicine* 44: 397, 1965

128. Burnell JM, Teubner EJ, Wergedal JE, Sherrard DJ: Bone crystal maturation in renal osteodystrophy in uremia. *J Clin Invest* 53: 52, 1974

129. Nichols G Jr, Nichols N: Effect of parathyroidectomy on content and availability of skeletal sodium in the rat. *Am J Physiol* 198: 749, 1960

130. Dent CE, Hodson CJ: Radiological changes associated with certain metabolic bone diseases. *Br J Radiol* 27: 605, 1954

131. Stanbury SW, Lumb GA: Metabolic studies of renal osteodystrophy. I: Calcium, phosphorus, and nitrogen metabolism in rickets, osteomalacia and hyperparathyroidism complicating chronic uremia and the osteomalacia of the adult Fanconi syndrome. *Medicine* 41: 1, 1962

132. Stanbury SW: Bone disease in uremia. *Am J Med* 44: 714, 1968

133. Barzel US, Jowsey J: The effects of chronic acid and alkali administration on bone turnover in adult rats. *Clin Sci* 36: 517, 1969

134. Kraut JA, Mishler DR. Singer FR and Goodman WG: The effects of metabolic acidosis on bone formation and bone resorption in the rat. *Kidney Int* 30: 694, 1986

135. Teitelbaum SL, Bergfeld MA, Freitag J, Hruska KA, Slata-

polsky E: Do parathyroid hormone and 1,25 dihydroxyvitamin D modulate bone formation in uremia? *J Clin Endocrinol Metab* 51: 247, 1980

136. Kraut JA, Shinaberger JH, Singer FR: Parathyroid gland responsiveness to acute hypocalcemia in dialysis osteomalacia. *Kidney Int* 23: 725, 1983

137. Bourdeau AM, Plachot JJ, Cournot-Witmer G, Pointillart A, Balsan S, Sachs C: Parathyroid response to aluminum in vitro: Ultrastructural changes and PTH release. *Kidney Int* 31: 8, 1987

138. Matthews M, Stauffer M, Cameron EC, Maloney N, Sherrard DJ: Bone biopsy to diagnose hyperoxaluria in patients with renal failure. *Ann Intern Med* 90: 777, 1979

139. Julian BA, Faugere MC, Malluche HH: Oxalosis in bone causing a radiographical mimicry of renal osteodystrophy. *Am J Kidney Dis* 9: 436, 1987

140. Ott SM, Andress DL, Sherrard DJ: Bone oxalate in a long-term hemodialysis patient who ingested high doses of vitamin C. *Am J Kidney Dis* 8: 450, 1986

141. Ahmad S, Hatch M: Hyperoxalemia in renal failure and the role of hemoperfusion and hemodialysis in primary oxalosis. *Nephron* 41: 235, 1985

142. Ono K: Secondary hyperoxalemia caused by vitamin C supplementation in regular hemodialysis patients. *Clin Nephrol* 26: 239, 1986

143. Worcester EM, Nakagawa Y, Bushinsky DA, Coe FL: Evidence that serum calcium oxalate supersaturation is a consequence of oxalate retention in patients with chronic renal failure. *J Clin Invest* 77: 1888, 1986

144. Parfitt AM: The quantitative approach to bone morphology. A critique of current methods and their interpretation. in: *Clinical Aspects of Metabolic Bone Disease,* edited by Frame B, Parfitt AM, Duncan H, Amsterdam, Excerpta Medica, 1973, p 86

145. Frost HM: The origin and nature of transient in human bone remodeling dynamics. in: *Clinical Aspects of Metabolic Bone Disease,* edited by Frame B, Parfitt AM, Duncan H, Amsterdam, Excerpta Medica, 1973, p 124

146. Frost HM: Tetracycline-based histologic analysis of bone remodeling. *Calcif Tissue Res* 3: 211, 1969

147. Ellis HA, Peart KM: Azotaemic renal osteodystrophy, a quantitative study on iliac bone. *J Clin Pathol* 26: 83, 1973

148. Sherrard DJ, Baylink DJ, Wergedal JE, Maloney N: Quantitative histological studies on the pathogenesis of uremic bone disease. *J Clin Endocrinol* 39: 119, 1974

149. Ritz E, Malluche HH, Krempien B, Mehls O: Bone histology in renal insufficiency. in: *Perspectives in Nephrology and Hypertension.* edited by David DS, New York, John Wiley and Son, 1977, p 197

150. Pierides AM, Edwards WG Jr, Cullum UX Jr, McCall JT, Ellis HA: Hemodialysis encephalopathy with osteomalacia, fractures and muscle weakness. *Kidney Int* 18: 115, 1980

151. Ward MK, Parkinson LS: Aluminum toxicity in renal failure. in: *Replacement of Renal Function by Dialysis,* edited by Drukker W, Parsons FM, Maher JF, 2nd edition, The Hague, Martinus Nijhoff, 1983, p 811

152. Platts MM, Owen G, Smith S: Water purification and the incidence of fractures in patients receiving home dialysis supervised by a single centre: Evidence for 'safe' upper limit of aluminium in water. *Br Med J* 288: 969, 1984

153. Sherrard DJ, Coburn JW, Brickman AD, Singer FR and Maloney N: Skeletal response to treatment with 1,25-dihydroxyvitamin D in renal failure. *Contrib Nephrol* 18: 92, 1980

154. Jaffe MD, Wellis PW III: Multiple fractures associated with long-term sodium heparin therapy. *JAMA* 193: 152, 1965

155. Schott GD, Willis MR: Muscle weakness in osteomalacia. *Lancet* 1: 626, 1976

156. Schoenfeld PJ, Martin JH, Barnes B, Teitelbaum SL: Amelioration of myopathy with 25-hydroxyvitamin D_3 therapy [25(OH)D_3] in patients on chronic hemodialysis. *Abstracts Third Workshop on Vitamin D, Asilomar,* 1977, p 160

157. Coburn JW, Brickman AS, Sherrard DJ, Singer FR, Baylink DJ, Wong EGC, Massry SG, Norman AW: Clinical efficacy of 1,25–dihydroxyvitamin D_3 osteodystrophy. in: *Vitamin D: Biochemical, and Clinical Aspects Related to Calcium Metabolism,* edited by Norman AW, Schaefer K, Coburn JW, DeLuca HF, Fraser D, Grigoleit HG, Herrath DV, Berlin, W de Gruyter, 1977, p 657

158. Massry SG, Popovtzer MM, Coburn JW, Makoff DL, Maxwell MH, Kleeman CR: Intractable pruritus as a manifestation of secondary hyperparathyroidism in uremia. Disappearance of itching following subtotal parathyroidectomy. *N Engl J Med* 279: 697, 1968

159. Mehls O, Ritz E, Burkhard K, Gillis G, Link W, Willich E, Schärer K: Slipped epiphysis in renal osteodystrophy. *Arch Dis Child* 50: 545, 1975

160. Holliday MA: Calorie deficiency in children with uremia: Effect upon growth. *Pediatrics* 50: 590, 1972

161. Chesney RW, Hamstra A, Jax DK, Mazess RB, DeLuca HF: Influence of long term oral 1,25-dihydroxyvitamin D in childhood renal osteodystrophy. *Contrib Nephrol* 18: 55, 1980

162. Llach F, Pederson J: Acute joint syndrome and maintenance hemodialysis. *Proc Clin Dial Transplant Forum* 9: 17, 1979

163. Lotem M, Bernheim J, Conforty B: Spontaneous rupture of tendons: a complication of hemodialyzed patients treated for renal failure. *Nephron* 21: 201, 1978

164. Gipstein RH, Coburn JW, Adams DA, Lee DBN, Parsa KP, Sellers A, Suki WN, Massry SG: Calciphylaxis in man: A syndrome of tissue necrosis and vascular calcification in 11 patients with chronic renal disease. *Arch Intern Med* 136: 1273, 1976

165. Seyle H: Calciphylaxis. Chicago, University of Chicago Press, 1962

166. Arieff AI, Massry SG: Calcium metabolism of brain in acute renal failure. *J Clin Invest* 53: 387, 1974

167. Ball JH, Butkus DE, Madison DS: Effect of subtotal parathyroidectomy on dialysis dementia. *Nephron* 18: 151, 1977

168. Massry SG, Goldstein DA: The search for uremic toxin(s) 'X'. 'X' = PTH. *Clin Nephrol* 11: 181, 1979

169. Weinberg SG, Lubin A, Wiener SN, Deoras MP, Ghose MK, Kopelman RC: Myelofibrosis and renal osteodystrophy. *Am J Med* 63: 755, 1977

170. Better OS, Shasha SM, Windver J, Chaimovitz C: Improvement in the anemia of hemodialysis patients following parathyroidectomy. *Kidney Int* 10: 487, 1976

171. Meytes D, Bogin E, Ma A, Dukes PP, Massry SG: Effects of parathyroid hormone on erythrocytes. *J Clin Invest* 67: 1263, 1981

172. Drüeke TB, Lacour B, Touam M, Jucquel JP, Placot JJ, Cournot-Witmer G, Calle P: Effects of aluminum on hematopoiesis. *Kidney Int* 29 (Suppl 18): S45, 1986

173. Remuzzi G, Benigni A, Dodesini P, Schieppati A, Livio M, Poletti E, Mecca G, de Gaetano G: Parathyroid hormone inhibits human platelet function. *Lancet* 2: 1321, 1981

174. Bagdade JD, Porte D, Bierman EL: Hypertriglyceridemia: a metabolic consequence of renal failure. *N Engl J Med* 279: 181, 1968

175. Winkler AW, Durlacher SH, Hoff HE, Man EB: Changes in

lipid content of serum and of liver following bilateral renal ablation or ureteral ligation. *J Exp Med* 77: 473, 1943

176. Cantin M: Kidney, parathyroid hormone and lipemia. *Lab Invest* 14: 1691, 1965

177. Lindall A, Carmera R, Cohen S, Compty C: Insulin hypersecretion in patients on chronic hemodialysis: Role of parathyroids. *J Clin Endocrinol* 32: 653, 1971

178. London GM, Fabiani F, Marchais SJ, de Vernejoul MC, Guerin AP, Safar ME, Metevier, Llach F: Uremic cardiomyopathy: An inadequate left ventricular hypertrophy. *Kidney Int* 31: 973, 1987

179. Bogin E, Massry SG, Harary I: Effect of parathyroid hormone on rat heart cells. *J Clin Invest* 67: 1215, 1981

180. Drüeke T, Fauchet M, Fleury J, Lesourd P, Toure Y, LePailleur C, De Vernejoul P, Crosnier J: Effects of parathyroidectomy on left ventricular function in haemodialysis patients. *Lancet* 1: 112, 1980

181. Stanbury SW: The phosphate ion in chronic renal failure. in: *Phosphate Inorganique, Biologie et Physiopathologie* edited by Hioco DJ, Paris, International Symposium, Sandoz, 1970, p 187

182. Clarkson EM, Luck VA, Hynson WV, Baily RR, Eastwood JB, Woodhead JS, Clements VR, O'Riordan JLH, De Wardener HE: The effect of aluminium hydroxide on calcium, phosphorus and aluminum balances, the serum parathyroid hormone concentration and the aluminium content of bone in patients with chronic renal failure. *Clin Sci* 43: 519, 1972

183. Coburn JW, Hartenbower DL, Brickman AS, Massry SG, Kopple JD: Intestinal absorption of calcium, magnesium phosphorus in chronic renal insufficiency. in: *Calcium Metabolism in Renal Failure and Nephrolithiasis.* edited by David DS, New York, John Wiley and Sons, 1977, p 77

184. Massry SG, Coburn JW, Popovtzer MM, Shinaberger JH, Maxwell MH: Kleeman CR: Secondary hyperparathyroidism in chronic renal failure: The clinical spectrum in uremia, during hemodialysis and after renal transplantation. *Arch Intern Med* 124: 431, 1969

185. Shah S, Cruz C, Castillo W: Persistent hypophosphatemia in patients on chronic hemodialysis without phosphate binding gels. *Kidney Int* (Abstract) 10: 526, 1976

186. Burnell JM, Teubner E: Effects of decreasing magnesium in patients with chronic renal failure. *Proc Clin Dial Transplant Forum* 5: 191, 1976

187. Strong HF, Schatz BC, Shinaberger JH, Coburn JW: Measurement of dialysance and bi-directional fluxes of calcium in vivo using radiocalcium. *Trans Am Soc Artif Intern Organs* 17: 108, 1971

188. Ramen A, Chong YK, Sreenevasan GA: Effects of varying dialysate calcium concentration on the plasma calcium fractions in patients on dialysis. *Nephron* 16: 181, 1976

189. Bouillon R, Verberckmoes R, Moor PD: Influence of dialysate calcium concentration and vitamin D on serum parathyroid hormone during repetitive dialysis. *Kidney Int* 7: 422, 1975

190. Prior JC, Cameron EC, Ballan HS, Lirenman DS, Moriarty MV, Price JDE: Experience with 1,25-dihydroxycholecalciferol therapy in hemodialysis patients with progressive vitamin D_2-treated osteodystrophy. *Am J Med* 67: 583, 1979

191. Randall RE Jr, Cohen MD, Spray CC Jr and Rossmeisl EC: Hypermagnesemia in renal failure. Etiology and toxic manifestations. *Ann Intern Med* 61: 73, 1964

192. Alfrey AC, Solomons CC, Ciricillo J, Miller NL: Extraosseous calcification. Evidence for abnormal pryophosphate metabolism in uremia. *J Clin Invest* 57: 692, 1976

193. Alfrey AC, Solomons CC: Bone pyrophosphate in uremia and its association with extraosseous calcification. *J Clin Invest* 57: 700, 1976

194. Felsenfeld AJ, Llach F: Vitamin D and metabolic bone disease: A clinicopathological overview. *Pathol Annu* 17: 383, 1982

195. Raisz LG, Yajnik CH, Bockman RS, Bower BB: Comparison of avialable parathyroid hormone immunoassays in the differential diagnosis of hypercalcemia due to primary hyperparathyroidism. *Ann Intern Med* 91: 739, 1979

196. Nebeker HG, Coburn JW: Parathyroid hormone and chronic renal failure. *Am Assoc Clin Chem Endo: Endocrinol Metab* 3: 1, 1985

197. Mayer GP, Habener JF, Potts JT Jr: Parathyroid hormone secretion in vivo: Demonstration of a calcium-independent non-suppressible component of secretion. *J Clin Invest* 57: 678, 1976

198. Duursma SA, Van Kesteren RG, Visser WJ, Rvelofs JM, Raymaker JA: Serum alkaline phosphatase: Its relation to bone cells and its significance as an indicator for vitamin D treatment in patients with renal insufficiency. in: *Vitamin D and Problems Related to Uremic Bone Disease.* edited by Norman AW, Schaefer K, Grigoleit HG, Herrath DV, Ritz E: Berlin, Walter De Gruyter, 1975, p 167

199. Hart W, Duursma SA. Visser WJ, Njio LKF: The hydroxyproline content of plasma of patients with impaired renal function. *Clin Nephrol* 4: 104, 1975

200. Hamet P, Stouder DA. Ginn HE, Hardman JG, Liddle GW: Studies of the elevated extra-cellular concentration of cyclic AMP in uremic man. *J Clin Invest* 56: 339, 1975

201. Price PA, Williamson MK, Lothringer JW: Origin of the vitamin D dependent bone protein found in plasma and its clearance by kidney and bone. *J Biol Chem* 256: 12760, 1981

202. Delmas PD, Wahner HW, Mann KG, Riggs BL: Assessment of bone turnover in postmenopausal osteoporosis by measurement of serum bone Gla-protein. *J Lab Clin Med* 102: 470, 1984

203. Delmas PD, Wilson DM, Mann KG, Riggs BL: Effect of renal function on plasma levels of bone Gla-protein. *J Clin Endocrinol Metab* 57: 1028, 1983

204. Malluche HH, Faugere MC, Fanti P: Plasma levels of bone Gla-protein reflect bone formation in patients on chronic maintenance dialysis. *Kidney Int* 26: 869, 1984

205. Martinez ME, Selgas R, DePedro C, Balaguer G, Escuin F, Sanchez Sicilia, Llach F: Osteocalcin levels in uremic patients: Influence of dialysis type and short term 1,25(OH)$_2$D treatment. (In Press)

206. Alfrey AC: Aluminum. *Adv Clin Chem* 21: 69, 1983

207. Hercz G, Andress DL. Nebeker HG, Shinaberger JH, Sherrard DJ, Coburn JW: Reversal of aluminum-related bone disease after substituting calcium carbonate for aluminum hydroxide. *Am J Kidney Dis* (In Press)

208. Milliner DS, Nebeker HG, Ott SM, Andress DL, Sherrard DJ, Alfrey AC, Slatapolsky E, Coburn JW: Use of the deferoxamine infusion test in the diagnosis of aluminum-related osteomalacia. *Ann Intern Med* 101: 775, 1984

209. Malluche HH, Smith AJ, Abreo K, Faugere MC: The use of desferrioxamine in the management of aluminum accumulation in bone in patients with renal failure. *N Engl J Med* 311: 140, 1984

210. Andress DL, Nebeker HG. Ott SM, Endres DB, Alfrey AC, Slatopolsky EA, Coburn JW, Sherrard DJ: Bone histologic response to long-term treatment with deferoxamine for aluminum-related bone disease. *Kidney Int* 31: 1344, 1987

211. Parfitt AM: Clinical and radiographic manifestations of renal osteodystrophy. in: *Calcium Metabolism in Renal Failure and Nephrolithiasis,* edited by David DS, New York, John Wiley and Sons, 1976, p 150

212. Meema HE, Schatz DL: Simple radiologic demonstration of cortical bone loss in thyrotoxicosis. *Radiology* 97: 9, 1970

213. Meema HE, Rabinovich S, Meema S, Lloyd GJ, Oreopoulos DG: Improved radiological diagnosis of azotemic osteodystrophy. *Radiology* 102: 1, 1972

214. Doyle FH: Radiological patterns of bone disease associated with renal glomerular failure in adults. *Br Med Bull* 28: 220, 1972

215. Glassford DM, Remmers AR Jr, Sarles HE, Lindley JD, Scurry MT, Fish JC: Hyperparathyroidism in the maintenance dialysis patient. *Surg Gyn Obstet* 142: 328, 1976

216. Shimada H, Nakamura M, Marumo F: Influence of aluminum on the effect of 1-alpha-(OH)D₃ on renal osteodystrophy. *Nephron* 35: 163, 1983

217. Craven JD: Renal glomerular osteodystrophy. *Clin Radiol* 15: 210, 1964

218. Ellis K, Hochstim RJ: The skull in hyperparathyroid bone disease. *Am J Roentgenol* 83: 732, 1960

219. Meema HE, Oreopoulos DG, Rabinovich S, Husdan H, Rapaport A: Periosteal new bone formation (Periosteal Neostosis) in renal osteodystrophy. *Radiology* 110: 513, 1974

220. Ritz E, Krempien B, Mehls O, Malluche HH: Skeletal abnormalities in chronic renal insufficiency before and during maintenance hemodialysis. *Kidney Int* 4: 116, 1973

221. Norfray J, Calenoff L, Del Greco F, Krumlovsky FA: Renal osteodystrophy in patients on hemodialysis as reflected in the bony pelvis. *Am J Roentgenol Radium Ther Nucl Med* 125: 352, 1975

222. Bailey GL, Griffiths HJL, Mocelin AJ, Gundy DH, Hampers CL, Merrill JP: Avascular necrosis of the femoral head in patients on chronic hemodialysis. *Trans Am Soc Artif Intern Organs* 18: 401, 1972

223. Parfitt AM, Massry SG, Winfield AD: Osteopenia and fractures occurring during maintenance hemodialysis. A 'new' form of renal osteodystrophy. *Clin Orthop* 87: 287, 1972

2204 Letteri JM, Cohn SH: Total body neutron activation: Analysis in the study of mineral homeostasis in chronic renal disease. in: *Calcium Metabolism in Renal Failure and Nephrolithiasis.* edited by David DS, New York, John Wiley and Sons, 1977, p 249

225. Cochran M, Bulusu L, Horsman A, Stasiac L, Nordin BEC: Hypocalcemia and bone disease in chronic renal failure. *Nephron* 10: 113, 1973

226. Bone JM, Davison AM, Robson JS: Role of dialysate calcium concentration in osteoporosis in patients on haemodialysis. *Lancet* 1: 1047, 1972

227. Henderson RG, Russell RGG, Earnshaw MJ, Ledingham JGG, Oliver DO, Woods CG: Loss of metacarpal and iliac bone in chronic renal failure: Influence of haemodialysis, parathyroid hormone, type of renal disease, physical activity and heparin consumption. *Clin Sci* 56: 31F, 1979

228. Fleisch H, Russell RGG: Experimental clinical studies with pyrophosphate and diphosphonates. in: *Calcium Metabolism in Renal Failure and Nephrolithiasis.* edited by David DA, New York, John Wiley and Sons, 1979, p 293

229. Rosenthall L, Kaye M: Technetium-99m-pyrophosphate kinetics and imaging in metabolic bone disease. *J Nucl Med* 16: 33, 1975

230. Olgaard K, Heerfordt J, Madsen S: Scintigraphic skeletal changes in uremic patients on regular hemodialysis. *Nephron* 17: 325, 1976

231. Davis BA, Poulose KP, Reba RC: Scanning for uremic pulmonary calcifications. *Ann Intern Med* 85: 132, 1976

232. Massry SG, Coburn JW: Divalent ion metabolism and renal osteodystrophy. in: *Clinical Aspects of Uremia and Dialysis,* edited by Massry SG, Sellers AL, Springfield IL, Charles C. Thomas Co, 1976, p 304

233. Parfitt AM: Soft tissue calcification in uremia. *Arch Intern Med* 124: 544, 1969

234. Contiguglia SR Sr, Alfrey AC, Miller NL, Runnells DE, LeGeros RZ: Nature of soft tissue calcification in uremia. *Kidney Int* 4: 229, 1973

235. Dreher W, Shelp W: Atrioventricular block in a long term dialysis patient. Reversal after parathyroidectomy. *JAMA* 234: 954, 1975

236. Schwartz KV: Heart block in renal failure and hypercalcemia. *JAMA* 235: 1550, 1976

237. Conger JD, Hammond WS, Alfrey AC, Contiguglia SR, Standord RE, Huffer WE: Pulmonary calcification in chronic dialysis patients. Clinical and pathologic studies. *Ann Intern Med* 83: 330, 1975

238. Kraikitpanitch S, Haygood CC, Baxter DJ, Yunice AA, Lindeman RD: Studies on the pathogenesis of myocardial calcification in azotemia. *Abstracts Am Soc Nephrol* 8: 4, 1975

239. Ritz E, Mehls O, Bomer J, Schmidt-Gayk H, Fiegel P, Reitinger H: Vascular calcification under maintenance hemodialysis. *Klin Wochenschr* 55: 375, 1977

240. Kopple JD, Coburn JW: Metabolic studies of low protein diets in uremia. II. Calcium phosphorus and magnesium. *Medicine* 52: 597, 1973

241. Goldsmith RS, Furszyfer J, Johnson WJ, Fournier AE, Arnaud CD: Control of secondary hyperparathyroidism during long-term hemodialysis. *Am J Med* 50: 692, 1971

242. Rutherford WE, Mercado A, Hruska K, Harter H, Mason N, Sparks R, Klahr S, Slatopolsky E: An evaluation of a new and effective phosphorus binding agent. *Trans Am Soc Artif Intern Organs* 19: 446, 1973

243. Moriniere PH, Roussel A, Tahiri Y: Substitution of aluminium hydroxide by high doses of calcium carbonate in patients on chronic haemodialysis. Disappearance of hyperaluminaemia and equal control of hyperparathyroidism. *Proc Eur Dial Transplant Assoc* 19: 784, 1982

244. Salusky IB, Coburn JW, Foley J, Nelson P, Fine RN: Calcium carbonate as a phosphate binder in children on dialysis. *Kidney Int* 27: 185, 1985

245. O'Donovan R, Baldwin D, Hammer M, Moniz C, Parsons V: Substitution of aluminium salts by magnesium salts in control of dialysis hyperphosphataemia. *Lancet* 1: 880, 1986

246. Mahoney JF, Hayes JM, Ingham JP, Posen S: Hypophosphataemic osteomalacia in patients receiving haemodialysis. *Br Med J* 2: 142, 1976

247. Drüeke T, Bordier PJ, Man NK, Jungers P, Marie P: Effects on high dialysate calcium concentration on bone remodeling, serum biochemistry, and parathyroid hormone in patients with renal osteodystrophy. *Kidney Int* 11: 267, 1977

248. Raman A, Chong YK, Sreenevasan GA: Effects of varying dialysate calcium concentrations on the plasma calcium fractions in patients on dialysis. *Nephron* 16: 181, 1986

249. Clarkson EM, McDonald SJ, DeWardener HE: The effects of a high intake of calcium carbonate in normal subjects and patients with chronic renal failure. *Clin Sci* 30: 425, 1966

250. Meyrier A, Marsac J, Richet G: The influence of a high calcium carbonate intake on bone disease in patients undergoing hemodialysis. *Kidney Int* 4: 146, 1973

251. Eastwood JB, Bordier PJ, DeWardener HE: Some biochem-

ical, histological radiological and clinical features of renal osteodystrophy. *Kidney Int* 4: 128, 1973

252. Rao TKS, Friedman EA: Fluoride and bone disease in uremia. *Kidney Int* 7: 125, 1975

253. Taves DR, Terry R, Smith FA, Gardner DE: Use of fluoridated water in long-term hemodialysis. *Arch Intern Med* 115: 167, 1965

254. Posen GA, Marier JR, Jaworski ZF: Renal osteodystrophy in patients on long-term hemodialysis with fluoridated water. *Fluoride* 4: 114, 1971

255. Siddiqui JY, Simpson W, Ellis HA, Kerr DNS: Serum fluoride in chronic renal failure. *Proc Eur Dial Transplant Assoc* 7: 110, 1970

256. Oreopoulos DG, Taves DR, Rabinovich S, Meema HE, Murray T, Fenton SS, DeVeber GA: Fluoride and dialysis osteodystrophy. Results of a double-blind study. *Trans Am Soc Artif Intern Organs* 20: 203, 1974

257. Griffith GC, Nichols G Jr, Asher JD and Flanigan B: Heparin osteoporosis. *JAMA* 193: 91, 1965

258. Jaffe MD, Wellis PW III: Multiple fractures associated with long-term sodium heparin therapy. *JAMA* 193: 158, 1965

259. Voigts AL, Felsenveld AJ, Llach F: The effects of calciferol and its metabolites on patients with renal failure. I. Calciferol, dihydrotachysterol and calcifediol. *Arch Intern Med* 143: 960, 1983

260. Voigts AL, Felsenfeld AJ, Llach F: The effects of calciferol and its metabolites on patients with chronic renal failure. II. Calcitriol, 1 alpha hydroxyvitamin D$_3$. *Arch Intern Med* 143: 1205, 1983

261. Brickman AS, Sherrard DJ, Jowsey J, Singer FR, Baylink DJ, Maloney N, Massry SG, Norman AW, Coburn JW: 1,25-dihydroxycholecalciferol. Effect on skeletal lesions and plasma parathyroid hormone levels in uremic osteodystrophy. *Arch Intern Med* 134: 883, 1974

262. Pierides M, Ward MK, Alvarez-Ude F, Ellis HA, Peart KM, Simpson W, Kerr DNS, Norman AW: Long-term therapy with 1,25(OH)$_2$D$_3$ in dialysis bone disease. *Proc Eur Dial Transplant Assoc* 12: 237, 1976

263. Sherrard DJ, Coburn JW, Brickman AS, Baylink DJ, Norman AW, Maloney N: A histologic comparison of 1,25(OH)$_2$ vitamin D treatment with calcium supplementation in renal osteodystrophy. in: *Vitamin D: Biochemical, Chemical and Clinical Aspects Related to Calcium Metabolism*, edited by Norman AW, Schaefer K, Coburn JW, DeLuca HF, Fraser D, Grigoleit HG, Herrath DV, Berlin, W de Gruyter, 1977, p 719

264. Sherrard DJ, Coburn JW, Brickman AS, Singer FR, Maloney N: Skeletal response to treatment with 1,25-dihydroxyvitamin D in renal failure. *Contrib Nephrol* 18: 92, 1980

265. Kanis JA, Candy T, Earnshaw M, Henderson RG, Heynem G, Malk R, Russell RGG, Smith R, Woods CG: Treatment of renal bone disease with 1-alpha-hydroxylated derivatives of vitamin D$_3$. *Q J Med* 48: 289, 1979

266. Colodro IH, Brickman AS, Coburn JW: Effects of 25(OH)-vitamin D$_3$ on intestinal absorption of calcium in normal and uremic man. *Clin Res* 23: 430, 1975

267. Recker RR, Schoenfeld P, Slatopolsky E: 25-hydroxyvitamin D in renal osteodystrophy. Results of a six center trial. in: *Vitamin D: Biochemical, Chemical and Clinical Aspects Related to Calcium Metabolism*, edited by Norman AW, Schaefer K, Coburn JW, DeLuca HF, Fraser D, Grigoleit HG, Herrath DV, Berlin, W de Gruyter, 1977, p 649

268. Papapoulos SE, Brownjohn AM, Goodwin FJ, Hately W, Marsh FP, O'Riordan JLH: The effect of 1-alpha-hydroxycholecalciferol and secondary hyperparathyroidism of chronic renal failure. in: *Vitamin D: Biochemical, Chemical and Clinical Aspects Related to Calcium Metabolism*, edited by Norman AW, Schaefer K, Coburn JW, DeLuca HF, Fraser D, Grigoleit HG, Herrath DV, Berlin, W de Gruyter, 1977, p 693

269. Kanis JA, Earnshaw M, Henderson GR, Heymen G, Ledingham JGG, Naik RB, Russel DO, Smith R, Wilkinson R, Woods CG: Correlation of clinical, biochemical and skeletal responses to 1-alpha-hydroxycholecalciferol in renal bone disease. *Clin Endocrinol* 7 (Suppl): 45S, 1977

270. Pierides AM, Kerr DNS, Ellis HA, Peart KM, O'Riordan JLH, DeLuca HF: 1-alpha-hydroxycholecalciferol in haemodialysis renal osteodystrophy. Adverse effects of anticonvulsant therapy. *Clin Nephrol* 5: 189, 1976

271. Regan RJ, Peacock M, Rosen SM, Robinson PJ, Horsman A: Effect of dialysate calcium concentration on bone disease in patients on hemodialysis. *Kidney Int* 10: 246, 1976

272. Kaye M, Chatterjee G, Cohen GF, Sagar S: Arrest of hyperparathyroid bone disease with dihydrotachysterol in patients undergoing chronic hemodialysis. *Ann Intern Med* 73: 225, 1970

273. David DS: Mineral and bone homeostasis in renal failure. Pathophysiology and management. in: *Calcium Metabolism in Renal Failure and Nephrolithiasis*, edited by David DS, New York, John Wiley and Sons, 1976, p 1

274. Wells SA Jr, Gunnells JC, Schneider AB, Sherwood LM: Transplantation of the parathyroid glands in man. Clinical indications and results. *Surgery* 78: 34, 1975

275. Sicard GA, Wells SA Jr: Surgical treatment of secondary hyperparathyroidism. in: *Surgery of the Thyroid and Parathyroid Glands*, edited by Kaplan EL, Edinburgh, Churchill-Livingstone, 1983, p 243

276. Wang C, Mahaffey JE, Axelrod L, Perlman JA: Hyperfunctioning supernumerary parathyroid glands. *Surg Gynecol Obstet* 148: 711, 1979

277. Gordon HE, Coburn JW, Passaro E: Surgical management of secondary hyperparathyroidism. *Arch Surg* 104: 520, 1972

278. Felsenfeld AJ, Gutman RA, Llach F, Harrelson JM, Wells SA: Postparathyroidectomy hypocalcemia as an accurate indicator of preparathyroidectomy bone histology in the uremic patient. *Miner Electrolyte Metab* 10: 166, 1984

279. Sakai S, David D, Shoji H, Stenzel KH, Rubin AL: Bone injuries due to tetany or convulsions during hemodialysis. *Clin Orthop* 118: 118, 1976

280. Robertson JA, Salusky IB, Norris KC, Coburn JW: Aluminum absorption in man: Comparison of sucralfate and aluminum hydroxide. *Kidney Int* 31: 214, 1987

281. Stummvoll HK, Graf H, Meisinger V: Effect of desferrioxamine on aluminum kinetics during hemodialysis. *Miner Electrolyte Metab* 10: 263, 1984

282. Ackrill P, Ralston AJ, Day JP, Hodge KC: Successful removal of aluminium from a patient with dialysis encephalopathy. *Lancet* 2: 692, 1980

283. Felsenfeld A, Rodriguez M, Coleman M, Ross D, Llach F: The effect of desferrioxamine (DFO) on aluminum bone disease and parathyroid hormone (PTH). *Abstracts Am Soc Nephrol* 20: 74A, 1987

284. Blake DR, Winyard P, Lunec J, Williams A, Good PA, Crewes SJ, Gutteridge JMC, Rowley D, Halliwell B, Cornish A, Hider RC: Cerebral and ocular toxicity induced by desferrioxamine. *Q J Med, New Series* 56: 345, 1985

285. Rahi AHS, Hungerford JL, Ahmed AI: Ocular toxicity of desferrioxamine: Light microscopic histochemical and ultrastructural findings. *Br J Opthalmol* 70: 373, 1986

286. Mofenson HC, Caraccio, Sharieff N: Iron sepsis: Yersinia

enterocolitica septicemia possible caused by an overdose of iron. *N Engl J Med* 316: 1092, 1987

287. Kanis JA, Earnshaw M, Heynen G, Russell RGG, Wood CG: The possible role of calcitonin deficiency in the development of bone disease due to chronic renal failure. *Calcif Tissue Res* 22 (Suppl): 147, 1977

288. Delano BG, Baker R, Gardner B, Wallach S: A trial of calcitonin therapy in renal osteodystrophy. *Nephron* 11: 287, 1973

289. Zucchelli P, Fusaroli M, Fabbri L, Pavlica P, Casanova S, Viglietta G, Sasdelli M: Treatment of ectopic calcification in uremia. *Kidney Int* 13 (Suppl 12): S86, 1978

290. Fleisch H, Bonjour JP: Diphosphanate treatment in bone disease. *N Engl J Med* 289: 1419, 1973

291. Zingraff J, Drüeke T, Roux JP, Rondon-Nucete M, Man NK, Jungers P: Bilateral fracture of the femoral neck complicating uremic bone disease prior to chronic hemodialysis. *Clin Nephrol* 2: 73, 1974

292. Brickman AS, Coburn JW, Norman AW, Massry SG: Short-term effects of 1,25 dihydroxycholecalciferol on disordered calcium metabolism of renal failure. *Am J Med* 57: 28, 1974

293. Brickman AS, Jowsey J, Sherrard DJ, Friedman G, Singer FR, Baylink DJ, Maloney N, Massry SG, Norman AW, Coburn JW: Therapy with 1,25-dihydroxyvitamin D_3 in the management of renal osteodystrophy. in: *Vitamin D and Problems Related to Uremic Bone Disease,* edited by Norman AW, Schaefer K, Grigoleit HG, Herrath DV, Ritz E, Berlin, W de Gruyter, 1975, p 241

294. Coburn JW, Brickman AS, Hartenbower DL, Norman AW: Intestinal phosphate absorption in normal and uremic man: Effects of $1,25(OH)_2$-vitamin D_3. in: *Phosphate Metabolism* edited by Massry SG, Ritz E, New York, Plenum Press, 1977, p 549

ENDOCRINE CHANGES IN CHRONIC DIALYSIS PATIENTS

FRANCISZEK KOKOT and ANDRZEJ WIĘCEK

INTRODUCTION

There are at least six reasons why endocrine abnormalities may be expected in patients with chronic renal failure (CRF).

1. The kidneys are an important endocrine organ where erythropoietin, angiotensin I and II, 1,25-dihydroxycholecalciferol, kinins, prostaglandins and other hormones are synthesised. As CRF is characterized by a decrease of functioning parenchyma, altered biosynthesis of renal hormones may be expected.

2. The kidneys are the target organ of many hormones (e.g. parathyroid hormone, calcitonin, aldosterone, vasopressin and angiotensin), involved in the regulation of its excretory and endocrine function. As function of the kidneys is deeply impaired in CRF, endocrine abnormalities evoked by feedback mechanisms may be expected.

3. The kidneys are an important excretory (e.g. cortisol, aldosterone, catecholamine, thyroid hormones, sex hormones) and biodegradating organ of hormones (e.g. PTH, calcitonin, insulin and other polypeptide hormones). Impaired excretion and (or) biodegradation of hormones may influence their biosynthesis and secretion in their organs.

4. CRF causes significant alterations of the internal environment, which in turn may influence the secretory control of hormones (e.g. hyperkalaemia stimulates aldosterone and suppresses renin secretion), their transport, the amount of free and protein-bound hormone in blood plasma, transformation and degradation of hormones and the responsiveness of hormone receptors at the cellular or subcellular level.

5. CRF is characterized by a catabolic metabolic constellation which, per se, may influence the function of many endocrine organs.

6. Finally the type of dietary, pharmacological and dialytic treatment used in patients with CRF may influence the function of endocrine organs.

From the above it follows that endocrine abnormalities in patients with CRF should be related to the severity and duration of uraemia, as well as to the kind of medical and dietary treatment.

In patients with CRF some endocrine abnormalities are of clinical relevance. Among these are alterations of vitamin D, carbohydrate and lipid metabolism, secondary hyperparathyroidism, relative erythropoietin deficiency, suppression of gonadal function, diminished growth and abnormalities in blood pressure regulation.

Other endocrine abnormalities detectable by specific methods are of minor clinical consequences or their importance in the pathogenesis of the chronic uraemic syndrome is unknown or poorly clarified.

Endocrine abnormalities associated with chronic renal

failure have been reviewed recently (1–6). In this chapter only more recent papers or those which contributed most to our understanding of endocrine abnormalities in chronic renal failure are cited. A more comprehensive list of references may be found in our previous papers (5, 7).

RENAL HORMONES IN CHRONIC RENAL FAILURE

Erythropoietin

Erythropoietin is a heat-stable polypeptide with a molecular weight of approximately 34,000 daltons. The primary site of renal erythropoietin production (glomerulus, renal medulla, juxtaglomerular apparatus or tubular cell) is unknown. When there is inadequate renal erythropoietin, extrarenal erythropoietin production is markedly increased. Because erythropoietin stimulates all steps of erythropoiesis, e.g. transformation of pluripotent haematopoietic stem cells (CFU-S) to cells giving rise to burst-forming units – erythroid (BFU-E) and transformation of erythroid progenitor cells-colony forming units – erythroid (CFU-E) to mature erythrocytes, anaemia may be expected in patients with chronic renal failure. Relative deficiency of erythropoietin seems to be only one of several factors involved in the development of anaemia in chronic renal failure (8, 9). In fact anaemia can be detected in patients with CRF once the plasma creatinine level exceeds 318 μmol/l (3.8 mg/dl) and can be effectively treated by human erythropoietin derived from recombinant DNA (10). In patients with end-stage renal insufficiency serum erythropoietin levels are usually normal or sometimes even elevated (11, 12). The levels of erythropoietin are usually below those expected for the degree of anaemia, but above those of normal individuals (9). In contrast to normals patients with CRF do not manifest an increase in plasma erythropoietin levels in response to physiological stimuli such as anaemia and hypoxia (13). The nature of the underlying kidney disease as well as concomitant independent diseases may influence the erythropoietin level in patients with CRF. Patients with congenital (14) or acquired polycystic disease (15) very often have higher plasma erythropoietin levels than those with other types of renal diseases. It is to be stressed that only some dialysed patients with acquired cystic disease manifest raised haematocrit levels. In most patients with end-stage renal failure the presence of acquired cystic disease of the kidneys has no effect on the haemoglobin concentration (16). In patients with CRF and concomitant liver or heart disease plasma erythropoietin levels are usually higher than in patients with 'pure' renal failure (17–19). After bilateral nephrectomy plasma erythropoietin levels are very low (11), which supports the notion, that plasma erythropoietin in CRF is predominantly of renal origin. The presence of marked secondary hyperparathyroidism has a suppressive effect on the plasma erythropoietin level (20, 21). Haemodialysis treatment seems to increase plasma erythropoietin only in patients with polycystic kidney disease (14, 22). Patients treated by continuous ambulatory peritoneal dialy-

sis (CAPD) tend to have higher plasma erythropoietin levels than those undergoing haemodialysis (23). After successful renal transplantation the haemoglobin concentration returns to normal in the majority of patients and normal plasma erythropoietin levels are found (24, 25). In some successfully transplanted patients inappropriately high plasma erythropoietin levels and erythrocytosis may be found (24, 25). In these patients enhanced production of erythropoietin by the residual native kidney has been proved (25).

Active vitamin D metabolites

Before exerting its biological action on target organs, 25-hydroxyvitamin D (25-OH-D) must be converted primarily by the kidney either to 1α,25-dihydroxyvitamin D [1,25(OH)$_2$-D] or 24,25-dihydroxyvitamin D [24,25(OH)$_2$-D) by the respective hydroxylases (26, 27). Therefore alterations in 1,25(OH)$_2$-D and 24,25(OH)$_2$-D biosynthesis in patients with chronic renal failure are not surprising. Serum 25-OH-D levels are usually normal even in advanced renal failure or may be increased in patients treated by vitamin D (28). In contrast to 25-OH-D, serum concentrations of 1,25(OH)$_2$-D are usually severely decreased or undetectable in end-stage renal failure (29–31) while 24,25(OH)$_2$-D levels are low but always detectable (28–31). In patients treated with CAPD considerable losses of both 1,25(OH)$_2$-D and 24,25(OH)$_2$-D into peritoneal dialysate have been reported (30, 32). These losses lead to low serum levels of these active vitamin D metabolites in CAPD patients and may be an important factor in exacerbating renal osteodystrophy (30). Administration of vitamin D to patients with end-stage renal failure treated by CAPD leads to a significant increase of serum 24,25(OH)$_2$-D levels (31). The presence of detectable serum 1,25(OH)$_2$-D and low 24,25(OH)$_2$-D levels in most patients with end-stage renal failure suggests synthesis of these active metabolites in extrarenal sites (for review see references 28, 31, 33). From data obtained in the last few years it appears, that deficiency of 1,25(OH)$_2$-D in chronic uraemic patients may be involved in the pathogenesis of hormonal, myopathic, cutaneous, cardiovascular, haematologic and immune dysfunctions of chronic uraemia (for a review see reference 33). As deficiency of 1,25(OH)$_2$-D in uraemic patients is accompanied by excess secretion of parathyroid hormone (PTH), and this hormone has been incriminated as an uraemic toxin (34), it remains to be elucidated, which of the two pathogenetic pathways deficient 1,25(OH)$_2$-D biosynthesis or secondary hyperparathyroidism is predominantly involved in the genesis of multiorgan disturbances in uraemia.

Prostaglandins

Patients with kidney disease and glomerular filtration rates below 25 ml/min show significant decreases in urinary PGE$_2$ and PGF$_{2\alpha}$ excretion (35). The urinary excretion rate of these prostaglandins (PG) is markedly diminished in patients with end-stage renal failure treated by chronic dialysis (35, 36). In some patients with chronic renal failure, however, normal (3) or even increased (37–39) urinary excretion of PGA, PGE_2 and $PGF_{2\alpha}$ have also been observed. The pathogenesis of altered urinary prostaglandins in CRF is not entirely clear and seems to depend upon the mass of residual renal parenchyma (35). The type of renal pathology also seems to influence urinary PG excretion. For example in patients with CRF caused by systemic lupus erythematosis (40) or chronic ischaemia (41) urinary excretion of PGE_2 is markedly elevated. As administration of nonsteroidal anti-inflammatory drugs to humans with CRF results in acute deteriorioration of the residual excretory kidney function (42) it seems that increased production of endogenous prostaglandins may be necessary for the maintenance of compensated renal function in advanced renal failure, by exerting a cytoprotective, diuretic, natriuretic and vasodilatory effect (43).

During haemodialysis elevated plasma levels of the prostaglandin PGE and the prostacyclin (PGI_2) metabolite 6-keto-$PGF_{1\alpha}$ have been found (38). Because the pulmonary endothelium is rich in prostaglandins (44), and lung damage occurs during haemodialysis (45) participation of PGI_2 in the pathogenesis of such haemodialysis induced circulatory disturbances as hypotension, headache and nausea seems very likely. The administration of the nonspecific cyclo-oxygenase inhibitor, indomethacin, however, does not influence haemodialysis induced hypotension (38), which does not support that concept.

The renin-angiotensin system

Depending upon fluid and electrolyte balance plasma renin activity (PRA) in patients with end-stage renal failure may be low, normal or high (46–51). Renin secretion responds to dietary sodium restriction and upright position in most uraemic patients (47, 48). After haemodialysis PRA may increase, diminish or remain unchanged depending upon dialysis-induced alterations of fluid and electrolyte balance (49, 52). In some haemodialysis patients PRA is largely uninfluenced by changes in sodium balance, posture or reduction in extracellular fluid volume (52–54). The reason for this unresponsiveness of the renin-angiotensin system to secretory stimuli is unclear. Administration of captopril, which is a potent converting enzyme inhibitor, to uraemic patients uniformly suppresses plasma angiotensin II and aldosterone concentrations associated with an increase in renin release and a fall in blood pressure (50). This suggests intactness of the renin-angiotensin system in patients with CRF and its importance in the regulation of blood pressure. In only a minority of patients with CRF is hypertension resistant to fluid removal by dialysis but controllable after bilateral nephrectomy, which seems to indicate renin dependency (51). The fall in blood pressure following dialysis observed in patients with high PRA seems to depend not only on the renin-angiotensin system, but also on a decline of other vasopressor mechanisms (46).

Serum angiotensin-converting enzyme (ACE) is significantly elevated in patients with end-stage renal disease (55–57), although contradictory results have been published

on this topic (58). After haemodialysis ACE increases significantly. This increase seems to be due to complement-mediated sequestration of leukocytes in the pulmonary vasculature leading to injury of the vascular endothelium, which is rich in ACE, with consequent interstitial oedema and a decrease in arterial oxygen tension (55).

Kallikrein-kinin system

Recent studies suggest that the renal kallikrein-kinin system is involved in the regulation of electrolyte and water transport by the distal part of the nephron. These effects could be due to direct action of kinins on sodium transport in the distal nephron, to changes in renal blood flow distribution, or to both (59). Several lines of evidence suggest the presence of complex interactions among the kallikrein-kinin, renin-angiotensin-aldosterone, vasopressin and prostaglandin systems of the kidneys (59).

In dialyzed patients with acute (60, 61) and chronic renal failure (62) the absolute amount of urinary kallikrein, which is a marker of the activity of the renal kallikrein-kinin system, is markedly decreased, while kallikrein excretion calculated per unit of residual GFR is significantly increased. It seems that the increased kallikrein secretion by the distal part of the residual nephrons is involved in the pathomechanism of increased fractional sodium and water excretion in these patients.

In patients with a functioning kidney transplant urinary kallikrein is decreased (63) as compared with normals. This could be due to the diminished functional tubular mass of these patients. Contrary to previous results, urinary kallikrein (estimated by radioimmunoassay) is not elevated during episodes of kidney graft rejection (64).

FUNCTION OF OTHER ENDOCRINE ORGANS IN DIALYZED AND NONDIALYZED PATIENTS WITH END-STAGE RENAL FAILURE

Because of the roles of the kidney in effecting hormonal action, end eliminating hormones and the effect of uraemic plasma on hormonal secretion and activity, a variety of endocrine abnormalities occur in CRF.

PITUITARY GLAND

Somatotropin (STH)-somatomedin-axis

In patients with end-stage renal failure elevated basal STH levels (65–68) and an exaggerated response to stimulatory agents (66, 68, 69, and for review see references 1 and 70) are usually found. Enhanced somatotropin secretion is neither affected significantly by protein intake (69) nor by haemodialysis (67). After successful renal transplantation plasma STH levels are in the normal range (71). Because the half disappearance time (T 1/2) of STH is normal in end-stage renal failure (72) high plasma levels of this hormone seem to be caused primarily by hypersecretion rather than by impaired renal clearance. Suppression of STH secretion after blockade of opioid receptors by naloxone (65) may suggest involvement of these receptors in the pathogenesis of elevated STH plasma levels. Despite intensive studies both the exact mechanism of abnormally elevated STH plasma levels and their pathophysiological importance remain to be elucidated. It can not be excluded that hypersecretion of STH is involved in the pathogenesis of carbohydrate intolerance and increased lipolysis encountered in CRF (for review see references 1, 2). As STH exerts a stimulatory effect on intestinal calcium absorption and on $1,25(OH)_2$-D biosynthesis (73, 74) increased STH secretion in CRF could be regarded as a purposeful mechanism counteracting the hypocalcaemia usually present in CRF.

As is well known, growth hormone acts peripherally stimulating synthesis of somatomedins by different organs, predominantly by the liver. Depending upon the technique of measurement (bioassay, radioreceptor assay or radioimmunoassay), differing levels of somatomedins have been reported in CRF. Bioassayable somatomedin levels are low in patients with end-stage renal failure (71, 75, 76). When using radioreceptor assay (77) or radioimmunoassays (76, 78, for review see reference 79) normal or elevated somatomedin levels have been reported. Using a specific radioimmunoassay for somatomedin I (IGF I) and a specific radioreceptor assay for somatomedin II (IGF II) suppressed plasma levels of IGF I and elevated concentrations of IGF II were noted in uraemic patients (80). Simultaneously an increased binding of somatomedins by uraemic serum was found (80). Finally an apparent small molecule has been found in the serum of uraemic patients that inhibits somatomedin (81, 82). These data suggest, that elevated somatomedin levels in uraemic serum may be due to enhanced protein binding and the presence of an somatomedin inhibitor.

Growth failure in uraemic children seems to be confounded by nutrional, metabolic and hormonal disturbances.

Prolactin

Hyperprolactinaemia is a frequent endocrine abnormality in patients with end-stage renal failure whether treated by haemodialysis or not (83–88 for review see reference 1). Although the kidneys are the main site of prolactin elimination (89), decreased renal biodegradation does not seem to be the main factor responsible for increased plasma prolactin levels. It seems, that hyperprolactinaemia associated with CRF is in part due to a decreased prolactin metabolic clearance rate, but is primarily caused by an increase in prolactin secretion (4). As hyperprolactinaemia in patients with CRF is suppressed by naloxone (88) it seems that opioid receptors may be involved in the mechanism of abnormally elevated prolactin levels in patients with CRF. After LH-RH administration a paradoxical increase of plasma prolactin levels can be noted (88). Because no correlation between plasma prolactin and PTH levels were observed (90) in CRF participation of enhanced PTH secretion in the pathogenesis of hyperprolactinaemia associated with

uraemia seems unlikely. Diminished responsiveness of prolactinaemia to both suppressive as well as stimulatory agents (83, 84, 86, 87) suggests a primary pituitary disorder involving either receptor binding or postreceptor phenomena, although the presence of a concomitant defect either in the hypothalamus or elsewhere in the central nervous system cannot be excluded. Haemodialysis treatment does not influence significantly the magnitude of hyperprolactinaemia (84). After successful renal transplantation normalization of prolactinaemia is observed (83, 84, 87).

The pathophysiological importance of hyperprolactinaemia in CRF is not clear. Hyperprolactinaemia may be involved in the pathogenesis of uraemic hypogonadism, and gynecomastia (for review see references 1, 2). As prolactin is a stimulant of $1,25(OH)_2$-D biosynthesis (91), hyperprolactinaemia could be a purposeful mechanism indirectly counteracting hypocalcaemia in CRF.

ACTH-cortisol axis

In patients with end-stage CRF plasma ACTH levels are most often normal or slightly increased (for review see reference 92).

Most data available in the literature confirm the intactness of the pituitary-adrenal feedback in CRF (93 for review see references 6, 70, 92), although abnormal function of the ACTH-cortisol axis has also been reported (94). Blockade of opioid receptors by naloxone is usually followed by an increased responsiveness of hypoglycaemia induced ACTH secretion (65).

Both in dialyzed and nondialyzed patients with CRF plasma cortisol levels are most often in the normal range (3, 93, 95–99). although elevated values have also been reported (94, 100, 101). The t 1/2 value of cortisol is usually prolonged as compared with normals (96). During haemodialysis plasma cortisol levels are not significantly changed (3, 94, 102) or show a tendency to fall at the beginning (99) or to rise at the end of the dialysis session (102). The decline of plasma cortisol at the beginning of haemodialysis seems to be evoked by transfer of free hormone into the dialysate (99, 103). This initial decline of plasma cortisol triggers ACTH secretion which explain the increase of cortisolaemia at the end of the dialysis session (99, 103). As may be expected dialysis treatment is followed by an abnormal diurnal pattern of cortisol secretion (102).

Pituitary-thyroid axis

The kidneys are an important organ of iodide elimination and of thyroid hormone biodegradation. Thus alterations of plasma TSH, iodide and thyroid hormones may be expected in patients with CRF (for review see references 104, 105). The magnitude of these alterations seems to be related to the degree of kidney failure (106). High plasma inorganic iodide levels are found in CRF despite increased extrarenal iodide elimination (107, 108). Iodine uptake by the thyroid gland is usually increased but incorporation of iodine into tyrosine and biosynthesis of active thyroid hormones are suppressed

(108). In haemodialyzed patients thyroidal iodine content is high, despite lower concentrations of active thyroid hormones in peripheral blood (109).

Plasma concentrations of thyroid hormones depend both on the degree of compromised excretory renal function (106) and the duration and type of dialysis treatment (110). In patients with CRF the plasma total thyroxine (TT_4) level is usually low (111, 112) but rarely is normal (113), while plasma free T_4 level (FT_4) is typically normal (104, 113). After long-term treatment by haemodialysis or haemofiltration plasma TT_4 levels tend to decline. Total triiodothyronine (TT_3) levels are usually in the low normal range irrespective of the type of dialysis treatment (104, 109, 113), while free T_3 concentrations are normal (113). This suggests altered conversion of T_4 to T_3 (109). Despite diminished conversion of T_4 to T_3 the total turnover rate of T_4 and 5-deiodination of T_4 to T_3 are normal in uraemic patients (104, 105, 109), which explains their normal total reverse T_3 (rT_3) levels (104). Plasma thyroxine binding globulin (TBG) levels are also normal in uraemic patients (112). In patients treated by CAPD or with the nephrotic syndrome plasma TBG levels may show a tendency to decline, however (114). After long-term treatment by a low protein, low phosphorus diet supplemented with essential amino acids and ketoanalogues a significant increase of total T_3 and T_4 and of their free fractions has been noted (115).

In spite of altered total plasma T_4 and T_3 levels the concentrations of TSH is most often normal both in haemodialyzed patients and in patients on CAPD (113, 116, 117). In contrast, a delayed or blunted response of TSH secretion to TRH may be found in patients with CRF irrespective of which type of dialysis treatment is used (70, 118, 119). These results contrast with those in which an abnormal TRH-TSH relationship was noted (120). Heparin which is used during haemodialysis, may displace T_4 from carrier proteins and cause of tachycardia or cardiac arrhythmia or both (70).

The alterations in plasma thyroid hormones described above are often accompanied by a significant increase of the thyroid gland volume (117). The exact reason of this increase of the thyroid volume is unknown. Among potential pathogenetic factors are increased iodine trapping by the thyroid gland (107) and the presence of strumigenic substances in uraemic plasma (117).

The pathophysiological importance of the above mentioned hormone abnormalitis is unknown. Signs of tissue hypothyroidism have been noted in only a few cases of CRF (109).

After successful renal transplantation normalization of all endocrine thyroid indices may be observed (121). In some transplanted patients elevated plasma TT_3 levels have even been noted (121).

In children treated by haemodialysis or by CAPD alterations of plasma thyroid hormones are similar to those seen in adults (122).

Hyperthyroidism is rarely found in dialyzed patients (123). The diagnosis of hyperthyroidism in uraemic patients is difficult due to similar signs and symptoms in these two pathological states.

Table 1 lists the most common abnormalities in plasma thyroid hormones in patients with CRF.

Pituitary gonadal axis

Abnormalities in sexual function are very frequent both in female and male patients with advanced renal failure. They are partially due to dysfunction of the hypothalamic-pituitary-gonadal axis (for review see references 1, 2, 124).

Pituitary-gonadal axis in men

In male patients with CRF basal plasma luteinizing hormone (LH) levels are usually markedly elevated (125–133). After administration of LH-releasing hormone (LH-RH), a subnormal, normal or even exaggerated response of plasma LH (126, 127, 130, 134 for review see reference 1) may be observed. Simultaneous administration of LH-RH with the opiate receptor blocker naloxone is followed by a significantly higher LH secretion than after LH-RH alone (134).

Basal plasma levels of follicle stimulating hormone (FSH) are most often elevated (125–130) in men with CRF al-

Table 1. Behaviour of indices of the pituitary-thyroid axis in patients with chronic renal failure on medical, haemodialysis and peritoneal dialysis treatment.

Plasma level		Medical management	Haemodialysis	Peritoneal dialysis
T_4	Total	Decreased or normal	Decreased or normal	Decreased
	Free	Normal	Normal	Normal or decreased
T_3	Total	Decreased	Decreased	Decreased
	Free	Decreased	Decreased	Decreased
rT_3	Total	Normal	Normal	Normal
	Free	Increased	Increased	Increased or normal
TSH	Basal	Normal	Normal	Normal
	after TRH administration	Blunted	Blunted	Blunted
TBG		Normal	Normal	Normal

though normal or even depressed concentrations have also been reported (for review see references 1, 70). After administration of LH-RH or clomiphene, a normal (1) or blunted (134) response of FSH secretion may be found. In hyporesponsive male patients administration of naloxone restores a normal FSH secretion pattern to LH-RH (134).

Chronic renal insufficiency is characterized by significantly depressed basal plasma testoterone levels in both sexes (125, 126, 128–130) and blunted or delayed response to human chorionic gonadotropin (HCG) (127) or LH-RH (134). Blocking opiate receptors by naloxone is usually followed by improvement of LH-RH-induced testosterone secretion (134). After long term treatment by a low protein, low phosphorus diet supplemented with essential amino acids and ketoanalogues restoration of blood levels of testosterone in male uraemic patients was noted (135).

Pituitary-gonadal axis in women

In female patients with CRF at the reproductive age predominantly normal or elevated LH levels have been reported (136). After administration of clomiphene a significant increase of plasma LH may be observed. In contrast, exogenous estrogens do not influence plasma LH levels which suggests the existence of a malfunctioning hypothalamic-pituitary-gonadal feedback (for review see references 1, 70).

In uraemic women within the reproductive age group normal or slightly elevated (136) but occasionally suppressed basal plasma FSH levels are found with a normal responsiveness to LH-RH or clomiphene respectively (for review see references 1, 70). In contrast to normal women, female patients with CRF do not show the normal cyclical changes in gonadotropin levels (136).

Ovarian function is also abnormal in women with end-stage renal failure. Plasma estrogens and progesterone usually are low (136). After administration of clomiphene, which stimulates gonadotropin secretion, no increase of plasma estrogen can be noted (136). This observation suggests ovarian resistance to the stimulatory action of gonadotropins.

Pathophysiological importance of pituitary-gonadal abnormalities in uraemic patients

From the above it follows that CRF is characterized by disturbances of gonadotropin, testosterone, estrogen and progesterone secretion. The presence of elevated plasma LH and FSH levels does not seem to be caused, or at least not exclusively, by suppressed renal clearance but rather is attributed to enhanced secretion of these hormones. Increased secretion of LH and FSH seems to be evidence of a persistently operative hypothalamic-pituitary-gonadal feedback triggered by primary gonadal dysfunction. In turn, the pathogenesis of gonadal dysfunction seems to be complex and multifactorial. Several lines of evidence suggest that secondary hyperparathyroidism, hyperendorphinism, hypersecretion of prolactin, deficiency of trace elements such as zinc, and unidentified uraemic toxins may be involved

(Figure 1) in the pathogenesis of the hormonal abnormalities of the hypothalamic-pituitary-gonadal axis in CRF (for review see references 124, 137). These hormonal abnormalities together with disturbances in the central and peripheral nervous system, i.e. uraemic encephalopathy and neuropathy, seem to be critical factors in the pathogenesis of uraemic hypogonadism. Parlodel treatment can improve sexual function and spermatogenesis in hypogonadal uraemic males (138). Hence, dysfunction of the hypothalamic-pituitary-gonadal axis in chronic renal failure seems to be due not only to the failing biodegrading and excretory function of the kidneys and compensatory mechanisms secondary to uraemia, but also to the altered internal environment, nutritional factors and organic alterations of the endocrine system.

Vasopressin

The kidneys are both the major target organ for vasopressin (AVP) and major site of metabolism of this peptide (139, 140). On the other hand, disturbances of fluid volume and tonicity are cardinal features of the uraemic syndrome. Hence, altered plasma AVP levels and metabolism are anticipated in patients with CRF. However, relatively few papers (139, 141–149) define the role, fate and regulation of antidiuretic hormone in patients with CRF. These reports suggest that plasma AVP is elevated in the majority of subjects with CRF (142, 145, 146, 149, 150). The elevated levels of AVP in CRF may be explained by abnormal volumetric or osmotic regulation of AVP secretion or both.

The metabolic clearance of synthetic AVP is significantly lower in uraemic patients on haemodialysis than in normal controls (140). The increase of plasma AVP level does not prove the presence of a physiological release of AVP to hyperosmolarity of plasma in patients with CRF. Results obtained in some studies showed the absence of a direct correlation between plasma osmolality and AVP in patients with CRF (145, 147) while in other studies such a correlation was found (142, 147, 148). Moreover, a positive correlation between blood pressure and plasma AVP levels before dialysis has been observed in patients with CRF (142) and recently such a correlation has been confirmed (147). Variability in salt and fluid intake, type of dialyzer and membranes and composition of the dialysis fluid may result in different influences, on AVP secretion explaining the often conflicting results obtained in patients with end-stage renal failure. For example while some authors found resistance of the uraemic patients AVP response to the stimulatory effect of volume contraction (151) others observed an increase in plasma AVP in uraemic patients undergoing volume contraction by ultrafiltration (146). In patients with CRF administration of physiological doses of angiotensin II (A II) have no stimulatory effect on AVP secretion (152). After blockade of the converting enzyme by captopril the volumetric regulation of AVP secretion is markedly blunted (153). In contrast to normals, calcium infusion is followed by an increase of AVP secretion (154). This increase seems to be mediated by parathyroid hormone (154).

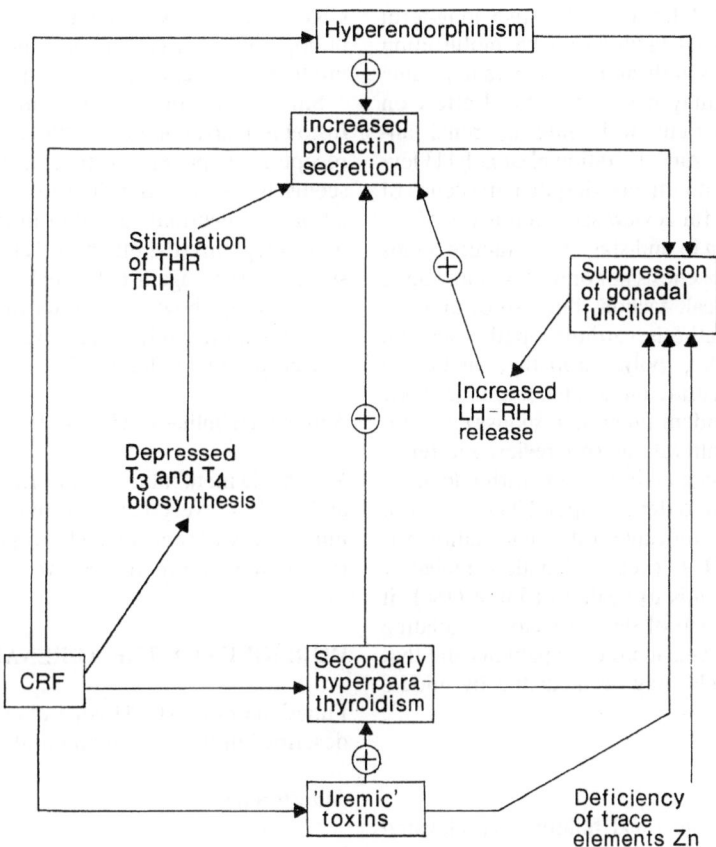

Figure 1. Relationship of different endocrine abnormalities in the pathogenesis of gonadal hypofunction in uraemic patients. CRF = chronic renal failure.

High levels of plasma AVP may decrease to normal after dialysis (147). Recent studies have shown that this post-dialytic fall of plasma AVP is caused by the transfer of this hormone through the dialyzing membrane into the dialysate (148). Summarizing, it seems that elevated plasma AVP levels in patients with CRF are caused by reduced renal clearance of this hormone, or by abnormalities in the volumetric and/or osmotic regulation of AVP secretion or both. After successful renal transplantation elevated plasma AVP levels usually decline to normal values (155).

HORMONES INVOLVED IN CALCIUM-PHOSPHATE METABOLISM

Parathyroid hormone (PTH)

Secondary hyperparathyroidism is a well known complication of CRF. Hypersecretion of PTH relates inversely to the glomerular filtration rate. Several factors seem involved in the pathogenesis of secondary hyperparathyroidism in patients with CRF. Among them are a decrease in the synthesis of 1,25-dihydroxycholecalciferol (156–158), skeletal resistance to the calcaemic action of PTH (159) phosphate retention (160, 161), elevated set point for calcium, regu-

lated PTH secretion (162) and impaired degradation of PTH by the decreased renal parenchyma (163). Contrary to previous opinions, hypocalcaemia may not be essential for the development of secondary hyperparathyroidism in CRF (164). After blockade of opioid receptors with naloxone the suppressive effect of calcium infusion on PTH secretion is significantly diminished (165). This suggests participation of opioid receptors in the pathogenesis of secondary hyperparathyroidism in end-stage renal failure.

The magnitude of secondary hyperparathyroidism is especially marked in patients with analgesic abuse nephropathy (166). Long-term administration of vitamin D of its active metabolites (167–173), of ketoacids (169, 171, 174), of a low phosphorus diet (169) and of aluminium hydroxide (172) has a suppressive effect on secondary hyperparathyroidism in chronic uraemia. No convincing effect of H_2-receptor blockade on the parathyroid status in uraemic man can be detected (175). Plasma PTH levels correlate positively with calcitonin levels (176) although other authors could not confirm such a correlation (177). PTH levels most often do not strictly correlate with the extent of bone abnormalities in patients with chronic renal failure (176, 178, 179 – see Chapter 44).

Long-term haemodialysis treatment using dialysis fluid with a high calcium concentration (2 mmol/l) has a suppressive effect on plasma PTH levels (180). Also long-term treatment of end-stage renal failure with haemofiltration (181) or CAPD (182, 183) significantly decreases in plasma PTH concentrations and may have a beneficial effect on renal osteodystrophy in patients with end-stage renal failure. After successful renal transplantation plasma PTH levels return to normal in most patients, despite persistence of bone alteration (179, 184, for review see reference 185).

Excessive PTH secretion in end-stage renal failure seems to be involved in the pathogenesis not only of uraemic bone disease and extraosseous calcifactions but also of uraemic anaemia, haemorrhagic diathesis, cardiomyopathy, skeletal myopathy, encephalopathy, polyneuropathy, metabolic (hyperlipidaemia, carbohydrate intolerance), immunologic (suppressed cellular dependent immune response) and endocrine (hypogonadism) alterations (for review see reference 137). Hyperprolactinaemia in patients with end-stage renal failure does not seem to depend upon PTH secretion, however (90). Because a significant positive correlation was found between plasma PTH levels and middle molecule fraction 2, which corresponds to peak 7 of Fürst (186), it seems likely that PTH is one of several factors regulating plasma middle molecule levels in uraemic patients and that some 'toxic' effects of PTH may be mediated by middle molecules.

Calcitonin

Most patients with end-stage renal failure have elevated plasma calcitonin concentrations (65, 176, 177, 187–190, for review see reference 92). Long-term administration of vitamin D or its metabolites is followed by an increase of calcitoninaemia in end-stage renal failure (167). Patients receiving CAPD show significantly lower calcitonin levels than patients on haemodialysis treatment (187). This may be caused by a significant loss of calcitonin into the peritoneal dialysate. Also haemoperfusion is followed by a suppression of plasma calcitonin caused by effective removal of this hormone by the charcoal column (191). After successful renal transplantation plasma calcitonin levels return to normal within few days when glomerular filtration improves, rising again during rejection episodes (189). Other authors reported only transitory decreases of calcitonin levels after renal transplantation (190).

Hypercalcitoninaemia in chronic uraemia may be due to accumulation or increased secretion or both. As the kidneys are one of the main organs degrading calcitonin (192) diminished destruction of this hormone by the failing kidneys could contribute to the increased concentrations of plasma calcitonin in patients with CRF. The absence of a significant correlation between serum calcitonin and serum creatinine concentrations (as an index of functionally active renal parenchyma) (187) seems to indicate, that decreased extraction and destruction of calcitonin by the kidneys are not the main or the only cause of hypercalcitoninaemia in patients with CRF. Participation of stimulatory agents of calcitonin secretion such as phosphates (193) or enterohormones (188) in the pathogenesis of hypercalcitoninaemia in patients with

CRF can not be excluded. Finally structurally abnormal but biologically inactive calcitonin molecules could also contribute to hypercalcitoninaemia in patients with CRF.

Since stimulation of calcitonin secretion by calcium infusion is nearly completely blunted after blockade of opioid receptors in patients with end-stage renal failure (65) it seems that hyperendorphinism, may be involved in the regulation of calcitonin secretion in these patients. Calcitonin may antagonize the effect of PTH and may thereby protect skeletal tissue against the reabsorptive action of PTH. A recent study, however, shows that endogenous calcitonin does not appreciably protect against hyperparathyroid bone disease in renal failure (177).

Active metabolites of vitamin D

Vitamin D metabolites play a critical role in mineral balance and the low levels that occur in uraemic patients contribute importantly to renal osteodystrophy as discussed in the section on renal hormones, above.

HORMONES OF THE ADRENAL CORTEX

Function of the ACTH-cortisol axis in patients with CRF is described in the section on pituitary abnormalities, above.

Aldosterone

Depending upon the water-electrolyte and acid-base status of uraemic patients, plasma aldosterone levels may be subnormal, normal or even extremely elevated. After successful renal transplantation plasma aldosterone levels are in the normal range (personal unpublished data, for review see references 70, 92 and 194). Plasma aldosterone levels seem to depend not only on the degree of hydration, and the plasma levels of hydrogen, sodium, potassium and magnesium, but also on the electrolyte composition of the dialysate and the administration of heparin during the dialysis (for review see references 70, 92). Before dialysis aldosterone secretion relates more closely to the activity of the renin-angiotensin system and to fluid and electrolyte balance than it does in dialyzed patients (194–199). Dialysis treatment abolishes the diurnal rhythm of aldosterone secretion (200, 201) and dissociates the relationship between the renin-angiotensin system and aldosterone secretion (47, 48). Increased plasma aldosterone levels observed in some uraemic patients function as a purposeful mechanism counteracting hyperpotassaemia by activation of extrenal potassium excretion (195, 198). Because heparin suppresses biosynthesis of steroids in the adrenal glands, drug-induced hypoaldosteronism may develop in some dialyzed patients.

Catecholamines

Plasma concentrations of catecholamines (CA) are usually elevated in patients with chronic renal failure (202, 203). Similarly basal norepinephrine (NE) levels in uraemic predialysis patients are significantly higher than in normals (203). In the upright posture a significantly greater rise in plasma NE levels occurs in patients with CRF than is observed in healthy subjects (203). The results of estimations of plasma levels in patients on maintenance haemodialysis are variable. Statistically significantly elevated levels of free dopamine (DA) and free NE, but normal levels of free epinephrine (EN) have been found in haemodialyzed patients (204). However careful analysis of data obtained in haemodialyzed patients revealed subgroups with either high, normal or low plasma free NE concentrations (204). This concentration heterogeneity could explain conflicting results and conclusions provided by previous reports (205, 206). Significantly elevated plasma levels of sulfo-conjugated CA and glucuro-conjugated EN, but normal concentrations of glucuro-conjugated DA and NE were noted in patients on maintenance haemodialysis treatment (204). Free tyrosine and sulfo-conjugated CA are effectively eliminated by the artificial kidney but glucuro-conjugated amines are not (204). Haemodialysis induced losses of tyrosine are about 200 fold greater than those of CA (204). Thus haemodialysis may effect CA synthesis by reducing the amount of available tyrosine, which is the precursor of CA. Despite considerable removal of tyrosine by the procedure, a 2 h haemodialysis does not influence the concentrations of tyrosine and free CA in arterial blood, suggesting large pools or rapid turnover, while DA sulfate and NE sulfate levels decline significantly (204).

The mechanisms responsible for the elevation in plasma levels of CA seem to be multiple, i.e. decreased renal clearance, diminished degradation of CA due to reduced catechol-O-methyl transferase, decrease in the neuronal uptake of NE, and increase in sympathetic nervous system activity caused by reduced baroreceptor sensitivity or by reduced end-organ response to NE (for review see references 202, 203).

The pathophysiologic significance of the abnormalities in plasma catecholamine concentrations in uraemia is not clear. Alterations of plasma CA concentrations as markers of sympathetic nervous system activity must be used with great caution in patients with end-stage renal failure due to the complex metabolic derangements in these patients (207). Participation of elevated CA levels in the pathogenesis of arterial hypertension in uraemic patients is likely (208). But it can not be excluded that elevated levels of CA are compensatory to a reduced pressor response to NE in uraemic patients (203). Secondary hyperparathyroidism is incriminated as one of the main factors responsible for reduced vasopressor responsiveness to CA (34).

HORMONES OF THE PANCREAS

Insulin

In patients with chronic renal failure hyperinsulinism has been observed by several authors (3, 209–211, for review see references 2, 5). After administration of glucose an exaggerated response of insulin secretion can usually be noted (209, 212). Despite increased plasma levels of insulin, carbohydrate intolerance may be present in uraemic patients. The pathogenesis of this metabolic abnormality is not entirely clear. Decreased cellular sensitivity to insulin (213), intracellular deficiency of potassium, metabolic acidosis, increased retention of magnesium, suppressed glucose utilization by peripheral tissues (214) and increase levels of hormones antagonizing the effects of insulin, i.e. somatotropin, glucagon, or secondary hyperparathyroidism, all seem to be involved in the pathogenesis of this metabolic abnormality (for review see references 5, 137, 209, 215). It can not be excluded that an increased secretion of biologically less acitive proinsulin may account for hyperinsulinaemia in patients with CRF (216).

Tissue resistance to insulin in chronic renal failure is especially marked in striated muscles (217), while fat tissue is normally responsive (for review see references 5 and 215).

Last but not least suppressed renal clearance of insulin by the residual renal parenchyma may be involved in the pathogenesis of hyperinsulinaemia in chronic uraemia (215).

After long-term haemodialysis treatment carbohydrate intolerance usually subsides, as a result of improved tissue sensitivity to insulin (209, 212, 218). Studies in patients treated by CAPD have reported both a deterioriation in glucose tolerance with a concomitant suppression of initially increased insulin secretion (219) as well as unchanged glucose tolerance (220) during CAPD. Recent results obtained in CAPD patients have shown that dialysate exchanges with 1.5% dextrose monohydrate solution had no effect on plasma insulin (221). In contrast, the 4.25% solution had a noticeable effect on plasma glucose concentration during the first 2 h. The rise in glucose was also paralleled by a marked insulin secretion in these CAPD patients (221).

Hyperinsulinism is also considered to be involved in the pathogenesis of hypertriglyceridaemia in uraemic patients (2).

Glucagon

Plasma glucagon levels are regularly increased in CRF and inversely correlated with residual creatinine clearance (211, 220, 222, for review see references 3 and 5). Glucagon secretion in advanced renal failure is responsive both to stimulatory and inhibitory factors (223). The elevated plasma levels of glucagon seems to be the consequence predominantly of a decreased metabolic turnover rate, and to a lesser degree to enhanced glucagon secretion (223). In patients on regular haemodialysis treatment similar plasma glucagon levels are found as in those not dialyzed. A single haemodialysis session usually does not significantly influence plasma glucagon levels (3, 222). In CAPD patients treated with dialysis fluid containing 4.25% dextrose (but not 1.5% dextrose solution) initial suppression of plasma glucagon was noted (221) similar to that found in both dialysed and nondialysed uraemic patients after an oral glucose tolerance test. In nondialyzed uraemic patients intravenous administration of exogenous glucagon is followed by a three to four fold greater hyperglycaemic effect than in dialyzed patients (224). After successful renal transplantation plasma glucagon levels are normal (225).

The pathophysiologic importance of increased glucagonaemia in CRF is not clear. Its role in the pathogenesis of carbohydrate intolerance in uraemic patients is questionable. After haemodialysis carbohydrate tolerance improves while plasma glucagon levels remain unchanged. This may be explained by the fact that elevated plasma levels of glucagon in CFR are mainly composed of a molecules of over 9,000 daltons, which are biologically inactive or less active than the physiological glucagon molecule of 3,485 daltons (5).

GASTROINTESTINAL HORMONES

Gastrointestinal disturbances such as anorexia, vomiting, haemorhages, erosions, gastritis and possibly peptic ulcer are very often found in patients with chronic renal failure (226). Some of these symptoms seem to be caused by abnormal secretion of gastrointestinal hormones influencing the motor and secretory function of the stomach, and intestine.

Gastrin

Hypergastrinaemia is present both in nondialyzed and dialyzed patients with chronic renal failure (188, 226–229). Serum gastrin levels usually correlate positively with plasma creatinine levels and are independent of the type of renal disease (226, 230, 231). Some authors, however, have not found any correlation between these two solute concentrations (227, 232, 233). Several authors found a strict correlation between the magnitude of atrophic mucosal changes in the stomach and the degree of hypergastrinaemia. Because the kidneys are the main sites of gastrin biodegradation and clearance (224), hypergastrinaemia is regarded as the consequence of reduced renal degradation of this hormone. Hypergastrinaemia in CRF may also be caused by overproduction of this hormone induced by hypo- or achlorhydria which is present in most patients with CRF (226). Finally, secondary hyperparathyroidism (235) and resistance of the gastric mucosa to gastrin (227) are believed to be involved in the pathogenesis of hypergastrinaemia in CRF. Depite the existence of hyperparathyroidism, the incidence of gastric ulcer in CRF and in primary hyperparathyroidism does not seem to be increased (233). Also no correlation between plasma gastrin and PTH levels has been found (226). Hypergastrinaemia in CRF is caused predominantly by big gastrin (G 34) molecules (227, 236) which are biologically six to eight times less active than little gastrin (G 17). In contrast, plasma levels of G 17 in CRF are comparable with those in normals (227). This may explain a 'normal' incidence of gastric ulcer in patients with CRF. These findings are in contrast to those of other authors, who observed hyperchlorhydria and an increased incidence of gastric ulcers in patients with CRF (237).

Long-term haemodialysis treatment most often does not influence elevated gastrin levels in patients with CRF (226, 238), although in some studies a decline in gastrinaemia was observed (227). Only trace amounts of gastrin could be detected in the dialysate (227). After successful renal transplantation plasma gastrin levels are normal (238–241), increasing markedly during rejection episodes (239).

Cholecystokinin

In patients with chronic renal failure plasma cholecystokinin levels are usually several times higher than in healthy subjects (242, 243). The pathophysiological importance of this finding is unknown.

Gastric inhibitory peptide (GIP)

Plasma GIP levels in patients with CRF are extremely elevated (231, 232, 242). This is mainly due to suppressed degradation and elimination of this hormone by the failing kidneys (232). The pathogenetic role of GIP, which seems to antagonize the action of gastrin on the gastric mucosa and cause hypo- or achlorhydria in patients with CRF (227) is not exactly known. After haemodialysis both an increase (231) and decline (232) of plasma GIP concentrations have been noted.

Pancreatic polypeptide (PP)

In chronic renal failure basal plasma PP levels are markedly elevated (211, 232, 244, 245). After administration of a test meal, a significant and prolonged increase in plasma PP levels has been observed (211). It remains to be elucidated whether increased plasma PP levels in CRF are caused by the decreased capability of the residual renal parenchyma to eliminate or degrade this hormone, or by an increased secretion of this polypeptide or both.

Other gastrointestinal hormones

In contrast to gastrin and pancreatic polypeptide, plasma levels of somatostatin and neurotensin are normal (232) in patients with CRF, while that of motilin is moderately increased (232). Both normal (232) and substantially elevated (245) levels of vasoactive intestinal polypeptide (VIP) have been reported in patients with CRF. Increased plasma VIP levels seem to be due not only to decreased renal and hepatic biodegradation but also to increased neuronal release, especially in the splanchnic system (246). The presence of normal plasma levels of stomatostatin and neurotensin and sometimes also normal levels of VIP seems to prove the existence of extra-renal sites of biodegradation of these hormones. No influence of haemodialysis on plasma VIP, somatostatin, motilin and neurotensin has been noted (232).

Basal plasma concentrations of secretin are significantly increased in both predialysis and dialysis (haemodialysis or CAPD) patients with CRF as compared to normals (243).

ATRIAL NATRIURETIC PEPTIDE

The atrial natriuretic peptide (ANP) is a potent diuretic, natriuretic and smooth muscle relaxing hormone, and is involved in the regulation of extracellular fluid volume, electrolyte balance and vascular tone (for review see references 247, 248). In patients with end-stage renal failure before haemodialysis or haemofiltration markedly elevated plasma ANP levels, two to four times higher values than in normals are found (249–251).

During isovolemic haemofiltration ANP levels do not change, yet ANP can be detected in haemofiltrates (249). After effective reduction of volume overload by haemodialysis or haemofiltration (249–251) ANP levels significantly decline. From data obtained in dialyzed or haemofiltered patients it follows that plasma ANP levels can be regarded as a sensitive indicator of fluid overload in uraemic patients (249–251). Experimental data indicate that ANP serves the purpose of effecting rapid adjustments to large alterations in circulating fluid volume (252) and that enhanced ANP secretion may play an important role in promoting the adaptive increase in sodium excretion per nephron observed in chronic renal failure (253).

ENDOGENOUS DIGITALIS-LIKE FACTORS

Endogenous inhibitors of the sodium pump have been implicated in the physiologic adaptation to chronic renal failure (for review see references 254, 255). In contrast to the atrial natriuretic peptide (ANP), Na^+, K^+-ATPase inhibitory activity is normal (256) or even low (257) in dialysis patients, but is increased in hypertensive patients with moderate renal insufficiency (256). During dialysis a significant rise in plasma Na^+, K^+-ATPase inhibitory activity can be observed (256). This increase is caused predominantly by a rise of fractions EI_1 and EI_3 of this inhibitor (256). Hence, haemodialysis may acutely raise plasma levels of Na^+, K^+-ATPase inhibitory activity, while long-term dialysis returns them to the normal range (256). The pathophysiologic importance of the presence of endogenous digitalis-like factors in chronic renal failure is not clear (258). It remains to be elucidated whether these factors are involved in the pathogenesis of hypertension and the adaptive increase in urinary sodium excretion per nephron in uraemic patients (258, 259).

OTHER HORMONES

In contrast to ACTH levels, which are normal or slightly elevated in CRF (see hormones of the ACTH-cortisol axis) other pituitary corticotrophic hormones, such as beta and gamma lipotropins are significantly elevated (260–262). Impaired clearance of β-lipotropins seems to be the major cause of the elevated plasma levels in dialyzed and non-dialyzed patients with end-stage chronic renal failure (262).

Plasma [Met]-enkephalin levels are markedly elevated in uraemic patients (263, 264) and directly correlated with plasma creatinine and urea concentrations (264). In contrast, plasma [Leu]-enkephalin levels are significantly lower in uraemic patients than in normals (264). After haemodialysis or haemofiltration a slight but statistically significant decline of plasma [Met]-enkephalin levels was noted, but no changes in [Leu]-enkephalin levels occurred (264). Plasma levels of [Met]-enkephalin estimated between haemodialysis or haemofiltration sessions are usually four times higher than in normals (264). These data (264, 265) as well as results obtained in our laboratory (65) suggest the presence of hyperendorphinism in uraemic patients with important pathophysiological consequences, participation in the pathogenesis of endocrine abnormalities and dysfunction of the autonomic nervous system.

Oxytocin levels are elevated in uraemic patients undergoing haemodialysis or CAPD (266).

SUMMARY

Endocrine alterations found in end-stage renal failure are caused mainly by 1) change of control of secretion, transport, peripheral transformation or binding to target cells of hormones and 2) impaired function of the kidneys as an endocrine, excretory and biodegrading organ of hormones as well as the most important organ involved in the maintenance of a stable internal environment. Among endocrine abnormalities, which are of clinical relevance, deficiency of erythropoietin $1,25(OH)_2$-D and gonadal hormones (testosterone and estrogens), hypersecretion of PTH, prolactin and endorphins and the presence of somatomedin inhibitors are notable. Other hormonal alterations, although present, contribute less to the pathogenesis of the chronic uraemic syndrome. All available types of dialysis therapy (haemodialysis, haemofiltration, peritoneal dialysis) exert minimal or no 'corrective' influence on endocrine alterations. Most of these alterations, but not all, are normalized after successful renal transplantation.

REFERENCES

1. Osten B, Kokot F, Klinkmann H: Endokrinologische Störungen bei chronischer Niereninsuffizienz und bei Dauerdialysebehandlung. Teil 1. Renale Hormone-Hypophyse. (Endocrine disorders in chronic renal failure and long-term dialysis treatment. Part I. Renal-hypophyseal hormones.) *Dtsch Gesundh-Wesen* 37: 2113, 1982
2. Osten B, Kokot F, Klinkmann H: Endokrinologische Störungen bei chronischer Niereninsuffizienz und bei Dauerdialysebehandlung. Teil 2. Schilddrüse-Nebenschilddrüse-Gastrin-Pancreas Nebenniere-Gonaden. (Endocrine disorders in chronic renal failure and long-term dialysis treatment. Part 2. Thyroid, parathyroid, gastrin, pancreas, adrenal, gonads.) *Dtsch Gesundh-Wesen* 37: 2196, 1982
3. Bonomini V, Orsoni G, Stefoni S, Vangelista A: Hormonal changes in uremia *Clin Nephrol* 11: 275, 1979
4. Czekalski S: Hormonal abnormalities in chronic uraemia – current nephrological problem. *Pol Arch Med Wewn* 61: 349, 1979

5. Kokot F: Endokrinologische Veränderungen bei chronischen Niereninsuffizienz. (Endocrine changes in chronic renal insufficiency.) *Z Gesamte Inn Med* 35: 34, 1980

6. Lim VS, Kathpalia SC, Henriquez C: Endocrine abnormalities associated with chronic renal failure. *Med Clin N Am* 62: 1341, 1978

7. Osten B, Kokot F, Klinkmann H: *Endokrinologische Störungen in Hämodialyse, Peritonealdialyse, Membranplasmapheres*, (Endocrine Disorders in Hemodialysis, Peritoneal Dialysis and Membrane Plasmapheresis,) edited by Wetzels E, Colombi A, Dittrich P, Gurland HJ, Kessel N, Klinkmann H, Berlin, Heidelberg, Springer-Verlag, 1986, p 468

8. Fisher JW: Mechanism of the anemia of chronic renal failure. *Nephron* 25: 106, 1980

9. McGonigle RJS, Wallin JD, Shaddusk RK, Fisher JW: Erythropoietin deficiency and inhibition of erythropoiesis in renal insufficiency. *Kidney Int* 25: 437, 1984

10. Winearls CG, Oliver DO, Pippard MJ, Reid C, Downing MR, Cotes PM: Effect of human erythropoietin derived from recombinant DNA on the anaemia of patients maintained by chronic haemodialysis. *Lancet* 2: 1175, 1986

11. Caro J, Brown S, Miller O, Murray TG, Erslev AJ: Erythropoietin levels in uremic nephric and anephric patients. *J Lab Clin Med* 93: 449, 1979

12. Radtke HW, Frei U, Erbes PM, Schoeppe W, Koch KM: Improving anemia by hemodialysis: Effect on serum erythropoietin. *Kidney Int* 17: 328, 1980

13. Mason C, Thomas TH: A model for erythropoiesis in experimental chronic renal failure. *Br J Haemat* 58: 729, 1984

14. Chandra M, Miller ME, Garcia JF, Mossey RT, McVicar M: Serum immunoreactive erythropoietin levels in patients with polycystic kidney disease as compared with other hemodialysis patients. *Nephron* 39: 26, 1985

15. Shalhoub RJ, Rajan UR, Kim VV, Goldwasser V, Kark JA, Antoniou LD: Erythrocytosis in patients on long term hemodialysis. *Ann Intern Med* 97: 686, 1982

16. Thompson BJ, Jenkins DAS, Allan PL, Elton RA, Winney RJ: Acquired cystic disease of the kidney in patients with end-stage chronic renal failure. *Nephrol Dial Transplant* 1: 38, 1986

17. Anagnostou A, Kurtzman NA: Hematological consequences of renal failure in *The Kidney*, edited by Brenner BM, Rector FC, Philadelphia, Saunders WB Co, 1986, p 1631

18. Brown S, Caro J, Erslev AJ, Murray TG: Spontaneous increase in erythropoietin and hematocrit value associated with transitent liver enzyme abnormalities in an anephric patient undergoing hemodialysis. *Am J Med* 68: 280, 1980

19. Simon P: Improvement of anemia in hemodialysed patients after viral and toxic hepatic cytolysis. *Br Med J* 280: 892, 1980

20. Meytes D, Bogin E, Andrew MA, Dukes PP, Massry SG: Effect of parathyroid hormone of erythropoiesis. *J Clin Invest* 67: 1263, 1981

21. Podjany E: Is anemia of chronic renal failure related to secondary hyperparathyroidism? *Arch Intern Med* 141: 453, 1981

22. Wallner SF, Vautrin RM: Evidence that inhibition of erythropoiesis is important in the anemia of chronic renal failure. *J Lab Clin Med* 97: 170, 1981

23. Zappacosta AR, Caro J, Erslev AI: Normalization of hematocrit in patients with end-stage renal disease on continuous ambulatory peritoneal dialysis: the role of erythropoietin. *Am J Med* 75: 53, 1982

24. Dagher FJ, Ramos E, Erslev AJ, Alongi SV, Karmi SA, Caro J: Are the native kidneys responsible for erythrocytosis in renal allografts? *Transplantation* 28: 296, 1979

25. Thevenod F, Radtke HW, Grützmacher P, Vincent E, Koch KM, Schoeppe W, Fassbinder W: Deficient feedback regulation of erythrocytosis in kidney transplant patients with polycythemia. *Kidney Int* 24: 227, 1983

26. Kawashima H, Kurokawa K: Metabolism and sites of action of vitamin D in the kidney. *Kidney Int* 29: 98, 1986

27. Fraser DR: Regulation of the metabolism of vitamin D. *Physiol Rev* 60: 551, 1980

28. Jongen MJM, van der Vijgh WJF, Lips P, Netelenbos JC: Measurements of vitamin D metabolites in anephric subjects. *Nephron* 36: 230, 1984

29. Rickers H, Christiansen C, Christensen P, Christensen M, Rødbro P: Serum concentrations of vitamin D metabolites in different degrees of impaired renal function. Estimation of renal and extrarenal secretion rate of 24,25-dihydroxyvitamin D. *Nephron* 39: 267, 1985

30. Shany S, Rapoport J, Goligorsky M, Yankowitz N, Zuili I, Chaimovitz C: Losses of 1-25- and 24,25-dihydroxycholecalciferol in the peritoneal fluid of patients treated by continuous ambulatory peritoneal dialysis. *Nephron* 36: 111, 1984

31. Shany S, Rapoport J, Zuili I, Yankowitz N, Chaimovitz C: Enhancement of 24,25-dihydroxyvitamin D levels in patients treated with continuous ambulatory peritoneal dialysis. *Nephron* 42: 141, 1986

32. Aloni J, Shany S, Chaimovitz C: Loss of 25-hydroxyvitamin D in peritoneal fluid: possible mechanisms for bone disease in patients treated with chronic ambulatory peritoneal dialysis. *Miner Eelectrolyte Metab* 9: 82, 1983

33. Merke J, Ritz E, Boland R: Are recent findings on 1,25-dihydroxycholecalciferol metabolism relevant for the pathogenesis of uremia? *Nephron* 42: 277, 1986

34. Massry SG: The toxic effect of parathyroid hormone in uremia. *Semin Nephrol* 3: 306, 1984

35. Lebel M, Grose JH: Abnormal renal prostaglandin production during the evolution of chronic nephropathy. *Am J Nephrol* 6: 96, 1986

36. Papanicolaou N, Mountokalakis T, Pallasides P, Palis M, Bariety J, Papavassillou J, Merikas G, Miliez P: Urinary prostaglandin in kidney disease. *Prostaglandins Med* 3: 47, 1979

37. Schneider M, Rathaus M, Shapiro J, Bernheim J: Urinary prostaglandins E_2 and $F_{2\alpha}$ in chronic renal failure. *Nephron* 40: 152, 1985

38. Borges MF, Kjellstrand CM: The effect of prostaglandins inhibition on the clinical course of chronic hemodialysis. *Nephron* 42: 122, 1986

39. Blum M, Bauminger S, Algneti A, Kisch E, Ayalen D, Aviram A: Urinary prostaglandin E in chronic renal disease. *Clin Nephrol* 15: 87, 1981

40. Kimberly RP, Gill JR, Bowden RE, Keiser HR, Plotz PH: Elevated urinary prostaglandins and the effects of aspirin on renal function in lupus erythematosus. *Ann Intern Med* 89: 336, 1978

41. McGiff JC, Crowshow K, Teroagno NA, Lonigro AJ, Svand JC, Williamson MA, Lee JB, Ng KKE: Prostaglandin-like substances appearing in canine renal venous blood during renal ischemia. Their partial characterization by pharmacologic and chromatographic procedures. *Circ Res* 27: 765, 1970

42. Berg KJ: Acute effects of acetylsalicylic acid in patients with chronic renal insufficiency. *Eur J Clin Pharmacol* 11: 111, 1977

43. Schlondorff D, Ardaillou R: Prostaglandins and other arachidonic acid metabolites in the kidney. *Kidney Int* 29: 108, 1986

44. Gryglewski RJ, Korbut R, Ocetkiewicz A: Generation of

prostacyclin by lungs in vivo and its release into the arterial circulation. *Nature* 273: 765, 1978

45. Craddock PR, Fehr J, Brigham KL, Kronenberg RS, Jacob HS: Complement and leukocyte-mediated pulmonary dysfunction in hemodialysis. *N Engl J Med* 296: 769, 1977

46. Batlle DC, von Riotte A, Lang G: Delayed hypotensive response to dialysis in hypertensive patients with end-stage renal disease. *Am J Nephrol* 6: 14, 1986

47. Kuska J, Kokot F, Libera T, Sledziński Z: The influence of upright position and sodium restriction in the diet on plasma renin activity (PRA) and aldosteronemia in patients with chronic nephritis. *Mater Med Pol* 9: 312, 1977

48. Kuska J, Kokot F, Panusz J: Regulation and significance of renin-angiotensin-aldosterone axis in patients with chronic nephritis. *Mater Med Pol* 10: 54, 1978

49. Kokot F, Kuska J: Plasma renin activity in patients with acute and chronic renal insufficiency treated by hemodialysis. *Proc Eur Dial Transplant Assoc* 8: 542, 1971

50. Kornerup HJ, Schmitz O, Danielsen H, Pedersen EB, Giese J: Significance of the renin-angiotensin system for blood pressure regulation in end-stage renal disease. *Contrib Nephrol* 41: 123, 1984

51. Weidmann P, Maxwell M: The renin-angiotensin-aldosterone system in terminal renal failure. *Kidney Int* 8 (Suppl 5): 219, 1975

52. Warren DJ, Ferris TF: Renin secretion in renal hypertension. *Lancet* 1: 159, 1970

53. d'Amore TF, Wauters JP, Waeber B, Brunner HR: Salt subtraction in patients on maintenance hemodialysis. Efficacy and limitations. *Am J Nephrol* 5: 275, 1985

54. Naik RB, Mathias CJ, Reid JL, Warren DJ: Effect of haemodialysis on the control of the circulation in patients with chronic renal failure. *Am J Nephrol* 5: 96, 1985

55. Nielsen AH, Knudsen F, Kristensen SD: Serum angiotensin-converting enzyme increases during hemodialysis. Evidence for injury of the pulmonary vascular endothelium. *Nephron* 40: 100, 1985

56. Silverstein E, Brunswick J, Rao TKS, Friedland J: Increased serum angiotensin-converting enzyme in chronic renal disease. *Nephron* 37: 206, 1984

57. Rumpf KW, Brat A, Armstrong V, Scheler F: Increased serum angiotensin-converting enzyme in end-stage renal disease. *Nephron* 40: 248, 1985

58. Le Treut A, Chevet D, Guenet L, Leray G, Afiouni N, Le Pogamp P, Le Gall JY: Serum angiotensin-converting enzyme levels in patients with chronic renal failure. *Path Biol (Paris)* 31: 182, 1983

59. Scicli AG, Carretero OA: Renal kallikrein-kinin system. *Kidney Int* 29: 120, 1986

60. Funaki N, Kuroda M, Sudo J, Takeda R: Urinary prostaglandin and kallikrein in the course of acute renal failure. *Pros Leuk Med* 9: 387, 1982

61. Mayfield RK, Margolius HS: Renal kallikrein-kinin system. *Am J Nephrol* 3: 145, 1983

62. Mitas JA, Lavy SB, Holle R, Frigon RP, Stone RA: Urinary kallikrein activity in the hypertension of renal parenchymal disease. *N Engl J Med* 299: 162, 1978

63. Brouhard BM, Cunningham RJ, Berger M, Petrusick TW, Travis LB: Urinary kallikrein excretion in renal transplant patients. *Clin Nephrol* 17: 241, 1982

64. Koolen MJ, van Brummelen P, Paul LC, Daha MR, van Es LA: Excretion of urokallikrein in renal transplant patients. *Transplantation* 37: 471, 1984

65. Grzeszczak W, Kokot F, Dulawa J: Effects of naloxone ad-

ministration on endocrine abnormalities in chronic renal failure. *Am J Nephrol* 7: 93, 1987

66. Kuska J, Kokot F, Sledzinski Z: Secretion of growth hormone after L-dopa stimulation in patients with renal failure treated with dialysis. *Acta Med Pol* 20: 217, 1979

67. Ijaya K: Pattern of growth hormone response to insulin, arginine and haemodialysis in uraemic children. *Eur J Pediatr* 131: 185, 1979

68. Kokot F, Kuska J: Das Verhalten des Wachstumshormons nach Insulin-Stimulierung bei chronischer Niereninsuffizienz. (Behavior of growth hormone following insulin stimulation in chronic renal failure.) *Z Gesamte Inn Med* 27: 207, 1972

69. Davidson MB, Fisher MB, Dabir-Vaziri N, Schaffer M: Effect of protein intake and dialysis on the abnormal growth hormone, glucose and insulin homeostasis in uremia. *Metabolism* 25: 455, 1976

70. Bundschu HD: Endokrine Störungen bei Niereninsuffizienz. (Endocrine disorders in renal insufficiency.) In: *Blutreinigungsverfahren* (Methods of Blood Purification), edited by Franz HE, Stuttgart, New York. G. Thieme Verlag, 1981, p 222

71. Saenger P, Wiedemann E, Schwartz E, Korth-Schutz S, Levy JE, Ribbio RR, Rubin A, Stenzel KH, New MI: Somatomedin and growth after renal transplantation. *Pediatr Res* 8: 164, 1974

72. Pimstone BL, Le Roith D, Epstein S, Kronheim S: Disappearance rates of plasma growth hormone after intravenous somatostatin in renal and liver disease. *J Clin Endocrinol Metab* 41: 392, 1975

73. Spanos E, Barrett D, MacIntyre I, Pike JW, Safilian EE, Haussler MR: Effect of growth hormone on vitamin D metabolism. *Nature* 273: 246, 1978

74. Eshildsen PC, Sørensen OH, Bishop JE, Norman AW: Acromegaly and vitamin D metabolism: effect of bromocriptine treatment. *J Clin Endocrinol Metab* 49: 484, 1979

75. Schüllerova M, Marek J, Schreiberova O, Tomasek R, Josifko M: Somatomedin in patients with chronic renal insufficiency. *Čas Lék Čes* 116: 519, 1977

76. Philips LS, Kopple JD: Circulating somatomedin activity and sulfate levels in adults with normal and impaired kidney function. *Metabolism* 30: 1091, 1981

77. Schriffrin A, Guyda H, Robitaille P, Posner B: Increased plasma somatomedin reactivity in chronic renal failure as determined by acid gel filtration and radioreceptor assay. *J Clin Endocrinol Metab* 46: 511, 1978

78. Bercu BB, Corden BJ, Schulman BJ, Rizzo WB, Reed GR: Circulating somatomedin-C levels in nephropathic cystinosis. *Isr J Med Sci* 20: 236, 1984

79. Phillips LS, Vassilopoulou: Sellin R: Somatomedins. *N Engl J Med* 302, 371, 438, 1980

80. Goldberg AC, Trivedi B, Delmez JA, Harter HR, Daughaday WH: Uraemia reduces serum insulin like growth factor I, increases insulinlike growth factor II, and modifies their serum protein binding. *J Clin Endocrinol Metab* 55: 1040, 1982

81. French CB, Genel M: Pathophysiology of growth failure in chronic renal insufficiency. *Kidney Int* 29 (Suppl 19): S59, 1986

82. Philips LS, Fusco AC, Unterman TG, Del Greco F: Somatomedin inhibotor in uremia. *J Clin Endocrinol Metab* 59: 764, 1984

83. Lim VS, Kathpalia SC, Frohman LA: Hyperprolactinemia and impaired pituitary response to suppression and stimulation in chronic renal failure: reversal after transplantation. *J Clin Endocrinol Metab* 48: 101, 1979

84. Ijaaiya K, Roth B, Schwenk A: Serum prolactin level in renal

insufficiency in children. *Acta Paediatr Scand* 69: 299, 1980

85. Grzeszczak W, Kokot F, Dulawa J: Influence of naloxone on prolactin secretion in patients with acute and chronic renal failure. *Clin Nephrol* 21: 47, 1984
86. Sievertsen GD, Lim VS, Nakawatase C, Frohman LA: Metabolic clearance and secretion rates of human prolactin in normal subjects and in patients with chronic renal failure. *J Clin Endocrinol Metab* 50: 846, 1980
87. Preces R, Horcajada C, Lopez-Novoa JM, Frutos MA, Casado S, Hernando L: Hyperprolactinemia in chronic renal failure. Impaired responsiveness to stimulation and suppression. Normalization after transplantation. *Nephron* 28: 11, 1981
88. Grzeszczak W, Kokot F, Dulawa J: Naloxone effect on the secretion of lutropin (LH) folitropin (FSH) prolactin and testosterone in patients with chronic renal failure. *Pol Arch Med Wewn* 73: 278, 1985
89. Bauer AGC, Wilson JHP, Lamberts SWJ: The kidney is the main site of prolactin elimination in patients with liver disease. *J Clin Endocrinol Metab* 51: 70, 1980
90. Kokot F, Grzeszczak W, Dulawa J: Besteht eine Beziehung zwischen der Parathormon- und Prolactinsekretion bei Kranken mit akutem und chronischem Nierenversagen? (Is there a relation between parathormone and prolactin secretion in patients with acute and chronic renal failure?) *Z Gesamte Inn Med* 39: 40, 1984
91. Spanos E, Coston KW, Ewans LMS, Galante LS, McAuley SJ, MacIntyre I: Effect of prolactin on vitamin D metabolism. *Mol Cell Endocrinol* 5: 163, 1976
92. Kokot F: Endokrinologische Veränderungen bei der chronischen Niereninsuffizienz. (Endocrine changes in chronic renal insufficiency.) *Z Gesamte Inn Med* 34: 743, 1979
93. Barbour GL, Sevier BR: Adrenal responsiveness in chronic hemodialysis. *N Engl J Med* 290: 1258, 1974
94. McDonald WJ, Golper TA, Mass RD, Kendall JW, Porter GA, Girard DE, Fischer MD: Adrenocorticotropin- cortisol axis abnormalities in hemodialysis patients. *J Clin Endocrinol Metab* 48: 92, 1979
95. Akmad M, Manziar AD: Simplified assessment of pituitary adrenal axis in a stable group of chronic hemodialysis patients. *Trans Am Soc Artif Intern Organs* 23: 703, 1977
96. Bacon GE, Kenny FM, Murdaugh HV, Richards C: Prolonged serum halflife of cortisol in renal failure. *J Hopkins Med J* 132: 127, 1973
97. Feldman H, Singer I: Endocrinology and metabolism in uremia and dialysis: a clinical review. *Medicine* 54: 345, 1974
98. Gilkes JJH, Eady RAJ, Rees LH, Munro DD, Moorhead JF: Plasma immunoreactive melantrophic hormones in patients on maintenance haemodialysis. *Br Med J* 1: 656, 1975
99. Knopp E, Staudinger E, v Dittrich P: Das Verhalten des freien Plasmakortisols während extrakorporaler Hämodialyse. (Behavior of free plasma cortisol during extracorporeal hemodialysis.) *Klin Wochenschr* 48: 1243, 1970
100. Ramirez G, Etheridge P, Meikle W, Jubiz W: Evaluation of the pituitary adrenal axis in patients with chronic renal failure. *Clin Res* 26: 148 (Abstract), 1978
101. Rosman PM, Benn R, Kay M, Rito J, Wallace EZ: Cortisol binding in uremic plasma. I. Absence of abnormal cortisol binding to corticosteroid-binding globulin. *Nephron* 37: 160, 1984
102. Bindeballe W, Drenkhahn E, Jüsgen W, Lahrtz H, Heybold K, Niedermayer W, Schemmel K: Der Einfluss der Hämodialyse auf den Hormonstatus bei terminaler Niereninsuffizienz. (The influence of hemodialysis on the hormone status in terminal renal failure.) *Dtsch Med Wochenschr* 98: 661, 1973

103. Kolbe K: Untersuchungen zur Kortisolproduktion bei Patienten mit terminaler Niereninsuffizienz während der Hämodialysebehandlung. (Investigation of cortisol production in patients with terminal renal failure undergoing hemodialysis treatment.) *Dissertation,* Aachen, 1979
104. Kapstein EM, Feinstein EJ, Nicoloff JT, Massry SG: Serum reverse triiodothyronine and thyroxine kinetics in patients with chronic renal failure. *J Clin Endocrinol Metab* 57: 181, 1983
105. Kaptein EM, Feinstein EI, Massry SG: Thyroid hormone metabolism in renal diseases. *Contrib Nephrol* 33: 122, 1982
106. Giordano C, DeSanto NG, Carella C, Capodicasa G, Amato G, Nuzzi F, Mioli V, Bazzato G, De Simone V, Tarchini A, Landini A, Coli U, Bordoni M, Mottola G, Capuano F: Thyroid status and nephron loss – a study in patient with chronic renal failure, end-stage renal disease and/or hemodialysis. *Int J Artif Organs* 7: 119, 1984
107. Beckers C, van Ypersele de Strihou C, Coche E, Troch R, Malvaux P: Iodine metabolism in severe renal insufficiency. *J Clin Endocrinol Metab* 29: 293, 1969
108. Kontras DA, Marketos SG, Rigopoulos GA, Melamos B: Iodine metabolism in chronic renal insufficiency. *Nephron* 9: 55, 1972
109. Lim VS, Fang VS, Katz AJ, Refetoff S: Thyroid dysfunction in chronic renal failure: a study of the pituitary thyroid axis and peripheral turnover kinetics of thyroxine and triiodothyronine. *J Clin Invest* 60: 522, 1977
110. Kalk WJ, Morley JE, Gold GH, Meyers A: Thyroid function tests in patients on regular hemodialysis. *Nephron* 25: 173, 1980
111. Beckett GJ, Henderson CJ, Elwes R, Seth J, Lambie AT: Thyroid status in patients with chronic renal failure. *Clin Nephrol* 19: 172, 1983
112. Inaba M, Nishizawa Y, Nishitani H, Miki T, Onishi Y, Mizutarii Y, Yamakawa M: Concentrations of thyroxine-binding globulin in sera and peritoneal dialysates in patients on chronic peritoneal ambulatory dialysis. *Nephron* 42: 58, 1986
113. Sennesal JJ, Verbeelen DL, Jonckeer MH: Thyroid dysfunction in patients on regular hemodialysis: Evaluation of the stable intrathyroidal iodine pool, incidence of goiter and free thyroid hormone concentration. *Nephron* 41: 141, 1985
114. Thysen B, Gatz M, Freeman R, Alpert BE, Charytan C: Serum thyroid hormone levels in patients on continuous peritoneal dialysis and regular hemodialysis. *Nephron* 33: 49, 1983
115. Ciardella F, Morelli E, Caprioli R, Casto G, Christu C, Rampa P, Petronio MG, Carbone C, Mantovanell A, Mazzotta L, Barsotti G: Restoration of thyroid secretion in uremic patients following a low protein, low phosphorus diet, supplemented with essential amino acids and keto analogues. *Contrib Nephrol* 53: 51, 1986
116. Czekalski S, Malczewska B, Sobieszczyk S, Kozak W, Eder M, Gryczyńska M, Bączyk K, Kosowicz J: Comparison of some circulating pituitary thyroid and gonadal hormone levels in nondialyzed and dialyzed males with chronic renal failure. *Dial Transplant* 10: 438, 1981
117. Hegedüs L, Andersen JR, Poulsen LR, Perrild H, Holm B, Gundtoft E, Hansen JM: Thyroid gland volume and serum concentrations of thyroid hormones in chronic renal failure. *Nephron* 40: 171, 1985
118. Czernichow P, Danzet MC, Brover M, Rappaport R: Abnormal TSH, PRL and GH in chronic uremia. *J Clin Endocrinol Metab* 43: 630, 1976
119. Semple CG, Beastall GH, Henderson JS, Thomsom MA, Kennedy AC: Thyroid function and continuous ambulatory

peritoneal dialysis. *Nephron* 32: 249, 1982

120. Davis FB, Spector DA, Davis PH, Hirsch BR, Walshe JJ, Yoshida K: Comparison of pituitary-thyroid function in patients with end-stage renal disease and in age- and sex matched controls. *Kidney Int* 21: 362, 1982

121. Vaziri ND, Gvinup C, Martin D, Seltzer J: Thyroid function in chronic renal failure after successful renal transplantation. *Clin Nephrol* 15: 131, 1981

122. DeSanto NG, Carella C, Fine RN, Lenmann E, Fine S, Amato G, Capodicasa G, Nuzzi F, Capasso G, Simone V, Lama G, Scoppa F: Thyroid function in uremic children – studies at various stages of nephron loss and during treatment with hemodialysis and/or CAPD. *Contrib Nephrol* 49: 56, 1985

123. Foley RJ, Hamner RW: Hyperthyroidism in end-stage renal disease. *Am J Nephrol* 5: 292, 1985

124. Massry SG, Goldstein DA, Procci WR, Kletzky OA: On the pathogenesis of sexual dysfunction of the uraemic male. *Proc Eur Dial Transplant Assoc* 17: 139, 1980

125. Czekalski S, Malczewska B, Sowinski J, Sobieszczak S, Kozak W, Eder M, Bączyk K: Serum concentration of pituitary, thryoid and gonadal hormone in nondialyzed and dialyzed males with chronic renal failure. *Proc Eur Dial Transplant Assoc* 15: 599, 1978

126. Distiller LA, Morely JE, Sagel J, Pokroy M, Rabkin R: Pituitary gonadal function in chronic renal failure. The effect of luteinizing releasing hormone and the influence of dialysis. *Metabolism* 24: 711, 1975

127. Holdsworth S, Atkins RC, Kretser DM de: The pituitary-testicular axis in men with chronic renal failure. *N Engl J Med* 296, 1245, 1977

128. Krolner B: Serum levels of testosterone and luteinizing hormone in patients with chronic renal disease. *Acta Med Scand* 205: 623, 1979

129. Lim VS, Fang WR: Gonadal dysfunction in uremic men. *Am J Med* 58: 655, 1975

130. Swamy AP, Woolf PD, Cestero RVM: Hypothalamic-pituitary-ovarian axis in uremic women. *J Lab Clin Med* 93: 1066, 1979

131. Mastrogiacomo I, De Besi L, Zucchetta P, Serafini E, Gasparotto ML, Marchini P, Pisani E, Dean P, Chini M: Effect of hyperprolactinemia and age on the hypogonadism of uremic men on hemodialysis. *Arch Androl* 12: 235, 1984

132. Joven J, Villabona C, Rubi es-Prat J, Espinel E, Galard R: Hormonal profile and serum zinc levels in uraemic men with gonadal dysfunction undergoing haemodialysis. *Clin Chim Acta* 148: 239, 1985

133. Van Coevorden A, Stolear J, Dhaene M, Van Herweghem JL, Mockel J: Effect of chronic oral testosterone undecannoate administration the pituitary-testicular axis of hemodialyzed male patients. *Clin Nephrol* 26: 48, 1986

134. Grzeszczak W, Kokot F, Więcek A: Importance of opioid receptors in the pathogenesis of endocrine abnormalities in chronic renal failure. *Contrib Nephrol* 78: 261, 1987

135. Barsotli G, Ciardella F, Morelli E, Fioretti P, Melis G, Paoletti A, Niosi F, Caprioli R, Fosso A, Carbone C, Giovanetti S: Restoration of blood levels of testosterone in male uremics following a low protein diet supplemented with essential amino acids and ketoanalogues. *Contrib Nephrol* 49: 63, 1985

136. Lim VS, Henriquez C, Sievertsen G, Frohman LA: Ovarian function in chronic renal failure: evidence suggesting hypothalamic anovulation. *Ann Intern Med* 93: 21, 1980

137. Massry SG: Current status of the role of parathyroid hormone in uremic toxicity. *Contrib Nephrol* 49: 1, 1985

138. Ermolenko UM, Kukhtewitch AV, Dedov II, Bunatian AF,

Melnichenko GA, Gitel EP: Parlodel treatment of uremic hypogonadism in men. *Nephron* 42: 19, 1986

139. Ardaillou R, Benmansour M, Roudeau E, Caillens H: Metabolism and secretion of antidiuretic hormone in patients with renal failure, cardiac insufficiency, and liver insufficiency. *Adv Nephrol* 13: 35, 1984

140. Ben Mausour M, Rainfray M, Paillard F, Ardaillou R: Metabolic clearance rate in immunoreactive vasopressin in man. *Eur J Clin Invest* 12: 475, 1982

141. Munoz EP, Easterling RE, Malvin RL: The effect of plasma calcium on plasma ADH level in anephric patients. *Nephron* 16: 49, 1976

142. Horky K, Sramkova J, Lachmanova J, Tomasek R, Dvorakova J: Plasma concentration of ADH in patients with chronic renal insufficiency on maintenance dialysis. *Horm Metab Res* 11: 241, 1979

143. Vaziri ND, Skowsky R, Warner A: Effect of isomolal volume reduction during hemofiltration on plasma ADH in patients with chronic renal failure. *Int J Artif Organs* 3: 322, 1980

144. Vaziri ND, Skowsky R, Saiki J, Warner A: Hemodialysis studies of antidiuretic hormone. *J Dial* 4: 185, 1980

145. Shimamoto R, Watari J, Miyahara M: A study of plasma vasopressin in patients undergoing chronic hemodialysis. *J Clin Endocrinol Metab* 45: 714, 1977

146. Caillens M, Pruszczyński W, Meyrier A, Ang KS, Rousselet F, Ardaillou R: Relationship between change in volemia at constant osmolality and plasma antidiuretic hormone. *Miner Electrolyte Metab* 4: 161, 1980

147. Jawadi MH, Ho LS, Dipette D, Ross DL: Regulation of plasma arginine vasopressin in patients with chronic renal failure maintained on hemodialysis. *Am J Nephrol* 6: 175, 1986

148. Iitake K, Kimura T, Matsui K, Ota K, Shoji M, Inoue M, Yoshinaga K: Effect of haemodialysis on plasma ADH levels, plasma renin activity and plasma aldosterone levels in patients with end-stage renal disease. *Acta Endocrinol* (Kbh) 110: 207, 1985

149. Fasanella d'Amore T, Wauter JP, Weber B, Nussberger J, Brunner HR: Response of plasma vasopressin to change in extracellular volume and/or plasma osmolality in patients on maintenance hemodialysis. *Clin Nephrol* 23: 299, 1985

150. Grzeszczak W, Kokot F, Dulawa J, Kuska J: Effect of naloxone on vasopressin secretion in patients with acute and chronic renal failure. *Pol Arch Med Wewn* 74: 176, 1985

151. Vaziri ND, Skousky R, Warner A: Effect of isoosmolar volume reduction during hemofiltration on plasma antidiuretic hormone in patients with chronic renal failure. *Int J Artif Organs* 3: 322, 1980

152. Hammer M, Olgaard K, Madsen S: The inability of angiotensin II infusion to raise plasma vasopressin levels in haemodialysis patients. *Acta Endocrinol* 95: 422, 1980

153. Ben Mansour M, Caillens H, Ardaillou R: The effect of inhibition of angiotensin II synthesis on the response of plasma antidiuretic hormone to the osmotic and volume dependent stimuli in uremic patients. *Nephrologie* 1: 109, 1980

154. Hammer M, Ladefoged J, Madsen S, Olgaard K, Tuegeaard E: Calcium-stimulated vasopressin secretion in uremic patients: an effect mediated via parathyroid hormone. *J Clin Endocrinol Metab* 51: 1070, 1980

155. Nieszporek T, Grzeszczak W, Kokot F, Szczechowska E, Więcek A: Renin-angiotensin aldosterone system and vasopressin secretion in renal transplant recipients treated by cyclosporin A or azathioprine with prednisone. *Pol Arch Med Wewn* 78: 261, 1987

156. Fraser DR, Kodicek E: Unique biosynthesis by kidney of a

biologically active vitamin D metabolite. *Nature* 228: 764, 1970

157. Silver J, Russell J, Sherwood LM: Regulation by vitamin D metabolites of messenger ribonucleic acid for preproparathyroid hormone in isolated bovine parathyroid cells. *Proc Natl Acad Sci USA* 82: 4270, 1985

158. Llach F, Massry SG: On the mechanism of secondary hyperparathyroidism in moderate renal insufficiency. *J Clin Endocrinol Metab* 61: 601, 1985

159. Massry SG, Tuma S, Dua S, Goldstein DA: Reversal of skeletal resistance to parathyroid hormone in uremia by vitamin D metabolites. *J Lab Clin Med* 94: 152, 1979

160. Rutherford WE, Bordier P, Marie P, Hruska K, Harter H, Greenwalt A, Blondin J, Haddad J, Bricker N, Slatopolsky E: Phosphate control and 25-hydroxycholecalciferol administration in preventing experimental renal osteodystrophy in the dog. *J Clin Invest* 60: 332, 1977

161. Slatopolsky ES, Caglar S, Gradowska L, Canterbury J, Reiss E, Bricker NS: On the prevention of secondary hyperparathyroidism in experimental chronic renal disease using 'proportional reduction' of dietary phosphorus intake. *Kidney Int* 2: 147, 1972

162. Brown EM, Wilkinson RE, Eastman RC, Pallotta J, Marynick SP: Abnormal regulation of parathyroid hormone release by calcium in secondary hyperparathyroidism due to chronic renal failure. *J Clin Endocrinol Metab* 54: 172, 1982

163. Freitag J, Marlin KJ, Hruska KA, Anderson C, Conrades M, Landenson J, Klahr S, Slatopolsky E: Impaired parathyroid hormone metabolism in patients with chronic renal failure. *N Engl J Med* 298: 29, 1978

164. Lopez-Hilker S, Galceran T, Chan YL, Rapp N, Martin KJ, Slatopolsky E: Hypocalcemia may not be essential for the development of secondary hyperparathyroidism in chronic renal failure. *J Clin Invest* 78: 1097, 1986

165. Grzeszczak W, Kokot F, Dulawa J: Einfluss von Naloxone auf die Parathormon- und Calcitoninsekretion bei Kranken mit akuter und chronischer Niereninsuffizienz. (Effect of naloxone on parathormone and calcitonin secretion in patients with acute and chronic renal failure.) *Z Klin Med* 41: 435, 1986

166. Jaeger P, Burckhardt P, Wauters JP, Trechsel U, Bonjour JP: Evidence for a particularly severe secondary hyperparathyroidism in analgesic abuse nephropathy. *Am J Nephrol* 5: 342, 1985

167. Fröhling PT, Kokot F, Verter K, Kaschube I, Lindenau K: Influence of vitamin D or its metabolites on the rate of progression of chronic renal failure. *Contr Nephrol* 53: 64, 1986

168. Pietrek J, Kokot F, Kuska J: Effects of 1-α-hydroxyvitamin D_3 on serum calcium and immunoreactive parathyroid hormone in patients with chronic renal failure. *Int Urol Nephrol* 10: 153, 1978

169. Fröhling PT, Schmicker P, Kokot F, Vetter K, Kaschube I, Götz K-H, Jacopian M, Lindenau K: Influence of phosphate restriction, ketoacids and vitamin D on the progression of renal failure. *Proc Eur Dial Transplant Assoc Eur Ren Assoc* 21: 561, 1984

170. Fröhling PT, Kokot F, Vetter K, Hohmann WD, Werber G, Grossmann T, Schmicker P, Lindenau K: Treatment of osteodystrophy in advanced renal failure during predialysis time. *Contrib Nephrol* 37: 62, 1984

171. Fröhling PT, Schmidt-Gayk H, Kokot F, Vetter K, Mayer E, Lindenau K: Influence of vitamin D and keto acids /KA/ on 1,25/OH/$_2$D levels in chronic renal failure. In: *Vitamin D, Biochemical and Clinical Update*, edited by Norman AW, Schaefer K, Grigoleit H-G, v. Herrath D, Berlin, Walter de Gruyter, 1985, p 952

172. Takamoto S, Onishi T, Mirimoto S, Imanaka S, Tsuchiya H, Seino Y, Yokokawa T, Lida N, Kumahara Y: Serum phosphate, parathyroid hormone and vitamin D metabolites in patients with chronic renal failure: effect of aluminium hydroxide administration. *Nephron* 40: 286, 1985

173. McGonigle RJS, Fowler MB, Timmis AB, Weston MJ, Parsons V: Uremic cardiomyopathy: potential role of vitamin D and parathyroid hormone. *Nephron* 36: 94, 1984

174. Fröhling PT, Kokot F, Schmicker R, Kaschube I, Lindenau K, Vetter K: Influence of ketoacids on serum parathyroid hormone levels in patients with chronic renal failure. *Clin Nephrol* 20: 212, 1983

175. Cunningham J, Segre GV, Slatopolsky E, Avioli LV: Effect of histamine H$_2$-receptor blockade on parathyroid status in normal and uraemic man. *Nephron* 38: 17, 1984

176. Kokot F, Kuska J, Sledziński Z, Białas B, Luciak M: Parathormon, Kalzitonin, 25-Hydroxykalziferol und Knochenhistologie bei Patienten mit chronischer Niereninsuffizienz. (Parathormone, calcitonin, 25-hydroxycalciferol and bone histology in patients with chronic renal insufficiency.) *Z Gesamte Inn Med* 34: 665, 1979

177. Malluche HH, Taugere MC, Ritz E, Caillens G, Wildberger D: Endogenous calcitonin does not protect against hyperparathyroid bone disease in renal failure. *Miner Electrolyte Metab* 12: 113, 1986

178. Zazgornik J, Kokot F, Pietrek J, Schmidt P, Kopsa H: Osteopathie, Parathormon- und 25-Hydroxycholekalziferol-Konzentrationen im Serum bei chronisch dialysierten Patienten. (Osteopathy, serum parathormone and 25-hydroxycholecalciferol levels in patients on long term hemodialysis.) *Wien Klin Wochenschr* 90: 496, 1978

179. Zazgornik J, Kokot F, Fürst K, Schmidt P, Pietrek J, Czembirek H, Kopsa H, Balcke P, Paietta E: Roentgenologic soft tissue and bone changes, parathyroid hormone, 25-hydroxycholecalciferol, calcium-phosphorus concentrations in serum in dialyzed and renal transplant patients. *Dial Transplant* 8: 389, 1979

180. Kokot F, Kuska J, Pietrek J: Das Verhalten der Parathormonsekretion bei hämodialysierten Patienten mit chronischer Niereninsuffizienz. (Behavior of parathyroid hormone secretion in hemodialysis patients with chronic renal failure.) *Z Gesamte Inn Med* 30: 443, 1975

181. Schaefer K, v. Herrath D, Pauls A, Hufler M: New insight into hemofiltration. *Semin Nephrol* 6: 161, 1986

182. Zucchelli P, Catizone L, Casanova S, Fusaroli M, Fabbri L, Ferrari G: Renal osteodystrophy in CAPD patients. *Miner Electrolyte Metab* 10: 326, 1984

183. Delmez JA, Fallon MD, Bergfeld MA, Gearing BK, Dougan CS, Teitelbaum SL: Continuous ambulatory peritoneal dialysis and bone. *Kidney Int* 30: 379, 1986

184. Kokot F, Zazgornik J, Pietrek J, Schmidt P, Fürst K, Czembirek H, Kopsa H: Parathormon- und 25-Hydroxycholekalziferol-Konzentrationen im Serum nierentransplantierter Patienten und ihr röntgenologisches Korrelation. (Parathormone and 25-hydroxycholecalciferol concentrations in the serum of renal transplant patients and their roentgenologic correlation.) *Z Gesamte Inn Med* 33: 516, 1978

185. Bonomini V, Campieri C, Feletti C, Orsoni G, Vangelista A: Hormonal abnormalities in renal transplantation. *Contrib Nephrol* 49: 70, 1985

186. Fröhling PT, Kokot F, Cernacek P, Vetter K, Kuska J, Spustova V, Kaschube I, Dziurik R: Relation between middle molecules and parathyroid hormone in patients with chronic renal failure. *Miner Electrolyte Metab* 7: 48, 1982

187. Martinez ME, Miguel JL, Gomez P, Selgas R, Salinas M,

Gentil M, Mateos F, Montero JL, Sicilia LS: Plasma calcitonin concentration in patients treated with chronic dialysis: differences between hemodialysis and CAPD. *Clin Nephrol* 19: 250, 1983

188. Kokot F, Kuska J, Mleczko Z, Szczechowska E, Pazera A: Über die Beziehung zwischen Gastrin- und Kalzitonin-Sekretion bei Kranken mit akuter und chronischer Niereninsuffizienz. (About the relationship between gastrin and calcitonin secretion in patients with acute and chronic renal insufficiency.) *Dtsch Gesundh-Wesen* 36: 429, 1981

189. Fuss M, Bergans A, Geurts J, Brauman H, Corvilain J: Effect of rapid variation of renal function on plasma calcitonin and parathyroid hormone in man. *Acta Endocrinologica (Kbh)* 92: 130, 1979

190. Nielsen HE, Olsen KJ: Serum calcitonin after renal transplantation. *Acta Med Scand* 205: 619, 1979

191. Kokot F, Nieszporek T: Influence of hemoperfusion on the concentrations of calcitonin, testosterone and cortisol in blood plasma. *Artif Organs* 3: 332, 1979

192. Ardaillou R, Sizonenko P, Meyner A, Valee G, Beaugas G: Metabolic clearance rate of radioiodinated human calcitonin in man. *J Clin Invest* 49: 2345, 1970

193. Heynen G, Franchimont P: Human calcitonin and serum phosphate. *Lancet* 1: 267, 1974

194. Weidmann P, Maxwell MH, de Lima J, Hirsch D, Franklin SS: Control of aldosterone responsiveness in terminal renal failure. *Kidney Int* 7: 351, 1975

195. Osten B, Wedler B: Untersuchungen zur Regulation und Funktion des Aldosterons unter besonderer Berücksichtigung der Nierenfunktion. (Investigation of the regulation and function of aldosterone with special attention to renal function.) *Dissertationsschrift* (Promotion B), Rostock, 1979

196. Schnurr E: Der Einfluss der Hämodialyse auf die Plasma-Aldosteron-Konzentration. Ein Beitrag zur Frage der Aldosteron-Regulation im Stadium der terminalen Niereninsuffizienz. (The influence of hemodialysis on plasma aldosterone concentration. A study concerning aldosterone regulation in states of renal insufficiency.) *Habilitationsschrift*, Düsseldorf, 1976

197. Vetter W, Haruba K, Armbruster H, Beckerhoff R, Nussberger J, Furrer J, Fontana A, Siegenthaler W: Control of plasma aldosterone during hemodialysis patients with terminal renal failure. *Nephron* 18: 114, 1977

198. Wedler B, Osten B, Schmidt R, Klinkmann H: Zum Verhalten des Serumaldosterons unter de Hämodialyse bei Patienten mit chronischer Niereninsuffizienz. (The behavior of serum aldosterone in patients with renal insufficiency undergoing hemodialysis.) *Dtsch Gesundh-Wesen* 32: 1912, 1977

199. Hene RJ, Roomans HA, Boer P, Roos JC, Dorhout Mees EJ: Relation between plasma aldosterone concentration and renal handling of sodium and potassium, in particular in patients with chronic renal failure. *Nephron* 37: 94, 1984

200. Rissmann K: Untersuchungen zur Aldosteronsekretion bei Patienten mit terminaler chronischer Niereninsuffizienz während der Hämodialysebehandlung. (Investigation of aldosterone secretion in patients with terminal renal failure undergoing hemodialysis treatment.) *Dissertation*, Aachen, 1979

201. Dordevi V, Kosti S, Stefanovi V: Study of plasma aldosterone in patients on chronic hemodialysis. *Acta Med Jugosl* 40: 49, 1986

202. Campese VM, Iseki K, Massry SG: Plasma catecholamines and vascular reactivity in uremic and dialysis patients. *Contrib Nephrol* 41: 90, 1984

203. Campese VM, Massry SG: Plasma catecholamines and vascular reactivity in acute and chronic renal failure. *Contrib Nephrol* 49: 128, 1985

204. Cuche J-L, Prinseau J, Selz F, Ruget G, Baglin A: Plasma free, sulfo- and glucuro-conjugated catecholamines in uremic patients. *Kidney Int* 30: 566, 1986

205. Lake CR, Ziegler MG, Coleman MD, Kopin IJ: Plasma levels of norepinephrine and dopamine-β-hydroxylase in CRF patients treated by dialysis. *Cardiol Med* 9: 1099, 1979

206. McGrath BP, Ledingham JGG, Benedict CR: Catecholamines in peripheral venous plasma in patients on chronic haemodialysis. *Clin Sci Mol Med* 55: 89, 1978

207. Brecht HM, Ernst W, Koch KM: Plasma noradrenaline levels in regular haemodialysis patients. *Proc Eur Dial Transplant Assoc* 12: 281, 1975

208. Zuccala A, Santoro A, Gaggi R, Chiarini C, Degli Eposti E, Sturani A, Zucchelli P: Relationship between plasma noradrenaline and blood pressure in uremia. *Contrib Nephrol* 49: 134, 1985

209. deFronzo RA, Andres R, Edgar P, Walker WG: Carbohydrate metabolism in uremia. A review. *Medicine* 52: 469, 1973

210. Kokot F, Kuska J: Das Verhalten der Insulinsekretion bei chronischer Niereninsuffizienz. (Behavior of insulin secretion in chronic renal insufficiency.) *Z Gesamte Inn Med* 28: 351, 1973

211. Wnuk R, Kokot F, Mleczko Z: Endocrine pancreatic function in patients with acute and chronic renal failure. *Pol Arch Med Wewn* 70: 111, 1983

212. Spitz IM, Rubenstein AN, Bersohn I, Abrahams C, Lowy C: Carbohydrate metabolism in renal disease. *Q J Med* 39: 201, 1970

213. Milutinovic S, Breyer D, Molnar V, Stefovic A, Jankovic N, Skrabalo Z, Rocic B: Changes in insulin binding during hemodialysis in uremic patients. *Nephron* 41: 307, 1985

214. Schmitz O: Insulin-mediated glucose uptake in nondialyzed and dialyzed uremic insulin-dependent diabetic subjects. *Diabetes* 34: 1159, 1985

215. Brech WJ: Urämische Glukoseintoleranz – Diabetes mellitus. (Uremic glucose intolerance – diabetes mellitus.) In: *Blutreinigungsverfahren – Technik und Klinik* (Blood Purification Treatment – Technik and Clinical Aspects), edited by Franz HE, Stuttgart, Hrsg Thieme, 1981, 0 167

216. Fisch HP: Funktionsstörungen endokriner Drüsen bei chronischer Niereninsuffizienz. (Endocrine gland functional disorders in chronic renal insufficiency.) *Med Klin* 74: 1363, 1979

217. Taylor R, Heaton A, Hetherington CS, Alberti KG: Adipocyte insulin binding and insulin action in chronic renal failure before and during continuous ambulatory peritoneal dialysis. *Metabolism* 35: 430, 1986

218. Davidson MB, Fister MB, Dabir-Vaziri N, Schaffer M: Effect of protein intake and dialysis on the abnormal growth hormone, glucose and insulin homeostasis in uremia. *Metabolism* 25: 455, 1976

219. Armstrong VW, Buschmann U, Ebert R, Fuchs C, Rieger J, Scheler F: Biochemical investigations of CAPD: plasma levels of trace elements and amino acids, and impaired glucose tolerance during the course of treatment. *Int J Artif Organs* 3: 327, 1980

220. Gahl GM: Medical management of continuous ambulatory peritoneal dialysis. In: *Continuous Ambulatory Peritoneal Dialysis*, edited by Legrain M, Excerpta Medica, Amsterdam, 1980, p 181

221. Armstrong VW, Creutzfeldt W, Ebert R, Fuchs C, Hilgers R, Scheler F: Effect of dialysate glucose on plasma glucose and

glucoregulatory hormones in CAPD patients. *Nephron* 39: 141, 1985

222. Bilbrey EL, Faloona GR, Withe MA, Knochel JP: Hyperglucagonemia of renal failure. *J Clin Invest* 53: 841, 1974

223. Sherwin RS, Bastl C, Finkelstein FO, Fisher M, Black H, Hendler R, Felig P: Influence of uremia and hemodialysis on the turnover and metabolic effects of glucagon. *J Clin Invest* 57: 722, 1976

224. Punz KK, Yeung CK, Yeung RTT: Effects of propranolol and metoprolol on glucose, cyclic AMP and insulin responses during pharmacologic hyperglucagonemia in hemodialysis patients. *Nephron* 39: 175, 1985

225. Duckworth WC, Heinemann M, Kemp I: Insulin and glucagon degradation by kidney. *Clin Res* 23: 318, 1975

226. El Ghonaimy E, Barsoum R, Soliman M, El Fikky A, Rashwan S, El Rouby O, Haddad S, El Khashab O, Abou Zeid M, Hassaballah N, Hassaballah A: Serum gastrin in chronic renal failure: morphological and physiological correlations. *Nephron* 39: 86, 1985

227. Muto S, Murayama N, Asano Y, Hosonda S, Miyata M: Hypergastrinemia and achlorhydria in chronic renal failure. *Nephron* 40: 143, 1985

228. Kokot F, Król Z, Mleczko Z, Pazera A, Szczechowska E: Der Einfluss von Cimethidin auf den Serumgastrinspiegel bei chronischem Nierenversagen. (The effect of cimetidine on serum gastrin levels in chronic renal failure.) *Dtsch Gesundh-Wesen* 36: 471, 1981

229. Kuska J, Kokot F, Gerlach J: Gastrinaemia after intravenous calcium load in patients with acute and chronic renal failure. *Pol Arch Med Wewn* 63: 149, 1980

230. Korman MG, Laver MC, Hansky J: Hypergastrinemia in chronic renal failure. *Br Med J* 1: 209, 1972

231. Owyang C, Miller LJ, Di Mango EP, Brennan LA, Go VLW: Gastrointestinal hormone profile in renal insufficiency. *Mayo Clin Proc* 63: 769, 1979

232. Sirinek KR, O'Dorlsio TM, Gaskill HV, Levine BA: Chronic renal failure: effect of hemodialysis on gastrointestinal hormones. *Am J Surg* 148: 732, 1984

233. Gold CH, Morley JE, Viljoen M, Tim LO, Fomseca M, Kalk WJ: Gastric acid secretion and serum gastrin levels in patients with chronic renal failure on regular hemodialysis. *Nephron* 25: 92, 1980

234. Grace SG, Davidson WD, State D: Renal mechanism for removal of gastrin from the circulation. *Surg Forum* 25: 323, 1974

235. Balman RM, Cooper WS, Garner SC, Munson PL, Wells SAJ: Stimulation of gastrin secretion in the pig by parathyroid hormone and its inhibition by thyrocalcitonin. *Endocrinology* 100: 1014, 1977

236. Taylor IL, Sells RA, Mc Connell RB, Dockray GO: Serum gastrin in patients with chronic renal failure. *Gut* 21: 1062, 1980

237. Sullivan SN, Tustanoff E, Slaughter DN: Hypergastrinemia and gastric acid hypersecretion in uremia. *Clin Nephrol* 5: 25, 1976

238. Wesdorp RIC, Falcao HA, Banks PB, Martino J, Fischer JE: Gastrin and gastric acid secretion in renal failure. *Am J Surg* 141: 334, 1981

239. Nielsen HE, Christensen CK, Brandsborg M, Brandsborg O: The effect of renal transplantation on basal serum gastrin concentration. *Acta Med Scand* 207: 85, 1980

240. Balcke P, Pointner H: Serumgastrin nach Nierentransplantation. (Serum gastrin after renal transplantation.) *Wien Klin Wochenschr* 92: 86, 1980

241. Żukowska-Szczechowska E, Kokot F, Grzeszczak W: Gastrinaemia in renal graft recipients treated by cyclosporine A or azathioprine with prednisone *Acta Med Pol* (in press)

242. Lauritzen JB, Lauritzen KB, Olsen ME, Timmerman I: Gastric inhibitory polypeptide (GIP) and insulin release in response to oral and intravenous glucose in uremic patients. *Metabolism* 9: 1096, 1982

243. Grekas DM, Raptis S, Tourkantonis AA: Plasma secretin, pancreozymin and somatostatin-like hormone in chronic renal failure patients. *Uremia Invest* 8: 117, 1984–1985

244. Lugari R, David S, Dall'Augine P, Nicolotti V, Parmeggiani A, Gnudi A, Luciani A, Toscani S, Zandomeneghi R: Human pancreatic polypeptide and somatostatin in chronic renal failure. *Proc Eur Dial Transplant Assoc Eur Ren Assoc* 21: 614, 1985

245. Boden G, Master RW, Owen OE, Rudnik MR: Human pancreatic polypeptide in chronic renal failure and cirrhosis of the liver: role of kidneys and liver in pancreatic polypeptide metabolism. *J Clin Endocrinol Metab* 51: 573, 1980

246. Henriksen JH, Staun-Olsen P, Borg Mogensen N, Fahrenkrug J: Circulating endogenous vasoactive intestinal polypeptide (VIP) in patients with uraemia and liver cirrhosis. *Eur J Clin Invest* 16: 211, 1986

247. Needleman P, Adams SP, Cole BR, Currie MG, Geller DM, Michener ML, Saper CB, Schwartz D, Standaert DG: Atriopeptins as cardiac hormones. *Hypertension* 7: 469, 1985

248. Needleman P, Greenwald JE: Atriopeptin: a cardiac hormone intimately involved in fluid, electrolyte, and blood pressure homeostatis. *N Engl J Med* 314: 828, 1986

249. Eisenhauer T, Talartschik ?, Scheler F: Detection of fluid overload by plasma concentration of human atrial natriuretic peptide (h-ANP) in patients with renal failure. *Klin Wochenschr* 64 (Suppl VI): 68, 1986

250. Rascher W, Tulassy T, Lang RE: Atrial natriuretic peptide in plasma of volume overloaded children with chronic renal failure. *Lancet* 2: 303, 1985

251. Hartter E, Pacher R, Frass M, Woloszczuk W, Leithner C: Plasma levels of atrial natriuretic peptide (ANP) in volume expanded patients: response to fluid removal by continuous pump driven hemofiltration. *Klin Wochenschr* 64 (Suppl VI): 112, 1986

252. Luft FC, Sterzel RB, Lang RE, Trabold EM, Veelken R, Ruskoaho H, Gao Y, Ganten D, Unger T: Atrial natriuretic factor determinations and chronic sodium homeostasis. *Kidney Int* 29: 1004, 1986

253. Smith S, Anderson S, Ballermann BJ, Brenner BM: Role of atrial natriuretic polypeptide in adaptation of sodium excretion with reduced renal mass. *J Clin Invest* 77: 1395, 1986

254. De Wardener HE, Clarkson EM: Concept of natriuretic hormone. *Physiol Rev* 65: 658, 1985

255. Buckalew VM, Gruber KA: Natriuretic hormone. *Annu Rev Physiol* 46: 343, 1984

256. Kelly RA, O'Hara DS, Mitch WE, Steinman TI, Goldszer RC, Solomon HS, Smith TW: Endogenous digitalis-like factors in hypertension and chronic renal insufficiency. *Kidney Int* 30: 723, 1986

257. Greenway DC, Nanji AA: Digoxin-like immunoreactive substance in renal failure: a reappraisal. *Nephron* 44: 108, 1986

258. Kramer HJ, Pennig J, Klingmüller D, Kipnowski J, Glänzer K, Düring R: Digoxin-like immunoreactivity substance(s) in the serum of patients with chronic uremia. *Nephron* 40: 297, 1985

259. Graves SW, Brown B, Waldes R: An endogenous digoxin-like substance in patients with renal impairment. *Ann Intern*

Med 99: 604, 1983

260. Gilkdes JJH, Eady RAJ, Rees LH, Monro DD, Moorhead JF: Plasma immunoreactive melantropic hormones in patients on maintenance hemodialysis. *Br Med J* 1: 656, 1975

261. Kuhn JM, Luton JP, Bricaire H: ACTH, β-endorphine, lipotropines: Études physiophahologiques chez l'homme. (ACTH, β endorphin, lipotropins: Pathophysiological studies in man.) *Ann Med Interne* 133: 148, 1982

262. Aronin N, Liotta AA, Shickmanter B, Schyssler GC, Krieger GT: Impaired clearance of β-lipotropin in uremia. *J Clin Endocrinol Metab* 53: 797, 1981

263. Smith R, Grossman A, Gaillard R, Clement Jones V, Ratter S, Mallinson J, Lowry PJ, Besser GM, Rees LH: Studies on circulating MET-enkephalin and β-endorphin: normal subjects and patients with renal and adrenal disease. *Clin Endocrinol* 15: 291, 1981

264. Zoccali C, Ciccarelli M, Mallamaci F, Maggiore Q: [MET]-enkephalin and [Leu]-enkephalin plasma levels in chronic renal failure *Nephrol Dial Transplant* 1: 219, 1987

265. Zoccali C, Ciccarelli M, Mallamaci F, Maggiore Q: Effect of naloxone on the defective autonomic control of heart rate in uraemic patients. *Clin Sci* 69: 81, 1985

266. Amico JA, Doll RB Jr, Finn FM, Ervin MG, Leake RD, Fisher DA, Ribonson AG: High pressure liquid chromatographic separation of an oxytocin/arginine vasotocin-like peptide from the plasma of patients with chronic renal failure. *J Clin Endocrinol Metab* 60: 644, 1985

NEUROLOGICAL ASPECTS OF DIALYSIS PATIENTS

FRANS G.I. JENNEKENS and AAGJE JENNEKENS-SCHINKEL

INTRODUCTION

Neurological complications in dialysis patients are manifold and frequent. Some relate to the persistence of a minor degree of uraemia, others complicate the dialysis procedure. A number of neurological disorders occur with relatively high frequency in patients requiring this form of therapy but do not relate to uraemia nor to the methods used for treatment.

For practical reasons, the various neurological changes are discussed according to the location of the lesion. Dialysis encephalopathy will not be discussed; this subject is dealt with in detail in chapter 50.

CEREBRAL DISORDERS

Uraemic encephalopathy

The clinical syndrome of uraemic encephalopathy is presently observed only rarely on the hospital wards, owing to the efficiency of dialysis therapy.

When dialysis treatment is not initiated, the signs and symptoms of uraemic encephalopathy may remain subclinical for a long time provided that (a) renal function decreases gradually, (b) water and electrolyte balance is maintained,

(c) blood pressure is kept within reasonable limits, (d) adequate food intake with protein restriction is observed and (e) iatrogenic intoxication is avoided. In some patients, however, renal insufficiency progresses rapidly and the course of the disease is complicated by unexpected or unavoidable factors. Encephalopathy in these patients is not necessarily due to 'uraemic intoxication' *per se* but to one or several other, often treatable conditions. It is often difficult to decide which manifestations result from uraemia and which from complicating disorders.

Clinical picture

The two main kinds of neurological changes to be distinguished in uraemic patients are those concerning complex mental functions and level of consciousness on the one hand and motor disturbances on the other hand. The initial neuropsychological changes involve decrease in alertness and attention span, inability to sustain attention and to concentrate on the tasks. Patients become irritable or apathic and incapable of performing their daily work. When the situation worsens, the sensorium becomes clouded and defects in orientation become apparent. Patients may be frightened and confused, and a delirious condition may develop. Often this can be attributed, however, to concomitant disturbances of electrolyte and water homeostasis. In the final stage, patients hardly react and become comatose (1).

The initial motor abnormality is *tremulousness*. This tremor is irregular in amplitude and has a frequency of 8 to 10/sec. It is only apparent during limb movements. The pathophysiology of this tremor is unknown. The second motor abnormality is called *asterixis* or flapping tremor. This phenomenon is not specific for uraemia but is also seen in other metabolic encephalopathies and occasionally in patients with focal brain lesions. Asterixis is caused by the inability to maintain a sustained position. When the hands are kept extended (or the feet dorsiflexed) a sudden interruption, lasting only a few moments, occurs, causing a downward flap. On electromyographic examination during this interruption there is electrical silence in the muscles involved which implies that the downward flap has to be attributed to a brief interruption of innervation (2). Malfunction of a hypothetical system concerned with maintenance of tonic postural contraction of muscle has been suggested as being responsible for the interruption (3). Bilateral and unilateral asterixis have been reported in patients with lesions in the pons, mesencephalon, thalamus and parietal lobe (4–8). *Myoclonus* is a third type of involuntary movement which develops in a late phase of uraemic encephalopathy. The term is used for twitchings occurring irregularly and asymmetrically in the limbs, trunk and head. At rest the muscle contractions are slight (fascicular) and cause only fine movements or none at all. During passive or active movements or both and sometimes in response to sensory stimuli, the contractions become stronger and are better described as jerks. In occasional patients the movements may even appear as ballistic. There are no concomitant specific EEG abnormalities. Patients in this condition have a clouded sensorium and are often stuporous. The jerks disappear after intravenous administration of clonazepam (0.75 to 1 mg in adults). Chadwick and French (9) called attention to the fact that uraemic myoclonus as described here resembles action (or intention) myoclonus and myoclonus in postanoxic encephalopathy. It has been suggested that this form of myoclonus is mediated by a spino-bulbarspinal reflex which is normally inhibited. The same authors point out that there is experimental evidence indicating that such myoclonus is caused by a functional disturbance of the reticular formation in the lower brain stem.

Generalised tonic and clonic convulsions are regularly seen in acute or advanced chronic renal failure. They are often indicative of non-uraemic complications as discussed later. In case of localised convulsions, focal brain lesions have to be considered. In the final stage patients are often mute and may be catatonic (10). The tendon reflexes may be brisk but in the terminal phase are often diminished.

Laboratory investigations and pathology

The cerebrospinal fluid (CSF) pressure is not raised, and the CSF protein content is often only slightly elevated. The CSF urea concentration is similar to that in serum. Pleocytosis has been reported previously but not in recent publications (11–14). Electro-encephalographic (EEG) changes develop concurrently with the clinical disorder and include disorganisation, slowing and loss of alpha frequency, diffuse slow wave bursts and specific paroxysmal discharges (15, 16). Visual and auditory evoked cortical responses are abnormal, that is response latencies are increased and peak amplitudes decreased (17–19).

The classical study by Olsen (20) did not detect specific structural changes within the brain by light microscopy.

Effect of dialysis; pathophysiology and pathogenesis

Little is definitely established about the pathophysiology and pathogenesis of uraemic encephalopathy. Several hypotheses have been introduced and rejected; others are being evaluated. Whatever the pathogenesis, the lesion(s) is (are) obviously rapidly reversible and, therefore, to a large extent functional and not structural. In this respect, the reaction to dialysis treatment and renal transplantation is instructive. Even when the clinical manifestations are severe, the whole syndrome clears up within days or weeks after the onset of adequate dialysis treatment. An equally rapid improvement of EEG abnormalities occurs (21, 22). Increase of dialysis frequency from two to three times weekly is reflected in further improvement of the EEG frequencies. Mild slowing of EEG waves which has been present for many months during dialysis treatment, may return to normal within 2 weeks following restoration of renal function by successful kidney transplantation (22).

Two differences between changes in uraemic encephalopathy and polyneuropathy should be noted. Firstly, as mentioned before, structural changes in the central nervous system (CNS) have not been observed whilst structural changes in the peripheral nervous system (PNS) are frequent and have been demonstrated by many investigators. Secondly, in contrast to the encephalopathy, the peripheral neuropathy shows little immediately favourable reaction to dialysis treatment. This unresponsiveness cannot be explained by the presence of structural lesions, as the response to restoration of kidney function by successful transplantation is excellent. Clearly the lesions in the central and the peripheral nervous systems cannot be lumped together. Differences between the blood-brain barrier and the blood-nerve barrier may result in a better protection from structural injury of the CNS than of the PNS.

Brain metabolism has been shown to be reduced in uraemia (23, 24) and O_2 utilisation is depressed. These changes may result from uraemic toxins, either by undue effects on neurotransmission (25) or by inhibition of enzyme activities. Activity of Na^+-K^+-ATPase in brain tissue of uraemic rats and activity of the Na^+-K^+-ATPase pump in brain synaptosomes of uraemic rats is decreased (26, 27). Inhibition of many other cerebral enzymes by constituents of uraemic dialysates has been demonstrated (28). The nature of the uraemic toxin(s) is still a matter of dispute. The available evidence points to effects of many 'toxic' substances, i.e. calcium and perhaps sodium, some amino acids, other small molecules, 'middle' molecules and hormones produced in excess (29). A case has been made for parathyroid hormone

(PTH) as one of the major uraemic toxins (see for review, 30). Plasma PTH levels have been reported to be raised even within 48 h of the onset of acute renal failure (31). PTH may affect cell processes in various ways. It increases calcium content of the brain and of other tissues. Intracellular calcium concentration affects regulation of many metabolic and enzymatic processes within the cell. Experimental investigations have demonstrated Ca^{++} accumulation in brain synaptosomes from uraemic rats and an effect of PTH on this accumulation has been reported (32). Increase of brain calcium content in acute experimental uraemia is associated with slowing of EEG waves. Increase in calcium content and changes in EEG frequencies are prevented by parathyroidectomy before the induction of uraemia (30). Changes closely resembling those associated with increase of brain calcium content in acute uraemia, are provoked in normal laboratory animals by administration of parathyroid extract. Patients with elevated plasma PTH have indeed a raised calcium concentration of brain tissue (31, 33).

Encephalopathy due to electrolyte disturbances and acidosis

Sodium imbalance

Experimental investigations have shown that the brain is protected to some extent against osmolar shifts; slow osmolar changes are tolerated better than rapid shifts (34). Acute hypo-osmolality or hyponatraemia may cause brain oedema because osmolality of brain tissue remains high in comparison to plasma osmolality attracting extracellular water (35). Subacute or chronic experimental hyponatraemia causes only a mild increase in brain water content, the osmolality of brain and plasma remaining equal. The critical factor for encephalopathy is probably the accumulation of water in the cells in the brain (36).

A rapid fall in the plasma sodium level in patients to less than 130 mmol/l may cause neurological changes whilst a slow decrease need not become apparent neurologically until values of 120 mmol/l have been reached. There are many causes of hypo-osmolality and hyponatraemia in patients with renal failure, e.g. congestive heart failure, the nephrotic syndrome, impaired water excretion, excessive water ingestion or dialysis. The manifestations are nonspecific and include headache, nausea, vomiting, drowsiness, muscle cramps, restless legs, asterixis, myoclonus, confusion, delirium, stupor and coma. Convulsions, either generalised or focal, are common. The CSF pressure is elevated and papilloedema may develop. The CSF protein is usually within normal limits.

Hypernatraemia and hyperosmolality cause brain shrinkage and are rare in patients with renal failure. They may occur accidentally during haemodialysis with high sodium dialysis fluid. Clinical manifestations include drowsiness, delirium, stupor or coma. Generalised or focal seizures and stroke-like motor deficits may occur.

Potassium imbalance

Potassium imbalance, either with hypo- or hyperkalaemia, causes neuromuscular and cardiac changes. Experimental investigations have elucidated that the mechanisms for potassium homeostasis in the CNS are highly efficient. This probably explains why potassium imbalance causes no clearly recognisable clinical manifestations of brain dysfunction (37).

Metabolic acidosis

Changes in pH profoundly affect cellular metabolism and function. The brain is protected by several mechanisms against arterial pH changes (38). The acid-base balance in the brain is reflected in the pH of the CSF. The blood-CSF barrier offers little resistance against diffusion of CO_2 but is relatively impermeable to bicarbonate. The decrease in the plasma bicarbonate level in metabolic acidosis is not followed by a similar decrease in the CSF. The compensatory fall in PCO_2 of the blood occurs rapidly; however, the final effect of these two events results in a relatively stable CSF pH, which initially even may show a temporary rise.

Correction of metabolic acidosis by intravenous administration of sodium bicarbonate solution is followed by a rise of PCO_2 in blood and CSF. The rise of CSF bicarbonate is much slower, however, causing a decrease of CSF pH which induces deterioration of brain function.

Chronic metabolic acidosis in advanced chronic renal failure resulting from retention of nonvolatile acids, does not cause clinically manifest effects on the central nervous system functions.

Rapidly developing severe metabolic acidosis, as occurs in acute renal failure, causes hyperventilation and substantial loss of CO_2 from the blood and the CSF. This is likely to be one of the factors causing confusion, stupor and eventually coma. Uraemic patients with convulsions are usually moderately or severely acidotic (39).

Calcium imbalance

Calcium ions play important roles in numerous cellular processes. It is, therefore, not surprising that calcium imbalance results in functional disturbances of many organ systems including the nervous system. Experimental evidence shows that the CSF calcium concentration remains relatively constant during alterations in plasma calcium concentration (40, 41). The homeostatic mechanisms involved, however, do not offer absolute protection. Following experimental parathyroidectomy, CSF calcium concentration decreases over a period of several weeks. It is, therefore, likely that brief changes in plasma calcium concentration induce only slight responses in CSF calcium concentration. An exchange between CSF and brain calcium has been demonstrated.

The total plasma calcium level in renal failure is characteristically depressed. Both the protein bound fraction and the ultrafiltrable portion decrease. Peripheral nervous system manifestations of hypocalcaemia present as tetany. Due to the protective action of the blood-brain barrier the CNS is, in general, less sensitive to hypocalcaemia than the PNS. The main signs of the CNS dysfunction are generalised or focal seizures and mental changes; PNS manifestations include paraesthesiae, muscle cramps, carpopedal spasms and laryngeal stridor. Trousseau's sign (carpal spasm within 3 min following inflation of a blood pressure cuff around the upper arm to above the systolic pressure) and the Chvostek sign (tapping on the facial nerve just in front of the ear elicits visible contractions in the facial musculature innervated by this nerve) may be positive. CNS manifestations of hypocalcaemia in uraemic patients are relatively small because the PTH levels are elevated and the calcium concentration in the brain is high (31, 33). Signs of peripheral nerve hyperexcitability are also observed only rarely, possibly because hypocalcaemia develops insidiously and peripheral nerve calcium concentrations remain relatively high.

Regardless of the cause, hypercalcaemic patients may present with evidence of encephalopathy such as impaired intellectual functioning, lethargy, confusion, hallucinations, delirium, stupor and coma (41, 42). Hypercalcaemia causes EEG changes strongly resembling those in other metabolic encephalopathies. Inappropriately high dialysis fluid calcium concentrations have been reported to cause hypercalcaemia in patients on maintenance dialysis (43). In addition to the changes already mentioned, these patients also developed dysarthria, myoclonic jerks and seizures.

Magnesium imbalance

Plasma magnesium levels are raised in severe chronic renal failure, usually without inducing any neurological manifestations (39, 44), but when magnesium levels reach two or three times normal values drowsiness may develop. Levels of this magnitude may occur by excessive magnesium administration to patients with renal failure (44). Hypermagnesaemia affects the neuromuscular junction by inhibiting acetylcholine release (39).

Disequilibrium syndrome

Manifestations of neurological dysfunction may become apparent during the course of a dialysis treatment, usually during its last hour or shortly thereafter (34, 45). Mild symptoms such as headache, nausea and muscle cramps occur in many patients. More severe manifestations such as restlessness, confusion and generalised convulsions tend to develop during rapid dialysis, often in the early stages of the dialysis procedure. With the exception of the muscle cramps, the syndrome was originally attributed to a rapid decrease of plasma urea concentration, leaving the brain with a relatively high urea concentration. This osmotic gradient causes a shift of water into the brain inducing cerebral oedema and brain swelling. Results of animal investigations, however, did not support the hypothesis that the osmotic gradient had to be attributed to urea or electrolytes (46, 47). Subsequently, the syndrome was considered to result from an osmotic gradient of unidentified, osmotically active agents and to

lowering of the pH of the CSF and the brain cell water (48). It was shown that during rapid dialysis of uraemic dogs the arterial pH rose slightly, whereas a fall was registered in brain and CSF pH. It has been suggested that organic acids accumulating during dialysis cause the decline in pH. These substances might be sufficiently osmotically active to cause brain swelling.

Prevention is possible by gradual correction of uraemia, particularly when initial blood urea concentrations are high. Intravenous use of osmotic agents such as glycerol can reduce the osmolar shift and may prevent neurological manifestations (49).

Intracranial neurological disorders tend to worsen during dialysis. When a presumed disequilibrium syndrome occurs in a patient fully adapted to a dialysis programme, a complicating intracranial disorder or errors in the composition of the dialysis fluid should be considered.

Wernicke syndrome and drug induced encephalopathy

A Wernicke syndrome may develop after frequent vomiting in uraemic patients with restricted food intake (50). This syndrome is characterised by ataxia and changes in ocular motility. The ocular manifestations include nystagmus, abducens palsy or palsy of conjugate gaze. Ocular disturbances are almost a prerequisite for this diagnosis (51). The Wernicke syndrome is frequently associated with a Korsakoff psychosis. Such patients have a defective recent memory, are confused and tend to confabulate. The ocular disturbances and ataxia respond to high doses of thiamin. The effect on the mental symptoms is less favourable.

Administration of drugs normally excreted by the kidneys, may cause neurotoxic effects in patients with renal failure. Penicillin is a well known example (52). In high doses it may cause myoclonus, hyperreflexia and coma. Cefazolin-induced encephalopathy in uraemia has been reported more recently (53).

Cerebrovascular disorders in dialysis patients

In the early 1970s reports of causes of death in patients treated with maintenance dialysis showed a high prevalence of vascular disorders, in particular ischaemic heart disease and cerebrovascular accidents (54, 55). It was suggested that the life span of dialysed patients was limited by accelerated atherosclerosis (54). Continued investigations raised doubt about this pessimistic view. It was argued that insufficient allowance had been made for pre-existing morbid conditions (56, 57). When patients known to have diabetes mellitus, atherosclerosis or a long history of hypertension prior to initiation of maintenance dialysis were excluded, and the age factor was sufficiently accounted for, the death rate due to atherosclerotic vascular diseases in dialysed patients was not significantly higher than in matched control populations. The accelerated atherosclerosis hypothesis remains unproven (58).

Cerebral lesions resulting from vascular disorders can be divided into two categories. The first category consists of diffuse or multifocal lesions or encephalopathies and the second comprises focal lesions. Among the diffuse lesions hypertensive encephalopathy is most frequent. Binswanger encephalopathy may be present in an occasional patient.

Hypertensive encephalopathy

Hypertensive encephalopathy is related to a sudden rise in blood pressure to severely high levels. Hypertension may be of primary or secondary origin; renal lesions are commonly present. The association of hypertensive encephalopathy with other conditions is well documented. Eclampsia is a special form of hypertensive encephalopathy.

Usually following an asymptomatic phase with moderate hypertension and proteinuria, patients develop an extremely high blood pressure (such as 250/150 mm Hg) and neurological and ophthalmological changes appear (59, 60) including severe headache with nausea and vomiting, drowsiness, confusion or agitation. Patients may have generalised or focal convulsions and an occasional patient may display neck stiffness. Some patients present evidence of persistent focal neurological lesions but these do not belong to the basic manifestations of the syndrome. Such lesions result from vascular damage and are due to haemorrhage or thrombosis. Ophthalmological investigation reveals papilloedema, retinal arteriolar abnormalities, 'cottonwool exudates' consisting of bundles of swollen axons (presumably resulting from ischaemia) and flame-shaped haemorrhages localised in the nerve fibre layer of the retina. The CSF pressure is raised and there may be a moderate rise in the CSF protein content. Lumbar puncture should, however, be avoided. Computed tomography of the brain often reveals brain swelling. If antihypertensive therapy is successful, the whole syndrome reverses rapidly with clearing of most manifestations, except for the focal changes. Anti-oedema therapy is often necessary in the acute phase.

The results of neuropathological investigations are of great interest. Apart from cerebral oedema and other changes present in brains from patients with and without malignant hypertension, three characteristic abnormalities are observed: (a) fibrinoid necrosis in the walls of intracerebral arterioles and small arteries, sometimes associated with fibrin thrombi, occluding the lumina, and with extravascular deposits of fibrin, (b) focal or segmental changes in the walls of arterioles and small arteries consisting of fibrous thickening and hyalinisation and sometimes occlusion of the lumina (c) micro-infarcts obviously associated with the vascular abnormalities described above. Because the clinical syndrome is entirely reversible, it is attributed by most authors to cerebral oedema, vasospasms and segmental dilatation of vessel walls. The latter are thought to be localised in parts of the vessels where muscular contractility of the wall has been surmounted by high intraluminar pressures (61). Changes in wall permeability of penetrating arterioles have been demonstrated within 90 sec after the onset of acute blood pressure elevation. For reasons unknown, small arteries and arterioles penetrating into the brain seem particularly liable to permeability changes at the level of the second and third cortical cell layers (62).

The predilection for changes in small vessels may be explained by the role these vessels have in auto-regulation of cerebral blood flow. A rise in blood pressure is immediately followed by an increase in cerebrovascular resistance localised mainly in the intracerebral small arteries. A breakdown of this auto-regulatory system occurring during hypertensive crises causes segmental dilatation of small vessels at sites where muscular contractility can not withstand intra-arterial blood pressure.

Binswanger encephalopathy (subcortical arteriosclerotic encephalopathy [SAE])

Interest in this type of vascular encephalopathy has been recently revived by reports of diagnostically characteristic computerised tomographic (CT) scan appearances (63, 64).

The SAE syndrome may develop in patients with a long history of hypertension or other disorders predisposing to vascular damage, e.g. diabetes mellitus (65–68). At middle age or in early senescence a slowly progressive dementia develops. There is loss of spontaneity, with sluggishness and perseveration. Aphasia, unilateral neglect or other neuropsychological defects are present. Memory loss is frequent but is not always predominant. At the same time, neurological manifestations of motor and sensory dysfunctions become apparent. Some of these may be due to cerebrovascular attacks but more often the neurological defects develop gradually over the course of many weeks or months. Periods of progression alternate with periods of stabilisation, lasting for months or years.

CSF pressure remains normal; the protein content is slightly elevated in some patients. CT scans show diffuse low attenuation in the white matter. Neuropathological investigations reveal diffuse and focal loss of brain with gliosis in the subcortical areas. Lacunes are often present in the basal ganglia, thalamus and pons (69). The white matter loss has been attributed to ischaemia and oedema. The preferential localisation of the changes in the subcortical regions is unexplained. Some authors are convinced that there is no essential difference between Bingswanger encephalopathy and multi-infarct dementia (70).

Transient ischaemic attack (TIA)

Transient ischaemic attacks (TIAs) are defined as temporary focal cerebral deficits, presumably related to ischaemia, lasting less than 24 h. TIAs are often associated with stenosis of extra- or intracranial arteries, they are predictors of cerebral infarcts and also of myocardial infarction (71–74). Thirty to 50% of patients with carotid territory TIAs have carotid occlusive disease. Carotid stroke from extracranial carotid occlusion is preceded in up to 50 to 70% by TIAs (75). TIAs may last a few seconds to several hours. Some patients have many attacks of exactly the same character, in others a stroke may follow the first TIA within days. Emboli, consisting of fibrin platelet material from atherosclerotic sites are considered to be the cause for most TIAs. Diagnosis is not always easy as TIAs may be mimicked by many other disorders including focal epilepsy, syncope, Stokes Adams attacks, migraine and vertigo. The clinical manifestations of the attack depend on which artery is involved. Carotid territory TIAs produce contralateral weakness and paraesthesiae and ipsilateral visual disturbances. There may be aphasia when the hemisphere dominant for speech is involved. The visual disturbances are characterised by unilateral visual transient loss or blurring of the upper or lower half of one visual field (amaurosis fugax). Homonymous hemianopia may occur in TIAs of the vertebrobasilar system. Strongly indicative for the latter are also diplopia or dysarthria and weakness or numbness on one or both sides of the body.

Cerebral infarct

Although a thrombotic stroke may present as a single sudden attack, a gradual or a 'stuttering' progressive course during several hours or days is not uncommon and this course is diagnostically helpful. The onset or progression occurs commonly during sleep or shortly after awakening.

The neurological picture is determined by the size and location of the infarct. When infarcts are large, cerebral oedema may develop which may be life-threatening. Nuclear magnetic resonance imaging demonstrates the ischaemic zone within hours after stroke, CT scanning within days.

In *cerebral embolism* the embolic material is derived commonly from a thrombus or an ulcerated atheromatous plaque in a carotid artery. The neurological defect appears suddenly, in a single attack. The brain region most commonly involved is the territory of the middle cerebral artery. A minority of the infarcts are haemorrhagic. The blood may reach the CSF but this is not usually the case. CT scans can demonstrate haemorrhagic infarcts.

Treatment of TIAs and infarcts

The aim of treatment is to prevent infarct or further infarcts. Patients with TIAs or thrombotic infarcts are treated with drugs that prevent clotting and reduce the tendency of platelets to aggregate. The infarct preventing effect of aspirin in such patients has been demonstrated (74); the optimal daily dose has, however, not yet been established. A positive effect has been obtained with two daily doses of 600 mg, but 300 mg per day or even less may be sufficient and lower doses have less side effects.

In patients with embolic infarcts the aim of treatment is to prevent further emboli. The heart is the main source of cerebral emboli and the most common cause is atrial fibrillation. Anticoagulants are effective in preventing embolism from heart disease (77), but anticoagulant therapy should be delayed for several days if the infarct is haemorrhagic.

Intracerebral haemorrhage and subdural haematoma

The two main causes of nontraumatic intracranial haemorrhage are hypertension and anticoagulant therapy (78).

Many dialysis patients have a long history of hypertension and periods of hypertension are not uncommon during maintenance dialysis. Administration of heparin is necessary to carry out extracorporeal circulation and some patients are treated with warfarin or anti-platelet agents to maintain angio-access patency. Hence, cerebral haemorrhage is a risk in patients treated with regular dialysis.

Hypertensive haemorrhages occur within the brain substance by ruptures of small penetrating arteries or arterioles with fibrinoid degeneration and microaneurysms. Extravasated blood forms an oval or roughly circular mass displacing and compressing adjacent brain tissue. Large haemorrhages may displace midline structures and vital centres may become compromised. Rupture or leakage through the cortical surface or into the ventricular system are common. The clinical picture is characterised by an abrupt onset and gradual or rapid evolution. CT scans accurately define and localise haemorrhages of 1.5 cm in diameter or larger, at least during the first 2 or 3 weeks after the onset of bleeding. During these weeks the X-ray absorption coefficient of the haematoma decreases and a phase will be entered in which the density is equal to that of the surrounding brain substance. If CT scanning is not possible, examination of the CSF is necessary for diagnosis. Usually the CSF will be bloody or xanthochromic. Apart from general medical care and anti-oedema treatment therapeutic possibilities are few. Surgical drainage of a large intracerebral supratentorial haematoma is usually considered futile in the acute phase. In acute or subacute cerebellar haemorrhages surgical drainage is the treatment of choice when the haematoma is large (more than 3 cm) and brain stem dysfunction is not yet severe and has lasted 12 h or less (79, 80). In general the prognosis is poor in patients with large haemorrhages. When the haematoma is small, restitution of function is often better than in patients with ischaemic infarcts, because the brain tissue is often more displaced than destroyed by the haematoma.

Intracranial haemorrhages occurring during anticoagulant therapy are infrequent. They are usually localised in the subdural space (81–83). Subacute or chronic subdural haematomata may cause pseudodementia, drowsiness, confusion and mild hemiparesis. When the possibility of a haematoma in this location is considered, confirmation of the diagnosis is usually easy. The haematoma or hygroma may be visualised by CT scanning or arteriography. Exceptionally, an epidural haematoma causing spinal cord compression with bilateral weakness of the legs and loss of sensibility in the lower limbs may occur in patients on anticoagulant therapy.

Central nervous system infections

Infections are frequent complications in dialysis patients (see Chapter 41). Among these, intracranial infections are rare, but often life-threatening (84, 85).

Intracranial infections may develop insidiously and patients may have few clinical symptoms. In patients with unusually severe headaches, meningitis should be considered. Signs of meningeal irritation (cervical rigidity and positive Kernig sign) should be sought and the cerebrospinal fluid should be examined. CT scanning is of great value in the diagnosis of brain abscesses. The presence of sources for a direct spread of infection to the meninges, particularly mastoiditis and infection of nasal air sinuses should be ruled out. Uncommon types of infections, such as fungal and cytomegalic virus infections, have been reported in patients treated with immunosuppressive drugs.

Management of epilepsy

Renal failure may influence the response to anticonvulsants by altering the distribution, metabolism and clearance of the drugs. In patients with renal insufficiency the plasma protein binding of acidic drugs is decreased, whilst for basic drugs it is normal or decreased (86). The diminished protein binding is not, or only partly, due to decreased plasma protein concentrations. Several hypotheses have been put forward to explain this change in binding capacity of proteins. Either the binding capacity is inhibited competitively by uraemic toxins, or it is decreased by changes in properties of the proteins. The first hypothesis is the more likely since the impaired protein binding is reversible. It may be caused by organic acids known to be retained in renal insufficiency (87).

So far studies of anticonvulsants in uraemic patients have been limited mainly to phenytoin and valproic acid. It has been demonstrated that steady state total plasma concentrations of these drugs were lower in uraemic than in nonuraemic patients (88, 89). Due to decreased protein binding, however, the free concentrations were relatively high. A further decrease in protein binding of valproic acid was observed during haemodialysis. This is possibly related to the administration of heparin which activates lipoprotein lipase (89). As a result the plasma level of non-esterified fatty acids increases and these compounds probably compete for binding sites with valproic acid.

Data presently available support the concept that no change in phenytoin and valproic acid dosages is required to treat epilepsy in uraemic patients. The lower steady state concentrations are compensated by higher free concentrations. Clinical experience conforms with this concept.

PERIPHERAL NEUROPATHIES

Uraemic polyneuropathy

Polyneuropathy is one of the principal and most frequent manifestations in chronic uraemia. At one time it was considered to be a potentially crippling disorder of patients on dialysis programmes, but it is now thought to be a calculable risk which can usually be prevented by early initiation of regular dialysis treatment. In a few patients, however, it may still cause serious problems.

Clinical features

Peripheral neuropathy is heralded by symptoms of dysfunction of lower motor neurones (LMN) or of primary sensory neurones. Whether or not muscle cramps in renal failure patients belong to this category is debated (90). Muscle cramps are recognised as early manifestations of LMN involvement in motor neurone disease (91) and many other neuropathies. They occur before the neurones have ceased to function, that is before muscle weakness occurs. Patients usually experience the cramps in the evening or late at night. The cramps are enhanced by preceding muscular exertion. Muscle cramps in chronic uraemia occur in a similar fashion. In favour of a relation with neuropathy is that the cramps occur predominantly in distal lower limb muscles. The nerve fibres innervating these muscles are the first to develop pathological changes.

The *restless legs syndrome* has been considered by some to be another symptom of peripheral neuronal dysfunction in uraemic patients (92). In the evening or when in bed, patients sense discomfort in the legs and feet and an urge to move the legs and to walk around. The syndrome has usually disappeared when clinical signs of neuropathy become apparent. The restless legs syndrome is, however, not a feature of LMN diseases and is absent in most other peripheral neuropathies. It has been reported in patients with a myoclonus syndrome. It responds favourably to clonazepam (0.5 mg at bedtime) in a similar way as action or intention myoclonus does. It is likely, therefore, that the site of origin is in the CNS (93).

When patients complain of paraesthesia (tingling or prickling) in the toes, feet or fingers, clinical signs of uraemic neuropathy are usually present and may even be severe (94). Burning feet occur only in a minority of patients (94, 95). Pain is absent in the early stages of neuropathy but may be prominent in advanced and severe neuropathy (96). Depressed or abolished ankle reflexes and impaired vibration perception of the halluces are early and initially the only clinical signs of peripheral neuropathy (97). In a minority of patients neuropathy progresses further. Atrophy and weakness of distal leg muscles may develop, as well as disturbance of all sensory modalities in a stocking-like distribution. Clinical signs of neuropathy in the upper limbs occur only in severe cases, which is in striking contrast to the changes in nerve conduction velocities (see below).

Although manifestations of autonomic neuropathy remain subclinical, laboratory investigations have shown that autonomic dysfunction is commonly present (98–103). Some evidence indicates that reflexes involving thin unmyelinated nerve fibres are less impaired than those of myelinated nerve fibres in the parasympathetic vagal nerve (104). Whether the fall in blood pressure during haemodialysis can be ascribed to autonomic neuropathy is as yet undecided. The relation between somatic and autonomic neuropathy is weak (102, 103).

In chronic uraemia increased susceptibility of peripheral nerves to pressure has not been demonstrated. Children with end-stage renal failure usually present no clinical evidence of peripheral neuropathy (105, 106).

Nerve conduction and quantitation of sensitivity

Electrophysiological investigations of patients with chronic uraemia have demonstrated slowing of conduction in all peripheral nerves studied (107, 108). Slowing occurs to almost the same degree in motor and sensory nerve fibres, in nerves of upper and lower limbs and in proximal and distal parts of limb nerves (107, 109–112). In the most severe cases conduction may fall to 60 or 50% of the normal values (13, 94). According to Nielsen (113) there is no critical degree of slowing of conduction indicating whether clinical signs of neuropathy will appear. Measurement of vibratory perception thresholds is more suitable to evaluate progression or recovery of uraemic neuropathy than is measurement of nerve conduction velocity (96, 114, 115). In a minority of the patients thermal sensitivity decreases before other sensory and motor functions are affected (116).

Neuropathy and the degree of renal insufficiency

Manifestations of peripheral neuropathy are part of the terminal uraemic syndrome. In patients regularly controlled in outpatient departments, signs of neuropathy are generally lacking as long as the creatinine clearance exceeds 6 ml/min (94). Exceptions to this rule occur, however. Septicaemia and catabolism may adversely affect the peripheral nerves and promote the development of neuropathy (117). In some patients the possibility of a pre-existing or iatrogenic neuropathy should be considered. It is only in a minority of the patients that a decrease of the creatinine clearance to less than 6 ml/min is accompanied by weakness of distal lower limb muscles and disturbance of sensation. In some this happens during a rapid exacerbation of chronic renal insufficiency. When it is possible to restore renal function to previous levels, the neuropathy persists and may now seem out of proportion to the degree of renal insufficiency (118).

Low protein, high calorie diet

Attempts have been made to prolong the non-dialysis period or the survival time of non-dialysable patients by prescribing low protein high calorie diets containing the minimal required amounts of essential amino acids. As far as neuropathy is concerned, a satisfactory result was claimed with a diet containing 15 to 20 g of protein and a supplement of essential amino acids and histidine (119, 120). Patients on these diets have a low plasma urea/creatinine ratio. It is conceivable that the toxin(s) inducing uraemic neuropathy accumulate(s) in the body fluids concomitantly with urea.

Effects of haemodialysis and continuous ambulatory peritoneal dialysis (CAPD)

In spite of variations in dialysis techniques and schedules there is general consensus as to the effect on peripheral neuropathy. Adequate haemodialysis prevents deterioration of neuropathy and may even induce a slow improvement (96, 121, 122). Much less favourable is the effect on reduced nerve conduction velocities. Neuropathy usually creates no problem in patients on CAPD treatment, though worsening has been reported in individual cases (123, 124). On the basis of a careful study Tegnér and Lindholm (125) concluded that haemodialysis and CAPD did not result in differences in the 'clinical score' of their patients.

Of great interest are the changes in nerve function which are recorded after a single dialysis. Nerve conduction velocity is not influenced to a measurable extent (126), but the following occur: (a) a slight fall in the vibratory perception threshold (127), (b) an increase in the amplitude of nerve (and muscle) action potentials (126), (c) a change in resistance of the sensory action potential threshold to ischaemia (128), and (d) a decrease in the relative refractory period (129) which is lengthened in these patients. All these changes point to a reversal of functional membrane abnormalities.

According to current opinion, serial measurements of nerve conduction velocity do not offer a reliable index for the adequacy of regular haemodialysis. If regular dialysis is obviously inadequate, as judged by the reappearance of uraemic symptoms, nerve conduction velocity does not necessarily worsen (130). Serial determinations of vibratory perception thresholds are, as stated before, more suitable in detecting changes in nerve function than nerve conduction studies are (96, 131).

The effect of transplantation

Succesful kidney transplantation is followed by a two-phase course of recovery of neuropathy. The first phase is brief and begins within a few days after transplantation. Nerve conduction velocity increases and an amelioration of clinical signs rapidly becomes apparent (132–134). The second phase occurs slowly and lasts many months (135, 136). Full clinical recovery is obtained in most patients and nerve conduction may attain normal levels, although persistance of some delay of conduction, particularly in lower limb nerves, is not unusual. Only in patients with very severe neuropathy do sequelae (of non-disabling nature) persist. There is no autonomic dysfunction in transplanted patients (103).

Pathology and pathophysiology of uraemic polyneuropathy

Although much remains to be elucidated, studies of the pathology and pathophysiology of uraemic neuropathy have been informative and relevant to the whole of that uraemic syndrome and to disorders of the peripheral nervous system in general.

Asbury, Victor and Adams (137) and Forno and Alston (138) demonstrated that degeneration of nerve fibres in uraemic neuropathy was characterised by (a) structural impairment of axons and myelin sheaths and (b) demyelination of apparently unimpaired axons. These observations were confirmed by others (139, 140). It was accepted that demyelination was due to a metabolic disorder in the Schwann cells (118, 141). It was also generally accepted that the slowing of nerve conduction could be explained by the demyelination. The classical concepts of the axon/Schwann cell relationships were questioned by Dyck and co-workers (142), however; they suggested that demyelination in uraemic polyneuropathy should be considered as secondary to a primary axonal lesion. The main reason for this hypothesis was that demyelination did not occur at random but clustered in selected bundles of fibres which frequently showed evidence of axonal degeneration. They reported similar findings in another type of neuropathy (Friedreich's ataxia) which was generally accepted as a primary neuronal disease. Electrophysiological findings agreed with the concept at uraemic neuropathy in dialysis patients was a primary axonal disorder with little tendency to regeneration (143).

Another major breakthrough was initiated by observations of the recovery process following renal transplantation.

The rapid increase in nerve conduction velocity within a few days after successful transplantation (134) could not be explained by remyelination and obviously also not by regeneration which occurs slowly. Functional disturbances caused by circulating toxins seemed to be implicated. The observations on changes in nerve function after a single dialysis confirmed the role of functional lesions. Although dialysis has a favourable effect, it had to be assumed that regular dialysis treatment does not completely remove these toxins. Functional alterations together with morphological changes are held responsible for the slowing of nerve conduction.

Pathogenesis

The aetiology of uraemic polyneuropathy is complex. At least three pathogenetic mechanisms must be distinguished: deficiency, intoxication and hormonal imbalance. We shall briefly summarize the current views.

1. Uraemic polyneuropathy is due to vitamin B deficiency
B_1 deficiency is the vitamin deficiency most likely implicated in view of the similarity of the neuropathies in uraemia and in conditions of B_1 shortage (144). Vitamin B_1 deficiency in uraemic patients with chronic renal failure has not been established, however, and there is no substantial loss of thiamin during dialysis, probably because of its binding to plasma proteins. Administration of vitamin B_1 neither cures nor prevents uraemic neuropathy (90).

2. Inhibition of enzyme activity by uraemic toxins causes polyneuropathy
Babb et al (145) suggested that a number of uraemic toxins had molecular masses in the 'middle' molecule range (300 to 2,000 daltons). Middle molecules would be less efficiently removed with haemodialysis than small molecules and accumulate in the body fluids. This hypothesis was supported by the observation that uraemic polyneuropathy was rarely seen in patients on long-term peritoneal dialysis (146), perhaps because the peritoneal membrane is more permeable for middle molecules. Although this theory is attractive, the search for neurotoxic middle molecules has been disappoint-

ing (147, 148). Experimental investigations have demonstrated neurotoxic effects of several smaller substances, such as methylguanidine and myoinositol. The main argument against a pathogenetic role of these compounds is the lack of correlation between the plasma levels and the severity of polyneuropathy (149, 150).

The search for enzymes inhibited in uraemia has not been without success. Transketolase is a thiamin-dependent enzyme with a role in the pentose phosphate pathway. This enzyme is present in Schwann cells and in the CNS. Sterzel et al (151) reported an increase of transketolase activity in post-dialysis erythrocytes compared to predialysis erythrocytes and postulated that this was secondary to the removal of an unknown inhibiting toxin. These findings, however, were not confirmed by others (152). Dobbelstein et al (153) reported excessive stimulation of erythrocyte glutamic oxalacetic transaminase by exogenous pyridoxal phosphate. This was interpreted as indicative of endogenous pyridoxal phosphate deficiency and was thought to be caused by inhibition of pyridoxal phosphate kinase. Clinical manifestations associated with pyridoxal phosphate deficiency are epilepsy and polyneuropathy.

Dialysable substances have been shown to inhibit ouabain sensitive, sodium stimulated, potassium dependent ATPase and inhibition of this enzyme has been demonstrated *in vivo* in uraemic rats (26). Inhibition of sodium transport across cell membranes results in slowing of conduction along these membranes. Renal transplantation is followed by a rapid increase in activity of this enzyme. Its inhibition may underlie the rapidly reversible component of decreased nerve conduction velocity (154). An interesting observation concerns the decrease of the specific sodium permeability of the nodal membrane in acute uraemia (155). It was suggested that this decrease might relate to elevated intracellular calcium or intra-axonal accumulation of cationic metabolites.

3. Raised PTH blood levels in uraemic patients may cause neuropathy (possibly by increase of the peripheral nerve calcium concentration)
This theory is supported by the following observations: (a) increased calcium concentrations in peripheral nerves and slowing of nerve conduction have been observed in uraemic dogs. Parathyroidectomy before the induction of uraemia prevented these changes (156). (b) In comparison with dialysis patients with normal or slightly elevated PTH levels, patients with high PTH blood levels show decreased motor nerve conduction velocities (157). Arguments against the role of PTH, however, are that (a) no correlation has been established in dialysis patients between four different immunochemically defined forms of PTH and nerve conduction velocity (158), (b) motor nerve conduction velocity in dialysis patients is not improved by parathyroidectomy (159), (c) polyneuropathy or slowing of nerve conduction is not a feature of hyperparathyroidism (160).

Mononeuropathy

A carpal tunnel syndrome (CTS) is a frequent complication

of long-term haemodialysis. Twenty to 50% of the patients dialysed for 10 years or longer are reported to have CTS (161). Though CTS has been stated to occur most frequently in limbs with arteriovenous shunts or fistulae (162–165), it is often bilateral (161). Its pathogenesis is likely to be multifactorial. All factors causing CTS in the normal population are also present in dialysed patients. Vascular access may be an additional factor. It leads to venous hypertension and in some cases to a certain degree of oedema in lower arm tissues which may narrow the carpal tunnel (162). Ischaemia due to a vascular steal mechanism may play a role in occasional patients. Aetiologically probably most important, however, are deposits of amyloid in the tissue surrounding the carpal tunnel. Amyloidosis is a complication of long-term haemodialysis. The precursor protein of this form of amyloid is β_2 microglobulin (166). The plasma levels of β_2 microglobulin are persistently raised, not only in patients on maintenance dialysis but also in patients on CAPD treatment (167).

Ulnar nerve palsies develop in occasional dialysis patients (168, 169). A relation with raised venous pressure, predisposing to nerve compression in narrow tunnels was suggested (170) before the discovery of amyloidosis in long-term dialysis. Severe nerve lesions obviously due to ischaemia have been reported in patients with bovine graft fistulae in the upper arm between the brachial artery and the cephalic vein (171).

SKELETAL MUSCLE DISEASE

There are at least two causes for muscle weakness in patients with chronic renal failure.

1. Muscle weakness due to wasting and malnutrition is not rare in uraemic patients (172–174). Such weakness is located predominantly in the proximal muscles and other anterior compartment muscles of the lower limbs. The histopathology of this condition is characterised by type II atrophy identical to that observed in cachexia (175). Biochemical investigations have disclosed a decrease in the energy rich phosphagens ATP and phosphocreatinine in muscle from uraemic patients (176).

2. Muscle weakness may be related to secondary hyperparathyroidism. A causal relation between primary hyperparathyroidism and proximal limb muscle weakness is well established (177). Secondary hyperparathyroidism commonly accompanies renal failure. Patients have bone pain and muscle atrophy. Microscopy reveals atrophy, predominantly of type II fibres. In transverse sections, the atrophic fibres are elongated in appearance as in neurogenic conditions. Serum creatine kinase activity is usually not raised.

Of interest is that carnitine levels in plasma and in muscle of dialysed patients may be decreased. Carnitine is a small molecule (165 daltons) which is easily lost in the dialysate during dialysis. This decrease in plasma levels is, however, restored within 6 to 8 h after dialysis (178–180). Storage of lipid droplets in type I fibres is considered to be the hallmark of a myopathy, caused by carnitine deficiency (181). No lipid storage has been observed in skeletal muscle biopsies from dialysed patients (172).

NEUROPSYCHOLOGICAL ASPECTS

A complete neuropsychological assessment is a prerequisite for accurate evaluation of the impairment of complex mental functioning. In most dialysis patients cognitive efficiency suffers. Using intelligence tests, such as Wechler's Adult Intelligence Scale, a deterioration of the total intelligence quotient (IQ) is found. This decline is partly due to slowness in performing the tests. In verbal tasks, requiring (over) learned knowledge, patients maintain their original level approximately. Performance IQ, as a measure of the ability to accomplish relatively new tasks with a visuo-spatial component under conditions of time pressure, deteriorates. Memory function is diminished particularly in registration, learning and reproduction of recently acquired data, the 'working memory' being more vulnerable than retrieval from long term memory store. A mild disturbance of language function may become manifest in the rather non-specific symptom of word finding difficulty. Written language may suffer from control errors (e.g. anticipations and perseverations). A clear-cut dyscalculia is seldom present. Patients may sometimes, however, lose grip of number structure, as becomes apparent in errors when writing dictated numbers. Gnosis and praxis are usually intact, although minor deviations may occur, e.g. left-right mirroring and mild constructional disorders. Although patients are usually capable of sufficient mental tracking during examination, many complain of problems in concentration which increase demonstrably during the intervals between dialysis treatments (182). Irritably and restlessness are prominent during the last hours of dialysis, and have to be considered as manifestations of the disequilibrium syndrome (183). The total neuropsychological picture is seen in encephalopathies of different aetiologies.

Few prospective studies comparing cognition before and during dialysis treatment have been published. Signs of a minor reduction in cognitive efficiency, possibly indicating cerebral dysfunction, present before the start of dialysis treatment, have been found to regress during the treatment period and to have disappeared after 12 months of successful dialysis. Higher general intellectual level and fewer marked signs of pre-treatment cognitive dysfunction seem to result in a more rapid adjustment to the treatment. However, these factors were of no predictive value after 12 months of treatment (184).

According to Teschan and coworkers (183) the adequacy of the dialysis treatment may be monitored by repeated neuropsychological measurements. Cognition-dependent indices vary directly with the degree of uraemia, choice reaction time and continuous performance tests being sensitive indices.

REFERENCES

1. Raskin NH, Fishman RA: Neurological disorders in renal failure (first of two parts). *N Eng J Med* 294: 143, 1976
2. Leavitt S, Tyler HR: Studies in asterixis. *Arch Neurol* 10: 370, 1964
3. Shahani BT, Young RR: Asterixis – a disorder of the neural mechanisms underlying sustained muscle contraction. in *The Motor System: Neurophysiology and Muscle Mechanisms*, edited by Shahani M, Amsterdam, Elsevier Scientific Publishing Company, 1976, p 301
4. Young RR, Shahani BT: Unilateral asterixis produced by a discrete CNS lesion. *Trans Am Neurol Assoc* 101: 306, 1976
5. Ericson G, Warren SE, Gribik M: Unilateral asterixis in a dialysis patient. *JAMA* 240: 671, 1978
6. Degos JD, Verroust J, Bochareine A, Serdaru M, Barbizet J: Asterixis in focal brain lesions. *Arch Neurol* 36: 705, 1979
7. Donat JR: Unilateral asterixis due to thalamic haemorrhage. *Neurology* 30: 83, 1980
8. Kudo Y, Fukai M, Yamadori A: Asterixis due to pontine haemorrhage. *J Neurol Neurosurg Psychiatry* 48: 487, 1985
9. Chadwick D, French AT: Uraemic myoclonus: an example of reticular reflex myoclonus. *J Neurol Neurosurg Psychiatry* 42: 52, 1979
10. Steinman TI, Yager HM: Catatonia in uremia. *Ann Intern Med* 89: 74, 1978
11. Madonick MJ, Berke K, Schiffer I: Pleocytosis and meningeal signs in uremia: report on 62 cases. *Arch Neurol Psychiat* 64: 431, 1950
12. Schreiner GE, Maher JF: *Uremia, Biochemistry, Pathogenesis and Treatment*. Springfield IL, Charles C Thomas, 1961, p 256
13. Tyler HR: Neurologic disorders in renal failure. *Am J Med* 44: 734, 1968
14. Jennekens FGI, Dorhout Mees EJ, Van der Most van Spijk D: Clinical aspects of uraemic polyneuropathy. *Nephron* 8: 414, 1971
15. Jacob JC, Gloor P, Elwan H: Electroencephalographic changes in chronic renal failure. *Neurology* 15: 419, 1965
16. Luyten JAFM, Storm van Leeuwen W, Jennekens FGI: EEG in uraemic patients with neuropathy. *Electroencephalogr Clin Neurophysiol* 28: 423, 1970
17. Cohen SN, Syndulko K, Rever B, Krant J, Coburn J, Tourtelotte WW: Visual evoked potentials and long latency event-related potentials in chronic renal failure. *Neurology* 33: 1219, 1983
18. Komsuoglu SS, Mehta R, Jones LA, Harding GFA: Brainstem auditory evoked potentials in chronic renal failure and maintenance hemodialysis. *Neurology* 35: 419, 1985
19. Brown JJ, Sufit RL, Sollinger HW: Visual evoked potential changes following renal transplantation. *Electroencephalogr Clin Neurophysiol* 66: 101, 1987
20. Olsen S: The brain in uraemia. *Acta Psychiatr Scand* 36 (Suppl 156): 1, 1961
21. Kiley J, Hines O: Electroencephalographic evaluation of uremia, wave frequency evaluation on 40 uremic patients. *Arch Intern Med* 116: 67, 1965
22. Kiley JE, Woodruff MW, Pratt KL: Evaluation of encephalopathy by EEG frequency analysis in chronic dialysis patients. *Clin Nephrol* 5: 245, 1976
23. Heyman A, Patterson JL Jr, Jones RW Jr: Cerebral circulation and metabolism in uremia. *Circulation* 3: 558, 1951
24. Scheinberg P: Effects of uremia on cerebral blood flow and metabolism. *Neurology* 4: 101, 1954
25. Biasioli S, D'Andrea G, Feriani M, Chiarmante S, Fabris A,

Ronco C, La Greca G: Uremic encephalopathy: an updating. *Clin Nephrol* 25: 57, 1986
26. Minkoff L, Gaertner G, Darab M, Levin ML: Inhibition of brain sodium-potassium ATPase in uremic rats. *J Lab Clin Med* 80: 71, 1972
27. Fraser CL, Sarnacki P, Arieff AI: Abnormal sodium transport in synaptosomes from brain of uremic rats. *J Clin Invest* 75: 2014, 1985
28. Hicks JM, Young DS, Wootton IDP: The effects of uraemic blood constituents on certain cerebral enzymes. *Clin Chim Acta* 9: 228, 1964
29. Bergström J: Uremia is an intoxication. *Kidney Int* 28 (Suppl 17): S2, 1985
30. Massry SG: Neurotoxicity of parathyroid hormone in uremia. *Kidney Int* 28 (Suppl 17): S5, 1985
31. Cooper JD, Lasarowitz VC, Arieff AI: Neurodiagnostic abnormalities in patients with acute renal failure. Evidence for neurotoxicity of parathyroid hormone. *J Clin Invest* 61: 1448, 1978
32. Fraser CL, Sarnacki P, Arieff A: Calcium transport abnormalities in uremic rat brain synaptosomes. *J Clin Invest* 76: 1789, 1985
33. Alfrey AC, Mishell JM, Burks J, Contiguglia SR, Rudolph H, Lewin E, Holmes JH: Syndrome of dyspraxia and multifocal seizures associated with chronic hemodialysis. *Trans Am Soc Artif Intern Organs* 18: 257, 1972
34. Plum F, Posner JB: *The Diagnosis of Stupor and Coma*. Third edition, Philadelphia, FA Davis Co, 1980, p 250
35. Arieff AI, Llach F, Massry SG: Neurological manifestations and morbidity of hyponatremia: correlation with brain water and electrolytes. *Medicine* (Baltimore) 55: 121, 1976
36. Fishman RA: Neurological manifestations of hyponatremia. in *Handbook of Clinical Neurology*, vol 28, edited by Vinken PJ and Bruyn GW, Amsterdam, North Holland Publishing Company, 1976, p 495
37. Reynolds EH: Neurological aspects of potassium imbalance. in *Handbook of Clinical Neurology*, vol 28, edited by Vinken PJ and Bruyn GW, Amsterdam, North Holland Publishing Company, 1976, p 463
38. Lockman L: Neurological aspects of acid-base metabolism. in *Handbook of Clinical Neurology*, vol 28, edited by Vinken PJ and Bruyn GW, Amsterdam, North Holland Publishing Company, 1976, p 507
39. Tyler HR: Neurological disorders in renal failure. in *Handbook of Clinical Neurology*, vol 27, edited by Vinken PJ and Bruyn GW, Amsterdam, North Holland Publishing Company, 1976, p 321
40. Bradbury M: *The Concept of a Blood Brain Barrier*. New York, John Wiley and Sons, 1979
41. Davis FA, Schauf CL: Neurological manifestations of calcium imbalance. in *Handbook of Clinical Neurology*, vol 28, edited by Vinken PJ and Bruyn GW, Amsterdam, North Holland Publishing Company, 1976, p 527
42. Frame B: Neuromuscular manifestations of parathyroid disease. in *Handbook of Clinical Neurology*, vol 27, edited by Vinken PJ and Bruyn GW, Amsterdam, North Holland Publishing Company, 1976, p 283
43. Rivera-Vazques AB, Noriega-Sánchez A, Ramirez-Gonzalez R, Martinez-Maldonado M: Acute hypercalcemia in hemodialysis patients: distinction from 'dialysis dementia'. *Nephron* 25: 243, 1980
44. Durlach J: Neuromuscular manifestations of magnesium imbalance. in *Handbook of Clinical Neurology*, vol 28, edited by Vinken PJ and Bruyn GW, Amsterdam, North Holland Pub-

lishing Company, 1976, p 545

45. Kennedy AC, Linton AL, Luke RG, Renfrew S, Dinwoodi A: The pathogenesis and prevention of cerebral dysfunction during dialysis. *Lancet* 1: 790, 1964
46. Arieff AI, Massry SG, Barientos A, Kleeman CR: Brain water and electrolyte metabolism in uremia: effects of slow and rapid hemodialysis. *Kidney Int* 4: 177, 1973
47. Mann H, Stiller S: Elimination of sodium chloride as the cause of dialysis disequilibrium syndrome. *Kidney Int* 17: 401, 1980 (Abstract)
48. Arieff AI, Guisado R, Massry SG, Lazarowitz VC: Central nervous system pH in uremia and the effect of hemodialysis. *J Clin Invest* 58: 306, 1976
49. Arieff AI, Lazarowitz VC, Guisado R: Experimental dialysis disequilibrium syndrome: prevention with glycerol. *Kidney Int* 14: 270, 1978
50. Faris AA: Wernicke's encephalopathy a complication of chronic hemodialysis. *Arch Neurol* 18: 248, 1968
51. Victor M: The Wernicke Korsakoff syndrome. in *Handbook of Clinical Neurology*, vol 28, edited by Vinken PJ and Bruyn GW, Amsterdam, North Holland Publishing Company, 1976, p 243
52. Dukes MNG: Meyler's *Side Effects of Drugs*. Ninth edition, Amsterdam, Excerpta Medica, 1980, p 416
53. Schwankhaus JD, Massucci EF, Kurtzke JF: Cefazolin-induced encephalopathy in a uremic patient. *Ann Neurol* 17: 211, 1985
54. Lindner A, Charra B, Sherrard DJ, Scribner BH: Accelerated atherosclerosis and prolonged maintenance hemodialysis. *N Engl J Med* 290: 679, 1974
55. Lazarus JM, Lowrie EG, Hampers CL, Merrill JP: Cardiovascular disease in uremic patients on hemodialysis. *Kidney Int* 7 (Suppl 2): S167, 1975
56. Burke JF Jr, Francos GC, Moore LL, Cho SY, Lasker N: Accelerated atherosclerosis in chronic dialysis: another look. *Nephron* 21: 181, 1978
57. Rostand SG, Greter JC, Kirk KA, Rutsky EA, Andreoli TE: Ischemic heart disease in patients with uremia undergoing maintenance hemodialysis. *Kidney Int* 16: 600, 1979
58. Lundin AP, Friedman EA: Vascular consequences of maintenance hemodialysis. An unproven case. *Nephron* 21: 177, 1978
59. Dinsdale HB: Hypertension and the central nervous system. in *Current Neurology*, edited by Tyler HR, Dawson DM, Boston, Houghton Mifflin Publ, 1978, p 196
60. Dinsdale HB: Hypertensive encephalopathy. in *Stroke, Pathophysiology, Diagnosis and Management*, edited by Barnett HJM, Stein BM, Mohr JP, Yatsu FM, New York. Churchill Livingstone, 1986, p 896
61. Chester EM, Agamanolis DP, Banker BQ, Victor M: Hypertensive encephalopathy: a clinicopathologic study of 20 cases. *Neurology* 28: 928, 1978
62. Nag S, Robertson DM, Dinsdale HB: Cerebral cortical changes in acute experimental hypertension. An ultrastructural study. *Lab Invest* 36: 150, 1977
63. Rosenberg G, Kornfeld M, Stovring J, Bicknell JM: Subcortical arteriosclerotic encephalopathy (Bingswanger): computerized tomography. *Neurology* 29: 1102, 1979
64. Junck L, Herrick MK, Langston JW: CT-scan in subcortical arteriosclerotic encephalopathy. *Neurology* 30: 791, 1980
65. Olzewski J: Subcortical arteriosclerotic encephalopathy. *World Neurology* 3: 359, 1962
66. Biemond A: On Binswanger's subcortical arteriosclerotic encephalopathy and the possibility of its clinical recognition. *Psychiatr Neurol Neurosurg* 73: 413, 1970

67. Caplan LR, Schoene WC: Clinical features of subcortical arteriosclerotic encephalopathy. *Neurology* 28: 1206, 1978
68. Editorial (anonymous): Binswanger's encephalopathy. *Lancet* 1: 923, 1981
69. Nichols FT III, Mohr JP: Binswanger's subacute arteriosclerotic encephalopathy. in *Stroke, Pathophysiology, Diagnosis and Management*, edited by Barnett HJM, Mohr JP, Stein BM, Yatsu FM, New York, Churchill Livingstone 1986, p 875
70. De Reuck J, Crevits L, De Coster W, Sieben G., van der Eecken H: Pathogenesis of Binswanger chronic progressive subcortical encephalopathy. *Neurology* 30: 920, 1980
71. Reinmuth OM: Transient ischemic attacks. in Current Neurology, vol 1, edited by Tyler HR, Dawson DM, Boston, Houghton Mifflin Publ, 1978, p 166
72. Mohr JP, Pessin MS: Extracranial carotid artery disease. in *Stroke, Pathophysiology, Diagnosis and Management*, edited by Barnett HJM, Mohr JP, Stein BM, Yatsu FM, New York, Churchill Livingstone 1986, p 293
73. Toole JF, Yuson CP: Transient ischemic attacks with normal arteriograms. Serious or benign prognosis. *Ann Neurol* 1: 100, 1977
74. Pessin MS, Duncan GW, Mohr JP, Poskanzer DC: Clinical and angiographic features of carotid transient ischemic attacks. *N Engl J Med* 296: 358, 1977
75. Russo LS: Carotid system transient ischemic attacks: Clinical, racial and angiographic correlations. *Stroke* 12: 470, 1982
76. Barnett HJM: Antithrombotic therapy in cerebral vascular disease; antispasmodics and fibrinolysins. in *Stroke, Pathophysiology, Diagnosis and Management*, edited by Barnett HJM, Mohr JP, Stein BM, Yatsu FM, New York. Churchill Livingstone, 1986, p 989
77. Gates PC, Barnett HJM, Silver MD: Cardiogenic stroke. in *Stroke, Pathophysiology, Diagnosis and Management*, edited by Barnett HJM, Mohr JP, Stein BM, Yatsu FM, New York, Churchill Livingstone, 1986, p 1085
78. Caplan LR: Intracranial hemorrhage. in *Current Neurology*, edited by Tyler HR, Dawson DM, Boston, Houghton Mifflin Publ 1979, p 185
79. Little JR, Tubman DE, Ethier R: Cerebellar hemorrhage in adults: diagnosis by computerized tomography. *J Neurosurg* 48: 575, 1978
80. Crowell RM, Ojemann RG: Spontaneous brain hemorrhage, surgical considerations. in *Stroke, Pathophysiology, Diagnosis and Management*, edited by Barnett HJM, Mohr JP, Stein BM, Yatsu FM, New York, Churchill Livingstone, 1986, p 1191
81. Snyder M, Renaudin J: Intracranial hemorrhage associated with anticoagulation therapy. *Surg Neurol* 7: 31, 1977
82. Bechar M, Lakke JPW, Van der Hem GK, Beks JWF, Penning L: Subdural hematoma during long term hemodialysis. *Arch Neurol* 26: 513, 1972
83. Leonard A, Shapiro FL: Subdural hematoma in regularly hemodialyzed patients. *Ann Intern Med* 82: 650, 1975
84. Keane WF, Shapiro FL, Ray L: Incidence and type of infections occuring in 445 hemodialysis patients. *Trans Am Soc Artif Intern Organs* 23: 41, 1977
85. Nsouli KA, Lazarus JM, Schoenbaum SC. Gottlieb MN, Lowrie EG, Shocair M: Bacteremic infection in hemodialysis. *Arch Intern Med* 139: 1255, 1979
86. Reidenberg MM: The binding of drugs to plasma proteins and the interpretation of measurements of plasma concentration of drugs in patients with poor renal function. *Am J Med* 62: 466, 1977
87. Depner T, Gulyassy PF, Stanfel DA, Jarrard EA: Plasma

protein binding in uremia: extraction and characterization of an inhibitor. *Kidney Int* 18: 86, 1980

88. Reynolds F, Jones NF, Zikoyanis PN, Smith SE: Salivary phenytoin concentrations in epilepsy and in chronic renal failure. *Lancet* 2: 384, 1976

89. Bruni J, Wang LH, Marbury TC, Lee CS, Wilder BJ: Protein binding of valproic acid in uremic patients. *Neurology* 30: 557, 1980

90. Asbury AK: Uremic neuropathy. in *Peripheral Neuropathy,* edited by Dyck PJ, Thomas PK, Lambert EH, Philadelphia, WB Saunders Co, 1975, p 982

91. Mulder DW: Motor neuron disease. in *Peripheral Neuropathy,* edited by Dyck PJ, Thomas PK, Lambert EH, Philadelphia, WB Saunders Co, 1975, p 759

92. Callaghan N: Restless legs syndrome in uremic neuropathy. *Neurology* 17: 359, 1966

93. Boghen D: Successful treatment of restless legs with clonazepam. *Ann Neurol* 6: 341, 1979

94. Jennekens FGI, Dorhout Mees EJ, Van der Most van Spijk D: Uraemic polyneuropathy. *Nephron* 8: 414, 1971

95. Nielsen VK: The peripheral nerve function in chronic renal failure. I Clinical symptoms and signs. *Acta Med Scand* 190: 105, 1971

96. Nielsen VK: The peripheral nerve function in chronic renal failure. VII Longitudinal course during terminal renal failure and regular dialysis. *Acta Med Scand* 195: 155, 1974

97. Nielsen VK: The peripheral nerve function in chronic renal failure. An analysis of the vibratory perception threshold. *Acta Med Scand* 191: 287, 1972

98. Hennessy WJ, Siemsen AW: Autonomic neuropathy in chronic renal failure. *Clin Res* 16: 385, 1968

99. Kersch ES, Krohnfield SJ, Unger A, Popper RW, Cantor S, Cohn K: Autonomic insufficiency in uremia as a cause of hemodialysis-induced hypotension. *N Engl J Med* 290: 650, 1974

100. Röckel A, Henneman H, Sternagel-Haase A, Heidhand A: Uraemic sympathetic neuropathy after haemodialysis and transplantation. *Eur J Clin Invest* 9: 23, 1979

101. Zuchelli P, Sturani A, Zuccala A, Santoro A, Degli Esposti E, Chiarini C: Dysfunction of the autonomic nervous system in patients with end-stage renal failure. *Contr Nephrol* 45: 69, 1985

102. Solders G, Persson A, Gutierrez A: Autonomic dysfunction in non-diabetic terminal uraemia. *Acta Neurol Scand* 71: 321, 1985

103. Mallamaci F, Zoccali C, Cicarelli M, Briggs JD: Autonomic function in uremic patients treated by hemodialysis or CAPD and in transplant patients. *Clin Nephrol* 25: 175, 1986

104. Solders G: Autonomic function tests in healthy controls and in terminal uraemia. *Acta Neurol Scand* 73: 638, 1986

105. Mentser MI, Clay S, Malekzadeh MH, Pennisi AJ, Ettenger RB, Uittenbogaart CH, Fine RN: Peripheral motor nerve conduction velocities in children undergoing chronic hemodialysis. *Nephron* 22: 337, 1978

106. Chan JC, Eng G: Long-term hemodialysis and nerve conduction in children. *Pediat Res* 13: 591, 1979

107. Nielsen VK: The peripheral nerve function in chronic renal failure. V Sensory and motor conduction velocity. *Acta Med Scand* 194: 445, 1973

108. Van der Most van Spijk D, Hoogland RA, Dijkstra S: Conduction velocities compared and related to degrees of renal insufficiency. in *New Developments in Electromyography and Clinical Neurophysiology,* vol 2, edited by Desmedt JE, Basel, Karger, 1973, p 381

109. Panayiotopoulos CP, Lagos G: Tibial nerve H-reflex and F-wave studies in patients with uremic neuropathy. *Muscle Nerve* 3: 423, 1980

110. Lachman T, Shamani BT, Young RR: Late responses as aids to diagnosis in peripheral neuropathy. *J Neurol Neurosurg Psychiatry* 43: 156, 1980

111. Fierro B, Modica A, D'Arpa A, Santangelo R, Raimondo D: F-wave study in patients with chronic renal failure on regular haemodialysis. *J Neurol Sci* 74: 271, 1986

112. Fierro B, Modica A, D'Arpa A, Santangelo R, Raimondo D: Analysis of F-wave in metabolic neuropathies: a comparative study in uremic and diabetic patients. *Acta Neurol Scand* 75: 179, 1987

113. Nielsen VK: The peripheral nerve function in chronic renal failure. VI The relationship between sensory and motor function and kidney function, azotemia, age, sex and clinical neuropathy. *Acta Med Scand* 194: 455, 1973

114. Kominami N, Tyler HR, Hampers CL, Merrill JP: Variations in motor nerve conduction velocity in normal and uremic patients. *Arch Intern Med* 128: 235, 1971

115. Tegnér R, Lindholm B: Vibratory perception threshold compared with nerve conduction velocity in the evaluation of uremic neuropathy. *Acta Neurol Scand* 71: 284, 1985

116. Lindblom U, Tegnér R: Thermal sensitivity in uremic neuropathy. *Acta Neurol Scand* 71: 290, 1985

117. McGonigle RJS, Bewick M, Weston MJ, Parsons V: Progressive predominantly motor uraemic neuropathy. *Acta Neurol Scand* 71: 379, 1985

118. Dinn JJ, Crane DL: Schwann cell dysfunction in uraemia. *J Neurol Neurosurg Psychiatry* 33: 605, 1970

119. Bergström J, Lindblom U, Norée LO: Preservation of peripheral nerve function in severe uraemia during treatment with low protein, high calorie diet and surplus of essential amino-acids. *Acta Med Scand* 51: 99, 1975

120. Capelli P, Di Paolo B, Evangelista M, Di Marco T, Albertazzi A: Low protein diet supplemented with essential amino acids and keto analogues. Effects on uremic polyneuropathy and encephalopathy. *Contr Nephrol* 53, 58, 1986

121. Caccia MR, Mangili A, Mecca G, Ubiali E, Zanoni P: Effects of haemodialytic treatment on uremic polyneuropathy. *J Neurol* 217: 123, 1977

122. Cadilhac J, Mion C, Duday H, Dapres G, Georgesco M: Motor nerve conduction velocities as an index of the efficiency of maintenance dialysis in patients with end-stage renal failure. in *Peripheral Neuropathies,* edited by Canal N, Pozza G, Amsterdam, Elsevier, North Holland Biomedical Press, 1978, p 211

123. Kurts SB, Wong VH, Anderson CF, Vogel JP, McCarthy JT, Mitchell JC, Kumar R, Johnson WJ: Continuous ambulatory peritoneal dialysis. Three years' experience at the Mayo Clinic. *Mayo Clin Proc* 58: 633, 1983

124. Said G, Boudier L, Selva J, Zingraff J, Drüecke T: Different patterns of uremic polyneuropathy: clinicopathologic study. *Neurology* 33: 567, 1983

125. Tegnér R, Lindholm B: Uremic polyneuropathy: Different effects of hemodialysis and continuous ambulatory peritoneal dialysis. *Acta Med Scand* 218: 409, 1985

126. Stanley E, Brown JC, Pryor JS: Altered peripheral nerve function resulting from haemodialysis. *J Neurol Neurosurg Psychiatry* 40: 39, 1977

127. Edwards AE, Kopple JD, Kornfeld CM: Vibrotactile threshold in patients undergoing maintenance dialysis. *Arch Intern Med* 132: 706, 1973

128. Castaigne P, Cathala HP, Beaussart-Boulengé L, Petrover M:

Effect of ischaemia on peripheral nerve function in patients with chronic renal failure undergoing dialysis treatment. *J Neurol Neurosurg Psychiatry* 35: 631, 1972

129. Lowitzsch K, Göhring U, Hecking E, Köhler H: Refractory period, sensory conduction velocity and visual evoked potentials before and after haemodialysis. *J Neurol Neurosurg Psychiatry* 44: 121, 1981

130. Dyck PJ, Johnson WJ, Lambert EH, O'Brien PC, Daube JR, Ovratt KF: Comparison of symptoms, chemistry and nerve function to assess adequacy of hemodialysis. *Neurology* 29: 1361, 1979

131. Nielsen VK: The peripheral nerve function in chronic renal failure. A survey. *Acta Med Scand Suppl* 573: 8, 1975

132. Ibraham MM, Crosland JM, Honigsberger L, Barnes AD, Dawson-Edwards P, Newman CE, Robinson BHB: Effect of renal transplantation on uraemic neuropathy. *Lancet* 2: 739, 1974

133. Nielsen VK: The peripheral nerve function in chronic renal failure. IX Recovery after transplantation. Electrophysiological aspects (sensory and motor nerve conduction). *Acta Med Scand* 195: 171, 1974

134. Oh SJ, Clements RS, Lee YW, Diethelm AG: Rapid improvement in nerve conduction velocity following renal transplantation. *Ann Neurol* 4: 369, 1978

135. Nielsen VK: The peripheral nerve function in chronic renal failure. VII Recovery after renal transplantation. Clinical aspects. *Acta Med Scand* 195: 163, 1974

136. Bolton CF: Electrophysiologic changes in uremic neuropathy after successful renal transplantation. *Neurology* 26: 152, 1976

137. Asbury AK, Victor M, Adams RD: Uremic polyneuropathy. *Arch Neurol* 8: 413, 1963

138. Forno L, Alston W: Uremic polyneuropathy. *Acta Neurol Scand* 43: 640, 1967

139. Jennekens FGI, Dorhout Mees EJ, van der Most van Spijk D: Nerve fibre degeneration in uraemic polyneuropathy. *Proc Eur Dial Transplant Assoc* 6: 191, 1969

140. Thomas PK, Hollinrake K, Lascelles RG, O'Sullivan DJ, Baillod RA, Moorhead JF, Mackenzie JC: The polyneuropathy of chronic renal failure. *Brain* 94: 761, 1971

141. Dayan AD, Gardner-Thorpe C, Down PF, Gleadle RI: Peripheral neuropathy in uremia. *Neurology* 20: 649, 1970

142. Dyck PJ, Johnson WJ, Lambert EH, O'Brien PC: Segmental demyelination secondary to axonal degeneration in uremic neuropathy. *Mayo Clin Proc* 46: 400, 1971

143. Hansen S, Ballantyne JP: A quantitative electrophysiological study of uraemic neuropathy. *J Neurol Neurosurg Psychiatry* 41: 128, 1978

144. Pekelharing CA, Winkler C: Mittheilung über die Beriberi (Communication on beriberi). *Dtsch Med Wochenschr* 13: 845, 1887 (in German)

145. Babb AL, Popovich RP, Christopher TG, Scribner BH: The genesis of the square meter-hour hypothesis. *Trans Am Soc Artif Intern Organs* 17: 81, 1971

146. Tenckhoff H, Shilipetar G, Boen ST: One year's experience with home peritoneal dialysis. *Trans Am Soc Artif Intern Organs* 11: 11, 1968

147. Raskin NH, Fishman RA: Neurological disorders in renal failure (Second of two parts). *N Engl J Med* 294: 204, 1976

148. Merrill JP: The search for 'factor X'. *Clin Nephrol* 11: 56, 1979

149. Baker LRI, Marshall RD: A reinvestigation of methylguanidine concentration in sera from normal and uraemic subjects. *Clin Sci* 41: 563, 1971

150. Blumberg A, Esslen E, Bürgi W: Myoinositol – a uremic neurotoxin. *Nephron* 21: 186, 1978

151. Sterzel RB, Semar M, Lonergan ET, Treser G, Lange K: Relationship of nervous tissue transketolase to the neuropathy in chronic uremia. *J Clin Invest* 50: 2295, 1971

152. Kopple JD, Dirige OV, Jacob M, Wang M, Swenseid ME: Transketolase activity in red blood cells in chronic uremia. *Trans Am Soc Artif Intern Organs* 18: 250, 1972

153. Dobbelstein H, Körner WF, Mempel W, Grosse-Wilde H, Edel HH: Vitamin B6 deficiency in uremia and its implication for the depression of immune responses. *Kidney Int* 5: 233, 1974

154. Nielsen VK: Pathophysiological aspects of uraemic neuropathy. in *Peripheral Neuropathies*, edited by Canal N, Pozza G, Amsterdam, Elsevier/North Holland Biomedical Press, 1978, p 197

155. Brismar T, Tegnér R: Experimental uremic neuropathy. Part 2 (Sodium permeability decrease and inactivation in potential clamped nerve fibres). *J Neurol Sci* 65: 37, 1984

156. Goldstein DA, Chui LA, Massry SG: Effects of parathyroid hormone and uremia on peripheral nerve calcium and motor nerve conduction velocity. *J Clin Invest* 62: 88, 1978

157. Avram MM, Iancu M, Morrow P, Feinfeld D, Huatuco A: Uremic syndrome in man: new evidence for parathormone as a multisystem neurotoxin. *Clin Nephrol* 11: 59, 1979

158. Schaefer K, Offerman G, Von Herrath D, Schröter R, Stölzer R, Arntz HR: Failure to show a correlation between serum parathyroid hormone, nerve conduction velocity and serum lipids in hemodialysis patients. *Clin Nephrol* 14: 81, 1980

159. Drüeke T, Chkoff N, DiGiulo S, Zingraff J, Delons S, Man NK, Jungers P, Crosnier J: Absence of increased motor nerve conduction velocity after parathyroidectomy in dialysis patients. *Kidney Int* 15: 449, 1979 (abstract)

160. Layzer RB: *Neuromuscular Manifestations of Systemic Disease*. Philadelphia, FA Davis Co, 1985, p 112

161. Pagani C, Zoerle C, Guaita MC, Bazzi C, Sovgato G, Torgi G: Carpal tunnel syndrome in long-term dialyzed patients. *Contr Nephrol* 45: 72, 1985

162. Warren DJ, Otieno LS: Carpal tunnel syndrome in patients on intermittent haemodialysis. *Postgrad Med J* 51: 450, 1975

163. Bosanac PR, Bilder B, Grunberg RW, Banach SF, Kintzel JE, Stephens HW: Post-permanent access neuropathy. *Trans Am Soc Artif Intern Organs* 23: 162, 1977

164. Harding AE, LeFanu J: Carpal tunnel syndrome related to antebrachial Cimino-Brescia fistula. *J Neurol Neurosurg Psychiatry* 40: 511, 1977

165. Walts AE, Goodman MD, Matoru PA: Amyloid carpal tunnel syndrome and chronic hemodialysis. *Am J Nephrol* 5: 225, 1985

166. Chanard J, Lavaud S, Toupance O, Melin JP, Gillery P, Revillard JP: B2 microglobulin-associated amyloidosis in chronic haemodialysis patients. *Lancet* 1: 1212, 1986

167. Ballardie FW, Kerr DNS, Tennent G, Pepys MB: Haemodialysis versus CAPD: equal predisposition to amyloidosis. *Lancet* 1: 795, 1986

168. Hamilton DV, Evans DB, Henderson RG: Ulnar nerve lesion as complication of Cimino-Brescia arteriovenous fistula. *Lancet* 2: 1137, 1980

169. Ahmad R, Raichura N: Ulnar nerve lesions as complication of Cimino-Brescia arteriovenous fistula. *Lancet* 2: 1381, 1980

170. Bailey RR, Lynn KL: Arteriovenous shunts and nerve damage. *Lancet* 1: 211, 1981

171. Bolton CF, Driedger AA, Lindsay RM: Ischaemic neuropathy in uraemic patients caused by bovine arteriovenous shunt. *J Neurol Neurosurg Psychiatry* 42: 810, 1979

172. Ahonen RE: Light microscopic study of striated muscle in

uremia. *Acta Neuropathol (Berl)* 49: 51, 1980

173. Kopple JD: Abnormal amino acid and protein metabolism in uremia. *Kidney Int* 14: 340, 1983
174. Alvestrand A, Fürst P, Bergström J: Intracellular amino acids in uremia. *Kidney Int* 24 (Suppl 16): 9, 1983
175. Jennekens FGI: Disuse, cachexia and ageing. in *Skeletal Muscle Pathology,* edited by Mastaglia FL, Walton JN, Edinburgh, London, New York, Churchill-Livingstone, 1981, p 605
176. DelCanale S, Fiaccadori E, Ronda N, Söderlund K, Antonucci C, Guariglia A: Muscle energy metabolism in uremia. *Metabolism* 35: 981, 1986
177. Bethlem J: *Myopathies* Second edition, Amsterdam, Elsevier North Holland 1980, p 269
178. Böhmer T, Bergrem H, Eiklid K: Carnitine deficiency induced during intermittent haemodialysis for renal failure. *Lancet* 1: 126, 1978
179. Mingardi G, Bizzi A, Cini M, Licini R, Mecca G, Garatini S: Carnitine balance in hemodialyzed patients. *Clin Nephrol* 13: 269, 1980
180. Bizzi A, Cini M, Garattini S, Mingardi G, Licini R, Mecca G: L-carnitine addition to haemodialysis liquid prevents plasma carnitine deficiency during dialysis. *Lancet* 1: 882, 1979
181. DiMauro S, Trevisan C, Hays A: Disorders of lipid metabolism in muscle. *Muscle Nerve* 3: 369, 1980
182. West TPJ: A comparison of predialysis and postdialysis cognitive abilities. *Dial Transplant* 7: 809, 1978
183. Teschan PE, Ginn HE, Bourne JR, Ward JW: Neurobehavioral probes for adequacy of dialysis. *Trans Am Soc Artif Intern Organs* 23: 556, 1977
184. Hagberg B: A prospective study of patients in chronic hemodialysis III. Predictive value of intelligence, cognitive deficit and ego defense structures in rehabilitation *J Psychosom Res* 18: 151, 1974

OPHTHALMOLOGICAL COMPLICATIONS ASSOCIATED WITH HAEMODIALYSIS

BETTINE C.P. POLAK

VISUAL COMPLAINTS

Visual complaints are frequent in dialysis patients, especially at the onset of chronic haemodialysis treatment. Many experience visual disturbances or headache, that usually are not due to a disequilibrium syndrome, causing a relative increase of intraocular pressure. In some patients these complaints do not disappear, returning during each individual dialysis session.

Lesions of the anterior segment such as limbal calcifications or limbal haemorrhages are generally asymptomatic. With 'red eyes of renal failure' some itching of the irritated eyes may occur due to deposition of calcium crystals in the superficial layers of the conjunctiva often combined with an inadequate tear film. Lens opacities are uncommon in dialysis patients, and usually do not cause visual complaints. Retinal vascular accidents may occur in dialysis patients disturbing visual acuity.

Visual complaints may be caused by therapy-induced eye infections, e.g. cytomegaloviral retinitis, but these infections are more frequent in transplanted patients due to immunosuppressive treatment.

ANTERIOR SEGMENT

Conjunctival and corneal calcifications

Corneal and conjunctival deposition of calcium salts, a frequent complication of chronic renal failure, usually occurs in the limbal area exposed by the interpalpebral fissure. This is attributed to the relatively high alkalinity, resulting from the diffusion of CO_2 from the exposed eye surface, thus promoting deposition of calcium salts when the $Ca \times PO_4$ product is elevated, especially in the presence of hyperphosphataemia. The latter is generally thought to be the main pathogenic factor involved in ocular calcification.

Ocular calcifications are usually asymptomatic although conjunctival irritation due to crystal deposition in the most superficial layers of the conjunctiva, better known as 'red eyes of renal failure' may occur. It seems probable that such conjunctival deposits in combination with an inadequate tear film are responsible for this phenomenon (1). Improvement has been noted after reduction of the $Ca \times PO_4$ product (2). Corneal calcification, however, usually does not regress after reduction of this product, whether achieved by diet and phosphate-binding antacids or adequate dialysis or both (3). Regression of corneal calcification may be observed when the $Ca \times PO_4$ product is reduced after parathyroidectomy and after kidney transplantation (4, 5). Conjunctival and corneal calcifications can be evaluated by slit-lamp biomicroscopy and handlight examination, and are expressed in three grades of intensity:

Grade 0 No deposits

Grade 1 Conjunctival deposits, only visible with the slit-lamp

Grade 2 Conjunctival and strictly limbal deposits, visible with a hand light and the naked eye

Grade 3 Extensive conjunctival and corneal deposits, easily visible with diffuse illumination and the naked eye

Grade 3 calcification generally appears as white, coarse, superficial subepithelial deposits in the interpalpebral limbal region, both on the nasal and temporal sides.

This extensive calcification can be distinguished from Vogt's limbus girdle as the calcification markedly extends into the cornea and conjunctiva (Figure 1). Histopathologically these deposits are seen in the limbal region, mainly subepithelial and to a lesser extent in the basal epithelial layers. Light microscopy shows deposition of Von Kossa positive material, indicating calcium-phosphate deposits (Figure 2). Grade 2 calcification, however, cannot accurately be distinguished from Vogt's limbus girdle, since the absence of a clear cornea may occur in both conditions (6).

The incidence of pingueculae, histologically characterised by degeneration of elastic fibres, is significantly higher in dialysis patients than in healthy subjects (4). The high incidence of degenerative ocular lesions in the dialysed pa-

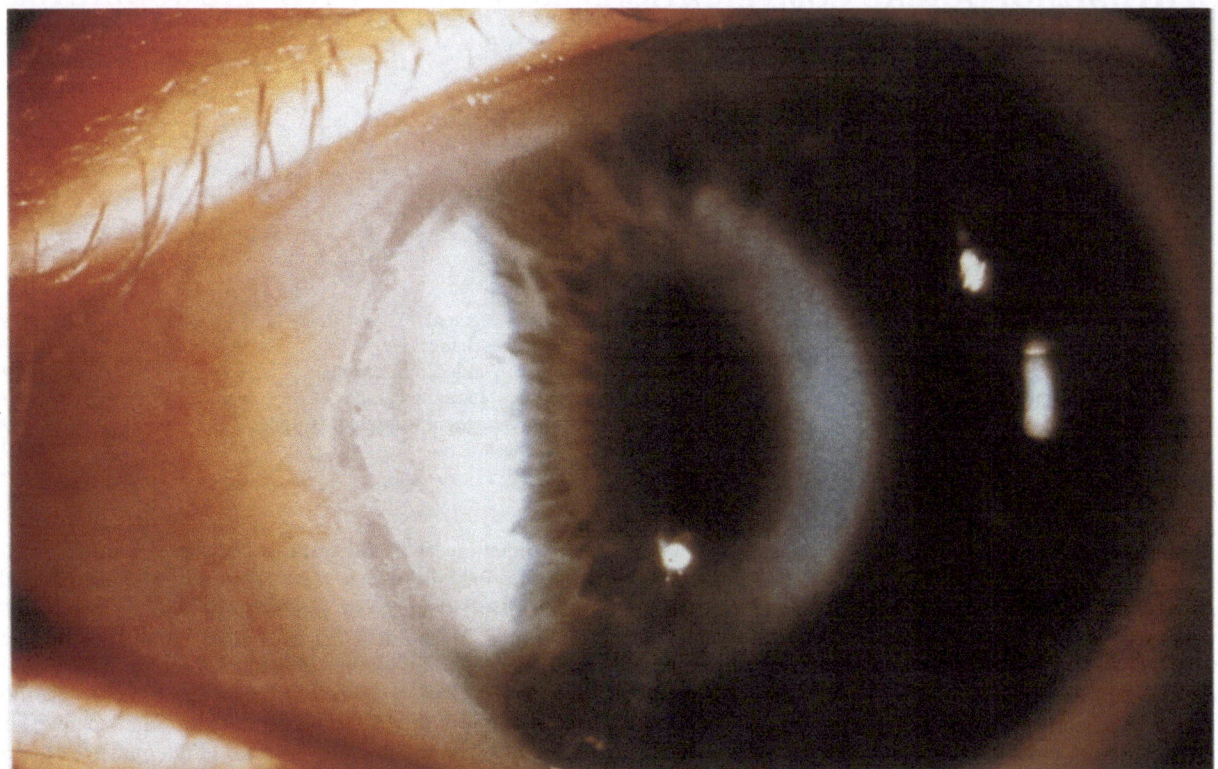

Figure 1. Slit-lamp picture of grade 3 calcification.

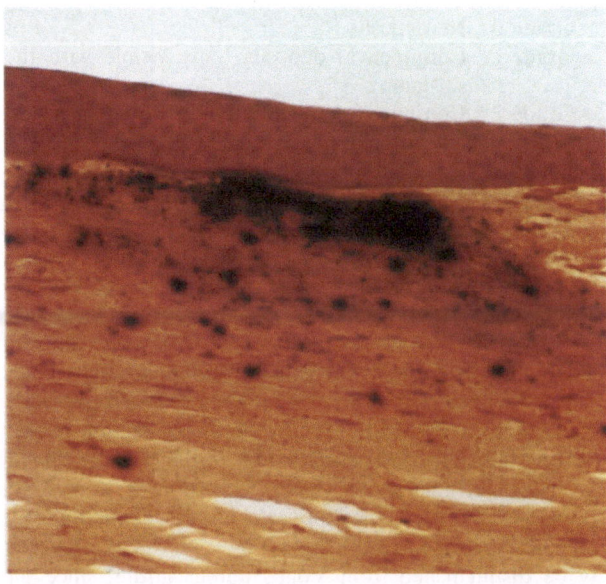

Figure 2. Histological section of the limbal area of the right eye of a 54 year-old patient with grade 3 calcification, deceased after 6 years of haemodialysis. Calcium deposits (black) in the limbal area are mainly located subepithelially, but also in the basal epithelial cells. Von Kossa's stain. Magnification 115×.

tients suggests that such lesions which are known to predispose to calcification, may promote calcification when the $Ca \times PO_4$ product is elevated. This suggests that both metastatic calcification as well as dystrophic factors contribute to the calciferous ocular lesions in dialysis patients.

Furthermore, ocular calcification correlates significantly with the duration of haemodialysis treatment and the patients' age (4). Because conjunctival and corneal calcifications can be detected prior to calcifications elsewhere in the body and the presence of calcium deposits gives useful clinical information, regular ophthalmological examination of each dialysis patient is recommended. It may alert the physician that certain therapeutic measures to reduce the $Ca \times PO_4$ product are indicated, such as administration of oral phosphate binders or parathyroidectomy.

Conjunctival haemorrhages

Conjunctival haemorrhages are sometimes seen in dialysis patients and may be attributable to a uraemic or heparin-induced haemorrhagic diathesis (7). The occurrence of small limbal bleedings may indicate that changes in the technique of dialysis treatment or other therapeutic measures are required; they may also be merely coincidental.

Lens opacities

In dialysis patients only a few cases of lens opacities have been reported (8, 9). The development of cataracts has been attributed to hypocalcaemia in some cases. Prior long term corticosteroid therapy for the primary kidney disease or for graft rejection may also have induced lens opacities in some dialysis patients. These lens opacities usually do not cause any visual complaints.

INTRAOCULAR PRESSURE

Patients undergoing haemodialysis sometimes complain of headache, nausea and fatigue, developing a few hours after haemodialysis has begun and disappearing some time after it is terminated. Sometimes these complaints develop in combination with a rise of intraocular pressure and a simultaneous increase of cerebrospinal fluid pressure. Changes in intraocular pressure, however, develop during each haemodialysis because of a disequilibrium between aqueous and plasma. The rise of intraocular pressure has been attributed to a delayed clearance of urea from the aqueous as compared to rapid initial clearance from plasma (10). The blood-aqueous barrier acts as a semipermeable membrane, which explains the delayed removal of urea from the aqueous and the increase of intraocular pressure which rises as plasma urea decreases generating an osmolar gradient promoting fluid flux into the aqueous (11). The cerebrospinal fluid pressure rises concomitantly with the increase of intraocular pressure during haemodialysis. This is induced by a similarly mediated increase of the blood-cerebrospinal fluid osmolar gradient. When the excess of urea from the aqueous diffuses into the plasma the intraocular pressure returns to normal. The urea-induced change in osmolarity can be counteracted by addition of dextrose to the dialysate (12). A gradual decrease of intraocular pressure could be demonstrated in patients who underwent dehydration by means of forced ultrafiltration without dialysis (4).

Because of the inevitable osmotically induced rise of intraocular pressure during each dialysis intraocular pressure should be measured, when possible, in each patient before the first dialysis is performed. It is also advisable to perform initially frequent short dialyses to avoid large fluctuations of plasma osmolarity and to prevent the development of a disequilibrium syndrome. The diagnosis of glaucoma, whether narrow-angle or open-angle in nature, is not a contraindication to perform dialysis. It is true that an attack of acute glaucoma during haemodialysis has occurred (13), but the rise in intraocular pressure is usually not noticeable by the patient and does not cause subjective complaints. Moreover, due to improved dialytic techniques and better uremia control a significant rise in intraocular pressure during dialysis rarely occurs anymore (14). In cases with an antecedent increase of intraocular pressure or when glaucoma has occurred in relatives, short dialysis has to be carried out at least three times each week, while the increase of intraocular pressure can be mitigated by the addition of

dextrose to the dialysis solution and by forced ultrafiltration. If a patient still develops an attack of glaucoma during dialysis treatment despite these measures, symptomatic therapy by means of miotic eye drops is indicated, if necessary, supplemented by use of a carbonic-anhydrase inhibitor.

POSTERIOR SEGMENT

Vascular changes

Retinal vascular abnormalities are frequently observed in renal disease because of hypertension or arteriosclerosis or both. The funduscopic changes in hypertensive and sclerotic retinopathy in association with renal disease have been evaluated by Scheie (15). Retinal vascular accidents, papiloedema, star-shaped macular oedema and spontaneous retinal haemorrhages may all occur in dialysis patients. Signs of hypertensive vasculopathy may gradually decrease or even disappear if hypertension is controlled. Hence, funduscopy at regular intervals may offer important clinical information. But, signs of arteriosclerosis of retinal and choroidal vessels persist, sclerosis of the choroidal vessels being more pronounced.

Pigmentary disintegration of pigment epithelium and choroid may be secondary to metabolic disturbances due to insufficient circulation in the choroid, but differentiation between such lesions and cicatricial lesions of viral origin may be difficult. At histopathological examination the retinal arterioles show slight sclerosis, which is mostly confined to thickening of the media of the vessel walls. The choroidal arterial walls, however, are found to be more sclerotic and thickened than the retinal vessel walls, and show mostly hyalinisation of the intima and occasional ruptures in the internal elastic membrane (Figure 3).

During regular dialysis treatment deterioration of diabetic retinopathy may occur, which has been attributed to iatrogenic (heparin-induced) haemorrhagic diathesis (16). To prevent progressive visual impairment in diabetic patients with terminal renal failure early renal transplantation should be considered, since stabilisation of the diabetic retinopathy and visual acuity is seen after transplantation. Alternatively regular peritoneal dialysis which obviates the use of heparin is preferred by many clinicians instead of regular haemodialysis.

Photocoagulation treatment and vitrectomy may be performed in dialysed diabetic patients without special complications.

Therapy-induced infections

With the increasing population of haemodialysis patients the number of patients with positive serological reactions for cytomegalovirus has increased (17). This infection may occur in dialysis patients, but occurs more frequently after kidney transplantation.

Early cytomegaloviral retinitis lesions appear either as

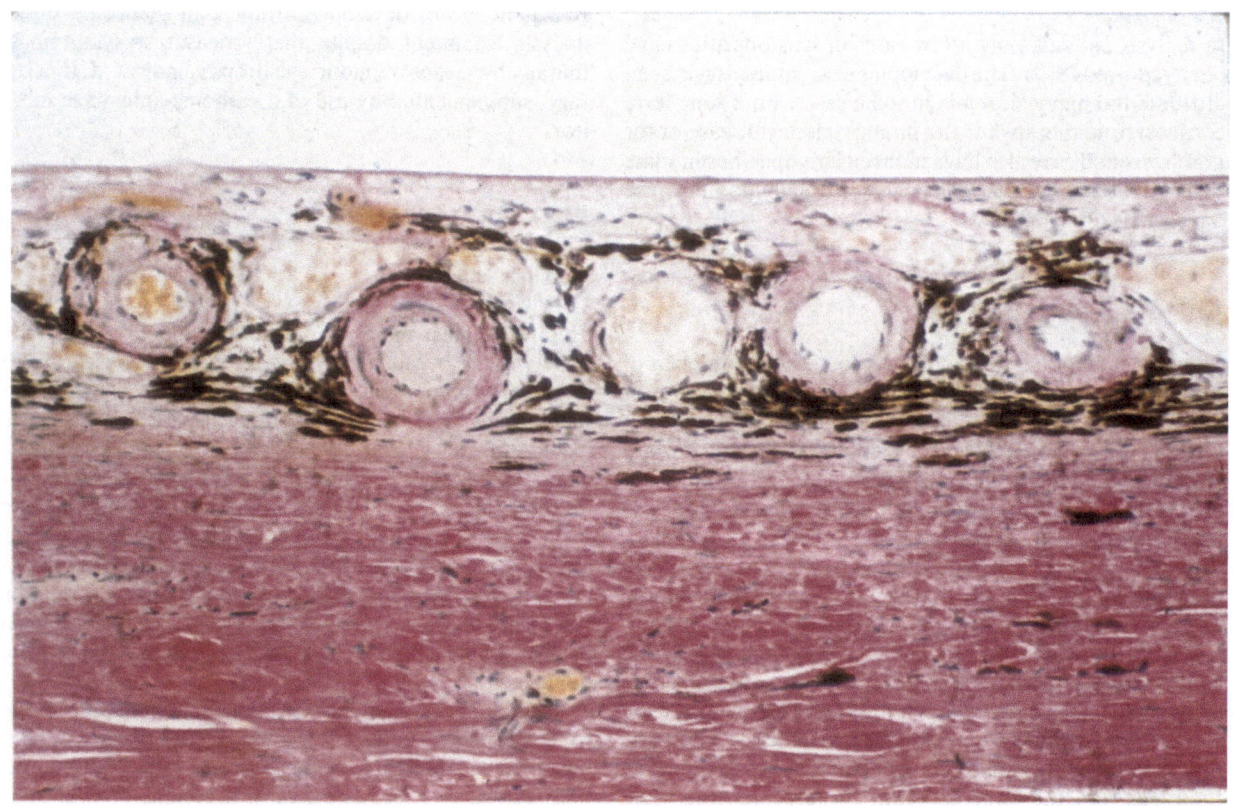

Figure 3. Choroidal arteriosclerosis, as observed at autopsy in all eyes of dialysis patients; 54 year-old woman (same patient as in Figure 2). Striking thickening of the arteriolar walls in the choroid. Von Gieson's stain. Magnification 115×.

scattered areas of retinal necrosis or white granular patches, while the retinal vessels in the involved area may be sheathed and retinal haemorrhages may occur (18). The ophthalmoscopic appearance of cytomegalic retinitis is not specific and may be attributed to a retinal vascular accident because of similar appearance or to vasculitis, giant cell arteriitis or neoplasm (4). In the presence of funduscopic findings suggesting a necrotising retinitis, the diagnosis cytomegalic retinitis may be considered if the results of laboratory tests are positive. Only when histopathological examination demonstrates the intraretinal presence of cytomegalic inclusion bodies is the diagnosis definitely established. There is no effective treatment for cytomegalic retinitis. Gamma globulin and cytosine arabinoside have been used without effect, whereas the effect of high doses of steroids is debatable (19). If indicated, vitrectomy may be performed in dialysed patients as in patients without renal disease.

Fluorescence angiography

The use of fluorescein in patients with terminal renal failure is not contraindicated because the dye (being water-soluble and having a small molecular mass [376 daltons]) is easily dialysable. Since fluorescence is maximal at normal blood pH and decreases with acidemia, the conditions for fluorescence are not optimal in patients with metabolic acidosis. Fluorescence increases in anaemia, however, because haemoglobin absorbs fluorescein. Therefore, in dialysis patients, who are usually anaemic, the fluorographic pictures will show satisfactory contrast.

The remarkable fact that the choroidal sclerotic changes in dialysis patients dominate those of the retina is confirmed by fluorographic findings. In contrast to the normal fluorogram, where the choroidal filling precedes the retinal filling by 0.5 to 1.0 second, the choroidal and retinal filling occur simultaneously and sometimes the arterial filling even precedes the appearance of the choroidal fluorescence. The sclerotic thickening of the choroidal vessel walls and the subsequent narrowing of the lumen increases flow resistance, retarding the flow through the choroidal vasculature, indicative of a choroidal perfusion disturbance in patients with renal failure.

OCULAR CHANGES IN TRANSPLANT PATIENTS

Because the graft function and the normalisation of the $Ca \times PO_4$ product determine whether and when regression of corneal and conjunctival calcification will occur in transplant recipients regular slit-lamp examination may provide important clinical information. Limbal calcifications usually do not change during the first post-transplant year.

Whereas lens opacities are uncommon during dialysis treatment, irreversible corticosteroid-induced posterior subcapsular cataracts are found in a high percentage of patients after renal transplantation. Glaucomatous visual field defects may develop without subjective complaints when blood pressure is reduced to normal. Regular control of the intraocular pressure is, therefore, also necessary after transplantation. Corticosteroid-induced ocular hypertension responds well to antiglaucomatous therapy.

Hypertensive vascular changes usually improve after successful transplantation, but deterioration may occur if hypertension persists or recurs.

Infections of the eye are more frequent in immunosuppressed, transplanted patients.

Thorough funduscopy should be performed during febrile episodes or with the occurrence of visual complaints in transplanted patients to detect any early signs of infections. If present the findings of the ophthalmologist may offer important information to the clinician.

REFERENCES

1. Porter R, Crombie AL: Corneal and conjunctival calcification in chronic renal failure. *Br J Ophthalmol* 57: 339, 1973
2. Berlyne GM, Shaw AB: Red eyes in renal failure. *Lancet* 1: 4, 1967
3. Parfitt AM: Soft-tissue calcification in uremia. *Arch Intern Med* 124: 544, 1969
4. Polak BCP: *Ophthalmological complications of haemodialysis and kidney transplantation.* MD Thesis, University of Leiden, The Netherlands. The Hague, Dr W Junk BV, 1980
5. Ehlers N, Kruse Hansen F, Hansen HE, Jensen OA: Corneo-conjunctival changes in uremia. Influence of renal allotransplantation. *Acta Ophthalmol* 50: 83, 1972
6. Sugar HS, Kobernick S: The white limbus girdle of Vogt. *Am J Ophthalmol* 72: 861, 1971
7. Pambor R, Pap I: Netzhautveränderungen unter der Hämodialyse (Retinal alterations during haemodialysis treatment). *Folia Ophthalmol* 2: 114, 1977 (in German)
8. Junceda Avello J: Catarata estelar reversible (complicacion de la dialisis extra-corporea) (Reversible stellate cataract complicating extracorporeal dialysis). *Arch Soc Oftalmol Hisp-Amer* 23: 817, 1963 (in Spanish)
9. Koch HR, Siedek M, Wiekenmeier P, Metzler U: Katarakt bei intermittierender Hämodialyse (Cataract associated with intermittent haemodialysis). *Klin Monatsbl Augenheilkd* 168: 346, 1976 (in German)
10. Gardner Watson A, Greenwood WR: Studies on the intraocular pressure during hemodialysis. *Canad J Ophthalmol* 1: 4, 1966
11. Galin MA, Davidson R, Pasmanik S: An osmotic comparison of urea and mannitol. *Am J Ophthalmol* 55: 244, 1963
12. Pambor R, Lachlein L, Dahse P: Das Verhalten des intraokularen Druckes unter der Hämodialyse (The course of intraocular pressure during haemodialysis). *Folia Ophthalmol* 1: 39, 1976 (in German)
13. Paul W, Bahlmann G: Chronische Hämodialyse und Augeninnendruck (Chronic haemodialysis and intraocular pressure). *Folia Ophthalmol* 1: 43, 1976 (in German)
14. Gutmann SM, Vaziri ND: Effect of hemodialysis on intraocular pressure. *Artif Organs* 8: 62, 1984
15. Scheie HG: Evaluation of ophthalmoscopic changes of hypertension and arteriolar sclerosis. *Arch Ophthalmol* 49: 117, 1953
16. Jansen JLJ: Therapeutische mogelijkheden bij patiënten met terminale nierinsufficiëntie als gevolg van diabetische nefropathie (Therapeutic possibilities in patients with terminal renal failure from diabetic nephropathy). *Ned Tijdschr Geneeskd* 123: 117, 1979 (in Dutch)
17. Coulson AA, Lucas ZJ, Condy M, Cohn R: An epidemic of cytomegalovirus disease in a renal transplant population. *West J Med* 120: 1, 1974
18. Venecia de G, Zu Rhein GM, Pratt MV, Kisken W: Cytomegalic inclusion retinitis in an adult. *Arch Ophthalmol* 86: 44, 1971
19. Carson S, Chatterjee SN: Cytomegalovirus retinitis: two cases occurring after renal transplantation. *Ann Ophthalmol* 10: 275, 1978

ORAL ASPECTS OF RENAL FAILURE

DAVID S. PRECIOUS

INTRODUCTION

In order to deliver high quality, effective health care to patients whose renal function has been replaced by dialysis, both physician and dentist should comprehend normal kidney physiology, some pathophysiology of renal disease, and the indications and treatment methods used both in the management of chronic renal disease and of dental disease. With the higher frequency of home dialysis, an increasing number of these patients seek care in general dental practice.

The major functions of the kidney include, elimination of metabolic end products, control of tissue fluid volume and pH, regulation of blood pressure and of red blood cell production and the metabolism of 25-OH cholecalciferol to $1,25(OH)_2$ cholecalciferol, the active form of vitamin D which controls calcium absorption in the small intestine (1).

Renal disease can be due to either glomerular or interstitial (tubular) lesions, both of which can lead to either acute or chronic renal failure. Acute renal failure is characterized by a sudden extreme reduction in glomerular filtration rate with consequent inability of the kidneys to maintain the internal physiologic milieu. Dialysis is indicated to stabilize the patient's biochemical state until his renal function can recover, which it frequently does after about 2 to 4 weeks. It is evident that no dental treatment other than that of a truly emergency nature, would be carried out for a patient in acute renal failure.

Chronic renal failure results from a gradual reduction in the total number of functioning nephrons (Figure 1). Clinical evidence of chronic renal failure often does not become manifest until 75% or more of the nephrons have been destroyed. Secondary hyperparathyroidism often develops early in the course. Inability to produce erythropoietin, bone marrow depression and a shortened red cell survival all contribute to the anemia which develops in patients with chronic renal failure. Platelet dysfunction associated with uremia may prolong bleeding although this is usually a late manifestation of the disease.

TIMING OF DENTAL TREATMENT

Prior to carrying out dental treatment for patients whose renal function has been replaced by dialysis, the dentist must consult the patient's physician. Most routine dental treatment can be accomplished on an outpatient basis between dialysis sessions.

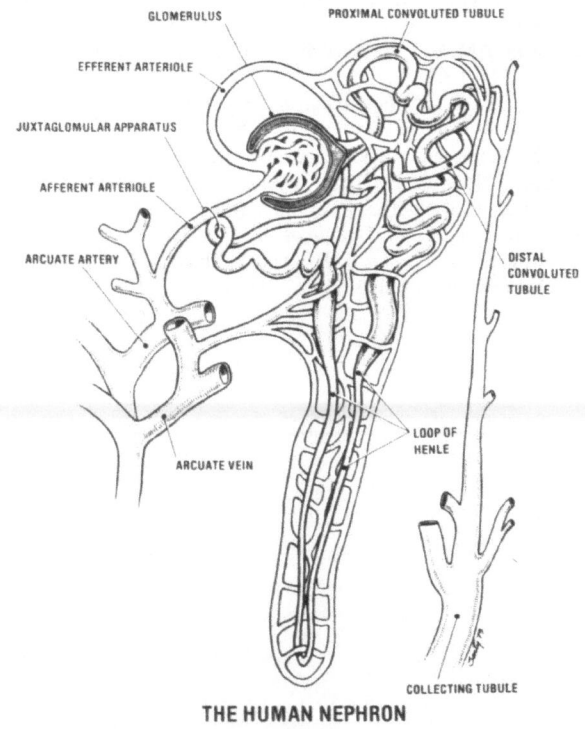

THE HUMAN NEPHRON

(After Smith, The Kidney, Oxford University Press)

Figure 1. Outline of microanatomy of the nephron.

Patients undergoing hemodialysis are given heparin to prevent thrombus formation while the patient's blood is in the dialyser. Heparin has a short duration of action (2 to 4 h). Therefore, dental treatment can be carried out safely on the day following dialysis when there is no danger of prolonged bleeding due to the presence of the anticoagulant, provided that an anticoagulant or antiplatelet aggregating agent is not used to maintain patency of the angioaccess.

CLINICAL AND RADIOGRAPHIC FINDINGS

It is very common to encounter conditions of oral neglect in that group of patients who are undergoing dialysis. This arises probably as a result not only of nonavailability of treatment because many dentists are reluctant to treat patients with severe systemic disease but also because the patients, themselves can assign a low priority to their dental needs.

When renal disease and its treatment have been present before puberty, the patients can demonstrate enamel hypoplasia and possibly tetracycline staining of the teeth. Alterations in growth of the dentofacial skeleton can produce dentofacial deformities of variable severity and sometimes frank malocclusions.

In adults with chronic renal failure undergoing dialysis, bone resorption leads to pathologic mobility of teeth and pocket formation associated with increased calculus formation and gingivitis (2). Decalcification also results in a softer than normal intact dentine. In children, however, there is resistance to dental caries which is attributed to the higher salivary pH and plaque pH, which has a blunted decrease in response to carbohydrate stimulation and to higher salivary fluoride (3, 4). Gingivitis is also decreased, the plaque index does not differ from that of normals and the calculus index is higher.

The increased rate of formation of dental calculus seen in this group of patients demands both close and increased frequency of supervision of general dental hygiene.

Secondary hyperparathyroidism is intimately involved in the radiographic findings of loss of lamina dura (Figure 2), the radiodense line which normally surrounds teeth, and the presence of osteolytic, lucent lesions of both the maxilla and the mandible (Figure 3).

There can also be generalized changes in radiodensity of the jaws and the periodontium.

Pallor of the oral mucous membranes is frequently observed in dialysis patients and is related to anemia, the etiology of which is discussed below.

Many patients complain of dry mouth (salivary flow is decreased in uremia), metallic taste (of uncertain cause) and relative macroglossia, which probably relates to the concomittant anemia.

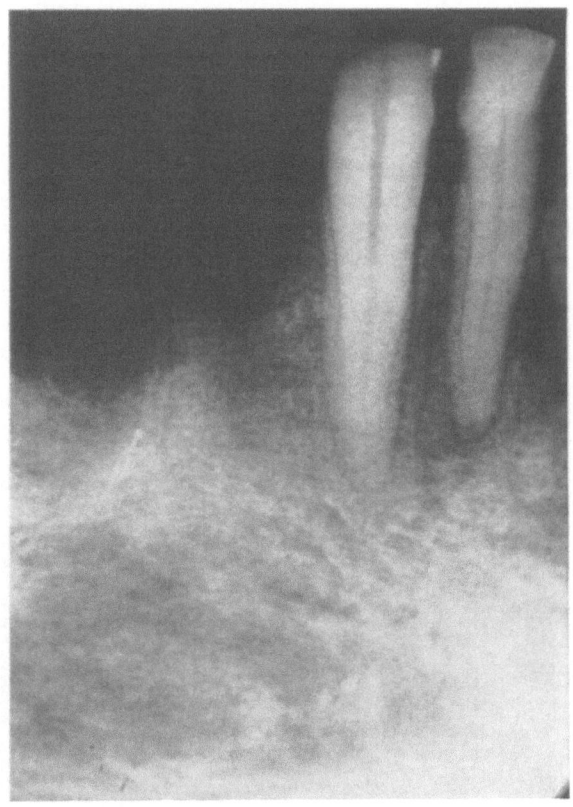

Figure 2. Loss of lamina dura of patient in chronic renal failure.

HEPATITIS B

Hepatitis B has been a frequent complication of dialysis in many centers, and special precautions are necessary when providing dental care for dialysis patients to prevent transmission of the disease to dental personnel (5).

Little evidence exists to substantiate the occurrence of infection other than by direct inoculation into the recipient's blood (6). One recent study failed to demonstrate the presence of hepatitis B antigen in aerosol created by the dentist's drill during work on patients whose blood was positive for hepatitis B antigen (7).

Keystone et al (8) recommend that instruments which have been used to treat hepatitis B carriers should be autoclaved. They disagree, however, with the recommendation that hepatitis B carriers be treated under virtual operating room conditions. They base their opinion on the paucity of evidence which implicates fomite transmission of the virus and they suggest 'that dentists can adequately protect themselves from acquiring hepatitis B virus by simple techniques: wearing gloves, a mask, and perhaps glasses when working on known hepatitis B carriers or those patients at high risk of infection'. Withers (9) states 'the wearing of gloves, a mask and protective eyewear will almost totally protect one from contracting the disease'.

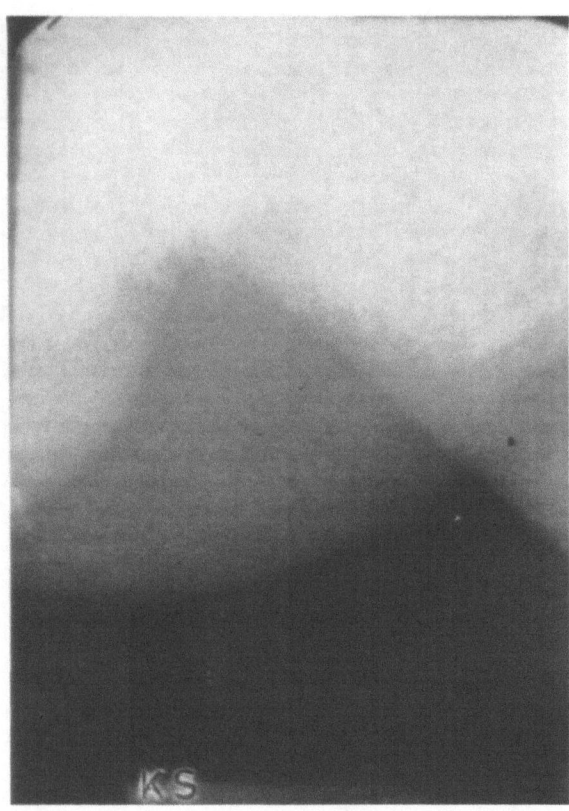

Figure 3. Osteolytic lesion of maxilla in patient with chronic renal failure.

With regard to the possibility of transmission of hepatitis B to other patients in the dental practice, Withers (9) recommends that 'all instruments should be sterilized and all environmental surfaces should be appropriately treated'. In a recent publication of the US Department of Health Education and Welfare (10) it is stated that 'thorough cleaning of environmental surfaces with detergents is the most important step in reducing the amount of virus on those surfaces'. This report also points out that there is no firm evidence of the transmission of hepatitis B from a carrier patient to a subsequent patient in the dental operatory.

It is advisable for dentists and related personnel to have a serum test performed which can identify hepatitis B antibody, because antibody positivity without the presence of hepatitis antigens can establish acquired immunity.

HYPERTENSION

Hypertension in patients with chronic renal failure is common. Dentists should use vasoconstrictor agents with care. Anxious patients can benefit from pre-treatment sedation with sodium pentobarbital or diazepam.

Digitalis is frequently used to treat the cardiac complica-

tions of hypertension and the dentist should know that digitalis in the presence of potassium depletion predisposes the patient to the development of serious cardiac dysrhythmias.

ANEMIA

Chronic renal failure is known to depress the production of erythropoietin, thereby decreasing both formation and rate of maturation of red blood cells. The severity of this anemia demands close cooperation among physician, anesthesiologist, and dentist if general anesthesia is deemed necessary to accomplish dental treatment (11).

PLATELET DYSFUNCTION

Platelet dysfunction results from uremia, and prevention of consequent bleeding following dental surgical treatment can usually be achieved using meticulous local measures which include atraumatic technique, the use of hemostatic sponges and proper home care instructions.

In the case of the patient who has undergone renal transplantation, in addition to the precautions mentioned above, there are the following considerations:

IMMUNOSUPPRESSION AND ANTIBIOTIC PROPHYLAXIS

Rejection is a potential hazard to the transplanted kidney. Almost all renal transplant recipients require lifelong immunosuppressive therapy. The principal immunosuppressive agents are azathioprine, a 6-mercaptopurine derivative and cyclosporin A, both of which can cause serious leukopenia unless the dose is monitored closely. Glucocorticoids such as prednisone and methylprednisolone are administered as adjunctive immunosuppressive agents.

Immunosuppression creates the potential for serious sepsis because naturally induced protective humoral and cellular immunity mechanisms are depressed, thus exposing the patients to greater risk from pathogenic microorganisms. For this reasons, renal transplant recipients should receive bacterial chemoprophylaxis when dental treatment which can produce bacteremia is performed. A prudent antibiotic regime is one which is similar to that recommended in the Guidelines of the American Heart Association for patients with rheumatic valvular heart disease (12). The dentist must also be ever wary in the immunosuppressed patient of myocotic and viral super-infections, such as oral candidiasis or herpes simplex virus stomatitis, either of which can progress to serious widespread local lesions, or more rarely, to generalized systemic disease (13).

Normally, steroids are given orally; but in the case where dental or oral surgical procedures are so extensive as to preclude the oral route, parenteral steroid administration is necessary to avoid the problems associated with acute steroid withdrawal.

SUMMARY

For the patient on chronic hemodialysis, important clinical considerations include timing of the dental treatment, the presence of hypertension and anemia, and the possibilities of hepatitis B and prolonged bleeding. In the case of the renal transplant recipient, bacterial chemoprophylaxis and prevention of acute steroid withdrawal are mandatory.

An understanding of some of the fundamental treatment methods and medications allows the dentist to communicate more knowledgeably with both patient and physician. Dentists are urged to consult with the patient's physician to aid in the delivery of safe, effective dental care. Physicians are urged to encourage their patients to seek dental evaluation and treatment.

REFERENCES

1. de Wardener HE: *The Kidney: An Outline of Normal and Abnormal Structure and Function.* Fourth Edition Edinburgh, Churchill-Livingstone, 1973

2. Löcsey L, Alberth M, Mauks G: Dental management of chronic haemodialysis patients. *Int Urol Nephrol* 18: 211, 1986

3. Peterson S, Woodhead J, Crall J: Caries resistance in children with chronic renal failure: plaque pH, salivary pH and salivary composition. *Pediat Res* 19: 796, 1985

4. Jaffe EC, Roberts GJ, Chantler C, Carter JE: Dental findings in chronic renal failure. *Br Dent J* 160: 18, 1986

5. Donaldson D: Homologous serum hepatitis and dental treatment of renal dialysis and kidney transplant patients. *Br Dent J* 132: 391, 1972

6. Maynard JE: Modes of hepatitis B virus transmission. in: *Hepatitis Viruses,* edited by Japan Medical Research Foundation, Tokyo, Univ Tokyo Press, 1978, p 125

7. Petersen NJ, Bond WW, Favero MS: Air sampling for hepatitis B surface antigen in a dental operatory. *J Am Dent Assoc* 99: 465, 1979

8. Keystone JS, Berris B, Blendis LM, Connon J, Love KR, Vellend H: Correspondence with Dr. J.E.H. Miller, Deputy Minister, Department of Health, Province of Nova Scotia, 1979

9. Withers JA: Hepatitis: a review of the disease and its significance to dentistry. *J Periodont* 51: 162, 1980

10. Council on Dental Therapeutics, Am Dent Assoc, Hepatitis Lab Div, Bur Epidemiol, Tuberculosis Control: Viral hepatitis type B, tuberculosis and dental care of Indochinese refugees. *MMWR* 29: 1, 1980

11. Stuart FP, Simonian SJ, Hill JL: Special considerations in surgical management of patients on hemodialysis and after successful kidney transplantation. *Surg Clin North Am* 56: 1, 1976

12. Kaye D: Prophylaxis for infective endocarditis: an update. *Ann Intern Med* 104: 419, 1986

13. Westbrook SDF: Dental management of patients receiving hemodialysis and kidney transplants. *J Am Dent Assoc* 96: 464, 1978

TRACE ELEMENTS AND REGULAR DIALYSIS

ALLEN C. ALFREY

INTRODUCTION

Although the emphasis on identifying uremic toxins has centered around organic compounds, it is now apparent that inorganic solutes also may be responsible for some of the symptomatology of the uremic state. The importance of such electrolyte disturbances as the cardiac and neuromuscular effects of hyperkalemia and hypermagnesemia, the extraskeletal calcification caused by hyperphosphatemia and hypertension induced by excess body sodium and water have been studied repeatedly. However, little attention has been directed toward trace element disturbances and their physiological consequences in dialyzed uremic patients.

A number of considerations suggest that trace element disturbances might occur in dialyzed uremic patients. As renal function declines, retention of certain trace elements normally excreted by the kidneys may occur. With proteinuria, those elements which are protein-bound might be excreted in increased amounts in the urine. As a result of the disturbances in vitamin D metabolism, the gastrointestinal absorption of some trace elements may also be affected. Finally, the dialysis procedure, per se, could appreciably alter the body burden of trace elements in that some may be removed, whereas others present as contaminants in the dialysis solution ccould be transferred to the patient.

EVALUATION OF BODY TRACE ELEMENTS

During the past decade analytical methods for trace element measurements have markedly improved. The more laborious and less sensitive colorimetric and gravimetric methods have largely been replaced by neutron activation analysis, x-ray fluorescence, flame and flameless atomic absorption techniques and, more recently, inductively coupled plasma emission spectroscopy. The ideal method for the determination of trace elements in biological specimens should be applicable to small sample sizes, have minimal preparatory steps and have adequate sensitivity and specificity for the element in question. Another consideration in regard to selecting the appropriate analytical technique is whether a single element or multiple elements in a biological sample require analysis. For single element analysis, the two commonly available systems are atomic absorption spectrophotometry and flameles atomic absorption spectrophotometry. For multiple elemental analyses, neutron activation analysis, x-ray fluorescence, electron microprobe analysis and inductively coupled plasma emission spectroscopy have largely replaced emission spectroscopy because of improved sensitivity and marked reduction or elimination of interferences. Although these techniques have been simplified and their sensitivity has improved, erroneous conclusions may be made if the investigator is not familiar with limitations of the methodology.

Another difficult problem in evaluating trace element disturbances is determining which tissue or fluid reflects satisfactorily the body burden of the trace element in question. Mertz (1) has divided tissues into four categories.

The *first group* include regulatory sites or tissues responsible for *maintaining homeostasis* by regulating absorption or excretion of an element such as the thyroid for iodide and the intestinal mucosa for iron.

The *second group* consists of tissues where the element under study has an *essential biological function*, i.e. for those elements which are essential co-factors of enzymes in specific organs or tissue. An example is zinc in carbonic anhydrase present in erythrocytes. Because of strong regulatory mechanisms, trace elements in such tissues may remain normal in concentration, despite total body depletion of the element in question. Thus, these tissues would not be good indicators of the body status of certain trace elements.

The *third group* comprises tissues involved in trace element *storage and transport*. Storage tissues, such as the bone marrow for iron, may sensitively reflect alterations in body stores of certain trace elements. Although blood serum and plasma are the most frequently analyzed samples, results may be difficult to interpret – for example, when elements are stored. Plasma trace element concentrations may be misleading when: 1) recently absorbed elements are transported to target organs, transiently elevating plasma concentrations, 2) the plasma is not in equilibration with important tissue stores, and 3) binding proteins are reduced, e.g. in such conditions as cirrhosis and the nephrotic syndrome with spurious lowering of the plasma concentrations of protein-bound trace elements.

The *fourth group* of tissues are the *sequestering tissues*. This group consists of the lungs, the kidneys, parts of the reticulo-endothelial system, nails, hair and the stratum corneum of the skin. These tissues can be used as indices of chronic exposure. Hair is especially useful for certain elements such as mercury and arsenic (in case of intoxication) and zinc and chromium (in case of deficiency).

TISSUE TRACE ELEMENTS IN UREMIA

The tissue most widely studied as an indicator of the status of the body burden of the various trace elements has been blood. Of the essential elements, blood vanadium has been reported to be both normal (2) and increased (3). Selenium (4, 5) and zinc (6) levels have largely been found to be decreased. Serum nickel levels have usually (7, 8), but not always (9), been found to be decreased in uremic patients. This reduction in serum nickel levels is felt to be a consequence of reduced nickel plasmin, an α-macroglobulin. Serum silicon levels have been found to be increased by a number of investigators (10–12). In general, plasma copper levels have been found to be normal. Inadequate information is available on three other essential trace elements: chromium, cobalt and manganese.

Regarding the non-essential elements, blood arsenic has been reported to be 10 times higher in uremic patients as compared to controls (13, 14), and plasma rubidium reduced by approximately 50% (15). Recently, plasma lithium levels have been shown to be increased by approximately five-fold in non-dialyzed uremic patients (16). This probably results from an inability to excrete this element because of compromised renal function. A final element shown to be increased in the blood of uremic patients is aluminum (17).

The meaning of the various blood trace element alterations must be interpreted with some caution, since the change may not reflect alterations in other tissues or necessarily the status of the total body burden of these various elements. In addition, the levels of most trace elements in blood are very low making their determination difficult, which probably accounts for some of the variations in levels reported above.

However, multiple tissue trace element profiles have been characterized in both dialyzed and non-dialyzed uremic patients. A number of trace element disturbances have been identified. These can be divided into three groups. The first group represents a similar disturbance in multiple tissues documenting an alteration in the total body burden of that element. Six elements belong to this group. Total body aluminum, tin, zinc and strontium are increased, whereas total body rubidium is decreased in dialyzed and non-dialyzed uremic patients. Total body bromine is decreased only in dialyzed uremic patients.

The second group of disturbances represents elements that may be increased or reduced in some tissues, whereas they are either normal or affected in the opposite direction in other tissues. Examples of this alteration are the increased liver and spleen iron concentrations in dialyzed uremic patients and the increased copper concentration in lungs associated with a reduced copper concentration in heart of both dialyzed and non-dialyzed uremic patients (18).

A third disturbance in trace elements would appear to be a translocation of an element from one organ to another. Two elements that fall into this group are cadmium and molybdenum, both of which are reduced in the diseased kidneys and increased in the liver.

Of the remaining essential elements, tissue selenium levels have been found to be normal in uremic patients (18). Iodine stores would seem to be adequate in most uremic patients as estimated by normal thyroid function (see Chapter 45). Silicon has been found to be increased in spleen and liver in patients with chronic renal failure (19). Bone fluoride has been found to be increased in patients who have been exposed to dialysis fluid contaminated with fluoride (20) (see Chapter 44). Tissue stores of lead (18, 19) and mercury (18) appear to be normal in most uremic patients. Uranium has been found to be increased in several dialyzed uremic patients (21). The most likely source for this perturbation is uranium contamination present in some water supplies.

MECHANISMS OF TRACE ELEMENT DISTURBANCES

It would appear that most trace element disturbances that occur in uremic patients are a result of uremia, per se, and not the dialysis procedure, since most elemental disturbances are shared by dialyzed and non-dialyzed uremic patients (18). However, the severity of the disturbance tends to be greater in the dialyzed patients. For most elements, this presumably occurs because of the longer duration of uremia in the dialyzed patient.

As a result of loss of renal function, strontium (22) and tin (23), which depend on the kidney for elimination, are probably retained, accounting for the increased body burden of these elements.

Another mechanism for some trace element disturbances is a translocation from one tissue to another in uremia. Normally, kidney cadmium content is considerably greater than that in other tissues. However, with chronic renal insufficiency, the cadmium content in the kidney decreases to extremely low levels, possibly as a consequence of reduction in binding proteins (metallothionine) in this diseased organ (18). The failure of the diseased kidney to bind and excrete cadmium may result in its displacement to the liver. A similar mechanism is proposed for the reduced renal content and increased hepatic content of molybdenum found in uremic patients.

Similarly, the high tissue zinc levels may also be a result of a translocation, since muscle (18), plasma (24, 25) and leu-

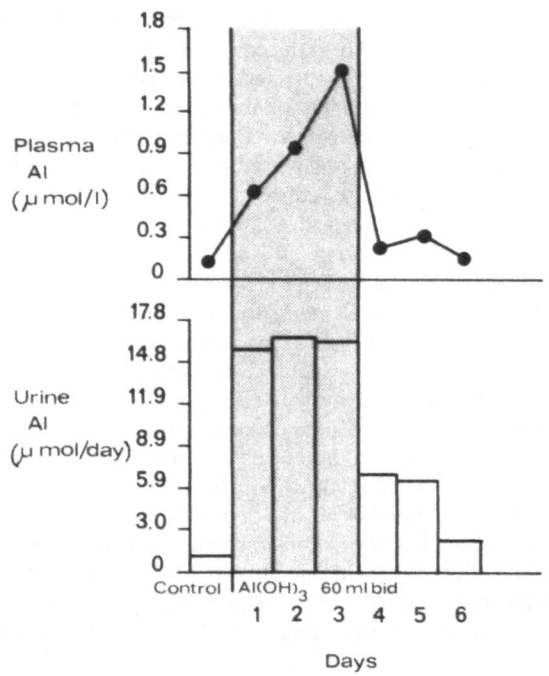

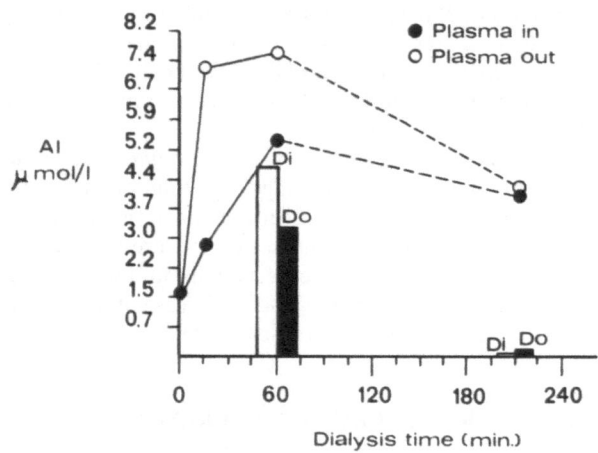

Figure 2. **Aluminum concentrations of plasma and dialysate during** hemodialysis of one patient. Di and Do refer to dialysis fluid entering or leaving the dialyzer. Filtered tap water was used to prepare the dialysate during the initial 60 min of study; water treated by reverse osmosis was used thereafter. Reprinted from *Kidney International* (17) with permission (slightly modified). Conversion μmol/l to μg/l: multiply by 27.

Figure 1. Plasma and urine aluminum concentrations in a control subject who received oral aluminum hydroxide for 3 days.

kocyte (6) concentrations tend to be low in association with the increased zinc levels in other tissues. This is further supported by the finding that zinc absorption and retention have been found to be normal in uremic patients (6). Furthermore, it would appear that the reduced zinc levels in certain tissues may be more a result of starvation than of the uremic state.

The most difficult trace element alteration to understand is rubidium depletion. It has largely been assumed that rubidium metabolism is similar to potassium metabolism. However, rubidium depletion in non-dialyzed uremic patients is far in excess of potassium depletion which may or may not be present. Thus, it would appear that in association with loss of renal function, rubidium excretion is somehow enhanced.

Other mechanisms of trace element disturbances are medications given to uremic patients and the dialysis procedure. The amount of increased total body aluminum found in some non-dialyzed uremic patients cannot be ascribed to the retention of the small amount of aluminum normally absorbed and excreted. A more likely explanation is that, with the loss of renal function, aluminum is retained after it is absorbed from the administration of phosphate-binding gels, which are commonly given to uremic patients. Aluminum has been shown to be absorbed from these aluminum-containing, phosphate-binding gels (25–27). In 13 normal subject, urinary aluminum excretion increased from a mean of 16 to 259 μg/day (0.6 to 9.6 mol/day) during the time the individuals ingested 60 ml of Al(OH)$_3$ twice daily. The changes in

plasma concentration and urinary excretion of aluminum in one patient ingesting Al(OH)$_3$ (120 ml/day) are shown in Figure 1. Although the increase in urinary aluminum seems small, if excretion was prevented because of renal failure, in one year's time this would result in an increase in the total body burden of aluminum of approximately 94 mg (3.5 mmol). Since the normal body aluminum content is probably less than 30 mg (1.1 mmol) this would represent a major increase in total body aluminum.

A second source of aluminum in dialyzed uremic patients is aluminum-contaminated dialysis solution. Aluminum has been shown to cross the dialyzing membrane readily (17). In addition, aluminum is bound in plasma to a non-dialyzable constituent – most likely a protein; therefore, virtually any aluminum contamination present in the dialysate acts as an effective gradient from the dialysate to the blood (17, 28). Furthermore, because of plasma's binding of aluminum even when dialysate aluminum is negligible, aluminum is not removed from plasma. The effect of aluminum contamination of dialysis fluid on plasma aluminum levels is shown in Figure 2. It can be appreciated that plasma aluminum levels rapidly increase during the first hour when dialysis is performed with aluminum-contaminated dialysate. However, following removal of aluminum from the dialysis solution, aluminum was not extracted from plasma as determined by measuring post-dialyzer dialysate and plasma aluminum levels. Another study carried out in patients from two dialysis units, one having aluminum-free dialysis fluid and the second having aluminum-contaminated dialysis fluid further supports the transfer of aluminum from dialysate to plasma (17). In those receiving dialysis with aluminum-free dialysis fluid, plasma aluminum levels, although elevated, were less than values found in patients dialyzed

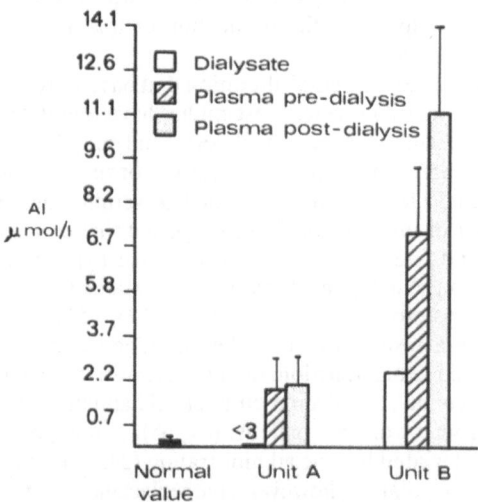

Effect of dialysate aluminum
on plasma aluminum levels

☐ Dialysate
▨ Plasma pre-dialysis
☐ Plasma post-dialysis

Al
μmol/l

Figure 3. Plasma aluminum concentrations in a control population and two groups of dialyzed uremic patients. Patients in Unit A had been maintained on low aluminum dialysate, whereas Unit B had inadequate water treatment and aluminum-contaminated dialysis fluid.

with aluminum-contaminated dialysis solution. In contrast to the latter group where postdialysis plasma aluminum values were significantly higher than predialysis values, there was little difference between pre- and postdialysis plasma aluminum levels in the former group of patients (Figure 3). If the dialysis fluid is free of aluminum, a small amount of aluminum may gradually be removed (see also Chapter 50). The dialysis procedure also tends to intensify rubidium depletion and creates the bromide deficiency which is found only in dialyzed uremic patients (18). Provided that concentration of these elements in dialysis fluid is low enough, as is usual, they will be extracted by the hemodialyzer and removed. This contrasts with normal renal handling which results in conservation of these elements by tubular reabsorption as occurs, for example, with chloride. Otherwise, the dialysis procedure could not be incriminated in the production of any of the other chronic trace element disturbances found in uremic patients (18). The only trace element disturbance improved by dialysis is cadmium excess.

PHYSIOLOGICAL CONSEQUENCES OF TRACE ELEMENT DISORDERS

Acute intoxication

A number of accidental intoxications have been described in dialyzed uremic patients. These have resulted from unexpected trace element contamination of the dialysate resulting from either the dialysis equipment or improper water treatment. To date, no naturally occurring trace element in water supplies has induced any acute toxicity. One patient on home dialysis in Australia had attacks of nausea, vomiting and fever during dialysis. Water used for the preparation of the dialysate was stored in a galvanized tank, and the patient was subsequently shown to have high plasma and erythrocyte zinc concentrations (29), which were presumably leached from the galvanized tank. The symptoms were alleviated by performing dialysis using properly pre-treated water. Acute copper intoxication characterized by hemolysis, leukocytosis, metabolic acidosis and gastrointestinal symptoms has been described in a number of dialysis patients (30–36). It was subsequently shown that copper was leached from copper tubing in the delivery system. Most of these intoxications occurred when the anion exchange column became depleted rendering the water acidic. We recently had the opportunity of studying a group of patients who experienced headache, dizziness, nausea and vomiting during dialysis. High nickel levels were present in the plasma of these patients and the dialysate. The source of the nickel was found to be a stainless steel heating unit used to warm the water after reverse osmosis treatment (35).

A common factor in these acute intoxications is that the elements involved – copper, zinc and nickel – are all bound to large plasma molecules. Thus, virtually any concentration of these elements in the dialysate would result in their transfer to the patient. It might be anticipated that under certain conditions other elements used in plasticizers or alloys such as mercury, iron, cadmium, tin and chromium could also be introduced into the dialysate and transferred to the patient, resulting in acute or chronic intoxication.

Acute fluoride intoxication occurred in one group of dialysis patients as a consequence of a malfunction in a municipal water treatment facility which increased the fluoride content of the water 50 times normal. All patients developed gastrointestinal symptoms and one patient died of cardiac arrest (36). Another potential source of large fluoride exposures during dialysis is an exhausted anion column previously exposed to water containing fluoride. Under these circumstances, the fluoride can be displaced from the resin and will enrich the dialysate (37).

Chronic intoxication and depletion

It is much more difficult to determine what chronic toxicity might result from trace element disturbances in dialyzed uremic patients. It should be appreciated that trace element disturbances in dialyzed uremic patients have not been fully characterized. In addition, geographic variations could also occur. Listed in Table 1 are some of the well established trace element alterations found in uremic patients and some of the clinical consequences that may be associated with these disturbances.

Probably the strongest evidence to date suggesting that trace elements may be responsible for some of the symptomatology in chronic dialysis patients is the association between aluminum excess and dialysis dementia. It was initially shown in 1976 that patients with this syndrome had significantly higher brain gray matter aluminum levels than dialysis patients who died of other causes (38). Subsequently, other investigators have confirmed this finding (39–41). There is also strong epidemiological evidence incriminating aluminum in the pathogenesis of dialysis dementia (42, 43). A number of studies have shown that high concentrations of aluminum can be toxic to the nervous system. Experimentally chronic subarachnoid injection of aluminum salts causes a progressive encephalopathy (44). In addition, two nonuremic patients with a chronic dementing neurological disease attributed to aluminum intoxication have been described (45, 46). Finally, Crapper and colleagues (47) have found elevated brain aluminum levels in patients with Alzheimer's disease and suggested that aluminum toxicity may be involved in the pathogenesis of this disease.

Because of the high incidence of osteomalacia in patients with dialysis dementia and the finding of high aluminum levels in bone, it has also been suggested that this may be an additional manifestation of aluminum intoxication (48, 49). Aluminum has also been implicated in the pathogenesis of porphyria cutanea tarda which occasionally occurs in dialyzed uremic patients (50) and in the production of a microcytic hypochromic anemia in association with normal iron stores.

One well-documented case of cobalt-induced cardiomyopathy, characterized by extensive myocardial necrosis, has been reported in a dialysis patient receiving cobaltous chloride for treatment of anemia (51). High levels of cobalt were found in the myocardium of an additional four patients, but the histological features were much less distinctive (52).

Other trace element disturbances could also be important in the pathogenesis of renal osteodystrophy in dialyzed uremic patients. Fluoride intoxication has been associated with

an increased incidence of osteomalacia in some dialysis centers (53). This is covered in greater detail in Chapter 44. Strontium (54) and possibly cadmium (55) can inhibit production of $1,25(OH)_2$ cholecalciferol, which in turn could further compromise the production of this hormone by a diseased kidney.

The second elemental alteration that has received considerable attention is zinc. Most studies have found decreased levels of zinc in serum, leukocyte and muscle of uremic patients (56–63); all other tissue stores of zinc are normal or increased (18). On the basis of low serum zinc levels, a number of investigators have suggested that certain symptoms and findings in renal failure such as hypogeusia, anorexia, impotence, and hormonal alterations (for example, low testosterone levels and increased LH, FSH and prolactin) are a result of zinc depletion. Zinc supplementation improved sexual function, increased testosterone levels and sperm counts, and decreased FSH, LH and prolactin levels in a group of dialysis patients (64, 65), and impotence has been alleviated by zinc administration (24, 66). In a similar patient population, however, zinc replacement had no effect on sexual function, testosterone levels or gonadotrophin levels (66), and this absence of effect on sexual function was substantiated by others (67, 68). Findings about zinc regarding smell, taste and appetite have also been conflicting (25, 68–70).

Little is known about the toxicity of excess tin. Alkyl tin compounds have been shown to induce an encephalopathy in animals. This encephalopathy is characterized by muscle weakness, tremulousness and eventually loss of ability to ambulate and death (71). Intoxication with organic tin resulting in a fatal neurological disease has been described in man (72). More recently, tin has been shown to be a potent inducer of heme oxygenase activity in the kidney (73) suggesting that excess tin may have considerable biological importance.

There are five known molybdenum metalloenzymes: nitrogenase, xanthine oxidase, nitrate reductase, aldehyde oxidase and sulfite oxidase (74). It also has been shown that xanthine oxidase activity varies directly with molybdenum intake (75). It thus appears possible that the excess liver molybdenum in dialyzed uremic patients could be associated with increased xanthine oxidase activity and in turn with overproduction of uric acid.

The depletion of bromide and rubidium would appear to have little, if any, importance in view of their current status of being non-essential trace elements. Increasing attention has been given, however, to the consideration that bromide may be an essential trace element. Under a number of experimental conditions, bromide repletion has been shown to induce a significant growth response (76, 77).

Studies have shown that rubidium and lithium may have contrasting biochemical properties and electroencephalographic effects (78). Rubidium may increase the release of neuronally stored norepinephrine and increase normetanephrine activity (76). Because of this effect on brain amines, it is possible that rubidium depletion, in association with lithium excess, could be responsible for some of the neur-

Table 1. Trace element disturbances in uremic patients.

Trace element	Possible clinical importance
Increased tissue burden	
Aluminum	Porphyria cutanea tarda
	Dialysis dementia
	Osteomalacia
	Anemia
Fluoride	Osteomalacia
Molybdenum	Gout
Silicon	Unknown
Cadmium	Zinc deficiency
Strontium	Reduced $1,25(OH)_2D_3$
Tin	Impairment of drug and toxin metabolism
Zinc	Unknown
Decreased tissue burden	
Bromide	Unknown
Rubidium	Impairment of neurological function

ological and electroencephalographic abnormalities associated with the uremic state.

The status of other essential trace elements which could be important in the uremic symptomatology has not been established. Experimental vanadium deficiency produces hypertriglyceridemia (80) and chromium deficiency in man has been associated with glucose intolerance (81). Thus, depletion of these elements, if present, could be involved in the pathogenesis of the altered carbohydrate and lipid metabolism found in uremic patients.

Similarly, the status of body copper stores in uremic patients needs to be evaluated more fully. Copper is required for lysyl oxidase activity which is necessary for cross-linking of collagen (82). Thus, a reduction in bone copper could be responsible for the abnormal bone matrix previously described in experimental uremia (83).

SUMMARY

It can only be concluded that the importance of trace element disturbances in producing disease in dialyzed uremic patients has not been fully defined. In spite of the paucity of studies, it is becoming increasingly apparent that a variety of trace element disturbances do exist in both dialyzed and non-dialyzed uremic patients. Acute intoxications due to nickel, copper, zinc and fluoride contamination of the dialysate have been well documented in a number of dialysis patients, but the chronic effects of trace element disturbances on the health of the dialyzed uremic patients has been more difficult to define. However, increasing evidence has been presented which strongly suggests that aluminum intoxication is responsible for the dialysis-associated encephalopathy syndrome (dialysis dementia), osteomalacia and anemia. It seems likely that some of the other trace element disturbances may also be responsible for some of the clinical disorders that can occur in dialyzed uremic patients. There is obviously a need for additional studies in this field.

REFERENCES

1. Mertz W: Trace element nutrition in health and disease: contributions and problems of analysis. *Clin Chem* 21: 468, 1975
2. Sprague SM, Fregene A, Wilkinson G, Costantino J, Rosenbaum RW, Mayor GH: Serum vanadium (V) concentration in chronic renal failure (CRF). *Abstracts Am Soc Nephrol* 13: 108A, 1980
3. Bello-Reuss EN, Grady TP, Mazumdar DC: Serum vanadium levels in chronic renal disease. *Ann Intern Med* 91: 743, 1979
4. Kallistratos A, Evangelou A, Seferiadis P, Vezyraki P, Barboutis K: Selenium and haemodialysis: serum selenium levels in healthy persons, non-cancer and cancer patients with chronic renal failure. *Nephron* 41: 217, 1985
5. Dworkin B, Weseley S, Rosenthal WS, Schwartz EM, Weiss L: Diminished blood selenium levels in renal failure patients on dialysis: correlations with nutritional status. *Am J Med Sci* 293: 6, 1987
6. Muirhead N, Kertesz A, Flanagan PR, Hodsman AB, Hollomby DJ, Valberg LS: Zinc metabolism in patients on mainte-

nance hemodialysis. *Am J Nephrol* 6: 422, 1986
7. McNeely MD, Sunderman FW Jr, Michay MW, Levine H: Abnormal concentrations of nickel in serum in case of myocardial infarction, stroke, burns, hepatic cirrhosis and uremia. *Clin Chem* 17: 1123, 1971
8. Hosokawa S, Nishitani H, Umemura K, Tomoyoshi T, Sawanishi K, Osamu Y: Serum and corpuscular nickel and zinc in chronic hemodialysis patients. *Nephron* 45: 151, 1987
9. Drazniowsky M, Parkinson IS, Ward MK, Channon SM, Kerr DNS: A method for the determination of nickel in water and serum by flameless atomic absorption spectrometry. *Clin Chim Acta* 145: 219, 1985
10. Dobbie JW, Smith MJB: The silicon content of body fluids. *Scott Med J* 27: 17, 1982
11. Berlyne G, Dudek E, Adler AJ, Rubin JE, Seidman M: Silicon metabolism: The basic facts in renal failure. *Kidney Int* 28 (Suppl 17): S-175, 1985
12. Adler AJ, Berlyne GM: Silicon metabolism. II. Renal handling in chronic renal failure patients. *Nephron* 44: 36, 1986
13. Brune D, Samasahl K, Wester PO: A comparison between the amounts of As, Au, Br, Cu, Fe, Mo, Se and Zn in normal and uraemic human whole blood by means of neutron activation analysis. *Clin Chim Acta* 13: 285, 1966
14. Bergström J, Wester PO: The effect of dialysis on the arsenic content of blood and muscle tissue from uraemic patients. *Proc Eur Dial Transplant Assoc* 3: 38, 1966
15. Rudolph H, Alfrey AC, Smythe WR: Muscle and serum trace element profile in uremia. *Trans Am Soc Artif Intern Organs* 19: 456, 1973
16. Alfrey AC, Durr JA, Miller N: The determination of endogenous lithium (Li) as a marker of proximal tubular Na and H_2O handling. *Clin Nephrol* 19: 32A, 1986
17. Kaehny WD, Alfrey AC, Holman RC, Schorr WJ: Aluminum transfer during hemodialysis. *Kidney Int* 12: 361, 1977
18. Smythe WR, Alfrey AC, Craswell PW, Crouch CA, Ibels LS, Kubo H, Nunnelley LL, Rudolph H: Trace metal abnormalities in chronic uremia. *Ann Intern Med* 96: 302, 1982
19. Indraprasit S, Alexander GV, Gonick HC: Tissue composition of major and trace elements in uremia and hypertension. *J Chronic Dis* 27: 135, 1974
20. Cordy PE, Gagnon R, Taves DR, Kay M: Bone disease in hemodialysis patients with particular reference to the effect of fluoride. *Trans Am Soc Artif Intern Organs* 20: 197, 1974
21. Alfrey AC, Smythe WR, Ibels LS, Nunnelley LL: *Trace Element Abnormalities in Chronic Uremia.* 2nd Annu Prog Report, Springfield, VA, National Technical Information Service, 1976, p 35
22. Spencer H, Lewin I, Belcher MJ, Scamachson J: Inhibition of radiostrontium absorption. *Int J Appl Radiat Isot* 20: 507, 1969
23. Nunnelley LL, Smythe WR, Alfrey AC, Ibels LS: Uremic hyperstannum: elevated tissue tin levels associated with uremia. *J Lab Clin Med* 91: 72, 1978
24. Antoniou LD, Shalhoub RJ, Sudhakar T, Smith JC Jr: Reversal of uraemic impotence by zinc. *Lancet* 2: 895, 1977
25. Atkin-Thor E, Goddward BW, O'Nion J, Stephen RL, Kolff WJ: Hypogeusia and zinc depletion in chronic dialysis patients. *Am J Clin Nutr* 31: 1948, 1978
26. Kaehny WD, Hegg AP, Alfrey AC: Gastrointestinal absorption of aluminum from aluminum containing antacids. *N Engl J Med* 296: 1839, 1977
27. Gorsky JE, Dietz AA, Spencer H, Osis D: Metabolic balance of aluminum studied in six men. *Clin Chem* 25: 1739, 1979
28. Kovalchik MT, Kaehny WD, Jackson T, Alfrey AC: Aluminum kinetics during hemodialysis. *J Lab Clin Med* 92: 712, 1978

29. Gallery ED, Blomfield J, Dixon SF: Acute zinc toxicity in haemodialysis. *Br Med J* 4: 331, 1972

30. Ivanovich P, Manzler A, Drake R: Acute hemolysis following hemodialysis. *Trans Am Soc Artif Intern Organs* 15: 316, 1969

31. Klein WJ, R, Metz EN, Price AR: Acute copper intoxication. *Arch Intern Med* 129: 578, 1972

32. Manzler AD, Schreiner AW: Copper-induced acute hemolytic anemia. *Ann Intern Med* 73: 409, 1970

33. Matter BJ, Pederson J, Psimenos G, Lindeman RD: Lethal copper intoxication in hemodialysis. *Trans Am Soc Artif Intern Organs* 15: 309, 1969

34. Lyle WH, Payton JE, Jui M: Hemodialysis and copper fever. *Lancet* 1: 1324, 1976

35. Webster JD, Parker TF, Alfrey AC, Smythe WR, Kubo H, Neal G, Hull AR: Acute nickel intoxication by dialysis. *Ann Intern Med* 92: 631, 1980

36. Mitchell G, Cirksena W, Samaras G, Wax C: Acute fluoride intoxication in hemodialysis patients. *Abstracts Am Soc Nephrol* 13: 47A, 1980

37. Johnson WJ, Taves DR: Exposure to excessive fluoride during hemodialysis. *Kidney Int* 5: 451, 1974

38. Alfrey AC, LeGendre GR, Kaehny WD: The dialysis encephalopathy syndrome. Possible aluminum intoxication. *N Engl J Med* 294: 184, 1976

39. McDermott JR, Smith AI, Ward MK, Fawcett RWP, Kerr DNS: Brain-aluminium concentration in dialysis encephalopathy. *Lancet* 1: 901, 1978

40. Cartier F, Allain P, Gary J, Chatel M, Menault F, Pecker S: Encephalopathie myoclonique progressive des dialyses. Role de l'eau utilisee pour l'hemodialyse. (Progressive myoclonic dialysis encephalopathy. Significance of the water utilized for preparation of dialysis fluid.) *Nouv Presse Med* 7: 97, 1978

41. Crapper DR, Quittkat S, Krishnan SS, Dalton AJ, DeBoni U: Intranuclear aluminum content in Alzheimer's disease, dialysis encephalopathy and experimental aluminum encephalopathy. *Acta Neuropathol* 50: 19, 1980

42. Parkinson IS, Ward MK, Feest TG, Fawcett RWP, Kerr DNS: Fracturing dialysis osteodystrophy and dialysis encephalopathy. An epidemiological survey. *Lancet* 1: 406, 1979

43. Platts MM, Goode GC, Hislop JS: Composition of the domestic water supply and the incidence of fractures and encephalopathy in patients on home dialysis. *Br Med J* 2: 657, 1977

44. Klatzo I, Wisniewski H, Streicher E: Experimental production of neurofibrillary degeneration. I. Light microscopic observations. *J Neuropathol Exp Neurol* 24: 187, 1965

45. Lapresle J, Duckett S, Galle P, Cartier L: Documents cliniques, anatomiques et biophysiques dans une encephalopathie avec presence de depots d'aluminum. (Clinical anatomical and biophysical data of a case of encephalopathy with accumulation of aluminum.) *C R Soc Biol (Paris)* 169: 282, 1975

46. McLaughlin AIG, Kazantzis G, King E, Teare D, Porter RJ, Owen R: Pulmonary fibrosis and encephalopathy associated with the inhalation of aluminum dust. *Br J Ind Med* 19: 282, 1975

47. Crapper DR, Krishman SS, Dalton AJ: Brain aluminum distribution in Alzheimer's disease and experimental neurofibrillary degeneration. *Science* 180: 511, 1973

48. Pierides AM, Edwards WG, Jr, Cullum UX, Jr, McCall JT, Ellis HA: Hemodialysis encephalopathy with osteomalacic fractures and muscle weakness. *Kidney Int* 18: 115, 1980

49. Hodsman AB, Sherrard DJ, Brickman AS, Alfrey AC, Goodman WG, Maloney N, Lee DBN, Coburn JW: Bone aluminum in osteomalacic renal osteodystrophy correlation with excess osteoid. *Abstracts Am Soc Neprhol* 13: 20A, 1980

50. Buchet JP, Lauwerys R, Hassoun A, Dratwa M, Wens R, Collart F, Tielemans C: Effect of aluminum on porphyrin metabolism in hemodialyzed patients. *Nephron* 46: 360, 1987

51. Manifold IH, Platts MM, Kennedy A: A cobalt cardiomyopathy in a patient on maintenance haemodialysis. *Br Med J* 2: 1609, 1978

52. Pehrsson K, Lins LE: Cobalt in uremic cardiomyopathy. *Lancet* 2: 51, 1978

53. Posen GA, Taves DR, Marier JR, Jaworski ZF: Renal osteodystrophy in long-term hemodialysis with fluoridated water. *Abstracts Am Soc Nephrol* 2: 51, 1968

54. Omdahl JL, DeLuca HF: Strontium induced rickets: metabolic basis. *Science* 174: 949, 1971

55. Piscator M: The chronic toxicity of cadmium. in: *Trace Elements in Human Health and Disease,* edited by Prasad AS, New York, Academic Press, 2, 1976, p 431

56. Blendis LM, Ampil M, Wilson DR, Kiwan J, Labranche J, Johnson M, Williams C: The importance of dietary protein in the zinc deficiency of uremia. *Am J Clin Nutr* 34: 2658, 1981

57. Bodgen JD, Oleske JM, Weiner B, Smith LG Jr, Smith LG, Najem GR: Elevated plasma zinc concentrations in renal dialysis patients. *Am J Clin Nutr* 33: 1088, 1980

58. Kiilerich S, Christiansen C, Crisensen MS, Naestoft J: Zinc metabolism in patients with chronic renal failure during treatment with 1,25-dihydroxy-cholecalciferol: a controlled therapeutic trial. *Clin Nephrol* 15: 23, 1981

59. Michael J, Hilton PJ, Jones NF: Zinc and the sodium pump in uremia. *Am J Clin Nutr* 31: 1945, 1978

60. Mountokalakis T, Dakanlis D, Boukis D, Virvidakis K, Voudiklari S, Koutselinis A: Hair zinc compared with plasma zinc in uremic patients, before and during regular hemodialysis. *Clin Nephrol* 12: 206, 1979

61. Paniagua-Sierra JR, Perez-Lopez A, Diaz-Bensussen S, Solis-Alpuche L, Saavedre-Guatemala H, Exaire-Murad JE: Zinc and copper concentration in plasma and erythrocytes of patients with chronic renal failure. *Arch Invest Med (Mex)* 12: 69, 1981

62. Siegler RL, Eggert JV, Udokesmalee E: Diagnostic indices of zinc deficiency in children with renal disease. *Ann Clin Lab Sci* 11: 428, 1981

63. Zumkley H, Bertram HP, Lison A, Knoll O, Losse H: Aluminum, zinc and copper concentrations in plasma in chronic renal insufficiency. *Clin Nephrol* 12: 18, 1979

64. Mahajan SK, Abassi AA, Prasad AS, Rabbini P, Briggs WA, McDonald FD: Effect of oral zinc therapy on gonadal function in hemodialysis patients: a double blind study. *Ann Intern Med* 97: 357, 1982

65. Mahajan SK, Hamburger RJ, Flamenbaum W, Prasad AS, McDonald FD: Effect of zinc supplementation on hyperprolactinaemia in uraemic men. *Lancet* 2: 758, 1985

66. Antoniou LD, Shalhoub RJ: Zinc and sexual dysfunction. *Lancet* 8: 1034, 1980

67. Brook AC, Johnston DG, Ward MK, Watson MJ, Cook DB, Kerr DN: Absence of a therapeutic effect of zinc in the sexual dysfunction of haemodialyzed patients. *Lancet* 2: 618, 1980

68. Joven J, Villabona C, Rubies-Prat J, Espinel E, Galard R: Hormonal profile and serum zinc levels in uraemic men with gonadal dysfunction undergoing haemodialysis. *Clin Chim Acta* 148: 239, 1985

69. Zetin M, Stone RA: Effects of zinc in chronic hemodialysis. *Clin Nephrol* 13: 20, 1980

70. Sprenger KBG, Bundschu D, Lewis K, Spohn B, Schmitz J, Franz H-E: Improvement of uremic neuropathy and hypogeusia by dialysate zinc supplementation: A double blind study.

Kidney Int 24 (Supll 16): S315, 1983

71. Stoner HB, Barner JM, Duff JI: Studies on the toxicity of alkyl tin compounds. *Br J Pharmacol* 10: 16, 1955

72. Alajouanine T, Derobert L, Thieffry S: Etude clinique d'ensemble de 210 cas d'intoxication par les sels organiques d'etain. (Clinical study of 210 cases of intoxication by organic tin compounds.) *Rev Neurol (Paris)* 98: 85, 1973

73. Kappas A, Maines TD: Tin: A potent inducer of heme oxygenase in kidney. *Science* 192: 60, 1976

74. Stiefel EJ: Proposed molecular mechanism for the action of molybdenum in enzymes: coupled proton and electron transfers. *Proc Natl Acad Sci USA* 70: 988, 1973

75. Higgins ES, Reichert DA, Westerfeld WW: Molybdate deficiency and tungstate inhibition studies. *J Nutr* 59: 539, 1956

76. Bosshardt DK, Huff JS, Barner RH: Effect of bromine on chick growth. *Proc Soc Exp Biol Med* 92: 219, 1956

77. Huff JW, Bosshardt DK, Miller OP, Barner RH: A nutritional requirement for bromine. *Proc Soc Exp Biol Med* 92: 216, 1956

78. Carroll BJ, Sharp PT: Rubidium and lithium: opposite effects on amine-mediated excitement. *Science* 172: 1355, 1971

79. Fieve RR, Meltzer H, Dunner DL, Levitt M, Mendlewicz J, Thomas A: Rubidium: biochemical, behavioral and metabolic studies in humans. *Am J Psychiat* 130: 55, 1973

80. Hopkins LL Jr, Mohr HE: Vanadium as an essential nutrient. *Fed Proc* 33: 1773, 1974

81. Levine RA, Steeten DHP, Doisy RJ: Effects of oral chromium supplementation on the glucose tolerance test in the elderly. *Metabolism* 17: 114, 1968

82. O'Dell BL: Biochemistry and physiology of copper in vertebrates. in: *Trace Elements in Human Health and Disease*, edited by Prasad AS, New York, Academic Press, I, 1976, p 391

83. Russell JE, Avioli LV: Effect of progressive end-stage renal insufficiency on bone mineral-collagen maturation. *Kidney Int* 7 (Suppl 2): S97, 1975

ALUMINIUM TOXICITY IN RENAL FAILURE

CHARLES R.V. TOMSON and MICHAEL K. WARD

INTRODUCTION

There is now no doubt that aluminium contamination of water supplies used for the preparation of dialysis fluid can lead to encephalopathy, vitamin D resistant fracturing osteomalacia and microcytic anaemia in patients receiving haemodialysis. Although the introduction of adequate water treatment to remove aluminium has effectively stopped the epidemics of these diseases which made them the major cause of death in some dialysis units in the 1970's, sporadic occurrences of identical syndromes have also been described in patients who have never received dialysis, have been trated exclusively with peritoneal dialysis or have received haemodialysis using water known to have a very low aluminium content. In these patients other sources of aluminium have been implicated, the oral administration of aluminium salts used as phosphate-binding agents and contamination of parenteral fluids being the culprits. The rate of aluminium accummulation, which has marked effects on the distribution within the body, has been slower with oral administration. Thus, a new pattern of aluminium-related disease with a different epidemiology is emerging in patients with renal failure. This has ensured that the prevention, detection and treatment of aluminium toxicity will continue to be an important part of nephrological practice for many years.

To appreciate the devastating effect that Al accumulation can have on brain and bone in patients with renal failure, we will present a historical description of encephalopathy and vitamin D resistant aluminium-induced osteomalacia and discuss the other clinical syndromes of anaemia and acute toxicity from peritoneal dialysis contamination, before commenting on Al metabolism in relation to sources of aluminium, body distribution, excretion, effects on metabolic functions, the detection of Al overload and the use of deferoxamine (desferrioxamine) in management.

ENCEPHALOPATHY

Clinical features in adults

In 1972 Alfrey and colleagues (1) reported the development of a unique neurological syndrome in five adult patients receiving dialysis with untreated Denver tap water. Other dialysis units described a remarkably similar picture (2–10). Characteristic speech disturbances, motor disturbances, seizures, and intellectual deterioration were described in all of these reports.

Speech and language disturbances

The speech disturbance is present in nearly all patients and is often the presenting feature. Nurses and relatives often describe this as 'stuttering' or 'stammering', although detailed analysis of speech patterns (11) reveals that the predominant abnormality is a combination of dysarthria and speech dyspraxia, worsened by embarrassment and by attempting to speak long sentences or at speed. True dysphasia is rare (11, 12). At first the patient may be able to disguise the problem by speaking unusually slowly or in short sentences. 'Speech arrest' may respond dramatically to intravenous benzodiazepenes in the early stages (13) and electroencephalography during attacks have shown seizure activity. With time, speech becomes increasingly unintelligle and mutism is common in the later stages. Dysgraphia and dyslexia may be part of a generalised language disturbance.

Motor disturbances

Two types of abnormality are described. Myoclonic jerking movements are typical and may interfere considerably with activity. These jerking movements may become generalised. Myoclonic contraction of the facial muscles causes 'facial grimacing'. The second type of abnormality of motor function, which is less common, is motor apraxia which may render the patient immobile, despite normal muscle power.

Seizures

Although the distinction from myoclonic jerking without loss of consciousness may be difficult, true epileptic fits are common, particularly in the later stages.

Intellectual deterioration

Intellectual deterioration in terms of symptomatic progressing dementia is present in a minority of patients at presentation (12) but frank dementia develops in most patients, often with preservation of insight until very late in the disease.

Other features

Profound fatigue, behavioural changes with or without frank psychotic features and the development of primitive reflexes are common. Localised neurological signs and peripheral neuropathy are no more common than in dialysed patients without aluminium-related encephalopathy. Alfrey (14) has suggested that presenting features in patients developing encephalopathy due to prolonged oral exposure are atypical: three such patients had vivid visual hallucinations as a presenting feature. With prolonged exposure to aluminium at lower levels, long-term survivors with renal failure managed by dialysis and transplantation may develop neurological features not yet recognised as aluminium-related. Bone disease was strongly associated with the syndrome in some reports (4, 5, 9, 16) but this association was either not present or not mentioned by other investigators.

Precipitating factors

Immobilisation, particularly after surgery, steroids, hypercalcaemia and hypophosphataemia have all been reported to precipitate or worsen the features of dialysis encephalopathy (16). These factors may act by increasing mobilisation of aluminium from bone.

Investigations

Serum Al levels are raised (90 to 600 μg/l [3.3 to 22.2 μmol/l]) but overlap considerably with levels of unaffected patients (17), suggesting that serum concentrations reflect recent exposure and not tissue burden. Measurement of cerebrosphinal fluid (CSF) Al concentration has been proposed (18) but not widely used. CSF cell count, protein and glucose content are normal. Radiological studies are normal or show non-specific cortical thinning on computerised tomographic (CT) scans. Reports of abnormal CSF dynamics (19) have not been confirmed. Electroencephalography (EEG) is abnormal in all cases. The record shows intermittent spiky, high voltage activity superimposed on a background of diffuse slowing; EEG abnormalities precede clinical disturbances (20, 21). However, a similar EEG picture may be found in a variety of other conditions and should not be used as the sole diagnostic criterion.

Epidemiology

As originally described, dialysis encephalopathy was an epidemic disease affecting only at most 10% of all dialysis units (22). This geographical inequality in the occurrence of the disease was shown to relate closely to the aluminium content of the water supply in Britain (23–25). Use of water with an Al content >50 μg/l (1.9 μmol/l) for dialysis without adequate treatment was associated with a high 'attack rate' of dialysis encephalopathy. In the USA (26) information on the Al content of municipal water was much less readily available (26). A retrospective analysis of the occurrence of cases in Denver, Salt Lake City, Chicago, Minneapolis and Alma, MI, however, revealed a close relationship between the risk of dialysis encephalopathy and the use uf alum-treated water without deionisation or reverse osmosis (27). In two centres for which adequate information was available a close relationship between the attack rate and cumulative exposure to aluminium through the dialysis fluid was found (27). In addition, analysis within several affected centres showed a close temporal relationship between the incidence of dialysis encephalopathy and the Al content of the water used to prepare the dialysis fluid (8, 9, 26) or a drop in incidence after introduction of adequate water treatment

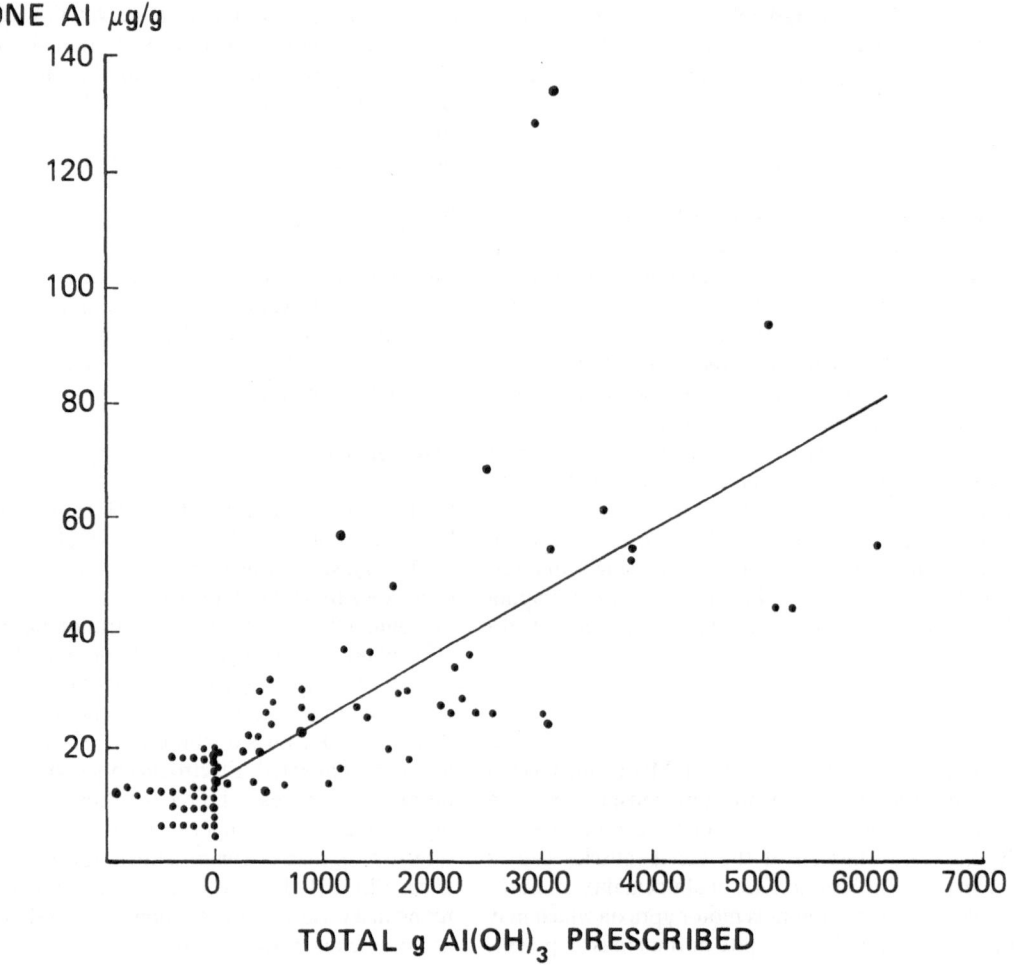

Figure 1. Correlation of bone aluminium content in μg/g of dry weight related to total quantity of aluminium hydroxide prescribed.

(14, 16, 17, 25, 28). Perhaps the most convincing single piece of evidence comes from Eindhoven in Holland, where an epidemic of dialysis encephalopathy occurred in one of two dialysis units using the same water supply (5). Water in the affected unit was heated in a tank in which two aluminium anodes had been installed as an anti-corrosion device. These had gradually dissolved, causing aluminium contamination of the dialysis fluid. New cases stopped occurring when these anodes where removed and several patients improved when moved to a new unit.

Not all cases of dialysis encephalopathy can be explained by contamination of dialysis fluid water with aluminium. Typical dialysis encephalopathy occurred in 14 patients in Nashville, despite the use by all but one patient of water treatment which was shown to remove all but trace amounts of aluminium (10). Three of these patients improved dramatically after discontinuation of oral aluminium salts, although there was no difference in cumulative prescribed dose of aluminium between affected patients and 14 unaffected matched controls. Oral aluminium salts have been implicated in the pathogenesis of encephalopathy in adults

not receiving dialysis (10, 29–32) and in adults receiving haemodialysis with adequately treated water (14) or peritoneal dialysis (33).

Pathology

Histopathological examination of the brain in patients dying with aluminium-related encephalopathy reveals little or no abnormality (12, 15). A striking loss of Purkinje cells from the cerebellum was reported in Newcastle (4) but has not been confirmed by other centres. The Al content of both grey and white matter is increased (5, 34, 35) with a more marked increment in the grey matter. Comparison of the Al content of 'whole brain' between those with encephalopathy and unaffected dialysis patients may fail to show such clear differences (23, 36, 37).

Treatment

Although benzodiazepenes help relieve some of the symptoms (12, 13), they do not influence the natural history of the disease. Some cases stabilise or improve after withdrawal of all sources of aluminium. Phosphate repletion, tried before the causative role of aluminium was established, appeared to lead to temporary benefit (38) but further studies failed to confirm this. Renal transplantation may be of benefit in the early stages (39–41) but may actually precipitate the syndrome in previously unaffected patients (42, 43) or accelerate it in affected patients. One case report, widely quoted, suggested that parathyroidectomy was beneficial (44), but a retrospective analysis of 21 patients showed no effect of parathyroid status or parathyroidectomy on outcome (45). The only treatment which can confidently be expected to improve the outcome is chelation with deferoxamine (46–48) and reduction in aluminium exposure from dialysis fluid and oral therapy.

Encephalopathy in children

Neurological abnormalities in children with renal failure associated with intoxication from orally administered aluminium salts have been reported by several groups (49–53). Neurodevelopmental delay, seizures, myoclonus, ataxia and an abnormal EEG have been associated with a raised brain aluminium content. The features are not as clear-cut as those of adult encephalopathy. In an international survey of 61 centres managing 728 children with end-stage renal failure, 24 cases of unexplained encephalopathy were identified. All had received oral aluminium and 23 had secondary hyperparathyroidism (53).

ALUMINIUM BONE DISEASE

This subject is dealt with in depth in Chapter 44.

Clinical features

The diagnosis of aluminium-related osteomalacia is strongly suggested by the occurrence of bone pain at rest or on weight-bearing, spontaneous fractures and a proximal myopathy. Hypercalcaemia is common, particularly after treatment with Vitamin D derivatives which are ineffective in relieving symptoms. Serum alkaline phosphatase activity is low (at least in the 'epidemic' form of the disease) and the syndrome is usually associated with low PTH concentrations in serum (54, 55).

Natural history

This depends on whether the patient continues to be exposed to aluminium and if so, at what rate. If exposure continues the disease may progress rapidly with the development of multiple fractures and immobility due to severe myopathy (54).

Investigations

Radiographic studies show fractures and decreased bone density. Features of hyperparathyroidism are uncommon. Isotope bone scans are abnormal, but the discriminatory value of this test has not been established. As in patients with encephalopathy, serum Al levels are usually raised but because of the close dependence of serum Al levels on current exposure, there is no 'cut-off' level at which aluminium-related bone disease may be predicted by serum levels (17). The diagnostic value of increments of serum aluminium after deferoxamine is discussed later. This test may help to identify patients with raised total bone Al content but does not predict bone histology. Similarly, a raised total bone Al content is highly specific for aluminium-related bone disease but may also be found in patients with hyperparathyroidism (56, 57). Bone histology is the accepted 'gold standard' for the diagnosis of this disorder and shows increased osteoid volume, decreased bone formation rates and stainable aluminium at the interface between osteoid and mineralised bone. If double tetracycline labels have been administered, absence of tetracycline deposition at the mineralisation front is observed where Al staining is positive. Inverse relationships may be shown between the extent of stainable aluminium at the mineralisation front and osteoblast number (58), osteoblast activity (59) and mineralisation rate (60).

Epidemiology

As with aluminium-related encephalopathy, the geographical distribution of fracturing osteodystrophy was uneven, although recognition of this was delayed by lack of distinction of this syndrome from hyperparathyroidism (24). A close association between fracturing osteodystrophy with myopathy and encephalopathy was also noted by some (4, 5, 9, 22, 23, 61, 62) but not all (10, 19, 27) centres. As early as 1972 it was observed that deionisation of the water used to prepare dialysis fluid prevented new cases occurring and stabilised established cases (63), suggesting a water-borne agent. In 1977 a report from Sheffield described the geographical distribution of fracturing osteodystrophy and encephalopathy in Yorkshire and showed that both syndromes were associated with water with a high Al content and a low calcium and fluoride content (23). In 1978 a report from Newcastle showed that both syndromes were prevented by dialysis with deionised water and provided strong suggestive evidence that the agent removed by deionisation was aluminium (54). Definitive epidemiological evidence of an association between the incidence of fracturing osteodystrophy and the Al content of the water used to prepare dialysis fluid was provided in the United Kingdom by Parkinson et al (24). This association was not as strong as that with encephalopathy, probaly because of variations between centres in diagnostic criteria and the frequency with which bone biopsies were performed.

Response to treatment

Unlike encephalopathy, aluminium-related bone disease usually responds well to transplantation (64), suggesting that aluminium may be mobilised more easily from bone, or at least from the mineralisation front. Following preliminary reports (65), chelation therapy with deferoxamine has become widely used to treat aluminium-related bone disease (66). Long-term follow-up of patients treated with (up to 18 months) courses of deferoxamine shows improvement of histological appearance and reduction of Al content (67). The degree of improvement relates to the parathyroid hormone level at the start of treatment. Patients who have undergone prior parathyroidectomy are less likely to improve (67, 68).

OTHER TOXIC EFFECTS OF ALUMINIUM

Acute poisoning

Two instances of acute aluminium poisoning have been reported, both associated with contaminated peritoneal dialysis fluid and plasma Al levels over $450 \mu g/l$ (69, 70). Clinical features included anorexia, nausea, vomiting, abdominal cramps and weight loss.

Anaemia

Microcytic hypochromic anaemia without evidence of iron deficiency preceding the development of aluminium-related encephalopathy was reported in some (7, 71–73) but not all of the centres which reported epidemic bone disease and encephalopathy as a result of aluminium-contaminated water supplies. Serum ferritin levels were normal or high and there was no response to iron supplementation. Serum Al levels have been $>400 \mu g/l$ in most of the patients reported. The mechanism by which aluminium exerts its toxic effects on the bone marrow is uncertain but a direct effect on enzymes involved in haem synthesis seems likely (74, 75). The anaemia improves after transfer to aluminium-free dialysis fluid (71, 72) or deferoxamine treatment (76).

There is an improvement of normochromic normocytic anaemia after deferoxamine treatment in patients with relatively low serum Al levels, with a high increment of serum aluminium after deferoxamine but no other evidence of toxicity (77). This normochromic normocytic anaemia related to aluminium is relatively resistant to erythropoietin (78), suggesting that aluminium exerts effects on haematopoiesis even at lower concentrations.

Parathyroid gland function

The effects of aluminium intoxication on parathyroid function are controversial (79, 80). Aluminium is known to accumulate in the parathyroid gland in primary hyperparathyroidism (81) and a negative correlation between gland weight and peak plasma Al concentration in uraemic patients undergoing parathyroidectomy has been reported (82). Aluminium in concentrations similar to those seen *in vivo* can interfere directly with parathyroid function *in vitro*, possibly by interfering with diglyceride synthesis (83). It is more difficult to prove that aluminium suppresses parathyroid activity *in vivo*. Two studies have suggested that chronic aluminium intoxication is associated with decreased parathyroid responsiveness to acute hypocalcaemia (84, 85) but in both of these studies several patients had undergone prior parathyroidectomy. Acute aluminium poisoning in dogs (86) and man (87) causes hypercalcaemia. Hence, it is impossible to be sure whether hypercalcaemia or hyperaluminaemia was responsible for the suppression of parathyroid activity observed. Transfer of patients from a high-aluminium dialysis fluid to a low-aluminium dialysis fluid was associated with a rise in parathyroid activity (88) but calcium concentrations were also altered. Removal of aluminium by deferoxamine has effects on bone metabolism which make reports of altered parathyroid hormone (PTH) secretion (67, 68, 89) difficult to interpret. At present it is not possible to reach firm conclusions regarding the effect of aluminium intoxication on parathyroid function.

ALUMINIUM METABOLISM

Distribution within the body

Aluminium is widely distributed, initially into a volume twice that of plasma (86). Prolonged hyperaluminaemia and raised urinary excretion after withdrawal of aluminium loading or after successful transplantation (90, 91) suggest a second compartment within tissues from which aluminium is slowly mobilised. Normal subjects have a total aluminium burden of around 30 mg, most of which is found in the lungs (43 to $67 \mu g/kg$ dry weight), bone (3.3 to $5.6 \mu g/kg$ dry weight) and liver ($4.1 \mu g/kg$ dry weight); brain content is $<4 \mu g/kg$ dry weight and serum concentration $<10 \mu g/l$ (35). The Al content of lungs rises with ages and probably relates to inhalation of aluminosilicate dust. In renal failure total aluminium burden may rise to several grams, with marked increases in bone, liver and brain content and in serum concentration (35). Rapid aluminium loading appears to favour accumulation within the brain, suggesting that bone uptake is rate-limited (27, 35, 92). Hyperparathyroidism appears to protect bone and liver from Al accumulation (79, 93, 94), possibly at the expense of increased brain and serum levels (79). Parathyroidectomy in the presence of significant aluminium loading leads to rapid accumulation in bone associated with a low turnover state (95–99).

The mechanism by which these and other factors affect aluminium distribution is unknown.

Oral absorption

Numerous reports of aluminium-related toxicity syndromes after the administration of aluminium compounds to patients with chronic renal failure who have not received dialysis and in whom no other source of aluminium could be identified (30, 31, 49–53, 100, 101) have made it clear that significant amounts of aluminium can be absorbed from orally administered aluminium hydroxide. Originally recognised by Berlyne et al (102), only since the elimination of aluminium-contaminated dialysis fluid has it been possible to clarify this relationship in patients receiving dialysis. Several studies in patients not exposed to aluminium-contaminated dialysis fluid have shown close correlations between serum Al levels and current dose (50, 101, 103–107) or cumulative dose (106, 108–110) of aluminium hydroxide. Heaf and Nielsen (106), using multiple linear regression, found that both cumulative and current dose made independent contributions to the variance of serum Al levels. Several studies also reported a significant correlation between total bone aluminium and cumulative dose of aluminium hydroxide (109, 111–113) (Figure 1). Oral administration of aluminium salts may also lead to increased brain Al in non-uraemic patients undergoing craniotomy (114).

The study of aluminium absorption has been limited by the lack of suitable isotopes. Balance experiments (115, 116) have given estimates of Al absorption which are much higher than would be consistent with the relatively small increase in total body Al content found in patients with renal failure. Methodological flaws and binding of aluminium within intestinal mucosal cells may explain these discrepancies.

Sources of aluminium

Aluminium compounds

Aluminium salts are widely used as antacids and are the most important source of bioavailable aluminium in the normal population. Dihydroxyaluminium aminoacetate is best absorbed, followed by aluminium hydroxide and aluminium carbonate; aluminium phosphate is poorly absorbed (117).

Foodstuffs

Exposure to aluminium from the use of aluminium pans (118, 119) for food preparation and from imbibed wine, beer and water (120) are minimal by comparison but may account for the small increases in serum Al found in patients with chronic renal failure in whom no other source can be implicated. Bioavailability of aluminium from environmental sources has usually been regarded as minimal.

Infant formulae

Proprietary milk for infant feeding has been shown to have a high aluminium content (121, 122) which was implicated in the development of aluminium-related encephalopathy in two infants with renal failure (121). The Al content of human breast milk is low (123).

Factors affecting aluminium absorption

Effect of gastric pH

On theoretical grounds (124), absorption of aluminium should be minimal in the acid milieu of the stomach, although the effect of this should be minimised (and the phosphate-binding effect maximised) by simultaneous ingestions of food. The effect on Al absorption of iatrogenic alteration in gastric pH has not been studied.

Effect of age

Many of the reports of toxicity from orally administered aluminium have been in children (50–53, 101, 105, 121, 125). This could be due to the higher dose (expressed as dose/kg body weight) required to maintain normophosphataemia in children, better compliance than in adults or increased aluminium absorption in the immature gut. Aluminium absorption has not been studied directly in children. By multiple linear regression analysis of factors predicting serum Al concentration in 12 children with chronic renal failure all of whom were taking aluminium hydroxide Andreoli et al (101) showed a negative partial correlation of serum Al levels with body weight which was independent of the positive partial correlation with the dose (expressed as dose/kg body weight). Sedman and colleagues (123) found urinary aluminium: creatinine ratios in normal infants to be six times higher than in adults, again suggesting increased Al absorption. In contrast, no information is available on Al absorption in the elderly.

Effects of parathyroid status and vitamin D

There seems little doubt that these interconnected factors influence aluminium handling in experimental animals and man, although some controversy remains (78, 79). In rats Al absorption is increased by administration of 1,25 dihydroxyvitamin D (126, 127) possibly by means of increased activity of a saturable transport mechanism for which aluminium competes with calcium (126). Conflicting results have been reported in human studies (128). Vitamin D may also affect Al distribution (94, 129) making interpretation of clinical studies difficult.

Similar difficulties attend the interpretation of experiments in rats on the effect of parathyroid hormone on Al absorption. Exogenous parathyroid hormone increases whole carcass Al content in non-uraemic rats fed aluminium (130), suggesting increased absorption, but also prevents the decrease in whole carcass aluminium when oral aluminium is withdrawn. This latter observation could be due to effects on distribution of Al within the body or to decreased excretion, although parathyroid hormone does not influence renal excretion of Al in uraemic rats (93).

Other factors

The effects of iron loading on Al absorption remain controversial (131, 132). Aluminium absorption is increased by low doses of fluoride but decreased by higher doses (133) and increased substantially by citrate (134). Preliminary evidence (135) suggests that intra-individual differences in Al absorption may predispose to aluminium-related disease.

Alternatives to aluminium-containing compounds

Calcium carbonate (107, 136–138) magnesium hydroxide (139–142) and magnesium carbonate (143) have been used for control of hyperphosphataemia in patients requiring dialysis and calcium carbonate has been used in patients with chronic renal failure not yet requiring dialysis (144, 145). Use of calcium carbonate has been limited by the frequent development of hypercalcaemia, attributable to increased Ca absorption (146), in all of the reported studies, with the attendant risk of exacerbation of ectopic and vascular calcification. The use of a low-calcium dialysis fluid solves this problem but is associated with a significantly increased incidence of hypotension during haemodialysis (138). Although calcium carbonate binds phosphate as effectively as milli-equivalent doses of aluminium hydroxide (146), larger numbers of tablets are required to achieve this dose and this may reduce compliance.

Magnesium salts also bind phosphate and have been shown to permit reduction of aluminium hydroxide dosage (139, 140, 143), although gastrointestinal side-effects (141) and interference with the action of potassium-binding resins (137, 147) may limit their use.

Sucralfate (a complex of sulphated sucrose and aluminium hydroxide) is an effective phosphate binder, but on a gram-for-gram basis appears to be absorbed as well as pure aluminium hydroxide (148). The suggestion that equivalent phosphate binding can be achieved by a smaller dose of sucralfate than aluminium hydroxide (149) deserves further investigation.

Calcium and iron heteropolyuronides (150) have been shown to be effective phosphate binding agents *in vitro* and in small scale clinical studies (151) but are not yet available for clinical use.

Transfer from dialysis fluid

Aluminium uptake from the dialysis fluid against an apparent concentration gradient has been described in numerous studies (152, 153–156) and is due to tight binding of Al to plasma proteins. Transferrin is the main plasma protein to which aluminium is bound (157–159); disagreement exists on whether Al also binds to albumin or to other plasma constituents. *In vivo* ultrafiltrable aluminium is between 20% (153) and 28% (155). Two independent techniques have shown an inverse relationship between the ultrafiltrable and the total serum Al level (155, 156), suggesting increased protein binding at higher concentrations. Graf (153) has shown that transfer of aluminium relates linearly to the gradient between the calculated ultrafilterable Al and the total dialysis fluid Al level. In practice, Ackrill and colleagues (154) have shown that dialysis fluid Al content should be below 14 μg/l and the European Economic Community Health Directorate, following a series of workshops, recommend that the water content of aluminium should be below 10 μg/l and the dialysis fluid below 20 μg/l with an aim to reducing this to below 10 μg/l has been recommended by several countries for the water used to prepare dialysis fluid.

As the Al content of raw water can vary from supply to supply from day to day in the same supply, depending on rainfall and pH, attention to detail as regards method of water treatment for each individual water supply is essential if appropriate treatment is to be used and maintained to achieve the recommended aluminium content for the preparation of dialysis fluid (see Chapter 7).

Contamination of parenteral fluids

High levels of aluminium have been detected in plasma derivatives (161–163) and parenteral nutrition solutions (90, 122, 123, 164). Contamination of haemofiltration replacement solutions has also been reported (165), although this is no longer a problem. The clinical importance of this contamination is minimal when use of the solutions is short-term, but significant accumulation of aluminium in bone in patients with normal renal functions has been reported after long-term parenteral nutrition (123, 166) and in patients with impaired renal function after long-term plasma exchange (163). Important sources of contamination include filters used in fractionation of plasma (161), casein hydrolysates (90) and intravenous calcium and phosphate supplements (122, 123).

One report has also shown Al contamination of deferoxamine solutions (167). To our knowledge this remains an important and unrecognised potential source of aluminium.

Absorption across peritoneal membrane

Experiences with peritoneal dialysis fluid contaminated with aluminium have shown that the peritoneum is potentially an important route of Al absorption (69, 70, 87), although such contamination is rare. Gilli et al (168) suggested that the low pH of peritoneal dialysis fluid increased Al dialysance by increasing solubility and suggested that the higher Al levels found in their patients treated by intermittent peritoneal dialysis were due to absorption from the dialysis fluid, which had an initial Al concentration between 10 and 50 μg/l. Using commercially prepared dialysis solutions with an Al concentration of 18 μg/l Gokal et al (169) showed that patients undergoing continuous ambulatory peritoneal dialysis (CAPD) not exposed to oral aluminium salts show an increase of serum Al levels to between 30 and 40 μg/l, again probably due to absorption of aluminium. This would be consistent with the known effect of protein binding on Al transfer across dialysis membranes. Conversely, patients with higher serum levels due to previous exposure show transfer of aluminium to peritoneal dialysate and a reduction in serum levels (70, 169, 170).

Aluminium excretion

Renal handling

Aluminium clearance in patients with normal renal function has been estimated at between 2.5 and 15.2 ml/min (59, 90, 152). Residual renal function markedly affects serum Al levels even in those requiring dialysis; Al clearance in these patients has been estimated at 30% of creatinine clearance (110). Estimates of Al clearance in dogs vary between 3% (86) and 50% (170) of creatinine clearance, the lower figure being obtained at very high serum levels. In rats micropuncture studies have shown an inverse relationship between ultrafiltrable and total serum Al and significant proximal tubular reabsorption (171).

Biliary excretion

In experiments on acute aluminium loading in dogs, Kovalchik et al (170) found that biliary Al clearance was less than 1% of total clearance. This study has often been quoted to justify the use of urinary Al excretion as an indicator of gastrointestinal absorption. Serum Al levels rise, however, in patients with jaundice (172) and high post-deferoxamine increments are found in patients with hepatitis (173), but these may have been due to redistribution of aluminium rather than decreased excretion (172). However, a report of aluminium-related bone disease in two patients with liver disease and of significant biliary excretion of aluminium after administration aluminium-containing antacids to patients with T-tubes in the common bile duct after biliary surgery raises the possibility that this may be an important route of excretion of orally administered aluminium in the human (174).

PRE-CLINICAL DETECTION OF ALUMINIUM ACCUMULATION

A review of the techniques available to measure Al concentrations is beyond the scope of this chapter but it is important to note that accurate determination of low concentrations has only been possible in the last decade or so (175). Electrothermal (flameless) atomic absorption spectrophotometry is the method most widely used, but even with this method quality control schemes show major disagreements between laboratories (176). Assuming that these problems can be overcome, how may the patient at risk from aluminium toxicity be identified?

Serum levels

Serum Al levels are affected mainly by current exposure (106, 109, 156, 162), although cumulative exposure (84, 106), residual renal function (110) and factors affecting tissue distribution (see above) may also contribute. These measurements are therefore useful for detecting acute episodes of Al exposure, for example from contaminated dialysis fluid in patients treated by haemodialysis (104) or peritoneal dialysis (69, 70). Their usefulness for predicting encephalopathy or aluminium-related bone disease is now much less certain and depends on the relative contribution of the factors mentioned above. Patients who developed these diseases because of high levels of exposure from dialysis fluid invariably had high levels and no 'cut-off' level could

be defined which satisfactorily separated patients with and without significant bone disease or encephalopathy. In patients exposed to long-term low-level accumulation serum levels are lower, yet there may be equally high tissue burdens of aluminium and correlation between serum and bone levels are poor. In a series of 56 patients receiving haemodialysis a serum level of >100 μg/l was highly specific (95%) for the detection of raised bone aluminium content (177). However, sensitivity was only 50%, no data were available on dialysis fluid aluminium, and it is unclear how these patients were selected. Nevertheless, it is reasonable to evaluate all patients with a serum aluminium level persistently above 100 μg/l for aluminium-related bone disease, encephalopathy and anaemia, and to withdraw any potential sources of aluminium, including oral aluminium hydroxide. This policy alone will fail to identify many patients with significant tissue deposits, however. It has led to interest in ways to identify those who have significant aluminium deposits in the brain or bone with low serum levels, a situation most likely to be seen following prolonged low exposure in patients now maintained by dialysis for many years.

Deferoxamine tests

Several groups have compared the rise in serum Al level after an infusion of deferoxamine, which appears to reflect 'mobilisable' aluminium, to the bone Al content (112, 125, 178–181). As originally proposed (178), 40 mg/kg is given after haemodialysis over 2 h and serum aluminium measurements are taken at 0, 24 and 36 h. In a series of 122 patients (selected either because of symptomatic bone disease or long-term haemodialysis) undergoing this test there were close correlations between the peak serum Al level and both stainable bone aluminium and total trabecular bone Al content (182). Ninety four per cent of the patients with histologically defined aluminium-related bone disease and 52% of those without these features showed an increment in serum Al of >200 μg/l. The combination of an increment of >200 μg/l with a low serum immunoreactive PTH level improved the predictive value. Other, smaller, studies have given higher doses of deferoxamine (180, 181) or smaller doses at the start of haemodialysis (179), making comparison of the results difficult. In addition, the value of the test depends on the prevalence of aluminium-related bone disease in the population under study and the results of small studies in patients undergoing bone biopsy because of symptomatic bone disease (179, 181) cannot necessarily be extrapolated to less selected populations.

From the information available it is reasonable to conclude that low serum Al levels by themselves are now of limited value in excluding the presence of aluminium toxicity as the cause of bone disease, anaemia or encephalopathy. If serum aluminium shows no rise after a deferoxamine test as described (178, 182) significant bone disease is extremely unlikely. Patients with high baseline serum Al levels (>100 μg/l) or an increment after deferoxamine of >200 μg/l or both may or may not have aluminium-related bone disease. In these patients a bone biopsy is the only rational way of deciding management. Patients with smaller Al increments should be followed carefully and biopsied if there is a clinical suspicion of bone disease. The diagnostic value of the test has not been established in children, who have a smaller 'bone reservoir' from which aluminium may be mobilised (125).

Pre-clinical detection of patients at risk of encephalopathy is also difficult. Biochemical tests are of limited value and biopsy of tissues other than brain would be unlikely to predict brain levels with sufficient accuracy. Encephalopathy attributable to aluminium has been reported in a patient with unremarkable bone and serum Al levels but a marked increment after deferoxamine (183) but no other information exists on the use of deferoxamine tests in this situation. Cerebrospinal fluid Al concentrations may be helpful (18).

Measurements of Al concentration in hair (114), red blood cells and leucocytes have not been shown to add to the information derived from serum levels. Erythrocyte dihydropteridine reductase activity correlates inversely with serum Al concentration (184) but its relationship to tissue Al content or to the risk of clinical toxicity has not been established.

TREATMENT WITH DEFEROXAMINE

All sources of aluminium, including oral aluminium phosphate binders, should be withdrawn. This in itself may lead to considerable improvement (28, 55, 185). Renal transplantation is beneficial in aluminium-related bone disease (64) and in early, but not late, encephalopathy. Small amounts of aluminium may be removed by dialysis against water with an Al concentration lower than 20% of the serum level (153) or by haemofiltration with aluminium-free replacement fluid (186). Charcoal haemoperfusion also increases Al clearance (187). Conversion to CAPD may allow negative Al balance in heavily intoxicated patients. All of these methods are relatively inefficient due to the small fraction of plasma Al which is freely exchangeable. Administration of deferoxamine increases this fraction by formation of a low molecular weight aluminium-deferoxamine complex (188, 189) and leads to increased Al removal. The amount of aluminium bound to transferrin remains unchanged in the presence of deferoxamine, implying that deferoxamine mobilises aluminium from tissues (66). Serum total Al concentration rises slowly after deferoxamine administration and reaches a peak 24 to 48 h later; maximal Al removal can therefore be expected if deferoxamine is given 48 h before dialysis, otherwise the drug may be removed without complexed aluminium. Intravenous administration has been used by most workers, but intraperitoneal administration is also effective (190–192). The aluminium-deferoxamine complex is readily dialysable across cuprophan membranes and highly permeable polyacrilonitrile membranes (193, 194).

Side-effects of deferoxamine include hypotension, visual and auditory neurotoxicity (66, 195). Deferoxamine also chelates iron. By acting as a siderophore, deferoxamine may also increase the risk of Yersiniosis (196, 197) and Mucormycosis (198, 199). Deferoxamine may also lead to temporary worsening of aluminium-related encephalopathy.

CONCLUSION

Aluminium accumulation in patients with renal failure causes encephalopathy, vitamin D resistant osteomalacia and anaemia. Every effort must be made to minimise aluminium exposure through dialysis fluid (adequate water treatment and reduction in the contamination of the chemical concentrates by aluminium) by using a dialysis fluid with the lowest possible Al levels. Many countries have established standards or recommendations regarding the maximum allowed Al concentration in water used to produce dialysis fluid (10 μg/l aluminium). The Health Directorate of the European Economic Community has also recommended a maximum dialysis fluid aluminium of 10 μg/l.

No completely satisfactory alternative yet exists to the use of aluminium compounds as phosphate binders. The continued use of these compounds and resulting slow accumulation of aluminium in patients maintained by dialysis ensures that the aluminium toxicity syndrome is likely to continue appearing for a considerable number of years to come and may present in unrecognised ways.

REFERENCES

1. Alfrey AC, Mishell JM, Burks J, Contiguglia SR, Rudolph H, Lewin E, Holmes JH: Syndrome of dyspraxia and multifocal seizures associated with chronic hemodialysis. *Trans Am Soc Artif Intern Organs* 18: 257, 1972
2. Mahurkar SD, Dhar SK, Salta R, Meyers L, Smith EC, Dunea G: Dialysis dementia. *Lancet* 1: 1412, 1973
3. Platts MM, Moorhead PJ, Grech P: Dialysis dementia. *Lancet* 2: 159, 1973
4. Ward MK, Pierides AM, Fawcett P, Shaw DA, Perry RH, Tomlinson BE, Kerr DNS: Dialysis encephalopathy syndrome. *Proc Eur Dial Transplant Assoc* 13: 348, 1976
5. Flendrig JA, Kruis H, Das HA: Aluminium intoxication: the cause of dialysis dementia? *Proc Eur Dial Transplant Assoc* 13: 355, 1976
6. Chokroverty S, Bruetman ME, Berger V, Reyes MG: Progressive dialytic encephalopathy. *J Neurol Neurosurg Psychiatry* 39: 411, 1976
7. Elliott HL, MacDougall AI: Aluminium studies in dialysis encephalopathy. *Proc Eur Dial Transplant Assoc* 15: 157, 1978
8. Rozas VV, Port FK, Easterling RE: An outbreak of dialysis dementia due to aluminum in the dialysate. *J Dial* 2: 459, 1978
9. Pierides AM, Edwards WG, Cullum UX, McCall JT, Ellis HA: Hemodialysis encephalopathy with osteomalacic fractures and muscle weakness. *Kidney Int* 18: 115, 1980
10. Dewberry FL, McKinney TD, Stone WJ: The dialysis dementia syndrome: report of fourteen cases and review of the literature. *asaio J* 3: 102, 1980
11. Barron J, Whiteley SJ, Horn AC, Ralston AR, Ackrill P: A new approach to the early detection of dialysis encephalopathy. *Br J Disorders Comm* 15: 75, 1980

12. Bates D, Parkinson IS, Ward MK, Kerr DNS: Aluminium encephalopathy. *Contr Nephrol* 45: 29, 1985
13. Nadel AM, Wilson WP: Dialysis encephalopathy: a possible seizure disorder. *Neurology* 26: 1130, 1976
14. Alfrey AC: Dialysis encephalopathy. *Kidney Int* 29 (suppl 18): S53, 1986
105 Burks JS, Alfrey AC, Huddlestone J, Norenberg M, Lewin E: A fatal encephalopathy in chronic haemodialysis patients. *Lancet* 1: 764, 1976
16. Platts MM, Anastassiades E: Dialysis encephalopathy: precipitating factors and improvement in prognosis. *Clin Nephrol* 15: 223, 1981
17. Parkinson IS, Ward MK, Kerr DNS: Dialysis encephalopathy, bone disease and anaemia: the aluminium intoxication syndrome during regular haemodialysis. *J Clin Path* 34: 1285, 1981
18. Brancaccio D, Bugiani O, Pacini L, Berlin A, Bisceglia J, Gallieni M, Surian M, Costantini S, Giordano R, Rizzica M: Spinal fluid aluminium in haemodialysed uraemic patients. *Proc Eur Dial Transplant Assoc-Eur Renal Assoc* 22: 354, 1985
19. Mahurkar SD, Meyers L, Cohen J, Kamath RV, Dunea G: Electroencephalographic and radionuclide studies in dialysis dementia. *Kidney Int* 13: 306, 1978
20. Noriega-Sanchez A, Martinez-Maldonado M, Haiffe RM: Clinical and electroencephalographic changes in progressive uremic encephalopathy. *Neurology* 28: 667, 1978
21. Hughes JR, Schreeder MT: EEG in dialysis encephalopathy. *Neurology* 30: 1148, 1980
22. Wing AJ, Brunner FP, Brynger H, Chantler C, Donckerwolckce RA, Gurland HJ, Jacobs C, Kramer P, Selwood NH: Dialysis dementia in Europe. *Lancet* 2: 190, 1980
23. Platts MM, Goode GC, Hislop JS: Composition of the domestic water supply and the incidence of fractures and encephalopathy in patients on home dialysis. *Br Med J* 2: 657, 1977
24. Parkinson IS, Ward MK, Feest TG, Fawcett RWP, Kerr DNS: Fracturing dialysis osteodystrophy and dialysis encephalopathy. An epidemiological survey. *Lancet* 1: 406, 1979
25. Davison AM, Walker GS, Oli H, Lewins AM: Water supply aluminium concentration, dialysis dementia, and effect of reverse-osmosis water treatment. *Lancet* 2: 785, 1982
26. Dunea G, Mahurkar SD, Mamdani B, Smith EC: Role of aluminum in dialysis dementia. *Ann Intern Med* 88: 502, 1978
27. Schreeder MT, Favero MS, Hughes JR, Petersen NJ, Bennett PH, Maynard JE: Dialysis encephalopathy and aluminum exposure: an epidemiologic analysis. *J Chron Dis* 36: 581, 1983
28. Platts MM, Owen G, Smith S: Water purification and the incidence of fractures in patients receiving home hemodialysis supervised by a single centre: evidence for 'safe' upper limit of aluminium on water. *Br Med J* 288: 969, 1984
29. Boukari M, Rottembourg J, Jaudon MC, Clavel JP, Legrain M, Galli A: Influence de la prise prolongee de gels d'alumine sur les taux seriques d'alumine chez les patients atteints d'insuffisance renale chronique. (Influence of long-term intake of aluminium gels on the serum aluminum concentrations in patients with chronic renal failure.) *Nouv Presse Med* 7: 85, 1978
30. Kerr DNS, Ward MK, Parkinson IS: Dialysis encephalopathy: questions and answers. in: *Proceedings of the Chronic Renal Disease Conference, 1980,* edited by Cummings NB, NIH, Washington, DC, Dept Health, Education and Welfare, 1981
31. Mehta RP: Encephalopathy in chronic renal failure appearing before the start of dialysis. *Can Med Assoc J* 120: 1112, 1979
32. Marsden SNE, Parkinson IS, Ward MK, Ellis HA, Kerr DNS: Evidence for aluminium accumulation in renal failure. *Proc Eur Dial Transplant Assoc* 16: 588, 1979
33. Smith DB, Lewis JA, Burks JS, Alfrey AC: Dialysis encephalopathy in peritoneal dialysis. *JAMA* 244: 365, 1980
34. McDermott JR, Smith AI, Ward MK, Parkinson IS, Kerr DNS: Brain-aluminium concentration in dialysis encephalopathy. *Lancet* 1: 901, 1978
35. Alfrey AC, Hegg A, Craswell P: Metabolism and toxicity of aluminum in renal failure. *Am J Clin Nutr* 33: 1509, 1980
36. Arieff AI, Cooper JD, Armstrong D, Lazarowitz VC: Dementia, renal failure, and brain aluminium. *Ann Intern Med* 90: 741, 1979
37. Geary DF, Fennell RS, Andriola M, Gudat J, Rodgers BM, Richard GA: Encephalopathy in children with chronic renal failure. *J Pediatr* 96: 41, 1980
38. Pierides AM, Ward MK, Kerr DNS: Haemodialysis encephalopathy: possible role of phosphate depletion. *Lancet* 1: 1234, 1976
39. Sullivan PA, Murnaghan DJ, Callaghan N: Dialysis dementia: recovery after transplantation. *Br Med J* 2: 740, 1977
40. Silke B, Fitzgerald GR, Hanson S, Carmody M, O'Dwyer WF: Dialysis dementia and renal transplantation. *Dial Transplant* 7: 486, 1978
41. Mittal VK, Sharma MJ, Toledo-Pereyra LH, Baskin S, McNichol LJ: Complete recovery from dialysis dementia following kidney transplantation. *Dial Transplant* 10: 41, 1981
42. Mattern WD, Krigman MR, Blythe WB: Failure of successful renal transplantation to reverse the dialysis-associated encephalopathy syndrome. *Clin Nephrol* 7: 275, 1977
43. Davison AM, Giles GR: The effect of transplantation on dialysis dementia. *Proc Eur Dial Transplant Assoc* 16: 407, 1979
44. Ball JH, Butkus DE, Madison DS: Effect of subtotal parathyroidectomy on dialysis dementia. *Nephron* 18: 151, 1977
45. de Gencarelli NC, Cournot-Witner G, Zingraff J, Drüeke T: The role of parathyroid function and parathyroidectomy in the outcome of aluminium-related dialysis encephalopathy. *Nephrol Dial Transplant* : 192, 1986
46. Ackrill P, Ralston AJ, Day JP, Hodge KC: Successful removal of aluminium from patient with dialysis encephalopathy. *Lancet* 2: 1980
47. Milne FJ, Sharf B, Bell P, Meyers AM: The effect of low aluminium water and desferrioxamine on the outcome of dialysis encephalopathy. *Clin Nephrol* 20: 202, 1983
48. Ackrill P, Ralston AJ, Day JP: Role of desferrioxamine in the treatment of dialysis encephalopathy. *Kidney Int* 29 (Suppl 18): S104, 1986
49. Baluarte HJ, Gruskin AB, Hiner LB, Foley CM, Grover WD: Encephalopathy in children with chronic renal failure. *Proc Clin Dial Transplant Forum* 7: 95, 1977
50. Sedman AB, Miller NL, Warady BA, Lum GM, Alfrey AC: Aluminum loading in children with chronic renal failure. *Kidney Int* 26: 201, 1984
51. Nathan E, Pedersen SE: Dialysis encephalopathy in a nondialysed uraemic boy treated with aluminium hydroxide orally. *Acta Paediatr Scand* 69: 793, 1980
52. Randall ME: Aluminium toxicity in an infant not on dialysis. *Lancet* 2: 1327, 1983
53. Polinsky MS, Gruskin AB: Aluminum toxicity in children with chronic renal failure. *J Pediatr* 105: 758, 1984
54. Ward MK, Feest TG, Ellis HA, Parkinson IS, Kerr DNS, Herrington J, Goode GL: Osteomalacic dialysis osteodystro-

phy: evidence for a aetiological water-borne agent, probably aluminium. *Lancet* 1: 841, 1978

55. Kerr DNS, Ward MK, Arze RS, Ramos JM, Grekas D, Parkinson IS, Ellis HA, Owen JP, Simpson W, Dewar J, Martin AM, McHugh MF: Aluminum-induced dialysis osteodystrophy: The demise of 'Newcastle bone disease'? *Kidney Int* 29 (Suppl 18): S58, 1986

56. McCarthy JT, Kurtz SB, McCall JT: Elevated bone aluminum content in dialysis patients without osteomalacia. *Mayo Clin Proc* 60: 315, 1985

57. Cournot-Witmer G, Zingraff J, Plachot JJ, Escaig F, Lefevre R, Boumati P, Bourdeau A, Garabedian M, Galle P, Bourdon R, Drüeke T, Balsan S: Aluminum localization in bone from hemodialyzed patients: relationship to matrix mineralization. *Kidney Int* 20: 375, 1981

58. Dunstan CR, Evans RA, Hills E, Wong SYP, Alfrey AC: Effect of aluminum and parathyroid hormone on osteoblasts and bone mineralization in chronic renal failure. *Calcif Tissue Int* 36: 133, 1984

59. de Vernejoul MC, Belenguer R, Halkidou H, Buisine A, Bielakoff J, Miravet L: Histomorphometric evidence of deleterious effect of aluminum on osteoblasts. *Bone* 6: 15, 1985

60. Nilsson P, Melsen F, Malmaeus J, Danielson BG, Mosekilde L: Relationships between calcium and phosphorus homeostasis, parathyroid hormone levels, bone aluminum, and bone histomorphometry in patients on maintenance hemodialysis. *Bone* 6: 21, 1985

61. Leather HM, Lewin IG, Calder E, Braybrooke J, Cox RR: Effect of water deionisers on 'fracturing osteodystrophy' and dialysis encephalopathy in Plymouth. *Nephron* 29: 80, 1981

62. Prior JC, Cameron EC, Knickerbocker WJ, Sweeney VP, Suchowersky O: Dialysis encephalopathy and osteomalacic bone disease. A case controlled study. *Am J Med* 72: 33, 1982

63. Posen GA, Gray DG, Jaworski ZF, Couture R, Rashid A: Comparison of renal osteodystrophy in patients dialyzed with deionized and non-deionized water. *Trans Am Soc Artif Intern Organs* 18: 405, 1972

64. Pierides AM, Ellis HA, Peart KM, Simpson W, Uldall PR, Kerr DNS: Assessment of renal osteodystrophy following renal transplantation. *Proc Eur Dial Transplant Assoc* 11: 481, 1974

65. Brown DJ, Dawborn JK, Ham KN, Xipell JM: Treatment of dialysis osteomalacia with desferrioxamine. *Lancet* 2: 343, 1982

66. Ackrill P: Aluminium removal by desferrioxamine: clinical practice 1985. in: *Aluminium and Other Trace Elements in Renal Diseases*, edited by Taylor A, London, Balliere Tindall, 1986, p 193

67. Andress DL, Nebeker HG, Ott SM, Endres DB, Alfrey AC, Slatoplosky EA, Coburn JW, Sherrard DJ: Bone histologic response to deferoxamine in aluminum-related bone disease. *Kidney Int* 31: 1344, 1987

68. Charhon SA, Chavassieux P, Boivin G, Parisien M, Chapuy M-C, Traeger J, Meunier PJ: Deferoxamine-induced bone changes in haemodialysis patients: a histomorphometric study. *Clin Sci* 73: 227, 1987

69. Cumming AD, Simpson G, Bell D, Cowie J, Winney RJ: Acute aluminium intoxication in patients on continuous ambulatory peritoneal dialysis. *Lancet* 1: 103, 1982

70. Rottembourg J, Gallego JL, Jaudon M-C, Clavel J-P, Legrain M: Serum concentration and peritoneal transfer of aluminium during treatment by continuous ambulatory peritoneal dialysis. *Kidney Int* 25: 919, 1984

71. Short AIK, Winney RJ, Robson JS: Reversible microcytic

hypochromic anaemia in dialysis patients due to aluminium intoxication. *Proc Eur Dial Transplant Assoc* 17: 226, 1980

72. O'Hare JA, Murnaghan DJ: Reversal of aluminum-induced hemodialysis anemia by a low-aluminum dialysate. *N Engl J Med* 306: 654, 1982

73. Touam M, Martinez F, Lacour B, Bourdon R, Zingraff J, diGiulio S, Drüeke T: Aluminium-induced, reversible microcytic anemia in chronic renal failure: clinical and experimental studies. *Clin Nephrol* 19: 295, 1983

74. McGonigle RJS, Parsons V: Aluminium-induced anaemia in haemodialysis patients. *Nephron* 39: 1, 1985

75. Buchet JP, Lauwerys R, Hassoun A, Dratwa M, Wens R, Collart F, Tielemans C: Effect of aluminum on porphyrin metabolism in hemodialysis patients. *Nephron* 46: 360, 1987

76. Tielemans C, Collart F, Wens R, Smeyers-Verbeeke J, van Hooff I, Dratwa M, Verbeelen D: Improvement of anemia with deferoxamine in hemodialysis patients with aluminum-induced bone disease. *Clin Nephrol* 24: 237, 1985

77. Praga M, Andres A, de la Serna J, Ruilope LM, Nieto J, Estenoz J, Millet VG, Arnaiz F, Rodicio JL: Improvement of anaemia with desferrioxamine in haemodialysis patients. *Nephrol Dial Transplant* 2: 243, 1987

78. Casali S, Passerini P, Campise MR, Graziani G, Cesana B, Perisic M, Ponticelli C: Benefits and risks of protracted treatment with human recombinant erythropoietin in patients having haemodialysis. *Br Med J* 295: 1017, 1987

79. Mayor GH: The case for parathyroid hormone. *Am J Kidney Dis* 6: 306, 1985

80. Alfrey AC: The case against aluminium affecting parathyroid function. *Am J Kidney Dis* 6: 309, 1985

81. Cann CE, Prussin SG, Gordan GS: Aluminum uptake by the parathyroid glands. *J Clin Endocrin Metab* 49: 543, 1979

82. Mendes V, Jorgetti V, Nemeth J, Lavergne A, Lecharpentier Y, Dubost C, Cournot-Witner C, Bourdon R, Bourdeau A, Zingraff J, Drüeke T: Secondary hyperparathyroidism in chronic renal failure: a clinico-pathological study. *Proc Eur Dial Transplant Assoc* 20: 731, 1983

83. Morrissey J, Slatoplosky E: Effect of aluminum on parathyroid hormone secretion. *Kidney Int* 29 (Suppl 18): S41, 1986

84. Andress D, Felsenfeld AJ, Voigts A, Llach F: Parathyroid hormone response to hypocalcemia in hemodialysis patients with osteomalacia. *Kidney Int* 24: 364, 1983

85. Kraut JA, Shinaberger JH, Singer FR, Sherrard DJ, Saxton J, Miller JH, Kurokawa K, Coburn JW: Parathyroid gland responsiveness to acute hypocalcemia in dialysis osteomalacia. *Kidney Int* 23: 725, 1983

86. Henry DA, Goodman WG, Nudelman RK, DiDomenico NC, Alfrey AC, Slatopolsky E, Stanley TM, Coburn JW: Parenteral aluminium administration in the dog: 1. Plasma kinetics, tissue levels, calcium metabolism and parathyroid hormone. *Kidney Int* 25: 362, 1984

87. Cannata JB, Briggs JD, Junor BJR, Fell GS, Beastall G: Effect of acute aluminium overload on calcium and parathyroid-hormone metabolism. *Lancet* i: 501, 1983

88. O'Hare JA, Murnaghan DJ: Evidence of increased parathyroid activity on discontinuation of high-aluminum dialysate in patients undergoing hemodialysis. *Am J Med* 77: 229, 1984

89. Fanti P, Faugere MC, Smith AJ, Malluche HH: Increased blood levels of 1,25 vit D after aluminum removal in haemodialysed patients. *Neph Dial Transplant* 2: 406, 1987

90. Klein GL, Alfrey AC, Miller NL, Sherrard DJ, Hazlet TK, Ament ME, Coburn JW: Aluminum loading during total parenteral nutrition. *Am J Clin Nutr* 35: 1425, 1982

91. Boukari M, Jaudon MC, Rottembourg PFJ, Luciani J, Legrain M, Galli A: Kinetics of serum and urinary aluminium after renal transplantation. *Lancet* 1: 1044, 1978

92. Norris KC, Crooks PW, Nebeker HG, Hercz G, Milliner DS, Gerszi K, Slatopolsky E, Andress DL, Sherrard DJ, Coburn JW: Clinical and laboratory features of aluminum-related bone disease: differences between sporadic and 'epidemic' forms of the syndrome. *Am J Kidney Dis* 6: 342, 1985

93. Alfrey AC, Sedman A, Chan Y-L: The compartmentalization and metabolism of aluminum in uremic rats. *J Lab Clin Med* 105: 227, 1985

94. Drüeke T, Lacour B, Touam M, Basile C, Bourdon R: Oral aluminium administration to uremic, hyperparathyroid, or vitamin-D supplemented rats. *Nephron* 39: 10, 1985

95. Felsenfeld AJ, Harrelson JM, Gutman RA, Wells SA, Drezner MK: Osteomalacia after parathyroidectomy in patients with uremia. *Ann Intern Med* 96: 34, 1982

96. Ellis HA: Aluminum and osteomalacia after parathyroidectomy. *Ann Intern Med* 96: 533, 1982

97. Charhon SA, Berland YF, Olmer MJ, Delawari E, Traeger J, Meunier PJ: Effects of parathyroidectomy on bone formation in hemodialyzed patients. *Kidney Int* 27: 426, 1985

98. de Vernejoul MC, Marchais S, London G, Morieux C, Bielakoff J, Miravet L: Increased bone aluminum deposition after subtotal parathyroidectomy in dialyzed patients. *Kidney Int* 27: 758, 1985

99. Andress DL, Ott SM, Maloney NA, Sherrard DJ: Effect of parathyroidectomy on bone aluminum accumulation in chronic renal failure. *N Engl J Med* 312, 468, 1985

100. Kaye M: Oral aluminium toxicity in a non-dialyzed patient with renal failure. *Clin Nephrol* 20: 208, 1983

101. Andreoli SP, Bergstein JM, Sherrard DJ: Aluminum intoxication from aluminum-containing phosphate binders in children with azotemia not undergoing dialysis. *N Engl J Med* 310: 1079, 1984

102. Berlyne GM, Ben-Ari J, Post D, Weinberger J, Stern M, Gilmore GR, Levine R: Hyperaluminaemia from aluminium resins in renal failure. *Lancet* 1: 494, 1970

103. Hosakawa S, Kohira S, Tomoyoshi T: Aluminum transfer in chronic renal failure patients during hemodialysis. *Blood Purif* 1: 62, 1983

104. Winney RJ, Cowie JF, Robson JS: Role of plasma aluminium in the detection and prevention of aluminium toxicity. *Kidney Int* 29 (Suppl 18): S91, 1986

105. Salusky IB, Coburn JW, Paunier L, Sherrard DJ, Fine RN: Role of aluminum hydroxide in raising serum aluminum levels in children undergoing continuous ambulatory peritoneal dialysis. *J Pediatr* 105: 717, 1984

106. Heaf JG, Nielsen LP: Serum aluminium in haemodialysis patients: relation to osteodystrophy, encephalopathy and aluminium hydroxide consumption. *Miner Electrolyte Metab* 10: 345, 1984

107. Gonella M, Calabrese G, Vagelli G, Pratesi G, Lamon S, Talarico S: Effect of high CaCO₃ supplements on serum calcium and phosphorus in patients on regular hemodialysis treatment. *Clin Nephrol* 24: 147, 1985

108. Masselot JP, Adhemar JP, Jaudon MC, Kleinknecht D, Galli A: Reversible dialysis encephalopathy: role for aluminium-containing gels. *Lancet* 2: 1386, 1978

109. Channon SM, Mawhinney WHB, Rodger RSC, Goodship THJ, Ellis HA, Wilkinson R, Ward MK: Accumulating aluminium deposition in bone due to aluminium hydroxide ingestion in patients with renal failure. in: *Aluminium and Other Trace Elements in Renal Disease*, edited by Taylor AP, London, Balliere Tindall, 1986, p 118

110. Altmann P, Butter KC, Plowman D, Chaput de Saintoigne DM, Cunningham J, Marsh FP: Residual renal function in hemodialysis patients may protect against hyperaluminemia. *Kidney Int* 32: 710, 1987

111. Raidt H, Vischedyck M, Kellinghaus H, Stenhausen D, Graefe U: Aluminium containing oral phosphorus binders and the aluminium content of bone. *Proc Eur Dial Transplant Assoc-Eur Renal Assoc* 22: 369, 1985

112. Sebert JL, Fournier A, Leflon P, Fohrer P, de Fremont JF, Moriniere P, Galy C, Marie A, Demontis R, Boudalliez B, Gueris J, Dkhissi H, Garabedian M, Lambrey G: Comparative evaluation of bone aluminium content and bone histology in patients on chronic hemodialysis and hemofiltration. *Nephron* 42: 34, 1986

113. Heaf JG, Podenphant J, Andersen JR: Bone aluminium deposition in maintenance dialysis patients treated with aluminium-free dialysate: role of aluminium hydroxide consumption. *Nephron* 42: 210, 1986

114. Winterberg B, Bertram HP, Roedig M, Kisters K, Raidt H, Spieker C, Zumkley H: Brain aluminium level and aluminium content of antacids in patients with normal renal function. *Nephrol Dial Transplant* 2: 408, 1987

115. Clarkson EM, Luck VA, Hynson WV, Bailey RR, Eastwood JB, Woodhead JS, Clements VR, O'Riordan JLH, de Wardener HE: The effect of aluminium hydroxide on calcium, phosphorus and aluminium balances, the serum parathyroid hormone concentration and the aluminium content of bone in patients with chronic renal failure. *Clin Sci* 43: 519, 1972

116. Gorsky JE, Dietz AA, Spencer H, Osis D: Metabolic balance of aluminium studied in six men. *Clin Chem* 25: 1739, 1979

117. Kaehny WD, Hegg AP, Alfrey AC: Gastrointestinal absorption of aluminum from aluminum-containing antacids. *N Engl J Med* 296: 1389, 1977

118. Trapp GA, Cannon JB: Aluminum pots as a source of dietary aluminum. *N Engl J Med* 304: 172, 1981

119. Ott SM: Aluminum accumulation in individuals with normal renal function. *Am J Kidney Dis* 6: 297, 1985

120. Knoll O, Lahl H, Bockmann J, Hennig H, Unterhalt B: Aluminum contamination of tap water and food. *Trace Element Med* 3: 172, 1986

121. Freundlich M, Zilleruelo G, Abitbol C, Strauss J, Faugere M-C, Malluche HH: Infant formula as a cause of aluminium toxicity in neonatal uraemia. *Lancet* 2: 527, 1985

122. McGraw M, Bishop N, Jameson R, Robinson MJ, O'Hara M, Hewitt CD, Day JP: Aluminium content of milk formulae and intravenous fluids used in infants. *Lancet* 1: 157, 1986

123. Sedman AB, Klein GL, Merritt RJ, Miller NL, Weber KO, Gill WL, Anand H, Alfrey AC: Evidence of aluminum loading in infants receiving intravenous therapy. *N Engl J Med* 312: 1337, 1985

124. Gacek EM, Babb AL, Uvelli DA, Fry DL, Scribner BH: Dialysis Dementia: the role of dialysate pH in altering the dialyzability of aluminum. *Trans Am Soc Artif Intern Organs* 25: 409, 1979

125. Roodhoft AM, van de Vyver FL, d'Haes PC, van Acker KJ, Visser WJ, de Broe ME: Aluminum accumulation in children on chronic dialysis: predictive value of serum aluminum levels and desferrioxamine test. *Clin Nephrol* 28: 125, 1987

126. Adler AJ, Berlyne GM: Duodenal aluminum absorption in the rat: Effect of vitamin D. *Am J Physiol* 249 (2 part 1): G209, 1985

127. Burnatowska-Hledin MA, Doyle TM, Eadie MJ, Mayor GH: 1,25-dihydroxyvitamin D₃ increases serum and tissue accumulation of aluminum in rats. *J Lab Clin Med* 108: 96, 1986

128. Alfrey AC, Hegg A, Miller N, Berl T, Berns A: Interrelationship between calcium and aluminum metabolism in dialyzed uremic patients. *Miner Electrolyte Metab* 2: 81–87, 1979

129. Fournier A, Demontis R, Tahiri Y, Moriniere P, Leflon A, Abdull-Massih Z, Atok H, Benelmouffok S: 1 OH Vitamin D$_3$ increases plasma aluminium in haemodialysis patients taking Al(OH)$_3$. *Proc Eur Dial Transpl Assoc* 21: 390, 1984

130. Mayor GH, Sprague SM, Hourani MR, Sanchez TV: Parathyroid hormone-mediated aluminum deposition and egress in the rat. *Kidney Int* 17: 40, 1980

131. Cannata JB, Suarez CS, Cuesta V, Roza RR, Allende MT, Herrera J, Llanderal JP: Gastrointestinal aluminium absorption: is it modulated by the iron absorptive mechanism? *Proc Eur Dial Transpl Assoc-Eur Renal Assoc* 21: 354, 1984

132. Blaehr H, Madsen S, Andersen JR: Effect of iron-loading on intestinal aluminium absorption in chronic renal insufficiency. in: *Aluminium and Other Trace Elements in Renal Disease,* edited by Taylor A, London, Balliere Tindall, 1986, p 71

133. Parsons V, O'Donovan R, Gibson M, Goode GC, Baldwin D: Aluminium and fluoride in uraemic bone: a possible interrelationship. in: *Aluminium and Other Trace Elements in Renal Disease,* edited by Taylor A, London, Balliere Tindall, 1986, p 57

134. Weberg R, Berstad A: Gastrointestinal absorption of aluminium from single doses of aluminium containing antacids in man. *Eur J Clin Invest* 16: 428, 1986

135. Boyce BF, Mocan MZ, Halls DJ, Cowan RA, Forwell M, Junor BJR: Aluminium-related osteomalacia due to oral aluminium: can patients at risk be identified by an aluminium absorption test? in: *Aluminium and Other Trace Elements in Renal Disease,* edited by Taylor A, London, Balliere Tindall, 1986, p 108

136. Slatopolsky E, Weerts C, Lopez-Hilker S, Norwood K, Zink M, Windus D, Delmez J: Calcium carbonate as a phosphate binder in patients with chronic renal failure undergoing dialysis. *N Engl J Med* 315: 157, 1986

137. Fournier A, Moriniere P, Sebert JL, Dkhissi H, Atik A, Leflon P, Renaud H, Gueris J, Gregoire I, Idrissi A, Garabedian M: Calcium carbonate, and aluminum-free agent for control of hyperphosphataemia, hypocalcaemia and hyperparathyroidism in uremia. *Kidney Int* 29 (Suppl 18): S114, 1986

138. Mactier RA, van Stone J, van Stone M, Twardowski Z: Calcium carbonate is an effective phosphate binder when dialysate calcium concentration is adjusted to control hypercalcemia. *Clin Nephrol* 28: 222, 1987

139. Guillot AP, Hood VL, Runge CF, Gennari FJ: The use of magnesium-containing phosphate binders in patients with end-stage renal disease on maintenance hemodialysis. *Nephron* 30: 114, 1982

140. Wheeler DC, Smith B, Walls J: Substitution of aluminium salts by magnesium salts in control of dialysis hyperphosphataemia. *Lancet* 1: 1380, 1986

141. Jennings AE, Bodvarsson M, Galicka-Piskorska G, Diedendorf AS, Simon GM, Levey AS: Use of magnesium hydroxide and low magnesium dialysate does not permit reduction of aluminum hydroxide during continuous ambulatory peritoneal dialysis. *Am J Kidney Dis* 8: 192, 1986

142. Shah GM, Winer RL, Cutler RE, Arieff AI, Goodman WG, Lacher JW, Schoenfeld PY, Coburn JW, Horowitz AM: Effects of a magnesium-free dialysate on magnesium metabolism during continuous ambulatory peritoneal dialysis. *Am J Kidney Dis* 10: 268, 1987

143. O'Donovan R, Baldwin D, Hammer M, Miniz C, Parsons V: Substitution of aluminium salts by magnesium salts in control of dialysis hyperphosphataemia. *Lancet* 1: 880, 1986

144. Makoff DL, Gordon A, Franklin SS, Gerstein AR, Maxwell MH: Chronic calcium carbonate therapy in uremia. *Arch Intern Med* 123: 15, 1968

145. Mak RHK, Turner C, Thompson T, Powell H, Haycock GB, Chantler C: Suppression of secondary hyperparathyroidism in children with chronic renal failure by high dose phosphate binders: Calcium carbonate versus aluminium hydroxide. *Br Med J* 291: 623, 1985

146. Ramirez JA, Emmett M, White MG, Fathi N, Santa Ana CA, Morawski SG, Fordtran JS: The absorption of dietary phosphorus and calcium in hemodialysis patients. *Kidney Int* 30: 753, 1986

147. Oe PL, Lips P, van der Meulen J, de Vries PMJM, van Bronswijk H, Donker AJM: Long-term use of magnesium hydroxide as a phosphate binder in patients on hemodialysis. *Clin Nephrol* 28: 180, 1987

148. Leung ACT, Henderson IS, Halls DJ, Dobbie JW: Aluminium hydroxide versus sucralfate as a phosphate binder in uraemia. *Br Med J* 86: 1379, 1983

149. Sherman RA, Hwang ER, Walker JA, Eisinger RP: Reduction in serum phosphorus due to sucralfate. *Am J Gastroenterol* 78: 210, 1983

150. Shneider HW, Kulbe KD, Weber H, Streicher E: In vitro and in vivo studies with a non-aluminum phosphate-binding compound. *Kidney Int* 29 (Suppl 18): S120, 1986

151. Schneider H: Alternatives to aluminium-containing phosphate binders. in: *Aluminium and Other Trace Elements in Renal Disease,* edited by Taylor A, London, Balliere Tindall, 1986, p 127

152. Kaehny WD, Alfrey AC, Holman RE, Schorr WJ: Aluminum transfer during hemodialysis. *Kidney Int* 12: 361, 1977

153. Graf H, Stummvoll HK, Meisinger V, Kovarik J, Wolf A, Pinggera WF: Aluminum removal by hemodialysis. *Kidney Int* 19: 587, 1981

154. Hodge KC, Day JP, O'Hara M, Ackrill P, Ralston AJ: Critical concentrations of aluminium in water used for dialysis. *Lancet* 2: 802, 1981

155. Hosakawa S, Imai T, Okumura T, Tomoyoshi T, Kawamura J, Sawanashi K, Yoshida O: Aluminum transfer during hemodialysis. *Trace Element Med* 1: 59: 1984

156. Rahman H, Channon SM, Skillen AW, Ward MK, Kerr DNS: Aluminum transfer during hemodialysis and its relation to serum ultrafilterable aluminum. *Trace Element Med 1985; 2:* 143, 1985

157. Trapp GA: Plasma aluminum is bound to transferrin. *Life Sci* 33: 311, 1983

158. Savory J, Wills MR: Dialysis fluids as a source of aluminum accumulation. *Contrib Nephrol* 38: 12, 1984

159. Rahman H, Channon SM, Skillen AW, Ward MK, Kerr DNS: Protein binding of aluminium in normal subjects and in patients with chronic renal failure. *Proc Eur Dial Transpl Assoc-Eur Renal Assoc* 21: 360, 1984

160. Berlin A: Prevention and monitoring of aluminium exposure during dialysis in the European Community, 1985. in: *Aluminium and Other Trace Elements in Renal Failure,* edited by Taylor A, London, Balliere Tindall, 1986, p 167

161. Milliner DS, Shinaberger JH, Shuman P, Coburn JW: Inadvertent aluminum administration during plasma exchange due to aluminum contamination of albumin-replacement solutions. *N Engl J Med* 312: 165, 1985

162. Maher ER, Brown EA, Curtis JR, Phillips ME, Sampson B: Accumulation of aluminium in chronic renal failure due to administration of albumin replacement solutions. *Br Med J* 292: 306, 1986

163. Maharaj D, Fell GS, Boyce BF, Ng JP, Smith GD, Boulton-Jones JM, Cumming RLC, Davidson JF: Aluminium bone disease in patients receiving plasma exchange with contaminated albumin. *Br Med J* 295: 693, 1987

164. Robinson MJ, Ryan SW, Newton CJ, Day JP, Hewitt CD, O'Hara M: Blood aluminium levels in preterm infants fed parenterally or with cows' milk formulae. *Lancet* 2: 1206, 1987

165. Mason JC, Jones NF, Hilton PJ: Aluminium in haemofiltration solutions. *Lancet* 1: 762, 1983

166. Ott SM, Maloney NA, Klein GL, Alfrey AC, Ament ME, Coburn JW, Sherrard DJ: Aluminum is associated with low bone formation in patients receiving chronic parenteral nutrition. *Ann Intern Med* 98: 910, 1983

167. Wagner K, Lenz T, Keller F, Neumayer HH, Fitzner R, Pipenhagen U, Dulce HJ, Distler A, Molzahn M: Does desferrioxamine induce aluminium load in patients on chronic haemodialysis? *Proc Eur Dial Transpl Assoc-Eur Renal Assoc* 22: 388, 1985

168. Gilli P, Farinelli A, Fagioli F, de Bastiani P, Buoncristiani U: Serum aluminium levels in patients on peritoneal dialysis. *Lancet* 2: 742, 1980

169. Gokal R, Ramos JM, Ellis HA, Parkinson I, Sweetman V, Dewar J, Ward MK, Kerr DNS: Histological renal osteodystrophy and 25 hydroxycholecalciferol and aluminium levels in patients on continuous ambulatory peritoneal dialysis. *Kidney Int* 23: 15, 1983

170. Kovalchik MT, Kaehny WD, Hegg AP, Jackson JT, Alfrey AC: Aluminum kinetics during hemodialysis. *J Lab Clin Med* 92: 712, 1978

171. Burnatowska-Hledin MA, Mayor GH, Lau K: Renal handling of aluminum in the rat: clearance and micropuncture studies. *Am J Physiol* 249: F192, 1985

172. Anderson K-J, Julshamn K, Schjoensby H: Increased serum aluminum levels in patients with jaundice. *N Engl J Med* 301: 728, 1979

173. Simon P, Allain P, Mauras Y, Ang KS: Hyperaluminemia test by desferrioxamine for the determination of tissue aluminum overload in hemodialysis patients. Aggravating factor of chronic infections by B and non-A, non-B virus. *Kidney Int* 21: 900, 1982

174. Williams JW, Vera SR, Peters TG, Luther RW, Bhattacharya S, Spears H, Graham A, Pitcock JA, Crawford AJ: Biliary excretion of aluminum in aluminum osteodystrophy with liver disease. *Ann Intern Med* 104: 782, 1986

175. Berlyne GM, Adler AJ: Serum aluminum cannot be measured accurately. *Am J Kidney Dis* 6: 288, 1985

176. Taylor A, Starkey BJ, Walker AW: Determination of aluminum in serum: findings of an external quality assessment scheme. *Ann Clin Biochem* 22: 351, 1985

177. Charhon SA, Chavassieux PM, Meunier PJ, Accominotti M: Serum aluminium concentration and aluminium deposits in bone in patients receiving hemodialysis. *Br Med J* 290: 1613, 1985

178. Milliner DS, Nebeker HG, Ott SM, Andress DL, Sherrard DJ, Alfrey AC, Slatopolsky E, Coburn JW: Use of the deferoxamine infusion test in the diagnosis of aluminum-related osteodystrophy. *Ann Intern Med* 101: 775, 1984

179. Malluche HH, Smith AJ, Abreo K, Faugere M-C: The use of deferoxamine in the management of aluminum accumulation in bone in patients with renal failure. *N Engl J Med* 311: 140, 1984

180. Berland Y, Charhon SA, Olmer M, Meunier PJ: Predictive value of desferrioxamine infusion test for bone aluminium deposits in hemodialyzed patients. *Nephron* 40: 433, 1985

181. Hodsman AB, Hood SA, Brown P, Cordy PE: Do serum aluminum levels reflect underlying skeletal aluminum accumulation and bone histology before or after chelation by deferoxamine? *J Lab Clin Med* 106: 674, 1985

182. Nebeker HG, Andress DL, Milliner DS, Ott SM, Alfrey AC, Slatopolsky E, Sherrard DJ, Coburn JW: Indirect methods for the diagnosis of aluminum bone disease: plasma aluminum, the desferrioxamine test and serum iPTH. *Kidney Int* 29 (Suppl 18): S96, 1986

183. Sprague SM, Corwin HL, Wilson RS, Mayor GH, Tanner CM: Encephalopathy in chronic renal failure responsive to deferoxamine therapy. Another manifestation of aluminum toxicity. *Arch Intern Med* 146: 2063, 1986

184. Altmann P, Al-Salihi F, Butter K, Cutler P, Blair J, Leeming R, Cunningham J, Marsh F: Serum aluminum levels and erythrocyte dihydropteridine reductase activity in patients on hemodialysis. *N Engl J Med* 317: 80, 1987

185. Smith GD, Winney RJ, McLean A, Robson JS: Aluminium-related osteomalacia: response to reverse osmosis water treatment. *Kidney Int* 32: 96, 1987

186. Bettinelli A, Buratti M, Colombi A, Aghemio A, Edefonti A: Aluminum loading in children on chronic hemofiltration. *Int J Artif Organs* 1: 131, 1987

187. Slatopolsky E, Weerts C, Finch J, Lee W, Windus D, Delmez J: The use of microencapsulated carbon in the removal of aluminium in dialysis. *Kidney Int* 29: 226, 1986

188. Stumvoll H-K, Graf H, Meisinger V: Effect of desferrioxamine on aluminum kinetics during hemodialysis. *Miner Electrolyte Metab* 10: 263, 1984

189. Bertholf RL, Savory J, Wills MR: Desferrioxamine decreases protein-bound aluminum in serum. *Trace Element Med* 3: 157, 1986

190. Payton CD, Junor BJR, Fell GS: Successful treatment of aluminium encephalopathy by intraperitoneal desferrioxamine. *Lancet* 1: 1132, 1984

191. Warady BA, Ford DM, Gaston CE, Sedman AB, Huffer WE, Lum GM: Aluminum intoxication in children: treatment with intraperitoneal desferrioxamine. *Pediatrics* 78: 651, 1986

192. O'Brien AAJ, McParland C, Keogh JAB: The use of intravenous and intraperitoneal desferrioxamine in aluminium osteomalacia. *Nephrol Dial Transplant* 2: 117, 1987

193. Bonal J, Montoliu J, Pedret JL, Bergada E, Andrew L, Bachs M, Revert L: Desferrioxamine induced aluminium removal in haemodialysis. *Proc Eur Dial Transplant Assoc-Eur Renal Assoc* 21: 366, 1984

194. Muirhead N, Hollomby DJ, Leung FY, Mitton R, Henderson AR, Keown PA, Stiller CR: Removal of aluminum during hemodialysis: effect of different dialyzer membranes. *Am J Kidney Dis* 8: 51, 1986

195. Olivieri NF, Buncic JR, Chew E, Gallant T, Harrison RV, Keenan N, Logan W, Mitchell D, Ricci G, Skarf B, Taylor M, Freedman MH: Visual and auditory neurotoxicity in patients receiving subcutaneous deferoxamine infusions. *N Engl J Med* 314: 869, 1986

196. Robins-Browne RM, Prpic JK: Desferrioxamine and systemic yersiniosis. *Lancet* 2: 1372, 1983

197. Boyce N, Thomson NM, Wood C, Atkins RC, Holdsworth S: Life-threatening sepsis complicating heavy metal chelation therapy with desferrioxamine. *Aus NZ J Med* 15: 654, 1985

198. Eiser AR, Slifkin RF, Neff MS: Intestinal mucormycosis in hemodialysis patients following deferoxamine. *Am J Kidney Dis* 10: 71, 1987

199. Goodill JJ, Abuelo JG: Mucormycosis – a new risk of deferoxamine therapy in patients with aluminum or iron overload? *N Engl J Med* 317: 54, 1987

PHARMACOLOGICAL CONSIDERATIONS FOR RENAL FAILURE AND DIALYSIS

JOHN F. MAHER

In patients with renal failure, especially those treated by dialysis, pharmacological considerations represent an area of increasing complexity, importance and expanding knowledge. These considerations involve such topics as pharmacokinetics, nephrotoxicity, effects of drugs on elimination kinetics, dialysis of poisons, depletion of drugs by dialysis and dosage modifications. The abundant literature includes several recent reviews of these subjects (1–14). The inexperienced physician can readily encounter numerous potential therapeutic pitfalls leading inappropriately to therapeutic nihilism. Even with experience prescribing errors are made to a population demanding and receiving many drugs. The typical patient treated by dialysis takes eight drugs, some of which are duplicates and a few of which are contraindicated (15).

DRUGS AND RENAL FAILURE

The incidence of adverse drug reactions in uremic patients is high (1, 2, 8, 9). It relates to decreased elimination of the unchanged drug or of toxic metabolites, alterations in drug distribution or protein binding, drug associated metabolic loads, synergism of drug toxicity and metabolic abnormalities, or possibly increased target organ susceptibility. In hospitalized patients, coexistent azotemia doubles the incidence of drug toxicity (16). The susceptibility may be even higher than recognized since toxicity can masquerade as uremia, and toxic drugs are often avoided or given in inappropriately low dosage to patients with renal failure (17, 18).

Pharmacokinetics

Drugs are absorbed to various extents, distributed to body tissues where pharmacologic actions and toxic reactions occur, and eliminated by one or more of several processes at various rates. Abnormalities in any of these factors may occur in uremia and be affected by dialysis. To avoid toxicity, guidelines can be followed, e.g. avoid unfamiliar drugs, verify maintenance doses or reduce dosage according to the decreased creatinine clearance. Pharmacokinetics in renal failure are often too complicated, however, for crude guidelines to achieve non-toxic therapy reliably. Physicians should not rely blindly on nomograms. Accordingly, some pharmacokinetic principles are outlined below and several reviews are recommended (1–4, 7–14, 19–23).

Bioavailability

When administered orally most drugs are incompletely absorbed. Many undergo some metabolic biotransformation during absorptive passage through the liver (19, 24). The amount of the drug that reaches the left ventricle in its pharmacologically active form is the bioavailable drug, usually expressed as a fraction of that administered. This fraction varies according to the drug. It also varies according to the dose of a given drug because of saturation of first-pass hepatic metabolic processes. Drugs with extensive first-pass metabolism include imipramine, lidocaine, meperidine, pentazocine, phenacetin, propoxyphene, propranolol and terbutaline (24).

There has been little study of bioavailability of drugs in renal failure. Impaired absorption of calcium owing to 1,25 vitamin D deficiency is well known, however. Antacids can bind not only phosphate but iron as well (25), decreasing absorption. Moreover, changes in gastric pH accompanying uremia can decrease absorption by influencing non-ionic diffusion. Bioavailability of propranolol may be increased in patients with renal failure, possibly because of a decrease in first-pass hepatic metabolism (19). Sulfonamide bioavailability is unchanged but furosemide and pindolol absorption decrease (19). The absorption of d-xylose is less complete and much slower in patients with chronic renal failure compared to normals (26), but experimental renal failure increases the absorption of sulfanilic acid (27). Hence, drug bioavailability cannot be universally predicted. Coexistent heart failure, cirrhosis or gastrointestinal motility disorders can also affect bioavailability.

Distribution space

Once absorbed, a drug distributes into tissues as determined by lipophilicity and solubility characteristics and plasma and tissue binding affinities. The rate and extent of distribution vary according to physical properties of the drug. Distribution (α phase) occurs predominantly by diffusion, usually rapidly, and if the rate varies with uremia it is likely to be faster because of increased capillary permeability. The distribution space of a drug is calculated as the amount of drug in the body at steady state divided by the steady state plasma concentration. After distribution equilibrium the plasma concentration decreases as a function of the elimination rate. The plasma concentration that would occur at the moment of bolus injection, if distribution equilibrium occurred instantaneously, can be back calculated from the elimination half-life. This concentration can be used in the equation:

$$V = \frac{I}{p}$$

(volume equals quantity administered, divided by plasma concentration at time zero)

to determine distribution volume. For unbound water soluble solutes, the distribution space may approximate extracellular fluid volume or total body water. Plasma protein binding decreases the apparent volume of distribution, whereas tissue protein binding increases it. Lipid soluble solutes often have high apparent volumes of distribution due to sequestration in tissues, including body fat (Figure 1).

By knowing the distribution volume of a given drug, its clearance can be related to this volume. Even if the clearance is a high absolute value, should it be a low fraction of the distribution volume the plasma concentration will decline slowly. For example, chlorpromazine clearance is 600 ml/min but the distribution volume exceeds 1400 l, so the half-life is about 30 h. Similarly, a large distribution volume limits removal by dialysis (28).

The removal rate by dialysis may be so rapid that it exceeds the intercompartmental transfer rate clearing only a small volume (29). This results in a transient rapid decline in the plasma concentration followed by an increment as equilibrium is slowly reestablished (30).

For many drugs both pharmacologic and toxic effects correlate with the concentration at the site of action. This site can be the interstitial fluid at the cell surface and the concentration usually equals that in plasma water. Yet because many drugs circulate bound to plasma or tissue proteins or both, the plasma water concentrations are lower than those of plasma or tissues (Figure 1).

Protein binding

A portion of most drugs normally binds to albumin or other plasma proteins. Such protein binding limits the concentration in the compartments that induce pharmacologic and toxic effects and ordinarily restricts the quantity available for elimination (Figure 1). In general, the more protein binding and the larger the distribution space of a drug, the lower is the plasma water concentration for a given quantity administered, but the pharmacologic effect is longer because the large reservoir outside of plasma water prolongs the elimination.

Decreased plasma protein binding of many drugs occurs in uremia (13, 20, 24, 28, 31–33) as listed in Table 1. The decrease in binding increases the fraction filtered so the removal rate may not decrease as rapidly as the decline in renal function. For drugs that are eliminated by extrarenal routes, such as phenytoin and diazepam, a greater fraction of free drug is delivered, for example to the liver, so the removal rate is faster than normal. Removal by hemodialysis is less impeded when protein binding is lower (28) so dialyzer clearances may be higher than in normal subjects. The distribution space increases when plasma protein binding is impaired and after a single dose, therapeutic and toxic effects may be greater than normal because of the higher plasma water concentration.

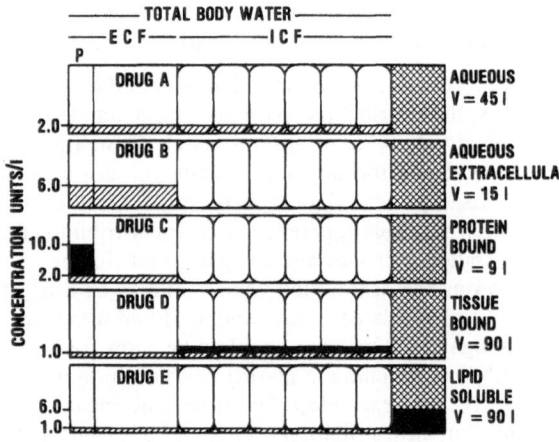

TYPES OF DISTRIBUTION AFTER INFUSION
(NET OF 90 UNITS TO 75 kg MAN)

Figure 1. Net infusion of the same quantity of different solutes yields different plasma concentrations because solutes distribute differently. A) total body water distribution, unbound; B) extracellular, unbound; C) extracellular with plasma protein binding; D) total body water with tissue protein binding; E) preferential distribution in body fat.

The decrease in protein binding is due, at least in part, to competition for the binding site by one or more retained metabolites. A major binding inhibitor is dialyzable, water soluble, heat stable, can be extracted in acid pH by organic solvents or by charcoal, and has been characterized as a propanoic acid derivative (34–37). Yet, the decreased binding of phenytoin does not correct with extensive *in vivo* dialysis, suggesting that a change in protein composition also occurs in uremia (38). During hemodialysis heparin releases

Table 1. Renal failure decreases protein binding of these drugs.

1. Cephalosporins	5. Penicillins
Cefazolin	Cloxacillin
Cefotixin	Dicloxacillin
Cephalexin	Nafcillin
Cephalothin	Penicillin G
2. Cardiac glycosides	6. Clofibrate
Digoxin	7. Diazepam
Digitoxin	8. Diazoxide
3. Sulfonamides	9. Doxycycline
Sulfadiazine	10. Furosemide
Sulfamethazole	11. Hippurate
Sulfamethoxazole	12. Insulin
Sulfisoxazole	13. Morphine
4. Barbiturates	14. Phenylbutazone
Amobarbital	15. Phenytoin
Pentobarbital	16. Salicylates
Thiopental	17. Thyroxine
	18. Triamterene
	19. Valproic acid
	20. Warfarin

free fatty acids which impede the binding of drugs to albumin.

In the case of digoxin, tissue protein binding decreases in uremia, which reduces the distribution space considerably (39). Because the distribution space is smaller, the plasma half-life would be expected to be shorter. Because the dominant mechanism of elimination, renal clearance, is more markedly decreased the half-life is increased, nevertheless (40).

Elimination rate

The elimination rate (mass per unit time) is usually corrected for plasma concentration and expressed as clearance. The plasma (drug) clearance is the sum of all mechanisms of elimination and is expressed as volume/time, customarily milliliters/minute, but sometimes as liters/hour/kilogram. Solutes may be eliminated by a single route or concurrently by several routes. If the plasma clearance is predominantly renal, the dose of the drug in question must be reduced considerably when severe renal failure develops.

When the plasma clearance per unit time is a high fraction of the distribution volume, the plasma concentration declines rapidly. Conversely, with a low fractional clearance due either to a low absolute clearance or a high volume of distribution, the plasma level will decline slowly. Since the rate of decline of the plasma concentration correlates directly with the plasma clearance, any slowing of this decline in uremic patients will be mostly determined by the fractional decrease in total clearance that results from renal failure. Conversely, the additional clearance by dialysis considered as a fraction of the total clearance rather than as an absolute value defines the augmentation attributed to dialysis.

Half-life

The biologic half-life is the time interval required to eliminate half of the body burden or of the administered dose of a drug. It can be expressed by the formula:

$$T\,1/2 = \frac{0.693}{r}$$

where r is the elimination rate. Under steady state conditions, e.g. at cessation of a continuous infusion that has reached equilibrium, the biologic half-life equals the interval required for the plasma concentration to decrease by 50%. After a single bolus dose, however, disappearance from plasma is determined by a combination of distribution and elimination. During the distributive (α) phase the plasma concentration declines faster than the true elimination half-life (Figure 2), so the elimination half-life (β) can only be determined in the post distributive phase. The plasma half-life is an easily determined, popularly used, and conveniently obtained variable that is related to the elimination rate by

$$T\,1/2 = \frac{0.693 \times V}{C}$$

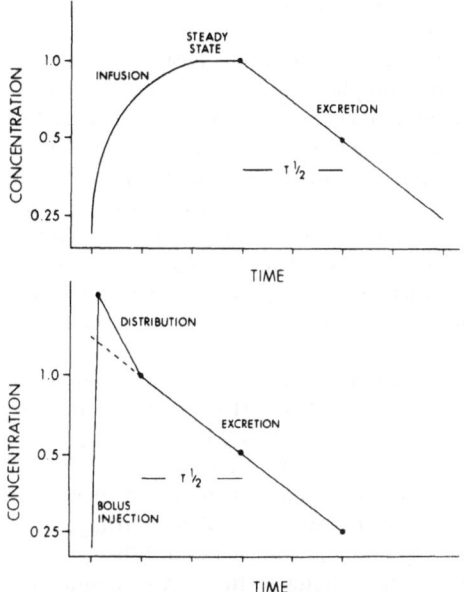

Figure 2. Plasma concentrations achieve steady state equilibrium during continuous infusion (upper half). Infused solute (minus that excreted) divided by steady state concentration equals distribution. After cessation of the infusion, plasma concentrations decrease exponentially. Plasma levels decrease by 50% in the interval, $T^{1}/_{2}$. With rapid ('bolus') injection, plasma levels are higher and decline more rapidly until the solute has distributed and then decrease exponentially. The plasma concentration projected to time zero can be used to estimate solute distribution.

where V is the apparent volume of distribution and C is the plasma clearance.

By this formula, it can be appreciated that the half-life increases, i.e. drugs persist in plasma, as clearance decreases. The extent of prolongation of the half-life in renal failure is a good guideline for the necessary lengthening of the dosing interval for such patients.

Mechanisms of drug elimination

Drugs may be excreted unchanged by the kidney, skin or

Table 2. Drugs with active metabolites.

Drug	Metabolite	Effect
Acetohexamide	1-OH hexamide	Hypoglycemia
Adriamycin	Adriamycinol	Tumor lysis
Allopurinol	Oxypurinol	Nephrolithiasis
Daunorubicin	Daunorubicinol	Tumor lysis
Clofibrate	Cl-phenoxyisobutyric acid	Rhabdomyolysis
Diazepam	Oxazepam	Encephalopathy
Flurazepam	Dexalkylflurazepam	Encephalopathy
Meperidine	Normeperidine	Convulsions
Succinylcholine	Succinylmonocholine	Paralysis

bowel, or if volatile, by the lung. Many drugs are lipid soluble allowing their penetration into cells. This increases the distribution space, decreasing the fraction in circulation and limiting the quantity available for excretion by mechanisms involving ultrafiltration or diffusion which effectively eliminate water soluble compounds. Biotransformation in tissues such as the liver promotes elimination of many compounds. Metabolic processes that biotransform drugs are oxidations, reductions, hydrolyses, acetylations and conjugations such as esterifications, e.g. with sulfate or synthesis of a glycine or glucuronide compound. Such biotransformed compounds are usually more water soluble and thus readily excreted by the kidney. Their pharmacologic activity or toxicity may be more pronounced, the same, less or nonexistent. Examples of drugs with active metabolites (24) are shown in Table 2. Renal failure often causes retention of such drug metabolites and biotransformation may be decreased, unchanged or even increased in uremia (1).

Renal handling of drugs

Renal elimination of drugs may occur by several possible mechanisms (41). A few substances such as mannitol or iothalamate are only filtered by the glomerulus and are neither secreted nor reabsorbed, and not synthesized or degraded. Their renal clearance equals that of inulin and closely approximates glomerular filtration rate under all circumstances. Renal handling of most drugs has not been thoroughly studied, however, and cannot be assumed to equal the filtration rate. Some high molecular weight solutes such as insulin, glucagon and other hormones are removed by the kidney by molecular biotransformation during the reabsorptive process after filtration. When glomerular filtration rate declines, the rate of such removal decreases (42–44). The excretion of such drugs as salicylates involves combined glomerular filtration and passive tubular reabsorption. With nephron loss, fractional reabsorption may decrease so that the drug clearance decreases less than glomerular filtration does, and renal cortical accumulation may be less than anticipated from the reduced elimination. Passive reabsorption may involve simple diffusion gradients as exemplified by urea. Reabsorption by nonionic diffusion also may occur as a function of pH since ionized solutes are poorly reabsorbed unlike the unionized fraction. Excretion of passively reabsorbed solutes is also flow dependent, correlating with urinary volume as well as glomerular filtration rate. Active transport is the mechanism whereby such drugs as mercurials and bromide are reabsorbed. Their excretion is maintained despite marked reduction in glomerular filtration as fractional reabsorption decreases. The renal tubule also actively secretes many drugs, such as penicillins and cephalosporins. This is the major mechanism of renal excretion of highly protein bound, poorly filterable solutes. With those drugs for which maximal tubular transport considerably exceeds that at therapeutic concentrations, nephron loss and decreased glomerular filtration may correlate poorly with the excretory rate, which is limited mostly by the renal blood flow rate. Whenever possible, the drug clearance should be determined rather than assumed to be a constant fraction of the residual glomerular filtration rate.

Metabolic effects of drugs

Whether eliminated normally or not, certain drugs have important metabolic effects. These may result from the drug composition itself. For example, the magnesium content of antacids may accumulate causing hypermagnesemic coma. A metabolic product of a drug may cause complications such as paraldehyde-induced acidoses. An effect on metabolism, such as the antianabolic effect of tetracyclines, may aggravate azotemia. Anionic drug salts such as the penicillins can affect mineral and acid base balance by renal excretion of the nonreabsorbable anion or alternatively by metabolism of the anion. An influence on a hormonal or renal mechanism, e.g. controlling water elimination, may result from drugs such as lithium or chlorpropamide. Table 3 lists some drugs with important metabolic effects.

End organ alterations

Because renal failure has important effects on the sites of therapeutic or toxic action, alterations in end organ response to drugs may occur. For drugs that affect the urinary tract, two modified responses occur. With a decreased nephron mass, the response to diuretics will be quantitatively less at any given dose although the fractional change in salt and water excretion may be higher than occurs in health. Limited responsiveness can lead to the use of higher doses, increasing the incidence of toxicity (45). Decreased excretion of certain antibiotics not only leads to higher plasma concentrations but also lower urinary concentrations, with which therapeutic response of urinary infection correlates (46).

Table 3. Examples of drug-induced metabolic abnormalities.

Hyperkalemia: Salt substitutes, Penicillin G, Spironolactone, Triamterene, Mannitol

Hypermagnesemia: Antacids, Laxatives

Hypercalcemia: Antibiotics, Thiazides, Hydroxylated vitamin D

High sodium load: Kayexalate, Carbenicillin, Ampicillin, Cephalothin

Azotemia: Ammonium chloride, Urethane, Tetracyclines, Adrenal corticosteroids

Acidosis: Phenformin, Paraldehyde, Nitrofurantoin, Methenamine mandelate, Ammonium chloride, Acetazolamide, Isoniazid

Alkalosis: Absorbable antacids, Carbenicillin, Large doses of penicillin G, Viomycin

Water retention: Acetaminophen, Barbiturates, Chlorpropamide, Clofibrate, Cyclophosphamide, Indomethacin, Morphine, Phenylbutazone, Vincristine

Water loss: Demeclocycline, Lithium, Fluoride anesthetics

Nephrotic syndrome: Oxazoladines, Heavy metals, Captopril, Chelates, Probenecid, Tolbutamide, Nonsteroidal anti-inflammatory drugs

---

Hence, these drugs may achieve toxicity without therapeutic effectiveness.

Uremic gastritis can contribute to the frequency of nausea and vomiting complicating therapy in uremic patients (18). The high ammonia content of uremic gastrointestinal fluid secondary to degradation of increased lumenal urea will be reduced as bacterial urease decreases with antibiotic therapy. This lowers gastric pH and thereby can affect drug absorption and induce peptic ulcers. In selected renal failure patients, antacid therapy may be required during antibiotic treatment. Increased susceptibility to peptic ulceration may relate more to other factors such as high concentrations of gastrin in uremic patients, however. These factors that affect the gastric mucosa increase the possibility of drug-induced gastrointestinal hemorrhage in uremic patients when drugs such as salicylates are used.

The high incidence of dermal drug reactions in renal failure may be misinterpreted as uremic dermatitis and frequently leads to excoriation and hemorrhage as pruritus accompanying uremia is exaggerated. Whether trace metal accumulation contributes to the greyish dermal discoloration that some dialyzed patients acquire is uncertain.

Myocardial irritability in uremic patients (47) is often aggravated by direct action of drugs like digitalis. Acute increases in plasma ionized calcium or potassium depletion complicating laxative or diuretic therapy may augment this risk.

Central nervous system depressants may cause or aggravate lethargy or coma in uremic patients not only because of drug accumulation but also because of increased susceptibility. Thiopental anesthesia, the short duration of which is because this lipid soluble barbiturate promptly distributes out of plasma into body fat, is prolonged in renal failure (48). Because urea facilitates the transport of dyes into the central nervous system, it may be anticipated that drug narcosis may be exaggerated in uremic patients. The demonstrated alteration in the blood cerebrospinal fluid barrier in uremic patients (49) may also contribute to higher cerebral concentrations of drugs or toxins that can cause central nervous system depression, easily misinterpreted as uremia.

ADVERSE EFFECTS OF DRUGS ON THE KIDNEY

Nephrotoxicity, a clinically important problem of remarkably high frequency, is a particular hazard for patients with preexisting renal disease (50–53). Careful drug surveillance and prevention of superimposed nephrotoxicity may delay the progression of chronic renal failure. Increased vulnerability of the kidney to toxins (relative to other organs) relates to the high renal blood flow rate and oxygen consumption, considerable enzyme activity, the large epithelial surface area, tubular transcellular transport mechanisms that often involve uncoupling of toxins from protein ligands and the interstitial and intratubular concentration gradients established by the countercurrent multiplication system (5).

Direct tubular damage may occur from heavy metals, for example from retention of bismuth, mercurial, antimony, platinum or iron compounds used therapeutically. When organic mercurial excretion is decreased because of preexisting renal disease, increased metabolic conversion to inorganic toxic products occurs potentially aggravating renal failure. Toxic tubular injury now most frequently occurs as a complication of antibiotic therapy, notably with the aminoglycosides. Other important classes of drugs causing nephrotoxicity are the organic iodides, hemolysins such as quinine and pigment producers such as phenazopyridine. Decrements in renal function may be irreversible and misinterpreted as progression of the underlying disease. Tubular injury from gold or mercury may chronically release renal tubular epithelial cell antigens, an immunologic reaction to which causes membranous nephropathy.

The papillary necrosis that follows prolonged ingestion of high doses of mixed analgesics (54) relates to accumulation of the phenacetin metabolite, N-acetyl-p-aminophenol, in the renal medulla and papilla. This leads to oxidant injury aggravated by salicylate induced uncoupling of oxidative phosphorylation and inhibition of prostaglandin synthetase. Renal function continues to deteriorate as abusive analgesic intake persists and may stabilize or improve with cessation of ingestion (55). Even after advanced irreversible disease has occurred, analgesic abuse should be avoided because of the risk of uroepithelial malignancy (56).

Acute hypersensitivity interstitial nephritis is often preceded by exposure to drugs including penicillins, sulfonamides, cephalosporins, phenytoin, cimetidine, phenedione, polymyxin, rifampin, allopurinol, phenylbutazone, furosemide and nonsteroidal anti-inflammatory agents (57–59). Nephrotic syndrome may occur with hypersensitivity to the oxazolidine anticonvulsants, chelates, nonsteroidal anti-inflammatory drugs, captopril, or probenicid. Less frequently, drug hypersensitivity causes an acute renal angiitis or glomerulonephritis.

Obstructive uropathy may result from precipitation of a drug such as methotrexate or sulfonamide crystals, from a metabolite such as oxalate derived from methoxyflurane, or from drug induced uricosuria. Methysergide therapy of migraine headaches may be complicated by retroperitoneal fibrosis causing periureteral obstruction. Alternatively, drugs may lead to interstitial calcification in the kidney as exemplified by the milk alkali syndrome and hypervitaminosis D.

Indirect mechanisms potentially causing nephrotoxicity are the hemodynamic effects of hypotension for example, complicating antihypertensive drugs or extracellular fluid depletion due to diuretic or laxative excess. Similarly, drug-induced potassium depletion may cause tubular injury. A precipitous fall in renal blood flow can occur when prostaglandin synthetase is inhibited by such drugs as aspirin or indomethacin in patients that depend on prostaglandin medicated vasodilation to offset vasoconstrictor effects of angiotensin or catecholamines (60).

The importance of nephrotoxicity in patients with preexisting renal disease is magnified by a potentially higher incidence as human exposure to an array of biologically active compounds increases. Radiation nephritis is another byproduct of scientific progress. Some forms of nephrotoxicity can be prevented by quantitatively decreasing or eliminating exposure. Further, toxin removal can reverse many functional and histologic abnormalities. Hence, correction of toxic nephropathy may delay or obviate the need of renal replacement therapy or may allow easier management of advanced renal failure by preserving some residual function.

DRUG-DIALYSIS INTERACTIONS

The interactions of drugs and dialysis include depletion of therapeutic concentrations when dialysis is undertaken for such purposes as therapy of renal failure, therapeutic removal of drug excess by dialysis, effects of drugs on dialysis kinetics and effects of dialysis induced metabolic alterations on pharmacologic activity. There are marked differences between the removal rates of drugs by hemodialysis, hemofiltration, hemoperfusion and peritoneal dialysis. Moreover, the elimination rate varies according to the species of hemodialyzer, the membrane permeability and the flow rates achieved (61, 62).

Determinants of dialyzer clearances

During dialysis, solutes are removed from blood by diffusion through the semipermeable dialysis membrane along chemical concentration gradients. The removal process, customarily expressed as a clearance, varies inversely with the square root of molecular size or approximately of molecular weight (63). Because the molecular size of drugs varies, so does the clearance for any species of dialyzer. Hence, clearance must be measured or at least predicted based on the known physical properties of the drug. The relation of dialyzer clearance to molecular weight is illustrated in Figure 3. As molecular size increases, the resistance to diffusive transport of solutes contributed by the dialysate becomes less important and membrane resistance becomes the more important impediment to diffusive transport (64). Newer more permeable membranes and improved blood flow geometry with thinner blood films increase clearances of high molecular weight drugs. Further, ultrafiltration does not discriminate according to molecular size until membrane permeability limits are reached. Thus, ultrafiltration becomes a mechanism for solute removal of increasing importance as solute size increases (65). Hemofiltration achieves high clearances of high molecular weight drugs. The kinetics of drug removal by dialysis and the determinants thereof have been reviewed recently (4, 11, 62, 66, 67).

In vitro dialyzer clearance measurements often translate poorly into the transport characteristics during clinical dialysis. Solute diffusion and filtration occur from plasma water. Accordingly, protein binding limits solute transport unless equilibrium is rapid between the free and bound moieties (Figure 4). *In vitro* studies using plasma as the perfusate offsets this error somewhat. The use of blood flow rates in clearance calculations assumes that plasma concentrations equal whole blood concentrations and that diffusion from cells occurs readily during dialysis. These assumptions have not been proved for most solutes and the evidence favors

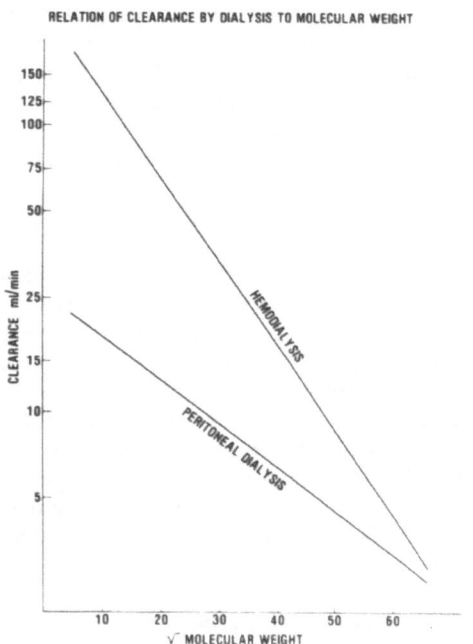

RELATION OF CLEARANCE BY DIALYSIS TO MOLECULAR WEIGHT

Figure 3. Clearance by hemodialysis or peritoneal dialysis is illustrated as inversely proportional to the square root of solute molecular weight.

diffusion, predominantly from plasma water during extracorporeal transit (68). It is customary to measure the extraction rate of a solute from plasma and factor that value by the flow rate of whole blood through the dialyzer. The error in such a calculation (69) is not as critical with most pertinent endogenous metabolites as it is with drugs. The validity of the clearances can be verified by measuring the quantity recovered in the dialysate and dividing it by the plasma concentration. Increased protein concentration and hematocrit also affect viscosity and therefore hydrostatic pressure and ultrafiltration rates, but decrease the water fraction of plasma or of whole blood. Protein-solute binding is highly dependent on plasma protein concentrations and solute concentration and cannot be regarded as a constant fraction when these parameters vary or when heparin affects free fatty acid concentrations. While a metal such as tin is bound far below saturation at physiologic concentrations, remaining almost completely protein bound despite a three-fold decrease in protein concentration or a one-hundred-fold increase in tin concentration (70), solutes such as iodide demonstrate saturation of the binding at low concentrations. Accordingly, the plasma clearance increases as iodide concentration increases (71). Toxic concentrations of many drugs will have lower fractional protein binding and thus higher clearances than those measured at therapeutic levels. The dialyzer clearance of several barbiturates correlates inversely with the fractional protein binding (Figure 5), while slight variations in molecular weight do not noticeably

EFFECT OF PROTEIN BINDING AND HEMATOCRIT ON DIALYZER SOLUTE CLEARANCE

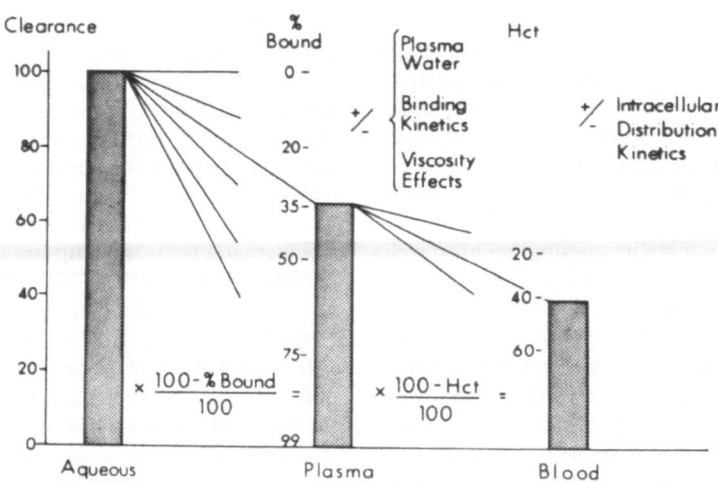

Figure 4. Compared to dialyzer clearances, *in vitro* (aqueous) clearances during clinical dialysis are lower because of protein binding and red blood cells limiting solute delivery to the membrane. (Reprinted from Maher (73) with permission).

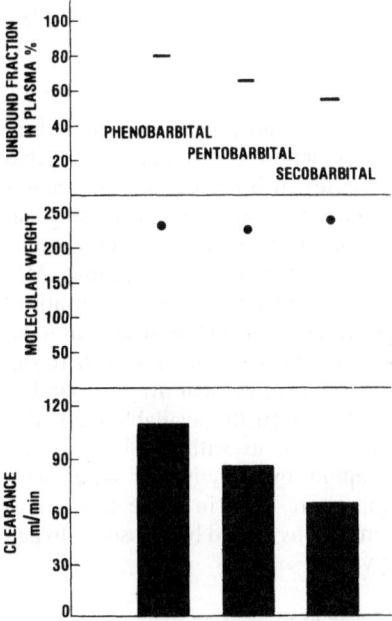

PROTEIN BINDING DECREASES DIALYZER CLEARANCE

Figure 5. The clearance of three barbiturates differs not because of differing molecular weights, but because of varying degrees of protein binding.

affect clearance (72). The low peritoneal clearance of digoxin is also explained in part by protein binding. Corrected to plasma water concentration, the removal rate is more appropriate for the molecular size (73). For highly bound solutes influx during dialysis may proceed at a high rate while efflux is impeded (63, 70).

As a general guideline, those solutes that are excreted by glomerular filtration will have high dialyzer clearances. However, renal elimination often interposes tubular transport, after ultrafiltration and therefore does not necessarily correlate with dialyzer clearance. For example, the dialyzer rapidly clears bromide but slowly clears phenolsulfophthalein, a large, slowly diffusible solute. In contrast, the renal tubule reabsorbs bromide almost completely, but renal excretion of phenolsulfophthalein is rapid because of tubular secretion. When measurements are not available, hemodialyzer clearance can be very crudely estimated by dividing the molecular weight into 12,000 ml/min and multiplying the product by the unbound fraction of the drug. With intermittent peritoneal dialysis the clearance will be about 12% that of hemodialysis, but somewhat higher for larger solutes because of the higher permeability of the peritoneum (63). Clearances of drugs by continuous ambulatory peritoneal dialysis are predictably low because of the low dialysate flow rate (74). Except for aminoglycosides and a few other drugs these low clearances do not affect appreciably the elimination kinetics even in patients with renal failure (74–76).

Influence of dialysis on half-life

Clearance is simply a removal rate corrected for the plasma concentration. To assess the effect of dialysis on the biologic half-life of a drug the dialyzer clearance must be considered in relation to the distribution volume. At any given clearance the half-life will correlate directly with the distribution volume. Because endogenous clearance of plasma continues during dialysis the effect of dialysis on total plasma clearance must also be assessed. Provided that intercompartmental transfer is sufficiently rapid that concentration disequilibrium does not occur, i.e. the distribution space remains constant during dialysis, and that dialysis does not affect the endogenous clearance by renal and extrarenal routes, the fractional increment in clearance should predict the change in half-life. For example, doubling the total body clearance decreases the half-life by 50%. Drugs and toxins have been considered dialyzable if the procedure removes a high fraction of the body burden of a drug in a reasonable period of time, but poorly dialyzable if a low fraction (14, 66). Such guidelines are helpful but by ignoring the concurrent endogenous clearance may overestimate or underestimate the contribution of dialysis. For example, hemodialysis adds considerably to the removal rate and significantly decreases the half-life of the slowly metabolized methanol but it changes the declining plasma concentration slope of the rapidly metabolized ethanol only slightly despite comparable dialyzer clearance (77). By contrast, a low dialyzer clearance may add considerably to the physiologic removal rate under conditions that impede the normal mechanism of elimination. For example, dialyzer removal of aminoglycosides from the anuric patient exceeds considerably the plasma clearance, but the same removal rate adds little when renal function is normal.

In relating dialyzer clearance to the physiologic clearance the effect of the drug itself on its own elimination must be considered. Comparisons of the half-life during shock and dialysis with the half-life data obtained on healthy subjects exposed to low drug concentrations may be meaningless. Similarly, dialyzer removal rates of toxins from uremic patients should not be compared to physiologic data from normals. To illustrate, the plasma half-life of glutethimide in intoxicated patients is prolonged with shock. It also increases as the plasma concentration increases, independent of changes in blood pressure, consistent with a rate limited metabolic degradation (78). Dialysis adds less to the relatively rapid removal rate at low plasma concentrations than to the slower removal rate at high levels because dialyzer clearance is not concentration dependent, unlike metabolic clearance. Clearances of some solutes may be higher in uremic patients than those achieved in normals because of decreased protein binding and because anemia increases the fraction of plasma in the extracorporeal circulation.

Dialyzer clearances must also be related to those achieved by other therapeutic modalities. Dialysis may be required to improve the half-life and clinical course of severely barbiturate intoxicated patients with circulatory insufficiency, or with advanced renal failure unresponsive to forced diuresis in contrast to those mildly intoxicated (79). Similarly, the high dialyzer clearance of bromide may be an unnecessary addition to the removal rate of intoxicated, otherwise normal, subjects (80), whereas those unresponsive to diuretics or intolerant of salt loading as occurs with heart failure or end stage renal disease, have a prolonged predialysis half-life that improves considerably with dialysis.

The distribution volume of a solute is a determinant of the fraction of the body burden removed by dialysis. For solutes such as digoxin, propoxyphene or glutethimide, the distribution space is very large due to such factors as tissue binding or a high lipid partition coefficient. Although the dialyzer clearance may be high, the low fraction of body digoxin in plasma means that little is presented to the dialysis membrane. Unless plasma and tissue stores rapidly equilibrate, it is fallacious to expect that enhanced removal, by using lipid or protein in the dialysate or by charcoal or resin hemoperfusion, will change materially the removal from tissue reservoirs. Even a rapidly diffusible solute like bromide can be removed from plasma faster than equilibration occurs with such extravascular pools as cerebrospinal fluid (81). Clinical drug effects correlate with concentrations in a particular extravascular compartment. This concentration will bear a constant relationship with plasma concentrations, except after an acute load is administered or after a process of rapid elimination is initiated. If distribution into plasma keeps pace with the removal rate, the plasma concentration will continue to reflect pharmacologic or toxic manifestations. When equilibration does not keep pace, the plasma concentration decreases rapidly during the procedure, suggesting therapeutic success. But the clinical response may be less than anticipated and an inappropriately small distribution volume is estimated (30) using either the formula

amount removed/delta plasma concentration

or

plasma clearance × half-life/0.693.

A secondary rebound increment in the plasma concentration will occur because the decrement in the concentration within the extravascular space was smaller. Under this circumstance an accurate half-life cannot be calculated from clearance data because the volume cleared cannot be determined precisely.

Dialysis has been criticized as a therapeutic modality for some intoxications, because the quantity removed is a small fraction of the dose ingested and presumably absorbed and thus of the body burden. It is assumed that the entire body burden of the drug is pharmacologically active. There are examples to the contrary, however, such as thiopental, the pharmacologic and toxic actions of which correlate with plasma, rather than body fat concentration (82). Such reasoning would also incorrectly argue that therapeutic removal of potassium expressed as a fraction of total body potassium is low and could not improve potassium intoxication clinically, contradicting the obvious clinical experience. In which space does the drug concentration determine therapeutic and toxic effects? For most drugs the answer is unknown.

In the final analysis, the most important parameter by which to judge the effect of dialytic removal of a drug may be the clinical response, often difficult to quantify accurately.

Depletion by dialysis

When patients undergo repetitive dialysis for therapy of renal failure, depletion of drugs such as antibiotics and of physiologic solutes such as vitamins and amino acids may occur requiring repletion (83). Drug assay methods may have insufficient sensitivity to detect therapeutic concentrations as accurately as toxic concentrations. Moreover, the clinical considerations for determining insufficient therapy are often less accurate than clinical signs of toxicity. Depletion of water soluble vitamins has been recognized (84), however, and removal of such drugs as antibiotics is well documented. Based on the available data, the drugs frequently used in patients with renal failure and removed sufficiently rapidly by dialysis that supplemental therapy may be required are listed in Table 4. Whenever possible serum concentrations should be measured to guide replacement therapy.

Metabolic effects of dialysis on drug action

Dialysis may affect profoundly the pharmacologic activity of a drug despite changing the serum concentration only slightly. The frequently recognized and extensively studied example of this effect is the precipitation or aggravation of digitalis intoxication as dialysis corrects hyperkalemia, hypocalcemia, hyponatremia and acidosis. Whether metabolic alterations of dialysis affect the activity of other drugs is largely unknown. Changes in osmolality, pH, protein, urea or glucose concentrations can influence pharmacologic activity. Because there are many drug interactions, lowering the concentration of one drug can affect the action of another poorly dialyzable drug. For example, decreasing qui-

Table 4. Drugs that usually require supplemental doses post dialysis.

Aminoglycosides: Amikacin, Gentamicin, Kanamycin, Netilmicin, Streptomycin, Tobramycin
Cephalosporins: Cephacetrile, Cefadroxil, Cefamandole, Cefazolin, Cefotixin, Cefuroxime, Cephalexin, Cephalothin, Cephradine, Ceforanide, Cefroxadine, Cefsulodin, Ceftazole, Ceftazedine, Moxalactam
Penicillins: Amoxicillin, Ampicillin, Azlocillin, Carbenicillin, Penicillin G, Ticarcillin
Other antibiotics: Chloramphenicol, Cycloserine, Ethambutol, Flucytosine, Fosfomycin, Isoniazid, Sulfonamides, Trimethoprim
Vasoactive drugs: Theophylline, Methyldopa, Procainamde, Quinidine, Atenolol
Immunosuppressive drugs: Azathioprine, Cyclophosphamide, 5-fluorouracil, Methylprednisolone
Vitamins: Ascorbic acid, Folic acid, Pyridoxine, Thiamin
Miscellaneous: Salicylates, Barbital, Phenobarbital, Lithium

nidine concentrations by dialysis may affect digoxin concentrations and pharmacodynamics. Moreover, improvement by dialysis of such lesions as uremic colitis may decrease the toxicity that ensues from a given excess of a specific drug.

Reverse dialysis and factors affecting unidirectional flux

Transport by diffusion during dialysis should occur at the same rate from plasma water to dialysate as in the opposite direction. Ultrafiltration, a more important transport mechanism for larger than for smaller solutes, will increase net flux in the direction of filtration. As the unidirectional flux is a function of concentration gradients, solutes added to or contaminating dialysate may manifest higher influx than efflux, if protein bound in plasma. Rapid binding of solutes to plasma proteins decreases plasma water concentrations, maintaining influx gradients, while measured efflux from plasma is decreased by protein binding. Preferential distribution into tissue, if rapid, also maintains influx gradients, whereas slow equilibration with a tissue pool limits efflux as well as decreasing more rapidly the influx gradient. The binding of trace metals and drugs to hemodialysis membranes (85, 86) can favor inward transport, contribute to solute removal and create errors in calculations of transport kinetics. Special considerations apply to peritoneal dialysis, although inward transport also exceeds efflux for bound drugs and back diffusion must be taken into account for accurate calculations (87). Solutes can accumulate in dialysate not only from plasma water but also from adjacent tissue as exemplified by fatty acids which are generated locally and enter peritoneal fluid directly, rather than via circulating blood (88). Moreover, because hepatic clearance rates may exceed absorptive rates from the peritoneum, it is possible to add locally drugs with potential systemic toxicity without achieving measurable systemic concentrations (89).

Hemofiltration

Hemofiltration has been developed as an alternative to treat uremia (90), and because simultaneous filtration-dialysis is often poorly tolerated hemodynamically, sequential filtration-dialysis has been introduced as a procedural variant (91). Unlike dialysis, the transport by hemofiltration does not discriminate by molecular size (until sieving occurs). Hence, the clearances of larger solutes can be much higher than occurs with hemodialysis. The considerable loss of large peptide hormones by hemofiltration (92) attests to this. Despite little study of pharmacokinetics during hemofiltration, clearances are predictable. With the post-dilution technique clearance should approximate the rate of ultrafiltration multiplied by the unbound fraction in plasma for all but the largest of drugs, e.g. vancomycin, which may be sieved somewhat. Predilution may allow some diffusion of drugs from erythrocytes or transfer from plasma protein to plasma water, so the clearance may be slightly higher than half the ultrafiltration rate corrected for binding.

Hemoperfusion

Cleansing of blood by direct perfusion through columns of sorbents or exchange resins has gained considerable popularity for removal of drugs and poisons (93–96). Because of direct contact of plasma with the sorbent (except for an ultrathin highly porous coating), extraction rates and consequently clearances are very high. Often the sorbent has a higher binding affinity for a drug than plasma proteins do, so the clearance of many drugs approaches the blood or plasma flow rate despite protein binding. As hemoperfusion proceeds, however, the sorbent approaches saturation and the extraction rate declines. Nevertheless, hemoperfusion removes many protein bound drugs rapidly. Despite the high clearance, the clinical results may not be favorable and the mortality may remain high because of the large distribution spaces and the low intercompartmental transfer rates, tissue binding and delays in initiating treatment (95, 97). Despite such limitations it is prudent to be aware of the capability of this technique to remove poisons and drugs. Amberlite resin perfusion removes lipid soluble nonpolar drugs better than polar compounds, and charcoal perfusion clears each type of drug equally well (98).

Another technique of detoxification recently described is an on-line plasma separator in which plasma perfuses a device wherein toxins diffuse into a channel containing cofactors and enzymes and detoxified solutes then diffuse back into circulation (99). Because uremia is characterized by a nondialyzable inhibitor of the enzyme thiopurine-methyltransferase (100), which is involved in the metabolism of 6-mercaptopurine, azathiprine and 6-thioguanine, such a system could be useful in selected uremic patients should they become so intoxicated.

Peritoneal dialysis

It is naive to consider the peritoneum inert like hemodialysis membranes. Although solute removal occurs predominantly by diffusion along electrochemical gradients, as with extracorporeal hemodialysis, there are many important transport differences (101–103). Convection contributes fractionally more to total mass transport, and membrane permeability is higher than with hemodialysis, so relatively higher transport rates of large solutes occur. Blood and dialysate flow rates are much lower than with hemodialysis, however. Diffusion equilibrium is not reached within an hour even for the smallest solutes, so predictably, maximal clearances are below the dialysate flow rate of 30 ml/min. Moreover, the diffusion barrier is living and its ionic charges restrict somewhat the passage of charged solutes. Lithium, phosphate and potassium transport rates are slower than predicted by solute size (63), and transport of cationic or anionic drugs such as penicillins should also be impeded. The diffusion barrier and the blood flow rate respond to pathologic, physiologic and pharmacologic influences. Numerous drugs, hormones and prostaglandins can alter transport kinetics both in patients with normal and abnormal vasculature (104). In general, transport can be augmented when certain drugs are instilled locally, selectively dilate the splanchnic vasculature or correct abnormal systemic hemodynamics (105, 106). Transport can also be augmented by increasing convection, by increasing the osmotic gradient (107), raising capillary hydrostatic pressure (108) or increasing the hydraulic permeability of the capillary, e.g. with secretin (109). Augmentation of the transport of specific drugs may be increased by adding appropriate agents such as chelates, albumin, tris buffer or lipid (104). In addition to the intentional use of drugs to accelerate transport, the physician must be aware that drugs used for other purposes can influence mesenteric blood flow and peritoneal transport rates. For example, the vasoconstrictor, norepinephrine, given intravenously significantly decreases peritoneal transport rates (108). In contrast, intravenous dopamine in high doses increases transport by virtue of adrenergic receptor-mediated somatic vasoconstriction, raising perfusion pressure, and dopaminergic receptor-mediated splanchnic vasodilation.

With continuous ambulatory peritoneal dialysis (CAPD), small solutes reach virtual concentration equilibrium between plasma and dialysate before the fluid is replaced (110). Since dialysate flow rate averages about 8 ml/min, clearances do not exceed that value. Except for the rare drug with a very low elimination rate, such low transfer rates during continuous peritoneal dialysis do not add significantly to the total plasma clearance.

MODIFICATION OF DRUG DOSAGE IN RENAL FAILURE

The margin of safety in therapeutics is the range between the effective dose or plasma concentration and the one that induces toxic reactions. For some drugs there is considerable latitude between these levels. For example, the dose of penicillin that results in neuromuscular toxicity may be as much as several hundred times the minimal effective dose. Unless massive dosage is used, for example to treat endocarditis, the dose calculation need not be precise. On the other hand, the cardiac glycosides have a narrow margin of safety. Unless the dosage is calculated carefully, plasma concentrations may be too low to achieve the desired effect or so high as to cause dose-related toxicity.

In adjusting dosage for patients with renal failure, usually the initial loading dose needs little or no reduction from the normal. A few notable exceptions include digoxin and morphine because of changes in distribution volume and sensitivity. After the initial dose achieves the peak plasma concentration, the plasma level decreases more slowly, i.e. the half-life is prolonged in proportion to the severity of renal failure as reflected by the increase in the plasma creatinine concentration or the decrease in glomerular filtration rate (Figure 6). It must be stressed that with renal failure the serum creatinine, when increasing, underestimates the severity of renal functional loss because it has not reached equilibrium concentration. The prolonged half-life means that the plasma concentration will be higher than usual when the next dose is due.

A marked reduction in dosage is required when the kid-

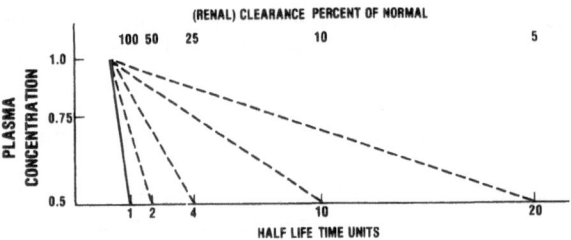

Figure 6. The half-life in time units (e.g. hours) increases as an inverse function of renal clearance expressed as percent of normal, so plasma concentrations decline more gradually.

ney is the only route of excretion of a drug and renal failure is severe. Obviously, the half-lives of those drugs eliminated predominantly by extrarenal routes are affected little by renal failure and intermediate effects result when elimination is partially renal (Figure 7). The fractional elimination by the kidney (the renal clearance as a fraction of total plasma clearance) determines the extent of dosage adjustment required in renal failure. This is the predominant basis whereby drugs are categorized as requiring little or no dosage modification in renal failure, modest adjustment or marked reduction.

Administration of the usual maintenance dose to a patient at the usual interval despite prolongation of half-life by renal failure results in accumulation of the drug in plasma, because the concentration is higher when the subsequent dose is added (Figure 8). The plasma concentration will eventually reach a level almost as many times higher than normal as the half-life is prolonged and the high equilibrium concentration will be approached after about five half-lives.

Therapeutic concentrations can be maintained by administering a lower dose at the usual interval or the usual dose at a prolonged interval. Because it is often difficult to fractionate the dose it is customary to increase the dosing interval. Moreover, it has been shown that fractionation of aminoglycoside dosage results in more toxicity than administering the same total maintenance dose at prolonged intervals (111). Nevertheless, prolongation of the dosing interval to longer than 48 h may allow concentrations to fall to suboptimal levels and remain so for too long a duration.

Obviously when renal failure is severe or when combined with hepatic failure, doses must be calculated most carefully. Unless clearance values for the specific drug are available, dosage reduction can be guided by the formula (112):

$$\text{Patient's dose} = \text{Normal dose} \times \frac{\text{FE } (C - 1) + 1}{1}$$

where FE is the fraction of the drug elimination normally contributed by renal excretion, and C is the patient's creatinine clearance as a fraction of the normal. The dosing interval may be calculated by the inverse equation:

EFFECT OF FRACTIONAL RENAL EXCRETION ON HALF LIFE IN RENAL FAILURE

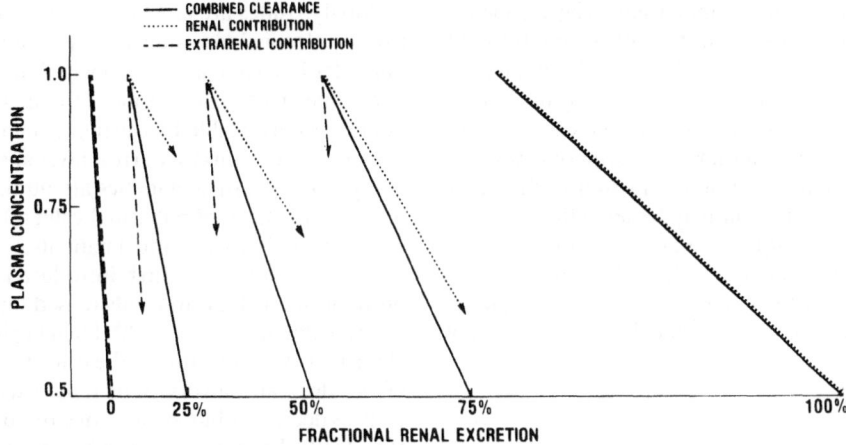

Figure 7. At any given level of impaired renal function, the rate of decrease of plasma concentration of a solute depends on the fraction eliminated by the kidney. When the renal contribution to total elimination is low, plasma concentrations may decrease rapidly despite renal failure provided that metabolic clearance is maintained. For solutes that depend mostly on renal excretion, elimination is very prolonged with renal failure.

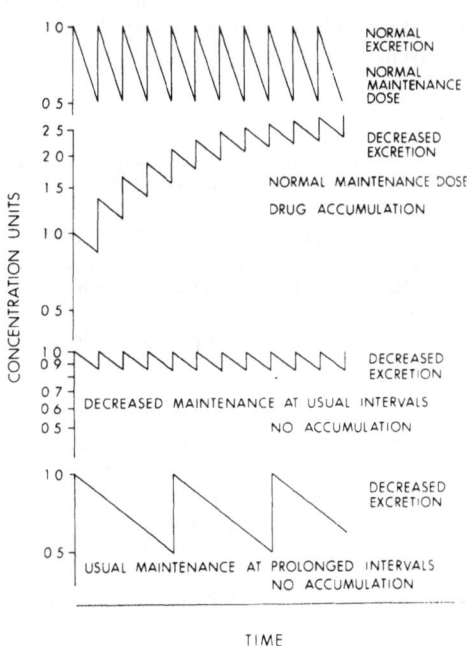

Figure 8. Repetitive administration of half the dose of a drug after half has been eliminated maintains appropriate concentrations. With slower elimination, the usual maintenance dose causes drug accumulation, while acceptable concentrations can be achieved with lower maintenance dosage or longer dosing intervals.

Patient's dosing interval =

$$\text{Normal interval} \times \frac{1}{\text{FE }(C - 1) + 1}$$

with a drug excreted 80% by the kidney and clearance reduced to 10% of normal, the dosing interval should be 1/0.8 (0.1–1) + 1 or 1/0.28 times the normal interval.

Because of the potential inaccuracies in dosage calculations, recommendations for drug therapy of patients with renal failure include (8):

1. Restrict drug use to definite indications.
2. If established, follow a previously determined regimen for renal failure dosage of a given drug.
3. A rough estimate of the proper dose may be calculated by formulae that use an assay of renal function factored by the renal contribution to normal elimination.

SPECIFIC DRUGS

Given these problems in the interpretation of interactions of drugs with dialyzers and with disturbances of normal pathways of elimination in renal failure and methods for calculating dosage adjustments, we can consider the available knowledge about specific compounds. The data can only provide guidelines; patient monitoring and clinical judgement must supersede nomograms and guidelines.

Antimicrobials

Nephrotoxicity has become a major complication of antibiotic therapy, particularly in patients with underlying renal insufficiency (5). Often, antibiotic nephrotoxicity is misinterpreted as infection or conversely is incriminated when hemodynamic effects of infection or pyelonephritis decrease renal function. In patients treated by dialysis, neurotoxicity, ototoxicity, hematological, cardiopulmonary, or gastrointestinal toxicity may be more important. The frequency, severity and mechanism of nephrotoxicity arising from different antibiotics varies considerably. Many have a narrow margin of safety and, since most are excreted by the kidney, their accumulation in renal failure can increase toxicity. Unfortunately, at any plasma level the urinary concentration is lower when renal function is impaired so that treatment of urinary tract infection may be less effective when blood levels are necessarily maintained below the toxic range (46). On the other hand, the diffusion of a toxic antibiotic across a dialysis membrane can decrease plasma concentrations below toxic and even below therapeutic levels.

Aminoglycosides

The aminoglycoside antibiotics are noted for their nephrotoxicity and ototoxicity. Neomycin is the most nephrotoxic and streptomycin is the least toxic of this class of drugs. The aminoglycosides are filtered at the glomerulus and a variable fraction is reabsorbed by proximal tubules, leading to renal cortical accumulation and proximal tubular injury manifested by tubular transport abnormalities and depression of glomerular filtration rate (113). Nephrotoxicity is more likely with advancing age, prior renal dysfunction or exposure to other nephrotoxins and follows renal cortical accumulation of the aminoglycosides, from which the elimination half-life is normally several days (114). To avoid aminoglycoside toxicity, adjust the dose pharmacokinetically and limit the duration of treatment (115). The high in-

cidence of hearing loss among patients with chronic renal failure may relate in part to exposure to ototoxins, of which aminoglycosides are most notorious (116). Aminoglycoside toxicity also includes a myasthenic syndrome due to neuromuscular blockade associated with impaired release of acetylcholine. This toxicity is more frequent in those with renal failure, is correctable by calcium administration, and often presents as a respiratory arrest after anesthesia (117). Aminoglycoside pharmacokinetics are outlined in Table 5. The data are the mean of published values for adults and do not apply precisely to individual patients.

Streptomycin when first introduced sometimes caused proteinuria, cylindruria, decreased urea clearance and, rarely, tubular necrosis (118). Such nephrotoxicity has been abolished by purification of the drug. Ototoxicity, a function of the dose and inversely of renal excretion, improves as dialysis decreases blood levels of streptomycin by more than 50% (119). Elimination is predominantly renal, by glomerular filtration, and the maintenance dose must be reduced substantially (Table 5) from the normal 0.5 g (0.86 mmol) every 12 h as renal failure prolongs the half-life (3, 13). Dialyzer clearance exceeds 40 ml/min despite 35% protein binding, reducing the half-life sufficiently to warrant a supplemental dose after dialysis.

Neomycin, like other aminoglycosides, is poorly absorbed. It can be used orally or by local application with relative impunity. When absorbed, it is very toxic, causing vestibular damage, deafness and proximal tubular necrosis. High dosage, enhanced absorption or impaired renal excretion contribute to the toxicity that sometimes complicates oral use, causing anuria and a high mortality rate (120). Hemodialysis removes neomycin rapidly enough (Table 5) to be useful in

Table 5. Aminoglycoside pharmacokinetics.

Drug (mol. wt).	% Bound in plasma	DV (l/kg)	Clearance (ml/min)			Half-life (h)			Dose (mg/kg)		
			N	A	H	N	A	H	N	A	H*
Amikacin (586)	4	0.25	90	4.0	37	2.2	50	5.3	5/8 h	2/24 h	4
Dibekacin (452)	12	0.20	90	4.3	60	2.2	42	4.0	1/8 h	0.5/36 h	1
Gentamicin (477)	< 10	0.25	92	4.0	31	2.3	54	7.0	1.2/8 h	0.7/72 h	0.7
Kanamycin (484)	0	0.26	88	4.0	30	2.5	55	6.0	5/8 h	4/72 h	4
Neomycin (615)	–	–			–	2.3	24	9.0	15/8 h (oral)	Avoid	–
Netilmicin (475)	< 10	0.23	80	5.0	35	2.5	40	5.5	1.2/8 h	0.7/72 h	0.7
Sisomicin (448)	0	0.20	85	4.3	–	2.5	50	–	0.8/8 h	–	–
Streptomycin (582)	35	0.26	80	2.5	42	2.7	80	5.0	10/12 h	7/72 h	4
Tobramycin (468)	10	0.25	80	4.0	32	2.2	55	5.9	1.2/8 h	1.2/72 h	0.5

Average of published values, DV = distribution volume, N = normal, A = anephric, H = hemodialysis.
* Dose to be added (mg/kg) after dialysis to the usual dose for the anephric patient.

the treatment of inadvertent systemic administration of neomycin (121), although renal elimination is faster.

Kanamycin sulfate was found to be an effective aminoglycoside antibiotic with a broader antibacterial spectrum than streptomycin, but its use was complicated by proteinuria, microhematuria, granular or hyaline cylindruria, and azotemia in 10 to 20% of patients at a dosage of 25 to 50 mg (57 to 113 μmol)/kg/day (122). Prolonged use, for example in chemotherapy of tuberculosis, usually causes proteinuria and cylindruria after 15 mg (34 μmol)/kg/day and oliguric renal failure in about 10% of patients so treated. Overt ototoxicity is infrequent and is also dose related. Kanamycin accumulates both in the renal cortex and in the middle ear, from which sites it is slowly eliminated (123). Because kanamycin is eliminated predominantly by the kidney, it accumulates in body fluids of patients with renal failure and the dose must be reduced substantially (Table 5). The half-life in hours may be roughly estimated by multiplying the serum creatinine concentration (mg/dl) by 3 (124). Hemodialysis removes kanamycin rapidly enough that a supplemental dose is required thereafter (125), while the clearance by intermittent peritoneal dialysis is 5 to 8 ml/min which reduces the half-life to about 16 h (126, 127). With CAPD the clearance should not exceed 5 ml/min and the half-life remains about 24 h (74). Supplemental doses of 100 mg (225 μmol) may be given daily during peritoneal dialysis if the plasma concentration decreases to 1 μg/ml (2 μmol/l) or less.

Gentamicin was introduced as a potentially safer, alternative aminoglycoside with a wider antibacterial spectrum. Unfortunately, the incidence of nephrotoxicity and ototoxicity is comparable to that of kanamycin. Nephrotoxicity, characterized by decreased glomerular filtration and proteinuria and often preceded by saluresis and enzymuria, occurs in 10 to 30% of patients receiving 2.0 mg (4 μmol)/kg daily for more than one week (128, 129). Proximal tubular necrosis with acute renal failure occurs occasionally, particularly after prolonged high doses, with preexisting renal disease, advanced age, prior nephrotoxin exposure or during concurrent therapy with cephalosporins (129, 130). Elimination, which is predominantly renal, decreases as the glomerular filtration rate declines. The half-life in hours is approximately 4 times the equilibrium plasma creatinine concentration (mg/dl) (131) but the half-life of gentamicin in the renal cortex is 112 h (132). Unless dosage is reduced substantially in patients with end-stage renal disease, a 30% incidence of vestibular toxicity occurs, correlating with duration of treatment and total dose (133). Although the dose should not raise the peak plasma concentration above 10 μg/ml (22 μmol/l) (134), nephrotoxicity correlates more with the minimal (predose) concentration, which should be kept below 2 μg/ml (4 μmol/l) by appropriate spacing of doses (111, 135). When plasma concentrations are higher, as many as one third of patients develop overt nephrotoxicity. Hemodialysis shortens the half-life considerably (Table 5) so toxicity is lessened and supplemental doses are required to maintain therapeutic concentrations (131, 136). Gentamicin transfers slowly out of tissues, however, so there may be a rebound increment in plasma concentrations. Binding of gentamicin amino groups to sulfite radicals of the polyacrylonitrile membrane of the dialyzer can augment the removal rate during the beginning of dialysis. With hemoperfusion, clearances exceed 100 ml/min and the half-life is reduced to the normal value of 2 h (137). The clearance by intermittent peritoneal dialysis is 10 ml/min which reduces the half-life to about 14 h (138). With CAPD the clearance is 3.0 ml/min and the half-life is 35 h (139). About 50% of an intraperitoneal dose is absorbed.

Amikacin is a semisynthetic, less toxic kanamycin derivative that is also eliminated predominantly by the kidney, thereby requiring dosage reduction in patients with renal failure (Table 5). Nephrotoxicity and ototoxicity occur in about 9% and 5%, respectively, of patients treated with amikacin, increasing in incidence with the same risk factors as for other aminoglycosides (140). The prolonged half-life in patients with renal failure is decreased considerably by hemodialysis (141) which affects the normal elimination half-life only slightly (142). During intermittent peritoneal dialysis, the half-life is about 20 h (141) and with CAPD it is about 30 h (74).

Tobramycin has antimicrobial activity and pharmacokinetic properties similar to those of gentamicin but a slightly lower incidence of nephrotoxicity. Renal failure prolongs the normally 2.2 h half-life which correlates with plasma creatinine concentration (143). In the renal cortex the half-life is 146 h (132). Hemodialysis removes tobramycin rapidly, decreasing the half-life considerably (Table 5). The reduced dosage used for uremic patients must be supplemented after dialysis (143, 144). The clearance to tobramycin by intermittent peritoneal dialysis is about 10 ml/min (half of the urea clearance) which reduces the half-life to 16 h (145). With CAPD the clearance is about 4.0 ml/min and the half-life is about 36 h (74, 146).

Sisomicin is a gentamicin derivative that has pharmacokinetics comparable to it (147) but may be less toxic. The elimination of sisomicin is about 75% renal, its half-life is prolonged in renal failure (Table 5) and the drug is removed by hemodialysis (148).

Netilmicin, ethyl sisomicin, is a semisynthetic aminoglycoside (149). The elimination rate is about 70% of the glomerular filtration rate (Table 5) and the half-life in hours is approximately 3 times the serum creatinine concentration (mg/dl) (150). Netilmicin accumulates readily in the kidney where its half-life is 198 h (132). It may be intrinsically less toxic than other aminoglycosides. Hemodialysis removes netilmicin fast enough to lower the half-life substantially (150). With hemodiafiltration and high flux membranes the clearance exceeds 100 ml/min and the half-life is reduced to normal (151). With CAPD the clearance is about 4 ml/min and the half-life is about 22 h (74), and somewhat faster elimination occurs with rapid exchange of peritoneal dialysate.

Dibekacin, 3', 4' dideoxykanamycin, is also eliminated mostly by the kidney at a rate proportional to the glomerular filtration rate (152). With renal failure the distribution volume of dibekacin increases. Nevertheless, hemodialysis lowers the half-life almost to normal.

Paromomycin is an amebicidal aminoglycoside that is used orally. It is poorly absorbed but accumulates in patients with renal failure. The half-life increases from the normal 2 h to about 40 h in anuric patients. Dosage adjustments for renal failure and dialysis pharmacokinetics have not been defined precisely (153).

Verdamicin is a new broad spectrum aminoglycoside, the pharmacokinetics and toxicity of which have not been precisely defined (154).

Lividomycin, which has not had much clinical use, depends on renal excretion and accumulates in renal failure, the half-life increasing from 2 to 44 h (155). Dialysis pharmacokinetics have not been defined.

Habekacin (567 daltons) is more nephrotoxic than dibekacin, achieving a higher renal cortical/plasma concentration ratio than other aminoglycosides. The normal half-life of 0.7 h is prolonged with renal failure (156).

Ribostamicin accumulates in renal failure, the half-life increasing from 2 h to over 48 h, but it can be removed by hemodialysis (12).

Cephalosporins

As a group the cephalosporins have a broad antibacterial spectrum, are chemically similar to the penicillins, and are excreted predominantly by the kidney by filtration and secretion (157). A rapid succession of new semisynthetic cephalosporin analogues have been developed during the past decade. Successive generations of cephalosporins have been increasingly useful for the treatment of gram negative infections so frequently encountered in patients with renal failure (158).

Cephaloridine (416 daltons) frequently causes dose-related renal tubular injury. It accumulates in patients with renal failure, whereas the normal renal clearance of 150 ml/min rapidly depletes plasma concentrations (159). With renal failure the half-life increases from 1.3 h to 20 h, but hemodialysis decreases it to 4 h despite 30% binding to plasma proteins (160). Peritoneal dialysis decreases the half-life to 7 h (161). This drug has largely been replaced by newer analogues and should be avoided in those with preexisting renal insufficiency because of the risk of further renal impairment. In anephric patients it could be acceptable, however.

Cephalothin clearance is quite high, due mostly to secretion by the kidney since a large fraction of plasma cephalothin is protein bound (157, 159). After the normal dose of 1,000 mg (2.5 mmol) intramuscularly, the peak plasma concentration of about 20 µg/ml (50 µmol/l) declines rapidly (157). With severe renal failure cephalothin persists in plasma despite the high extrarenal clearance (Table 6). The half-life is reduced to 6 h by peritoneal dialysis and to 3.3 h by hemodialysis (159, 161, 162). The low clearances by dialysis can be explained by protein binding which, however, is decreased somewhat in uremic patients (20). Hemoperfusion achieves clearances as high as 150 ml/min (137). Very high plasma concentrations of cephalothin may cause myoclonic seizures. Cephalothin can cause reversible acute renal

failure (163) but verification of the diagnosis can be difficult amid the many other potential causes of renal impairment in severely ill patients. Increased susceptibility to cephalothin nephrotoxicity should be anticipated in patients who receive excessive dosage (over 6.0 g (15 mmol/day), who have preexisting renal impairment, the elderly, those who suffer from intercurrent cephalosporin or penicillin sensitivity, or those treated concurrently with other potential toxins or with potent diuretics such as furosemide or ethacrynic acid (157, 164). By blocking tubular secretion probenecid can be protective to the kidney but will cause greater accumulation in plasma (165).

Cefaclor is rapidly absorbed from the gastrointestinal tract and fractional elimination by the kidney is less than that of other cephalosporins (Table 6), so that accumulation in patients with renal failure is only minimal (166, 167). Removal of cefaclor by hemodialysis is not rapid, presumably because of protein binding (166, 167).

Cefadroxil is a derivative of cephalexin. It is well absorbed from the gastrointestinal tract and eliminated almost exclusively by the kidney (168). The half-life increases considerably with renal failure but is reduced by hemodialysis (Table 6). The dose of cefadroxil should be reduced as the glomerular filtration rate declines and a supplemental dose should be added after dialysis.

Cefamandole is another new cephalosporin that is particularly effective against certain gram negative organisms. Despite considerable protein binding, it normally has a short half-life (Table 6) and depends mostly on renal elimination (13, 169). The prolonged half-life of cefamandole in patients with renal failure is reduced substantially by hemodialysis but only lowered to 7.2 h by intermittent peritoneal dialysis and to 10.4 h by CAPD (169-171).

Cefazolin reaches higher peak plasma concentrations than cephalothin, has a smaller distribution space and a longer half-life, in part because it is more highly bound to plasma proteins (157). Renal excretion is largely by secretion and bactericidal urinary concentrations can be maintained despite moderate renal failure (172). Cephazolin accumulates in plasma of patients with renal failure (Table 6), as the half-life in hours is approximately 3 times the serum creatinine concentration (mg/dl) (173-175). Hemodialysis reduces the half-life considerably (173, 174). Despite only a modest reduction of protein binding in patients with renal failure, binding is markedly decreased during hemodialysis (176). With CAPD the clearance is only 1.0 ml/min and the half-life is reduced only minimally (177).

Cefixime, a new cephalosporin analogue, distributes in a large volume (1.1 l/kg), is cleared at 164 ml/min and has a half-life of 3.2 h (178). With renal failure the clearance decreases to 41 ml/min and the half-life is prolonged to 11.5 h, the distribution space diminishing. Hemodialysis achieves a clearance of about 30 ml/min, reducing the half-life to 8.2 h, but the CAPD clearance is less than 1.0 ml/min which does not lower the half-life.

Cefmenoxime (530 daltons) is a third generation cephalosporin similar in antibacterial spectrum to cefotaxime. It is 77% bound to plasma proteins and distributes in 0.23 l/kg

(179). The clearance is about 250 ml/min, largely due to glomerular filtration and tubular secretion, and decreases to 30 ml/min with severe renal failure, increasing the half-life from about 1.1 h to 15 h. Hemodialysis clears cefmenoxime at 52 ml/min, reducing the half-life to 4.5 h (179) while CAPD clears it at the rate of 1.9 ml/min (180). With renal failure the dose should be reduced from about 100 mg (189 μmol)/kg/day to about 10 mg/kg/day.

Cefmetazole (472 daltons) is a new cephamycin derivative that is eliminated mostly (70%) by the kidney with a renal clearance of 110 ml/min (181). Its distribution volume, 0.19 l/kg, is unaffected by renal failure, which prolongs the half-life from 0.8 h to 15 h (181). Its antibacterial spectrum resembles that of cefoxitin.

Cefonicid is highly protein bound and eliminated more slowly than other cephalosporins, allowing once or twice daily dosing in normal subjects (182, 183). Renal failure prolongs the half-life mandating dosage reduction (Table 6). The low hemodialyzer clearance should reduce the half-life only minimally and the peritoneal clearance is less than

Table 6. Cephalosporin pharmacokinetics.

Drug (mol. wt.)	% Bound in plasma	DV (1/kg)	Clearance (ml/min)			Half-life (h)			Dose (mg/kg)		
			N	A	H	N	A	H	N	A	H*
Cephalothin (396)	70	0.26	450	30	–	0.6	12	3.3	15/8 h	15/24 h	7
Cefaclor (386)	25	0.30	240	90	75	0.8	2.6	1.6	15/6 h	15/12 h	4
Cefadroxil (381)	20	0.31	170	12	18	1.4	22	3.3	15/12 h	7/24 h	7
Cefamandole (463)	70	0.18	250	18	30	1.0	12	6.0	30/6 h	10/12 h	10
Cefazolin (476)	80	0.13	65	5.0	8.0	2.0	35	7.0	15/8 h	4/24 h	6
Cefonicid (565)	98	0.11	23	2.0	3.4	4.8	60	–	15/12 h	3/72 h	–
Cefoperazone (668)	90	0.20	80	65	–	2.0	2.6	2.1	40/8 h	40/12 h	–
Ceforanide (520)	80	0.16	46	6.0	–	2.7	25	12	15/12 h	7/24 h	4
Cefotaxime (477)	40	0.18	250	100	–	1.1	2.6	1.8	30/4 h	30/8 h	–
Cefotetan (576)	88	0.17	40	15	–	3.5	18	7.5	–	–	–
Cefoxitin (427)	75	0.20	350	13	40	0.8	18	4.0	40/6 h	15/24 h	10
Cefroxadine (365)	10	0.25	200	5	–	1.0	40	3.4	–	–	–
Cefsulodin (555)	15	0.28	120	16	40	1.8	12	2.6	–	–	–
Ceftazidime (547)	17	0.23	125	11	55	1.8	32	3.6	30/12 h	7/24 h	–
Ceftizoxime (405)	35	0.37	160	12	–	1.6	28	–	50/8 h	25/24 h	–
Ceftriaxone (559)	85	0.18	15	11	–	8.0	15	12	30/12 h	15/12 h	–
Cefuroxime (424)	40	0.19	165	12	–	1.4	17	3.3	30/8 h	10/24 h	10
Cephalexin (347)	15	0.26	250	17	–	1.0	28	5.0	15/6 h	7/24 h	7
Cephapirin (445)	50	0.16	270	80	–	0.8	2.5	1.8	15/6 h	15/12 h	3
Cephradine (349)	14	0.25	360	25	–	1.0	15	–	–	–	–
Moxalactam (564)	50	0.24	95	14	42	2.4	19	3.9	30/8 h	15/24 h	10

Average of published values, DV = distribution volume, N = normal, A = anephric, H = hemodialysis.
* Dose to be added (mg/kg) after dialysis to the usual dose for the anephric patient.

Cefoperazone is third generation cephalosporin that is slowly cleared from plasma, mostly by extrarenal routes (185–187). The half life increases minimally with renal failure (Table 6). Because cefoperazone is highly protein bound, plasma concentrations are only minimally influenced by hemodialysis and the peritoneal clearance is much less than the extrarenal clearance.

Ceforanide resembles cefamandole structurally and antibacterially but is eliminated more slowly (Table 6). With renal failure, the half-life increases but it is reduced by hemodialysis despite 80% protein binding of the drug (188, 189). Peritoneal dialysis should affect ceforanide pharmacokinetics only minimally.

Cefotaxime, a third generation cephalosporin, has a high clearance about half accounted for by renal excretion and the rest by metabolism to desacetyl cefotaxime (190, 191). Cefotaxime has a short half-life even in uremic patients, but the dose should be reduced with renal failure, nevertheless, since the half-life of the desacetyl metabolite increases from about 1.4 h to 14 h (Table 6). Bioassay values of cefotaxime may be spuriously high because of the metabolite. Hemodialyzer clearance of cefotaxime is less than the nonrenal clearance, so that half-life decreases only modestly. With CAPD cefotaxime clearance is about 2.0 ml/min and the metabolite clearance is about 3.0 ml/min (192, 193).

Cefotetan is a cephamycin with activity similar to that of cefotaxime. It is retained in patients with renal failure (Table 6). Although the clearance by hemodialysis is not high it exceeds the extrarenal clearance, thereby lowering the half-life (194, 195). With CAPD the clearance is 1.8 ml/min and the half-life is 15.5 h (195).

Cefotiam (599 daltons) distributes in 0.35 l/kg and is cleared at about 250 ml/min, mostly by the kidney (196). With renal failure the half-life increases from 0.9 h to 8.0 h as the clearance decreases to 27 ml/min dialysis clears this drug at about 50 ml/min, lowering the half-life to 2.7 h.

Cefoxitin is a semisynthetic cephamycin derivative. It is normally rapidly cleared by the kidney (197) and accumulates in patients with renal failure (Table 6), but not as much as anticipated because decreased protein binding of cefoxitin in uremia augments hepatic clearance (198). Although decreased binding should increase the clearance by dialysis, the distribution volume increases considerably with renal failure (199). Nevertheless, the half-life of cefoxitin decreases substantially with hemodialysis (14). With CAPD the clearance is 4.0 ml/min or less, insufficient to lower the half-life appreciably (200). The clearance by hemofiltration is 53 ml/min, reducing the half-life to 3.4 h (201).

Cefpiramide is a third generation antipseudomonal drug with a normal half-life of about 4 h (158).

Cefroxadine persists in plasma of patients with renal failure because the clearance falls markedly (Table 6), but it is rapidly removed by hemodialysis (202).

Cefsulodin, an effective antipseudomonal and antistaphylococcal is eliminated mostly by the kidney, accumulates in renal failure (Table 6) and is rapidly removed by hemodialysis (203, 204).

Ceftazidime is eliminated mostly by the kidney (205, 206). Hence it accumulates in renal failure, but is cleared rapidly by hemodialysis. The clearance by intermittent peritoneal dialysis is 8.5 ml/min, which reduces the half-life to below 9 h (205).

Ceftezole (440 daltons) is distributed in about 0.20 l/kg has low fractional binding, predominant excretion by the kidney at a clearance of 220 ml/min and a normal half-life of 0.6 h that increases to 11 h with renal failure (207).

Ceftizoxime has an antibacterial spectrum similar to cefotaxime but is eliminated more slowly, almost exclusively by the kidney (Table 6). It accumulates in patients with renal failure and is rapidly removed by hemodialysis (208, 209). Ceftizoxime is rapidly absorbed from the peritoneum and is cleared at a rate of 3.1 ml/min during CAPD which lowers the half-life to about 10 h (209).

Ceftriaxone normally slowly eliminated, is retained only minimally in patients with renal failure (210, 211). Hemodialysis lowers the half-life minimally because clearance is impeded by protein binding (Table 6). With CAPD the clearance is below 1.0 ml/min and the decrease in half-life is negligible (211).

Cefuroxime depends on renal elimination (158) and accumulates in plasma of patients with renal failure (Table 6). Hemodialysis decreases the half-life to about twice the normal value, but the clearance by CAPD (about 4.0 ml/min) lowers the prolonged half-life only slightly (212).

Cephacetrile (361 daltons) has a half-life of less than an hour after parenteral use (157). With renal failure, the half-life increases to 26 h and it decreases with hemodialysis to about 2 h. The recommended dose of cephacetrile, 15 mg (40 μmol)/kg/8 h, should be reduced to 7 mg/kg/24 h in uremic patients but a supplement of 10 mg/kg should be added after dialysis. Accumulation in plasma can cause a reversible encephalopathy that improves with hemodialysis (213).

Cephalexin is effective orally, achieving plasma concentrations of almost 20 μg/ml (60 μmol/l) with standard dosage (157). Thereafter, plasma concentrations decline rapidly but elimination is almost entirely renal, so cephalexin accumulates in those with renal failure (67, 159, 162, 175). The prolonged half-life of cephalexin in uremic patients (Table 6) is reduced by hemodialysis (159). With CAPD the clearance is 2.5 ml/min and the half-life is 8.6 h (177). Nephrotoxicity can occur with high plasma concentrations of cephalexin (214).

Cephaloglycin (405 daltons) is also effective orally, but absorption is poor and the drug has largely been replaced. Nevertheless, as excretion is mostly renal, it accumulates in patients with renal failure (158).

Cephanone is cleared from plasma at 56 ml/min, 95% of which occurs by renal excretion (175). In plasma 88% of the drug is bound and its distribution volume is 0.18 l/kg. The normal elimination half-life is 2.5 h.

Cephapirin has a short half-life (Table 6) that increases only modestly with renal failure since a considerably fraction of its elimination is extrarenal (13, 157). The half-life is reduced only minimally by hemodialysis, presumably because a high fraction is protein bound (215).

Cephradine is almost completely absorbed after oral administration, is rapidly cleared, mostly by the kidney (Table 6) and accumulates in patients with renal failure (13, 216). Because of minimal protein binding it should be rapidly cleared by hemodialysis.

Moxalactam is a structurally unique beta lactam antibiotic related to third generation cephalosporins with a broad antimicrobial spectrum. It consists of two epimers that have similar pharmacokinetics. Moxalactam depends mainly on renal excretion, is retained in plasma with renal failure (217–220) and is removed rapidly by hemodialysis (Table 6). With high flux dialysis the half-life is reduced to 3.0 h (220). The peritoneal clearance during CAPD averages 1.2 ml/min reducing the half-life to about 17.7 h (217). With renal failure protein binding of moxalactam decreases increasing the apparent volume of distribution.

Aztreonam (435 daltons) is a beta lactam antibiotic that distributes in 0.20 l/kg and is eliminated predominantly by the kidney at a clearance of about 100 ml/min (221, 222). With renal failure the half-life is prolonged from about 2.0 h to about 8 h as the plasma clearance decreases to 24 ml/min, mandating a decrease to 25% of the usual maintenance dose. The hemodialysis clearance of 19 ml/min lowers the half-life to 2.7 h while the peritoneal clearance during CAPD of 2.1 ml/min reduces it to 7.1 h. The metabolite is inactive.

Carumonam (484 daltons), a beta lactam antibiotic that is about 18% protein bound, distributes in extracellular fluid and is eliminated by the kidney (223). With renal failure the half-life increases from 1.7 h to 11.3 h.

Imipenim is a beta lactam antibiotic that is eliminated by nonrenal metabolism and by the kidney where it undergoes hydrolysis. The distribution space is about 0.3 l/kg and the plasma clearance is 250 ml/min. With renal failure the half-life increases from 1.0 h to about 3.0 h as the clearance decreases to 55 ml/min (224, 225). The hemodialyzer clearance of about 75 ml/min reduces the half-life to about 1.5 h.

Cilastin inhibits renal brush border dehydropeptidase (224, 225). Hence, it increases urinary imipenem but does not prolong its half-life in plasma. Cilastin distributes in 0.24 l/kg and is cleared at 200 ml/min, about half by the kidney. With renal failure the half-life is prolonged from 0.9 h to about 15 h and the dose should be reduced. The hemodialyzer clearance of 44 ml/min reduces the half-life to about 3 h.

Penicillins

The penicillins remain antibiotics of choice for many infectious diseases. An infrequent but serious complication of penicillin therapy is acute hypersensitivity interstitial nephritis. Patients often manifest skin rash, eosinophilia, hematuria, leukocyturia (including eosinophiluria), proteinuria, cylindruria, enlarged tender kidneys and impaired renal function with or without oliguria (226). Interstitial accumulation of mononuclear cells and eosinophils accompanies an intense immune response at the tubular basement membrane to a penicilloyl haptene (226). The lesion does not depend on the dose or elimination rate but occurs more often with higher doses and with the synthetic penicillins, methicillin and ampicillin (227). Acute hypersensitivity angiitis and glomerulonephritis may also complicate penicillin therapy (228).

An increased incidence of hypersensitivity skin reactions, but not of gastrointestinal toxicity, complicates penicillin therapy when renal failure preexists (229). Massive dosage, especially with concurrent probenecid therapy blocking renal tubular secretion of penicillin or with antecedent renal failure may be complicated by neurotoxicity with myoclonic seizures and coma (230). The potassium content of penicillin G, 1.7 mEq/million units, can be potentially toxic. Alternatively, sodium retention with resultant fluid overload may result from massive doses of the sodium salts of penicillin (1.7 mEq/million units), ampicillin (3 mEq/g) or carbenicillin or ticarcillin (5 mEq/g). High doses of penicillins can also impair hemostasis by inducing abnormalities of platelet function and a heparin-like effect (231). Penicillin kinetics in dialysis patients have been reviewed recently (231).

Penicillin G is excreted mostly unchanged by the kidney by filtration and secretion at a clearance approaching renal plasma flow. The phenoxymethyl derivative, *penicillin V*, is better absorbed, but bioavailability is not known to be impaired in uremia. After absorption, these drugs bind loosely to albumin, distribute in a large volume and are rapidly eliminated (Table 7). Renal failure prolongs the half life substantially but unless massive doses are used, e.g. for septicemia, dosage adjustment need not be very precise because of the wide margin of safety (8, 17, 216). When the dose exceeds 20 million units daily (1.6 million units equals one gram), or considerably less in patients with renal failure, penicillin can cause lethargy, coma, multifocal myoclonus or eleptiform seizures (158). Abnormalities in the blood cerebrospinal fluid barrier in uremia (49) which normally maintains a 20:1 penicillin gradient can contribute to this complication which is responsive to hemodialysis. About 30% of absorbed penicillin can be removed by hemodialysis (232) and a supplemental dose can be required thereafter. Little is removed by peritoneal dialysis, however. Charcoal hemoperfusion can achieve a penicillin clearance of 140 ml/min (233). Combined with hemodialysis, hemoperfusion is superior to dialysis, alone, for treatment of penicillin intoxication. *Sulbenicillin*, α sulfabenzyl penicillin (414 daltons) is also rapidly eliminated by the kidney. With renal failure the half-life increases from 0.5 h to 7 h, so the usual dose of one gram should be given every 12 h rather than every 6 h (234).

Ampicillin, the prototype of the aminopenicillins, has a broad antibacterial spectrum. It causes hypersensitivity reactions, including interstitial nephritis, more often than penicillin G. Because ampicillin elimination is predominantly by the kidney (Table 7), the normal short half-life increases substantially in patients with renal failure (3, 67, 232, 235). Accordingly, the dose should be decreased in uremic patients to avoid ampicillin neurotoxicity. Hemodialysis removes ampicillin sufficiently rapidly to decrease the half-life so that dosage should be supplemented after dialysis (67, 236). Peritoneal dialysis does not affect plasma ampicillin concentrations or half-life appreciably (237), although ampicillin absorption occurs across the peritoneum.

Amoxicillin is closely related chemically and pharmacologically to ampicillin. Pharmacokinetic parameters in health, with renal failure and during hemodialysis (Table 7) are also similar for these two aminopenicillins (158, 238–240) except that because of better absorption from the gastrointestinal tract, amoxicillin reaches higher peak plasma concentrations and a greater fraction is eliminated by the liver.

Hetacillin is also a chemical modification of ampicillin to which it is metabolized (158). Accordingly, the pharmacokinetics of this well-absorbed drug become those of ampicillin. *Pivampicillin* is another ester of ampicillin with enhanced absorption and comparable pharmacokinetics after metabolic conversion. Other similar semisynthetic aminopenicillins are *bacampicillin, talampicillin, epicillin* and *cyclacillin* (158).

Methicillin is a semisynthetic penicillinase resistant penicillin administered parenterally because of poor gastrointestinal absorption. It is rapidly eliminated (Table 7) mostly by the kidney (67, 241), requiring modest dosage reduction in patients with renal failure. Hemodialysis reduces the half-life only slightly so supplementation after dialysis can be minimal if any, and peritoneal dialysis does not alter elimination kinetics appreciably. Methicillin causes acute interstitial nephritis (226, 242) more often than other penicillins. As many as 17% of patients given high doses of methicillin develop detectable renal abnormalities. Restoration of renal function is more likely and occurs faster with prednisone therapy (242). Occasionally, methicillin-induced renal failure is so severe as to require hemodialysis.

Nafcillin is a semisynthetic penicillinase resistant penicillin that is partially absorbed after oral administration (158). Its elimination is mostly extrarenal (Table 7) and as it is highly protein bound and distributed in a large volume, its elimination kinetics are not appreciably affected by dialysis (243). Large doses of sodium nafcillin may induce metabolic alkalosis.

Oxacillin is an oral semisynthetic penicillinase resistant penicillin. It is eliminated rapidly both by renal excretion and hepatic degradation (Table 7). The dose must be modified only slightly, if at all, in patients with renal failure (244). Because it is highly protein bound, little removal occurs by peritoneal dialysis and supplemental doses are not required (232, 237). Removal by peritoneal dialysis is also

Table 7. Penicillin pharmacokinetics.

Drug (mol. wt)	% Bound in plasma	DV (l/kg)	Clearance (ml/min)			Half-life (h)			Dose (mg/kg)		
			N	A	H	N	A	H	N	A	H*
Penicillin (356)	60	0.35	420	36	40	0.5	12	4.0	20/6 h	5/12 h	5
Ampicillin (349)	20	0.25	270	30	30	1.3	12	4.5	7/6 h	4/6 h	5
Amoxicillin (365)	18	0.37	310	40	60	1.4	13	4.0	10/8 h	7/12 h	7
Methicillin (402)	40	0.31	425	60	–	0.6	4.0	–	15/6 h	7/12 h	3
Nafcillin (436)	90	0.35	410	200	14	0.7	2.0	2.0	7/6 h	7/6 h	0
Oxacillin (442)	90	0.33	400	200	–	0.5	1.6	1.6	15/6 h	7/12 h	0
Cloxacillin (436)	90	0.15	150	–	–	0.6	1.2	1.2	7/6 h	7/8 h	0
Dicloxacillin (470)	95	0.12	110	50	–	0.7	1.3	1.2	4/6 h	4/6 h	0
Carbenicillin (378)	50	0.16	100	11	50	1.2	20	6.2	50/4 h	30/12 h	15
Ticarcillin (496)	55	0.20	120	16	43	1.2	12	2.2	40/4 h	30/12 h	20
Azlocillin (461)	30	0.23	180	60	15	1.3	5.4	2.6	50/8 h	20/12 h	20
Mezlocillin (540)	30	0.20	400	100	–	1.0	6.0	2.2	50/8 h	20/12 h	15
Mecillinam	–	0.59	400	75	–	1.0	3.8	2.3	10/4 h	–	–
Piperacillin (540)	18	0.18	260	50	–	0.9	3.5	2.5	30/6 h	30/8 h	15

Average of published values, DV = distribution volume, N = normal, A = anephric, H = hemodialysis.
* Dose to be added (mg/kg) after dialysis to the usual dose for the anephric patient.

minimal. Oxacillin has caused hypersensitivity interstitial nephritis (245) and neurotoxicity (246).

Cloxacillin is another isoxazolyl penicillin that is highly protein bound with pharmacokinetics similar to those of oxacillin (Table 7). Although protein binding decreases somewhat with uremia, hemodialysis removes too little cloxacillin to affect the half-life measurably (247).

Dicloxacillin has pharmacokinetics that are similar to those of oxacillin (Table 7). Because of extensive protein binding little dicloxacillin is removed by hemodialysis (248).

Floxacillin (454 daltons) is also more than 90% bound in plasma, distributes in 0.13 l/kg and is cleared at 140 ml/min, mostly by hydroxylation (249). With renal failure the half-life increases from 0.9 to 2.7 h and the metabolite is comparably retained. Dialysis removes little floxacillin (250).

Carbenicillin, a synthetic penicillin particularly effective against Pseudomonas species, distributes in a small volume and in plasma, about half is protein bound (251). Excretion is rapid and predominantly renal (Table 7). In uremic patients the plasma half-life increases substantially (13, 232, 252). As hepatic degradation contributes to the elimination, combined renal and hepatic failure prolongs the half-life even more (to 24 h). To avoid neurotoxicity the dosage should be decreased and the dosing interval increased to 12 h with oliguria and to 24 h with associated hepatic failure (251). Hemodialysis decreases the half-life by about 50% and a dosage supplement is required after dialysis, while the peritoneal clearance of 6 to 7 ml/min affects the half-life somewhat less (251–253). In patients retaining salt the sodium content of carbenicillin can contribute to fluid overload. Large doses in sodium restricted patients can cause hypokalemic alkalosis because the carbenicillin anion is poorly reabsorbed by the tubule, promoting potassium and hydrogen ion loss (254). Massive doses of penicillin can cause the same problem (255). High plasma concentrations of carbenicillin can also cause neurotoxicity (256), hepatotoxicity (257) and abnormalities of coagulation (231, 258) including platelet dysfunction, impaired conversion of fibrinogen to fibrin and heparin-like activity. Carbenicillin is administered parenterally. *Carbenicillin indanyl* is an ester that is rapidly absorbed from the small intestine and is hydrolyzed to carbenicillin, and thereafter has the same pharmacokinetics (259). Absorption of an oral dose is somewhat delayed in uremic patients but a higher peak plasma concentration is reached since the half life is prolonged considerably. Hemodialysis reduces the half-life of the absorbed carbenicillin by about 50%.

Ticarcillin is a semisynthetic penicillin with pharmacologic properties similar to carbenicillin but greater bactericidal activity (260–262). Because dosage is lower, less toxicity is anticipated. Nevertheless, renal failure prolongs the half-life sufficiently (261, 262) to warrant dosage reduction (Table 7) to avoid neurotoxicity (263). Hemodialysis removes ticarcillin rapidly enough to justify post dialysis supplementation, but the peritoneal clearance of 6 ml/min only reduces the half-life to 9 h.

Temocillin is a carbenicillin derivative that binds highly to plasma proteins, distributes in 0.22 l/kg and is eliminated more slowly at a clearance of 44 ml/min, about half renal (264, 265). With renal failure the clearance decreases to 10 ml/min and the half-life increases from about 4.5 h to about 20 h. The dose should be reduced from 1.5 g/24 h to 1 g/48 h in anuric patients. The clearance by hemodialysis lowers the half-life to about 8 h, while with CAPD it is 13.4 h.

Azlocillin, an acylureido penicillin, resembles carbenicillin pharmacologically. Normally it is rapidly eliminated by the kidney (Table 7) and is retained in renal failure (266, 267). Hemodialysis removes 30 to 45% of administered azlocillin, reducing the half-life substantially (266, 267). Thus, dosage must be reduced in uremic patients and a supplement is required after dialysis.

Mezlocillin is another new, extended-spectrum penicillin that is pharmacologically similar to carbenicillin. It is normally eliminated rapidly by renal and extrarenal mechanisms (Table 7), although the latter may demonstrate saturation at high plasma concentrations. Because mezlocillin elimination decreases with renal failure, the half-life is prolonged and modest reduction of the dose is required (268–271). Hemodialysis decreases the half-life sufficiently to warrant a supplemental dose thereafter, whereas during peritoneal dialysis the half-life is about 3 h and little or no supplementation is required (269, 270).

Piperacillin, another extended spectrum penicillin, is a piperazine derivative which is very effective against Pseudomonas species and other gram negative organisms. It is excreted mostly by the kidney (Table 7) but the half-life increases only modestly with renal failure and is reduced by hemodialysis which removes about half of an administered dose in 4 h (272–274).

Mecillinam, the first of the amdinopenicillins, has bactericidal effects against a variety of gram negative organisms but not Pseudomonas. The plasma clearance is high and the half-life is short (Table 7). With renal failure both renal and extrarenal clearances decrease prolonging the half-life (275, 276). The elimination rate of mecillinam is approximately doubled by hemodialysis so the half-life decreases by 50%, but peritoneal dialysis does not affect the half-life appreciably.

Clavulanic acid (175 daltons) is a beta lactamase inhibitor that augments the pharmacodynamics of beta lactam antibiotics (158). It is available in combination with amoxicillin or ticarcillin. In normals the plasma clearance is about 200 ml/min, the distribution volume 0.22 l/kg and the half-life about 1.1 h (238, 261). With renal failure the clearance falls to about 60 ml and the half-life increases to 4 h. Hemodialysis reduces the half-life to normal.

Tetracyclines

The tetracyclines are broad-spectrum bacteriostatic agents that should be avoided, when possible, in patients with renal failure because their antianabolic effects considerably increase azotemia, negative nitrogen balance, acidosis and serum phosphate, and their gastrointestinal toxicity frequently induces fluid and electrolyte depletion with attendant decrements in renal function (277–279). There is little evidence of direct nephrotoxicity, although massive doses of *tetracycline* infused acutely decrease inulin and PAH clearances (280). *Demeclocycline,* which impairs renal conservation of water by inhibiting cyclic AMP action and release (281), causes reversible renal failure, especially in cirrhotic patients without inducing overt extracellular volume depletion (282, 283). *Doxycycline* appears to be the least likely of these drugs to aggravate azotemia (284). Outdated tetracyclines degrade to anhydro-metabolites that can cause a reversible Fanconi syndrome (285).

The tetracyclines are bound in plasma to a variable extent, have large distribution volumes and rather long elimination half-lives in health (Table 8). *Chlortetracycline* and *minocycline* have the lowest fractional elimination by the kidney. Only modest retention of minocycline and doxycycline occur in plasma of patients with renal failure (284, 286, 287) and little dosage modification if any is needed to avoid excessive plasma concentrations. Nevertheless, toxicity may occur even when the dose has been adjusted (288). The half-lives of demeclocycline, *oxytetracycline* and tetracycline are prolonged substantially in uremic patients (216). *Methacycline* also is excreted in large part by the kidney. Hemodialyzer clearances of most tetracyclines exceed 20 ml/min (289) but because of the large distribution spaces the half-lives remain long, decreasing by only 10 to 25% (279). Binding of doxycycline to dialysis membranes can contribute to the removal during the procedure (86). Hemoperfusion should achieve higher clearances than hemodialysis but elimination would nevertheless be slow because of the large distribution volume. Peritoneal clearance of tetracycline is only about 5 ml/min, which does not reduce plasma concentrations appreciably. Considerable absorption can occur from dialysis fluid, however (126, 290).

Polymyxins

Renal and neural toxicity are major drawbacks to therapy with polymyxins, a group of polypeptide antibiotics of which *polymyxin B* may be the least toxic. Toxicity is negligible at doses below 2 mg (2 μmol)/kg/day but higher doses or impaired excretion cause tubular injury and azotemia (291).

Polymyxin B (1200 daltons) is excreted predominantly by the kidney without metabolic change (292). Severe renal failure prolongs the half-life (Table 9) and the dose must be decreased from 0.8 mg/kg/8 h to 0.8 mg (0.7 μmol)/kg every 3 to 4 days (3). The extent of protein binding of polymyxin B is controversial. Dialysis removes very little of this large solute and dosage supplementation after dialysis is not warranted.

Sodium *colistimethate* (968 daltons) was introduced with the expectations of greater safety than polymyxin B with which it has a comparable antibacterial spectrum and pharmacokinetics. Toxicity at therapeutic blood levels of 5 to 10 μg/ml (4 to 8 μmol/l) is not well established. But renal failure complicates higher levels, which are more likely in the elderly, those with preexisting renal impairment or after high doses (293–295). Neuromuscular blockade, potentially causing apnea, is also more frequent with antecedent renal disease (117, 296). Colistin, which is identical to polymyxin E, is excreted unchanged by the kidney. The plasma half-life increases with severe renal failure (Table 9) and the dose must be decreased from the normal 2.5 mg (2 μmol/kg every 12 h to 2.0 mg/kg every 72 h or less (296). About half of the drug is bound in plasma and the distribution volume is about 0.45 l/kg. Hemodialysis accelerates the disappearance rate of colistin from plasma somewhat while peritoneal clearances are less than 10 ml/min, influencing the half-life insufficiently to recommend a dosage supplement thereafter (297, 298). Occasionally, acute hypersensitivity interstitial nephritis has also complicated therapy with the polymyxins (299).

Sulfonamides

Sulfonamides (249 to 314 daltons) absorb well from the gastrointestinal tract (70 to 100%), bind highly to plasma proteins (50 to 90%) and distribute in volumes ranging from 0.15 to 0.60 l/kg (13). Elimination is predominantly renal, both of the free sulfonamide and after acetylation to the more active, less soluble metabolite (1). The renal clearance of sulfonamides ranges from about 20 to 30 ml/min and is increased by alkalinization of the urine (13). Renal failure decreases the elimination rate considerably, prolonging the

Table 8. Tetracycline pharmacokinetics.

Drug	Mol. Wt.	% Bound in plasma	DV (1/kg)	% Renal excretion	Half-life (h)	
					N	A
Chlortetracycline	479	60	1.4	15	6.0	8.0
Demeclocycline	465	80	1.5	20	13	80
Doxycycline	444	85	0.9	40	16	23
Methacycline	442	80	1.0	50	12	60
Minocycline	458	75	0.3	10	16	24
Oxytetracycline	460	30	1.7	30	9.0	60
Tetracycline	444	60	1.6	60	8.0	70

Average of published values, DV = distribution volume, N = normal, A = anephric.

half-lives of *sulfamethoxazole, sulfisoxazole* and *sulfadiazine* (Table 9), *sulfamethizole* from 8 to 18 h and *sulfacytine* from 4 h to more than 24 h, thereby increasing concentrations in plasma (1, 13, 20, 300–302). Persistence of free sulfonamide in plasma (partly due to some impairment of acetylation rate) (303, 304) allows increased availability for conversion to the acetylated form which is normally fractionally bound to a greater extent. Nevertheless, protein binding of sulfonamides decreases in patients with renal failure (32, 33, 305, 306). Appropriate dosage of sulfonamides for uremic patients has not been precisely defined but should be reduced to about 25% of normal (14). Hemodialysis clears sulfonamides at a rate of about 20 ml/min, decreasing the prolonged half-life (Table 9) by about 50% (300, 301, 307), and dialysis increases the impaired protein binding of sulfonamides toward normal (306). Sulfonamides are cleared at about 2.0 ml/min with CAPD or higher when peritonitis occurs (308).

Nephrotoxicity is a serious adverse reaction to sulfonamides that was very frequent before the development of more soluble congeners, sulfonamide mixtures and alternative antibiotics (309). After high dosage, especially with acidosis or dehydration, characteristic sulfonamide crystals may be identified in the urinary sediment or distal tubule, often accompanied by tubular injury. Sulfonamides may also impair renal function by acute hypersensitivity interstitial nephritis, focal or diffuse granulomatous nephritis or tubular necrosis without demonstrable crystallization (310). Rarely, sulfonamide derivatives such as acetazolamide have also crystallized in the urinary tract (311). Deterioration in renal function with azotemia and tubular necrosis has also occurred with *cotrimoxazole*, a preparation of sulfamethoxazole and trimethoprim (312). Interstitial fibrosis with irreversible renal failure can occur with this combination or reversible acute interstitial nephritis can develop (313).

Other antibiotics

Chloramphenicol (323 daltons) is eliminated in part by renal excretion of the unchanged drug, but mostly by hepatic conjugation to the glucuronide and renal excretion of this conjugate. With renal failure, protein binding of chloramphenicol normally about 55% (13, 66) decreases slightly but significantly, an abnormality that dialysis corrects (314). The distribution space of chloramphenicol is about 0.9 l/kg. Nevertheless, because of rapid hepatic elimination the half-life is only 3.0 h. It increases slightly in uremic patients (Table 9) but is much longer in those with hepatic failure (315). The glucuronide conjugate persists in uremic patients with a half-life of about 100 h. This metabolite is not known to contribute to hematologic toxicity, but the bone marrow in uremic patients may be more susceptible to inhibition. Nevertheless, therapeutic concentrations can only be achieved in uremic patients with full doses of chloramphenicol. With hepatic failure the dose must be reduced or the drug avoided. The clearance of chloramphenicol by hemodialysis is about 50 ml/min which affects the half-life only slightly in uremic patients but, by doubling the elimination rate, decreases the half-life considerably in those with combined renal and hepatic failure. Hemoperfusion rapidly removed chloramphenicol from an inadvertently intoxicated child (316).

Clindamycin (425 daltons), an especially useful drug for anaerobic infections, is about 95% bound in plasma and distributed in a volume of 0.66 l/kg from which it is rapidly cleared, mostly by the liver (13). The half-life in plasma is prolonged only slightly by renal failure (20, 83, 317) and is unaffected by dialysis which removes negligible amounts of clindamycin (Table 9). The clearance by hemoperfusion ranges from 55 to 125 ml/min (137).

Lincomycin, an analogue of clindamycin, is not as active an antibiotic and has more side effects, but a similar antibacterial spectrum and pharmacokinetics. Lincomycin (407 daltons) is highly protein bound and eliminated mostly by hepatic metabolism. Renal failure prolongs the half-life (Table 9) and removal by dialysis is minimal (318).

Erythromycin, a rather large solute (734 daltons), is moderately well absorbed from the gastrointestinal tract, about 70% protein bound in plasma and distributed in a volume of 0.6 l/kg (13). Elimination clearance exceeds 500 ml/min, mostly by the liver, and the half-life is prolonged only moderately in patients with renal failure (Table 9) from the normal value of 1.8 h (20, 319). Hemodialysis lowers plasma erythromycin concentrations minimally because of the large molecular size, the high fractional protein binding and the high distribution volume which even increases in uremia. Little or no dosage reduction is recommended in uremic patients but erythromycin may cause ototoxicity (320) or acute interstitital nephritis (59).

Vancomycin (about 1800 daltons) is an antistaphylococcal

Table 9. Miscellaneous antimicrobials: half-lives.

Drug	N	A	H
Colistimethate	4.0	15	14
Polymixin B	4.0	36	35
Sulfadiazine	8.0	22	11
Sulfisoxazole	6.0	11	6.0
Sulfamethoxazole	11	24	14
Chloramphenicol	3.0	4.5	4.3
Clindamycin	3.0	3.2	3.2
Lincomycin	4.5	12	10
Erythromycin	1.8	4.8	4.6
Vancomycin	6.0	200	100
Fosfomycin	1.5	20	3.0
Ciprofloxacin	4.5	10	3.2
Amphotericin B	24	24	24
5-Fluorocytosine	5.0	100	8.0
Ketoconazole	2.4	2.2	2.2
Metronidazole	7.2	8.5	3.0
Amantadine	14	200	24
Acyclovir	2.7	20	5.5
Trimethoprim	12	24	22

Average of published values, N = normal, A = anephric, H = hemodialysis.

antibiotic that is about 10% protein bound in plasma and slowly distributes into a volume of about 0.6 l/kg. Elimination is almost exclusively renal at 70% of the filtration rate (13). Vancomycin accumulates in plasma in patients with renal failure as the half-life is prolonged from 6 to 200 h (Table 9), and small amounts of this large solute are removed by hemodialysis but the half-life is reduced since the low dialyzer clearance equals or exceeds the very low clearance (about 4 ml/min) in anuric patients (321, 322). Accordingly, the dose should be decreased in uremic patients from the normal 1.0 g (about 600 μmol) every 12 h to 1.0 g every 7 days and this dose is also reasonable for hemodialysis patients. Transport across the peritoneum is measurable and the clearances (6.0 ml with intermittent peritoneal dialysis and 2.0 ml with CAPD) are comparable to those achieved with hemodialysis (323, 324). Hemofiltration achieves a clearance of about 140 ml/min and a half-life of 4 h, but only a central compartment is cleared and plasma concentrations rebound to values close to pretreatment levels (325). Overdosage of vancomycin can cause direct nephrotoxicity and ototoxicity.

Very little *novobiocin* (613 daltons) is excreted unchanged by the kidney and dialysis is not known to decrease appreciably its plasma concentration so no dosage modification is recommended for uremic patients (1).

Fosfomycin (182 daltons), a broad-spectrum antistaphylococcal antibiotic, distributes in 0.3 l/kg, is unbound in plasma, retained in renal failure (Table 9) and rapidly removed by hemodialysis (12, 326, 327). The dose should be decreased from 1.0 g every 6 h to 1.0 g every 24 h and a supplement of 800 mg should be given after hemodialysis.

Bacitracin (1411 daltons) is so nephrotoxic that its use is restricted to local application. If absorbed, this large poorly dialyzable solute is excreted mostly by the kidney at a clearance normally of 100 ml/min (328).

Urinary Antiseptics

Treatment of urinary tract infections with *nitrofurantoin* is less efficacious as renal failure decreases the normally high renal excretion and thus urinary concentration. Peripheral neuropathy and metabolic acidosis are complications that make it preferable to avoid nitrofurantoin in patients with renal failure (329). Although 60% protein bound in plasma, dialysance of nitrofurantoin (238 daltons) approaches 80 ml/min (71). *Nalidixic acid* (232 daltons), highly protein bound and eliminated by both hepatic metabolism and renal excretion, persists in plasma of uremic patients. Therapeutic efficacy of nalidixic acid diminishes with renal failure, side effects are more frequent, metabolic acidosis may be aggravated and dialytic removal has not been studied (330). *Pipemidic* acid (303 daltons) is related to nalidixic acid, distributes in a volume exceeding 2.0 l/kg and is cleared at 384 ml/min (214 ml/min renal); the half-life normally 4.6 h, increases with renal failure (331). Similarly, *methenamine mandelate* (292 daltons), normally rapidly excreted by the kidney with a half-life in plasma of 3 to 6 h (8), also presumably accumulates in renal failure. As it may exaggerate metabolic

acidosis, mandelamine should be avoided in uremic patients. Dialysis pharmacokinetics have not been studied. *Phenazopyridine* (Pyridium) is potentially nephrotoxic (332). Its elimination is delayed in renal failure and it should be avoided when possible in uremic patients. *Cinoxacin* is a synthetic organic compound used for the treatment of urinary tract infections. The normal half-life of 1.6 h increases to 12 h when the creatinine clearance is below 20 ml/min, consistent with decreased urinary concentrations and efficacy in uremia (333). *Norfloxacin*, an analogue of cinoxacin, is 40% renally eliminated, the half-life increasing from 4 h in normal subjects to 8 h in those with renal failure (334). *Ciprofloxacin*, another carboxyquinolone, is cleared at 600 ml/min (230 ml/min renal) from a distribution space of 2.1 l/kg and is retained in renal failure, the half-life increasing from about 4.5 h to about 10.0 h (335). The dose should be reduced by 50% with renal failure and the hemodialyzer clearance is 57 ml/min, which lowers the half-life to normal (Table 9). *Ofloxacin* also has a distribution volume exceeding 2.0 l/kg and is cleared at 241 ml/min (197 ml/min renal), the half-life increasing from the normal 7.9 h to 37 h with renal failure (336). Removal by dialysis is minimal. *Pefloxacin* also has a large distribution volume and a long half-life that is not appreciably influenced by hemodialysis (337).

Tuberculostatic drugs

Because of long-term use, excessive accumulation of tuberculostatic drugs may induce chronic toxicity. *Isoniazid* (137 daltons) is minimally bound in plasma (Table 10), distributed in a large volume and excreted in the urine at a clearance of about 40 ml/min partly unchanged, but mostly after acetylation (338). The acetylation rate varies among patients as genetically determined and also as influenced by hepatic function. Thus, the normal half-life varies from about 1.2 to 5 h. Renal failure prolongs the half-life to about 3 to 9 h, so the dose should not exceed 150 to 200 mg (1 to 1.5 mmol) daily (1–3, 83). Excessive dosage can be removed by hemodialysis which doubles the elimination rate, by peritoneal dialysis or by hemoperfusion (339–342). After dialysis, a supplemental dose of about 3 mg (22 μmol)/kg should be given (83, 342). *Rifampin*, a large solute (823 daltons), distributes in a large volume and is highly bound to plasma proteins (Table 10). Only a small fraction is eliminated by the kidney. Neither renal failure nor dialysis affect elimination kinetics sufficiently to warrant dosage modification (1, 8, 13). Acute hypersensitivity interstitial nephritis may occur, especially with intermittent rifampin therapy (343). This lesion may be insidious in onset and follow a prolonged course terminating with interstitial fibrosis (344). Rifampin can also induce digoxin and digitoxin metabolism, decreasing plasma levels and precipitating heart failure (345). *Ethambutol* (204 daltons) is minimally protein bound, but also distributes in a large volume (Table 10). It is excreted mostly unchanged by the kidney at a clearance exceeding 400 ml/min (346). Renal failure prolongs the half-life and the dose should be reduced. Hemodialyzer clearance is about 50 ml/

min which decreases the half-life in uremic patients to about 5 h, requiring a dosage supplement of about 5 mg (25 μmol)/ kg after dialysis. Since most *cycloserine* is excreted unchanged by the kidney, dosage reduction is advised in uremic patients if the drug must be used (1). This minimally bound small drug (102 daltons) should be removed rapidly by dialysis. Overdosage has been successfully treated by peritoneal dialysis with removal of 17% of the ingested dose (347). *Para-aminosalicylate* is excreted mostly by the kidney, partly unchanged and partly after acetylation or glycine conjugation. With renal failure, the half-life normally one hour, is prolonged to about 20 h and although some free para-aminosalicylate is removed by dialysis, the dose should not exceed 2 g/day (2, 3). *Pyrazinamide* (129 daltons) is excreted predominantly by the kidney so dosage reduction is advisable in uremic patients, whereas *ethionamide* elimination is mostly extrarenal and rapid (348). *Viomycin* is also eliminated mostly into the urine (148), but pharmacokinetics of each of these drugs during renal failure or dialysis has not been studied in detail. Both viomycin and *capreomycin* are potentially nephrotoxic (148).

Fungicides

Antifungal therapy with the insoluble polyene antibiotic, *amphotericin B,* is often limited by dose dependent and potentially reversible nephrotoxicity characterized by cylindruria, decreased renal blood flow and filtration rate, tubular acidosis, tubular necrosis and interstitial calcification (349, 350). The kidney eliminates only a small fraction of amphotericin B and preexisting renal failure does not demand dosage reduction, but the development of azotemia is an indication to discontinue the drug or decrease the dose. Salt depletion aggravates the fall in renal blood flow and filtration rate induced by amphotericin B while sodium loading attenuates it (351). Amphotericin B has a very large distribution space (4.0 l/kg), slow intercompartmental transfer and a normal half-life (Table 9) of about 24 h (14). Negligible amounts of amphotericin B (about 1,000 daltons and 90% protein bound in plasma) are removed by dialysis (352). Intraperitoneal administration is painful because of the irritant vehicle, sodium desoxycholate, and amphotericin increases the rate of peritoneal ultrafiltration (353).

Eliminated largely unchanged by the kidney at a clearance about two thirds that of creatinine, *5-fluorocytosine* (129 daltons) distributes in a volume of 0.6 l/kg and only about 5% is bound in plasma (354, 355). Renal failure prolongs the half-life from about 5 h to 100 h (14, 83, 355), increasing the likelihood of bone marrow suppression and hepatotoxicity. In uremic patients, the dosage must be decreased from 35 mg (270 μmol)/kg every 6 h to about 5 mg (40 μmol)/kg/24 h and the patient must be monitored carefully for toxicity. Hemodialysis achieves clearances of 85 ml/ min (144) and decreases the half-life to about 8 h (Table 9) so a maintenance dosage of 20 mg (150 μmol) after each dialysis is recommended (352, 355). The peritoneal clearance is close to that of urea (about 15 ml/min) and decreases the half-life by more than 50%.

Miconazole is an imidazole fungicide that is more than 90% bound in plasma and is eliminated mostly by the liver, so the normal half-life of about 24 h does not change appreciably in uremic patients (356, 357). Protein binding should inhibit removal by dialysis. *Ketoconazole* is 99% protein bound is plasma and cleared from a large distribution volume at more than 500 ml/min. The half-life of 2.4 h does not change appreciably with renal failure (357, 358). Hemodialysis removes negligible amounts of ketoconzaole and little penetrates into the peritoneum. *Fluconazole* is cleared slowly (0.5 ml/min) mostly by the kidney (70%) from a volume of 0.8 l/kg with a half life of 25 h. Because protein binding is minimal, some removal by dialysis is anticipated.

Miscellaneous Antimicrobials

Chloroquin (320 daltons) is 55% bound in plasma and highly bound in tissue. It is normally slowly eliminated from a large volume partly by biotransformation and partly unchanged by the kidney at a clearance approximately half that of creatinine and has a plasma half-life of about 60 h. The chloroquin clearance decreases when creatinine clearance does, but short courses of therapy for acute malaria do not require dosage modification (1, 359). With a glomerular filtration rate below 30 ml/min the half-life approaches 200 h, prolonged treatment should be avoided if possible and dosage should be limited to 100 mg (300 μmol)/day for the first 2 weeks and 50 mg daily thereafter (359). The hemodialyzer

Table 10. Pharmacokinetics of tuberculostatic drugs.

Drug	% Bound in plasma	DV (l/kg)	% Renal excretion	Half-life (h)		Dose (mg/kg)	
				N	A	N	A
Isoniazid	<10	0.7	15*	2.5	6.0	4.0/24h	3.0/24h
Rifampin	80	1.4	10	3.0	4.0	9/24h	9/24h
Ethambutol	20	1.2	80	3.0	9.0	20/24h	5/24h
P-Aminosalicylate	–	0.6	80	1.0	20	150/24h	Avoid
Cycloserine	<10	0.6	65	–	–	4/12h	–

Average of published values, DV = distribution volume, N = normal, A = anephric.
* After acetylation, most isoniazid is excreted in the urine.

clearance of 60 ml/min is only about 15% of total plasma clearance (360). *Chloroguanide,* a smaller molecule, is also bound in plasma but considerably less in tissue. Accordingly, renal excretion of the unchanged drug which accounts for 40 to 60% of elimination normally decreases plasma concentrations to negligible levels within 24 h, raising the possibility of slowed elimination in uremic patients (361). *Pyrimethamine* (249 daltons) has a renal clearance of about 3 ml/min and a plasma half-life of 4 to 6 days (362). The effect of renal failure and of dialysis on its pharmacokinetics needs further study. *Trimethoprim* is rapidly absorbed, is about 50% protein bound in plasma and distributed to a volume of 1.5 l/kg (14). About half of trimethoprim (290 daltons) is eliminated by the kidney at a clearance of 200 ml/min. The normal half-life of 12 h increases to 24 h in uremic patients (20, 302). Hemodialysis should lower the half-life only modestly and peritoneal dialysis achieves a clearance of about 4.0 ml/min (308). *Primaquine* (259 daltons) is rapidly biotransformed, little of the unchanged drug normally appearing in the urine. The hemolytic effect on sensitive erythrocytes and the antimalarial effect depend on the metabolite, the elimination kinetics of which need to be studied in uremic and hemodialysis patients (363). After virtually complete absorption, *quinine* (324 daltons) is distributed in tissue and in plasma is 70% bound. Largely biotransformed by hepatic hydroxylation, less than 5% of quinine is excreted unchanged by the kidney (363). The half-life of 4 to 6 h probably is unaffected by renal failure and little, if any, dose modification is required. Dose related toxicity includes hemolysis and tubular necrosis. Peritoneal clearance of quinine is 8 ml/min or less, below the normal renal clearance and much lower than achieved by hemodialysis *in vitro* (364). Quinine amblyopia improves with dialysis despite only modest reduction in plasma quinine concentrations (365).

Pentamidine (593 daltons), which is effective against Pneumocystis carinii, disappears rapidly from plasma into tissues where it persists for months (14). Because excretion is at least partially renal, modest dosage reduction is recommended with concurrent severe renal failure and nephrotoxicity is a potential complication (366).

Metronidazole (171 daltons) is a trichamonacidal antibiotic that is also effective against anaerobic organisms. In plasma about 20% binds to proteins. Metronidazole distributes in a 0.7 l/kg volume from which it is eliminated at a clearance of about 80 ml/min mostly by nonrenal mechanisms, predominantly hydroxylation to metabolites some of which are active. The normal half-life of about 7.2 h increases minimally with renal failure (Table 9) but is reduced by hemodialysis (which clears it at 60 ml/min) to about 3.0 h (11, 14, 367, 368). The hydroxymetabolites are retained in renal failure and comparably removed by dialysis. Peritoneal clearance (high flow) is 16 ml/min reducing the half-life to 5.2 h, while the clearance during CAPD is 5.2 ml/min which affects the half-life minimally (369). Overdosage can cause vestibular toxicity and symptoms that mimic uremia.

Tinidazole, a similar antiprotozoal drug, is about 10% bound in plasma, distributes in 0.7 l/kg and is cleared mostly by metabolism at about 35 ml/min (370). The half-life increases from about 14.5 h to about 16 h with renal failure but is reduced to 4.3 h by hemodialysis which clears it at 60 ml/min.

Ornidazole has similar kinetics; 10% is bound in plasma, the distribution volume is 0.7 l/kg, the normal clearance is 90 ml/min, of which 5 ml/min is renal, and the half-life is 12 h (371). The clearance decreases to 46 ml/min with renal failure but the half-life is not prolonged, so presumably the distribution volume decreases. The hemodialyzer clearance is 64 ml/min and peritoneal clearance during CAPD is 3.0 ml/min (371).

Mebendazole is about 90% bound in plasma, eliminated by hepatic metabolism and not appreciably removed by hemodialysis (372).

Thiabendazole, used for treatment of strongyloidiasis, is rapidly metabolized at about 1800 ml/min ($T^{1/2} = 1.2$ h) by the liver, so its elimination is unimpaired in uremic patients, but the hydroxymetabolite and glucuronide and sulfate esters may accumulate causing vomiting (373, 374). Removal of both thiabendazole and its metabolite by hemodialysis is minimal (clearances 14 to 19 ml/min) and dosage adjustment is not advised except that it is preferred to keep therapeutic courses brief. Hemoperfusion removes thiabendazole at 300 ml/min and the metabolites at 73 to 282 ml/min (374).

Dapsone (248 daltons), a sulfone used for therapy of leprosy, is distributed throughout body water and is about 50% bound in plasma (348). The normal half-life averages 28 h. Since about 70% of excretion is renal, dosage reduction has been recommended for uremic patients (8). With overdosage, dapsone elimination can be accelerated by hemodialysis or by oral charcoal treatment (375). Other drugs used for leprosy include *sulfoxane,* a substituted dapsone, and *amithiozone,* a thiosemicarbazone, both of which are likely to be retained in renal failure and *clofazimine,* a phenazine congener that has a large distribution volume and a long half-life and is less likely to be affected by impaired renal function. Dialysis pharmacokinetics of these drugs need to be studied.

Amantidine (109 daltons), an antiviral agent that is 60% bound in plasma, is eliminated by the kidney, normally at a clearance of about 400 ml/min from a very large distribution space (4.5 l/kg) with a resultant half-life in plasma of about 14 h (376, 377). It accumulates in patients with renal failure and can cause cardiac arrhythmias and neuropsychiatric toxicity (377). The half-life equals 14 × plasma creatinine concentration plus 3.4 h. Hemodialysis clears amantidine at 67 ml/min, reducing the extremely prolonged half-life in uremic patients (Table 9) to about 24 h (378). In uremic patients the dose should be decreased from 100 mg every 12 h to 100 mg every 7 days.

Acyclovir (225 daltons), an antiviral agent, distributes in 0.7 l/kg; it is about 20% bound in plasma. Elimination is mostly renal at a clearance of about 200 ml/min. The half-life, normally 2.7 h, increases to 20 h with renal failure (Table 9) and is reduced to 5.5 h by hemodialysis which achieves a clearance of about 100 ml/min (379, 380). With CAPD the peritoneal clearance is 4.0 ml/min, which lowers the half-life modestly (380). Overdosage can cause acute renal failure and coma (381).

Vidarabine (267 daltons) is eliminated by both renal and hepatic mechanisms, the half-life increasing from 1.5 h to 5 h with renal failure and only minimal dosage reduction being required (14).

Interferon pharmacokinetics are not affected appreciably by renal failure or by dialysis (382). The half-life is about 15 h.

Cardiovascular Drugs

Digitalis glycosides

Digitalis toxicity is a frequent and serious problem especially in patients with renal failure. Whenever possible, the therapeutic emphasis in dialysis patients should be on control of salt and water balance by restriction of intake and removal of excess by dialysis so that digitalis can be avoided or used in modest dosage.

Ouabain (585 daltons) is rapidly excreted by the normal kidney and the plasma half-life, normally 14 h, increases to 60 h in anuric patients (383). Little if any is bound in plasma and the distribution space is large. About 15% of a dose can be eliminated by dialysis. In contrast, *digitalis* (powdered leaf) is excreted more slowly but like ouabain is retained in renal failure, increasing the likelihood of intoxication.

Digitoxin and digoxin have been studied more extensively and because of shorter half-lives than digitalis and greater understanding of their kinetics, are preferred in patients with renal failure (384, 385). Aluminum hydroxide can decrease bioavailability of the cardiac glycosides (386).

Digoxin (781 daltons) is well absorbed, about 25% protein bound in plasma and distributed in a large volume, equivalent to about 9 l/kg because of considerable binding in tissue. Absorption is slower in uremic patients but higher plasma concentrations are obtained because tissue binding decreases with renal failure or hyperkalemia, reducing the volume of distribution by about 50% (39, 387). Hence, a full loading dose of digoxin can be hazardous and a dose of 10 μg (13 nmol)/kg has been recommended (388). Excretion is primarily by the kidney as unchanged digoxin at a clearance close to that of creatinine (384, 389). Digoxin half-life (Table 11) increases from 42 h to 120 h with advanced renal failure (13, 20, 83). There is also evidence that digoxin is partially reabsorbed and that excretion is flow rate dependent at low rates of urine flow (40). Optimal serum digoxin concentrations are 0.5 to 2.0 ng/ml (1 to 3 nmol/l). While toxicity may occur at these concentrations in association with such metabolic abnormalities as hypercalcemia and hypokalemia, toxicity is much more frequent with levels above 3.0 ng/ml (384). The maintenance dose for uremic patients should be reduced to about one-third of the usual. There are, however, considerable individual differences among uremic patients in digoxin bioavailability, distribution volume, clearance and sensitivity, and patients must be monitored carefully (390). Because of the narrow margin of safety, the dose should be calculated carefully and serum

concentrations assayed. The maintenance dose may be calculated from the equation, μg/kg/day = 0.06 Ccr + 1.3 (389). The creatinine clearance (Ccr) should not be assumed to be a simple reciprocal of serum creatinine concentration in the elderly, in those with decreased lean body mass or in dialyzed patients. Yet despite using formulae, many patients with renal failure can't be given the correct dose of digoxin because of such variables as the change in distribution volume, and in the number of binding sites and their affinity for the drug. Although digoxin traverses dialysis membranes, Clearances of only about 20 ml/min (386) do not affect the elimination half-life appreciably (although plasma levels may decrease transiently), supplemental dosage should not be given and potassium removal by dialysis may precipitate digitalis intoxication (391, 392). With hemofiltration, digoxin clearances are about 45 ml/min (386). Digoxin clearances of 50 to 100 ml/min have been achieved by hemoperfusion decreasing the half-life (393, 394), but only a small fraction of the absorbed drug is removed and the observed clinical improvement may relate to other factors. During continuous ambulatory peritoneal dialysis peritoneal digoxin clearance is 2.0 ml/min, which is much less than the endogenous removal rate (386, 395).

Digitoxin (765 daltons) is almost completely absorbed and is extensively metabolized by hepatic microsomal enzymes. The kidney excretes mostly cardioinactive metabolites and only about 10% unchanged digitoxin. Optimal serum concentrations are 10 to 35 ng/ml (15 to 50 nmol/l) and toxicity is usually associated with concentrations above 40 ng/ml (389). The volume of distribution of this lipophilic drug is about 0.5 l/kg (13, 83, 396), decreasing somewhat with renal failure. Renal failure prolongs the half-life only slightly (Table 11) from about 150 to 170 h (13, 20, 397). Accordingly, the dose requires little reduction in uremic patients (about 70% of the usual maintenance of 0.1 to 0.2 mg/day) but maximal loading doses may be hazardous. With severe coexistent liver failure, the dose of digitoxin must be reduced further. The metabolism of digitoxin may be accelerated by drugs such as phenobarbital and rifampin that induce microsomal enzymes (345). As digitoxin is about 90% protein bound in plasma, little is removed by dialysis. The long half-life, even in patients with normal elimination rates, portends a prolonged episode of digitalis intoxication, once it occurs. Hemoperfusion, however, can double the elimination rate of experimentally intoxicated dogs and may be useful clinically (398).

Mibrinone, a new nonglycosidic inotropic agent with vasodilator properties, has a normal renal clearance of 288 ml/min and a half-life of 1.0 h that increases to 3.0 h with renal failure (399).

Antiarrhythmic agents

Procainamide (272 daltons) is well absorbed and distributes rapidly to tissues where it is bound. About 20% is bound in plasma and the distribution volume is about 2.0 l/kg (13, 14, 400). Therapeutic plasma concentrations are 4 to 8 μg/ml (15 to 30 μmol/l). Elimination is partly by acetylation at a genetically determined rate and partly by renal excretion of the unchanged drug (400). Nonrenal clearance in slow acetylators is 240 ml/min and in fast acetylators is 350 ml/min, while renal clearance is normally 370 ml/min regardless of acetylator type (14, 401). Despite lowering the distribution volume, renal failure increases the half-life to 10 to 16 h from the normal 2.5 to 3.5 h (Table 11) and the dosing interval should be increased to 12 to 24 h from the usual 4 to 6 h, or the drug should be avoided (14, 83, 401, 402). The N-acetyl metabolite is pharmacologically active, depends highly on renal elimination and is retained in renal failure as the half-life increases from 6 h to 41 h (401, 403). The hemodialyzer clearance is about 60 ml/min for both procainamide (and its metabolite) which reduces the half-life to about 6 h, justifying a small supplement thereafter (402–404). The clearance by hemoperfusion is about 125 ml/min. Peritoneal clearances during CAPD are below 6.0 ml/min and do not abbreviate the half-life (405).

Quinidine is almost completely absorbed from the gastrointestinal tract and in plasma 80% is bound at therapeutic concentrations of 2 to 5 μg/ml (6 to 15 μmol/l). Quinidine (324 daltons) distributes in a large volume (2.5 l/kg) because of binding by tissue proteins (13, 14). Elimination occurs mostly by hepatic hydroxylation at a clearance of about 300 ml/min with a half-life of 7 h which is not appreciably prolonged by renal failure (Table 11), but excretion of the metabolites is delayed (406). Intoxication with quinidine manifesting resistant shock has been treated by hemodialysis which achieves a clearance of 20 ml/min, reduces plasma concentrations by 25%, shortens the half-life slightly and induces clinical improvement (407). Because hypokalemia protects against quinidine intoxication, low potassium dialysate is recommended. During CAPD the peritoneal clearance is only about 1.0 ml/min which does not affect the half-life appreciably (408).

Disopyramide (340 daltons), a well absorbed antiarrhythmic drug, distributes in a volume of 0.8 l/kg. Plasma protein binding correlates inversely with drug concentration and is about 40% at therapeutic plasma levels of 3 μg/ml (9 μmol/l) (13). Elimination occurs by the kidney, both as unchanged drug and as the dealkylated metabolite. The clearance decreases from 106 ml/min to about 50 ml/min with renal failure (409). The elimination half-life correlates with creatinine clearance, increasing with renal failure (410), but is lowered by dialysis (Table 11).

Lidocaine is eliminated almost entirely by the liver at a clearance of about 600 ml/min. Renal failure does not alter the distribution volume (1.5 l/kg), protein binding in plasma (60%), or elimination half-life (2 h) and no change in dosage is required (13, 14, 411, 412). Heart failure decreases both the distribution volume and the clearance, so peak concentrations are higher, but the half-life is not prolonged. The hemodialyzer clearance of about 20 ml/min is insufficient to warrant dosage adjustment (413).

Tocainide is an orally active lidocaine analogue normally distributed in 1.6 l/kg, 10% bound in plasma and cleared at 180 ml/min, 40% of which is by the kidney (414). The half-life increases from about 13 h to 24 h with renal failure as the clearance falls to about 100 ml/min, but the distribution volume increases. Hemodialysis shortens the half-life to 8.5 h.

Mexilitine is also effective orally, is 60% bound to plasma proteins, and distributes in a very large volume, 8.0 l/kg, from which it is normally cleared at more than 500 ml/min. The half-life of 10.4 h increases to about 17.3 h as the clearance falls to 300 ml/min with renal failure. Neither hemodialysis nor peritoneal dialysis remove appreciable quantities of mexilitine (415, 416).

Lorcainide is about 70% bound in plasma and eliminated with a half-life of 5.1 h that increases to 7.0 h with renal failure (417). Only about 10% is removed by hemodialysis which does not decrease the half-life.

Bretylium, an adrenergic neuronal blocker that has potent anti-arrhythmic action, distributes in a very large volume and is excreted mostly unchanged by the kidney with a half-life of about 8 h (418). In uremic patients the half-life is prolonged to about 30 h but decreases to 13 h with hemodialysis.

Amiodarone is orally effective and shares some properties of bretyllium. It is highly bound in plasma, has a very large distribution volume and a low renal clearance and is not recovered in hemodialysate (419). The half-life of 6.1 h is not affected by renal failure.

Cibenzoline has a very large distribution volume and a high clearance, mostly renal. Renal failure prolongs the half-life from about 7 h to 13 h (420).

The calcium channel blockers are discussed below, beta blockers are discussed under antihypertensive drugs, and phenytoin is discussed under anticonvulsants.

Calcium channel blockers

Verapamil (454 daltons) is about 90% bound in plasma, distributes in about 5 l/kg, and is metabolized with a half-life of 5.0 h to norverapamil, a less potent agent with a half-life

Table 11. Half-lives of cardiovascular drugs.

Drug	Half-life		
	N	A	H
Digoxin	42	120	90
Digitoxin	150	170	160
Procainamide	3.0	13	6.0
Quinidine	7.0	10	9.0
Disopyramide	7.0	17	13
Lidocaine	2.0	2.0	2.0
Tocainide	13	24	8.5
Mexilitine	10.4	17.3	17
Bretylium	8.0	30	13
Verapamil	5.0	3.7	3.7
Nifedipine	3.0	3.0	3.0
Diltiazem	5.0	3.5	3.5

Average of published values, DV = distribution volume, N = normal, A = anephric, H = hemodialysis.

of about 10 h (421, 422). With renal failure the half-life is somewhat shorter, presumably due to a smaller distribution space. Hemodialysis removes only small amounts of verapamil and its metabolite.

Nifedipine (346 daltons) is more than 90% bound to plasma proteins, has a large distribution volume (over 3 l/kg), a hepatic clearance above 1.1 l/min, and a half-life of about 3.0 h. The metabolites are inactive. Neither renal failure nor dialysis affect the half-life (423–425). Hemodialyzer clearances are less than 5.0 ml/min. Hemoperfusion does not add impressively to total plasma clearance.

Diltiazem (410 daltons) is also eliminated from a volume of about 4 l/kg by metabolism. The deacetylated metabolite has about half the activity of the parent compound. The normal half-life of about 5.0 h may be shorter in patients with renal failure and the metabolite does not accumulate (426). Plasma protein binding of about 80% inhibits removal by dialysis.

Nitrendipine has a half-life of about 4.8 h which is unrelated to renal function (427).

Antihypertensives

In uremic patients, hypertension is a frequent problem, often responsive to dietary sodium restriction, diuretics, and dialysis. Whereas excessive salt depletion may precipitate reversible uremia in patients with preterminal renal failure, once terminal oliguria occurs therapy of hypertension must stress control of sodium balance. Some patients only respond after hemofiltration, continuous ambulatory peritoneal dialysis or use of potent antihypertensive drugs, which should not substitute for sodium homeostasis and should be titrated carefully against blood pressure (see also Chapter 34).

Reserpine therapy may be complicated by bradycardia, peptic ulceration, nasal congestion, depression, diarrhea and extrapyramidal disturbances. Partially absorbed, reserpine distributes in a large volume including body fat and is about 40% bound in plasma. It rapidly depletes catecholamines. Reserpine is eliminated partially unchanged by the kidney and partially after metabolic hydrolysis (428). The half-life, normally 48 to 96 h, increases non-linearly as creatinine clearance decreases and little reserpine (609 daltons) should be removed by dialysis because of its large size and large distribution volume.

Hydralazine, a peripheral vasodilator, may cause tachycardia, headache, neuropathy, anemia, retroperitoneal fibrosis (429) and a lupus like syndrome. Peak plasma concentrations of hydralazine may exceed 1 µg/ml normally and the kidney excretes a small fraction of the drug while most undergoes hepatic acetylation at a clearance of about 400 ml/min (430). Hydralazine is about 85% protein bound in plasma, distributes in a volume of 1.9 l/kg with an elimination half-life (Table 12) of about 2.5 h, only minimally affected by the acetylation rate (13). Increased plasma concentrations in uremic patients (430) may represent a retained metabolite. Plasma protein binding (85%) limits removal of this small solute (160 daltons) by dialysis.

Prazosin, also a sympatholytic vasodilator, is about 95% bound in plasma and distributes in a 0.6 l/kg volume (13, 431). The elimination half-life of about 3 h increases minimally in patients with renal failure (Table 12) because less than 1.0% is excreted by the kidney. The blood pressure response may be augmented and prolonged in patients with renal failure in association with increased bioavailability, higher peak plasma concentrations and a change in the distribution volume (432). Because of the high fractional protein binding, little prazosin (391 daltons) should be removed by dialysis.

The metabolic fate of other pertinent α adrenergic blockers such as *phentolamine, phenoxybenzamine* and *dibenamine* is unknown. Renal failure is not known to affect their pharmacokinetics. *Tolazoline* is rapidly excreted by the kidney, however, via the organic base secretory pathway (433) and dosage reduction should be indicated in uremic patients. The distribution volume is 1.6 l/kg; the half-life increases from 4.4 h to 8.3 h with renal failure (434).

Doxazosin distributes in 1.0 l/kg; it is cleared at 88 ml/min with a normal half-life of 9.5 h that increases to 13.3 h with renal failure (435). The antihypertensive effect is prolonged by renal failure and 98% protein binding in plasma inhibits removal by dialysis. *Urapadil* is 94% bound in plasma, is cleared at 200 ml/min mostly by nonrenal mechanisms and has a normal half-life of 3.7 h (436). *Indoramin* is 85% bound in plasma, distributes in 7.4 l/kg and has a hepatic clearance of about 1500 ml/min with a normal half-life of 5.5 h (437). *Terazosin* is eliminated mostly by nonrenal

Table 12. Hlf-lives of antihypertensive, vasodilator and diuretic drugs.

Drug	Half-life		
	N	A	H
Hydralazine	2.5	11	10
Prazosin	3.0	3.6	3.6
Methyl Dopa	6.0	15.6	9.5
Clonidine	12	40	20
Minoxidil	4.0	4.0	–
Captopril	1.5	32	4.0
Propranolol	3.8	3.6	3.6
Sotalol	5.0	50	7.0
Practolol	9.0	60	14
Acebutolol	4.0	4.0	3.6
Atenolol	6.0	50	6.0
Metoprolol	4.0	4.0	–
Labetalol	4.5	5.5	5.0
Chlorothiazide	1.5	5.0	–
Furosemide	0.9	4.0	3.0
Bumetanide	1.5	2.0	–
Triamterene	4.2	10	–
Amiloride	6.0	100	–
Theophylline	8.0	8.0	2.5
Dyphylline	2.0	12.0	5.5

Average of published values, N = normal, A = anephric, H = hemodialysis.

mechanisms and the normal 10 h half-life is not prolonged by renal failure (438).

Methyldopa is excreted predominantly by the kidney, but most of the drug is first conjugated by the liver to the ortho-methyl sulfate. The distribution space of α methyldopa is about 0.4 l/kg; elimination is biphasic with half-lives of about 2 h (Table 12). With renal failure methyldopa accumulates (439), but the rate of hepatic conjugation increases. Toxicity includes drowsiness, impotence, hemolytic anemia, hepatic dysfunction and retroperitoneal fibrosis. Dialysis removes 30 to 40% of an administered dose of methyldopa (211 daltons) at a dialysance one-third that of urea (440).

Clonidine, an imidazoline derivative, also lowers blood pressure by altering central nervous sympathetic activity. The drug is well absorbed, about 30% bound in plasma and distributed in a big volume, about 3 l/kg (13, 14). More than half of administered clonidine is excreted by the kidney and the removal rate, normally about 200 ml/min, correlates with creatinine clearance (441). The normal half-life of about 12 h increases (Table 12) to about 40 h with severe renal failure (41, 441, 442). The clearance of clonidine (230 daltons) by hemodialysis averages about 40 ml/min which removes 5% of an administered dose but decreases the half-life. Only minimal reduction of the maintenance dose is advised for uremic patients as determined by the blood pressure response.

Guanfacine (252 daltons) is an antihypertensive with properties similar to clonidine. The total plasma clearance is about 360 ml/min and the half-life is 12 h. Although 80% is excreted by the kidney, renal failure does not result in retention of the drug because the metabolic clearance rate increases in uremic patients (443, 444). About 15% is unbound in plasma and the hemodialyzer clearance of 53 ml/min does not lower the half-life very much (443).

Guanethidine (198 daltons), a potent postganglionic blocker, is excreted mostly by hepatic metabolism. The renal clearance is 300 ml/min but the normal half-life of guanethidine is long, consistent with a large distribution space (445). Although small amounts of the drug persist for days because of tissue uptake, urinary excretion appears to be an important pathway for elimination of guanethidine, the side effects of which include postural hypotension, bradycardia, impotence, diarrhea, and nasal congestion. Dialysis kinetics of this small solute have not been studied.

Since elimination of hexamethonium, a ganglionic blocker, is mostly renal at a clearance approximating that of inulin, retention would be anticipated in uremic patients and dosage reduction required (446). Similarly, *mecamylamine* excretion by the kidney is decreased with renal failure and blood pressure should be titrated with lower doses (447). *Tetraethylammonium* is rapidly and quantitatively eliminated by the kidney by secretion via the organic base pathway. Caution is advised in treating uremic patients since elimination is delayed (448).

Plasma clearance of *minoxidil*, a potent vasodilator, approaches 600 ml/min, most of which is by hepatic glucuronide conjugation (449). The distribution volume approaches 3 l/kg; the half-life is 4 h (Table 12). Little unchanged minoxidil appears in the urine, and accumulation is not expected in uremic patients. The remarkably potent antihypertensive effect of minoxidil is sometimes accompanied by unanticipated improvement in renal function that justifies its use in severe hypertension. Minoxidil (212 daltons), which is not protein bound, should cross dialysis membranes readily but the dialyzer clearance shouldn't decrease the half-life appreciably because of the large distribution volume. Side effects include salt retention, hypertrichosis and an increased incidence of pericardial effusion (450).

Diazoxide achieves a peak therapeutic concentration of 20 μg/ml (90 μmol/l), 95% of which is protein bound and distributes in 0.25 l/kg; its half-life is about 24 h (451). The potent vasodilator effect of this salt retaining thiazide correlates with the unbound fraction. About 30% of renal excretion is as the unchanged drug at a clearance of 25 ml/min, while the metabolites are cleared at 100 ml/min. Uremia does not change the half-life appreciably, but decreases the bound fraction to 85% while the pharmacologic activity of a given blood level or dose is not increased (452). Despite the protein binding, the clearance by hemodialysis is 25 ml/min and peritoneal dialysis shortens the half-life (453).

Nitroprusside is eliminated by metabolism, but the metabolite, thiocyanate depends on renal elimination, can cause psychosis and hypothyroidism and is rapidly removed by dialysis (454). When given systemically, nitroprusside does not preferentially dilate the mesenteric vasculature or increase peritoneal clearances, but it does when administered intraperitoneally (104, 105).

Captopril (217 daltons) is about 30% bound in plasma, and distributes in 0.7 l/kg; its clearance is about 800 ml/min, half of which is renal (13, 455, 456). The normal half-life is about 1.5 h, increasing to 32 h with severe renal failure (Table 12). Hemodialysis achieves a clearance of 112 ml/min, reducing the half-life to below 4 h (456). The antihypertensive effect is prolonged with renal failure. Captopril can induce proteinuria, membranous glomerulopathy and reversible renal failure (457). *Enalopril* (464 daltons) is hydrolyzed to the decarboxylic acid enalaprilate, the active compound which has a renal clearance of 111 ml/min and a half-life of 8.4 h, prolonged to 10.9 h with renal failure (458).

β adrenergic blockers

The β adrenergic blocking agents, useful for the treatment of hypertension, angina pectoris and cardiac arrythmias, have pharmacokinetics that vary considerably among the different congeners (459). *Propranolol* (259 daltons), the prototype, undergoes first pass hepatic metabolism, which may be reduced in uremia, and is then about 93% bound in plasma and distributed in a volume of 3.6 l/kg (13, 14, 459). Hepatic clearance of 800 ml/min biotransforms propranolol to 4-hydroxypropranolol, napthoxylactic acid and unidentified metabolites (460, 461). The half-life, normally 3.8 h, is not prolonged by renal failure (Table 12), but the metabolites persist at high concentrations with a half-life of 120 h (461, 462). Hemodialysis clears propranolol at 15% of the urea clearance which doesn't reduce the half-life, but the metabolites are cleared rapidly by dialysis, reducing the half-life to 5 h (442, 460). Cimetidine, which decreases hepatic blood flow, reduces the elimination rate of propranolol by about 30% (463).

Other nonselective β adrenergic blockers include *Nadolol* (307 daltons), which has a 16 h half-life normally that is prolonged to 45 h with renal failure (14). Its elimination correlates with glomerular filtration rate and it is removed by hemodialysis (464).

Pindolol, about 50% bound in plasma and distributed in a volume of 2 l/kg, is normally cleared at 540 ml/min, half of which is by the kidney (459, 465). Its half-life, normally 3.5 h, is not appreciably prolonged in patients with renal failure. The half-life of the hydroxy-metabolite is 8 h.

Mepindolol (methyl pindolol) is eliminated by nonrenal mechanisms and does not accumulate in renal failure (466). Its half-life is 4 h.

Sotalol elimination is predominantly renal at a clearance of 110 ml/min and correlates with creatinine clearance (467). With renal failure, its half-life increases from about 5 h to 50 h (Table 12) but it is reduced by hemodialysis to 7 h (464, 467, 468). Because of rebound from the large distribution volume (2.4 l/kg), plasma concentrations increase after dialysis.

The half-life of *timolol* (4 h) is not prolonged by renal failure since elimination is mostly hepatic from a distribution volume of 1.6 l/kg (464).

Oxprenol distributes in 1.2 l/kg, is 80% bound in plasma and has a normal half-life of 2.0 h with a clearance of 600 ml/min (459). Neither renal failure nor dialysis should affect elimination kinetics extensively. Retroperitoneal fibrosis is a potential risk (469).

Alprenol is 85% bound in plasma, distributes into a volume of 3.3 l/kg and is metabolized at 1200 ml/min with a half-life of about 3 h (459). The hydroxy-metabolite is active. Renal failure should not cause drug retention and protein binding should inhibit removal by dialysis.

Practolol, the prototype of the cardioselective β adrenergic blockers, depends on renal elimination. The normal half-life of 9 h increases to about 60 h with severe renal failure (Table 12) but it is reduced to 14 h by hemodialysis (470). Fractional binding in plasma is low and the distribution space is 1.6 l/kg. Epithelial cell toxicity such as retroperitoneal fibrosis limits its use.

Acebutolol is 26% protein bound, distributes in volume of 1.2 l/kg and is eliminated at a clearance of about 600 ml/min, mostly by biotransformation to a N-acetylmetabolite (13, 459, 471, 472). Renal failure does not increase the half-life, normally about 4 h (Table 12), but prolongs the half-life of its metabolite, normally 8 h, to 32 h. Hemodialysis clears acebutolol at a rate of about 42 ml/min, decreasing the half-life of both the drug and its metabolite (471).

Atenolol (266 daltons) distributes in 0.7 l/kg; it is eliminated predominantly by the kidney at a clearance about 80% that of creatinine (473). Protein binding is minimal. The elimination half-life increases from 6 h to about 50 h when renal failure occurs (Table 12) and the dose must be decreased to about 25% of the usual 100 mg (0.4 mmol)/d (442, 473–475). Hemodialysis reduces the half-life to about 6 h so supplemental dosage is needed thereafter (442, 474). With peritoneal dialysis the half-life is about 24 h (475) and the peritoneal clearance is 2.5 ml/min. Atenolol and other β adrenergic blocking agents can cause retroperitoneal fibrosis (469).

Metoprolol (253 daltons) is about 12% bound in plasma, distributes in about 5.0 l/kg; and is eliminated at a clearance of 1,100 ml/min by α hydroxylation (13, 459). The half-life of 4 h is not increased by renal failure (Table 12) which does prolong the half-life of the active hydroxymetabolite to 72 h or longer (442, 476). Hemodialysis reduces the half-life of the metabolite to 5 h.

Labetalol is about 50% bound in plasma, distributes in about 8.0 l/kg and has a high hepatic clearance, about 1500 ml/min unaffected by renal failure (13, 459, 477). The half-life is 4.5 h normally, 5.5 h with renal failure and 5.0 h during hemodialysis (Table 12). The hemodialyzer clearance is 30 ml/min and the peritoneal clearance is 2.0 ml/min.

Tolamolol distributes in 3.2 l/kg; it is about 90% bound in plasma. Its clearance is 1,000 ml/min and its half-life is about 3 h (459). Neither renal failure nor dialysis should influence its elimination kinetics to a great extent.

Betaxolol clearance, normally 132 ml/min, decreases by 50% with renal failure and the half-life increases from about 18 h to about 32 h (478). Its distribution space is about 8.2 l/kg.

Butofilolol has a normal half-life of 19 h unaffected by renal failure (479).

Diuretics

As renal failure progresses, potent diuretics become less effective, most agents are clinically ineffective and the risk of drug toxicity increases.

Mannitol is distributed extracellularly and cleared by glomerular filtration. With renal failure the half-life of mannitol increases to 36 h from 1.3 h, prolonging the expansion of extracellular fluid volume, potentially precipitating heart failure, hyponatremia and hyperosmolar coma (480). Little osmotic diuresis ensues. In anephric patients, the plasma clearance of mannitol is only 2 ml/min (481). With peritoneal dialysis the half-life is 21 h and with hemodialysis it is 6 h, but rapid dialysis should be avoided to prevent disequilibrium.

Organic *mercurials* are bound in tissue, particularly renal tubular cells, and rapidly excreted by the kidney. Renal failure increases the half-life from the normal 2.5 h to more than 24 h, and with preexisting renal insufficiency mercurials should be avoided (14, 482). Shortly after a massive dose, sufficient mercury may be in circulation that slow dialytic removal may add to the impaired total elimination rate.

After nearly complete gastrointestinal absorption, *acetazolamide* (222 daltons) is 80% protein bound in plasma, tightly bound in tissues to carbonic anhydrase and excreted by the kidney with a normal half-life of 8 h. It is retained in renal failure and may aggravate acidosis (1). The clearance by hemodialysis is 22 ml/min (483).

Thiazides, distributed extracellularly and 20 to 95% bound in plasma, are excreted unchanged by the kidney within a few hours by filtration and secretion. Patients with heart failure or impaired renal function excrete chlorothiazide more slowly, prolonging the half-life from about 1.5 h to 5 h (1, 13, 14). Hydrochlorothiazide has a normal half-life of 2.5 h and is similarly retained. *Chlorthalidone* normally has a half-life of about 44 h which increases with renal failure (13, 484). *Indapamide* has a half-life of 21 h. It doesn't accumulate in renal failure and is not removed by dialysis (485). An extrarenal effect of thiazides may be potentiation of parathyroid hormone activity increasing serum calcium and magnesium in maintenance dialysis patients (486). Most thiazide complications, however, are either those of diuresis or related to hypersensitivity, e.g. acute interstitial nephritis (59, 487).

Despite renal failure, *ethacrynic acid* may induce saluresis but often only after high doses with attendant ototoxicity, hyperuricemia and gastrointestinal disturbances (45, 488). Elimination of ethacrynic acid at a half-life of about 3 h is partly hepatic and partly renal. This highly bound drug is secreted by the organic acid pathway after which some pH dependent back diffusion occurs. High doses of either *metalozone* or *furosemide* can also induce a clinically effective diuresis despite several renal failure (489, 490). The half-life of metolazone is normally 4 h which should increase in uremic patients (484). About 90% of furosemide is bound is plasma. With renal failure binding decreases to 70% (491). It is distributed in 0.3 l/kg, excreted by the kidney at a clearance close to that of creatinine and retained in renal failure and cirrhosis (492, 493). With renal failure the half-life increases from 0.9 h to 4.0 h (494). Toxicity includes gastrointestinal disturbances, hyperuricemia, hyperglycemia, and deafness (488). Acute interstitial nephritis has rarely been attributed to furosemide or thiazides (495). *Bumetanide* distributes in 0.12 l/kg, is cleared at 160 ml/min and has a half-life of 1.5 h which rises to 2.0 h with renal failure (496). *Muzolamine* is also effective despite renal impairment. Higher doses are required but the half-life (1.5 h) is prolonged (484). *Torasemide* has a half-life of 3.2 h uninfluenced by renal failure, hemodialysis or hemofiltration (497). *Etozolin* has a half-life of about 8.0 h unaffected by renal failure (498). *Piretanide,* another potent loop diuretic, is 95% bound in plasma, distributes in 0.2 l/kg and cleared at 240 ml/min, about half renal (499, 500). With renal failure the half-life increases from 1.0 h to 2.2 h and protein binding decreases to 90%. Potent diuretics influence tubular transport of toxins and can aggravate renal ischemia secondary to extracellular volume depletion. The new uricosuric saluretic, *ticrynafen,* has induced renal failure frequently, due to tubular degeneration, interstitial nephritis or acute uric acid precipitation (501).

With renal failure the aldosterone antagonist, *spironolactone,* is less effective but the risk of hyperkalemia is increased because extrarenal potassium loss decreases (8). Spironolactone is rapidly biotransformed by the liver to active metabolites that may be retained in renal failure (502). *Triamterene* also may cause hyperkalemia. Normally that drug is about 50% bound in plasma, distributes in a volume of 2.5 l/kg and is cleared mostly by metabolism with a half-life of 4.2 h and to a lesser extent by the kidney by filtration and secretion (503). The hydroxymetabolites may be pharmacologically active. Trimaterene can induce immune hemolytic anemia with reversible oliguric renal failure (504). *Amiloride* elimination correlates with creatinine clearance. Renal failure prolongs the half-life from 6 h to over 100 h (505). There are limited data on the effect of dialysis on plasma concentrations of most diuretics, although protein binding limits the diffusion of most of these drugs.

Other vasoactive drugs

Since *theophylline* is eliminated mainly by hepatic oxidation, the half-life, normally 8 h, does not increase in uremia (13). Because theophylline is rapidly removed from a distribution volume of 0.5 l/kg by peritoneal dialysis (9.5 ml/min), hemodialysis (80 ml/min) or hemoperfusion (140 ml/min), supplemental dosage may be required after these procedures to maintain therapeutic levels (506–511). The half-life with peritoneal dialysis is 5.5 h and with hemodialysis 2.5 h. *Dyphylline* distributes in 0.8 l/kg, has a high renal clearance and half-life of 2.0 h. Renal failure prolongs the half-life to 12 h and hemodialysis lowers it to 5.5 h (512).

Nitroglycerin does not depend on the kidney for elimination (13). *Isosorbide dinitrate* has a normal half-life of 4 h that increases minimally with renal failure. The volume of distribution and the clearance are very high and the hemodialyzer clearance of 92 ml/min does not affect the plasma level (513). *Amphetamine, ephedrine* and *phentermine* are partially excreted unchanged and partially metabolized (1). Accumulation of these drugs may occur in patients with renal failure, but other sympathomimetic amines are largely metabolized. More than half of *neostigmine* is excreted by the kidney and renal failure prolongs the half-life from 1.3 h to 3.0 h (514). *Buflomedil* distributes in 1.4 l/kg, is mostly metabolized and has a half-life of 3.1 h which increases to 5.4 h with renal failure (515).

Sedatives, tranquilizers, and psychotherapeutic drugs

Barbiturates that have a longer duration of activity have lower fractional protein binding and lipid solubility and higher renal excretion and dialyzer clearances than short-acting congeners (79). *Barbital* (184 daltons) is not concentrated in body fat, is only 5% bound in plasma and is excreted predominantly by the kidney at a clearance well below the filtration rate due to passive back diffusion. It may accumulate in uremic patients (516). Renal excretion of *phenobarbital* (232 daltons) also occurs by filtration with pH dependent back diffusion, accounting for 25% of its elimination, increasing with alkaline osmotic diuresis to a maximum of 17 ml/min (517). The remainder is inactivated by hepatic microsomal enzymes. In plasma about 20% of phenobarbital is protein bound at therapeutic concentrations. Because of a lipid partition coefficient of 3:1, the distribution space is about 0.9 l/kg (13). The normal half-life is about 90 h (Table 13). Retention of phenobarbital may aggravate uremic lethargy and coma, and with renal failure the dose should be decreased and the patient monitored for oversedation (18). Peritoneal clearance of phenobarbital (255 daltons) is 5 to 10 ml/min, but increases by as much as 30 percent with an alkaline buffer or protein in the dialysate (518). Intraperitoneal furosemide increases peritoneal clearance of phenobarbital from 6 to 16 ml/min (519). Hemodialyzer clearances exceeding 50 ml/min improve acute intoxication but at low plasma concentrations higher fractional binding may limit depletion (79). With hemoperfusion the clearance is 138 ml/min, reducing the half-life to about 8.0 h (520). In contrast to these barbiturates, *thiopental* is ultrashort-acting because its very high lipid partition coefficient causes rapid distribution out of plasma into a 1.9 l/kg volume. It is about 80% bound in plasma and has a normal half-life of about 10 h. Although eliminated by metabolism rather than by renal excretion, thiopental narcosis is prolonged by uremia (48). *Secobarbital* and *pentobarbital*, preferentially distributed in body fat and about 40 and 30% bound in plasma, are short-acting and eliminated predominantly by hepatic biotransformation (521). Protein binding of pentobarbital decreases when renal failure occurs (522). Clearances of these barbiturates by forced diuresis and peritoneal dialysis do not exceed 5 ml/min despite alkaline, osmotic diuresis or intraperitoneal alkali or albumin, and the half-lives are affected only slightly (79, 523). Hemodialyzer clearances above 30 ml/min decrease the half-life of severely intoxicated patients from 35 to 20 h (79). With renal failure the half-life is about 45 h (Table 13). *Amobarbital* and *butabarbital* are intermediate in their elimination rates by dialy-

Table 13. Half-lives of sedatives, tranquilizers and analgesics.

Drug	Half-life		
	N	A	H
Phenobarbital	90	144	8.0
Pentobarbital	35	45	20
Diazepam	40	40	–
Oxazepam	8.0	22	–
Glutethimide	40	–	15
Chlorpromazine	30	30	30
Imipramine	18	18	18
Nortriptyline	31	31	31
Bromide	24	–	2.0
Lithium	22	40	6.0
Ethosuccimide	50	–	3.5
Salicylic acid	3.8	8.1	4.9
Acetaminophen	2.5	2.5	1.6
Ibuprofen	2.0	2.0	2.0
Naproxen	15	15	15
Sulfinpyrazone	2.5	9.5	9.5

Average of published values, N = normal, A = anephric, H = hemodialysis.

sis, protein binding, lipid partition and duration of action. Lipid soluble barbiturates are cleared more rapidly (120 to 140 ml/min) by hemoperfusion through charcoal or resin columns (520, 524–526).

The benzodiazepines are all more than 80% bound in plasma and are biotransformed by the liver. *Chlordiazepoxide* (300 daltons) distributes into a volume of 0.3 l/kg and *diazepam* (285 daltons) into 1.1 l/kg (13, 527). In uremic patients, protein binding of diazepam decreases, which may increase its pharmacologic effect (528). Benzodiazepine pharmacokinetics are complex with active metabolites excreted by the kidney and half lives of about 10 h (chlordiazepoxide) and 40 h (diazepam), but the drugs are generally well tolerated by uremic patients (1, 67, 529). Little removal occurs with dialysis (Table 13), but pharmacokinetics have not been studied in detail (530). *Lorazepam* and *oxazepam* distribute into 1.1 l/kg and 1.0 l/kg volumes and are eliminated with half-lives of 14 h and 8 h (Table 13) by conjugation to metabolites that are inactive, unlike the other benzodiazepines (13, 67, 527). With renal failure oxazepam half-life increases to 22 h (531). *Flurazepam* has a distribution volume of 3.4 l/kg and a half-life of about 72 h that depends in small part on renal elimination (13, 14, 527). Nevertheless, a metabolic encephalopathy can occur from retention of a poorly dialyzable flurazepam metabolite in uremic patients treated with the usual dose (532). *Temazepam* is metabolized with a normal half-life of 10 h that increases to 21 h with renal failure (533). *Clonazepam* is biotransformed with a half-life exceeding 30 h that should not be prolonged with renal failure (14). The half-life of *midazolam* increases from 4.6 h to 4.9 h with renal failure as the clearance decreases from 800 ml/min to 470 ml/min, but the distribution volume is reduced from 3.8 l/kg to 2.2 l/kg, and protein binding decreases from 96% to 94% (534). The clearance of benzodiazepines by hemodialysis ranges from 5 ml/min to 60 ml/min which doesn't affect plasma levels appreciably (535), while hemoperfusion clearances should exceed 100 ml/min.

Chloral hydrate circulates about 50% bound to plasma protein and is biotransformed to trichlorethanol, an active metabolite eliminated by the liver and the kidney with a half-life of about 8 h (536). Overdosage responds clinically to dialysis, which achieves trichlorethanol clearances above 150 ml/min, decreasing the plasma half-life to less than 4 h (537). Hemodialysis clears chloral hydrate at 120 ml/min, decreasing the half-life from 35 h to 6 h (538) and chloral hydrate is also removed rapidly by hemoperfusion (539).

Normally, *ethchlorvynol* (145 daltons), about 40% protein bound in plasma and distributed in 4 l/kg, is eliminated slowly (half-life 25 h) by hepatic metabolism and to a lesser extent by renal clearance of 23 ml/min (14). Peritoneal clearances of 19 ml/min and hemodialyzer clearances of 64 ml/min decrease the half-life to less than 24 h (540). Resin hemoperfusion achieves clearances above 200 ml/min, decreasing the half-life to about 4 h (541, 542).

Glutethimide, about 50% bound in plasma and eliminated mostly by hepatic metabolism, has a very high lipid partition coefficient and a large distribution volume (about 3 l/kg). It should not accumulate in renal failure and is removed slowly by forced diuresis or peritoneal dialysis (78, 543). Its half-life is concentration dependent because of saturation kinetics (78). Hemodialyzer clearances of glutethimide (217 daltons) may exceed 90 ml/min, decreasing the plasma half-life (Table 13) from 40 h to 15 h (78, 543). Clearances of 120 to 200 ml/min can be achieved by hemoperfusion (526, 544–546).

Meprobamate is readily absorbed from the gastrointestinal tract, distributes in 0.7 l/kg, is about 20% bound in plasma and is excreted predominantly by the liver with a half-life of about 12 h (14). Only 20% of meprobamate is excreted unchanged by the kidney at a clearance below 40 ml/min. Forced diuresis may increase the clearance. Drug retention should be anticipated with renal failure, but only modest reduction of the dose is required. As peritoneal clearance of meprobamate (218 daltons) approaches 20 ml/min and hemodialyzer clearance may exceed 100 ml/min, severe intoxication with meprobamate may improve with dialysis (547, 548). With hemoperfusion, clearances exceed 100 ml/min (520, 526, 546).

Little *methyprylon* is excreted unchanged, and renal clearance remains below 10 ml/min despite forced diuresis. It does not accumulate with renal failure and major modification of dosage is not necessary. Acute intoxication with methyprylon (183 daltons) can improve with dialysis as peritoneal clearances of 15 to 20 ml/min and hemodialyzer clearances of 50 ml/min may be achieved (549), but improvement could relate to removal of a toxic metabolite. With severe intoxication, the half-life is longer because of saturation kinetics or shock (550). Hemoperfusion clears methyprylon at 50 to 160 ml/min (526, 544, 546).

Methaqualone intoxication also responds to charcoal hemoperfusion (544, 546) which clears it at about 200 ml/min, or to dialysis which achieves a peritoneal clearance of 7.5 ml/min and a hemodialyzer clearance of 23 ml/min (551). Methaqualone is about 80% bound in plasma, distributes in about 6 l/kg and is eliminated mostly by the liver (14, 67).

Ethinamate intoxication has been successfully treated by hemodialysis, but the pharmacokinetics need further study (552). It is normally eliminated by hepatic metabolism.

Clinical improvement has accompanied dialysis for *paraldehyde* intoxication, but this may have resulted from correction of the metabolic acidosis (553). Some paraldehyde (132 daltons) is eliminated unchanged by the lung but most is metabolized by the liver. Uremia increases susceptibility to paraldehyde acidosis.

The phenothiazines include such drugs as *fluphenazine, acetophenazine, chlorprothixine, thiolhixine, promethazine, chlorpromazine, triflupromazine, prochlorperazine, perphenazine,* and *thioridazine*. After absorption of an unpredictable fraction, phenothiazines avidly bind to plasma proteins and rapidly distribute to all body tissues, and because of marked lipophilicity, have distribution volumes as high as 20 l/kg (13, 14). They are slowly eliminated by metabolism (Table 13). Although renal elimination is minimal, uremic patients may be more susceptible to phenothiazine toxicity, including extrapyramidal myoclonus and toxic psychosis (1,

554). Because of avid tissue binding, phenothiazine removal by dialysis or hemoperfusion has a negligible effect on half-life.

Imipramine, desimipramine, nortriptyline, protriptyline, amitriptyline and *doxepin* are dibenzazepines that also bind more than 90% to plasma proteins, are very lipophilic and distribute into spaces of 10 l/kg or more and are then eliminated primarily by hepatic metabolism with half-lives (Table 13) of 16 to 80 h (13, 14). Renal failure does not prolong their half-lives but conjugated hydroxymetabolites accumulate (555). Dialysis removes minimal amounts of the tricyclic antidepressants (556–558) and despite high clearances by hemoperfusion, only a small fraction is removed from the large distribution volume (98, 539, 559, 560). *Trazadone* has a half-life of 4.1 h that is probably not prolonged by renal failure or abbreviated by hemodialysis (561).

Monoamine oxidase inhibitors include *phenelzine, pargyline, tranylcypromine, isocarboxazid* and *nialamide*. Their pharmacologic effects persist after the drugs or their active metabolites are eliminated. Retention of these drugs which are eliminated by acetylation does not occur with renal failure and although clinical improvement has occurred with dialysis, there are no pharmacokinetic data to provide a basis for such therapy (6).

Sodium *bromide*, distributes in extracellular fluid and normally is excreted by the kidney at a clearance below 2 ml/min. It accumulates when sodium is retained as in heart failure, nephrotic syndrome or cirrhosis, potentially causing a toxic psychosis. The normal half-life in plasma may exceed 24 h (Table 13). It is not prolonged by renal failure until oliguria occurs. Saline diuresis decreases the half-life of bromide to about 12 h. Potent diuretics clear bromide at up to 14 ml/min, decreasing the half-life to below 6 h (80). The peritoneal clearance of bromide is 14 ml/min and the hemodialyzer clearance exceeds 100 ml/min, decreasing the half-life to below 2 h, faster than distribution equilibrium occurs (80, 81).

Lithium salts, in popular psychotherapeutic use, have a narrow margin of safety, potentially causing neuromuscular irritability and distal tubular injury when plasma concentrations exceed 2.0 mEq/l (5,562). Dose dependent nephrogenic diabetes insipidus is due to inhibition of vasopressin stimulated water transport at a site biochemically proximal to that of cyclic AMP (563). Renal excretion of lithium by filtration with proximal tubular reabsorption at a clearance of 15 to 25 ml/min, is increased by osmotic diuresis, acetazolamide or bicarbonate therapy. Chronic lithium therapy can induce irreversible renal failure with chronic interstitial nephritis, tubular atrophy and medullary fibrosis (564). Lithium accumulates in renal failure (Table 13) causing toxic coma which improves with hemodialysis, decreasing the half-life from over 40 h to less than 6 h (565, 566). Peritoneal clearance of lithium of about 12 ml/min can exceed renal clearance and reduce the half-life to 17 h (567). Symptoms correlate better with the calculated total body pool of lithium than with the plasma level, however (566). Lithium can be efficaciously and safely used in maintenance hemodialysis patients by following pharmacokinetic principles (568).

Anticonvulsants

Phenytoin (diphenylhydantoin) is eliminated mostly by oxidation followed by glucuronide conjugation of the metabolite and renal excretion of the conjugate. Phenytoin (252 daltons), about 90% protein bound in plasma, distributes in 0.64 l/kg and has a concentration dependent elimination half-life that averages 16 h (13). Renal failure decreases the protein binding to about 65% because of a compositional change in plasma proteins in uremia and competitive binding by a uremic metabolite (38, 569, 570). An any given dose, less protein binding allows greater distribution to sites of action and metabolism. Accordingly, the half-life decreases in renal failure to about 8 h (Table 13). No dosage modification is recommended and phenytoin is usually well tolerated in uremic patients. Conjugated 4-hydroxyphenytoin is retained in the plasma of uremic patients (571). Osteomalacia may complicate chronic use and acute interstitial nephritis is a potential hazard (57, 572). Decreased protein binding allows a dialyzer clearance of about 12 ml/min in uremic patients, but only a small fraction is removed from the large distribution volume and the half-life is 15 h (573). Both peritoneal dialysis and hemodialysis have been clinically effective in treating massive overdosages of phenytoin (574, 575) despite low clearances (23% of peritoneal dialysate flow rate [576] and 31 ml/min [577] by hemodialysis). The clearance with CAPD is 2.0 ml/min.

Liver injury increases the potency and duration of action of oxazolidine anticonvulsants, *trimethadione* and *paramethadione*, but nephrectomy prolongs and potentiates only paramethadione activity in the rat (578). These small solutes are not highly bound in plasma, distribute in 0.6 l/kg, and are cleared by hepatic microsomes to active metabolites with long half-lives. Hypersensitivity to the oxazolidines may be manifested by nephrotic syndrome with minimal glomerular changes (579).

Valproic acid, normally about 80% protein bound in plasma, distributes in a volume of about 0.6 l/kg; it is eliminated by concentration dependent β oxidation with a clearance of 8 ml/min and a half-life of 12 h (13, 580). Renal failure decreases the concentration dependent protein binding to about 70% but does not delay the elimination, so dosage adjustment is not necessary (580). Hemodialyzer clearance of about 35 ml/min decreases the half-life but the peritoneal clearance of 2.2 ml/min has little effect (580–582).

Carbamazepine, an analeptic, also used for treatment of trigeminal neuralgia, has caused reversible acute renal failure (583). It is normally eliminated slowly (half-life 15 h) and the clearance by hemodialysis (54 ml/min) can exceed endogenous plasma clearance (28 ml/min) despite 70% protein binding in plasma (584). With hemoperfusion carbamazepine half-life is about 8 h and clinical improvement occurs (585).

Ethosuximide (141 daltons) is unbound in plasma, distributes in about 0.7 l/kg and has a normal half-life of about 50 h with a clearance of about 10 ml/min, mostly hepatic (13, 586). Hemodialysis clears it at 140 ml/min, reducing the half-life to 3.5 h (586).

Analgesics

Salicylates are small solutes (137 to 180 daltons) distributed in a volume of 0.15 l/kg; as much as 50% is bound in plasma (13). Plasma clearance decreases from 60 to about 14 ml/min as concentrations increase and the half-life increases from 2.4 to 19 h (13). The kidney excretes unchanged salicylates and the metabolites, salicyluric acid, salicylic phenolic and acyl glucuronides and gentisic acid. Free salicylate excretion increases when the urine is rendered alkaline. Plasma salicylate at any given dose is higher with a decreased glomerular filtration rate or decreased proximal tubular secretion. Plasma protein binding decreases with high salicylate concentrations, hypoproteinemia or renal failure (587). Major clinical signs of salicylate intoxication include tinnitus, acid base disturbances, gastric ulceration, bleeding tendencies, central nervous system depression and nephrotoxicity (5). Only a small fraction of patients with salicylate intoxication (i.e. after massive overdosage, with plasma concentrations above 80 mg/dl, with concurrent disease or clinical deterioration) should be considered for dialysis (81). Hemodialyzer clearance exceeds 100 ml/min decreasing the plasma half-life in intoxicated patients from about 16 h to 4 h (588). Comparable clearances are achieved by hemoperfusion (525, 526). Peritoneal clearances are much lower but increase with an alkaline buffer or albumin in the dialysate and can improve clinical intoxication (589). Maintenance of therapeutic plasma concentrations in uremic patients requires dosage reduction, but susceptibility to toxicity is high nevertheless. Because salicylates inhibit prostaglandin synthetase, they can depress renal blood flow in patients with congestive heart failure, lupus erythematosus or other conditions that stimulate the renin angiotensin system (20). *Salsalate* has a normal half-life of 1.2 h that increases to 2.1 h with renal failure. The half-life of its metabolite, salicylic acid, increases from the normal 3.8 h to 8.1 h in uremic patients (Table 13), but is reduced to 4.9 h by hemodialysis (590).

Diflunisal, a difluorophenyl salicylate, is normally more than 99% protein bound in plasma. Dose dependent metabolic elimination with a half-life of about 10 h yields an unstable metabolite. Uremia decreases the binding to 54% because of a lower association constant and competitive binding, an abnormality that hemodialysis corrects (591).

Phenacetin and its major metabolite, *acetaminophen*, are rapidly absorbed, only minimally bound to plasma proteins and readily diffuse into a 0.9 l/kg volume (14, 67). Chronic high dosage is associated with papillary necrosis and chronic interstitial nephritis and, acutely, acetaminophen may cause hepatic necrosis (5, 54, 592). Analgesic nephrophathy accounts for 3 to 30% of patients requiring regular dialysis for end-stage renal disease and may be complicated by uroepithelial malignancy so excessive doses should be avoided in dialysis patients (593, 594). These small solutes are cleared by hemodialysis at more than 100 ml/min, decreasing the plasma half-life below that of conventional therapy (595). Peritoneal clearances are only 3 ml/min (596). The half-life of acetaminophen (paracetamol) in normals and anephric patients is about 2.5 h (Table 13) as hepatic clearance of

330 ml/min yields the conjugates acetaminophen glucuronide and acetaminophen sulfate which accumulate in uremic plasma (597). Hemodialysis clears acetaminophen at 80% of urea clearance, reducing the half-life slightly (to 1.6 h), and the metabolites at 50 to 70% of urea clearance representing 60% of the removal rate. Hemoperfusion clearances of 120 ml/min decrease to 30 ml/min with saturation of the charcoal column but the procedure decreases the half-life (598) and may be the most efficient method for rapid removal of acetaminophen (525). Treatment by N acetyl cysteine is the most important measure for acute overdosage but hemoperfusion may have an additive role (599).

Propoxyphene is eliminated mainly by hepatic metabolism. In anephric patients, first-pass metabolism is decreased raising peak plasma concentrations, but the terminal half-life is not increased (600). Hepatic clearance normally is about 800 ml/min and the half-life is about 18 h (14, 600). Overdosage can cause coma and respiratory arrest, responsive to narcotic antagonists. Peritoneal clearance is 8 ml/min and hemodialyzer clearance varies from 7 to 100 ml/min (600, 601). The metabolite, norpropoxyphene, is cleared at 16 ml/min. Since the distribution volume is 10 to 25 l/kg, less than 10% of ingested propoxyphene (339 daltons and 80% protein bound) is recovered in dialysate.

The half-life of *antipyrine* is significantly shorter in uremic patients (7.3 h) than in normals (13.2 h), a paradox explained by induction of hepatic metabolism as the volume of distribution remains unchanged (602). Metabolites persist in uremic plasma, however.

Azapropazone (apazone) is more than 95% bound in plasma, distributes in 0.15 l/kg and is cleared at about 10 ml/min, 60% of which is via the kidney. With renal failure the half-life increases from 12 h to 32 h (603).

Pentazocine rapidly disappears from plasma mostly by oxidation and conjugation in the liver (604). The half-life is 2 to 3 h, dosage modification is not required in uremic patients and dialysis pharmacokinetics await study.

The *opiates* distribute rapidly in a large tissue volume and are removed by dealkylation and hydrolyses in the liver and excreted in the urine (605). About 35% of *morphine* is bound in plasma, the distribution volume is 3 l/kg and the half-life is about 2.5 h, increasing slightly with renal failure (13, 527). Most morphine is glucuronide conjugated, while about 10% appears in the urine, unchanged, by filtration and secretion at an increasing rate as the urine is acidified. The active glucuronide metabolite half-life is 4 h, which increases to 41 h in renal failure contributing to respiratory depression (606). Increased sensitivity to a single dose standard dosage also may occur in uremic patients. Blood levels can be decreased by dialysis, but pharmacokinetics require further study (607). *Codeine* elimination resembles that of morphine. Conventional doses may cause narcosis in uremic patients and peak plasma codeine levels are higher than normal at a later time (608). About 10% of *meperidine* is excreted in the urine unchanged, while most of the drug undergoes rapid hepatic degradation to normeperidine which can induce convulsions (609). *Methadone* can be used in patients on dialysis without complications. It is about 85%

protein bound in plasma and is eliminated by hepatic biotransformation (610). *Bupremorphine*, a semisynthetic lipophilic opioid, is 96% protein bound and eliminated by hepatic dealkylation with a normal half-life of 3 h, not appreciably affected by renal failure (611). *Alfentanil* and *fentanil* are highly bound in plasma, distribute in large volumes, and are eliminated by the liver with half lives of 1.6 h and 3.7 h respectively, unaffected by renal failure (13).

Antirheumatic and anti-inflammatory drugs

Most nonsteroidal anti-inflammatory drugs do not depend much on renal elimination. They are highly bound in plasma and can displace other compounds from binding sites. In addition to salicylates, these drugs include acetic acids, propionic acids, anthranilic acids, oxicams and pyrazoles. The nonsteroidal drugs block prostaglandin synthetase and can cause renal ischemia, hyperkalemia, nephrotic syndrome, interstitial nephritis and renal failure (612, 613).

Well absorbed, *indomethacin* is eliminated predominantly by hepatic biotransformation with some enterohepatic recycling and renal excretion (13). Renal excretion of indomethacin decreases with blockade of tubular secretion or renal failure. The biphasic half-life, normally 1 and 9 h, does not increase, and dosage modification is not required in uremic patients. Dialysis should not remove much indomethacin (357 daltons) because about 95% is bound in plasma.

Sulindac (356 daltons) is about 95% bound in plasma and has biphasic hepatic elimination with half-lives of 8 and 16 h (14). Some of the metabolites are active but rapidly eliminated.

Phenylbutazone is well absorbed and more than 95% bound in plasma. It is eliminated slowly by hepatic metabolism from a small distribution volume. With renal failure, protein binding of phenylbutazone decreases and the half-life, normally 70 h, decreases slightly (614). Nevertheless, binding inhibits removal by dialysis. Hemoperfusion rapidly removes phenylbutazone reducing the half-life to 6 h (615).

Ibuprofen, naproxen, fenbufen, ketoprofen, fenoprofen and *benoxaprofen* are propionic acid derivatives that inhibit prostaglandin synthetase. Ibuprofen (206 daltons) is 99% protein bound, distributed in 0.15 l/kg, and eliminated by metabolism with a half-life (Table 13) of about 2 h (616). No accumulation occurs in renal failure but protein binding decreases to 95% or less (617, 618). The hemodialyzer clearance of about 26 ml/min does not decrease the half-life (618). Hydroxy- and carboxy-metabolites accumulate in renal failure with half-lives of 24 h or more. Naproxen is also 99% protein bound and is eliminated partly by metabolism and partly by renal excretion of the unchanged drug with a half-life (Table 13) of about 15 h (616). The half-life is not prolonged by renal failure nor decreased by hemodialysis, so dosage adjustments are not required (619, 620). The metabolite, desmethylnaproxen, has a 18 h half-life unchanged by renal failure. Fenoprofen (559 daltons) is 99% protein bound and eliminated mostly by hydroxylation with a half-life of 3 h (616). Fenbufen also is biotransformed and its elimination half-life of 11 h is not prolonged by renal failure (621). Ketoprofen is 99% bound in plasma, distributes in 0.1 l/kg and is eliminated by metabolism with a 2 h half-life that increases to 3.2 h with renal failure (622). Benoxaprofen is highly protein bound and depends in part on renal elimination. The half-life increases from 27 h normally to 73 h with renal failure (623). About 90% of *mefenamic acid*, is protein bound in plasma and the half-life, normally 4 h, is not prolonged by renal failure nor decreased by hemodialysis which achieves clearances of only 8 to 16 ml/min (624). *Meclofenamate* has a normal half-life of 2 h. *Tolmetin* is eliminated rapidly in part by the kidney with a half-life of 0.8 h (14). Uremia decreases plasma protein binding of tolmetin, an abnormality that hemodialysis corrects (625). *Piroxicam* is about 99% protein bound, eliminated by hepatic metabolism and has a half-life of 45 h, uninfluenced by renal failure (14, 616). *Tenoxicam* is hydroxylated by the liver. With renal failure the half-life decreases from 64 h to 50 h as protein binding decreases from 99.3% to 98.7% (626).

Colchicine is rapidly absorbed and distributes into a very large volume from which most is metabolized and about 20% is excreted into the urine unchanged. The half-life is about 2 h and does not increase with renal failure (8, 14). Gastrointestinal irritation may preclude high doses or prolonged use in renal failure. Dialysis pharmacokinetics need study, but colchicine is removed by hemoperfusion, although little clinical benefit ensues (95).

Gold salts, often effective antirheumatic drugs, are excreted slowly mainly by the kidney, augmented by such chelates as penicillamine and dimercaprol. Almost completely protein bound in plasma, little removal by dialysis occurs even with chelation and accumulation would be likely in patients with renal failure. Toxicity includes cutaneous hypersensitivity reactions, bone marrow depression and nephrotoxicity, heralded by proteinuria and microhematuria, potentially leading to nephrotic syndrome or acute renal failure (627).

Probenecid, by blocking active tubular reabsorption (large doses) causes uricosuria. This effect and blockade of secretion of such organic acids as uric acid (by small doses) and penicillin quantitatively decrease as renal failure progresses. About 80% protein bound in plasma, the half-life of probenecid (285 daltons) is between 6 and 12 h with elimination mostly by extrarenal metabolism (14). Toxicity includes recurring nephrotic syndrome and chronic renal failure (628).

Sulfinpyrazone (404 daltons), a uricosuric and antiplatelet aggregating agent, is highly protein bound in plasma and eliminated mostly by renal secretion. The half-life increases from about 2.5 h to 9.5 h with severe renal failure and it is not appreciably affected by hemodialysis (629). Sulfinpyrazone can cause acute interstitial nephritis (50).

Allopurinol (135 daltons) is rapidly metabolized (half-life 0.7 h) to oxipurinol (alloxanthine), thereby inhibiting xanthine oxidase. Oxipurinol is excreted by the kidney with a plasma half-life of 28 h (630). Accumulation of this metabolite occurs with renal failure and the dose should not exceed 300 mg (22 mmol)/day or the drug avoided. A vasculitic type toxic syndrome can complicate allopurinol therapy in patients with renal failure (631). Oxipurinol is not appreciably protein bound and hemodialysis removes about 40% of the drug from the body (631).

Immunosuppressive and antineoplastic agents

Adrenal corticosteroids are well absorbed and about 90% protein bound in plasma. Elimination occurs by hepatic metabolism with renal excretion of inactive metabolites. Half-lives are 0.5 to 4 h. Neither renal failure nor dialysis affect the half-lives appreciably (Table 14). Hemodialyzer clearances correlate with the dose but range from only 15 to 40 ml/min, yet dialysis removes cortisol metabolites (632–634).

Azathioprine is well absorbed and distributed in total body water with about 30% protein binding in plasma. It is cleaved nonenzymatically to 6-mercaptopurine and oxidized (14). Renal failure decreases the rate of elimination of azathioprine metabolites but does not modify biologic activity, probably because very rapid metabolic inactivation of the biologically active metabolites limits the duration of activity (635). The dose should be reduced only slightly with renal failure. The incidence, precocity and duration of leukopenia is unaffected by renal failure and immunosuppressive activity also remains unchanged despite inhibition of thiopurine methyl transferase, the enzyme pertinent to metabolic disposition (100). High doses of *6-mercaptopurine* may cause crystalluria and hematuria (636). Concurrent allopurinol therapy delays elimination of the purine analogs. The dialyzer clearance of azathioprine is close to the uric acid clearance and the half-life during dialysis is 4 h, only slightly below the normal value (637).

Cyclosporine A (1202 daltons) binds extensively to plasma proteins is lipophilic and distributes slowly into and from a 3.5 l/kg volume (638, 639). It is eliminated by metabolism with a clearance of about 500 ml/min and a normal half-life of 27 h that decreases to 16 h with renal failure. Hemodialysis removes less than 1% of the drug (Table 14).

Cyclophosphamide distributes into a volume of about 0.5 l/kg and is less than 20% protein bound in plasma (14). About 90% of cyclophosphamide is biotransformed in the liver. One or more of the metabolites may function as an alkylating agent (640). Cyclophosphamide impairs free water clearance but is not nephrotoxic. Hemorrhagic cystitis is attributed to the excretion of a metabolite. The normal half-life of 7 h increases somewhat with renal failure, favoring avoidance of the drug or dosage reduction with careful hematologic monitoring. Hemodialysis clears cyclophosphamide (261 daltons) reducing the half-life (Table 14) to about 2.5 h (641, 642). Other alkylating agents such as *chlorambucil, mechlorethamine, melphalan* and *busulfan* have undergone less study in renal failure, but disappear rapidly from plasma by metabolism with half-lives of less than 2 h. Their plasma concentrations should not be influenced appreciably by dialysis or renal failure, and dosage requires little or no modification in these circumstances (643).

Bredinin is a new imidazole-derived immunosuppressive

drug that undergoes little metabolism and depends mostly on renal elimination. With renal failure the half-life increases from 4.8 h to 155 h (644). Hemodialysis removes 43% of the drug is 4 h (Table 14).

The nitrosoureas include *streptozocin, carmustine* (BCNU), *lomustine* (CCNU) and *semustine* (methyl CCNU) which are degraded within minutes (14), but their metabolites may have prolonged half-lives in uremic patients. Streptozocin can cause reversible proximal tubular injury and renal failure (645) while treatment with methyl CCNU can be followed by progressive renal atrophy, interstitial fibrosis and renal failure (646).

The pyrimidine analogs, *5-fluorouracil* and *cytosine arabinoside*, are rapidly distributed and biotransformed. Renal failure does not affect this metabolic elimination rate and normally little unchanged drug appears in the urine and no dosage adjustment is necessary (643). Hemodialysis removes 37% of the 5-fluorouracil (130 daltons) that perfuses the dialyzer allowing safe regional chemotherapy perfusion, but probably affects systemic therapy considerably less because of the larger distribution volume (642).

Methotrexate is about 50% bound to plasma proteins and distributes in a volume of about 0.5 l/kg (13, 14). This folic acid analog is eliminated biphasically with half-lives of about 2 h and 7 h, mainly by renal excretion (647). Plasma accumulation occurs in uremic patients, but dosage modification to achieve a normal plasma concentration is complicated by the fact that plasma protein binding decreases, increasing the biologically active fraction (648). Renal failure prolongs the half-life to about 12 h (Table 14). It is not decreased appreciably by hemodialysis or peritoneal dialysis, which achieve clearances of 37 and 5 ml/min, respectively (649, 650). Hemoperfusion, especially with uncoated charcoal, achieves higher clearances lowering the half-life to about 4 h, but delayed intercompartmental transfer causes postperfusion rebound increments (651, 652). In addition to bone marrow suppression, toxicity may include acute tubular necrosis (650).

With renal failure, *bleomycin* clearance decreases from 117 ml/min to 27 ml/min and the half-life increases from about 3 h to 24 h (653). Dermal fibrosis, interstitial pneumonitis, ataxia and episodic loss of consciousness are more likely with renal failure (654). There is no measurable removal by hemodialysis (655). *Doxorubicin* distributes in a very large volume and is rapidly eliminated, mostly by hepatic metabolism (14). This antineoplastic antibiotic has caused progressive glomerular lesions, tubular atrophy, interstitial nephritis and renal failure (656). Care must be taken in administering these drugs since necrosis of the hand can result from retrograde flow in an arteriovenous fistula (657). No major reduction in the dosage of *actinomycin D, daunorubicin, busulfan, melphalan, mitomycin C, vincristine* or *vinblastine* should be required for patients with renal failure (14, 643), but metabolites may accumulate. *Mithramycin* dosage should be reduced by 50% (14, 643).

Dose dependent nephrotoxicity is the major hazard limiting the use of the potent antitumor agent *cis-platinum* (658). More than 90% of cis-platinum in plasma is protein bound, so hemodialysis removes very little and although only a portion of its elimination occurs via the urine, renal failure prolongs the half-life from about 60 h to 240 h (659).

Hypoglycemic agents

Insulin metabolism is discussed extensively in Chapter 45. Resistance to insulin characterizes renal failure, but since the elimination rate decreases by as much as 50% and body mass and caloric intake may decrease, dosage reduction is often required. Hemodialysis does not affect the elimination rate of insulin (42, 660). Insulin absorption from peritoneal dialysis fluid allows control of carbohydrate metabolism in diabetic patients, despite the high load of glucose (661).

The sulfonylureas and biguanides are hypoglycemic agents to which uremic patients have increased sensitivity. *Tolbutamide*, a sulfonylurea, is about 90% protein bound in plasma and eliminated with a half-life of 5 h by oxidation to inactive metabolites normally excreted by the kidney (662). As neither renal failure nor dialysis affect plasma concentrations appreciably, it is the preferred oral hypoglycemic for uremic patients. The metabolites of *tolazamide* and *acetohexamide* cause hypoglycemia and are excreted by the kidney. *Chlorpropamide*, about 90% protein bound in plasma, is slowly excreted, unchanged by the kidney (662). Renal failure prolongs the half-life from 35 h to as long as 200 h (Table 14). Delayed excretion correlates better with loss of tubular function than of glomerular filtration, and the half-life increases with concurrent therapy with drugs such as probenecid, chloramphenicol and to a lesser extent, allopu-

Table 14. Half-lives of miscellaneous drugs.

Drug	Half-life		
	N	A	H
Prednisolone	3.2	4.6	4.6
Cyclosporin A	27	16	16
Cyclophosphamide	7.0	8.0	2.5
Bredinin	4.8	155	5.0
Methotrexate	2.0	12	12
Chlorpropamide	35	200	–
EDTA	2.2	7.4	–
Gallamine	2.2	12.5	7.0
Atracurium	0.3	0.4	–
Pancuronium	2.2	4.3	–
Propylthiouracil	2.0	9.0	–
Methimazole	14	50	–
Organic iodides	1.0	30	4.0
Clofibrate	17	100	–
Bezafibrate	2.0	19.5	–
Fenofibrate	20	150	–
Cimetidine	1.9	4.3	2.5
Ranitidine	3.0	7.0	4.3
Metoclopramide	3.5	14	14

Average of published values, DV = distribution volume, N = normal, A = anephric, H = hemodialysis.

rinol and clofibrate (663). Severe recurrent hypoglycemic coma can complicate renal retention of chlorpropamide (664). As plasma protein binding decreases with increased concentrations of chlorpropamide, dialysis can contribute to removal of excessive dosage (665). Chlorpropamide may induce water retention with hyponatremia and reversible and reproducible features of the syndrome of inappropriate antidiuretic hormone secretion (666).

The biguanides, *buformin* and *phenformin* have normal half-lives of 2 to 3 h. They are excreted into the urine unchanged and faster in alkaline urine, although phenformin is in part metabolized (667). Phenformin should be avoided in uremic patients not only because of potential retention in plasma, but also because of the increased tendency to lactic acidosis. Although little phenformin is removed by dialysis, lactic acidosis can be improved (668, 669).

Vitamins

Nutrition in uremic patients, which is discussed in Chapter 53, usually includes vitamin supplementation. The fat soluble *vitamin A* circulates bound to protein, is extensively stored in tissues notably the liver, and is degraded metabolically. In renal failure, plasma vitamin A increases from 1.4 to 3.6 μmol/l (84, 670). Yet, vitamin A is normally absent in urine and only appears coincident with proteinuria. The increment in measured vitamin A levels is largely due to an increase in retinol binding protein (which should be low in hypervitaminosis A) and does not cause increased levels in tissues including bone (671). High levels correlate with increases in β carotene, cholesterol and triglyceride concentrations in plasma. Plasma retinol and retinol binding protein concentrations increase considerably in uremic patients and decrease, but not to normal, with discontinuation of vitamin supplements (672). Yet, excessive supplements can cause toxicity including osteolytic hypercalcemia (673). Plasma vitamin A levels are reduced only minimally by hemodialysis (674, 675). As discussed in greater detail in Chapter 44, *vitamin D* is converted by the kidney to the metabolically active form, 1,25 dihydroxycholecalciferol. Accordingly, vitamin D resistance occurs in renal failure, inducing hypocalcemic osteodystrophy. Because of awareness that overdosage can precipitate or aggravate renal failure (676, 677), vitamin D has been used cautiously in uremic patients. The 1,25 (OH)$_2$ metabolite and potent analogues have been valuable adjunctive treatments of renal osteodystrophy but can cause hypercalcemia and further deterioration of renal function (678, 679).

Thiamin (265 daltons), a water soluble B vitamin, is stored in tissues and metabolically degraded, appearing in urine only when tissue depots are saturated. Plasma concentrations increase slightly with renal failure and decrease with hemodialysis (which clears it at 15 to 40 ml/min), but only by about 10% because of protein binding (680–682). Nevertheless, unless supplemented, maintenance dialysis patients may have low plasma concentrations (84). About 10% of *riboflavin* (376 daltons) is excreted into the urine and the metabolic fate of the remainder is unknown. Plasma ribofla-

vin concentrations increase significantly with renal failure and dialyzer clearance is about 35 ml/min (681–683). With adequate dietary intake, little (2 mg/day) or no supplement should be required with dialysis. *Nicotinic acid* and *nicotinamide* are eliminated mainly by metabolism, but the kidney contributes more importantly to elimination when very high doses are given. Plasma levels decrease minimally with dialysis and may be decreased in uremic patients (684). *Pyridoxine* (169 daltons), a small solute, is eliminated metabolically. Deficiency of pyridoxine in uremic patients associated with low dietary intake, renal or dialyzer losses or incomplete metabolic activation, can manifest decreased erythrocyte transaminase activity, diminished reactivity of lymphocytes and neuropathy (84, 685). A supplement of 50 mg/day is recommended (686). The clearance by hemodialysis is 55 ml/min (681). *Pantothenic acid* is excreted primarily by the kidney. Elevated plasma concentrations in uremic patients are decreased by about 30% by hemodialysis, which clears it at 30 ml/min (682, 685). As *biotin* is also excreted by the kidney, increased plasma concentrations may occur with renal failure (685). Plasma concentrations decrease by 30% with hemodialysis, which clears it at 45 ml/min (682). *Folic acid* is partially bound is plasma and at low concentrations, little appears in urine. High plasma concentrations are mainly excreted by the kidney. Maintenance dialysis patients may become depleted as the dialyzer clearance can exceed 50 ml/min, but tissue storage limits removal. Dialyzer losses are comparable to normal urinary excretion and plasma concentrations usually remain above 7 ng/ml (16 nmol/l) (687, 688). Cessation of supplements does not induce hematological changes (689). *Cyanocobalamin* is stored in the liver, excreted by the kidney, and cleared very slowly by dialysis because of its large size and partial protein binding (684). Hemofiltration can remove it more rapidly. Dietary vitamin B$_{12}$ should keep most patients from deficiency, maintaining plasma concentrations between 200 and 900 pg/ml (150 and 660 pmol/l). Without dialysis the levels are high in uremic patients (682). *Ascorbic acid* (176 daltons) is mostly metabolized but high doses are excreted by the kidney. One of the metabolites, oxalate, may accumulate in tissues of uremic patients, including kidney, potentially accelerating renal failure (690, 691). The supplemental dose should not exceed 200 mg/day to avoid oxalosis (693). As hemodialysis clears ascorbic acid at 100 ml/min and decreases plasma levels by about 40%, supplements are required (689, 692). The peritoneal clearance is about 16 ml/min (682). Maintenance dialysis patients may have low plasma *vitamin E* concentrations (84).

Metals and chelates

Pharmacokinetics of organic gold salts, platinum and mercury have been discussed under antirheumatics, antineoplastics and diuretics, respectively. *Iron*, which may gain access to the circulation from dialysate (85), is net removed during dialysis as blood is lost leading to iron deficiency, discussed in detail in Chapter 40. Oral iron is satisfactorily absorbed in uremic patients and can improve iron deficiency anemia (25,

694). Parenteral iron dextran also repletes iron stores but may not be utilized as well and can be followed by hemosiderosis (25, 695). Indeed, increased serum ferritin levels and splenic siderosis correlate with the amount of iron dextran administered to dialysis patients (696). Removal of iron during dialysis usually requires the addition of the chelate, deferoxamine (697). The treatment of renal osteodystrophy (Chapter 44) with *aluminum* hydroxide phosphate binding gels can lead to hyperaluminumemia (698), one of the trace metal abnormalities discussed in Chapter 50. Contamination of dialysate water, however, is usually the predominant source of aluminum, the protein binding of which inhibits removal by dialysis (699). Chelation with deferoxamine mobilizes aluminum stores and increases the ultrafilterable fraction that can be removed by dialysis (697). *Phosphate* depletion may result from excessive use of oral sorbents leading not only to osteomalacia but also to an encephalopathy, possibly also related to aluminum intoxication (700, 701). The *magnesium* content of antacids and of laxatives also may accumulate, leading to an encephalopathy. *Cobalt* toxicity may occur in maintenance dialysis patients treated with cobaltous chloride and this metal normally eliminated by the kidney, should be avoided in uremic patients (702). Organic *antimonials* are also excreted primarily by the kidney and may accumulate in patients with renal failure when treated for protozoal infections (703). *Arsenicals* and *bismuth* preparations are not only dangerous in patients with renal disease because of their retention, but also because of potential nephrotoxicity aggravating renal failure (5). In general, protein binding limits removal of metals during hemodialysis but they may enter the blood from the dialysate (70, 704). With the addition of a chelate, the complexed metals may diffuse out of blood, usually slowly, but often faster than the removal rate by the injured kidney (289, 705). Although measurable quantities of $^{67}gallium$ citrate are found in hemodialysate, removal rates are low and do not interfere with imaging techniques (706). *Thallium* is removed much faster by hemodialysis or by hemoperfusion than the kidney clears it (707).

Chelating agents tightly bind metal ions and these metallocomplexes are excreted unchanged by the kidney. Renal failure impairs their therapeutic effectiveness. *Dimercaprol* binds those metals that have affinity for sulfhydryl groups. It accumulates in patients with renal failure, potentially causing hypoglycemia and can be removed slowly by dialysis (708). Excreted by both glomerular filtration and tubular secretion, *calcium disodium edetate* accumulates in renal failure patients (Table 14), the half-life increasing from 2.2 h to 7.4 h (709). It can cause nephrotoxicity related at least partly to transtubular transport of the dissociable metallocomplexes (710). *Penicillamine*, rapidly excreted into the urine, effectively binds such metals as copper, lead and mercury, and potentially accumulates in renal failure. Hypersensitivity toxic reactions include nephrotic syndrome (711). The clearance of *diethylenetriamine-pentaacetic acid*, 50 ml/min with hemodialysis and 14 ml/min with peritoneal dialysis, provides a mechanism for treating hemosiderosis in uremic patients (144, 289, 712). *Deferoxamine,* another iron chelate, is also excreted by the kidney and is cleared at 4 ml/min with cuprophane hemodialysis or at 40 ml/min with high flux membranes (697). Deferoxamine has induced acute renal failure (713). The mercury chelate, *2,3 dimercaptosuccinic acid*, is 50% extracted during passage through a hemodialyzer and lowers mercury half-life substantially (714).

Miscellaneous drugs

The anticoagulant, *heparin*, is not removed by dialysis. More than 8,000 daltons and extensively protein bound, heparin is eliminated by enzymatic degradation with a half-life of less than 2 h, unaffected by renal failure (13, 14). *Bishydroxycoumarin* is more than 99% bound in plasma and eliminated by hepatic metabolism. Renal failure does not prolong the effect on prothrombin time (715). Dialysis does not remove it. *Sodium warfarin,* which is about 97% protein bound in plasma, is eliminated slowly by metabolism, with a normal half-life of about 40 h (13, 14). Protein binding decreases with renal failure and the half-life may be somewhat shorter, i.e. 30 h. Dialysis does not affect its kinetics. *Phenindione* therapy is occasionally complicated by sensitivity reactions including severe dermatitis, leukocytosis, proteinuria, edema and tubular necrosis (716). Caution is advised with the use of oral anticoagulants, not because of increased responsiveness but because of the bleeding diathesis and lesions of uremia (717).

Antiplatelet aggregating agents, including *dipyridamole* and *prostacyclin*, have been used to maintain shunt patency, reduce heparin dose or eliminate it or augment peritoneal transport rates (106, 718). Their pharmacokinetics are not appreciably influenced by uremia or by dialysis.

The muscle relaxant, *gallamine* (892 daltons), is eliminated almost exclusively by the kidney. With renal failure the half-life (Table 14) increases from 2.2 h to 12.5 h as the clearance falls from 84 ml/min to 17 ml/min (719). It should be avoided in patients with renal failure because prolonged neuromuscular blockade can occur. It can be removed by hemodialysis at a clearance of 13 ml/min, which reduces plasma levels by 63% achieving a half-life of about 7 h (720, 721). Hemodialysis also lowers plasma *d-tubocurarine* levels by about 50%. This drug is also cleared mostly by the kidney at about 200 ml/min and the half-life, normally 1.5 h; increases with renal failure (722). *Atacurium* (983 daltons) decomposes noneyzymatically at a clearance of about 480 ml/min with a half-life of 0.3 h (Table 14), not appreciably affected by renal failure (722, 723). The metabolites do not cause neuromuscular blockade but a major metabolite, *laudanosine* accumulates in renal failure and is a central stimulant. Most *metocurine* is eliminated by unknown mechanisms but the half-life increases in renal failure from 6 h to 11.4 h (724). But in uremic patients higher serum concentrations are required for 90% inhibition of myogenic responses. The half-life of *pancuronium* increases from 2.2 h to 4.3 h with renal failure, while that of its analogue, *norcuron*, increases from 1.3 h to 1.6 h (722, 725). The clearance of *vecuronium* is 210 ml/min which is mostly nonrenal. Renal failure increases the half-life from 1.3 h to 1.6 h. The half-life of *fazadinium*, normally 0.9 h, is not prolonged by renal failure (726).

The cholinesterase inhibitors, *neostigmine* and *pyridostigmine*, may have prolonged action in uremic patients, allowing a more persistent effect of succinyl choline (727). Up to 50% of *atropine* is excreted by the kidney with a half-life of 2.5 h and caution is advised when atropine is used in uremic patients (728). It is not removed by dialysis (729). In choosing an anesthetic it should be recalled that preexisting renal functional impairment may predispose to further loss of renal function due to the toxic effects of the fluorinated anesthetics, *enflurane* and *methoryflurane* (730). A detailed discussion of anesthesia for uremic patients is given in Chapter 52.

Since *propylthiouracil* is excreted in part by the kidney, the half-life is prolonged from about 2 h to about 9 h and dosage should be reduced (8, 731). Protein binding should inhibit removal by dialysis (Table 14). *Methimazole* is also partly excreted by the kidney and partly metabolized. Dosage reduction is recommended as renal failure prolongs the half-life (Table 14) from 14 to 50 h (1, 8).

Iodide is excreted by the kidney by filtration and reabsorption in competition with thyroidal uptake (732). Because protein binding is minimal with high dosage, dialysis removes iodide. Accumulation of povidone-iodine used topically may contribute to increased plasma iodine levels (733). The iodinated radiographic contrast media normally excreted by the kidney, with half-lives of less than an hour (Table 14), accumulate in patients with renal failure as the half-life is prolonged to about 30 h (734). Hemodialysis decreases the half-life to 4 h. Hemodialyzer clearances exceed 50% of urea clearances and peritoneal clearance is 7 ml/min (735). Nephrotoxicity, the most important complication of iodide radiography, occurs with a variety of contrast media as a function of the structural configuration of the organic iodide, the percentage of iodine, the dose used, the site of injection, and prior renal function (736, 737). Care should be taken to avoid dehydration or manipulations that decrease renal blood flow prior to iodide radiography, particularly in those with preexisting impairment of renal function. Acute renal failure, a recognized complication of infusion pyelography, can easily be misinterpreted as natural progression of the underlying renal disease.

The kidney excretes *clofibrate* (242 daltons), in part unchanged and also after hepatic conjugation. As the half-life increases from 17 h to 100 h with renal failure (Table 14), significant dosage reduction is mandatory (738, 739). Removal of clofibrate by dialysis is limited by 95% protein binding, which decreases somewhat in uremic patients. The dose should be lowered from 1.5 to 2.0 g/day to 1.0 to 1.5 g (4 to 6 mmol) per week to avoid toxicity including ataxia, muscle weakness, gastrointestinal disturbances and increased creatinine phosphokinase, while maintaining the lipid lowering effect (738, 739). Acute interstitial nephritis with renal failure also may complicate therapy (740). *Bezafibrate* (351 daltons) has a normal clearance of 100 ml/min which is predominantly renal. It accumulates in patients with renal failure, the half-life increasing from 2 h to 19.5 h (Table 14), and the peritoneal clearance of only 0.2 ml/min contributes negligibly to its elimination (741). *Fenofibrate*, another hypolipemic drug, is more than 99% bound in plasma and excreted mostly by the kidney with a half-life of 20 h that increases to 150 h with renal failure and is not abbreviated by hemodialysis (742). *Acipimox* depends virtually entirely on renal elimination. Renal failure prolongs its half-life considerably beyond the normal 2 h, but hemodialysis lowers it to 2.6 h (743).

Cimetidine (252 daltons), a reversible competitive antagonist of histamine H_2 receptor action, is excreted mostly by the kidney. About 20% of cimetidine is protein bound in plasma and the distribution volume is 2.1 l/kg (13). With renal failure, the elimination half-life increases from 1.9 h to 4.3 h (Table 14) as the elimination rate correlates with creatinine clearance (744, 745). Cimetidine increases plasma creatinine concentrations possibly by decreasing secretion but does not decrease glomerular filtration rate or other parameters of renal function (746). In uremic patients, cimetidine dosage must be reduced to 300 mg (1.2 mmol)/12 h, half of the usual dose, to prevent toxicity consisting of drowsiness, dizziness, confusion, flushing, sweating, diarrhea, muscular pain and rash (747), symptoms that can mimic uremia. Cimetidine decreases hepatic blood flow, impairing metabolism of drugs such as diazepam, antipyrine and propranolol (463, 748). Cimetidine also reversibly lowers circulating levels of immunoreactive parathyroid hormone without affecting serum concentrations of calcium, phosphorus or magnesium (749). Hemodialysis clears cimetidine at 40 ml/min, reducing the half-life to 2.5 h (745, 746, 750, 751) and reducing plasma concentrations by about 70% (747), but rebound increments occur thereafter. Peritoneal clearance of cimetidine ranges from 3 to 10 ml/min, insufficient to affect pharmacokinetics appreciably (751, 752). With hemoperfusion the clearance is 85 ml/min which exceeds the nonrenal clearance of 36 ml/min (751). The half-life of the sulphoxide metabolite increases from 1.7 h to 14.4 h with renal failure (744). It may be toxic and is removed by hemodialysis. *Ranitidine* distributes in 1.8 l/kg, is normally cleared at about 750 ml/min mostly by the kidney, with a normal half-life of about 3 h that increases to 7.0 h with renal failure and is reduced to about 4.3 h (Table 14) by hemodialysis (753, 754). *Omeprazole*, which inhibits gastric acid secretion, is eliminated by hepatic metabolism with a half-life of 0.6 h that doesn't increase with renal failure (755). Extensive protein binding should inhibit removal by dialysis.

Metoclopramide (354 daltons), an antiemetic normally cleared at 875 ml/min with a half-life of 3.5 h, is retained in patients with renal failure because of a fall in nonrenal as well as renal clearance, prolonging the half-life to 14 h (756). Neither hemodialysis nor peritoneal dialysis reduces the half-life (Table 14) appreciably (757).

Doxapram, a central nervous stimulant, normally distributes in 1.8 l/kg and is cleared at 320 ml/min with a half-life of 2.4 h (758). The half-life of the metabolite is 4.8 h. These values are not affected by renal failure.

CONCLUSIONS

In choosing a drug for the uremic patient, it is preferable when possible to select one that normally does not depend primarily on renal excretion, one that is little affected by changes in plasma protein binding, distribution volume or receptor sensitivity and one that is not complicated by active or toxic metabolites (464). For example, diazepam is preferable to barbiturates, alkylating agents are preferable to methotrexate and synthetic penicillins are preferable to tetracyclines and aminoglycosides.

Pharmacokinetic principles must be followed in caring for uremic patients. The physician who must rely blindly on nomograms and 'cookbook' style guidelines to adjust dosage in the treatment of renal disease has no business administering potentially toxic drugs to patients with impaired renal function (23).

ACKNOWLEDGEMENT

The opinions and assertions contained herein are the private views of the author and should not be construed as official or as necessarily reflecting the views of the Uniformed Services University of the Health Sciences or Department of Defense. Their is no objection to publication.

Because data are acquired rapidly in this field the reader is advised to check package inserts and current literature for pertinent new findings. Care of individual patients must be guided by clinical and laboratory findings. The data cited have been checked carefully but cannot supersede clinical judgement.

The extensive and excellent secretarial assistance of Mrs. Barbara Fitzgerald is greatly appreciated.

REFERENCES

1. Reidenberg MM: *Renal Function and Drug Action*. Philadelphia, WB Saunders Co, 1971
2. Fabre J, Balant L, Chavaz A: Recent drug management advances in renal insufficiency. *Adv Nephrol* 4: 223, 1974
3. Whelton A: Antibacterial chemotherapy in renal insufficiency. A review. *Antibiot Chemother* 18: 1, 1974
4. Dedrick RL: Pharmacokinetic and pharmacodynamic considerations for chronic hemodialysis. *Kidney Int* 7 (Suppl 2): S7, 1975
5. Maher JF: Toxic and irradiation nephropathies. in *Strauss and Welt's Diseases of the Kidney* edited by Earley LE, Gottschalk CW, Boston, Little, Brown and Co, 1979, p 1431
6. Winchester JF, Gelfand MC, Knepshield JH, Schreiner GE: Dialysis and hemoperfusion of poisons and drugs – update. *Trans Am Soc Artif Intern Organs* 23: 762, 1977
7. Seyffart G: Drugs in renal failure: dosing guidelines for frequently used drugs in end-stage renal disease and dialysis patients. *Blood Purif* 3: 140, 1985
8. Anderson RJ, Bennett WM, Gambertoglio JG, Schrier RW: Fate of drugs in renal failure. in the *The Kidney* edited by Brenner BM, Rector FC Jr, 2nd edn, Philadelphia, WB Saunders Co, 1981, p 2659
9. Maher JF: Pharmacokinetics in patients with renal failure. *Clin Nephrol* 21: 39, 1984
10. Gibson RP: Renal disease and drug metabolism: an overview. *Am J Kidney Dis* 8: 7, 1986
11. Lee CC, Marbury TC: Drug therapy in patients undergoing haemodialysis; clinical pharmacokinetic considerations. *Clin Pharmacokinet* 9: 42, 1984
12. La Greca G, Biasioli S, Borin D, Brendolan A, Chiaramonte S, Fabris A, Feriani M, Pisani E, Ronco C: Drugs and dialysis. *Int J Artif Organs* 6: 139, 1983
13. Benet LZ, Sheiner LB: Design and optimization of dosage regimens; pharmacokinetic data. in *Goodman and Gilman's The Pharmacological Basis of Therapeutics* edited by Gilman AG, Goodman LS, Rall TW, Murad F, 7th edn, New York, MacMillan Publ Co, 1985, p 1663
14. Bennett WM, Aronoff GR, Morrison G, Golper TA, Pulliam J, Wolfson M, Singer I: Drug prescribing in renal failure: dosing guidelines for adults. *Am J Kidney Dis* 3: 155, 1983
15. Anderson RJ, Melikian DM, Gambertoglio JG, Berns AS, Cadnapaphornchai P, Egan DJ, Goldberg JP, Henrich WL, Hicks DL, Kovalchik MT, Olin DB: Prescribing medication in long-term dialysis units. *Arch Intern Med* 142: 1305, 1982
16. Smith JW, Seidl LG, Cluff LE: Studies on the epidemiology of adverse drug reaction. V. Clinical factors influencing susceptibility. *Ann Intern Med* 65: 629, 1966
17. Cutler RE, Christopher TG, Forrey AW, Blair AD: Modification of drug therapy in chronic dialysis patients. *Kidney Int* 7 (Suppl 2): S16, 1975
18. Schreiner GE, Maher JF: *Uremia: Biochemistry, Pathogenesis and Treatment.* Springfield, IL, Charles C. Thomas Co, 1961
19. Atkinson AJ Jr, Kushner W: Clinical pharmacokinetics. *Annu Rev Pharmacol Toxicol* 19: 105, 1971
20. Welling PG, Craig WA: Pharmacokinetics in disease states modifying renal function. in *The Effect of Disease States on Pharmacokinetics* edited by Benet LZ, Washington, Am Pharm Assoc Acad Pharm Sci, 1976, p 155
21. Dettli L: Drug dosage in renal disease. *Clin Pharmacokinet* 1: 126, 1976
22. Fabre J, Balant L: Renal failure, drug pharmacokinetics and drug action. *Clin Pharmacokinet* 1: 99, 1976
23. Levy G: Pharmacokinetics in renal disease. *Am J Med* 62: 461, 1977
24. Muther RS, Bennett WM: Drug therapy in renal failure. *Compr Ther* 8(5): 44, 1982
25. Parker A, Izard MW, Maher JF: Therapy of iron deficiency in patients on maintenance dialysis. *Nephron* 23: 181, 1979
26. Craig RM, Murphy P, Gibson TP, Quintanilla A, Chao GC, Cochrane C, Patterson A, Atkinson AJ Jr: Kinetic analysis of d-xylose absorption in patients with chronic renal failure. *J Lab Clin Med* 101: 496, 1983
27. Kimura T, Ikeda K, Kobayashi A, Nakayama T: Effect of experimental acute renal failure on intestinal barriers to drug absorption. *Chem Pharm Bull* (Tokyo) 32: 2471, 1984
28. Keller F, Wilms H, Schultze G, Offerman G, Molzahn N: Effect of plasma protein binding, volume of distribution and molecular weight on the fraction of drugs eliminated by hemodialysis. *Clin Nephrol* 19: 201, 1983
29. Schindhelm K, Skalsky M, Mahoney JF, Farrell PC: Creatinine transfer between interstitial and intracellular fluid: a comparison between normal and uremic subjects. *asaio J* 2: 25, 1979
30. Maher JF: Interrelation of hemoperfusion, plasma clearance and half life. in *Artificial Kidney, Artificial Liver and Artificial Cells* edited by Chang TMS, New York and London, Plenum Press, 1978, p 297
31. Boobis SW: Alteration of plasma albumin in relation to de-

creased drug binding in uremia. *Clin Pharmacol Ther* 22: 147, 1977

32. Reidenberg MM: The binding of drugs to plasma proteins and the interpretation of measurements of plasma concentrations of drugs in patients with poor renal function. *Am J Med* 62: 467, 1977

33. Gulyassy PF, Depner TA: Impaired binding of drugs and endogenous ligands in renal diseases. *Am J Kidney Dis* 2: 578, 1983

34. Lichtenwalner DM, Suh B, Lorber B, Rudnick MR, Craig WA: Partial purification and characterization of the drug-binding-defect inducer in uremia. *J Lab Clin Med* 97: 72, 1981

35. Depner TA, Gulyassy PF: Plasma protein binding in uremia: extraction and characterization of an inhibitor. *Kidney Int* 18: 86, 1980

36. Bowmer CJ, Lindup WE: Investigation of the drug-binding defect in plasma from rats with glycerol-induced acute renal failure. *J Pharmacol Exp Ther* 210: 440, 1979

37. Mabuchi H, Nakahashi H: Isolation and characterization of an endogenous drug-binding inhibitor present in uremic serum. *Nephron* 44: 277, 1986

38. Reidenberg MM, Odar-Cederlöf I, von Bahr C, Borga ML, Sjoqvist R: Protein binding of diphenylhydantoin and desmethylimipramine in plasma from patients with poor renal function. *N Engl J Med* 285: 264, 1971

39. Jusko WJ, Weintraub M: Myocardial distribution of digoxin and renal function. *Clin Pharmacol Ther* 16: 449, 1974

40. Halkin H, Skeiner LB, Peck CC, Melman KL: Determinants of renal clearance of digoxin. *Clin Pharmacol Ther* 17: 385, 1975

41. Weiner IM: Mechanisms of drug absorption and excretion. *Annu Rev Pharmacol* 7: 39, 1967

42. Navalesi R, Pilo A, Lenzi S, Donato L: Insulin metabolism in chronic uremia and in the anephric state: effect of the dialytic treatment. *J Clin Endocrinol Metab* 40: 70, 1975

43. Hall CL, Hardwicke J: Low molecular weight proteinuria. *Annu Rev Med* 30: 199, 1979

44. Emmanuel DS, Lindheimer MD, Katz AI: Uremia in rats with normal kidneys: a model for the study of renal function in a uremic environment. *Kidney Int* 11: 209, 1977

45. Maher JF, Schreiner GE: Studies on ethacrynic acid in patients with refractory edema. *Ann Intern Med* 62: 15, 1965

46. Kunin CM: Limitations upon the use of antibiotics imposed by renal insufficiency. *Modern Treatment* 7: 355, 1970

47. Bailey GL, Hampers CL, Merrill JP: Reversible cardiomyopathy in uremia. *Trans Am Soc Artif Intern Organs* 13: 263, 1967

48. Richards RK, Taylor JD, Kueter KE: Effect of nephrectomy on the duration of sleep following the administration of thiopental and hexobarbital. *J Pharmacol Exp Ther* 108: 461, 1953

49. Freeman RB, Sheff MF, Maher JF, Schreiner GE: The blood-cerebrospinal fluid barrier in uremia. *Ann Intern Med* 56: 233, 1962

50. Roxe BM: Toxic nephropathy from diagnostic and therapeutic agents. Review and commentary. *Am J Med* 69: 759, 1980

51. Schreiner GE: Drug related nephropathy. *Contrib Nephrol* 10: 30, 1978

52. Taliercio CP, Vlietstra RE, Fischer LD, Burnett JC: Risks for renal dysfunction with cardiac angiography. *Ann Intern Med* 104: 501, 1986

53. Smith CR, Moore RD, Leitman RD: Studies of risk factors for aminoglycoside nephrotoxicity. *Am J Kidney Dis* 8: 308, 1986

54. Dawborn JD, Fairley KF, Kincaid-Smith P, King WE: The association of peptic ulceration, chronic renal disease and analgesic abuse. *Q J Med* 35: 69, 1966

55. Nanra RS, Fairley KF, Kincaid-Smith P: Recovery renal function in patients with analgesic nephropathy. *Aust Ann Med* 19: 195, 1970

56. Gonwa TA, Corbett WT, Schey HM, Buckalew VM Jr: Analgesic associated nephropathy and transitional cell carcinoma of the urinary tract. *Ann Intern Med* 93: 249, 1980

57. Heptinstall RH: Interstitial nephritis: a brief review. *Am J Path* 83: 214, 1976

58. Adler SG, Cohen AH, Border WA: Hypersensitivity phenomena and the kidney: role of drugs and environmental agents. *Am J Kidney Dis* 5: 75, 1985

59. Linton AL, Clark WF, Driedger AA, Turnbull DI, Lindsay RM: Acute interstitial nephritis due to drugs. Review of the literature with a report of nine cases. *Ann Intern Med* 93: 735, 1980

60. Kimberly RP, Bowden RE, Keiser HR, Plotz PH: Reduction of renal function by newer nonsteroidal anti-inflammatory drugs. *Am J Med* 64: 804, 1978

61. Lanao JM, Dominguez-Gil A, Taberno JM, Macias JF: Influence of the type of dialyzer on the pharmacokinetics of amikacin. *Int J Clin Pharmacol Ther Toxicol* 21: 197, 1983

62. Gibson TP: Principles of drug dose adjustment during hemodialysis. *Am J Kidney Dis* 3: 110, 1983

63. Lasrich M, Maher JM, Hirszel P, Maher JF: Correlation of peritoneal transport rates with molecular weight: a method for predicting clearances. *asaio J* 2: 107, 1979

64. Colton CK, Smith KA, Merrill EW, Farrell PC: Permeability studies with cellulosic membranes. *J Biomed Mater Res* 5: 459, 1971

65. Nolph KD, Nothum RJ, Maher JF: Ultrafiltration: a mechanism for removal of intermediate molecular weight substances in coil dialyzers. *Kidney Int* 6: 55, 1974

66. Talki S, Gambertoglio JG, Honda DH, Tozer TN: Pharmacokinetic evaluation of hemodialysis in acute drug overdose. *J Pharmacokinet Biopharm* 6: 427, 1978

67. Gibson TP, Nelson HA: Drug kinetics and artificial kidneys. *Clin Pharmacokinet* 2: 403, 1977

68. Nolph KD, Bass OE, Maher JF: Acute effects of hemodialysis on removal of intracellular solutes. *Trans Am Soc Artif Intern Organs* 20: 622, 1974

69. Bass OE, Nolph KD, Maher JF: Dialysance and clearance measurements during clinical dialysis – a plea for standardization. *J Lab Clin Med* 86: 378, 1975

70. Maher JF, Montero G, Chieffo S: Tin protein binding kinetics in normal and uremic plasma and its effect on dialysis fluxes. *Trans Am Soc Artif Intern Organs* 22: 149, 1976

71. Maher JF, Schreiner GE, Marc-Aurele J: Methodologic problems associated with in vitro measurements of dialysance. *Trans Am Soc Artif Intern Organs* 5: 120, 1959

72. Maher JF: Selective dialysis for removal of large solutes, a reappraisal. *Kidney Int* 7 (Suppl 3): S361, 1975

73. Maher JF: Principles of dialysis and dialysis of drugs. *Am J Med* 62: 475, 1977

74. Maher JF: Influence of continuous ambulatory peritoneal dialysis on elimination rate of drugs. *Peritoneal Dial Bull* 7: 159, 1987

75. Paton TW, Cornish WR, Manuel MA, Hardy BG: Drug therapy in patients undergoing peritoneal dialysis. Clinical pharmacokinetic considerations. *Clin Pharmacokinet* 10: 404, 1985

76. Janknegt R, Koks CHW: Pharmacokinetic aspects during continuous ambulatory peritoneal dialysis: a literature review. *Pharm Weekbl (Sci)* 6: 229, 1984

77. Marc-Aurele J, Schreiner GE: The dialysance of ethanol and methanol: a proposed method for the treatment of massive intoxication by ethyl or methyl alcohol. *J Clin Invest* 39: 892, 1960

78. Maher JF: Determinants of serum half life of glutethimide in intoxicated patients. *J Pharmacol Exp Therap* 174: 450, 1970

79. Setter JF, Freeman RB, Maher JF, Schreiner GE: Factors influencing the dialysis of barbiturates. *Trans Am Soc Artif Intern Organs* 10: 340, 1964

80. Schmitt GW, Maher JF, Schreiner GE: Ethacrynic acid enhanced bromuresis. A comparison with peritoneal and hemodialysis. *J Lab Clin Med* 68: 913, 1966

81. Schreiner GE: The role of hemodialysis (artificial kidney) in acute poisoning. *Arch Intern Med* 102: 896, 1958

82. Brodie BB, Bernstein E, Mark LC: The role of body fat in limiting the duration of action of thiopental. *J Pharmacol Exp Ther* 105: 421, 1952

83. Keller F, Offerman G, Lode H: Supplementary dose after hemodialysis. *Nephron* 30: 220, 1982

84. Kopple JD, Swendseid ME: Vitamin nutrition in patients undergoing maintenance hemodialysis. *Kidney Int* 7 (*Suppl* 2): S79, 1975

85. Maher JF, Freeman RB, Schmitt G, Schreiner GE: Adherence of metals to cellophane and removal by whole blood. A mechanism for solute transport during hemodialysis. *Trans Am Soc Artif Intern Organs* 11: 104, 1965

86. Rumpf KW, Rieger J, Ansorg R, Doht B, Scheler F: Binding of antibiotics by dialysis membranes and its clinical relevance. *Proc Eur Dial Transplant Assoc* 14: 607, 1977

87. Janicke DM, Morse GD, Apicella MA, Jusko WJ, Walshe JJ: Pharmacokinetic modelling of bidirectional transfer during peritoneal dialysis. *Clin Pharmacol Ther* 40: 209, 1986

88. Maher JF, Hirszel P, Hohnadel DC, Abraham J, Lasrich M: Fatty acid removal during peritoneal dialysis: mechanisms, rates and significance. *asaio J* 1: 8, 1978

89. Dedrick RL, Myers CE, Bungay PM, De Vita VT JR: Pharmacokinetic rationale for peritoneal drug administration in the treatment of ovarian cancer. *Cancer Treat Rep* 62: 1, 1978

90. Henderson LW: Hemofiltration. *Kidney Int* 13 (*Suppl* 8): S145, 1978

91. Bergström J, Asaba H, Fürst P, Oules R: Dialysis, ultrafiltration and blood pressure. *Proc Eur Dial Transplant Assoc* 13: 293, 1977

92. Kramer P, Matthaei D, Fuchs C, Arnold R, Ebert R, McIntosh C, Schauder P, Schwinn G, Scheler F, Ludwig H, Spittelu G: Assessment of hormone loss through hemofiltration. *Artif Organs* 2: 128, 1978

93. Chang TMS: Hemoperfusion alone and in series with ultrafiltration or dialysis for uremia, poisoning and liver failure. *Kidney Int* 10, (*Suppl* 7): S305, 1976

94. Rosenbaum JL, Kramer MS, Raja R, Winsten S, Dalal F: Hemoperfusion for acute drug intoxication. *Kidney Int* 10 (*Suppl*) 7): S341, 1976

95. Bismuth C, Conso F, Wattel F, Gosselin B, Lambert H, Genestal M: Coated activated charcoal hemoperfusion. Experience of French antipoison centers in 60 cases. *Vet Hum Toxicol* 2: 81, 1979

96. Winchester JF: Evolution of artificial organs: extracorporeal removal of drugs. *Artif Organs* 10: 59, 1986

97. Farrell PC: Acute drug intoxication and extracorporeal intervention. *asaio J* 3: 39, 1980

98. Pond S, Rosenberg J, Benowitz NL, Takki S: Pharmacokinetics of haemoperfusion for drug overdose. *Clin Pharmacokinet* 4: 329, 1979

99. Sofer S, Wills RA, Van Wie BJ: A model enzymic extracorporeal detoxification system. *Artif Organs* 3: 147, 1979

100. Pazmiño P, Sladek SL, Weinshilboum RM: Thio-s-methylation in uremia: Erythrocyte enzyme activities and plasma inhibitors. *Clin Pharmacol Ther* 28: 356, 1980

101. Nolph KD, Popovich RP, Ghods AJ, Twardowski ZJ: Determinants of low clearances of small solutes during peritoneal dialysis. *Kidney Int* 13: 117, 1978

102. Nolph KD: The first hemodialyzer. *asaio J* 1: 2, 1978

103. Maher JF: Characteristics of peritoneal transport: physiological and clinical implications. *Miner Electrolyte Metab* 5: 201, 1981

104. Maher JF: Peritoneal transport rates: mechanisms, limitations and methods for augmentation. *Kidney Int* 18 (*Suppl* 10): S117, 1980

105. Nolph KD, Ghods AJ, Brown PA, Twardowski ZJ: Effects of intraperitoneal nitroprusside on peritoneal clearances in man with variations of dose, frequency of administration and dwell times. *Nephron* 24: 114, 1979

106. Maher JF, Hirszel P, Lasrich M: An experimental model for study of pharmacologic and hormonal influences on peritoneal dialysis. *Contr Nephrol* 17: 131, 1979

107. Zelman A, Gisser D, Whittam PJ, Parsons RH, Schuyler R: Augmentation of peritoneal dialysis efficiency with programmed hyper/hypo-osmotic dialysates. *Trans Am Soc Artif Intern Organs* 23: 203, 1977

108. Hirszel P, Lasrich M, Maher JF: Augmentation of peritoneal mass transport by dopamine. Comparison with norepinephrine and evaluation of pharmacologic mechanisms. *J Lab Clin Med* 94: 747, 1979

109. Maher JF, Hirszel P, Lasrich M: Effects of gastrointestinal hormones on transport by peritoneal dialysis. *Kidney Int* 16: 130, 1978

110. Popovich RP, Moncrief JW, Nolph KD, Ghods AJ, Twardowski ZJ, Pyle WK: Continuous ambulatory peritoneal dialysis. *Ann Intern Med* 88: 449, 1979

111. Bennett WM, Plamp CE, Gilbert DN, Parker RA, Porter GA: The influence of dosage regimen on experimental gentamicin nephrotoxicity: dissociation of peak serum levels from renal failure. *J Infect Dis* 140: 576, 1979

112. Tozer TN: Nomogram for modification of dosage regimens in patients with chronic renal function impairment. *J Pharmacokinet Biopharm* 2: 13, 1974

113. Humes HD, Weinberg JM, Knauss TC: Clinical and pathophysiologic aspects of aminoglycoside toxicity. *Am J Kidney Dis* 2: 5, 1982

114. Cronin RE: Aminoglycoside nephrotoxicity: pathogenesis and prevention. *Clin Nephrol* 11: 251, 1979

115. Brogard JM, Comte F, Spach MO: Nephrotoxicity of aminoglycosides. Effects on pharmacokinetics and prevention. *Contr Nephrol* 42: 182, 1984

116. Henrich WL, Thompson P, Bergstrom G, Lum SM: Effect of dialysis on hearing acuity. *Nephron* 18: 348, 1977

117. McQuillen MP, Cantor HE, O'Rourke JR: Myasthenic syndromes associated with antibiotics. *Arch Neurol* 18: 402, 1968

118. McDermott W: Toxicity of streptomycin. *Am J Med* 2: 491, 1947

119. Edwards KDG, Whyte HM: Streptomycin poisoning in renal failure. *Br Med J* 1: 753, 1959

120. DeBeukelaer MM, Travis LB, Dodge WF, Guerra FA: Deafness and acute tubular necrosis following parenteral administration of neomycin. *Am J Dis Child* 121: 250, 1971

121. Krumlovsky FA, Emmerman J, Parker RH, Wisgerhof M, Del Greco F: Dialysis in treatment of neomycin overdosage.

Ann Intern Med 76: 443, 1972

122. Yow EM, Abu-Nasser H: Kanamycin: a reevaluation after three years experience. *2nd Int Symposium Chemother* 1: 148, 1963

123. Toyoda Y, Tachibana M: Tissue levels of kanamycin in correlation with oto and nephrotoxicity. *Acta Otolaryngol* 86: 9, 1978

124. Cutler RE, Orme BM: Correlation of serum creatinine concentration and kanamycin half life. *JAMA* 209: 539, 1969

125. Danish M, Schultz R, Jusko WJ: Pharmacokinetics of gentamicin and kanamycin during hemodialysis. *Antimicrob Agents Chemother* 6: 841, 1974

126. Greenberg PA, Sanford JP: Removal and absorption of antibiotics in patients with renal failure undergoing peritoneal dialysis. Tetracycline chloramphenicol, kanamycin and colistimethate. *Ann Intern Med* 66: 465, 1967

127. Atkins RC, Mion C, Despaux E, Van-Hai N, Julien C, Mion H: Peritoneal transfer of kanamycin and its use in peritoneal dialysis. *Kidney Int* 3: 391, 1973

128. Wilfert JN, Burke JP, Bloomer HA, Smith CB: Renal insufficiency associated with gentamicin therapy. *J Infect Dis* 124: S148, 1971

129. Milman N: Renal failure associated with gentamicin therapy. *Acta Med Scand* 196: 87, 1974

130. Gary NE, Buzzeo L, Salaki J, Eisinger RP: Gentamicin-associated acute renal failure. *Arch Intern Med* 136: 1101, 1976

131. Christopher TG, Korn D, Blair AD, Korrey AW, O'Neill MA, Cutler RE: Gentamicin pharmacokinetics during hemodialysis. *Kidney Int* 3: 38, 1974

132. Brier ME, Mayer PR, Brier RA, Visscher D, Luft FC. Aronoff GR: Relationship between rat renal accumulation of gentamicin, tobramycin and netilmicin and their toxicities. *Antimicrob Agents Chemother* 27: 812, 1985

133. Gailiunas P, Dominguez-Moreno M, Lazarus JM, Lowrie EG, Gottlieb MN, Merrill JP: Vestibular toxicity of gentamicin. Incidence in patients receiving long-term hemodialysis therapy. *Arch Intern Med* 138: 1621, 1978

134. Dahlgren JG, Anderson ET, Hewitt WL: Gentamicin blood levels: a guide to nephrotoxicity. *Antimicrob Agents Chemother* 8: 58, 1975

135. Hull HG, Sarubbi FA: Gentamicin serum concentrations: pharmacokinetic predictions. *Ann Intern Med* 85: 183, 1976

136. Letourneau-Saheb L, Lapierre L, Daigneault R, Prud-'Homme M, St-Louis G, Sirois G: Gentamicin pharmacokinetics during hemodialysis in patients suffering from chronic renal failure. *Int J Clin Pharmacol Biopharm* 15: 116, 1977

137. Rosenbaum JL, Levine J, Falk B, Raja R, Kramer MS: Effect of hemoperfusion on clearance of gentamicin, cephalothin and clindamycin from plasma of normal dogs. *J Infect Dis* 136: 801, 1977

138. Indraprasit S, Ukaravichien V, Pummangara C, Kaojarern S: Gentamicin removal during intermittent peritoneal dialysis. *Nephron* 44: 18, 1986

139. Pancorbo S, Comty C: Pharmacokinetics of gentamicin in patients undergoing continuous ambulatory peritoneal dialysis. *Antimicrob Agents Chemother* 19: 605, 1981

140. Lane AZ, Wright GE, Blair DC: Ototoxicity and nephrotoxicity of amikacin. An overview of phase II and phase III experience in the United States. *Am J Med* 62: 911, 1977

141. Madhavan T, Yaremchuk K, Levin N, Pohlad D, Burch K, Fisher E, Cox F, Quinn EL: Effect of renal failure and dialysis on the serum concentration of the aminoglycoside amikacin. *Antimicrob Agents Chemother* 10: 464, 1976

142. Ho PWL, Pien FD, Kominami N: Massive amikacin 'overdose'. *Ann Intern Med* 91: 227, 1979

143. Pechere J, Dugal R: Pharmacokinetics of intravenously administered tobramycin in normal volunteers and in renal-impaired and hemodialyzed patients. *J Infect Dis* 134: S118, 1976

144. Christopher TG, Blair AD, Forrey AW, Cutler RE: Hemodialyzer clearances of gentamicin, kanamycin, tobramycin, amikacin, ethambutol, procainamide and flucytosine with a technique for planning therapy. *J Pharmacokin Biopharm* 4: 427, 1976

145. Malacoff RF, Finkelstein FD, Andriole VT: Effect of peritoneal dialysis on serum levels of tobramycin and clindamycin. *Antimicrob Agents Chemother* 8: 574, 1975

146. Bunke CM, Aronoff GR, Brier ME, Sloan SR, Luft FC: Tobramycin kinetics during continuous ambulatory peritoneal dialysis. *Clin Pharmacol Ther* 34: 110, 1983

147. Rodriguez V, Bodey GP, Valdivieso M, Feld R: Clinical pharmacology of sisomicin. *Antimicrob Agents Chemother* 7: 38, 1975

148. Appel GV, Neu HC: The nephrotoxicity of antimicrobial agents, *N Engl J Med* 296: 663, 1977

149. Luft FC, Block R, Sloan RS, Yum MN, Costello R, Maxwell DR: Comparative nephrotoxicity of aminoglycoside antibiotics in rats. *J Infect Dis* 138: 541, 1978

150. Luft FC, Brannon DR, Stropes LL, Costello RJ, Sloan RS, Maxwell DR: Pharmacokinetics of netilmicin in patients with renal impairment and in patients on dialysis. *Antimicrob Agents Chemother* 14: 403, 1978

151. Basile C, Di Maggio A, Curino E, Scatizzi A: Pharmacokinetics of netilmicin in hypertonic hemodiafiltration and standard hemodialysis. *Clin Nephrol* 24: 305, 1985

152. Leroy A, Humbert G, Fillastre JP: Pharmacokinetics of dibekacin in normal subjects and in patients with renal failure. *J Antimicrob Chemother* 6: 113, 1980

153. Navarini A, Montanari A, Bruschi G, Rossi E, Borghetti A, Migone L: The kinetics of aminosidine in renal patients with different degrees of renal failure. *Clin Nephrol* 4: 23, 1975

154. Weinstein MJ, Wagman GH, Marquez JA, Testa RT, Waitz JA: Verdamycin, a new broad spectrum aminoglycoside antibiotic. *Antimicrob Agents Chemother* 7: 246, 1975

155. Fillastre JP, Humbert G, Daufresne MF, Dubois D, Leroy A: Pharmacodynamics of lividomycin in renal failure. *Proc Eur Dial Transplant Assoc* 10: 547, 1973

156. Stewens J, Marre R, Englebart K, Schulz E, Sack K: Habekacin: nephrotoxicity pharmacokinetics and prophylactic efficacy in rats. *Arzneimittel Forschung* 35: 1440, 1985

157. Moellering RC Jr, Swartz MN: The newer cephalosporins. *N Engl J Med* 294: 24, 1976

158. Mandell GL, Sande MA: Antimicrobial agents: penicillins, cephalosporins and other beta-lactam antibiotics. in *Goodman and Gilman's The Pharmacological Basis of Therapeutics* edited by Gilman AG, Goodman LS, Rall TW, Murad F, 7th edn, New York, MacMillan Publ Co, 1985, p 1115

159. Kirby WMM, deMaine JB, Serrill WS: Pharmacokinetics of the cephalosporins in healthy volunteers and uremic patients. *Postgrad Med J* 47: S41, 1971

160. Curtis JR, Marshall MJ: Cephaloridine serum levels in patients on maintenance haemodialysis. *Br Med J* 2: 149, 1970

161. Perkins RL, Smith EM, Saslow S: Cephalothin and cephaloridine: comparative pharmacodynamics in chronic uremia. *Am J Med Sci* 257: 116, 1969

162. Craig WA, Welling PG, Jackson TC, Kunin CM: Pharmacology of cephazolin and other cephalosporins in patients with renal insufficiency. *J Infect Dis* 128: S347, 1973

163. Engle JE, Drago J, Charlin B, Schoolwerth AC: Reversible acute renal failure after cephalothin. *Ann Intern Med* 83: 222, 1975

164. Carling PC, Idelson BA, Casano A, Alexander EA, McCabe WR: Nephrotoxicity associated with cephalothin administration. *Arch Intern Med* 135: 797, 1975

165. Tune BM, Wu KY, Longerbeam DF, Kempson RL; Transport and toxicity of cephaloridine in the kidney. Effect of furosemide, p-aminohippurate and saline diuresis. *J Pharmacol Exp Ther* 202: 472, 1977

166. Berman SJ, Boughton WH, Sugihara JG, Wong EGC, Sato MM, Siemsen AW: Pharmacokinetics of cefaclor in patients with end-stage renal disease and during hemodialysis. *Antimicrob Agents Chemother* 14: 281, 1978

167. Gartenberg G, Meyers BR, Hirschman SZ, Srulevitch E: Pharmacokinetics of cefaclor in patients with stable renal impairment and patients undergoing hemodialysis. *J Antimicrob Chemother* 5: 465, 1979

168. Humbert G, Leroy A, Fillastre JP, Godin M: Pharmacokinetics of cefadroxil in normal subjects and in patients with renal insufficiency *Chemotherapy* 25: 189, 1979

169. Gambertoglio JG, Aziz NS, Len ET, Grausz H, Naughton JL, Benet LZ: Cefamandole kinetics in uremic patients undergoing hemodialysis. *Clin Pharmacol Ther* 26: 592, 1979

170. Ahern MJ, Finkelstein FO, Andriole VT: Pharmacokinetics of cefamandole in patients undergoing hemodialysis and peritoneal dialysis. *Antimicrob Agents Chemother* 10: 457, 1976

171. Pancorbo S, Comty C: Pharmacokinetics of cefamandole in patients undergoing continuous ambulatory peritoneal dialysis. *Peritoneal Dial Bull* 3: 135, 1983

172. Eastwood JB, Gower PPE, Curtis JR: The serum half life and urine concentrations of cefazolin sodium in patients with terminal renal failure: effect of haemodialysis. *Scot Med J* 20: 240, 1975

173. Hiner LB, Baluarte J, Polinsky MS, Gruskin AB: Cefazolin in children with renal insufficiency. *J Pediat* 96: 335, 1980

174. Brogard JM, Pinget M, Brandt C, Lavillaureix J: Pharmacokinetics of cefazolin in patients with renal failure; special reference to hemodialysis. *J Clin Pharmacol* 17: 225, 1977

175. Kirby WMM, Regamy C: Pharmacokinetics of cefazolin compared with four other cephalosporins. *J Infect Dis* 128: S341, 1973

176. Greene DS, Tice AD: Effect of hemodialysis on cefazolin protein binding. *J Pharm Sci* 66: 1508, 1977

177. Bunke CM, Aronoff GR, Brier ME, Sloan RS, Luft FC: Cefazolin and cephalexin kinetics in continuous ambulatory peritoneal dialysis. *Clin Pharmacol Ther* 33: 66, 1983

178. Guay DRP, Meatherall RC, Harding GK, Brown GR: Pharmacokinetics of cefixime (CL 284, 635; FK 027) in healthy subjects and patients with renal insufficiency. *Antimicrob Agents Chemother* 30: 485, 1986

179. Gambertoglio JG, Alexander DP, Barriere SL: Cefmenoxime pharmacokinetics in healthy volunteers and subjects with renal insufficiency and on hemodialysis. *Antimicrob Agents Chemother* 26: 845, 1984

180. Sica DA, Polk RE, Kerkering TM, Patterson P, Baggett J: Cefmenoxime kinetics during continuous ambulatory peritoneal dialysis. *Eur J Clin Pharmacol* 30: 713, 1986

181. Ohkawa M, Orito M, Sugata T, Shimamura M, Sawaki M, Nakashita E, Kuroda K, Sasahara K: Pharmacokinetics of cefmetazole in normal subjects and in patients with impaired renal function. *Antimicrob Agents Chemother* 18: 386, 1980

182. Barriere SL, Gambertoglio JG, Alexander DP, Stagg RJ, Conte JG Jr: Pharmacokinetic disposition of cefonicid in patients with renal failure and receiving hemodialysis. *Rev Infect Dis* 6 (*Suppl* 4): S809, 1984

183. Fillastre JP, Fourtillan JB, Leroy A, Ramis N, Lefevre MA, Reumont G, Humbert G: Pharmacokinetics of cefonicid in uremic patients. *J Antimicrob Chemother* 18; 203, 1986

184. Morse GD, Lane T, Nairn DK, Deterding J, Curry J, Gal P: Peritoneal transport of cefonicid. *Antimicrob Agents Chemother* 31: 292, 1987

185. Balant L, Dayer P, Rudhardt M, Allaz AF, Fabre J: Cefoperazone: Pharmacokinetics in humans with normal and impaired renal function and pharmacokinetics in rats. *Clin Ther* 3: 50, 1980

186. Spyker DA, Richmond JD, Scheld WM, Bolton WK: Pharmacokinetics of multiple-dose cefoperazone in hemodialysis patients. *Am J Nephrol* 5: 355, 1985

187. Hodler JE, Galeazzi RL, Rudhardt M, Seiler AG: Pharmacokinetics of cefoperazone in patients undergoing chronic ambulatory peritoneal dialysis: clinical and pathophysiological implications. *Eur J Clin Pharmacol* 26: 609, 1984

188. Hess JR, Berman SJ, Boughton WH, Sugihara JG, Musgrave JE, Wong EGC, Siemsen AM: Pharmacokinetics of ceforanide in patients with end-stage renal disease on hemodialysis. *Antimicrob Agents Chemother* 17: 251, 1980

189. Hawkins SS, Alford RH, Stone WJ, Smyth RD, Pfeffer M: Ceforanide kinetics in renal insufficiency. *Clin Pharmacol Ther* 30: 468, 1981

190. Matzke GR, Abraham PA, Halstenson CE, Keane WF: Cefotaxime and desacetyl cefotaxime kinetics in renal impairment. *Clin Pharmacol Ther* 38: 31, 1985

191. Ohkawa M, Okasho A, Motoi I, Tokunaga S, Shoda R, Kawaguchi S, Sawaki M, Shimamura M, Hirano S, Kuroda K, Awazu S: Elimination kinetics of cefotaxime and desacetyl cefotaxime in patients with renal insufficiency and during hemodialysis. *Chemotherapy* 29: 4, 1983

192. Albin HC, Demotes-Mainard FM, Bouchard JL, Vincon GA, Martin-Dupont C: Pharmacokinetics of intravenous and intraperitoneal cefotaxime in chronic ambulatory peritoneal dialysis. *Clin Pharmacol Ther* 38: 259, 1985

193. Heim KL, Halstenson CE, Comty CM, Affrime MB, Matzke GR: Disposition of cefotaxime and desacetyl cefotaxime during continuous ambulatory peritoneal dialysis. *Antimicrob Agents Chemother* 30: 15, 1986

194. Smith BR, LeFrock JL, Thyrum PT, Doret BA, Yeh C, Onesti G, Schwartz A, Zimmerman JJ: Cefotetan pharmacokinetics in volunteers with various degrees of renal function. *Antimicrob Agents Chemother* 29: 887, 1986

195. Browning MJ, Holt HA, White LO, Chapman ST, Banks RA, Reeves DS, Yates RA: Pharmacokinetics of cefotetan in patients with end-stage renal failure on maintenance dialysis. *J Antimicrob Chemother* 18: 103, 1986

196. Konishi K, Ozawa Y: Pharmacokinetics of cefotiam in patients with impaired renal function and in those undergoing hemodialysis. *Antimicrob Agents Chemother* 26: 647, 1984

197. Humbert G, Fillastre JP, Leroy A, Godin M, Van Winzum C: Pharmacokinetics of cefoxitin in normal subjects and in patients with renal insufficiency. *Rev Infect Dis* 1: 118, 1979

198. Sasano H, Fujimato T, Une T, Tachizawa H, Ogawa H: Cefoxitin, a semisynthetic cephamycin antibiotic. Metabolism in rats with renal insufficiency. *Arzneimittel Forschung* 28: 1596, 1978

199. Garcia MJ, Dominguez-Gil A, Tabernero JM, Bondia Roman A, Pharmacokinatics of cefoxitin in patients undergoing hemodialysis *Int J Clin Pharmacol Biopharm* 17: 366, 1979

200. Arvidsson A, Alvan G, Tranaeus A, Malmborg AS: Pharma-

cokinetic studies of cefoxitin in continuous ambulatory peritoneal dialysis. *Eur J Clin Pharmacol* 28: 333, 1985

201. Garcia MJ, Dominguez-Gil A, Taberno JM, Diaz Molina M: Pharmacokinetics of cefoxitin during haemofiltration. *Eur J Clin Pharmacol* 25: 395, 1983

202. Nieto MJ, Lanao JM, Dominguez-Gil A, Taberno JM Macias JF: Elimination of cefroxadine (CGP-9000) from patients undergoing dialysis. *Eur J Clin Pharmacol* 24: 109, 1983

203. Gibson RP, Granneman GR, Kallai JE: Cefsulodin kinetics in renal impairment. *Clin Pharmacol Ther* 31: 602, 1982

204. Matzke GR, Keane WF: Cefsulodin pharmacokinetics during hemodialysis. *Trans Am Soc Artif Intern Organs* 28: 324, 1982

205. Nikolaidis P, Tourkantonis A: Effect of hemodialysis on ceftazidine pharmacokinetics. *Clin Nephrol* 24: 142, 1985

206. van Dalen R, Vree TB, Baars AM, Termond E: Dosage adjustment for ceftazidine in patients with impaired renal function. *Eur J Clin Pharmacol* 30: 597, 1986

207. Ohkawa M, Kuroda K: Pharmacokinetics of ceftezole in patients with normal and impaired renal function. *Chemotherapy* 26: 242, 1980

208. Ohkawa M, Okasho S, Sugata T, Kuroda K: Elimination kinetics of ceftizoxime in humans with and without renal insufficiency. *Antimicrob Agents Chemother* 22: 308, 1982

209. Gross ML, Somani P, Ribner BS, Raeader R, Freimer EH, Higgins JT: Ceftizoxime elimination kinetics in continuous ambulatory peritoneal dialysis. *Clin Pharmacol Ther* 34: 673, 1983

210. Ti TY, Fortin L, Kreeft MH, East DS, Ogilvie RI, Somerville PJ: Kinetic disposition of intravenous ceftriazone in normal subjects and patients with renal failure on hemodialysis or peritoneal dialysis. *Antimicrob Agents Chemother* 25: 83, 1984

211. Albin H, Ragnaud JM, Demotes F, Vincon G, Couzineau M, Wone C: Pharmacokinetics of intravenous and intraperitoneal ceftriaxone in chronic ambulatory peritoneal dialysis. *Eur J Clin Pharmacol* 31: 479, 1986

212. Chan MK, Browning AK, Poole CJM, Matheson LA, Li CS, Baillod RA, Moorhead JF: Cefuroxime pharmacokinetics in continuous and intermittent peritoneal dialysis. *Nephron* 41: 161, 1985

213. Heinecke G, Hoffler MJ, Finke K: Reversible encephalopathy following cephacetrile therapy in high doses in a patient on chronic intermittent hemodialysis. *Clin Nephrol* 5: 45, 1976

214. Verma S, Kieff E: Cephalexin related nephropathy. *JAMA* 234: 618, 1975

215. McCloskey RV, Terry HE, McCracken AW, Sweeney MJ, Forland MF: Effect of hemodialysis and renal failure on serum and urine concentrations of cephapirin sodium. *Antimicrob Agents Chemother* 1: 90, 1972

216. Bryan CS, Stone WJ: Antimicrobial dosage in renal failure: a unifying nomogram. *Clin Nephrol* 7: 81, 1977

217. Morse G, Janicke D, Cafarell R, Piontek K, Apicella M, Jusko WJ, Walshe JJ: Moxalactam epimer disposition in patients undergoing continuous ambulatory peritoneal dialysis. *Clin Pharmacol Ther* 38: 150, 1985

218. Srinivason S, Neu H: Pharmacokinetics of moxalactam in patients with renal failure and during hemodialysis. *Antimicrob Agents Chemother* 20: 398, 1981

219. Aronoff GR, Sloan RS, Mong SA, Luft FC, Kleit SA: Moxalactam pharmacokinetics during hemodialysis. *Antimicrob Agents Chemother* 19: 575, 1981

220. Jacobson EJ, Zahrowski JJ, Nissenson AR: Moxalactam kinetics in hemodialysis. *Clin Pharmacol Ther* 30: 487, 1981

221. Fillastre JP, Leroy A, Baudoin C, Humbert G, Swabb EA, Vertucci C, Godin M: Pharmacokinetics of aztreonam in pa-

tients with chronic renal failure. *Clin Pharmacokinet* 10: 91, 1985

222. Gerig JS, Bolton N, Swabb EA, Scheld WM, Bolton WK: Effect of hemodialysis and peritoneal dialysis on aztreonam pharmacokinetics. *Kidney Int* 26: 308, 1984

223. Horber F, Egger HJ, Weidekamm E, Dubach UC, Frey FJ, Probst PJ, Stoeckel K: Pharmacokinetics of carumonam in patients with renal insufficiency. *Antimicrob Agents Chemother* 30: 116, 1986

224. Verpooten GA, Verbist L, Buntinx AP, Entwistle CA, Jones KH, DeBroe ME: The pharmacokinetics of imipenim (thienamycin-formamidine) and the renal dehydropeptidase inhibitor cilastin sodium in normal subjects and patients with renal failure. *Br J Clin Pharmacol* 18: 183, 1984

225. Gibson TP, Demetriades JL, Bland JA: Impenim/cilastin: pharmacokinetic profile in renal insufficiency. *Am J Med* 78 (*Suppl* 6A): 54, 1985

226. Baldwin DS, Levine BB, McCluskey RT, Gallo GR: Renal failure and interstitial nephritis due to penicillin and methicillin. *N Engl J Med* 279: 1245, 1968

227. Woodroffe AJ, Thomson NM, Meadows R, Lawrence JR: Nephropathy associated with methicillin administration. *Aust NZ J Med* 4: 256, 1974

228. Schrier RW, Bulger RJ, Van Ardsel PP Jr: Nephropathy associated with penicillin and homologues. *Ann Intern Med* 64: 116, 1966

229. Tourkantonis A, Friedrich H, Heinze V: Ampicillin-Nebenwirkungen bei Patienten mit Niereninsuffizienz. (Ampicillin-side effects in patients with renal insufficiency.) *Med Klin* 66: 1154, 1971

230. Bloomer HA, Barton LJ, Maddock RK Jr: Penicillin induced encephalopathy in uremic patients. *JAMA* 200: 121, 1967

231. Andrassy K, Ritz E: Antimicrobial therapy in dialysis patients. I. Penicillins and cephalosporins. *Blood Purif* 3: 94, 1985

232. Barza M, Weinstein L: Pharmacokinetics of the penicillins in man. *Clin Pharmacokinet* 1: 297, 1976

233. Wickerts CJ, Asaba H, Gunnarson B, Bygdeman S, Bergström J: Combined carbon haemoperfusion and haemodialysis in treatment of penicillin intoxication. *Br Med J* 1: 1254, 1980

234. Montanari A, Borghi L, Canali M, Coruzzi P, Novarini A, Borghetti A; The influence of renal function on the elimination kinetics of sulbenicillin in man. *Int J Clin Pharmacol Ther Toxicol* 18: 225, 1980

235. Kunin CM, Finkelberg Z: Oral cephalexin and ampicillin: antimicrobial activity, recovery in urine and persistence in blood of uremic patients. *Ann Intern Med* 72: 349, 1970

236. Jusko WJ, Lewis GP, Schmitt GW: Ampicillin and hetacillin pharmacokinetics in normal and anephric subjects. *Clin Pharmacol Ther* 14: 90, 1973

237. Reudy J: Effects of peritoneal dialysis on physiologic disposition of oxacillin, ampicillin and tetracycline in patients with renal disease *Can Med Assoc J* 94: 257, 1966

238. Horber FF, Frey FJ, Descoaedres C, Murray AT, Reubi FC: Differential effects of impaired renal function on the kinetics of clavulanic acid and amoxicillin. *Antimicrob Agents Chemother* 29: 614, 1986

239. Franke EL, Appel GB, Neu HC: Kinetics of intravenous amoxicillin in patients on long-term dialysis. *Clin Pharmacol Ther* 26: 31, 1979

240. Humbert G, Spyker DA, Fillastre JP, Leroy A: Pharmacokinetics of amoxicillin: dosage nomogram for patients with impaired renal function. *Antimicrob Agents Chemother* 15: 28, 1979

241. Bulger RJ, Lindholm DD, Murray JS, Kirby WMM: Effect of uremia on methicillin and oxacillin blood levels. *JAMA* 187: 319, 1964

242. Galpin JE, Shinaberger JH, Stanley TM, Blumenkrantz MJ, Bayer AS, Friedman GS, Montgomerie JZ, Guze LB, Coburn JW, Glassock RJ: Acute interstitial nephritis due to methicillin. *Am J Med* 65: 756, 1978

243. Rudnick M, Morrison G, Walker B, Singer I: Renal failure, hemodialysis and nafcillin kinetics. *Clin Pharmacol Ther* 20: 413, 1977

244. Rosenblatt JE, Kind AC, Brodie JL, Kirby WMM: Mechanisms responsible for the blood level differences of isoxazolyl penicillins. *Arch Intern Med* 121: 345, 1968

245. Tillman DB, Oill PA, Guze LB: Oxacillin nephritis. *Arch Intern Med* 140: 552, 1980

246. Malone AJ Jr, Field S, Rosman J, Shermerdiak WP: Neurotoxic reaction to oxacillin. *N Engl J Med* 296: 453, 1977

247. Nauta EH, Mattie H: Pharmacokinetics of flucloxacillin and cloxacillin in healthy subjects and patients on chronic intermittent haemodialysis. *Br J Clin Pharmacol* 2: 111, 1975

248. McCloskey RV, Hayes CP: Plasma levels of dicloxacillin in oliguric patients and the effect of hemodialysis. *Antimicrob Agents Chemother* 7: 770, 1967

249. Thijssen HHW, Wolters J: The metabolic disposition of flucloxacillin in patients with impaired kidney function. *Eur J Clin Pharmacol* 22: 429, 1982

250. Oe PL, Simonian S, Verhoef J: Pharmacokinetics of the new penicillins; amoxacillin and flucloxacillin in patients with terminal renal failure undergoing hemodialysis. *Chemotherapy* 19: 279, 1973

251. Hoffman TA, Cestero R, Bullock WE: Pharmacodynamics of carbenicillin in hepatic and renal failure. *Ann Intern Med* 73: 173, 1970

252. Latos DL, Bryan CS, Stone WJ: Carbenicillin therapy in patients with normal and impaired renal function. *Clin Pharmacol Ther* 17: 692, 1975

253. Eastwood JB, Curtis JR: Carbenicillin administration in patients with severe renal failure. *Br Med J* 1: 486, 1968

254. Klastersky J, Vanderkelen B, Daneau N, Mathieu M: Carbenicillin and hypokalemia. *Ann Intern Med* 78: 774, 1973

255. Brunner FP, Frick PG: Hypokalemia, metabolic alkalosis and hypernatremia due to massive penicillin therapy. *Br Med J* 4: 550, 1968

256. Whelton A, Carter CG, Garth MA: Carbenicillin-induced acidosis and seizures. *JAMA* 218: 1942, 1971

257. Wilson FM, Belamaric J, Lauter CB, Lerner AM: Anicteric carbenicillin hepatitis. *JAMA* 232: 818, 1975

258. Brown CH III, Natelson EA, Bradshaw MW, Williams TW Jr, Alfrey CP Jr: The hemostatic defect produced by carbenicillin. *N Engl J Med* 291: 265, 1974

259. Bailey RR, Eastwoord JB, Vaughan RB: The pharmacokinetics of an oral form of carbenicillin in patients with renal failure. *Postgrad Med J* 48: 422, 1972

260. Libke RD, Clarke JT, Ralph ED, Luthy RP, Kirby WMM: Ticarcillin vs carbenicillin: clinical pharmacokinetics. *Clin Pharmacol Ther* 17: 441, 1975

261. Dalet F, Amado E, Cabrera E, Donate T, del Rio G: Pharmacokinetics of the combination of ticarcillin with clavulanic acid in renal insufficiency. *J Antimicrob Chemother* 17 (*Suppl* C): 57, 1986

262. Wise R, Reeves DS, Parker AS: Administration of ticarcillin, a new antipseudomonal antibiotic in patients undergoing dialysis. *Antimicrob Agents Chemother* 5: 119, 1974

263. Kallay MC, Taberchian H, Riley GR, Chessin LN: Neurotox-

icity due to ticarcillin in patients with renal failure. *Lancet* 1: 608, 1979

264. Boelaert J, Daneels R, Schurgers M, Mellows G, Swaisland AJ, Lambert AM, Van Landuyt HW: Effects of renal function and dialysis on temocillin pharmacokinetics. *Drugs* 29 (*Suppl* 5): 109, 1985

265. Leroy A, Humbert G, Fillastre JP, Borsa F, Godin M: Pharmacokinetics of temocillin in subjects with normal and impaired renal function. *J Antimicrob Chemother* 12: 47, 1983

266. Aletta JM, Francke EF, Neu HC: Intravenous azlocillin kinetics in patients on long-term hemodialysis. *Clin Pharmacol Ther* 27: 563, 1980

267. Leroy A, Humbert G, Godin M, Fillastre JP: Pharmacokinetics of azlocillin in subjects with normal and impaired renal function. *Antimicrob Agents Chemother* 17: 344, 1980

268. Kosmidis J, Doundoulaki P, Stathakis C, Zerefos N, Bounia A, Daikos GK: Elimination kinetics of mezlocillin in normal and impaired renal function including effects of dialysis. *Arzneimittel Forschung* 29: 1960, 1978

269. Francke E, Mehta S, Neu HC, Appel GB: Kinetics of intravenous mezlocillin in chronic hemodialysis patients. *Clin Pharmacol Ther* 26: 228, 1979

270. Kampf D, Schurig R, Weihermüller K, Förster D: Effects of impaired renal function, hemodialysis and peritoneal dialysis on the pharmacokinetics of mezlocillin. *Antimicrob Agents Chemother* 18: 81, 1980

271. Janicke DM, Mangione A, Schultz RW, Jusko WJ: Mezlocillin disposition in chronic hemodialysis patients. *Antimicrob Agents Chemother* 20: 590, 1981

272. Francke EL, Appel GB, Neu HC: Pharmacokinetics of intravenous piperacillin in patients undergoing chronic hemodialysis. *Antimicrob Agents Chemother* 16: 788, 1979

273. Thompson MIB, Russo ME, Matsen JM, Atkin-Thor E: Piperacillin pharmacokinetics in subjects with chronic renal failure. *Antimicrob Agents Chemother* 19: 450, 1981

274. Giron JA, Meyers BR, Hirschman SZ, Srulevitch E: Pharmacokinetics of piperacillin in patients with moderate renal failure and in patients undergoing hemodialysis. *Antimicrob Agents Chemother* 19: 279, 1981

275. Bailey K, Cruickshank JG, Bisson PG, Radford BL: Mecillinam in patients on hemodialysis. *Br J Clin Pharmacol* 10: 177, 1980

276. Patel IH, Bornemann LD, Brocks VM, Fang LST, Talkoff-Rubin NE, Rubin RH: Pharmacokinetics of intravenous amdinocillin in healthy subjects and patients with renal insufficiency. *Antimicrob Agents Chemother* 28: 46, 1985

277. Shils ME: Renal disease and the metabolic effects of tetracycline. *Ann Intern Med* 58: 489, 1963

278. Orr LH Jr, Rudisill E Jr, Brodkin R, Hamilton RW: Exacerbation of renal failure associated with doxycycline. *Arch Intern Med* 138: 793, 1978

279. Morgan T, Ribush N: The effect of oxytetracycline and doxycycline on protein metabolism. *Med J Aust* 1: 55, 1972

280. Clausen G, Nagy Z, Szaloy L, Aukland K: Mechanisms in acute oliguric renal failure induced by tetracycline infusion. *Scand J Clin Lab Invest* 35: 625, 1975

281. Singer I, Rotenberg D: Demeclocycline induced nephrogenic diabetes insipidus. In vivo and in vitro studies. *Ann Intern Med* 79: 679, 1973

282. Carrilho F, Bosch J, Arroyo V, Mas A, Viver J, Rodes J: Renal failure associated with demeclocycline in cirrhosis. *Ann Intern Med* 87: 195, 1977

283. Oster JR, Epstein M, Ulano HB: Deterioration of renal function with demeclocycline administration. *Curr Ther Res* 20: 794, 1976

284. Stenback O, Myhre E, Berdal BD: The effect of doxycycline on renal function in patients with advanced renal insufficiency. *Scand J Infect Dis* 5: 199, 1973

285. Frimpter GW, Timpanelli AE, Eisenmenger WJ, Stein HS, Ehrlich LI: Reversible 'Fanconi Syndrome' caused by degraded tetracycline. *JAMA* 184: 111, 1963

286. Allen JC: Minocycline. *Ann Intern Med* 85: 482, 1976

287. Heaney D, Eknoyan G: Minocycline and doxycycline kinetics in renal failure. *Clin Pharmacol Ther* 24: 233, 1978

288. George CRP, Guiness NDG, Lark DJ, Evans RA: Minocycline toxicity in renal failure. *Med J Aust* 1: 640, 1973

289. Maher JF, Freeman RB, Setter JG, Rubin M, Schreiner GE: Dialysance studies of varied solutes and biochemical changes during hemodialysis. *Trans Am Soc Artif Intern Organs* 10: 332, 1964

290. Rose HD, Roth DA, Koch ML: Serum tetracycline levels during peritoneal dialysis. *Am J Med Sci* 250: 66, 1965

291. Yow EM, Moyer JH, Smith CP: Toxicity of polymyxin B. II. Human studies with particular reference to evaluation of renal function. *Arch Intern Med* 92: 248, 1953

292. Hoeprich PD: The polymyxins. *Med Clin North Am* 54: 1257, 1970

293. Adler S, Segal DP: Non-oliguric renal failure secondary to sodium colistimethate: a report of four cases. *Am J Med Sci* 262: 109, 1971

294. Koch-Weser J, Sidel VW, Federman EB, Kanarek P, Finer DC, Eaton AE: Adverse effects of sodium colistimethate. *Ann Intern Med* 72: 857, 1970

295. Wolinsky E, Hines JD: Neurotoxic and nephrotoxic effects of colistin in patients with renal disease. *N Engl J Med* 266: 759, 1962

296. MacKay DN, Kaye D: Serum concentrations of colistin in patients with normal and impaired renal function. *N Engl J Med* 270: 394, 1964

297. Curtis JR, Eastwood JB: Colistin sulfomethate sodium administration in the presence of severe renal failure and during haemodialysis and peritoneal dialysis. *Br Med J* 1: 484, 1968

298. Goodwin NJ, Friedman EA: The effects of renal impairment, peritoneal dialysis and hemodialysis on sodium colistimethate levels. *Ann Intern Med* 68: 984, 1968

299. Beirne GJ, Hansing CE, Octaviano GN, Burns RO: Acute renal failure caused by hypersensitivity to polymyxin B sulfate. *JAMA* 202: 62, 1967

300. Baethke R, Golde G, Gahl G: Sulfamethoxazole/trimethoprim: pharmacokinetic studies in patients with chronic renal failure. *Eur J Clin Pharmacol* 4: 233, 1972

301. Adam WR, Dawborn JK: Urinary excretion and plasma levels of sulfonamides in patients with renal impairment. *Australas Ann Med* 3: 250, 1970

302. Bergan T, Brodwall EK, Vik-Mo H, Anstad U: Pharmacokinetics of sulfadiazine, sulfamethoxazole and trimethoprim in patients with varying renal function. *Infection* 7 (Suppl 4): S382, 1979

303. Fine A, Sumner D: Alteration of hepatic acetylation in uraemia. *Proc Eur Dial Transplant Assoc* 11: 433, 1974

304. Reidenberg MM, Kostenbauder H, Adams WP: Rate of drug metabolism in obese volunteers before and during starvation and in azotemic patients. *Metabolism* 18: 209, 1969

305. Anton AH: The effect of disease, drugs and dilution on the binding of sulfonamides in human plasma. *Clin Pharmacol Ther* 9: 561, 1968

306. Kawamura T, Yagi N, Sugawara H, Yamahata K, Takada M: Efficacy of hemodialysis and the effects of certain displacing agents on plasma protein binding of sulfamethoxazole and sulfaphenazole in patients with chronic renal failure. *Chem Pharmacol Bull* (Tokyo) 28: 268, 1980

307. Skimming LH, Knies PT, Anthony MA, Melerango ES: Hemolytic anemia caused by sulfamethoxypyridazine. Report of a case successfully treated by hemodialysis. *Ohio Med J* 57: 280, 1961

308. Halstenson CE, Blevins RB, Salem NG, Matzke GR: Trimethoprimsulfamethoxazole pharmacokinetics during continuous ambulatory peritoneal dialysis. *Clin Nephrol* 22: 239, 1984

309. Weinstein L, Maddoff MA, Samet CCM: The sulfonamides. *N Engl J Med* 263: 793, 1960

310. Lehr D: Clinical toxicity of sulfonamides. *Ann NY Acad Sci* 69: 417, 1957

311. Glushein AS, Fisher ER: Renal lesions of sulfonamide type after treatment with acetazolamide (Diamox). *JAMA* 160: 204, 1956

312. Kalowski S, Nanra RS, Mathew TH, Kincaid-Smith P: Deterioration in renal function in association with co-trimoxazole therapy. *Prog Biochem Pharmacol* 9: 129, 1974

313. Smith EJ, Light JA, Filo RS, Yum N: Interstitial nephritis caused by trimethoprim-sulfamethoxazole in renal transplant recipients. *JAMA* 244: 360, 1980

314. Grafnetterova J, Vodrazka Z, Jandova D, Schuck O, Tomasek R, Lachmanova J: The binding of chloramphenicol to serum proteins in patients with chronic renal insufficiency. *Clin Nephrol* 6: 448, 1976

315. Kunin CM, Glasko AJ, Finland M: Persistence of antibiotics in blood in patients with acute renal failure. II. Chloramphenicol and its metabolic products in the blood of patients with severe renal disease or hepatic cirrhosis. *J Clin Invest* 38: 1498, 1959

316. Mauer SM, Chavers BM, Kjellstrand CM: Treatment of an infant with severe chloramphenicol intoxication using charcoal-column hemoperfusion. *J Pediat* 96: 136, 1980

317. Peddie BA, Dann E, Bailey RR: The effect of impairment of renal function and dialysis on the serum and urine levels of clindamycin. *Aust NZ J Med* 5: 198, 1975

318. Reinarz JA, McIntosh DA: Lincomycin excretion in patients with normal renal function, severe azotemia and with hemodialysis and peritoneal dialysis. *Antimicrob Agents Chemother* 5: 232, 1965

319. Kunin CM, Finland M: Persistence of antibiotics in the blood of patients with acute renal failure. III Penicillin, streptomycin, erythromycin and kanamycin. *J Clin Invest* 38: 1509, 1958

320. Mery A, Kanfer A: Hearing loss and erythromycin pharmacokinetics in patients receiving hemodialysis. *Ann Intern Med* 144: 419, 1984

321. Lindholm DD, Murray JS: Persistence of vancomycin in the blood during renal failure and its treatment by hemodialysis. *N Engl J Med* 274, 1047, 1966

322. Nielsen HE, Hansen HE, Korsager B, Skov PE: Renal excretion of vancomycin in kidney disease. *Acta Med Scand* 197: 261, 1975

323. Pancorbo S, Comty C: Peritoneal transport of vancomycin in 4 patients undergoing continuous ambulatory peritoneal dialysis. *Nephron* 31: 37, 1982

324. Morse GD, Farolino DF, Apicella MA, Walshe JJ: Comparative study of intraperitoneal and intravenous vancomycin pharmacokinetics during continuous ambulatory peritoneal dialysis. *Antimicrob Agents Chemother* 31: 173, 1987

325. Matzke GR, O'Connell MB, Collins AJ, Keshaviah PR: Disposition of vancomycin during hemofiltration. *Clin Pharmacol Ther* 40: 425, 1986

326. Revert L, Lopez J, Pons J, Olag T: Fosfomycin in patients subjected to periodic hemodialysis. *Chemotherapy* 23 (Suppl 1): 204, 1977

327. Bouchet JL, Quentin C, Albin H, Vincon G, Guillin J, Martin-Dupont P: Pharmacokinetics of fosfomycin in hemodialyzed patients. *Clin Nephrol* 23: 218, 1985

328. Zintel HA, Ma RA, Nichols AC, Ellis H: The absorption, distribution, excretion, and toxicity of bacitracin in man. *Am J Med Sci* 218: 439, 1949

329. Felts JH, Hayes DM, Gergen JA, Toole JF: Neural, hematologic and bacteriologic effects of nitrofurantoin in renal insufficiency. *Am J Med* 51: 331, 1971

330. Adam WR, Dawborn JK: Plasma levels and urinary excretion of nalidixic acid in patients with renal failure. *Aust NZ J Med* 2: 126, 1971

331. Mannista P, Solkinen A, Mantyla R, Gordin A, Salo H, Hanninen U, Nunisto L: Pharmacokinetics of pipemidic acid in healthy middle-aged volunteers and elderly patients with renal insufficiency. *Xenobiotica* 14: 339, 1984

332. Alano FA, Webster GD: Acute renal failure and pigmentation due to phenazopyridine (Pyridium). *Ann Intern Med* 72: 89, 1970

333. Szwed JJ, Brannon DE, Sloan RS, Luft FC: Pharmacokinetics of cinoxacin in patients with renal failure. *J Antimicrob Chemother* 4: 451, 1978

334. Arrigo G, Cavaliere G, D'Amico G, Passarella E, Broccali G: Pharmacokinetics of norfloxacin in chronic renal failure. *Int J Clin Pharmacol Ther Toxicol* 23: 491, 1985

335. Boelaert J, Valcke Y, Schurgers M, Daneels M, Rosseel MT, Bogaert MG: The pharmacokinetics of ciprofloxacin in patients with impaired renal function. *J Antimicrob Chemother* 16: 87, 1985

336. Fillastre JP, Leroy A, Humbert G: Ofloxacin pharmacokinetics in renal failure. *Antimicrob Agents Chemother* 31: 156, 1987

337. Montay G, Jacquot C, Bariety J, Cunci R: Pharmacokinetics of pefloxacin in renal insufficiency. *Eur J Clin Pharmacol* 29: 345, 1985

338. Jenne JW, Beggs WH: Correlation of *in vitro* and *in vivo* kinetics with clinical use of isoniazid, ethambutol and rifampin. *Am Rev Respir Dis* 107: 1013, 1973

339. Hagstam KE, Lindholm T: Treatment of exogenous poisoning with special regard to the need for artificial kidney in severe complicated cases. *Acta Med Scand* 175: 507, 1964

340. Cocco AE, Pazourek LJ: Acute isoniazid intoxication-management by peritoneal dialysis. *N Engl J Med* 269: 852, 1963

341. Königshausen T, Altrogge G, Hein D, Grabansee B, Putter D: Hemodialysis and hemoperfusion in the treatment of most severe INH-poisoning. *Vet Hum Toxicol* 21: 12, 1979

342. Gold CH, Buchanan N, Tringham V, Viljoen M, Strickwold B, Moodley GP: Isoniazid pharmacokinetics in patients in chronic renal failure. *Clin Nephrol* 6: 365, 1976

343. Campese VM, Marzullo F, Schema FP, Coratelli P: Acute renal failure during intermittent rifampicin therapy. *Nephron* 10: 256, 1973

344. Bansal VK, Bennett D, Molnar Z: Prolonged renal failure after rifampin. *Am Rev Respir Dis* 116: 137, 1977

345. Novi C, Bissoli F, Simonati V, Volpini T, Baroli A, Vignati G: Rifampin and digoxin: possible drug interaction in a dialysis patient *JAMA* 244: 2521, 1980

346. Christopher TG, Blair A, Forrey A, Cutler RE: Kinetics of ethambutol elimination in renal disease. *Proc Clin Dial Transplant Forum* 3: 96, 1973

347. Atkins R, Cutting CJ, Mackintosh TF: Acute poisoning by cycloserine. *Br Med J* 1: 907, 1965

348. Mandell GL, Sande MA: Antimicrobial agents: drugs used in the chemotherapy of tuberculosis and leprosy. in *Goodman and Gilman's The Pharmacological Basis of Therapeutics*, edited by Gilman AG, Goodman LS, Rall TW, Murad F, 7th edn, New York, Macmillan Publ Co, 1985, p 1199

349. Butler WT, Bennett JE, Alling DW, Wertlake PT, Utz JP, Hill GJ: Nephrotoxicity of amphotericin B. *Ann Intern Med* 61: 175, 1964

350. Burgess JL, Birchall R: Nephrotoxicity of amphotericin B with emphasis on changes in tubular function. *Am J Med* 53: 77, 1972

351. Gerkins JF, Branch RA: The influence of sodium status and furosemide on canine acute amphotericin B nephrotoxicity. *J Pharmacol Exp Ther* 214: 306, 1980

352. Block ER, Bennett JE, Levoti LG, Klein WJ, MacGregor RR, Henderson L: Flucytosine and amphotericin B: Hemodialysis effects on the plasma concentration and clearance. *Ann Intern Med* 80: 613, 1974

353. Maher JF, Hirszel P, Bennett RR, Chakrabarti E: Amphotericin selectively increases peritoneal ultrafiltration. *Am J Kidney Dis* 4: 285, 1984

354. Dawborn JK, Page MD, Schiavone DJ: Use of 5-fluorocytosine in patients with impaired renal function. *Br Med J* 3: 382, 1973

355. Rault RM, Hulme B, Davies RR: 5-Fluorocytosine treatment of candidiasis on a patient receiving regular hemodialysis. *Clin Nephrol* 3: 225, 1973

356. Stevens DA, Levine HB, Deresinski SC: Miconazole in coccidioidomycosis. II. Therapeutic and pharmacologic studies in man. *Am J Med* 60: 199, 1976

357. Keller F, Lode H, Offerman G: Antimicrobial therapy in dialysis patients. II. Remaining antibiotics and antimicrobial agents. *Blood Purif* 3: 104, 1985

358. Johnson RJ, Blair AD, Ahmad S: Ketoconazole kinetics in chronic peritoneal dialysis. *Clin Pharmacol Ther* 37: 325, 1985

359. Fabre J, de Freudenreich J, Duckert A, Pitton JS, Rudhardt M, Virieux C: Influence of renal insufficiency on the excretion of chloroquin phenobarbital, phenothiazines and methacycline. *Helv Med Acta* 33: 307, 1976

360. Akintonwa A, Odutula TA, Edeki T, Mabadeje AFB: Hemodialysis clearance of chloroquin in uremic patients. *Ther Drug Monit* 8: 285, 1986

361. Smith CC, Ihrig J, Menne R: Antimalarial activity and metabolism of biguanides. *Am J Trop Med Hyg* 10: 694, 1961

362. Smith CC, Ihrig J: Persistent excretion of pyrimethamine following oral administration. *Am J Trop Med Hyg* 8: 60, 1959

363. Webster LT: Drugs used in the chemotherapy of protozoal infections: malaria. in *Goodman and Gilman's The Pharmacological Basis of Therapeutics*, edited by Gilman AG, Goodman LS, Rall TW, Murad F, New York, MacMillan Publ Co 1985, p 1029

364. Donadio JV, Whelton A, Gilliland PF, Cirksena WJ: Peritoneal dialysis in quinidine intoxication. *JAMA* 204: 274, 1968

365. Floyd M, Hill AVL, Ormston BJ, Menzies R, Porter R: Quinine amblyopia treated by hemodialysis. *Clin Nephrol* 2: 44, 1974

366. Walzer PD, Perl DP, Krogstad DJ, Rawson PG, Schultz MG: Pneumocystis carinii pneumonia in the United States. Epidemiologic, diagnostic and clinical features. *Ann Intern Med* 80: 83, 1974

367. Somogyi A, Kong C, Sabto J, Gurr FW, Spicer WJ, McLean AJ: Disposition and removal of metronidazole in patients undergoing haemodialysis. *Eur J Clin Pharmacol* 25: 683, 1983

368. Roux AF, Moirot E, Delhotal B, Leroy J, Bonmarchand GP, Humbert G, Flouvat B: Metronidazole kinetics in patients with acute renal failure on dialysis: a cumulative study. *Clin Pharmacol Ther* 36: 363, 1984

369. Guay DR, Meatherall RC, Baxter H, Jacyk WR, Penner B: Pharmacokinetics of metronidazole in patients undergoing continuous ambulatory peritoneal dialysis. *Antimicrob Agents Chemother* 25: 306, 1984

370. Flouvat BL, Imbet C, Dubois DM, Temperville BP, Roux AF, Chevalier GC, Humbert G: Pharmacokinetics of tinidazole in chronic renal failure and in patients on haemodialysis. *Br J Clin Pharmacol* 15: 735, 1983

371. Merdjan H, Baumelou A, Diquet B, Chick O, Singlas E: Pharmacokinetics of ornidazole in patients with renal insufficiency; influence of haemodialysis and peritoneal dialysis. *Br J Clin Pharmacol* 19: 211, 1985

372. Allgayer H, Zähringer J, Bach P, Bircher J: Lack of effect of haemodialysis on mebendazole kinetics: studies in a patient with echinococcosis and renal failure. *Eur J Clin Pharmacol* 29: 243, 1984

373. Schumaker JD, Band JD, Lensmeyer GL, Craig WA: Thiabendazole treatment of severe strongyloidiasis in a hemodialyzed patient. *Ann Intern Med* 89: 644, 1978

374. Bauer LA, Raisys VA, Watts MT, Ballinger J: The pharmacokinetics of thiabendazole and its metabolites in an anephric patient undergoing hemodialysis and hemoperfusion. *J Clin Pharmacol* 22: 276, 1982

375. Neuvonen PJ, Elonen E, Haapanen EJ: Acute dapsone intoxication: clinical findings and effect of oral charcoal and haemodialysis on dapsone elimination. *Acta Med Scand* 214: 215, 1983

376. Aoki FY, Sitar DS, Ogilvie RI: Amantidine kinetics in healthy young subjects after long-term dosing. *Clin Pharmacol Ther* 26: 729, 1979

377. Wu MJ, Ing TS, Soung LS, Daugirdas JT, Hano JE, Gandhi VC: Amantadine hydrochloride pharmacokinetics in patients with impaired renal function. *Clin Nephrol* 17: 19, 1982

378. Soung L, Ing TS, Daugirdas JT, Wu M, Gandhi VC, Ivanovich PT, Hano JE, Viol GW: Amantadine pharmacokinetics in hemodialysis patients. *Ann Intern Med* 93: 46, 1980

379. Krasny HC, Liao SH, DeMiranda P, Laskin OL, Welton A, Lietman PS: Influence of hemodialysis on acyclovir pharmacokinetics in patients with chronic renal failure. *Am J Med* 73: 202, 1982

380. Shah GM, Winer RL, Krasny HC: Acyclovir pharmacokinetics in a patient on continuous ambulatory peritoneal dialysis. *Am J Kidney Dis* 7: 507, 1986

381. Spiegel DM, Lau K: Acute renal failure and coma secondary to acyclovir therapy. *JAMA* 255: 1882, 1986

382. Hirsch MS, Tolkoff-Rubin NE, Kelly AP, Rubin RH: Pharmacokinetics of human and recombinant interferon in patients with chronic renal failure who are undergoing hemodialysis. *J Infect Dis* 148: 335, 1983

383. Selden R, Haynie G: Ouabain plasma level kinetics and removal by dialysis in chronic renal failure. A study in fourteen patients. *Ann Intern Med* 83: 15, 1975

384. Doherty JE: Digitalis glycosides. Pharmacokinetics and their clinical implications. *Ann Intern Med* 79: 229, 1973

385. Finkelstein FO, Goffinet JA, Hendler ED, Lindenbaum J: Pharmacokinetics of digoxin and digitoxin in patients undergoing hemodialysis. *Am J Med* 58: 525, 1975

386. Rambausek M, Ritz E: Digitalis in chronic renal insufficiency. *Blood Purif* 3: 4, 1985

387. Ohnhaus EE, Vozeh S, Neusch E: Absolute bioavailability of digoxin in chronic renal failure. *Clin Nephrol* 11: 302, 1979

388. Gault MH, Churchill DN, Kalra J: Loading dose of digoxin in renal failure. *Br J Clin Pharmacol* 9: 593, 1980

389. Gault MH, Jeffrey JR, Chiruto E, Ward LL: Studies of digoxin dosage, kinetics and serum concentrations in renal failure and review of the literature. *Nephron* 17: 161, 1976

390. van der Vijgh WJF, Oe PL: Pharmacokinetic aspects of digoxin in patients with terminal renal failure. IV. Clinical implications of own observations with a recent review of literature. *Int J Clin Pharmacol Biopharm* 16: 540, 1978

391. Ackerman GL, Doherty JE, Flanigan WJ: Peritoneal dialysis and hemodialysis of tritiated digoxin. *Ann Intern Med* 67: 718, 1967

392. van der Vijgh WJF, Oe PL: Pharmacokinetic aspects of digoxin in patients with terminal renal failure. II. On hemodialysis. *Int J Clin Pharmacol Biopharm* 15: 255, 1977

393. Carvallo A, Ramirez B, Honig H, Knepshield J, Schreiner GE, Gelfand MC: Treatment of digitalis intoxication by charcoal hemoperfusion. *Trans Am Soc Artif Intern Organs* 22: 718, 1976

394. Gibson TP, Lucas SV, Nelson HA, Atkinson AJ Jr, Okita GT, Ivanovich P: Hemoperfusion removal of digoxin from dogs. *J Lab Clin Med* 91: 673, 1978

395. Pancorbo S, Comty C: Digoxin pharmacokinetics in continuous peritoneal dialysis. *Ann Intern Med* 93: 639, 1980

396. Graves PE, Fenster PE, MacFarland RT, Marcus FI, Perrier D: Kinetics of digitoxin and the bis- and monodigitoxides of digitoxigenin in renal insufficiency. *Clin Pharmacol Ther* 36: 607, 1984

397. Jeliffe RW, Buell J, Kalaba R, Sridhar R, Rockwell R, Wagner JG: An improved method of digitoxin therapy. *Ann Intern Med* 72: 453, 1970

398. Shah G, Nelson HA, Atkinson AJ Jr, Okita GT, Ivanovich P, Gibson TP: Effect of hemoperfusion on the pharmacokinetics of digitoxin in dogs. *J Lab Clin Med* 93: 370, 1979

399. Larsson R, Liedholm H, Andersson KE, Keane MA, Henry G: Pharmacokinetics and effects on blood pressure of a single oral dose of milrinone in healthy subjects and in patients with renal impairment. *Eur J Clin Pharmacol* 29: 549, 1986

400. Koch-Weser J: Pharmacokinetics of procainamide in man. *Ann NY Acad Sci* 179: 301, 1979

401. Gibson TP, Atkinson AJ Jr, Matusik E, Nelson LD, Briggs WA: Kinetics of procainamide and N-acetylprocainamide in renal failure. *Kidney Int* 12: 422, 1977

402. Nattel S, Ogilvie RI, Kreeft J, Sitar DS, Graham DN, Rangno RE, Dufresne LR, Barre PE: Procainamide acetylation and disposition in dialysis patients. *Clin Invest Med* 2: 5, 1979

403. Stec GP, Atkinson AJ Jr, Nevin MJ, Thenot JP, Ruo TI, Gibson TP, Ivanovich P, Del Greco F: N-acetylprocainamide pharmacokinetics in functionally anephric patients before and after perturbation by hemodialysis. *Clin Pharmacol Ther* 26: 618, 1979

404. Atkinson AJ, Krumlovsky FA, Huang CM, Del Greco F: Hemodialysis for severe procainamde toxicity. Clinical and pharmacokinetic observations. *Clin Pharmacol Ther* 20: 585, 1976

405. Raehl CL, Moorthy AV, Beirne GJ: Procainamide pharmacokinetics in patients on continuous ambulatory peritoneal dialysis. *Nephron* 44: 191, 1986

406. Kessler KM, Lowenthal DT, Warner H, Gibson T, Briggs W, Reidenberg MM: Quinidine elimination in patients with congestive heart failure or poor renal function. *N Engl J Med* 290: 706, 1974

407. Woie L, Øyri A: Quinidine intoxication treated with hemo-

dialysis. *Acta Med Scand* 195: 237, 1974

408. Chin TWF, Pancorbo S, Comty C: Quinidine pharmacokinetics in continuous ambulatory peritoneal dialysis. *Clin Exp Dial Apheresis* 5: 391, 1981

409. Francois B, Mallein R, Randolet J, Lussignol M: Pharmacokinetics of disopyramide in patients with chronic renal failure. *Eur J Drug Metab Pharmacokinet* 8: 85, 1983

410. Johnston A, Henry JA, Warrington SJ, Hamer NAJ: Pharmacokinetics of oral disopyramide phosphate in patients with renal impairment. *Br J Clin Pharmacol* 10: 245, 1980

411. Thomson PD, Melmon KL, Richardson JA, Cohn K, Steinbrunn W, Cudihee R, Rowland M: Lidocaine pharmacokinetics in advanced heart failure, liver disease and renal failure in humans. *Ann Intern Med* 78: 499, 1973

412. Collinsworth KA, Strong JM, Atkinson AJ Jr, Winkle RA, Perlroth F, Harrison DC: Pharmacokinetics and metabolism of lidocaine in patients with renal failure. *Clin Pharmacol Ther* 18: 59, 1975

413. Vaziri ND, Saiki JK, Hughes W: Clearance of lidocaine by hemodialysis. *South Med J* 72: 1567, 1979

414. Wiegers U, Hanrath P, Kuck KH, Pottage A, Graffner C, Augustin J, Runge M: Pharmacokinetics of tocainide in patients with renal dysfunction and during haemodialysis. *Eur J Clin Pharmacol* 24: 503, 1983

415. Wang T, Wuellner D, Woosley RL, Stone WJ: Pharmacokinetics and nondialyzability of mexilitine in renal failure. *Clin Pharmacol Ther* 37: 649, 1985

416. Jones TE, Reece RA, Fisher GC: Mexilitine removal by peritoneal dialysis. *Eur J Clin Pharmacol* 25: 839, 1983

417. Somani PK, Simon V, Gupta RK, King P, Shapiro RS, Stockard H: Lorcainide kinetics and protein binding in patients with end-stage renal disease. *Int J Clin Pharmacol Ther Toxicol* 22: 121, 1984

418. Josselin J, Narang PK, Adir J, Yacobi A, Sandler JH: Bretylium kinetics in renal insufficienty. *Clin Pharmacol Ther* 33: 144, 1983

419. Bonati M, Galletti F, Volpi A, Cumetti C, Rumolo R, Tognoni S: Amiodarone in patients on long-term dialysis. *New Engl J Med* 308: 906, 1983

420. Canal M, Flouvat B, Aubert P, Guedon J, Prinseau J, Baglin A: Pharmacokinetics of cibenzoline in patients with renal impairment. *J Clin Pharmacol* 25: 197, 1985

421. Shah GM, Winer RL: Verapamil kinetics during maintenance hemodialysis. *Am J Nephrol* 5: 338, 1985

422. Mooy J, Schols M, v Baak M, v Hoof M, Muytjens A, Rahn KH: Pharmacokinetics of verapamil in patients with renal failure. *Eur J Clin Pharmacol* 28: 405, 1985

423. Martre H, Sari R, Taburet AM, Jacobs C, Singlas E: Haemodialysis does not effect the pharmacokinetics of nifedipine. *Br J Clin Pharmacol* 20: 155, 1985

424. Kleinbloesem CH, von Brummelin P, Woitliez AJ, Faber H, Breimer DD: Influence of haemodialysis on the pharmacokinetics and hemodynamic effects of nifedipine during continuous infusion. *Clin Pharmacokinet* 11: 316, 1986

425. Spital A, Scandling JD: Nifedipine in continuous ambulatory peritoneal dialysis. *Arch Intern Med* 143: 2025, 1983

426. Pozet N, Brazier JL, Hadj Aissa A, Khenfer D, Faucon G, Apoil E, Traeger J: Pharmacokinetics of diltiazem in severe renal failure. *Eur J Clin Pharmacol* 24: 635, 1983

427. Aronoff GR: Pharmacokinetics of nitrendipine in patients with renal failure: comparison to normal subjects. *J Cardiov Pharmacol* 6 (*Suppl* 7): S974, 1984

428. Zsotér TT, Johnson GE, DeVeber GA, Paul H: Excretion and metabolism of reserpine in renal failure. *Clin Pharmacol*

Ther 14: 325, 1973

429. Curtis JR: Drug-induced renal disease. *Drugs* 18: 377, 1979

430. Koch-Weser J: Hydralazine. *N Engl J Med* 295: 320, 1976

431. Lowenthal DT, Hobbs D, Affrime MB, Twomey TM, Martinez EW, Onesti G: Prazosin kinetics and effectiveness in renal failure. *Clin Pharmacol Ther* 27: 779, 1980

432. Chaignon M, Le Roux E, Aubert P, Lucsko M, Safar M, Fluovat B, Guedon J: Clinical pharmacology of prazosin in hypertensive patients with chronic renal failure. *J Cardiov Pharmacol* 3: 151, 1981

433. Weiner N: Drugs that inhibit adrenergic nerves and block adrenergic receptors. in *Goodman and Gilman's The Pharmacological Basis of Therapeutics*, edited by Gilman AG, Goodman LS, Rall TW, Murad F, 7th edn, New York, MacMillan Publ Co, 1985, p 181

434. Ward RM, Daniel CH, Kendig JW, Wood MA: Oliguria and tolazoline pharmacokinetics in the newborn. *Pediatrics* 77: 307, 1986

435. Carlson RV, Bailey RR, Begg EJ, Cowlishaw MG, Sharmon JR: Pharmacokinetics and effect on blood pressure of doxazosin in normal subjects and patients with renal failure. *Clin Pharmacol Ther* 40: 561, 1986

436. Hellberg OK, Vlaho M: Pharmacokinetik von Urapadil bei hypertonen Patienten mit eingeschrankter Nierenfunktion. Pharmacokinetics of Urapidil in patients with impaired renal function. *Med Welt* 34: 1407, 1983

437. Holmes B, Sorkin EM: Indoramin; a review of its pharmacodynamic and pharmacokinetic properties and therapeutic efficacy in hypertension and related vascular cardiovascular and airway diseases. *Drugs* 31: 467, 1986

438. Jungers P, Ganeval D, Pertuiset N, Chauveau P: Influence of renal insufficiency on the pharmacokinetics and pharmacodynamics of terazosin. *Am J Med* 80 (*Suppl* 5B): 94, 1986

439. Myhre E, Stenbaek Ø, Rugstad HE, Arnold E, Hansen T: Pharmacokinetics of methyldopa in renal failure and bilaterally nephrectomized patients. *Scand J Urol Nephrol* 16: 257, 1982.

440. Yeh BK, Dayton PG, Waters WC III: Removal of alpha-methyldopa (Aldomet) in man by dialysis. *Proc Soc Exp Biol Med* 136: 840, 1970

441. Hulter HN, Licht JH, Ilnicki LP, Singh S: Clinical efficacy and pharmacokinetics of clonidine in hemodialysis and renal insufficiency *J Lab Clin Med* 94: 223, 1979

442. Niedermayer W, Seiler KU, Wasserman O: Pharmacolkinetics of antihypertensive drugs (atenolol, metoprolol, propranolol and clonidine) and their metabolites during intermittent haemadialysis in humans. *Proc Eur Dial Transplant Assoc* 15: 607, 1978

443. Kirch W, Kohler H, Axthelm T: Pharmacokinetics of guanfacine in patients undergoing haemodialysis. *Eur J Drug Metab Pharmacokinet* 7: 277, 1982

444. Kiechel JR: Pharmacokinetics of guanfacine in patients with impaired renal function and in some elderly patients. *Am J Cardiol* 57: 18E, 1986

445. McMartin C, Randel RK, Vinter J, Allan BR, Humberstone M, Leishman AWD, Sandler G, Thirkettle JL: The fate of guanethidine in two hypertensive patients. *Clin Pharmacol Ther* 11: 423, 1970

446. Young IM, De Wardener HE, Miles BE: Mechanism of renal excretion of methonium compounds. *Br Med J* 2: 1500, 1951

447. Milne MD, Rowe GG, Somers K, Muehrcke RC, Crawford MA: Observations on the pharmacology of mecamylamine. *Clin Sci* 16: 599, 1957

448. Rennick BR, Moe GK, Lyons RH, Hoobler SW, Neligh R:

Absorption and renal excretion of the tetraethylammonium ion. *J Pharmacol Exp Ther* 91: 210, 1947

449. Gottlieb TB, Thomas RC, Chidsey CA: Pharmacokinetic studies of minoxidil. *Clin Pharmacol Ther* 13: 436, 1972

450. Zarate A, Gelfand MC, Horton JD, Winchester JF, Gottlieb MJ, Lazarus JM, Schreiner GE: Pericardial effusion associated with minoxidil therapy in dialyzed patients. *Int J Artif Organs* 3: 15, 1980

451. Pruitt AW, Faraj BA, Dayton PG: Metabolism of diazoxide in man and experimental animals. *J Pharmacol Exp Ther* 188: 248, 1974

452. Pohl JEF, Thurston H: Use of diazoxide in hypertension with renal failure. *Br Med J* 4: 142, 1971

453. Sellers RM, Koch-Weser J: Protein binding and vascular activity of diazoxide. *N Engl J Med* 281: 1141, 1969

454. Danzig LE: Dynamics of thiocyanate dialysis. The artificial kidney in the therapy of thiocyanate intoxication. *N Engl J Med* 252: 49, 1955

455. Guidicelli JF, Chaegnon M, Richer C, Giroux B, Guedon J: Influence of chronic renal failure on captopril pharmacokinetics and clinical and biological effects in hypertensive patients. *Br J Clin Pharmacol* 18: 749, 1984

456. Duchin KL, Pierides AM, Heald A, Singhvi SM, Rommel AJ: Elimination kinetics of captopril in patients with renal failure. *Kidney Int* 25: 942, 1984

457. Farrow PR, Wilkinson R: Reversible renal failure during treatment with captopril. *Br Med J* 2: 1680, 1979

458. Shionoiri H, Miyayaki N, Yasuda G, Sugimoto K, Uneda S, Kaneko Y: Blood concentration and urinary excretion of enalapril in patients with chronic renal failure. *Nippon Jinzo Gakkai Shi* 27: 1291, 1985

459. Tjandramaga TB: Altered pharmacokinetics of β adrenoceptor blocking drugs in patients with renal insufficiency. *Arch Int Pharmacodyn Ther* 248 (*Suppl*): 38, 1980

460. Lowenthal DT, Briggs WA, Gibson TP, Nelson H, Cirksena WJ: Pharmacokinetics of oral propranolol in chronic renal disease. *Clin Pharmacol Ther* 16: 761, 1974

461. Thompson FD, Joekes AM, Foulkes DM: Pharmacokinetics of propranolol in renal failure. *Br Med J* 2: 434, 1972

462. Stone WJ, Walle T: Massive propranolol metabolite retention during maintenance hemodialysis. *Clin Pharmacol Ther* 28: 449, 1980

463. Feely J, Wilkinson JR, Wood AJJ: Reduction of liver blood flow and propranolol metabolism by cimetidine. *N Engl J Med* 304: 692, 1981

464. Fabre J, Fox HM, Dayer P, Balant L: Differences in kinetic properties of drugs: implications as to the selection of a particular drug for use in patients with renal failure with special emphasis on antibiotics and β adrenoceptor blocking agents. *Clin Pharmacokinet* 5: 441, 1980

465. Safar ME, Chau NP, Levenson JA, Simon AC, Weiss YA: Pharmacokinetics of intravenous and oral pindolol in hypertensive patients with chronic renal failure. *Clin Sci Mol Med* 55: 275S, 1978

466. Krauss W, Kampf D, Fischer HC: Pharmacokinetics of mepindolol in patients with chronic renal failure. *Eur J Clin Pharmacol* 27: 429, 1984

467. Berglund G, Descaps R, Thomas JA: Pharmacokinetics of sotalol after chronic administration to patients with renal insufficiency. *Eur J Clin Pharmacol* 18: 321, 1980

468. Tjandramaga TB, Thomas J, Verbeek R, Verbesselt R, Verbeckmoes R, De Schepper PJ: The effect of end-stage renal failure and haemodialysis on the elimination kinetics of sotalol. *Br J Clin Pharmacol* 3: 259, 1976

469. McCluskey DR, Donaldson RA, McGeown MG: Oxprenolol and retroperitoneal fibrosis. *Br Med J* 2: 1429, 1980

470. Harvengt C, Desager JP, Muschart JM, Tjandramaga TVM, Verbeeck R, Verbeckmoes R: Influence of hemodialysis on the half-life of practolol in patients with severe renal failure. *J Clin Pharmacol* 15: 605, 1975

471. Roux A, Aubert P, Guedon J, Flouvat B: Pharmacokinetics of acebutolol in patients with all grades of renal failure. *Eur J Clin Pharmacol* 17: 339, 1980

472. Smith RS, Warren DJ, Renwick AG, George CF: Acebutolol pharmacokinetics in renal failure. *Br J Clin Pharmacol* 16: 253, 1983

473. McAinsh J, Holmes BF, Smith S, Hood D, Warren D: Atenolol kinetics in renal failure. *Clin Pharmacol Ther* 28: 302, 1980

474. Domart M, Goupil A, Baglin A: Pharmacokinetics of atenolol in patients with terminal renal failure and influence of haemodialysis. *Br J Clin Pharmacol* 9: 379, 1980

475. Campese V, Feinstein EI, Gura V, Mason WD, Massry SG: Pharmacokinetics of atenolol in patients treated with chronic hemodialysis or peritoneal dialysis. *J Clin Pharmacol* 23: 393, 1985

476. Seiler KU, Schuster KJ, Meyer GF, Niedermayer W, Wasserman O: The pharmacokinetics of metoprolol and its metabolites in dialysis patients. *Clin Pharmacokinet* 5: 192, 1980

477. Wood AJ, Ferry DG, Bailey RR: Elimination kinetics of labetalol in severe renal failure. *Br J Clin Pharmacol* 13 (*Suppl*): 81S, 1982

478. Palminteri R, Assael BM, Bianchetti G, Gomeni R, Claris-Appiani A, Edelfonti A, Morselli PL: Betaxolol kinetics in hypertensive children with normal and abnormal renal function. *Clin Pharmacol Ther* 35: 141, 1984

479. Jeanniot JP, Hocein G, Ledudal P, Cautreels W, Guidicelli CP, Tillement JP: Butofilolol pharmacokinetics in chronic renal insufficiency. *Int J Clin Pharmacol Res* 4: 165, 1984

480. Borges H, Hocks J, Kjellstrand CM: Mannitol intoxication in patients with renal failure. *Arch Intern Med* 142: 63, 1982

481. Young TK, Lee SC, Tai LN: Mannitol absorption and excretion in uremic patients regularly treated with gastrointestinal perfusion. *Nephron* 25: 112, 1980

482. Freeman RB, Maher JF, Schreiner GE, Mostofi FK: Renal tubular necrosis due to nephrotoxicity of organic mercurial diuretics. *Ann Intern Med* 57: 34, 1962

483. Vaziri ND, Saiki J, Barton CH, Rajudin M, Ness RL: Hemodialyzability of acetazolamide. *South Med J* 73: 422, 1980

484. Klooker P, Bommer J, Ritz E: Treatment of hypertension in dialysis patients. *Blood Purif* 3: 15, 1985

485. Acchiardo SR, Skoutakis VA: Clinical efficacy, safety and pharmacokinetics of indapamide in renal impairment. *Am Heart J* 106: 237, 1983

486. Koppel MH, Massry SG, Shinaberger JH, Hartenbower DL, Coburn JW: Thiazide-induced rise in serum calcium and magnesium in patients on maintenance hemodialysis. *Ann Intern Med* 72: 895, 1970

487. Magil A, Baloon HS, Cameron EC, Rae A: Acute interstitial nephritis associated with thiazide diuretics. Clinical and pathologic observations in three cases. *Am J Med* 69: 939, 1980

488. Levin NW: Furosemide and ethacrynic acid in renal insufficiency. *Med Clin North Am* 55: 107, 1971

489. Dargie HJ, Allison MEM, Kennedy AC, Gray MJB: High dosage metolazone in chronic renal failure. *Br Med J* 4: 196, 1972

490. Gregory LF Jr, Durrett RR, Robinson RR, Clapp JR: The short term effect of furosemide on electrolyte and water excretion in patients with severe renal disease. *Arch Intern Med*

125: 69, 1970

491. Goto S, Yoshitomi H, Miyamoto A, Inoue K, Nakano M: Binding of several loop diuretics to serum albumin and human serum from patients with renal failure and liver disease. *J Pharmacobiodyn* 3: 667, 1980

492. Huang CM, Atkinson AJ, Levin M, Levin NW, Quentanilla A: Pharmacokinetics of furosemide in advanced renal failure. *Clin Pharmacol Ther* 16: 659, 1974

493. Beermann B, Dalén E, Lindstrom B: Elimination of furosemide in healthy subjects and in those with renal failure. *Clin Pharmacol Ther* 22: 70, 1977

494. Riva E, Fossali E, Bettinelli A: Kinetics of furosemide in children with chronic renal failure undergoing regular haemodialysis. *Eur J Clin Pharmacol* 21: 303, 1982

495. Lyons H, Pin VW, Cortell S, Cohen JJ, Harrington JT: Allergic interstitial nephritis causing reversible renal failure in four patients with idiopathic nephrotic syndrome. *N Engl J Med* 288: 124, 1973

496. Lau HSH, Hyneck ML, Berardi RR, Swartz RD, Smith DE: Kinetics, dynamics and bioavailability of bumetanide in healthy subjects and patients with chronic renal failure. *Clin Pharmacol Ther* 39: 635, 1986

497. Loute G, Adam A, Ers P, Heremans C, Willems B: The influence of haemodialysis and haemofiltration on the clearance of torasemide in renal failure. *Eur J Clin Pharmacol* 31 (Suppl): 53, 1986

498. Knauf H, Liebig R, Schollmeyer P, Rosenthal J, Kolle EU, Mutechler E: Pharmacodynamics and kinetics of etozolin/ozolinone in hypertensive patients with normal and impaired kidney function. *Eur J Clin Pharmacol* 26: 687, 1984

499. Brazier JL, Pozet N, Faucon G, Traeger J, Hadj-Haissa A: Kinetics of a high dose of piretanide in renal failure. *Eur J Clin Pharmacol* 21: 307, 1982

500. Walter U, Röckel A, Lahn W, Heidland A, Heptner W: Pharmacokinetics of the loop diuretic piretanide in renal failure. *Eur J Clin Pharmacol* 29: 337, 1985

501. Cohen LH, Norby LH, Champion C, Spargo B: Acute renal failure from ticrynafen. *N Engl J Med* 301: 1180, 1979

502. Karim A, Zagarella J, Hribar J, Dooley M: Spironolactone I. Disposition and metabolism. *Clin Pharmacol Ther* 19: 158, 1976

503. Pruitt AW, Dayton PG, Steinhorst J: Fate of triamterene in man. *Clin Res* 22: 77A, 1974

504. Takahashi H, Tsukada T: Triamterene- induced haemolytic anemia with acute intravascular haemolysis and acute renal failure. *Scand J Haematol* 23: 169, 1979

505. George CF: Amiloride handling in renal failure. *Br J Clin Pharmacol* 9: 94, 1980

506. Weinberger M, Hendeles L: Role of dialysis in the management and prevention of theophylline toxicity. *Dev Pharmacol Ther* 1: 26, 1980

507. Lawyer C, Aitchison J, Sutto J, Bennett W: Treatment of theophylline neurotoxicity with resin hemoperfusion. *Ann Intern Med* 88: 516, 1978

508. Maher JF, Cassetta M, Shea C, Hohnadel DC: Transperitoneal theophylline flux and peritoneal permeability. *Nephron* 20: 18, 1978

509. Levy G, Gibson TP, Whitman W, Procknal J: Hemodialysis clearances of theophylline. *JAMA* 237: 1466, 1977

510. Lee CSC, Peterson JC, Marbury TC: Comparative pharmacokinetics of theophylline in peritoneal dialysis and hemodialysis. *J Clin Pharmacol* 23: 274, 1983

511. Russo ME: Management of theophylline intoxication with charcoal hemoperfusion. *N Engl J Med* 300: 24, 1979

512. Lee CC, Wang LH, Majeske BL, Marbury TC: Pharmacokinetics of dyphylline elimination by uremic patients. *J Pharmacol Exp Ther* 217: 340, 1981

513. Bauer H, Laufen H, Franz HE: Isosorbide dinitrate in plasma and dialysate during haemodialysis. *Eur J Clin Pharmacol* 30: 187, 1986

514. Cronnelly R, Stanski DR, Miller RD, Sheiner LB, Sohn YJ: Renal function and the pharmacokinetics of neostigmine in anesthetized man. *Anesthesiology* 51: 222, 1979

515. Rey E, d'Atkis F, Richard MO, Fillastre JP, Olive G: Pharmacokinetics of buflomedil in patients with chronic renal failure. *Int J Clin Pharmacol Ther Toxicol* 22: 648, 1984

516. Cameron JS, Toseland PA, Read JF, Bewick M, Ogg CS, Ellis FG: Accumulation of barbitone in patients on regular haemodialysis. *Lancet* 1: 912, 1970

517. Myschetsky A, Lassen NA: Urea induced osmotic diuresis and alkalization of urine in acute barbiturate intoxication. *JAMA* 185: 936, 1963

518. Campion DS, North JD: Effect of protein binding of barbiturates on their rate of removal during peritoneal dialysis. *J Lab Clin Med* 66: 549, 1965

519. Exaire E, Treviño-Becerra A, Monteon F: An overview of treatment with peritoneal dialysis in drug poisoning. *Contrib Nephrol* 17: 39, 1979

520. DeBroe ME, Verpooten GA, Christiaens MA, Rustaert RJ, Holvoet J, Nagler J, Heyndrickx A: Clinical experience with prolonged combined hemoperfusion-hemodialysis treatment of severe poisoning. *Artif Organs* 5: 59, 1981

521. Goldbaum LR, Smith PK: The interaction of barbiturates with serum albumin and its possible relation to their disposition and pharmacologic actions. *J Pharmacol Exp Ther* 111: 197, 1954

522. Ehrnebo M, Odar-Cederlöf I: Binding of amobarbital, pentobarbital and diphenylhydantoin to blood cells and plasma proteins in healthy volunteers and uraemic patients. *Eur J Clin Pharmacol* 8: 445, 1975

523. Knochel JP, Barry KG: THAM dialysis; an experimental method to study diffusion of certain weak acids in vivo II. Secobarbital. *J Lab Clin Med* 65: 361, 1965

524. Rosenbaum JL, Kramer MS, Raja R: Resin hemoperfusion for acute drug intoxication. *Arch Intern Med* 136: 263, 1976

525. Gelfand MC, Winchester JF, Knepshield JH, Hanson KM, Cohan SL, Strauss BS, Geoly KL, Kennedy AC, Schreiner GE: Treatment of severe drug overdosage with charcoal hemoperfusion. *Trans Am Soc Artif Intern Organs* 23: 599, 1977

526. Koffler A, Bernstein M, LaSette A, Massry SG: Fixed-bed charcoal hemoperfusion. Treatment of drug overdose. *Arch Intern Med* 138: 1691, 1978

527. Forycke Z, Martens F, Thalhofer S, Ibe K: Tranquilizers, analgetics and antidepressants in patients treated with hemodialysis. *Blood Purif* 3: 109, 1985

528. Kangas L, Kanto J, Forsström J, Iisalo E: The protein binding of diazepam and N demethyldiazepam in patients with poor renal function. *Clin Nephrol* 5: 114, 1976

529. DeSilva JAF, Koechlin BA, Bader G: Blood level distribution patterns of diazepam and its major metabolite in man. *J Pharm Sci* 55: 692, 1966

530. Cruz IA, Kramer NC, Parrish AE: Hemodialysis in chlordiazepoxide toxicity. *JAMA* 202: 438, 1967

531. Ochs HR, Greenblatt DJ, Klehr U: Disposition of oxazepam in patients on maintenance hemodialysis. *Klin Wochensch* 62: 765, 1984

532. Taclob L, Needle M: Drug induced encephalopathy in patients on maintenance hemodialysis. *Lancet* 2: 704, 1976

533. Kroboth PD, Smith RB, Rault R, Silver MR, Sorkin MI, Puschett JP, Juhl RP: Effect of end-stage renal disease and aluminum hydroxide on temazepam kinetics. *Clin Pharmacol Ther* 37: 453, 1985

534. Vinik HR, Reves JF, Greenblatt DJ, Abernathy DR, Smith LR: The pharmacokinetics of midizolam in chronic renal failure patients. *Anesthesiology* 59: 390, 1983

535. Balogh A, Fünfstück R, Demme U, Kangas L, Sperschneider H, Traeger A, Stein G, Pekearinen A: Dialyzability of benzodiazepines by haemodialysis and controlled sequential ultrafiltration (CSU) in vitro. *Arch Pharmacol Toxicol* 49: 174, 1981

536. Breimer DD: Clinical pharmacokinetics of hypnotics. *Clin Pharmacokinet* 2: 93, 1977

537. Vazari ND, Kumar KP, Mirahamadi K, Rosen SM: Hemodialysis in treatment of chloral hydrate poisoning. *South Med J* 70: 377, 1977

538. Stalker NE, Gambertoglio JG, Fukumitsu CJ, Naughton JL, Benet LZ: Acute massive chloral hydrate intoxication treated with hemodialysis. *J Clin Pharmacol* 18: 136, 1978

539. Heath A, Wickström I, Ahlmen J: Hemoperfusion in tricyclic antidepressant poisoning. *Lancet* 1: 155, 1980

540. Teehan BP, Maher JF, Carey JJH, Flynn PD, Schreiner GE: Acute ethchlorvynol (Placidyl®) intoxication. *Ann Intern Med* 72: 875, 1970

541. Lynn RI, Honig CL, Jatlow PI, Kliger AS: Resin hemoperfusion for treatment of ethchlorvynol overdose. *Ann Intern Med* 91: 549, 1979

542. Zmuda MJ: Resin hemoperfusion in dogs intoxicated with ethchlorvynol (Placidyl®). *Kidney Int* 17: 303, 1980

543. De Myttenaere M, Schoenfeld L, Maher JF: Treatment of glutethimide poisoning; a comparison of forced diuresis and dialysis. *JAMA* 203: 885, 1968

544. Chang TMS, Coffey JD, Lister C, Taroy E, Stark A: Methaqualone, methypyrlon and glutethimide clearance by the ACAC microcapsule artificial kidney: in vitro and in patients with acute intoxication. *Trans Am Soc Artif Intern Organs* 19: 87, 1973

545. De Myttenaere MH, Maher JF, Schreiner FE: Hemoperfusion through a charcoal column for glutethimide poisoning. *Trans Am Soc Artif Intern Organs* 13: 190, 1967

546. Rosenbaum JL, Kramer MS, Raja RM: Amberlite hemoperfusion in the treatment of acute drug intoxication. *Int J Artif Organs* 2: 316, 1979

547. Maddock RK, Bloomer HA: Meprobamate overdosage; evaluation of severity and methods of treatment. *JAMA* 201: 999, 1967

548. Lobo PI, Spyler D, Surratt P, Westervelt FB Jr: Use of hemodialysis in meprobamate overdosage. *Clin Nephrol* 7: 73, 1977

549. Yudis M, Swartz C, Onesti G, Ramirez O, Snyder D, Brest A: Hemodialysis for methyprylon (Noludar) poisoning. *Ann Intern Med* 68: 1301, 1968

550. Pancorbo AS, Palagi PA, Piecoro JJ, Wilson HD: Hemodialysis in methyprylon overdose; some pharmacokinetic considerations. *JAMA* 237: 470, 1977

551. Proudfoot AT, Noble J, Nimmo J, Brown SS, Cameron JC: Peritoneal dialysis and haemodialysis in methaqualone (Mandrax) poisoning. *Scott Med J* 13: 232, 1968

552. Langecker H, Neuhaus G, Ibe K, Kessel M: Ein Suicid-Versuch mit Valamin mit einem Beitrag zur Elimination und Therapie. (A suicide attempt with Valmid with a contribution to removal and therapy). *Arch Toxicol* (Berl) 19: 293, 1962

553. Gutman RA, Burnell JM, Solak F: Paraldehyde acidosis. *Am J Med* 42: 455, 1967

554. Berger M, White J, Travis LB, Browhard BH, Cunningham RJ III, Patnode R, Petrusick T: Toxic psychosis due to cyproheptadine in a child on hemodialysis: a case report. *Clin Nephrol* 7: 43, 1977

555. Lieberman JA, Cooper TB, Suckow RF, Steinberg H, Borenstein M, Brenner R, Kane JM: Tricyclic antidepressant and metabolite levels in chronic renal failure. *Clin Pharmacol Ther* 37: 301, 1985

556. Dawling S, Lynn K, Rosser R, Braithwaite R: Nortriptyline metabolism in chronic renal failure: metabolite elimination. *Clin Pharmacol Ther* 32: 322, 1982

557. Faulkner RD, Senekjian HO, Lee CS: Hemodialysis of doxepin and desmethyldoxepin in uremic patients. *Artif Organs* 8: 151, 1984

558. Dawling S, Lynn K, Rosser R, Braithwaite R: The pharmacokinetics of nortriptyline in patients with chronic renal failure. *Br J Clin Pharm* 12: 39, 1981

559. Trafford JAP, Jones RH, Evans R, Sharp P, Sharpstone P, Cook J: Haemoperfusion with R-004 amberlite resin for treating acute poisoning. *Br Med J* 2: 1453, 1977

560. Winchester JF, Gelfand MC, Tilstone WJ: Hemoperfusion in drug intoxication: clinical and laboratory aspects. *Drug Metab Rev* 8: 69, 1978

561. Doweiko J, Fogel BS, Goldberg RJ: Trazadone and hemodialysis. *J Clin Psychiat* 45: 361, 1984

562. Davis JM, Fan WE: Lithium. *Annu Rev Pharmacol* 11: 285, 1971

563. Singer I: Lithium and the kidney. *Kidney Int* 19: 324, 1981

564. Hansen HE, Hestbech J, Sorensen JL, Norgaard K, Heilskov J, Amdisen A: Chronic interstitial nephropathy in patient on long-term lithium treatment. *Q J Med* 48: 577, 1979

565. Amdisen A, Skjoldborg: Haemodialysis for lithium poisoning. *Lancet* 2: 213, 1969

566. Jaeger A, Sauder P, Kopferschmitt J, Jaegle ML: Toxicokinetics of lithium intoxication treated by hemodialysis. *J Toxicol Clin Toxicol* 23: 501, 1986

567. Brown EA, Pawlinkowski TRB: Lithium intoxication treated by peritoneal dialysis. *Br J Clin Pract* 35: 90, 1981

568. Port F, Kroll PD, Rosenzweig J: Lithium therapy during maintenance hemodialysis. *Psychosomatics* 20: 130, 1979

569. Letteri JM, Mellk H, Louis S, Kutt H, Durante P, Glazko A: Diphenylhydantoin metabolism in uremia. *N Engl J Med* 285: 648, 1971

570. Steele WH, Lawrence JR, Elliott HL, Whiting B: Alterations of phenytoin protein binding with in vivo haemodialysis in dialysis encephalopathy. *Eur J Clin Pharmacol* 15: 69, 1979

571. Borgå O, Hoppel C, Odar-Cederlöf I, Garle M: Plasma levels and renal excretion of phenytoin and its metabolites in patients with renal failure. *Clin Pharmacol Ther* 26: 306, 1979

572. Agarwal BN, Cabebe FG, Hoffman BI: Diphenylhydantoin-induced acute renal failure. *Nephrol* 18: 249, 1977

573. Martin E, Gambertoglio JG, Adler DS, Tozer TN, Roman LA, Grausz H: Removal of phenytoin by hemodialysis in uremic patients. *JAMA* 238: 1750, 1977

574. Tenckhoff H, Sherrard DJ, Hickman RO: Acute diphenylhydantoin intoxication. *Am J Dis Child* 116: 422, 1968

575. Thiel GB, Richter RW, Powell MR, Doolan PD: Acute Dilantin poisoning. *Neurology* 11: 138, 1961

576. Czajka PA, Anderson WH, Christoph RA, Banner W Jr: A pharmacokinetic evaluation of peritoneal dialysis for phenytoin intoxication. *J Clin Pharmacol* 20: 565, 1980

577. Rubinger D, Levy M, Roll D, Czaczkes JW: Inefficiency of haemodialysis in acute phenytoin intoxication. *Br J Clin Pharmacol* 7: 405, 1979

578. Swinyard EA, Schiffman DO, Goodman LS: Effects of liver injury and nephrectomy on the anticonvulsant activity of oxazolidine 2,4 diones. *J Pharmacol Exp Ther* 105: 365, 1952

579. Bergstrand A, Bergstrand CG, Engstrom N, Herrlin KM: Renal histology during treatment with oxazolidine – diones (trimethadione, ethadione and paramethadione). *Pediatrics* 30: 601, 1962

580. Marbury TC, Lee CS, Bruni J, Wilder BJ: Hemodialysis of valproic acid in uremic patients. *Dial Transplant* 9: 961, 1980

581. Mortensen RB, Hansen HE, Pedersen B, Hartmann-Andersen F, Husted SE: Acute valproate intoxication: biochemical investigations and hemodialysis treatment. *Int J Clin Pharmacol Ther Toxicol* 21: 64, 1983

582. Orr JM, Farrell K, Abbott FS, Ferguson S, Godolphin WJ: The effects of peritoneal dialysis on the single dose and steady state pharmacokinetics of valproic acid in a uremic epileptic child. *Eur J Clin Pharmacol* 24: 387, 1983

583. Nicholls DP, Yasin M: Acute renal failure from carbamazepine. *Br Med J* 4: 490, 1972

584. Lee CS, Wang LH, Marbury TC, Bruni J, Perchalski RJ: Hemodialysis clearance and total body elimination of carbamazepine during chronic hemodialysis. *Clin Toxicol* 17: 429, 1980

585. Gary NE, Brya WM, Eisinger RP: Carbamazepine poisoning: treatment by hemoperfusion. *Nephron* 27: 202, 1981

586. Marbury TC, Lee CC, Perchalski RJ, Wilder BJ: Hemodialysis clearance of ethosuximide in patients with chronic renal disease. *Am J Hosp Pharm* 38: 1757, 1981

587. Borgå O, Odar-Cederlöf I, Ringberger V, Norlin A: Protein binding of salicylate in uremic and normal plasma. *Clin Pharmacol Ther* 20: 464, 1976

588. Schreiner GE, Maher JF, Argy WP Jr, Siegel L: Extracorporeal and peritoneal dialysis of drugs in Brodie BB, Gillette JR: *Concepts in Biochemical Pharmacology, Handbook of Experimental Pharmacology,* Vol 28, Berlin, Springer-Verlag, 1971, p 403

589. Summitt RL, Etteldorf JN: Salicylate intoxication in children; experience with peritoneal dialysis and alkalinization of the urine. *J Pediat* 64: 803, 1964

590. Williams ME, Weinblatt M, Rosa RM, Griffin VL, Goldlust B, Shang SF, Harrison LI, Brown RS: Salsalate kinetics in patients with chronic renal failure undergoing hemodialysis. *Clin Pharmacol Ther* 39: 420, 1986

591. Verbeek RK, De Schepper PJ: Influence of chronic renal failure and hemodialysis on diflusinal plasma protein binding. *Clin Pharmacol Ther* 27: 628, 1980

592. Boyer TD, Rouff SL: Acetaminophen induced hepatic necrosis and renal failure. *JAMA* 218: 440, 1971

593. Bengtsson U, Johansson S, Angervall L: Malignancies of the urinary tract and their relation to analgesic abuse. *Kidney Int* 13: 107, 1978

594. Gonwa TA, Hamilton RW, Buckalew VM Jr: Chronic renal failure and end stage renal disease in northwest North Carolina. Importance of analgesic associated nephropathy. *Arch Intern Med* 141: 462, 1981

595. Faird NR, Glynn JP, Kerr DNS: Haemodialysis in paracetamol self-poisoning. *Lancet* 2: 396, 1972

596. Maclean D, Peters DJ, Brown RAG, McCathie M, Baines GF, Robertson PGC: Treatment of acute paracetamol poisoning. *Lancet* 2: 849, 1968

597. Øie S, Lowenthal DT, Briggs WA, Levy G: Effect of hemodialysis on kinetics of acetaminophen elimination by anephric patients. *Clin Pharmacol Ther* 18: 680, 1975

598. Rigby RJ, Thomson NM, Parkin GW, Cheung TPF: The treatment of paracetamol overdose with charcoal haemoperfusion and cysteamine. *Med J Austr* 1: 396, 1978

599. Winchester JF, Gelfand MC, Helliwell M, Vale JA, Goulding R, Schreiner GE: Extracorporeal treatment of salicylate or acetaminophen poisoning – is there a role? *Arch Intern Med* 141: 370, 1981

600. Giacomini KM, Gibson TP, Levy G: Effect of hemodialysis on propoxyphene and norpropoxyphene concentrations in blood of anephric patients. *Clin Pharmacol Ther* 27: 508, 1980

601. Gary NE, Maher JF, De Myttenaere MH, Liggero SH, Scott KG, Matusiak W, Schreiner GE: Acute propoxyphene hydrochloride intoxication. *Arch Intern Med* 121: 453, 1968

602. Maddocks JL, Wake CJ, Harber MJ: The plasma half life of antipyrine in chronic uraemic and normal subjects. *Br J Clin Pharmacol* 2: 339, 1975

603. Breuing KH, Gilfrich HJ, Meinertz T, Wiegand UW, Jahnchen E: Disposition of azapropazone in chronic renal and hepatic failure. *Eur J Clin Pharmacol* 20: 147, 1981

604. Berkowitz B: Influence of plasma levels and metabolism on pharmacological activity: pentazocine. *Ann NY Acad Sci* 179: 269, 1971

605. Way EL, Adler TK: The pharmacologic implications of the fate of morphine and its surrogates. *Pharmacol Rev* 12: 383, 1960

606. Säwe J, Svensso J, Odar-Cederlöf I: Kinetics of morphine in patients with renal failure. *Lancet* 2: 211, 1985

607. Zabinska K, Smólenski O, Hanicki Z, Bogdal J, Paczek Z, Wiernikowski A, Hirszel P: Ostre zatrucia leczone dialysa. (Severe intoxications treated with dialysis). *Przegl Lek* 23: 717, 1967

608. Barnes JN, Williams AJ, Tomson MJF, Toseland PA, Goodwin FJ: Dihydrocodeine in renal failure: further evidence for an important role of the kidney in the handling of opioid drugs. *Br Med J* 290: 740, 1985

609. Szeto HH, Inturrisi CE, Houde R, Saal S, Cheigh J, Reidenberg MM: Accumulation of normeperidine, an active metabolite of meperidine in patients with renal failure or cancer. *Ann Intern Med* 86: 738, 1977

610. Glazer WM, Cohn GL: Methadone maintenance in a patient on chronic hemodialysis. *Am J Psych* 134: 931, 1977

611. Summerfield RJ, Allen MC, Moore RA, Sear JW, McQuay HJ: Buprenorphine in end stage renal failure. *Anaesthesia* 40: 914, 1985

612. Henrich WL: Nephrotoxicity of nonsteroidal anti-inflammatory agents. *Am J Kidney Dis* 2: 478, 1983

613. Carmichael J, Shankel SW: Effects of nonsteroidal anti-inflammatory drugs on prostaglandins and renal function. *Am J Med* 78: 992, 1985

614. Held H, Enderle C: Elimination and serum protein binding of phenylbutazone in patients with renal insufficiency. *Clin Nephrol* 6: 388, 1976

615. Strong JE, Wilson J, Douglas JF, Coppel DL: Phenylbutazone self-poisoning treated by charcoal haemoperfusion. *Anaesthesia* 34: 1038, 1979

616. Flower RJ, Moncada S, Vane JR: Analgesic-antipyretics and anti-inflammatory agents; drugs employed in the treatment of gout. in Goodman and Gilman's The Pharmacological Basis of Therapeutics, edited by Gilman AG, Goodman LS, Rall TW, Murad F, New York, MacMillan Publ Co, 1985, p 674

617. Ochs HR, Greenblatt DJ, Verburg-Ochs B: Ibuprofen kinetics in patients with renal insufficiency who are receiving maintenance hemodialysis. *Arthritis Rheum* 28: 1430, 1985

618. Antal EJ, Wright CE III, Brown BL, Albert KS, Aman LC, Levin NW: The influence of hemodialysis on the pharmacoki-

netics of ibuprofen and its major metabolites. *J Clin Pharmacol* 26: 184, 1986

619. Anttila M, Haataja M, Kasanen A: Pharmacokinetics of naproxen in subjects with normal and impaired renal function. *Eur J Clin Pharmacol* 18: 263, 1980

620. Weber SS, Troutman WG, Trujeque L: Effect of hemodialysis on plasma naproxen concentration. *Am J Hosp Pharm* 36: 1567, 1979

621. Rogers HJ, Savitsky JP, Glenn B, Spector RG: Kinetics of single doses of fenbufen in patients with renal insufficiency. *Clin Pharmacol Ther* 29: 74, 1981

622. Stafanger G, Larsen HW, Hansen H, Sorensen K: Pharmacokinetics of ketoprofen in patients with chronic renal failure. *Scand J Rheumatol* 10: 189, 1981

623. Aronoff GR, Ozawa T, DeSante KA, Nash JF, Ridolfo AS: Benoxaprofen kinetics in renal impairment. *Clin Pharmacol Ther* 32: 190, 1982

624. Wang LH, Lee CS, Marbury TC: Hemodialysis of mefenamic acid in uremic patients. *Am J Hosp Pharm* 37: 956, 1980

625. Pritchard JF, O'Neill PJ, Affrime MB, Lowenthal DT: Influence of uremia and hemodialysis on the plasma protein binding of tolmetin. *Pharmacology* 29: 312, 1984

626. Horber FF, Guentert TW, Weidelkamm E, Heizmann P, Descoeudres C, Frey FJ: Pharmacokinetics of tenoxicam in patients with impaired renal function. *Eur J Clin Pharmacol* 29: 697, 1986

627. Silverberg DS, Kidd EG, Shnitka TK, Ulan RA: Gold nephropathy. A Clinical and pathologic study. *Arthritis Rheum* 13: 812, 1970

628. Scott JJ, O'Brien PK: Probenecid, nephrotic syndrome and renal failure. *Ann Rheum Dis* 27: 249, 1968

629. Bern M, Cavaliere BM, Lucas G: Plasma levels and effects of sulfinpyrazone in patients requiring chronic hemodialysis. *J Clin Pharmacol* 20: 107, 1980

630. Elion GB, Yu T, Gutman AB, Hitchings GH: Renal clearance of oxipurinol, the chief metabolite of allopurinol. *Am J Med* 45: 69, 1968

631. Hande KR, Noone RM, Stone WJ: Severe allopurinol toxicity. Description and guidelines for prevention in patients with renal insufficiency. *Am J Med* 76: 47, 1984

632. Sherlock JE, Letteri JM: Effect of hemodialysis on methylprednisolone plasma levels. *Nephron* 18: 208, 1977

633. Bergrem H: Pharmacokinetics and protein binding of prednisolone in patients with nephrotic syndrome and patients undergoing hemodialysis. *Kidney Int* 23: 876, 1983

634. Deck KA, Fischer B, Hillen H: Studies on cortisol metabolism during haemodialysis in man. *Eur J Clin Invest* 9: 203, 1979

635. Bach JF, Dardenne M: The metabolism of azathioprine in renal failure. *Transplantation* 12: 253, 1971

636. Duttera MJ, Carolla RL, Gallelli JF, Gullion DS, Leim DE, Henderson ES: Hematuria and crystalluria after high dose 6-mercaptopurine administration. *N Engl J Med* 287: 292, 1972

637. Schusziarra V, Ziekursch V, Schlamp R, Siemensen HC: Pharmacokinetics of azathioprine under haemodialysis. *Int J Clin Pharmacol Biopharm* 14: 298, 1976

638. Follath F, Wenk M, Vozeh S, Thiel G, Brunner F, Loertschen R, Lemaire M, Nussbaumer K, Niederberger W, Wood A: Intravenous cyclosporin kinetics in renal failure. *Clin Pharmacol Ther* 34: 638, 1983

639. Ptachcinski RJ, Venkataramanan R, Burckart GJ: Clinical pharmacokinetics of cyclosporin. *Clin Pharmacokinet* 11: 107, 1986

640. Cohen JL, Jao JY, Jusko WJ: Pharmacokinetics of cyclophos-

phamide in man. *Br J Pharmacol* 43: 677, 1971

641. Milsted RAV, Jarman N: Haemodialysis during cyclophosphamide treatment. *Br Med J* 1: 820, 1978

642. Galletti PJ, Pasqualino A, Geering RG: Hemodialysis in cancer chemotherapy. *Trans Am Soc Artif Intern Organs* 12: 20, 1966

643. Raymond JR: Nephrotoxicity of antineoplastic and immunosuppressive agents. *Curr Probl Cancer* 8: 1, 1984

644. Takada K, Yoshikawa H, Muranishi S, Takahara S, Naganon S, Fukinishi T, Sonoda T, Ichikawa Y: Elimination characteristics of bredinin from patients serum in hemodialysis. *Int J Clin Pharmacol Ther Toxicol* 23: 197, 1985

645. Holt S, Naysmith S, Reid J, Buist TAS: Hazards of hepatic artery infusion of streptozocin. *Scott Med J* 23: 163, 1979

646. Harmon WE, Cohen HJ, Schneeberger EE, Grupe WE: Chronic renal failure in children treated with methyl CCNU. *N Engl J Med* 300: 1200, 1979

647. Henderson ES, Adamson RH, Oliverio VT: The metabolic fate of tritiated methotrexate. II. Absorption and excretion in man. *Cancer Res* 25: 1018, 1965

648. Bryan CW, Henry P: Methotrexate clearance in rats with impaired renal function. *Clin Res* 21: 817, 1973

649. Hande KR, Balow JE, Drake JC, Rosenberg SA, Chabner BA: Methotrexate and hemodialysis. *Ann Intern Med* 87: 495, 1977

650. Ahmad S, Shen F, Bleyer WAL: Methotrexate induced renal failure and ineffectiveness of peritoneal dialysis. *Arch Intern Med* 138: 1146, 1978

651. Gibson TP, Reich SD, Krumlovsky FA, Ivanovich P: Hemoperfusion for methotrexate removal. *Clin Pharmacol* 23: 351, 1978

652. Molina R, Fabian C, Cowley B: Use of charcoal hemoperfusion with sequential hemodialysis to reduce methotrexate levels in a patient with acute renal insufficiency. *Am J Med* 82: 350, 1987

653. Petrilli ES, Castaldo TW, Matutat RJ, Ballon SC, Gutierrez ML: Bleomycin pharmacology in relation to adverse effects and renal function in cervical cancer patients. *Gynec Oncol* 14: 350, 1982

654. Perry DJ, Weiss RB, Taylor HG: Enhanced bleomycin toxicity during acute renal failure. *Cancer Treat Rep* 66: 592, 1982

655. Crooke ST, Luft F, Broughton A, Strong J, Casson K, Einhorn L: Bleomycin serum pharmacokinetics as determined by radioimmunoassay and a microbiologic assay in a patient with compromised renal function. *Cancer* 39: 1430, 1977

656. Burke JF, Laucius F, Brodovsky HS, Soriano RZ: Doxorubicin hydrochloride-associated renal failure. *Arch Intern Med* 137: 385, 1977

657. Dragon LH, Braine HG: Necrosis of the hand after daunorubicin infusion distal to an arteriovenous fistula. *Ann Intern Med* 91: 58, 1979

658. Madias NE, Harrington JT: Platinum nephrotoxicity. *Am J Med* 65: 307, 1978

659. Prestayko AW, Luft FC, Einhorn L, Crooke ST: Cisplatin pharmacokinetics in a patient with renal dysfunction. *Med Pediat Oncol* 5: 183, 1978

660. Fuss M, Bergans A, Brauman H, Toussaint C, Vereerstraeten P, Franckson M, Corvilain J: ^{125}I-insulin metabolism in chronic renal failure treated by renal transplantation. *Kidney Int* 5: 372, 1974

661. Shapiro DJ, Blumenkrantz MJ, Levin SR, Coburn JW: Absorption and action of insulin added to peritoneal dialysate in dogs. *Nephron* 22: 174, 1977

662. Smith DL, Vecchio TI, Forist AA: Metabolism of antidiabetic

sulfonylureas in man. *Metabolism* 14: 229, 1965

663. Petitpierre B, Perrin L, Rudhardt M, Herrera A, Fabre J: Behaviour of chlorpropamide in renal insufficiency and under the effect of associated drug therapy. *Int J Clin Pharmacol* 6: 120, 1972

664. Rothfield EL, Crews AH Jr, Ribot S, Bernstein A: Severe hypoglycemia. Result of renal retention of chlorpropamide. *Arch Intern Med* 115: 468, 1965

665. Graw RG, Clarke RR: Chlorpropamide intoxication treatment with peritoneal dialysis. *Pediatrics* 45: 106, 1970

666. Weissman PN, Shenkman L, Gregerman RJ: Chlorpropamide induced hyponatremia. Drug induced inappropriate antidiuretic hormone activity. *N Engl J Med* 284, 65, 1971

667. Beckmann R: The fate of biguanides in man. *Ann NY Acad Sci* 148: 820, 1968

668. Ewy G, Pabico RC, Maher JF, Mintz DH: Lactic acidosis associated with phenformin therapy and localized tissue hypoxia. Report of a case treated by hemodialysis. *Ann Intern Med* 59: 878, 1963

669. Tobin M, Mookerjee BK: Hemodialysis for phenformin associated lactic acidosis. *J Dial* 2: 273, 1978

670. Werb R, Clark WR, Lindsay RM, Jones EOP, Linton AL: Serum vitamin A levels and associated abnormalities in patients on regular dialysis treatment. *Clin Nephrol* 12: 63, 1979

671. Stein G, Schone S, Geinitz D, Abendroth K, Kokot F, Fünfstück R, Sperschneider H, Keil E: No tissue level abnormality of vitamin A concentration despite elevated serum vitamin A of uremic patients. *Clin Nephrol* 25: 87, 1986

672. Stewart WK, Fleming LW: Plasma retinol and retinol binding protein concentration in patients on maintenance haemodialysis with and without vitamin A supplements. *Nephron* 30: 15, 1982

673. Farrington K, Miller P, Varghese Z, Baillod RA, Moorhead JF: Vitamin A toxicity and hypercalcaemia in chronic renal failure. *Br Med J* 282: 1999, 1981

674. Ellis S, DePalma J, Cheng A, Capozzalo P, Dombeck D, Discala VA: Vitamin A supplements in hemodialysis patients. *Nephron* 26: 215, 1980

675. Gotloib L, Sklan D, Mines M: Hemodialysis; effect on plasma levels of vitamin A and carotenoid. *JAMA* 239: 751, 1978

676. Chaplin H Jr, Clark LD, Ropes MW: Vitamin D intoxication. *Am J Med* 221: 269, 1951

677. Nolph KD, Stoltz M, Maher JF: Calcium free peritoneal dialysis. Treatment of vitamin D intoxication. *Arch Intern Med* 128: 809, 1971

678. Berl T, Berns AS, Huffer WE, Hammill K, Alfrey AC, Arnaud CD, Schrier RW: 1,25 dihydroxycholecalciferol effects in chronic dialysis. A double-blind controlled study. *Ann Intern Med* 88: 774, 1978

679. Christiansen C, Rodbro P, Christensen MS, Hartnack B, Transbol I: Deterioration of renal function during treatment of chronic renal failure with 1,25 dihydroxycholecalciferol. *Lancet* 2: 700, 1978

680. Niwa T, Ito T, Matsui E: Plasma thiamine levels with hemodialysis. *JAMA* 218: 885, 1971

681. Marumo F, Kamata K, Okubo M: Deranged concentrations of water soluble vitamins in the blood of undialyzed and dialyzed patients with chronic renal failure. *Int J Artif Intern Organs* 9: 17, 1986

682. Stein G, Sperschneider H, Koppe S: Vitamin levels in chronic renal failure and need for supplementation. *Blood Purif* 3: 52, 1985

683. Ito T, Niwa T, Matsui E: Vitamin B_2 and vitamin E in long-term hemodialysis. *JAMA* 217: 699, 1971

684. Lasker N, Harvey A, Baker H: Vitamin levels in hemodialysis and intermittent peritoneal dialysis. *Trans Am Soc Artif Intern Organs* 9: 51, 1963

685. Dobbelstein H, Korner WF, Mempel W, Grosse-Wilde H, Edel HH: Vitamin B_6 deficiency in uremia and its implications for the depression of immune responses. *Kidney Int* 5: 233, 1974

686. Kopple JD, Mercurio K, Blumenkrantz MJ, Jones MR, Tallos J, Roberts C, Card B, Saltzman R, Casciato DA, Swenseid ME: Daily requirement for pyridoxine supplements in chronic renal failure. *Kidney Int* 19: 694, 1981

687. Whitehead VM, Comty CH, Posen GA, Kaye M: Homeostasis of folic acid in patients undergoing maintenance hemodialysis. *N Engl J Med* 279: 970, 1968

688. Skoutakis VA, Acchiardo SR, Meyer MC, Hatch FE: Folic acid dosage for chronic hemodialysis patients. *Clin Pharmacol Ther* 18: 200, 1975

689. Ramirez G, Chen M, Boyce HW Jr, Fuller SM, Butcher DE, Brueggemeyer CD, Newton JL: The plasma and red cell vitamin B levels of chronic hemodialysis patients: a longitudinal study. *Nephron* 42: 412, 1986

690. Reznik VM, Griswold WR, Brams MR, Mendoza SA: Does high dose ascorbic acid accelerate renal failure. *N Engl J Med* 302: 1418, 1980

691. Balcke P, Schmidt P, Zaggornik J, Kopsa H, Haulenstock A: Ascorbic acid aggravates secondary hyperoxalemia in patients on chronic hemodialysis. *Ann Intern Med* 101: 344, 1984

692. Sullivan JF, Eisenstein AB, Mottola OM, Mittal AK: The effect of dialysis on plasma and tissue levels of vitamin C. *Trans Am Soc Artif Intern Organs* 18: 277, 1972

693. Pönkä A, Kuhlbäck B: Serum ascorbic acid in patients undergoing chronic hemodialysis. *Acta Med Scand* 213: 305, 1983

694. Eschbach JW, Cook JD, Scribner BH, Finch CA: Iron balance in hemodialysis patients. *Ann Intern Med* 87: 710, 1977

695. Ali M, Fayemi O, Rigolosi R, Frascino J, Marsden T, Malcolm D: Hemosiderosis in hemodialysis patients; an autopsy study of 50 cases. *JAMA* 244: 343, 1980

696. Murray JA, Slater DN, Parsons MA, Fox M, Smith S, Platts MM: Splenic siderosis and parenteral iron dextran in maintenance haemodialysis patients. *J Clin Pathol* 37: 59, 1984

697. Chang TMS, Barre P: Effect of desferrioxamine on removal of aluminum and iron by coated charcoal haemoperfusion and haemodialysis. *Lancet* 2: 1051, 1983

698. Berlyne GM, Ben Ari J, Pest D, Weinberger J, Stern M, Gilmore GR, Levine R: Hyperaluminaemia from aluminum resins in renal failure. *Lancet* 2: 494, 1970

699. Kaehny WD, Alfrey AC, Holman RE, Shorr WJ: Aluminum transfer during hemodialysis. *Kidney Int* 12: 361, 1977

700. Pierides AM, Ward MK, Kerr DNS: Haemodialysis encephalopathy; possible role of phosphate depletion. *Lancet* 1: 1234, 1976

701. Alfrey AC, Le Gendre GR, Kaehny WD: The dialysis encephalopathy syndrome. Possible aluminum intoxication. *N Engl J Med* 294: 184, 1976

702. Curtis JR, Goode GC, Herrington J, Urdaneta LE: Possible cobalt toxicity in maintenance hemodialysis patients after treatment with cobaltous chloride: a study of blood and tissue cobalt concentration in normal subjects and patients with terminal renal failure. *Clin Nephrol* 5: 61, 1976

703. Rees PH, Keating MI, Kager PA, Hockmeyer WT: Renal clearance of pentavalent antimony (sodium stibogluconate). *Lancet* 2: 226, 1980

704. Salvadeo A, Minola C, Segagni S, Villa S: Trace metal changes in dialysis fluid and blood of patients on hemodialysis. *Int J*

Artif Organs 2: 17, 1979

705. Gilberson A, Vaziri ND, Mirahamadi K, Rosen SM: Hemodialysis of acute arsenic intoxication with transient renal failure. *Arch Intern Med* 136: 1303, 1976

706. Marlette JM, Ma KW, Shafer RB: Effect of hemodialysis on gallium-67-citrate scanning. *Clin Nucl Med* 5: 401, 1980

708. De Backer W, Zachee P, Verpooten GA, Majelyne W, Vanheule A, De Broe ME: Thallium intoxication treated with combined hemoperfusion-hemodialysis. *J Toxicol Clin Toxicol* 19: 259, 1982

708. Doolan PD, Hess WC, Kyle LH: Acute renal insufficiency due to bichloride of mercury. Observations on gastrointestinal hemorrhage and BAL therapy. *N Engl J Med* 249: 273, 1953

709. Osterloh J, Becker CE: Pharmacokinetics of CaNa$_2$ EDTA and chelation of lead in renal failure. *Clin Pharmacol Ther* 40: 686, 1986

710. Foremen H, Finnegan C, Lushbaugh CC: Nephrotoxic hazard from uncontrolled edathamil calcium disodium therapy. *JAMA* 160: 1042, 1956

711. Ross JH, McGinty F, Brewer DG: Penicillamine nephropathy. *Nephron* 26: 184, 1980

712. Wainer E, Boner G, Lubin E, Rosenfeld JB: Clearance of Tc^{99-m} DTPA in hemodialysis and peritoneal dialysis: concise communication. *J Nucl Med* 22: 768, 1981

713. Batey R, Scott J, Jain S, Sherlock S: Acute renal insufficiency occurring during intravenous desferrioxamine therapy. *Scand J Haematol* 22: 277, 1979

714. Kostyniak PJ: Mobilization and removal of methylmercury in the dog during extracorporeal complexing hemodialysis with 2,3 dimercaptosuccinic acid (DMSA). *J Pharmacol Exp Ther* 221: 63, 1982

715. Sacho JJ, Henderson RR: Use of bishydroxycoumarin (Dicoumarol) in the presence of impaired renal function. *JAMA* 148: 839, 1952

716. Wright JS: Phenindione sensitivity with leukaemoid reaction and hepatorenal damage. *Postgrad Med J* 46: 452, 1970

717. O'Reilly RA, Aggler PM: Determinants of the response to oral anti-coagulant drugs in man. *Pharmacol Rev* 22: 35, 1970

718. Turney JH, Williams LC, Fenwell MR, Parsons V, Weston MJ: Platelet protection and heparin sparing with prostacyclin during regular dialysis therapy. *Lancet* 2: 219, 1980

719. Ramzan MI, Shanks CA, Triggs EJ: Gallamine disposition in surgical patients with chronic renal failure. *Br J Clin Pharmacol* 12: 141, 1981

720. Singer MM, Dutton R, Way WL: Untoward results of gallamine administration during bilateral nephrectomy: treatment with haemodialysis. *Br J Anaesth* 43: 404, 1971

721. Cozantis D, Haapenen E: Studies on muscle relaxants during haemodialysis. *Acta Anaesth Scand* 23: 225, 1979

722. Bevan DR, Donati F, Gyasi H, Williams A: Vecuronium in renal failure. *Can Anaesth Soc J* 31: 491, 1984

723. Castagnoli K, Hennis PJ: The pharmacokinetics and pharmacodynamics of atracurium in patients with and without renal failure. *Anesthesiology* 61: 699, 1984

724. Brotherton WP, Matteo RS: Pharmacokinetics and pharmacodynamics of metocurine in humans with and without renal failure. *Anesthesiology* 55: 273, 1981

725. Fahey MR, Morris RB, Miller RD, Nguyen TL, Upton RA: Pharmacokinetics of Org NC 45 (Norcuron) in patients with and without renal failure. *Br J Anaesth* 53: 1049, 1981

726. Bevan DR, D'Souza J, Rouse JM, Caldwell J, Smith RL: Clinical pharmacokinetics and pharmacodynamics of fazadinium in renal failure. *Eur J Clin Pharmacol* 20: 293, 1981

727. Bishop MJ, Hornbein TF: Prolonged effect of succinylcholine

after neostigmine and pyridostigmine administration in patients with renal failure. *Anesthesiology* 58: 384, 1983

728. Gosselin RE, Gabourel JD, Wills JH: Fate of atropine in man. *Clin Pharmacol Ther* 1: 597, 1960

729. Worth DP, Davison AM, Roberts TG, Lewins AM: Ineffectiveness of haemodialysis in atropine poisoning. *Br Med J* 286: 2023, 1983

730. Mazze RI: Fluorinated anaesthetic nephrotoxicity: an update. *Can Anaesth Soc J* 31 (*Suppl*): S16, 1984

731. Alexander WD, Evans V, MacAulay A, Gallagher TF Jr, Londono J: Metabolism of ^{35}S-labelled antithyroid drugs in man. *Br Med J* 2: 290, 1969

732. Bricker NS, Hlad CJ: Observations on the renal clearance of I^{131}. *J Clin Invest* 34: 1057, 1955

733. Gardner DF, Mars DR, Thomas RG, Bumrungsup C, Misbin RI: Iodine retention and thyroid dysfunction in patients on hemodialysis and continuous ambulatory peritoneal dialysis. *Am J Kidney Dis* 7: 471, 1986

734. Hansson R, Lindholm T: Elimination of hypaque (sodium 3,5 diacetamido-2, 4, 6 triiodobenzoate) and the effect of hemodialysis in anuria. A clinical study and an experimental investigation on rabbits. *Acta Med Scan* 174: 611, 1963

735. Ackrill P, McIntosh CS, Nimmon C, Baker LRI, Cattell WR: A comparison of the clearance of urographic contrast medium (sodium diatrizoate) by peritoneal and haemodialysis. *Clin Sci Mol Med* 50: 69, 1976

736. Byrd L, Sherman RL: Radiocontrast-induced acute renal failure: a clinical and pathophysiologic review. *Medicine* 58: 270, 1979

737. Gomes AS, Baker JD, Martin-Paredo V, Dixon SM, Takiff H, Machleder HI, Moore WS: Acute renal dysfunction after major arteriography. *Am J Roentgenol* 145: 1249, 1985

738. Goldberg AP, Sherrard DJ, Haas LB, Brunzell JD: Control of clofibrate toxicity in uremic hypertriglyceridemia. *Clin Pharmacol Ther* 21: 317, 1977

739. Gugler R, Körten JW, Jensen CJ, Klehr U, Hartlapp J: Clofibrate disposition in renal failure and acute and chronic liver disease. *Eur J Clin Pharmacol* 15: 341, 1979

740. Cumming A: Acute renal failure and interstitial nephritis after clofibrate treatment. *Br Med J* 2: 1529, 1980

741. Williams AJ, Walls J: The pharmacokinetics of bezafibrate in patients undergoing continuous ambulatory peritoneal dialysis. *Peritoneal Dial Bull* 6: 69, 1986

742. Desager JP, Costermans J, Verbeckmoes R, Harvengt C: Effect of hemodialysis on plasma kinetics of fenofibrate in chronic renal failure. *Nephron* 31: 51, 1982

743. Bonadonna A, Cascone C, Muinaretto G, De Luca M, Bruno R, Maggi E, Tomassia V: A pilot study of the pharmacokinetics and triglyceride lowering activity of acipimox in dialyzed uremic patients. *Int J Clin Pharmacol Ther Toxicol* 23: 112, 1985

744. Larsson R, Erlanson P, Bodemar G, Walan A, Fransson L, Norlander B: The pharmacokinetics of cimetidine and its sulphoxide metabolite in patients with normal and impaired renal function. *Br J Clin Pharmacol* 13: 163, 1982

745. Larsson R, Bodemar G, Norlander B: Oral absorption of cimetidine and its clearance in patients with renal failure. *Eur J Clin Pharmacol* 15: 153, 1979

746. Ma KW, Brown DC, Masler DS, Silvis SE: Effects of renal failure on blood levels of cimetidine. *Gastroenterology* 74: 473, 1978

747. Jones RH, Lewin MR, Parsons V: Therapeutic effect of cimetidine in patients undergoing haemodialysis. *Br Med J* 1: 650, 1979

748. Klotz U, Reimann I: Delayed clearance of diazepam due to cimetidine. *N Engl J Med* 302: 1012, 1980

749. Jacob AI, Lanier D, Canterbury J, Bourgoinie JJ: Reduction by cimetidine of serum parathyroid hormone levels in uremic patients. *N Engl J Med* 302: 671, 1980

750. Bjoeldager PAL, Jensen JB, Nielsen LP, Larsen NE, Hvidberg EF: Pharmacokinetics of cimetidine in patients undergoing hemodialysis. *Nephron* 34: 159, 1983

751. Pizzella KM, Moore MC, Schultz RW, Walshe J, Schentag JJ: Removal of cimetidine by peritoneal dialysis, hemodialysis and charcoal hemoperfusion. *Ther Drug Monit* 2: 273, 1980

752. Vaziri ND, Ness RL, Barton CH: Peritoneal dialysis clearance of cimetidine. *Am J Gastroenterol* 71: 572, 1979

753. Garg DC, Baltodano N, Jallad NS, Perez G, Oster JR, Eshelman FN, Weidler DJ: Pharmacokinetics of ranitidine in patients with renal failure. *J Clin Pharmacol* 26: 286, 1986

754. Roberts AP, Harrison C, Dixon GT, Curtis JR: Plasma ranitidine concentration after intravenous administration in normal volunteers and haemodialysis patients. *Postgrad Med J* 59: 25, 1983

755. Naesdal J, Andersson T, Bodemar G. Larsson R, Regårdh CG, Skanberg I, Walan A: Pharmacokinetics of [^{14}C] omeprazole in patients with impaired renal function. *Clin Pharmacol Ther* 40: 344, 1986

756. Bateman DN, Gokal R, Dodd TRP, Blain PG: The pharmacokinetics of single doses of metoclopramide in renal failure. *Eur J Clin Pharmacol* 19: 437, 1981

757. Berardi RR, Cornish LA, Hyneck ML: Metoclopramide removal during continuous ambulatory peritoneal dialysis. *Drug Intell Clin Pharm* 20: 154, 1986

758. Baker JR, Peck CC, Raybuck BD, Owens EL, Schuster BG: Normal pharmacokinetics of doxapram in a patient with renal failure and hypothyroidism. *Br J Clin Pharmacol* 11: 305, 1981

ANAESTHESIA AND MAJOR SURGERY IN PATIENTS WITH RENAL FAILURE

JOHN E. UTTING

In the last few years there has been, thanks to advances in nephrology, a complete change in the fields of anaesthesia and surgery in relation to patients with renal failure. It is, for example, no longer the rule that they come to the operating room for renal transplantation showing major patho-physiological features of uraemia, such, for example, as gross metabolic acidosis, a bleeding tendency and a high plasma potassium. Now their blood pressure is generally well-controlled, they are not suffering from gross overhydration and their general condition is frequently good. As nephrology has advanced, so has anaesthesia become simpler. A simple summary of the practical problems which face the surgeon and the anaesthetist are given in Table 1.

Occasionally patients with chronic renal failure present for surgery which is completely unconnected with the condition, which is found incidentally; this is probably increasingly so as the population becomes older. In some cases it will be suspected because of the nature of the lesion; patients presenting with prostatic symptoms, for example, not infrequently show some degree of renal failure.

The common major surgical operations on those treated by dialysis are, of course, renal transplant, graft nephrectomy, vagotomy and gastric drainage before renal transplantation and nephrectomy; the establishment of some of the newer types of fistulae may also be regarded as major surgery. Those presented for graft nephrectomy can be in poor physical condition: this is also true of patients who have developed acute renal failure after surgery or accident and who are being treated in the intensive care unit (ICU).

EFFECTS OF ANAESTHESIA ON THE KIDNEY

Much of the work on the effects of anaesthesia on renal function is difficult to interpret. For example, changes due to anaesthesia may not be entirely separable from those due to concomitant manipulations or, indeed, to surgery. Almost all of the investigations into renal blood flow (RBF) under anaesthesia have involved the use of p-aminohippurate (PAH), and the well-known difficulties in using this agent are compounded by a paucity of knowledge on the effect of anaesthesia on the clearance of the substance; halothane in high concentrations is, indeed, known to inhibit PAH transport (1); this would cause renal blood flow to be underestimated.

Any changes in renal function induced by anaesthesia reverse rapidly when the agents are withdrawn, with the possible exception of di-ethyl ether, which may give longer lasting changes (2). There is one obviously nephrotoxic anaesthetic, methoxyflurane, but its use is now very limited. The effects of anaesthesia are generally additive to the effects of surgery, but very much more rapidly reversible; anaesthesia is not associated, for example, with prolonged salt and water retention; indeed, in some circumstances, it probably protects the kidney from the effects of surgery, because sympathetic activity and catecholamine release, secondary to surgical trauma, are reduced.

There is little information about potential damage to the failing kidney by anaesthetic agents other than by specific toxicity. Clinical evidence would suggest that patients with advanced deterioration in renal function can be safely anaesthetised if the technique is appropriate, the anaesthetist is skillful, fluid therapy is carefully controlled and gross hypotension and hypertension are avoided.

Volatile and gaseous agents

In the intact human subject the weight of evidence supports the view that the general anaesthetic agents increase renal vascular resistance and decrease both RBF and glomerular filtration rate (GFR); but the effect on the former is greater than the latter and the filtration fraction tends to increase, whilst urinary volume declines and urinary osmolarity increases. Early work on this subject has been summarised and annotated (3). Unfortunately, however, it is often difficult in this early work to separate the effects of anaesthesia from those of surgery.

That the effects can be due to anaesthesia alone is suggested by work in young, fit volunteers who were not subject to surgery during investigation (4–6). This work covered cyclopropane, halothane and unsupplemented nitrous oxide anaesthesia with a muscle relaxant. Renal blood flow decreased and renal vascular resistance rose.

The decrease in GFR was less marked and in this study the filtration fraction was not significantly increased (except in the case of halothane). All three techniques were associated with a marked antidiuresis; urinary volume (V) fell, U_{Osm} increased and so did the ratio U_{Osm}/P_{Osm}, whilst there was a change from the excretion of solute free water (C_{H_2O}) to tubular reabsorption (T_{H_2O}). The antidiuresis was blocked by ethanol, suggesting that an increased secretion of antidiuretic hormone (ADH) was responsible, except in the case of the nitrous oxide/relaxant technique, in which the response was not blocked. This pattern of reduction in RBF, GFR and urinary volume found with halothane is also typical of isoflurane (7) and enflurane (8).

Studies of dogs (9) previously implanted with flow-meters, however, showed that halothane decreased RBF only slightly, if at all, and that renal vascular resistance was decreased. Certainly, work with the isolated kidney (10) showed that halothane increased renal blood flow (and urinary volume, sodium excretion and osmolal clearance) but in these circumstances, of course, the kidney is free from haemodynamic, neural and extra-renal hormonal influences. In the isolated kidney preparation halothane does not seem to abolish autoregulation (11) when arterial perfusion pressure varies between 75 and 125 mm Hg.

Analgesic drugs

The analgesic agents are not properly anaesthetic agents but their use pre-operatively and post-operatively warrants their inclusion herein. Morphine has been investigated in the dog; in one study (12) a decrease in RBF was found and in another a slight increase (13). Morphine is associated with decreased urine production. It has been suggested that the increase in ADH associated with its administration is due to concomitant surgery (14). In the human, neuroleptanalgesia has caused little change in haemodynamic variables and only a moderate alteration in solute clearance and in sodium and water excretion (15). The technique involved the use of the analgesic fentanyl together with the butyrophenone derivative, dehydrobenzperidol which has some alpha-adrenergic blocking activity.

Induced hypotension

Ganglion blocking agents cause an initial decrease in RBF that soon returns to near normal levels, presumably as further vasodilatation occurs. Glomerular filtration rate, however, remains low as long as blood pressure is reduced (16). In the dog, hypotension induced by sodium nitroprusside (which directly affects vessels, mainly arterioles) is associated with an increased RBF, but renal vascular resistance remains unchanged; when trimetaphan is used, however, blood flow decreases (17). Hypotension due to halothane is mainly caused by a decrease in cardiac output; during the period of low blood pressure there is renal vasodilatation

Table 1. A list of problems *commonly* of importance to anaesthetist and surgeon when dealing with patients with chronic renal failure.

Electrolyte distrubances	*Pulmonary complications*
overhydration	oedema
underhydration	uraemic lung
low plasma potassium	infections
raised plasma potassium	
metabolic acidosis	*Endocrine abnormalities*
	osteoporosis
Haematological disturbances	
anaemia	*Gastro-intestinal tract*
bleeding tendency	full stomach
platelet malfunction	bleeding
others	hepatitis
Cardio vascular disturbances	*Neurological abnormalities*
hypertension	altered consciousness
left ventricular hypertrophy	convulsions
+/− strain	'drug sensitivities'
congestive cardiac failure	
coronary artery disease	*Immune system*
conduction defects	immunosuppression
cardiomyopathy	
pericarditis	
effectss of drug therapy	

Drugs
anti-hypertensive agents
  beta blockers
  alpha blockers
  alpha and beta blockers (labetalol)
  diuretics
  peripheral vasodilators
insulin and other anti-diabetic drugs

but vasoconstriction may occur during recovery (18).

In clinical practice induced hypotension may be associated with renal failure even in normal subjects. Renal dysfunction must be regarded as a relative contra-indication even when the dysfunction is mild. It is probably absolutely contra-indicated in severe renal failure.

Renal toxicity of inhalation agents

Methoxyflurane, a volatile anaesthetic agent, can itself cause renal failure, usually when high doses have been used for long periods (19). This failure is associated with a high urinary output and is unresponsive to vasopressin; it usually becomes evident within 24 h of anaesthesia, may last a few days or several weeks and can be fatal, or at least permanent (20, 21). It is, in fact, metabolites which are responsible, the fluoride ion being primary and oxalic acid probably contributing to the damage (22). The renal toxicity of methoxyflurane is increased by the aminoglycoside antibiotics (23, 24) and by tetracyclines (25). Enzyme induction, with for example, phenobarbitone, can also increase toxicity by increasing the rate of metabolic breakdown (26). Clearly this agent is contra-indicated in renal failure.

Enflurane is also metabolised to fluoride ions but to a lesser extent than methoxyflurane is (8). However, there have been at least three reports of post-operative renal deterioration in patients with pre-existing renal disease (27–29) though evidence against the agent in this respect could not be regarded as conclusive. Opinions differ as to whether it should be used in patients with renal failure. Isoflurane produces less fluoride than enflurane, and halothane probably least of all (30, 31).

The effects of mechanical ventilation

Most major surgery performed on patients with renal dysfunction is accompanied by anaesthesia in which muscle relaxants are used and, in consequence, artificial pulmonary ventilation instituted. The effect or artificial ventilation on renal function has been studied in some detail in both animals and in man. Most studies, however, are directed towards resolving the difficulties which occur in the ICU where, of course, artificial ventilation may be kept up for many days rather than for hours. Nevertheless, artificial ventilation during surgery will have an effect on renal function even if it be a minor one.

In the operating theatre artificial ventilation is by intermittent positive pressure (IPPV). In the ICU, however, it is not infrequent for continuous positive pressure ventilation (CPPV) to be used; here the airway pressure is kept above atmospheric for the entire respiratory cycle, to keep open both airways and alveoli and so improve oxygenation.

CCPV is mainly irrelevant to the operating theatre, but it probably affords a number of indications of the tendency in changes of renal function which are seen in IPPV. It is for this reason that it is mentioned here. Recently the subject has been reviewed (32) and much of what follows is taken from their account.

Renal blood flow was reduced when IPPV was established in one study in animals (33); most studies showed a decline in RBF when IPPV is changed to CPPV. GFR was unchanged in the only study in which this variable was compared during spontaneous ventilation and IPPV (34). However, when CPPV was compared to IPPV it was usually found that GFR declined when CPPV was established. *Urinary sodium excretion* has been found to diminish (or remain unchanged) when IPPV was established (35), but when the change from IPPV and CPPV was investigated, most studies showed a decline in sodium excretion.

Urinary volume went down in four studies when IPPV was established after spontaneous ventilation (34, 36–38), but in two studies it increased (39, 40). Again this variable was reduced in every study of CPPV compared to IPPV.

Water clearance and osmolal clearance did not differ in spontaneous ventilation and IPPV (34, 38, 40) but during CPPV, as compared to IPPV, it would seem that C_{H_2O} is unchanged or goes up and C_{Osm} is unchanged or goes down.

Results of studies of *plasma or urinary anti-diuretic hormone* which compared spontaneous ventilation with IPPV have been equivocal: some studies demonstrated it to go up (36, 38), to go down (39, 40) or remain the same (34). During CPPV, ADH levels have usually been higher than during IPPV.

The pattern of decreased RBF, GFR, V and $U_{Na}V$ which seems to be associated with CPPV and, to a lesser extent, perhaps, with IPPV could be due simply to increased renal sympathetic activity and there is, indeed, some evidence to show that this is how it is caused; the changes do not seem to occur in the dennervated kidney (41).

The changes, with intermittent positive pressure at least, are not great and must, of course, be compared with those changes produced by the volatile and gaseous agents and by local analgesic techniques. For short periods, as during surgery, it would seem that this factor can be ignored.

REGIONAL TECHNIQUES

Many would consider that brachial plexus bloock was the anaesthetic of choice when an arterio-venous fistula is being established, but this can hardly be considered to be major surgery. Nevertheless, it is worth noting that the duration of the block in patients with renal disease can be substantially shorter than in normal patients (42, 43). It is possible that bupivicaine may be more toxic in the patient with chronic renal failure than in the normal subject. In any local technique in which adrenaline is used the toxic effects of that agent also must be considered (44).

Spinal and epidural analgesia

The most widely used and relevant techniques as far as major surgery is concerned are spinal and epidural block. There are accounts of the successful use of both for renal transplantation (45–47). More recently there has been another favourable account of the use of regional techniques in patients with renal disease (48). Some authorities would not regard technique contra-indicated in uraemic neuropathy, though most anaesthetists probably would. It should be added that epidural haematoma formation, which is a potential hazard, does not in practice seem to be a great problem, providing, of course, there is not platelet dysfunction. The onset of subarachnoid block may be faster in patients with chronic renal failure than in normal subjects (43).

Circulatory effects

Both epidural and spinal analgesia cause considerable circulatory upset. The kidney itself receives its sympathetic nerve supply from spinal segments T4 to L1 (inclusive) but sympathetic nerve block of the kidney in itself probably has little effect, certainly in the absence of changes in blood pressure. V and C_{H_2O} reportedly go down with spinal and up with epidural analgesia (49), but the differences may not be fundamental.

However, spinal and epidural analgesia both cause venular and arteriolar dilation. In the fit patient a restricted block will not cause significant hypotension, especially if he or she has been pre-loaded with fluid before the block is instituted. The cardiac output will increase to compensate for the decrease in peripheral resistance. However, this does not necessarily apply to the unfit patient and certainly does not apply to any patient when the sympathetic block extends to the cardiac accelerator fibres which arise from segments T1 and T4 (inclusive). If these are involved in the block their positive chronotropic and inotropic effect will be lost and the arterial blood pressure will fall.

These principles are common to both epidural and spinal techniques but two other factors are especially important in epidural analgesia where, in addition to vasodilatation and cardiac depression with a 'high' block there are also the problems of cardiorespiratory depression due to the absorption of the local analgesic solution and beta-sympathetic stimulation due to the absorption of adrenaline should this be used with the local (50). It is worth noting that at least bupivicaine may be more toxic in patients with renal failure than in normal patients (51), and in acidotic and hyperkalaemic patients, when adrenaline is given concurrently, the risk of arrythmias may be very considerable (52).

Clinical aspects

The depression of renal function during spinal and epidural analgesia seems to be less than during general anaesthesia (53–57). Despite this it is not a popular method of tackling the problem of anaesthesia in patients with severe renal dysfunction.

It is largely fruitless to speculate as to why this should be. In some circumstances it may be because the anaesthetist is not familiar with the techniques involved. The main factors, however, are probably unrelated to this. Many patients do not wish to be awake during surgical procedures. Not only that but the anaesthetist may not wish to have the patient awake because such operations as renal transplantation are

not lacking in crises which are usually best handled when the patient is asleep.

Finally, the control over the patient's physiological variables is better under general anaesthesia than under local and recent advances in general anaesthesia such, for example, as the introduction of new muscle relaxants, has made the management of patients with little or no renal function under general anaesthesia considerably easier.

EFFECT OF SURGERY ON THE KIDNEY

In general, the effects of both surgery and anaesthesia on the kidney are in the same direction. The most obvious effect of surgery (with anaesthesia) is to produce oliguria. Surgery, however, seems to differ from anaesthesia, since it greatly increases the secretion of ADH (58), and it is tempting to ascribe the diminution of urine flow to this factor.

Oliguria of surgery

Increased ADH secretion is not the only, nor even the pre-eminent cause of oliguria, because such urine as is produced is poorly concentrated (59). Furthermore, even if exogenous ADH is administered to the surgical patient, the urine seldom becomes more concentrated than plasma (60). An alternative explanation must, therefore, be sought.

Surgical trauma causes sympathetic discharge, and an increase in the levels of circulating catecholamines and anaesthesia only partly protects against this. It seems likely that the effect of both together is to divert blood from cortex to medulla in addition to reducing the absolute flow through the organ (61). Alternatively, the high levels of ADH might themselves divert blood flow in the same direction (62). The effect of such a diversion would, of course, be the production of urine of a low concentration.

The oliguria can be reduced and urine flow raised by increasing fluid administration during surgery but this manoeuvre loads to a cumulative positive balance fot both salt and water (63). In patients with renal dysfunction the dangers of fluid overload are even greater than they are in normal subjects.

Hypovolaemia is not, or should not be, a feature of surgery. However, the kidney, especially the renal cortex, takes a full part in the generalised vasoconstriction, caused by sympathetic stimulation and the circulatory disorder, which characterises the shock syndrome. From this even the normal kidney may not recover and, though hard scientific evidence on the subject is sparse, it would seem very likely that the failing kidney, from whatever cause, is more sensitive to ischaemia than is the normal one.

That anaesthetist and surgeon must make sure that a diminution in RBF because of hypovolaemia does not occur. This statement would seem to be so obvious as to be unnecessary. However, in a situation in which fuller accounts of relatively minor matters are recorded such, for example, as the effect of general anaesthesia, this must be emphasised.

The 'third space'

It is now over 25 years since it was first claimed that major surgery induced an apparent reduction in the volume of extracellular fluid (ECF) (64). It was suggested that this was due to sequestration of fluid at traumatised regions, into a 'third space', but other factors, such as evaporation of fluid from the wound, were also involved. The infusion of large quantities of fluid similar to ECF (Hartmann's solution, Ringer-lactate) during surgery certainly led to an increase in urine production and of sodium excretion. This, however, was at the expence of an often very considerable positive balance of both water and salt.

It has been shown that the sequestration of extracellular fluid and the development of the so-called third space is not as great a factor as had originally been thought since methodological difficulties were involved (65). Nevertheless, it is generally accepted that surgical trauma does cause considerable loss of fluid and that fluid is needed during surgery if blood pressure and urine output are to be maintained.

This obviously poses considerable problems for the anaesthetist who is caring for a patient with renal failure during an extensive operation. Administration of too much fluid can lead to oedema, even to pulmonary oedema, since left ventricular function is often depressed, and too little to cessation of urine flow with the consequent possibility that further degrees of renal failure will occur. In this circumstances the use of a central venous pressure line is only a partial answer.

Hormonal changes

Adrenocortical hormone secretion, both glucocorticoid and mineralocorticoid, increases during surgery and in the postoperative period. This would appear to contribute to, but is not entirely responsible for, the water and salt retention, which occurs after surgery. A full account of adrenocortical physiology is beyond the scope of this chapter.

Renin secretion is increased by surgery but not, to any great extent, by anaesthesia (66, 67). It is quite possible that the angiotensin so produced is responsible for some of the sodium retention both by stimulating the production of aldosterone and by a direct renal effect.

Other hormones such as the natriuretic hormone, prostaglandins and kallikrein-bradykinin may well be important in the response to surgery, but their place has not yet been assessed.

THE EFFECTS OF RENAL FAILURE ON SOME ANAESTHETIC DRUGS

Anaesthetic agents and the drugs used in anaesthesia both influence renal function and are influenced by it. There follows a short account of the main agents used in anaesthetic practice which are influenced greatly by reduced renal function (See also Chapter 51). There are, of course, many more which the anaesthetist might administer which would

be so influenced. These, however, are probably the most important.

Narcotics

Though narcotics are mainly metabolised in the liver to non-polar compounds, these products may have pharmacological effects. Meperidine, for example, is partly metabolised to normeperidine and this may accumulate in patients with renal failure and give rise to epileptiform convulsion (68).

Less morphine appears to be bound to plasma protein in the patient with renal failure than in the normal subject (69). Whatever the cause of sensitivity to morphine may be, it should be administered with caution to uraemic patients who may show a considerable degree of sensitivity to it. Codeine, pentazocine and naloxone, however, can be used without dose modification in renal failure (70).

Thiopentone

It has been known for some time that uraemic patients require a lower dose of thiopentone than normal patients do (71). It is possible that this may be due to a concomitant decrease in the plasma albumen concentration or, alternatively, to displacement of the drug from protein by substances accumulating in the plasma during renal failure (72). It may also be that the so-called blood-brain barrier is more permeable in the uraemic state (73).

Neuromuscular blocking agents

Non-depolarising agents

The older non-depolarising muscle relaxants such, for example, as tubocurarine, gallamine, pancuronium, alcuronium and metocurine suffered from the disadvantage that they were mainly excreted by the kidney. Though they depend, to a large extent, on distribution for the termination of action, especially when one dose has been used, it is quite possible to cause prolonged curarisation with these agents, expecially if several doses are given. The literature on this subject is voluminous (60) and there is no doubt that the problem was a real one, with curarisation sometimes lasting for several days.

The advent of two new agents, atracurium and vecuronium, has largely eliminated this problem. Atracurium is eliminated largely by molecular breakdown (by the Holffmann reaction) and vecuronium by metabolism (mainly in the liver); in neither case would the kidney seem to be involved, though if very large doses of vecuronium are administered over a long period, as in the ICU, delayed recovery from curarisation can occur (74). The use of these agents in clinically anephric patients has been described; both atracurium (75) and vecuronium (76) proving satisfactory.

Depolarising agents

There is only one depolarising agent in common use, i.e. suxamethonium. It has the virtue of giving the most rapid relaxation of any of the muscle relaxant drugs and is the agent of choice when a rapid endotracheal intubation is required as, for example, when there is thought to be gastric residue which might be inhaled.

Suxamethonium is broken down by pseudocholinesterase and is not, to any important extent, excreted by the kidney. Unfortunately, however, its use is attended by a rise in the potassium concentration, a rise of up to 0.5 mmol/l in normal subjects. In patients with renal failure and a high plasma potassium to start with, this could be dangerous. A single dose seems not to cause a higher rise in potassium in patients with renal failure than in normal patients (77). There is some evidence that, with repeated doses, the rise can be very high (77, 78), though this view is not unanimous.

Anticholinesterase agents and atropine

The half-life of neostigmine is prolonged in renal failure because a significant proportion is excreted by the kidney (79). Atropine too, is excreted by the kidney. However, this does not seem to militate against the use of small doses of these agents in patients with renal failure. It has been suggested that the use of the anticholinesterase agents may prolong the effect of succinylcholine in patients with renal failure (50).

PERI-OPERATIVE MANAGEMENT

This section is based on the use of general anaesthesia; there is no further account of regional techniques other than that already given. Much of what is written here, however, applies to the use of regional as it does to general anaesthesia.

There are three different types of problems when dealing with the peri-operative management of renal failure patients. No practitioner could possibly confuse them but the fact that they are different tends to reduce the clarity of writing.

Firstly: there is the patient with no useful renal function at all who is on dialysis. It is sometimes true that such patients may be sick and it is always true that the abnormal behaviour of the anephric patient with regard to drugs must be kept in mind, but the anaesthetist does not have the duty of preserving residual and marginal renal function.

Secondly: there is the patient presented for renal transplant. Here the anaesthetist must make sure that the conditions for renal function are as good as possible when the graft is inserted; thereafter optimal conditions for graft survival and function must be provided.

Thirdly: there is the patient with marginal renal function who is not on dialysis, including patients with grafts which are failing. Here the anaesthetist must make sure that there is no further deterioration. To do this he must make sure that urine output continues; peri-operative oliguria and anuria invite further renal damage.

Pre-operative assessment

The anaesthetist can usually rely on there being a great deal of information available about a patient who is in chronic renal failure when he or she makes a pre-operative visit. The problems likely to be encountered have been outlined in Table 1. It is perhaps worthwhile outlining the bare essentials of assessment; these are summarised in Table 2.

Potassium levels can change very rapidly and should be measured within 4 to 6 h of surgery, when this be appropriate. In diabetic patients there is a need for frequent estimations of both plasma glucose and potassium, since very rapid changes can take place in both.

Pre-operative preparation

In general, drugs which have been administered to the patient pre-operatively should be continued. This is especially true of the anti-hypertensive agents since withdrawing these

Table 2. Features the anaesthetist will find important in the pre-operative visit.

History	*Physical examination*
possibility of 'full stomach'	signs of cardiac failure
exercise tolerance	state of hydration
attacks of left ventricular failure	psychological state
dialysis history	venous access
water and salt intake	state of dentition
corticosteroid therapy	(?) difficult intubation
hepatitis	
	Chest X-Ray
Electrocardiogram	heart size
Left ventricular hypertrophy	pulmonary congestion
and strain	intercurrent pathology
digitalis toxicity	(e.g. pneumonia)
arrhythmias	
(e.g. atrial fibrillation)	*Biochemical*
	Serum electrolytes,
Haematology	especially K+
haemoglobin and haematocrit	serum creatinine and blood
clotting	urea nitrogen
platelet count	full acid-base & blood gas
prothrombin time	analysis (if specially
partial thromboplastin time	indicated)

Drug intake
digitalis (overdose not uncommon)
beta-blockers (association with bradycardia during anaesthesia)
other anti-hypertensive agents (labile blood pressure under anaesthesia)
diuretics (associated with hypokalaemia)
anti-arrhythmic drugs (underlying cardiac arrhythmias)
calcium channel blockers (associated with bradycardia and hypotension during anaesthesia)
corticoids (appropriate dose fixed pre-operatively)
immunosuppressive (danger of sepsis)

agents may be associated with gross hypertension and cardiac ischaemia on induction of anaesthesia and endotracheal intubation.

As surgery is performed on the fasting patient and as patients with renal dysfunction can rapidly become both water and salt depleted, it may be necessary to give some intravenous fluid before induction of anaesthesia since the dehydration will increase the tendency towards oliguria inherent in surgery and anaesthesia and may thus predispose towards the development of acute renal failure. It has in fact been shown that the administration of saline before major surgery in patients with chronic renal failure preserves renal function (81).

Gross hyperkalaemia may have to be corrected and it is also generally considered wrong to induce anaesthesia if the serum K^+ exceeds 5.5 mmol/l. If there is urgency and the potassium is high, cation exchange resin or glucose and insulin may be required whilst as a 'first-aid' treatment the use of calcium will tide patients over an acute emergency.

Most patients present for renal transplantation with a haemoglobin concentration of 7 to 8 g/dl, but the level may be as low as 4 g/dl. Transfusion is generally avoided because of the well-known factors of marrow suppression and possible HLA sensitization but since it is possible that cadaver transplant survival may be improved by preoperative transfusion (82–84) has meant that this approach has been questioned.

Premedication

Narcotics cause a decrease in GFR (see above) and their metabolism is affected by renal failure; they are not, for these reasons, considered to be good premedicant drugs in this type of patient unless he or she is in pain. Pharmacologically a small dose of a phenothiazine might be preferable for reasons already given. The newer, shorter-acting, diazepines, such as temazepam, have been suggested to be suitable (85).

No premedication substitutes for adequate psychological management and, in practice, a light medication with any of the usual agents will do no harm, provided the patient is not very ill. Once the premedication has been given, however, there is a need for close observation.

Insulin infusion and corticoid administration may be considered to be part of premedication in those patients who require such treatment. They will not be dealt with further.

Induction of anaesthesia

Induction of anaesthesia with inhalation agents can be a stormy procedure and it is usual to induce with an intravenous agent. Of these thiopentone probably remains the best; certainly there is no evidence that any other agent is conspicuously better. However, to avoid hypotension the dose of thiopentone should be kept small and the drug given slowly.

Spontaneous and controlled ventilation

There are basically two techniques of general anaesthesia available, general anaesthesia with a volatile agent and spontaneous ventilation or general anaesthesia with a muscle relaxant and controlled ventilation. Most anaesthetists would use the former technique for, say, a short cystoscopy on a patient with renal dysfunction and most would use the latter for a longer operation, and certainly when muscular relaxation is required. However, there are a number of situations in which there would be a difference of opinion.

Spontaneous ventilation

Here it might well be that the choice would lie between nitrous oxide supplemented with halothane, isoflurane or enflurane. Of these the first probably gives the best conditions; though doubts have arisen about its hepatotoxicity there is no rational case for abandoning its use completely. Repeated anaesthesia with this agent should be avoided, however. As has been stated, isoflurane, like halothane, generates very little fluoride; however, it is not an ideal agent for spontaneous ventilation. Enflurane may be considered more suitable; its use for brief periods in patients with renal dysfunction seems to be safe.

Controlled ventilation

Anaesthesia can be considered to be a tetrad – of narcosis, reflex suppression, muscular relaxation and controlled apnoea. *Narcosis* may conveniently be obtained using nitrous oxide and oxygen; unfortunately, however, this may lead to 'awareness under anaesthesia', and it is now usual to supplement its use with a low concentration of a volatile agent; in patients with renal failure, isoflurane would seem to be the most suitable. *Reflex* suppression is, to a large degree, provided by the nitrous oxide and the volatile agent. However, the use of relatively small doses of analgesic agents has a great deal to commend it; not only does it tend to obtund rises in blood pressure, but it tends to make the awakening process more pleasant by providing some residual analgesia at the end of surgery In this respect the use of fentanyl with droperidol has already been mentioned, and is dealt with in more detail below. *Muscular relaxation* can now be provided by the new muscle relaxants atracurium or vecuronium. The residual action should usually be reversed with anti-cholinesterase. Finally, a discussion of *controlled apnoea* by intermittent positive pressure ventilation has already been undertaken. The inspired oxygen concentration should be adequate (at least 30%) and normocapnia should be attempted.

The narcotic agents and droperidol

Fentanyl has been recommended as being suitable for use during anaesthesia because it is said to be short acting. This is not entirely true; the respiratory depression produced by fentanyl may last for a long time, (86). The newer agent, sufentinil, has caused respiratory depression post-operatively in a patient with renal failure (87).

Droperidol in combination with fentanyl has been recommended as suitable for patients with renal dysfunction (88) and certainly its use is widespread. It has even been suggested that these agents should be used in high dosage as the sole anaesthetic agents and that this combination attenuates the stress response, with resulting lower levels of catecholamines; in this way the myocardial depressant effects of nitrous oxide also can be avoided. There are, however, difficulties both with regard to awareness during anaesthesia (these drugs are not true anaesthetic agents) and with regard to post-operative respiratory depression; in fact, the post-operative course can be dangerous unless impeccable post-operative care is available.

Reversal of neuromuscular block
The reversal of residual neuromuscular block should be undertaken with a small dose of neostigmine together with atropine, if there be any doubt about full recovery. The use of the drugs in this way is not contra-indicated by renal failure.

Intra-operative management

The management of the patient during major surgery is as important as the anaesthetic technique. A good deal of what must be regarded as management, however, can only be considered to be personal opinion and not scientifically attested fact. What follows must be viewed in this light.

Monitoring

This is a contentious subject. Many anaesthetists believe that intensive monitoring is the best approach to patient safety; others, however, believe that too many variables can cause confusion and danger, especially in a crisis. Here points only of specific importance to patients with renal failure will be considered.

The electrocardiogram
There can be few groups of patients in which electrocardiographic monitoring is more important. A bradycardia sometimes leading to a cardiac arrest is not unknown in patients on large doses of beta-blocking drugs. Signs of potassium toxicity may appear during anaesthesia especially, for example, when diabetic patients are being treated, and even signs of digoxin overdosage have appeared during surgery.

Blood pressure
Few would deny the importance of taking the blood pressure in patients with renal failure, even for the shortest procedures. Some variation of the Riva Rocci method such, for example, as the oscillometer may be used but an automated blood pressure measuring device, like the Dynamap, has much to commend it since it enables the anaesthetist to keep

a good record, and to perceive trends without being slavishly attached to the apparatus.

Intra-arterial monitoring must be viewed in the light on the fact that these patients frequently have gross arterial disease and that fistulae may, at some time, have to be established. If arterial cannulation is thought necessary, an artery like the dorsalis pedis may be chosen.

Central venous pressure
A central venous pressure (CVP) line is often considered desirable during major surgery but during renal transplant it must be regarded as mandatory since the CVP is of especial importance in that operation. If inserted centrally, the dangers of a pneumothorax must be kept in mind.

Pulmonary artery catheterisation
In general this is of use in the critically ill, in some patients presented for graft nephrectomy, for example. It also gives a better indication of optimum fluid load during renal transplant than does the CVP (see below).

Electrolyte estimations, urinary volume
If the pre-operative K^+ is high it will be necessary to monitor it during surgery. It is especially important to monitor both glucose and K^+ in anephric diabetic patients since glucose induced hyperkalaemia may occur (89). Urine volume is a crucial measurement, but urinary osmolality during surgery is generally low and its measurement may not give much useful information.

Intra-operative fluid therapy

Prophylactic administration of fluids to patients with chronic renal failure before major surgery, has already been mentioned. During surgery urine output should be kept up if at all possible. It may sometimes be wiser to risk pulmonary congestion than further renal failure, since the former is more easily treated than the latter. Hartmann's solution is usually suitable for infusion if the plasma K^+ is not elevated, for though it does contain potassium, the amount in it is low. Saline will, in practice, be very suitable, and if the plasma Na^+ is high, the use of dextrose should be considered.

The administration of adequate fluid is of especial importance in surgery for renal transplantation. There is evidence of a correlation between immediate graft function and the state of the circulation as evidenced by the pulmonary end-capillary wedge pressure and, to a lesser extent, with the CVP (90). Because immediate graft function seems to protect against the subsequent development of acute tubular necrosis, this is a matter of importance. Many would suggest that the CVP should be high when the graft is inserted. This may mean considerable volumes of fluid being administered if the patient has been recently and rigorously dialysed. The possibility of pulmonary congestion, or even of frank pulmonary oedema, must, however, always be kept in mind.

During renal transplant mannitol (e.g. 0.5 to 1.0 g/kg) is frequently given rapidly after the graft has been inserted in an attempt to stimulate urine production. It may sometimes be indicated in other patients in renal failure who are having major surgery, and who show severe oliguria or anuria, with adequate fluid loading. Repeated doses have to be avoided if renal function does not improve lest pulmonary oedema ensue.

Blood loss should be replaced with fresh whole blood or with packed red cells. Because of the low haemoglobin in these patients blood replacement should be commenced at an earlier stage than would be the case in a patient with normal renal function. Colloid infusions, with the exception of albumen when specifically indicated, are best avoided.

Intra-operative changes in pulse rate and blood pressure

Bradycardia, often of considerable degree, is not infrequently seen in these patients and is especially likely to occur in patients treated with beta-blocking drugs. It responds to atropine.

Tachycardia is less frequent. Should it occur in the absence of hypovolaemia it may well be due to the fact that anaesthesia is too light. However, not infrequently there is no immediately obvious cause, and in that situation, sepsis should be suspected.

Hypotension may be accompanied by bradycardia, in which case it will frequently respond to atropine. If this is not the case hypovolaemia, sepsis or cardiac failure should be considered and appropriate treatment instigated. The use of peripheral vasoconstrictors is generally contra-indicated since the renal vasculature will share in the vasoconstriction.

Hypertension may be difficult to control and may be accompanied by electromyographic signs of ischaemia. If too light anaesthesia is not the cause, treatment with such drugs as hydralazine and diazoxide should be considered.

Dopamine

Dopamine in low dosage has been known for some time to lower renal vascular resistance. Low dose dopamine has certainly been of use in oliguric states in which it may cause an increase in urine flow. Its routine use, however, remains controversial.

Post-operative care

As it has been suggested that intra-operative fluid therapy should be generous, there is a need to be cautious in the immediate post-operative period and skilled nursing is required to make sure that an overdose of fluid is not given accidentally. Frequent plasma electrolyte measurements are required. Skilled nursing and medical attention is required too, in respect of the use of the analgesic agents. Here small doses administered intravenously may be safer and more effective than larger doses given intramuscularly. The need for caution has already been stressed.

Oxygen therapy should be continued for some 4 to 6 h into the post-operative period. The need for continued pulmonary ventilation due to persistent curarisation should, with the new muscle relaxants, be a feature of the past.

REFERENCES

1. Bastron RD, Perkins FM, Kaloyanides GI: In vitro inhibition of p-aminohippurate transport by halogenated anesthetics. *J Pharmacol Exp Ther* 200: 75, 1977
2. Jacobsen E, Christiansen AH, Lunding M: The role of the anaesthetist in the management of acute renal failure. *Br J Anaesth* 40: 442, 1968
3. Mazze RI, Schwartz FD, Slocum HC, Barry MG: Renal function during anesthesia and surgery; the effects of halothane anesthesia. *Anesthesiology* 24: 279, 1963
4. Deutsch S, Goldberg M, Stephen GW, Wu WH: Effects of halothane anesthesia on renal function in normal man. *Anesthesiology* 27: 793, 1966
5. Deutsch S, Pierce EC Jr, Vandam LD: Cyclopropane effects on renal function in normal man. *Anesthesiology* 28: 547, 1967
6. Deutsch S, Bastron RD, Pierce EC Jr, Vandam LD: The effect of anaesthesia with thiopentone, nitrous oxide, narcotics and neuromuscular blocking drugs on renal function in normal man. *Br J Anaesth* 41: 807, 1969
7. Mazze RI, Cousins MJ, Barr GA: Renal effects and metabolism of isoflurane in man. *Anesthesiology* 40: 536, 1974
8. Cousins MJ, Greenstein LR, Hitt BA, Mazze RI: Metabolism and renal effects of enflurane in man. *Anesthesiology* 44: 44, 1976
9. Vatner SF, Smith NT: Effects of halothane on left ventricular function and distribution of regional blood flow in dogs and primates. *Circ Res* 34: 155, 1974
10. Bastron RD, Pyne JL, Inagaki M: Halothane induced renal vasodilation. *Anesthesiology* 50: 125, 1979
11. Bastron RD, Perkins RM, Pyne JL: Autoregulation of renal blood flow during halothane anesthesia. *Anesthesiology* 46: 142, 1977
12. Miller RL, Forsyth RR, Melmon KL: Morphine induced redistribution of cardiac output in the unanesthetized monkey. *Pharmacology* 7: 138, 1972
13. Priano LL, Vatner SF: Morphine effects on cardiac output and regional blood flow distribution in conscious dogs. *Anesthesiology* 55: 236, 1981
14. Don HF, Dieppa RA, Taylor P: Narcotic analgesics in anuric patients. *Anesthesiology* 42: 745, 1975
15. Gorman HM, Craythorne NWB: The effects of a new neurolept-analgesic agent (Innovar) on renal function in man. *Acta Anaesth Scand* Suppl 24: 111, 1966
16. Miles BE, de Wardener HE, Churchill-Davidson HC, Wylie WD: The effect of the renal circulation of pentamethonium bromide during anaesthesia. *Clin Sci* 11: 73, 1952
17. Wang HH, Lui LMP, Katz RL: A comparison of the cardiovascular effects of sodium nitroprusside and trimethaphan. *Anesthesiology* 46: 40, 1977
18. Engelman RM, Guy HH, Smith SJ, Boyd AD, Narbay RD, Turndorf H: The effect of hypotensive anesthesia on renal haemodynamics. *J Surg Res* 18: 293, 1975
19. Crandell WB, Pappas SG, Macdonald A: Nephrotoxicity associated with methoxyflurane anesthesia. *Anesthesiology* 27: 591, 1966
20. Panner BJ, Freeman RB, Rath-Mayo IA: Toxicity following methoxyflurane anesthesia. Clinical and pathological observations in two fatal cases. *JAMA* 214: 86, 1970
21. Hollenberg NK, McDonald FD, Cotran R: Irreversible acute oliguric renal failure; a complication of methoxyflurane anesthesia. *N Eng J Med* 286: 877, 1972
22. Frascino JA, Venamee P, Rosen PP: Renal oxalosis and azotaemia after methoxyflurane anesthesia. *N Engl J Med* 283: 676, 1970

23. Mazze RI, Cousins MJ: Methoxyflurane nephrotoxicity – a study of dose-response in man. *JAMA* 225: 1611, 1973

24. Barr GA, Mazze RI, Cousins MJ, Kose KJ: An animal model for combined methoxyflurane and gentamicin nephrotoxicity. *Br J Anaesth* 45: 306, 1973

25. Kuzucu EY: Methoxyflurane, tetracycline, and renal failure. *JAMA* 211: 1162, 1970

26. Cousins MJ, Mazze RI: Anaesthesia, surgery and renal function, immediate and delayed effects. *Anaesth Intensive Care* 1: 355, 1973

27. Harnett MN, Lane W, Bennett WM: Non-oliguric renal failure and enflurane. *Ann Intern Med* 81: 560, 1974

28. Lockning R, Mazze RI: Possible nephrotoxicity from enflurane in patient with severe renal disease. *Anesthesiology* 40: 203, 1974

29. Eichorn JH, Hedley-Whyte J, Steinman TI, Kaufmann JM, Laasberg LH: Renal failure following enflurane anesthesia. *Anesthesiology* 45: 557, 1976

30. Mazze RI, Cousins MJ, Barr GA: Renal effects and metabolism of isoflurane in man. *Anesthesiology* 40: 536, 1974

31. Mazze RI, Sievenpiper TS, Stevenson J: Renal effects of enflurane and halothane in patients with abnormal renal function. *Anesthesiology* 60: 161, 1984

32. Priebe HJ, Hedley-White J: Respiratory support and renal function in *International Anesthesiology Clinics*, 22, No 1, edited by Priebe HJ, Boston, Little Brown and Co, 1984

33. Moore ES, Galvez MB, Paton JB, Fisher DE, Behrman RE: Effects of positive pressure ventilation on intrarenal blood flow in infant primates. *Prediatr Res* 8: 792, 1974

34. Hemmer M, Viquerat CE, Suter PM, Vallotton MB: Urinary antidiuretic hormone excretion during mechanical ventilation and weaning in man. *Anesthesiology* 52: 395, 1980

35. Gett PM, Jones ES, Shepherd GF: Pulmonary oedema associated with sodium retention during ventilator treatment. *Br J Anaesth* 43: 460, 1971

36. Tarak TK, Chaudhury RR: The mechanism of positive pressure respiration induced antidiuresis in rats. *Clin Sci* 28: 407, 1965

37. Sladen A, Laver MD, Pontoppidan H: Pulmonary complications and water retention in prolonged mechanical ventilation. *N Engl J Med* 279: 448, 1968

38. Khambatta HJ, Baratz RA: IPPB, plasma ADH, and urine flow in conscious man. *J Appl Physiol* 33: 362, 1972

39. Verma YS, Gupta KK, Mehta S, Chaudhury RR: A study of plasma antidiuretic activity before and during intermittent positive pressure respiration in human subjects. *Indian J Med Res* 56: 73, 1968

40. Baratz RA, Philbin DM, Patterson RW: Urinary output and plasma levels of antidiuretic hormone during intermittent positive-pressure breathing in the dog. *Anesthesiology* 32: 17, 1970

41. Fewell JE, Bond GC: Renal denervation eliminates the renal response to continuous positive pressure ventilation. *Proc Soc Exp Biol Med* 161: 574, 1979

42. Bromage PR, Gertel M: Brachial plexus anesthesia in chronic renal failure. *Anesthesiology* 36: 488, 1972

43. Orko R, Pitkanen M, Rosenberg PH: Subarachnoid anaesthesia with 0.75% bupivacaine in patients with chronic renal failure. *Br J Anaesth* 58: 605, 1986

44. Rooke NT, Milne B: Acute pulmonary edema after regional anesthesia with lidocaine and epinephrine in a patient with chronic renal failure. *Anesth Analg* 63: 636, 1984

45. Vandam LD, Harrison JH, Murray JE, Merrill JP: Anesthesia aspects of renal homotransplantation in man. *Anesthesiology* 23: 783, 1962

46. Wyant GM: The anaesthetist looks at tissue transplantation: three years' experience with kidney transplants. *Can Anaesth Soc J* 14: 255, 1967

47. Merin RG, Linke CL: Regional anaesthesia for renal transplantation. *Reg Anaesth* 4: 13, 1979

48. Maddern PJ: Anaesthesia for the patient with impaired renal function. *Anaesth Intensive Care* 11: 321, 1983

49. Halperin BD, Feeley TV: The effects of anesthesia and surgery on renal function in *International Anesthesiology Clinics*, 22, no 1, edited by Prieb HF, Boston, Little Brown and Co, 1984

50. Bromage PR: Physiology and pharmacology of local analgesia. *Anesthesiology* 28: 592, 1967

51. Gould DB, Aldrete JA: Bupivacaine cardiotoxicity in a patient with renal failure. *Acta Anaesthesiol Scand* 27: 18, 1983

52. Weir PHC, Chung FF: Anaesthesia for patients with chronic renal disease. *Canad Anaesth Soc J* 31: 468, 1984

53. Lynn RB, Sancetta SM, Simeone FA, Scott RW: Observations on the circulation in high spinal anesthesia. *Surgery* 32: 195, 1951

54. Kennedy WF, Sawyer TK, Gerbershagen HV, Cutler RE, Allen GD, Bonica JJ: Systemic cardiovascular and renal hemodynamic alterations during peridural anesthesia in normal man. *Anesthesiology* 31: 414, 1969

55. Kennedy WF, Sawyer TK, Gerbershagen HV, Everett GB, Cutler RE, Allen GD, Bonica JJ: Simultaneous systemic cardiovascular and renal hemodynamic measurements during high spinal anesthesia in normal man. *Acta Anaesth Scand, Suppl* 37: 163, 1970

56. Sivarajan M, Avory DW, Lindblook LE, Schwettmann RS: Systemic and regional blood flow changes during spinal anesthesia in the Rhesus monkey. *Anesthesiology* 43: 78, 1975

57. Sivarajan M, Avory DW, Lindblook LE: Systemic and regional blood flow during epidural analgesia without epinephrine in the Rhesus monkey. *Anesthesiology* 45: 300, 1976

58. Moran WH, Miltenberger FW, Shuayb WA, Zimmermann B: The relationship of antidiuretic hormone to surgical stress. *Surgery* 56: 99, 1964

59. Zideman DA, Bevan DR, Dudley HAF: Osmolar output in the perioperative period. *Anaesthesia* 33: 788, 1978

60. Bevan DR: *Renal Function in Anaesthesia and Surgery*. London, Academic Press, New York, Grune and Stratton, 1979

61. Truniger B, Rosen SM, Grandchamp A, Strebel H, Kriek HR: Redistribution of renal blood flow in haemorrhagic hypotension. Role of renal nerves and catecholamines. *Eur J Clin Invest* 1: 277, 1971

62. Johnson MD, Park CS, Malvin RL: Antidiuretic hormone and the distribution of renal cortical flow. *Am J Physiol* 232: F111, 1977

63. Hutchin P, Terzi RG, Holandsworth LC: Renal response to intraoperative fluid administration. *Surg Gynec Obstet* 129: 794, 1969

64. Shire T, Williams J, Brown F: Acute changes in extracellular fluids associated with major surgical procedures. *Ann Surg* 154: 803, 1961

65. Roth E, Lax LC, Maloney JV: Ringer's lactate solution and extracellular fluid volume in the surgical patient: a critical analysis. *Ann Surg* 169: 149, 1969

66. Robertson D, Michelakis AM: Effect of anesthesia and surgery on plasma renin activity in man. *J Clin Endocrinol Metab* 34: 831, 1972

67. Bailey DR, Miller ED, Kaplan JA, Rogers PW: The renin-angiotensin-aldosterone system during cardiac surgery with morphine-nitrous oxide anesthesia. *Anesthesiology* 42: 538, 1975

68. Inturrisi CE: Disposition of narcotics in patients with renal disease. *Am J Med* 62: 528, 1977

69. Olsen GD, Bennett WM, Porter GA: Morphine and phenytoin binding to plasma proteins in renal and hepatic failure. *Clin Pharmacol Ther* 17: 677, 1977

70. Bennett WM: Prescribing drugs for patients with reduced renal function. in *Drugs and Renal Disease,* edited by Bennett WM, 2ⁿᵈ edition, New York, Edinburg, London, Melbourne Churchil Livingstone, 1986, p 26

71. Dundee JW, Richards RK: Effect of azotemia upon the action of intravenous barbiturate anesthesia. *Anesthesiology* 15: 333, 1954

72. Gnoneim MM, Pandya H: Plasma protein binding of thiopental in patients with impaired renal or hepatic function. *Anesthesiology* 42: 545, 1975

73. Freeman RB, Sheff MF, Maher JF, Schreiner GE: The blood-cerebrospinal fluid barrier in uremia. *Ann Intern Med* 56: 233, 1962

74. Smith CL, Hunter JM, Jones RS: Vecuronium infusions in patients with renal failure in an ITU. *Anaesthesia* 42: 387, 1987

75. Hunter JM, Jones RS, Utting JE: Use of atracurium in patients with no renal function. *Br J Anaesth* 54: 1251, 1982

76. Hunter JM, Jones RS, Utting JE: Comparison of vecuronium, atracurium and tubocurarine in normal patients and in patients with no renal function. *Br J Anaesth* 56: 941, 1984

77. Koide M, Waud BE: Serum potassium concentrations after succinylcholine in patients with renal failure. *Anesthesiology* 36: 142, 1972

78. Miller RD, Way WL, Hamilton WK, Layzer RB: Succinylcholine-induced hyperkalemia in patients with renal failure. *Anesthesiology* 36: 138, 1972

79. Cronnelly R, Stanski DR, Miller DR, Sheiner LB, Sohn YJ: Renal function and the pharmacokinetics of neostigmine in anesthetized man. *Anesthesiology* 51: 222, 1979

80. Bishop MJ, Hornbein TF: Prolonged effect of succinylcholine after neostigmine and pyridostigmine administration in patients with renal failure. *Anesthesiology* 58: 284, 1979

81. Tasker PRW, MacGregor GA, DeWardener HE: Prophylactic use of intravenous saline in patients with chronic renal failure undergoing major surgery. *Lancet* 2: 911, 1974

82. Morris PJ: Blood transfusions and transplantation. *Transplantation* 26: 276, 1978

83. Van Rood J: Blood transfusion and transplantation. *Transplantation* 26: 275, 1978

84. Opelz G, Terasaki PI: Dominant effects of transfusions on kidney graft survival. *Transplantation* 29: 153, 1980

85. Breimer DD, Jochemsen R, Von Albert HH: Pharmacokinetics of benzodiazepines. *Drug Research* 30: 875, 1980

86. Becker ID, Paulson BA, Miller RD, Severinghaus JW, Eger EI: Biphasic respiratory depression after fentanyl-droperidol or fentanyl alone used to supplement nitrous oxide anesthesia. *Anesthesiology* 44: 291, 1976

87. Wiggum DC, Cork RC, Weldon ST, Gandolfi AJ, Perry DS: Postoperative respiratory depression and elevated sufentanil levels in a patient with chronic renal failure. *Anesthesiology* 63: 708, 1985

88. Morgan M, Lumley J: Anaesthetic considerations in chronic renal failure. *Anaesth Intensive Care* 3: 218, 1975

89. Charters P: Renal transplantation in diabetes mellitus. *Anesthesiology* 63: 708, 1985

90. Carlier M, Squifflet JP, Pirson Y, Gribomont B, Alexandre GPJ: Maximal hydration during anaesthesia increases pulmonary artery pressure and improves function of human renal transplant. *Transplantation* 34: 201, 1982

91. Goldberg LJ: Dopamine – clinical uses of an endogenous catecholamine. *N Engl J Med* 291: 707, 1974

NUTRITION IN DIALYSIS PATIENTS

THEODORE I. STEINMAN and WILLIAM E. MITCH

INTRODUCTION

Contemporary concerns about nutrition in renal failure derive from the development of artificial organs. When dialysis was used initially, nutritional management was limited to a daily intravenous infusion of 100 g glucose. This amount maximally suppressed protein catabolism in fasting normal subjects. As solute and fluid loads can be more effectively removed with the newly developed, highly porous filtration membranes (e.g. solutes with mass of 10,000 daltons), there is increasing concern for maintaining adequate nutrition since protein and energy malnutrition and wasting have been noted in every nutritional survey of maintenance dialysis patients, affecting at least one-third of this population. The nutritional state generally deteriorates with time and home dialysis patients seem to do better than in-center patients (1). Fortunately, the use of short time, high flux hemodialysis does not appear to cause any additional adverse nutritional consequences over a 6-month period (2).

Although the mechanism(s) for wasting are complex, an important factor is the adequacy of the diet. The relationship between protein intake and morbidity and mortality in 98 non-diabetic patients undergoing maintenance hemodialysis showed that patients with the lowest net protein catabolic rate (0.63 g/kg/day) had the lowest protein intake, the greatest frequency of hospitalization and number of days in the hospital, and the highest mortality rate (3). The protein intake tended to correlate inversely with both the hospitalization rate and the mortality rate, suggesting that a low nutrient intake contributes to a poor prognosis in maintenance dialysis patients.

NUTRITIONAL ASSESSMENT

Nutritional status can be assessed in five ways: by estimates of protein and energy intake, biochemical measurements, anthropometry, electromagnetic estimates of body water and measurements of immune status (4: Table 1). Indices which have been used include: body weight, calorie and protein intakes, serum concentrations of albumin, retinol binding protein, pre-albumin (PA), transferrin, creatinine and triglycerides, hemoglobin concentration, total lymphocyte count, delayed hypersensitivity, muscle mass measured by forearm x-ray, measurement of muscle strength by grip, anthropometry, and body fat measured by bioelectrical impedance, double-labelled water ($D_2^{18}O$), computerized axial tomography (CT), magnetic resonance imaging (MRI), infrared interactance and ultrasonography.

Diet History

A dietary history is used to identify those patients with an inadequate intake. Poor dietary intake can develop for a variety of reasons, including anorexia, nausea and vomiting, food aversions, changes in smell and taste, socioeconomic problems, misunderstanding dietary instructions, and food fadism beginning before or with development of renal failure. Assessment of possible problems with chewing or swallowing, dysphagia, abdominal pain, early satiety, postprandial fullness, diarrhea or constipation should be made routinely in dialysis patients.

Anthropometry

Height and weight measurements are important indicators of somatic status. Weight can be expressed as absolute weight, weight for height, or most commonly, relative body weight (observed body weight/ideal body weight for patient's height and body frame). If a patient has lost 10% of his or her body weight in the previous 6 months, or weighs less than 90% of his or her ideal body weight, nutritional investigation and support are indicated.

The endogenous energy supply includes the two major organic fuels, triglycerides and protein; the small amount of glycogen is a neglible component of energy supply (5). Protein is included in the fat-free body mass and constitutes about 1/5 of non-fat weight. Nearly all of the remainder of the fat-free body mass is accounted for by water. Total body energy supply is, therefore, a function of fat and lean tissue mass and can be described by the following equation:

$$\text{Total body kcal} = [9.3 \times \text{total body fat (g)}] + [1.02 \times \text{fat-free body mass (g)}]$$

Anthropometry permits the body to be partitioned into fat and fat-free components (Table 2). The amount of and the rate of change in whole body energy supply and protein mass can be quantified and used with other indices of energy and protein metabolism to assess nutritional status (5, 6). Fat-free mass can be estimated from body weight and the sum of four skinfold thicknesses (7) (biceps, triceps, subscapular

and suprailiac sites); and total body fat is calculated from this estimate using appropriate equations for age and gender (8). For example, skin over the posterior aspect of the non-dominant arm, midway between the shoulder and elbow, is grasped and gently pulled away from the underlying muscle. Calipers are applied and the measurement can be compared to a standard set of values to determine whether fat depletion or obesity is present (Table 3) (9).

Percent body fat

Percent body fat (10) can be calculated from equation [1] which is a derived regression equation for the prediction of body density from the log of the sum of the triceps, biceps, and subscapular skinfold thicknesses in mm (X) and from equation [2] which relates body density to the proportion of fat in the body.

$$\text{Density} = 1.1689 - 0.0793 \, (X) \quad \text{Males age 17–72} \quad [1]$$
$$\text{or} = C - M \, (\log \text{skinfold thicknesses})$$

$$\% \, \text{Fat} = \left(\frac{4.95}{\text{Density}} - 4.5 \right) (100). \quad [2]$$

The coefficients (C and M) for the regression equation for body density are shown in Table 4 by age and sex groups.

Body frame size can be determined by elbow breadth (Table 5) using calipers to identify small-, medium- and large-framed males and females.

A widely accepted and clinically practical anthropometric method is arm muscle area (AMA). AMA is determined by two measurements: 1) triceps skinfold in mm (TSF) and 2) mid arm circumference in mm (MAC). The following formula is used to calculate arm muscle area (11):

$$\text{AMA} = \left(\frac{\text{MAC} - \pi \times \text{TSF}}{4\pi} \right)_2$$

Bone-free arm muscle area (also called available AMA) is calculated from the following formulae:

$$\text{Bone-free AMA (cm}^2) \text{ in males} = \text{AMA} - 19.0 \, \text{cm}^2.$$
$$\text{Bone-free AMA (cm}^2) \text{ in females} = \text{AMA} - 15.5 \, \text{cm}^2.$$

Table 1. Parameters to assess nutrition.

1. Nutrition intake
   a. Diet history
   b. Diet recall
   c. Urea nitrogen appearance (UNA)
2. Biochemistry
   a. Serum proteins
      1) Albumin
      2) Pre-albumin (PA)
      3) Retinol binding protein
      4) Transferrin
   b. Other serum chemistries
      1) Creatinine
      2) Triglycerides
      3) Cholesterol
      4) HDL cholesterol
3. Anthropometry (see Table 2)
4. Measurements of immune status
   a. Hemoglobin
   b. Total lymphocyte count
   c. Immunoglobulins (IgG)
   d. Acute phase proteins
   e. Delayed hypersensitivity

Table 2. Anthropometry.

1. Height and weight
2. Skin fold thickness
   a. Biceps
   b. Triceps
   c. Subscapular
   d. Suprailiac
3. Mid-arm muscle circumference
4. Arm muscle area (AMA)
5. Muscle strength measured by grip
6. Body fat/muscle mass measured by:
   a. Bioelectrical impedance
   b. Forearm X-ray
   c. Double-labelled water ($D_2^{18}O$)
   d. ^{40}K

Table 3. Percentiles for triceps skinfold for whites of the United States health and nutrition examination survey I of 1971 to 1974.

Age group	Triceps skinfold (mm) percentiles															
	n	5	10	25	50	75	90	95	n	5	10	25	50	75	90	95
	Males								Females							
1–1.9	228	6	7	8	10	12	14	16	204	6	7	8	10	12	14	16
2–2.9	223	6	7	8	10	12	14	15	208	6	8	9	10	12	15	16
3–3.9	220	6	7	8	10	11	14	15	208	7	8	9	11	12	14	15
4–4.9	230	6	6	8	9	11	12	14	208	7	8	8	10	12	14	16
5–5.9	214	6	6	8	9	11	14	15	219	6	7	8	10	12	15	18
6–6.9	117	5	6	7	8	10	13	16	118	6	6	8	10	12	14	16
7–7.9	122	5	6	7	9	12	15	17	126	6	7	9	11	13	16	18
8–8.9	117	5	6	7	8	10	13	16	118	6	8	9	12	15	18	24
9–9.9	121	6	6	7	10	13	17	18	125	8	8	10	13	16	20	22
10–10.9	146	6	6	8	10	14	18	21	152	7	8	10	12	17	23	27
11–11.9	122	6	6	8	11	16	20	24	117	7	8	10	13	18	24	28
12–12.9	153	6	6	8	11	14	22	28	129	8	9	11	14	18	23	27
13–13.9	134	5	5	7	10	14	22	26	151	8	8	12	15	21	26	30
14–14.9	131	4	5	7	9	14	21	24	141	9	10	13	16	21	26	28
15–15.9	128	4	5	6	8	11	18	24	117	8	10	12	17	21	25	32
16–16.9	131	4	5	6	8	12	16	22	142	10	12	15	18	22	26	31
17–17.9	133	5	5	6	8	12	16	19	114	10	12	13	19	24	30	37
18–18.9	91	4	5	6	9	13	20	24	109	10	12	15	18	22	26	30
19–24.9	531	4	5	7	10	15	20	22	1060	10	11	14	18	24	30	34
25–34.9	971	5	6	8	12	16	20	24	1987	10	12	16	21	27	34	37
36–44.9	806	5	6	8	12	16	20	23	1614	12	14	18	23	29	35	38
45–54.9	898	6	6	8	12	15	20	25	1047	12	16	20	25	30	26	40
55–64.9	734	5	6	8	11	14	19	22	809	12	16	20	25	31	36	38
65–74.9	1503	4	6	8	11	15	19	22	1670	12	14	18	24	29	34	36

From Frisancho (12).

Although mid-arm circumference is widely used as an index of lean body mass and correlates with total body nitrogen, it is not a good index of tissue repletion (12).

Bioelectrical impedance estimates lean body mass based on the principle that lean tissue, comprised primarily of electrolyte-containing water, readily conducts an applied electrical current; fat acts as an insulator and conducts little current (13). Therefore, electrical conductivity of fat-free tissue mass is far greater than that of fat. In the living organism intra- and extracellular fluids behave as electrical conductors and cell membranes act as electrical condensers. At low frequencies (approximately 1 kHz) the current passes mainly through the extracellular fluid while at higher frequencies (500 to 800 kHz) it passes through the extra- and intracellular fluids. In practice, an imperceptible current is passed between the foot and hand of the patient and an absolute value for impedance is calculated based on the resistance to electrical current. As fluid increases with a given height, impedance decreases. Bioelectrical impedance has been shown to be a reproducible and accurate assessment of total body water in normal subjects (14). Its use in dialysis patients with abnormalities in body fluid spaces has not been validated.

Measurement of total body potassium from ^{40}K enrichment also estimates fat-free body tissue (15). The rationale is that potassium and nitrogen distribute uniformly in fat-free tissue and that total body potassium can be reliably estimated by counting gamma rays from ^{40}K, a naturally occurring potassium radioisotope. The standard error of the estimate of total body potassium is approximately 3% (16, 17).

Table 4. Linear regression equations for the estimation of body density × 10^3 (kg/m^3) from the logarithm of the skinfold thickness (biceps + triceps + subscapular).

Age (years)	Males		Females	
	C	M	C	M
17–19	1.1643	0.0727	1.1509	0.0715
20–29	1.1593	0.0694	1.1605	0.0777
30–39	1.1213	0.0487	1.1385	0.0654
40–49	1.1530	0.0730	1.1303	0.0635
50+	1.1569	0.0780	1.1372	0.0710
Overall 17–72	1.1689	0.0793	1.1543	0.0756

From Durnin and Womersley (7).

Electromagnetic and sound waves

Computerized axial tomography (CT) can define the proportions of muscle, fat and bone in an upper or lower extremity because the cross-sectional area of fat, muscle, bone, or visceral organ can be established from the specifically designed software programs (Table 6). This method yields a good estimate of changes in lean body mass, but there are two important limitations (18–20). The first is the radiation exposure, which limits studies in children and pregnant women. The second is the relatively high cost of the study.

Magnetic resonance imaging (MRI) has also been used to define body fat and total body water in humans; the technique does not expose patients to ionizing radiation (21). When the patient is placed in an electromagnetic field, changes in the field proportional to the electrolyte content of the body are measured to yield an estimate of lean tissue (22). Although MRI is a safe method for evaluating human tissue mass and composition, its use is limited because of its high cost.

Infrared interactance has been used for the past 2 decades to determine the fat and moisture content of meat. Its use is based on the finding that when a molecule is subjected to infrared radiation, wavelengths corresponding to the natural vibrational frequencies of that molecule are absorbed; the remainder are reflected. The relation of the absorptive and reflective properties of the tissue depends upon its chemical composition. Available instruments consist of a fiber-optic probe that conducts the infrared beam from a generator and collects the resultant radiation; the ratio of energy reflected from the subject to that reflected by a standard reference is the interactance and the shape of the interactance spectrum permits a quantitative analysis of tissue water and fat. The percent body fat at each skinfold site determined with this method corresponds closely to standard anthropometry measurements (20). Total body fat can be estimated from the average of the fat content at five standard skinfold sites. The principal advantages of infrared interactance are safety, portability, and relatively low cost.

Ultrasonography of regional subcutaneous fat and skeletal muscle mass is based on the finding that the velocity of a sound wave in tissue depends upon the tissue density, often referred to as its acoustic impedance (20). When a transmitted sound wave reaches an interface between two media (i.e. tissues) of differing acoustic impedance, the wave changes its reflection and refraction. Differences in the sound wave configuration can be used to quantify fat-free body mass. While ultrasonography is far less expensive than either CT or MRI, it is not as sensitive or accurate as either technique.

Biochemical measurements

Plasma or serum protein concentrations will change with protein/calorie nutrition. This occurs because in humans nutrition is probably the most important factor regulating albumin synthesis (23, 24). However, by the time serum albumin falls to below normal, malnutrition can be advanced; serum transferrin will decrease earlier with undernutrition and is a better indicator. Transferrin concentration can either be measured directly or estimated from total iron binding capacity (TIBC) by the equation:

$$\text{transferrin} = 0.8 \times \text{TIBC} - 43.$$

Serum pre-albumin has been touted as the best indicator of changes in nutrition because it is the only parameter linked to body weight, arm muscle circumference, triceps skinfold thickness and serum albumin and creatinine concentrations (25). Pre-albumin levels, like acute-phase response proteins (fibrinogen, alpha-1-acid glycoprotein, alpha-1-antitrypsin and haptoglobin), are decreased in malnutrition (26).

Table 5. Frame size from height and elbow breadth.

Height (cm)	Elbow breadth		
	Small frame (mm)	Medium frame (mm)	Large frame (mm)
Men			
150–154	<62	62–71	>71
155–158	<64	64–72	>72
159–168	<67	67–74	>74
169–178	<69	69–76	>76
179–188	<71	71–78	>78
189–190	<74	74–81	>81
191–194	<76	76–82	>82
195–199	<78	78–83	>83
200–204	<79	79–85	>85
205–209	<80	80–88	>89
Women			
145–148	<56	56–64	>64
149–158	<58	58–65	>65
159–168	<59	59–66	>66
169–178	<61	61–68	>68
179–180	<62	62–69	>69
181–184	<63	63–70	>70
185–189	<64	64–71	>71
190–194	<65	65–72	>72
195–199	<66	66–73	>73

Height without shoes.
The medium frame elbow breadths for men <155 cm or ≥191 cm and women ≥181 cm were determined by extrapolation on a semilog graph.

Table 6. Electromagnetic and sound waves in nutritional assessment.

Computerized axial tomography
Magnetic resonance imaging
Infrared interactance
Ultrasonography

Immunologic function

Immunocompetence has been used as a functional index of nutritional status. Plasma immunoglobulin levels, antibody production, phagocytic function, inflammatory responses, complement function, secretory and mucosal immunity, and other defense mechanisms all may be impaired with inadequate nutrition. One of the most simple and reliable immunological indicators of nutritional status is the blood lymphocyte count. The percentage of T-cells in the peripheral blood is reduced in malnutrition, but the percentage of B-lymphocytes in malnutrition is normal or increased (26). The reduction in T cells parallels the severity of weight loss, impairment of delayed hypersensitivity, and the decrease in phytohemaglutinin-stimulated DNA synthesis by lymphocytes. The abnormalities reverse quickly and completely with nutritional improvement. Despite the fall in T lymphocytes, plasma IgG levels decrease slowly and progressively with malnutrition, and become subnormal only after about 5 weeks of undernutrition. In contrast, plasma levels of the third complement component decrease further and more rapidly (26).

Malnutrition depresses the delayed hypersensitivity response and this may be a major cause of the higher incidence of infections in malnourished patients. Patients who exhibit anergy have more infections and lower serum albumin values when compared to those who respond to skin testing (27). There can be reversal of skin test anergy when protein and calories are orally supplemented in the anergic patient undergoing maintenance hemodialysis (28).

Nutrition profile

To assess a patient's nutritional status, an estimate of the adequacy of the diet is critical. Urea nitrogen appearance can be used to calculate the protein and amino acid intake (29) and dietary interviews supplemented with dietary diaries can be used to estimate calorie, vitamin and mineral intake (30). A flow sheet including the following nutritional indices (Table 7) should be maintained: intake (oral, intravenous and dialysate), urea nitrogen appearance, height, body weight, relative body weight, biceps, triceps and subscapular skin fold thicknesses, percent body fat, mid arm muscle circumference, serum levels of total proteins, serum albumin, transferrin, pre-albumin, pre-dialysis serum calcium, phosphorus, potassium, creatinine and urea concentrations hematocrit, total blood lymphocyte count, and skin tests for delayed hypersensitivity (31).

ACUTE RENAL FAILURE

Mechanisms of protein degradation

Malnutrition in acute renal failure (ARF) is probably the most important reason why mortality in ARF has remained high in spite of dialysis (32). Malnutrition occurs because of the catabolic influence of ARF, the disease causing ARF,

changes in the normal hormonal milieu, physical inactivity, and infection (32, 33). Protein degradation in muscle increases in ARF, being more severe when complicated by sepsis, trauma or surgery. Serum levels of epinephrine, glucagon, and cortisone are generally high, and there may be resistance to the action of insulin (34–36) which promotes the intracellular degradation of protein. Protein loss and proteolysis cause increased formation of urea and other waste products, thereby aggravating the symptoms of uremia (37, 38). The enhanced flux of amino acids from muscle is probably a part of the protective response to stimulate the gluconeogenic pathway, but in hospital patients there is no apparent benefit from this flux. Stimulation of gluconeogenesis is consistent with the rise in plasma glucagon occurring in hypercatabolic acutely ill patients. Although pharmacologic levels of glucagon are needed to change protein degradation in muscle (32), this hormone may stimulate hepatic proteolysis since large doses of amino acids appear to suppress glucagon- induced hepatic autophagy (39).

In ARF blood glucose rises, and this has been shown in experimental ARF to be due to a post-insulin receptor defect in muscle glucose metabolism (40). In contrast, insulin-mediated uptake of amino acids by muscle is normal in ARF (41, 42). However, insulin-stimulated protein synthesis in

Table 7. Nutritional assessment profile.

1. General appearance
   Thin ——— Well nourished ——— Obese ———
   Edema ——— Other ———

2. Anthropometry
   Height
   Weight
   $$\text{Relative body weight} = \frac{\text{actual weight}}{\text{ideal weight}} \times 100.$$
   Biceps, triceps, subscapular skinfold (mm)
   Mid arm circumference
   Calculated values
       Body fat (%)
       Arm muscle circumference (cm²)

3. Biochemistry (serum)
   Total protein   (g/dl)
   Albumin   (g/dl)
   Tranferrin   (mg/dl)
   Pre-albumin   (g/l)
   Calcium   (mg/dl)
   Phosphorus   (mg/dl)
   Potassium   (mEq/l)
   Creatinine   (mg/dl)
   Urea   (mg/dl)
   Hematocrit, Hemoglobin
   Total lymphocyte count

4. Diet assessment
   Nutrition intake by diet history, recall, observation
       Oral, intravenous, from dialysate
   Urea nitrogen appearance

5. Skin tests for delayed hypersensitivity.

muscle is depressed (43). Thus, stimulation of protein degradation in muscle, plus a decrease in insulin-stimulated protein synthesis, leads to a sharp rise in protein loss (40, 44).

Recent reports note increased proteolytic activity in ultrafiltrates of plasma obtained from hypercatabolic ARF patients (45, 46). It has been suggested that the complement component, C_{5a}, is released during hemodialysis and may activate or release leukocyte proteases, leading to a catabolic state during hemodialysis (47). Although enhanced release of proteases or a reduction in protease inhibitors may play a role in the catabolic response to ARF, it is unlikely that plasma proteases play an important role in the enhanced intracellular proteolysis that leads to malnutrition.

Another possibility is that a circulating factor directly stimulates muscle proteolysis. For example, it was reported that a polypeptide appearing to be interleukin-1 enhances protein degradation in rat muscle (48). It was suggested that the circulating polypeptide stimulates muscle synthesis of prostaglandin E_2 (PGE_2), which then promotes muscle protein degradation. Inhibition of PGE_2 synthesis with indomethacin or the use of lysosomal thiol proteases, blocked the stimulatory effects of leukocyte pyrogens on-muscle protein degradation. In experimental conditions associated with muscle protein catabolism (e.g. burns and metabolic acidosis), there was no relation between muscle PGE_2 production and protein breakdown (49, 50).

Hemodialysis itself may contribute to malnutrition in ARF patients. Increased oxygen consumption occurs during hemodialysis (51), indicating an intradialytic hypermetabolic state. Nitrogen balance becomes sharply negative during dialysis, even when adjusted for changes in the urea pool (52). Metabolic acidosis is another mechanism for protein catabolism in ARF. In conditions associated with increased glucocorticoid production, such as ARF, muscle proteolysis is stimulated and dietary protein utilization is impaired. Also, losses of glucose, amino acids, proteins, and water soluble vitamins during hemodialysis or peritoneal dialysis can contribute to wasting. In catabolic ARF, an energy intake of about 50 kcal/kg/day provided by hypertonic glucose may be necessary to meet energy needs (53). Mortality of critically ill patients with ARF was higher in those with negative caloric balances compared to those with neutral to positive balances (33).

In summary, there is abundant evidence that protein catabolism is stimulated by ARF because of impaired energy utilization, acidosis, hemodialysis and probably circulating activators of proteolysis. Methods used to combat this include increasing calorie intake and correcting acidosis. Since dialysis is associated with negative nitrogen balance and has not improved mortality in ARF, its use should be for fluid overload or treating uremic symptoms. As will be discussed, there may be little benefit from infusing large amounts of amino acids because the rise in serum urea may necessitate dialysis.

Energy expenditure and measurement

In the critically ill patient with ARF, measurement of resting energy expenditure (REE) can help determine the nutritional requirements (54). Direct calorimetry measures energy expenditure in the form of heat generated from all sources, while indirect calorimetry refers to energy expenditure determined from measuring the amount of oxygen consumed and carbon dioxide produced (55). The latter is the more useful for clinical care.

The ratio of V_{CO_2} production to V_{O_2} utilization is the respiratory quotient ($RQ = V_{CO_2}/V_{O_2}$). The ratio is 1.0 when only carbohydrates are being oxidized, 0.80 when only amino acids are oxidized, and 0.707 when only lipids are oxidized.

When the contributions of V_{CO_2} and V_{O_2} from oxidation of amino acids (estimated from nitrogen excretion) are subtracted from the total V_{CO_2} and V_{O_2} values, the resulting ratio of CO_2 production to O_2 utilization from oxidation of fat and carbohydrates is termed the non-protein respiratory quotient (npRQ). Because more oxygen is consumed relative to the CO_2 production during oxidation of amino acids, the npRQ is generally larger than the RQ. Measurements of the npRQ will determine the relative contributions of fat and carbohydrates to overall production of energy or heat.

The REE is calculated as follows (54):

$$REE \ (kcal/min) = 3.827 \, V_{O_2} \ (4\,min) + 1.223 \, V_{CO_2}$$
$$(4\,min) - 1.994 \text{ urinary nitrogen } (N_2) \ (g/min)$$
$$REE \ (kcal/24\,h) = kcal/min \times 1440.$$

The non-protein respiratory quotient is calculated as follows:

$$npRQ = \frac{1.44 \, V_{CO_2} \ (ml/min) - 4.754 \text{ urinary } N_2 \ (g/24\,h)}{1.44 \, V_{O_2} \ (ml/min) - 5.923 \text{ urinary } N_2 \ (g/24\,h)}.$$

Regardless of the method, a ratio of total caloric intake to REE less than 1.0 is an inadequate calorie intake (54) and indicates that caloric intake should be increased. A ratio of caloric intake to REE greater than 1.0, with an npRQ greater than 1.0, indicates net lipogenesis. In these patients the total caloric intake should be reduced to avoid lipogenesis.

An accurate estimation of the fasting rate of oxygen consumption can also be used to predict the state of lean body mass depletion because the loss of body weight and the decline in oxygen consumption rate correlate directly (55).

From a practical, clinical standpoint, it is easy to estimate the REE from the Harris and Benedict (56) equation:

For men:
Heat production/day = 66.5 + (13.7 × weight in kg) + (5.0 × height in cm) − (6.8 × age in years)
For women:
Heat production/day = 65.1 + (9.6 × weight in kg) + (1.8 × height in cm) − (4.7 × age in years)

Activity contributions to energy expenditure can then be estimated to be:

Sedentary – 30% above REE
            (total energy = REE × 1.3)
Light   – 50% above REE
            (total energy = REE × 1.5)
Moderate   – 75% above REE
            (total energy = REE × 1.75)
Intense   – 100% above REE
            (total energy = REE × 2.0).

Nutritional management

The goals of nutritional therapy in ARF are to: 1) provide adequate nutrients to maintain nutritional status or improve it in depleted patients; 2) enhance wound healing and resistance to infection; 3) promote healing of the renal lesion. Optimal nutritional needs in ARF are not well defined (32). The lack of defined therapies is due mainly to the enormous disparity of causes of ARF and illnesses associated with ARF (57).

Suggested guidelines are as follows for patients with mild catabolism (e.g. nephrotoxin-induced ARF) and a urea nitrogen appearance 2 to 5 g above nitrogen intake: treatment with adequate calories (i.e. >35 kcal/kg/day) and the minimum daily protein requirement of 0.6 g protein/kg/day (at least 50% of the protein must be high quality protein). A water-soluble vitamin supplement and sufficient sodium bicarbonate to prevent metabolic acidosis should be given. The goal is to provide adequate nutrition without raising nitrogen intake to a level that will create or increase the need for dialysis to remove waste products. Obviously, sodium and fluid intake will depend on changes in body weight and serum sodium concentration.

For those patients with moderately severe catabolism (e.g. ARF from hypotension) and a urea nitrogen appearance of 8 to 10 g above nitrogen intake, the catabolic stress of the illness or recent surgery usually requires dialysis. In such patients intestinal feeding should be used if at all possible. With intestinal or intravenous feeding, the minimum fluid with maximum calories (i.e. >35 kcal/kg/day) should be given along with a mixture of essential amino acids at 10 to 20 g/day. The goal is to minimize the requirement for dialysis and thereby avoid the catabolic stress of dialysis. As a general rule, the BUN should be kept below 100 mg/dl to avoid complications.

For those patients with severe catabolism (e.g. ARF associated with sepsis, major burns or trauma) and a urea nitrogen appearance >10 g above nitrogen intake, there is not satisfactory therapy and mortality remains at 80 to 90%. In such severely catabolic patients there is often wasting and markedly negative nitrogen balance despite the intravenous administration of 21 to 42 g/day of amino acids (59). In several studies (59–62), total parenteral nutrition (TPN) with either a low-dose or high-dose of essential amino acids alone or a mixture of essential and non-essential amino acids plus glucose did not improve negative nitrogen balance, and there was no difference in survival. Although one prospective, controlled trial showed that recovery from ARF was improved in patients treated with essential amino acids plus

glucose compared to glucose alone, hospital mortality was only slightly and not significantly improved (63). However, other trials of similar regimens have not shown the same improved recovery of renal function (64).

In severely stressed patients, lipids may not be utilized as well as glucose to maintain nitrogen balance (58). During parenteral hyperalimentation, serial monitoring of protein catabolic rates by urea kinetic modeling permits continuous assessment of the effect of increasing caloric intake on protein sparing (65).

If TPN is used, vitamin supplementation is necessary. Vitamin E (10 IU), niacin (20 to 40 mg), thiamine (3 mg), riboflavin (3 mg), pantothenic acid (10 to 15 mg), pyridoxine (10 mg), ascorbic acid (100 mg) and biotin (100 to 200 mg) should be added to the supplementation. Folic acid (1 to 2 mg), vitamin B_{12} (5 μg), and vitamin K (5 to 10 mg) should also be given, but in a separate administration because of possible antagonistic reactions with other compounds (66).

Parenteral vitamin A should be eliminated unless TPN is continued for several weeks because serum retinol-binding protein (the vitamin A carrier protein) is elevated in patients with renal failure. Trace element supplementation remains to be defined. In the catabolic patient small amounts of zinc (2 to 4 mg/day) should be provided. Measuring zinc levels does not guard against total body deficits.

Electrolytes also need to be administered with the TPN solution, and it is recommended that the following be employed initially: 50 mEq sodium/l, 35 mEq potassium/day, 20 mEq phosphorus/day, 8 mEq magnesium/day and 10 mEq calcium/day. If plasma concentrations of any of these electrolytes are elevated, adjustments are necessary. Potential intravascular and intracellular deficits can occur when ARF begins to resolve and an anabolic phase occurs. Hypophosphatemia can become profound with TPN feedings, even in the patient with ARF. Inadequate phosphorus supplementation can occur when patients are receiving large amounts of carbohydrate (greater than 500 mg/day). Hypophosphatemia has been associated with decreased oxygen transport capacity, respiratory failure and muscular weakness. Hypokalemia can also occur during the anabolic phase in the renal failure patient receiving TPN. While hyperkalemia is of great concern, the converse must be also considered because hypokalemia can develop when cellular synthesis exceeds the availability of potassium ions.

When results of multiple studies were summarized (67), it was concluded that amino acid infusion usually results in a decrease in net urea production, but no consistent improvement in the rate of recovery of renal function. Although there is a suggestion that survival of the episode of ARF is improved by such treatment, overall hospital survival is not affected. Despite improvement in nutritional status, such catabolic patients continue to die from infection or non-renal complications of the condition that caused the ARF initially. The optimal regimen has not been identified. There is little justification for using very large amounts of amino acids in an attempt to promote more rapid protein utilization since this will undoubtedly raise the requirements for dialysis to remove waste products derived from metabolism of the infused amino acids. As noted above, dialysis itself is probably catabolic and such practice will only aggravate the already precarious state.

CHRONIC RENAL FAILURE

Evidence of protein-calorie undernutrition has been noted in virtually all nutritional surveys of dialysis patients (68). The National Cooperative Dialysis Study sponsored by the NIH indicated that nutritional status was the most abnormal in patients with subnormal serum cholesterol and very low BUN values, suggesting an inadequate intake (69). Those patients with average BUN values >100 mg/dl fared worse in terms of the frequency of hospitalization and complicating illnesses compared to patients with average BUN values below 80 mg/dl. Higher BUN levels are an index of accumulated waste products, whether they are due to inadequate dialysis or excessive protein intake (70). At present, no single waste product has been identified as the uremic toxin, but since catabolism of dietary and endogenous proteins is directly proportional to urea production, the BUN is an index of the accumulation of all putative uremic toxins.

Marked body protein depletion exists in chronic uremia, with decreased dietary protein intake and uremia-induced increased catabolism being major factors (71). There is no proportional increase in the albumin synthetic rate to compensate for the exaggerated catabolism. Patients with chronic renal failure and those undergoing hemodialysis have a relative body weight below the normal values obtained from the NHANES Survey (9). Additional evidence for wasting in this population are the subnormal values of skin fold thickness, mid-arm muscle circumference, total body nitrogen, serum protein (albumin and tranferrin concentrations) and a low total lymphocyte count. Serum complement (C3) may reflect early protein wasting in the chronic dialysis population since values are decreased when serum total proteins are still in the normal range (72).

Energy intake and expenditure

Energy expenditure by stable undialyzed chronic renal failure patients and those treated by hemodialysis is close to that of sedentary, normal subjects. Normal subjects in the U.S. engaged in sedentary to light physical activity have at least 60 to 70% of daily energy expenditure attributable to that calculated as resting expenditure (REE) plus that generated by eating (i.e. the specific dynamic action of food). Most of the remaining energy expenditure is related to obligatory activities of dressing, washing, shaving, sitting and standing. Energy expenditure at energy level of activity in the non-dialyzed and dialyzed uremic was directly correlated with the work performed, as in normal subjects (75). These data suggest that the energy requirements for dialysis patients are near those of sedentary normal subjects, certainly they are not below normal levels. Yet, in clinically stable dialysis patients, energy intake is often 20 to 25% below values of normal individuals of the same age and sex

(76, 77). In general, skin fold thickness measurements suggest that maintenance dialysis patients have a low body fat. Consequently, in the non-obese dialysis patient, an energy intake of 35 to 42 kcal/kg/day is recommended to meet metabolic needs (78).

Kopple et al (73) have shown the interdependence of protein and energy intakes. They demonstrated an improvement in body weight and serum albumin concentration at dietary protein intakes of 0.75 and 1.25 g/kg/day in dialyzed outpatients if caloric intake exceeded 35 kcal/kg/day compared to lower energy intakes. Although nitrogen balance will improve as protein intake increases to a value of approximately 1.1 to 1.2 g/kg/day, the improvement also depends on calorie intake.

Over a 2-year period, fat was found to increase while fat-free tissue decreased in stable chronic dialysis patients (74). Adherence to an adequate intake of protein and calories over a 2-year observation (monitored by diet records and periodic urea nitrogen appearance determinations) demonstrated that no malnutrition occurred in dialysis patients. The results show that an adequate intake can avoid malnutrition if intake is monitored carefully.

Hypoglycemia has been reported in hemodialysis patients taking propranolol. The suggested mechanism is that this beta blocker limits the availability of free fatty acids and may inhibit hepatic, glucagon-stimulated, glucose output (91). Metoprolol seems to exert less interference with energy substrates in hemodialysis patients under fasting conditions. Therefore, a cardiac-selective beta blocker may be preferred for the chronic dialysis patient.

Dialysis, hormonal changes and nutrition

Insulin is the most potent anabolic hormone, but there is resistance to its anabolic effects in muscle in chronic uremia (79). Plasma glucagon levels and serum growth hormone concentrations are increased in sera of uremic subjects. Somatomedins, which mediate the actions of growth hormone, tend to be normal or decreased in the sera of dialysis patients. Impaired somatomedin acitivity may promote wasting because the biological activity of somatomedins is noted to be reduced in children and adults with chronic renal failure (80, 81). Somatomedin activity appears to improve, at least transiently, with hemodialysis and may reflect an improved nutritional status.

Excess parathyroid hormone (PTH) production may also promote protein wasting because it affects energy utilization. In one study (82), parathyroidectomy led to improved nitrogen balance and in another study (83), injection of PTH or PTH extract into humans increased urinary nitrogen excretion and promoted negative nitrogen balance. PTH may also promote protein wasting by raising serum calcium and causing anorexia, nausea and vomiting or by limiting activity because of severe bone disease. In a controlled study in hemodialysis patients, it was shown that parathyroid hormone can be suppressed by treatment with a mixture of amino acids and ketoanalogues (84). The ketoacid treated patients showed a significant fall in PTH and plasma phosphate levels, while no changes in plasma 25-hydroxyvitamin D or plasma calcitonin were observed. It is possible that ketoacid administration in the chronic dialysis population may be beneficial with respect to control of secondary hyperparathyroidism and thus enhance nitrogen balance (Table 8).

Metabolic and endocrine activities of the kidney theoretically may promote or maintain nutrition. The kidney secretes renin, erythropoietin and 1,25 dihydroxycholecalciferol, and degrades many peptide hormones. The kidney also consumes and releases a number of amino acids into the blood, thereby contributing to the homeostasis of the body's amino acid pools (85). Severe kidney disease could cause a lack of 1,25 dihydroxycholecalciferol, carnitine deficiency, and contribute to aluminum toxicity. Each could contribute to proximal muscle weakness of chronically uremic patients, and this debility in turn would promote wasting. Since 25-hydroxycholecalciferol can stimulate muscle protein synthesis in vitro, it is possible that vitamin D deficiency in renal failure may promote protein wasting more directly.

Metabolic aspects of dialysis

Net protein degradation and negative nitrogen balance occur during hemodialysis. Among the possible causes for the catabolic response to hemodialysis are the removal of substrates such as amino acids, peptides, glucose metabolites (pyruvate, lactate) and glucose if a glucose-free dialysate is used. Fasting patients lose, on the average, about 7 g of free amino acids and about 2 to 3 g of peptides or bound amino acids during hemodialysis (86). Also, net protein degradation is reported to increase with hemodialysis, suggesting there might be a direct catabolic influence or an indirect one from increased energy expenditure (87). There are losses of 20 to 30 g of glucose per hemodialysis if a glucose-free dialysate is used. A small quantity of water-soluble vitamins is also lost with each hemodialysis (88). Since patients generally do not eat during hemodialysis, nutrient losses must be replaced from endogenous stores. For this reason and because of heparin use, lipolysis is stimulated. When energy levels are low, protein wasting may occur to stimulate gluconeogenesis.

Blood-membrane interactions might be another mechanism which accelerates protein catabolism during dialysis. In normal subjects undergoing a sham dialysis through a cuprophane membrane, net release of free tyrosine and phenylalanine from the leg increased approximately 100% (89). Since these amino acids are not metabolized by muscle, the results suggest that dialysis enhanced catabolism of leg muscle protein. The increased release of aromatic amino acids was prevented by indomethacin, suggesting that the protein breakdown was mediated by prostaglandins (90).

A potential way to reverse some of the catabolic effects of dialysis is to dialyze against a bicarbonate instead of an acetate bath. This practice reportedly increased body mass and improved nutrition. It was noted that patients were able to eat more normally after a bicarbonate dialysis than after an acetate dialysis. Since metabolic acidosis stimulates muscle protein catabolism in experimental chronic renal failure (92), it was postulated that better regulation of metabolic acidosis accounted for the beneficial effects of bicarbonate dialysis (93). For example, correction of metabolic acidosis and maintenance of serum bicarbonate above 20 mEq/l has been associated with an increase in arm muscle circumference when compared to a similar patient group with more severe acidosis (94). Experimental studies have shown that chronic metabolic acidosis in chronic renal failure stimulates protein catabolism and branched-chain amino acid (BCAA) decarboxylation in skeletal muscle, possibly contributing to the reduced intra- and extracellular concentrations of BCAA (95). When dietary regimens are restricted in BCAA intake, it is important to maintain plasma bicarbonate levels near normal.

Water soluble vitamins

It is common practice to provide dialysis patients with vitamin C because water soluble vitamins are dialyzable. Oxalic acid is a bicarboxylic acid derived from the metabolism of amino acids and vitamin C. In spite of significant oxalate removal with dialysis, plasma oxalate levels are elevated with as little as 500 mg of vitamin C supplement per day (96, 97). Moreover, dialyzed chronic renal failure patients appear to develop a greater oxalate burden than uremic patients not on dialysis (98). It is possible that oxalate accumulation can have long-term adverse consequences, including soft tissue deposition of calcium oxalate and interference with vitamin B_{12} metabolism. Consequently, only 100 mg of vitamin C per day is recommended. If vegetables are soaked or excessively boiled to decrease their potassium content, the content of water soluble vitamins is also decreased and the supplement should be doubled.

All water soluble vitamins are removed by dialysis so a supplement containing the recommended daily allowance (RDA) should be provided (99). Although this is recommended, it should be pointed out that in a longitudinal study, chronic dialysis patients were able to maintain normal plasma and red blood cell levels of some water-soluble vitamins without daily supplementation (100). An exception is pyridoxine (vitamin B_6). Pyridoxine deficiency occurs in approximately 70% of patients with chronic renal failure. Suggested mechanisms are malabsorption or interaction with drugs, such as hydralazine, penicillamine and diphenylhydantoin, which form inactive compounds with the vita-

Table 8. Hormonal influences on nutrition in renal failure.

Anabolic	Catabolic
Insulin	Epinephrine
Growth Hormone	Cortisone
Somatomedins	Glucagon
Vitamin D	Proteases
Carnitine	Polypeptide-?Interleukin-1
	Parathyroid Hormone

min. However, because there are many similarities between the syndromes of chronic uremia and vitamin B_6 deficiency, it is recommended that uremic patients take 10 mg/day of pyridoxine HCl (101), approximately 5 times the RDA for non-pregnant, non-lactating subjects.

Pantothenic acid is essential for the formation of co-enzyme A, and low levels of this vitamin, in conjunction with pyridoxine deficiency, can markedly decrease antibody response, and depress cellular and humoral immunity (102). Pantothenic acid deficiency could, therefore, be a factor in the altered immune state of chronic renal failure. Riboflavin, thiamin, biotin, niacin, and tryptophan deficiencies are rare, but could contribute to an impaired antibody response. Deficiencies of these vitamins could represent a particular danger in the elderly and in the chronically ill.

Lipid soluble vitamins

Vitamin A and E supplements are not needed by uremic patients. In predialysis subjects and hemodialysis patients, plasma levels of vitamin A are, in fact, high because vitamin A is bound to retinol binding protein in a 1 : 1 molar ratio (103). This protein is high even when there is loss in the dialysate in some patients on continuous ambulatory peritoneal dialysis (CAPD), suggesting increased production of the binding protein. Despite elevated plasma levels of vitamin A in uremia, vitamin A stores are probably not increased and do not account for the problems of uremia (104, 105). Persistently elevated chloramine levels in dialysis water can cause an oxidant-induced, hemolytic anemia. Patients so affected are noted to have low vitamin E levels, which might contribute both to hemolysis and to an altered immunological state. Removing chloramine from the dialysis water will increase vitamin E levels towards normal and correct the hemolysis; the influence on immunologic status is less clear (106, 107). Although vitamin E has been advocated for the treatment of lipoprotein disorders in uremia, short-term vitamin E administration at the high dose of 600 IU/day did not raise HDL cholesterol. Active forms of vitamin D often need to be supplemented (see Chapter 45).

NUTRITION IN PERITONEAL DIALYSIS

A strong correlation exists between nitrogen balance and energy intake, emphasizing the importance of an adequate energy intake in the prevention of long-term negative nitrogen balance in uremic patients (108). Anthropometric measurements showed patients on CAPD were anabolic when the diet provided 1.4 g protein/kg/day and at least 35 kcal/kg/day (8). In contrast, when CAPD patients ate less than 1.0 g protein/kg/day and 30 kcal/kg/day, there was evidence of mild to moderate wasting; values of body weight, skinfold thickness and mid-arm muscle circumference were decreased. Establishing the usual pre-uremic weight is a reasonable goal in therapy for CAPD patients, although long-term CAPD patients will frequently have an increase in body fat and weight gain above their ideal body weight.

Presumably the increase in body fat is related to glucose absorbed from the dialysate and will be associated with changes in triceps skinfold thickness, serum triglycerides, and cholesterol (109). Total caloric intake from the diet and glucose absorbed from the dialysis should be in the range of 35 to 40 kcal/day to prevent protein wasting (110).

Based on nitrogen balance measurements, it is recommended that CAPD patients eat 1.2 to 1.5 g protein/kg/day (Table 9); and at least 50% of the protein be of high biological value (110). However, in one study, CAPD patients remained in positive nitrogen balance despite eating slightly less protein than prescribed (111). In this latter study, the average protein losses into the dialysate were 13.3 g/day while patients were eating a daily average of 1.03 g protein/kg and 32 kcal/kg. In spite of this, the triceps skinfold thickness and mid arm muscle circumference remained in the normal range for most patients. Thus, the ideal protein intake for CAPD patients has not been settled. Studies have shown most patients do not eat as much as 1.4 g protein/kg/day (112, 113), and some studies have noted an increase in body fat and muscle mass in both males and females treated long-term by CAPD (6, 114). Potassium balance correlates directly with nitrogen balance, and high fecal potassium losses help maintain normal serum potassium concentrations (115).

A non-linear correlation exists between the molecular weight of a protein and its peritoneal loss during CAPD. However, peritoneal permeability to proteins remains stable after 3 to 4 years on CAPD and during long-term therapy, albumin, alpha-1-antitrypsin and transferrin show the greatest losses with CAPD. Peritonitis has a markedly adverse influence on serum albumin, vitamin B_{12} and folate levels. With peritonitis, average protein losses into the dialysate increase to more than 15 g/day. With antibiotic treatment, protein losses fall, but may remain elevated for many days to weeks. Although increasing the diet may combat these losses, it is unlikely that neutral nitrogen balance can be achieved. Obviously, the mainstay of therapy is appropriate antibiotics.

Glucose as an energy source

Glucose absorbed from the dialysate is a major source of energy for CAPD patients (115–117). There is close correlation ($r = 0.91$) between the amount of glucose absorbed each day and the dialysate glucose infused (118). This permits calculation of the glucose absorbed per liter of dialysate ($r = 0.96$) by the formula (119):

g glucose absorbed/l dialysate = 11.3 × dialysis fluid dextrose monohydrate concentration (g/dl) − 10.9.

A detailed study (119) calculated that 192 ± 61 g/day of glucose were absorbed from a dialysate content that averaged 252 ± 62 g/day. Glucose absorbed contributed 8.4 ± 2.7 kcal/kg/day (an average 500 to 600 kcal/day) to the patient's energy intake. Consequently, the total caloric intake (from diet and dialysate), can be calculated as approximately 50% from carbohydrates, 30% from fat and 20% from

Table 9. Recommended daily dietary intake for CAPD patients.

Protein	1.2 to 1.5 g/kg/day standard body weight
Calories	35 to 40 kcal/kg/day standard body weight (energy source and dialysate)
Carbohydrate	35% of calorie intake (oral)
Fat	Remainder of non-protein calorie oral intake
Polyunsaturated/Saturated fatty acid ratio 1.5/1.0	
Total fiber	20 to 25 g
Calcium	1.0 to 1.5 g
Phosphorus	0.8 to 1.1 g
Magnesium	200 to 300 mg
Potassium	2 to 3 g
Sodium	adjusted as to blood pressure, serum sodium and edema-free weight (average 2 to 3 g)
Vitamin supplements:	Vitamin B_{12} — $3 \mu g$
	Vitamin B_6 — 10 mg
	Vitamin B_1 — 2 mg
	Vitamin C — 100 mg
	Vitamins A, E, K — (none unless specifically indicated)
	Other water soluble vitamins (riboflavin, niacin, etc.) — RDA for normals
	Vitamin D — as dictated by serum Ca and P values and bone disease
	Folic acid — 1 mg
	Biotin — unknown

Adapted from Kopple and Blumenkrantz (116, 118).
During episodes of peritonitis increase protein intake to 1.5 to 1.8 g/kg.

protein (120). On the down side, the absorption of glucose may decrease appetite and reduce food intake, with glucose making up an even larger proportion of calories in CAPD patients (121).

Amino acids

The pattern of almost all amino acids, and especially the essential amino acids, in the plasma of uremic patients is markedly abnormal, resembling the pattern found in malnourished, non-uremic patients (122, 123).

For this reason and to increase intake, a dialysis solution containing amino acids as an osmotic agent has been suggested as a substitute for glucose in the CAPD patient (124–126). In each week the CAPD patient loses 10 to 30 g of amino acids into the dialysate (116, 127–130). Protein and amino acid losses correlate directly with dwell time in both CAPD and continuous cycling peritoneal dialysis (CCPD), but are independent of the dextrose concentration in the dialysis solution. In CAPD patients, amino acid losses correlate with post-absorptive plasma concentrations, so there is approximately a 29% loss of total essential amino acids (89). Of the 8 to 13 g protein/day loss into the dialysate, approximately 6 g are albumin, 3 g are total amino acids, with IgG losses averaging 1.25 ± 0.20 g/day (Table 10) (129, 131). High vs low protein diets have no effect on dialysate protein losses, and there is no relationship between the daily volume of dialysate and the protein lost.

Substituting a 1% or 2% mixture of essential and non-essential amino acids for glucose in the dialysis solution will result in 80 to 90% of the amino acids being absorbed over 6 hours (Table 11). One hour after instilling the dialysate, plasma amino acid concentrations increased two- to three-

fold and returned to pre-instillation values by 6 hours (132), suggesting the absorbed amino acids were used for protein synthesis or degraded. A 2% amino acid dialysis solution has an osmolality which approximates a dialysis solution of 4.25 g/dl of dextrose without amino acids (133). When amino acids were used alternately with glucose as an osmotic agent during a 3-month period, there was no detectable change in the metabolism of glucose, fat and protein, but the plasma concentration of the branched-chain amino acids (leucine, isoleucine, valine) increased (125). Since branched-chain amino acid concentrations are often low in plasma and muscle of non-dialyzed uremic and CAPD patients, this change presumably represents an improvement.

Instillation of amino acids into the peritoneal cavity is well

Table 10. Plasma protein and amino acid values and losses in CAPD.

	Serum or plasma	CAPD losses/24 h
Total Protein	6.6 ± 0.1 g/dl	8–13 g
Albumin	3.5 ± 0.1 g/dl	5–6 g
Transferrin	228 ± 11 mg/dl	310–350 mg
IgG	14 ± 0.12 g/dl	1.1–1.5 g
IgA	220 ± 18 mg/dl	150–190 mg
IgM	234 ± 36 mg/dl	50–90 mg
C3	107 ± 6 mg/dl	65–75 mg
C4	32 ± 2 mg/dl	19–23 mg
Total amino acids	$3415 \pm 134 \mu mol/l$	3.0–3.7 g
Essential/Non-essential ratio	0.48 ± 0.03	0.55–0.65

Adapted from Kopple et al (129), Blumenkrantz et al (131).

tolerated. Serum concentrations of cholesterol, HDL cholesterol, LDL cholesterol, triglycerides, glucose, albumin, transferrin, phosphorus, and glycosylated hemoglobin are unchanged after amino acid dialysis fluid is used. The extra nitrogen does not increase the plasma ammonium concentration, although the urea nitrogen level does increase slightly. Serum triglycerides remain elevated, so it has been recommended that the diet contains a polyunsaturated/saturated fat ratio of 1.5 : 1.0.

NUTRITION IN HEMODIALYSIS

Based on numerous nitrogen balance studies, the hemodialysis patient should ingest between 1.0 to 1.2 g protein/kg/day of desired body weight (136, 137). At least half of the protein should be of high biological value, and caloric intake should be at least 35 kcal/kg/day of desired body weight if the patient is not obese. Phosphorus intake should be in the range of 800 mg/day (Table 12). Even with this reduced phosphorus intake, phosphorus binders, preferably non-aluminum-containing compounds, should be used to prevent a rise in serum phosphorus and secondary hyperparathyroidism. Calcium intake should be approximately 1,500 mg/day. However, a rise in the serum calcium × phosphorus product above 55 mg^2/dl^2 must be avoided. Therefore, a calcium supplement should be delayed until the serum phosphorus is in the normal range. Approximately 200 mg/day of magnesium should be prescribed along with about 2 g/day of potassium. Dietary sodium should be adjusted for blood pressure control; an average amount is 2 g/day. Dietary sodium must be restricted if there is any excessive interdialytic weight gain or hypertension. As with CAPD patients, pyridoxine HCl 10 mg/day, vitamin C 100 mg/day, folic acid 1 mg/day and the RDA of other water soluble vitamins for healthy adults should be given (136).

Supplements

Constipation in dialysis patients can be caused by a low dietary fiber or fluid intake, lack of exercise, iron supplementation, and/or the daily use of phosphate binders. Wheat bran is a concentrated form of fiber that may help reduce constipation. While wheat bran is high in potassium and protein, its use does not seem to aggravate hyperkalemia or azotemia when taken daily; perhaps these products are excreted because of the greater fecal bulk.

Fish oil

A fish oil supplement may be useful for hemodialysis patients because of beneficial effects on lipids, platelets and blood pressure. It has been shown that 8 weeks of a dietary supplement of eicosapentaenoic acid caused a 35% fall in triglycerides, a 10% rise of high-density lipoproteins (HDL) cholesterol, a 36% rise of HDL$_2$ cholesterol fraction and a 54% rise of the HDL$_2$: HDL$_3$ cholesterol ratio (137). In

Table 12. Recommended daily dietary intake for hemodialysis patients.

Nutrient	
Protein	1.0 to 1.2 g/kg desired body weight at least 50% high biological value
Calories	25 to 45 kcal/kg desired body weight
Carbohydrate	35% of caloric intake
Fat	Remainder of non-protein caloric intake
Vitamins	
Vitamin A	No additional recommended
Vitamin E	No additional recommended
Vitamin D	Individualized
Vitamin B (Thiamine)	1.5 to 2.0 mg
Riboflavin	1.8 mg
Vitamin B$_6$ (Pyroxidine)	10 mg
Vitamin B$_{12}$	3 μg
Panthothenic Acid	5 mg
Vitamin C	100 mg
Folic Acid	1 mg
Biotin	unknown
Minerals	
Sodium	Individualized (average 2 to 3 g)
Potassium	Individualized (average 2 to 3 g)
Calcium	1 to 2 g elemental calcium
Phosphorus	0.8 to 1.1 g
Zinc	unknown (may improved appetite)
Iron	Individualized (depending on serum ferritin)
Fluid	500 ml plus daily urine output
Fiber	20 to 25 g
Fish Oil	Individualized (3 to 4 g)

If the patient is overweight, 25 kcal/kg; if underweight, 45 kcal/kg. Give calcium supplementation only with serum phosphorus 5 mg/dl or less.

Table 11. Amino acid composition in amino acid dialysate (10 g/l).

	mg/100 ml	μmol/l
Threonine	42	3530
Proline	42	3650
Glycine	213	27735
Alanine	213	23370
Valine	46	3930
Methionine	58	3895
Isoleucine	48	3665
Leucine	62	4735
Tyrosine	4	220
Phenylalanine	62	3760
Lysine	58	3975
Histidine	44	2840
Tryptophan	18	880
Arginine	104	5975

Adapted from Oren et al (133).

addition, platelet aggregation in response to ADP or collagen was significantly reduced. The activated, whole blood clotting time was prolonged from 41 to 153 sec and 69% of the patients had a reduction in factor VIII-related antigen. This antigen is usually elevated in hemodialysis patients and is thought to be a marker of endothelial damage. Finally, blood pressure was noted to fall with the fish oil supplement. Although the supplement appears to be a panacea (for hemodialysis patients), long-term studies have not demonstrated a decline in cardiovascular mortality.

Amino acids and glucose

Amino acid supplements in the chronic hemodialysis population have been advocated because of amino acid losses during dialysis and continuous arteriovenous hemofiltration (138–141). A double blind study (140) showed that an oral essential amino acid (EAA) supplement decreased the catabolic effects of dialysis when compared to an isocaloric supplement. Hematocrit, serum total protein, albumin, and transferrin, and cortical/trabecular bone density improved with the EAA supplement, but not in the calorie supplement patients. Although it seems that nutrient losses occurring with dialysis can be replaced to alleviate the catabolic stress of the procedure (142), stabilized hemodialysis patients exhibit cellular malnutrition even though they are given supplemental amino acid infusions for 3 months (143). The cellular amino acid imbalance could not be corrected despite the 10% mixture of amino acids given after each dialysis, providing a total of 1.6 to 1.8 kg of free amino acids over the 3-month interval. Hemodialysis patients are in positive net protein balance on non-dialysis days, whether they are eating a higher or low protein content. However, on hemodialysis treatment days protein balance is negative, although somewhat less with a high protein diet (134).

The resting transmembrane potential of skeletal muscle is abnormally low in uremic patients and reversed by chronic dialysis. An oral EAA supplement can restore the resting membrane potential to normal when dialysis time was reduced to the point of lowering the transmembrane potential (144), suggesting that the EAA supplement may permit a reduction of dialysis time in certain compliant patients if resting transmembrane potential is used as an endpoint.

Nutritional hemodialysis has been advocated for the undernourished patient. When nutrients such as 5% glucose plus 0.4% amino acids are added to the dialysis fluid, efficient uptake can be enhanced by reducing the dialysate flow rate. At dialysate flow rates of 50 to 60 ml/min, urea and creatinine dialysance approach dialysate flow rate, and net glucose and amino acid absorption varies directly with the dialysate flow rate. Uptakes of 78% over 3 to 5 h can be achieved at this very low flow rate, leading to a mean caloric intake of about 200 kcal/h (142). In order to control hyperglycemia, continuous, low-dose insulin infusion is required (Table 13). Because of the low urea and creatinine dialysances, additional dialysis time will be required to prevent uremic symptoms. Consequently, the advantages of adding amino acids to hemodialysis baths are not clear.

Another method of providing extra nutrition in malnourished hemodialysis patients who eat or digest food poorly is to infuse amino acids. Two caveats should be emphasized. First, as discussed previously, the impact of such therapy on morbidity, mortality and recovery of renal function is marginal in patients with acute renal failure (57). Second, such therapy obligates infusion of water and nitrogen which can dictate increased dialysis treatment time (to combat fluid overload, hyponatremia and azotemia) and hence add to the catabolic stress from hemodialysis. On the other hand, intravenous amino acids are not simply removed by the dialysis procedure. Wolfson et al (86) infused 40 g of amino acids during each hemodialysis treatment of stable, maintenance hemodialysis patients and found that about 90% of the amino acids were retained. If adequate calories are provided, retained amino acids should promote more positive nitrogen balance. Because infused amino acids will also increase the fluid load and urea production, such therapy must be carefully and repeatedly monitored to ensure that the net effect is beneficial, i.e. that the calculated urea appearance rate is less than total nitrogen intake (134).

DIABETES AND DIALYSIS

The diabetic patient treated by CAPD presents a difficult nutritional problem. Blood glucose values increase because of the glucose load from the dialysis solution. A bloated sensation from the infusate can decrease the patient's appetite and the patient should be instructed to eat when dialysate is removed from the abdomen. The patient can also suffer from constipation from phosphate binders, diarrhea from diabetic enteropathy, and nausea and vomiting from diabetic gastroparesis. Understandably, these conditions can result in the patient being fearful of eating. Frequent small feedings may be the only method of ensuring an adequate intake of nutrients.

It is recommended that the diabetic CAPD patient eat 1.2 to 1.5 g protein/kg ideal body weight/day, at least 60% of the protein being of high biological value (117). Since utilization of dietary protein is influenced directly by the total energy intake, the patient should eat 35 kcal/kg/day (145). The more active the individual, the higher the required energy intake should be, and with infection or other catabolic

Table 13. Nutritional hemodialysis.

Dialysis solution 5% dextrose and 0.4% amino acids
Dialysis fluid flow rate (Q_d): 5 to 50 ml/min
Blood flow rate (Q_b): 200 ml/min
Urea and creatinine clearances directly relate to dialysis fluid flow rate
Net glucose and amino acid absorption at Q_d 27 ml/min over 3 to 5 h: 78% and 78%
Mean caloric intake: 199 kcal/h
Insulin infusion needed to control hyperglycemia

Adapted from Feinstein (142).

stresses, the energy intake should be doubled.

Diabetic patients may require a protein supplement to ensure an adequate intake. When nausea and vomiting are present, the patient should be placed on a clear liquid diet for a short time and then advanced to a full liquid diet. Use of an enteral feeding solution delivered by an intestinal tube should be considered if nausea and vomiting attributable to gastroparesis persist. Total parenteral nutrition should be the last consideration for patients unable to take in a sufficient amount of protein and calories (146). A TPN solution containing 4.5 to 6.5% amino acids (60 to 80 g protein/day), 17.5 to 40% glucose concentration (depending upon fluid volume limitations), and 10% vegetable oil emulsion supplying essential fatty acid requirements can provide adequate protein for anabolism while limiting urea production (147). Nitrogen balance can become positive withing 2 weeks of beginning TPN when energy requirements of 40 to 45 kcal/kg body weight are met. Homeostatic blood sugar control can be achieved by a constant infusion of insulin along with the dextrose and protein input. Caution is recommended in continuing phosphate- or potassium-binding drugs during the initial phases of nutritional therapy because patients show additional requirements for these electrolytes.

If protein and calorie goals conflict or are incompatible, then it is important to set priorities. The first priority is to achieve an adequate protein intake (i.e. 1.2 to 1.5 g/kg/day for CAPD patients). Secondly, carbohydrate and fat intake should be adjusted to achieve the energy requirement, approximately 45% of total calories from carbohydrates and approximately 35% from fat.

NUTRITION IN THE ELDERLY

The patient over 65 years of age with chronic renal failure represents a special problem because of the nutritional deficiencies that may occur in the elderly (Table 14). Protein-calorie malnutrition is more frequent with increasing age, in part attributed to a decrease in physical activity and basal oxygen consumption. A reduced metabolic rate with age is a result of a declining body mass (148). Protein-calorie malnutrition, vitamin deficiency and deficiencies of trace elements also can adversely affect the immune system.

Hypodipsia occurs commonly in elderly patients, even when they seem fully capable of obtaining water. Although

Table 14. Nutrition problems in the elderly.

Decreased caloric intake
Decreased physical activity
Decreased basal oxygen consumption
Hypodipsia
Osteopenia
Iron deficiency
Folate and other vitamin deficiencies
Zinc deficiency

the mechanism of a thirst deficit in the elderly is unclear, hypodipsia could exacerbate hypotension during dialysis.

Age-related osteopenia is common in the elderly and can be exacerbated by decreased calcium absorption. Lower plasma levels of 1,25 dihydroxyvitamin D_3 have been noted even in non-uremic elderly patients, and this factor plus a high-fiber diet, given to control constipation, can reduce calcium absorption. The above factors combined with physical inactivity lead to negative calcium balance in the elderly patient and would augment the abnormalities of calcium metabolism associated with renal failure (149).

Iron and folate deficiency are common in the elderly because of decreased intake. These deficiencies are greatly augmented by dialysis, and supplements (1 mg folate/day, 200 mg iron/day) are recommended. In addition, folate stores can be affected by drugs used in the dialysis population including trimethoprim, phenytoin, barbiturates, cholestyramine, and aspirin. Folate deficiency may contribute to impaired antibody synthesis and cellular immunity.

Serum zinc levels decrease with aging, probably due to long-term, marginal intake of zinc. Low levels can be aggravated by increased zinc excretion in patients with type II diabetes mellitus. Zinc is necessary for functioning of T-lymphocytes and cellular and humoral immunity (150), and hypozincemia might contribute to the progressive deterioration in T-lymphocyte function with aging. Zinc deficiency in uremic patients has also been associated with disturbances in taste and sexual performance. However, in CAPD patients, red cell zinc levels are normal even though serum zinc levels are significantly below normal (151). Thus, the importance of a low serum level is unclear and an excess of dietary zinc can cause abnormal copper metabolism despite a normal copper intake. Dietary copper supplementation has led to a rapid recovery of low levels of IgA and IgG levels, but IgM tends to remain depressed for many months. Consequently, supplements of different trace metals should be given only for specific indications and carefully monitored (see Chapter 49).

NUTRITION IN CHILDREN

An abnormal plasma aminogram has been noted in uremic children treated by dietary manipulation or by hemodialysis; the pattern is similar to that noted in adults with chronic renal failure. Dialysis does not correct the abnormal plasma amino acid pattern in uremic children, and more worrisome, free amino acid losses during hemodialysis could not be fully compensated for by children eating an adequate protein intake (152). Oral supplements of essential amino acids or ketoanalogues only partially corrected the amino acid abnormalities, and no biochemical improvement in protein metabolism was observed in children receiving regular hemodialysis. Plasma methionine and 3-methyl-histidine levels were elevated by the supplement, but apparently without ill effects.

Children with end-stage renal disease who do not ingest adequate calories have increased insulin binding to red blood cell receptors. Therefore, in uremia there may be two independent causes for abnormalities in insulin binding. The end result is removal of an anabolic hormone. Failure to consider energy intake and nutritional status, especially in children, may result in a wide variety of disorders (153). Supplementing the protein intake with amino acid and keto acid supplements may help correct the insulin resistance in uremic children. Children on CAPD tend to gain edema-free weight, with serum cholesterol and triglyceride levels increasing to abnormal values during treatment. However, this population still is prone to protein depletion as noted by plasma total protein, albumin, transferrin and C3 levels being lower than normal controls (154). Energy intake tended to be more suppressed than protein intake. Nutritional parameters were more abnormal in children less than 10 years old as compared to older children, but both groups displayed reduced height, weight, and mid arm muscle circumference. During the course of treatment with CAPD, the serum total proteins slowly decreased. Low protein and energy intake and dialysate protein losses may contribute to the decreased stature and poor nutritional status of these children (155).

EFFECT OF EXERCISE ON NUTRITION

Patients maintained on chronic dialysis are sedentary; they have a poor degree of physical fitness and reduced maximum aerobic capacity (156). Improved carbohydrate metabolism, lowering of hypertriglyceridemia and an increase in high-density lipoprotein cholesterol concentration in hemodialysis patients is noted with exercise (157–160). Regular exercise training is associated with a reduction in fasting glucose by 5.4%, an improvement in the glucose disappearance curve by 20.4% and a decrease in the plasma insulin levels by 35% (159). In some patients exercise is associated with a reduction in the doses of antihypertensive medications, decrease in phosphate binder therapy, and an increase in hematocrit/hemoglobin, while body weight and diet remain the same. An additional benefit of exercise training in hemodialysis patients is on the psychological status, with an improvement in depression, hostility, anxiety, social interaction and outlook for the future (160). In chronically uremic rats, increased proteolysis in muscle can be reduced by exercise training (161).

In a controlled study of healthy young adults it was shown that the plasma insulin concentration declined and plasma epinephrine and norepinephrine levels increased substantially during exercise (162). In contrast, plasma insulin did not fall and the epinephrine and norepinephrine levels increased only slightly in dialysis patients after exercise. However, these differences between the two groups were not significant and the plasma glucagon concentration did not change significantly from baseline in either the control or uremic groups during exercise. The changes in response to exercise plus their normally sedentary existence probably contribute to the impaired glucose tolerance, insulin resistance, hyperinsulinemia, hyperlipidemia, and an accelerated rate of atherosclerosis in dialysis patients. Unfortunately, few dialysis patients will take advantage of the beneficial effects of exercise even though it is not necessary for the exercise to be vigorous to achieve metabolic benefits. It remains to be determined whether the decreased participation is psychological, due to limited enthusiasm by the physician or chronic fatigue caused by malnutrition. Perhaps widespread use of recombinant DNA-produced erythropoietin will provide an answer to this question. Regardless, the remarkable potential benefits of exercise (156) should make an exercise program an integral part of any dialysis therapy.

REFERENCES

1. Teschan PE: Nutrition in renal failure. *Artif Organs* 10: 301, 1986
2. Rubin JE, Friedman P, Berlyne GM: Rapid blood flow short dialysis does not adversely affect clinical, biochemical or nutritional status of patients. *Trans Am Soc Artif Intern Organs* 32: 377, 1986
3. Acchiardo SR, Moore LW, Latour PA: Malnutrition as the main factor in morbidity and mortality of hemodialysis-patients. *Kidney Int* 24 (Suppl 16): S199, 1983
4. Cianciaruso B, Capuano A, Marcuccio F, Auciello A, Reed LA, Laviano A, Contaldo F, Borrelli R, Nastasi A, Andreucci VE: Reliability of clinical evaluation of nutritional status of patients undergoing hemodialysis (HD). *4th Int Congr Nutr Metab in Renal Dis* (Abstract), 1985
5. Heymsfield SB, Casper K: Anthropometric assessment of the adult hospitalized patient. *JPEN J Parenter Enteral Nutr* 11: 36S, 1987
6. Bennett SE, Wilson JM, Walls J: Serial assessment of nutritional status in continuous ambulatory peritoneal dialysis. *Peritoneal Dial Bull* 4: S5, 1984
7. Durnin JVGA, Womersley J: Body fat assessed from total body density and its estimation from skinfold thickness: measurements on 481 men and women aged from 16 to 72 years. *Br J Nutr* 32: 77, 1974
8. Giordano C, De Santo NG, Pluvio M, Di Leo VA, Capodicasa G, Cirillo D, Esposito R, Damiano M: Protein requirement of patients on CAPD: A study of nitrogen balance. *Int J Artif Organs* 3: 11, 1980
9. Frisancho AR: New standards of weight and body composition by frame size and height for assessment of nutritional status of adults and the elderly. *Am J Clin Nutr* 40: 808, 1984
10. Lohman SG: Skinfolds and body density and their relationship to body fatness: a review. *Human Biol* 53: 181, 1981
11. Heymsfield SB, McManus C, Smith J, Stevens V, Nixon DW: Revised equations for calculating bone-free arm muscle area. *Am J Clin Nutr* 36: 680, 1982
12. Frisancho AR: New norms of upper limb fat and muscle areas for assessment of nutritional status. *Am J Clin Nutr* 34: 2450, 1981
13. Presta E, Wang J, Harrison GG, Bjorntorp P, Harker WH, Van Itallie TB: Measurement of total body electrical conductivity: a new method for estimation of body composition. *Am J Clin Nutr* 37: 735, 1983
14. Lukaski HC, Johnson PE, Bolonchuk WW, Lykken GI: Assessment of fat-free mass using bioelectrical impedance measurements of the human body. *Am J Clin Nutr* 41: 810, 1985

15. Burkinshaw L, Morgan DB, Silverton NP, Thomas RD: Total body nitrogen and its relation to body potassium and fat free mass in healthy subjects. *Clin Sci* 61: 457, 1983

16. Burkinshaw L: Sex dependent calibration factor of a whole body radiation counter. *Int J Appl Radiat Isot* 29: 387, 1978

17. Stelin G, Ahlmen J, Morelli B, Tylen U: Computed tomography and total body potassium measurements of patients on continuous ambulatory peritoneal dialysis. *asaio J* 8: 46, 1985

18. Heymsfield SB, Olafson RP, Kutner MH, Dixon DW: A radiographic method of quantifying protein calorie undernutrition. *Am J Clin Nutr* 32: 693, 1979

19. Maughan RJ, Watson JS, Weir J: The relative proportion of fat, muscle, and bone in the normal human forearm as determined by computed tomography. *Clin Sci Mol Med* 66: 683, 1984

20. Heymsfield SB, Rolandelli R, Casper K, Settle RG, Koruda M: Application of electromagnetic and sound waves in nutritional assessment. *JPEN J Parenter Enteral Nutr* 11: 64S, 1987

21. Lewis DS, Rollwitz WL, Bertrant HA, Masoro EJ: Use of NMR for measurement of total body water and estimation of body fat. *J Appl Physiol* 60: 836, 1986

22. Presta E, Segal KR, Rutin B, Harrison GG, Van Itallie TB: Comparison in man of total body electrical conductivity and lean body mass derived from body density: validation of a new body composition method. *Metabolism* 22: 524, 1983

23. Rothschild MA, Horatz M, Schreiber SS: Albumin synthesis (first of two parts). *N Engl J Med* 286: 748, 1972

24. Rothschild MA, Horatz M, Schreiber SS: Albumin synthesis (second of two parts). *N Engl J Med* 286: 816, 1972

25. Cano N, Fernandez JP, Lacombe P, Lankester M, Pascal S, Defayolle M, Labastie J, Saingra S: Statistical selection of nutritional parameters in hemodialysed patients. *Kidney Int* 32 (Suppl 22): S178 1987

26. Dominioni L, Dionigi R: Immunological function and nutritional assessment. *JPEN J Parenter Enteral Nutr* 11: 70S, 1987

27. Twomey P, Ziegler D, Rombeau J: Utility of skin testing in nutritional assessment: A critical review. *JPEN J Parenter Enteral Nutr* 6: 50, 1982

28. Hak LJ, Leffell MS, Lamanna RW, Teasley KM, Bazzarre CH, Mattern WD: Reversal of skin test anergy during maintenance hemodialysis by protein and calorie supplementation. *Am J Clin Nutr* 36: 1089, 1982

29. Maroni BJ, Steinman TI, Mitch WE: A method for estimating nitrogen intake of patients with chronic renal failure. *Kidney Int* 27: 58, 1985

30. Wetstein L: Dietary considerations in the treatment of renal disease. in *Nutrition and the Kidney*, edited by Mitch WE, Klahr S, Boston, Little Brown and Co, 1988, p 299

31. Kopple JD: Nutritional therapy in kidney failure. *Nutr Rev* 39: 193, 1981

32. Mitch WE, Milmore DW: Nutritional considerations in the treatment of acute renal failure. in *Acute Renal Failure*, edited by Brenner BM, Lazarus JM, New York, Churchill Livingstone, 1988, p 618

33. Mault JR, Bartlett RH, Dechert RE, Clark SF, Swartz RD: Starvation a major contribution to mortality in acute renal failure? *Trans Am Soc Artif Intern Organs* 29: 390, 1983

34. Wilmore DW: Mechanisms of catabolism in acutely stressed patients. *4th Int Congr Nutr Metab in Renal Dis* (Abstract), 1985

35. Mitch WE, May RC, Clark AS, Maroni BJ, Kelly RA: Influence of insulin resistance and amino acid supply on muscle protein turnover in uremia. *Kidney Int* 32 (Suppl 22): S104, 1987

36. Salusky IB, Slugel-Link RM, Jones MR: Effects of acute uremia on protein degradation and amino acid release in the rat hemicorpus. *Kidney Int* 24 (Suppl 16): S43, 1983

37. Mitch WE, Clark AS: Muscle protein turnover in uremia. *Kidney Int* 24 (Suppl 16): S2, 1983

38. Allman MA, Stewart PM, Tiller DJ, Horvath JS, Duggin GG, Johnson J, Hall BM: Haemodialysis patients: Protein and energy nutrition. *4th Int Congr Nutr Metab in Renal Des* (Abstract), 1985

39. Schworer CM, Mortimore GE: Glucagon-induced autophagy and proteolysis in rat liver: mediation by selective deprivation of intracellular amino acids. *Proc Natl Acad Sci USA* 73: 3169, 1979

40. May RC, Clark AS, Goheer A, Mitch WE: Identification of specific defects in insulin-mediated muscle metabolism in acute uremia. *Kidney Int* 23: 490, 1985

41. Maroni BJ, Karapanos G, Mitch WE: System A amino acid transport in incubated muscle: Effect of insulin and acute uremia. *Am J Physiol* 251: F74, 1986

42. Maroni BJ, Karapanos G, Mitch WE: System ASC and Na-independent neutral amino acid transport in muscle of uremic rats. *Am J Physiol* 251: F81, 1986

43. Feinstein EI: Parenteral nutrition in acute renal failure. *Am J Nephrol* 5: 145, 1985

44. Clark AS, Mitch WE: Muscle protein turnover and glucose uptake in acutely uremic rats: Effects of insulin and the duration of renal insufficiency. *J Clin Invest* 72: 836, 1983

45. Heidland A, Weipert J, Schaefer RM, Heidbreder E, Peter G, Hörl WH: Proteases and other catabolic factors in renal failure. *Kidney Int* 32: 594, 1987

46. Hörl W, Wanner C, Schollmeyer P: Proteinases in catabolism and malnutrition. *JPEN J Parenter Enteral Nutr* 11: 988, 1987

47. Schaefer RM, Heidland A, Hörl WH: Leucocyte proteinases and proteinase inhibitors in the catabolism of acute renal failure. *Kidney Int* 32 (Suppl 22): S100, 1987

48. Baracos V, Rodemann P, Dinarello CA, Goldberg AL: Stimulation of muscle protein degradation and prostaglandin E$_2$ release by leukocytic pyrogen (interleukin-1). *New Eng J Med* 308: 553, 1983

49. Clark AS, Kelly AS, Mitch WE: Systemic response to thermal injury in rats: increased protein degradation and altered glucose utilization in muscle. *J Clin Invest* 74: 888, 1984

50. May RC, Kelly RA, Mitch WE: Metabolic acidosis stimulates protein degradation in rat muscle by a glucocorticoid-dependent mechanism. *J Clin Invest* 77: 614, 1986

51. Mault JR, Dechert RE, Bartlett RH, Swartz RD, Ferguson SK: Oxygen consumption during hemodialysis for acute renal failure. *Trans Am Soc Artif Intern Organs* 28: 510, 1982

52. Mitch WE, Saper DW: An evaluation of reduced dialysis frequency using nutritional therapy. *Kidney Int* 20: 122, 1981

53. Spreiter SC, Myers BD, Swenson R: Protein energy requirements in subjects with acute renal failure receiving intermittent hemodialysis. *Am J Clin Nutr* 33: 1433, 1980

54. Anderson CF, Loosbrock LM, Motness MS: Nutrient intake in critically ill patients: Too many or too few calories? *Mayo Clin Proc* 61: 853, 1986

55. Kinney J: Indirect calorimetry in malnutrition: nutritional assessment of therapeutic reference? *JPEN J Parenter Enteral Nutr* 11: 98S, 1987

56. Harris JA, Benedict FG: *A Biometric Study of Basal Metabolism in Man*. Washington, DC, Carnegie Institute of Washington, 1919

57. Feinstein EI, Massry SG: Nutritional therapy in acute renal failure. in *Nutrition and the Kidney*. edited by Mitch WE,

Klahr S, Boston, Little Brown and Co, 1988, p 80

58. Blumenkrantz MJ, Kopple JD, Koffler A, Kamdar AK, Healy MD, Feinstein EI, Massry SG: Total parenteral nutrition in the management of acute renal failure. *Am J Clin Nutr* 31: 1831, 1978

59. Pelosi G, Proietti R: Acute renal failure: Parenteral nutrition with essential and non-essential amino acids. *Nutr Supp Serv* 2: 22, 1982

60. Tescher M, Heidland A: Nutrition in acute renal failure. *Blood Purif* 3: 170, 1985

61. Feinstein EI, Blumenkrantz MJ, Healy M, Koffler A, Silberman H, Massry SG, Kopple JD: Clinical and metabolic responses to parenteral nutrition in acute renal failure – a controlled double-blind study. *Medicine* 60: 124, 1981

62. Feinstein EI, Kopple JD, Silberman H, Massry SG: Total parenteral nutrition with high or low nitrogen intake in patients with acute renal failure. *Kidney Int* 24 (Suppl 16): S319, 1983

63. Abel RM, Beck CH, Abbott WM, Ryan JA Jr, Barnett GO, Fisher JE: Improved survival from acute renal failure after treatment with intravenous essential L-amino acids and glucose. Results of a prospective double-blind study. *New Eng J Med* 288: 695, 1973

64. Leonard CD, Luke RG, Siegel RR: Parenteral essential amino acids in acute renal failure. *Urology* 6: 154, 1975

65. Kosanovich JM, Dumler F, Horst M, Quandt C, Sargent JA, Levin NW: Use of urea kinetics in the nutritional care of the acutely ill patient. *JPEN J Parenteral Enteral Nutr* 9: 165, 1985

66. Kouba J: Vitamin, electrolyte, and trace minerals in patients with renal failure requiring total parenteral nutrition. *ADA RDPG Newsletter* 5: 7, 1986

67. Wesson DE, Mitch WE, Wilmore DW: Nutritional considerations in the treatment of acute renal failure. in *Acute Renal Failure*, edited by Brenner BM, Lazarus JM, Philadelphia, WB Saunders Co, 1983, p 618

68. Kopple JD: Causes of catabolism and wasting in acute or chronic renal failure. *Proc Int Congr Nephrol* 9: 1498, 1984

69. Lowrie EG, Laird NM, Parker TF, Sargent JA: Effect of the hemodialysis prescription of patient morbidity: Report from the National Cooperative Dialysis Study. *N Engl J Med* 305: 1176, 1981

70. Kelly RA, Mitch WE: Creatinine, uric acid, and other nitrogenous waste products: Clinical implication of the imbalance between their production and elimination in uremia. *Semin Nephrol* 3: 286, 1983

71. Bianchi R, Mariani G, Toni MG, Carmassi F: The metabolism of serum albumin in renal failure on conservative and dialysis therapy. *Am J Clin Nutr* 31: 1615, 1978

72. Falkenhagen D, Falkenhagen U, Schmicker R, Tessenow W, Holtz M, Schmidt R, Schmitt E, Klinkmann H: Serum complement and protein metabolism in chronic dialysis patients. *Int J Artif Organs* 2: 65, 1979

73. Kopple JD, Shinaberger JH, Coburn JW, Sorensen MK, Rubini ME: Optimal dietary protein treatment during chronic hemodialysis. *Trans Am Soc Artif Intern Organs* 15: 302, 1969

74. Carvounis CP, Carvounis G, Hung MH: Nutritional status of maintenance hemodialysis patients. *Am J Clin Nutr* 43: 946, 1986

75. Monteon FJ, Laidlaw SA, Shaib JK, Kopple JD: Energy expenditure in patients with CRF. *Kidney Int* 30: 741, 1986

76. Kluthe R, Luttgen FM, Capetiann T, Heinze V, Katz N, Sudhoff A: Protein requirements in maintenance hemodialysis. *Am J Clin Nutr* 31: 1812, 1978

77. Wolfson J, Strong CJ, Minturn D, Gray DK, Kopple JD:

78. Slomowitz L, Monteon F, Lam C, Laidlaw S, Kopple J: Energy requirements in hemodialysis patients. *Abstracts Am Soc Nephrol* 19: 89A, 1986

79. Davidson MB, Fisher MB, Dabir-Vaziri N, Schaffer M: Effect of protein intake and dialysis on the abnormal growth hormone, glucose, and insulin homeostasis in uremia. *Metabolism* 25: 455, 1976

80. Phillips LS, Pennisi AJ, Belosky DC: Somatomedin activity and inorganic sulfate in children undergoing dialysis. *J Clin Endocrinol Metab* 46: 165, 1978

81. Phillips LS, Kopple JD: Circulating somatomedin activity and sulfate levels in adults with normal and impaired kidney function. *Metabolism* 30: 1019, 1981

82. Massry SG: Pathogenesis of uremic toxicity. in *Textbook of Nephrology*, edited by Massry SG, Glassock RJ, Baltimore, Williams and Wilkins, 1983, vol 2, p 73

83. Kopple JD, Cianciaruso B, Massry SG: Does parathyroid hormone cause protein wasting? *Contr Nephrol* 20: 138, 1980

84. Lindenau K, Kokot F, Froehling PT: Suppression of parathyroid hormone by therapy with a mixture of keto analogues/amino acids in hemodialysis patients. *Nephron* 43: 84, 1986

85. Kopple JD, Fukuda S: Effects of amino acid infusion and renal failure on the uptake and release of amino acids by the dog kidney. *Am J Clin Nutr* 33: 1363, 1980

86. Wolfson M, Jones WR, Kopple JD: Amino acid losses during hemodialysis with infusion of amino acids and glucose. *Kidney Int* 21: 500, 1982

87. Farrell PC, Hone PW: Dialysis-induced catabolism. *Am J Clin Nutr* 33: 1417, 1980

88. Kopple JD, Swendsied ME: Vitamin nutrition in patients undergoing maintenance hemodialysis. *Kidney Int* 7 (Suppl 2): S79, 1975

89. Fürst P, Alvestrand A, Bergström J: Effects of nutrition and catabolic stress on intracellular amino acid pools in uremia. *Am J Clin Nutr* 33: 1387, 1980

90. Alvestrand A, Gutierrez A, Wahren J, Bergström J: Blood-membrane interaction without dialysis induces increased protein catabolism in normal man. *4th Int Congr Nutr Metab in Renal Dis* (Abstract), 1985

91. Pun KK, Yeung CK, Chak W, Ho PWM, Chan MK, Lin JH, Yeung RTT: Effects of selective and non-selective beta-blockers on the alanine and free fatty acid responses to glucagon challenge in hemodialysis patients. *Clin Nephrol* 26: 222, 1986

92. May RC, Kelly RA, Mitch WE: Mechanisms for abnormal muscle protein turnover in chronic uremia: The influence of metabolic acidosis. *J Clin Invest* 79: 1099, 1987

93. Seyffart G, Ensminger A, Scholz R: Significant increase of body mass during long-term bicarbonate hemodialysis. *4th Int Congr Nutr Metab in Renal Dis* (Abstract), 1985

94. Stefanidis CJ, Patrikarea A, Neofotistou V, Ziroyiannic P, Papadoyannakis N: Metabolic acidosis and protein metabolism in uremia. *4th Int Congr Nutr Metab in Renal Dis* (Abstract), 1985

95. Hara Y, May RC, Kelly RA, Mitch WE: Acidosis, not azotemia, stimulates branched-chain, amino acid catabolism in uremic rats. *Kidney Int* 32: 808, 1987

96. Yamauchi A, Fujii M, Shirai D, Mikami H, Okada A, Imai E, Ando A, Orita Y, Kamada T: Plasma concentration and peritoneal clearance of oxalate in patients on continuous ambulatory peritoneal dialysis (CAPD). *Clin Nephrol* 25: 181, 1986

97. Ono K, Hisasue Y, Morimatsu M: Should vitamin C supple-

mentation be restricted in regular dialysis patients? *ASAIO Trans* 32: 111, 1986

98. Pru C, Eaton J, Kjellstrand C: Vitamin C intoxication and hyperoxalemia in chronic hemodialysis patients. *Nephron* 39: 112, 1985

99. Mydlik M, Derzsiova K, Valek A, Szabo T, Dandar V, Takac M: Vitamins and continuous ambulatory peritoneal dialysis (CAPD). *Int Urol Nephrol* 17: 281, 1985

100. Ramirez G, Chen M, Boyce HW, Fuller SM, Butcher DE, Brueggemeyer CD, Newton JL: The plasma and red cell vitamin B levels of chronic hemodialysis patients: A longitudinal study. *Nephron* 42: 41, 1986

101. Wolfson M, Kopple JD: The effects of vitamin B_6 deficiency in chronically azotemic and sham-operated rats. *Kidney Int* 32 (Suppl 22): S162, 1987

102. Dunnell EG, Teschan PE, Wilson PC: Vitamin levels in dialysis patients. *4th Int Congr Nutr Metab in Renal Dis* (Abstract), 1985

103. Henderson IS, Leung ACT, Shenkin A: Vitamin status in continuous ambulatory peritoneal dialysis. *Peritoneal Dial Bull* 4: 143, 1984

104. Stein G, Schone S, Geinitz D, Abendroth K, Kokot F, Funfstuck R, Sperschneider H, Keil E: No tissue level abnormality of vitamin A concentration despite elevated serum vitamin A of uremic patients. *Clin Nephrol* 25: 87, 1986

105. Vahlquist A, Berne B, Danielson BG, Grefberg N, Berne C: Vitamin A losses during continuous ambulatory peritoneal dialysis. *Nephrol* 41: 179, 1985

106. Cohen JD, Viljoen M, Clifford D, De Oliveira AA, Milne FJ: Plasma vitamin E levels in a chronically hemolyzing group of dialysis patients. *Clin Nephrol* 25: 42, 1986

107. Taccone-Gallucci M, Giardini O, Ausiello C, Piazza A, Spagnoli GC, Bandino D, Lubrono R, Taggi F, Evangelista B, Monaco P, Tabilio MR, Valeri M, Citti G, Casciani CU: Vitamin E supplementation in hemodialysis patients: Effects on peripheral blood mononuclear cells, lipid peroxidation and immune response. *Clin Nephrol* 25: 81, 1986

108. Blumenkrantz MJ, Roberts CE, Card B, Coburn JW, Kopple JD: Nutritional management of the adult patient undergoing peritoneal dialysis. *J Am Diet Assoc* 73: 251, 1978

109. O'Connell PJ, Ibels LS, Thomas MA, Harris DCH, Kesselhut J, Heathcote K: Nutritional assessment in patients on long-term continuous ambulatory peritoneal dialysis. *Kidney Int* 30: 617, 1986

110. Diamond SM, Henrich WL: Nutrition and peritoneal dialysis. in *Nutrition and the Kidney*, edited by Mitch WE, Klahr S, Boston, Little Brown and Co, 1988, p 80

111. Acchiardo S, Moore L, Kraus A, LaHatte G: Nutritional evaluation of CAPD patients. *Peritoneal Dial Bull* 4: S1, 1984

112. Flynn MA: Nutritional problems in continuous ambulatory peritoneal dialysis. *Peritoneal Dial Bull* 4: S142, 1984

113. Gahl GM, Baeyer HV, Averdunk R, Riedinger H, Borowzak B, Schurig R, Becker H, Kessel M: Outpatient evaluation of dietary intake and nitrogen removal in continuous ambulatory peritoneal dialysis. *Ann Intern Med* 94: 643, 1981

114. DeSanto NG, Capodicasa G, Capasso G, Nuzzi F, Giordano G: Body composition in uremic children on CAPD and hemodialysis. in *Frontiers in Peritoneal Dialysis*, edited by Maher JF, Winchester JF, New York, Field, Rich and Assoc, 1986, p 443

115. Blumenkrantz MJ, Kopple JD, Moran JK, Coburn JW: Metabolic balance studies and dietary protein requirements in patients undergoing continuous ambulatory peritoneal dialysis. *Kidney Int* 21: 849, 1982

116. Kopple JD, Blumenkrantz MJ: Nutritional requirements for patients undergoing continuous ambulatory peritoneal dialysis. *Kidney Int* 24 (Suppl 16): S18, 1984

117. Haber MO, Pettit JM: Nutritional considerations in the diabetic patient on continuous ambulatory peritoneal dialysis. *Peritoneal Dial Bull* 2: S50, 1982

118. Kopple JD, Blumenkrantz MJ: Nutrition in adults on continuous ambulatory peritoneal dialysis. *Perspect Peritoneal Dial* 2: 1, 1984

119. Grodstein GP, Blumenkrantz MJ, Kopple JD, Moran JK, Coburn JW: Glucose absorption during continuous ambulatory peritoneal dialysis. *Kidney Int* 19: 564, 1981

120. DiMaio G, Carozzi S, Nasini G, Lamperi S: Serum lipids patterns in uremic patients after 48 months on CAPD. *Peritoneal Dial Bull* 4: S18, 1984

121. Lindholm B, Ahlberg M, Alvestrand A, Fürst P, Tranaeus A, Bergström J: Nitrogen balance and protein and energy intake during CAPD. *4th Int Congr Nutr Metab in Renal Dis* (Abstract), 1985

122. Flugel-Link RM, Jones MR, Kopple JD: Red cell and plasma amino acid concentrations in renal failure. *JPEN J Parenter Enteral Nutr* 7: 450, 1983

123. Dombros N, Oren A, Marliss EB: Plasma amino acid profiles and amino acid losses in patients undergoing CAPD. *Peritoneal Dial Bull* 2: 27, 1982

124. Khanna R, Wu G, Rodella H, Oreopoulos DG: Use of amino acid containing solution in CAPD patients. *Peritoneal Dial Bull* 4: S121, 1984

125. Pederson FB, Bragsholt C, Laier E, Frifelt JJ, Trostmann AF, Ekelund S, Paaby P: Alternate use of amino acid and glucose solutions in CAPD. *Peritoneal Dial Bull* 5: 215, 1985

126. Oreopoulos DG, Marliss E, Anderson GH, Oren A, Dombross N, Williams P, Khanna R, Rodella H, Brandes L: Nutritional aspects of CAPD and the potential use of amino acid containing dialysis solutions. *Peritoneal Dial Bull* 3: S10, 1983

127. Poisetti PG, Fontena F, Ballocchi S, Zanazzi MA, Scarpioni L: Protein losses in long-term continuous ambulatory peritoneal dialysis (CAPD). *Peritoneal Dial Bull* 5: 271, 1985

128. Sandoz P, Vallance D, Winder AF, Walls J: Protein and amino acid losses from the peritoneum during CAPD and CCPD. in *Frontiers in Peritoneal Dialysis*, edited by Maher JF, Winchester JF, New York, Field, Rich and Assoc, 1986, p 446

129. Kopple JD, Blumenkrantz MJ, Jones MR, Moran JK, Coburn JW: Plasma amino acid levels and amino acid losses during continuous ambulatory peritoneal dialysis. *Am J Clin Nutr* 36: 395, 1982

130. Young GA, Brownjohn AM, Parsons FM: Protein losses in patients receiving continuous ambulatory peritoneal dialysis. *Nephron* 45: 196, 1987

131. Blumenkrantz MJ, Gahl GM, Kopple JD, Kamdar AV, Jones MR, Kessel M, Coburn JW: Protein losses during peritoneal dialysis. *Kidney Int* 19: 593, 1981

132. Williams P, Marliss E, Anderson GH, Oren A, Stein A, Khanna R, Pettit J, Brandes L, Rodella H, Mupas L, Dombros N, Oreopoulos DG: Amino acid absorption following intraperitoneal administration in CAPD patients. *Peritoneal Dial Bull* 2: 124, 1982

133. Oren A, Wu G, Anderson GH, Marliss E, Khanna R, Pettit J, Mupas L, Rodella H, Brandes L, Roncari DA, Kakis G, Harrison J, McNeil K, Oreopoulos DG: Effective use of amino acid dialysate over four weeks in CAPD patients. *Peritoneal Dial Bull* 3: 66, 1983

134. Borah MF, Schoenfeld PY, Gotch FA, Sargent JA, Wolfson

M, Humphreys MH: Nitrogen balance during intermittent dialysis therapy of uremia. *Kidney Int* 14: 491, 1978

135. Alvestrand A: Nutritional requirements of hemodialysis patients. in *Nutrition and the Kidney,* edited by Mitch WE, Klahr S, Boston, Little Brown and Co, 1988, p 180

136. Feinstein EI, Kopple JD: Severe wasting and malnutrition in a patient undergoing maintenance dialysis [clinical conference]. *Am J Nephrol* 5: 398, 1985

137. Rylance PB, Gordge MP, Saynon R, Parsons V, Weston MJ: Fish oil modifies lipids and reduces platelet aggregatability in hemodialysis patients. *Nephron* 43: 196, 1986

138. Paganini EP, Flaque J, Whitman G, Nakamoto S: Amino acid balance in patients with oliguric acute renal failure undergoing slow continuous ultrafiltration (SCUF). *Trans Am Soc Artif Intern Organs* 28: 615, 1982

139. Quarto di Palo F, Buccianti G, Valenti GF, Miradoli R, Polli EE: Nutritive hemodialysis in renal failure. *Dial Transplant* 7: 457, 1978

140. Acchiardo S, Moore L, Cockrell S: Effect of essential amino acids on chronic hemodialysis patients. *Trans Am Soc Artif Intern Organs* 28: 608, 1982

141. Heidland A, Kult J: Long-term effects of essential amino acids supplementation in patients on regular dialysis treatments. *Clin Nephrol* 3: 234, 1975

142. Feinstein EI: Nutritional hemodialysis. *Kidney Int* 32 (Suppl 22): S167, 1987

143. Metcoff J, Dutta S, Burns G, Pederson J, Matter B, Rennert O: Effects of amino acid infusions on cell metabolism in hemodialyzed patients with uremia. *Kidney Int* 24 (Suppl 16): S 87, 1983

144. Cotton JR, Woodward T, Knochel JP: Correction of uremic cellular injury with a protein-restricted amino acid-supplemented diet. *Am J Kidney Dis* 5: 233, 1985

145. Nath KA, Hostetter TH: Nutritional requirements of diabetics with nephropathy. in *Nutrition and the Kidney,* edited by Mitch WE, Klahr S, Boston, Little Brown and Co, 1988, p 250

146. Miller DG: Use of total parenteral nutrition in patients with renal failure. *Nutr Supp Serv* 1: 14, 1981

147. Batist G, Bistrian BR, Kaldany A, Phinney S, Busick EJ, Miller DG, D'Elia JA: Intravenous total parenteral nutrition in diabetic renal failure. *Nephron* 28: 244, 1981

148. Morley JE: Nutritional status of the elderly. *Am J Med* 81: 679, 1986

149. Hruska KA: Requirements for calcium, phosphorus and vitamin D. in *Nutrition and the Kidney,* edited by Mitch WE, Klahr S, Boston, Little Brown and Co, 1988, p 104

150. Antoniou LD, Shalhoub RJ: Zinc-induced enhancement of lymphocyte function and viability in chronic uremia. *Nephron* 40: 13, 1985

151. Wallaeys B, Cornelis R, Mees L, Lameire N: Trace elements in serum, packed cells, and dialysate of CAPD patients. *Kidney Int* 30: 599, 1986

152. Bulla M, Bremer HJ, Ronda-Vidozola R, Roth B: The effect of oral essential amino acids and their keto analogues on children receiving regular hemodialysis. *Int J Ped Nephrol* 7: 73, 1986

153. Arnold WC, Hill DE, Boughter M: Relationship of nutritional status to erythrocyte insulin receptors in adults and children with uremia. *Kidney Int* 32 (Suppl 22): S202, 1987

154. Salusky IB, Fine RN, Nelson P, Blumenkrantz MJ, Kopple JD: Nutritional status of children undergoing continuous ambulatory peritoneal dialysis. *Am J Clin Nutr* 38: 599, 1983

155. Kohaut EC: Growth in children with end-stage renal disease treated with continuous ambulatory peritoneal dialysis for at least one year. *Peritoneal Dial Bull* 2: 159, 1982

156. Davis TA, Klahr S: Exercise and nutrition in patients with renal disease. in *Nutrition and the Kidney,* edited by Mitch WE, Klahr S, Boston, Little Brown and Co, 1988, p 277

157. Kolker JD, Galligan E, Trebbin WM, Solomon RJ, Herbert PN, Weinberg MS: Reduction of hyperlipidemia in continuous ambulatory peritoneal dialysis. *Peritoneal Dial Bull* 4: S34, 1984

158. Kettner A: Exercise in dialysis patients. *Int J Artif Organs* 5: 83, 1982

159. Goldberg AP, Hagberg J, Delmez JA, Carney RM, McKevitt PM, Ehsani AA, Harter HR: The metabolic and psychological effects of exercise training in hemodialysis patients. *Am J Clin Nutr* 33: 1620, 1980

160. Painter PL, Nelson-Worel JN, Hill MM, Thornberry DR, Weinstein AB: Effects of exercise training during hemodialysis. *Nephron* 43: 87, 1986

161. Davis TA, Karl IE, Goldberg AP, Harter HR: Effects of exercise training on muscle protein catabolism in uremia. *Kidney Int* 24: 5, 1983

162. Castellino P, Bia M, DeFronzo RA: Metabolic response to exercise in dialysis patients. *Kidney Int* 32: 877, 1987

MANAGEMENT OF THE UREMIC DIABETIC PATIENT

ELI A. FRIEDMAN

INTRODUCTION: SCOPE OF PROBLEM OF UREMIA IN DIABETES

According to the National Diabetes Data Group, there are approximately 5.8 million people in the United States who have been diagnosed by a physician as being diabetic. An additional 4 to 5 million people have undiagnosed diabetes (1). The prevalence of diabetes is rising despite a falling incidence, due to a 19% decline in deaths caused by diabetes from a peak of 300 per 100,000 population in 1973, to 230 per 100,000 in 1981. Diabetes is the seventh leading underlying cause of death. In 1982, 34,583 deaths were attributed to diabetes. Individuals with diabetes have a higher than normal risk for macro- and microvascular disease, diabetic coma and fetal or maternal death complicating pregnancy. Diabetes is responsible for 5,800 new cases of blindness, 4,500 perinatal deaths, 40,000 lower extremity amputations and 3,000 deaths in diabetic coma (ketotic and hyperosmolar). By conservative estimate, about 4,000 new cases of end-stage renal disease (ESRD) are caused by diabetes annually (2). Because etiologies other than diabetes are less securely diagnosed, Mauer and Chavers contend that 'Diabetes is the most important cause of ESRD in the Western world' (3). We concur.

In 1922, when Banting et al (4) administered pancreatic extracts to seven diabetic patients observing that 'Patients report a complete relief from the subjective symptoms of the disease', they had no knowledge of the myriad vascular complications which accompany long-term life prolongation in this formerly fatal disorder. As diabetic patients survived beyond 10 years, they manifested a peculiar triopathy (neuropathy, retinopathy, nephropathy) (5) apparently unresponsive to any treatment regimen. After learning to juggle insulin, diet, and activity, about one-half of diabetics who benefited from 'Banting's miracle' lost vision and died unseeing and in renal failure. Other diabetic patients whether treated with insulin or by a dietary regimen, suffered an inordinately high prevalence of fatal heart attacks and cerebrovascular disease.

For 20 years, clinicians vigorously debated whether renal and other vascular complications of diabetes were – like glucose intolerance – genetically predetermined, and therefore unavoidable, or a result of hyperglycemia, and potentially preventable. Confounding efforts to elucidate the natural history of vasculopathy was unrecognized confusion between the two major subtypes of diabetes, each presenting as hyperglycemia.

To address this problem, expert committees were convened by the World Health Organization (6) and the National Diabetes Data Group (NDDG) (7). Their reports suggest that the name 'insulin-dependent diabetes mellitus (IDDM)' be used for a condition 'characterized by abrupt onset of symptoms, insulinopenia, dependence on injected insulin to sustain life, and proneness to ketosis.' Confirmation of IDDM, according to the NDDG, is provided by demonstrating low plasma insulin levels, circulating islet cell antibody (ICA) titers and characteristic HLA DR types (DR3, DQ and DR4). When attempting to classify new onset diabetic patients it is evident that the majority (80 to 95% depending on race) have noninsulin dependent diabetes (NIDDM). Patients with NIDDM are usually older at onset of hyperglycemia, typically obese, and have 'normal' circulating insulin levels to which their tissues are 'resistant.' IDDM and NIDDM are also designated as Type I and Type II diabetes respectively.

Utilizing the NDDG guidelines, Wilson et al (8) classified 100 consecutive newly diagnosed diabetic patients aged 13 to 70 years at the time of starting insulin. In their series, 70 patients who were diagnosed under the age of 40 years fit the NDDG stereotype for IDDM relatively well; 88% of those who were under 20 years at diagnosis were ICA positive, one-third were DR3/DR4 heterozygotes and only 6% had

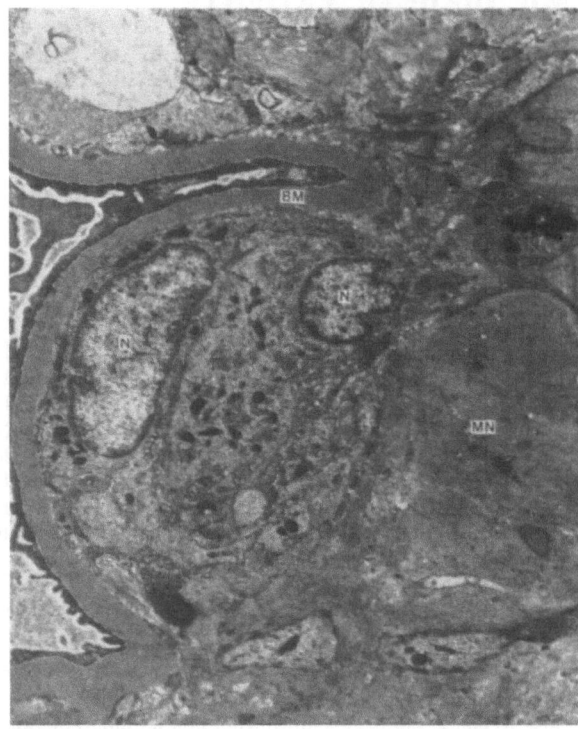

Figure 1. Electron photomicropgraph of glomerulus obtained by biopsy from a proteinuric diabetic patient showing a thick glomerular basement membrane (BM) and an expanded mesangium forming a nodule (MN). The capillary loop is filled with endothelial cells in which nuclei are marked (N).

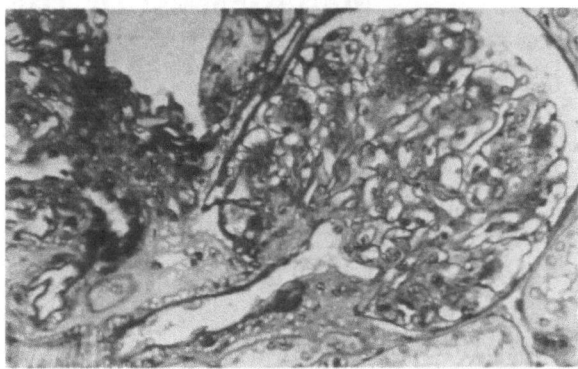

Figure 2. Light photomicropgraph of glomerulus from an asymptomatic diabetic patient showing mesangial expansion and early nodular glomerulosclerosis.

neither high risk antigen. NDDG guidelines do not permit classification of many diabetic patients who are older than 40 years of age at diagnosis; only one-fifth of whom are ICA positive and less than one-third are DR3/DR4 heterozygotes.

Approximately 15 years after Banting's introduction of insulin, Kimmelsteil and Wilson (9) recognized a specific, diabetes-induced nodular intercapillary glomerulosclerosis (KW nodule) in kidneys from NIDDM patients studied at autopsy. KW nodules, now considered the hallmark of diabetic nephropathy, occur in both IDDM and NIDDM, and represent expansion of glomerular mesangial matrix into single or multiple spherical lesions (Figure 1) which encroach on patent capillary loops reducing glomerular blood flow. Equally prevalent in both diabetes types is diffuse intercapillary glomeruslosclerosis, a thickened glomerular basement membrane, associated with an enlarged mesangium filled with periodic acid-Schiff staining material (Figure 2).

Clinical nephropathy develops in about 30% of patients with IDDM and 10% of patients with NIDDM. Its course is well documented in IDDM but only partially characterized in NIDDM. Nephropathy is first manifested by microalbuminuria (minimal quantities of albuminuria) followed after months to a decade or longer by fixed proteinuria, and progressive azotemia and renal death (10).

NATURAL HISTORY OF DIABETIC NEPHROPATHY

Carefully studied series of NIDDM and IDDM patients have extended our concept of the onset of diabetic nephropathy from a disease defined by proteinuria and azotemia, to a disorder beginning a decade earlier with subtle deviations from normal renal function. What was formerly termed 'early diabetic nephropathy' (proteinuria of about 1 g/24 h with or without serum creatinine elevation to about 2 mg/dl [177 μmol/l]) is now regarded as a correlate of extensive histopathologic renal injury. Renal functional perturbations precede development of glomerulosclerosis by as long as a decade. The evolution of diabetic glomerulosclerosis can be followed in biopsies of kidneys transplanted from nondiabetic donors to diabetic recipients. Glomerular basement membrane (GBM) thickening and mesangial expansion are evident within a year, and in some patients typical KW nodules are present by the third year (11). The course of diabetic glomerulopathy has also been inferred from studies in animal models. Whether it is valid to extrapolate from the streptozotocin-induced diabetic rat and alloxan-induced diabetic dog to human diabetic nephropathy is undetermined.

Abnormalities noted in hyperglycemic IDDM patients include a supranormal glomerular filtration rate (GFR), increased renal plasma flow (RPF) and enlargement of the whole kidney and glomerulus. Reduction in renal size and a decrease in GFR to normal can be effected by normalization of plasma glucose by subcutaneous administration of insulin by a programmed pump. The mechanism for increased glomerular size (hypertrophy) in diabetes is not understood. There is a linear relationship between the duration of diabetes and the number of glomeruli sufficiently occluded by glomerulosclerosis to be obsolescent. With progressive loss of glomerular function, there occurs compensatory hypertrophy in residual glomeruli; the most pronounced hupertrophy is noted in least effected glomeruli. Immunglobulin and albumin are deposited in a ribbon-like pattern along tubular basement membranes and Bowman's capsule in some diabetic kidneys, probably reflecting passive entrapment of plasma proteins rather than an active immune process. Albumin deposition in a linear pattern has also been observed by fluorescence microscopy in skin and muscle though its significance is equally obscure (12).

PATHOGENESIS OF DIABETIC NEPHROPATHY

Debate over the relative importance of capillary hypertension and hyperglycemia in the pathogenesis of diabetic glomerulopathy has recently been diverted by new interest in the sorbitol end-path of glucose metabolism. Winegrad (13) challenged the view that 'some factor common to diverse types of diabetes mellitus apparently confers risks for progressive disease and clinical manifestations in a characteristic group of susceptible sites'. He states the 'case for myoinsoitol' as important to diabetic end-organ damage based on: 1) Hyperglycemia causes increased polyol activity in peripheral nerve axons and Schwann cells associated with decreases in nerve myoinositol and motor nerve conduction velocity (14). 2) Diabetic rats treated with an aldose reductase inhibitor do not accumulate sorbitol in nerves and thereby preserve their myoinositol content and electrical conductivity. 3) Feeding rats a 1% myoinositol diet prevents electrical injury to nerves by induced-diabetes even though hyperglycemia and increased nerve sorbitol levels are present (15). 4) Glomeruli isolated from streptozotocin-induced diabetic rast exhibit elevated hexitol (probably sorbitol), small decreases in myoinositol, and significant decreases in $Na^+ - K^+$-ATPase (16); inhibition of aldose reductase prevents these changes. 5) Lastly, aldose reductase inhibition blocks the 40% increase in GFR caused by hyperglycemia without decreasing blood pressure or the level of blood glucose (17). Feeding a 1% myoinositol diet reduced elevated GFR in streptozotocin-induced diabetic rast without lowering blood glucose or blood pressure.

Some complications of diabetes result from 'a complex pattern of chronic structural modification that is site specific and not unique to diabetes' while others have 'significant site-specific aspects of the vascular pathology in the so-called microangiopathic complications', Winegrad theorizes that hyperglycemia activates a series of perturbations which decrease $Na^+ - K^+$-ATPase activity in peripheral nerve, kidney, and retina. Hyperglycemia, he reasons, inhibits a recently identified metabolic regulatory system which uses receptor stimulated phosphatidylinositol turnover to control a major component of the tissue's $Na^+ - K^+$-ATPase activity. Phosphatidylinositol synthesis, which is necessary for the system's maintenance selectivity uses myoinositol. At normal plasma levels of myoinositol, hyperglycemia acts through increased polyol pathway activity to impair the maintenance of small myoinositol pools, inhibits phosphatidylinositol synthesis dependent on these pools, and prevents

maintenance of pools used to control the activity of a component of $Na^+ - K^+$-ATPase Decreased $Na^+ - K^+$-ATPase activity in vascular smooth muscle is a potential cause of derangements in regulation of intraglomerular vascular tone and of altered responses to vasoactive neurotransmitters and hormones (13). This mechanism may be the basic perturbation in glomerular hemodynamics in diabetes.

As an alternative explanation for diabetic complications, kidney transplantation has generated compelling evidence that hyperglycemia is a major if not sole determinant of diabetic glomerulopathy. Firstly, recurrent intercapillary glomerulosclerois and renal failure can destroy kidneys obtained from nondiabetics when transplanted into diabetics (18). Secondly, kidneys transplanted into recipients who have developed diabetes show characteristic KW nodules. Thirdly, early glomerulopathy is sometimes reversible in a euglycemic environment as shown by disappearance of glomerulosclerosis in two cadaveric donor kidneys obtained from a diabetic after transplantation into nondiabetic recipients (19).

Understandably, judgment as to which of three (hyperglycemia, hemodynamic, myoinositol) pathogenetic schools of diabetic complications is correct may be withheld pending further data. Furthermore, inferences from experiments in the induced-diabetic rat suggest that small vessel injury may, under defined circumstances, be associated with plasma hyperviscosity, elevated circulating thromboxane and platelet-derived growth factor(s) alone or in combination. For current patient management, normalization of hypertensive blood pressures and establishment of euglycemia are desirable clinical objectives no matter which biochemical-hemodynamic basis for diabetic complications is uncovered.

RENAL FUNCTIONAL IMPAIRMENT

Diabetic nephropathy is a silent disorder during its first decade. In NIDDM, its onset is often discovered by a laboratory report of proteinuria during treatment for some other illness. While the metabolic consequences of IDDM are usually recognized during efforts to sustain euglycemia, GFR and RPF may be continuously supernormal for years without detection until proteinuria or azotemia supervene. Retinal microvasculopathy, discoverable as leakage of intravenously injected fluorescein into the vitreous chamber, is also asymptomatic for years until vitreous hemorrhage prompts eye consultation.

Proteinuria is the most constant sign of diabetic glomerulopathy. Elevated urinary albumin excretion (>1 g/24 h) at any time in the course of diabetes signals a likelihood of progression of renal disease; the risk of renal insufficiency is approximately 20 times greater in diabetic patients with even small amounts of urinary albumin excretion than in those free of this finding (20). It is now helpful to distinguish between macro- and microalbuminuria. The Albustix@ test detects protein excretion greater than 250 mg/24 h, about 50% of which is albumin. Another commonly employed test for macroproteinuria, the heat and acetic acid test, is positive only when total urinary protein excretion increases to 3 to 4 times normal, of which albumin is the main component (about 50%) in diabetic nephropathy. Over the past 5 years, Mogensen has demonstrated that in both IDDM (21) and NIDDM (22) the leakage of small amounts of urinary albumin presages subsequent renal insufficiency. Healthy individuals excrete albumin in a range of 2.5 to 26 mg/24 h, with a geometric mean of about 9.5 mg/24 h; almost all values (92%) fall below 18 mg/24 h (23). Microalbuminuria, defined as an albumin excretion rate of between 26 and 250 mg/24 h, and measured by radioimmunoassay, is a marker of future serious nephropathy.

Nephropathy in diabetes is characterized by a slow, continuous increase in albumin excretion from microalbuminuria to a nephrotic syndrome (>3.5 g/24 h). Sustained proteinuria occurs in about one-half of all IDDM patients by the 20th year of insulin treatment; its prevalence in NIDDM is unclear. Proteinuria greater than 1 g/day in IDDM connotes the probable onset of azotemia within 1 to 5 years. The meaning of fixed proteinuria in NIDDM is less interpretable because this subset of diabetics is older and therefore prone to nephrosclerosis, in itself a cause of proteinuria. Remission, fluctuation and progression of proteinuria may occur repeatedly in the same individual.

NEPHROTIC SYNDROME

Urinary protein excretion in diabetes usually increases after 5 or more years of fixed proteinuria to more than 3.5 g/day inducing hypoalbuminemia, a reduced plasma oncotic pressure, and massive edema, the nephrotic syndrome. Nephrotic patients may gain 10 to 30 kg, over weeks to months, due to retention of salt and water. A markedly expanded intravascular volume often is mistaken for congestive failure due to intrinsic heart disease. While cardiomyopathy is not infrequent in long-term diabetes, the most common explanation for massive anasarca, dyspnea, and pulmonary edema in a nephrotic diabetic is nephrogenic rather than cadiogenic fluid retention. A fluid overloaded nephrotic diabetic patient should be treated with diuretics (furosemide plus metolazone) before administering digoxin. The diagnosis of diabetic glomerulosclerosis can be inferred after observing a transition from microalbuminuria, through fixed proteinuria, to a nephrotic syndrome. A universal finding (95%) in nephrotic diabetics is the presence of coincident diabetic retinopathy. So closely are retinopathy and nephropathy linked, in a renal-retinal syndrome, that failure to detect retinopathy in a diabetic patient with a renal disorder is reason to suspect a cause other than diabetes. Resort to kidney biopsy to establish a renal diagnosis is unnecessary in most nephrotic diabetics. Biopsy may prove helpful, however, in nephrotic patients with findings atypical for diabetic nephropathy such as normal fundi, small kidneys, or red cell casts.

Nephrotic diabetics have advanced histopathologic glomerulopathy. Within approximately 6 months to 1 year following the onset of nephrotic range proteinuria, azotemia indicative of a GFR below 25 ml/min develops. There is wide variability in the rate at which proteinuric diabetic patients lose renal function. Uremia therapy can be anticipated in an individual patient by plotting the inverse (reciprocal) of the serum creatinine concentration against time. Although past experience indicates that uremia follows nephrosis within 1 to 3 years, therapeutic optimists, including the author, believe current efforts to regulate blood pressure will blunt the slope of renal functional decline thereby extending this interval. A 'worst case' projection of the impact of proteinuria was provided by Caird (24), in 1961, who found that only 28% of patients with IDDM survived for 10 years after onset of 'clinical' proteinuria in an era when neither dialysis nor kidney transplantation was available.

Signs and symptoms of renal insufficiency begin earlier in a diabetic than in a nondiabetic patient. As GFR declines below 20 ml/min, azotemic diabetic patients (both NIDDM and IDDM) suffer reduction in muscle mass and diminished tolerance to minor intercurrent disorders. A simple viral respiratory infection, for example, easily tolerated by a diabetic patient with normal renal function, may confine an azotemic diabetic patient to bed for a week. The clinical expression of visceral autonomic neuropathy intensifies as renal function deteriorates. Alternating hypotension when erect and hypertension when supine confounds blood pressure regulation. Concurrent bowel malfunction (periodic obstipation cycling with explosive noctural diarrhea), and accelerating vision loss amplify morbidity. Daily living becomes an admixture of panic and futility in a patient who is clearly failing. Maintenance of euglycemia is challenging when GFR is falling; renal catabolism of administered insulin in IDDM and endogenous insulin (and other small peptide hormones) in NIDDM is inconsistant from day to day. As a consequence, profound hypoglycemia may result from formerly safely tolerated doses of insulin or oral hypoglycemic agents.

Conservative therapy must be supplanted by either dialysis or a kidney transplant at a higher residual creatinine clearance in a diabetic than in a nondiabetic patient. Maintenance hemodialysis, though rarely required in a nondiabetic patient whose creatinine clearance is above 5 ml/min (approximately equivalent to a serum creatinine of 10 to 15 mg/dl [885 to 1327 μmol/l]), is often forced in a diabetic whose creatinine clearance falls to 10 ml/min (serum creatinine concentration of approximately 5 mg/dl [442 μmol/l]).

As a generalization, it takes between 15 and 20 years for a diabetic patient to manifest uremia. In our Brooklyn series, the mean interval between diagnosis of diabetes and performance of first hemodialysis was 14.9 ± 9.3 years. The longest interval between onset of diabetes and initiation of hemodialysis (20.5 ± 5.9 years) was noted in IDDM patients who became diabetic before the age of 20 years. Type I diabetics with onset after the age of 20 years initiated hemodialysis after a mean of 15.3 ± 8.6 years, which was not different from the mean of all 232 diabetic patients in the study.

HYPERTENSION

Hypertensive blood pressures should be corrected in every diabetic patient at all levels of renal function. Normalizing hypertensive blood pressures protects against retinal hemorrhage (25), and slows the rate of loss of GFR. Few data describe survival of diabetic patients on dialysis as a function of blood pressure control. It has been demonstrated, however, that uncontrolled hypertension adds a significant risk to patient and kidney graft survival in diabetic kidney transplant recipients (26). Effective drug regimens for blood pressure reduction can now avoid the side-effects of unbearable somnolence, crippling orthostatic hypotension, or bladder and bowel paralysis. Tailoring a combination of diuretics, vasodilators, calcium channel blockers, and renin antagonists to the individual diabetic may take weeks to months of trial and error. Angiotensin converting enzyme (ACE) inhibitors are particularly beneficial to management of hypertensive diabetics (27). Our objective in blood pressure reduction is a systolic pressure no higher than 130 mm Hg and a diastolic pressure of 80 mm Hg or below. Diuretics are vital to attainment of blood pressure control in most diabetic patients because intravascular volume expansion usually contributes to hypertension. Doses of furosemide as high as 480 mg daily are required to maintain a nephrotic diabetic patient free of edema when the creatinine clearance is less than 20 ml/min. Metolazone, a long acting thiazide, in daily doses of 5 to 20 mg, given in combination with furosemide, often effects diuresis in an hypoalbuminemic nephrotic azotemic patient who has been unresponsive to furosemide alone.

Experience suggests that enalapril alone, or in combination with transdermal clonidine (and a loop diuretic such as furosemide) will normalize blood pressure in previously difficult-to-regulate patients. ACE inhibitors reduce intrarenal hypertension, by relaxing efferent glomerular arterioles, attenuating intraglomerular hypertension, a key pathogenetic mechanism responsible for glomerular damage. We have found that about 10% of patients are unable to tolerate this regimen because of hypotension. Should there be inadequate blood pressure control, addition of transdermal clonidine or oral nifedipine usually is effective. For persistent diastolic pressures above 110 mm Hg, minoxidil in morning plus afternoon doses totaling as much as 75 mg/day is added. An important signal that the limit of conservative care has been reached in an azotemic diabetic patient is the inability to normalize blood pressure as renal insufficiency progresses.

PROTEIN RESTRICTION

The potential beneficial effect of a protein restricted diet on the course of progressive renal disease is periodically rediscovered. In 1949, Addis (28) observed 'We can improve the condition of small-kidney rats by giving them little protein and can make them uremic by giving them a lot of protein'. In dietary experiments with Masugi nephritis, Ad-

dis found that: 'On the low protein diet all the rats were markedly improved or wholly recovered, whereas all the rats that were given a high protein diet quickly died in uremia.' In insightful experiments, repeated and confirmed 30 years later, Addis removed three-quarters of renal mass and then fed protein diets which were deficient (3.7%), adequate (22.6%) or higher (64.1%) than needed for proper nutrition in the rat. Mortality varied inversely with dietary protein content, and was 38% on the high, 13% on the adequate, and 0% on the low protein diet. Addis commented that in rats with renal insufficiency, 15 g of protein a day would provide, 'a protein content just adequate for maintenance and growth.'

Pursuing this line of inquiry, Hostetter et al (29) demonstrated that the severity of glomerulosclerosis in rats with remnant kidneys or streptozotocin-induced-diabetes could be reduced by dietary protein restriction. The mechanism by which a high protein intake accelerates glomerulosclerosis has been related to hemodynamic abnormalities including increased glomerular perfusion and hyperfiltration (30). Giordano and coworkers (31) advocate low protein nutrition as 'a powerful tool in a preventive strategy for end-stage renal disease, a goal which has been missed during the last 20 years'. These investigators reported that in uremic patients matched for age, sex, renal diagnosis, and degree of hypertension who started with a mean plasma creatinine of 225 μmol/l (2.5 mg/dl), 'progression to terminal uremia was complete in 16 months in patients on free diets while it took 7.6 years for patients on low protein nutrition.' Whether the rate of intercapillary glomerulosclerosis in diabetes can be slowed by adherence to a low protein diet is unknown. Attman et al (32) prescribed a protein-reduced diet (20 to 30 g/day) for a mean of 5 months in 21 diabetic patients with renal failure and observed, 'Most patients experienced considerable amelioration of their uremic symptoms'. Until a definitive trial of dietary protein restriction is conducted in diabetic patients with decreased renal reserve, the prudent clinician is well advised to limit the daily protein allotment to 40 g/day in every diabetic patient with a lower than normal GFR. Whether this prescription should be extended to diabetics with normal or supernormal GFR is speculative, though the logistics of attempting dietary modification for 12% of the American population would require an enormous economic, cultural, and educational effort.

EYES AND FEET

For the diabetic patient in the midst of progressive nephropathy, continuation of employment, function within school and home environments, and rehabilitation after the onset of renal failure are contingent on preservation of sight and limbs. Diabetes is the leading cause of blindness in the 41 to 60 year old age group (33). When recognized prior to development of extensive vitreous hemorrhaging, diabetic retinopathy regresses and stabilizes following panretinal photocoagulation with an argon laser (34); vision that would otherwise surely have been lost can be preserved. A similar approach to defensive foot care, as advocated by Levin and Davidson (35) will unquestionably avoid lower limb amputations. The reality learned by nephrologists and kidney transplant surgeons is that diabetics require extensive and comprehensive services beyond what is usually encompassed by the specialty of nephrology. It is enervating to establish a functioning renal allograft in a patient unable to perform previous duties because of preventable blindness and limb-loss. A team approach, including a podiatrist and ophthalmologist, to overall care will minimize the probability of such unfavorable outcomes. Preventive medicine is also vital during hospitalizations for vascular access, intercurrent disease, or kidney transplantation, when the patient's head should be elevated to reduce intraocular pressure and soft coverings ('booties') should cover the heels to protect against pressure necrosis.

UREMIA THERAPY

Diabetic nephropathy is the most prevalent correctly diagnosed cause of renal failure in the United States. The rise in the proportion of Medicare supported diabetics on dialysis has been startling. Only a decade ago, diabetic patients who developed uremia were excluded from kidney transplant and home hemodialysis programs in the mistaken belief that their survival was poor and rehabilitation was unobtainable. In 1975, only 198 of 15,921 (1.2%) reported kidney transplant recipients were diabetic (36). By contrast, in 1985, diabetic nephropathy was the listed diagnosis in 1,765 of 9,047 (20%) recipients of cadaver donor kidney transplants performed in the United States. A smaller, yet substantial proportion (about 10%) of European kidney transplant recipients are diabetic. Diabetes is the reported cause of renal failure in 31% of newly treated patients on continuous ambulatory peritoneal dialysis (CAPD) (37). Of new patients currently starting maintenance hemodialysis in the United States, approximately 28% are diabetic.

Demographics of uremia due to diabetic nephropathy

The rate at which renal failure develops in IDDM (30%) is much higher than in NIDDM. NIDDM has about nine times the prevalence of IDDM. In Brooklyn, the majority of newly evaluated, inner city, diabetic uremic patients beginning maintenance hemodialysis, are blacks with NIDDM. Several surveys have shown higher rates for both diabetes and uremia in blacks as compared to whites (38); approximately one-quarter of black women older than 55 years are diabetic (39). There are, however, no reported analyses of ESRD therapy which segregate patients by both race and diabetes type. We conducted a point prevalence analysis of the race and sex of 232 diabetics (a subset [16%] of a total of 1,450 patients) undergoing maintenance hemodialysis at 14 centers in Brooklyn in 1986 (Table 1). Black women comprised 37.5% of the total study population. In our study, the majority of diabetic patients on hemodialysis 139 (59.9%) had NIDDM. Despite study of each subject's course, we were unable to assign diabetes type in 24 (10.3%) of subjects.

OPTIONS IN THERAPY

Hemodialysis

Misconceptions of the potential for survival of diabetics treated by maintenance hemodialysis persisted through the end of the 1970s. Prestigious investigators reported that as many as four of five diabetics die within 1 year of starting

Table 1. Race, sex and diabetes type of hemodialyzed diabetics in Brooklyn.

	Black		White		Hispanic		Total	
	n	(%)	n	(%)	n	(%)	n	(%)
Men	51	(21.9)	35	(15.1)	15	(6.5)	101	(43.5)
Women	87	(37.5)	24	(10.3)	20	(8.6)	131	(56.5)
Total	138	(59.5)	59	(25.4)	35	(15.1)	232	

Type of diabetes	Number	Age diabetic (years)	Current age (years)	Interval (years of diabetes)*
IDDM	12	10.2 ± 5.1	32.1 ± 4.8	20.5 ± 5.9
NIDDM	139	46.3 ± 12.7	63.1 ± 8.9	13.3 ± 13.3
Probably IDDM	19	35.5 ± 9.9	53.0 ± 9.3	15.3 ± 8.6
Probably NIDDM	38	40.0 ± 11.1	60.6 ± 8.3	17.2 ± 8.4
Indeterminate	24	36.6 ± 11.5	56.1 ± 8.3	17.2 ± 7.6
All patients	232	41.5 ± 14.4	59.6 ± 11.2	14.9 ± 9.3

* Number of years between diagnosis of diabetes and first hemodialysis.

maintenance hemodialysis. With regulation of hypertension and hyperglycemia, survival improved progressively. By 1980, it was evident that maintenance hemodialysis will sustain life for the majority of uremic diabetics for at least 2 years. Consequent to provision of Medicare funding, fear of imposing an unjustifiable monetary burden on a diabetic's family was removed as a barrier to acceptance for uremia therapy. Although strong prejudice against starting diabetic patients on hemodialysis persists in Great Britain, in the United States, one quarter of all newly treated ESRD patients are diabetic, and 80% of all uremic diabetics are managed solely by hemodialysis.

There are substantive problems in proffering hemodialysis to diabetics (Table 2). Creating a satisfactory vascular access, for example, may prove to be a major surgical feat due to atherosclerosis of limb arteries and thrombosis of veins. An innovative vascular surgeon, however, nearly always is successful in developing an access by employment of prosthetic grafts (Teflon or bovine carotid artery) or insertion of metallic devices (40). Regulation of blood glucose during dialysis necessitates limitation of dialysate glucose concentration to 100 mg/dl, or use of a glucose-free dialysis solution. With reduction in duration of dialysis from 12 to 16 h in the 1960s to 3 to 5 h, IDDM patients need have little interruption in meal schedule or insulin administration on dialysis days.

The ranking causes of death in hemodialyzed diabetics are macrovascular disease of the heart and brain. Reducing hypertensive blood pressures and minimizing the quantity of saturated dietary lipids limits these risks. Overall, management of metabolic control for a diabetic on dialysis is little different from that advocated for diabetic patients with normal renal function.

Every comparative study of diabetic and nondiabetic patients on maintenance hemodialysis shows the diabetic to have inferior survival. Underscoring this point is the account by Kjellstrand, Goetz, and Najarian (41) who found half-time survival of diabetics on hemodialysis to be 3 years while nondiabetic patients had a half-time of $7^1/_2$ years. By applying blood pressure and blood glucose control measures and extracting excess intravascular volume by ultrafiltration during dialysis, Shapiro and Comty (42) improved survival in both hemodialyzed younger, Type II diabetics and Type I diabetics of all ages. Concern that repetitive infusions of heparin during hemodialysis would intensify vitreous hemorrhaging due to diabetic retinopathy has been assuaged. Prospective studies of visual acuity in diabetics hemodialyzed for as long as 3 years indicate that heparinization during hemodialysis does not adversely effect diabetic retinopathy (43).

No specific schedule for insulin administration in IDDM patients on hemodialysis has been identified. As a generalization, we prefer two doses (pre-breakfast and pre-dinner) of a mixture of intermdiate (NPH) and regular insulin with supplemental pre-meal doses of regular insulin administered as determined by three or more finger-stick blood glucose measurements made by the patient. For diabetic patients with reduced vision, arrangements have to be made for glucose testing and insulin injection by a family member or friend.

While survival of diabetics on maintenance hemodialysis has improved, dialytic therapy does not restore full vigor to a diabetic patient. We studied 232 diabetic patients on maintenance hemodialysis in 14 dialysis units in Brooklyn in 1986 and observed absymal rehabilitation; only seven patients had resumed full-time employment. Indeed, only 24% of hemodialyzed diabetics were capable of any activity beyond caring for themselves. Whether normalization of red blood cell mass by treatment with recombinant DNA synthesized erythropoietin will improve rehabilitation for hemodialyzed diabetics is currently being determined.

Peritoneal dialysis

Peritoneal dialysis, performed intermittently, or as continuous ambulatory peritoneal dialysis (CAPD) is enthusiastically proposed by some investigators as the preferred treatment for uremic diabetics (44). Advantages presumed for CAPD over hemodialysis for diabetics include avoidance of heparin, more consistent correction of uremic dysmetabolism and intraperitoneal administration of insulin (Table 3).

Table 2. Concerns in initiating maintenance hemodialysis in a uremic diabetic patient.

Vascular access
  Bovine heterograft
  Teflon graft
  Metallic device
Propensity to hypotension
  Minimize intradialytic weight gain
  Bicarbonate dialysate
  Gradual ultrafiltration
Preservation of vision
  Collaboration with ophthamologist
  Low heparin dosage
  Two or more pillows for head elevation
Avoidance of limb amputation
  Heel 'booties'
  Collaboration with podiatrist
Obstipation
  Prescribe detergent with antacid gel
  Question about bowel habits
Depression
  Membership in patient organizations
  Full explanation of therapy

Table 3. Advantages of CAPD for diabetic patients.

Rapid establishment as home therapy
Partner not essential
Few profound hypotensive episodes
Insulin regimen simplified
Enthusiastic patient acceptance
Minimal stress on cardiovascular system
Superior (to hemodialysis) mobilization of plasma lipids

Disadvantages of CAPD, however, are considerable (Table 4). Pending prospective controlled trials of CAPD versus maintenance hemodialysis, the popularity of CAPD is evident in Medicare statistics which show that CAPD now accounts for about 16% of all dialysis in the United States. According to the NIH CAPD registry, approximately one in three new patients begun on CAPD is diabetic. By contrast with home hemodialysis which takes weeks to months to master, motivated patients, including blind diabetics, can learn to perform CAPD at home within 10 to 15 days. Technical aspects of CAPD are discussed in Chapter 25. Legrain et al (44) who have extensive personal experience in treating diabetics with both home hemodialysis and CAPD though considering home hemodialysis preferable (75% survival at 3 years in 67 patients younger than 50 years), also designate CAPD as 'a first choice treatment'.

Survival for Type I diabetics after 1 and 2 years of CAPD is 92 and 75%, respectively (45). In the few studies reporting outcome after 2 years, survival drops to about 50% by the third year, which is approximately equivalent to that attained by maintenance hemodialysis. As is true for hemodialysis, diabetics on CAPD, have a greater death rate than age and sex matched nondiabetics. If over 60, a diabetic on CAPD faces a 6 times greater risk of dying than a nondiabetic patient. The NIH CAPD registry report for 1985 listed diabetes, black race, and age over 60 as variables adding to the risk of death (46). CAPD has social advantage, including freedom from a machine and electrical outlets and facility in travel, which must be weighed against its disadvantages of unremitting attention to fluid exchange, constant risk of peritonitis, and disappearing exchange surface. Election of CAPD for a uremic diabetic is an individualized decision dependent on thoughtful evaluation of all treatment options (Table 5).

Hemofiltration

Several reports describe the course of uremic diabetics maintained by hemofiltration, a uremia therapy discussed by Henderson in Chapter 13 and by Baldamus in Chapter 14. Although hemofiltration was devised in the United States, its clinical application has been most extensively evaluated in Europe. In Italy, for example, Segoloni and coworkers (47), conducted a multicenter retrospective study of the 'potentialities' of hemofiltration for diabetics in ESRD. In a series of 13 diabetics, 10 IDDM, and 3 NIDDM, these workers amassed a total experience of 171 patient-months of follow-up noting 'surprisingly few complications when compared to the high incidence of major clinical complications seen in conventional hemodialysis.' While the number of treated patients is small, Segoloni et al attained an encouraging actuarial survival rate of 91% at 1 year, and 61% at 2 years. There have been few recent reports of the value of hemofiltration for diabetic nephropathy, reflecting the technique's greater expense and complexity as compared to hemodialysis.

Kidney transplantation

In terms of survival and rehabilitation for diabetics, renal transplantation from either a cadaver or live donor is distinctly superior to either CAPD or maintenance hemodialysis. Our first kidney transplants in diabetics were performed 15 years ago because of discontent with poor survival on hemodialysis. At first, seemingly unavoidable excessive morbidity and mortality indicated no advantage for the diabetic transplant recipient. Other groups had similar difficulty with transplants in diabetics as illustrated by the 1978 series of 49 diabetic patients treated by hemodialysis and transplantation in which 2 year survival for dialysis patients was 74% compared to only a 54% 2 year survival for 22 transplant recipients (48). It was only after Najarian's Minnesota team devoted a decade to fine tuning surgical and immunosuppressive regimens that cumulative patient survival for diabetic recipients was improved at 4 years to 95, 83, and 67% in kidneys from HLA identical siblings, other relatives, or cadaver donors respectively (49). Results in Minnesota prompted Sutherland et al (49) to conclude that: 'Virtually every diabetic patient with renal failure referred to the University of Minnesota was accepted for transplantation, regardless of age, associated complications, or availability of a related donor. Kidney transplantation should be the treatment of choice for the uremic diabetic patient'.

Composite national data compiled in the recent report of the University of California at Los Angeles Transplant Reg-

Table 4. Disadvantages of CAPD for diabetic patients.

Catheter related
  Pain, bleeding, dialysate leak
  Obstruction
  Perforation of abdominal viscus
Mechanical
  Abdominal hernia
  Hydrothorax, ascites
Peritoneal
  Peritonitis
  Peritoneal thickening (sclerosis)
Neuropsychiatric
  Depression
  Boredom with regimen
Time commitment

Table 5. Options in therapy for the uremic diabetic patients.

Hemodialysis
  Home dialysis
  Facility hemodialysis
Peritoneal dialysis
  Intermittent (IPD)
  Continuous Ambulatory (CAPD)
  Continuous Cyclic (machine) (CCPD)
Kidney transplantation
  Living donor kidney
  Cadaver donor kidney
Hemofiltration (Europe)

istry supports this view documenting that in recipients of cadaver donor first kidney grafts: 'the remarkable transition of diabetes as a high-risk factor to diabetes becoming no different from any other original disease with regard to both patient as well as graft survival rates' (50). During the past decade, our own results improved steadily (Table 6); currently, cyclosporine treated diabetics have survival at 1 and 2 years equivalent to that in nondiabetic recipients, but kidney graft survival is about 10% lower in diabetics. We encourage a kidney transplant as the first therapy to be considered in newly evaluated diabetics with ESRD. Several teams are exploring the value of partial pancreas grafts prior to, at the time of, or following a kidney transplant (51, 52). While 1 year allograft survival has reached 60 to 80% in selected recipients (53), I believe that the dual surgical problems of vascularizing the engrafted organ and diverting its exocrine secretions will limit the utility of pancreas transplants. More promising are islet allografts, or a hybrid bionic device with islets either polymer coated or encased in hollow fibers (54).

CO-MORBID RISK FACTORS

Longevity during uremia therapy in diabetic nephropathy is contingent on co-morbid variables resulting from diabetic neurpathy and vasculopathy (Table 7). A schema for quantifying extrarenal diseases which may alter morbidity and mortality during treatment is listed in Table 8. A constant concern in every uremic diabetic patient is the threat to the heart, brain and other organs posed by occlusive vascular disease. The major cause of death in diabetics post-transplant or on dialysis, is cardiovascular and cerebrovascular catastrophe. Occlusive vascular disease accounted for 19 (46%) of 41 deaths in a series of diabetic kidney transplant recipients, of which 16 were due to coronary disease (55). In the report by Rao and Andersen (56), the incidence of occlusive vascular disease was compared in 99 diabetic and 283 nondiabetic recipients of cadaver kidney transplants. Prior to transplantation, diabetics had a higher prevalence of clinical vascular disease (33%) than did the nondiabetics (13%). Post-transplant vascular disease was significantly

more frequent in diabetics (33%) than in nondiabetic patients (13%). Amputations (18%), and strokes were many times more likely to occur in diabetic recipients than in nondiabetic recipients. Asymptomatic coronary artery disease in uremic diabetics had a very poor prognosis in a 1978 study by Bennett et al (57) who reported that of 11 consecutive diabetic patients without clinical evidence of coronary artery disease, every patient had 'multifocal atherosclerotic coronary disease' and eight patients died within a mean of 19.8 months.

Heart disease imparts a serious risk to the uremic diabetic. Of seven transplant recipients with severe coronary artery disease reported by D'Elia et al (58), three had a myocardial infarction, two had a cerebrovascular accident, and two patients with sustained allograft function died suddenly 29 and 62 months post-transplant. Thallium stress testing will identify diabetics likely to manifest symptomatic coronary artery disease (59). Of 13 recipients with a positive thallium stress test, six (46%) subsequently had cardiovascular events, two of which were fatal, whereas of 47 recipients with negative stress tests, only 13 (28%) later had a cardiovascular event, four of which were fatal. Stress testing to aid in selection for living donor kidney transplantation, sharply reduced perioperative mortality, achieving a recipient survival rate at 2 years of 94%. Survival in poor cardiac risks who were relegated to receive cadaveric donor kidneys, not surprisingly, had a 2 year patient survival of only 66%.

To establish 'guidelines for the cardiac evaluation of diabetics prior to renal transplantation', Philipson et al (60) studied 60 diabetics being considered for a kidney transplant and concluded that 'patients with diabetes and end-stage renal disease who are at highest risk for cardiovascular events can be identified, and these patients probably should not undergo renal transplantation'. Applying these guide-

Table 6. State University of New York, Health Science Center at Brooklyn. Diabetic and nondiabetic recipients of kidney transplants. Patient and graft actuarial survival: 1984–1986.

	Patients survival		Graft survival	
	1 yr	2 yr	1 yr	2 yr
Nondiabetics				
Live donor (n = 38)	95%	91%	82%	77%
Cadaver donor (n = 137)	90%	83%	83%	64%
Diabetics				
Live donor (n = 25: 22 IDDM, 3 NIDDM)	93.4%	91.6%	73.3%	69.2%
Cadaver donor (n = 41: 31 IDDM, 10 NIDDM)	88.0%	81.4%	68.0%	54.6%

Table 7. Co-morbid factors influencing outcome of uremia therapy in diabetes.

1) Angina or myocardial infarction.
2) Other cardiovascular problems, hypertension, congestive heart failure, cardiomyopathy.
3) Respiratory disease.
4) Gastrointestinal problems, gastroparesis, obstipation, nocturnal diarrhea.
5) Neurologic problems, cerebrovascular accident or stroke residual.
6) Musculoskeletal disorders, including renal bone disease.
7) Infections excluding vascular access-site or peritonitis.
8) Hepatitis, hepatic insufficiency.
9) Hematologic problems other than anemia.
10) Spinal abnormalities, lower back problems or arthritis.
11) Vision loss.
12) Limb amputation.
13) Mental or emotional illness (psychosis, neurosis, depression).

Each factor can be scored from 0 to 3 (0 = absent, 1 = mild – of minor import to patient's life, 2 = moderate, 3 = severe). By proportional hazard analysis, the relative significance of each variable can be isolated from the other 12.

lines, of the seven patients who had a negative thallium stress test, four received a transplant, without subsequent 'cardiovascular events'. In 53 diabetics with positive or non-diagnostic stress thallium tests, cardiac catheterization was employed to identify 26 patients with mild or no coronary disease or left ventricular dysfunction; 16 patients in this group received transplants with no cardivascular events. Notably, moderate heart disease was found in ten patients, of whom eight received transplants and two died of heart disease. In the group of 13 patients with severe coronary artery disease, or left ventricular malfunction, eight died before receiving a transplant, three from cardiovascular disease. It is pertinent to the management of uremia in diabetes to appreciate that in this series the overall prevalence of coronary artery disease was 38%.

We now include coronary angiography, a procedure imposing substantive risk (61), in our pre-transplant evaluation of all diabetic patients. Acknowledging the serious significance of heart disease in a uremic diabetic, we nevertheless do not agree with Libertino et al (62) who stated (in an era preceding generally available coronary angioplasty) that 'Chronic hemodialysis should be recommended for those patients who have severe coronary artery disease'. Corry et al (63) depend on the results of coronary angiography to assign potential recipients to either a combined pancreas-kidney transplant if no evidence of coronary artery disease is discerned, or a kidney transplant after reparative cardiac surgery. Dialysis is the elected therapy when significant coronary artery occlusion is discovered and uncorrected. Our approach to the management of severe coronary artery disease is to revascularize the myocardium by either coronary angioplasty or a coronary artery bypass, as an enabling procedure prior to performance of a kidney transplant.

CONCLUSIONS

Diabetes is a ubiquitous disorder responsible for at least one-quarter of new cases of uremia in the United States. Life prolongation can be achieved by peritoneal dialysis, maintenance hemodialysis, or a kidney transplant. No prospective controlled trial comparing these therapies has been reported. We have found that a functioning kidney transplant proffers the uremic diabetic higher probability for

Table 8. Quantifying co-morbid risk factors in uremia therapy for diabetic patients.

1)	Cystometrogram, urine culture, residual volume.
2)	Electrocardiogram, excercise stress test.
3)	Coronary angiography.
4)	Vital capacity.
5)	Visual acuity, fluorescein angiography.
6)	Metabolic radiographic bone survey.
7)	Podiatric assessment.
8)	Dental assessment.
9)	Social worker and nurse educator's assessment of potential for self-care.

survival with good rehabilitation than does either CAPD or maintenance hemodialysis. No matter how treated, macrovascular disease, particularly of the coronary arteries poses a threat to long-term survival of diabetics in ESRD. Preliminary trial indicates that screening intended transplant recipients with coronary angiography will identify coronary artery disease in many patients which may then be corrected pre-transplant. Whether treated by CAPD, hemodialysis, or a transplant, vigorous treatment of hypertension is a key component of management. Multiple small advances in understanding of the pathogenesis of extrarenal vasculopathic complications coupled with safer immunosuppression have improved patient and graft survival in diabetic kidney graft recipients to the degree that – in two large series – they are now equivalent to results attained in nondiabetics.

Diabetes, a disorder of high prevalence, extensive morbidity, and substantive early mortality, is yielding to a combined basic-science-clinical team effort. At its onset, IDDM may be halted or reversed by immunomodulation with cyclosporine or azathioprine. Midway in its course, biochemical and hemodynamic intervention slows the previously inexorable progress of microvasculopathy, and after organ destruction, bionics and transplant medicine are forestalling death while improving – in an increasing minority – rehabilitation. By the next edition of this work, it is safe to predict, that the diabetic's lot will be better still.

REFERENCES

1. U.S. Dept. of Health and Human Services: *Diabetes in America. Diabetes Data Compiled in 1984.* NIH Publication No. 85-1468, 1985
2. Mazze RS, Sinnock P, Deeb L, Brimberry JL: An epidemiological model for diabetes mellitus in the United States: five major complications. *Diabetes Res Clin Pract* 1: 185, 1985
3. Mauer SM, Chavers BM: A comparison of kidney disease in type I and type II diabetes. *Adv Exp Med Biol* 189: 299, 1985
4. Banting FG, Best CH, Collip JB, Campbell WR, Fletcher AA: Pancreatic extracts in the treatment of diabetes mellitus. Preliminary report. *Canad Med Assoc J* 12: 141, 1922
5. Root HF, Pote WH, Frehner H: Triopathy of diabetes. Sequence of neuropathy, retinopathy, and nephropathy in one hundred fifty-five patients. *Arch Intern Med* 94: 931, 1954
6. WHO Expert Committee on Diabetes Mellitus, second report: *WHO Technical Report Series, No. 546,* Geneva: World Health Organisation, 1980
7. National Diabetes Data Group. Classification and diagnosis of diabetes mellitus and other categories of glucose intolerance: *Diabetes* 16: 283, 1979
8. Wilson RM, Van der Minne P, Deverill I, Heller SR, Gels. thorpe K, Reeves WG, Tattersall RB: Insulin dependence: problems with the classification of 100 consecutive patients. *Diabetic Med* 2: 167, 1985
9. Kimmelsteil P, Wilson C: Intercapillary lesions in the glomeruli of the kidney. *Am J Path* 2: 83, 1936
10. Mogensen CE, Christensen CK, Vittinghus E: The stages in diabetic renal disease. With emphasis on the stage of incipient diabetic nephropathy. *Diabetes* 32: 943, 1983
11. Mauer SM, Barbosa J, Vernier RL, Kjellstrand CM, Busselmeier, Simmons RL, Najarian JS, Goetz FC: Development of

diabetic vascular lesions in normal kidneys transplanted into patients with diabetes mellitus. *N Eng J Med* 295: 916, 1976

12. Miller K, Michael AF: Immunopathology of renal extracellular membranes in diabetes mellitus. Specificity of tubular basement-membrane immunofluorescence. *Diabetes* 25: 701, 1976

13. Winegrad AI: Banting Lecture 1986. Does a common mechanism induce the diverse complications of diabetes? *Diabetes* 36: 396, 1987

14. Greene DA, Winegrad AI: Effects of acute experimental diabetes on composite energy metabolism in peripheral nerve axons and Schwann cells. *Diabetes* 30: 967, 1981

15. Greene DA, Lattimer SA: Impared rat sciatic nerve sodium-potassium adenosine triphosphatase in acute streptozotocin diabetes and its correction by dietary myoinositol supplementation. *J Clin Invest* 72: 1058, 1983

16. Cohen MP: Aldose reductase, glomerular metabolism, and diabetic nephropathy. *Metabolism* 35 (Suppl 1): 55, 1986

17. Goldfarb S, Simmons DA, Kern EFO: Amelioration of glomerular hyperfiltration in acute experimental diabetes by dietary myoinositol and by aldose reductase inhibitor (Abstract). *Clin Res* 34: 725A, 1986

18. Maryniak RK, Mendoza N, Clyne D, Balakrishnan K, Weiss MA: Recurrence of diabetic nodular glomerulosclerosis in a renal transplant. *Transplantation* 39: 35, 1985

19. Abouna GM, Adnani MS, Kumar MSA, Samhan SA: Fate of transplanted kidneys with diabetic nephropathy. *Lancet* 1: 622, 1986

20. Grenfell A, Watkins PJ: Clinical diabetic nephropathy: natural history and complications. *Clin Endocrin of Metab* 15: 783, 1986

21: Mogensen CE, Christensen CK: Predicting diabetic nephropathy in insulin-dependent patients. *N Engl J Med* 311: 89, 1984

22. Mogensen CE: Microalbuminuria predicts clinical proteinuria and early mortality in maturity onset diabetes. *N Engl J Med* 310: 356, 1984

23. Mogensen CE: Microalbuminuria and incipient diabetic nephropathy. *Diabetic Nephropathy* 3: 75, 1984

24. Caird RI: Survival of diabetics with proteinuria. *Diabetes* 10: 178, 1961

25. Hanna AK, Roy M, Zinman B, McCulloch JC, Mortimer C, Falk JA, Chipman M, Gordon AS, Marliss EB: An evaluation of factors associated with proliferative diabetic retinopathy. *Clin Invest Med* 8: 109, 1985

26. Friedman EA, Chou LM, Beyer MM, Butt KMH, Manis T: Adverse impact of hypertension on diabetic recipients of transplanted kidneys. *Hypertension* 7 (6 Pt 2): 1131, 1985

27. Passa P, LeBlanc H, Marre M: Effects of enalapril in insulin-dependent diabetic subjects with mild to moderate uncomplicated hypertension. *Diabetes Care* 10: 200, 1987

28. Addis T: *Glomerular Nephritis Diagnosis and Treatment*, New York, MacMillan Publ Co, 1949

29. Hostetter TH, Olson JL, Rennke HG, Venkatachalam MA, Brenner BM: Hyperfiltration in remnant nephrons: a potentially adverse response to renal ablation. *Am J Physiol* 24: F85, 1985

30. Zatz R, Brenner BM: Pathogenesis of diabetic microangiopathy. *Am J Med* 80: 443, 1986

31. Giordano C, Capodicasa G, De Santo NG: Effects of various diets on the progression of human and experimental uraemia. *Proc Eur Dial Transplant Assoc* 21: 549, 1984

32. Attman PO, Bucht H, Larsson O, Uddebom G: Protein-reduced diet in diabetic renal failure. *Clin Nephrol* 19: 217, 1983

33. Little HL, Jack RL, Patz A, Forsham PH: *Diabetic Retinopathy,* New York, Thieme Medical Publisher Inc, 1983

34. Diabetic Retinopathy Study Research Group: Photocoagulation treatment of proliferative diabetic retinopathy: The second report of diabetic retinopathy study findings. *Am J Ophtalmol* 85: 82, 1978

35. Levin M: Pathophysiology of diabetic foot lesions. In *Clinical Diabetes Mellitus* edited by Davidson JK, New York, Thieme Medical Publishers Inc, 1986, p 383

36. The 12th Report of the Human Renal Transplant Registry: *JAMA* 233: 787, 1975

37. *Report of the National CAPD Registry of the National Institutes of Health.* January 1, 1981 through August 31, 1985. National Institute of Arthritis, Diabetes, and Digestive and Kidney Diseases January 1986

38. Friedman EA: Race and diabetic nephropathy. *Transplant Proc* 19 (Suppl 2): 77, 1987

39. Harris MI, Hadden WC, Knowler WC, Bettett PH: Prevalence of diabetes and impaired glocuse tolerance and plasma glucose levels in U.S. population aged 20–74 yr. *Diabetes* 36: 523, 1987

40. Kaplan AA, Grant J, Galler M, Galen MA, Longnecker RE: Regional experience with the hemasite no-needle access device. *Trans Am Soc Artif Intern Organs* 29: 369, 1983

41. Kjellstrand CM, Goetz FC, Najarian JS: Transplantation and dialysis in diabetic patients: an update. In *Diabetic Renal Retinal Syndrome* edited by Friedman EA, L'Esperance FA, New York, Grune & Stratton, 1980, p 345

42. Shapiro FL, Comty CM: Hemodialysis in diabetics – 1981 update. In *Diabetic Renal-Retinal Syndrome 2 Prevention and Management* edited by Friedman EA, L'Esperance FA, New York, Grune & Stratton, 1982, p 309

43. Ramsay RC, Cantrill HL, Knobloch WH, Shapiro FL, Comty CM, Kjellstrand CM: Visual parameters in diabetic patients on chronic dialysis. *Diabetic Nephropathy* 2: 30, 1983

44. Legrain M, Rottembourg J, Bentchikou A, Poignet JL, Issad B, Barthelemy A, Strippoli P, Gahl GM, de Groc F: Dialysis treatment of insulin dependent diabetic patients: ten years experience. *Clin Nephrol* 21: 72, 1984

45. Amair P, Khanna R, Liebel B, Pierratos A, Vas S, Meema E, Blair G, Chisolm L, Vas M, Zingg W, Digenis G, Oreopoulos D: Continuous ambulatory peritoneal dialysis in diabetic end-stage renal disease. *N Engl J Med* 306: 625, 1982

46. Steinberg SM, Cutler SJ, Novak JW, Nolph KD: *Report of the National CAPD Registry of the National Institutes of Health.* NIADDKD, Bethesda, 1986

47. Segoloni GP, Pacitti A, Salomone M, Verceloon A: Hemofiltration in diabetic uremic patients. *Diabetic Nephropathy* 3: 21, 1984

48. Mitchell JC, Frohnert PP, Kurtz SB, Anderson CF: Chronic peritoneal dialysis in juvenile-onset diabetes mellitus: a comparison with hemodialysis. *Mayo Clin Proc* 53: 775, 1978

49. Sutherland DER, Fryd DS, Simmons RL, Kjellstrand CM, Ramsay RC, Goetz FC, Mauer SM, Najarian JS: Long-term diabetic renal transplants. In *Diabetic Renal Retinal Syndrome* edited by Friedman EA, L'Esperance FA, New York, Grune & Stratton, 1980, p 353

50. Terasaki PI, Himaya NS, Cecka M, Cicciarelli J, Cook DJ, Ito T, Iwaki Y, Mickey MR, Takiff H, Tiwari JL, Toyotome A: Overview. in *Clinical Transplants 1986* edited by Terasaki PI, Los Angeles, UCLA Tissue Typing Laboratory, 1986, p 367

51. Sutherland DER, Goetz FC, Moudry KC, Abouna GM, Najarian JS: Use of recipient mesenteric vessels for revasculaization of segmental pancreas grafts: technical and metabolic considerations. *Transplant Proc* 19: 2300, 1987

52. Toledo-Pereyra, Mittal VK: Complications of pancreas transplantation-effect of technique. *Transplant Proc* 19: 2319, 1987

53. Sutherland DER, Moudry KG: Clinical pancreas and islet transplantation. *Transplant Proc* 19: 113, 1987

54. Araki Y, Solomon BA, Basile RM, Chick WL: Biohybrid artificial pancreas. Long-term insulin secretion by devices seeded with canine islets. *Diabetes* 34: 850, 1985

55. Okiye SE, Engen DE, Sterioff SS, Frohnert PP, Johnson WJ, Offord KP, Zincke H: Primary and secondary renal transplantation in diabetic patients. *JAMA* 249: 492, 1983

56. Rao KV, Anderson RC: The impact of diabetes on vascular complications cadaver renal transplantation. *Transplantation* 43: 193, 1987

57. Bennett WM, Kloster F, Rosch J, Barry L, Porter GA: Natural history of asymptomatic coronary arteriographic lesions in diabetic patients with end-stage renal disease. *Am J Med* 65: 779, 1978

58. D'Elia JA, Weinrauch LA, Kaldany A, Libertino KA, Leland OS Jr, Healy RW, Miller DG: Improving survival after renal transplantation for diabetic patients with severe coronary artery disease. *Diabetes Care* 4: 380, 1981

59. Morrow CE, Schwartz JS, Sutherland DE, Simmons RL, Ferguson RM, Kjellstrand CM, Najarian JS: Predictive value of thallium stress testing for coronary and cardiovascular events in uremic diabetic patients before renal transplantation. *Am J Surg* 146: 331, 1983

60. Philipson JD, Carpenter BJ, Itzkoff J, Hakala TR, Rosenthal JT, Taylor RJ, Puschett JB: Evaluation of cardiovascular risk for renal transplantation in diabetic patients. *Am J Med* 81: 630, 1986

61. Weinrauch LA, Healy RW, Leland OS Jr., Goldstein HH, Kassissieh SD, Libertino JA, Takacs FJ, D'Elia JA: Coronary angiography and acure renal failure in diabetic azotemic nephropathy. *Ann Intern Med* 86: 56, 1977

62. Libertino JA, Zinman L, Salerno R, D'Elia J, Kaldany A, Weinrauch LA: Diabetic renal transplantation. *J Urol* 124: 593, 1980

63. Corry RJ, Nghiem DD: Evolution of technique and results of pancreas transplantation at the University of Iowa. *Clin Transplant* 1: 52, 1987

PREVENTION OF RENAL FAILURE

JOHN M. BURKART, ROBERT W. HAMILTON and VARDAMAN M. BUCKALEW Jr.

INTRODUCTION

The social burden of treating large numbers of patients with end stage renal disease (ESRD) by dialysis and transplantation has prompted renewed efforts toward prevention and treatment of this catastrophic illness. Despite these efforts, the number of patients entering ESRD treatment continues to mount (1). Progress in control of this major public health problem will require a combination of basic research into the mechanisms of the disease processes which cause ESRD, a better understanding of the epidemiology of ESRD, clinical trials of promising therapies and the application of relevant public health measures to populations at highest risk. A discussion of these larger issues is beyond the scope of this chapter. Our purpose is to discuss the more narrow issues relating to individual patients with chronic renal failure (CRF).

Every patient with CRF is a potential dialysis patient since all chronic renal diseases, no matter what their cause, have the potential to progress to ESRD. The first responsibility of

physicians is to determine whether these patients have one of the conditions listed in Table 1. If these conditions were prevented or treated adequately, the risk of developing ESRD would be reduced. In this chapter we will discuss the general approach to some of those conditions. A discussion of preventing progression of CRF by dietary means which can be applied to renal disease of all etiologies is presented in chapter 53.

HYPERTENSION AND RENAL DISEASE

A complex relationship exists between hypertension and the kidney. Considerable evidence suggests that an inherited defect in renal sodium handling is a basic cause of primary essential hypertension (2) with chronic renal parenchymal disease being the most common cause of secondary hypertension (accounting for 2 to 5% of all hypertension [3]). Most important for purposes of this chapter, however, is the fact that hypertension is a major risk factor in the development of CRF and ESRD.

Renal damage from hypertension may be evident very early. For example, urinary excretion of N-acetyl-b-glucosamidase, a sensitive indicator of proximal renal tubular damage, may be increased in hypertensive patients with no other evidence of renal disease (4). Furthermore, most patients with hypertension of more than 5 years duration have arteriographic evidence of vascular damage in the interlobar and arcuate arteries (5) even though renal excretory function remains normal. Those patients who develop any degree of proteinuria or a BUN above 20 mg/dl (7.14 mmol/l) have an increased risk of death (6, 7).

Prevalence and incidence

Estimates of the prevalence and incidence of renal disease resulting from hypertension show geographical variation. Hypertension nephropathy was diagnosed in 17.4% of 88,968 patients developing ESRD from 1973 to 1979 in 20 states in the eastern United States, and was the second most prevalent disease after glomerulonephritis (GN) (28.4%). The incidence of hypertensive nephropathy rose steadily each year, however, to 13 per million person-years in 1979, a rate equal to the incidence of GN in that year (8). Data from the Medicare ESRD program for the years 1978-1980 show a similar trend (9). The prevalence of hypertensive nephropathy rose from 16 in 1979 to 19 per million person-years in 1980 while the prevalence of GN changed only from 15 to 16 per million person-years. Thus, a potentially preventable condition appears to have emerged as the leading cause of ESRD in the United States. This trend may be due to the increasing age of the dialysis population; however, other factors not yet identified may also be important.

Hypertensive nephropathy is not as significant a cause of ESRD in Europe. In 1979 it accounted for only 7.6% of cases, and was sixth in rank behind GN, interstitial nephritis, multisystem disease and cystic disease (10). The incidence in 1982 appeared to be similar to that in 1979 (11). The reason for the large difference in prevalence of this condition between the United States and Europe is probably due to the higher proportion of black patients in the United States (see below).

Hypertensive nephropathy is less prevalent in the transplant population. In a series of 7,935 patients transplanted from 1983 to the present time in 300 centers from across the United States, hypertension-induced renal disease was the primary cause of renal failure in 3.5% of whites and 15.4% of blacks, with an overall prevalence of 5.2% (12). The lower prevalence of hypertensive nephropathy in transplant patients compared to the entire population of patients with ESRD is probably due to the fact that ESRD from hypertensive nephropathy develops more frequently in patients too old for transplantation. The higher prevalence in black transplant patients compared to whites suggests that blacks develop hypertensive renal disease at a younger age than whites.

Clinical patterns of renal involvement

The severity and rate of development of CRF in primary hypertension varies widely. Most patients with primary essential hypertension and renal damage have a slow deterioration of renal function over many years which does not progress to ESRD (13). But in about 10 to 20% of patients, renal function deteriorates slowly (over 10 to 20 years), resulting in ESRD (3). In another group of perhaps 20%, renal function deteriorates more rapidly (3). This group tends to have higher blood pressures and may have an increased susceptibility to renal damage from hypertension. Finally, rapid deterioration of renal function is seen in patients with accelerated or malignant hypertension, many of whom do not recover sufficiently to avoid dialysis (14, 15).

Prevention of hypertension-associated renal disease

There has been general agreement for many years that treatment of accelerated or malignant hypertension reduces the risk of CRF. This concensus has been confirmed by the improved survival rates for patients with renal insufficiency who were treated with the modern, more effective antihypertensive drugs. In the study by Guelpa et al (16), 5-year survival rates for patients with malignant hypertension and CRF improved from 35% during 1966–1977 to 72% during 1977–1982.

The preventability of CRF associated with mild to moderate hypertension has only recently been demonstrated by two epidemiologic studies. In the Veterans Administration cooperative study of morbidity and mortality in patients with diastolic blood pressures between 90 and 114 mm Hg, three cases of renal damage were seen in the placebo group versus none in the treated group (17). In the Veterans Administration study of patients with diastolic blood pressures between 115 and 129 mm Hg, two patients developed renal damage in the placebo group and none in the treated group (18).

Despite the fact that CRF can be prevented by the treatment of mild and moderate hypertension, there is no evidence as yet of a decline in ESRD from this cause. It is possible that patients developing ESRD from hypertension derive from the pool of patients whose hypertension is poorly controlled, or whose hypertension is discovered too late for intervention to be effective.

Table 1. Preventable or treatable causes of CRF and ESRD.

1. Hypertensive renal disease
2. Obstructive uropathy
3. Interstitial nephritis due to
   a. drugs
   b. heavy metals
   c. hypercalcemia
4. Glomerulonephritis associated with
   a. systemic lupus erythematosus
   b. Wegener's granulomatosus
   c. Goodpasture's syndrome
5. Idiopathic glomerular disease
   a. membranous nephropathy
   b. crescentic GN

The pathophysiology of renal damage from hypertension is poorly understood. There is reason to believe that such damage from hypertension is mediated, at least in part, by an elevation of pressure in glomerular capillaries (19). Furthermore, studies in experimental animals show that drugs which lower systemic pressure but have no effect on glomerular capillary pressure may not prevent progression of renal damage (21). Angiotensin converting enzyme (ACE) inhibitors lower glomerular pressure by causing efferent arteriolar dilation and are particularly effective in reducing hypertensive renal damage in rats (20, 21). Clinical trials are now in progress to evaluate the relevance of these observations to humans.

CRF in subsets of the hypertensive population

Diabetes mellitus

The beneficial effects of treatment of hypertension on the development of CRF is illustrated in several small studies of patients with diabetes mellitus. In six diabetic men with proteinuria and moderate hypertension, treatment with beta blockers and other drugs such as hydralazine and diuretics reduced protein excretion and the rate of decline of renal function (22). Likewise, treatment of 14 patients with diabetic nephropathy reduced the rate of deterioration of glomerular filtration rate (23), and treatment with captopril reduced renal protein excretion in 16 insulin-dependent diabetic patients (24).

Blacks

The prevalence of hypertension nephropathy in the black population is about 6 to 7 times that in the white population (10, 11). it is also clear that blacks with hypertension have more renal disease than whites with hypertension (25–27). It would be expected, therefore, that early and adequate treatment of blacks with hypertension would have a major impact on the incidence of ESRD. However, this expectation has not yet been demonstrated.

Bilateral renal artery stenosis

Bilateral renal artery stenosis or renal artery stenosis in a solitary kidney is often overlooked as a cause of reversible CRF (28). In most patients with bilateral disease, one side is more severely impaired than the other, and most such patients will be improved by surgical repair (29, 30). Dean et al (29) reported improvement or cure of hypertension in 24 of 25 such patients with an increase in creatinine clearance from 3 to 67 ml/min in 21 of these patients. Equally good results were reported by Novick et al (30) in a series of patients with stenosis of the renal artery in a solitary kidney.

The diagnosis of bilateral renal artery disease in patients with CRF requires renal arteriography. Most of the patients have generalized arteriosclerosis and are in the older age groups (30). In our experience, these patients have difficult-to-control hypertension and epigastric and/or flank bruits are present in more than 75% (31). Most have femoral and/or carotid bruits as well.

Summary

Hypertension, a risk factor for the development of ESRD, can be treated more succesfully now than at any time in the past, and future prospects are for even greater advances. Extra effort should be made by physicians to control hypertension in those patients who are at higher risk of developing ESRD, namely blacks and patients with CRF or any cause, especially those with diabetes mellitus and hypertension-induced nephrosclerosis.

OBSTRUCTIVE UROPATHY

Prevalence, incidence and causes

Obstructive uropathy may be caused by many conditions, the most common of which are listed in Table 2. The overall prevalence of obstructive uropathy in ESRD has not been reported in large populations. It was approximately 3.5% in California in 1975 (32) and 8% in northwest North Carolina in 1974–1976 (33). The prevalence of obstructive uropathy in ESRD was not reported in the European data and must have been included under a different diagnosis, probably pyelonephritis (10). Neither is the prevalence of conditions which cause obstructive uropathy well defined. Reflux nephropathy was responsible for 5 to 15% of ESRD in two small series of selected patients (34, 35). Nephrolithiasis accounted for 2.4% of ESRD in 1980–1982 in Europe (11), and 0.9% in Minneapolis, Minnesota over an 18-year period (36).

Diagnosis

Obstruction of the urinary tract may be classified according to duration (acute, subacute or chronic), location (renal

Table 2. Most common causes of urinary tract obstruction.

1. Intrinsic Causes
   a. Intraluminal obstruction
      Calculi, renal papillae, blood clots
   b. Neurogenic bladder
      Congenital, acquired
   c. Ureteral dysfunction
   d. Anatomical
      Tumor, infections, strictures, trauma

2. Extrinsic Compression
   a. Reproductive system-related
      Female – pregnancy, tumor, endometriosis
      Male – benign prostatic hypertrophy,
      carcinoma of the prostate
   b. Vascular causes
   c. Retroperitoneal
      Inflammatory, tumor, infectious

tubular, upper urinary tract or lower urinary tract) and degree (complete or partial). Fortunately, there are some clinical manifestations of urinary tract obstruction that, when present, are sufficient to point towards the diagnosis (Table 3). However, at other times, the patient may have only nonspecific symptoms or may even be asymptomatic. Progressive renal insufficiency may occur, therefore, before the diagnosis of obstruction is made.

Obstruction of urine flow is almost always diagnosed by radiologic imaging. Intravenous urography (IVP), computed tomographic scanning (CT scanning), ultrasonography and radionuclide scintigraphy can all be used to make the diagnosis. Acute obstruction is diagnosed best by intravenous urography or CT scanning (37) which shows delayed excretion. The obstructed kidney may have a higher density than that of the normal kidney, and the site of obstruction may be demonstrated as a cut-off of contrast along the path of the ureter.

With chronic obstruction, dilatation of the ureters, collecting system and renal pelvis are seen with IVP or CT scanning; ultrasonic examination shows dilatation of the collecting system along with thinning of the renal cortex (38); radionuclide scintigraphy shows diminished blood flow to the kidneys with isotope persistence in the collecting system and ureters (39).

The most important preventable disease states which cause obstructive uropathy, reflux nephropathy and nephrolithiasis are discussed in the remainder of this section.

Reflux nephropathy

Reflux nephropathy is primarily a disease of childhood. Unfortunately, it is often asymptomatic and the renal damage leading to CRF and ESRD is usually established by the time of the diagnosis. At present, the only early clinical marker for the disease is complicated, recurrent urinary tract infections.

Prevalence and incidence

The prevalence of asymptomatic bacteriuria in neonates is 1% (40). Over an 8-year period, Shannon (41) detected bacteriuria in 1.5% of infants admitted to a pediatric service,

Table 3. Clinical signs and symptoms and laboratory manifestations suggestive of obstructive uropathy.

1. Pain
2. Abdominal mass
3. Changes in urine output
4. Recurrent urinary tract infections
5. Infections refractory to treatment
6. Impairment of renal function
7. Polycythemia
8. Hypertension
9. Gross hematuria
10. Hyperchloremic hyperkalemic metabolic acidosis
11. Hypernatremia

most of whom were asymptomatic. Of these children, 49% were found to have vesicoureteral reflux and 8% had radiologic evidence of renal damage. It is thought that about one half of all infants with documented urinary tract infection under the age of one year have a radiologically demonstrable abnormality of their urinary tract (42, 43). The most frequently demonstrated abnormality is vesicoureteral reflux, although an occasional obstructive lesion amenable to urologic intervention is demonstrated. Screening for prevention of chronic renal insufficiency from this type of obstructive uropathy must be done during the first 2 to 3 years of life.

Screening

At present, vesicoureteral reflux is best demonstrated by voiding cystourethrography. A voiding cystourethrogram has the added benefit of being able to classify the degree of scarring. Radionucleotide micturating cystography has been proven to be a simple, reliable non-invasive screening test; however, it does not allow grading of the severity of reflux (44). A screening test (radionucleotide, or voiding cystourethrogram) should be done in any child under the age of 3 years who has one well documented urinary tract infection, or who has proteinuria. In females older than 3 years, screening tests may be postponed until there have been two or three documented urinary tract infections. In males over 3 years of age screening tests should be done after one infection.

Treatment and prevention

The treatment of vesicoureteral reflux is controversial and involves urologic surgery. It is helpful in preventing renal scarring and progression towards ESRD if performed within the first few years of life (45, 46). Of note is the fact that surgical treatment has not been shown to decrease the incidence of recurrent urinary tract infections (45), and there is no evidence that surgery can halt the progression towards ESRD in children with severe scarring or in those operated on later in life (47). Hyperfiltration in residual nephrons may determine progression once significant renal damage has occurred (47–49) (see Chapter 53). Therefore, antireflux surgery is probably indicated only at an early age for children with severe reflux or in patients with progressive severity of reflux or progressive renal scarring.

Nephrolithiasis

Recurrent nephrolithiasis is another preventable cause of obstructive uropathy and ESRD which occurs in all age groups. It was not many years ago that, for lack of insight into pathophysiology, nephrolithiasis was said to be idiopathic in most cases. Treatment consisted of a low calcium diet and forced fluids. This did little to prevent recurrence of stones or their subsequent complications. Recent research has provided new insight into the pathogenesis of the disease so that the outlook for these patients has improved considerably. An identifiable cause can be found in at least 90% of patients with nephrolithiasis (50), and a specific course of treatment can be designed which will significantly decrease recurrence rates and prevent many of the complications.

Prevalence and incidence

The incidence of nephrolithiasis in the general population has increased over the past 20 years to its present rate of 0.7 to 1.6 per thousand in the United States (51). It is the third most common disorder of the urinary tract in hospitalized patients and occurs in 12% of white males by 70 years of age (52). One-third of patients will require cystoscopy and up to one-third will require hospitalization (53) despite recent advances in extracorporeal shock-wave lithotripsy (54). As mentioned previously, up to 2.4% of ESRD may be due to renal nephrolithiasis (11).

Pathophysiology

CRF from nephrolithiasis is a result of recurrent infection, chronic obstruction or a complication of urologic instrumentation. Eighty percent of kidney stones contain calcium (51). Most stones contain predominantly calcium oxalate, while an occasional stone contains mainly calcium phosphate. Other less common stones are formed of magnesium ammonium phosphate, uric acid and cystine. All stone types are potentially preventable.

Currently, there are three theories of calcium stone formation: oversaturation of calcium salts; deficiency of inhibitors of calcium salt precipitation; and increased amount of organic matrix in urine (55–57). These theories are not mutually exclusive, and more than one of these mechanisms is probably operative during stone formation; a detailed discussion of these theories is beyond the scope of this chapter. The most dramatic difference between people who form calcium oxalate tones and those who do not lies in the higher urinary calcium levels in the stone-former (58). The most common cause of hypercalciuria is increased intestinal absorption of calcium (absorptive hypercalciuria) (59). Other metabolic defects demonstrated in stone-formers are renal hypercalciuria, absorptive hypercalciuria, hyperuricosuria, hyperoxaluria, hypocitraturia, cystinuria, a persistently high or low urinary pH and Type I renal tubular acidosis (RTA). It is the discovery and understanding of these metabolic defects that has revolutionized treatment of stone disease.

Treatment and prevention

Treatment of an acute attack of nephrolithiasis entails a combination of urologic and medical therapies. At times treatment requires instrumentation and/or hospitalization. Once the acute illness has subsided, treatment ahould be directed toward prevention of recurrence and subsequent complications. Pak et al (60) have shown a dramatic decrease in the number of stones formed after selective treatment designed to correct the underlying metabolic derange-

ments in 128 patients with known recurrent nephrolithiasis. A brief review of present recommendations for workup and treatment options has been recently reported (61). Examples of specific therapy include the following: the use of sodium cellulose phosphate for absorptive hypercalciuria Type I; calcium restriction and high fluid intake for absorptive hypercalciuria Type II; orthophosphate for absorptive hypercalciuria Type III; thiazides for renal hypercalciuria; allopurinol for hyperuricosuric calcium oxalate nephrolithiasis; potassium citrate for enteric hyperoxaluria; and potassium citrate for hypocitraturia.

INTERSTITIAL NEPHRITIS

Prevalence and causes

Tubulo-interstitial inflammation may occur in association with a variety of primary glomerular diseases. Interstitial nephritis without primary glomerular disease (IN) is a major cause of CRF, with a prevalence of 10 to 25% in the ESRD population in the United States (8, 9, 33) and Europe (10). It may be due to a variety of preventable insults, including chronic exposure to environmental toxins such as lead and other heavy metals; drugs including analgesics, lithium, diuretics and antiepileptics; chronic urinary obstruction; intermittent obstruction due to recurrent nephrolithiasis; metabolic disturbances such as potassium depletion, hyperuricemia and hypercalcemia; and chronic infection (33).

Obstructive uropathy and its major causes are discussed elsewhere in this chapter. Of the remaining preventable causes of IN, the most important are abuse of over-the-counter antipyretic analgesics, chronic lead nephropathy and hypercalcemic nephropathy.

Analgesic nephropathy

Prevalence and incidence

Some controversy continues to exist, but most authorities now accept the concept of analgesic nephropathy (AN) as a real entity. The prevalence of this condition in patients with ESRD demonstrates marked geographic variability with a high of about 30% in Queensland and New South Wales in Australia, to a low of about 1% in the northeastern United States (64). The highest prevalence in the United States is in the southeast where in certain areas up to 10% of ESRD may be due to AN (33). The overall prevalence in the United States is about 1% (8, 9, 63). In Europe the highest prevalences are in Belgium (18%), Switzerland (17.2%) and Germany and Scotland (5%) (10).

Relative risk

Individuals at risk for AN are those who consume analgesics daily (62). In these individuals, the relative risk of developing ESRD is approximately 4 compared to individuals who consume no analgesics or only occasionally consume analgesics (62). It has been estimated that the threshold dose for increased risk is 2 to 3 kg of index analgesic (63). This is the equivalent of taking 4 to 6 tablets or powders containing 300 mg/day of index analgesic for 3 to 5 years.

Which analgesic?

Most epidemiologic studies indicate that increased risk of ESRD is associated with the daily consumption of analgesic mixtures containing phenacetin (62). This impression is supported by the apparent decline in incidence of AN in several Scandinavian coutries, Scotland and Canada upon removal of phenacetin from over-the-counter analgesics (62). A ban on use of phenacetin in Australia, however, has had no effect on the incidence of AN in patients developing ESRD (64, 65). The data from Australia, where compound analgesic consumption is very high, and where phenacetin has been replaced in the popular preparations with either salicylamide or acetaminophen, suggest these newer analgesic combinations may be nephrotoxic. In support of this possibility, we have recently reported three cases of apparent AN in patients taking preparations containing aspirin and acetaminophen or ones containing acetaminophen alone (66).

Diagnosis

The diagnosis of AN requires a high index of suspicion and a recognition of the typical features of the syndrome. In our experience, patients with AN may present in a variety of ways including mild renal failure of undetermined etiology, a history of recurrent urinary tract infections, or with nephrolithiasis. The patient is about two to six times more likely to be female than male (63, 67). (In Australia, patients present most commonly with clinical evidence of papillary necrosis [68]). Anemia out of proportion to the renal failure is common. Tubular dysfunction causing metabolic acidosis out of proportion to the renal failure is also common (68). Urinalysis may be unremarkable, or contain some protein (usually not more than 2.5 g/24 h) or sterile pyuria or both.

Obtaining the history of habitual analgesic ingestion in patients with the typical clinical picture is the key to diagnosis. It is well documented that many patients with AN deny analgesic consumption on direct questioning (69). In our experience, the best approach is to question the patient concerning those conditions for which analgesics are usually consumed, most commonly headache. Patients with chronic pain syndromes are usually not reluctant to describe their condition in detail.

Prevention

The prevention of ESRD due to AN depends on making the diagnosis at a relatively early stage of the disease and convincing patients to discontinue their harmful practice. In a study of 48 patients, we found that 12 presented initially to our center with ESRD, while 34 remained stable and only two progressed to ESRD over a 1 to 3-year period of follow-up (33). Other studies have indicated a similarly low incidence of progression when analgesic abuse was curtailed (65, 70, 71).

Complete abstinence from analgesic consumption may not be attainable in most cases. We have found that the best approach for patients who must take analgesics is to take those containing only one drug, to avoid those which inhibit renal prostaglandin synthesis and to take them less often. In addition, frequent monitoring for further rises in the serum creatinine or for evidence of urinary tract infection is important since many patients have a tendency to return to heavy consumption of their favorite analgesic compound despite advice to the contrary and their own best intentions.

Lead nephropathy

Prevalence and incidence

The concept that CRF and ESRD may be caused by lead exposure is based on indirect evidence and is still controversial. Two scenarios have been proposed. Epidemiologic studies from Australia suggest that excessive exposure to lead in early childhood may lead to chronic interstitial nephritis and ESRD in adulthood (72). In addition, epidemiologic studies of adults with occupational lead exposure or with lead exposure from environmental sources such as moonshine whiskey and lead ore smelters suggest an increased risk of CRF and ESRD (73-75).

Because of the controversial nature of the concept, and because there are no generally accepted diagnostic criteria, there are no reliable estimates of the prevalence and incidence of lead nephropathy in the population of patients with CRF and ESRD. In a population in northwest North Carolina where the ingestion of lead contaminated moonshine whiskey is prevalent, we estimated that lead nephropathy was the cause of 7% of CRF due to IN and approximately 3% of ESRD (33). Because of geographic variation in lead exposure, however, it would be expected that the prevalence of lead nephropathy in North Carolina would not be typical of other geographic areas.

Lead nephropathy does not appear as a category in large population surveys of causes of ESRD. However, it has been suggested that some portion of patients with so-called 'gouty nephropathy' may have, in reality, lead nephropathy (76) (see below). The prevalence of gouty nephropathy in the ESRD population is less than 1% (9). It has also been suggested that some patients with hypertensive nephropathy may, in fact, have lead nephropathy (77). The potential significance of this intriguing suggestion has not yet been fully evaluated.

Diagnosis

The diagnosis of lead nephropathy should be suspected in adults with CRF due to IN who have a history of excessive lead exposure, either in childhood or as adults. Many patients with lead nephropathy have hyperuricemia and a history of acute gouty arthropathy, so called 'saturnine gout' (78). Some patients may present with hyporeninemic hypoaldosteronism and Type IV RTA (79). Most have hypertension.

The renal biopsy shows IN without features to distinguish lead nephropathy from other causes of IN. Changes of chronic hypertension in renal arterioles are usually present. Immunoglobulin deposits in glomerular capillaries and tubular basement membranes have also been reported (74).

The most important diagnostic test is measurement of renal lead excretion for 24 h following the administration of two 0.5 g doses of ethylenediamine tetra acetic acid (EDTA) 12 h apart (77). This 'lead mobilization test' demonstrates the presence of an increased body burden of lead and documents a previous excessive lead exposure. A positive test in the presence of chronic IN is presumptive evidence for a diagnosis of lead nephropathy.

Prevention and treatment

Excessive lead exposure in children continues to be a problem (80). If the concept of lead nephropathy outlined above is correct, it would be expected that public health measures designed to reduce this exposure would decrease the incidence of ESRD in the adult population eventually.

It is not yet clear whether treating adults with putative lead nephropathy with EDTA will prevent progression to ESRD. There is no doubt that EDTA treatment can reduce the body store of lead by promoting renal excretion. Furthermore, Weeden et al (74) showed that EDTA treatment of a group of patients with high body lead stores caused an increase in GFR. Since no adverse effects are apparent (81), treatment with EDTA in patients with IN suspected of having lead nephropathy is recommended.

Hypercalcemic nephropathy

Chronic hypercalcemia can produce a variety of structural and functional abnormalities of the kidney. These include the following: renal tubular defects such as sodium, potassium, magnesium or phosphorus wasting, acid-base disorders, nephrogenic diabetes insipidus, nephrolithiasis, nephrocalcinosis and most importantly, acute and chronic renal failure (82). Patients with chronic hypercalcemia associated with primary hyperparathyroidism, multiple myeloma, metastatic bone disease, sarcoidosis or vitamin D intoxication are especially prone to develop these problems. Hypercalcemic nephropathy is characterized initially by an acute reversible prerenal component due to a concentrating defect, renal sodium losses and subsequent volume depletion. Eventually, if left untreated, progressive CRF will slowly develop (83).

Chronic hypercalcemic nephropathy has the pathologic characteristics of IN. Vascular and glomerular calcifications may occasionally be seen. As the renal disease progresses the serum calcium concentration becomes normal and may patients are therefore classified as having IN. Consequently, the prevalence of hypercalcemic nephropathy in ESRD populations is uncertain, but was reported to be 0.28% in European populations (10, 11).

The diagnosis is suggested if hypercalcemia is accompanied by a renal concentrating defect, renal failure and radiologic evidence of nephrocalcinosis. Prevention of progressive CRF is directed initially toward identifying and treating the cause of hypercalcemia. The underlying disease state should be treated when possible; if not, the hypercalcemia should be treated nonspecifically in an attempt to prevent further renal complications. Although some authors have demonstrated improvement in renal function with correction of the hypercalcemic state (84), others have shown continued progression to ESRD (85).

GLOMERULONEPHRITIS

Prevalence, incidence and causes

Disorders of glomerular structure and function can be secondary to a multitude of systemic diseases but may also be idiopathic. Prevalence rates of GN were reported at 28.6% of ESRD patients in the United States (1981) (9) compared to 46.6% in European populations (1976) (86). Interestingly, the incidence of GN in the ESRD population in the United States has decreased from 36.4% in 1973 to 19.7% in 1980 (9) with a similar direction of change noted in Europe (10). Despite the reported decrease in incidence, GN remains the most prevalent cause of ESRD in most dialysis populations.

Preventing diseases in which secondary GN occurs is of more importance in underdeveloped parts of the world where malaria, schistosomiasis and other chronic infections are endemic. In developed countries, the most treatable systemic diseases causing progressive GN are systemic lupus erythematosus (SLE), Wgener's granulomatosus and Goodpasture's syndrome. Treatment of idiopathic membranous GN and idiopathic crescentic GN may also prevent progression to ESRD in some cases.

Systemic lupus erythematosus

Both our perception and approach to SLE have slowly evolved although the disease itself probably has not changed. In the pre-steroid era, most patients died from toxic SLE before the development of renal disease (87). Now, the systemic manifestations of lupus are fairly well controlled by the use of corticosteroids. Paradoxically, this treatment allows patients to live longer and thus develop CRF and ESRD (88).

The median survival for patients with SLE and CRF was less than 1 year in the 1940s (89). It improved to a median survival of 5 years by 1970. The most recent NIH reports show a median survival of 15 years, with minimal progression to ESRD in patients treated under various therapeutic protocols (90). Improvement in survival is most likely due to better control of hypertension, less dependence on high dose corticosteroid therapy, availability of medical intensive care units and intervention with cytotoxic drugs. Although only about 1% of ESRD is secondary to SLE (86), the historical data noted above and reports from a 1987 NIH conference (91) suggest that this is a preventable form of ESRD.

Pathophysiology

Renal disease from SLE may present in a variety of ways. Most patients have systemic manifestations such as arthritis, rash, pleuritis, fever and serologic abnormalities. An occasional patient will present with renal disease alone, the earliest finding of which may be nothing more than an increase in white blood cells or red blood cells in the urine sediment (92, 93). These patients may have only a positive serologic test for anti-nuclear antibodies and a renal biopsy suggestive of SLE. What is important to note is that CRF in SLE is a dynamic process. Not only does the urinalysis change, but the renal pathology has been documented to change over time (94). Patients found initially to have a benign lesion may have a more malignant lesion on subsequent biopsies.

The central pathologic process in the pathogenesis of SLE is the uncontrolled production of autoantibodies. It is these antibodies, along with the subsequently formed immune complexes, that cause the organ damage of SLE.

Diagnosis

Systemic lupus erythematosus should be considered in the work-up of any patient with GN. One should especially suspect the disease in black females. Usually, systemic symptoms such as fever, arthritis, facial rash, and weight loss combined with certain laboratory findings are sufficient to make the diagnosis. Laboratory tests helpful in making the diagnosis are the urinalysis; 24-hour urine protein studies; antinuclear antibodies, particularly antidouble-stranded DNA antibody levels; C3,C4 and CH50 levels; circulating immune complexes; cryoglobulin levels; and renal biopsy.

The subject of renal biopsy in SLE is somewhat controversial. We recommend biopsy in most patients for several reasons. First, as mentioned above, pathologic findings are not always predictable. Secondly, the treatment varies according to the lesion found on renal biopsy (see below). Thirdly, prognostic information can be acquired which may predict response to therapy and the natural history of the disease. Lastly, the chronicity of the illness can be determined so the relative risk/benefit ratio of treatment can be discerned.

Treatment

Although lupus nephritis is not preventable, treatment directed toward prevention of subsequent renal damage may be successful. There is, however, no general agreement about whom to treat or the form of treatment. Kant and Pollak (95) suggest that no treatment other than conservative therapy and observation is needed if the renal biopsy shows a normal kidney, mesangioproliferative, or membranous lesions. For the proliferative lesions, they suggest treatment with various combinations of prednisone and a cytotoxic drug such as cyclophosphamide, azathioprine or nitrogen mustard. Although early studies did not show a clear benefit from cytotoxic drugs, Austin and colleagues (96) have shown recently that intravenous 'pulse' cyclophosphamide significantly reduces the risk of ESRD and has fewer side effects than prednisone alone. In their study, patients with active SLE were randomized to receive either prednisone, cytotoxic therapy, or both. All biopsy types of SLE were present in each patient group.

High dose intravenous methylprednisolone (97) is probably also useful in a subset of patients with diffuse proliferative lesions on biopsy and recent rapid deterioration of renal function. Kimberly et al (97) demonstrated a rapid return of renal function with this therapy, but the long-term preventive effects are unknown. Studies by the Lupus Nephritis Collaborative Study Group show that plasmapheresis has no beneficial effect on the clinical, renal or serologic manifestations of SLE with nephritis (98).

In summary, conservative therapy can be chosen in patients with mild forms of lupus nephritis who do not seem to have active systemic disease. Patients must be observed closely for new signs of active disease which, if noted, suggest that progression to ESRD may occur. Prevention of this complication may be accomplished by treating the patient with pulse cyclophosphamide and low dose prednisone as described by Austin et al (96).

Wegener's granulomatosis

Wegener's granulomatosis is a systemic vasculitis characterized by pulmonary angitis with granuloma formation (99). The classical clinical triad includes involvement of upper airways, lungs and kidneys (100). Other clinical features suggestive of the disease are fever, weight loss, nonproductive cough, pleuritic chest pain, hemoptysis, dypsnea on exertion, sinus complaints, dermatologic findings and occular involvement. The mean age at onset is about 40 and males are affected slightly more often than females.

Renal disease is the major cause of morbidity and mortality in Wegener's granulomatosis. Prior to the introduction of corticosteroids and cytotoxic drugs the disease was rapidly progressive, with 80% of patients dying within 1 year of the diagnosis (101). However, with the use of cytotoxic agents, several series have shown a markedly improved outlook for these patients with reported 1-year survival rates of from 72 to 100% (102). The prevalence of Wegener's granulomatosis in ESRD is unknown but probably represents no more than 1 to 2% of chronic dialysis populations.

Pathophysiology

The etiology of Wegener's granulomatosis is unknown. The lung is involved pathologically most often (94% of patients) with granulomas and vasculitis almost invariably seen (103). Eighty-five percent of patients have well-documented renal disease. The histologic changes found in the kidneys range from mild focal segmental GN to a fulminant diffuse necrotizing GN with proliferative and crescentic changes. Granulomas and arteritis are seldom seen in renal biopsy specimens.

Diagnosis

Most patients present with clinical signs and symptoms suggestive enough to make a presumptive diagnosis. The definitive diagnosis of Wegener's granulomatosis requires evidence of disease in upper airways, lung and kidney. In such patients the pathognomonic finding is non-caseating granulomas in upper airways or lung.

Treatment

The treatment consists of cyclophosphamide and prednisone as outlined by Fauci et al (103), initiating therapy with daily dosing. As soon as possible the prednisone is changed to alternate-day therapy and gradually tapered after 6 months to 1 year of therapy. Cyclophosphamide is continued for at least a full year after a patient is in complete remission and then gradually tapered. It is important to establish the diagnosis of Wegener's early in order to begin the treatment that could prevent irreversible organ damage and, most importantly, progression toward ESRD.

Goodpasture's syndrome and related diseases

The term Goodpasture's syndrome refers to the triad of pulmonary hemorrhage, GN and circulating antiglomerular basement membrane (anti-GBM) antibodies. Pulmonary symptoms usually dominate the clinical presentation, but an occasional patient may have covert pulmonary disease detected only by chest x-ray or arterial blood gas testing. The glomerular disease may be asymptomatic and manifested only by an abnormal urinalysis, but a majority of cases have a rapidly progressive and fulminant course. The disorder is most common in males and tends to occur in young adults. It accounts for 1 to 2% of all cases of GN and probably accounts for less than 1% of ESRD populations (86).

Pathophysiology

The glomerular injury of Goodpasture's disease is mediated by interaction of the circulating autoantibodies to intrinsic GBM glycoproteins resulting in activation of complement and infiltration of the glomerulus by polymorphonucleocytes and monocytes (104). Coagulation mechanisms and monocytes then actively participate in the subsequent generation of crescents (105). The stimulus for production of these anti-GBM antibodies is unknown, although there is some association of the disease with inhalation of environmental toxins causing autoantigen release from the pulmonary alveolar walls (106). The pulmonary disease is probably mediated via mechanisms similar to those of the glomerular disease, but there is no correlation between pulmonary symptoms and anti-GBM antibody titers (105). Furthermore, pulmonary hemorrhage also occurs in other

non-anti-GBM mediated disease states such as the vasculitides, SLE and Henoch Schönlein purpura.

Diagnosis

Goodpasture's disease should be considered in any patient who presents with both pulmonary and renal disease. A microcytic hypochromic anemia due to iron loss from the pulmonary hemorrhage is often found (107). Circulating anti-GBM antibodies are present in more than 90% of patients at the onset of their disease (108). Renal biopsy may show focal and segmental glomerular hypercellularity with segmental necrosis of glomerular tufts, but most often reveals crescentic GN (109). The hallmark of anti-GBM antibody related GN is linear deposits of IgG and, less frequently, IgA outlining the peripheral capillary loops (108).

Course and treatment

Although the natural history of the disease is somewhat unpredictable, the majority of untreated patients with anti-GBM mediated crescentic GN will progress to ESRD and require maintenance-dialysis (110). The literature suggests that aggressive treatment with plasmapheresis, cytotoxic drugs and prednisone is not helpful in preventing progression to ESRD in patients with severe crescentic disease (>50% crescents), oliguria and the need for dialysis at time of presentation (111). However, it has been shown in subgroups of patients who are neither dialysis-dependent nor oliguric and who have less than 50% crescents on renal biopsy that intensive plasma exchange, daily cytotoxic drugs and pulse methlprednisolone therapy followed by daily steroids control both the pulmonary hemorrhage (104) and prevent progression to ESRD (112).

Primary glomerulonephritis

The primary glomerulonephritides are a heterogeneous collection of diseases in which patients present with GN without manifestations of systemic disease. They may present with acute GN, rapidly progressive or chronic GN, nephrotic syndrome or with asymptomatic abnormalities on urinalysis. The glomerular lesions found on renal biopsy are minimal change, focal and segmental sclerosis, membranous, membranoproliferative, mesangioproliferative and crescentic GN. Although there are anecdotal reports of responses to various therapeutic modalities for all these disease entities, the best documented treatments with efficacious results are for minimal change disease, membranous and crescentic GN (113). Of these, only membranous and crescentic GN are likely to progress to ESRD if left untreated.

Idiopathic membranous glomerulonephritis

Idiopathic membranous GN is probably the most common cause of nephrotic syndrome in adults, accounting for at least 30% of cases (114), but is rare in children. Eighty percent of adults so affected present with nephrotic syndrome and about one-third each with hypertension or chronic renal failure. The prevalence and incidence of progression to ESRD shows geographic variability. In the United States, 29% to 40% of patients spontaneously remit (115, 116), while the likelihood of complete or partial remission was 54% among untreated patients in France (115). Progression to ESRD ranged from 4 to 50% in selected populations (116, 117). The survival rate of patients with membranous GN at 5, 10 and 15 years was 94%, 83% and 69%, respectively, suggesting a slow rate of progression (118). Those destined to progress to ESRD show signs during the first 5 years of clinically apparent disease (119).

The prevalence of membranous GN in ESRD was 0.43% in Europe in 1977 (86). In a select group of patients who underwent transplantation and subsequent native nephrectomy, 2% were clearly identified as having membranous GN (120).

Diagnosis

The diagnosis is made only by renal biopsy. The typical features of membranous GN by light microscopy include diffuse and uniform thickening of the capillary wall usually without any significant proliferation of mesangial, endothelial or epithelial cells (121). Subepithelial spikes can be seen on silver staining while immunoflorescence studies characteristically reveal fine granular deposits of IgG, C3 and other immunoglobulins along the subepithelial surface of the peripheral capillary loops. Secondary causes must be ruled out before it is assumed that the disease is idiopathic and treatment initiated.

Course and treatment

Most nephrologists treat adult patients with serum creatinine concentration of less than 3 mg/dl (265 µmol/l) and nephrotic syndrome in one of two ways. The National Collaborative Study of Adult Idiopathic Nephrotic Syndrom has shown a probable reduction in progression to ESRD using high dose alternate-day steroids alone (122). Ponticelli et al (123), using a therapeutic regimen which consisted of intravenous and oral steroids, alternating with oral chlorambucil on a monthly basis, found a statistically signficant reduction in progression to ESRD in patients who received treatment versus those given only supportive therapy.

Idiopathic crescentic glomerulonephritis

Idiopathic crescentic GN is a descriptive histopathologic term applied to a group of glomerular lesions in which crescents of Bowman's capsule involves at least 50% of glomeruli (124). Crescents are also found in patients with poststreptococcal GN, SLE, polyarteritis nodosa, various vasculitides, Goodpasture's Syndrome and chronic infections, among others (125). Most patients with crescentic GN of any cause have a rapid deterioration in renal function and hence the confusing term 'rapidly progressive GN' (RPGN). RPGN, however, is purely descriptive and is not absolutely synonymous with crescentic GN. Twenty to fifty percent of

patients with crescents will have the idiopathic form (124). Without treatment, approximately 80 to 90% of such patients will progress to ESRD. Most patients are dialysis-dependent within 6 months of the diagnosis if left untreated (125). The prevalence of idiopathic crescentic GN was reported to be 1.7% of the European ESRD population in 1976 (85).

Typically, patients are middle-aged males who occasionally have a history of an antecedent upper respiratory infection or recent hydrocarbon exposure and an insidious onset. The urinalysis is abnormal, but other serologic testing, such as complement studies, rheumatoloogy screening and cryoglobulins are normal. There are no associated signs of systemic diseases.

Diagnosis

Idiopathic crescentic GN represents a true emergency. The diagnosis should be considered in any patient who presents with GN and a rapidly progressive deterioration in renal function. The diagnosis is made by renal biopsy which shows predominantly fibrocellular crescents on light microscopy. Electron microscopy is nonspecific and the findings on immunofluorescent studies are the basis of further subclassification of the disease.

Course and treatment

The treatment and prognosis varies according to the immunofluorescent findings on renal biopsy. Linear deposition of IgG is pathognomonic of Type I crescentic GN. Granular deposition represents Type II and absence of immunofluorescent staining is representative of Type III.

Type I is due to anti-GBM antibody production unassociated with pulmonary hemorrhage. Treatment consists of quadruple therapy, i.e. pulse steroids, plasmapheresis, cytotoxic drugs and antithrombotic drugs (113, 123). If treatment is initiated early, one can probably prevent the progression to ESRD; in the absence of treatment, the vast majority of these patients will progress to ESRD.

Type II is associated with granular immune-complex deposition on immunofluorescent studies (125), and is, by definition, idiopathic in origin. Without treatment, most patients will progress to ESRD. However, Bolton (126) has reported a remarkable improvement in renal function in 70 to 80% of patients treated with 'pulse' methylprednisolone therapy followed by daily prednisone.

Type III is associated with the absence of immune complex deposition on immunofluorescent staining. This probably represents a vasculitis and is a common cause of RPGN in elderly patients. Couser (127) has demonstrated a beneficial result when using 'pulse' methulprednisolone therapy in patients with this disease.

ACUTE DETERIORATION OF RENAL FUNCTION

No chapter on prevention of renal disease would be complete without a discussion of the patient who presents with an accelerated deterioration of renal function. Our purpose

Table 4. Causes of acute deterioration of renal function in chronic renal failure.

1. Volume depletion
2. Urinary tract infection
3. Superimposed nephrotoxicity, e.g. due to nonsteroidal anti-inflammatory drugs, iodinated contrast agents or aminoglycosides
4. Poorly controlled hypertension
5. Natural history

here is not to discuss acute renal failure comprehensively, but to call attention to these reversible causes of acute renal failure listed in Table 4 which commonly occur in patients with otherwise stable CRF.

The first four conditions, volume depletion, urinary tract infection, nephrotoxic drugs and poorly controlled hypertension, should be considered in all patients with acute renal failure. However, these conditions are more likely to cause irreversible, dialysis-dependent renal failure in patients with some underlying chronic parenchymal renal disease, and must not be overlooked in such patients. Occasionally, patients with chronic renal failure will develop a rapidly accelerated, downhill course with no apparent cause. In those cases, rapid deterioration appears to be a manifestation of the natural history of the disease.

SUMMARY

It can be estimated from the foregoing discussion that approximately 15 to 30% of ESRD is, at least theoretically, preventable. It is incumbent upon nephrologists and other physicians to investigate thoroughly patients presenting with renal failure so that, with proper intervention, the development of ESRD from certain conditions can be prevented. One goal of future research and education should be a reduction in the number of patients who become dialysis-dependent as a result of these conditions.

REFERENCES

1. Blagg CR: The end stage renal disease program: here are some of the data. *JAMA* 257: 662, 1987
2. De Wardener HE, MacGregor GA: Dahl's hypothesis that a saluretic substance may be responsible for a sustained rise in arterial pressure: its possible role in essential hypertension. *Kidney Int* 18: 1, 1980
3. Kaplan NM: *Clinical Hypertension* Fourth Edition, Baltimore, Williams & Wilkins, 1986
4. Alderman MH, Melcher L, Drayer DE, Reidenberg MM: Increased excretion of urinary N-acetyl-b-glucosaminidase in essential hypertension and its decline with antihypertensive therapy. *N Engl J Med* 309: 1213, 1983
5. Hollenberg NK, Epstein M, Basch RI, Merrill JP: 'No man's land' of the renal vasculature: an arteriographic and hemodynamic assessment of the interlobar and arcuate arteries in essential and accelerated hypertension. *Am J Med* 47: 845, 1969
6. Kannel WB, Stampfer MJ, Castelli WP, Verter J: The prognostic significance of proteinuria: the Framingham study. *Am Heart J* 108: 1347, 1984
7. Bauer GE, Humphery TJ: The natural history of hypertension with moderate impairment of renal function. *Clin Sci Mol Med* 45: 191s, 1973
8. Sugimoto T, Rosansky SJ: The incidence of treated end stage renal disease in the eastern United States: 1973–1979. *Am J Pub Health* 74: 14, 1984
9. Eggers PW, Connerton R, McMullen M: The Medicare experience with end stage renal disease: trends in incidence, prevalence and survival. *Health Care Financing Review* 5: 69, 1984
10. Brynger H, Brunner FP, Chantler C, Donckerwolcke RA, Jacobs C, Kramer P, Selwood NH, Wing AJ: Combined report on regular dialysis and transplantation in Europe, X, 1979. *Proc Eur Dial Transplant Assoc* 17: 2, 1980
11. Broyer M, Brunner FP, Brynger H, Donckerwolcke RA, Jacobs C, Kramer P, Selwood NH, Wing AJ: Combined report on regular dialysis and transplantation in Europe, XIII, 1982. *Proc Eur Dial Transplant Assoc* 20: 5, 1983
12. Cook DJ, Takiff H: Original disease of the recipient. *Clinical Kidney Transplants 1986*. Los Angeles, UCLA Tissue Typing Laboratory, 1986
13. Bulpitt CJ, Breckenridge A: Plasma urea in hypertensive patients. *Br Heart J* 38: 689, 1976
14. Lawton WJ: The short-term course of renal function in malignant hypertensives with renal insufficiency. *Clin Nephrol* 17: 277, 1982
15. Isles CG, McLay A, Boulton Jones JM: Recovery in malignant hypertension presenting as acute renal failure. *Q J Med* 53: 439, 1984
16. Guelpa G, Lucsko M, Chaignon M, Guedon J: Hypertension arterielle maligne, aspect semilogique et pronostique. (Malignant arterial hypertension; clinical and prognostic aspects.) *Schweiz Med Wochenschr* 114: 1870, 1984
17. Veterans Administration Cooperative Study Group on Antihypertensive Agents: Effects of treatment on morbidity in hypertension. II. Results in patients with diastolic blood pressure averaging 90 through 114 mm Hg. *JAMA* 213: 1143, 1970
18. Veterans Administration Cooperative Study Group on Antihypertensive Agents: *JAMA* 202: 1028, 1970
19. Brenner BM, Meyer TW, Hostetter TH: Dietary protein intake and the progressive nature of kidney disease: the role of hemodynamically mediated glomerular injury in the pathogenesis of progressive glomerular sclerosis in aging, renal ablation, and intrinsic renal disease. *N Engl J Med* 307: 652, 1982
20. Anderson S, Rennke HG, Brenner BM: Therapeutic advantage of converting enzyme inhibitors in arresting progressive renal disease associated with systemic hypertension in the rat. *J Clin Invest* 77: 1993, 1986
21. Meyer TW, Anderson S, Rennke HG, Brenner BM: Converting enzyme inhibitor therapy limits progressive glomerular injury in rats with renal insufficiency. *Am J Med* 79(3c): 31, 1985
22. Mogensen CE: Long-term antihypertensive treatment inhibiting progression of diabetic nephropathy. *Br Med J* 285: 685, 1982
23. Bjorck S, Nyberg G, Mulec H, Granerus G, Herlitz H, Aurell M: Beneficial effects of angiotensin converting enzyme inhibition on renal function in patients with diabetic nephropathy. *Br Med J* 293: 471, 1986
24. Hommel E, Parving HH, Mathiesen E, Edsberg B, Nielsen

MD, Giese J: Effect of captopril on kidney function in insulin-dependent diabetic patients with nephropathy. *Br Med J* 293: 467, 1986

25. Gillum RF, Liu KC: Coronary heart disease mortality in United States blacks, 1940–1978: trends and unanswered questions. *Am Heart J* 108: 728, 1984

26. Levy SB, Talner LB, Coel MN, Holle R, Stone RA: Renal vasculature in essential hypertension: racial differences. *Ann Intern Med* 88: 1, 1978

27. Frohlich ED, Messerli FH, Dunn FG, Oigman W, Ventura HO, Sundgaard-Riise K: Greater renal vascular involvement in the black patient with essential hypertension: a comparison of systemic and renal hemodynamics in black and white patients. *Miner Electrolyte Metab* 10: 173, 1984

28. Ying CY, Tifft CP, Gavras H, Chobanian AV: Renal revascularization in the azotemic hypertensive patient resistant to therapy. *N Engl J Med* 311: 1070, 1984

29. Dean RH, Lawson JD, Hollifield JW, Shack RB, Polterauer P, Rhamy RK: Revascularization of the poorly functioning kidney. *Surgery* 85: 44, 1979

30. Novic AC, Pohl MA, Schreiber M, Gifford RW, Vidt DG: Revascularization of renal function in patients with atherosclerotic renovascular disease. *J Urol* 129: 907, 1983

31. Graves JW, Buckalew VM Jr: Prospective evaluation of the renal artery bruit in atherosclerotic renovascular hypertension (ARVH). *Kidney Int* 1987 (in press)

32. Mann MM, Strauss DP: A medical and demographic description of 2,395 chronic hemocialysis patients in California. *California Kidney Information Service*, 1975

33. Gonwa TA, Hamilton RW, Buckalew VM Jr: Chronic renal failure and end-stage renal disease in northwest North Carolina. *Arch Intern Med* 141: 462, 1981

34. Salvatierra O Jr, Tanagho EA: Reflux as a cause of end stage kidney disease: report of 32 cases. *J Urol* 117: 441, 1977

35. Hodson J: Reflux nephropathy. *Med Clin North Am* 62: 1201, 1978

36. Smith CL: When should the stone patient be evaluated? Early evaluation of single stone formers. *Med Clin North Am* 68: 455, 1984

37. Newhouse JH, Pfister RC: The nephrogram. *Radiol Clin North Am* 17: 213, 1979

38. Pfister RC, Newhouse JH: Interventional percutaneous pyeloureteral techniques. I. Antegrade pyelography and ureteral perfusion. *Radiol Clin North Am* 17: 341, 1979

39. Joekes AM: Obstructive uropathy. *Semin Nucl Med* 4: 187, 1974

40. McCarthy JM, Pryles CV: Clean, voided and catheter neonatal urine specimens. *Am J Dis Child* 106: 473, 1963

41. Shannon FT: Urinary tract infection in infancy. *NZ Med J* 75: 282, 1972

42. Drew JH, Acton CM: Radiological findings in newborn infants with urinary infection. *Arch Dis Child* 51: 628, 1976

43. Rolleston GL, Shannon FT, Utley WLF: Relationship of infantile vesicoureteric reflux to renal damage. *Br Med J* 1: 460, 1970

44. Blaufox MD, Gruskin A, Sandler P, Goldman H, Ogwo JE, Edelmann CM: Radionuclide scintigraphy for detection of vesicoureteral reflux in children. *J Pediatr* 79: 239, 1971

45. McRae CU, Shannon FT, Utley WLF: Effect on renal growth of reimplantation of refluxing ureters. *Lancet* 1: 1310, 1974

46. Willscher MK, Bauer SB, Zammuto PJ, Retik AB: Renal growth and urinary infection following anti-reflux surgery in infants and children. *J Urol* 115: 722, 1976

47. Babcock JR, Keats GK, King LR: Renal changes after an uncomplicated antireflux operation. *J Urol* 115: 720, 1976

48. Torres VE, Velosa JA, Holley KE, Kelalis PP, Stickler GB, Kurtz SB: The progression of vesicoureteral reflux nephropathy. *Ann Intern Med* 92: 776, 1980

49. Cotran RS: Glomerulosclerosis in reflux nephropathy. *Kidney Int* 21: 528, 1982

50. Pak CYC, Britton F, Peterson R, Ward D, Northcutt C, Breslau NA, McGuire J, Sakhaee K, Bush S, Nicar M, Norman DA, Peters P: Ambulatory evaluation of nephrolithiasis. *Am J Med* 69: 19, 1980

51. Abraham PA, Smith CL: Medical evaluation and management of calcium nephrolithiasis. *Med Clin North Am* 68: 281, 1984

52. Johnson CM, Wilson DM, O'Fallon WM, Malek RS, Kurland LT: Renal stone epidemiology: A 25 year study in Rochester, Minnesota. *Kidney Int* 16: 624, 1979

53. Coe FL, Keck J, Norton ER: The natural history of calcium urolithiasis. *JAMA* 238: 1519, 1977

54. Chaussy C, Schmiedt E, Jocham D, Brendel W, Forssmann B, Walther V: First clinical experience with extracorporeally induced destruction of kidney stones by shock waves. *J Urol* 127: 417, 1982

55. Breslau NA, Pak CYC: Urinary saturation, heterogeneous nucleation, and crystallization inhibitors in nephrolithiasis. in *Contemporary Issues in Nephrology. Nephrolithiasis*, Vol 5, edited by Coe FL, Brenner BM, Stein JH, New York, Churchill Livingstone, 1980, p 13

56. Fleisch H: Inhibitors and promotors of stone formation. *Kidney Int* 13: 361, 1978

57. Malagodi MH, Moye HA: Physical and chemical characteristics of renal stone matrix. *Urol Surv* 31: 87, 1981

58. Robertson WG, Morgan DB: The distribution of urinary calcium excretion in normal persons and in stone formers. *Clin Chim Acta* 27: 503, 1973

59. Coe F: Treatment of hypercalciuria. *N Engl J Med* 311: 116, 1984

60. Pak CYC, Peters P, Hurt G, Kadesky M, Fine M, Reisman D, Splann F, Caramela C, Freeman A, Britton F, Sakhaee K, Breslau NA: Is selective therapy of recurrent nephrolithiasis possible? *Am J Med* 71: 615, 1981

61. Pak CYC: New developments in the diagnosis and management of patients with renal stone disease. *Mediguide Nephrol* 1: 1, 1986

62. Buckalew VM Jr, Schey HM: Renal disease from habitual antipyretic analgesic consumption: an assessment of the epidemiologic evidence. *Medicine* 65: 291, 1986

63. Murray T, Goldberg M: Analgesic abuse and renal disease. *Annu Rev Med* 26: 537, 1975

64. Disney APS, Row PG: Australian maintenance dialysis survey. *Med J Aust* 2: 651, 1974

65. Stewart JH, McCarthy SW, Storey BG, Roberts BA, Gallery E, Mahony JF: Diseases causing end-stage renal failure in New South Wales. *Br Med J* 1: 440, 1975

66. Burkart JM, Buckalew VM Jr: Nephropathy associated with habitual ingestion of acetaminophen. *Kidney Int* 31: 192, 1987

67. Nanra RS, Stuart-Taylor J, de Leon AH, White KH: Analgesic nephropathy: Etiology, clinical syndrome, and clinicopathologic correlations in Australia. *Kidney Int* 13: 79, 1978

68. McCredie M, Stewart JH, Mahony JF: Is phenacetin responsible for analgesic nephroppathy in New South Wales? *Clin Nephrol* 17: 134, 1982

69. Murray T, Goldberg M: Chronic interstitial nephritis: etiologic factors. *Ann Intern Med* 82: 453, 1975

70. Murray TG, Goldberg M: Analgesic associated nephropathy

in the USA; epidemiologic clinical and pathogenetic features. *Kidney Int* 13: 64, 1978

71. Gault MH, Rudwal TC, Engles WD, Dossetor JB: Syndrome associated with the abuse of analgesics. *Ann Intern Med* 68: 906, 1968

72. Emmerson BT: Chronic lead nephropathy. *Kidney Int* 4: 1, 1973

73. Bennett WM: Lead nephropathy. *Kidney Int* 28: 212, 1985

74. Weeden RP, Mallik DK, Batumen V: Detection and treatment of occupational lead nephropathy. *Arch Intern Med* 139: 53, 1979

75. Morgan JM, Hartley MW: Etiologic factors in lead nephropathy. *South Med J* 69: 1445, 1976

76. Beck L: Requiem for gouty nephropathy. *Kidney Int* 30: 280, 1986

77. Batumen V, Landy E, Maesaka JK, Weeden RP: Contribution of lead to hypertension with renal impairment. *N Engl J Med* 309: 17, 1983

78. Emmerson BT: The clinical differentiation of lead gout from primary gout. *Arthritis Rheum* 11: 623, 1968

79. Morgan JM, Burch HB: Comparative tests for the diagnosis of lead poisoning. *Arch Intern Med* 130: 335, 1972

80. Landrigan PJ: Occupational and community exposures to toxic metals: lead, cadmium, mercury and arsenic. *West J Med* 137: 531, 1982

81. Weeden RP, Batumen V, Landy E: The safety of EDTA lead mobilization test. *Environ Res* 30: 58, 1983

82. Ferris T, Kashgarian M, Levithin H, Brandt I, Epstein FH: Renal tubular acidosis and renal potassium wasting acquired as a result of hypercalcemic nephropathy. *N Engl J Med* 265: 924, 1961

83. Hellstromn J: Primary hyperparathyroidism: observations in a series of 50 cases. *Acta Endocrinol* 16: 30, 1954

84. Lins LE: Reversible renal failure caused by hypercalcemia. *Acta Med Scand* 203: 309, 1978

85. Schrier RW: Hypercalcemic nephropathy. in *Textbook of Medicine*, edited by Wyngaarden JB, Smith LH, Philadelphia, WB Saunders Co, 1982, p 562

86. Jacobs C, Brunner FP, Chantler C, Donckerwolcke RA, Gurland HJ, Hathway RA, Selwood NH, Wing AJ: Combined report on regular dialysis and transplantation in Europe, VII, 1976. *Proc Eur Dial Transplant Assoc* 14: 4, 1977

87. Bell ET: *Renal Diseases*, 2nd edition, Philadelphia, Lea and Febiger, 1950.

88. Pollak VE, Pirani CL, Kark RM: Effect of large doses of prednisone on the renal lesions and life span of patients with lupus glomerulonephritis. *J Lab Clin Med* 57: 495, 1961

89. Soffer IJ, Southren AL, Weiner HE, Wolf RL: Renal manifestations of systemic lupus erythematosus: A clinical and pathologic study of 90 cases. *Ann Intern Med* 54: 215, 1961

90. Steinberg AD: The treatment of lupus nephritis. *Kidney Int* 30: 769, 1986

91. Balow JE, Austin HA III, Tsokos GC, Antonovych TT, Steinberg AD, Klippel JH: Lupus nephritis. *Ann Intern Med* 106: 79, 1987

92. Ascer K, Walker JA, Lief PD, Barland P, Bank N: Triad of glomerulonephritis, antinuclear antibodies and positive skin immunofluorescence. Variant of systemic lupus erythematosus. *Am J Med* 74: 83, 1982

93. Hollcraft RM, Dubois EL, Lundberg GD, Chandor SB, Gibert SB, Quismorio FB, Barbour BH, Friou GJ: Renal damage in systemic lupus erythematosus with normal renal function. *J Rhematol* 3: 251, 1976

94. Hill GS, Hinglais N, Tron F, Bach JF: Systemic lupus erythe-

matosus: morphologic correlations with immunologic and clinical data at the time of biopsy. *Am J Med* 64: 61, 1978

95. Kant KS, Pollak VE: Multisystem diseases. Nephritis in systemic lupus erythematosus. in *Current Therapy in Nephrology and Hypertension 1984–1985*, edited by Glassock RJ, Philadelphia, BC Decker, 1984, p 139

96. Austin HA III, Klippel JH, Balow JE, Le Riche NGH, Steinberg AD, Plotz PH, Decker JL: Therapy of lupus nephritis. Controlled trial of prednisone and cytotoxic drugs. *N Engl J Med* 314: 614, 1986

97. Kimberly RP, Lockshin MD, Sherman RL, McDougal JS, Inman RD, Christian CL: High-dose intravenous methylprednisolone pulse therapy in systemic lupus erythematosus. *Am J Med* 70: 817, 1981

98. Hebert L, Nielsen E, Phol M, Lachin J, Hunsicker L, Lewis E: Clinical course of severe lupus nephritis during the controlled clinical trial of plasmapheresis therapy (PPT). *Kidney Int* 31: 201, 1987

99. Fauci AS, Haynes BF, Katz P: The spectrum of vasculitis: clinical, pathologic, immunologic and therapeutic considerations. *Ann Intern Med* 89: 660, 1978

100. Fahey JL, Leonard E, Churg J, Godman G: Wegener's granulomatosis. *Am J Med* 17: 168, 1954

101. Walton EW: Giant-cell granuloma of the respiratory tract (Wegener's granulomatosis). *Br J Med* 2: 265, 1958

102. Reza MJ, Dornfeld L, Goldberg LS, Bluestone R, Pearson CM: Wegener's granulomatosis: Long-term follow-up patients treated with cyclophosphamide. *Arthritis Rheum* 18: 501, 1975

103. Fauci AS, Haynes BF, Katz P, Wolff SM: Wegener's granulomatosis: Prospective clinical and therapeutic experience with 85 patients for 21 years. *Ann Intern Med* 98: 76, 1983

104. Leatherman JW, Davies DF, Hoidal JR: Alveolar hemorrhage syndromes: Diffuse microvascular lung hemorrhage in immune and idiopathic disorders. *Medicine* 63: 343, 1984

105. Atkins RC: The macrophage in human rapidly progressive glomerulonephritis. *Lancet* 1: 830, 1976

106. Zimmerman SW, Groehler K, Beirne GJ: Hydrocarbon exposure and chronic glomerulonephritis. *Lancet* 2: 199, 1975

107. Benoit FL, Rulon DB, Theil GB, Doolan PD, Watten RH: Goodpasture's syndrome: a clinicopathologic entity. *Am J Med* 37: 424, 1964

108. Wilson CB, Dixon FJ: Renal injury from immune reactions involving antigens in or of the kidney. in *Contemporary Issues in Nephrology. Immunologic Mechanisms of Renal Disease* Vol 3, edited by Brenner BM, Stein J, New York, Churchill-Livingstone, 1979, p 35

109. Glassock RJ, Cohen AH, Adler S, Ward H: Secondary glomerular diseases. in *The Kidney*, edited by Brenner BM, Rector FC, Philadelphia, WB Saunders Co, 1986, p 1014

110. Wilson CB, Dixon FJ: Anti-glomerular basement membrane antibody-induced glomerulonephritis. *Kidney Int* 3: 74, 1973

111. Johnson JP, Moore J Jr, Austin HA, Balow JE, Antonovych TT, Wilson CT: Therapy of anti-glomerular basement membrane antibody disease: Analysis of prognostic significance of clinical, pathologic and treatment factors. *Medicine* 64: 219, 1985

112. Peters DK, Rees AJ, Lockwood CM, Pusey CD: Treatment and prognosis of anti-basement membrane antibody mediated nephritis. *Transplant Proc* 14: 513, 1982

113. Glassock RJ, Cohen AH, Adler S, Ward H: Primary glomerular diseases. in *The Kidney*, edited by Brenner BM, Rector FC, Philadelphia, WB Saunders Co, 1986, p 929

114. Pollak VE, Rosen S, Pirani CL, Muehrcke RC, Kark RM:

Natural history of lipoid nephrosis and membranous glomerulonephritis. *Ann Intern Med* 69: 1171, 1968

115. Johnson RJ, Couser WG: Membranous nephropathy. in *Current Therapy in Nephrology and Hypertension 1984–1985*, edited by Glassock RJ, Philadelphia, BC Decker, 1984, p 207

116. Coggins CH, Frommer JP, Glassock RJ: Membranous nephropathy. *Semin Nephrol* 2: 264, 1982

117. Glassock RJ: Corticosteroid therapy is beneficial in adults with idiopathic membranous glomerulopathy. *Am J Kidney Dis* 1: 376, 1982

118. Honkanen E: Survival in idiopathic membranous glomerulonephritis. *Clin Nephrol* 25: 122, 1986

119. Kida H, Asamoto T, Yokoyama H, Tomosugi N, Hattori N: Long-term prognosis of membranous nephropathy. *Clin Nephrol* 25: 64, 1986

120. Schwartz MM, Cotran RS: Primary renal disease in transplant recipients. *Hum Pathol* 7: 455, 1976

121. Heptinstall RH: *Pathology of the Kidney*, 3rd edition, Boston, Little Brown and Co, 1983, p 519

122. Collaborative Study of the Adult Idiopathic Nephrotic Syndrome. A controlled study of short-term prednisone treatment in adults with membranous nephropathy. *N Engl J Med* 301: 1301, 1979

123. Ponticelli C: Prognosis and treatment of membranous nephropathy. *Kidney Int* 29: 927, 1986

124. Lewis EJ, Schwartz MM: Idiopathic crescentic glomerulonephritis. *Semin Nephrol* 2: 193, 1982

125. Glassock R: A clinical and immunopathologoc dissection of rapidly prograssive glomerulonephritis. *Nephron* 22: 253, 1978

126. Bolton WK: Crescentic glomerulonephritis. in: *Current Therapy in Nephrology and Hypertension 1984–1985*, edited by Glassock RJ, Philadelphia, BC Decker, 1984, p 213

127. Couser WG: Idiopathic rapidly progressive glomerulonephritis. *Am J Nephrol* 2: 57, 1982

PROLONGED SURVIVAL ON HEMODIALYSIS

A. PETER LUNDIN, III

INTRODUCTION

When maintenance hemodialysis (HD) began to be used to treat end-stage renal disease (ESRD) over 25 years ago, the long-term survival of the treated patients was scarcely considered, because their short-term survival seemed so chancy. Much has changed since those early days. Despite the fact that our knowledge of toxic factors and deficiencies that cause the uremic syndrome is far from complete, we see growing numbers of patients surviving on HD for 10 or more years. These long surviving hemodialysis patients (LSHP) represent one of the best successes of modern medical technology.

There is no single definition of long survival; it has been applied to patients on hemodialysis for a relatively short time, even less than one year. For the purpose of this chapter I would like to consider the LSHP to be those on hemodialysis for at least 10 years, but the scarcity of information on this special population would make a very short work. Patients who have survived a long time after the failure of their kidneys do not constitute a homogeneous population, because they may drift from one to another of the various methods of treatment for ESRD. Those who have remained on hemodialysis for longer than 10 years have not been studied frequently, either because their numbers are few in individual centers, because their physicians wish not to bother those who have survived the rigors of dialysis for so many years, or because having survived the gauntlet of medical care, the patients themselves prefer to be left alone.

Study of the pathobiology of LSHP is useful for delineating the limits of life expectancy for HD patients. Adverse reactions from many years of exposure to incompletely corrected uremia and accumulated contaminants may first become manifest in the LSHP. Physical and psychological factors that enhance or limit long survival could be pinpointed in retrospective cohort studies of LSHP and other comparable patients who began HD at the same time but did not survive. Complicating conditions present in deceased

patients and absent in LSHP might suggest that control or elimination of these conditions contributes to long survival.

Human physiology impaired by uremia has been described 1) in chronic renal failure, 2) under conditions where the uremic effect has been moderated to a greater or lesser degree by dialysis, and 3) after the reversal of uremia by kidney transplantation. This sequence suggests that uremia-induced abnormalities of hormonal function, cardiac physiology and bone disease, among others, can be improved by efficient HD and reversed by transplantation. The relatively normal lifestyle of many dialysis patients shows adaptation to the uremic state with recovery when the uremic condition is reversed by transplantation. The fact that transplantation can reverse the controlled uremic abnormalities in dialysis patients demonstrates the lack of permanent damage. Which of these uremic-induced abnormalities might lead to permanent disability with long-term dialysis and which can be reversed even after long impairment is still unclear. Several studies have identified hypertension as an important risk factor in early cardiovascular death and implicated control of blood pressure as crucial to long survival (1–3).

Two international conferences in Capri (1981) and New York (1982) have been held to explore the pathobiology of LSHP. Data from these meetings provide the bulk of available information on risk factors for long survival and the condition of LSHP.

POTENTIAL FOR LONG-TERM DIALYSIS SURVIVAL

Select dialysis patients can live at least 20 years despite multiple metabolic abnormalities of incompletely corrected uremia. Their prospect for long survival is improving because of advances in at least three areas causing dialysis morbidity. Improvements in dialysis technology have led to shorter, more comfortable and more efficient treatments. Better understanding of the pathophysiology of renal osteodystrophy make prevention or treatment of renal bone disease more probable. Genetic reproduction of erythropoietin and its injection into dialysis patients may reverse the complications of chronic anemia (4). The necessary physical prerequisites for long survival are an absence of life-threatening illness and preserved function of other vital organs. In addition, prevention or control of conditions that could lead to vital organ failure such as hypertension, smoking, abnormal calcium-phosphate metabolism, bone disease, infections and repeated access failure must be achieved both in the time preceding the need for dialysis, and after its initiation. Other risks to be avoided, most probably including accumulation of toxic substances from dialyzers, tubing and untreated water, will become apparent with time. The patient's medical condition when beginning HD will help indicate the individual's chances for long-term survival.

Long survival on HD requires more than a healthy body. The patient must also find an acceptable lifestyle and be able to envision a positive future. For this the patient must come to see dialysis and its associated restrictions as a means to an end, rather than an end in itself. Success requires a suitable personality with the will to go on despite the obstacles. It is clear that the patient's adaptation, rehabilitation and participation in his or her own care are helpful for long survival. Vital to this adaptation is the patient's feeling that he has some control over his life. Health professionals need to realize that the patient involved in his own care will have a better attitude toward his illness and a greater motivation to solve his health problem. For example, normalization of blood pressure and calcium-phosphate regulation, both necessary for long survival, are possible only with the cooperation of the patient.

For the psychologically adaptable patient whose health problems are limited to simple kidney failure, an optimal hemodialysis treatment is crucial for an acceptable life, as well as for keeping the patient in good physical shape for the desired kidney transplant. The difficulty in defining adequacy of dialysis, however, has permitted a wide spectrum of dialysis prescription, some clearly suboptimal. The inadequately dialyzed patient is subject to recurrence of such uremic complications as pericarditis, protein-calorie malnutrition and greater susceptibility to infection. Many of the cardiovascular deaths in these patients could be a result of failure to remove excess fluid (5). Such patients look and act as if they were ill, never really feel well, and will rarely, if ever, adapt to dialysis, since it is for them merely a prolongation of illness.

The number of patients worldwide now alive and sustained by HD or transplant for more than 10 years is not available. European Dialysis and Transplant Association (EDTA) statistics for 1980 reveal that over 3,000 of nearly 9,000 patients who began renal failure treatment in Europe before 1970 were still alive at least a decade later (6). A third of the surviving patients have never been transplanted and half have been transplanted only once, but it is not apparent how many of the transplanted patients are back on hemodialysis. In Italy there are 328 living 10-year HD patients (7). What percent of the total number starting dialysis these survivors represent is not obtainable, since records were not kept prior to 1972. Not surprisingly, the majority of these survivors were between 20 and 40 years of age when they began HD, and it is probable that they had few other medical problems.

The percentage of patients alive after 5 and 10 years in several individual renal programs can be obtained from a review of the literature (Table 1). Five year survival is about 70% (58 to 87%), while after 10 years about 50% (40 to 67%) of patients are still alive. The most recent experience indicates that 5 year survival for younger, uncomplicated patients on HD is better than 90% (8–10). Results for longer survival with individual ESRD therapies in groups of patients are adulterated by the frequent shifting between these therapies (11). Comparisons between individual treatments such as HD or transplant are also made difficult by the prognostic dissimilarities between patients before starting. Most LSHP began hemodialysis therapy before 1970, when for the most part only those with the best prognosis (youngest and healthiest) were accepted. Thus, it might be assumed that these survival rates represent the best that can be expected. But it must be pointed out that an adequate control of blood pressure and calcium-phosphate metabolism was not obtained in many of these early patients months before and years after they started dialysis (1, 12). Most of the cardiovascular deaths reported in HD patients in Seattle and Brooklyn were seen in patients in whom hypertension was predominant throughout their dialysis course (1, 13). Cigarette smoking appears to have a lethal effect, seen within 2 years in some HD patients. In the study by Haire et al (14) 72% of 38 normotensive smokers survived for 2 years and 40% for 6 years. When smoking was combined with hypertension the results were, as expected, considerably worse. Beyond 10 years on hemodialysis, absence of cardiovascular disease in the normotensive patient is noteworthy (13). As important as initial good health and avoidance of complications for survival of dialysis patients is the learning curve of

Table 1. Survival during maintenance hemodialysis in uncomplicated patients.

Author (year)	5 yr (%)	10 yr (%)	Mean age at start (n)
Lewis (1969)	57.8	–	35 ± 12 (302)
Moorhead (1970)	80.7	–	–
Johnson (1973)	70	–	38 (98)
Lindner (1974)	61.5	40.2	37 ± 0.5 (39)
Henari (1977)	68.4	57.7	39.2 (200)
Price (1978)	60	40	37.5
Kries (1978)	75	–	–
Wing (1978)	70	60	15–34
	60	40	35–44
Lundin (1980)	87	67	32.8 ± 9.7 (42)
Shapiro (1983)	97	–	46 (209)
	84	–	61 (362)
Charra (1983)	90	85	34.4 ± 9.3 (44)
Hellerstedt (1984)	78	–	21–45 (351)
Hutchinson (1987)	80	–	43

the medical professionals caring for them. This is demonstrated in the stepwise improvement in survival seen with time in several large dialysis programs (8–10), despite the fact that new patients tended to be older and sicker over time.

The major cause of death for the 10+ year dialysis patient in Brooklyn as well as in London has been sepsis (15). While infection is a frequent complication of HD, in our LSHP it has been seen largely in center-based patients. The home-based patients' personal responsibility for cleansing the skin and inserting the needles is a plausible explanation for their avoidance of infection.

PHYSICAL STATUS OF LONG-SURVIVING HEMODIALYSIS PATIENTS

Cardiovascular

It is unusual to find symptoms of coronary artery disease in a 10+ year HD patient. Scribner (13) reports negative findings in 11 patients alive for more than 15 years (six dialysis, five transplant). Nine of the 11 patients also had no symptoms for peripheral vascular disease. Others have also found symptomatic heart disease to be infrequent in the long-surviving patients (Table 2) (13, 16, 17). Using echo and phonocardiography, non-invasive measures of cardiac function, seven patients treated by HD for more than 10 years were compared with a group treated for less than 4 years. Although end-diastolic diameter, end-systolic diameter and ejection fraction were found to be abnormal in both groups when compared with normals, the only significant differences between the patient groups were aortic root diameter and left ventricular posterior wall thickness. From this study it appears that deterioration of systolic ventricular function in dialysis patients can be slow to develop.

These observations do not exclude the presence of asymptomatic coronary artery atherosclerosis, however. In a population infrequently exposed to vigorous exercises, evidence of myocardial ischemia might be seen only with exertion. To test for the presence of underlying asymptomatic heart disease in LSHP, ten patients on dialysis for a mean of 8.4 years were subjected to stress testing, a method widely used for detecting the presence of coronary artery disease (19). The findings were negative. These negative results gain significance in a population for which there is a high expectation of abnormality. In addition, the exercise in these patients was not limited by signs of heart failure but rather by leg fatigue. A marker of developing cardiac disease besides angina pectoris or exercise-limiting congestive heart failure would be the new onset of cardiac arrythmias. Although not uncommon in new dialysis patients, there is no evidence that arrythmias have become a particular problem in most LSHP.

It appears, then, that most of those exposed to major cardiovascular risk factors will succumb in less than 10 years of dialysis. The cardiovascular prognosis for the others will depend on the severity and duration of exposure to lesser risk factors, such as hypertriglyceridemia, low levels of high-density lipoprotein cholesterol, and atherogenic polyamines (20, 21). Triglyceride levels are lower in long-surviving patients than in those more recently starting HD (22). Whether having lower triglycerides is a function of time on dialysis or a selective advantage for long-term patients from the beginning is not clear. Adverse effects of possible vasculopathic substances, such as polyamines and some amino acid metabolites, may depend on the efficiency of removal by hemodialysis.

Metastatic calcification of peripheral blood vessels, periarticular tissue, skin and tissues of the eye are frequently seen to occur in uremic patients both before and after the beginning of dialytic treatment (23, 24). less commonly observed, but more life-threatening, are diffuse calcium deposits in visceral organs such as heart and lung (25, 26). These deposits have been discovered by postmortem examination in many patients who exhibited no signs and symptoms of them before death. Important etiologic factors for tissue calcification besides supersaturated plasma levels of calcium and phosphate may be parathyroid disease, acid-base status, and ingestion of active forms of vitamin D.

Neither visceral nor peripheral calcification is a necessary or inevitable concomitant of long-term HD. Nine of 10 of our longest surviving patients have no deposits found on x-ray, although this test does not exclude their presence. One of 10 of our patients, more than 13 years on dialysis, has had diffuse vascular calcification for many years without complications. Such deposits are usually located in the media of the vessels without narrowing of the lumen, and thus may not have an adverse prognosis. Cardiac calcification was found in only one of the 10 LSHP studied by

Table 2. Cardiovascular findings in long-term hemodialysis survivors.

	Mean age	Previous MI or symptoms angina	Cardiomegaly (LVH)	Ischemic EKG changes	Symptomatic peripheral vascular disease
Scribner (n = 6)	44.8	0	–	–	1
Baillod (n = 28)	–	1 (3.5%)	2 (7%)	9 (32%)	–
Zingraff (n = 40)	42.5	3 (7.5%)	10 (25%)	–	–
Lundin (n = 10)	39.3	–	4 (40%)	1 (10%)	0

Abramowitz et al (18). Eleven of 28 LSHP followed by Baillod et al (16), included among them the two longest survivors, also have no obvious vascular calcifications. This complication is closely related to the patient's age when dialysis was started, 25 years for those without deposits and 37 years for those with. Prognosis depends on the severity of organ or vascular impairment, as well as on the potential for reabsorption of calcium. Control of hyperphosphatemia and administration of physiologic rather than pharmacologic doses of Vitamin D analogs are likely to be of importance in the prevention of metastatic calcification.

Osteodystrophy and complications of the joints

After cardiovascular disease, progressive bone damage may be the most important limitation to long life for the dialysis patient. According to EDTA statistics, disabling bone disease (defined as bone pain requiring analgesics with fractures on x-ray, major deformity, aseptic necrosis and slipped epiphyses) occurs in 4.7% of first year dialysis patients, increases to 18.6% of those on dialysis for over 5 years and is found in 19% at 10 years (6, 27). Piccoli et al (28) found that 100% of their 10-year patients had osteomalacia and 80% had changes of secondary hyperparathyroidism (osteitis fibrosa). Lindergard et al (29) noticed that most of the bone mineral loss in their LSHP had occurred before the onset of dialysis, with little further change during recent years. Most of their patients (80%) continue to have subnormal bone mineral content with minimal improvement after parathyroidectomy or treatment with 1 alpha hydroxyvitamin D_3.

In Seattle three of the six longest surviving patients (>15 years) have bone problems described as 'disabling' while the condition of the others is 'moderate' (13). One of 10 Brooklyn patients has incapacitating osteomalacia. None of the others are severely affected, but all have lost at least one inch of height over 10 years as a result of asymptomatic compaction of spinal vertebrate. Osteopenia is seen on x-ray in most of the patients, suggesting osteomalacia or osteoporosis.

Although there are a number of useful treatments for osteitis fibrosa (an increase in the levels of dialysis fluid calcium to exceed the ionized fraction, better control of hyperphosphatemia, surgical parathyroidectomy, or treatment with active vitamin D metabolites) these interventions appear to have little effect on osteomalcia. Removing Al with the iron chelator, deferoxamine, has led to improvement (30). Considerable evidence has accumulated over the past 6 to 7 years strongly implicating aluminum (Al) derived from dialysis solution water or phosphate binders or both as a major cause of osteopenia and disabling bone disease in hemodialysis patients. In patients followed for 10 years on dialysis it was found that osteopenia was prevented when parathyroid hormone (PTH) concentrations were greater than 600 pg/ml (31). This last observation raises some concern about total suppression of parathyroid activity, whether through active vitamin D metabolites or by parathyroidectomy. These actions, along with the continued use of Al phosphate binders, might bring about the conditions that lead to Al osteomalacia (32–33).

Uncontrolled hyperparathyroidism has adverse effects, nevertheless. PTH-induced damage to nerves, bone marrow, red cells, muscle and heart may lead to severe incapacititation of the long-term patient (34). Avram et al (35) found that their living long-term patients had lower PTH levels (mean 523 pg/ml) than had the 10-year patients who died (mean 672 pg/ml). It is uncertain whether parathyroid hormone contributed to the death of patients in the latter group. Some balance needs to be found between exuberant parathyroid function and complete suppression.

Disabling joint complications are common in LSHP. Wrist, shoulder and hip joints are frequently affected. Joint pain with periarticular calcification, boney erosion and morning stiffness occur in 50 to 90% of patients up to and beyond the 10th year of hemodialysis (36, 37). Carpal tunnel syndrome (CTS) from median nerve compression is particularly frequent in LSHP, although it can also be found in those on HD for only a few years (13, 38, 39). The CTS seen in LSHP is associated with cystic bone lesions and deposition in tendon sheaths of amyloid-like material which does not react with antibodies to known amyloid proteins (40, 41). The source of this amyloid-like protein appears to be $beta_2$-microglobulin (42). Deposition in joint tissues in LSHP could be the consequence of loss of renal catabolism or increased production in response to a bio-incompatible extracorporeal circuit.

Arthropathy causing pain and stiffness in the shoulders is seen with increasing frequency in LSHP (43). The cause may be the same as that seen in CTS. The shoulder pain seems to be particularly troublesome during dialysis or at night, interfering with sleep.

Endocrinologic dysfunction

Apart from hyperparathyroidism and erythropoietin deficiency, hemodialysis patients rarely exhibit signs or symptoms of hormonal dysfunction, despite abnormalities in blood levels, feedback control, peripheral function, and metabolism of many hormones. There have been no reports of the state of endocrine function in long-term patients, although it is well described in short-term ones. We recently studied the pituitary gland reserve of patients on dialysis a mean of 8.8 years, using a combined stimulation test of insulin, thyrotropin releasing hormone and luteinizing hormone releasing hormone (LHRH). Subnormal pituitary reserve was found, most commonly for adrenocorticotropic hormone (ACTH) and prolactin and less often for luteinizing hormone and thyroid stimulating hormone (TSH). These findings are not different from those found in short-term patients, suggesting that pituitary gland function is not significantly affected by length of time on dialysis. It should also be noted that all of our 10+ year patients also have normal fasting glucose levels.

Hematologic and immunologic complications

Some dialysis patients, particularly those who have undergone nephrectomy, have difficulty maintaining a hematocrit above 20% and may even require frequent transfusions. Their morbidity is substantial, and long survival is the exception rather than the rule. Four groups of observers have reported mean hematocrits in long-term patients to range from 28 to 34% (13, 16, 17, 35). None of the patients studied currently are transfusion-requiring. During the first several years they were on dialysis, most long-term patients had lower hematocrits, requiring occasional transfusions. Coratelli et al (44) found that globulin synthesis was more effective in patients dialyzed for 10 years when compared with those only one year on dialysis. An explanation for their higher hematocrits was improved globin synthesis, a possible consequence of increased production of erythropoietin from acquired renal cysts (see below). No deterioration was noted in the coagulation system in a dozen patients on dialysis a decade or more (45).

Abnormalities of the immune system in uremia, particularly cell mediated immunity, have been well explored (46, 47). Deficits in immunologic function do not progressively worsen with long-term HD (49). Long-term patients do not show a greater susceptibility to viral complications due to deficiencies of cell mediated immunity than would be expected in normal individuals. Most of the patients begun on hemodialysis in the 1960s have been exposed to hepatitis B antigen from frequent transfusions, but few have become hepatitis B antigen carriers. One adverse consequence of long-term cellular immunosuppression would be malignancy. Whether or not chronic renal failure predisposes to malignancy is unclear from the literature. Common solid tumors are the most frequent cause of cancer in these patients, as opposed to the epithelial and lymphopoliferative cancers seen in transplant patients. Whether the uremic propensity for cell-mediated immunosuppression can be ameliorated or worsened by dialysis is unclear, but except for the possibility of malignant transformation in the acquired renal cycts, cancer does not seem to be frequent in the LSHP.

Bacterial infection was the major cause of death in our long-term patients, and it was seen exclusively in center dialyzed patients. Seven of 10 long-term patients dialyzed at home have not had bacterial infections in the years since their external shunts were replaced by AV fistulas or grafts. Considering the frequency of exposure to bacterial infection with each needle puncture, this experience does not indicate a decreased resistance to bacterial infection.

Neurologic complications

Incapacitating peripheral neuropathy was once felt to be an inevitable complication of long-term hemodialysis. This has been shown to be untrue, since progression can be halted when adequate dialysis is given. In Paris, 8 of 40 long-term patients had signs of lower limb neuropathy early in their course without further progression (17). In three of these patients preventable causes were determined to be treatment with isoniazid for tuberculosis, complications of heroin addiction, and inadequate dialysis.

Dementia is a frightening and usually fatal complication

seen in dialysis patients, most frequently where water aluminum levels are high (49). In these high level areas dementia is associated with length of exposure, but in other places long-term hemodialysis has not been associated with any signs of CNS dysfunction (50).

Gastrointestinal abnormalities

There is an increased incidence of peptic ulceration in uremic patients (51). A probable contributory cause is the higher mean gastrin levels seen in many of these patients due to a decrease of renal catabolic capability (52). Major upper gastrointestinal complications, however, have not been frequent in LSHP. It could be presumed that this group should be suffering from prolonged exposure to elevated gastrin levels, although in a group of LSHP gastrin levels were found to be lower than those measured in new patients (53). Whether the lower levels of gastrin represent impaired gastric excretion or just more normal physiology is not known.

Hepatomegaly is reported to occur after several years of dialytic therapy (54). Others have seen hepatic inflammatory reactions due to refractile particles presumed to be silicone from the blood tubing pump segment (55). A connection between these observations has not been established, but longer exposure to elutable dialysis materials might be expected to lead to hepatic enlargement with liver dysfunction. This has not been observed in any of our patients, although several have splenomegaly detected by radionuclide scanning.

Another possible gastrointestinal complication of LSHP is colonic diverticulosis due to frequent episodes of phosphate binder-induced constipation. None of our LSHP has had manifestations of diverticular disease, and in the one patient studied with contrast material only a single diverticulum of the transverse colon was seen.

Vascular access

Perhaps the most essential ingredient for long-term dialysis success is a reliable vascular access. Few dialysis associated problems are more psychologically and physically devastating than access complications. Most of our earliest patients began dialysis with the external shunt and suffered frequent shunt failure. Some underwent surgery up to 30 times in order to preserve old or create new access to the circulation. The greatest number of surgical access procedures in a single patient that I recall was somewhere between 65 and 70; it is not hard to lose count. The majority of LSHP have achieved stable blood access; they probably would otherwise no longer be on HD or alive. Patients who continue to experience occasional problems are those with bovine implants or grafts of artificial materials. Their inability to have a stable functioning fistula appears to be related to the number of previous access operations with consequent loss of veins and arteries. Three of four LSHP have had the same fistula for over 18 years, indicating the superiority of an A-V fistula as a blood access for dialysis.

Acquired renal cysts

Although the kidneys in dialysis patients are shrunken and bereft of most vital functions, they may still produce enough erythropoietin to maintain the hematocrit at a low but stable level. This function provides more than sufficient rationale for not removing this otherwise useless tissue except under urgent conditions. The prospect of such an urgent condition is becoming increasingly apparent in LSHP with the identification of cystic degeneration and tumor formation in the scarred remnants of what used to be kidneys (56, 57). Acquired (as opposed to congenital) cysts occur in as many as one third of the patients on HD. The number of patients with cysts increases in proportion to length of time on hemodialysis, with cysts found in 92% of patients on for more than 8 years (58). Complications from these cysts include bleeding with hematuria and flank pain, adenomatous formation and malignant degeneration. Metastases from renal cancers have been reported and should be of concern when the tumor is more than 3.0 cm in diameter. It is recommended that every patient on dialysis for more than 3 years have a sonographic or CT evaluation of the kidneys. Aspiration cytology may be indicated, since it is often difficult to determine radiographically if a tumor is malignant (59). The cysts appear to regress after successful renal transplantation (60), but the potential for cancerous growth, particularly under immunosuppressive therapy, has not been evaluated. This concern may provide a rationale for nephrectomy in LSHP, particularly with the advent of commercially available erythropoietin.

PSYCHOLOGICAL FACTORS CONTRIBUTING TO LONG-TERM SURVIVAL

LSHP have been described as 'givers of ulcers rather than getters of ulcers' (61). Their most important personality trait is the strong desire for independence and control of the dialysis regimen. This trait can be readily seen both in the LSHP remaining in centers and in those who dialyze at home. These patients are usually perceived as stubborn or aggressive as a result of their frequently challenging or ignoring professional advice and instructions, particularly during their early years on dialysis. In the later dialysis years, advice is usually sought only when new and potentially serious medical problems arise. The frequently exhibited aloofness and desire for isolation is not selfishness as often described, but rather a mark of independence from exclusive professional control of their dialysis. The majority of our LSHP are closely involved with other patients or willing to become so if necessary. Their long survival is undeniable proof of the beneficial effects of their attitude. Rather than attempting to dominate or control the dialysis regimen themselves, health professionals should be encouraging patient independence and self-control. To do this, they must themselves become comfortable with both the idea and the reality of independence in their patients.

CONCLUSION

The capacity of HD to support life for more than 10 years has been clearly demonstrated. Control of hypertension, prevention of infection and good vascular access are probably the most important longevity factors, but the additional requirement for an aggressive and independent personality in the patient should not be underestimated.

Major limitations on even longer survival have been defined (renal osteodystrophy, atherosclerosis) or remain speculative (persistent uremic abnormalities, dialysis related contaminants). Most of these problems are also likely to be amenable to control with optimal dialysis treatment and yet to be defined adjunctive therapies. Adverse effects of trace elements, carcinogens and other water contaminants and blood contacting dialysis materials should be preventable by water treatment and development of bio-compatible materials. The objective of any dialysis prescription should be to keep the HD patient alive and well until the problems with transplant rejection are finally eliminated. Anticipating that a universally acceptable transplant solution will be available within 10 years, the life expectancy of the uncomplicated young patient (<40 years of age) beginning HD today should be normal.

REFERENCES

1. Lundin AP, Adler AJ, Feinroth MV, Berlyne GM, Friedman EA: Maintenance hemodialysis, survival beyond the first decade. *JAMA* 244: 38, 1980
2. Rostand SG, Kirk KA, Rutsky EA: Relationship of coronary risk factors to hemodialysis-associated ischemic heart disease. *Kidney Int* 22: 304, 1982
3. Charra B, Calemard E, Cuche M, Laurent G: Control of hypertension and prolonged survival on maintenance hemodialysis. *Nephron* 33: 96, 1983
4. Eschbach JW, Egrie JC, Downing MR, Browne JK, Adamson JW: Correction of the anemia of end-stage renal disease with recombinant human erythropoietin: result of phase I and II clinical trial. *N Engl J Med* 326: 73, 1987
5. Plough AL, Salem S: Social and contextual factors in the analysis of mortality in end-stage renal disease patients. *Am J Public Health* 72: 1293, 1982
6. Jacobs C, Broyer M, Brunner FA, Brynger H, Donckerwolcke RA, Kramer P, Selwood NH, Wing AJ: Combined report on regular transplantation in Europe XI 1980. *Proc Eur Dial Transplant Assoc* 18: 2, 1981
7. Gabardini FP, Surian M, Colussi G: Uremic patients under dialysis and/or transplantation for more than ten years in Italy. in: *Uremia: Pathobiology of Patients Treated for 10 Years or More*, edited by Giordano C, Friedman EA, Milan, Wichtig Editore, 1981, p 41
8. Blagg CR, Wahl PW, Lamers JU: Treatment of chronic renal failure at the Northwest Kidney Center, Seattle from 1960 to 1982. *asaio J* 6: 170, 1983
9. Shapiro F, Umen A: Risk factors in hemodialysis patient survival. *asaio J* 6: 176, 1983
10. Mion CM, Murad G, Canaud B, Chong G: Maintenance dialysis: A survey of 17 years' experience in Languedoc-Roussillon with a comparison of methods in a 'Standard Population.' *asaio J* 6: 205, 1983

11. Hutchinson TA, Harvey CE: Survival with different forms of dialysis treatment. *asaio J* 8: 13, 1985

20. Pendras JP: Parathyroid disease in long-term maintenance hemodialysis. *Arch Intern Med* 124: 312, 1969

13. Scribner BH: The long-term Seattle hemodialysis and transplant survivors. in: *Uremia: Pathobiology of Patients Treated for 10 Years or More,* edited by Giordano C, Friedman EA, Milan, Wichtig Editore, 1981, p 32

14. Haire HM, Sherrard DJ, Scardapane D, Curtis FK, Brunzell JD: Smoking, hypertension and mortality in a maintenance dialysis population. *Cardiovasc Med* 3: 1163, 1978

15. Bradley JR, Evans DB, Calne R: Long-term survival in hemodialysis patients. *Lancet* 1: 295, 1987

16. Baillod RA, Varghese Z, Fernando ON, Moorhead JF: Review of 71 patients receiving renal replacement for greater than 10 years. in: *Uremia: Pathobiology of Patients Treated for 10 Years or More,* edited by Giordano C, Friedman EA, Milan, Wichtig Editore, 1981, p 35

17. Zingraff J, Man NK, Drüeke T, Jungers P, Crosnier J, Funck-Brentano JL: Long-term results in forty uremic patients treated by hemodialysis for more than 10 years. in: *Uremia: Pathobiology of Patients Treated for 10 Years or More,* edited by Giordano C, Friedman EA, Milan, Wichtig Editore, 1981, p 50

18. Abramowitz EM, Musunuru RSK, Scarpa WJ, Mandel G: Cardiovascular effects of a decade or longer of maintenance hemodialysis. in: *Prevention of Kidney Disease and Long-Term Survival,* edited by Avram MM, New York, Plenum, 1982, p 177

19. Lundin AP, Stein RA, Frank F, LaBelle P, Berlyne GM, Krasnow N, Friedman EA: Cardiovascular status in long-term hemodialysis patients: An exercise and echocardiographic study. *Nephron* 28: 234, 1981

20. Brunzell JD, Albers JJ, Haas LB, Goldberg AP, Agadoa L, Sherrard DJ: Prevalence of serum lipid abnormalities in chronic hemodialysis. *Metabolism* 26: 903, 1977

21. Bagdade JD, Subbaiah PV, Pantos D, Bartos F, Campbell RA: Polyamines: An unrecognized cardiovascular risk factor in chronic dialysis. *Lancet* 1: 412, 1979

22. Frank WM, Rao TKS, Manis T, Delano BG, Avram MM, Saxena AK, Carter AC, Friedman EA: Relationship of plasma lipids to renal function and length of time on maintenance hemodialysis. *Am J Clin Nutr* 31: 1886, 1982

23. Parfitt AM: Soft tissue calcification in uremia. *Arch Intern Med* 124: 544, 1969

24. Kuzela DL, Hoffer WE, Conger JD, Winter SD, Hammond WS: Soft tissue calcification in chronic dialysis patients. *Am J Path* 86: 406, 1977

25. Terman DS, Alfrey AC, Hammond WS, Donndelinger T, Ogden DA, Holmes JH: Cardiac calcification in uremia. A clinical, biochemical and pathologic study. *Am J Med* 50: 744, 1971

26. Conger JD, Hammond WS, Alfrey AC, Contiguglia SR, Stanford RE, Huffer WE: Pulmonary calcification in chronic dialysis patients, clinical and pathologic studies. *Ann Intern Med* 83: 330, 1975

27. Brynger H, Brunner FP, Chantler C, Donckerwolke RA, Jacobs C, Kramer P, Selwood NH, Wing AJ: Combined report on regular dialysis and transplantation in Europe X, 1979 *Proc Eur Dial Transplant Assoc* 17: 2, 1980

28. Piccoli G, Giachino G, Jeantet A, Quarello F, Bossi P, Squiccimarro G, Zatteri R, Rossi P, Vercellone A: Bone disease in hemodialyzed patients treated for 10 years or more. in: *Uremia: Pathobiology of Patients Treated for 10 Years or More,* edited by Giordano C, Friedman EA, Milan, Wichtig Editore, 1981, p 89

29. Lindergard B, Lindholm T, Sandstrom S, Johnell O: Renal osteodystrophy in patients dialyzed for 10 years or more. in: *Uremia: Pathobiology of Patients Treated for 10 Years or More,* edited by Giordano C, Friedman EA, Milan, Wichtig Editore, 1981, p 83

30. Ott SM, Andress DL, Nebeker HG, Milliner DS, Maloney NA, Coburn JW, Sherrard DJ: Changes in bone histology after treatment with desferrioxamine. *Kidney Int* 29 (Suppl 18): S108, 1986

31. Main J, Velasco N, Catto GRD, Fraser RA, Edward N, Adami S, O'Riordan JLH: The effect of hemodialysis, vitamin D metabolits and renal osteodystrophy on the skeletal demineralization associated with renal osteodystrophy. *Clin Nephrol* 26: 279, 1986

32. Andress DL, Ott SM, Maloney NA, Sherrard DJ: Effect of parathyroidectomy on aluminum accumulation in chronic renal failure. *N Engl J Med* 312: 468, 1985

33. Charhon SA, Berland YF, Olmer MJ, Delawari E, Traeger J, Meunier PJ: Effects of parathyroidectomy on bone formation and mineralization in hemodialyzed patients. *Kidney Int* 27: 426, 1985

34. Massry SG: Is parathyroid hormone a uremic toxin? *Nephron* 19: 125, 1977

35. Avram MM, Pahilan A, Gan A, Rizvi SA, Slater P, Fein P, Avram R, Iancu M: Factors influencing longevity of patients over 10 years on hemodialysis treatment. Role of parathyroid hormone (PTH) and serum phosphate (P). in: *Uremia: Pathobiology of Patients Treated for 10 Years or More,* edited by Giordano C, Friedman EA, Milan, Wichtig Editore, 1981, p 53

36. Tatler GLV, Baillod RA, Varghese Z, Young WB, Farrow S, Wills MR, Moorhead MF: Evolution of bone disease over 10 years in 135 patients with terminal renal failure. *Br Med J* 4: 315, 1973

37. Gelfand GF, Bienenstock H, Avram MM, Rosenblum D: Musculoskeletal abnormalities of the 10-year hemodialysis patient. in: *Prevention of Kidney Disease and Long-Term Survival,* edited by Avram MM, New York, Plenum, 1982, p 223

38. Scardapane D, Halter S, De Lisa JA, Sherrard DJ: Hand dysfunction due to carpal tunnel syndrome: A common sequela of dialysis. *Proc Clin Dial Transplant Forum* 9: 15, 1979

39. Schwarz A, Keller F, Seyfert S, Poll W, Molzahn M, Distler A: Carpal tunnel syndrome: a major complication in long-term hemodialysis patients. *Clin Nephrol* 22: 133, 1984

40. Morita T, Suzuki M, Kamimura A, Hirasawa Y: Amyloidosis of a possible new type in patients receiving long-term hemodialysis. *Arch Pathol Lab Med* 109: 1029, 1985

41. Feaves AZ, Emmett M, White MG, Greenway G, Michaels DB: Carpal tunnel syndrome with cystic bone lesions secondary to amyloidosis in chronic hemodialysis patients. *Am J Kidney Dis* 7: 130, 1986

42. Casey TT, Stone WJ, DiRaimondo CR, Brontley BD, DiRaimondo CV, Gorevic PD, Page DL: Tumoral amyloidosis of bone of beta$_2$-microglobulin origin in association with long-term hemodialysis. *Human Path* 17: 731, 1986

43. Brown EA, Arnold IR, Gower PE: Dialysis arthropathy: complications of long-term treatment with hemodialysis. *Br Med J* 292: 166, 1986

44. DiPillo FW, Gandhi H: Over decade maintenance hemodialysis: Its effect on uremic anemia and coagulation. in: *Prevention of Kidney Disease and Long-Term Survival,* edited by Avram MM, New York, Plenum, 1982, p 191

45. Coratelli P, Corciulo R, Izzo P, Amerio A: Globin synthesis of patients on regular dialysis treatment for more than 10 years. in: *Uremia: Pathobiology of Patients Treated for 10 Years or*

More, edited by Giordano C, Friedman EA, Milan, Wichtig Editore, 1981, p 138

46. Dobbelstein H: Immune system in uremia. *Nephron* 17: 409, 1976

47. Wilson WEC, Kirkpatrick CH, Talmage DW: Suppression of immunologic responsiveness in uremia. *Ann Intern Med* 62: 1, 1965

48. Vercellone A, Segoloni GP, Giacchino F, Canavese C, Mess-ina M, Pozzato M, Rotunno M, Squiccimarro G, Thea A, Camussi G, Piccoli G: Immune responsiveness versus dialytic age. in: *Uremia: Pathobiology of Patients Treated for 10 Years or More*, edited by Giordano C, Friedman EA, Milan, Wichtig Editore, 1981, p 273

49. Dunea G, Mahurkar SD, Mamdani B, Smith EC: Role of aluminum in dialysis dementia. *Ann Intern Med* 88: 502, 1978

SOCIAL, ETHICAL, AND LEGAL ISSUES INVOLVED IN CHRONIC MAINTENANCE DIALYSIS

NANCY BOUCOT CUMMINGS

INTRODUCTION

The treatment of end-stage renal disease (ESRD) raises many of the ethical issues and dilemmas associated with therapy of chronic, irreversible diseases and of catastrophic illness, and with the use of life-sustaining technologies. The thorniest problems which trouble nephrologists in dealing with ESRD include the multiple issues surrounding initiating treatment and terminating treatment. Concerned nephrologists, citizens, politicians and bureaucrats worry about the high cost of the long-term therapy, the cost-benefit and the allocation of scarce resources since provision of care for one expensive governmentally funded medical program often means cuts in another program (1). Hard choices in therapy may be influenced by forces outside the medical professions including politicians, lawyers, ethicists, clergy and lay persons.

The specific details of socio-economic, political and medical, as well as moral and ethical issues, vary from country to country, but the generic issues raised by dialysis treatment of chronic renal failure (CRF) are similar. An appreciation of the inability of low-income countries to provide tertiary care, of which dialysis is one example, helps clarify the potential issues for high-income countries should funding need to be curtailed in times of severe economic stringency. While industrialized countries have been able to provide a wide range of tertiary care for their citizens, the specter of increasing national debt and concomitant increases in costly health technologies is bound to force hard economic choices as governments are obliged to determine how scarce resources are to be allocated.

Comparative costs

The average annual cost of dialysis treatments for one individual exceeds the average family income in the United States (Table 1). The total annual federal expenditures for ESRD treatment of over two billion dollars are comparable to expenditures for coronary by-pass surgery, but are more visible because they are a budgetary cost for the government. Expenditures for personal consumption of potato chips in the United States in 1985 were three billion dollars (2), and the sum the American public spent on tobacco products alone was fourteen times the government's payment for ESRD therapy in 1986 (3).

Geographic patterns

Before 1972, in the United States major financial barriers limited the provision of ESRD therapy to patients with CRF. The passage of the ESRD amendment to Public Law (PL) 92–603 removed those barriers and entitled well over 90% of the population to treatment by dialysis or transplantation or both. The United Kingdom's provision of ESRD treatment has been strongly influenced by cost-controls imposed by setting budget allocations in advance, whereas, in the United States unlimited funding after treatment has been provided has been the usual practice. In the Federal Republic of Germany, France, Italy, and Spain, ESRD treatment is funded by insurance, and the predominant assumption is that all patients are entitled to medically indicated treatment (4). Most of the Western European countries, Australia, Canada, Israel, Japan, New Zealand,

and the United States provide ESRD coverage for a sizeable proportion of patients with CRF (Table 2). The coverage for ESRD treatment in countries included in the European Dialysis and Transplant Association (EDTA) Registry shows a roughly linear correlation between the number of ESRD patients treated per million population (PMP) and the gross national product (GNP) per capita (5).

In the countries which now provide nearly universal ESRD coverage, the age and disease restrictions in force in the 1960s have been removed. Often care was limited to 15 to 45 year old patients with a single, uncomplicated disease, a situation which raised major ethical issues about who should receive this expensive, scarce therapy. In most high-income countries, this obstacle has been removed, but other problems have arisen. Physicians in the United States have been concerned about the high incidence of malpractice suits and, as a result, often practice 'defensive medicine.' Issues raised throughout the medical community about initiation and termination of life-sustaining technologies for the critically or chronically ill or both have resulted in new laws, regulations, and bureaucratic hassles for the health care team. Nephrologists have not been immune from these concerns, which have led to both legal problems and court hearings. It is the goal of this chapter to give a brief overview of the social, ethical, and legal issues which surround provision of compassionate medical care to CRF patients requiring dialysis treatment.

DEMOGRAPHICS

A global perspective of health resources

For industrialized, high-income countries, medical resources are more plentiful and allow for the provision of tertiary care for a reasonable percentage of their populations; but for low-income countries, even the provision of minimal primary care is a strain on their limited economic resources. Distribution of resources for health care reflects not only the ability of a society to care for the individual but also the priorities of the government tailored by its financial capabilities. A governmental role in the health sector takes into account three situations: health for special groups or for groups of critical economic importance, programs to control the spread of diseases; and improvement of most people's health (6). In allocating primary health care funds, three broad approaches to the evaluation of human life which have been considered are individual willingness to pay for decreased risk of death, a human capital method based on lifetime earnings, and values placed on human life (7). There is a vast difference in the availability of funds for primary and tertiary care between those in the developed countries (industrial market economies) and developing countries (non-market industrial economies). In the low-income countries, where funds for even primary care are severely limited, the per capita average public expenditure for health was $11 in 1983 (Table 3); and 16 countries had per capita public expenditures of $2 or less (8). Public expenditures for health ranged from $0.5 to $1,122 per capita in 1983. This contrast emphasizes the industrialized countries' potential to provide sizable sums of money for health care of individuals – a luxury which is virtually impossible in low-income countries.

To understand the social, ethical, and legal issues confronting the treatment of dialysis patients, it is helpful to have an understanding of the composition of a given population. The EDTA Registry provides detailed data about its member countries (Chapter 31), while the United States' ESRD Program Management and Medical Information System (ESRD PMMIS) of the Health Care Finance Adminis-

Table 1. Medicare reimbursements, by enrollees and per capita reimbursements for persons with end stage renal disease: 1974–84.

Year	Reimbursements		Enrollment		Reimbursement per enrollee	
	Amount in millions	Percent change	Number thousand	Percent change	Amount $	Percent change
1974	228.5	–	16.0	–	14,300	–
1975	361.1	58.0	22.7	41.9	15,900	11.2
1976	512.2	41.8	28.9	27.3	17,720	11.4
1977	641.3	25.2	34.8	20.4	18,420	3.9
1978	800.0	24.7	43.5	25.0	18,390	– 0.2
1979	1,010.7	26.3	54.4	25.1	18,579	1.0
1980	1,252.2	23.8	61.9	13.8	20,229	8.9
1981	1,476.2	17.9	70.4	13.7	20,969	3.7
1982	1,660.9	12.5	77.9	10.7	21,321	1.7
1983	1,893.6	14.0	86.5	11.0	21,891	2.7
1984	1,953.5	3.2	92.8	7.3	21,051	– 3.8
ACRG[1]	–	23.9	–	19.2	–	– 3.9

[1] Annual compound rate of growth, all calculations are based on unrounded numbers.
NOTE: Data are incomplete for most recent years due to continual updating of the payment files.
SOURCE: Health Care Financing Administration, Bureau of Data Management and Strategy: Weekly health insurance merge record, June 1986.

tration (HCFA) provides patient-specific information about billing records and incidence-specific medical information for the United States.

Patterns of dialysis therapy provided in the United States

An increasing rate of new persons on dialysis, an apparent increase in severity as indicated by both age distribution and number of patients with diabetes, an increasing percent of patients on continuous ambulatory peritoneal dialysis (CAPD), an increasing rate of kidney transplantation, and an increase in reuse of dialysis filter elements are noted in the FY 1987 ESRD Renal Disease Research Report (9). In 1984, there were 23,979 new ESRD beneficiaries. Patterns of this group were: 71.6% 45 years of age or over; 55.2% male; and 31.9% non-white races. From 1979 to 1984, the program incidence increased from 76 PMP to 102 PMP, a 5.9 percent annual increase (Table 4). Incidence rates were strongly age-related: from 17 PMP in the 0 to 25 age group to 286 PMP for the group 65 years of age and over. The ESRD population distribution by age in 1984 was: 6.5% in the under-25 age group; 28.1% in the 25 to 44 years age group; 39.9% in the 45 to 64 age group; and 25.5% in the group 65 years of age and over. Fifty-five percent were male, and 67% were white. Medicare ESRD enrollment (rates per million) increased from 242 in 1979 to 393 in 1984, a 10.2% annual increase. The highest enrollment rates were in the age groups 45 to 64 years of age (827 per million); and 65 years of age and over (845 per million). The greatest increase in enrollment has occurred for patients with renal failure secondary to diabetes, a 23.5% annual increase.

Treatment trends for the years 1980 to 1985 reported in the ESRD Facility Survey (Medicare and non-Medicare-entitled patients included) show an increase in the number of dialysis patients from 52,364 to 84,797, an average annual growth rate of 10.1%. In 1985, 79.7% of all dialysis patients received 'in unit' hemodialysis, while the remainder were dialyzed at home or were in self-dialysis training (Table 5). Since 1980, the home dialysis population declined 3.4%. By 1985 home hemodialysis patients represented 4.7% of the total dialysis population and 23.9% of the total home population, and CAPD accounted for 92% of the total increase in self-dialysis.

Table 2. New end-stage renal disease patients per million population, by selected countries: 1979–1982.

Country	Number of patients per million				Annual percent increase	Percent change 1981–1982
	1979	*1980*	*1981*	*1982*		
Czechoslovakia	13	15	17	20	13.3	14.7
West Germany	43	47	51	52	7.2	3.4
France	36	42	44	41	4.5	− 6.2
East Germany	18	20	22	26	12.0	18.4
Israel	51	58	52	62	6.7	20.5
Italy	34	38	43	43	7.6	− 1.2
Poland	6	6	6	7	3.9	16.1
Spain	32	38	40	42	9.7	5.0
Sweden	39	47	47	53	11.0	12.8
England	22	25	28	31	11.7	12.2
United States[1]	76	82	83	89	5.1	7.5
White	61	67	68	72	5.7	6.4
All other	167	176	169	184	3.3	9.2

[1] Includes only Medicare-entitled end-stage renal disease (ESRD) patients. Of all ESRD patients in the U.S., 7 to 10% are not Medicare eligible.
SOURCE: *European Dialysis and Transplant Association Annual Report: 1983;* Health Care Financing Administration, Bureau of Data Management and Strategy: Data from the Program Management and Medical Information System, 1979–1982.

Table 3. Health as a social indicator, 1983.

	Public Health expenditures per capita U.S. dollars	*GNP million U.S. dollars*	*GNP per capita U.S. dollars*	*Population 1000*	*Calories % of requirements*	*Population with safe water, %*
World	119	13,087,979	2,839	4,691,102	111	62
Developed	454	10,518,183	9,417	1,116,969	132	97
Developing	11	2,569,796	736	3,574,133	104	51

From Sivard RL: *World Military and Social Expenditures 1986,* 11th Edition, World Priorities, Washington, DC.

In 1984 there were 78,769 patients on dialysis, comprising 79.6% of all ESRD Medicare beneficiaries, and 5,820 (5.9%) received kidney transplants. Patients 55 years or over made up 55% of the total ESRD beneficiary population. Persons 65 years of age and older were hospitalized 40% more than patients 15 to 24 years of age and required 86% more inpatient days. Elderly dialysis patients are the fastest growing group of dialysis patients in most industrialized countries except in the United Kingdom, which has stringent financial constraints limiting universal provision of such treatment modalities. The elderly tolerate dialysis reasonably well, and their treatment is prescribed in a fashion similar to that for patients of all ages in most of the world's high-income countries. By the end of 1985, 51% of renal facilities were freestanding (i.e. not affiliated with hospitals). Proprietary facilities accounted for 42% of renal facilities and were almost exclusively freestanding (Table 6). Nonprofit renal facilities were mainly hospital-owned and -operated.

Table 4. Medicare end-stage renal disease program incidence rates per million population by age, sex, and race: 1979–1984.

Age, sex, and race	1979	1980	1981	1982	1983	1984	Average annual percent increase	1983–84 percent increase
			Number of enrollees per million population					
Total	76	82	83	89	98	102	5.9	3.2
Age								
Under 25 years	15	16	16	17	16	17	2.1	7.3
25–44 years	66	70	68	71	72	73	2.3	1.3
45–64 years	165	176	181	192	195	204	4.3	4.5
65 years or older	174	193	189	210	284	286	10.4	0.8
Sex								
Male	87	95	94	101	111	115	5.7	4.0
Female	66	71	71	77	87	89	6.1	2.3
Race								
White	61	67	68	72	79	81	5.8	3.5
All other	167	176	169	184	213	217	5.4	1.8

SOURCE: Health Care Financing Administration, Bureau of Data Management and Strategy: Data from the Program Management and Medical Information System, 1979–1984, and Census Population Estimates-Series P-25, No 965.

Table 5. End-stage renal disease (ESRD) dialysis population, by type and place of dialysis: 1980–1985.[1]

Type and place of dialysis	1980	1981	1982	1983	1984	1985	Average annual percent increase	Percent change 1984–85
Total	52,364	58,924	65,765	71,987	78,483	84,797	10.1	8.0
In-unit hemodialysis	43,271	48,011	52,559	57,029	62,462	67,559	9.3	8.2
In-unit peritoneal	911	944	885	745	603	588	− 8.4	− 3.0
Home hemodialysis	4,715	4,481	4,394	4,323	4,125	3,983	− 3.3	− 3.4
Home peritoneal[2]	612	646	816	790	259	231	− 17.7	− 10.8
CAPD[3]	2,334	4,347	6,523	8,532	9,995	11,236	37.0	12.4
CCPD[4]	–	–	–	–	859	953	10.9	10.9
Self-training	521	495	588	568	481	569	− 1.8	− 18.3

[1] Counts are as of December 31 of each year from ESRD Facility Surveys.
[2] This figure decreased significantly in 1984, partially because of CCPD[4] patients being counted in this category in previous years. A CCPD[4] category was added to the ESRD Facility Survey in 1984.
[3] Continuous ambulatory peritoneal dialysis.
[4] Continuous cycling peritoneal dialysis. CCPD rate of growth is calculated from 1984.
NOTE: Self training figures include in-unit hemodialysis, in-unit peritoneal, CAPD, and CCPD patients.
SOURCE: Health Care Financing Administration, Bureau of Data Management and Strategy: Data from the ESRD Facility Survey, 1980–85.

Table 6. Number and percent of certified end-stage renal disease providers, by type of ownership: 1982–1985.

Ownership	1982		1983		1984		1985	
	Number	Percent	Number	Percent	Number	Percent	Number	Percent
Total	1,218	100.0	1,309	100.0	1,368	100.0	1,463	100.0
Proprietary	437	35.9	504	38.5	552	40.4	616	42.1
Hospital-based	14	1.1	14	1.1	23	1.7	26	1.8
Freestanding	423	34.7	490	37.4	529	38.7	590	40.3
Nonprofit	781	64.1	805	61.5	816	59.6	847	57.9
Hospital-based	677	55.6	668	51.0	677	49.4	689	47.1
Freestanding	104	8.5	137	10.5	139	10.2	158	10.8

SOURCE: Health Care Financing Administration, Bureau of Data Management and Strategy: Data from the Program Management and Medical Information System, 1982–1985.

QUALITY OF LIFE

Assessment

It is often extremely difficult to assess the 'quality of life.' Health care professionals and patients may have very different views of what constitutes a 'good' or an 'unsatisfactory' quality of life (10, 11). Because of the elusive nature of evaluating the parameters involved, research in this area has been relatively 'soft.' The majority of the published works has been undertaken by psychiatrists, social workers, and nephrology nurses, with occasional collaboration of nephrologists. Nurses (12–14) and social workers spend a greater amount of time with patients than do other members of the professional team and, hence, have developed a variety of research 'instruments' to assess quality of life. They have endeavored to develop mechanisms for alleviating the evident distress that they observe on the unit and which they hear reported from the home and social environment. There has been a tendency for nephrologists to consult with psychiatrists when they find evidence of any of a number of psychological or psychiatric symptoms among dialysis patients. Consequently, psychiatrists (15–20) have developed an interest in the problems of dialysis patients and have contributed to the literature on the subject.

ESRD patients are a therapeutic challenge because of the chronicity of their disease and their total dependence upon a machine and upon the health professionals responsible for treatment by these machines; their very existence constantly reminds them of the delicate balance between life and death that is supported by this life-sustaining technology. While physicians are concerned primarily with the medical aspects of chronic renal failure, they are also acutely aware that social and psychological factors (21–23) have a major influence upon patients' lives. These social and psychological factors affect the degree of compliance with prescribed treatments and the amount of support that families and friend are able to provide. Studies which assess the impact of various parameters upon the patients' well-being and quality of life have considered such social factors as: education, religion (24, 25), occupation, family structure (26–28), and

rehabilitation (29); the strength and impact of such support systems as the dialysis team, the family, friends, and community; adjustment and coping mechanisms, which include restrictions, losses, defense mechanisms, denial, conflict, handling of changes in the balance between dependence vs independence; and the presence of constant stress, especially that related to fear of failure of equipment and of death.

A prospective study of quality of life

A prospective study (30), The National Kidney Dialysis and Transplantation (NKDT) Study, evaluated: 1) quality of life, 2) quality of care, 3) disability and health status, 4) rehabilitation and 5) cost of treatment in a survey of over 1,000 patients from 11 dialysis and/or transplant centers balanced by characteristics. The study provides unique information including responses of about 859 patients, 347 who were in-center dialysis patients, 81 who were on CAPD or CCPD, and 144 who had received kidney transplants. This sample provides a singular body of information on the largest group ever analysed for these parameters. The average age of in-center dialysis patients was 52 years, and the average educational level was over 12 years. In-center patients were sicker than patients on other treatment modalities and had other health problems in addition to CRF. Sixteen percent of dialysis patients were 65 or older, and this age group accounted for 21.4% of in-center dialysis patients. There was an average of 1.1 co-morbid conditions per patient, with in-center patients averaging 1.55 co-morbid conditions each. The percentage distributions of co-morbid conditions and of 'total sickness impact profile score' for those over and under 65 years were within one-to-two percentage points. The patients' overall functional status was rated by the Karnofsky Index (31), which has 11 categories covering all possible levels of function from completely normal to dead, along with questions adapted from the Rand Health Insurance Study which fit the unique experiences of ESRD patients. 'Based on established standards of quality of life for the normal population, ESRD patients, despite their illness, appear to have adjusted reasonably well, even though they assess their quality of life to be somewhat lower than that of the general population' concludes the NKDT study. In a comparison of 24 indices or variables, there were 14 with statistically significant differences in dialysis patients under 65 years as compared to those 65 and older. The older group had a higher well-being index than did the under-65 group: more positive feelings, less negative feelings, greater satisfaction with their marriages, greater satisfaction with their family life, greater satisfaction with their savings and investments, greater satisfaction with their standard of living, a feeling that their life was easier. Nevertheless, persons over 65 also felt their health was poorer than that of others of the same age, that they had greater functional impairment, had markedly less ability to work, and had a much lower current-employment rate.

Psychosocial factors

Research examining psychological and psychosocial effects of chronic dialysis (32) has raised numerous controversial issues, such as the role of denial (33) in emotional adjustment and the relationship of intelligence (34, 35) to vocational rehabilitation in dialysis patients. Inconsistent findings leading to controversies are partially attributable to variance in research design and to shortcomings in methodology and reporting of data. Methodological criticisms focus on subject selection, subject description, illness measures, assessment procedures, conditions of testing, comparison groups and data analysis. The conclusion is that consideration of these factors in the design and conduct of studies will greatly enhance the quality of research in this area. The literature of the decades from the 1960s to 1980s describes the psychosocial, psychiatric, and neuropsychiatric status of uremic and chronic dialysis patients. It examines various psychological stresses of and reactions to ESRD; predicts emotional adjustment and rehabilitation of pre-existing emotional personality, cognitive and social factors; considers denial either as a potential killer or a factor contributing to successful adjustment to chronic dialysis and defines predictive factors in rehabilitation. 'The frequent failure of published studies to meet minimum standards of research design or reporting limits the certainty with which conclusions on the psychological aspects of dialysis can be asserted. Further efforts in this field should be directed toward maintaining as much scientific rigor as possible within the constraints of the problem under scrutiny.' (36).

Stresses

Chronic disease poses a constant strain for all patients, and those patients who have ESRD have additional stresses: dependencies upon medical machinery and personnel; the constant threat of death and of reduced life expectancy, and decreased physical stamina and strength (37–39). Dialysis treatment demands significant blocks of time, repetitively, so that patients are tied to a fairly rigid schedule. For those patients who are being dialysed in-center, there is the additional burden of commuting to and from a center, a situation which also may require arranging for transportation to the center if the patient cannot cope on his own. Stringent fluid and dietary restrictions impose a special sacrifice. The broad range of responses which patients have reported to the rigors of dialysis is noteworthy. 'Despite all these problems there is a striking variation in how well patients cope with ESRD; many lead active, fulfilling family, professional and personal lives, while others stop work, abnegate responsibilities, neglect themselves and become angry and irritable.' (40)

Studies in several different countries detail aspects of the stresses placed upon dialysis patients. A Canadian study of 70 dialysis and transplant patients has shown that there is a strong correlation between low levels of perceived control over a variety of life dimensions and increased feelings of helplessness and depression (41). Losses frequently identified with ESRD treatment that add to the emotional stresses include reducing or giving up active participation in valued activities, such as work, household and/or school duties, and leisure activities. These intrusions threaten the individual's security and enjoyment of life and contribute to a loss of sense of personal prestige, self-respect, esteem, and the usual quality of life. This Canadian group also reviewed the literature (40) and identified a number of problem areas that need more incisive research: mood-depression, suicide, rehabilitation, marital and sexual dysfunction, quality of life, course of adjustment, compliance, dialysis unit environment, and sensory cognitive deficits. They corroborated the multiplicity of stresses associated with ESRD: uncertainty about survival; machine dependency; major changes in staff or in organization of treatment delivery causing signficiant emotional stress; a conflict of dependency with the goals of rehabilitation and resumption of predialysis activities; severe dietary and fluid restrictions; time demands; patient mobility and opportunities for travel; potential problems such as income or job loss; conflict between treatment schedules and work time; general feelings of malaise; side effects of medication; limited reproductive capacity; strains in family life (42) and friendships and a lack of time, energy, and resources to continue hobbies and leisure time activities.

'Considering the stressful nature of dialysis, it is easy to lose sight of the fact that the majority of patients adapt relatively successfully' was a conclusion of a study of psychiatric symptoms in patients undergoing chronic dialysis in Royal Infirmary, Edinburgh, Scotland (43). This evaluation of 85 chronic HD patients showed that symptoms were more frequent in women than in men, in those on home dialysis, in those living in rural areas, in unemployed men, and in those with a disturbed nuclear family. Analysis of symptoms showed six factors that surprisingly were not associated with affective illness: general dissatisfaction, thoughts of suicide, confidence and well-being, usefulness and enjoyment, concentration and alertness, and sleep disturbance. Moreover, there was a high incidence of general distress, anxiety, and sexual dysfunction. Suicidal thoughts were found to be common, and it was considered that 'they probably arise from the existential crisis posed by a life-threatening illness that forces abandonment of many hopes and aspirations that the patients may have had for their life and from their concern about the effects of the illness and its treatment on their families.'

Levy, an American psychiatrist (44, 45), and long an observer of dialysis and its stresses, concurs with other researchers about the major stress of machine dependency and its psychological complications. These stresses include: dependency-independency conflicts, chronic illness, the dialysis procedure itself, unrealistic expectations made of patients, stress from multiple losses; specific psychological complications, such as depression and dementia; and suicide, sexual dysfunction, rehabilitation problems and uncooperativeness. The potential for psychosocial intervention such as short-term therapy or group sessions with nurses and other personnel caring for patients is frequently recommended by Levy, and results indicate varying rates of success. Such sessions can facilitate staff discussions of personal problems involved in patient care and social maneuvers that may assist patient adjustment.

The stress of total adjustment to new limitations is most evident in requirements for shifts in occupational patterns. The ability to work, for men especially, but also for women, is closely linked with gender identity, self-esteem, and prestige. Work is the means to earn money. The loss of personal freedom, detailed above, and especially the loss of life expectancy, have marked effects on rehabilitation. The socioeconomic aspects of rehabilitation are even more evident in patients with manual occupations and less flexible jobs.

Suicide

Since the inception of chronic dialysis, there have been reports (46) of increases in the incidence of suicide, although no prospective study comparing suicides among dialysis patients with those of patients having other similarly stressful chronic diseases has been done. The incidence of suicide among dialysis patients has been reported to range from 4 to 400 times that of the general population. Statistics in this area are fuzzy. Suicide is often not reported; there are opportunities for patients to end their lives during the course of routine therapy; and withdrawal from dialysis therapy is no longer considered to be suicide. Two retrospective questionnaire studies of suicide have been conducted, one in Switzerland and one in the United States. Questionnaires (47) involving 3,478 dialysis patients were completed by 127 of the 201 American centers that were solicited. There were 20 successful and 17 unsuccessful suicide attempts committed by exsanguination, overdosage, or 'food-drink' binges. The incidence of successful suicides reported in the American study was more than 400 times that in the general American population. The Swiss study (48) provides data from questionnaires returned by 25 of the 30 dialysis and 6 transplant centers to which they were sent. Of 574 deaths reported in the period 1965 to 1978, ten (1.74%) were due to suicide and 16 to refusal of further therapy, giving a total of 4.52% of deaths that stemmed from suicide or refusal to continue therapy. The study reported that in 1978 the suicide and refusal-of-treatment death rate was 25 times the

suicide rate in the Swiss general population. Explanations for this increased rate include impaired quality of life, many readily available ways and possibilities to end life, the relatively high average age of patients on dialysis, and additional problems of systemic diseases, such as diabetes mellitus and malignancies.

Support systems

The support systems that are important for all human beings are especially vital for dialysis patients in helping them to adapt to a complex and limiting lifestyle. A Canadian psychologist (40) who studied these stresses notes, 'despite all these problems there is a striking variation in how well patients cope with ESRD. Many lead active, fulfilling family, professional, and personal lives while others stop work, abnegate responsibilities, neglect themselves, and become angry and irritable.' Numerous authors have corroborated the importance of family, the dialysis team, friends, work environment, and other types of support in helping the patient to adapt to ESRD therapy. Frequently, the gravity of the condition appears to be denied by caregivers, family members, and even the patients themselves in order to facilitate the task of daily living. The life-threatening illness and its complex treatment modalities are routinized, with both positive and negative effects for patients (49). A positive outcome is the patient's ability to carry on with life in as satisfactory a manner as possible. Negative consequences may result from an overzealous attempt to normalize the situation, prohibiting the expression of healthy emotional reactions such as anger, anxiety, and frustration at the truly overwhelming life restrictions and stresses imposed by the illness and its treatment modalities.

Family

Notable problems may occur for the families of ESRD patients as well. Family goals may have to be modified; role reversal can occur, laying weighty and unexpected role behaviors and responsibilities upon a spouse or child; disorganization or even disintegration of the family as a functional system may result. For the physician, it may be necessary to make complex medical-ethical decisions that are influenced by and have an impact on both the patient and his family. One must be concerned with the needs of the community as financial resources targeted for health care balloon and are more widely perceived as excessively burdensome. The conceptual framework must take into account preventive care needs, sustenance and restorative care, rehabilitative needs, sociological and community problems affecting patient care, changes in financial status, changes in social and emotional lifestyle (50), psychological difficulties, greater stresses upon the family than upon the patient (51), reduced coping abilities (52), role changes (53, 54), the family's experiencing of numerous stressors related to the condition of CRF and maintenance hemodialysis (55), and the fact that family support is a critical variable in adjustment of patients on hemodialysis.

Adjustment and rehabilitation

The nursing and social work literature is replete with articles discussing factors involved in patients' adjustment to dialysis (56–59). Compliance trends in a pilot study of 35 in-center hemodialysis patients, ages 29 to 74, mean age 55, 63% male, 60% married, 60% black, showed positive treatment regimen compliance in the areas of medications and general physicians' orders and moderate noncompliance relative to diet and medications. Self-care activities were rated fair to good; social functioning was rated poor to moderate. Distribution of patients by sickness impact was: lower 40%; moderate 37%; and more serious 23%. Those with fewest illness-related deficits had problems primarily in social interaction; those with moderate deficits experienced emotional and behavioral difficulties; and the largest number of illness deficits involved alertness behavior, communication, and home management. There was some correlation between respondents with fewer deficits and stronger social support. Overall social functioning ranged from fair to poor. Significant factors identified were family support, role reversal, and relationships with caregivers, as well as items related to religious faith, sexual functioning, and decision-making.

Rehabilitation has decreased as the average age of dialysis patients and the multiplicity of systemic and co-morbid diseases among this group has increased. This must be viewed in light of the age of retirement, existence of part-time work, and women's ability to work in the home. In the United States the data on patients returning to work may be under-reported because of the fear of potential loss of disability payments. One rehabilitation study (60) of 18 dialysis centers involving 2,481 patients indicated a large proportion of dialysis patients are severely debilitated. 'Only 60 percent of nondiabetic patients and 23 percent of diabetic patients were capable of a level of activity beyond that of caring for themselves.'

Patients do remarkably well on dialysis, but it is a rigorous, demanding, and stressful therapy. The literature is replete with statements alluding to the intrusive and deleterious effect of dialysis upon quality of life. 'Maintaining life by means of machinery prompts some opinions that the quality of an individual's life can be greatly diminished, even to the point that death may be preferrable. Such an attitude has far-reaching moral, ethical, and legal implications, especially for nurses with dialysis patients.' (61) 'Technology has given us the ability to prolong life (defeat the enemy for a time), but also robs patients of solemnity in their final moments.' (62) The importance of support systems is alluded to frequently, but, again, there are few prospective, objective studies (63, 64).

Home dialysis

Home dialysis has been associated with medical observations that patients are in better health, and some studies have shown that home-dialysis patients are better rehabilitated. However, there are a few studies of families which indicate that home dialysis has a negative impact on family life (65–

68). A Monroe, Louisiana, study (69) which had 50 completed interviews of 22 spouses of hospital dialysis patients and 28 spouses of home dialysis patients showed that home dialysis spouses viewed ill husbands and wives as more dependent on them than did center spouses. Home dialysis spouses were more resentful. In addition, home dialysis spouses, compared with hospital-dialysis patients' spouses, were less satisfied with the location of dialysis; resented dialysis more strongly; reported lower levels of family functioning and marital happiness, including a greater decrease in marital happiness since dialysis began; perceived patients as being more dependent on them and others and reported more negative changes in children since dialysis began.

In another context, two sociologists, Parsons and Fox (70), concluded that the nuclear family is not generally equipped to cope effectively with illness in the home because of the extra stresses it places on relationships. Another study focussed on 15 children in Philadelphia families in which one parent was undergoing home dialysis (71). They were studied by means of the Minnesota Multiphasic Personality Inventory, human figure drawings, and family interviews. All of the children were found to be clinically depressed, some were hypochondriacal, two-thirds of them had a history of being referred by teachers to school counselors and psychiatrists for behavioral problems in school; all referred children showed disorders of psychomotor activity and reduced academic achievement; and most of the disturbed children seemed to be responding to depressed parents or to partial object loss.

ETHICAL ISSUES AND DILEMMAS

Remarkable scientific and technologic advances in medicine in the past 50 to 75 years have been accompanied both by an unanticipated ability to prolong lives and by the intrusion of ethical and moral problems never envisioned in the time of Hippocrates or even in the nineteenth century. The development and empiric application of dialysis in treatment of acute renal failure during World War II and the feasibility and application of kidney transplantation in CRF patients provided an early focus on ethical issues such as the use of living related kidney donors in the 1950's and the allocation of the limited funding for dialysis therapy in the 1960s. Such ethical issues, along with many others in the fields of medicine, biomedical research, and genetics, were seminal in the development of the field of biomedical ethics about two decades ago. These ethical issues in the area of kidney disease and treatment are gaining increasing attention, especially in this decade.

Principles and models

Consciously or unconsciously, those making decisions about treatment consider one or more of a number of principles to be ethically binding. These include truth, the value of life, freedom, justice, and benefit, which has two aspects: not harming, and helping people. In the decision-making process, several models influencing treatment decisions have been identified. These include: the warrior, parent, contractual, and covenantal models (72). These models, respectively, take approaches that consider medical treatment as a battle against death; the physician being in a parental role of knowing what is best for the patient; two people developing an explicit contract in which the health professional is the giver and the patient is the recipient of services; and lastly, medical care arrangements being a covenant in which there are mutual commitments. It is of great importance to the therapeutic relationship for the patient and his caregiver to have a similar view of the treatment process. This is achieved most felicitously with the covenantal model, in which both patient and caregiver are involved in decision-making (73).

Initiation and withdrawal of dialysis treatment

The ethical issues raised by the use of dialysis are prototypic of those raised by the use of many of the dramatic life-sustaining technologies developed in this last half century. The specific issues may vary according to the country involved. The success of dialysis in extending lives has been excellent. However, not all is positive. With the increased use of dialysis, a wider spectrum of patients who have more complex diseases, multisystem complications, and serious co-morbid conditions, as well as being older are utilizing ESRD therapy. This remarkable technology has become a burden for some patients and the question of whether to withdraw dialysis therapy has posed one of the weightiest problems for the kidney health care team (74). There is limited, often anecdotal, information about how decisions to withhold or to withdraw dialysis therapy are made, and there is no uniform mechanism for making such decisions. A patient care team in Rochester (75) addressed such decisions against a background of medical data and a number of social, legal, and ethical tenets. The team requires agreement among three qualified physicians and the patient, if the patient is competent, or the legal next of kin if the patient is not. The patient is allowed freedom of choice or, if the patient is not competent, documentation about what the patient would desire is required before therapy can be discontinued. In any patient's situation where there is even the slightest hint of litigation were ESRD therapy to be terminated, every possible measure to treat the patient is followed in spite of the personal or collective conviction of the medical professionals that treatment is not appropriate.

An issue of critical concern to patients is their quality of life. Judge Benjamin Cardozo, at the time a member of the New York State Supreme Court, affirmed the broader right to privacy in a statement interpreted by many courts to include the right to make health care decisions for oneself. Cardozo declared that, 'Every human being of adult years and sound mind has a right to determine what shall be done with his own body and cannot be subjected to medical treatment without his consent (76).' The frequently discussed ethical principle of autonomy requires that the patient be allowed to decide if he or she wishes to make a

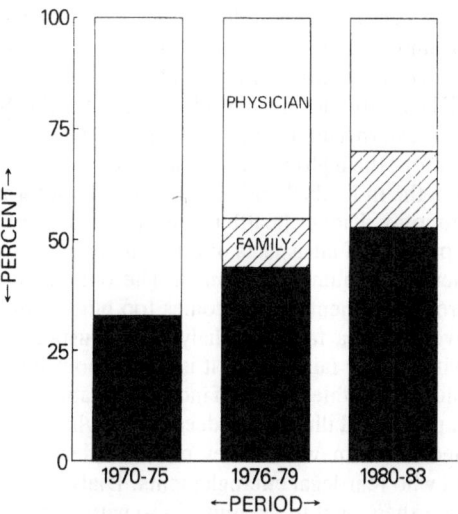

Figure 1. Distribution of Decision Makers Initiating Discontinuation of Dialysis, According to Study Period. In the early 1970s physicians initiated discontinuation in 66 percent of cases. In the early 1980s families and patients initiated discontinuation in 70 percent of cases; decision making by physicians had declined significantly (P<0.005). From Neu and Kjellstrand (81).

committment to such a long-term treatment as chronic dialysis and whether or not the committment is worth the trade-off. Studies of perceptions of quality of life, as observed by the health care team and as evaluated by the patient, often show a marked difference in the two viewpoints. Because it is difficult for a patient to comprehend what dialysis therapy may entail, patients frequently may be allowed a trial period on dialysis, both to see if it will be beneficial, and to allow the patient the opportunity to adapt to the therapy or even to decide that he does not wish to endure the demanding nature of the therapy. The Ann Arbor, Michigan, VA Medical Center has an ESRD Committee which assesses patients' desires to stop dialysis therapy. Port (77) notes that health professionals have a responsibility not only to aid patients in their rehabilitation, but also to provide support for patients and their families should withdrawal from dialysis be desired by and/or recommended for their patients. He adds: 'I believe that very rigid criteria for acceptance to chronic dialysis care may be more harmful by excluding patients who might benefit from therapy than an open acceptance policy that includes the willingness to discontinue dialysis according to a patient's request when there is no hope for reversibility (77).'

A Canadian nephrologist (78) states that 'when patients have decided to start treatment, we should provide every guarantee that if things do not go well, they can discontinue it.' This Canadian group believes it should provide appropriate support to deal with the consequences of whatever decision is made. If the treatment were to be withdrawn, the patient and family should have the reassurance that appropriate care and comfort will be provided and that there is 'hope even if it is for those who survive,' including help with costs and insurance.

Allocation decisions other than those based purely on medical grounds are made, albeit subtly in some situations and only in certain countries. Most analyses of ethical issues about ESRD treatment are considered against the background of Western culture and of high-income countries which can afford the high costs and which tend to place great weight upon the individual and his rights of self-determination or autonomy. Kidney health teams make a major effort to inform patients of all aspects of this complex technology so that they are genuinely informed. The option of withdrawing from treatment, if it becomes too burdensome, is usually given. It is a fact that dialysis can sustain life in patients with kidney failure, but it is not without its drawbacks. Holden (79) states, 'Even if individual patients prefer death to a prolonged illness, the decisions might be denied by the medical team which does not consider death an option and who fear legal entanglements. Dialysis patients who exercise their right to die must do so with many subtle harassments. For a great majority of dialysis patients, a meaningful life is an increasingly reachable goal. Each person should be able to choose and should be assisted in making an independent choice by having adequate information and demonstration of emotional support. The presence of alternatives may tend to reinforce an individual's feeling that life, even with difficulty, is worth living as long as one is in control of the human decision-making process.'

The experience in the United Kingdom has differed from that of most high-income countries because of its more stringent budget for health expenditures and especially that available for ESRD. A prospective study (80) of patients suffering from renal failure in Northern Ireland was carried out during a 3-year period, 1968 to 1970. Patients were 'followed until death, acceptance for regular dialysis, or the end of the survey period, and assessed for their suitability for treatment.' While criteria of acceptance of patients may have changed over this period, it is of interest to note which patients were deemed unacceptable in times of marked fiscal constraint. In addition to medical criteria used for exclusion of patients from treatment, 37% were considered unsuitable because of mental disease, low IQ, or the designation 'uncooperative patient.'

Decision-making has evolved from the more paternalistic authoritarian pattern of earlier decades to a situation characterized by a greater degree of autonomy for the patient. With this has come a great emphasis upon the importance of 'informed consent' accompanied by substantive discussions about how informed can a patient be and what methods can be used to achieve a genuinely well-informed patient who is able to make a reasonable decision about his or her care on the basis of available options. In the United States threats of costly malpractice suits and concern about possible litigation and medical liability have resulted in major efforts by physicians and other members of the delivery team to avoid litigation regardless of cost, even though recognizing that cost containment should be a part of their responsibility.

An assessment of decisions related to withdrawal of dialysis therapy was the focus of a retrospective study (81) of 1,766 patients who entered the Regional Kidney Disease Center, Hennepin Country, Minnesota, between its inception, January 1, 1966, and July 1, 1983. Of 704 patients who died, there were 155 patients who died because dialysis was stopped before a biologic cause of death supervened. This group included 45 diabetic and 110 nondiabetic patients. Dialysis was discontinued in 16.8% of nondiabetic patients over 60 years of age. In all age groups except the oldest, dialysis was stopped 3 to 5 times more often among diabetic patients. Half of the 132 patients whose charts contained notes about the competence of the patients and the decision-making process, were judged to be competent and half incompetent. No apparent complication triggered the decision in 39.4% of the competent patients, but new medical complications preceded the withdrawal decision in all the incompetent patients. Physicians suggested to families of 73.4% of incompetent patients that dialysis be stopped, while families took the initiative in 26.6%. Increasingly, patients and families initiated discussions about these decisions (Figure 1). Almost three-fourths of patients in whom the decision to discontinue dialysis was made were on in-center dialysis. When dialysis was terminated, 67% of patients lived at home with their families. However, 64% of the patients died in a medical center, and only 13% died at home. Hennepin County Medical Center's bioethics committee, established in 1972, was never involved in a review of a decision to withdraw dialysis therapy.

A preliminary study (77) of 2,564 deaths in dialysis patients reported to the Michigan Kidney Registry, 1980 to 1984, indicated that 227 (8.9%) had discontinued dialysis without a return of renal function. Of this group of 227 patients, 11.0% were white and 4.5% were black. Dialysis was withdrawn more frequently in patients over 65 years of age than in those under 65.

Selection criteria and allocation of scarce resources

Deliberations about treatments differ when viewed against a background of unlimited resources as compared to one of economic stringency. Involved in considerations of resource allocation in times of stringency are two key questions: 1) What factors should be considered? Among these are the need, likelihood of success, possible choices, social worth, responsibility, ability to pay, and constraints; 2) Who should decide how to allocate scarce resources? Should physicians, patients, patients' families, the committee process, the judicial process, administrative policy, or the hospital fiscal office make the decision? (82)

There exist few objective studies of how decisions involving patient selection for ESRD treatment are made. The technical feasibility of chronic dialysis opened a Pandora's box of economic and ethical issues. The inordinate annual costs to provide even the least costly type of dialysis were beyond the reach of most people. The Admissions and Policy Committee of the Seattle Artificial Kidney Center, known as the 'God Committee,' (83) conducted patient reviews to decide who should be provided with the limited resources. These reviews highlighted the somber social, ethical, and economic issues that accompanied provision of these limited resources. Committees responsible for selecting patients to be treated with dialysis were forced to develop selection criteria with which most committee members were extremely uncomfortable. Some of the criteria selected were: age, family responsibilities, employment, sex, and 'social worth.' Since 1972, with government funding for 80% of the costs for dialysis, selection criteria are primarily medical. Nevertheless, the troubling decisions about who, when, and how long to treat have given sleepless nights to nephrologists. Many centers in the United States have formed committees composed of nephrologists; health professionals, such as nurses, social workers, and dialysis technicians; ethicists, clergy, and lawyers; and patients and their families who are given the charge to determine the most appropriate therapy to recommended to patients, including a possible recommendation of no ESRD therapy.

A survey of 86 stable, chronic dialysis patients conducted in West Virginia indicated that 94% of the patients approved of discussion of the topics of withdrawal of cardiopulmonary resuscitation (CPR) or of dialysis (84). If there were brain injury and coma, 41% would request withdrawal of dialysis and 68% withdrawal of CPR. In a situation of acute illness, 93% of patients would want to be informed of the situation and 71% wished to participate in medical decision-making.

Availability of funds for dialysis treatments, for which the individual costs range from (US) $20,000 to 30,000/year, limits ability to provide care in different countries of the world. In the United States, because of virtual universal ESRD coverage, almost no one is excluded from chronic dialysis. Belding Scribner has noted that the primary sociomedical issue of chronic dialysis in the 1980s is 'negative selection' (85). Fox (86) stated, 'It is as though physicians have suspended all biomedical, as well as psychological and social, criteria of judgment concerning who should be dialyzed and who should not; perhaps they believe they have no right to make decisions of this sort.' The availability of life-sustaining technologies for treatment of chronic diseases in those industrialized countries with broad federal health programs and social security programs has made it possible to treat patients whose financial limitations make it impossible for them to pay for treatment. However, there is often a selection process at work that may militate against referral of patients for dialysis, such as that noted in the study of decision-making in the United Kingdom (87).

The history of chronic renal failure treatment is replete with examples of the ethical issues that arise when patients develop irreversible life-threatening illnesses which may be ameliorated by scarce and inordinately expensive therapies. The age restrictions applied to dialysis have been lifted in most Western European Countries, Canada, Australia, New Zealand, Japan and the United States, and today the elderly are increasingly being provided ESRD treatment. About 25% of ESRD patients are over 65 years of age in these high-income countries (88), except for the United Kingdom. While the elderly are considered to tolerate dialysis reasonably well, one of the special problems in this age group is co-morbidity.

The selection processes involved are both formal and informal. ESRD therapy initially may be considered by a family physician who refers his patient to an internist or nephrologist, or by a nephrologist who has followed the patient with renal disease for a long period of time and recognizes when ESRD treatment is indicated. While many centers and countries do not commit to writing the criteria used for selection for and continuation of chronic dialysis, the Section on Renal Disease, University of Arizona Health Sciences Center has spelled out its policy (89), which is representative of many tacit lists of criteria used in other centers (Table 7).

The importance attached to selection criteria for ESRD patients has been evaluated in a recent study (90) that utilized questionnaires completed by 373 dialysis center directors in the United States (slightly over 40% of the total number) and by 80 transplantation center directors (slightly over 50%). In priority order, a study of criteria considered very important by 95 to 97% of the respondents were medical benefit, likelihood of medical benefit, qualitative prognosis, willingness, and quantitative prognosis (Table 8). Questioned about the use of five selection criteria in situations of unlimited vs limited resources, the directors' responses differed as follows: use of quantitative prognosis

Table 7. Criteria for selection for and continuation of chronic dialysis.

Section on Renal Disease.
Health Sciences Center.
University of Arizona.

1) All patients shall be provided chronic dialysis therapy who:
   1. Grant fully informed consent; and
   2. Have chronic, irreversible end-stage renal disease; and
   3. Have a reasonable expectation of a quality of life acceptable to themselves; and
   4. Desire and can cooperate with such therapy; and
   5. Are legal residents of, or can establish legal residence in, the State of Arizona.
2) Patients will not be provided chronic dialysis therapy who suffer from a simultaneously present invariably rapidly fatal disease.
3) No patient shall be denied therapy on the basis of psychological, economic, or social factors, or on the basis of age, sex, ethnic origin of disability if criteria #1–5 above are otherwise met.
4) Patients shall have the right, and be informed of the right, to continue chronic dialysis, once initiated, if they so desire. Chronic dialysis may not be terminated against a patient's stated will.
5) Patients shall have the right, and be informed of the right, to discontinue chronic dialysis at any time they so desire by simply failing to appear for their scheduled treatments.
6) Chronic dialysis may be terminated in the event a patient is unable to state his will and cannot be reasonably expected to regain the ability to state his will, upon recommendation of the patient's physician with the consent of the legal next-of-kin, or, upon recommendation of the patient's physician and the consent of his legal guardian.

January 2, 1984

changed from 71 to 96%; qualitative prognosis from 44 to 79%; ability to pay from 4 to 45%; medical benefit from 62 to 95%; and age from 10 to 85%. The responses to this questionnaire indicate that over half of center directors would evaluate social values of patients' lives and that less than a third would use an egalitarian system of random selection. It is also of interest that when resources are not scarce, facility directors are less critical about assessing medical benefit. The response of the directors to the age question in the face of scarcity is comparable to the situation in the United Kingdom, where there is tacit discrimination against the elderly.

Strong Memorial Hospital, a tertiary care center for the Rochester, New York area, analyzed all patients treated for renal failure during 1983 and 1984 to identify steps in their decision-making process (75). Of the 228 patients admitted in renal failure, 42% were not known to have renal disease by either the medical staff or the referring physician at the outset. Appropriate emergency kidney treatment was initiated immediately and after the acute crisis was controlled, and definitive studies were undertaken to determine if the kidney failure were reversible. Ultimately, 12.6% of this group were started on chronic dialysis, in 24% a decision to withdraw treatment was made, 34% had a return of renal function, and 34% died.

Bioethecists, Lo and Jonsen (91), delineate four critical criteria for the differential decision about whether a therapy is prolonging life or death. They suggest: 1) evaluate if the treatment is useless or futile, recognizing that a therapeutic trial is often indicated; 2) since the patient might be ambivalent and change his or her mind, a wish to decline treatment should be considered only after proper disclosure to, and comprehension by, the patient; 3) only the patient's criteria and standards can be used to evaluate quality of life; 4) costs of care and extent of resources must be evaluated. Society itself and the patient can limit care for cost, but not the individual physician, who should always have the best interest of the patient in mind, not the cost to society. At such times, there needs to be a great concern for family involvement, especially since families need to work out complex feelings of sadness, denial, and anger.

In June 1980 Health, Education, and Welfare (HEW) Secretary Patricia Harris withdrew tentative authorization of government funds to cover heart transplants and commented that authorization of funds no longer could depend solely on safety, effectiveness, and acceptance of technology by the medical community. A new technology must be evaluated also in terms of its 'social consequences.' High costs have surfaced as a significant social factor, and the possibility of another expensive program like the ESRD program has produced marked bureaucratic and congressional caution in the United States.

Informed consent and competency

In order to provide the patient autonomy in making medical decisions, one must have informed consent. Ideally, informed consent, within the spectrum of the ability to com-

Table 8. Importance attached to selected criteria.

*Average importance-scores**	*Percent who would consider criterion*
Very important	*Virtually all would consider*
Medical Benefit (4.2)	Qualitative Prognosis (97%)
Likelihood of Medical Benefit (4.0)	Psychological Stability (97%)
Qualitative Prognosis (3.8)	Likelihood of Medical Benefit (96%)
Willingness (3.7)	Quantitative Prognosis (96%)
Quantitative Prognosis (3.6)	Medical Benefit (95%)
Somewhat important	*Very large majority would consider*
Psychological Stability (3.2)	Willingness (89%)
Age (2.7)	Age (88%)
Unique Moral Duties (2.5)	
	Majority would consider
Slightly important	Unique Moral Duties (69%)
Disproportionate Resources (2.2)	Disproportionate Resources (66%)
Progress of Science (2.0)	Environment (61%)
Social Value (2.0)	Progress of Science (58%)
Environment (2.0)	Social Value (56%)
Ability to Pay (1.8)	
	Very large minority would consider
Virtually unimportant	Ability to Pay (43%)
Sex (1.0)	Random Selection (31%)
Constituency (1.4)	Constituency (27%)
	Very large majority would consider
	Sex (1%)

* Criteria are scored on a 5-4-3-2-1- scale reflecting decreasing importance. 'Average' here refers to the 'mean.'
From Kilner (90).

prehend, enables the patient to understand the details and significance of proposed treatments, risks, benefits, alternatives, etc. so that he or she may make a rational decision. Four elements of informed consent have been delineated (92): 1) disclosure, 2) comprehension of information and 3) voluntary consent of a 4) competent patient. According to the context, the concept of competence can be relative. Technically, 'competency' is a legal term referring to a court determination (93), whereas 'capacity to consent' and 'decision-making capacity' are terms applicable to a patient's ability to make decisions regarding his health care. The President's Commission (94) analyzed legal and ethical issues involved in decisional incapacity and endorsed traditional methods of determining capacity by the attending physician in consultation with family, close friends, and caregivers. Resort to the courts should be necessary only when conflict, or uncertainty, about the patient's capacity arises. The commission identified three facets of capacity for health care decision-making: ability to understand the nature of the treatment choice presented, appreciation of the implications of various alternatives and making and communicating a reasoned choice. The issues of competence vs incompetence and informed consent are relevant for the patient in delineating his health care wishes by use of a living will and a durable power of attorney, as noted in the next section.

LEGAL ISSUES

Background

The emergence of legal issues in the field of dialysis therapy is largely a phenomenon in high-income, developed countries, which also have the highest number of ESRD patients on dialysis therapy. To place the legal situation in perspective, one needs to consider the number and distribution of lawyers in the world* (95). Medical-legal issues are raised more frequently in the United States, which has the greatest number of lawyers of any country in the world. The Amer-

* There is no source of current information about the number of lawyers in the world or in individual countries. To provide a sense of the pattern of distribution of legal practitioners throughout the world who have different types of responsibilities and different titles, an analysis was made of the 1978 reference *Law and Judicial Systems of Nations* (94). Practitioners of the law profession in different countries have markedly different responsibilities and titles. Of the 141 countries listed, according to the limited data available, 6 had no equivalent of lawyers, 65 had numbers listed, and 70 countries had no numbers listed. Thus, in this 1978 publication, there were approximately 754,691 lawyers, or equivalents, reported, of which the United States had 424,980 (December, 1976), or fifty-six percent. The next largest groups of legal practitioners, in descending order of numbers and ranging from 40,000 to 16,000, were in the United Kingdom, Italy, Hungary, Philippines, Mexico, Argentina, and Egypt. (Canada and France did not report numbers.)

ican Bar Association (96) listed 676,584 practicing lawyers as of January 1987, a 60% increase over the preceding decade. These figures highlight the potential litigational capabilities and propensities of countries. The United States alone had over ten times the number of lawyers that the United Kingdom had in the 1970s and about 56% of the reported lawyers in the world. Most of the literature related to legal issues in dialysis relates to American situations. Since legal precedents are set by cases, three cases reaching State supreme courts and two cases heard in lower courts which involved patients' rights to be treated are presented below, as well as a summary of an English case in the literature.

Termination of dialysis: three State Supreme court cases

One of the ethical issues addressed above is the right of a patient to determine that he or she will no longer be treated or will determine under what circumstances, should he or she be unable to voice his or her wishes, a surrogate may make such a decision on his or her behalf. The issue of termination of dialysis, either in comatose patients at the request of families or in the case of a blind diabetic patient who had found existence too painful to continue, is addressed in the three State supreme court cases. These highlight legal, ethical, and medical issues decision-makers must consider when it is deemed medically appropriate to terminate dialysis treatment. These decisions are prototypic for most of the life-sustaining technologies, especially in situations where patients are no longer mentally competent to make decisions about their own treatment. The other three cases indicate problems arising with patients who cannot comply with the rigorous requirements of dialysis treatment, both on the renal units and in adhering to therapeutic regimens.

The question 'To what extent should aggressive medical treatment be administered to preserve life after life itself, for reasons beyond anyone's control, has become irreversibly burdensome?' was asked by Judge Christopher Armstrong of the Massachusetts Appellate Court, who heard Earle Spring's case (97). Withdrawal of life-prolonging dialysis was requested for Earle Spring, a 77-year-old patient suffering from advanced senility and ESRD, by his wife of 55 years and his only son. This case took over 15 months of hearings, appeals, reversals, and stays before the Massachussetts Supreme Judicial Court issued its opinion, upholding a probate court judgment that the temporary guardian not authorize further life-prolonging treatments. During this protracted period of time and before the final opinion was rendered the patient died. The Supreme Court acknowledged the 'fearful strain' placed upon Mr. Spring's family by the lengthy judicial process and stressed the desirability of 'expediting such cases.' The court further noted (98) that even a court order cannot guarantee total immunity because, whenever a physician in good faith decides that a particular treatment is not indicated, there is always a risk 'that in subsequent litigation the omission will be found to have been negligent.' Earle Spring's nephrologist has commented, 'The way I practice medicine is very much determined by what the courts tell me to do.'

The case of Peter Cinque, heard in the New York Supreme Court (99), is illustrative of the major efforts often required by patients or their families who desire to terminate treatment. Cinque, a 41-year-old blind, diabetic amputee being dialysed thrice weekly, had numerous complications and experienced pain requiring medication. While still alert, he requested that dialysis be stopped and that he be allowed to die at home. After initial concurrence of his nephrologist and hospital authorities with his request to stop dialysis, treatment was continued, and a court order compelling his continued dialysis was obtained by the hospital. Cinque then had a respiratory arrest, became comatose, and was sustained on a respirator. His guardian ad litem recommended that his request to end treatment be granted, and the trial court ruled that the hospital discontinue treatment.

The legal guardian of James Robert Smith (100), a comatose patient on hemodialysis, petitioned on Smith's behalf that dialysis be stopped after the family, his physician, the hospital staff and the court-appointed religious visitor unanimously agreed that Smith would have chosen this course had he been able make his own decision. The New Mexico Right-to-Die Act of 1977 provided that a physician would be immune from legal liability if he or she honored a patient's written instructions directing that 'maintenance medical treatment' not be used if the patient had been certified terminally ill in compliance with the act (97). After the lower court ruled that dialysis could be discontinued, the Supreme Court of New Mexico reversed the ruling in an opinion stating that New Mexico had no statute empowering a guardian to request or authorize ending dialysis of an incompetent person. The New Mexico legislature amended the Right-to-Die Act to allow a physician to remove life-sustaining medical treatment from an incompetent patient certified as terminally ill or in an irreversible coma if all family members who can be reached after reasonable effort agree that the patient, if competent, would have chosen such a course (97).

Court decisions about dialysis treatment of noncompliant patients

During chronic dialysis therapy, health care teams occasionally have found that continued treatment of a given disruptive patient interferes with the ability of the team to function appropriately in providing care to other patients on the dialysis unit. Two American cases illustrate legal actions and outcomes. The first case, Payton v. Weaver (101), was instituted by Brenda Marie Payton, who alleged that the physician and hospital had wrongfully refused to provide her with regular hemodialysis treatment. Payton, in addition to a confessed addiction to heroin and barbiturates for over 15 years, had alcohol, weight, and emotional problems. In her lucid moments, she was noted to be marvelously sympathetic and articulate, but her behavior at other times made it extremely difficult to provide the medical care of which she was in need. Dr. Weaver, who had treated her since 1975,

sent her a letter stating that he would no longer permit her to be treated in the outpatient dialysis unit because of her 'persistent uncooperative and antisocial behavior for more than 3 years, her persistent refusal to adhere to reasonable constraints of hemodialysis, the dietary schedules and medical prescriptions, the use of barbiturates and other illicit drugs and because all this resulted in disruption of our program.' After the County Superior Court denied her writ of mandate, the patient appealed. The Court of Appeal held that: 1) no legal obligation to provide dialysis treatment arose from the physician's obligation to abandon the patient only after due notice and ample opportunity afforded to secure presence of other medical attendants; and 2) while ESRD is an extremely serious and dangerous disease which can create imminent danger of loss of life if not properly treated, need for continued treatment is not a condition qualifying for mandatory emergency services. The court held that 'a hospital contains a unique, or scarce, medical resource needed to preserve life, it is arguably in the nature of a public service enterprise' and should not be permitted to withhold its services arbitrarily or without reasonable cause. While disruptive conduct on the part of a patient may constitute good cause of an individual hospital to refuse continued treatment, since it would be unfair to impose serious inconvenience upon a hospital simply because such a patient selected it, it may be that there exists a collective responsibility on the part of providers of scarce health resources in a community, enforceable through equity, to share the burden of difficult patients over time through an appropriately devised contingency plan. The trial court found that Brenda's disruptive conduct was, at least to some extent, within her power to control, or modify, and, by implication at least, that absent such control or modification, her conduct was of such a nature as to justify respondent hospitals refusing her access to their facilities. Various types of conservatorships were discussed and the appeal court suggested that the trial court's order requiring Dr. Weaver to provide dialysis treatment to Brenda, pending appeal, remain in effect until the court's decision became final. The local networks' dialysis units informally arranged to provide dialysis care for Brenda in rotation so that the burden would not fall unduly upon a single unit. (Within a month of the time this arrangement was made, Brenda Payton was hit by a bus and killed, September 1982).

The responsibility of a patient to participate in his own care was the issue raised in the suit, Brown v. Bower (102). Michael Brown is a noncompliant patient who was treated at the University of Mississippi's Medical Center (UMC) until he voluntarily left Jackson to be treated at Pascagoula, Mississippi. This 28-year-old patient's dialysis treatment was started at age 18. From the beginning of his treatment, he showed an inability to adapt to the constraints imposed by his condition and an almost complete failure to cooperate with his treatment regimen. He had two failed transplants because he did not take his antirejection drugs. He was given an opportunity to try peritoneal dialysis, but this too was unsuccessful because of his failure to follow necessary instructions. Brown persistently failed to comply with dietary and fluid requirements of his treatment, thus contributing to numerous medical crises. His behavior on the dialysis unit was abusive and threatening, compromising delivery of care to other patients. When Brown sought treatment at the UMC on his return to Jackson, Dr. Bower refused, and Brown was returned to Pascagoula by ambulance for each dialysis session. The Fifth Circuit Court order mandated that Brown's right to treatment was conditional on his improved cooperation with treatment; that he be accompanied by some member of his family during the entire time he is receiving treatment; that he shall not engage in abusive speech or conduct while receiving treatment; and that he shall conform to the reasonable regimen for self-treatment and diet prescribed by the treating physician. The aspect of Brown's defense which has stood firm was his entitlement to treatment at UMC under the Hill-Burton Act, 42 USC S291 et seq, requiring that services be made available to all persons residing in the area of hospitals which have accepted federal grants. The Court concluded that Brown had not established a right to treatment against Dr. Bower, but that UMC is obligated to provide dialysis treatment under the Community Assurance required by the Hill-Burton Act.

There have been marked limitations to provision of dialysis therapy in the United Kingdom, but very few instances of court cases such as those that arose in the United States. In early 1984, under pressure from the social services and hostel staff, the Churchill Hospital, Oxford, England (103), offered dialysis to a high-risk patient, a 42-year-old man with a history of psychiatric illness and severe mental impairment as well as advanced renal disease, after having cared for him for about a year. His behavior was increasingly disruptive, and he required sedation while being dialysed to prevent him from removing the blood lines from his arm. 'By degrees the staff of the renal unit came to the view that treatment by dialysis was a failure and would ultimately have to be discontinued. The dialysis sessions were proving a torment to both patient and medical staff and the unit's capacity to deal with other patients was being affected.' The renal unit took the ultimate decision to discontinue treatment, after which the hostel's director summoned the aid of the British Kidney Patient Association (BKPA), which offered to pay for private care. The BKPA had been on record as saying that it would pay for private treatment for a patient who had been refused treatment under NHS and would send the bill to the health authority. In 1980, the Court of Appeal had taken the position that it could not be supposed that the Secretary of State for Social Services had to provide all the latest equipment. Further, it was added that it could not be pronounced that the Secretary of State had to provide all the kidney machines asked for or all the new developments for every patient who would benefit from them. 'The Court held that the limitation of health resources had to be determined in the light of current Government economic policy.' It is stated that 'though limitation of resources was not a dominant factor in this case, fair and sensible allocation of the unit's resources had to be taken into account, if justice was to be done to other patients, and treatment given to those most likely to benefit from it.' The Court further noted that,

'As with any incurable and progressive condition, treatment to the bitter end may not be in the patient's best interest.'

Advance health care directives: 'living will' and durable power of attorney

The three State Supreme Court cases discussed above illustrate the difficulties which arise when there has not been advanced written communication by patients indicating their wishes about treatment options should they become unable to make decisions because of physical or mental incapacity. Family members, caregivers, judges, and legal representatives are the persons usually given the responsibility for making treatment decisions when adults are incapacitated. Without prior discussion with the patient, decision-makers may have difficulty not only in determining what the patients might have wanted, but also they may not agree. Gradually into this morass, in the United States, have come options for two types of written directives that can be used to avoid difficulties by allowing the patient: 1) to provide specific instructions about how he wishes to be treated or not treated in specific situations; and 2) to appoint an agent to make health care decisions should the patient become mentally incapacitated.

These two types of advance directives about health care, which are recognized legally, are 'living wills' and durable power of attorney. By September 1986, all but twelve States had enacted laws recognizing living wills, often referred to as declarations or directives, created in accordance with the State's Natural Death Act. These directives document a patient's wishes about health care should he or she have a terminal illness and be unable to provide further instructions. A durable power of attorney allows the power of attorney to endure even if the individual making it becomes incompetent. Durable powers of attorney are recognized throughout the United States except in the District of Columbia, which had a bill pending before council as of November 1987. The durable power of attorney can be used for designating whether treatments are to be continued or to be discontinued in specific circumstances.

A 1982 Harris survey (94) revealed that only about one out of every three persons of the general population had given instructions to anyone about their treatment wishes should they become incompetent and, of these, only about one out of every four had provided written instructions. Later studies have shown that physicians often have not discussed these matters with patients. Members of the groups (nurses, social workers, clergy, etc.) who would counsel patients about such procedures are often not as conversant about the options as they should be ideally.

Physicians and other health care providers cannot treat a patient without his consent except in the case of an emergency, when the law permits implied consent. Not only does a patient have the right of autonomy or self-determination in regard to his choices, but the physician can refuse to treat a patient if the result of the patient's exercise of self-determination conflicts with the physician's personal beliefs or values. In general, capacity for wise health care decision-making usually entails the patient's ability to understand the nature of the treatment choice presented, his or her appreciation of the implications of various alternatives, and making and communicating of a reasoned choice.

SUMMARY

Dialysis is a remarkable, life-sustaining technology whose broad availability in most high-income countries has enabled legions of patients with chronic renal failure to survive. Many patients are able to enjoy a reasonable quality of life in the face of the rigorous schedule of dialysis and of its accompanying stresses. However, the virtually universal funding for dialysis in developed countries has brought with it new issues. Social, ethical, and legal issues delineated in the dialysis field are prototypic of issues raised by other types of chronic diseases and by other life-sustaining technologies. Social concerns arise because of the impact of both the treatment and its high costs on the family, the community, the state, and economies of countries, both those able to provide the largesse for dialysis funding and those that cannot provide adequate funds for even minimal primary health care. There is a paucity of objective studies and of prospective studies about social and ethical issues in the field of dialysis.

With the wide application of this therapy has come treatment of patients whose quality of life may not be felicitous. Increasingly, patients (or families of incompetent patients acting on behalf of the patient) are exerting their right of autonomy and making their own health care decisions, often even if it requires going to court. The health care teams have had to face hard ethical questions related to initiation and withdrawal of dialysis therapy in complex medical situations. In the United States, which has become increasingly litigious, physicians and hospitals worry about legal entanglements and practice defensive medicine, although there have been greater concerns about the possibility of lawsuits in dialysis practice than there have been actual lawsuits. One must view with great optimism the fact that patients, families, and health care teams are beginning to grapple with these hard social, ethical and legal concerns, which are not easy but must be confronted. Solutions to some of the problems raised should have applicability to other facets of chronic medical care.

REFERENCES

1. *The Price of Life: Ethics and Economics. Report of the Task Force on: The Affordability of New Technology and Highly Specialized Care: Life at any Price?,* Graven D (Chair), Minnesota Coalition of Health Care Costs, December, 1984
2. Reid TR: The chips are up in the snack food industry. *Washington Post,* March 17, 1987, p A3
3. US Department of Commerce, Bureau of Economic Analysis, Survey of Current Business 67: 32, 1987
4. Halper T: Life and death in a welfare state: end-stage renal disease in the United Kingdom. *Milbank Mem Fund Q* 63: 52, 1985
5. Jacobs C, Broyer M, Brunner FP, Brynger H, Donckerwolcke R, Kramer P, Selwood NH, Wing AJ, Blake PH: Combined report on regular dialysis and transplantation in Europe, XI, 1980. *Proc Eur Dial Transplant Assoc* 18: 14, 1981
6. Golladay F: *Health Sector Policy Paper.* Washington DC, World Bank, 1982, p 34
7. Creese AL, Henderson RH: Cost-benefit analysis and immunization programmes in developing countries. *Bull WHO* 58: 491, 1980
8. Sivard RL: World military and social expenditures 1986, 11th Edition. *World Priorities,* Washington DC, 1986
9. *Health Care Financing Research Report; End-Stage Renal Disease 1985:* US Dept. Health and Human Services, Sept 1987, Baltimore, MD, Health Care Financing Administration Publ No 03274
10. Johnson JP, McCauley CR, Copley JB: The quality of life of hemodialysis and transplant patients. *Kidney Int* 22: 286, 1982
11. Kaplan De-Nour A, Shanan J: Quality of life of dialysis and transplanted patients. *Nephron* 25: 117, 1980
12. Hay D, Oken D: The psychological stresses of intensive care nursing. *Psychosom Med* 34: 109, 1972
13. Huber JW: Criteria for good adjustment to chronic hemodialysis: nurse-patient differences. *Rehabil Psychol* 29: 147, 1984
14. Rhodes LM: Social climate perception and depression of patients and staff in a chronic hemodialysis unit. *J Nerv Ment Dis* 169: 169, 1981
15. Abram HS: The psychiatrist, the treatment of chronic renal failure, and the prolongation of life: II. *Am J Psychiatry* 126: 157[43], 1969
16. Abram HS: Psychiatry and medical progress: therapeutic considerations. *Int J Psychiatry Med* 6: 203, 1975
17. Abram HS: Survival by machine: the psychological stress of chronic hemodialysis. in: *Psychiatric Medicine, Coping with Physical Illness,* edited by Moss RH, New York, Plenum Medical Book Co, 1977
18. Anderson K: The psychological aspects of chronic hemodialysis. *Can Psychiatry Assoc J* 20: 385, 1975
19. Crammond WA, Knight PR, Lawrence JR: The psychiatric contribution to a renal unit undertaking chronic haemodialysis and renal homotransplantation. *Br J Psychiatry* 113: 1201, 1967
20. Stewart RS: Psychiatric issues in renal dialysis and transplantation. *Hosp Community Psychiatry* 34: 623, 1983
21. Blodgett C: A selected review of the literature of adjustment to hemodialysis. *Int J Psychiatry Med* 11: 97, 1981–82
22. Blodgett CJ: The process of adjustment in chronic renal failure and hemodialysis. *Disserta Abstr Int* 44: 905-B, 1983
23. Hilbert GA: An investigation of the relationship between social support and compliance of hemodialysis patients. *Am Nephrol Nurs Assoc J* 12: 133, 1985
24. Garvin RB, Hollandsworth Jr JG, Gersch HA: Identifying reinforcers for hemodialysis patients: importance of religious and social factors. *J Psychol Christianity* 1: 40, 1982
25. O'Brien ME: Religious faith and adjustment to long-term hemodialysis. *J Religion Health* 21: 68, 1982
26. Hill MN: When the patient is the family. *Am J Nurs* 81: 536, 1981
27. Levenberg SB: Studies in family-oriented crisis intervention with hemodialysis patients. *Int J Psychiatry Med* 9: 83, 1978–79
28. Polk GC: Crisis theory: application and utilization with hemodialysis patients and family. *Nephrol Nurs* 4: 8, 1982
29. Hagberg B: A prospective study of patients in chronic hemodialysis. III. Predictive value of intelligence, cognitive deficit

and ego defence structures in rehabilitation. *Psychosom Res* 18: 151, 1974

30. Evans RW, Manninen DL, Garrison LP, Hart LG: *The Treatment of End-Stage Renal Disease in the US: Selected Findings from the National Kidney Dialysis and Kidney Transplantation Study*, Seattle, WA, Battelle Human Affairs Research Centers, 1985

31. Karnofsky DA, Burchenal JHK: The clinical evaluation of chemotherapeutic agents in cancer. in: *Evaluation of Chemotherapeutic Agents*, edited by MacLeod CM, New York, Columbia University Press, 1949, p 191

32. Osberg JW III, Meares GJ, McKee DC, Burnett GB: Research issues in psychological studies of chronic dialysis. *Psychiatry Res* 3: 307, 1980

33. Goldstein AM: Denial and external locus of control as mechanisms of adjustment in chronic medical illness. *Essence* 1: 5, 1976

34. Olsen CA: A statistical review of variables predictive of adjustment in hemodialysis patients. *Nephrol Nurs* 5(6): 16, 1983

35. Osberg JW, Meares GJ, McKee DC, Burnett GB: Intellectual functioning in renal failure and chronic dialysis. *J Chron Dis* 35: 445, 1982

36. Malmquist A: A prospective study of patients in chronic hemodialysis. I. Method and characteristics of the patient group. *J Psychosom Res* 17: 333, 1973

37. Baldree KS, Murphy SP, Powers MJ: Stress identification and coping patterns in patients on hemodialysis. *Nurs Res* 31: 107, 1982

38. Lamping DL: *Psychosocial Adaptation and Adjustment to the Stress of Chronic Illness*. Unpublished PhD Thesis. Harvard University, May 1981

39. Nichols KA, Springford V: The psycho-social stressors associated with survival by dialysis. *Behav Res Ther* 22: 563, 1984

40. Binik YM: Coping with chronic life-threatening illness: psychosocial perspectives on end-stage renal disease. *Can J Behav Sci/Rev Can Sci Comp* 15: 373, 1983

41. Devins GM, Binik YM, Hollomby DJ, Barre PE, Guttmann RD: Helplessness and depression in end-stage renal disease. *J Abnorm Psychol* 90: 531, 1981

42. Chowanec GD, Binik YM: End stage renal disease (ESRD) and the marital dyad. A literature review and critique. *Soc Sci Med* 16: 1151, 1982

43. Livesley NJ: Factors associated with psychiatric symptoms in patients undergoing chronic hemodialysis. *Can J Psychiatry* 26: 562, 1981

44. Levy NB: Psychological reactions to machine dependency: hemodialysis. *Psychiatr Clin North Am* 4: 351, 1981

45. Levy NB: Psychological complications of dialysis. Psychonephrology to the rescue. *Bull Menninger Clin* 48: 237, 1984

46. Gerber KE, Nehemkis AM, Farberow NL, Williams J: Indirect self-destructive behavior in chronic hemodialysis patients. *Suicide Life Threat Behav*, 11: 31, 1981

47. Abram HS, Gordon L, Moore MD, Westervelt Jr FB: Suicidal behavior in chronic dialysis patients. *Am J Psychiatry* 127: 1199, 1971

48. Haenel T, Brunner F, Battegay R: Renal dialysis and suicide: occurrence in Switzerland and in Europe. *Compr Psychiatry* 21: 140, 1980

49. O'Brien ME, Donley R, Flaherty MJ, Johnstone B: Therapeutic options in end-stage renal disease: a preliminary report. *Am Nephrol Nurs Assoc J* 13: 313, 1986

50. Piening S: Family stress in diabetic renal failure. *Health Soc Work* 31: 134, 1984

51. Brown TM, Feins A, Park RG, Paulus DC: Living with long-term home dialysis. *Ann Intern Med* 81: 165, 1974

52. Shanan J, Kaplan De-Nour A, Garty I: Effects of prolonged stress on coping style in terminal renal failure patients. *J Human Stress* 2: 19, 1976

53. Kaplan De-Nour A, Czaczkes JW: Bias in assessment of patients on chronic dialysis. *Psychosom Res* 18: 217, 1974

54. Streltzer J, Finklestein F, Feigenbaum H, Kitsen J, Cohn G: The spouse's role in home hemodialysis. *Arch Gen Psychiatry* 33: 55, 1976

55. Steinglass P, Gonzalez S, Dosovitz I, Reiss D: Discussion groups for chronic hemodialysis patients and their families. *Gen Hosp Psychiatry* 4: 7, 1982

56. Dimond M: Social support and adaptation to chronic illness: the case of maintenance hemodialysis. *Res Nurs Health* 2: 101, 1979

57. Kossoris P: Family therapy as an adjunct to hemodialysis and transplantation. *Am J Nurs* 70: 1730, 1970

58. O'Brien ME: Effective social environment and hemodialysis adaptation: a panel analysis. *J Health Soc Behav* 21: 360, 1980

59. Palmer SE, Canzoma L, Wai L: Helping families respond effectively to chronic illness: home dialysis as a case example. *Soc Work Health Care* 8: 1113, 1982

60. Gutman RA, Stead WW, Robinson RR: Physical activity and employment status of patients on maintenance dialysis. *New Engl J Med* 304: 309, 1981

61. Martin MA: Dialysis decision: unsolved controversy. *J Nephrol Nurs* 2: 5, 1985

62. Barrocas A: Death and dying: a team approach to care. *Postgrad Med* 69: 175, 1981

63. Foster FG, McKegney FP: Small group dynamics and survival on chronic hemodialysis. *Int J Psychiatry Med* 8: 105, 1977–78

64. Gerber KE, Nehemis AM: Designing a problem of psychological consultation to nurses in a dialysis setting. *J Am Assoc Nephrol Nurs Tech* 7 (1): 249, 1980

65. Brachney BE: The impact of home hemodialysis on the marital dyad. *J Marit Fam Ther*, January 1979, p 55

66. Farmer CJ: The prevalence of psychiatric illness among patients on home haemodialysis. *Psychol Med* 9: 509, 1979

67. Peterson KJ: Integration of medical and psychosocial needs of the home hemodialysis patient: implications for the nephrology social worker. *Soc Work Health Care* 9(4): 33, 1984

68. Reichwalt-Klugger E, Tieben-Heibert A, Korn R, Stein L, Weck K, Maiwald G, Mehls O, Diekmann L, Muller-Wiefel DE, Jochmus I, Schärer K: Psychosocial adaptation of children and their parents to hospital and home hemodialysis. *Int J Pediatr Nephrol* 5: 45, 1984

69. McGee MG: Familial response to chronic illness: the impact of home versus hospital dialysis. *J Am Nephrol Nurs Tech* 8(4); 9, 1981

70. Parsons T, Fox R: Illness, therapy and the modern urban American family. *J Soc Issues* 13: 3144, 1952

71. Tsaltas MO: Children of home dialysis patients. *JAMA* 236: 2764, 1976

72. May WF: *The Physician's Covenant*, Philadelphia, Westminster, 1983

73. Kilner JF: Ethical issues and the ESRD patient. *Am J Kidney Dis* (in press)

74. Kay M, Lella JW: Discontinuation of dialysis therapy in the demented patient. *Am J Nephrol* 6: 75, 1986

75. Freeman RB: *Renal Dialysis Decision-Making*. Prepared by contract to the University of Rochester for the Office of Technology Assessment, US Congress, Washington DC, March 1986

76. Schloendorff v New York Hospital, 211 NY 125, 105 NE 92, 93

[1914] (New York State Supreme Court decision)

77. Port FK: Death and survival in patients with end-stage renal failure. *Am J Kidney Dis* (in press), 1988

78. Oreopoulos DG: Should we let them die? The moral dilemmas of economic restraints on life-support treatments [Editorial]. *Can Med Assoc J* 126: 745, 1982

79. Holden MO: Dialysis or death: the ethical alternatives. *Health Soc Work* 5: 18, 1980

80. McGeown MG: Chronic renal failure in Northern Ireland, 1968–70. *Lancet* 1: 307, 1972

81. Neu S, Kjellstrand CM: Stopping long-term dialysis: an empirical study of withdrawal of life-supporting treatment. *New Engl J Med* 314: 14, 1986

82. Cummings NB: Uremia therapy: the resource allocation dilemma from a global perspective. *Kidney Int* 28 (Suppl 17); S133, 1985

83. Alexander S: They decide who lives, who dies. *Life Magazine* November 9, 1962, p 102

84. Holley J, Finucane F, Moss A: Attitudes regarding cardiopulmonary resuscitation and withdrawal of dialysis by a population of chronic dialysis patients. *Abstracts Am Soc Nephrol* 20: 77A, 1987

85. Fox RC: The medical profession's changing outlook on hemodialysis (1950–1976). in: *Essays in Medical Sociology,* New York, John Wiley & Sons, 1979, p 122

86. Fox RC (Moderator): Exclusion from dialysis: a sociologic and legal perspective (Nephrology Forum). *Kidney Int* 19: 739, 1981

87. Challah S, Wing AJ, Bauer R, Morris RW, Schroeder SA: Negative selection of patients for dialysis and transplantation in the United Kingdom. *Br Med J* 288: 1119, 1984

88. Dialysis for chronic renal failure in *Life-Sustaining Technologies and the Elderly,* US Congress, Office of Technology Assessment, OTA-BA-306 Washington, DC, US Government Printing Office, July, 1987

89. University of Arizona Health Sciences Center, Department of Internal Medicine, Section on Renal Disease, Policy on Criteria for Patient Selection, January 1984

90. Kilner JF: Selecting patients when resources are limited, A study of U.S. medical directors of kidney dialysis and kidney transplantation facilities. *Am J Publ Health* 77: 144, 1988

91. Lo B, Jonsen AR: Clinical decisions to limit treatment. *Ann Intern Med* 93: 764, 1980

92. Beauchamp TL, Childress JF: *Principles of Biomedical Ethics,* 2nd Edition, New York, Oxford University Press, 1983

93. *A Matter of Choice, Planning Ahead for Health Care.* (Information paper prepared for use by the chairman and ranking minority member of the Special Committee on Aging, US Senate) Washington, DC, Am Assoc Retired People, PF3861, December 1986

94. *President's Commission for the Study of Ethical Problems in Medicine and Biomedical and Behavioral Research, Making Health Care Decisions,* Vol 2, Appendix B, 1982

95. Rhyned CS: *Law and Judicial Systems of Nations,* 3rd Edition, Washington DC, The World Peace Through Law Center, 1978

96. American Bar Association Internal Report, January 1987

97. *In re Spring,* 380 Mass 629, 405 NE 2d 115, (1980)

98. *Right-to-Die Court Decisions.* New York, Society for the Right to Die, Inc, 1987

99. *In re Lydia E Hall Hospital,* 116 Misc 2d 477, 455 NYS 2d 706 (Supreme Court, Nassau County 1982)

100. New Mexico ex rel Smith v Fort, No 14, 768 (NM 1983)

101. Payton v Weaver, 131 Cal App 3d 38, App 182 Cal Report 225

102. Brown v Bower, US District Court, Southern District, of Mississippi, Jackson Division, Civil Action No. J 86–8759 (B), filed 12/21/87

103. Brahams D: When is discontinuation of dialysis justified? *Lancet* 1: 176, 1985

INDEX OF SUBJECTS